Principles and Methods
of Toxicology

Second Edition

Editor

A. Wallace Hayes, Ph.D., DABT, ACT

Corporate Toxicologist and
Vice-President
Center for Toxicology
RJR Nabisco, Inc.
Winston-Salem, North Carolina

Raven Press New York

Raven Press, 1185 Avenue of the Americas, New York, New York 10036

Made in the United States of America

Library of Congress Cataloging-in-Publication Data

Principles and methods of toxicology.

Includes bibliographies and index.
1. Toxicology. 2. Toxicity testing. I. Hayes, A. Wallace (Andrew Wallace), 1939–   . [DNLM: 1. Toxicology. 2. Toxicology—methods.   QV 600 P957]
RA1211.P74   1988   615.9   85-42509
ISBN 0-88167-439-7

The material contained in this volume was submitted as previously unpublished material, except in the instances in which some of the illustrative material was derived.

Great care has been taken to maintain the accuracy of the information contained in the volume. However, neither Raven Press nor the editor can be held responsible for errors or for any consequences arising from the use of the information contained herein.

Materials appearing in this book prepared by individuals as part of their official duties as U.S. Government employees are not covered by the above-mentioned copyright.

9 8 7 6 5 4 3 2 1

Preface

The First Edition of this textbook was designed primarily for courses dealing with an evaluation of toxicologic data with a particular emphasis on those methodologies used in toxicology. This Second Edition has been expanded to include a more systematic approach to toxicology without losing its methodological basis. This edition describes current testing procedures, offers useful guidelines on data interpretation, and highlights major areas of controversy. Every effort has been made to keep the book simple and suitable for use as a textbook for graduate teaching.

Since toxicology is the study of the harmful action of chemicals on biologic tissues, it necessitates an understanding of biologic mechanisms as well as the methods employed to examine these mechanisms. However, the vastness of the field of toxicology and the rapid accumulation of data preclude the possibility of any one individual absorbing and retaining more than a fraction of these techniques. There are, however, specific methods that are applicable to a large number of chemicals. An understanding of the principles underlying these methods is not only manageable but essential. Thus, individuals who are not directly involved with the day-to-day activity of toxicology, or who have not yet entered a specialized field in toxicology, will find this book a valuable resource in acquiring a broad understanding of toxicological approaches available.

This volume has been designed to serve as a textbook for, or adjunct to, courses in general as well as advanced toxicology. The overall framework of the Second Edition follows that of the initial volume with the exception that major sections on principles related to toxicology have been added. A number of new authors have been added to this edition to broaden input and provide coverage of the ever-changing field of toxicology. New chapters have been added on metabolism, food-borne toxins, solvents, pesticides, and on the regulatory process as it relates to toxicology.

The only true "facts" in biology are the results of individual experiments carried out under control conditions by carefully defined methodology. Although it is not the purpose of this volume to catalog or to discuss these biologic "facts," it is the purpose of this book to present those methodologies which can generate these facts. Achievement of this goal requires the more or less arbitrary resolution to select methods and testing protocols from the current literature. The bibliography of each chapter will carry the reader beyond the techniques and methods presented in the book.

This volume has been organized to best facilitate its use. The first section covers basic toxicologic principles including the philosophies underlying testing strategies. The second section covers basic toxicologic testing methods and includes most of the testing procedures now required to meet regulatory standards. The third section deals with specific organ systems and contains chapters on kinetics and effects on cellular organelles and target organs. Each method or procedure is discussed from the standpoint of technique and interpretation of data. A state-of-the-art approach is emphasized as are the various problems and pitfalls encountered. Each chapter contains information that allows a person to perform an experiment or test a protocol, and also provides insight into the rationale behind the experiment.

Principles and Methods of Toxicology, Second Edition, will be useful as both a text for introductory courses in toxicology and as a valuable, timely review for the practicing toxicologist. Research scientists who have used the first edition as a reference source will find updated material in areas of their special or peripheral interest.

A. Wallace Hayes

Preface to the First Edition

This volume has been designed primarily as a textbook for courses dealing with an evaluation of toxicologic data. It provides a thorough, systematic introduction to toxicology. It describes the most current testing procedures, offers useful guidelines on data interpretation, and highlights major areas of controversy. Every effort has been made to keep the book simple and suitable for use as a textbook for graduate teaching.

Since toxicology is the study of the harmful action of chemicals on biologic tissues, it must of necessity involve an understanding of biologic mechanisms, which can only be accomplished through an understanding of the appropriate methods. However, the vastness of the subject, as well as the rapid accumulation of data, precludes the possibility that any one individual can absorb and retain more than a small fraction of these techniques. It is evident, however, that certain specific methods are applicable to a large number of chemicals, and an understanding of the principles underlying each method is essential. For those individuals not directly involved with the day-to-day activity of toxicology or who have not yet entered a specific field in toxicology, this book will be a valuable resource to select from the many representative approaches available.

The only true "facts" in biology are the results of individual experiments carried out under control conditions by carefully defined methodology. Although it is not the purpose of this book to catalog and discuss these biologic "facts," it *is* the purpose of this book to present those methodologies that can generate these facts. Achievement of this goal requires the more or less arbitrary resolution to select from the current literature the methods and testing protocols that will allow this goal to be readily achieved. In addition, the bibliography of each chapter will carry the reader beyond the techniques and methods presented in the book.

This volume has been organized to best facilitate its use. The first section covers basic toxicologic testing methods and includes most of the testing procedures now required to meet regulatory standards. The second section deals with specific organ systems and contains chapters on kinetics, metabolism, and effects on cellular organelles and target organs. Each method or procedure is discussed from the standpoint of technique and interpretation of data. The "state-of-the-art" approach is emphasized as are the various problems and pitfalls encountered. Each chapter contains information that not only allows a person to perform an experiment or test a protocol, but also provides insight into the rationale behind the experiment.

Principles and Methods of Toxicology will be useful as both a text for introductory courses in toxicology and as a valuable, timely review for the practicing toxicologist.

A. Wallace Hayes

Acknowledgments

Appreciation is warmly expressed to the many people who contributed knowingly and otherwise to this book. The editor thanks the authors, who revised chapters and who prepared new chapters, for keeping in mind that thoughtfully worded information is greatly appreciated by the reader. I am especially indebted to the contributors, whose combined expertise made a volume of this breadth possible, and to Sandra J. Smith and Donna Lynn Tuttle, who skillfully edited the manuscripts. The responsibility for any errors remains with the editor. Credit for eliminating those that have gone rests with the various authors, with Ms. Smith and Ms. Tuttle, and with the editorial staff at Raven Press.

Contents

Specific Organ Systems

Contributors

Paul D. Anderson, Ph.D.   *ERT/Resource Engineering Co., 696 Virginia Road, Concord, Massachusetts 01742*

Paul H. Ayres, Ph.D.   *Toxicology Research Division, Building 611-9, R. J. Reynolds Tobacco Company, Bowman Gray Technical Center, Winston-Salem, North Carolina 27102*

Barbara D. Beck, Ph.D.   *Gradient Corporation, 44 Brattle Street, Cambridge, Massachusetts 02138*

William O. Berndt, Ph.D.   *Department of Pharmacology, University of Nebraska Medical Center, Conkling Hall 5009, 42nd Street and Dewey Avenue, Omaha, Nebraska 68105*

David J. Brusick, Ph.D.   *Hazleton Laboratories America, Inc., Suite 400, 5516 Nicholson Lane, Kensington, Maryland 20895*

Gary T. Burger, D.V.M.   *R. J. Reynolds Tobacco Company, Bowman Gray Technical Center, Winston-Salem, North Carolina 27102*

Edward J. Calabrese, Ph.D.   *Division of Public Health, University of Massachusetts, Amherst, Massachusetts 01003*

Ping Kwong (Peter) Chan, Ph.D.   *Research Laboratories, Toxicology Department, Rohm and Haas Company, 727 Norristown Road, Spring House, Pennsylvania 19477*

Eric D. Clegg, Ph.D.   *Reproductive and Developmental Toxicology Branch, Office of Health and Environmental Assessment, Office of Research and Development, U. S. Environmental Protection Agency, REAG-RD 689, 401 M Street, Washington, D.C. 20460*

Joel B. Cornacoff, Ph.D., D.V.M.   *Sterling-Winthrop Research Institute, 81 Columbia Turnpike, Rensselaer, New York 12144*

Mary E. Davis, Ph.D.   *Department of Pharmacology and Toxicology, West Virginia University Medical Center, Morgantown, West Virginia 26506*

Jack H. Dean, Ph.D.   *Department of Toxicology, Sterling-Winthrop Research Institute, 81 Columbia Turnpike, Rensselaer, New York 12144*

J. Donald deBethizy, Ph.D.   *Toxicology Research Division, R. J. Reynolds Tobacco Company, Bowman Gray Technical Center, Winston-Salem, North Carolina 27102*

Randy Deskin, Ph.D.   *Toxicology and Product Safety Department, American Cyanamid Company, 1 Cyanamid Plaza, Wayne, New Jersey 07470*

John J. Fenoglio, Jr., M.D.   *Department of Pathology, Columbia University College of Physicians and Surgeons, New York, New York 10032*

Bruce A. Fowler, Ph.D.   *Director, Toxicology Program, University of Maryland, 660 West Redwood Street, Baltimore, Maryland 21201*

Shayne C. Gad, Ph.D.   *Director of Toxicology, G. D. Searle & Co., 4901 Searle Parkway, Skokie, Illinois 60077*

Michael A. Gallo, Ph.D.   *Department of Environmental and Community Medicine, University of Medicine and Dentistry of New Jersey, Robert Wood Johnson Medical School, 675 Hose Lane, Piscataway, New Jersey 08854-5635*

F. Peter Guengerich, Ph.D.   *Department of Biochemistry, Vanderbilt School of Medicine, 21st and Garland Avenue, Nashville, Tennessee 37232*

Robert M. Harrington, Ph.D.   *R. J. Reynolds Tobacco Company, Bowman Gray Technical Center, Winston-Salem, North Carolina 27102*

A. Wallace Hayes, Ph.D.   *Corporate Toxicologist, and Vice-President, Center for Toxicology, RJR Nabisco, Winston-Salem, North Carolina 27102*

Johnnie R. Hayes, Ph.D.   *R. J. Reynolds Tobacco Company, Bowman Gray Technical Center, Winston-Salem, North Carolina 27102*

William R. Hewitt, Ph.D.   *Department of Investigative Toxicology, Smith Kline & French Laboratories, Philadelphia, Pennsylvania 19101*

I. K. Ho, Ph.D. *Department of Pharmacology and Toxicology, University of Mississippi Medical Center, 2500 North State Street, Jackson, Mississippi 39216*

David G. Hoel, Ph.D. *National Institute of Environmental Health Sciences, National Institutes of Health, Research Triangle Park, North Carolina 27709*

Michael D. Hogan, Ph.D. *National Institute of Environmental Health Sciences, National Institutes of Health, Research Triangle Park, North Carolina 27709*

Beth Hoskins, Ph.D. *Department of Pharmacology and Toxicology, University of Mississippi Medical Center, 2500 North State Street, Jackson, Mississippi 39216*

Y. J. Kang, Ph.D. *Director, Reproductive and Developmental Toxicology, Smith Kline & French Laboratories, P.O. Box 7929, Philadelphia, Pennsylvania 19101*

Gerald L. Kennedy, Jr., B.S. *Haskell Laboratory for Toxicology and Industrial Medicine, E. I. DuPont de Nemours & Company, Elkton Road, Newark, Delaware 19711*

Perry J. Kurtz, Ph.D. *Health and Molecular Sciences Department, Battelle Columbus Division, 505 King Avenue, Columbus, Ohio 43201*

George W. Lucier, Ph.D. *National Institute of Environmental Health Sciences, National Institutes of Health, Research Triangle Park, North Carolina 27709*

Michael T. Luster, Ph.D. *Head, Immunotoxicology Section, National Toxicology Program, National Institute of Environmental Health Sciences, National Institutes of Health, P.O. Box 12233, Research Triangle Park, North Carolina 27709*

Howard Maibach, M.D. *Department of Dermatology, University of California, San Francisco, California 94143-0989*

Jeanne M. Manson, Ph.D. *Smith Kline & French Laboratories, Research and Development Division, P.O. Box 1539, L 60, King of Prussia, Pennsylvania 19406-0939*

Harihara M. Mehendale, Ph.D. *Department of Pharmacology and Toxicology, University of Mississippi Medical Center, 2500 North State Street, Jackson, Mississippi 39216-4505*

L. Cheryl Miller, M.S. *Clinical Immunology, Sandoz, Ltd., CH-4002, Basel, Switzerland*

Arnold T. Mosberg, Ph.D. *Center for Toxicology, RJR Nabisco, Inc., Winston-Salem, North Carolina 27102*

Stata Norton, Ph.D. *Department of Pharmacology, Toxicology and Therapeutics, University of Kansas Medical Center, 39th and Rainbow Boulevard, Kansas City, Kansas 66103*

Esther Patrick, Ph.D. *Department of Dermatology, University of California, San Francisco, California 94143*

Timothy D. Phillips, Ph.D. *Department of Veterinary Public Health, Texas A&M University, College Station, Texas 77843-4468*

Gabriel L. Plaa, Ph.D. *Département de pharmacologie, Faculté de médecine, Université de Montréal, Montréal, Québec, Canada H3C 3J7*

Walter W. Piegorsch, Ph.D. *National Institute of Environmental Health Science, National Institutes of Health, P.O. Box 1233, Research Triangle Park, North Carolina 27709*

Chada S. Reddy, D.V.M., Ph.D. *Department of Veterinary Biomedical Sciences, College of Veterinary Medicine, University of Missouri, Columbus, Missouri 65211*

Andrew Gordon Renwick, Ph.D. *Department of Clinical Pharmacology, University of Southampton, Medical and Biological Sciences Building, Bassett Crescent East, Southampton, S09 3TU, United Kingdom*

Jane Robens, Ph.D. *USDA/ARS, Beltsville Agricultural-Research Center West, Building 005, Beltsville, Maryland 20705*

Gary J. Rosenthal, Ph.D. *Chemical Industry Institute of Toxicology, P.O. Box 12137, Research Triangle Park, North Carolina 27709*

R. L. Schueler, Ph.D. *6271 Old Washington Road, Sykesville, Maryland 21784*

Kent R. Stevens, Ph.D. *Berlex Laboratories, 110 East Hannover Avenue, Cedar Knolls, New Jersey 07927*

Robert L. Suber, Ph.D. *Center for Toxicology, RJR Nabisco, Inc., Bowman Gray Technical Center, Winston-Salem, North Carolina 27102*

W. David Taylor, B.S. *Center for Toxicology, RJR Nabisco, Inc., Bowman Gray Technical Center, Winston-Salem, North Carolina 27102*

Dori J. Thomas, Ph.D. *Department of Pharmacology and Toxicology, West Virginia University Medical Center, Morgantown, West Virginia 26506*

John A. Thomas, Ph.D. *Department of Pharmacology, The University of Texas Medical Center at San Antonio, 7703 Floyd Curl Drive, San Antonio, Texas 78284*

Michael J. Thomas, M.D., Ph.D. *Department of Pharmacology and Toxicology, West Virginia University Medical Center, Morgantown, West Virginia 26506*

Bernard M. Wagner, M.D. *Deputy Director, The Nathan S. Kline Institute for Psychiatric Research, Orangeburg, New York 10962*

Carol T. Walsh, M.D. *Department of Pharmacology and Experimental Therapeutics, Boston University School of Medicine, 80 East Concord Street L-603, Boston, Massachusetts 02118*

Carrol S. Weil, M.S. *Consultant, 4326 McCaslin Street, Pittsburgh, Pennsylvania 15217*

Harold Zenick, Ph.D. *Reproductive and Developmental Toxicology Branch, Office of Health and Environmental Assessment, Office of Research and Development, U. S. Environmental Protection Agency, REAG-RD 689, 401 M Street, SW, Washington, D.C. 20460*

Principles and Methods of Toxicology, Second Edition, edited by A. Wallace Hayes, Raven Press, Ltd., New York © 1989.

CHAPTER 1

The Use of Toxicology in the Regulatory Process

*Barbara D. Beck, **Edward J. Calabrese, and †Paul D. Anderson

*Gradient Corporation, Cambridge, Massachusetts 02138; **Division of Public Health, University of Massachusetts, Amherst, Massachusetts 01003; †ERT/Resource Engineering Co., Concord, Massachusetts 01742*

BACKGROUND

Since ancient times, man has attempted to reduce or eliminate the risk of disease from toxic materials. Early regulatory authorities focused much of their attention on adulterated food and drugs. Undoubtedly, this reflected the relative ease in associating acute health effects, such as food poisoning, with exposure to contaminants in the diet or in medications. Thus Hutt (59) quotes Pliny the Elder, writing in the 1st century A.D., as stating, "So many poisons are employed to force wine to suit our taste—and we are surprised that it is not wholesome!"

Recently, particularly during the last 20 years, government agencies have increased their efforts to develop and implement legislation to protect people from toxic chemicals. The increase in effort is due to several factors:

1. The realization that the presence of environmental chemicals is pervasive. The publication of *Silent Spring* by Rachel Carson in 1962 (26), detailing the presence of the pesticide DDT in the environment and its effects on wildlife, has had a major influence here.
2. The additional realization of the vast number of environmental chemicals to which man has been exposed, especially since World War II. Of the more than 5,000,000 known chemicals, approximately 70,000 are in commercial use today (45).
3. The establishment of a causal relationship between certain diseases and environmental exposure. The asbestos-induced diseases—asbestosis, lung cancer, and mesothelioma—are examples of the types of debilitating illnesses that are attributed to environmental exposure.
4. The reduction in microbial disease, which is a result of improved sanitation, has altered the focus of society to other causes of ill health. As the standard of living has improved, the public has demanded greater protection from chemically induced disease than in the past.

At the federal level in the United States, four agencies bear most of the direct responsibility for the regulation of toxic chemicals—the Food and Drug Administration (FDA), the Occupational Safety and Health Administration (OSHA), the Consumer Product Safety Commission (CPSC), and the Environmental Protection Agency (EPA). Table 1 describes the acts that empower these and several other agencies.

It is clear from Table 1 that there is a broad range of chem-

TABLE 1. *Federal laws related to exposures to toxic substances*

Legislation	Agency	Area of concern
Food, Drug and Cosmetics Act (1906, 1936, amended 1958, 1960, 1962, 1968, 1976)	FDA	Food, drugs, cosmetics, food additives, color additives, new drugs, animal and food additives, and medical devices
Federal Insecticide, Fungicide and Rodenticide Act (1948, amended 1972, 1975, 1978)	EPA	Pesticides
Dangerous Cargo Act (1952)	DOT, USCG	Water shipment of toxic materials
Atomic Energy Act (1954)	NAC	Radioactive substances
Federal Hazardous Substances Act (1960, amended 1981)	CPSC	Toxic household products
Federal Meat Inspection Act (1967); Poultry Products Inspection Act (1968)	USDA	Food, feed, color additives, and pesticide residues
Egg Products Inspection Act (1970); Occupational Safety and Health Act (1970)	OSHA, NIOSH	Workplace toxic chemicals
Poison Prevention Packaging Act (1970, amended 1981)	CPSC	Packaging of hazardous household products
Clean Air Act (1970, amended 1974, 1977)	EPA	Air pollutants
Hazardous Materials Transportation Act (1972)	DOT	Transport of hazardous materials
Clean Water Act (formerly Federal Water Control Act; 1972, amended 1977, 1978)	EPA	Water pollutants
Marine Protection, Research and Sanctuaries Act (1972)	EPA	Ocean dumping
Consumer Product Safety Act (1972, amended 1981)	CPSC	Hazardous consumer products
Lead-based Paint Poison Prevention Act (1973, amended 1976)	CPSC, HEW (HHS), HUD	Use of lead paint in federally assisted housing
Safe Drinking Water Act (1974, amended 1977)	EPA	Drinking water, contaminants
Resource Conservation and Recovery Act (1976)	EPA	Solid waste, including hazardous wastes
Toxic Substances Control Act (1976)	EPA	Hazardous chemicals not covered by other laws, includes premarket review
Federal Mine Safety and Health Act (1977)	DOL, NIOSH	Toxic substances in coal and other mines
Comprehensive Environmental Response, Compensation, and Liability Act (1981); Superfund Amendments and Reauthorization Act (1986)	EPA	Hazardous substances, pollutants and contaminants

Adapted from ref. 86.

ical exposures with which regulatory authorities are concerned. Chemicals may be regulated by an environmental medium (e.g., air and water), by usage (e.g., food and consumer products), and by the type of environment (e.g., workplace). While the acts in Table 1 represent 80 years of legislative history, 14 of the 19 have been written since 1970.

The language, philosophy, and historical context of the different acts have had an important influence on how agencies function in establishing exposure limits for environmental chemicals or other activities relevant to their mission (e.g., setting priorities for hazardous waste-site clean-up). For example, Section 109 of the EPA's Clean Air Act, which forms the basis for setting ambient air quality standards, focuses solely on the protection of public health. Section 109 states that the EPA must set "ambient air quality standards the attainment and maintenance of which in the judgment of the Administrator, based on such criteria and allowing an *adequate margin of safety,* are requisite to protect the public health" (emphasis added) (116). Congress did not define "an

adequate margin of safety" nor did it specify that the EPA should consider feasibility or costs in standard setting.

In contrast, Section 6 of the Toxic Substances Control Act (TOSCA; 18) states that for chemicals which "present(s) an unreasonable risk of injury to health or the environment" the EPA needs to "protect adequately against such risk using the least burdensome requirement." Here, the focus is not only on the protection of public health, but also on the costs associated with such protection.

While "adequate margin of safety" and "unreasonable risk of injury to health" have not been clearly defined, over the past six or seven years agencies have generally interpreted this language as requiring a qualitative, and frequently quantitative, estimate of the health risks associated with an exposure and the reduction in risks resulting from regulatory action. A major factor in the increased use for risk analysis was the Supreme Court decision in 1980 in the case of Industrial Union Department, AFL-CIO v. American Petroleum Institute. In this case, OSHA proposed lowering the occupational standard for benzene from 10 to 1 ppm on the basis that benzene was a carcinogen, that any reduction in exposure would result in a reduction in risks, and that 1 ppm was technologically feasible. The Supreme Court did not find for the Union, stating that "Before he can promulgate any permanent health or safety standard, the Secretary [of Labor] is required to make a threshold finding that a place of employment is unsafe—in the sense that *significant risks* are present and can be eliminated or lessened by a change in practices" (emphasis added) (59a). The Court left the decision of what constitutes a "significant risk" to OSHA. This landmark decision has had a major impact on agencies in addition to OSHA, resulting in an increase in the development and use of tools to quantify risks from exposure to environmental chemicals.

The primary focus of this chapter is on the use of regulatory toxicology at the federal level. However, recent activities in the state of California regulating exposure to carcinogens and reproductive toxins in food, drinking water, and other media merit discussion. In 1986, California passed the "Safe Drinking Water and Toxic Enforcement Act of 1986," commonly referred to as Proposition 65. This act contains two major provisions—one prohibiting the "discharge or release [of] a chemical known to the state to cause cancer or reproductive toxicity into water" and the other, a labeling requirement, mandating that no person expose another individual to any carcinogen or reproductive toxin without providing "clear and reasonable warning." Exemptions for carcinogens are provided for exposure levels that pose "no significant risk assuming lifetime exposure" and, for reproductive toxins, for exposures at 1/1000 the observed effect level.

The broadness of the language of the act has created much concern among both the environmental community and the regulated industries. Issues include the information required to label a chemical as a carcinogen or a reproductive toxin, distinctions between naturally occurring and added toxins, and the regulatory authority of the state versus the federal government. In theory, the regulation could be applied to a very large number of chemicals under many exposure scenarios. However, the latitude with which the act will be interpreted and its eventual magnitude of impact are still unclear. Many of the issues raised are similar to those debated in the federal regulatory arena, for example, regarding the relevance of animal response to human response and the definition of significant risk levels.

There are four main agencies with authority to regulate chemicals at the federal level, but other governmental and nongovernmental agencies can influence the regulatory process as well. The American Conference of Governmental Industrial Hygienists (ACGIH) sets exposure limits based solely on health protection for approximately 600 workplace chemicals. These exposure limits, known as Threshold Limit Values or TLVs (4), do not carry any regulatory weight, but it is not uncommon for workplaces to adhere to the TLVs for chemicals that OSHA does not regulate or which have an exposure limit that has not been revised since the inception of OSHA in 1970. The TLVs have also been used by several state environmental agencies to derive acceptable ambient levels for toxic air pollutants (119).

Agencies in the Department of Health and Human Services that influence the regulatory process include the National Cancer Institute; the National Institute of Environmental Health Sciences, in particular the National Toxicology Program; the National Institute for Occupational Safety and Health (NIOSH) and the Center for Environmental Health (part of the Centers for Disease Control, CDC); and the Agency for Toxic Substances and Disease Registry (114). These agencies affect the process in several ways, ranging from decisions on which chemicals to test in long-term cancer bioassays to defining principles for evaluating carcinogens, and to site-specific (as with a hazardous waste site) and chemical-specific risk assessments. International organizations such as the World Health Organization (WHO) and the International Agency for Research on Cancer (IARC) also have had a significant role in the use of information by regulatory agencies.

INFORMATION USED IN THE REGULATORY PROCESS

Three categories of scientific information are employed by agencies in the evaluation and regulation of toxic chemicals in the environment: (a) epidemiology, (b) controlled clinical exposures, and (c) animal toxicology.

In vitro studies and evaluation of structure–activity relationships are also employed by regulatory agencies, although to a lesser extent than the three main categories cited above. *In vitro* studies and structure–activity relationships are often used to support the interpretation of information from the three major categories.

Epidemiology, studies of clinical exposures, and animal toxicology provide qualitatively different information, with unique advantages and limitations. Environmental epidemiology studies, which attempt to associate disease or other adverse outcomes with an environmental exposure, have the advantage of measuring an effect in humans at exposure conditions that are by definition realistic. The first demonstration that benzene was a carcinogen came from epidemiological studies of rubber workers (60). It wasn't until several years after these studies (68) that benzene was shown to cause cancer in animal studies. Studies of the London smog pollution episode in 1952 demonstrated that high levels of pollution from coal combustion could cause mortality, particularly in the very young, the elderly, and those individuals with pre-existing cardiopulmonary disease (66). Evaluation of similar effects in animal studies would be difficult, given the complexity of the exposure in London and the lack of good animal models for certain susceptible populations, such as asthmatics. In general, epidemiology has been particularly helpful in the evaluation of working environments or other environments where exposure concentrations are relatively high.

Several factors limit the use of epidemiological studies by regulatory agencies. One of the major limitations is the lack of good exposure information, for both chemical species and for actual concentrations. The lack of good exposure information limits the ability to quantify the effects of ambient air pollution in the United States. The Harvard University Six City Study has shown that outdoor NO_2-monitoring devices are inadequate in accurately assessing exposure to NO_2, due to the importance of indoor exposure (95).

Another limitation is that epidemiological studies of worker populations may be unsuitable for prediction of health effects in the general population. The general population is more heterogeneous than the worker population and, for some pollutants, may exhibit a greater range in susceptibility. Thus, studies of lead workers would greatly underestimate the toxicity of this pollutant in the population of concern for ambient exposures, namely children under the age of 5 years (120).

Epidemiology studies are frequently limited by the need for a relatively large increase in disease incidence (twofold or more), given the sample sizes generally available to such investigations. For example, Enterline (41) notes that it would require a large population (1000 deaths using the Peto model) to detect a 50% excess in deaths from lung cancer at an asbestos level of 2 f/cm^3.

Lastly, epidemiological investigations can show a correlation between an exposure and an effect in the population only after the harm has occurred. From a public health perspective, this is disadvantageous, since such studies would not prevent the occurrence of disease. Recent efforts to utilize biological markers of exposure or effect of exposure, such as DNA adducts and urinary mutagens (91), as part of epidemiology studies may result in preventive actions before the occurrence of disease.

Controlled clinical studies of humans exposed to pollutants address some of the difficulties of epidemiology studies. The exposures can be controlled and quantified, the effects are observed in humans, and the exposed population can be chosen to consist of susceptible individuals, such as asthmatics or exercising individuals. Thus, changes in airway resistance in asthmatics exposed to SO_2 during exercise (12,99) have been important in the EPA's evaluation of the National Ambient Air Quality Standard (NAAQS) for this pollutant, both in terms of the appropriate exposure concentration and the relevant averaging time. Given the subtlety of these changes (nonsymptomatic bronchoconstrictions) and the fact that they occur only in a selected subset of the general population (asthmatics constitute about 4% of the total population), these effects would not have been detectable in the general population.

However, one of the advantages of controlled clinical exposure studies is that they are performed with humans, and this is also their major limitation. Since these studies must be limited to short-term effects that are readily reversible, they cannot be used to evaluate the potential of a chemical to cause chronic disease. Furthermore, because of the mildness of the changes observed in these studies, one may question their clinical significance. For example, how does one interpret the change in resistance observed with SO_2 exposure, given that, if not perceptible, the relationship to physical performance may be questionable (51)? Also, although some susceptible populations, such as mild asthmatics, can be tested, individuals with a greater degree of impairment, such as asthmatics who require continual medication, are usually not considered to be appropriate subjects for these studies because of the greater potential for harm during exposure.

Animal toxicology studies constitute the third major source of information for assessing the toxicity of chemicals. Animal toxicology studies allow the investigator the greatest degree of control over the exposure conditions, the population exposed, and the effects measured. One can readily evaluate the very subtle effects of acute and chronic exposure. For example, recent studies demonstrated morphological and numerical changes in the pulmonary type I and type II cell populations in rats exposed to 0.12 ppm O_3 (32). It would have been very difficult to describe this effect with other approaches, and yet the effect is clearly of concern for humans who are exposed at comparable concentrations in the ambient environment, although for shorter time periods.

The ability to manipulate the experimental conditions permits the evaluation of many variables on the response to toxic chemicals. Thus, Elsayed and Mustafa (40) were able to demonstrate the protective effect of vitamin E on the acute toxicity of NO_2 in mice. The role of metabolism in susceptibility to polycyclic aromatic hydrocarbon-induced carcinogenesis has been evaluated in studies of genetic variants in mice (65). Such studies can be important in predicting modifiers of toxicity in humans and in predicting the susceptible human populations.

Lastly, animal toxicology studies are uniquely suited to the study of novel pollutants for which epidemiology studies are premature and for which clinical exposure studies would be unethical, due to uncertainties about the potential health effects. Using an animal bioassay, Beck and Brain (10) were able to demonstrate that emissions from residential coal-burning stoves were highly toxic and that emissions from wood-burning stoves were moderately toxic to the lungs as compared with the potent pneumotoxin, alpha-quartz.

The limitations of animal studies fall into two broad categories: (a) those due to difficulties in extrapolating from animals to humans, and (b) those due to difficulties in extrapolating from the high exposures in animal studies to the lower exposures typically experienced by humans. Interspecies extrapolation is complicated by the greater homogeneity of laboratory animals than humans, the controlled conditions of housing and diet, innate genetic factors, and other variables. The relevance of trichloroethylene (TCE)-induced hepatocarcinogenesis in the mouse to humans has been questioned on the basis of differences in peroxisomal proliferation in the liver in the two species (1,39). Similarly, it is possible that effects may occur at the high exposure concentrations typically used in animal studies that are not relevant to effects predicted at ambient exposure concentrations, where detoxification pathways are not saturated. Large collections of macrophages with unusual appearance are observed in rats exposed to high concentrations of diesel particulates (127), under conditions where particle clearance mechanisms from the lungs are probably overwhelmed. Such macrophages are not observed in rats at lower exposure concentrations, and their significance to humans who are exposed to diesel particulates in orders of magnitude lower than those employed in the animal studies is of question. A summary comparing the differences between epidemiology, controlled clinical exposure, and animal toxicology studies is provided in Tables 2–4.

We can conclude from the preceding discussion that there is no "best" source of information for regulatory agencies.

TABLE 2. *Advantages and disadvantages of epidemiological studies*

Advantages	Disadvantages
Exposure conditions realistic	Costly and time consuming
Occurrence of interactive effects among individual chemicals	Post facto, not protective of health
Effects measured in humans	Difficulty in defining exposure, problems with confounding exposure
Full range in human susceptibility frequently expressed	Increase in risk must be ~2× to be detected
	Effects measured often relatively crude (morbidity, mortality)

TABLE 4. *Advantages and disadvantages of animal toxicology studies*

Advantages	Disadvantages
Readily manipulated exposure conditions	Uncertainties in relevance of animal response to human response
Ability to measure many types of responses	Controlled housing, diet, etc., of questionable relevance to humans
Ability to assess effect of host characteristics (e.g., gender, age, genetics) and other modifiers (e.g., diet) of response	Exposure concentrations and time frames often very different from those experienced by humans
Potential to evaluate mechanisms	

The rational approach is to examine all sources of information in the evaluation of toxic chemicals. Some kinds of information may be especially useful in *hazard identification,* the likelihood that a chemical will be toxic to humans, whereas other types of information will be more appropriately applied to the estimation of the exposure–response relationship.

RISK ASSESSMENT PARADIGM

In response to a directive from the United States Congress, the FDA contracted with the National Research Council of the National Academy of Sciences to evaluate the risk assessment process in the federal government and to make recommendations on how the process could be improved. As a result of this effort, the Committee on the Institutional Means for Assessment of Risks to Public Health published a book in 1983 entitled *Risk Assessment in the Federal Government: Managing the Process* (78). The book summarizes past experiences, and although it does not propose new ways to evaluate environmental chemicals it has nevertheless had an important effect on the use of scientific information by regulatory agencies in its codification of the risk assessment process.

TABLE 3. *Advantages and disadvantages of controlled clinical studies*

Advantages	Disadvantages
Well-defined, controlled exposure conditions	Costly
Responses measured in humans	Relatively low exposure concentrations and short-term exposures
Potential to study subpopulations (e.g., asthmatics)	Limited to relatively small groups (usually <50 individuals)
Ability to measure relatively subtle effects	Limited to short-term, minor, reversible effects
	Usually most susceptible group not appropriate for study

The report has been particularly influential in two areas: (a) the separation of the risk assessment process from the risk management process, and (b) the classification of the risk assessment process into four broad components—*hazard identification, dose–response assessment, exposure assessment,* and *risk characterization.*

The Committee defined risk assessment as the "characterization of the potential adverse health effects of human exposure to environmental hazard," and noted that risk assessment also involved "characterization of the uncertainties inherent in the process of inferring risk" (78). Given the uncertainties in the data base (e.g., the relevance of an animal model to humans or the choice of model for low-dose extrapolation), the Committee described the need to develop a risk assessment policy in the choice of "inference options," which represent scientifically plausible options for the interpretation and application of scientific data.

The risk management process is the mechanism whereby regulatory agencies evaluate alternative regulatory options and choose among them. Risk management utilizes the information derived from risk assessment, and it also incorporates "political, social, economic and engineering information in the decision process." The Committee noted that the distinction between risk assessment and risk management was critical. The influence of risk management issues, such as the economic significance of a product, on the risk assessment process would seriously undermine the credibility of the risk assessment. This concern is not novel, and is exemplified in the separation between NIOSH and OSHA. NIOSH is located in the Department of Health and Human Services and is responsible for recommending standards for workplace exposures to OSHA, located in the Department of Labor. As the federal agency responsible for setting standards for workplace exposures and for implementing them, OSHA also is required to consider feasibility in the choice of exposure limits. It is not uncommon to find that exposure levels permissible by OSHA are different from the NIOSH recommended exposure levels (115).

Of course, the distinction between risk assessment and risk management is not nearly so clear in practice. For example, the choice of a low-dose extrapolation model for carcinogens, which leads to a higher estimate of risk than other models, represents a risk management decision as much as a science policy decision. That is, the approach is conservative and provides the regulator with a greater level of confidence that the true risk to the human population is likely to be less than that expressed through the model. This approach would be consistent with prudent public health policy.

The first component of risk assessment, *hazard identification,* involves an evaluation of whether a particular chemical can cause an adverse health effect in humans. The types of information used in hazard identification include all categories described in the previous section. In hazard identification, the risk assessor must evaluate the quality of the studies (choice of appropriate control groups, sufficient numbers of animals, etc.), the severity of the effect described, the relevance of the toxic mechanisms in animals to those in humans, and many other factors.

The result is a scientific judgment that the chemical can, at some exposure concentrations, cause an adverse health effect in humans. Usually the result is not a simple yes-or-no evaluation but a weight-of-evidence estimation of the likelihood that the particular chemical is toxic. For example, studies showing that ozone can suppress pulmonary defenses against microbial agents in several species of animals (70), and information on similarities in pulmonary defenses between humans and animals (49), would lead to the conclusion that ozone exposure in humans could, under certain conditions, result in an increased susceptibility to infection.

The hazard identification process has been codified mainly for carcinogens as exemplified in the classification schemes from a variety of agencies including IARC (62), the EPA (122), and OSHA (83).

Dose–response evaluation, the second component of the risk assessment process, involves the characterization of the relationship between the dose of a chemical administered or received and the incidence of an adverse health effect in the exposed population. Characterizing the dose–response relationship involves a determination of the importance of the intensity of exposure, concentration × time relationships, whether a chemical has a threshold, and the shape of the dose–response curve. The metabolism of a chemical at different doses, its persistence over time, and an estimate of the similarities in disposition of a chemical between humans and animals also are involved. While the National Academy of Science report considers dose–response estimates mostly in terms of carcinogens, the evaluation of the dose–response relationships has long been a key component of pharmacology and toxicology for many chemicals (78). For example, in Chapter 6 of this book, methods are described on the use of analytical techniques for describing LD_{50} studies.

In *exposure assessment,* the third component of the risk assessment process, a determination is made of the amount of a chemical to which humans are exposed. Data are frequently very limited in exposure assessment. Measures of chemicals in environmental media, such as air or soil, or in food may be available; however, the extrapolation of those levels to a dose received by humans has many uncertainties. Models exist that can describe the movement of chemicals through a particular medium and assumptions can be made regarding inhalation, ingestion, or dermal contact rates and the bioavailability of the chemical. This information can then be used to derive an estimate of the dose taken up by humans.

Host factors, such as exercise, the use of certain consumer products, or the consumption of particular foodstuffs, will complicate the exposure assessment as will concomitant exposure to chemicals that may interact with the chemical of concern. The use of biological monitoring—measurement of volatile organic chemicals in exhaled breath for example (125)—as well as personal sampling devices, such as respirable particulate monitors (112), represent new ways in which the uncertainties of exposure assessment can be reduced.

The last stage of the risk assessment process, *risk characterization,* involves a prediction of the frequency and severity of effects in the exposed population. Information should be provided on both the risk to individuals and the aggregate risk of the exposed population. It is critical that the risk characterization describes the biological and statistical uncertainties in the final estimation and identifies which component of the risk assessment process (hazard identification, dose–response, or exposure) involved the greatest degree of uncertainty. Unfortunately, there is a tendency to focus solely on the *number* in the risk characterization, such as 2000 cancer deaths from toxic air pollutants in the United States each year (52), and not on the uncertainties and assumptions used in the derivation of the number. In this example, the uncertainties include the use of the upper 95% confidence of the linearized multistage model for carcinogenesis, the assumption of a 24-hr/day lifetime exposure at a ventilation rate of 20 m^3/day, and other variables. Because the degree of uncertainty varies greatly among risk assessments for different chemicals, the lack of consideration of uncertainty can lead to inappropriate levels of concern for different chemicals.

EVALUATION OF CARCINOGENS

Background

The evaluation of carcinogens by regulatory and other agencies currently represents the most developed use of animal toxicology, as compared with the evaluation of systemic toxicants for either short- or long-term effects. This is a reflection of several factors, such as the availability of more sophisticated models for cancer than for noncancer effects and the response of regulatory agencies to the great public concern for carcinogens in the environment. In this chapter, we describe some of the key issues that agencies address in the interpretation and application of scientific data on carcinogens. These issues fall into the categories of hazard identification and dose–response assessment (78). Hazard identification for carcinogens addresses two questions: (a) What is the evidence that a particular chemical is an animal carcinogen? and (b) What is the likelihood that an animal carcinogen is a human carcinogen?

The evidence that a chemical is an animal carcinogen frequently derives from long-term animal bioassays. Such studies usually consist of exposing groups of about 50 animals (typically rats or mice) to two concentrations of a chemical over the lifetime of the animals. Sex- and age-matched unexposed animals constitute the control group. At termination of the bioassay, the animals are killed and the number of tumor-bearing animals and the number and type of tumors per animal are quantified. Interim examinations may be performed, particularly on animals that appear moribund.

Dose Selection

Dose selection plays a key issue in the design and interpretation of the animal bioassay. Animals are usually exposed at two dose levels: the maximum tolerated dose (MTD) and $\frac{1}{2}$ MTD. The MTD is predicted from subchronic toxicity studies as the dose that "causes no more than a 10% weight decrement, as compared to the appropriate control groups, and does not produce mortality, clinical signs of toxicity or pathologic lesions (other than those related to a neoplastic response) that would be predicted [in the long-term bioassay] to shorten an animal's natural lifespan" (106). The MTD is not a nontoxic dose and is expected to produce some level of acceptable toxicity to indicate that the animals were sufficiently challenged by the chemical and to increase the sensitivity of the bioassay (55).

An objection to the use of MTDs has been that metabolic overloading may occur at high dose levels leading to an abnormal handling of the test compound (74). For example, metabolites could be produced as a consequence of saturation of detoxification pathways. Organ toxicity could occur that might not happen at lower concentrations of the chemical (69), particularly at those concentrations to which humans are typically exposed leading to "secondary carcinogenesis." Haseman (55), in an evaluation of the use of the MTD in the National Toxicology Program (NTP), concluded that for such arguments to be relevant to the interpretation of a particular study, it is important to demonstrate not only that metabolic overloading or organ toxicity occurred, but also that these phenomena are mechanistically related to the process of carcinogenesis. He further notes that reducing the MTD to $\frac{1}{2}$ MTD for the high dose would have resulted in more than two-thirds of the carcinogenic effects in NTP feeding studies being undetected.

Tumor Types

Another key issue in the evaluation of animal bioassays is the analysis of the tumors themselves. Considerations include the categorization of benign tumors and whether tumor analysis should be site-specific or based on all sites. The position of IARC (61) is that "few, if any, chemicals exist which produce only benign tumors and no malignant tumors in any species" and that chemicals which cause a marked increase in the number of benign tumors" are now viewed with almost as much suspicion as potential human hazards as they would have been if the induced tumors had been malignant." Thus, it has been the general policy of regulatory agencies to accord almost the same weight to benign tumors as to malignant tumors, especially if there is evidence that the benign tumors could progress to malignancy (122).

It is sometimes stated that one should consider only the overall incidence of tumors, since, from a public health perspective, the concern is with total cancer risk for humans rather than risk at any one site. While this position has an innate appeal, it is not tenable in practice for two main reasons:

1. This approach greatly decreases the ability of the bioassay to detect a positive effect, given the high background incidence of some tumor types in rodents. For example, testicular tumors can be as high as 82% in rats and liver tumors can be as high as 25% in mice (54).
2. The grouping of tumor types that do not share a common cellular origin is of questionable biological relevance, since the mechanisms involved in the production of the different tumor types could differ. Furthermore, the metastatic potential of different tumor types is highly variable and would have an important influence on the lethality of a particular type of cancer.

Illustrative of the problems of the grouping approach, Haseman and co-workers (56) observed that of 45 chemicals classified as carcinogens using a site-specific analysis, less than half showed an increase in the overall incidence of tumors. Thus, the practice of regulatory and other agencies has been to perform analyses on a site-specific basis in most cases.

Weight of Evidence

The decision to classify as an animal carcinogen also involves a weight-of-evidence determination. This reflects the judgment that the data showing positive evidence of carcinogenicity are sufficient for a chemical to be classified as an animal carcinogen. The EPA uses three criteria to make a finding of "sufficient evidence of carcinogenicity" (122). A chemical is considered carcinogenic for animals when it causes an increase in malignant or combined malignant and benign tumors in (a) "multiple species or strains," or (b) "multiple experiments (e.g., with different routes of administration or using different dose levels)," or (c) "to an unusual degree in a single experiment with regard to high incidence, unusual site or type of tumor, or early age at onset."

"Limited evidence of carcinogenicity" is found when the positive experiments involve only a single species, strain, or experiment or when the experiments had inadequacy in design or conduct such as the lack of adequate follow-up time. "Inadequate evidence" applies to experiments that have major limitations so that they are not interpretable as to the presence or absence of carcinogenicity.

The EPA (122). IARC (62), and other agencies conclude that a chemical demonstrating sufficient evidence of carcinogenicity from animal experiments is a potential human carcinogen. This conclusion is supported by evaluation of known human carcinogens in animal bioassays. For the 26 chemicals or processes associated with cancer indication in humans by IARC (111), 20 of the 23 for which the tests are described as adequate also have been positive in animal bioassays (54,68) (Table 5). Hematite is described as negative in animal bioassays, although it is likely that the actual carcinogen for hematite miners is not the hematite itself but radon, a radioactive gas known to cause lung cancer in uranium miners, which is also found in hematite mines (96). Benzene has more recently been found to be carcinogenic

TABLE 5. Chemicals or industrial processes associated with cancer induction in humans: Comparison of target organs and main routes of exposure in animals and humans

Chemical or industrial process	Humans			Animals		
	Main type of exposure[a]	Target organ	Main route of exposure[b]	Animal	Target organ	Route of exposure
Aflatoxins	Environmental, occupational[c]	Liver	p.o., inhalation[c]	Rat	Liver, stomach, colon, kidney	p.o.
				Fish, duck, marmoset, tree shrew, monkey	Liver	p.o.
				Rat	Liver, trachea	i.t.
				Rat	Liver	i.p.
				Mouse, rat	Local	s.c. injection
				Mouse	Lung	i.p.
4-Aminobiphenyl	Occupational	Bladder	Inhalation, skin, p.o.	Mouse, rabbit, dog	Bladder	p.o.
				Newborn mouse	Liver	s.c. injection
				Rat	Mammary gland, intestine	s.c. injection
Arsenic compounds	Occupational, medicinal, and environmental	Skin, lung, liver[c]	Inhalation, p.o., skin	Mouse, rat, dog	Inadequate, negative	p.o.
				Mouse	Inadequate, negative	Topical, i.v.
Asbestos	Occupational	Lung, pleural cavity, gastrointestinal tract	Inhalation, p.o.	Mouse, rat, hamster, rabbit	Lung, pleura	Inhalation or i.t.
				Rat, hamster	Local	Intrapleural
				Rat	Local	i.p., s.c. injection
					Various sites[c]	p.o.
Auramine (manufactured)	Occupational	Bladder	Inhalation, skin, p.o.	Mouse, rat	Liver	p.o.
				Rabbit, dog	Negative	p.o.
				Rat	Local, liver, intestine	s.c. injection
Benzene	Occupational	Hemopoietic system	Inhalation, skin	Mouse	Inadequate	Topical, s.c. injection
Benzidine	Occupational	Bladder	Inhalation, skin, p.o.	Mouse	Liver	s.c. injection
				Mouse	Liver	p.o.
				Rat	Zymbal gland, liver, colon	s.c. injection
				Hamster	Liver	p.o.
				Dog	Bladder	p.o.
Bis(chloromethyl)ether	Occupational	Lung	Inhalation	Mouse, rat	Lung, nasal cavity	Inhalation
				Mouse	Skin	Topical
					Local, lung	s.c. injection
				Rat	Local	s.c. injection
Cadmium-using industries (possibly cadmium oxide)	Occupational	Prostate, lung[c]	Inhalation, p.o.	Rat	Local, testis	s.c. or i.m. injection
Chloramphenicol	Medicinal	Hemopoietic system	p.o., injection		(No adequate tests)	
Chloromethyl methyl ether (possibly associated with bis(chloromethyl) ether	Occupational	Lung	Inhalation	Mouse	Initiator	Skin
					Lung[c]	Inhalation
				Rat	Local, lung[c]	s.c. injection
					Local[c]	s.c. injection

Chromium (chromate-producing industries)	Occupational	Lung, nasal, cavities[c]	Inhalation	Mouse	Local	s.c. or i.m. injection
				Rat	Lung	Intrabronchial implantation
Cyclophosphamide	Medicinal	Bladder	p.o., injection	Mouse	Hemopoietic system, lung	i.p., s.c. injection
				Mouse	Various sites	p.o.
				Rat	Bladder[c]	i.p.
				Rat	Mammary gland	i.p.
				Rat	Various sites	i.v.
Diethylstilbestrol	Medicinal	Uterus, vagina	p.o.	Mouse	Mammary	p.o.
				Mouse	Mammary, lymphoreticular, testis, vagina	s.c. injection, s.c. implantation
				Rat	Local	s.c. implantation
				Hamster	Mammary, hypophysis[c], bladder	s.c. injection
				Hamster	Kidney	s.c. implantation
				Squirrel monkey	Uterine serosa	s.c. implantation
Hematite mining (? radon)	Occupational	Lung	Inhalation	Mouse, hamster, guinea pig	Negative	Inhalation, i.t.
				Rat	Negative	s.c. injection
Isopropyl oils	Occupational	Nasal cavity, larynx	Inhalation	(No adequate tests)		(No adequate tests)
Melphalan	Medicinal	Hemopoietic system	p.o., injection	Mouse	Initiator	Skin
				Mouse	Lung, lymphosarcomas	i.p.
				Rat	Local	i.p.
Mustard gas	Occupational	Lung, larynx	Inhalation	Mouse	Lung	Inhalation, i.v.
					Local, mammary	s.c. injection
2-Naphthylamine	Occupational	Bladder	Inhalation, skin, p.o.	Hamster, dog, monkey	Bladder	p.o.
				Mouse	Liver, lung	s.c. injection
				Rat, rabbit	Inadequate	p.o.
Nickel (nickel refining)	Occupational	Nasal cavity, lung	Inhalation	Rat	Lung	Inhalation
				Mouse, rat, hamster	Local	s.c., i.m. injection
				Mouse, rat	Local	i.m. implantation
N,N-bis(2-chloroethyl)2-naphthylamine	Medicinal	Bladder	p.o.	Mouse	Lung	Inhalation
				Rat	Local	s.c. injection
Oxymetholone	Medicinal	Liver	p.o.	(No adequate tests)		(No adequate tests)
Phenacetin	Medicinal	Kidney	p.o.	(No adequate tests)		(No adequate tests[e])
Phenytoin	Medicinal	Lymphoreticular tissues	p.o., injection	Mouse	Lymphoreticular tissues	p.o., i.p.
Soot, tars, and oils	Occupational, environmental	Lung, skin (scrotum)	Inhalation, skin	Mouse, rabbit	Skin	Topical
Vinyl chloride	Occupational	Liver, brain[c], lung[c]	Inhalation, skin	Mouse, rat	Lung, liver, blood vessels, mammary, zymbal gland, kidney	Inhalation

[a] The main types of exposure mentioned are those by which the association has been demonstrated; exposures other than those mentioned may also occur.
[b] The main routes of exposure given may not be the only ones by which such effects could occur.
[c] Indicative evidence.
From ref. 111, with permission.

in animals (68). There remains no good animal model of arsenic-induced cancer for oral exposure. Recent studies provide evidence of arsenic-induced lung cancer in animals exposed by intratracheal distillation (92,93). Tests have been inadequate for oxymetholone, phenacetin, and isopropyl oils.

Table 6 presents an illustration of the EPA's weight-of-evidence scheme for carcinogens based on animal and human data. It is similar to IARC's classification scheme, except that an additional category is included for "no evidence" (meaning good nonpositive studies). Squire (107) has proposed a ranking scheme for animal carcinogens which incorporates elements of the weight-of-evidence (hazard identification) determination and of the dose–response relationship which is presented in Table 7.

Low-dose Extrapolation

One of the most contentious aspects of the evaluation of animal carcinogens by regulatory agencies is the dose–response relationship. Animals are typically exposed to carcinogens at levels that are orders of magnitude greater than those likely to be encountered by humans in the environment. It would be impossible to perform animal experiments with a large enough number of animals to directly estimate the level of risk at low exposure levels. Thus, to obtain a quantitative estimate of the risks humans are likely to encounter at ambient exposures requires the use of "low-dose extrapolation models." Quantitative risk assessment for carcinogens has been broadly used in the United States (85), but less so in other countries (105).

The choice of mathematical model depends on two factors: (a) the hypothesis for the mechanism of carcinogenesis for a particular chemical, and (b) the science policy decision to choose, in the absence of data firmly supporting one model or another, the more conservative model (of several biologically plausible models).

Genetic Versus Epigenetic Mechanisms

The determination of whether carcinogenesis is a threshold or nonthreshold phenomenon has been a key determinant in the choice of model. The evidence for carcinogenesis being a nonthreshold phenomenon derives from studies showing that carcinogenesis proceeds through stages, the first of which—*initiation*—represents an alteration in the DNA of a cell by a chemical carcinogen. (For a detailed review of carcinogenesis, see refs. 42 and 124.) This lesion, which may be a mutation, chromosomal rearrangement, or other alteration, is irreversible and can, over time, result in that particular cell losing its ability to respond to normal growth control mechanisms, becoming transformed, dividing, and eventually progressing to tumor development. The latter stages of carcinogenesis, after initiation, are termed promotion and progression. Promotion is less well defined than initiation and represents the process by which an initiated cell develops a growth advantage over uninitiated cells. It was demonstrated initially in skin painting experiments in mice (11) and later in models of carcinogenesis in the liver (89). Most chemicals that have been shown to have initiating activity also have promoting activity, and thus are classified as complete carcinogens.

Promotion involves only initiated cells and is composed of at least two stages, the first of which is reversible. Later, the process of promotion is believed to be irreversible (103). The mechanisms of promotion are poorly understood. Alterations in cell membrane phenomena, including activation of various enzyme systems and changes in intercellular communication patterns, appear to be key events. Progression, the process by which a benign tumor progresses to a malignant tumor, is also poorly defined. Several steps may be involved, such as oncogene activation or changes in host immune defenses (81).

There is relative agreement that carcinogenesis is likely to be a nonthreshold phenomenon for the classical carcinogens, such as benzo[a]pyrene and vinyl chloride, which are electrophilic agents and are known to interact with DNA (126); however, there is much debate over whether carcinogenesis is a threshold phenomenon for chemicals that do not interact with the genome and which may induce cancer through epigenetic (outside the genome) mechanisms. Included in this category are chemicals such as 2,3,7,8-tetrachlorodibenzo-*p*-dioxin (TCDD, also referred to as dioxin) and TCE, which have been hypothesized by some investigators to cause cancer through "epigenetic mechanisms," as yet poorly defined,

TABLE 6. *Illustrative categorization of evidence based on animal and human data[a]*

Human evidence	Animal evidence Sufficient	Limited	inadequate	No data	No evidence
Sufficient	A	A	A	A	A
Limited	B1	B1	B1	B1	B1
Inadequate	B2	C	D	D	D
No data	B2	C	D	D	E
No evidence	B2	C	D	D	E

[a] The above assignments are presented for illustrative purposes. There may be nuances in the classification of both animal and human data indicating that different categorizations than those given in the table should be assigned. Furthermore, these assignments are tentative and may be modified by ancillary evidence. In this regard all relevant information should be evaluated to determine if the designation of the overall weight of evidence needs to be modified. Relevant factors to be included along with the tumor data from human and animal studies include structure–activity relationships, short-term test findings, results of appropriate physiological, biochemical, and toxicological observations, and comparative metabolism and pharmacokinetic studies. The nature of these findings may cause an adjustment of the overall categorization of the weight of evidence.
From ref. 122.

TABLE 7. *Proposed system for ranking animal carcinogens*

Factor	Score
A. Number of different species affected	
Two or more	15
One	5
B. Number of histogenetically different types of neoplasms in one or more species	
Three or more	15
Two	10
One	5
C. Spontaneous incidence in appropriate control groups of neoplasms induced in treated groups	
<1%	15
1–10%	10
10–20%	5
>20%	1
D. Dose–response relationships (cumulative oral dose equivalents per kilogram of body weight per day for 2 years)[a]	
<1 μg	15
1 μg–1 mg	10
1 mg–1 g	5
>1 g	1
E. Malignancy of induced neoplasms	
>50%	15
25–50%	10
<25%	5
No malignancy	1
F. Genotoxicity, measured in an appropriate battery of tests	
Positive	25
Incompletely positive	10
Negative	0

[a] Based on estimated consumption of 100 g of diet per kilogram of body weight. Scoring could also be developed for inhalation or other appropriate routes.
From ref. 107, with permission.

which would be reversible (90,129). Relevant mechanisms might include stimulation of cell division and alterations in membrane properties.

For example, Reddy and Lalwai (97) have proposed that a relationship may exist between the proliferation of peroxisomes (subcellular organelles) and the development of hepatocellular carcinoma induced by some hyperlipidemic drugs, halogenated solvents, and plasticizers via the involvement of reactive oxygen species such as H_2O_2. Thus mice, which are more susceptible to TCE-induced liver cancer than rats, show a high degree of liver peroxisomal proliferation in response to TCE. The reason TCE is a potent peroxisome proliferator in mice, but not in rats, relates to the observations that TCE displays linear kinetics for trichloroacetic acid (TCA) formation, the principal TCE metabolite, whereas the reaction achieves saturation in rats. Thus, as the dose of TCE is increased, proportionally more TCA is produced in mice than in rats. Since TCA is believed to be the agent responsible for TCE-induced peroxisome proliferation, these metabolic differences could explain the increased susceptibility of mice to TCE-induced liver cancer (109).

The extent to which human peroxisomes proliferate in response to chemicals is unclear. Individuals on long-term hyperlipidemic therapy do have histopathological changes in the liver consistent with peroxisomal proliferation (97). However, *in vitro* experiments suggest that human cells may be less responsive than rodent cells (1). In any case, since this response involves enzyme induction, it would, in theory, involve a threshold and be occurring through an epigenetic mechanism. Low-dose extrapolation in this case could involve a different modeling approach than that for the "genotoxic" carcinogens.

The decision to evaluate a chemical as a genotoxic or an epigenetic carcinogen has a major impact on the final standards for that chemical. In the United States, TCDD has been considered a genotoxic carcinogen. The CDC has estimated an acceptable level for TCDD intake to be approximately 600 fg/kg/day (63). In contrast, Canada considers TCDD to be a nongenotoxic carcinogen and, using a safety factor approach, has estimated 10,000 fg/kg/day to be an acceptable intake (87). Tables 8 and 9 describe the main arguments in favor of and against the use of thresholds in describing carcinogenesis (54).

Mathematical Models

The choice of the low-dose extrapolation model can have a major impact on the estimate of risk at low exposure levels. Figure 1 shows the estimate of risk from 2-acetylaminoflu-

TABLE 8. *Major arguments in favor of threshold dose (no-effect level)*

1. Assumption of some critical level of exposure below which the carcinogenic process will not be initiated.
2. Chemical carcinogenesis is a multistage process involving exposure, absorption, distribution, activation, deactivation, and elimination of the chemical per se or products formed from it. Interference with any of these processes may constitute a threshold. Possibility that activation of the system which leads to the carcinogenic products will not be initiated at low dose levels.
3. Small quantities of environmental chemicals may not reach their receptor because the rate of elimination or metabolic degradation is relatively more effective with smaller doses.
4. The possibility exists of a relatively greater effectiveness of repair mechanisms including DNA repair and immunosuppression at low doses.
5. Where effective repair processes are present, even if a substance interacts with the receptor, it need not necessarily produce an adverse effect.
6. Although carcinogenic and mutagenic chemicals may have special properties with regard to the nature and characteristics of their adverse effects, they are subject to the same physiochemical and biological interactions that are considered to result in a threshold dose for other chemicals.
7. Concept of proper detoxification and adequate repair systems including DNA repair and immunosuppression.
8. Possibility that activation of the system which leads to the carcinogenic products will not be initiated at low dose levels.

From ref. 54, with permission.

TABLE 9. *Major arguments against threshold dose (no-effect levels)*

1. For toxic effects such as neoplastic disease or mutations of genetic material, a single molecule of a chemical is sufficient to initiate a process that may progressively lead to an observed, irreversible, harmful effect so that it may not be possible to demonstrate a "threshold dose" for a carcinogen or a mutagen.
2. There are no known chemical carcinogens that can produce tumors that are not found to occur in the absence of that chemical. The threshold hypothesis requires the assumption that the carcinogen in question acts by some novel mechanism, independent of all ongoing processes on the target organ or site.
3. Experiments on radiation induced cancer have not revealed a threshold within the realm of statistical reliability.
4. Mathematically derived conclusions suggest that it is impossible to demonstrate no-effect levels experimentally. A *no effect* level for a group of animals may occur because the dose is really below the theoretical no-effect level (e.g., below the threshold) or because the number of animals is too small or because the time of observation was too short (e.g., as in cancer with a long latent period between exposure and appearance of tumors).
5. Even if a threshold is postulated, there is presently no empirical or theoretical basis for determining the dose at which it may occur.
6. The human population is a very diverse, genetically heterogenous group that is exposed in varying degrees to a large variety of toxicants. Assumption of one threshold is unrealistic. If thresholds do exist, not all members of the population have the same one.

From ref. 54, with permission.

orene at low exposure levels using different models. The level of risk varies by many orders of magnitude at the same exposure level, depending on the model chosen. The model most commonly used by regulatory agencies in the United States is the linearized multistage model (5). The EPA uses the upper 95% confidence limit of this model on the basis of its biological plausibility (it assumes a nonthreshold) and its conservatism (it is unlikely to underestimate risk at low exposure levels) (122).

One difficulty with the use of the upper 95% confidence limit is that this approach basically reduces the model to worst-case curve fitting and does not take basic carcinogenic mechanisms into account. Thus, while Cook et al. (29a) have stated that if the multistage model, as they defined it, of carcinogenesis were correct, then the value of k, or the number of stages of cellular transformation, would generally be from four to six (29a). However, the algorithm used in the calculation of cancer risk by the EPA for the multistage model requires k to assume a value not greater than the number of dose levels used in the study. Because three dose levels are usually employed—the MTD, $\frac{1}{2}$ MTD, and controls—the value of k is restrained to be, at most, equal to three.

Furthermore, when the MTD dose has been overestimated and excessive mortality occurs, the MTD cannot be used for risk assessment, thereby reducing k from three to two. Al-

lowing the value of k to be determined by the number of dose levels in a study, rather than on an understanding of the process of carcinogenesis, results in risk estimations of the multistage model that have reduced biologic relevance. In fact, the term multistage is itself somewhat misleading in this context. Alternative models are being developed that address this issue, and which take into account cell initiation, proliferation, and transformation (73).

Physiologically Based Pharmacokinetic Models

One of the areas of recent regulatory attention is that of physiologically based pharmacokinetic (PB-PK) models and their potential use in risk assessment. This issue is discussed in depth in *Chapter 30* by Renwick (*this volume*), but it is important to discuss the topic here as well to put it into a regulatory context.

PB-PK models are essentially mechanistic models that try to describe quantitatively the pharmacokinetic processes affecting the disposition of a chemical and its metabolism from the time it is absorbed to the interaction with different and various body tissues. Once it is determined whether the parent compound or its metabolites is the cause of a carcinogenic response, a PB-PK model may be developed to quantify the magnitude and the time course of exposure to this agent at the critical target site in the animal model. After the estimates of target tissue dose in the animal model have been made and validated, the information can then be scaled to the human to obtain an estimate of target organ dose in humans. This estimate may then be used to predict human cancer risk under different exposure conditions. It should be emphasized that the PB-PK model neither offers an explanation of what the mechanism of cancer initiation is nor predicts or differentiates the sensitivity of one target organ over another or one species over another (6,24). Furthermore, full validation of the model at the relatively low levels of environmental chemicals to which humans are exposed is extremely difficult, if not impossible.

Despite these limitations, PB-PK modeling does offer an important tool for researchers and regulators alike. Even though PB-PK models are not able to provide interspecies differential susceptibility for target organs, the models have been able to quantify target organ doses between species. Of added significance is that new information about the pharmacokinetics of a chemical can be incorporated into the model without affecting the basic structure of the model, thus enhancing its predictive capability.

The use of PB-PK models also provides important advantages over conventional pharmacokinetic analyses (6,24). In typical pharmacokinetic modeling, time-course curves are determined for the concentration of the administered agent or its metabolite(s) in blood or some other body compartment. The resulting curves are then described by curve-fitting biostatistical techniques. The approach of conventional pharmacokinetics may be criticized for being more dependent on the mathematical model than on the biological system it purports to represent. However, PB-PK models are designed to predict kinetic behavior over a wide range of doses and exposure conditions, and are based on basic physiologic and

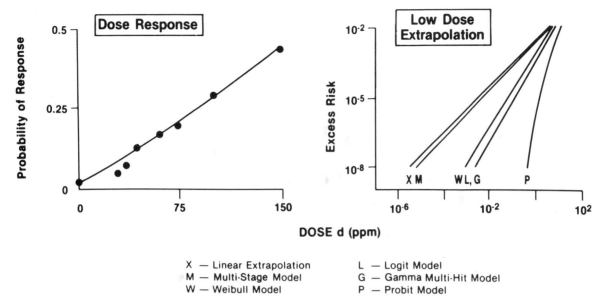

X — Linear Extrapolation
M — Multi-Stage Model
W — Weibull Model

L — Logit Model
G — Gamma Multi-Hit Model
P — Probit Model

FIG. 1. Low-dose extrapolation for 2-acetylaminofluorene under several mathematical models. (From ref. 14, with permission.)

metabolic parameters. This modeling requires many data on anatomical and physiological parameters, the partitioning of test agents into selected tissues, and the biochemical constants for tissue binding and metabolism in various organs. From these data, a series of mass balance differential equations can be written to describe the interactions between the chemical and the animal model.

PB-PK modeling has been applied to several agents including methylene chloride and ethylene dichloride (6,24). A look at the methylene chloride case will illustrate the powerful implications of this approach. Anderson et al. (6) developed a PB-PK model based on data indicating two routes of metabolism, one dependent on oxidation by mixed function oxidase (MFO) and the other dependent on glutathione s-transferase (GST) in four species (mouse, rat, hamster, human). Models were designed to quantify the contributions of the two metabolic pathways in the lung and liver and to allow for extrapolation from rodents to humans. Kinetic constants for the model were obtained from experiments or the literature, with model validation involving a comparison of predicted blood concentration time-course data in rats, mice, and humans with experimental data from these species.

The capacity of methylene chloride to cause tumors in mice was associated with the target tissue dose and was closely related to the amount of methylene chloride metabolized by the GST but not the MFO pathway. Using the PB-PK model, the target tissue doses in humans exposed to low concentrations of methylene chloride were between approximately 50- and 200-fold lower than would have been predicted by the linear extrapolation and body surface area factors used in conventional risk assessment methods. Thus, the PB-PK analysis suggests that conventional risk analysis greatly overestimates the risk to humans exposed to low levels of methylene chloride. One of the major uncertainties, however, is the metabolic capacity of the body at low exposure levels where metabolism may not be saturated. Also, the dominant

pathway for methylene chloride metabolism at other organ sites has not been determined. Still, the PB-PK approach represents an attractive development since it can increase the biological plausibility of predictive approaches while still incorporating biomathematical approaches for low-dose risk prediction.

Biologically Relevant Dose

Quantitative estimates of cancer risk at low exposure levels can be markedly enhanced by information on the delivered dose to the critical tissue (7,16,31,33). Hoel et al. (58) stated that it is likely to be "biologically more meaningful to relate tumor response to concentrations of specific DNA adducts in the target tissue than it is to relate tumor response to administered dose of a chemical." Despite the number of cancer bioassays for hundreds of chemicals, such quantitative relationships between administered and delivered doses are known for very few agents [i.e., vinyl chloride (48), dimethylnitrosamine, benzo[a]pyrene (58), and formaldehyde (108)].

Given the fact that the data needed to determine biologically relevant doses for cancer risk assessments are insufficient, it is usually accepted that the administered dose is proportional to this measure of exposure. The treatment dose is assumed to be a "valid" linear estimate for the unknown delivered dose, varying from it by not more than a constant scaling factor.

This assumption was strongly criticized by Hoel et al. (58), who demonstrated that this approach was frequently extremely conservative in that it overstates the cancer risk at low doses when the relationship between the delivered dose and the administrative dose is sublinear. It should also be noted that the degree of conservatism will vary for different chemicals; thus this approach could lead to an inappropriate ranking of different chemicals. Development of the biologically relevant dose approach requires a good understanding of the metabolism of the chemicals as well as characterization of the DNA adduct which is relevant to carcinogenesis.

Relative Potency Across Species

Another issue in the low-dose extrapolation approach is the question of whether carcinogenic potencies derived from this approach are likely to reflect the potencies in man. In other words, are there differences in the metabolism of chemicals or the tissue response such that quantitative extrapolation from carcinogenic potency in animals to potency in humans would be inappropriate? In general, comparison of potencies across species for known human carcinogens has indicated relative concordance. For example, in Table 10, the potencies for human carcinogens are similar to the potencies for rodent carcinogens, at least within an order of magnitude. Thus, the relative ranking across species of these carcinogens would be the same with aflatoxin B_1 being very potent and vinyl chloride of much lower potency. However, it is impossible to assess the converse of this issue, that is, does the potency of chemicals that have been shown to be animal carcinogens correlate well with their human carcinogenicity? In the absence of scientific confirmation, the prudent public policy has been to assume a similar ranking across species unless there is convincing evidence to assume otherwise. The uncertainties in mechanisms of carcinogenesis are usually so great as to preclude doing otherwise; however, relevant types of evidence might be as follows:

1. The demonstration of basic metabolic differences between rodents and humans such that a carcinogenic metabolite would be present at much lower concentrations in hu-

mans, as may occur with methylene chloride (see *Low Dose Extrapolation* section).
2. The demonstration of fundamental differences in the responsiveness of target cells such that the hyperplastic response does not occur.

One of the major debates regarding the relevance of cancer potency estimates derived from rodent bioassays to human cancer risk has been with mouse liver cancer. After several hundred cancer bioassays, it has become evident that the B6C3F1 mice responds much more sensitively than the Fisher 344 rat (the other commonly used rodent for cancer bioassays) to the development of pollutant-induced liver cancer (82). In a review of 85 chronic exposure assays, the mouse model developed hepatomas in 45 studies whereas the rat developed these tumors in 15 studies.

As a result of such interspecies differences in response, as well as the possibility that the mouse is uniquely sensitive to developing hepatomas, the Nutrition Foundation (82) organized an ad hoc review panel to assess the predictive relevance of the mouse hepatoma. One of the important conclusions derived from their appraisal is that the mouse, in contrast to the rat, develops tumors in the NTP bioassay from agents that have been found to be nongenotoxic in mutagenicity assays. While this area remains under intense investigation, the panel offered the suggestion that this mouse model may possess preinitiated cells in the liver in that "nongenotoxic" carcinogens are actually acting not as initiators but as cancer promoters. As discussed earlier, this conclusion would be particularly relevant with respect to the choice of low-dose extrapolation model. Another issue would be the extent to which humans possess preinitiated cells at different organ sites.

TABLE 10. *Comparison of potencies: animal and human*

Chemical	Potency[a]			
	Mouse	Rat	Dog	Human[b]
AN	—	0.06	—	<0.3
Aflatoxin, B_1	130[c]	500–1300	—	200 (3)
As	1.5–30	<0.01	—	15 (3)
Benzene	~0.0008	~0.0008	—	0.001 (3)
Benzidine	0.08	130–2500[d]	0.2	34 (10)
Chlornaphazine	20	—	—	2 (10)
Chloroform	0.01	0.002	—	<0.001
DCB	0.006	0.025	0.14	≤5
Diethylstilbestrol[e]	14	—	—	1[c] (10)
EDB	6	6	—	0.8 (10)
Lead acetate	0.001	0.007	—	<2.5
Saccharin	—	0.0003[c]	—	<0.04
Vinyl chloride	0.004	0.01	—	0.02 (3)
Radiation $(rem/yr)^{-1}$	0.01	—	—	0.02 (3)
Smoking $(no./d \times kg)^{-1}$	0.06	—	—	0.6 (3)

[a] Values are $kg \times d/mg$ except where noted.

[b] Number in parentheses next to human potency is our estimate of the accuracy of the number.

[c] Includes intrauterine exposure.

[d] Oral administration. Value for s.c. injection is 0.06 in rat and 0.08 in mouse.

[e] Women ingesting pills in pregnancy, resulting in cancer in daughters.

From ref. 32a, with permission.

Less Than Lifetime Exposure

A common situation for regulators occurs when exposure to elevated levels of carcinogens happens for up to several years but less than a lifetime. While lifetime cancer risk estimates are usually performed by the EPA with the linearized multistage model to determine excess lifetime cancer risk, the Carcinogen Assessment Group (CAG) of the EPA has adapted the Multistage–Weibull model to address the issue of less than lifetime exposure. This approach assumes that the earlier in life exposure starts the greater the ultimate risk, since there will be longer time available for the cancer to be expressed. The model also assumes that even if the exposure is stopped. the risk will still continue to accrue.

These assumptions have been challenged by the observation that postexposure accrual of risk for certain carcinogens may be markedly diminished (e.g., smoking-related lung cancer, nickel-related nasal cancer, DDT-induced liver cancer in mice, and benzo[a]pyrene-induced skin cancer in mice). These results demonstrate that even carcinogens that interact with DNA have potent tumor promoting activity. Freni (47) stated that "a model that does not recognize the potential of reduced additional incremental risk accrued after cessation of exposure is a model with an inherent safety factor of unknown magnitude." Given the widespread practical importance of this problem, more research is needed to determine quantitative methods to validate this approach.

In conclusion, the process by which regulatory agencies evaluate and set standards for carcinogens is clearly a combination of science and science policy. Regulators must make decisions based on incomplete information. When data are lacking, the policy has been to act conservatively so that the true risks from a chemical are not likely to be greater than those estimated. Unfortunately, the uncertainties in the risk assessment process and the use of upper bound levels have frequently not been well communicated to the risk managers and to the general public, giving the final risk assessment numbers a greater weight than may be warranted. In general, the risk assessment values for carcinogens are, at best, "order of magnitude" estimates.

A Case Study

Introduction

The preceding discussion demonstrates some of the major uncertainties in risk assessment for carcinogens by regulatory agencies and the role of science policy in choosing different options. In this section we provide a case study on risk assessment for 2,3,7,8-tetrachlorodibenzo-p-dioxin (TCDD, commonly referred to as dioxin). We hope that this example will help clarify the distinction between science and regulatory policy.

As has been presented elsewhere in this chapter, excess lifetime cancer risk can be estimated by combining the carcinogenic potency of a given compound with exposure information. Differences in excess lifetime cancer risk estimates, therefore, arise from either alternative exposure estimates, alternative potency estimates, or more typically both. Exposure estimates are often thought to be the major contributor

to differences among cancer risk estimates; however, derivation of potency estimates can contribute as much, if not more, than exposure estimates.

This case study explores how much uncertainty surrounds the estimate of TCDD cancer potency, where some of this uncertainty arises, how much various sources contribute and how United States regulatory agencies differ in their assessment of TCDD cancer potency. The approach taken was to compile TCDD cancer potency estimates and compare them with respect to dose–response model, rodent bioassay, and selection and treatment of bioassay results (5).

Approach

Previously published cancer potency estimates for TCDD by United States federal agencies were reviewed. Excluded from the comparison were potency estimates from Canada, Europe, and state agencies. Inclusion of some of these would have led to greater uncertainty surrounding TCDD potency estimate. For example, all United States agencies use nonthreshold dose–response models whereas the Canadian government uses a threshold model. At very low doses, all United States agency models predict a response in humans; the Canadian model does not.

Only existing potency estimates were compared. New potency estimates of greater variation could have been generated. These were not performed, since the intent of the case study was to demonstrate the range of the uncertainty in the risk assessment process of federal agencies today and the basis for the uncertainty.

Each potency estimate was converted to a unit risk by multiplying the potency estimate by a constant dose of 10 fg of TCDD per kilogram body weight per day (10 fg/kg/day). This dose was chosen to facilitate the presentation of the results. Since the same dose is used to derive all the unit risks, differences between the unit risks are therefore due to differences between potency estimates. In the remainder of the case study, *unit risk* and *potency estimate* are used interchangeably.

In comparing the potency estimates in the case study, we asked three questions:

1. How much of the difference between potency estimates is due to the choice of dose–response model?
2. How much of the difference between potency estimates is due to the choice of bioassay?
3. How much of the difference between potency estimates is due to the choice of data set?

The case study makes a distinction between a *bioassay* and a *data set*. *Bioassay* is defined as the unanalyzed results of an experimental animal cancer study. *Data set* is defined as the individual data that were used to generate a particular potency estimate, and encompasses how the results of one or more bioassays were selected, analyzed, and treated. Agencies could differ in which tumor sites were selected, how dose was converted from rodents to humans, whether pharmacokinetic information was employed, and so on. Clearly, many data sets can be developed from a single bioassay. The steps in the data selection process that contribute most of the uncertainty are discussed in the case study.

It should be noted that since dose–response curves predicted by a high- to low-dose extrapolation model are frequently nonlinear, the difference in unit risk estimates reported in the case study will change with changing dose. Further, the differences due to bioassay or dose–response model are not independent of each other. For example, the magnitude of the difference between two potency estimates as a result of bioassay selection depends on whether the Weibull model or the linearized multistage model is used.

Results

Eleven potency estimates for TCDD were compared. Eight of the potency estimates were derived by the United States

EPA (119), two were derived by the CDC (63), and one was derived by the FDA (72).

Unit risk values vary from 1.3×10^{-3} to 7.7×10^{-18}, a difference of 1.7×10^{14} (Fig. 2A). However, the potency estimates used for standard setting by the agencies (indicated by closed circles) are all within an order of magnitude of one and another (range: 1.9×10^{-7} to 1.6×10^{-6}) (Fig. 2A).

Effect of dose–response model

A plot of the unit risks using an identical data set (119), but different high- to low-dose models reveal that choice of response model accounts for more than 10^{13}-fold of this difference (compare Figs. 2A and 2B). For the particular dose

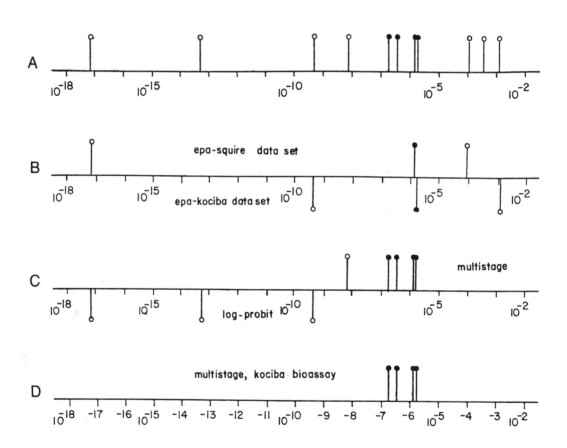

EXCESS LIFETIME CANCER RISK (10 fg/kg/day)

FIG. 2. A–D. Unit risks for TCDD, calculated by multiplying TCDD potency estimates by a lifetime dose of 10 fg dioxin kg/day, are plotted. The axes are log scale (to the base 10) and the units are excess individual lifetime cancer risk. Potency estimates used by agencies for standard setting are marked with a *black circle*. **A:** All 11 unit risk values are plotted. **B:** Unit risks are plotted that were calculated using the same data set but different models (Weibull, multistage, log probit). **C:** Unit risks are plotted that were derived using the multistage model but different bioassays. **D:** The unit risks plotted were derived using the multistage model and the same bioassay (64), thus the differences between potency estimates are due entirely to treatment of bioassay results.

and bioassay used to generate the unit risks, the Weibull model predicted the highest potency estimates; the log probit model, the lowest; and the multistage predicted intermediate potency estimates. Interestingly, the choice of dose–response model accounts for none of the differences between potency estimates actually used by agencies for standard setting (Fig. 2B) because all agencies used the linearized multistage or one hit model for standard setting.

This result could be due to a stronger scientific basis for the choice of one model over another. Alternatively, the choice of relatively similar dose–response models could reflect policy concerns by federal regulatory agencies. The use of vastly differing potency estimates for a single carcinogen by different regulatory agencies within the same country could represent an untenable public policy.

Effects of bioassay

A plot of unit risks using the linearized multistage model but different bioassays indicates that choice of bioassay contributes to the differences between TCDD potency estimates derived by different agencies (Fig. 2C). All agencies used results from at least the Kociba et al. (64) rat bioassay. The CDC also used results from the NTP (80) to estimate a lower limit on the range of excess lifetime cancer risk due to TCDD exposure. Since the higher CDC estimate is usually used to estimate allowable soil levels, and not the lower estimate, all agencies used the same model and same bioassay to derive TCDD potency estimates for standard setting.

Effect of data set

As was shown above, neither dose–response model nor choice of bioassay contributed to the order of magnitude difference from potency estimates used for standard setting. The difference arises, instead, from how agencies select and treat the results of bioassays (Fig. 2D). Several steps contribute to the order of magnitude difference observed between TCDD potency estimates. The largest difference, more than fivefold, is due to alternate ways of converting dose between animals and man. Some agencies converted dose on the basis of surface area rather than on the basis of body weight. Smaller differences arise when different tumor sites are selected (up to threefold); when tumor incidence is plotted against administered dose instead of dose measured in the liver (up to twofold); when an adjustment is, or is not, made for early mortality; and finally when the two pathologists quantified the incidence of tumors in tissue observed in cross-section differently (less than twofold).

Conclusions

The case study has revealed that for dioxin, the order of magnitude difference in the potency estimates used by federal agencies for standard setting arises entirely from how bioassay results are selected, analyzed, and interpreted. The choice of which bioassay and dose–response model to use has the potential to cause much larger, i.e., many orders of magnitude,

difference, but does not do so because all agencies use the same bioassay and similar dose–response models.

Larger differences between potency estimates could have arisen had agencies consistently selected parameters at each step of the potency estimation process that increased or decreased the potency estimate. No agency did this. Agencies made conservative assumptions at some steps, and less conservative assumptions at other steps. Nevertheless, in most steps the EPA used assumptions that were more conservative than those of the CDC or FDA, and thus developed a higher potency estimate for dioxin.

The difference between the potency estimates is reducible, but it probably cannot be eliminated. Differences in judgment by experts—for example, different tumor counts by two pathologists examining the same cross-sectional slides—will never be entirely eliminated. On the other hand, further research could lead to a reduction in the uncertainty and differences. For example, if we knew which dose–response model was most representative of the mechanism of carcinogenesis or if we knew how dose in rodents is related to dose in humans, uncertainty could be greatly reduced.

Use of *science policy* decisions is another way to reduce the difference between potency estimates. In effect, the agencies have already done this for dose–response model selection by basing excess lifetime cancer risk estimates on the linearized multistage model. While such decisions reduce differences between agencies, they have the disadvantage of hiding true uncertainty. For dose–response models, this uncertainty is very large, since there is currently no overwhelming scientific basis for the choice of one dose–response model over another. Furthermore, for dioxin, the linearized multistage model may be inappropriate given the limited genotoxicity of this chemical as compared with its cancer potency (101). It is important for regulators to recognize how much uncertainty may be hidden by science-policy decisions, and how this hidden uncertainty could affect the regulatory process.

EVALUATION OF SYSTEMIC TOXICANTS

In its broadest sense, systemic toxicity refers to all adverse effects, but in general it is applied only to chemicals that cause some type of adverse effect through a threshold mechanism. That is, for these chemicals, there is a level of exposure below which there is minimal, if any, chance for an adverse effect. The effects range from skin and eye irritation to subchronic or chronic damage to any organ system, such as pulmonary fibrosis.

The underlying mechanism is that multiple cells must be injured before an adverse effect is experienced, and that the injury must occur at a rate that exceeds the rate of repair. This contrasts with carcinogenesis, in which a genotoxic insult in a single cell is theoretically sufficient to allow that cell to grow to a malignant tumor (124). An example of a threshold-type injury can be seen with pulmonary fibrosis due to mineral dust exposure. Fibrotic areas may be present and observed as radiographic or histopathologic changes in the lungs of miners as a consequence of mineral dust exposure in the absence of any physiological impairment such as reduced FEV_1 or in the absence of changes in lung volume. Physiological impairment will occur as the fibrosis increases and the fibrotic areas begin to coalesce (131).

The general approach for setting exposure limits for systemic toxicants thus differs from that commonly used for carcinogens. When animal studies are used to derive limits, uncertainty factors are applied to the dose levels in the animal experiments to account for the lack of information on how to extrapolate from the animal species to humans. While these factors have traditionally been termed "safety" factors, "uncertainty" factors more accurately describes their use, which is to account for uncertainties in the relationship between exposure to a chemical in an animal study and a particular effect, and in the relationship between lifetime daily exposure to the same chemical in the general population of humans and the likelihood of a particular effect. The application of the appropriate uncertainty factors to an experimental exposure yields a level defined as the *acceptable daily intake* (ADI), which represents a daily intake level of a chemical in humans which is associated with no risk of adverse effects. The ADI is expressed in terms of milligrams of chemical per kilogram of body weight per day (79).

Recently, the EPA has decided to refer to such an exposure level as the risk reference dose or RfD. The basis for the change in terminology is that the ADI does not represent a magic dividing line between safe and nonsafe but is an exposure level, derived through a consistent methodology, at which the chance of adverse effects is low. It is still possible that there are some humans who, because of special susceptibility, could suffer an adverse effect at the RfD level. Thus, the use of the word "acceptable" is really not appropriate.

The history as well as the experimental support for uncertainty factors has been described by Dourson and Stara (38). Basically these authors describe four categories of uncertainty factors:

1. A 10-fold uncertainty factor to account for variations in susceptibility in humans. This would be the only factor applied to human studies in which exposure to a chemical resulted in no observed adverse effects, i.e., a *No Observed Adverse Effect Level,* or NOAEL, could be defined from this study. (If the study population consisted of humans known to constitute the susceptible population and a NOAEL was defined with a lifetime exposure, no uncertainty factor would be required.) In the following section we discuss in detail the variability in human responsiveness to environmental pollutants and its relevance to the regulatory process.
2. A 10-fold uncertainty factor to extrapolate from animal data to human data. The assumption here is that some humans may be more susceptible than experimental animals to a particular chemical, but that the magnitude of the increased susceptibility is within a factor of 10.
3. A 10-fold uncertainty factor to extrapolate from a subchronic exposure to a chronic exposure. The assumption is that if a chemical were given over the lifetime of the animal rather than over a fraction of the lifetime, a smaller amount of chemical would result in the same NOAEL.
4. An uncertainty factor between 1 and 10 to extrapolate from a *Lowest Observed Adverse Effect Level* (LOAEL)— the lowest level of exposure at which an adverse effect was observed—to a NOAEL. This factor is a matter of toxicological judgment, taking into account the severity of effect observed at the LOAEL as well as the shape of the dose–response curve. In a recent EPA publication on the RfD (123), a value of 10 is described to apply to LOAEL studies. However, a modifying factor greater than zero, but less than 10, can also be utilized.

Uncertainty factors are used multiplicatively. Thus, to determine the RfD:

1. An uncertainty factor of 100 is applied to the NOAEL in chronic animal studies.
2. An uncertainty of 1000 is applied to the NOAEL in subchronic studies.
3. An uncertainty factor between 1000 and 10,000 is applied to the LOAEL subchronic animal studies (where a NOAEL was not defined).

The RfD approach represents a generally accepted (NAS, FDA, and EPA among others) method for setting lifetime exposure limits for humans and the use of the 10-fold uncertainty factors has some experimental support (38). For example, the ratio between the subchronic and chronic NOAEL or LOAEL for 52 chemicals was less than 10 in 96% of the cases. Thus, the uncertainty factor of 10 would not be adequate with only 4% of these chemicals.

However, there are several limitations in the RfD approach, the net result of which is that the same RfD does not imply the same level of risk for all chemicals, and that excursions above the RfD do not represent the same increase in risk for all chemicals. First of all, the choice of a LOAEL or a NOAEL does not take into consideration the greater experimental confidence associated with, for example, studies using more experimental animals. An exposure concentration defined as a NOAEL could turn out to be a LOAEL, had more experimental animals been used. This approach may reward poorer experiments, since fewer animals would result in a higher RfD than studies with larger numbers of animals (34).

Additionally the RfD approach does not make use of dose-response information, which is a key determinant in assessing the likelihood of effects. Thus, a chemical with a steep dose-response curve would be associated with a greater likelihood of effects as exposure increased above the RfD and a smaller likelihood of effects with exposure below the RfD than would a chemical with a more shallow dose–response curve (37).

There are other approaches that can be used, in addition to the modifying factor approach, that can address the issues of experimental quality and the shape of the dose–response curve. Dourson (37) has proposed a *Mathematical Model Approach* for estimating RfDs that incorporates information on the level of confidence in the LOAEL or the NOAEL and on the shape of the dose–response curve. Although other procedures have been presented (34), we will describe only the method of Dourson to provide an example of how improvements could be made in the derivation of RfDs.

With this method, an adverse effect level is defined as a certain percent of adverse response above background and the lower 95% confidence limit on dose associated with this level is calculated. The uncertainty factors are applied to this confidence limit. Since the lower confidence limit applies to a LOAEL, rather than to a NOAEL, uncertainty factors can be applied that reflect the severity of effect as well as the shape of the dose–response curve. Thus, a steeper dose–response curve would result in a smaller uncertainty factor than would a more shallow dose–response curve. Also, the use of the lower 95% confidence limit for dose rewards better experiments.

In the example provided in Fig. 3, an uncertainty factor of 10 is applied to the LOAEL to estimate a NOAEL using dog data, because the effect (liver necrosis) is relatively adverse and is accompanied by a relatively shallow dose–response curve. In contrast, an uncertainty factor of 1 is applied to the rat data because of the mildness of the response (slight body weight decrease) and the steep dose–response curve.

An additional difficulty with the RfD approach revolves around the basis for the uncertainty factor used for extrapolating from animals to humans. Dourson and Stara (38) consider the interspecies uncertainty factor as basically a scaling factor, assuming that different species are equally sensitive to a chemical when the dose is expressed on a dose-per-unit surface area, which is really a reflection of metabolic differences across species (22). In this case, one could normalize data based on a surface area correction factor (body weight $\frac{2}{3}$) and eliminate the 10-fold uncertainty factor.

In fact, the reason that the uncertainty factor of 10 works is that most animal experiments on which toxicological risk assessments are based utilize rats and mice, and that metabolic differences (which usually scale according to a surface area function) frequently account for species differences in toxicity (22). In these cases, a scaling factor of about 8 for rats and 13 for mice would account for differences in the surface area to body weight ratios. An uncertainty factor of 10 applied to experiments using tree shrews would not be adequately protective, and an uncertainty factor of 10 applied to experiments using elephants would be overly protective.

The basis for the interspecies uncertainty factor assumes that differences across species are primarily due to differences in the exposure–dose relationship and that this difference can be expressed as a function of surface area. If, through pharmacokinetic modeling, as has been described by Anderson et al. (6), or through the use of measures of biologically effective dose, such as benzo[a]pyrene–DNA adducts in target cells (91), we define exactly the relationship between exposure

and dose across species, the conclusion would be that this uncertainty factor could be eliminated.

In fact, while species differences frequently are a consequence of differences in the exposure–dose relationship, differences may also occur in the ability of different animal species to respond to the same level of metabolite at the target cell. Thus, macrophages of different animal species, when exposed to the fibrogenic mineral dust, alpha-quartz, do not demonstrate the same response in terms of levels or characteristics of fibroblast stimulating factor (53,57) which is consistent with differences in response to intratracheally instilled alpha-quartz (2,17,50).

It would be more appropriate to consider the interspecies extrapolation as two factors: one to account for scaling differences across species (22,35), and one to account for innate differences in responsiveness. For derivation of an RfD, both a scaling factor and an uncertainty factor should be applied. Data are generally not available now to make such a determination, but this distinction could help in the design of modeling studies and in future experiments to address the basis for differences across species.

ROLE OF HIGH RISK GROUPS

In the previous section, we described the RfD concept as used by regulatory agencies to estimate acceptable levels for noncancer effects. One of the factors in the derivation of this level was to account for variations in population susceptibility. The purpose of this section is to expand upon that issue, to describe the basis for variations in susceptibility and the magnitude of that variation, and to demonstrate the relationship of this issue to the regulatory process. (For more detail the reader is referred to refs. 15, 18, and 19.)

There is a high degree of variability in the response of humans to different exposure levels of air and water pollutants (19,30). In fact, the variability in the dose–response relationship in a heterogeneous population makes difficult the estimate of an acceptable level for chemical contaminants that

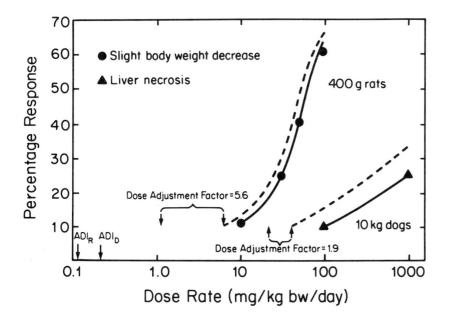

FIG. 3. Hypothetical dose–response data for slight body weight decrease (*circles*) or liver necrosis (*triangles*) in rats and dogs, respectively. *Solid lines* indicate hypothetical data. *Dashed lines* represent lower 95% confidence limits (CLs). An ADI has been estimated from the dog data (ADI_D) by a dose adjustment factor of 1.9 to the lower 95% confidence limit and a 100-fold uncertainty factor. An ADI has been estimated from the rat data (ADI_R) by a dose adjustment factor of 5.6 and a 10-fold uncertainty factor. (From ref. 37, with permission.)

would be protective of the whole population. Perhaps the most critical question is not what is a "safe" numerical standard, but how many individuals are adversely affected at different levels of exposure (25).

Knowing which groups of individuals are at high risk with respect to pollutants is very important in answering this question, since these individuals will be the first to experience morbidity and mortality as pollutant levels increase. If the high risk segments are protected, then the entire population also is protected. Information concerning both the identification and quantification of high risk groups should play an integral role in the derivation of environmental health standards, including how the United States EPA has attempted to utilize this knowledge in setting ambient air and drinking water standards.

Noncancer Endpoints

The Clean Air Act Amendments of 1970 specifically require that primary air quality standards completely protect the public's health and that the standards incorporate sufficient safety margins. There is an implicit assumption in the Clean Air Act Amendments that a "no-effects" level exists for every pollutant and for each adverse health effect (43). Despite the enhanced susceptibility of high risk subpopulations to the toxic effects of pollutants, Finklea et al. (43) stated that high risk groups were not, to any great extent, considered in any quantitative or analytic sense in the derivation of the original NAAQS. The rationale of the EPA was that "adequate protection for the larger susceptible population segments and the margins of safety included would also ensure protection for the large number of relatively small susceptible segments of the population for which we have little or no quantitative exposure information" (43). Thus, high risk segments of the population were often not specifically considered in the standard derivation process because there was not enough evidence to offer a precise assessment of risk, and because it was thought that they made up only a negligible percentage of the population. In contrast, recent analyses by the EPA, as with the NAAQS for lead, utilize the concept of high risk population in a more quantitative way by estimating the fraction of the susceptible subpopulation (children) that would be protected at different air levels of lead (120).

In trying to assess the role of high risk groups in the derivation of environmental health standards, it is useful to consider the extent to which the EPA has utilized the concept of high risk groups within the standard setting process. Perhaps the most common approach utilized by the EPA and other regulatory agencies has been the implementation of safety (or uncertainty) factors. While this approach implicitly recognizes that certain people are more sensitive to pollutants than others, it is inherently imprecise. The precise difference in sensitivity between a statistically "normal" individual and groups at increased risk will vary for the different causes of the high risk condition and for different pollutants.

The EPA has utilized the uncertainty factor approach in attempting to deal with protecting the high risk individuals, as illustrated by the national drinking water standards for noncarcinogenic chlorinated hydrocarbon insecticides and herbicides (18). These substances were tested in two animal species, the rat and dog. Chronic toxicity testing provided an estimate of the lowest level of pollutant (on a milligram of dose per kilogram of body weight) that the animal could ingest with either minimal or no toxic effects. In the absence of data to indicate a basis for an alternative choice, the species that was the most sensitive to the substances was chosen to derive the standard, implying that humans are as sensitive as the most sensitive animal species. In the absence of supporting human exposure data (as with most cases, with the exception of methoxychlor), an uncertainty factor of 500 was applied to the minimally toxic dose in the most sensitive animal species (i.e., the minimally toxic dose was divided by 500). It should be noted that this methodology differs from that of the RfD approach described earlier, in which case a factor of 100 would have been applied. This number was taken to be the total amount of insecticide (or herbicide) to which a human could be exposed each day over an unspecified period of time without suffering any adverse health effects.

Next, amounts of the chlorinated hydrocarbons normally consumed via the diet were derived from market basket surveys. If this amount were substantially less than $\frac{1}{500}$ of a known toxic dose in the most sensitive animal species tested (i.e., the assumed acceptable level of intake for humans), then a drinking water limit was established that would permit 20% of the safe limit to be consumed via water.

Several questions occur when evaluating such a methodological scheme. For example, on what basis can we assume that the most sensitive humans have the same degree of responsiveness as the most sensitive animals? Why was 500 chosen as a safety factor? What assurances exist that it would provide sufficient protection for the general population as well as high risk groups for these chemicals? Who, in fact, are the groups considered at increased risk?

The main problem with such an approach is its lack of specificity in identifying susceptible subpopulations, the extent of their susceptibility, and, very importantly, what fraction is protected by different standard levels. It should also be realized, however, that when only limited data are available, imprecise safety factors are the only realistic options available. Still, this approach will result in uncertain levels of protection. Alternative approaches must be developed to reduce the magnitude of that uncertainty.

The EPA has specifically evaluated the increased sensitivity of specific high risk groups with respect to several toxic substances including carbon monoxide, lead, nitrates, nitrogen dioxide, ozone, and sulfur dioxide (Table 11). Following is a detailed description of the EPA's consideration of high risk groups in the derivation of drinking water standards for nitrates and cadmium. The role of high risk groups in deriving standards for carcinogens is also discussed.

Nitrates in Drinking Water

The drinking water standard of 10 mg nitrate (NO_3^{-2}) as mg nitrogen per liter is designed to prevent the formation of elevated levels of methemoglobin (MetHb) in infants. In the presence of nitrite (NO_2^{-1}), formed from nitrate in infants, hemoglobin is oxidized to MetHb, which is not able to re-

TABLE 11. *High risk groups in the derivation of standards by the United States EPA*

A. Drinking Water Standards

Substance	High risk condition considered
Arsenic	None
Barium	No specific groups; but a safety factor of two incorporated to account for variation (or increased susceptibility) within the human population.
Cadmium	None
Fluoride	Children—to prevent mottling of teeth
Lead	Children—to prevent neurological disorders
Mercury	Based on humans who exhibited toxicity at the lowest level of exposure from a group of mercury poisoned adults
Nitrate	Infants—to protect against methemoglobinemia
Selenium	None
Sodium (no standard)	Individuals with heart and kidney disease
Chlorinated hydrocarbon insecticides (noncarcinogenic)	None
Chlorophenoxy herbicides (noncarcinogenic)	None

B. National Ambient Air Quality Standard

Substance	Original group	Groups currently considered
Carbon monoxide	Individuals with neurological or visual impairment	Adults with heart disease (angina, coronary artery disease)
Lead	Children—to protect against neurological and hematological impairment	Same
Nitrogen dioxide	Children—to protect against respiratory infections, also concern for changes in lung structure	Same
Ozone	Asthmatics	Exercisers, individuals with pre-existing disease
Particulates	Elderly, individuals with cardiopulmonary disease	Same
Sulfur dioxide	Elderly, individuals with cardiopulmonary disease	Asthmatics

versibly combine with oxygen. Levels of 1–2% and 2–5% MetHb are typical in the blood of adults and infants, respectively. When concentrations are less than 5% MetHb, there are no obvious indications of toxicity. However, with levels of MetHb from 5 to 10%, clinical signs of toxicity (e.g., cyanosis) may appear (18).

Infants are at considerable risk to nitrate-related toxicity as compared with adults. Factors that predispose infants to the development of MetHb formation include:

1. The incompletely developed ability to secrete gastric acid. This permits the gastric pH to be high enough (5–7 pH) to permit the growth of nitrate-reducing bacteria in the gastrointestinal tract, thereby converting the nitrate to nitrite before absorption into the circulation (113).
2. The higher levels of fetal hemoglobin in infants. This form of hemoglobin is more susceptible than adult hemoglobin to oxidation to MetHb (13).
3. The diminished enzymatic capability of infants to reduce MetHb to hemoglobin (100).

Research has revealed that levels of nitrate beyond 20 mg/l resulted in a marked upshift in the frequency of methemoglobinemia in infants but not among adults (18). Consequently, a standard of 10 mg/l is principally designed to prevent the occurrence of elevated levels of MetHb in infants. Concentrations twice as great would still protect adults.

Cadmium

Studies with rats show that at a kidney concentration of 200 ppm cadmium (Cd) (117), renal damage is initiated. The

EPA calculated that humans would need to ingest 50 μg Cd/day for 50 years to reach a level of 200 ppm in their kidneys. In the derivation of the Cd drinking water standard, the EPA assumed a daily Cd exposure of 75 μg from the diet and 20 μg from water. This 20 μg Cd/day from drinking water would occur at a level of 0.01 mg/l. The total daily Cd exposure is therefore approximately 95 μg Cd/day, and thus a safety factor of 4 was assumed.

In proposing their drinking water standard for cadmium, the EPA requested feedback from the public as to whether the standard should include additional protection for cigarette smokers, since smoking is a source of appreciable cadmium exposure (e.g., approximately 1.5 μg Cd/cigarette) (19). It is interesting to note that of the 52 comments received by the EPA on this issue, only three suggested that this standard be modified to include protection for the cigarette smokers. The EPA decided not to incorporate additional safety factors to protect smokers (122). Thus, this example describes a situation in which protection of a high risk group was not taken into account in derivation of a standard.

Standards for Carcinogens: Role for High Risk Groups?

In general, setting of levels for carcinogen exposure has not addressed the role of population variability in susceptibility to carcinogens. Consequently, groups at high risk to environmental carcinogens, with the obvious exceptions of smoking as a risk factor for exposure to asbestos, uranium, and coke-oven emission-related cancer, have not generally been addressed. It should be noted, however, that the conservatism of the cancer risk assessment process might result in adequate protection of high risk groups.

Still, there is evidence that development, genetics, nutrition, and other factors can play an important role in enhancing susceptibility to environmentally related cancer (for further discussion, see refs. 15, 20, and 43). For example, individuals with the inherited disease, xeroderma pigmentosum, which is characterized by a significantly reduced capacity to repair UV-induced damage to DNA, are at exceptionally high risk to UV-induced skin cancer (27,28). Lower (67) has proposed that, based on animal models and limited human epidemiological data, individuals who are slow acetylators of arylamines may be at increased risk of bladder cancer following exposure to these dyes. The role of diet and certain types of cancer is shown in studies demonstrating an inverse relationship between amount of vitamin A in the diet and susceptibility to hydrocarbon-induced epithelial cancers (29). It is likely that, even given the same exposure to a carcinogen, individuals are not equally susceptible to the induction of cancer and in many cases the differential susceptibility may be very large.

The role of population variability should be considered by regulatory agencies in risk assessments for carcinogens. Identification and quantification of susceptible population could provide decision-makers with a theoretical framework on which to base regulatory action. Tamplin and Gofman (110) have employed knowledge of susceptible populations in predicting the incidence of cancer from drinking water to help define acceptable levels of exposure. Tamplin and Gofman (110) assumed that the latency period is shorter for *in utero* exposure (i.e., five years versus 15 years for all radiation exposure beyond birth). Consideration of the increased susceptibility of the fetus to radiation-induced cancer resulted in greater estimates of cancer risk as compared with traditional methodological approaches which predict carcinogenic effects at low doses based on high levels of exposure in adults (98).

IMPLICATIONS OF CHEMICAL INTERACTIONS FOR THE REGULATORY PROCESS

One of the major difficulties in current environmental public health practice is that the focus is on a limited number of environmental contaminants with little consideration of interactive effects among pollutants (77). In fact, the number of environmental pollutants in different media is large, making it difficult to estimate the degree of public health protection afforded by our present regulatory apparatus. Still, it is clear that the scientific and regulatory communities must address the issue of multiple chemical exposures. In fact, animal models and human epidemiological studies show that interactions do occur among chemicals and that this can result in greater-than-additive effects. For example, uranium miners who do not smoke have a fourfold greater risk of lung cancer than the general nonsmoking population. Smokers have an approximately 10-fold greater risk of cancer than nonsmokers. However, uranium miners who smoke display a 40-fold greater cancer risk than the general population of nonsmokers. A similar magnitude of interaction occurs with occupational asbestos exposure and smoking.

While environmental toxicologists are now addressing the issue of chemical interactions, such interactions have been studied for many years by the drug industry, insecticide manufacturers, and forensic/clinical toxicologists. Given the widespread use of multiple drug therapy, the need to anticipate possible interactions has been essential.

Chemical interactions have been broadly classified by three general terms: *Addition* (additivity)—when the toxic effect produced by two or more chemicals in combination is equivalent to that expected by simple summation of their individual effects; *antagonism*—when the effect of a combination is less than the sum of the individual effects; and *synergism*—when the effect of the combination is greater than would be predicted by summation of the individual effects. Other terms have been used such as indifference and potentiation, which represent specialized aspects of antagonism and synergism, respectively.

In testing for possible interactions, several important considerations must be addressed. These include temporal (time) factors and response–end point considerations.

Time Factor

While most screening tests for interactions employ simultaneous exposure, this type of exposure approach has the chance of reducing the likelihood of detecting some potential interactions. For example, two agents may affect the same cellular mechanism but have markedly different times of onset to expression. If a critical threshold of reversible cellular injury is required for the adverse effect, tests of acute toxicity of combinations given simultaneously may show antagonism, whereas an additive action would be observed if the dosing and observation periods were spaced to cause the maximum effect.

Toxic Effect

Since most toxic substances have multiple toxic effects, the nature of any chemical interaction may vary depending on the measured responses. For example, since chlorinated insecticides and halogenated solvents produce liver injury independently, it is reasonable to expect that they would act in an additive or synergistic manner when combined. However, the insecticide is likely to be a central nervous system stimulant, whereas the solvent may be a central nervous system depressant. Thus, as measured by neurological tests, these chemicals could interact in an antagonistic way.

Predictive Models

Development of predictive models of chemical interaction must rely on an understanding of the basic toxicological principles concerning kinetics of reactions of chemicals with primary sites of action (tissue receptor sites) and with secondary tissue sites of reaction. Four factors have been identified as of central importance:

1. Relative affinities of the individual chemicals for sites of action (e.g., target enzymes, cellular membranes, etc.);
2. Relative affinities for sites of loss of the chemical (e.g., detoxifying enzymes, nonvital tissue binding sites, pathways of excretion, and storage sites);
3. Intrinsic activity of the agents at their sites of action; and
4. Sites of bioactivation.

While many of the examples are derived from the pharmacology literature, similar interactions could occur among environmental chemicals.

Pharmacokinetic Drug/Pollutant Interactions

The above four factors allow us to predict how toxicological interactions may occur. The biological damage caused by a toxic agent is proportional to the amount of the biologically active form of the agents able to react with critical cellular macromolecules. An interaction may occur when the availability of an active chemical is altered by the presence of another agent, or when its reactivity with critical macromolecules is altered by the presence of another agent. The first case involves a site of loss of active chemical whereas the second involves an interaction at a site of action. Thus, considerable research activity has investigated the capacity of a chemical to affect the absorption, distribution, metabolism, and excretion of another chemical.

Absorption

Absorption of an agent may be affected by a second drug which alters pH or gut motility. For example, aspirin is absorbed more rapidly at low pH because more of the drug is present in the readily diffusible nonionized lipid soluble form. Agents taken simultaneously that cause an increase in the pH will slow down the gastric absorption of aspirin. Similarly, the absorption of tetracycline is reduced by aluminum hydroxide gels and readily ionized salts of calcium and magnesium. In contrast, the gastrointestinal absorption of acetaminophen is enhanced in the presence of sorbitol.

Protein binding

Drugs may compete for the same protein binding sites in plasma. When this occurs, the effective biological concentrations of the displaced drug can rise markedly. For example, usually 98% of the anticoagulant drug warfarin is bound to the plasma protein albumin so that only 2% of the total drug in the plasma is biologically active. If the effect of another drug competing for the same plasma albumin site is to reduce the binding of warfarin from 98 to 96%, the concentration of pharmacologically active warfarin would be doubled. This interaction would have approximately the same effect on clotting time as would doubling the dose of the anticoagulant. This type of interaction with an anticoagulant drug has resulted in a number of clinical incidents, with some resulting in fatal hemorrhagic complications.

Metabolism

Many chemicals including drugs and environmental contaminants enhance the metabolic capacity of the liver. Other chemicals may diminish the metabolic capacity of the liver. These interactions could have profound implications. In fact, it is now recognized that several of the insecticide synergists (i.e., agents that, when administered along with insecticides, markedly enhance the insecticide's ability to kill insects) act by blocking the enzymes normally affecting insecticide detoxification (128). For example, the toxicity of the insecticide carbaryl against susceptible female houseflies is enhanced by over 200-fold by certain chemical synergists. This knowledge has been used to develop more effective insecticide formulations.

In the above example, the investigators used the concept of synergism to enhance toxicity and develop more efficient insecticidal formulations. The concern of public health agencies has been, of course, to reduce human exposures to potentially dangerous mixtures. Insecticides provide another example of how agencies use information on chemical interactions.

In 1957, Frawley et al. (46) reported the first synergistic interaction of two organophosphate insecticides (i.e., malathion and ethyl p-nitrophenyl phenyl phosphonothionate or EPN) which led to the development of the FDA requirement that all newly registered organophosphate insecticides be evaluated for possible synergisms against all the already registered organophosphate insecticides. As more organophosphate insecticides were developed, this regulatory requirement became an extreme testing burden. However, with elucidation of the biochemical mechanism[1] for this interaction, it became possible to assess possible interactions of organophosphate insecticides via biochemical means and thereby circumvent the time-consuming and costly toxicological testing of whole animals. In both examples, that of making a more efficient insecticidal preparation and that of predicting adverse public health effects from multiple agent exposures, predictions of chemical interactions were markedly enhanced with a clear understanding of the mechanisms of toxicity.

The examples given above represent ideal situations since the mechanisms of toxicity of the insecticides were very well characterized. More frequently, little information is available on toxic mechanisms. Regulatory agencies need to develop approaches in such situations when reasonable mechanistic predictions cannot be made. To this end, Finney (44) developed a theoretical mathematical approach for predicting the degree of toxicity derived from various types of chemical interactions. Pozzani et al. (94) indicated that only two of the 36 pairs of mixtures of industrial vapors tested for acute toxicity in rats deviated significantly from the calculations of Finney's theoretical approach for additive joint toxicity. According to Smyth (104), the study by Pozzani et al. (94) supported the hypothesis that the acute toxicity of chemical mixtures randomly chosen has a high likelihood of being accurately predicted by Finney's theoretical formula for additive joint toxicity. In an attempt "to evaluate the overall confidence that can be placed on the prediction of the joint toxicity of many chemical pairs," Smyth et al. (104) studied the toxicity of 27 industrial chemicals in all possible pairs to rats. Their results were consistent with the prediction of Finney (44) that most interactions should be considered as additive until proven otherwise. Smyth et al. (104), in agreement with the general findings of Pozzani et al. (94), concluded that approximately 5% of the various combinations tested exhibited more or less than additive effects.

While synergy among chemicals may be relatively rare, given the large number of chemicals in commerce, the potential for such interactions is still a source of concern. For instance, if there are N potentially toxic chemicals in commerce today and if we assume there is a total of 12,000 chemicals, then the number of potential pairs is $N(N - 1)/2$. Consequently, of the $12,000 \times 11,999/2$ pairs, 2.5% or 1.8 million pairs may act synergistically. Thus, even though the majority of interactions would be additive, there would still be a very large number of synergistic interactions.

Most studies have evaluated synergism at only very high or acute levels of exposure. It is important, however, to ask whether synergisms would occur at lower (more realistic) concentrations. While the former Chief of NIOSH's Toxicology Division, Dr. Herbert Stokinger, has stated that the interactions of substances at low levels of exposure would be "physiologically inconsequential," there are actually very few data on which to make judgments. A recent theoretical assessment of the consequences of exposures to low levels of multiple carcinogens concluded that current predictions of low-dose carcinogen risk using linear dose–response assumptions are not worst case estimates of risk but may underestimate risk, since the predicted slope of the dose–response curve is steeper at low level exposures that at the higher levels of exposure (8,9).

The gist of Murphy's (75) thesis and that of others, such as deBruin (36) and Calabrese (18,24), is that the number of possible combinations of exposures is multiplicative and far exceeds the capacity of the toxicological community to assess even a very small percentage of the permutations for but a few toxic endpoints. The most plausible way out of this societal dilemma is to gain a better understanding of cellular mechanisms and chemical disposition of individual agents so that biologically/chemically realistic models for predictions can be developed and tested for their validation. Murphy (75) concluded that "creative application of data obtained in the molecular toxicology laboratory may enable us to examine the laundry list of chemicals from varied dump sites and make reasonable predictions as to whether there is increased risk because of likelihood of toxicological interactions."

While Murphy (75) has laid out a general research agenda, the OSHA (83) carcinogen hearings tried to establish the potential importance of carcinogen interactions. Many leading scientists testified at these hearings on the widespread occurrence of synergism amongst carcinogens. For example, Dr. Richard Griesemer of the National Cancer Institute (83) testified that synergism amongst carcinogens was not only widespread but also was a frequent phenomenon. However, it must be understood that carcinogen interaction may also result in antagonistic effects and, as in the case of synergisms, antagonisms are widespread and also frequent. For example, the suppressive effects of polycyclic aromatic hydrocarbons on carcinogenicity are well known (36).

Predicting the potential interaction of multiple chemical agents is a major regulatory concern of international and United States advisory and regulatory agencies such as OSHA (83,84), the ACGIH (3), WHO (130) and, most recently, the EPA (121). In their perspective on the subject, the EPA (121) identified several areas of concern.

1. While most information known about toxicant interactions is based on acute toxicity studies using animals with mixtures of two compounds, the EPA has questioned the toxicological framework whereby chronic responses can be inferred from the acute interaction studies. The EPA claimed that the major problem in this regard was the need to prove that the mechanism(s) of the interaction from the acute study would apply to the low-dose chronic exposure.
2. The EPA feels that the use of information from two component mixtures to predict the interactions of greater than two compounds has problems as far as developing an inherent mechanistic perspective. The EPA stated that if two agents interact because of the effects of one agent on the kinetics of the other, the addition of a third compound, which modified the kinetics of one of the two agents, may markedly change the degree of toxicologic interaction.
3. The EPA expressed concern that interspecies differences

---

[1] EPN inhibits the nonspecific enzyme carboxyesterase that detoxifies malathion. Thus, in the presence of EPN, malathion is more persistent and causes a greater effect as a cholinesterase inhibitor than would have occurred had enzymatic detoxification mechanisms not been affected.

are difficult enough to understand when only a single toxicant is used. It is possible that the magnitude of any interaction in animals will be significantly different in humans.

4. The EPA asserted that none of the models employed for describing chemical interactions is able to predict the magnitude of toxicant interactions without considerable data.

The role of chemical interactions in the standard-setting process in the United States remains to be seen. Common sense demands that interactions be considered in the development of health-based standards. The question naturally arises whether some of our present standards should be modified in light of recent evidence concerning synergistic interactions of various pollutants. Shy et al. (102) were of the opinion that the present ambient air standards should not be revised as a result of knowledge derived from new laboratory studies that include various combinations of pollutants. Since the present air standards were primarily derived from epidemiological studies, chemical interactions were occurring even though only single pollutants were specifically related to health effects. Similar reasoning could probably be used for epidemiologically based industrial standards as well. However, for standards that are based primarily on toxicological data, the role of interactions must be addressed.

CONCLUSIONS

The function of toxicology in the regulatory process is to predict effects in humans at ambient exposure concentrations. When the level of uncertainty is high, for example with low-dose extrapolation of carcinogens, the policy decision is to choose an approach that may err on the side of conservatism. The determination of how conservative is conservative enough and when enough information is available to choose other options represents critical science-policy decisions for regulatory authorities. It is extremely important for regulatory bodies to clearly articulate the basis for decisions on toxic chemicals and describe how much is based on science and how much on science policy.

Using the risk assessment paradigm of the National Academy of Sciences described earlier in this chapter, the two central subject areas of toxicology in the regulatory process are hazard identification and assessment of dose–response relations. With hazard identification, the use of regulatory toxicology is to provide a weight-of-evidence evaluation of the likelihood that a particular chemical will produce a response in humans that is comparable to the response observed in animals. Other components of hazard identification include identification of susceptible populations and an assessment of how responses of the susceptible group may differ from the general population. Also important are interactive effects between the chemical of interest and other environmental chemicals.

With dose–response assessment, regulatory toxicology seeks to predict effects in humans at exposure concentrations that are typically much lower than those utilized in animal studies. Historically, a distinction has been made between carcinogens and noncarcinogens. This distinction is based on the assumption that any exposure to a carcinogen carries some level of risk. Many carcinogens interact with DNA, and the alteration of DNA in even a single cell could result in that cell becoming transformed and eventually malignant. Noncarcinogens are assumed to cause injury through a threshold mechanism. That is, multiple cells must be injured at a rate that exceeds the rate of repair for an adverse effect to be expressed.

Recently, this distinction has become less clear. Some carcinogens, such as TCDD, may function through nongenotoxic mechanisms and would, therefore, exhibit a sublinear dose–response at low doses. In contrast, the setting of a threshold level for some noncarcinogens, such as lead, has become difficult as methodologies to quantify physiological alterations become more refined and responses are observed at very low levels of exposure.

Ultimately, improvement of how toxicology is used in the regulatory process requires better understanding of basic cellular mechanisms involved in responses to toxic chemicals. Mechanisms are typically evaluated in *in vitro* or *in vivo* animal models. However, verification of toxicological mechanisms using human cells *in vitro* or with preclinical indicators of response in humans must also be research priorities for toxicologists.

ACKNOWLEDGMENTS

This work was partially supported by Grant CR-807809 to the Interdisciplinary Programs in Health from the EPA. The section entitled "Implications of Chemical Interactions for the Regulatory Process" was based in large part on work by E. J. Calabrese (23).

REFERENCES

1. Allen, K. L., Green, C. E., and Tyson, C. A. (1987): Comparative studies of peroxisomal enzyme induction in hepatocytes from rat, cynomolugus monkey and human by hypolipidemic drugs. *Toxicologist,* 7:63.
2. Allison, A. C., Harington, J. S., and Birbeck, M. (1966): An examination of the cytotoxic effects of silica on macrophages. *J. Exp. Med.,* 124:141–154.
3. American Conference of Governmental Industrial Hygienists (1983): *TLVs: Threshold Limit Values for Chemical Substances and Physical Agents in the Work Environment with Intended Charges for 1983-1984.* American Conference of Governmental Industrial Hygienists, Cincinnati, Ohio, p. 58.
4. American Conference of Governmental Industrial Hygienists (1986): *Documentation of the Threshold Limit Values,* 5th ed. American Conference of Governmental Industrial Hygienists, Cincinnati, Ohio.
5. Andersen, P. (1986): *Ninth Symposium on Statistics and the Environment,* October, 1986. Sponsored by the National Academy of Sciences, Washington, D.C.
6. Andersen, M. E., Clewell III, H. J., Gargas, M. L., Smith, F. A., and Reitz, R. H. (1987): Physiologically based pharmacokinetics and the risk assessment process for methylene chloride. *Toxicol. Appl. Pharmacol.,* 87:185–205.
7. Anderson, M. E., Hoel, D. G., and Kaplan, N. L. (1980): A general scheme for the incorporation of pharmacokinetics in low-dose risk estimation for chemical carcinogenesis: Example—vinyl chloride. *Toxicol. Appl. Pharmacol.,* 55:154–161.
8. Barenbaum, M. C. (1981): Criteria for analyzing interaction between biologically active agents. *Adv. Cancer Res.,* 35:269–335.

9. Barenbaum, M. C. (1985): Consequences of synergy between environmental carcinogens. *Environ. Res.*, 38:310–318.

10. Beck, B. D., and Brain, J. D. (1982): Prediction of the pulmonary toxicity of respirable combustion products from residential wood and coal stoves. In: *Residential Wood and Coal Combustion*, pp. 264–280. Air Pollution Control Association, Pittsburgh, Pennsylvania.

11. Berenblum, I. (1941): The cocarcinogenic action of croton resin. *Cancer Res.*, 1:44–48.

12. Bethel, R. A., Epstein, J., Sheppard, D., Nadel, J. A., and Boushey, H. A. (1983): Sulfur dioxide-induced bronchoconstriction in freely breathing exercising, asthmatic subjects. *Am. Rev. Respir. Dis.*, 128:987–990.

13. Betke, J., Kleihaver, E., and Lipps, M. (1956): Vergleichende Untersucheg uber Sportanoxydation von Nabelschnur und Erwachsenenhamoglobin. *Ztschr. Kinderh.*, 77:549.

14. Bickis, M., and Krewski, D. (1985): Statistical design and analysis of the long-term carcinogenicity bioassay. In: *Toxicological Risk Assessment, Vol. I*, edited by D. B. Clayson, D. Krewski, and I. Munro, pp. 125–147. CRC Press, Boca Raton, Florida.

15. Brain, J. D., Beck, B. D., Warren, J., and Shaikh, R., editors (1988): *Variations in Susceptibility to Inhaled Pollutants.* Johns Hopkins University Press, Baltimore, Maryland.

16. Brown, C. C. (1976): Mathematical aspects of dose–response studies. Carcinogenesis—The concept of thresholds. *Oncology*, 33:62–65.

17. Burns, C. A., Zarkower, A., and Ferguson, F. G. (1980): Murine immunological and histological changes in response to chronic silica exposure. *Environ. Res.*, 21:298–307.

18. Calabrese, E. J. (1978): Chemical interactions in the standard deviation process. In: *Methodological Approaches to Deriving Environmental and Occupational Health Standards*, pp. 73–105. Wiley, New York.

19. Calabrese, E. J. (1978): *Pollutants and High Risk Groups.* Wiley, New York.

20. (Deleted.)

21. Calabrese, E. J. (1979): The role of high risk groups in the derivation of environmental health standards. *Rev. Environ. Health*, 3(2):131–147.

22. Calabrese, E. J. (1983): *Principles of Animal Extrapolation.* Wiley, New York.

23. Calabrese, E. J. (1986): Chemical interactions and their implications for primary drinking water standards. *Water Res. Q.*, 5(1):9–12.

24. Calabrese, E. J. (1987): Animal extrapolation: A look inside the toxicologist's black box. *Environ. Sci. Technol.*, 21:618–623.

25. Carnow, B. W. (1976): Panel discussion on TLV's—Lead. In: *Health Effects of Occupational Lead and Arsenic Exposure: A Symposium*, edited by B. W. Carnow, p. 197. U.S. PHS, NIOSH, Washington, D.C.

26. Carson, R. (1962): *Silent Spring.* Houghton Mifflin, Boston, Massachusetts.

27. Cleaver, J. E. (1968): Defective repair replication of DNA in xeroderma pigmentosum. *Nature*, 218:652–656.

28. Cleaver, J. E., and Carter, P. M. (1973): Xeroderma pigmentosum: Influence of temperature on DNA repair. *J. Invest. Dermatol.*, 60:29–32.

29. Colditz, G. A., Stampfer, M. J., and Green, L. C. (1988): Diet. In: *Variations in Susceptibility to Inhaled Pollutants*, edited by B. D. Brain, A. J. Waven, and R. A. Shaiker, pp. 314–331. Johns Hopkins University Press, Baltimore, Maryland.

29a.Cook, P. J., Doll, R., and Fellingham, S. A. (1969): A mathematical model for the age distribution of cancer in man. *Int. J. Cancer*, 4:93–112.

30. Cooper, W. C. (1973): Indicators of susceptibility to industrial chemicals. *J. Occup. Med.*, 15(4):355.

31. Cornfield, J. (1977): Carcinogenic risk assessment. *Science*, 198:696–698.

32. Crapo, J. D., Barry, B. E., Chang, L.-Y., and Mercer, R. R. (1984): Alteration in lung structure caused by inhalation of oxidants. *J. Toxicol. Environ. Health*, 13:301–321.

32a.Crouch, E., and Wilson R. (1979): Interspecies comparison of carcinogenic potency. *J. Toxicol. Environ. Health*, 5:1095–1118.

33. Crump, K. S. (1979): Dose response problems in carcinogenesis. *Biometrics*, 16(4):357–367.

34. Crump, K. S. (1984): A new method for determining allowable daily intake. *Fund. Appl. Toxicol.*, 4:854–871.

35. Davidson, I. W. F., Parker, J. C., and Beliles, R. P. (1986): Biological basis for extrapolation across mammalian species. *Regul. Toxicol. Pharmacol.*, 6:211–237.

36. deBruin, A. (1976): Synergism and antagonism between organicals. In: *Biochemical Toxicology of Environmental Agents*, pp. 383–419. Elsevier/North Holland, New York.

37. Dourson, M. L. (1986): New approaches in the derivation of acceptable daily intake (ADI). *Comments Toxicol.*, 1:35–48.

38. Dourson, M. L., and Stara, J. F. (1983): Regulatory history and experimental support of uncertainty (safety) factors. *Regul. Toxicol. Pharmacol.*, 3:224–238.

39. Elcombe, C. R., Rose, M. S., and Pratt, I. S. (1985): Biochemical, histological, and ultrastructural changes in rat and mouse liver following the administration of trichloroethylene: Possible relevance to species differences in hepatocarcinogenicity. *Toxicol. Appl. Pharmacol.*, 79:365–376.

40. Elsayed, N. M., and Mustafa, M. G. (1982): Dietary antioxidants and the biochemical response to oxidant inhalation. I. Influence of dietary vitamin E on the biochemical effects of nitrogen dioxide exposure in rat lung. *Toxicol. Appl. Pharmacol.*, 66:319–328.

41. Enterline, P. E. (1983): Epidemiologic basis for the asbestos standard. *Environ. Health Perspect.*, 52:93–97.

42. Farber, E. (1982): Chemical carcinogenesis, a biological perspective. *Am. J. Pathol.*, 106:271–296.

43. Finklea, J. F., Shy, C. M., Moran, S. B., Nelson, W. C., Larsen, R. I., and Akland, G. G. (1975): The role of environmental assessment in the control of air pollution. In: *Advances in Environmental Science and Technology*, vol. 7, edited by J. N. Pitts and R L. Metcalf, pp. 315–389.

44. Finney, D. J. (1952): *Probit Analysis.* Cambridge University Press, London.

45. Fishbein, L. (1980): Potential industrial carcinogenesis and mutagenic alkylating agents. In: *Safe Handling of Chemical Carcinogens, Mutagens, Teratogens, and Highly Toxic Substances*, Vol. I. Ann Arbor Science, Ann Arbor, Michigan, pp. 329–363.

46. Frawley, J. P., Fuyat, H. N., Hagan, E. C., Blake, J. R., and Fitzhugh, O. G. (1957): Marked potentiation in mammalian toxicity from simultaneous administration of two anti-cholinesterase compounds. *J. Pharmacol. Exp. Ther.*, 121:96.

47. Freni, S. C. (1985): Issues in the use of cancer risk estimates: An epidemiologic approach. (*Unpublished manuscript.*)

48. Gehring, P. J., Watanabe, P. G., and Park, C. N. (1978): Resolution of dose–response toxicity data for chemicals requiring metabolic activation: Example—Vinyl chloride. *Toxicol. Appl. Pharmacol.*, 44:581–591.

49. Green, G. M., Jakab, G. J., Low, R. B., and Davis, G. S. (1977): Defense mechanisms of the respiratory membrane. *Am. Rev. Respir. Dis.*, 115:479–514.

50. Gross, P., de Villiers, A. J., and de Treville, R. T. P. (1967): Experimental silicosis: The "atypical reaction" in the Syrian hamster. *Arch. Pathol.*, 84:87–94.

51. Hackney, J. D., and Linn, W. S. (1983): Controlled clinical studies of air pollutant exposure: Evaluating scientific information in relation to air quality standards. *Environ. Health Perspect.*, 52:187–191.

52. Haemisegger, E., Jones, A., Steigerwald, B., and Thomson, V. (1985): The air toxics problem in the United States. U.S. Environmental Protection Agency, no. 450/1-85-001. Washington, D.C.

53. Harington, J. S., Ritchie, M., King, P. C., and Miller, K. (1973): The *in-vitro* effects of silica-treated hamster macrophages on collagen production by hamster fibroblasts. *J. Pathol.*, 109:21–37.

54. Hart, R. W., and Fishbein, L. (1985): Interspecies extrapolation of drug and genetic toxicity data. In: *Toxicological Risk Assessment*, Vol. I, edited by D. B. Clayson, D. Krewski, and I. Munro, pp. 3–40. CRC Press, Boca Raton, Florida.

55. Haseman, J. K. (1985): Issues in carcinogenicity testing: Dose selection. *Fund. Appl. Toxicol.*, 5:66–78.

56. Haseman, J. K., Tharrington, E. C., Huff, J. E., and McConnell, E. E. (1986): Comparison of site-specific and overall tumor incidence analyses for 81 recent National Toxicology Program Carcinogenicity studies. *Regul. Toxicol. Pharmacol.*, 6:155–170.

57. Heppleston, A. G. (1984): Pulmonary toxicology of silica, coal and asbestos. *Environ. Health Perspect.*, 55:111–127.

58. Hoel, D. G., Kaplan, H. L., and Andersen, M. E. (1983): Implication of nonlinear kinetics on risk estimation in carcinogenesis. *Science*, 219:1032–1037.

59. Hutt, P. B. (1985): Use of quantitative risk assessment in regulatory decision making under federal health and safety statutes. In: *Risk Quantitation and Regulatory Policy,* edited by D. G. Hoel, R. A. Merrill, and F. P. Perera, pp. 15–29. Cold Spring Harbor Laboratory, Cold Spring Harbor, New York.

59a. Industrial Union Department (1980): AFL-CIO v. American Petroleum Institute, 448 U.S. 60165 L. Ed. 2d 1010, 100 S. Ct. 2844.

60. Infante, P. F., and White, M. C. (1983): Benzene: Epidemiologic observation of leukemia by cell type and adverse health effects associated with low level exposure. *Environ. Health Perspect.,* 52: 75–82.

61. International Agency for Research on Cancer (1980): *Long-term and Short-term Screening Assays for Carcinogens: A Critical Appraisal.* IARC Monographs, Supplement 2. International Agency for Research on Cancer, Lyons, France.

62. International Agency for Research on Cancer (1982): *Evaluation of Carcinogenic Risk of Chemicals to Humans.* IARC Monographs, Supplement 4. International Agency for Research on Cancer, Lyons, France.

63. Kimbrough, R., Falk, H., Stehr, P., and Fries, G. (1984): Health implications of 2,3,7,8-tetrachlorodibenzo-*p*-dioxin (TCDD) contamination of residential soil. *J. Toxicol. Environ. Health,* 14:47–93.

64. Kociba, R. J., Keyes, D. G., Beyer, J. E., Carron, R. M., Wade, C. E., Dittenber, D. A., Kalnins, R. P., Frauson, L. E., Park, C. N., Barnard, S. D., Hummel, R. A., and Humiston, C. G. (1978): Results of a two-year chronic toxicity and oncogenicity study of 2,3,7,8-tetrachlorodibenzo-*p*-dioxin in rats. *Toxicol. Appl. Pharmacol.,* 46:273–303.

65. Kouri, R. E., and Nebert, D. W. (1977): Genetic regulation of susceptibility to polycyclic hydrocarbon induced tumors in the mouse. In: *Origins of Human Cancer,* edited by H. H. Hiatt, J. D. Watson, and J. A. Winstyen, pp. 811–835. Cold Spring Harbor Laboratory, Cold Spring Harbor, New York.

66. Lipfert, F. W. (1980): Sulfur oxides, particulates and human mortality: Synopsis of statistical correlations. *J. Air Pollut. Control Assoc.,* 30:366–371.

67. Lower, G. (1979): Genetic susceptibility to arylamine induced bladder cancer. *Environ. Health Perspect.,* 29:71–79.

68. Maltoni, C., Conti, B., and Cotti, G. (1983): Benzene: A multipotential carcinogen. Results of long-term bioassays performed at the Bologna Institute of Oncology. *Am. J. Ind. Med.,* 4:589–630.

69. Melnick, R. L., Boorman, G. H., Haseman, J. K., and Huff, J. (1984): Toxicity and carcinogenicity of melamine in F344 rats and B6C3F1 mice. *Toxicol. Appl. Pharmacol.,* 72:292–303.

70. Miller, F. J., Illing, J. W., and Gardner, D. E. (1978): Effect of urban ozone levels on laboratory-induced respiratory infections. *Toxicol. Lett.,* 2:163–169.

71. Deleted.

72. Miller, S. A. (1983): Prepared statement. In: *Dioxin—The Impact on Human Health,* Vol. 78. Hearings before the Subcommittee on Natural Resources, Agriculture Research and Environment. Committee on Science and Technology, U.S. House of Representatives. Washington, D.C., pp. 78–88.

73. Moolgavkar, S. (1986): Carcinogenesis modelling: From molecular biology to epidemiology. *Ann. Rev. Public Health,* 1:151–169.

74. Munro, I. C. (1977): Considerations in chronic toxicity testing: The chemical, the dose, the design. *J. Environ. Pathol. Toxicol.,* 1: 183–197.

75. Murphy, S. D. (1983): General principles in the assessment of toxicity of chemical mixtures. *Environ. Res.,* 48:141–144.

76. National Research Council (1977): *Drinking Water and Health,* Vol. 1. National Academy Press, Washington, D.C.

77. National Research Council (1980): *Principles of Toxicological Interactions Associated with Multiple Chemical Exposures.* National Academy Press, Washington, D.C.

78. National Research Council (1983): *Risk Assessment in the Federal Government: Managing the Process.* National Academy Press, Washington, D.C.

79. National Research Council (1986): *Drinking Water and Health,* Vol. 6. National Academy Press, Washington, D.C.

80. National Toxicology Program (1982): Carcinogenesis bioassay of 2,3,7,8-tetrachlorodibenzo-*p*-dioxin (CAS No. 1746-01-6) in Osborne Mendel rats and B6C3F1 mice (Gavage study). NTP Technical Report Series, Issue 209, p. 135 NTP.

81. Nilsson, K., and Klein, G. (1982): Phenotypic and cytogenetic characteristics of human B-lymphoid cell lines and their relevance for the etiology of Burkitt's lymphoma. *Adv. Cancer Res.,* 37:319–380.

82. Nutrition Foundation (1983): The relevance of mouse liver hepatoma to human carcinogenic risk. A Report of the International Expert Advisory Committee, Washington, D.C., p. 34.

83. Occupational Safety and Health Administration (1980): Identification, classification, and regulation of potential occupational carcinogens. *Fed. Reg.,* 45:5002–5296.

84. Occupational Safety and Health Administration (1983): General Industry Standards, Subpart 2, Toxic and Hazardous Substances. Code of Federal Regulations. 40:1910.1000 (d) (2) (i). Chapter XVII—Occupational Safety and Health Administration, p. 667.

85. Occupational Safety and Health Administration (1986): Occupational exposure to asbestos, tremolite, anthophyllite, and actinolite; final rules. *Fed. Reg.,* 51:22612–22790.

86. Office of Science and Technology Policy (1985): Chemical carcinogens; A review of the science and its associated principles. *Fed. Reg.,* 50:10372–10442.

87. Ontario Ministry of the Environment (1984): Polychlorinated dibenzo-*p*-dioxins (PCDDs) and polychlorinated dibenzofurans. Scientific Criteria Document for Standard Development, No. 4-84 September.

88. Overton, J. H., Jr., and Miller, F. J. (1984): Dosimetry by ozone and nitrogen dioxide in man and animals. EPA publ. no. EPA-600/D-84-126.

89. Peraino, C., Fry, R. J. M., and Staffeldt, E. (1971): Reduction and enhancement by phenobarbital of hepatocarcinogenesis induced in the rat by 2-acetyl-aminofluorene. *Cancer Res.,* 31:1506–1512.

90. Perera, F. P. (1984): The genotoxic/epigenetic distinction: Relevance to cancer policy. *Environ. Res.,* 34:175–191.

91. Perera, F. P., and Weinstein, I. B. (1982): Molecular epidemiology and carcinogen-DNA adduct detection: New approaches to studies of human cancer causation. *J. Chronic Dis.,* 35:581–600.

92. Pershagen, G., and Bjorklund, N. E. (1985): On the pulmonary tumorigenicity of arsenic trisulfide and calcium arsenate in hamsters. *Cancer Lett.,* 27:99–104.

93. Pershagen, G., Noraberg, G., and Bjorklund, N. E. (1984): Carcinomas of the respiratory tract in hamsters given arsenic trioxide and/or benzo-*a*-pyrene by the pulmonary route. *Environ. Res.,* 37: 425–432.

94. Pozzani, U. S., Weil, C. S., and Carpenter, C. P. (1959): The toxicological basis of TLVs: 5. The experimental inhalation of vapor mixtures by rats, with notes upon the relationship between single dose inhalation and single dose oral data. *Am. Ind. Hyg. Assoc. J.,* 20:364–369.

95. Quakenbush, J. J., Kanarek, M. S., Spengler, J. D., and Letz, R. (1982): Personal monitoring for nitrogen dioxide exposure: Methodological considerations for a community study. *Environ. Int.,* 8: 249–258.

96. Radford, E. P., and Renard, K. G. S. C. (1984): Lung cancer in Swedish iron miners exposed to low doses of radon daughters. *N. Engl. J. Med.,* 310:1485–1494.

97. Reddy, J. K., and Lalwai, N. D. (1983): Carcinogenesis by hepatic peroxisome proliferators: Evaluation of the risk of hypolipidemic drugs and industrial plasticizers to humans. *CRC Crit. Rev. Toxicol.,* 12:1–58.

98. Riddiough, C. R., Musselmann, R., and Calabrese, E. J. (1977): Is EPA's radium-226 drinking water standard justified? *Med. Hypotheses,* 3(5):111.

99. Roger, L. J., Kehrl, H. R., Hazucha, M., and Horstman, D. H. (1985): Bronchoconstriction in asthmatics exposed to sulfur dioxide during repeated exercise. *J. Appl. Physiol.,* 59:784–791.

100. Ross, J. D., and Des Forges, J. F. (1959): Reduction of methemoglobin by erythrocytes from cord blood. Further evidence of deficient enzyme activity in newborne period. *Pediatrics,* 23:218.

101. Shu, H. P., Paustenbach, D. J., and Murray, F. J. (1987): A critical evaluation of the use of mutagenesis, carcinogenesis, and tumor promotion data in a cancer risk assessment of 2,3,7,8-tetrachlorodibenzo-*p*-dioxin. *Regul. Toxicol. Pharmacol.,* 7:57–88.

102. Shy, C. M., Alarie, Y., Bates, D. V., Frank, R., Hackney, J. D., Horvath, S. M., and Nadel, J. A. (1974): Synergism or antagonism of pollutants producing health effects. Report to the U.S. Senate Committee of Public Works, pp. 483–499. NAS, Washington, D.C.

103. Slaga, T. J. (1983): Overview of tumor promotion in animals. *Environ. Health Perspect.,* 50:3–14.
104. Smyth, H. F., Jr., Weil, C. S., West, C. P., and Carpenter, J. S. (1969): An exploration of joint toxic action: 27 Industrial chemicals in rats in all possible pairs. *Toxicol. Appl. Pharmacol.,* 14:340–347.
105. Somers, E. (1986): The weight of evidence: Regulatory toxicology in Canada. *Regul. Toxicol. Pharmacol.,* 6:391–398.
106. Sontag, J. M., Page, N. P., and Safiotti, U. (1976): Guidelines for carcinogen bioassays in small rodents. DHHS publ. (NIH) 76-801. National Cancer Institute, Bethesda, Maryland.
107. Squire, R. A. (1981): Ranking animal carcinogens: A proposed regulatory approach. *Science,* 214:877–880.
108. Starr, T. B., and Buck, R. D. (1984): The importance of delivered dose in estimating low-dose cancer risk from inhalation exposure to formaldehyde. *Fund. Appl. Toxicol.,* 4:740–753.
109. Stott, W. T., Quast, J. F., and Watanabe, P. G. (1982): The pharmacokinetics and macromolecular interactions of trichloroethylene in mice and rabbits. *Toxicol. Appl. Pharmacol.,* 62:137–151.
110. Tamplin, A. R., and Gofman, J. W. (1970): *Population Control Through Nuclear Pollution.* Nelson-Hill, Chicago, Illinois.
111. Tomatis, L., Agthe, C., Bartsch, H., Huff, J., Montesano, R., Saracci, R., Walker, E., and Wilbourn, J. (1978): Evaluation of the carcinogenicity of chemicals: A review of the monograph program of the International Agency for Research on Cancer (1971–1977). *Cancer Res.,* 38:877–885.
112. Tosteson, T., Spengler, J. D., and Weber, R. A. (1982): Aluminum, iron, and lead content of respirable particulate samples from a personal monitoring system. *Environ. Int.,* 2:265–268.
113. U.S. Department of Health, Education and Welfare, Public Health Service (1962): Public Health Drinking Water Standards. Rockville, Maryland.
114. U.S. Department of Health and Human Services (DHHS) (1985): Risk assessment and risk management of toxic substances. Report to the Secretary of DHHS from the Executive Committee of the DHHS Committee to Coordinate Environmental and Related Programs. Washington, D.C.
115. U.S. Department of Health and Human Services (1986): NIOSH recommendations for occupational safety and health standards. *Morbid. Mortal. Weekly Rep.,* 35:1S–33S.
116. U.S. Environmental Protection Agency (1970): Section 109 of the Clean Air Act. Clean Air Amendments of 1970, PL-91-604. Washington, D.C.
117. U.S. Environmental Protection Agency (1975): Interim primary drinking water standards. *Fed. Reg.,* 40(51):11990–11998.
118. U.S. Environmental Protection Agency (1976): Toxic Substances Control Act, PL-94-46a, Oct. 11, 1976. Washington, D.C.
119. U.S. Environmental Protection Agency (1985): Health Assessment Document for Polychlorinated Dibenzo-*p*-dioxins. Office of Health and Environmental Assessment, EPA/600/8-84/014F, Washington, D.C.
120. U.S. Environmental Protection Agency (1986): Air Quality Criteria for Lead, Vols. I–IV, EPA-600/8-83/028adf. Washington, D.C.
121. U.S. Environmental Protection Agency (1986): Guidelines for the health risk assessment of chemical mixtures. *Fed. Reg.,* 51(185): 34013–34025.
122. U.S. Environmental Protection Agency (1986): Guides for carcinogen risk assessment. *Fed. Reg.,* 51:33992–34003
123. U.S. Environmental Protection Agency (1987): Reference dose (RfD): Description and use in health risk assessments. Appendix A of Integrated Risk Information System Supportive Documentation, Vol. I, EPA/600/8-86/032a. Washington, D.C.
124. U.S. Interagency Staff Group on Carcinogens (1986): Chemical carcinogens: A review of the science and its associated principles. *Environ. Health Perspect.,* 67:201–282.
125. Wallace, L. A., Pellizzari, E. D., Hartwell, T. D., Sparacino, C., and Zelon, H. (1983): Personal exposure of volatile organics and other compounds indoors and outdoors: The TEAM study. *Proceedings of the 76th Annual Meeting of the Air Pollution Control Association.* Air Pollution Control Association, Pittsburgh, Pennsylvania.
126. Waring, M. J. (1981): DNA modification and cancer. *Annu. Rev. Biochem.,* 50:159–192.
127. White, H. J., and Garg, B. D. (1981): Early pulmonary response of the rat lung to inhalation of high concentration of diesel particles. *J. Appl. Toxicol.,* 1:104–110.
128. Wilkinson, C. F. (1971): Effects of synergists on the metabolism and toxicity of anticholinesterase. *Bull. WHO,* 40:171–190.
129. Williams, G. M. (1985): Identification of genotoxic and epigenetic carcinogens in liver culture systems. *Regul. Toxicol. Pharmacol.,* 5:132–144.
130. World Health Organization (1981): Health effects of combined exposures in the work environment. WHO Technical Report Series 662. Washington, D.C., pp. 5–76.
131. Ziskind, M., Jones, R. N., and Weil, H. (1976): Silicosis. *Am. Rev. Respir. Dis.,* 113:643–665.

Principles and Methods of Toxicology, Second Edition, edited by A. Wallace Hayes, Raven Press, Ltd., New York © 1989.

CHAPTER **2**

Metabolism: A Determinant of Toxicity

J. Donald deBethizy and Johnnie R. Hayes

Toxicology Research Division, R. J. Reynolds Tobacco Company, Bowman Gray Technical Center, Winston-Salem, North Carolina 27102

Biological Oxidation
    Cytochrome P-450-Dependent Monooxygenase System • Microsomal Flavin-Containing Monooxygenase • Cooxidation of Xenobiotics by Prostaglandin Endoperoxide Synthetase
Biochemical Conjugations
    Glucuronidation: Uridine Diphosphate-Glucuronosyltransferase • Sulfate Conjugations • Glutathione *S*-transferases • Methylation • Amide Synthesis
Hydrolysis
    Epoxide Hydrolase • Esterases and Amidases

Microfloral Metabolism
    Xenobiotic Biotransformation by Microbes Colonizing Mammals • Role of Diet in Modulating Microfloral Metabolism • Examples of Xenobiotics Whose Toxicity is Dependent on Microfloral Metabolism • Cyclamate
Integration of Metabolic Pathways
    Bromobenzene • Multiple Pathways for Xenobiotic Activation
References

As the first macromolecules began to organize into complex arrays with the basic attributes of life, environmental factors were present that represented disruptive forces. These forces were not only physical but chemical as well. Chemicals existed in the early milieu of life that interacted with these life forms, disrupting the delicate balances through which they maintained their integrity. Those life forms that developed protective mechanisms, such as the cell membrane and the ability to store energy and motility, were able to survive. It does not stretch the imagination to hypothesize that these early life forms manufactured molecules capable of reacting with environmental chemicals, thereby decreasing their biological activity. An example of such a molecule that exists in mammals today is the nucleophile glutathione, which can react nonenzymatically with many electrophilic chemicals to reduce their toxicity. The next step in the development of protective mechanisms may have been the development of macromolecular catalysis to chemically alter disruptive chemicals. These macromolecular catalyses were the first detoxication enzymes. Evidence for such a scenario exists in the occurrence of certain detoxication enzymes in both animal and plant species ranging from simple, single cellular to complex, multicellular organisms.

An alternative to the hypothesis that the enzymes that metabolize foreign compounds (or xenobiotics, as they are often called) developed for this specific purpose is that they represent enzymes of normal anabolic and catabolic metabolism.

These enzymes, in addition to functioning in their normal biochemical role, also function in xenobiotic metabolism. Examples of such enzymes include the methyltransferases involved in DNA synthesis and in detoxication, such as the metabolism of nicotine. However, it would appear fortuitous that normal cellular metabolism could have evolved to metabolize the broad array of chemical structures that are foreign to organisms. Another factor which diminishes the confidence in the latter hypothesis is that many of the xenobiotic metabolizing enzymes can rapidly respond with increased activity to the presence of xenobiotics and environmental change. This would be unlikely if they simply represented enzymes of normal metabolism with the ability to metabolize alternative substrates. Many of the enzymes involved in xenobiotic metabolism are also involved in specific aspects of the metabolism of normal cellular biochemical constituents. However, generally these enzymes are isozymes with higher substrate specificity for the endogenous compounds than the isoenzymes involved in xenobiotic metabolism. This could as likely represent a process by which the cell utilized a preexisting xenobiotic metabolizing enzyme for metabolism of endogenous substrates, instead of vice versa.

An alternative view is these enzymes underwent parallel evolution with some developing toward metabolism of endogenous compounds and others developing toward xenobiotic metabolism. Whatever the evolutionary source of the xenobiotic metabolizing enzymes, it is obvious that they represent a distinct mechanism for metabolizing the thousands of naturally occurring and synthetic chemicals to which cells and cellular systems are exposed. Since xenobiotic metabolism does not always represent detoxication, the term *biotransformation* has come into general use to denote the actions of xenobiotic metabolizing enzymes, although it is still not semantically specific for xenobiotic metabolism.

The majority of organisms studied has biotransformation enzymes, although there is diversity in the occurrence, function, and rates of specific enzymes. Certain bacteria contain more primitive or less highly developed systems and may lack certain pathways altogether. Even mammals demonstrate diversity in the activity or rates of specific systems and, as would be expected of genetically controlled functions, there are species and individual differences. This diversity extends to the organ level in multicellular organisms. Specific organs show different levels of activity and specific cell types within organs demonstrate variation in biotransformation. There is even subcellular diversity in that certain of these enzymes are compartmentalized whereas others are free in the cytoplasm.

The wide variety of chemicals to which organisms may be exposed requires that the biotransformation enzymes have broad substrate specificity. This is a characteristic that is not shared by the majority of enzymes involved in anabolic and catabolic metabolism. Also, the types of reactions catalyzed are diverse. These include oxidation, reduction, epoxidation, deamination, hydroxylation, sulfoxidation, desulfuration, dehalogenation, and conjugation with endogenous compounds, to name a few.

Biotransformation has been divided into two distinct phases. Phase I reactions result in *functionalization,* the addition or the uncovering of specific functional groups that are required for subsequent metabolism by phase II enzymes. Phase II reactions are biosynthetic. These phase I and II reactions are often coordinated, with the product of one reaction becoming the substrate of the other. A commonality of biotransformation reactions is the conversion of hydrophobic xenobiotics into more polar, more easily excreted compounds. Since the composition of cells is more lipid than their environment, nonpolar compounds tend to accumulate. This would lead to bioconcentration of chemicals within the cell to levels higher than that of the environment and increase the likelihood of a cytotoxic event. However, conversion of nonpolar chemicals to more polar metabolites allows them to be more easily excreted by the cell. Conjugation of a xenobiotic with an endogenous compound, a phase II reaction, results in not only greater water solubility, but in some cases the added chemical group is recognized by specific carrier proteins or proteins involved in facilitated diffusion or active transport. This increases the cell's ability to remove the xenobiotic.

There are many diverse examples of xenobiotics whose toxicity is directly dependent upon the activity of the biotransformation enzymes. For most chemicals, increases in the activity of these enzymes result in decreases in toxicity whereas decreases in activity result in increased toxicity. However, there are also examples in which the product of xenobiotic metabolism is more toxic than the parent compound. Conversion of a foreign compound to a more toxic metabolite is termed *metabolic activation.* For example, the

majority of genotoxic chemicals require metabolic activation before initiating genotoxicity. The enzymes that protect the animal from the toxicity of certain compounds may be responsible for toxicity of others. An organism's susceptibility to the toxicity of a particular chemical is dependent, in many cases, upon the delicate balance between detoxication and metabolic activation that exists during exposure to the xenobiotic. Due to the sensitivity of the enzymes of xenobiotic biotransformation to both endogenous and exogenous factors, this balance may differ among individuals and at different points in time.

The enzyme systems that metabolize xenobiotics are affected by the physiologic state of the animal and by the environment. Activity varies during the perinatal development of the animal with different activities appearing at different stages of development, both before and after birth. During the perinatal period and continuing throughout the life of the animal, many of the enzymes associated with xenobiotic metabolism can be influenced by the animal's environment. Diet can alter activity, through both the chemicals in the diet and nutritional quality. Exposure to dietary contaminants and to chemicals in the water and air can decrease or increase the activity of biotransformation enzymes toward specific chemicals. These factors, among others, alter an animal's susceptibility to specific toxic compounds.

The diversity of enzymes that has been implicated in xenobiotic metabolism is illustrated in Table 1. Some of these enzymes appear predominately involved in xenobiotic metabolism; others such as alcohol dehydrogenase metabolize xenobiotics as alternatives to their endogenous substrates. Other enzymes are more difficult to classify, such as super-

TABLE 1. *Examples of types of reaction and enzymes that participate in xenobiotic metabolism*

Oxidation	Ester hydrolysis
Cytochrome	Carboxylesterases
P-450-dependent	Amidases
monooxygenase	Methylation
Xanthine oxidase	O-methyltransferases
Peroxidases	N-methyltransferases
Amine oxidase	S-methyltransferases
Monoamine oxidase	Acetylation
Dioxygenases	N-acetyltransferase
Reduction	Acyltransferases
Cytochrome	Others
P-450-dependent	Thiosulfate
reductases	sulfurtransferase
Keto-reductase	(rhodanese)
Glutathione peroxidases	Alcohol dehydrogenases
Hydration	Aldehyde dehydrogenases
Epoxide hydrolase	Superoxide dismutase
Conjugation	
Glucuronosyltransferase	
Sulfotransferase	
Glutathione S-transferase	
Glucosyltransferase	
Thioltransferase	
Amide synthesis	
(transacylase)	

oxide dismutases, which detoxify reactive oxygen generated during normal cellular metabolism.

BIOLOGICAL OXIDATION

Cytochrome P-450-Dependent Monooxygenase System

The cytochrome P-450-dependent monooxygenase system is central to the metabolism of many xenobiotics. Not only is it the primary enzymatic system for metabolism of many xenobiotics but it is also involved as the initial step in the further metabolism of many others. As a result, cytochrome P-450 plays key roles in several areas of research including pharmacology, toxicology, physiology, and biochemistry. Several names for the system exist in the literature. The names most commonly encountered are as follows:

1. Mixed function oxidase
2. Cytochrome P-450 system
3. Cytochrome P-450-dependent monooxygenase system.

These names are generally related to either a specific function or are descriptive of a biochemical mechanism. This system is a *monooxygenase* because it incorporates one atom of oxygen into its substrates.

Components of Cytochrome P-450 System

The history of the discovery of cytochrome P-450 and the elucidation of its functions and mechanisms of action are intriguing. Cytochrome P-450 was first described independently in 1958 by Klingenberg (60) and Garfinkel (29) in microsomes isolated from rat liver homogenates and pig liver homogenates, respectively. Klingenberg noted that G. R. Williams first observed the pigment during 1955 in the laboratory of Britton Chance at the Johnson Foundation. The name cytochrome P-450 derived from the occurrence of a pigment which when reduced and treated with carbon monoxide yielded a spectrophotometric Soret band at 450 nm. Six years after the publication of the original description of the P-450 peak in hepatic microsomes, Omura and Sato (89,90) published their pivotal papers describing cytochrome P-450 as a b-type hemocytochrome. Their work illustrated that the cytochrome was located in hepatic microsomes, which form from the endoplasmic reticulum upon cellular disruption. Upon isolation from the membrane using proteases, cytochrome P-450 is converted to a form whose reduced carbon monoxide complex produces a peak at 420 nm. This form was termed *cytochrome P-420* and was found to be inactive in metabolism. Conversion of cytochrome P-450 to the inactive cytochrome P-420 upon isolation from the membrane was one of the major limitations encountered in early attempts to understand the mechanism of this membrane-bound monooxygenase.

Before the discovery of cytochrome P-450, Julius Axelrod and his colleagues in the Laboratory of Chemical Pharmacology at the National Heart Institute were involved with studies of the metabolic disposition of drugs (4). They found that oxidative metabolism of amphetamine required the cofactor NADPH and the presence of oxygen. An important publication by Estabrook et al. (25) brought together studies of cytochrome P-450 biochemistry and studies of drug bio-

transformation. They established that cytochrome P-450 was the terminal oxidase involved with the C-21 hydroxylation of steroids in adrenal cortical microsomes. This was followed by a study from Cooper et al. (17) that demonstrated the involvement of cytochrome P-450 in both steroid and drug metabolism by hepatic microsomes. Many individuals and laboratories have played major roles in the development of the current knowledge concerning cytochrome P-450, and the interested reader who becomes acquainted with the original literature will no doubt recognize the role of these pioneers in the development of a new field of study—that of xenobiotic biotransformation.

It became obvious that although cytochrome P-450 played a major role in the activity of the monooxygenase, it did not act alone. In 1950, Horecker (43) isolated a flavoprotein from the liver, but no function was identified. This flavoprotein utilized reducing equivalents from NADPH and was later named *NADPH-cytochrome c reductase* (EC 1.6.2.4). Williams and Kamin (119) and Phillips and Langdon (95) reported in 1962 that NADPH-cytochrome c reductase occurred in the hepatic endoplasmic reticulum and might be involved in drug and steroid oxidation. In 1955, La Du et al. (62) showed that cytochrome c could inhibit dealkylation of aminopyrine. This was followed by a more comprehensive set of studies by Gillette et al. (30) in 1957 that presented additional evidence that cytochrome c reductase was involved in xenobiotic metabolism. Further proof for the involvement of the flavoprotein came in 1969 when it was shown that antibodies to the reductase inhibited xenobiotic metabolism (61,88) and Lu et al. (68,69) demonstrated its requirement in monooxygenase activity reconstituted from isolated components.

One confusing aspect concerning this flavoprotein is its nomenclature. As previously mentioned, it is generally known as NADPH-cytochrome c reductase. However, no cytochrome c occurs in the endoplasmic reticulum and cytochrome c is not its normal substrate. A more appropriate name used for this flavoprotein is *NADPH-cytochrome P-450 reductase,* indicating its natural substrate and function.

Although the major components of the cytochrome P-450-dependent monooxygenase system appear to be cytochrome P-450 and cytochrome P-450 reductase, other components may also be involved with metabolism of specific xenobiotics. *Cytochrome b5 reductase* has been proposed to participate in monooxygenase activity through electron transport to *cytochrome b5* and subsequently to cytochrome P-450. However, several systems of electron transport in the endoplasmic reticulum and isolated microsomes, as well as other activities, such as peroxidation, have greatly complicated the elucidation of the role of cytochrome b5. Cytochrome b5 may affect cytochrome P-450-mediated xenobiotic metabolism by shunting electrons either toward or away from P-450 (82). An elucidation of the role of cytochrome b5 must await further understanding of the complex electron transfer pathways that exist in the endoplasmic reticulum.

Substrate Specificity

Although the catalytic activity of the monooxygenase systems appears to require only two proteins, NADPH⁻ cytochrome P-450 reductase and cytochrome P-450, it is capable of carrying out a variety of different reactions with a large number of substrates. This ability is based not only upon the occurrence of a variety of cytochrome P-450 *isozymes*[1] but upon the basic reaction mechanism of the cytochrome and its unique lack of substrate specificity. The nonspecificity of the monooxygenase provides important flexibility to the xenobiotic metabolism capability of the organism, but this flexibility comes with a price. Generally, the enzymatic reactions of anabolism and catabolism are both extremely specific in substrate specificity and catalytically efficient, resulting in high activity and high turnover number. The turnover number and efficiency of the cytochrome P-450-dependent monooxygenase are considerably lower than most enzymes. This is probably related to inefficiency in substrate binding, oxygen activation, and electron transport. However, inefficiency of metabolism is more than made up for by the ability to metabolize a wide variety of chemical structures and the ability to catalyze a variety of reactions. An additional factor that compensates for the relatively low turnover number is the high concentration of the system in organs important in detoxication. Before a discussion of the various reactions catalyzed by cytochrome P-450, a discussion of the catalytic cycle is appropriate. A knowledge of the catalytic cycle will assist in understanding the various reactions catalyzed by the system and in predicting metabolic pathways for specific xenobiotics.

Catalytic Cycle of the P-450-Dependent Monooxygenase System

The reaction catalyzed by the cytochrome P-450-dependent monooxygenase system and its stoichiometry are illustrated in Fig. 1.

One molecule of substrate reacts with one molecule of molecular oxygen and NADPH to yield the oxidized substrate containing one atom from molecular oxygen, water (containing the other oxygen atom), and oxidized NADPH. The incorporation of one oxygen atom from molecular oxygen into the substrate is the source of the name *monooxygenase.* The oxidation of substrate and concomitant reduction of one atom of oxygen to water is the source of the name *mixed function oxidase.* Although the stoichiometry of the reaction appears simple, obtaining this stoichiometry in the laboratory is a difficult task (33). The main difficulty is the number of oxidation–reduction reactions that occur simultaneously in the endoplasmic reticulum. These reactions utilize both oxygen and NADPH and may yield water and oxidized NADP. Accounting for these diverse reactions is difficult, but when such attempts have been successful, the predicted stoichiometry has been obtained.

It is recommended that the reader carefully follow the reaction sequence illustrated in Fig. 2 during this discussion of the catalytic cycle. The initial step of the cycle is the binding of the substrate (represented by S in Fig. 2) to cytochrome P-450. As previously mentioned, cytochrome P-450 exists as a series of closely related isozymes, each of which demon-

$$RH + O_2 + NADPH + H^\oplus \longrightarrow ROH + H_2O + NADP^\oplus$$

FIG. 1. Reaction and stoichiometry of cytochrome P-450-dependent monooxygenase.

strates a degree of substrate specificity. This substrate specificity is not absolute and some overlapping is evident. At any point in time several isozymes of cytochrome P-450 exist in the endoplasmic reticulum. This is dependent upon the specific environmental and physiologic conditions of the organism. Therefore, the binding of the substrate to the active site of the cytochrome P-450's may represent binding to a single isozyme predominantly, but not exclusively. The activity of the catalytic process, as well as the specific metabolites produced, is a function of the particular isozyme profile. Although our understanding of the structure of the active site of P-450 is developing, more needs to be learned. From the chemical nature of the substrates metabolized, it is obvious that the active site must be predominately hydrophobic in nature. However, the active site cannot be simply a fatty pool in which a variety of lipophilic substrates can bind, since metabolism is site specific with respect to substrate and is not random. Therefore, the substrate must have a specific orientation within the active site.

As occurs with many other enzymes, the binding of the substrate to the hemoprotein appears to produce conformational alterations in the enzyme that assist its catalytic activity. For instance, substrate binding results in cytochrome P-450 being more easily reduced by cytochrome P-450 reductase. The available data indicate that the heme moiety of the hemoprotein exists in very close proximity to the substrate binding site. It is also a constituent of the active site. Upon binding of the substrate to the active site, changes in the absorption spectrum of the cytochrome are detected. Since the oxidized heme iron is paramagnetic, the technique of electron paramagnetic resonance (EPR) can be applied to probe its environment in the heme. These studies have revealed alterations in the EPR signal that correlate with the spectra changes observed upon substrate binding. Both the EPR and visible spectra changes are thought to result from the substrate binding in close proximity to the heme iron with a concomitant displacement of a water molecule. The heme is transformed from the low-spin form to the high-spin form and the substrate is bound in close spatial proximity to the oxygen activation site on the heme. The exact relationships between the spin state of the cytochrome and substrate binding is more complex than described here. The reader is referred to the discussion of changes in spin state of cytochrome P-450 by Sligar and Murray (105).

The next step in the catalytic cycle following substrate binding is the one-electron reduction of the substrate–P-450 binary complex. As mentioned, substrate binding and concomitant alterations in cytochrome P-450 may facilitate this reduction step. The ferric (Fe^{+3}) hemocytochrome P-450–substrate complex is reduced by a single electron to the ferrous (Fe^{+2}) hemocytochrome P-450–substrate complex. This electron is provided by NADPH through the action of the flavoprotein, NADPH-cytochrome P-450 reductase. This flavoprotein contains two flavins, flavin adenine dinucleotide (FAD) and flavin mononucleotide (FMN). The flavoprotein appears to exist in its half-reduced (one-electron reduced) form and on reaction with NADPH is fully reduced (two-

---

[1] The term "isozyme" is used somewhat loosely in the context of cytochrome P-450 since certain isozymes appear to predominately catalyze certain types of reactions and other isozymes predominately catalyze other reactions.

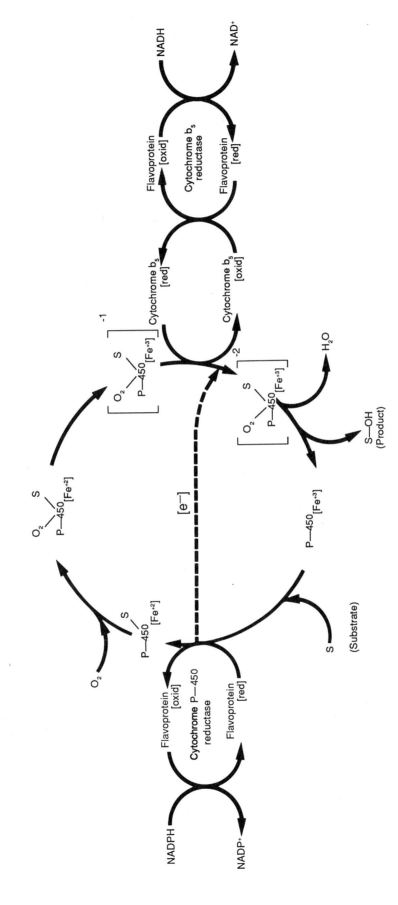

FIG. 2. Catalytic cycle of the cytochrome P-450-dependent monooxygenase.

electron reduced). The intramolecular electron flow appears to be from FAD to FMN. It is interesting that whereas the flavoprotein is a one-electron donor, its substrate, NADPH, provides two electrons. The mechanism for the two-electron shuttle by the one-electron donor flavoprotein is incompletely understood.

The flavoprotein has at least two domains, one of which is imbedded in the membrane and the other is above the plane of the membrane on the cytosolic side. The domain solubilized in the membrane consists mainly of hydrophobic amino acids. The actual interaction with NADPH and oxidation–reduction probably takes place outside the membrane. Another interesting aspect of cytochrome P-450 reductase is that the quantity of P-450 is in large excess to the quantity of reductase (as much as 20-fold or more, depending upon conditions). This means that each flavoprotein must reduce several cytochrome P-450 molecules, indicating that the interaction between the reductase and P-450 is an important consideration as discussed in more detail below.

Upon reduction of the ferric hemocytochrome P-450–substrate binary complex to the ferrous state by the reductase, the complex binds oxygen. This results in the ternary complex ferrous hemocytochrome P-450–substrate-oxygen shown in Fig. 2. The oxygen binds at the free ligand of the heme iron and is thought to be oriented spacially with the substrate-binding portion of the active site. Under anaerobic conditions and in the presence of carbon monoxide, the P-450-carbon monoxide complex is formed instead of the oxygen complex. This produces the characteristic spectral peak at 450 nm. Uncoupling (interrupting the flow of electrons) the catalytic cycle at this point can produce oxidized ferric cytochrome P-450 and a reduced form of oxygen, the superoxide radical.

At this stage of the catalytic cycle highly critical reactions take place that are still incompletely understood. The major event is the activation of the oxygen molecule. The ternary complex accepts a second electron; the source of which is either NADH or NADPH, depending upon the mediator of electron transport. Since the semipurified reconstituted system consisting of isolated P-450, cytochrome P-450 reductase, and phospholipid requires only the presence of NADPH, NADPH-dependent cytochrome P-450 reductase can mediate this step. However, as previously mentioned, in some systems it appears that cytochrome b_5 can mediate the electron transfer, employing reducing equivalents from NADH through NADH-cytochrome b_5 reductase. Whichever the source of the second electron, it results in the production of the peroxycytochrome P-450–substrate complex, which has a net charge of (−2).

Of the variety of mechanisms proposed for oxygen activation and insertion into the substrate, two appear to be generally accepted. The first hypothesis states that an oxinoid species is produced by protonation and removal of water. The activated oxygen or oxinoid species then reacts with substrate to yield incorporation of an oxygen atom. The second hypothesis states that a hydroxyl radical is formed with the insertion of the oxygen atom preceded by a radical mediated mechanism. Whatever the mechanism, an oxidized substrate is formed with the concomitant production of water. The oxidized substrate and water are released, regenerating the oxidized ferric cytochrome P-450, which can again initiate the catalytic cycle.

It must be emphasized, however, that the other pathways of electron transport in the endoplasmic reticulum can have significant impact on the catalytic activity of the monooxygenase by altering the availability of reducing equivalents. The interested reader is encouraged to consult other sources (e.g., see Ortiz de Montellano, ref. 92) for a more comprehensive discussion of these pathways.

The catalytic cycle just described appears to be common for cytochrome P-450-dependent monooxygenase activity associated with xenobiotic metabolism in a variety of organs and among different species. However, certain of these monooxygenases, especially the more specific forms associated with anabolic and catabolic metabolism, have different mediators of electron transport. For example, the adrenal cortex mitochondrial system utilizes a nonheme iron protein in addition to cytochrome P-450 reductase in the electron transport chain, as does the monooxygenase in certain microorganisms.

The P-450 system is not totally independent and its activity is affected by a number of factors. One of these is the availability of reducing equivalents. The monooxygenase is primarily dependent upon NADPH, and possibly to a lesser extent upon NADH. NADPH is generated from the pentose-phosphate shunt, isocitrate dehydrogenase, and the malate enzyme. Under most conditions these pathways provide saturating levels of NADPH. However, certain conditions can stress the ability of the cell to provide NADPH and it may become rate limiting. Under conditions of high monooxygenase activity, starvation may reduce the activity toward certain substrates due to reduced levels of NADPH. It is generally believed that the decreased activity due to limiting NADH is an unlikely condition. A discussion of these and other factors that regulate monooxygenase activity can be found in the review by Thurman et al. (112).

An additional factor that influences monooxygenase activity is the endoplasmic reticulum membrane. NADPH cytochrome P-450 reductase, NADH cytochrome b_5 reductase, and cytochrome b_5 are bound to the membrane by tails of hydrophobic amino acids. On the other hand, cytochrome P-450 appears to be an integral hemoprotein that exists within the membrane, as opposed to being attached to it. Earlier efforts to isolate this enzyme system with proteolytic enzymes resulted in cleaving the reductases at the hydrophobic tail, producing purified reductases with activity, albeit with lower molecular weights. This indicates that the reactions of electron transport probably take place at the cytosolic face of the endoplasmic reticulum (46). These early attempts at purification did not result in the release of catalytically active cytochrome P-450. With the advent of detergent-based solubilization techniques that allowed the gentle disruption of the phospholipid matrix, it became possible to free active cytochrome P-450 from the membrane (68,69). The apparent requirement for a phospholipid fraction (generally phosphatidylcholine) for the reconstitution of an active form of the monooxygenase indicates the importance of the lipid environment. Since substrates of the enzyme system are somewhat lipid soluble and cytochrome P-450 exists within the membrane, substrates dissolve in the membrane to reach the active site of cytochrome P-450.

The asymmetric nature of the protein components of the system with respect to the membrane surface, coupled with the disproportionality of the concentrations of the components (i.e., a 1:20–40 ratio between the flavoprotein and cytochrome P-450) indicates an interesting topology and interaction between the components. Several hypotheses have been proposed to reconcile these factors into a unified reaction scheme, but none has been totally successful.

One hypothesis states that the flavoprotein and cytochrome P-450 exist in fixed aggregates during metabolism with a single reductase serving to reduce a number of closely associated cytochrome P-450 molecules (26,93). This allows a catalytic advantage from the close association of components. These supramolecular complexes within the bulk lipid of the membrane may be only transient, occurring during steady state metabolism and may disaggregate upon depletion of substrate.

Another hypothesis states that the components of the monooxygenase can freely diffuse laterally within the plane of the membrane. Electron transport would take place during random productive collisions within the membrane (123). Such lateral diffusion would be influenced by lipid–protein and protein–protein interactions.

For example, if the protein content of the membrane increases, protein–protein interactions may decrease the lateral diffusion (57). This could result in a diffusion-limited reaction rate; however, this does not appear to be the case. It does appear that cytochrome P-450 may form a transient complex with the reductase that has an extremely short, non-rate-limiting half-life (38). In artificial membranes, the components of the monooxygenase appear to be randomly distributed and interact by lateral diffusion (111). Whether or not this is true in the endoplasmic reticulum with its mixture of lipids and proteins is unknown. It is possible that the monooxygenase exists in a lipid domain different from the bulk lipid of the membrane. Care must be utilized in the interpretation of data obtained from purified enzymes reconstituted in artificial lipid vesicles or micelles and even isolated microsomes, since such systems may not reflect the complexity of the endoplasmic reticulum in the living cell.

Reactions Catalyzed by the Cytochrome P-450-Dependent Monooxygenase System

On first inspection it appears that cytochrome P-450 can catalyze a bewildering number of reactions (Table 2). However, on closer inspection there is a degree of commonality among these reactions. The first area of commonality is that

TABLE 2. *Major oxidative reactions catalyzed by the cytochrome P-450-dependent monooxygenase system*

Aliphatic hydroxylation
Aromatic hydroxylation
Epoxidation
N-Dealkylation
O-Dealkylation
Deamination
Sulfoxidation
N-Oxidation

most of the reactions represent oxidations. Second, the reactions convert lipophilic substrates to more hydrophilic products. Third, many of the reactions can be represented as hydroxylations as pointed out by Mannering (63).

Aliphatic hydroxylation

Examination of aliphatic hydroxylation reactions is illustrative of several important aspects of monooxygenase activity. The reaction mechanism, which may be common to several other types of monooxygenase reactions, appears to occur by a radical abstraction mechanism (35). Oxygen activation produces an iron peroxide at the heme of cytochrome P-450. Hydrogen abstraction results in a hydroperoxide (OOH^-) free radical and carbonium ion formation. This free radical interacts with substrate to yield hydroxylation. Another important aspect is that the radical abstraction mechanism is site selective resulting in a nonrandom hydroxylation. The specific hydroxylation site is determined by substrate structure and the specific spacial orientation of the substrate at the active site. Different isozymes of cytochrome P-450 show different degrees of site selectivity. For example, *n*-hexane hydroxylation can occur at C-1, C-2, C-3, and C-4. Isozymes of P-450 induced by the barbiturate phenobarbital metabolized *n*-hexane to yield a 4–5-fold increase in the 2-, 3-, and 4-hydroxylated metabolites and only a slight increase at the 1 position. On the other hand, isozymes induced by benzo[*a*]pyrene (BP) result in decreased yields of the 1- and 2-hydroxylated products, but increased yields of the 3- and 4-hydroxylated products (27). Hydroxylation of aliphatic compounds is generally considered to be detoxication because of the greater water solubility of the products, but one must be cautioned against overgeneralization, since more toxic products could be produced by subsequent metabolism.

Aromatic oxidation

Aromatic oxidation can occur by two mechanisms, direct oxygen insertion into the C—H bond and by addition of oxygen to the C=C double bond (i.e., epoxide formation). The latter appears to be the predominate mechanism.

An example of a compound that is hydroxylated by both direct insertion of oxygen at the C—H bond and oxygen addition at the C=C bond is *p*-chlorobenzene. Both 3- and 4-chlorobenzene oxides are formed by the addition reaction to yield the arene epoxides. These spontaneously rearrange to form *o*-chlorophenol and *p*-chlorophenol. The occurrence of *m*-chlorophenol as a metabolite is an example of the direct insertion reaction. The production of arene oxides has been widely studied due to their importance in the formation of epoxide ultimate carcinogens. These epoxides can also be formed in nonaromatic systems yielding reaction products as illustrated by the metabolism of aflatoxin B_1. This mycotoxin is metabolized to a number of hydroxylated products and also to the 2,3-epoxide. It is generally agreed that this epoxide is the ultimate carcinogen of aflatoxin B_1.

Oxidative dealkylation and reductive reactions

Oxidative dealkylation at nitrogen atoms is a monooxygenase-catalyzed reaction by which a variety of primary, secondary, and tertiary amines are metabolized. The products of this reaction consist of the alcohol form of the substrate and an aldehyde. For example, formaldehyde is produced from *N*-demethylation reactions. The mechanism for *N*-dealkylation reactions has been proposed to be either carbon oxidation to yield the carbinolamine intermediate or through oxidation at the nitrogen atom to produce the *N*-oxide. Current evidence suggests that the former mechanism is more likely.

Ether compounds can also be dealkylated. Ether *O*-dealkylation is similar to *N*-dealkylation and is thought to proceed through the initial oxidation of the carbon adjacent to oxygen (i.e., carbon oxidation). The products of this reaction are again an alcohol and an aldehyde, analogous to those produced by *N*-dealkylation.

Other oxidative reactions that have received attention are nitrogen oxidation, oxidative desulfuration, oxidative dehalogenation, and oxidative denitrification. An interesting series of reactions in which cytochrome P-450 appears to participate under special conditions are reductive reactions. Examples of such reactions are nitro reduction, azo reduction, arene oxide reduction, and reductive dehalogenation. These reactions are generally studied *in vitro* under anaerobic conditions in the presence of isolated microsomes and NADPH. Since these reactions require low oxygen tension to progress, their role in *in vivo* metabolism is not understood. Whether or not these reactions represent simply a curious phenomenon associated with cytochrome P-450 or a viable metabolic pathway is not known. It may be possible that under certain cellular conditions of low oxygen tension these reactions may take place *in vivo*. Also note that cytochrome P-450 reductase can catalyze certain reductions.

Role of Cytochrome P-450-Dependent Monooxygenase in Toxicity

The toxicity of any agent is dependent upon its concentration at its target site. This is a function of many factors including the route of exposure, the pharmacokinetics of the xenobiotic, the excretion of both the parent compound and its metabolites, and the sensitivity of the target site. The ability of the organism to clear the xenobiotic through excretion will have a profound influence on the concentration at the target site. Directly associated with the ability to clear many xenobiotics is the ability to metabolize the xenobiotic to more water soluble metabolites.

Without doubt, the cytochrome P-450-dependent monooxygenase plays a pivotal role in the metabolism of xenobiotics. It is the prime metabolic route for the majority of xenobiotics, acting either directly in detoxication or indirectly by priming the xenobiotic for further metabolism through functionalization as illustrated in other sections of this chapter.

Although the original interest in the P-450 system was associated with its ability to metabolize drugs and decrease both their toxicity and duration of action, it soon became evident that in certain cases this enzyme system converted certain drugs from pharmacologically inactive forms to active forms. Examples of the metabolic activation of toxicants, such as the *in vivo* conversion of the inactive insecticide parathion to its active form paraoxon were soon encountered and the metabolic activation of benzo[a]pyrene (BP) as shown in Fig. 3. Further studies have indicated that metabolic activation plays an important role in the toxicity of a large number of compounds (37).

Species Differences in Metabolism

Since the activity of the cytochrome P-450-dependent monooxygenase plays a central role in the expression of the toxicity of the majority of xenobiotics, the study of its activity is important. Knowledge of the rates at which a xenobiotic is metabolized and the chemical and biologic nature of its metabolites assist in understanding not only its toxicity but its mechanism of action. This then provides essential information required to enable the toxicologist to predict its toxicity. However, one factor that complicates the ability to extrapolate the toxicity of a xenobiotic between species is the differences in how species metabolize xenobiotics. Generally, the basic reactions and major metabolites of a xenobiotic are similar among species. However, subtle differences in metabolism can lead to major differences in susceptibility to toxicity.

A variety of mechanisms can be associated with differences between species in their response to a xenobiotic. These include the following:

1. Absorption
2. Distribution
3. Organ differences in metabolic capacity
4. Quantitative differences in metabolism
5. Excretion
6. Sensitivity of either the target organ or biochemical target site

Although all of these factors may be more or less important in understanding species differences in the susceptibility to the same xenobiotic, it appears that one of the dominant factors is xenobiotic metabolism. The following mechanisms may account for species differences:

1. A lack of, or genetic "defect" in, a particular metabolic pathway,
2. Differences in the K_m and V_{max} of specific enzymes,
3. The existence of different isozymes and differences in the ratios of specific isozymes of important enzymes, such as cytochrome P-450,
4. Differences in the ratio of activities of separate enzyme systems that act together to metabolize a specific xenobiotic.

Either the lack of a specific pathway or a defect in a pathway will make a species or individual organism susceptible to xenobiotics that are detoxicated via that pathway. Conversely, when the xenobiotic is metabolically activated by that pathway the species will be resistant. Although there does not appear to be a mammalian example of the lack of the monooxygenase system, examples exist for other enzymes, such as the lack of glucuronidation in cats. A more common explanation of species difference is the variation in the activity (K_m, V_{max}) and substrate specificity of isozymes associated with xenobiotic metabolism. At low doses or environmental exposures, these differences will be expressed in detoxication and species susceptibility. Caution needs to be utilized in both the design and interpretation of studies to investigate species differences. Low doses, below enzyme saturation, may not reveal species differences. However, as the dose increases and begins to saturate the enzyme's ability to detoxicate the xenobiotic toxicity may become evident. Care must be utilized when investigating these differences *in vitro* since this activity may not reflect *in vivo* activity for a number of reasons.

When one metabolite represents a metabolically activated form and another a detoxicated form, the ratio of these metabolites can be reflected in a species susceptibility to a xenobiotic. This type of species difference is most commonly encountered when the cytochrome P-450-dependent monooxygenase acts in coordination with another pathway. Species may differ in either the initial monooxygenase priming reaction or in the activity of the secondary pathway. This is illustrated by the metabolic activation of BP (see Fig. 3) in rats and mice. The metabolic activation of BP requires initial epoxidation by the P-450-dependent monooxygenase at the 7,8-position followed by hydration of the epoxide by epoxide hydrolase to yield the 7,8-dihydrodiol. The dihydrodiol is then epoxidated by the monooxygenase to yield the ultimate carcinogen of BP, the 7,8-dihydrodiol 9,10-oxide.

When mouse hepatic microsomes were used for metabolic activation in the Ames assay for mutagenicity, BP was highly mutagenic, indicating a high degree of metabolic activation. However, when rat hepatic microsomes were employed in the same assay only slight mutagenicity was evident. This indicated a significantly lower ability for the rats to metabolically activate BP *in vitro* (87). Although mice metabolize BP to a greater extent than rats, rats have 6–7-fold more epoxide hydrolase activity. Further studies (85,86) indicated that both species have adequate monooxygenase activity to metabolically activate BP and that higher epoxide hydrolase activity in the rat may have been responsible for the lower mutagenicity. Therefore, the species differences in the secondary pathway, epoxide hydrolase, may have controlled the mutagenicity, as opposed to differences in the monooxygenase activity.

Just as species demonstrate differences in metabolism that alter toxicity, different strains of the same species may demonstrate differences in metabolism and toxicity. For instance, if a different strain of mouse had been used in the studies described above, the data may have been different. It is important to recognize these strain differences when designing toxicologic studies. The mechanisms associated with strain differences may be diverse. As with any genetically controlled activity, differences in metabolism are not unusual. However, laboratory animals are generally bred in distinct groups, and without extensive outbreeding, strain differences can develop quite rapidly. In the wild it would be less likely to encounter such strain differences, but individual differences may be greater. Other factors (e.g., diet and environment) may result in what appears to be strain differences.

Species differences in metabolism and consequently susceptibility lead to an important concept in toxicology—that of *selective toxicity*. Ideally, a pesticide should be toxic only to the organism against which it is directed. This concept of selective toxicity has resulted in efforts to develop selective pesticides. For these activities to be fruitful, it is important that species differences in metabolism are understood and that this information is utilized. For further discussions of species differences, the reader is directed to the articles by Walker and Oesch (115) and that by Caldwell (13).

For the toxicologist, the species differences of major importance are those between humans and those species used in toxicologic testing. Without an understanding of these species differences it will be difficult to extrapolate toxicologic studies performed with animals to humans. Studies of species differences in animals are difficult to design and interpret, and those involving humans are even more complex. This complexity results from the large differences in xenobiotic biotransformation found in humans. Many factors contribute to these individual differences in metabolism:

1. Humans are free-living and have few restraints to reproductive diversity, thus diminishing the development of small genetic pools that result in genetically less diverse, more homogeneous control of metabolism.
2. Environmental factors such as diet, nutrition, and xenobiotic exposure are diverse among humans.
3. Humans generally have more control and probably more interest in the consumption of various nonnutritive materials such as alcohol and drugs which can alter metabolism.

These, as well as other factors, result in a large diversity in susceptibility to xenobiotic exposure. This is, in part, why such large safety factors are employed in risk or hazard assessments of xenobiotics to which humans may be exposed. These safety factors are utilized in an attempt to protect the vast majority of individuals at risk. An excellent discussion of intraindividual and interindividual variation can be found in the monograph by Vesell and Penno (113).

Induction of Cytochrome P-450

When animals are exposed to certain xenobiotics their ability to metabolize a variety of xenobiotics is increased. This phenomenon produces a transitory resistance to the toxicity of many compounds. However, this may not be the case with compounds that require metabolic activation. The exact toxicologic outcome of this increased metabolism will be dependent upon the specific xenobiotic and its specific metabolic pathway. Since the toxicologic outcome of a xenobiotic exposure can depend upon the balance between those reactions that represent detoxication and those that represent activation, increases in metabolic capacity may, at times, produce unpredictable results.

One of the initial reports of increased metabolic capacity associated with xenobiotic exposure suggests how induction may provide a survival advantage. Brown et al. (11) in 1954 were studying the metabolism of methylated aminoazo dyes and found that xenobiotics in the animal diets enhanced the monooxygenase-dependent demethylation of these com-

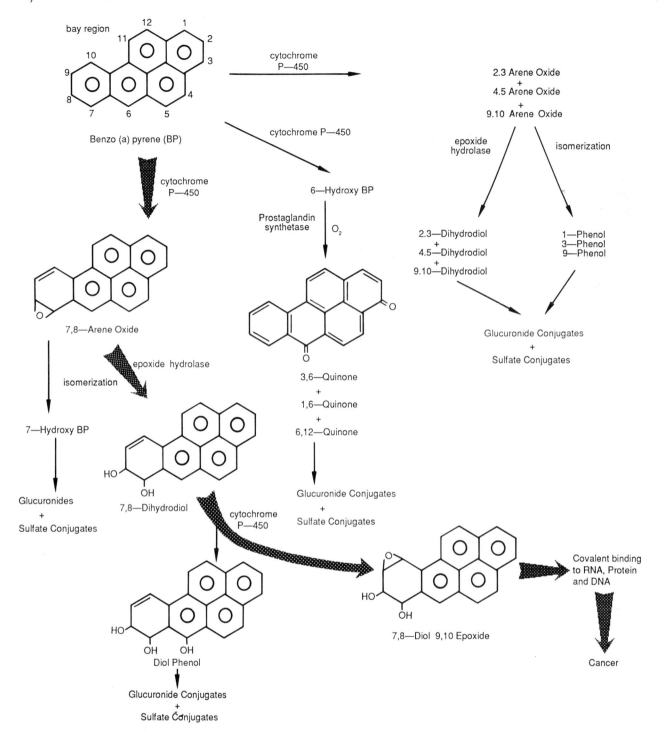

FIG. 3. Biotransformation and metabolic activation (indicated by heavy arrows) of the carcinogen benzo[a]pyrene (BP).

pounds. Free-living animals consume a variety of foods that may contain toxic constituents. If the animal can respond rapidly to these toxic compounds by developing resistance, it can continue to utilize the food source. One mechanism of rapidly developing such resistance is through increased detoxication resulting from stimulation of enzyme activity.

Conney published a pivotal review in 1967 which indicated that more than 200 chemicals caused a stimulation of cytochrome P-450-dependent metabolism and that most of these chemicals were monooxygenase substrates (16). This

increase in cytochrome P-450 activity has been termed *induction*. In most cases, the increase in activity is a true enzyme induction that requires *de novo* protein synthesis. Although the induction of the P-450 system has been most intensively investigated, other enzymes of biotransformation can be induced, such as glucuronidation. Many studies have been directed toward the mechanisms associated with induction; yet, this mechanism is still not completely understood.

At least one inducer, BP, appears to induce cytochrome P-450 by binding to a specific receptor protein in the nucleus.

This binding initiates a series of events leading to the production of specific mRNAs that result in *de novo* protein synthesis. Induction of monooxygenase activity is a coordinated process that may involve several enzymes. For instance, not only is the quantity of cytochrome P-450 generally increased but also the quantity of cytochrome P-450 reductase. Other enzymes may also be induced, such as the enzymes involved in heme synthesis. Also, certain inducers increase the total quantity of endoplasmic reticulum in the cell. A thorough discussion of induction is beyond the scope of this chapter, but induction studies have been a major factor in our understanding of not only the mechanisms associated with biotransformation but also the role of biotransformation in modifying the toxicity and action of xenobiotics.

Currently, one of the most active areas of research on cytochrome P-450 is investigations of the various P-450 isozymes induced by a variety of inducers. These studies have revealed that specific inducers alter the profile of constitutive isozymes. Specific isozymes are detected after induction that cannot be detected in the uninduced animals. The occurrence of these isozymes is transitory and they disappear when the animal is no longer exposed to the inducer. At any one moment, the ability of the animal to metabolize a specific xenobiotic is dependent upon the spectrum of isozymes that occur in the animal. For a more detailed discussion of the different forms of cytochrome P-450, the reader is referred to Chapter 28 (this *volume*) and to the recent books on mammalian cytochromes P-450 edited by Guengerich (36).

Microsomal Flavin-Containing Monooxygenase

Since 1960 it has been apparent that a microsomal monooxygenase other than cytochrome P-450 could catalyze the oxygenation of nucleophilic nitrogen and sulfur compounds. Purification to homogeneity indicated it was a flavin-containing monooxygenase free of cytochrome that requires NADPH. This enzyme (EC 1.14.13.8) has been referred to as amine oxidase, Ziegler's enzyme, dimethylaniline monooxygenase, and flavin-containing monooxygenase.

This microsomal enzyme catalyzes the oxidative attack on the nucleophilic nitrogen and sulfur heteroatom of a variety of xenobiotics. It was once thought that oxidations of basic aliphatic and tertiary aromatic amines were carried out by the flavin-containing monooxygenase and primary aromatic amines, and the acidic nitrogens of amides were catalyzed by cytochrome P-450, while secondary amines were oxidized by both enzyme systems. More recent studies with the purified enzymes have demonstrated that there is no clear division between the types of substrates preferred by the two enzymes. Therefore, the metabolism of each nitrogen-containing xenobiotic must be considered on an individual basis. The thermal instability of the flavin-containing monooxygenase in the absence of NADPH had made it relatively easy to separate the activity of this enzyme *in vitro* from that of cytochrome P-450.

Many nitrogen and sulfur containing xenobiotics are metabolized by this phase I enzyme. *N*-oxidation of tertiary amines yields amine oxides which form *N*-hydroxy ammo-nium ions. Primary and secondary amines are oxidized to hydroxylamines.

Cooxidation of Xenobiotics by Prostaglandin Endoperoxide Synthetase

Pathways other than the microsomal monooxygenases may be involved in xenobiotic oxidation. Marnett et al. (75) demonstrated that prostaglandin synthetase, an enzyme system responsible for prostaglandin biosynthesis, was capable of oxidizing BP to quinones. Oxidation resulted from a one-electron pathway involving an oxidizing agent produced during the hydroperoxidase catalyzed reduction of prostaglandin G_2 to the hydroxy endoperoxide, prostaglandin H_2. Prostaglandin synthetase is a major source of alkyl hydroperoxides produced during normal metabolism (74). Tissues possessing prostaglandin synthetase activity are capable of oxidizing certain xenobiotics, even though they are low in cytochrome P-450 content. In fact, acetaminophen, which is activated to a reactive intermediate by cytochrome P-450 (Fig. 4), can also be activated by prostaglandin synthetase in the medulla of the kidney (Fig. 5). This tissue is low in cytochrome P-450 activity, but in the presence of arachidonic acid the medulla activates acetaminophen to a reactive intermediate that covalently binds to tissue macromolecules (8).

The bladder also possesses high prostaglandin synthetase activity. Mattammal et al. (76) proposed that several structurally diverse renal and bladder carcinogens are metabolically activated by prostaglandin synthetase. For example, the bladder carcinogen 2-amino-4-(5-nitro-2-furyl)thiazole is thought to be activated by prostaglandin synthetase cooxidation in bladder transitional epithelium to metabolites ca-

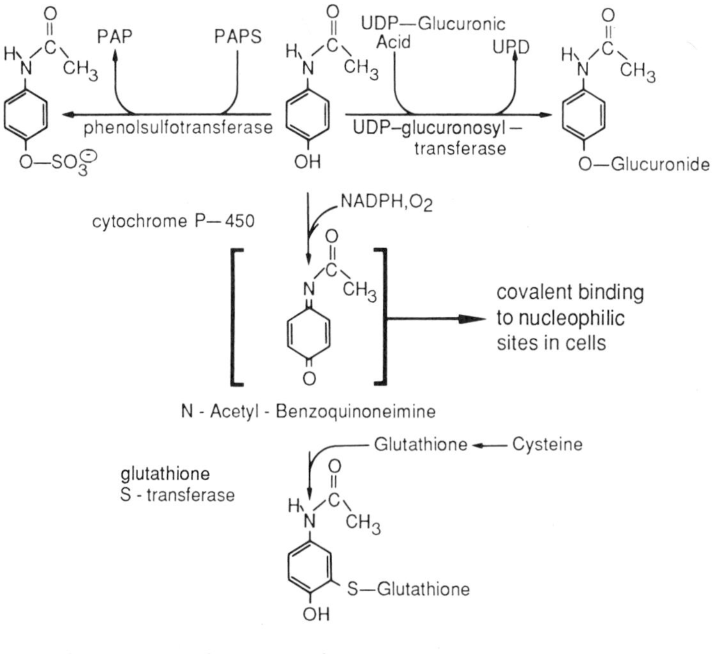

FIG. 4. Biotransformation of the analgesic acetaminophen.

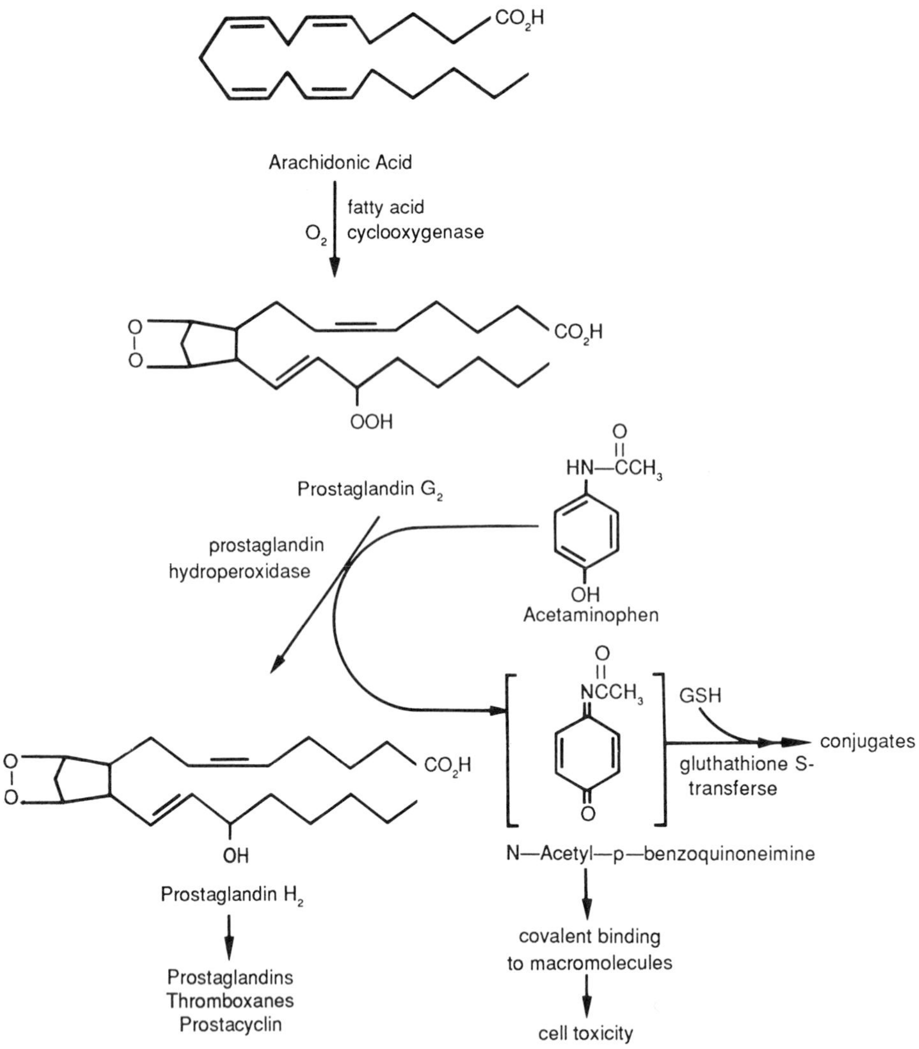

FIG. 5. Cooxidation of acetaminophen by prostaglandin endoperoxide synthetase.

pable of covalently binding RNA and DNA. Feeding aspirin to rats inhibits the bladder lesion produced by the carcinogen 5-nitrofuran, which suggests that prostaglandin synthetase is involved in the metabolic activation of 5-nitrofuran, since aspirin inhibits prostaglandin synthetase.

Use of the analgesic *p*-phenetidine has declined because of reports of kidney damage in humans following prolonged use. Andersson et al. (3) proposed a mechanism by which phenetidine is activated by kidney prostaglandin synthetase. The primary amine nitrogen of phenetidine undergoes a one-electron oxidation similar to that shown in Fig. 5 for acetaminophen. This leads to hydrogen abstraction to yield the reactive nitrenium radical. This radical is postulated based on its rate of reaction with reduced glutathione.

BIOCHEMICAL CONJUGATIONS

Mammals can synthesize xenobiotic conjugates that are more polar and readily excreted than the parent compound. Conjugate synthesis is finely controlled through various feedback pathways. Two major reactants are required for conjugate synthesis: a xenobiotic with the appropriate functional group and a cosubstrate that can be conjugated with the xenobiotic. If the xenobiotic does not have a functional group amenable to conjugation, such as a hydroxyl group, it may be oxidized (functionalized) by cytochrome P-450. The oxidized product and the cosubstrate must be simultaneously available for conjugation. Both functions must be tightly integrated for rapid excretion of the xenobiotic. Although the forthcoming sections will discuss each conjugating system as a separate entity, it must be emphasized that *in vivo* metabolism is integrated. Examples showing the integration of the conjugating system with related pathways will be described.

Glucuronidation: Uridine Diphospho-Glucuronosyltransferase

Cytochrome P-450-dependent monooxygenase is the principal phase I oxidative enzyme. Similarly, uridine diphospho(UDP)-glucuronosyltransferase is the principal phase II enzyme. Glucuronosyltransferases can utilize monooxygenase products to form glucuronides. However, it is not a necessity for substrates of the glucuronosyltransferase to be monooxygenase products. Significant numbers of xenobiotics and a few endogenous compounds possess the necessary functional groups for glucuronidation and do not require functionalization.

Whereas the multienzyme complex of the monooxygenase is termed a "system" because the enzymes are closely linked, the multiple enzymes of glucuronidation are not linked, but are interdependent. The general mechanism of conjugating enzymes involves the activation of an endogenous molecule to yield a high energy form. Subsequent reaction of this activated high energy form of the endogenous molecule with the xenobiotic produces the conjugate. Activation to the high energy form may occur in a different cellular compartment than conjugation, as is the case with glucuronidation.

Although the products of the cytochrome P-450-dependent monooxygenase are more water soluble that their parent compounds, some still possess considerable lipophilicity. Subsequent conjugation produces metabolites with higher water solubility. These metabolites can generally be readily excreted in the bile or in the urine. An additional method by which glucuronidation produces less toxic metabolites is via the addition of a bulky moiety to the xenobiotic. This can result in both the shielding of reactive portions of the xenobiotic and also in the blocking of reactions between the xenobiotic and its toxigenic receptor responsible for the toxicologic sequelae. Although in some cases the product of glucuronidation has more biological activity than the parent compound and can be considered metabolically activated, examples are far fewer than with monooxygenase oxidation.

History of the discovery of glucuronidation and the glucuronosyltransferases is interesting and the reader is directed to R. T. Williams' classic book on detoxication mechanisms (120) and the comprehensive discussions of this enzyme by Dutton (23) and Gorski and Kasper (32).

Biochemistry of Glucuronidation

Glucuronidation (illustrated in Fig. 6) requires the availability of three reactants:

1. UDP-α-D-glucuronic acid (UDPGA) generated in the cytoplasm,
2. UDP-glucuronosyltransferase (EC 2.4.1.17) bound to the membranes of the endoplasmic reticulum,
3. A suitable substrate with the requisite functional group.

Maximal enzyme activity is dependent upon optimal concentrations of these reactants at the membrane site of catalysis.

D-Glucose is the original precursor of UDPGA. During anabolic metabolism D-glucose is converted to α-D-glucose-1-phosphate. This compound serves as substrate for UDP-glucose pyrophosphorylase (EC 2.7.7.9), which catalyzes its reaction with uridine triphosphate to yield the high energy phosphate containing UDP-D-glucose and pyrophosphate (Fig. 6). UDP-D-glucose then reacts with nicotine adenine dinucleotide (NAD) catalyzed by UDP-glucose dehydrogenase (EC 1.1.1.22) to yield UDP-D-glucuronic acid, which completes glucose activation. This compound is termed the *glycone* indicating its source. The xenobiotic is termed the *aglycone*. The activation of glucose occurs in the cytoplasm; whereas glucuronidation occurs within the endoplasmic reticulum.

The formation of UDP-glucuronic acid within the cytoplasm and its water solubility raise the question as to how it can penetrate the lipid environment of the membrane for reaction with the enzyme. Several hypotheses have been presented including a membrane-bound carrier and even transfer of the glucuronic acid moiety to another intermediate. Additional studies may clarify this question.

By whatever mechanism, UDP-glucose and the aglycone (xenobiotic) substrate must be present for the reaction to be initiated. As previously mentioned, in many cases the xenobiotic substrate for glucuronidation is a hydroxylated product of monooxygenase metabolism. It has been suggested that there is a direct linkage of the monooxygenase and transferase. Although this would increase the catalytic efficiency of this type of detoxication, there is little evidence for direct linkage.

On the other hand, both enzymes are bound within the lipid–protein matrix of the membrane and may be in close proximity. The monooxygenase product would not have to diffuse from the membrane for subsequent glucuronidation, increasing the efficiency of sequential metabolism. It is possible that release of the monooxygenase product is vectorial toward the transferase. This would not require linkage of the enzymes, but would increase the overall efficiency of the reactions.

Little is known concerning the events that take place at the active site of UDP-glucuronosyltransferase. Various studies have generated a number of hypotheses, but the difficulties of studying the enzyme in its natural environment have made confirmation of mechanism difficult. It is known that that there is inversion at the anomeric carbon of glucuronic acid β-D-glucuronide. Glucuronides could be produced by nucleophilic displacement with the aglycone displacing UDP with resulting inversion. The displacement may proceed through a S_N2 mechanism.

The number of xenobiotics that have been shown to be substrates for UDP-glucuronosyltransferase is large and continues to grow. The major functional groups forming glucuronides are: (a) hydroxyl, (b) carboxyl, (c) amino, and (d) sulfhydryl. The substituents to which these functional groups are attached can be quite variable. Similar to the substrate requirements for the monooxygenase, the aglycone must be somewhat lipid soluble to be a substrate for the transferase. This may be meaningful with respect to the active site of the enzyme, but could simply reflect the necessity for the substrate to be soluble in the endoplasmic reticulum.

Endogenous compounds associated with normal metabolism and homeostasis are also substrates for the transferase. Endogenous substrates include bilirubin, catechols such as 3-O-methyladrenaline, serotonin, and 17-hydroxy-containing steroids. An example of the importance of the glucuronidation of endogenous compounds is illustrated by a hereditary disease termed *Crigler–Najjar syndrome*. The severe form of the disease appears autosomal and recessive. It is characterized by high bilirubin blood levels and no hepatic UDP-glucuronosyltransferase metabolism of bilirubin. Hyperbilirubinemia produces kernicterus and results in death

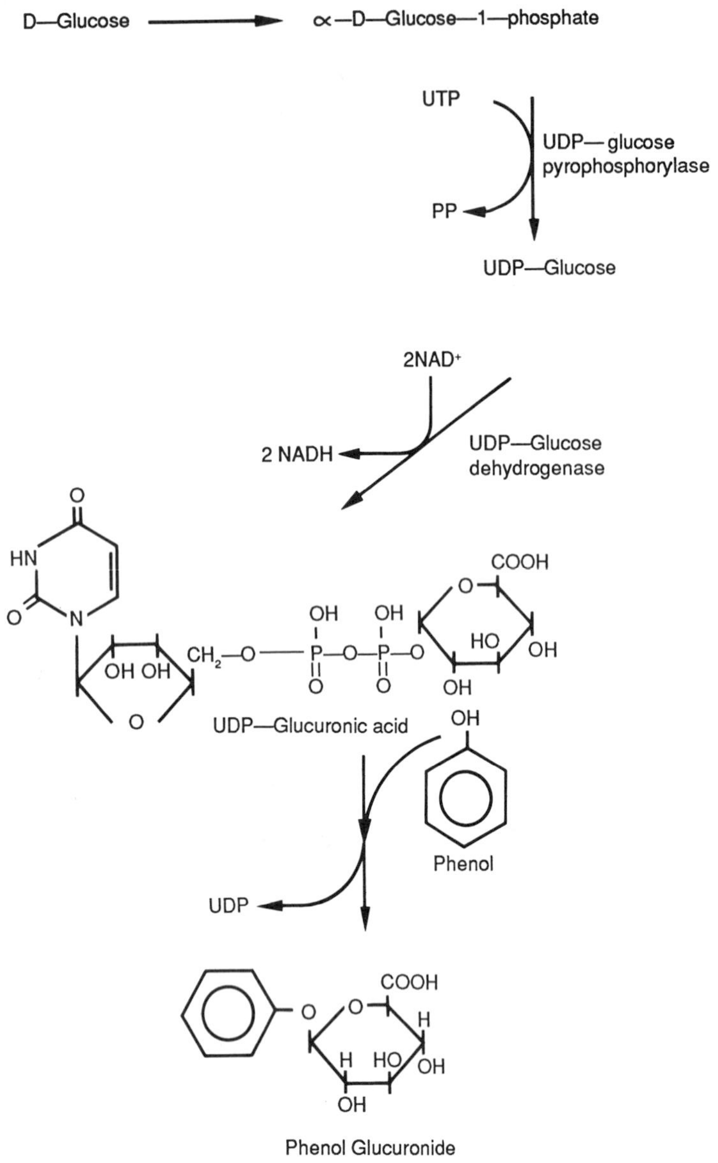

D—Glucose ⟶ ∝—D—Glucose—1—phosphate

UTP

UDP—glucose
pyrophosphorylase

PP

UDP—Glucose

2NAD⁺

2 NADH

UDP—Glucose
dehydrogenase

UDP—Glucuronic acid

Phenol

UDP

Phenol Glucuronide

FIG. 6. Glucuronidation of phenol: An example of the pathway leading to production of glucuronic acid conjugates.

in early childhood. Milder forms of the disease may respond to induction of transferase activity by phenobarbital.

The major physiochemical property of glucuronides that influences detoxication is the increased polarity and water solubility compared with the parent compound. An additional factor is that glucuronides are relatively strong acids with pka's of 3 to 4. Since the carboxyl group of the glycone portion of the molecule is unprotonated at physiologic pH, highly water soluble salts can be formed, increasing their ability to be excreted.

Like the monooxygenase, UDPGA-glucuronosyl-transferase is an integral part of the endoplasmic reticulum and deeply embedded, apparently more so than the monooxygenase. Also similar to the monooxygenase, its interaction with the phospholipids of the membrane has a strong influence on its activity. Two general theories prevail as to how it is associated with the membrane. One theory suggests the transferase is constrained by membrane lipids; the other suggests the enzyme is actually compartmentalized within the

membrane. Both theories were devised to explain certain characteristics of the enzyme activity. One of these characteristics that has puzzled investigators is the need for *in vitro* activation of the enzyme's activity in isolated microsomes. A variety of activation treatments, including sonication and detergent treatment will dramatically increase transferase activity. Various workers have suggested that these treatments remove constraints on the enzyme by making the membrane more permeable to substrates. The exact relationship between *in vitro* and *in vivo* activity is poorly understood. It appears as if *in vivo* activity is higher than unactivated *in vitro* activity.

The close association of the enzyme with the membrane confounded its isolation and purification. Recent attempts at purification of UDP-glucuronosyltransferase have been more successful. The breakthrough came with the use of detergent solubilization coupled with affinity chromatography (32). Purification of the transferase has been reviewed by Burchell (12). Although these studies have added to our understanding of the physiochemical nature of the protein, one of their important contributions has been a better understanding of the heterogeneity of the transferase. Earlier studies of substrate metabolism under a number of conditions suggested that several forms of the enzyme may exist. However, the number of factors that can or could affect enzyme activity in microsomal preparations raised questions concerning the validity of the heterogeneity. Although studies with the purified enzyme are also susceptible to artifacts, they do provide stronger evidence that the transferase proteins represent a family of isozymes that differ in substrate specificity. Heterogeneity may help explain such factors as species and strain differences in glucuronidation and the influence of environmental factors on metabolism.

An additional factor illustrated by the purification studies is the lipid dependency of the transferase. Studies of the microsomal-bound enzyme indicated that there appears to be a close association of phospholipid with the enzyme. Alterations in membrane phospholipids altered enzyme activity. Since the transferase appears to be deeply imbedded in the membrane, the importance of lipid–protein interaction would not be unexpected.

Attempts at purification of the enzyme indicated that various preparations had different quantities of phospholipid associated with them. The substrate specificity and activity of these preparations appeared, in part, to be related to this bound phospholipid leading to a "false" heterogeneity. When the lipid was stripped from the preparations and added back in controlled amounts, the true heterogeneity of the transferases was evident. Glucuronosyltransferase and the cytochrome P-450-dependent monooxygenase are examples of membrane-bound enzymes whose activity is controlled, in part, by lipid–protein interactions within the membrane.

Reactions Catalyzed by UDP-Glucuronosyltransferases

As with many of the detoxication enzymes, the glucuronosyltransferases have a low order of substrate specificity. This lack of substrate specificity makes them ideally suited as detoxication enzymes. Whether or not they evolved as detoxication enzymes or represent enzymes of normal metabolism whose lack of specificity make them suitable for detoxication is open to debate. Of interest in this respect is that they occur only in higher organisms. Glucuronosyltransferases have been found in all mammals, birds, and reptiles that have been investigated, although their specific activities toward selected substrates vary among different species and strains. Unlike the monooxygenase, they have not been found in bacteria and less highly developed species. This fact, among others, lends support to Dutton's hypothesis that these transferases evolved to metabolize endogenous compounds, such as bilirubin, catecholamines, and steroids, and not as detoxication enzymes (22). For a review of methods for assaying glucuronosyltransferases see reference 124.

Table 3 illustrates the functional groups that form glucuronides with examples of the reactions. The glucuronides formed from these functional groups have different properties. Stability is among the most important with respect to detoxication. Breakdown of the glucuronide can lead to reformation of the parent compound and in certain cases the

production of highly reactive electrophilic species. These reactive species may be responsible for the production of both acute and chronic toxicity by covalent binding to nucleophilic sites on tissue macromolecules.

Among the most commonly encountered glucuronides are those involving linkage of glucuronic acid and the xenobiotic through the oxygen atom. These *O*-glucuronides may form with a number of chemical classes including aryl, alkyl, and acyl compounds as illustrated in Table 3.

Aryl-*O*-glucuronides are formed through an ether bond and are highly stable compounds. Inductive effects of functional groups on the aglycone influence the stability of these glucuronides, as might be expected. They are highly stable in both acid and alkaline conditions. Stability aids in excretion and decreases the potential for breakdown and reformation of the aglycone.

The alkyl-*O*-glucuronides are ether-linked glucuronides that can form from a variety of primary, secondary, and tertiary alcohols. Although generally stable at physiologic conditions, they can be hydrolyzed under acidic conditions.

The enolic glucuronides are formed from aglycones without a free hydroxyl group. Glucuronides are formed from the enolized keto group. These conjugates lack the stability of ether glucuronides and are susceptible to both acid and alkaline hydrolysis. They are more stable at neutral and alkaline pH's than in acid conditions.

Ester glucuronides can be produced from a variety of carboxylic acids, including primary, secondary, and tertiary aliphatic acids and both aryl and heterocyclic compounds. They are generally stable in acidic conditions, but are susceptible to alkaline hydrolysis.

The chemical properties of *N*-glucuronides are different from *O*-glucuronides. One of the most important of these is their lack of stability. They are especially unstable at pH's below neutrality. The instability of these compounds may have important biologic consequences; examples are discussed in more detail below.

The *S*-glucuronides are not as commonly encountered as the *O*-glucuronides, but they represent important detoxication pathways for thiolic compounds. Their stability is similar to the *O*-glucuronides.

The *C*-glucuronides represent recently recognized conjugates and few examples are known. Generally, they appear to be formed by the transferase, but other possible mechanisms of formation have been suggested.

Role of UDP-Glucuronosyltransferases in Detoxication and Metabolic Activation

The foregoing discussion suggests that UDP-glucuronosyltransferases play a critical role in the metabolism and detoxication of xenobiotics. Many substrates require functionalization by the monooxygenase before metabolism by the transferase, whereas others can be directly conjugated. The conjugates are more water soluble compounds than the parent xenobiotic, and some readily form salts. Addition of the glycone may enable some of the conjugates to be more readily excreted through carrier-mediated mechanisms. Mechanisms other than increased excretion rates may also be important. The addition of the relatively bulky glycone may hide or

TABLE 3. *Functional groups forming glucuronides*

Functional group	Compound class	Example

Hydroxyl → *O*-glucuronide
 	
$-\overset{\|}{\underset{\|}{C}}-OH \rightarrow -\overset{\|}{\underset{\|}{C}}-O-$Glucuronic acid
	Alcohols
	  Aliphatic
	  Alicyclic
		
		Trichlorethanol
		Hexobarbital

	Benzylic Phenolic	Methylphenylcarbinol Phenol
$\overset{}{\underset{}{>}}$N—OH → $\overset{}{\underset{}{>}}$N—O—Glucuronic acid	Enols Hydroxyamines	4-Hydroxycoumarin *N*-hydroxy-2-acetylaminofluorene

Carboxyl → *O*-glucuronide
 	
$\overset{}{\underset{\|\|}{C}}-OH \rightarrow \overset{}{\underset{\|\|}{C}}-O-$Glucuronic acid
   O   O
	Carboxylic acids
	  Aliphatic
	  Aromatic
		
		2-Ethylhexanoic acid
		Benzoic acid

	Aryl-alkyl Heterocyclic	Phenylacetic acid Nicotinic acid

Amine → *N*-glucuronide
  N-glucuronic acid
     O H
	Aromatic	Aniline

$\|\|$ $\|$ —O—C—N-glucuronic acid (R)₃—N⁺—glucuronic acid	Carbamate Aliphatic tertiary Amine	Meprobamate Tripelennamine

R—SO₂—N—glucuronic acid
       $\|$
       H
	Sulfonamide	Sulfadimethoxine

	Heterocyclic	Sulfisoxazole
Sulfhydryl → *S*-glucuronide *O-S*-glucuronic acid	Arylthiol Dithiocarbamic acid	Thiophenol
C—S—glucuronic acid Carbon → C—glucuronide C—glucuronic acid	 1,3-Dicarbonyl system	 Phenylbutazone

Modified from ref. 64.

hinder the biologic reactivity of particular functional groups on the xenobiotic. Also, binding of the toxicant to particular receptors responsible for toxicity may be blocked. Overall, these mechanisms represent an efficient system for detoxication. On the other hand, glucuronidation of certain compounds facilitates metabolic activation by transporting the reactive metabolite to the target site.

Aromatic amines are some of the most studied examples of the role glucuronidation plays in metabolic activation of carcinogens. These glucuronides transport the proximate carcinogen to the target site where it decomposes to the species that reacts with cellular macromolecules producing the biochemical lesion responsible for generating the pathological lesion.

Several of the arylamines are potent bladder carcinogens including 4-aminobiphenyl, 1-naphthylamine, and benzidine. Metabolic activation of these carcinogens to the ultimate carcinogen appears similar and requires the action of UDP-glucuronosyltransferase. Metabolic activation begins with cytochrome P-450-dependent monooxygenase activation of the arylamine to the proximate carcinogen, an *N*-

hydroxyarylamine. Other specific ring hydroxylated forms may be produced and represent more stable products. The unstable *N*-hydroxyarylamines are then converted to more stable *N*-glucuronides. These *N*-glucuronides of the *N*-hydroxyarylamines are then transported to the bladder. In the bladder, the *N*-glucuronides are subject to β-glucuronidase activity, which splits off the glycone. They are also subject to hydrolysis in acidic urine producing the *N*-hydroxyarylamine. The *N*-hydroxarylamine spontaneously converts to the electrophilic arylnitrenium ion as illustrated in Fig. 7.

The electrophilic arylnitrenium ion can then react with nucleophilic centers on macromolecules of the bladder epithelium, especially DNA, to initiate tumor formation. The concentration of glucuronide in the bladder, in combination with the time the glucuronide remains in the bladder, can modify the potential for tumor formation. Glucuronides may function in this manner with a number of carcinogens and be important in explaining why certain target organs are susceptible to a specific carcinogen and others are not susceptible. In the above example, glucuronidation may protect the liver but make the bladder, the target organ, susceptible.

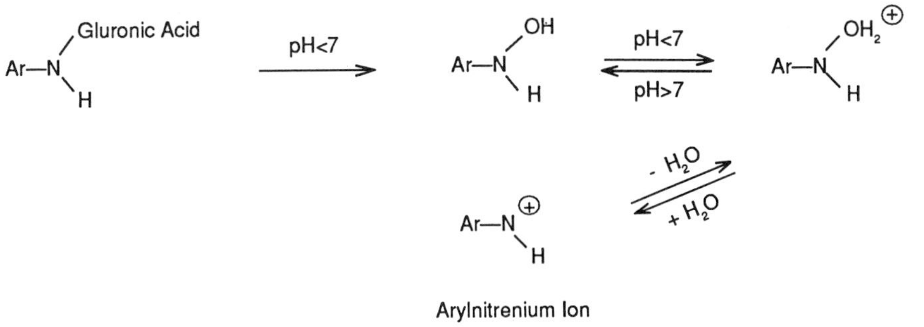

FIG. 7. Metabolic activation of aromatic amines via glucuronidation.

Species and Sex Differences in UDP-Glucuronosyltransferase Activity

Studies of species, strain, and sex differences in glucuronidation are complicated by a number of factors. Activity may be affected by age, hormonal status, exposure to dietary and environmental xenobiotics, and nutrition. Factors associated with the methodology to determine differences in glucuronidation also play a role including substrate, assay method, method of freeing latent activity, and the method of isolating the preparation employed to measure activity. This has led to a number of reports of differences in activity that could be artifactual. However, the large number of reports concerning differences in glucuronidation among species, strains, and the sexes indicate that certain of these differences are real.

There have been a few reports of lower animals producing glucuronides including prokaryotes and invertebrates, but no reports of their formation in plants. Fish and reptiles do demonstrate glucuronidation of xenobiotics, but vary dramatically in activity, which is generally 10-fold or more lower than mammalian activity. Birds have glucuronidation ability similar to mammals.

Differences among mammalian species in their ability to glucuronidate a xenobiotic may be quite large. However, as mentioned, in some cases this could be artifactual. The guinea pig generally has higher activity than most other laboratory species. This higher activity may be associated with less latent enzyme activity, since its UDPGA-glucuronosyltransferase can be activated by much more gentle methods than other species. Cats are well known for their extremely low transferase activity. Although capable of forming glucuronides with endogenous compounds, this genus forms only low levels or no glucuronides with xenobiotics. A well-known example of a strain difference is the almost complete lack of bilirubin glucuronidation in the Gunn rat. This strain also has low activity toward a number of xenobiotic substrates, but normal activity toward others. There is a genetic component to this, with the low activity being autosomally recessive.

Sex differences appear hormonally related and can be substrate dependent. Although it is sometimes stated that males have higher glucuronidation activity than females, this is substrate dependent and no general classification should be made. Like monooxygenase activity, activity may be sensitive to imprinting or programming during the neonatal period. As with species and strain differences, care must be taken

when extrapolating data obtained with one substrate to others.

Induction of Glucuronosyltransferases

UDP-glucuronosyltransferases appear to be inducible enzymes much like cytochrome P-450. They are inducible by many of the same inducers. Some believe induction of both enzymes is under the same or similar regulatory control. However, evidence of a true induction process involving *de novo* protein synthesis is not currently as strong as that for the P-450 system. For instance, care must be taken that the activation of UDP-glucuronosyltransferases is not confused with induction. Studies, such as those of Pfeil and Bock (103), indicating increases in the quantity of the transferase after administration of inducer, coupled with genetic studies indicating a common regulatory receptor for both the monooxygenases and the transferases (70) indicate a true induction. Few specific inducers of the transferases that do not also induce the monooxygenase are known. For example, *trans*-stilbene oxide and ethoxyquin appear only to induce the transferase, but more studies are needed to determine if this is a true induction.

In parallel with the monooxygenase, there appear to be two major classes of inducers, phenobarbital type and 3-methylcholanthrene type, but other classes probably exist. Induction of the transferases modifies the toxicity of xenobiotics in a manner similar to induction of the monooxygenase, as previously discussed.

Sulfate Conjugation

Description of the Pathway

As early as 1815, it was recognized that mammals excrete organic sulfates in their urine (40). The discovery that organic sulfates were esters produced by conjugation of endogenous organic compounds with inorganic sulfate came over 50 years later (5). The early workers believed the sulfate conjugates were ethers formed between aryl compounds and inorganic sulfate. Therefore, they called these metabolites *ethereal sulfates*. These metabolites are actually sulfuric acid esters and the term ethereal sulfate is only historical (83), although it is still sometimes used.

Conjugation with inorganic sulfate utilizes an activated sulfate cosubstrate, 3'-phosphoadenosine 5'-phosphosulfate (PAPS) (21). Inorganic sulfate is converted to PAPS in a series of reactions depicted in Fig. 8. Adenosine triphosphate (ATP) sulfurylase catalyzes the formation of adenosine-5'-phosphosulfate (APS) from ATP and sulfate. Since this is an exergonic reaction that liberates pyrophosphate, the APS must be reactivated by phosphorylation with an additional mole of ATP. This reaction is catalyzed by APS phosphokinase and produces PAPS and adenosine diphosphate (ADP). Sulfotransferases catalyze the electrophilic attack of the activated sulfur atom of PAPS on either the hydroxyl oxygen of alcohols, N-hydroxylamines, and phenols or the amine nitrogen of aryl amines to form O-sulfates and N-sulfates, respectively (116). The electrophilic attack of the electron-deficient sulfur of PAPS is illustrated in Fig. 9.

Sulfotransferases esterify a variety of endogenous substrates including steroids, carbohydrates, and proteins (44). The sulfated products are important constituents of cells; for example, chondroiton sulfate is a major component of connective tissue and cerebroside sulfate is found in nerve tissue. In addition to cellular constituents, sulfation plays a role in the disposition of hormones. Sulfation directs lipophilic compounds, such as steroidal hormones, to more polar environments including the active sites of enzymes and to body fluids. For example, sulfation enhances elimination of steroids from the adrenal gland (80).

Xenobiotic conjugation with sulfate is an important route for conversion of lipophilic xenobiotics to more readily excreted polar metabolites (54). Sulfation of xenobiotics with an aliphatic or aromatic hydroxyl group readily occur. For example, phenol is excreted as its sulfate conjugate. Often it is necessary for phase I metabolism to functionalize a xenobiotic with a hydroxyl group before it can be sulfated. For example, toluene is oxidized to benzyl alcohol before conjugation with sulfate (Fig. 10).

The sulfotransferases are divided into five groups according to the Nomenclature Committee of the International Union of Biochemistry (51) (Table 4).

Extrahepatic Metabolism

The liver is the principal organ of xenobiotic metabolism by virtue of its size and its central location in systemic circulation. Portal blood flow that drains the intestinal tract passes through the liver before the heart and systemic circulation. However, because sulfation is important in the metabolism of endogenous compounds, it has widespread distribution in mammalian tissue. For example, in the monkey the specific activity for isoprenalin sulfation by selected tissues is lung > kidney > small intestine > liver (121).

Species Differences

There is wide species variation in sulfation of two model substrates, isoprenalin and harmol. For example, the activity toward isoprenalin in the mouse liver is 10 times that in the monkey liver.

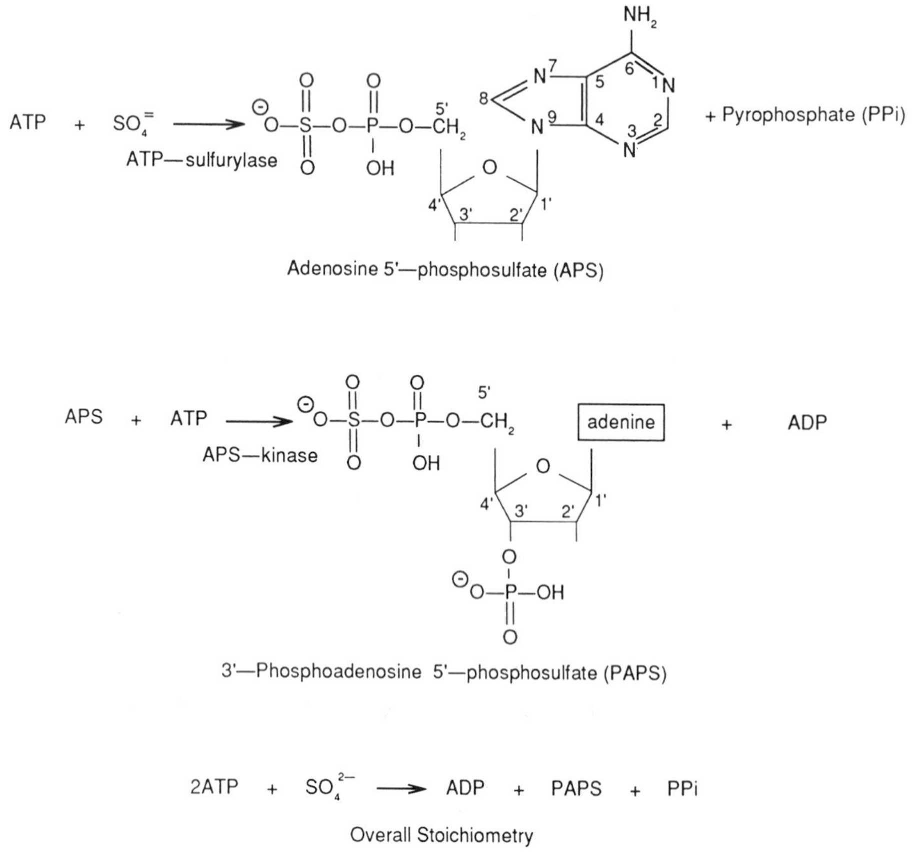

Adenosine 5'—phosphosulfate (APS)

3'—Phosphoadenosine 5'—phosphosulfate (PAPS)

$$2ATP + SO_4^{2-} \longrightarrow ADP + PAPS + PPi$$

Overall Stoichiometry

FIG. 8. Reactions catalyzing the formation of PAPS from inorganic sulfate and ATP.

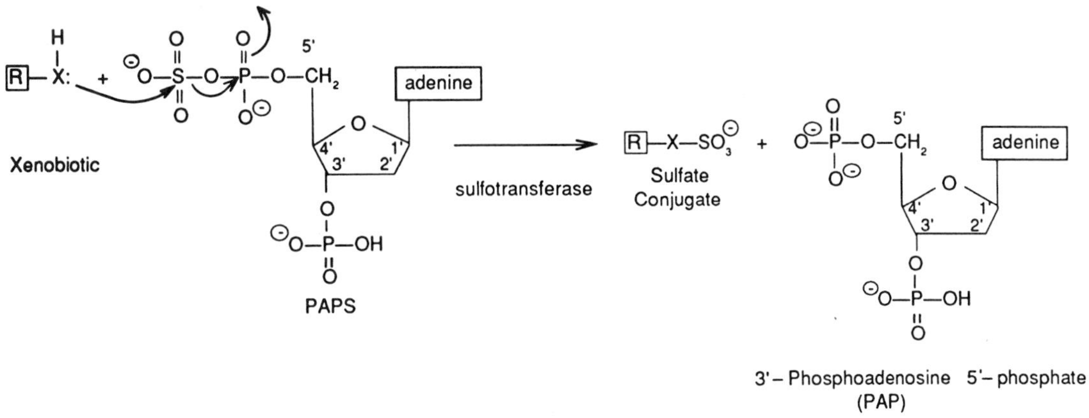

FIG. 9. Synthesis of a sulfate conjugate from a model xenobiotic by sulfotransferase.

Sulfation occurs in most species including mammals, birds, reptiles, amphibians, fish, and invertebrates. The most notable exception to this is the low sulfotransferase activity in the pig. Members of the cat family are deficient in glucuronyl transferase activity, but have high sulfotransferase activity. This balance of glucuronyl transferase and sulfotransferase must always be kept in mind when evaluating the activity of either enzyme system. A deficiency in one pathway can shift metabolism since similar functional groups are conjugated by these two enzyme systems. In addition, sulfation appears to have high affinity, but low capacity for phenols while glucuronidation has low affinity and high capacity for these substrates.

Factors Modifying Metabolism

Unlike other detoxication enzymes, sulfotransferases are not induced by the classical inducers phenobarbital and 3-methylcholanthrene. However, several inhibitors of sulfotransferase have been discovered and exploited experi-mentally to study these enzymes. Pentachlorophenol and 2,6-dichloro-4-nitrophenol are potent sulfotransferase in-hibitors. Only 0.2 μM pentachlorophenol is required for 50% inhibition of 2-chloro-4-nitrophenol sulfation by purified aryl sulfotransferase IV (51). Pentachlorophenol and 2,6-dichloro-4-nitrophenol are effective inhibitors because the *ortho* and *para* aromatic ring positions are substituted with electron withdrawing groups. This effect is consistent with the mechanism whereby the sulfotransferases facilitate electrophilic attack of the hydroxyl oxygen by the sulfur (Fig. 9).

Sex and Developmental Differences

There are major sex differences in the sulfate conjugation of steroid hormones. For example, female rats have five-fold higher activity for cortisol metabolism than do male rats (103). This sex difference in cortisol metabolism is apparently due more to suppression of sulfotransferase by male hormone levels than to the ovaries stimulating activity (102,104). Three steroid sulfotransferases have been isolated from rat liver and it is the relative amounts of these isozymes that account for

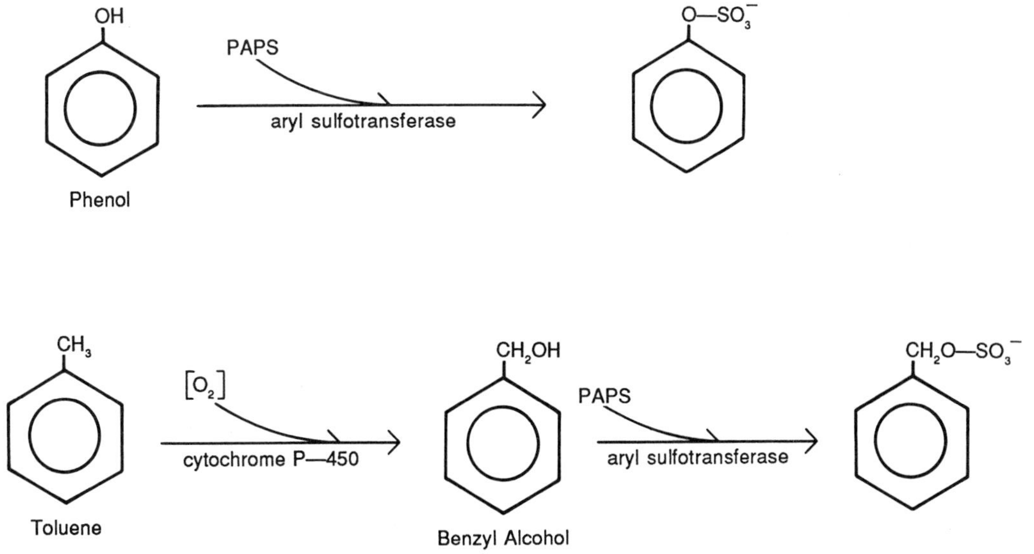

FIG. 10. Sulfotransferase catalyzed sulfation of phenol and toluene.

TABLE 4. *Sulfotransferases involved in the metabolism of xenobiotics*

EC No.	Name	Examples of substrates
2.8.2.1	Aryl sulfotransferase	2-Naphthol, phenol, substituted phenols, serotonin, acetaminophen
2.8.2.2	Alcohol sulfotransferase (also called, hydroxysteroid sulfotransferase)	Primary and secondary aliphatic alcohols, nonaromatic hydroxysteroids
2.8.2.4	Estrone sulfotransferase	Estrone and other aromatic hydroxysteroids
2.8.2.9	Tyrosine ester sulfotransferase	Tyrosine methyl ester, 2-cyanoethyl-N-hydroxythioacetamide
2.8.2.14	Bile-salt sulfotransferase	Conjugated and unconjugated bile acids

From ref. 59, with permission.

the large sex difference. Lower sulfotransferase activity observed in neonates has been attributed to sexual immaturity because as gonads develop, sulfotransferase activity increases. However, sulfation is not always greater in females than in males. For example, the hepatocarcinogen 2-acetylaminofluorene is sulfated to a greater extent in male rats.

Role of Sulfation in Metabolic Activation

One of the most studied examples of metabolic activation by sulfation is the activation of 2-acetylaminofluorene (2-AAF) illustrated in Fig. 11. *N*-hydroxylation of the amide nitrogen by the cytochrome P-450-dependent monooxygenase is followed by sulfation of the *N*-hydroxy group (a phase II metabolic reaction). The *N-O*-sulfate ester is unstable and decomposes to an electrophilic nitrenium ion-carbonium resonance ion which can form covalent adducts at nucleophilic sites on macromolecules. Support for the hypothesis that the sulfate conjugate of 2-AAF is the reactive metabolite comes from studies indicating factors that modulate sulfotransferase activity also modulate 2-AAF carcinogenicity. Male rats have higher sulfotransferase activity and develop more 2-AAF-induced tumors than females. Reduction of sulfotransferase activity in male rats by either castration, hypophysectomy, thyroidectomy, or steroid hormones reduces 2-AAF covalent adducts. These results are consistent with the hypothesis that sulfation of 2-AAF is required for covalent modification of DNA. This mechanism is at least partially responsible for the activation of several other xenobiotics including aromatic amines, mono- and dinitrotoluene, *N*-hydroxyphenacetin, 1'-hydroxysafrole, N₃-hydroxyxanthine, and other *N*-hydroxyarylamides (84). In addition to this mechanism, sulfation of a 7,12-dimethylbenzanthracene metabolite has been shown to produce a reactive metabolite capable of adduction with glutathione and protein (117).

Glutathione *S*-transferases

A collection of cytosolic enzymes known as glutathione *S*-transferases is capable of conjugating relatively hydrophobic electrophilic molecules with the nucleophile reduced glutathione (Fig. 12) (14). This conjugate is less lipophilic, more water soluble, and likely to be excreted in the urine. Another advantage of glutathione conjugation is that the conjugate is a larger molecule (M.W. 307) than the parent xenobiotic and

is likely to be secreted into the bile and excreted in the feces. It also will be less likely to react with toxicologic targets.

Glutathione *S*-transferases are cytosolic proteins that catalyze the conjugation of glutathione with a substrate bearing an electrophilic atom (48). The transferases facilitate the nucleophilic attack of *glutathione thiolate ion* (GS⁻) on the electron-deficient atom of the relatively hydrophobic electrophilic xenobiotic (Fig. 13). There is little specificity in the active site for the xenobiotic other than it must possess hydrophobic character.

In addition to catalyzing the conjugation of xenobiotics with glutathione, glutathione *S*-transferases are capable of binding the xenobiotic on the enzyme surface. This binding may or may not inhibit the catalytic activity of the enzyme, but does prevent the xenobiotic from interacting with critical cellular sites, such as proteins and nucleic acids. The glutathione *S*-transferase possessing this property has been termed *ligandin* (106,107).

Glutathione *S*-transferases can form covalent bonds between reactive xenobiotics and the enzyme's active site. Such binding inactivates the enzyme, but also inactivates the reactive xenobiotic and represents an additional detoxication mechanism (51). This process is called *suicide inactivation* and has been demonstrated for other detoxication enzymes.

Because of these three glutathione *S*-transferase activities, the enzymes have been called "a triple threat in detoxification" by Jakoby and Keen (50). This system can detoxify a broad spectrum of compounds that an organism may either encounter in its environment or generate during cellular metabolism (91). Although the system is not highly efficient (i.e., operates only at relatively high xenobiotic concentrations), it is capable of catalyzing or reacting with a number of reactive chemical groups.

Description of the Pathway

Although the urinary metabolites of glutathione conjugates, *mercapturic acids,* were first described in the nineteenth century (6,47), it was not until the 1950s that glutathione was identified as the source of cysteine in mercapturic acids (120). The intracellular concentration of reduced glutathione is relatively high in most tissues (1–10 μmole/g-wet tissue) (1). It is synthesized in the cytosol of most cells via the γ-glutamyl cycle, a series of tightly controlled, enzyme-catalyzed reactions (Fig. 14). The three amino acids that comprise

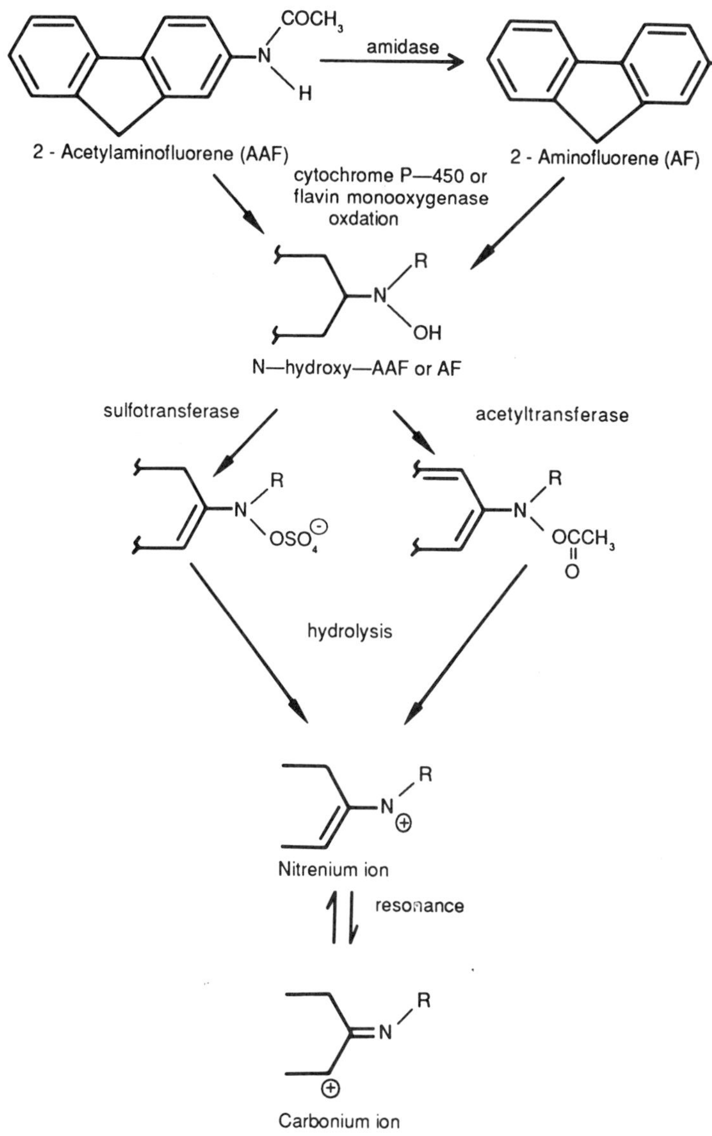

FIG. 11. Metabolic activation of 2-acetyl-aminofluorene to a reactive metabolite capable of covalent modification of macromolecules.

glutathione, cysteine, glycine, and glutamic acid, can enter the cycle from several biochemical pathways, even though the cycle depicts them arising from glutathione.

Xenobiotics that act as substrates for the glutathione *S*-transferases fall into four broad categories as depicted in Fig. 15: (a) reaction with electrophilic carbon, (b) nitrogen, (c) sulfur, and (d) oxygen (39,49,55).

Reaction with electrophilic carbon

Displacement of leaving groups such as halides, sulfates, sulfonates, phosphates, and nitro groups from saturated carbon or hetero atoms: Displacement is facilitated if the saturated carbon atom is allylic or benzylic. Displacement of halide or nitro groups on aromatic rings occurs if there are sufficient electron-withdrawing groups that predispose the ring system toward nucleophilic substitution. The rate of formation of a carbanion intermediate of the aromatic ring governs the overall rate of the reaction. Functional groups that

withdraw electrons stabilize the carbanion and are considered "good leaving groups." Those that donate electrons to the ring deactivate the ring making the displacement of the leaving group by glutathione less likely (Fig. 16).

Opening of strained rings such as epoxides and 4-membered lactones: As shown in Fig. 15, the 1,2-epoxide of naphthalene is opened resulting in a 1-naphthol conjugate of glutathione.

Addition to activated double bonds via Michael addition: The glutathione thiolate anion will also attack β-unsaturated xenobiotics due to the partial positive charge on the β-carbon as shown in Fig. 16 (addition reaction). Figure 15 illustrates the addition of glutathione to the β-carbon of an acrylate ester.

Reaction with electrophilic nitrogen

The reaction sequence and overall stoichiometry for the reaction of organic nitrate esters with glutathione is shown in Fig. 15. This reaction was once attributed to glutathione

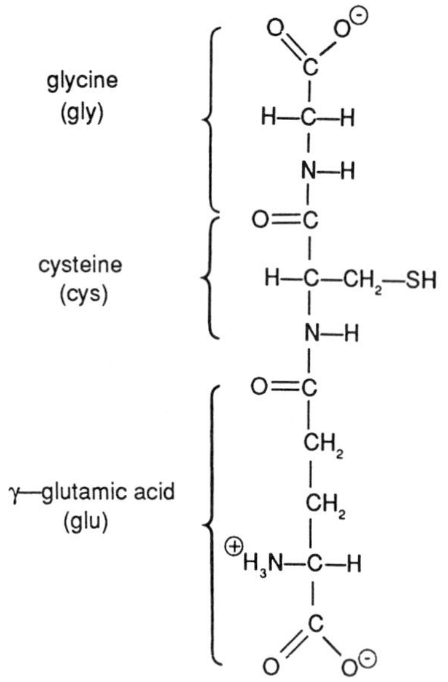

glycine
(gly)

cysteine
(cys)

γ—glutamic acid
(glu)

FIG. 12. Structure of reduced glutathione (MW 307).

reductase, but is now known to be catalyzed by glutathione S-transferases. The transferases catalyze the removal of nitrite from the ester generating an R—O—S conjugate with glutathione. The vasodilators nitroglycerin and erythrityl tetranitrate are two organic nitrate ester substrates for this reaction. The alcohol-glutathione conjugate can react with another reduced glutathione molecule, similar to reactions disulfides undergo, to yield an alcohol and oxidized glutathione.

Reaction with electrophilic sulfur

Alkyl and aryl thiocyanates are also substrates for glutathione S-transferase catalyzed conjugations as shown in Fig. 15. Products of nucleophilic attack of thiolate ion on the sulfur of the xenobiotic result in a mixed disulfide and hydrogen cyanide. The mixed disulfide can react with another molecule of glutathione to yield a thiol of the xenobiotic (RSH) and oxidized glutathione (GSSG).

Reaction with electrophilic oxygen

Figure 15 illustrates how glutathione reacts with organic hydroperoxides by a two-step sequence. The first step is catalyzed by glutathione S-transferase and forms an alcohol or phenol and a glutathione sulfenic acid intermediate (GSOH). Another glutathione reacts nonenzymatically with the sulfenic acid to form oxidized glutathione and water. Glutathione S-transferase 2-2 (formerly AA) purified from the rat possesses as much activity toward cumene hydroperoxide as it does toward the classical transferase substrate 1-chloro-2,4-dinitrobenzene.

Glutathione S-transferases Nomenclature

The glutathione S-transferases were originally named by their substrate specificity, such as S-epoxide transferase and S-alkyl transferase. When purification techniques and homogeneous preparations of the transferases became available, it was found that the transferases had overlapping substrate specificities. Nomenclature based on substrate specificities were no longer appropriate. Jakoby and his co-workers termed the transferases purified from rat liver in the inverse order of their elution from carboxymethylcellulose columns used to purify the proteins (52,63). The decision to name the proteins in the inverse order of elution rather than in the order of elution from the column resulted from an attempt to keep some ties with the older nomenclature system. The first of five peaks eluting from the column was known to possess epoxide transferase activity and the last, aryl transferase activity. It was convenient to name them transferases E, D, C, B, and A in the order of their elution from the column. This way the E peak corresponded with the epoxide transferase activity and the A peak corresponded with the

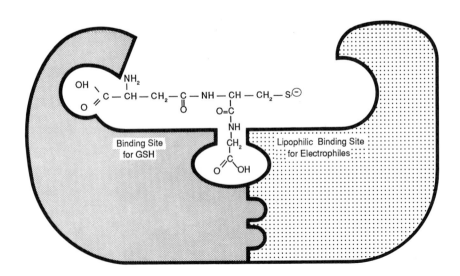

FIG. 13. Illustration of the active site of a glutathione S-transferase.

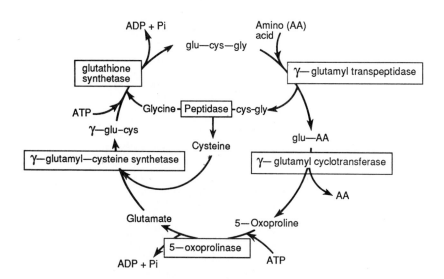

FIG. 14. The gamma-glutamyl cycle responsible for the biosynthesis of reduced glutathione. (From ref. 84, with permission.)

aryl transferase activity. However, with the advent of recombinant DNA techniques there was a need for a more systematic nomenclature that was sufficiently flexible to include new isozymes as they were characterized. This resulted in the establishment of a new system listed in Table 5.

Mercapturic Acid Formation

Mercaturic acids are *N*-acetylated *S*-substituted cysteine conjugates that arise from conjugation of a xenobiotic with glutathione (10).

The glutathione conjugates formed in the liver and other tissues as shown in pathway 1 of Fig. 17 are polar and partition into the aqueous phase of cells and blood. Since 25%

of the blood flow passes through the kidney, glutathione conjugates are transported to the kidney. There the glutathione-xenobiotic conjugate undergoes a series of reactions, shown in pathway 2 of Fig. 17, that result in mercapturic acid formation.

The initial step in mercapturic acid synthesis is cleavage of glutamic acid from cysteine catalyzed by γ-glutamyltranspeptidase (E.C.2.3.2.2). This enzyme is located in the brush border of the proximal tubules in the kidney (118). Evidence that this enzyme is involved in glutathione degradation comes from observations of pronounced glutathionemia and glutathionuria (high levels of glutathione in blood and urine, respectively) in patients who lack detectable γ-glutamyltranspeptidase. This enzyme not only hydrolyzes the glutathione moiety but transfers the γ-glutamyl group to a variety

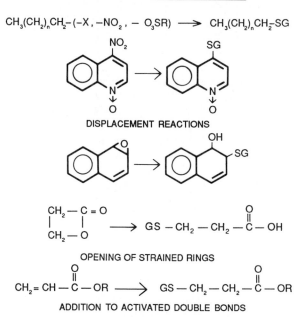

FIG. 15. Examples of the reactions catalyzed by the glutathione *S*-transferases.

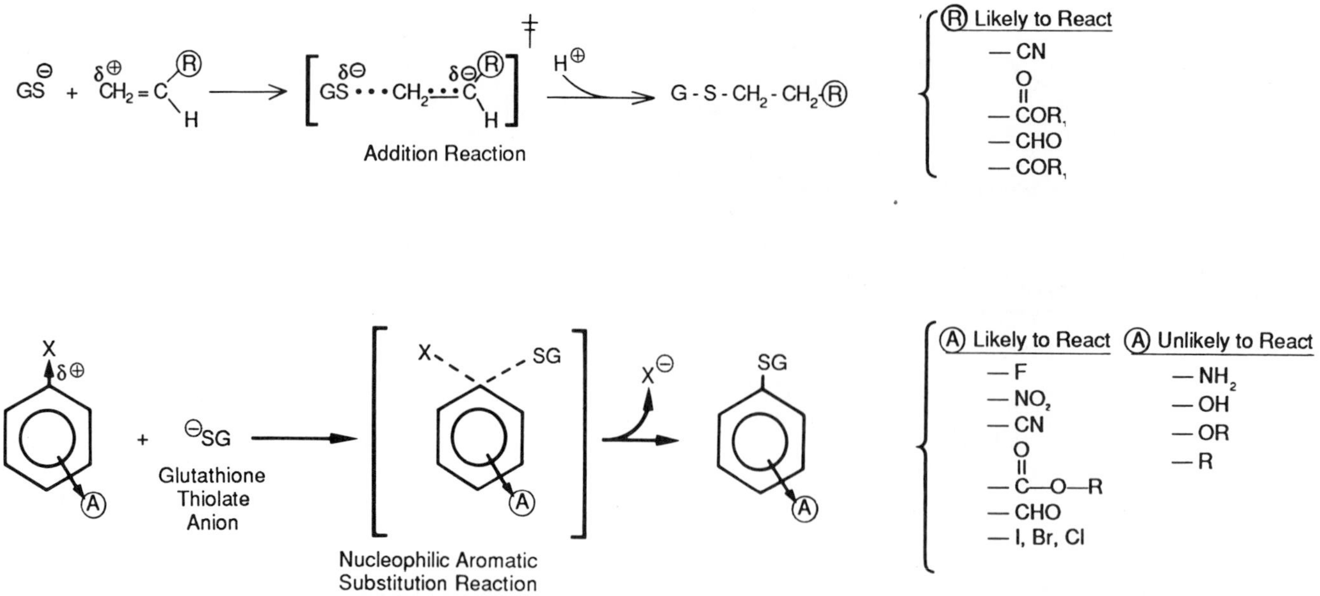

FIG. 16. Putative reaction mechanisms for the glutathione *S*-transferase-catalyzed nucleophilic attack of the glutathione thiolate anion on electrophilic xenobiotics where X represents a nalogen and ⓡ and ⓐ the listed substituents.

of amino acids and dipeptides. These two reactions have been shown to proceed at equivalent rates under physiologic conditions (122).

Next, the glycine group is cleaved from the resulting cysteinylglycine conjugate by aminopeptidase M yielding the *S*-substituted cysteine conjugate of the xenobiotic. The cysteine conjugate is a substrate for *N*-acetyl transferase that acetylates the free amino group of cysteine to yield the mercapturic acid, which is excreted in the urine (pathway 3, Fig. 17). These two enzymes, γ-glutamyltranspeptidase and aminopeptidase M, are also responsible for the normal turnover of glutathione in mammalian cells previously shown in Fig. 14.

At one time only those compounds that were conjugated to glutathione and excreted extensively in the urine as mercapturates were thought to yield this metabolite. With the advent of high pressure liquid chromatography (HPLC) and soft ionization techniques for mass spectroscopy, the presence of mercapturic acids as common metabolites of xenobiotics is well documented.

TABLE 5. *Nomenclature for the rat glutathione transferases*

New nomenclature	Previous nomenclature
Glutathione transferase 1-1	Ligandin, B1, YaYa, L2
Glutathione transferase 1-2	Ligandin, B, B2, YaYa, BL
Glutathione transferase 2-2	AA, YcYc, B2
Glutathione transferase 3-3	A, Yb1Yb1, A2
Glutathione transferase 3-4	C, Yb1Yb2, AC
Glutathione transferase 4-4	D, "D," Yb2Yb2, C2
Glutathione transferase 5-5	E
Glutathione transferase 6-6	Mt

From ref. 61, with permission.

Role of Glutathione *S*-transferases in Detoxification

Free reactive electrophilic intermediates of xenobiotics can produce damage to important cellular constituents. Reduced glutathione and the glutathione *S*-transferases protect cells from this damage by capturing reactive electrophiles before they react at nucleophilic sites critical to cell viability (34).

The metabolism of acetaminophen, an analgesic that at high doses can produce hepatic necrosis, serves as an example of this protective system. A large body of work has shown that one of the principal ways in which acetaminophen produces its hepatotoxicity is via the reactive intermediate, *N*-acetyl-*p*-benzoquinone imine, as shown in Fig. 4. This intermediate is apparently a soft electrophile that reacts readily with the strong, soft nucleophile glutathione. As long as the amount of glutathione present at the site of activation of acetaminophen is sufficient to bind the reactive intermediate, no toxicity ensues. However, as was demonstrated in a classic study by Mitchell et al. (79), when glutathione is depleted by pretreatment with diethyl maleate, the benzoquinone imine covalently binds to tissue proteins resulting in tissue necrosis. Mitchell et al. (79) were among the first to propose that glutathione plays a fundamental role in protecting tissues against electrophilic attack by xenobiotics.

Since these early studies demonstrating the protective role of glutathione, many compounds have been shown to form conjugates with glutathione. For a comprehensive review of these reactions, see Chasseaud (15).

Species Differences

Glutathione *S*-transferases have been found in many terrestrial species including reptiles, birds, insects, amphibians, and plants. The lack of glutathione *S*-transferase in fish sug-

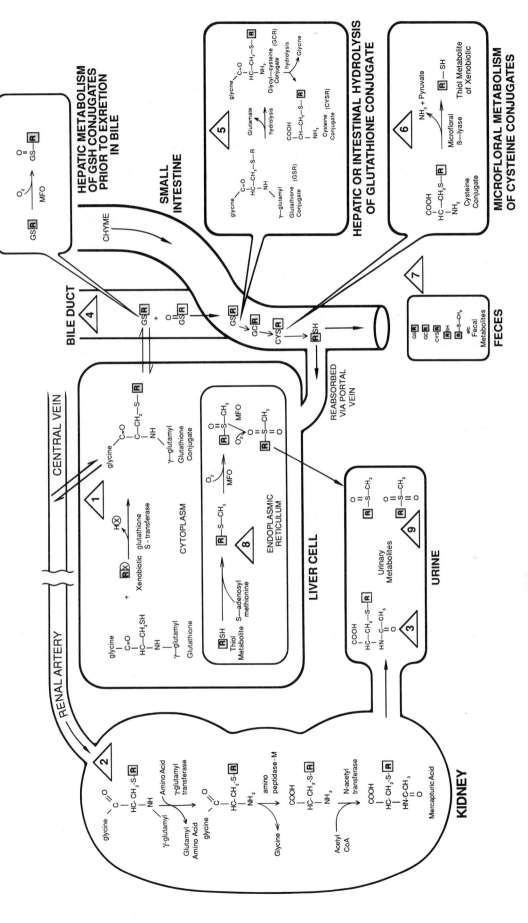

FIG. 17. Integration of glutathione conjugate disposition in mammals.

gests that these enzymes developed to protect terrestrial organisms from xenobiotics in the food and air. Aquatic organisms are bathed in a rich source of nucleophilic material, water, that can hydrolyze many reactive compounds reducing their toxicity. They also do not need the highly developed excretory systems found in terrestrial species.

Environmental Factors Affecting Metabolism

Factors that influence the availability of reduced glutathione drastically alter the effectiveness of glutathione S-transferases. As discussed above, the toxicity of acetaminophen is modulated by the availability of reduced glutathione. Most xenobiotics that react nonenzymatically with glutathione result in its depletion. Other mechanisms may also lower glutathione availability. For example, certain individuals have genetic defects in the γ-glutamyl cycle resulting in low tissue concentrations of glutathione. These individuals are generally anemic due to the lack of glutathione and the resulting oxidative damage to erythrocytes (77).

Nutritional factors that limit sulfur amino acid availability can decrease glutathione S-transferase activity by reducing glutathione availability (109). Methionine is an essential amino acid that can be used to synthesize cysteine and cystine via the transsulfuration pathway. If diets low in sulfur amino acids are fed, the availability of glutathione for conjugation with reactive intermediates of xenobiotics can be decreased.

Sex and Developmental Differences

Liver glutathione-S-transferase activities are low in prepubertal male and female rats. As rats reach sexual maturity between 30 and 50 days of age, glutathione conjugating activity toward dichloronitrobenzene is two- to threefold higher in males than females (65). This difference in glutathione-S-transferase activity was not related to sex steroids but was dependent on pituitary secretions. When male and female rats were hypophysectomized, glutathione S-transferase activity was increased. When pituitary secretions were reinitiated by implanting pituitaries in hypophysectomized rats, glutathione S-transferase activities were lowered to control levels. The search for the hypophyseal effector ruled out prolactin as the modulator of glutathione S-transferase activity, but suggested that growth hormone may play a role in establishing glutathione S-transferase activities (64).

These studies have suggested that growth hormone is important in regulating adult levels of glutathione S-transferase in the rat, but it appears that other factors also play a role. The student of toxicology should be aware of the multifaceted way that xenobiotics can affect organisms. For example, monosodium glutamate, which produces lesions in the arcuate nucleus of the hypothalamus, can lower the glutathione S-transferase activity in male rats. This could in turn increase the sensitivity of the organism to electrophilic chemicals.

Role of Glutathione S-transferases in Metabolic Activation

Glutathione conjugation does not always produce innocuous and readily excreted metabolites. Certain compounds are toxic only after conjugation with glutathione or cysteine. For example, Elfarra and Anders (24) compiled a list of 1,2-dihaloalkanes and halogenated alkenes whose glutathione or cysteine conjugates were nephrotoxic (Fig. 18). Glutathione reacts with the 1,2-dihaloalkanes via a glutathione-S-transferase-catalyzed reaction that yields sulfur mustards. An electrophilic episulfonium ion can be formed from the mustard when the second halogen atom is displaced by a cellular nucleophile. The episulfonium ion intermediate has been implicated in the toxicity of these chemicals. Recent evidence indicates that the major DNA adduct resulting from exposure to the carcinogen, 1,2-dibromoethane was S-2-N-7-guanylethylglutathione (45).

As shown in Fig. 17, glutathione and cysteine conjugates (GSR) formed in the liver (pathway 1) can be secreted in the bile (pathway 4). Glutathione conjugates can be hydrolyzed to cysteine conjugates by pancreatic peptidases in the small intestine (pathway 5). Cysteine conjugates originating from the bile and those formed by hydrolysis of glutathione conjugates are good substrates for microfloral β-lyase (pathway 6). β-Lyase, an enzyme found in liver, kidney, and intestinal microflora, cleaves thioether linkages in cysteine conjugates of xenobiotics (110). The resulting thiol compounds are more hydrophobic than the conjugates and can be readily absorbed in the small intestine. These thiol metabolites return to the liver via the portal circulation and act as substrates for thiol S-methyl transferase that methylates the thiol group (pathway 8). Enterohepatic circulation (pathways 1 → 4 → 5 → 6 → 8) of glutathione conjugates accounts for some of the unusual sulfur-containing metabolites (pathway 9) found in the urine of animals treated with xenobiotics, such as propachlor (96). A portion of the glutathione-derived sulfur-containing metabolites formed in the small intestine is excreted in the feces (pathway 7 of Fig. 17).

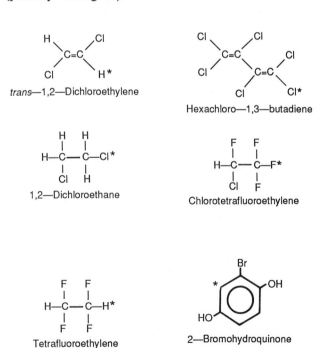

FIG. 18. Halogenated hydrocarbons that form glutathione and cysteine S-conjugates that are nephrotoxic. *Asterisks* indicate the position where the glutathione S-transferase catalyzed displacement (SN₂) occurs.

Reactions of glutathionyl and cysteinyl conjugates shown in Figs. 17 and 18 are thought to play a role in the nephrotoxicity of several xenobiotics. For example, the cysteinyl conjugate of trichloroethylene, S-(1,2-dichlorovinyl)-L-cysteine (DCVC), is a potent nephrotoxin and a β-lyase substrate. Inhibition of renal β-lyase with aminooxyacetic acid, an inhibitor of pyridoxyl phosphate-dependent enzymes, protected against DCVC-induced nephrotoxicity (24).

In general, glutathione conjugate synthesis results in readily excreted polar metabolites. However, in some cases (depicted in Fig. 17), the residence time of a glutathione conjugate in the body is prolonged. This can result in formation of metabolites that are more reactive than either the original, parent xenobiotic, or the glutathione conjugate. If these reactive metabolites interact with critical cellular sites, toxicity can ensue. For a recent review, see Anders (2).

Methylation

Xenobiotic methylation is a relatively minor pathway for eliminating chemicals from the body because it rarely results in a more polar metabolite. Those cases, such as methylation of nitrogen heterocycles, where methylation produces a quarternary base are exceptions. Methylation of endogenous substrates, such as histamine, amino acids, proteins, carbo-

hydrates, and polyamines, is important in regulation of normal cellular metabolism and accounts for the presence of this activity in mammalian cells. Only when a xenobiotic fits the requirements for the enzymes involved in these normal reactions does methylation become important in the metabolism of foreign compounds.

Methylation can be achieved by two routes. First and foremost is the methyl transferase-catalyzed methylation that requires S-adenosylmethionine (SAM) as a cosubstrate. Most biologic methylations require SAM as the methyl donor. However, there are methyl transferases that require SAM as a cosubstrate, but vary in other requirements for optimal activity (72). Reactions involving four of these SAM-dependent methyltransferases are shown in Fig. 19. Two enzymes catalyze nitrogen methylation: aromatic azaheterocycle N-methyltransferase and indolethylamine N-methyltransferase. Oxygen methylation is primarily catalyzed by catechol O-methyltransferase and sulfur methylation by thiol S-methyltransferase. A secondary source of methylation is N_5-methyltetrahydrofolate (5-CH$_3$-THF)-catalyzed methylation. This methylation is important in nucleic acid synthesis. However, 5-CH$_3$-THF is 1000 times less reactive toward the soft nucleophiles shown in Fig. 19 than SAM, suggesting that it plays a smaller role in xenobiotic methylation.

Nicotine methylation is a major route for its disposition in the guinea pig. The enzyme responsible for nicotine methylation is an aromatic azaherocycle N-methyltransferase that

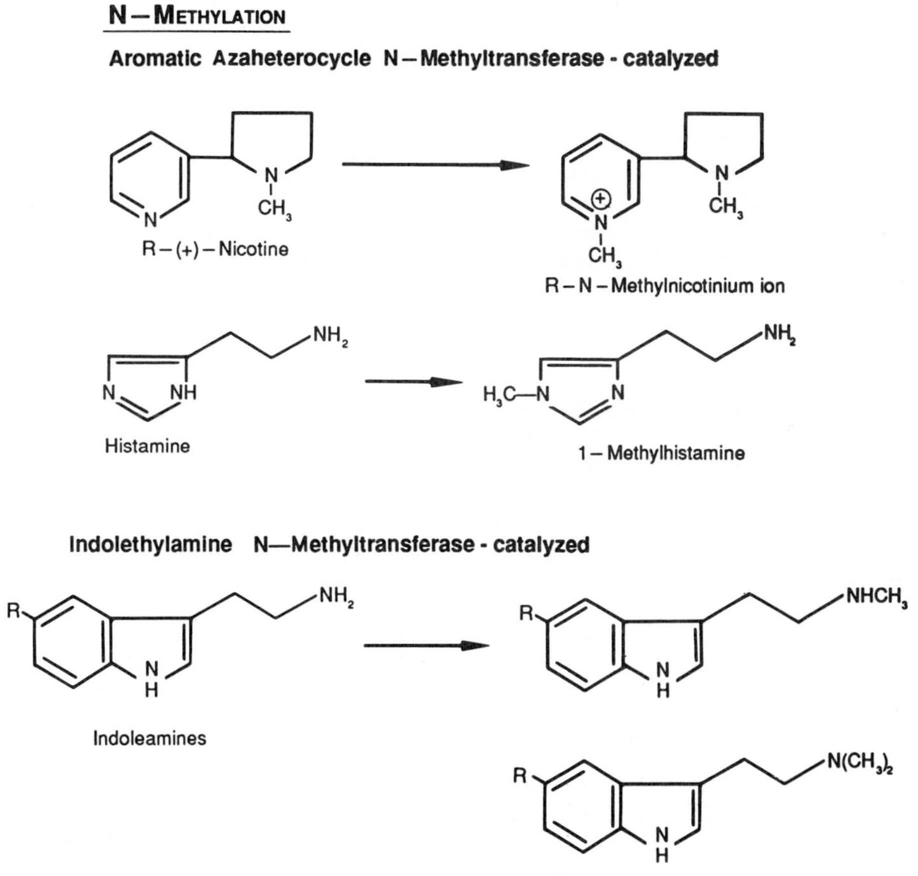

N—METHYLATION

Aromatic Azaheterocycle N—Methyltransferase - catalyzed

R—(+)—Nicotine

R—N—Methylnicotinium ion

Histamine

1—Methylhistamine

Indolethylamine N—Methyltransferase - catalyzed

Indoleamines

FIG. 19. Methylation reactions.

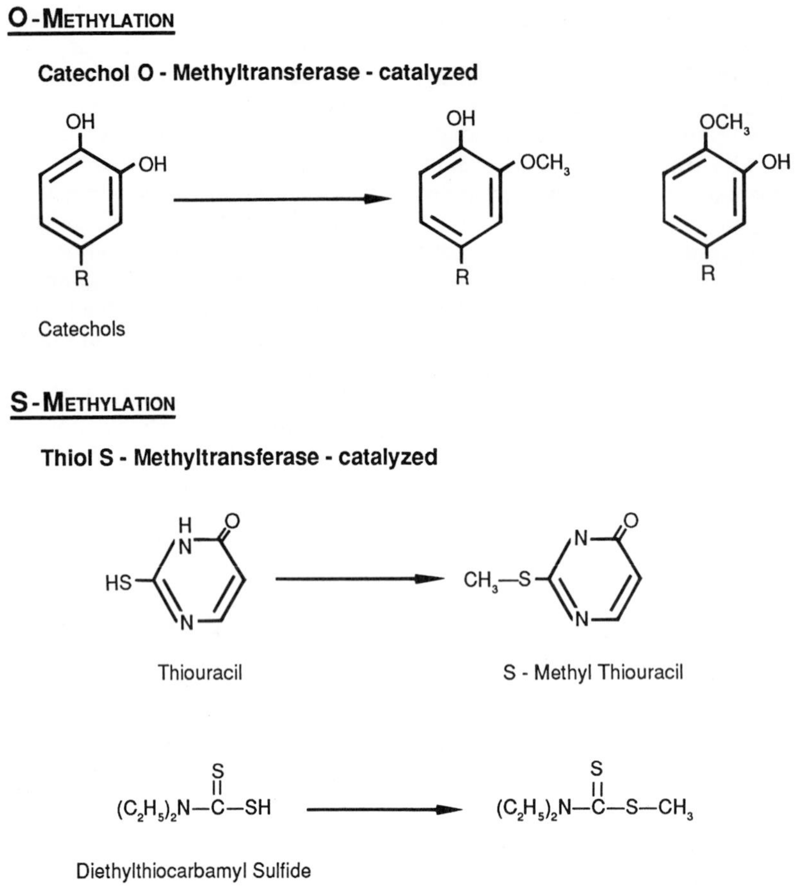

O-Methylation

Catechol O - Methyltransferase - catalyzed

Catechols

S-Methylation

Thiol S - Methyltransferase - catalyzed

Thiouracil   S - Methyl Thiouracil

Diethylthiocarbamyl Sulfide

FIG. 19. (*Continued.*)

normally methylates histamine (Fig. 19). Guinea pigs are well known for their ability to methylate histamine. This is why they are good animal models for studying xenobiotic methylation. Nicotine is an example of a xenobiotic that can be metabolized by an enzyme of normal cellular metabolism. Since nicotine is a weak base, methylation of the pyridyl nitrogen results in charges at both nitrogens at physiologic pH increasing water solubility and urinary excretion.

Methylation reactions can be stereoselective. For example, the R(+) enantiomer of nicotine is preferentially methylated over the S(−) enantiomer (18). Stereoselective metabolism of xenobiotics can be important in understanding the metabolic basis of toxicity. Since most biotransformation reactions are catalyzed by enzymes, there is always the possibility that the active site will select one orientation around a spiral center over another.

Amide Synthesis

Amide biosynthesis can take place via two principal routes:

1. Conjugation of a carboxylic acid-containing xenobiotic with the free amino group of an amino acid such as glycine;
2. The acetylation of a xenobiotic containing a primary amine ($-NH_2$).

Amide synthesis by either route requires the participation of the active form of the carboxylic acid group, acetyl coenzyme A (CoA). When the xenobiotic is a carboxylic acid, the acid must be activated in an energy requiring reaction, as shown in reactions 1 and 2 of Fig. 20. For example, the carboxylic acid of benzoic acid is activated to a thioester CoA intermediate that reacts with the primary amine of glycine to form the amide, hippuric acid. When a xenobiotic contains the primary amine (e.g., sulfanilamide in Fig. 20), the activated acetyl group is derived from acetyl CoA.

Glycine has historical significance in xenobiotic conjugation because it is one of the earliest reactions attributed to xenobiotic metabolism. Keller (59) administered benzoic acid to himself and then isolated and characterized the major metabolite, hippuric acid, a glycine conjugate. This reaction has been used as a liver function test in humans. The liver is the principal site of glycine conjugation. Amino acids other than glycine can also be used for conjugating aromatic and heterocyclic carboxylic acids. For example, arginine is used by arachnids, glutamine by chimpanzees, and ornithine by certain birds.

Acetylation is the principal pathway of amide formation for aromatic primary amines, endogenous primary aliphatic amines, anutrient amino acids, hydrazines, and hydrazides. Mercapturic acid formation in the kidney is an example of acetylation that has been presented. In this reaction, the primary amine group of the cysteine conjugate of the xenobiotic

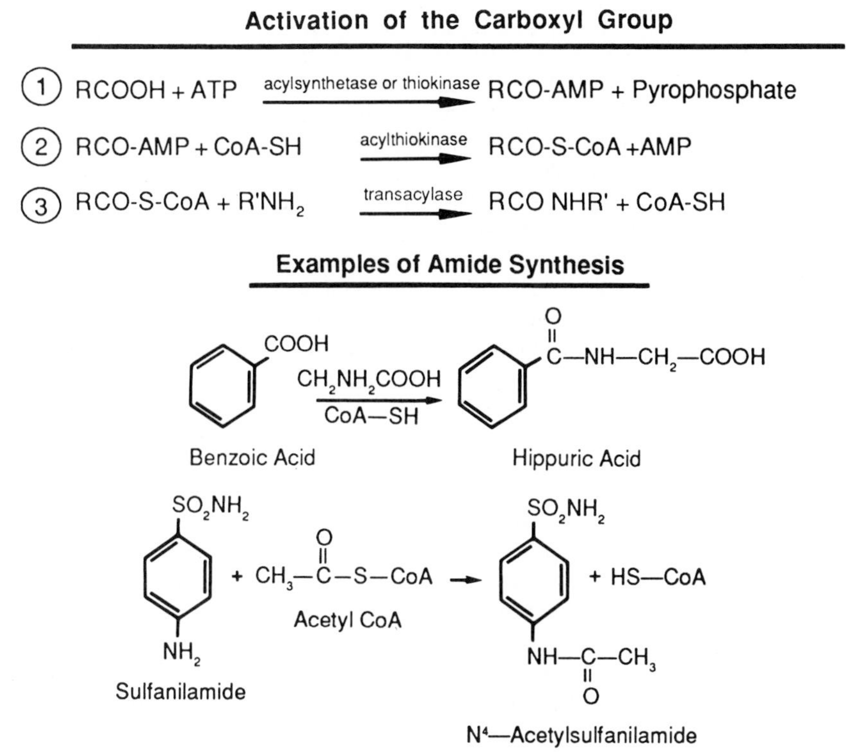

Activation of the Carboxyl Group

(1) RCOOH + ATP $\xrightarrow{\text{acylsynthetase or thiokinase}}$ RCO-AMP + Pyrophosphate

(2) RCO-AMP + CoA-SH $\xrightarrow{\text{acylthiokinase}}$ RCO-S-CoA + AMP

(3) RCO-S-CoA + R'NH$_2$ $\xrightarrow{\text{transacylase}}$ RCO NHR' + CoA-SH

Examples of Amide Synthesis

Benzoic Acid $\xrightarrow[\text{CoA—SH}]{\text{CH}_2\text{NH}_2\text{COOH}}$ Hippuric Acid

Sulfanilamide + Acetyl CoA (CH$_3$—C—S—CoA) → N^4—Acetylsulfanilamide + HS—CoA

FIG. 20. Series of reactions leading to amide formation from either a xenobiotic containing a carboxylic functional group (RCOOH) or a primary amine group (R'NH$_2$). (From ref. 80, with permission.)

is acetylated to form the mercapturic acid. It is worth noting that the use of the -uric suffix to denote an acidic urinary metabolite was once common. Mercapturic acids, hippuric acid, and salicyluric acid all share this common suffix that is probably derived from the fact that these acids and uric acid had similar characteristics and both were isolated from urine.

The main route of metabolism of isoniazid in humans is its conjugation with acetyl CoA to form the amide metabolite (63). Isoniazid is eliminated much faster from the body once it is acetylated. With the widespread use of isoniazid to control tuberculosis, it became obvious that there were major differences in the rates at which individuals eliminated the drug. Careful studies of hundreds of patients showed that there were two distinct populations, the fast and the slow acetylators. Slow acetylators inherited the trait as a homozygous recessive allele. Before chronic administration of certain drugs that require acetylation for detoxication and whose therapeutic index is low, it is important to know if a patient is a slow or a fast acetylator.

HYDROLYSIS

Many xenobiotics and their phase I metabolites contain either a carboxyl ester, an amide bond, or an epoxide that mask hydrophilic functional groups such as alcohols, carboxylic acids, and amines. The rate at which an organism can hydrolyze these bonds and unmask these functional groups can influence their toxicity. In fact, pesticides and therapeutic drugs have been synthesized with intent to modulate bioavailability of the active species by affecting the rate of hydrolysis of the parent compound.

Hydrolysis normally competes with other detoxication reactions. An example of competition is demonstrated by the metabolism of acrylate esters. Most acrylate esters either react with glutathione via a glutathione S-transferase catalyzed pathway or are hydrolyzed by B-esterases to acrylic acid and the corresponding alcohol (Fig. 23).

Epoxide Hydrolase

Organisms may be exposed to epoxides either from the environment as contaminants of food, water, and air or epoxides may be formed from the metabolism of specific xenobiotics. Epoxides are generally reactive electrophilic compounds due to the strained oxirane ring (Fig. 22). Excess strain energy can be released by ring opening in the presence of nucleophiles. Ring opening may follow either a S_N1 mechanism, with the formation of an intermediate with carbonium ion character, or an S_N2 mechanism, with bond formation with the attacking nucleophile. The latter case has important toxicologic consequences when the nucleophile is a critical tissue macromolecule, because it results in covalent modification of the macromolecule. This modification results in a biochemical lesion that may be the precursor to a number of pathologic lesions, including cancer.

The chemical reactivity and consequently the biologic activity of epoxides are influenced by the constituents attached to the oxirane ring carbons. Epoxides with asymmetric carbon atoms can exhibit optical activity and exist as enantiomers in a racemic mixture. Reaction of epoxides with nucleophiles with an asymmetrical center will produce diastereoisomers with different spatial orientations around the carbon center. Production of diastereoisomers is important in biological ac-

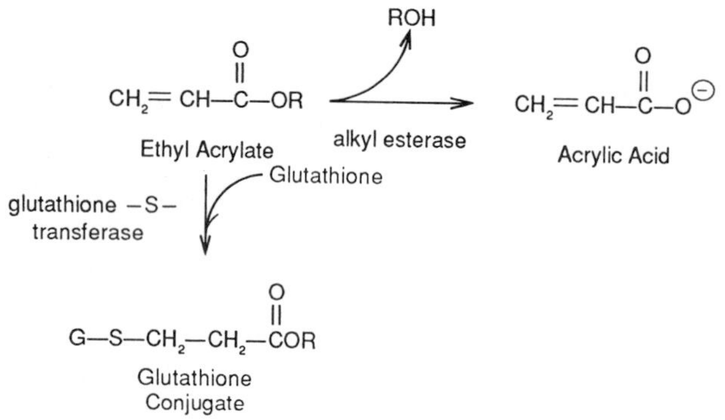

$$CH_2 = CH - \overset{\overset{\displaystyle O}{\displaystyle \|}}{C} - OR \xrightarrow[\text{alkyl esterase}]{\quad \overset{\displaystyle ROH}{\quad} \quad} CH_2 = CH - \overset{\overset{\displaystyle O}{\displaystyle \|}}{C} - O^{\ominus}$$

Ethyl Acrylate   Acrylic Acid

glutathione —S—transferase   ⌐ Glutathione

$$G - S - CH_2 - CH_2 - \overset{\overset{\displaystyle O}{\displaystyle \|}}{C}OR$$

Glutathione
Conjugate

FIG. 21. Routes of disposition of ethyl acrylate.

tivity with respect to both reaction at critical biochemical sites and subsequent metabolism. For instance, one isomer may react more efficiently at the toxigenic receptor and also be a poor substrate for subsequent metabolism when compared to another isomer.

Although not always the case, the epoxides that are formed *in vivo* appear to be more important than those that occur in the environment. Highly reactive epoxides would most likely interact with nucleophilic sites in the environment, such as proteins, in food, and not be absorbed in their active form. Epoxides formed *in vivo* are produced close to their sites of action and require only diffusion or short transport to their target. Epoxides most frequently formed *in vivo* represent alkene and arene oxides. Their efficient detoxication is important to cellular survival.

Detoxication of epoxides may follow several routes including the following:

1. Spontaneous decomposition,
2. Nonenzymatic reaction with glutathione,
3. Reaction with glutathione catalyzed by glutathione transferase,
4. Hydration by epoxide hydrolase,
5. Minor mechanisms, such as cytochrome P-450 hydrolysis.

Nonenzymatic and enzymatic conjugation with glutathione has been previously discussed.

A major route for biodisposition of epoxides is hydration catalyzed by epoxide hydrolase. This enzyme was previously referred to as epoxide hydrase and epoxide hydratase and readers will often encounter these terms still in use. This microsomal enzyme catalyzes the biotransformation of arene oxides and aliphatic epoxides to vicinal (Latin: *vicinalis*, neighboring) dihydrodiols. In most cases this enzymatic pathway results in less reactive metabolites that are more readily excreted from the organism either as the diol or as a glucuronide or sulfate conjugate of the diol.

Epoxide hydrolase is a membrane-bound protein located in the endoplasmic reticulum of most mammalian cells. The mechanism of the hydrolase catalyzed reaction appears to be a nucleophilic attack by water or hydroxyl ion on the side of the molecule opposite to the epoxide ring. This stereoselective attack usually results in the diols having a *trans* configuration.

Epoxide hydrolase has been found in a variety of tissues including liver, kidney, lung, skin, intestine, colon, testis,

ovary, spleen, thymus, heart, and brain. The activity of this enzyme in newborn rats is relatively low, increasing during neonatal development until adult males have about twice the activity of females. This sexual dimorphism is remarkably similar to that seen in the rat for cytochrome P-450. In addition, the activity of this enzyme is induced by the classical inducers of cytochrome P-450. Although *trans*-stilbene oxide has been shown to be an inducer of epoxide hydrolase, no specific inducer of epoxide hydrolase has been reported. Two widely used inhibitors of epoxide hydrolase are trichloropropane oxide and cyclohexene oxide.

Located in the endoplasmic reticulum, the enzyme is ideally situated to catalyze the detoxification of lipophilic epoxides formed by cytochrome P-450. For large hydrophobic molecules such as polyaromatic hydrocarbons, the dihydrodiol formed by epoxide hydrolase can be a substrate for an additional cytochrome P-450-catalyzed oxidation. This epoxidation, hydrolysis, epoxidation reaction sequence can result in the production of highly mutagenic metabolites.

One of the best described examples of metabolic activation is the biotransformation of benzo(a)pyrene to the ultimate mutagen benzo(a)pyrene trans-7,8-dihydrodiol-9,10-oxide, which is shown in Fig. 3 and described above under metabolic oxidations. These diol epoxides are poor substrates for further metabolism by epoxide hydrolase and, as shown in Fig. 3, react with critical cellular macromolecules.

An immunologically distinct epoxide hydrolase has also been identified in the cytosol of some species. This enzyme may play a role in hydrolysis of more water-soluble epoxides that partition out of the endoplasmic reticulum. As discussed earlier, this enzyme competes with glutathione transferases for cytosolic epoxides. The activity of the cytosolic epoxide hydrolase appears to be highest in mice and rabbits and relatively low in rats.

Esterases and Amidases

Hydrolysis of xenobiotics containing ester linkages and amide bonds is catalyzed by a group of enzymes with broad substrate specificity. In general, these enzymes perform endogenous functions and appear to metabolize xenobiotics that have structures similar to endogenous substrates.

The reactions carried out by this diverse group of enzymes are illustrated in Fig. 23. Recently, it has become apparent that the specificity of carboxylesterases depends on the nature of the R groups rather than on the atom (*O, N,* or *S*) adjacent to the carbonyl carbon (46,47). The esterases have been broadly grouped into three categories based on their reactivity with organophosphorous compounds (114). Those esterases preferring carboxylesters with aryl groups in the R position and that can utilize organophosphate esters as substrates are classified as A-esterases (Table 6). Those esterases preferring esters with alkyl groups in the R position and that are inhib-

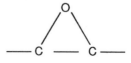

FIG. 22. An example of a strained epoxide oxirane ring.

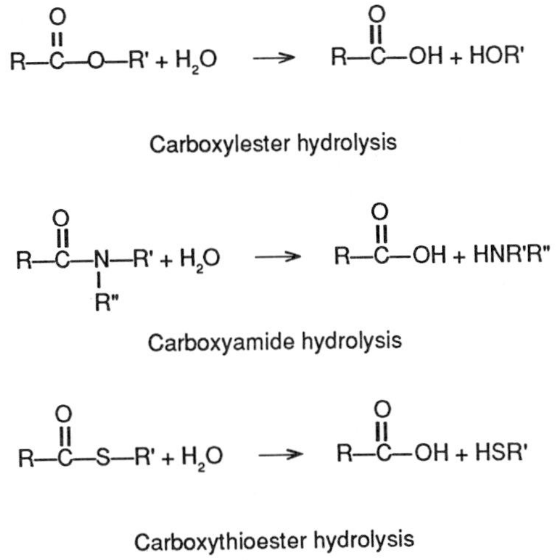

$$R-\overset{\overset{\displaystyle O}{\|}}{C}-O-R' + H_2O \longrightarrow R-\overset{\overset{\displaystyle O}{\|}}{C}-OH + HOR'$$

Carboxylester hydrolysis

$$R-\underset{\underset{\displaystyle R''}{|}}{\overset{\overset{\displaystyle O}{\|}}{C}}-N-R' + H_2O \longrightarrow R-\overset{\overset{\displaystyle O}{\|}}{C}-OH + HNR'R''$$

Carboxyamide hydrolysis

$$R-\overset{\overset{\displaystyle O}{\|}}{C}-S-R' + H_2O \longrightarrow R-\overset{\overset{\displaystyle O}{\|}}{C}-OH + HSR'$$

Carboxythioester hydrolysis

FIG. 23. Reactions catalyzed by esterases and amidases.

ited by organophosphate esters are classified as B-esterases. Another group of esterases that prefer acetate esters and do not interact with organophospates are referred to as C-esterases. This classification has been devised (7) to help organize this multifarious group of enzymes. It also has some practical value in toxicology. The mechanism of organophosphate and carbamate insecticide toxicity is inhibition of acetyl cholinesterase, a B-type esterase. Organophosphate insecticides, such as malathion are detoxified in mammals by A-esterase hydrolysis. Many insects have lower levels of A-esterases than mammals. The selective toxicity of malathion in birds and insects can be explained by the low activity of A-esterases compared to mammals (115).

MICROFLORAL METABOLISM

Xenobiotic metabolism by microorganisms can be divided into reactions occurring in the environment and reactions occurring inside the body (97). Metabolism of chemicals by microorganisms in the environment has become familiar through the use of microorganisms to degrade chemical spills. The *in vivo* metabolism of chemicals by microorganisms is not as familiar. Mammals are colonized by microorganisms [only those animals raised in a germ-free environment (gnotobiotic) are microbe-free]. The metabolic reactions carried out by these microorganisms are dependent upon the substrate and environment in which they are growing. Microbes growing in an aerobic environment are capable of cleavage of aromatic nuclei and can use these xenobiotics as sole carbon sources for biosynthetic reactions and growth. Microbes growing in an anaerobic environment are more likely to carry out reductive metabolism. The hallmark of metabolism by organisms colonizing the intestinal tract of mammals is reduction (Table 7).

Since the majority of microbes that colonize various surfaces of the mammalian body reside in the intestinal tract, most of this discussion will center around intestinal microflora metabolism. The intestinal microflora can alter xenobiotic bioavailability by metabolizing the parent compound to a metabolite that may be absorbed to a greater or lesser extent (9). Intestinal microflora can also metabolize products of xenobiotic biotransformation that are secreted into the intestine either directly from the blood or via the bile, saliva, or by swallowing respiratory tract mucus. Metabolism of secreted metabolites is a common mechanism by which microflora influence xenobiotic toxicity.

Xenobiotic Biotransformation by Microbes Colonizing Mammals

Anatomical Location

The intestinal tract of mammals contains a variety of microorganisms. The location, total number, and species diversity of microflora vary among mammals ranging from ruminants, which have evolved to be dependent on micro-

TABLE 6. *Classification of esterases by how they interact with organophosphates and substrate specificity*

Esterase	Interaction with organophosphates	Substrates	Examples
A-esterases (arylesterases)	Substrates	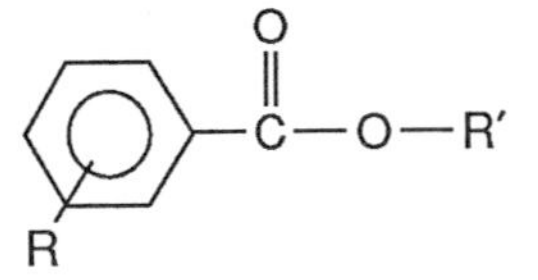 $$\overset{\overset{\displaystyle O}{\|}}{}\\ \text{Aromatic Esters}$$ Aromatic Esters	Organophosphate and carbamate insecticides
B-esterases (carboxyl esterases including cholinesterases)	Inhibitors	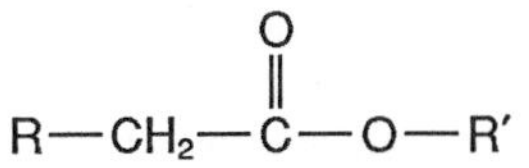 $$R-CH_2-\overset{\overset{\displaystyle O}{\|}}{C}-O-R'$$ Aliphatic Esters	Acetylcholine, acrylate esters, succinylcholine, propanidid
C-esterases (acetylesterases)	No interaction	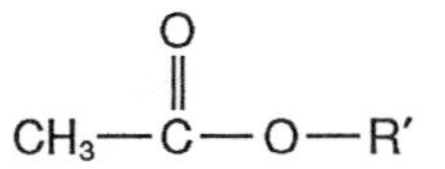 $$CH_3-\overset{\overset{\displaystyle O}{\|}}{C}-O-R'$$ Acetate Esters	p-Nitrophenyl acetate, n-propylchloroacetate

TABLE 7. *Types of metabolic reactions carried out by intestinal bacteria*

Hydrolysis	Reduction
Glucuronides	Double bonds
Other glycosides	Nitro groups
Sulfate esters	Azo groups
Amides	Aldehydes
Esters	Ketones
Sulfamates	Alcohols
Nitrates	N-oxides
	Arsonic acids
Dealkylation	Dehydroxylation
O-alkyl	
N-alkyl	
S-alkyl	
Metal-alkyl	
Deamination	Dehalogenation
Decarboxylation	Aromatization
Heterocyclic ring	Heterocyclic ring scission
Fission	
Scission	
Acetylation	Nitrosamine
	Formation
	Degradation
Esterification	

floral metabolism for energy needs, to monogastric mammals such as humans, which have great numbers of bacteria only in the large intestine. Because of this variation in location within the intestinal tract, the types of microorganism present and hence the types of microfloral metabolism vary with the mammalian species being studied.

Another factor that relates to the location of the microflora is the disposition of the xenobiotic and its microfloral metabolites. Chemicals metabolized by microflora located in the stomach will be distributed differently than chemicals metabolized in the large intestine.

The majority of mammals have a gradient of microflora that increases in numbers and species diversity along the intestinal tract from the foregut to the hindgut. Most research on microfloral metabolism has focused on microorganisms that colonize the large intestine of humans, since most of the research in toxicology is directed toward understanding the toxicity of chemicals in man.

Role of Diet in Modulating Microfloral Metabolism

The microflora colonizing the digestive tract of mammals play a major role in the digestion of plant cell wall constituents that are indigestible by mammalian enzymes. These dietary fibers provide energy substrates that support the large bacterial populations in the gut. These energy sources also influence the microfloral metabolism of xenobiotics. Certain types of dietary fiber such as the fermentable carbohydrate pectin, can influence the toxicity of xenobiotics that require microfloral metabolic activation by increasing the number of anaerobic bacteria colonizing the large intestine (20). This diet-induced elevation in the number of bacteria increases the total metabolic capacity of the large intestine for metab-

olizing xenobiotics. For an excellent review of this topic see Rowland and Wise (99).

Examples of Xenobiotics Whose Toxicity is Dependent on Microfloral Metabolism

Nitroaromatics

A body of literature has now accumulated indicating that the toxicity of many nitroaromatic compounds is dependent on microfloral metabolism. One of the most studied nitroaromatics is 2,6-dinitrotoluene (DNT) that is hepatocarcinogenic in male rats (66). Long and Rickert (67) have shown that DNT is metabolized to the 2,6-dinitrobenzylalcohol glucuronide conjugate that is preferentially excreted in the bile of male rats (Fig. 24). The glucuronide conjugate is hydrolyzed by gut microfloral β-glucuronidase, and one or both of the nitro groups are reduced by microfloral nitroreductase to a reduced aglycone. The resulting aminobenzyl alcohol is relatively nonpolar and reabsorbed in the intestine where it returns to the liver via the portal circulation. In the liver, the aglycone is activated to the putative proximate carcinogen by N-hydroxylation of the amine functional group followed by sulfation of the N-hydroxy group (58). Evidence that intestinal microflora were required for the activation of DNT was provided by Mirsalis and Butterworth (78) who showed that the genotoxicity of DNT in hepatocytes isolated from male rats treated with DNT was dependent on the presence of bacteria in the intestinal tract. Rats raised in a germ-free or gnotobiotic environment showed minimal levels of genotoxicity.

Long and Rickert (67) showed that the level of DNT-derived radioactivity covalently bound to DNA, RNA, and protein isolated from the livers of rats treated with DNT was also dependent on the presence of intestinal microflora. Dietary treatments that increased the microbial metabolic capacity of the rat's large intestine also increased the covalent binding of DNT-derived radioactivity to hepatic macromolecules.

Additional evidence emphasizing the role of microflora in the metabolic activation of DNT was the observation that DNT was not genotoxic when tested *in vitro* in isolated hepatocytes (78). These results indicated that liver metabolism was not sufficient to activate the molecule to the ultimate carcinogen. The genotoxicity of DNT to liver cells only occurred when the compound was administered to the animal and allowed to undergo enterohepatic circulation involving intestinal microflora.

The importance of complementary *in vitro* short-term toxicity tests with suitable *in vivo* tests for predicting a chemical's toxicity is well illustrated by this example where the toxicity of DNT was dependent on the disposition within the host rather than the metabolic activation within a single organ.

Cyclamate

The sodium and calcium salts of cyclamic acid (cyclohexyl sulfamic acid) were used as an artificial sweetening agent

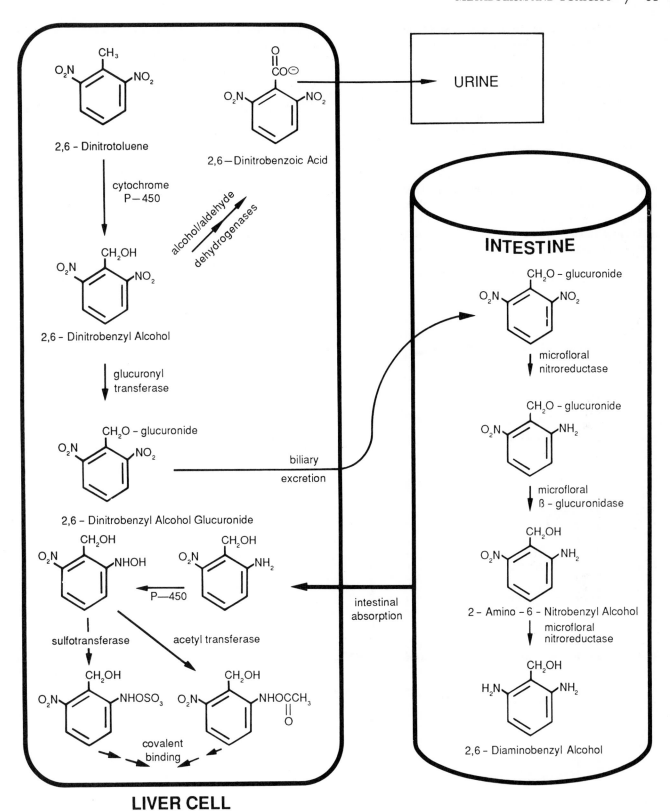

FIG. 24. Putative route of disposition of 2,6-dinitrotoluene.

until 1969 in the United States when it was removed from the market because a metabolite, cyclohexylamine, was suspected of being a bladder carcinogen.

Work by Renwick and Williams (98) has shown that most of the hydrolysis of cyclamate to cyclohexylamine takes place in the gut by the microflora as shown in Fig. 25. The cyclohexylamine is more lipophilic than the parent acid and is readily absorbed from the intestine and excreted in the urine. The minor urinary metabolites include cyclohexanol and *trans*-cyclohexane-1,2-diol.

Although only trace amounts of the cyclohexylamine could be detected in humans administered cyclamate, chronic exposure to the acid increased the capacity of the subjects to produce this metabolite (71). It was found that certain individuals possessed a greater capacity to metabolize cyclamate to cyclohexylamine. These individuals were called converters.

Thus, cyclamate is a good example of how prior exposure to a xenobiotic can alter the disposition of the xenobiotic. For additional reading on intestinal microflora xenobiotic metabolism, see Goldman (31) and Scheline (100).

INTEGRATION OF METABOLIC PATHWAYS

To understand a complex system, it is necessary to reduce it to basic components and study each component separately. After achieving an understanding of the components, it is important to integrate them back into the whole. Xenobiotic metabolism is a complex system. Now that the reader has examined many components of the system in detail, let us examine how they act in concert to protect an organism from toxic injury. Specific examples of integrated biotransformation will be presented.

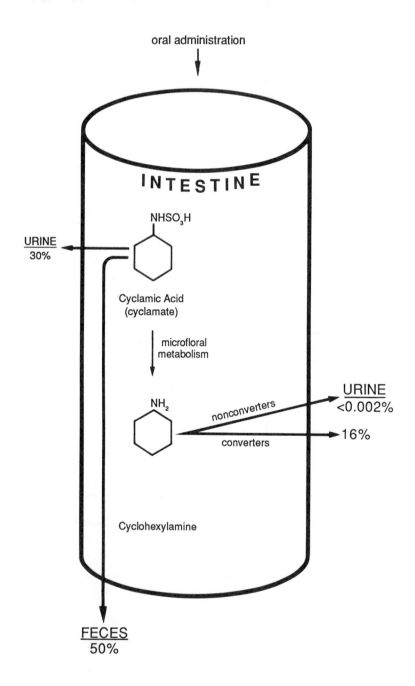

FIG. 25. Metabolic degradation of cyclamic acid by intestinal microflora.

Bromobenzene

Bromobenzene, an industrial solvent, produces centrilobular necrosis in the rat liver. Bromobenzene's hepatotoxicity results from metabolic activation of the parent compound via epoxidation (Fig. 26) catalyzed by cytochrome P-450-dependent monooxygenase. Bromobenzene 3,4-epoxide is relatively stable and diffuses from its site of formation in the endoplasmic reticulum. It can then follow several disposition routes depending on a variety of factors. The epoxide is a substrate for epoxide hydrolase, which would catalyze its hydration to the diol (Fig. 26). It is also a substrate for glutathione S-transferase 5-5 that catalyzes thioether formation. The glutathione conjugate is processed by the kidney to the mercapturic acid, which is excreted in the urine (see Fig. 17). The epoxide can also undergo spontaneous rearrangement to form p-bromophenol. This metabolite can cycle through oxidation by cytochrome P-450. If the phase II reactions do not trap the reactive epoxide metabolite formed from phase I metabolism of bromobenzene, the electrophilic carbon of the epoxide will react nonenzymatically with nucleophilic sites on cellular macromolecules. The ability of electrophilic metabolites to react covalently with critical cellular macromolecules is responsible for many chemical-induced toxicities, including chemical carcinogenicity. The delicate balance between detoxication and metabolic activation determines whether a chemical will be toxic to an organism and in what tissue. Toxic doses of bromobenzene produce centrilobular hepatic necrosis while BP, which is activated via a similar epoxidation mechanism is carcinogenic (Fig. 3). However, many compounds that are activated to mutagens and are tumorigenic are also cytotoxic.

Multiple Pathways for Xenobiotic Activation

Three different pathways by which chemicals can be nephrotoxic have been presented: oxidation by cytochrome P-450, formation of an episulfonium ion of a cysteine conjugate, and oxidation by prostaglandin synthetase. Very often a xenobiotic's toxicity results from more than one route of activation, even within the same organ. For example, acetaminophen has been associated with analgesic nephropathy. Acetaminophen can be activated by both cytochrome P-450 and prostaglandin synthetase to a reactive metabolite capable of binding to macromolecules (see Figs. 4 and 5). The realization that a pathway other than the well-characterized P-450 route was involved occurred through observations that acetaminophen was covalently bound in the kidney inner medulla of the rabbit, a site nearly devoid of P-450 activity (81). However, large in vivo doses of acetaminophen produce damage only in the kidney cortex, because prostaglandin synthetase is inhibited by these large doses. The cytochrome P-450 pathway is not inhibited and is responsible for cortical damage. Aspirin and indomethacin are specific inhibitors of prostaglandin synthetase. Analgesic preparations containing both aspirin and one of the analgesics known to be activated by prostaglandin synthetase would probably show consid-

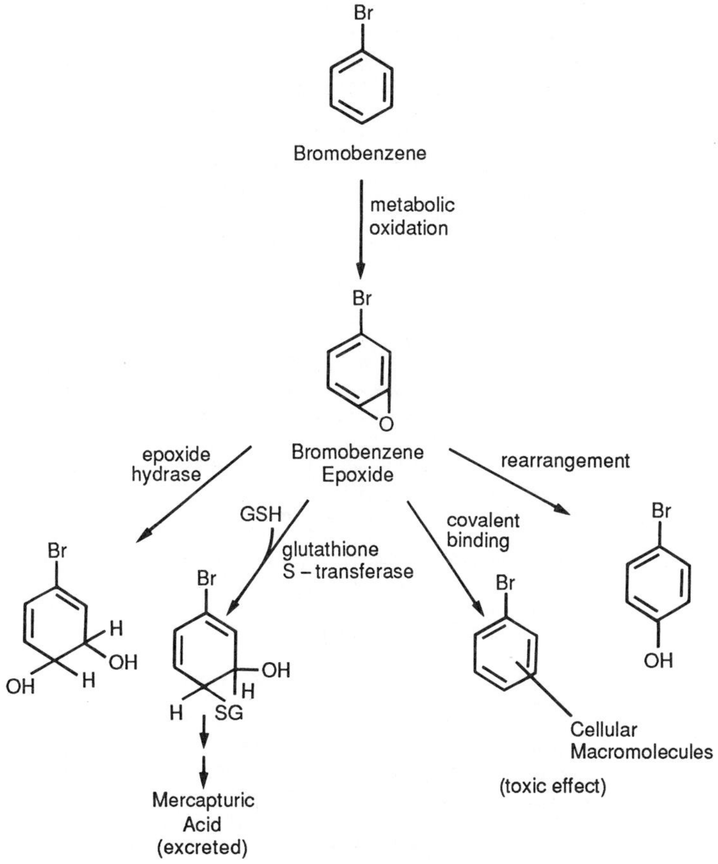

FIG. 26. Routes of disposition of bromobenzene. (From ref. 82, with permission.)

erably less toxicity to the kidney medullary tissue. This gradient of oxidation pathways across the kidney—with the cortex possessing higher monooxygenase activity than prostaglandin synthetase, the outer medulla being intermediate, and the inner medulla possessing higher prostaglandin synthetase activity—results in certain xenobiotics being more toxic to one region of the kidney than another (125). These examples stress the importance of understanding the metabolic activation of a toxicant in explaining its mechanism of action.

Another example of competing pathways is acrylate esters metabolism. Many acrylate esters are good substrates for both alkyl esterase and glutathione S-transferase, and can react with glutathione nonenzymatically. Depending on the dose and route of administration of these compounds, these pathways compete for acrylate metabolism. The alkyl esterase hydrolyzes the acrylate ester to acrylic acid and the corresponding alcohol (Fig. 22) and glutathione adds to the β-carbon of the acrylate ester. Both pathways are considered detoxication pathways. However, at high doses, glutathione can be depleted faster than it can be resynthesized. Elimination of the glutathione pathway can result in saturation of the esterase pathway and an accumulation of the acrylate ester at the site of administration producing tissue damage.

REFERENCES

1. Akerboom, T. P. M., and Sies, H. (1981): Assay of glutathione, glutathione disulfide, glutathione mixed disulfides in biological samples. In: *Methods in Enzymology, Vol. 77, Detoxication and Drug Metabolism: Conjugation and Related Systems*, edited by S. P. Colowick and N. O. Kaplan, p. 376. Academic Press, NY.
2. Anders, M. W. (1988): Glutathione-dependent toxicity: Biosynthesis and bioactivation of cytotoxic S-conjugates. *ISI Atlas Pharmacol.*, 2:99–104.
3. Andersson, B., Nordenskjold, M., Rahimtula, A., and Moldeus, P. (1982): Prostaglandin synthetase-catalyzed activation of phenacetin metabolites to genotoxic products. *Mol. Pharmacol.*, 22:479–485.
4. Axelrod, J. The discovery of the microsomal drug-metabolizing enzymes. In: *Drug Metabolism and Distribution: Current Reviews in Biomedicine 3*, edited by J. W. Lamble, pp. 1–6. Elsevier Biomedical Press, NY.
5. Baumann, E. (1876): Ueber sulfosauren im harn. *Ber. Dtsch. Chem. Ges.*, 9:54.
6. Braumann and Preusse, (1879): Ueber bromophenylmercaptursäure. *Ber. Dtsch. Chem. Ges.*, 12:806–810.
7. Bergmann, F., Segal, R., and Riman, S. (1957): New type of esterase in dog-kidney extract. *Biochem. J.*, 67:481–486.
8. Boyd, J. A., and Eling, T. E. (1981): Prostaglandin endoperoxide synthetase-dependent cooxidation of acetaminophen to intermediates which covalently bind *in vitro* to rabbit renal medullary microsomes. *J. Pharmacol. Exp. Ther.*, 219:659–664.
9. Boxenbaum, H. G., Bedersky, I., Jack, M. L., and Kaplan, S. A. (1979): Influence of gut microflora on bioavailability. *Drug Metab. Rev.*, 9:259–279.
10. Boyland, E., and Chasseaud, L. F. (1969): The role of glutathione and glutathione S-transferases in mercapturic acid biosythesis. *Adv. Enzymol.*, 32:173–219.
11. Brown, R. R., Miller, J. A., and Miller, E. C. (1954): The metabolism of methylated aminoazo dyes. IV. Dietary factors enhancing demethylation *in vitro*. *J. Biol. Chem.*, 209:211–217.
12. Burchell, B. (1981): Identification and purification of multiple forms of UDP-glucuronosyltransferase. In: *Reviews in Biochemical Toxicology 3*, edited by E. Hodgson, J. R. Bend, and R. M. Philpot, pp. 1–32. Elsevier/North-Holland, NY.
13. Caldwell, J. (1980): Comparative aspects of detoxication in mammals. In: *Enzymatic Basis of Detoxication*, edited by W. B. Jakoby, pp. 85–114. Academic Press, NY.
14. Chasseaud, L. F. (1973): The nature and distribution of enzymes catalyzing the conjugation of glutathione with foreign compounds. *Drug Metab. Rev.*, 2:185–220.
15. Chasseaud, L. F. (1978): The role of glutathione and glutathione S-transferases in the metabolism of chemical carcinogens and other electrophilic agents. *Adv. Cancer Res.*, 29:175–274.
16. Conney, A. H. (1967): Pharmacological implications of microsomal enzyme induction. *Pharmacol. Rev.*, 19:317–350.
17. Cooper, D. Y. (1964): Photochemical action spectrum of the terminal oxidase of mixed function oxidase systems. *Science*, 147:400–402.
18. Cundy, K. C., Sato, M., and Crooks, P. A. (1985): Stereospecific *in vivo* N-methylation of nicotine in the guinea pig. *Drug Metab.*, 13(2):175–185.
20. deBethizy, J. D., Sherrill, J. M., Rickert, D. E., and Hamm, Jr., T. E. (1983): Effects of pectin-containing diets on the hepatic macromolecular covalent binding of 2,6-dinitro-[³H]toluene in Fischer-344 rats. *Toxicol. Appl. Pharmacol.*, 69:369–376.
21. De Meio, R. H. (1975): Sulfate activation and transfer. In: *Metabolism Pathways, Vol. 7*, edited by D. M. Greenberg, 3rd ed., pp. 287–385. Academic Press, NY.
22. Dutton, G. J. (1971): Glucuronide-forming enzymes. In: *Handbook of Experimental Pharmacology, Part 2*, p. 378. Springer-Verlag, NY.
23. Dutton, G. J. (1980): *Glucuronidation of Drugs and Other Compounds*. CRC Press, Boca Raton, FL.
24. Elfarra, A. A., and Anders, M. W. (1984): Commentary: Renal processing of glutathione conjugates—Role in nephrotoxicity. *Biochem. Pharmacol.*, 33:3729–3732.
25. Estabrook, R. W., Cooper, D. Y., and Rosenthal, O. (1963): The light reversible carbon monoxide inhibition of the steroid C-21-hydroxylase system of adrenal cortex. *Biochem. Z.*, 338:741–755.
26. Franklin, M. R., and Estabrook, R. W. (1971): On the inhibitory action of mersalyl on microsomal drug oxidation: A rigid organization of the electron transport chain. *Arch. Biochem. Biophys.*, 143:318–329.
27. Frommer, U., Ullrich, V., Staudinger, H., and Orranius, S. (1972): The monooxygenation of *n*-heptane by rat liver microsomes. *Biochem. Biophys. Acta*, 280:487–494.
28. Fukami, J.-I. (1984): Metabolism of several insecticides by glutathione S-transferase. *Int. Encycl. Pharmacol. Ther.*, 113:223–264.
29. Garfinkel, D. (1958): Studies on pig liver microsomes. I. Enzymic and pigment composition of different microsomal fraction. *Arch. Biochem. Biophys.*, 77:493–509.
30. Gillette, J. R., Brodie, B. B., and La Du, B. N. (1957): The oxidation of drugs by liver microsomes: On the role of TPNH and oxidase. *J. Pharmacol. Exp. Ther.*, 119:532–540.
31. Goldman, P. (1978): Biochemical pharmacology of the intestinal flora. *Annu. Rev. Pharmacol.*, 18:523–539.
32. Gorski, J. P., and Kasper, C. B. (1977): Purification and properties of microsomal UDP-glucuronosyltransferase from rat liver. *J. Biol. Chem.*, 252:1336–1343.
33. Gorsky, L. D., Koop, D. R., and Coon, M. J. (1984): On the stoichiometry of the oxidase and monooxidase reaction catalyzed by liver microsomal cytochrome P-450. *J. Biol. Chem.*, 259:6812–6817.
34. Grover, P. L. (1982): Glutathione S-transferases in detoxification. *Biochem. Soc. Trans.*, 10:80–82.
35. Groves, J. R., McCusky, G. A., White, R. E., and Coon, M. J. (1978): Aliphatic hydroxylation by highly purified liver microsomal cytochrome P-450. Evidence for a carbon radical intermediate. *Biochem. Biophys. Res. Commun.*, 81:154–160.
36. Guengerich, F. P., Ed. (1985): *Mammalian Cytochromes P-450, Vols. 1 and 2*. CRC Press, Boca Raton, FL.
37. Guengerich, F. P., and Liebler, D. C. (1985): Enzymatic activation of chemicals to toxic metabolites. *CRC Crit. Rev. Toxicol.*, 14:259–307.
38. Gut, J. (1982): Rotation of cytochrome P-450 II. Specific interactions of cytochrome P-450 with NADPH-cytochrome P-450 reductase in phospholipid vesicles. *J. Biol. Chem.*, 257:7030–7036.
39. Habig, W. H. (1982): Glutathione S-transferases: Versatile enzymes of detoxification. In: *Radioprotectors and Anticarcinogens*, edited by O. F. Nygaard, pp. 169–190. Academic Press, NY.

40. Henry, W. (1815): *The Elements of Experimental Chemistry, Vol. II*, 7th ed., p. 352. Baldwin, Cradock, and Joy, London.
41. Heymann, E. (1980): Carboxylesterases and amidases. In: *Enzymatic Basis of Detoxication*, edited by W. B. Jakoby, pp. 291–323. Academic Press, NY.
42. Heymann, E. (1982): Hydrolysis of carboxylic esters and amides. In: *Metabolic Basis of Detoxication*, edited by W. B. Jakoby, J. R. Bend, and J. Caldwell, pp. 229–245. Academic Press, NY.
43. Horecher, B. L. (1950): Triphosphopyridine nucleotide cytochrome c reductase in liver. *J. Biol. Chem.*, 183:593–605.
44. Huttner, W. B. (1982): Sulphation of tyrosine residues—A widespread modification of proteins. *Nature*, 299(5880):273–276.
45. Inskeep, P. B., Koga, N., Cmarik, J. L., and Guengerich, F. P. (1986): Covalent binding of 1,2-dihaloalkanes to DNA and stability of the major DNA adduct, *S*-[2-(*N*7-guanyl)ethyl] glutathione. *Cancer Res.*, 46:2839–2844.
46. Ito, A., and Sato, R. (1969): Proteolytic microdissection of smooth-surfaced vesicles of liver microsomes. *J. Cell Biol.*, 40:179–189.
47. Jaffe (1879): Ueber die nach einführung von bromobenzol und chlorbenzol in organismus entstehenden Schwefelthaltigen sauren. *Ber. Dtsch. Chem. Ges.*, 12:1092–1098.
48. Jakoby, W. B. (1978): The glutathione *S*-transferases: A group of multifunctional detoxification proteins. *Adv. Enzymol. Relat. Areas Mol. Biol.*, 46:383–414.
49. Jakoby, W. B., and Habig, W. H. (1980): Glutathione transferases. In: *Enzymatic Basis of Detoxification, Vol. II*, edited by W. B. Jakoby, pp. 63–94. Academic Press, NY.
50. Jakoby, W. B., and Keen, J. H. (1977): A triple-threat in detoxification: The glutathione *S*-transferases. *Trends Biochem. Sci.*, 2:229–231.
51. Jakoby, W. B., Duffel, M. W., Lyon, E. S., and Ramaswamy, S. (1984): Sulfotransferases active with xenobiotics—Comments on mechanism. In: *Progress in Drug Metabolism, Vol. 8*, edited by J. W. Bridges and L. F. Chasseaud, pp. 11–33. Taylor and Frances, London.
52. Jakoby, W. B. (1976): Glutathione *S*-transferases: Catalytic aspects. In: *Glutathione: Metabolism and Function*, edited by I. M. Arias and W. B. Jakoby, pp. 189–211. Raven Press, NY.
53. Jakoby, W. B., Ketterer, B., and Mannervik, B. (1984): Commentary: Glutathione transferases: Nomenclature. *Biochem. Pharmacol.*, 33:2539–2540.
54. Jakoby, W. B. (1980): Sulfotransferases. In: *Enzymatic Basis of Detoxification, Vol. II*, edited by W. B. Jakoby, pp. 199–228. Academic Press, NY.
55. Jerina, D. M., and Bend, J. R. (1977): Glutathione *S*-transferases. In: *Biological Reactive Intermediates*, edited by D. J. Jollow, pp. 207–236. Plenum Press, New York.
56. Kasper, C. B., and Henton, D. (1980): Glucuronidation. In: *Enzymatic Basis of Detoxification, Vol. II*, edited by W. B. Jakoby, pp. 3–41. Academic Press, NY.
57. Kawato, S. (1982): Rotation of cytochrome P-450. I. Investigations of protein–protein interactions of cytochrome P-450 in phospholipid vesicles and liver microsomes. *J. Biol. Chem.*, 257:7023–7029.
58. Kedderis, G. L., Dyroff, M. C., and Rickert, D. E. (1984): Hepatic macromolecular covalent binding of the hepatocarcinogen 2,6-dinitrotoluene and its 2,4-isomer *in vivo*: Modulation by the sulfotransferase inhibitors pentachlorophenol and 2,6-dichloro-4-nitrophenol. *Carcinogenesis*, 5(9):1199–1204.
59. Keller, W. (1842): Ueber verwandlung der Benzöesäure in hippursäure. Justus Liebig's *Ann. Chem.* 43:108–111.
60. Klingenberg, M. (1958): Pigments of rat liver microsomes. *Arch. Biochem. Biophys.*, 75:379–386.
61. Kuriyama, Y., Omura, T., Sickevitz, and Palade, G. E. (1969): Effects of phenobarbital on the synthesis and degradation of the protein components of rat liver microsomal membranes. *J. Biol. Chem.*, 244:2017–2026.
62. La Du, B. N., Gaudette, L., Trousof, N., and Brodie, B. B. Enzymatic dealkylation of aminopyrine (Pyramidon) and other alkyamines. *J. Biol. Chem.*, 214:741–752.
63. Mannering, G. J. (1971): Microsomal enzyme systems which catalyze drug metabolism. In: *Fundamentals of Drug Metabolism and Drug Digestion*, edited by B. N. La Du, et al., pp. 206–252. The Williams and Wilkins Co., Baltimore.
64. Lamartiniere, C. A. (1981): The hypothalamic-hypophyseal-gonadal regulation of hepatic glutathione *S*-transferases in the rat. *Biochem. J.*, 198:211–217.
65. Lamartiniere, C. A., and Lucier, G. W. (1983): Endocrine regulation of xenobiotic conjugation enzymes. *Basic Life Sci.*, 24 (*Organ Species Specif. Chem. Carcinog.*):295–312.
66. Leonard, T. B., and Popp, J. A. (1981): Investigation of the carcinogenic initiation potential of dinitrotoluene: Structure–activity study. *Proc. Am. Assoc. Cancer Res.*, 22:82.
67. Long, R. M., and Rickert, D. E. (1982): Metabolism and excretion of 2,6-dinitro-[14C]toluene *in vivo* and in isolated perfused rat livers. *Drug Metab. Dispos.*, 10:455–458.
68. Lu, A. Y. N., Strobel, H. W., and Coon, M. J. (1969): Hydroxylation of benzphetamine and other drugs by a solubilized form of cytochrome P-450 from liver microsomes: Lipid requirement for drug demethylation. *Biochem. Biophy. Res. Commun.*, 36:545–551.
69. Lu, A. Y. H., Strobel, H. W., and Coon, M. J. (1970): Properties of a solubilized form of the cytochrome P-450-containing mixed-function oxidase of liver microsomes. *Mol. Pharmacol.*, 6:213–220.
70. Malik, N., Koteen, G. M., and Owens, I. S. (1979): Induction of UDP-glucuronosyl transferase (EC-2.4.1.17) activity in the Reuber H-4-II-E hepatoma cell culture. *Mol. Pharmacol.*, 16:950–960.
71. Mallett, A. K. (1985): Metabolic adaptation of rat faecal microflora to cyclamate *in vitro*. *Fd. Chem. Toxicol.*, 23:1029–1034.
72. Mandell, H. G. (1981): Pathways of drug biotransformation: Biochemical conjunctions. In: *Fundamentals of Drug Metabolism and Drug Disposition*, edited by B. N. La Du, H. G. Mandel, and E. L. Way, pp. 169–171. Robert E. Kreiger Publishing Co., Malabar, FL.
73. Mannering, G. T. (1971): Microsomal enzyme systems which catalyze drug metabolism. In: *Fundamentals of Drug Metabolism and Drug Disposition*, edited by B. N. La Du, pp. 206–252. The Williams and Wilkins Co., Baltimore.
74. Marnett, L. J., and Reed, G. A. (1979): Peroxidatic oxidation of benzo[*a*]pyrene and prostaglandin biosynthesis. *Biochemistry*, 18:2923–2929.
75. Marnett, L. J., Reed, G. A., and Johnson, J. T. (1977): Prostaglandin synthetase dependent benzo[*a*]pyrene oxidation: Products of the oxidation and inhibition of their formation by antioxidants. *Biochem. Biophys. Res. Commun.*, 79:569–576.
76. Mattammal, M. B., Zenser, T. V., and Davis, B. B. (1981): Prostaglandin hydroperoxidase-mediated 2-amino-4-(5-nitro-2-furyl)[14C]thiazole metabolism and nucleic acid binding. *Cancer Res.*, 41:4961–4966.
77. Meister, A., and Tate, S. S. (1976): Glutathione and related gamma-glutamyl compounds: Biosynthesis and utilization. *Annu. Rev. Biochem.*, 45:559–604.
78. Mirsalis, J. C., and Butterworth, B. E. (1982): Induction of unscheduled DNA synthesis in rat hepatocytes following *in vivo* treatment with dinitrotoluene. *Carcinogenesis*, 3:241–245.
79. Mitchell, J. R. (1973): Acetaminophen-induced hepatic necrosis. IV. Protective role of glutathione. *J. Pharmacol. Exp. Ther.*, 187:211–217.
80. Miyazaki, M., Yoshizawa, I., and Fishman, J. (1969): Directive *O*-methylation of estrogen catechol sulfates. *Biochemistry*, 8(4):1669–1672.
81. Mohandas, J., Duggin, G. G., Horvath, J. S., and Tiller, D. J. (1981): Metabolic oxidation of acetaminophen (paracetamol) mediated by cytochrome P-450 mixed-function oxidase and prostaglandin endoperoxide synthetase in rabbit kidney. *Toxicol. Appl. Pharmacol.*, 61:252–259.
82. Morgan, E. T., and Coon, M. J. (1984): Effects of cytochrome b5 on cytochrome P-450-catalyzed reactions: Studies with manganese-substituted cytochrome b5. *Drug Metab. Dispos.*, 12:358–364.
83. Mulder, G. J. (1981): Introduction. In: *Sulfation of Drugs and Related Compounds*, edited by G. J. Mulder, pp. 1–3. CRC Press, Boca Raton, FL.
84. Mulder, G. J. (1981): Generation of reactive intermediates from xenobiotics by sulfate conjugation—Their potential role in chemical carcinogenesis. In: *Sulfation of Drugs and Related Compounds*, edited by G. J. Mulder, pp. 213–226. CRC Press, Boca Raton, FL.
85. Oesch, F. (1980): Species differences in activating and inactivating enzymes related to *in vitro* mutagenicity mediated by tissue preparations from these species. *Arch. Toxicol.*, Suppl. 3:179–194.

86. Oesch, F., Bentley, P., and Glatt, H. R. (1970): Prevention of benzo[a]pyrene induced mutagenicity by homogenous epoxide hydratase. *Int. J. Cancer,* 18:448–452.

87. Oesch, F., and Glatt, H. R. (1976): Evaluation of the importance of enzymes involved in the control of mutagenic metabolites. *IARC Sci. Publ.,* 1232:255–274.

88. Omura, T. (1969): (Discussion). In: *Microsomes and Drug Oxidations,* edited by J. R. Gillette, pp. 160–161. Academic Press, NY.

89. Omura, T., and Sato, R. (1964): The carbon monoxide binding pigment of liver microsomes. I. Evidence for its hemoprotein nature. *J. Biol. Chem.,* 239:2370–2378.

90. Omura, T., and Sato, R. (1964): The carbon monoxide-binding pigment of liver microsomes. II. Solubilization, purification and properties. *J. Biol. Chem.,* 239:2379–2385.

91. Orrenius, S., and Moldeus, P. (1984): The multiple roles of glutathione in drug metabolism. *Trends Pharmacol. Sci.,* 5:432–435.

92. Ortiz de Montellano, P. R., Ed. (1986): *Cytochrome P-450 Structure, Mechanism and Biochemistry,* Plenum Press, NY.

93. Peterson, J. A. (1978): Parches and pockets: The microenvironments of a membrane bound hemeprotein. In: *Microenvironments and Metabolic Compartmentation,* edited by P. A. Srere and R. W. Estabrook, pp. 433–450. Academic Press, NY.

94. Pfeil, H., and Bock, K. W. (1983): Electroimmunochemical quantification of UDP-glucuronosyl transferase in rat liver microsomes. *Eur. J. Biochem.,* 131:619–623.

95. Phillips, A. H., and Langdon, R. G. (1962): Hepatic triphosphopyridine nucleotide-cytochrome reductase: Isolation, characterization, and kinetic studies. *J. Biol. Chem.,* 237:2652–2660.

96. Rafter, J. J. (1983): Studies on the reestablishment of the intestinal microflora in germ-free rats with special reference to the metabolism of N-isopropyl-alpha-choloracetanilide (propachlor). *Xenobiotica,* 13:171–178.

97. Renwick, A. G. (1977): Microbial metabolism of drugs. In: *Drug Metabolism: From Microbe to Man,* edited by D. V. Parke and R. L. Smith, pp. 169–189. Proceedings of the International Symposium, Guilford, England. Taylor and Francis, London.

98. Renwick, A. G., and Williams, R. T. (1972): The fate of cyclamate in man and other species. *Biochem. J.,* 129:869–879.

99. Rowland, I. R., and Wise, A. (1985): The effect of diet on the mammalian gut flora and its metabolic activities. *CRC Crit. Rev. Toxicol.,* 16:31–103.

100. Scheline, R. R. (1973): Metabolism of foreign compounds by gastrointestinal microorganisms. *Pharmacol. Rev.,* 25:451–523.

101. Sekura, R. D., Marcus, C. J., Lyon, E. S., and Jakoby, W. B. (1979): Assay of sulfotransferases. *Anal. Biochem.,* 95:82–86.

102. Singer, S. S., and Bruns, L. (1978): Enzymatic sulfation of steroids—VII. Hepatic cortisol sulfation and glucocorticoid sulfotransferases in old and young male rats. *Exp. Gerontol.,* 13:425–429.

103. Singer, S. S., Giera, D., Johnson, J., and Sylvester, S. (1976): Enzymatic sulfation of steroid—I. The enzymatic basis for the sex difference in cortisol sulfation by rat liver preparations. *Endocrinology,* 98:963–974.

104. Singer, S. S., and Sylvester, S. (1976): Enzymatic sulfation of steroids: II. The control of the hepatic cortisol sulfotransferase activity and of the individual hepatic steroid sulfotransferases of rats by gonads and gonadal hormones. *Endocrinology,* 99:1346–1352.

105. Sligar, S. G., and Murray, R. I. (1986): Cytochrome P-450cam and other bacterial P-450 enzymes. In: *Cytochrome P-450: Structure, Mechanism, and Biochemistry,* edited by P. R. Ortiz de Montellano, pp. 429–503. Plenum Press, NY.

106. Smith, G. J., and Litwack, G. (1980): Roles of ligandin and the glutathione S-transferases in binding steroid metabolites, carcinogens and other compounds. *Rev. Biochem. Toxicol.,* 2:1–47.

107. Smith, G. J., Ohl, V. S., and Litwack, G. (1977): Ligandin, the glutathione S-transferases, and chemically induced hepatocarcinogenesis: A review. *Cancer Res.,* 37:8–14.

108. Stirling, L. A. (1980): Microorganisms and environmental pollutants. In: *Introduction to Environmental Toxicology,* edited by F. E. Guthrie and J. J. Perry, pp. 329–342.

109. Tateishi, N., and Sakamoto, Y. (1983): Nutritional significance of glutathione in rat liver. In: *Glutathione: Storage, Transport and Turnover in Mammals,* edited by S. Y. Sakamoto, T. Higashi, and N. Tateishi, pp. 13–38. Japan Science Society Press, Tokyo/VNH Science Press, Utrecht.

110. Tateishi, M., Suzuki, S., and Shimizu, H. (1978): Cysteine conjugate beta-lyase in rat liver: A novel enzyme catalyzing formation of thiol-containing metabolites of drugs. *J. Biol. Chem.,* 253:8854–8859.

111. Taniguchi, H., Imai, Y., and Sato, R. (1984): Role of the electron transfer system in microsomal drug monooxygenase reaction catalyzed by cytochrome P-450. *Arch. Biochem. Biophys.,* 232:585–596.

112. Thurman, R. G. (1987): Regulation of monooxygenation in intact cells. In: *Mammalian Cytochromes P-450,* Vol. II, edited by F. P. Guengerich, pp. 131–152. CRC Press, Inc., Boca Raton, FL.

113. Vesell, E. S., and Penno, M. B. (1983): Intraindividual and interindividual variations. In: *Biological Basis of Detoxication,* edited by J. Caldwell and W. B. Jakoby, pp. 369–410. Academic Press, NY.

114. Walker, C. H., and Mackness, M. I. (1983): Esterases: Problems of identification and classification. *Biochem. Pharmacol.,* 32(22): 3265–3269.

115. Walker, C. H., and Oesch, F. (1983): Enzymes in selective toxicology. In: *Biological Basis of Detoxication,* edited by J. Caldwell and W. B. Jakoby, pp. 349–368. Academic Press, NY.

116. Watabe, T., Hiratsuka, A., and Okuda, H. (1985): Sulfate conjugations. *Tok. Foramu,* 8:264–277.

117. Watabe, T. (1985): Metabolic activation of 7,12-dimethylbenz[a]anthracene and 7-methylbenz[a]anthracene via hydroxymethyl sulfate esters by P-450-sulfotransferase. *Gann Monogr.,* 30: 125–139.

118. Wendel, A., Heinle, H., and Silbernagl, S. (1977): The degradation of glutathione derivatives in the rat kidney. *Curr. Probl. Clin. Biochem.,* 8:73–84.

119. Williams, C. H., Jr., and Kamin, H. (1962): Microsomal triphosphopyridine nucleotide-cytochrome c reductase of liver. *J. Biol. Chem.,* 237:587–595.

120. Williams, R. T. (1959) *Detoxication Mechanisms,* 2nd ed., Chapman and Hall, London.

121. Wong, K. P., and Yeo, T. (1982): Importance of extrahepatic sulphate conjugation. *Biochem. Pharmacol.,* 31:4001–4013.

122. Wood, J. L. (1970): Biochemistry of mercapturic acid formation. In: *Metabolic Conjugation and Metabolic Hydrolysis, Vol. 2,* edited by W. H. Fishman, pp. 261–299. Academic Press, NY.

123. Wu, E.-S., and Yang, C. S. (1984): Lateral diffusion of cytochrome P-450 in phospholipid bilayers. *Biochemistry,* 23:28–33.

124. Zakim, D., Hochman, Y., and Vessey, D. A. (1985): Methods for characterizing the function of UDP-glucuronyltransferases. In: *Biochemical Pharmacology and Toxicology,* edited by D. Zakim and D. A. Vessey, pp. 161–227. John Wiley, NY.

125. Zenser, T. V., Mattammal, M. B., and Davis, B. B. (1979): Demonstration of separate pathways for the metabolism of organic compounds in rabbit kidney. *J. Pharmacol. Exp. Ther.,* 208:418–421.

Principles and Methods of Toxicology, Second Edition, edited by A. Wallace Hayes, Raven Press, Ltd., New York © 1989.

CHAPTER 3

Food-Borne Toxicants

Chada S. Reddy and *A. Wallace Hayes

*Department of Veterinary Biomedical Sciences, College of Veterinary Medicine, University of Missouri, Columbia, Missouri 65211; and *R. J. R. Nabisco, Bowman Gray Technical Center, Winston-Salem, North Carolina 27102*

Natural Components
  Toxicants in Foods of Plant Origin • Toxicants in Foods of Animal Origin
Food Contaminants
  Bacterial Toxins • Mycotoxins • Metals

Food Additives
  Safety Assessment of Food Additives • Safety of Food Additives • Toxic Factors Produced During Processing
Conclusion
References

The chemical entities comprising those constituents of food that are pertinent to food safety encompass a wide spectrum of substances that are introduced into foods in several ways. These can be broadly categorized into three groups: (a) those present as naturally occurring components in foods; (b) those present as contaminants secondary either to microbial invasion of foods or to chemical contamination of the environment in which foods and feeds are produced and stored; and (c) those added by man in the course of food manufacture and preparation.

Sixty to eighty percent of all human cancers have been associated with our environment. A majority of environmental cancers are attributable to naturally occurring chemicals in the environment (49). Although accurate estimates are unavailable, up to 35% of environmental cancers may be caused by prolonged consumption of dietary carcinogens and cocarcinogens and are thus avoidable by practicable dietary modifications.

As toxicologists, we should not only concentrate our efforts in identifying deleterious dietary components, their mechanisms of action and therapeutic and/or preventive measures against such agents, but also aim at identifying dietary constituents capable of protecting against the adverse effects of food toxicants. Two examples of an increasing number of classes of food components that may negate the toxic effects of food-borne chemicals are the antimutagenic and anticarcinogenic effects of certain naturally occurring phenolics (224), and the anticancer effects of pentose polymers, which are abundant in unrefined cereal fiber and certain vegetables (14). The presence of such agents in human and animal diets, although extremely beneficial, has no doubt contributed to the lack of correlations between experimental animal data and epidemiologic human data. An understanding of the multitude of such agents and the magnitude of protection offered by these agents against specific toxicants is extremely important if realistic human risk estimations are to be made concerning food toxicants.

NATURAL COMPONENTS

This group of toxicants includes compounds that are naturally present in foods irrespective of microbial or other forms of contamination. Although a majority of toxic compounds in this group are derived from food and feed components of plant origin, examples exist of severe acute intoxications resulting from consumption of toxic animal products (e.g., puffer fish). Among the plants, those utilized in human foods and animal feeds are rarely associated with acute intoxications resulting from naturally present chemicals, in normal populations. Small segments of highly sensitive individuals in the human population have been reported to suffer from adverse reactions to selected classes of compounds, for example, favism in individuals deficient in glucose-6-phosphate dehydrogenase in their red blood cells (135). Acute toxicoses due to plant toxins are well known in domestic animals as well as in humans (mainly children) as a result of consumption of these plants during drought, due to ignorance, due to their presence in the diet, or for medicinal purposes (114). Long-term or delayed effects resulting from the consumption of various natural plant food components are extremely important from the standpoint of duration of exposure as well as the extent of the population exposed.

Accordingly, the discussion of natural toxins is subdivided into two sections. The first section deals with natural components of plant foods that make up human and animal diet. These compounds are generally not acutely toxic to normal populations. Evidence obtained, mostly from recent studies, indicates the possibility of deleterious effects following long-term intake. The group of natural constituents that are not a part of normal animal or human diet but which are consumed either accidentally or because other food sources are not available, will not be discussed here. The second section deals with toxins that are present in fishes consumed by human beings.

Toxicants in Foods of Plant Origin

Foods of plant origin account for most (70%) of the world's supply of protein. Although plants with obvious toxic effects have been excluded from human diet by trial and error, advances in the 20th century have identified groups of compounds in human diets that may exert deleterious (toxic as well as antinutritive) effects. Some of the important classes of such compounds are discussed below.

Enzyme Inhibitors

Substances capable of inhibiting the activity of digestive enzymes (proteases, amylases, and lipases) have been identified in many plant foods, particularly among legumes. Protease inhibitors are the most studied.

Protease inhibitors

Following the initial observations of Osborne and Mendel (172) that heat treatment improved the nutritive value of soybean protein, two broad classes of protease inhibitors were identified from the soybean with each class having several isoinhibitors (127). Kunitz inhibitor is the major member of the first class whose members have molecular weights (MW) between 20,000 and 25,000 and act principally against trypsin. The second class of inhibitors range in MW from 6000 to 10,000, have high proportion of disulfide bonds, are relatively heat stable, and inhibit both trypsin and chymotrypsin at independent binding sites (127). Bowman–Birk inhibitor is an example of this class.

Kunitz inhibitor is capable of inhibiting trypsin derived from cow, pig, salmon, stingray, barracuda, and turkey (111). Other enzymes affected by this inhibitor include bovine chymotrypsin, human plasmin, cocoonase, and plasma kallikrein. Human trypsin exists in two forms. The cationic form, which accounts for a majority of trypsin activity, is only weakly inhibited whereas the anionic form is fully inhibited (127). In addition, there appear to be 5 Bowman–Birk-like protease inhibitors, an insect protease inhibitor, and a papain inhibitor associated with raw soybeans. A number of varieties of beans, peas, cereal grains, and potatoes have also been shown to contain one or more protease inhibitors. A list of

inhibitors in a variety of plant foods and their specificity toward various enzymes has been compiled by Liener and Kakade (127).

The major effects of protease inhibitors in animal diets include growth depression and pancreatic hypertrophy. Resistance of raw soybean protein to proteolysis, low levels of sulfur-containing amino acids in soybean protein, and lower digestibility, absorption, and utilization of available nitrogen from the small intestine due to the presence of protease inhibitors, all appear to contribute to growth depression (76,127). Pancreatic hypertrophy is postulated to result from constant pancreatic hypersecretion necessitated by release of a humoral agent (possibly cholecystokinin pancreozymin) in the upper small intestine in response to the lack of free trypsin and chymotrypsin following binding with the inhibitor (76). Intestinal trypsin and chymotrypsin are proposed to be involved in the negative feedback inhibition of pancreatic secretion.

In humans, the extent of *in vivo* protease inhibition by inhibitors from various sources is unknown. Although any single source such as soybeans is unlikely to be consumed in quantities of toxicological significance, consumption of multiple sources of protease inhibitors can increase the risk of pancreatic hypertrophy and cancer (156).

Amylase inhibitors

Wheat, rye, kidney beans, taro root, and unripened mangoes and bananas contain proteinaceous inhibitors of pancreatic amylase acting in a noncompetitive fashion (76,249). Most of the inhibitors are highly specific with respect to the source of the amylase. A list of natural proteinaceous inhibitors of amylase and other carbohydrases is presented by Pressey (184).

Feeding large doses of amylase inhibitor with a starch-based diet reduced the growth rate in rats in spite of increased or normal feed intake (69,202). A decrease in the rate of starch hydrolysis in the small intestines, decreased absorption, attenuation of the rise in blood glucose and a fall in nonesterified fatty acids in animals and humans, and a decreased rate of ^{14}C-starch incorporation into lipid in humans (185) are events that are consistent with reduced growth rates. This starch-blocking effect of amylase inhibitors has generated enormous interest in their possible use to control obesity. In fact, it is estimated that over one million kidney-bean-derived starch-blocker tablets were consumed daily during the first part of 1982 (213). A recent study indicates that no significant reduction in the absorption of calories occurred across the human gastrointestinal mucosa in the presence of starch blockers compared with placebo (17). The normal human pancreas secretes 10 times the amount of amylase required for complete digestion of starch and the amount of amylase inhibitor present in starch blockers at the prescribed dose would at best inhibit only a fraction of the amylase present (76).

Lipase inhibitors

A protein from soybean cotyledons known to decrease lipolytic activity of pancreatic lipase has been shown to exert its action by adhering to the oil–water interface and effectively reduce substrate concentration *in vitro* (201). Gallaher and Schneeman (76) demonstrated the lipase-inhibiting effect of cellulose in the intestinal lumen, but neither pancreatic lipase nor the absorption of triacylglycerol were affected. The physiological significance of lipase inhibitors is, in a manner similar to those of amylase inhibitors, nullified by a large excess in the normal production of pancreatic lipase in man and animals.

Lectins

Lectins are plant proteins or glycoproteins that can interact specifically with certain carbohydrates such as those in cell membranes. Their ability to agglutinate red blood cells (RBC) of different species of animals as well as humans has been used to identify new lectins and has also resulted in this group being named *phytohemagglutinins*.

Lectins are capable of stimulating lymphocytes to undergo mitosis, and have been used extensively to study lymphocyte dynamics and function. Following the initial discovery of highly toxic ricin from castor bean, lectins have been detected in a number of edible plants (e.g., legume seeds, potatoes, wheat germ). A summary of edible plant lectins and their toxicity can be found in reviews by Jaffe (103,104).

Toxic effects of lectins are dependent on source, species, dose, and route. The nature of effects ranges from growth depression to lethality. Binding of lectins to cells in the crypts and villi of the intestines, followed by nonspecific inhibition of active and passive absorption of all nutrients including water across the intestinal mucosa, appears to account for growth depression and possibly death following long-term exposure to high levels (104). King *et al.* (113) demonstrated that bean lectins can cause necrosis of intestinal epithelial cells. Mortality following acute systemic lectin exposure is associated with impaired liver function, hepatocellular necrosis, and abnormal carbohydrate and respiratory metabolism (100). An indication that lectins may impair the immune system arises from the interesting observation that doses of lectin which were lethal to the Japanese quail were ineffective in germ-free birds that died following exposure to coliforms along with lectins. Several human intoxications, possibly from lectins in raw or partially cooked beans and bean products, are reviewed by Jaffe (103).

Glucosinolates

Glucosinolates (GS) are a group of nearly 80 flavor-imparting thioglucoside compounds found in all crucifer and related plants. Not only are the parent GS of horticultural crops (e.g., cabbage), oil seeds (e.g., rapeseed), condiments (e.g., mustard seed), and herbage (e.g., *Brassica,* kale) important but their products of enzymatic hydrolysis are important as well. The isothiocyanates, nitriles, oxazolidinethione (OZT), and thiocyanate ions formed either from fresh tissue that is crushed or during heating are the major products of hydrolysis (241). The enzyme thioglucosidase, which hydrolyzes GS, is present both in the plant itself and in bacteria in the digestive tract of man and animals (230).

Feeding rats a ration containing 0.85% (*S*)-2-hydroxy-3-butenyl GS (epiprogoitrin) resulted in enlargement of the thyroid, liver, and kidneys (241). At 2.6% of the diet, epiprogoitrin caused the death of all rats in 56 days. Oral dosing of rats and humans with the R isomer of GS (progoitrin) resulted in increased serum levels of OZT (goitrin) and a concomitant decrease in the uptake of radioiodine by the thyroid (241). Subsequently, thyroid enlargement (goiter) was shown to be related to the formation of OZT, and the liver and kidney damage related to the formation of nitriles during enzymatic hydrolysis of GS (241).

Isothiocyanates formed in foods and feeds as a result of enzymatic hydrolysis decompose into thiocyanate ion. Thiocyanate ion is capable of inhibiting uptake of iodine by the thyroid, ultimately resulting in depression of growth rate, hyperplasia, and hypertrophy of the thyroid. Thyroid enlargement is also produced following feeding of OZT to rats. Inhibition of the uptake of iodine by thyroid following thiocyanate ion exposure can be overcome by large amounts of iodine in the diet. OZT, however, presumably acts by inhibiting the incorporation of iodine into precursors of thyroxine and thus interferes with the secretion of thyroxine (141). This condition is not reversible by excess dietary iodine.

The nitrile fraction from GS-containing foods and feeds, when fed at a level of 0.2% of the diet, killed rats in 14 days, and, when fed at 0.1% of the diet for 106 days, rats had body weight gains equal to 17% of the control rats. Bile duct hyperplasia, hepatocyte necrosis, and megalocytosis of renal tubular epithelium were seen in these animals (231).

Although no direct evidence of human goiter resulting from dietary GS exists, the likelihood of accentuation of goiter due to iodine deficiency by high levels of goitrogens remains.

Cyanogens

Cyanogenic compounds are derived not only from plants but also from fungi, bacteria, and even members of the animal kingdom (155). More than 2000 plants are known to be cyanophoric, the main contributors to human and/or animal diets occurring in certain grasses, pulses, root crops, and fruit kernels (155,182). Some common sources for humans include cassava, sweet potatoes, yam, maize, millets, bamboo, sugarcane, peas, beans, almond kernel, lemon, lime, apple, pear, cherry, apricot, prune, and plum. Although more than 20 glycosides have been identified in edible plant varieties, only four (i.e., amygdalin, dhurrin, linamarin, and lotaustralin) are of practical toxicologic importance. The sources and hydrolysis products of cyanogenic glycosides are reviewed by Conn (42).

Toxic effects of cyanogenic glycosides are mediated by hydrogen cyanide (HCN) released during the hydrolysis of the glycoside. The hydrolysis is triggered by physical disruption (mastication, trampling, etc.) or stress (drought, frost, etc.), and is mediated by two enzymes, β-glucosidase and hydroxynitrile lyase, that are present within the plant or in bacteria in the gastrointestinal tract of man and animals (182). The scheme of breakdown and the hydrolysis products are presented in Fig. 1. β-Glucosidases within each plant are specific to the glycoside present in that plant. Hydroxyalanine

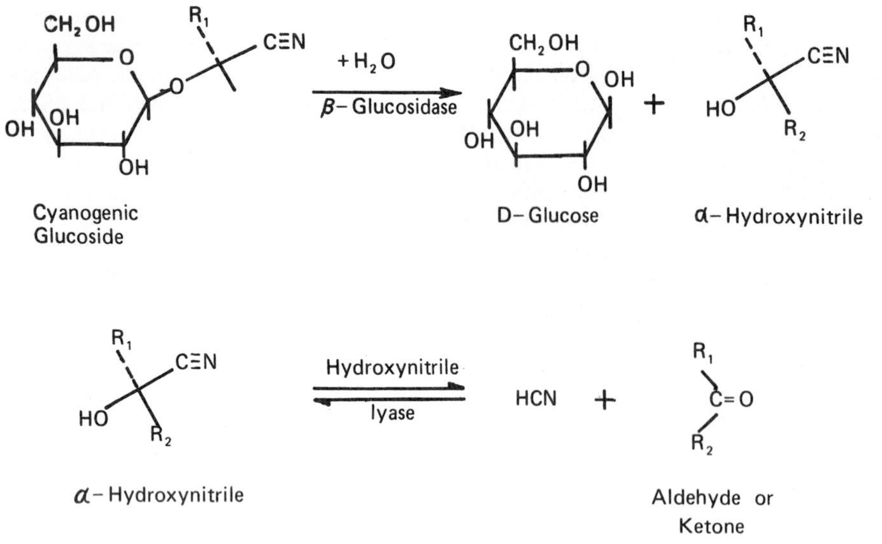

FIG. 1. Enzymatic hydrolysis of cyanogenic glycosides. Initially, the cyanogenic glucoside is hydrolyzed by a β-glucosidase, releasing D-glucose and an α-hydroxynitrile. The latter compound may dissociate either enzymatically or nonenzymatically to yield HCN and the corresponding aldehyde or ketone. (From ref. 182, with permission.)

lyase, however, is capable of hydrolyzing the bond between HCN and a great number of aldehydes (182).

Yields of HCN from common food and feed sources range from 0 to 910 mg/100 g (182). Animals have often been poisoned by young sorghum and arrow grass. Young bamboo shoots and tea made from peach leaves are examples of dietary sources of HCN poisoning in children. The minimal lethal dose of HCN in man and animals is 0.5–3.5 mg/kg and 2–10 mg/kg, respectively. Toxic effects of HCN result from its affinity toward metalloporphyrin-containing enzymes, more specifically cytochrome oxidase. Cyanide concentration of only 33 μM can completely block electron transfer through the mitochondrial electron transport chain and thus prevent O_2 utilization (182). Death results from generalized cytotoxic anoxia. Signs of acute cyanide poisoning in humans are hyperventilation, headache, nausea and vomiting, generalized weakness, coma, and death due to respiratory depression and failure.

Treatment of acute cyanide intoxication involves, in addition to artificial respiration, conversion of hemoglobin in the blood to methemoglobin with nitrites (sodium or amyl). Methemoglobin competes with cytochrome oxidase for HCN and binds to HCN to form cyanmethemoglobin. The simultaneous administration of sodium thiosulfate will convert free cyanide present in the blood to thiocyanate, which is eliminated. As free cyanide in the blood decreases, additional cyanide dissociates from the cyanmethemoglobin and is subsequently eliminated (36).

Although our knowledge of cyanogenic plants has led to the alleviation of acute cyanide intoxication in large part, recent evidence relates chronic cyanide intake to a number of human diseases. In addition to low levels of cyanide in the diet, exposure to HCN can occur via cigarette smoke (232) and bacterial action in the intestinal and the urinary tracts, and from industrial chemicals used in electroplating, metal refining, production of synthetic fibers, adhesives, plastics, and insecticides (182). A syndrome termed tropical ataxic neuropathy (TAN), which is characterized by my-

elopathy, bilateral optical atrophy, deafness, and polyneuropathy, has been linked to increased consumption of cassava diets in Nigeria (175). These diets were also poor in sulfur-containing amino acids which can detoxify HCN to thiocyanoalanine and subsequently to inert 2-amino-4-thiazolidine carboxylic acid (see ref. 182).

Major detoxification pathways of low levels of HCN are conversion of cyanide to thiocyanate using endogenous thiosulfate, and catalysis by ubiquitous enzyme rhodanese; to a minor extent, conversion is achieved by combining with endogenous hydroxycobalamin (Vit B_{12a}) to form cyanocobalamin (182). Higher incidence of goiter in TAN patients and the presence of endemic goiter in the Idjwl Island of eastern Zaire have been linked to high endogenous generation of goitrogenic thiocyanates from dietary cyanide. Low protein intake coupled with cassava or other cyanogenic diets also seems to be associated with cretinism and with pancreatic damage which may lead to diabetes. For details on the toxic effects of chronic cyanide exposure, see reviews by Montgomery (155) and Poulton (182). Other disease syndromes linked statistically to chronic cyanide exposure (not necessarily dietary) are tobacco amblyopia, retrobulbar neuritis in pernicious anemia, and Leber's optic atrophy.

A more recent problem with the use of *laetrile* as an anticancer agent stemmed from the initial belief that an amygdalin derivative, L-mandelonitrile-β-glucuronide (laetrile), was converted to large quantities of HCN by purportedly high levels of β-glucosidase in cancer cells (for review see ref. 50). Cancer cells were also believed to be deficient in rhodanese, thus allowing the HCN to selectively kill cancer cells. These assumptions have not been unequivocally proven. Also, most laetrile used in Mexico is not L-mandelonitrile-β-glucuronide but principally amygdalin, sometimes contaminated with bacteria. As reviewed by Poulton (182), intense testing of amygdalin by the National Cancer Institute and others failed to produce effective anticancer results in both experimental and clinical trials. Amygdalin toxicity is accentuated by simultaneous consumption of sources of β-

glucosidase in the diet. Finally, amygdalin is teratogenic and mutagenic, thus making laetrile unsuitable for cancer chemotherapy.

Toxic Proteins, Peptides, and Amino Acids

Although severe adverse reactions associated with excess protein consumption have seldom been reported, Stults (227) cites studies reporting hypertrophy of liver and kidneys in animals and increased calcium excretion in humans in conjunction with high protein ingestion. In the late 1970s several reports appeared documenting 225 nonlethal adverse reactions and 60 deaths associated with the use of partially hydrolyzed protein (liquid protein products) as the sole source of calories for rapid weight loss. Toxic signs in the first group of individuals ranged from nausea, vomiting, and diarrhea to myocardial infarction and anaphylaxis (227). Death was assumed to result from cardiac insult.

Protein toxicants such as hemagglutinins (lectins) and enzyme inhibitors have already been discussed. Proteins causing allergic reactions and microbial protein toxins are discussed in subsequent sections. Toxic peptides, thus far identified as important in animal and human health are for the most part derived from mushrooms.

Mushroom poisoning

There are about 5000 species of mushrooms with a history of food use of which about 100 may be toxic and 12 are known to contain lethal toxins (192). Recent reviews of mushroom toxins include those by Rodricks and Pohland (192), Lampe (122), and Wieland and Faulstich (250).

Toxicoses resulting from the consumption of mushrooms range in severity from mild to fatal, and in the latency of onset from less than 2 hr to greater than 72 hr. Despite the vast number of mushroom varieties, the differential diagnosis of mushroom poisoning is facilitated by the history and nature of the syndrome produced by the limited varieties of toxins. Two types of syndromes have been identified based on the latency period (rapid or delayed) for the onset of symptoms (123).

The rapid onset type usually manifests itself within 3 hr after consumption of the toxic mushroom or immediately after consumption of alcohol plus the toxic mushroom. Such intoxications are rarely serious and require only symptomatic treatment (123).

Mushrooms producing severe *gastroenteric irritation* include *Chlorophyllum molybdites, Entoloma lividum, Trichodoma pardinum, Omphalotus olearius,* and *Paxillus involutus.* A number of other mushrooms that produce mild and occasionally delayed onset (6–8 hr) of symptoms are listed by Lampe (122). Abdominal discomfort caused by emesis and diarrhea may sometimes persist in children who have consumed raw mushrooms. If untreated by fluid replacement, such persistent cases may prove fatal. Although cooking has been shown to inactivate these toxicants, the chemical nature of specific toxicants in most species remains unknown.

Muscarine poisoning with typical signs of *parasympathetic* stimulation progressively manifests as profuse sweating, nausea, vomiting, and abdominal pain; blurred vision, salivation, lacrimation, rhinorrhea, and diarrhea; and rarely, tremors, dizziness, and bradycardia. Manifestations are seen within 3 hr after the consumption of raw or cooked mushrooms that belong to the genera *Inocybe, Clitocybe, Omphalotus,* and occasionally *Amanita* and *Boletus* (122). Although atropine can be given to effect (until signs subside or dryness of the mouth develops), no treatment is usually required.

Two groups of mushrooms contain compounds known to *affect the central nervous system* (CNS). The first group is comprised of the genera *Psilocybe, Panaeolus, Copelandia, Gymnopilus, Conocybe,* and *Pluteus* and contains two related hallucinogenic compounds, psilocybin and psilocin. With increasing dose (6–12 mg of psilocybin required to induce hallucinations), these compounds are capable of causing weakness, drowsiness, altered temperature sensation, difficulty in focusing, changes in mood, distorted appearance of shapes and colors of objects, altered sense of hearing, paresthesis in the extremities, a dream-like state, and visual hallucinations. Death has been reported in small children, associated with mydriasis, hyperthermia, hallucinations, loss of conciousness, and convulsions (145). Signs of psilocybin intoxication can be reversed by diazepam or phenothiazine, and external cooling to combat hyperthermia.

The second group of mushrooms belongs to the genus *Amanita* (*A. pantherina* and *A. muscaria*) and contains the deliriant toxins muscimol and ibotenic acid as the principal components. It is presumed that ibotenic acid is decarboxylated *in vivo* to muscimol, the active form that antagonizes γ-aminobutyric acid (GABA) at the bicuculine-reactive postsynaptic receptors (123). The intoxication, referred to as the *Pantherine syndrome,* is characterized by periods of dizziness, drowsiness, and/or sleep alternating with periods of elation, increased motor activity, tremors, visual illusions, and delirium. In children, it may progress to coma and convulsions. Therapy is minimal and involves protection of adults from injury during episodes of manic excitement, and respiratory support with anticonvulsant therapy in children when needed.

Certain species of edible mushrooms belonging to the genus *Coprinus* contain coprine (1-cyclopropanol-1-N^5-glutamine), which is metabolized in the body to 1-aminocyclopropanol and then to the active compound cyclopropanone hydrate (253). Cyclopropanone hydrate reversibly inhibits the low K_m acetaldehyde dehydrogenase in the liver, resulting in acetaldehyde accumulation and toxicity following alcohol consumption. This increase in alcohol sensitivity occurs within 72 hr following the consumption of the toxic mushroom, and differs from that induced by disulfiram (Antabuse, a therapeutic agent against chronic alcoholism) in that coprine does not affect dopamine-β-decarboxylase and is a more potent alcohol sensitizer than disulfiram. Signs of alcohol sensitization include flushing, hypotension, tachycardia, palpitations, paresthesia, nausea, vomiting, and intense headache. Other mushrooms that are capable of producing alcohol-sensitization, but are not known to contain coprine, include *Clitocybe claviceps, Boletus luridus,* and *Verpa bohemica.*

The *delayed onset* type systemic toxicity of mushrooms usually appears later than 6 hr following consumption of the offending mushroom. Three distinct syndromes have been identified.

Mushrooms inducing *headache* are located mostly in eastern Europe and belong predominantly to the genus *Gyromitra. Gyromitra esulenta,* mistaken for edible morel by inexperienced collectors, contains a number of hydrazone derivatives of aldehydes. Gyromitrin, the acetaldehyde derivative of *N*-methyl-*N*-formyl hydrazone, and other prototoxins are hydrolyzed to form the active toxin monomethylhydrazine (MMH; 122). MMH and other hydrazines in mushrooms interfere with the action of pyridoxine. Due to the volatile nature of the MMH, which can be extracted into boiling water that could be discarded following cooking, cooks and personnel involved in the commercial preparation of cooked mushrooms are at risk of toxicosis. Characteristic signs of this sudden onset syndrome include an initial feeling of fatigue followed by severe headache, abdominal fullness, and persistent vomiting. MMH is carcinogenic in mice and hamsters, causing cancer of the lung, liver, gallbladder, and cecum following long-term exposure in water.

Emesis and profuse diarrhea followed by rapidly developing hepatic insufficiency (similar to acute hepatitis) are characteristic of poisoning by *A. phalloides* (green death cap) and related mushrooms. These species account for almost all mushroom-related fatalities in North America—approximately one-half of a mature cap of an *A. phalloides* being lethal for an adult (123). Among the two classes of thermostable peptide toxins in *A. phalloides,* the cyclic octapeptides, amatoxins (Fig. 2), appear to be responsible for all of the observed clinical effects (122), which begin to appear after a 12-hr latency period. Signs of hepatotoxicity include an increase in serum transaminases, decrease in blood glucose and clotting factors, and occasionally jaundice. Hepatic encephalopathy and renal failure may be present terminally. The lethal dose of amatoxins is estimated to be 0.1 mg/kg or lower (250). The fatality rate is about 10% even with intensive symptomatic care, which includes fluid replacement, activated charcoal hemoperfusion, forced diuresis, etc. A return toward normal factor V and fibrinogen is prognostic of recovery (123). Amatoxins inhibit RNA polymerase II by binding to the enzyme directly, and subsequently inhibit mRNA synthesis by blocking the formation of phosphodiester bonds at the elongation step, due to stabilization of ternary complex of template, enzyme, and the nascent ribonucleotide chain (240).

The second group of polypeptide toxins, the phallotoxins, are capable of causing hepatotoxic effects only at very high doses. These effects include swelling of the liver due to engorgement of hepatic sinusoids with blood, and depletion of blood in the peripheral circulation leading to hemodynamic shock. Cellular events leading to the final hepatotoxicity involve inhibition of cellular G-actin concentration by a combined effect of stimulated G-actin polymerization into F-actin, and inhibition of F-actin depolymerization. This leads to the loss of membrane elasticity and cell surface vesiculation and subsequent hepatocyte damage (250).

Several species of the genus *Cortinarius* have been shown in Europe to cause *nephropathy* that begins to manifest as polydypsia 3–17 days following consumption of a toxic dose. This leads to oliguria, and anuria in severe cases, and is often followed by nausea, headaches, muscular pains, and chills. Morphologic changes include renal tubular necrosis, fatty degeneration of liver, and intestinal inflammation. Although the heat stable toxin orellanine has been isolated, its structure is still in question (122).

Although several other mushroom species have been reported to be toxic and produce unique actions, additional confirmation and chemical and mechanistic studies need to

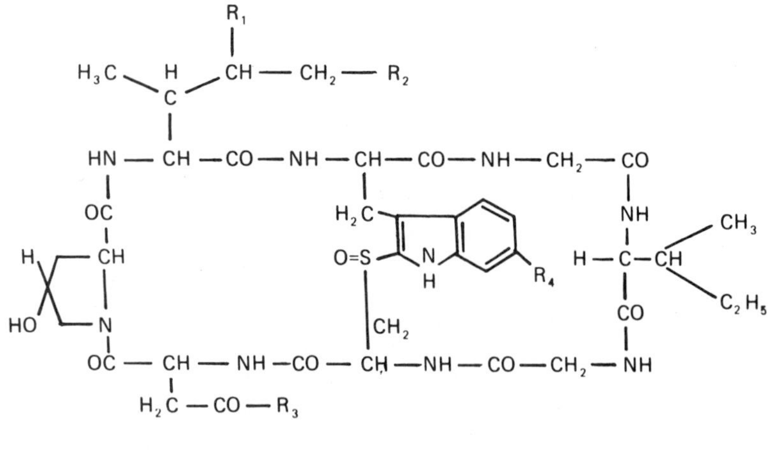

	R_1	R_2	R_3	R_4
α – Amanitin	•OH	•OH	•NH$_2$	•OH
β – Amanitin	•OH	•OH	•OH	•OH
γ – Amanitin	•CH	•H	•NH$_2$	•OH
ε – Amanitin	•OH	•H	•OH	•OH
Amanin	•OH	•OH	•OH	•H
Amanullin	•H	•H	•NH$_2$	•OH
Amaninamide	•OH	•OH	•NH$_2$	•H

FIG. 2. Structure of amatoxins.

be performed to better understand the nature of the toxicity. The risks of human intoxication resulting from commercial processing of *Gyromitra sp.* and possible testicular damage as well as carcinogenic effects resulting from the consumption of the edible mushrooms *Coprinus sp.* and *Gyromitra sp.* respectively, have been discussed. Other identified human conditions associated with mushroom production, commerce, and consumption are hypersensitivity to edible mushrooms in certain populations; hypersensitive allergic alveolitis and other pulmonary allergic changes in mushroom workers from spores of certain mushrooms (mushroom worker's lung); hemolytic reactions following consumption of mushrooms belonging to genera *Gyromitra, Boletus,* and *Paxillus;* and dermatitis (allergic) from contact with one or more species of the genera *Boletus, Lactarius, Clavaria,* and *Agaricus.*

Allergens

Most allergens in foods are normally nontoxic, large MW substances most often identified with the protein fraction. Their toxicity (allergenicity) is attributable to the abnormal sensitivity of the individual consuming it. All foods are capable of eliciting an allergic reaction. Allergy is a rather common affliction, affecting, for example, 20% of American schoolchildren (3). Common causes of food allergy are grains, milk, eggs, fish, crustaceans, tomatoes, strawberries, nuts, chocolate, and other beverages. Although any tissue of the body can be affected, the skin and the respiratory tract account for 90% of food allergies (179). Immunologic mechanisms in most food allergies are immediate hypersensitivity (type I) and delayed hypersensitivity (type IV) involving humoral and cell-mediated responses, respectively. Type I hypersensitivity is dependent on circulating antibodies of the IgE class (reagin) and the eventual release of vasoactive substances such as serotonin and histamine. Signs are elicited a few minutes after exposure and may be life-threatening. Type IV (delayed) hypersensitivity is dependent on specifically sensitized lymphocytes which are attracted to the site of antigen exposure by lymphokines released by already existing T-lymphocytes (144). Symptoms of allergic reaction from foods vary in the extent of systemic involvement and severity depending on the allergen involved. Eczema and urticaria are common signs involving the skin. Allergic rhinitis, pneumonitis, and asthma reflect involvement of the respiratory system; abdominal distress, vomiting, and diarrhea reflect gastrointestinal involvement; and headaches, convulsions, and behavioral problems reflect nervous system involvement (179).

Toxic amino acids

In general, foodstuffs do not contain individual amino acids of nutritional importance in amounts that cause adverse reactions. Although growth depression might result from high-level dietary supplementation of amino acids that are not seriously deficient in the diet, this is likely only if the diet is low in protein or deficient in one of the essential amino acids (87). Therapeutic use of amino acids on the other hand, can lead to adverse effects including mild gastric distress (essential amino acids); numbness over the back of the neck and the back, weakness, and palpitation lasting up to 2 hr (Chinese restaurant syndrome by monosodium glutamic acid; MSG) associated with eating Chinese food; nausea, febrile reaction, and/or headaches (methionine, isoleucine, and threonine); and disorientation in mental patients treated with monoamine oxidase (MAO) inhibitors (methionine and tryptophan). However, in general 10 times the required dose of the amino acid needs to be given, usually on an empty stomach, to elicit these reactions (87). MSG had long been used as a flavor enhancer in commercially processed foods. MSG as well as other acidic amino acids, but not basic or neutral amino acids, produced lesions in rats and mice in the arcuate nucleus of the hypothalamus and in other brain areas devoid of blood–brain barrier (170). In addition, MSG causes lesions in the retina and the lateral geniculate nucleus (170). Schwarcz and Coyle (206) proposed a mechanistic role for ionic imbalance caused by large doses of acidic amino acids in the causation of brain lesions.

A number of naturally occurring atypical amino acids of toxicologic importance have been reviewed by Liener (126). Hypoglycin A (β-methylene cyclopropyl alanine) and its γ-glutamyl conjugate, hypoglycin B, are components of the fruit of the plant, *Blighia sapida* (ackee in Jamaica and isin in Nigeria). In undernourished individuals consumption of this fruit, especially in the unripened stage, has been associated with hypoglycemia resulting from inhibition of gluconeogenesis. Inhibition of gluconeogenesis involves interference with the transfer of long-chain fatty acyl residues, by β-methylene cyclopropylacetyl CoA, a metabolite of hypoglycin A, from CoA to carnitine and thus with β-oxidation. Signs of intoxication include vomiting followed by convulsions, coma, and even death. Vomiting appears to be a central effect resulting from the accumulation of short-chain branched fatty acids secondary to inhibition of isovaleryl CoA (126).

The legume koa haoli (*Lenucaena leucocephala*) found in Hawaii has potentially high nutritive value for animals and humans (157). However, widespread use of this legume is precluded by the goitrogenic effect, in ruminants, of the metabolite (3,4-dihydroxypyridine) of an unusual amino acid mimosine, that is present in this plant. Mimosine, in both ruminants and nonruminants, also causes reversible destruction of hair follicle matrix (loss of hair) and growth depression. Due to the structural similarity of mimosine with tyrosine, antityrosine effect has been proposed as one of the possible mechanisms of toxicity (126). Mimosine is also known to inhibit pyridoxal-containing transaminases, tyrosine decarboxylase, several metal-containing enzymes, cystathionine synthetase, and cystathionase (126).

Djenkolic acid, which is an amino acid that is structurally similar to cystine, is present in the djenkol bean (*Pithocolobium lobatum*) in Sumatra and Java and neither substitutes for cystine nor is totally metabolized. Unmetabolized djenkolic acid crystallizes in the kidney, thus causing hematuria and crystalluria (126).

Favism, a hemolytic disease in persons genetically deficient in glucose-6-phosphate dehydrogenase (G6PD), results from the consumption of broad beans (*Vicia faba*) in the Mediterranean region and in the Middle East. The amino acid

3,4-dihydroxyphenylalanine is present in fava beans and has been given a causative role owing to its capability *in vitro* of lowering the reduced glutathione (GSH) content of RBC, which subsequently leads to hemolysis possibly accompanied by jaundice and hemoglobinuria. The instability of GSH in the susceptible RBC has been attributed to the inability of the G6PD-deficient cells to maintain an adequate supply of NADPH (38). Recent evidence, however, indicates that the pyrimidine aglycones of glucosides, vicine and convicine, in fava beans, produce greater effects on GSH levels in RBC than the 3,4-dihydroxyphenylalanine and are the more likely etiologic agents (38).

The etiology of the neurologic disease in cattle consuming cycads, which is still in question, could possibly be α-amino-β-methylaminopropionic acid (synonym: β-N-methylamino-L-alanine), an amino acid which was markedly neurotoxic to chicks and rats (see discussion on cycads).

Displacement of sulfur by selenium (Se) from amino acids in plants growing on high Se soils results in excessive levels of nonprotein seleno-amino acids such as methylselenocysteine and selenocystathionine, and protein amino acids such as selenocysteine and selenomethionine (126). The seleno-amino acid, when incorporated into structural animal proteins, results in defective hair and hooves that are eventually lost during longer term exposure in livestock. In human beings, toxic syndrome characterized by abdominal distress, nausea, vomiting, diarrhea, and loss of scalp and body hair had been reported following consumption of coco de mono (*Lecythis ollaria*) nuts containing high levels of selenocystathionine (5).

The amino acids L-2,4-diaminobutyric acid (DABA) and 3-N-oxalyl-L-2,3-diaminopropionic acid (ODAP) and related homologues, present in seeds of several species of *Lathyrus* used as food in the Indian subcontinent, have been implicated in the pathogenesis of a syndrome, neurolathyrism (59). The amino acids 3-cyanoalanine and 4-glutamylcyanoalanine, components of the seeds of *Vicia sativa* growing in areas where *L. sativus* is grown, also cause a neurologic syndrome (convulsions, rigidity, prostration, and death) in rats and chickens and may enhance the neurolathyrogenic potential of *L. sativus* (59). Humans exhibit signs of muscular rigidity, weakness, paralysis of leg muscles and, in extreme cases, death (177) following consumption of *L. sativus* seeds at a level of one-third to one-half of the daily diet for 3–6 months, a situation not uncommon in poorer families in certain areas in India and Bangladesh, especially during famine. The mechanism of action appears to involve the ODAP-mediated enhancement of glutamine release and inhibition of high-affinity reuptake of the neurotransmitter glutamine by the nerve terminal synaptasomes of the brain and spinal cord (177). Despite the governmental ban on the sale of *L. sativus* seeds in many states in India, problems continue to surface owing to the lack of an effective ban on its production and use.

Plant phenolics

Plant phenolics comprise a large array of substituted phenolic compounds that impart color and astringent taste to foods but are not essential for plant life. Major groups of phenolic compounds include phenolic acids and coumarins, and flavonoids including anthocyanidins (47). Although some plant phenols are quite toxic, serious human poisonings or loss of animals are mostly caused by phenolics uncommon in human food and animal feed (215).

Phenolic acids are derived from benzoic and cinnamic acids and usually occur as esters or conjugates. Important members of these groups include *p*-hydrobenzoic, protocatechuic, vanillic, gallic, syringic, *o*-hydroxy salicylic, and gentisic acids in the first, and *p*-coumaric, caffeic, ferrulic, and sinapic acid in the second groups. An account of the chemistry, biosynthesis, and occurrence of phenolic acids as well as flavonoids is presented by Deshpande *et al.* (47).

The flavonoids, most of which occur as glycosides, are by far the largest group and include a diverse range of plant phenolics such as red and blue anthocyanin pigments of flowers, the yellow flavones, flavonols, flavanols, aurones, chalcones, and isoflavones.

Additionally, two major groups of polyphenols, namely, tannin and lignin, also occur widely in plants. Tannins impart a dry, astringent taste to foods and are important in the food and tanning industries for their ability to bind proteins and prevent putrefaction. Lignins, on the other hand, contribute to the strength and rigidity of the higher plants. Other examples of potentially toxic phenols include nitrogenous phenols such as tyrosine and mescaline; mycotoxins such as aflatoxins; flavorings such as myristicin, coumarin, and safrole; hypericin and psolalen-related compounds as photosensitizers; and phenolic gossypol pigments.

Quantitatively and toxicologically, polymeric phenols appear to be the most important of the phenolic compounds that occur in cereals, millets, legumes, and fruits. Deleterious effects of these compounds (mainly tannins) include lower feed efficiency, reduced digestibility of foods and feeds, reduced protein utilization, diminished body weight gain, damage to the mucosal lining of the gastrointestinal tract, and cancer of the mouth and esophagus (47). Some of these effects may, at least to some extent, be the result of the strong protein and starch binding effect of tannins, which lead to a resistance in dietary components to digestive processes as well as to binding to, and inhibition of, digestive enzymes themselves. A decrease in body weight results from the above effects coupled with reduced food consumption due to the astringency of the tannins. Some of the direct toxic effects of oral tannins are increased secretion of gastric and duodenal mucus; increased excretion of mucoproteins, sialic acid, and glucosamine in the feces of rats; and sloughing off esophageal mucosa, subcutaneous edema, and thickening of the crop in chicks. An oral dose following epithelial damage or the application of a tannic acid gel to burns can lead to enhanced tannin absorption and systemic toxic effects including degenerative changes in liver and kidneys (47,215). Livestock losses can exceed $10 million annually, attributable to consumption of hydrolyzable oak tannins in the southwestern United States, when other forage is lacking (215).

The mutagenicity and carcinogenicity of plant phenolics have been reviewed by MacGregor (134), Stich and Powrie (222), and Stich et al. (223). Of the more than 2000 flavonoid phenolics, about 30 (typified by quercetin, kaempferol, and norwogonin) have been shown to be genotoxic in the Ames assay (134). Studies using other test systems have yielded conflicting results. It is still unclear whether these effects are a result of direct DNA modification or are secondary to changes in biochemical processes that affect DNA replication. Data on carcinogenicity are nonexistent even though there are populations that consume high levels of flavonoids, either as part of their daily diet or as daily supplements (rutin, skullcap, and bioflavonoid tablets) which are available through health food stores.

Recently, attention has been focused not on the genotoxic effects of phenols but rather on the antimutagenic and anticarcinogenic effects of plant phenolics, especially the nonflavonoids. Stich and Rosin (224) have reviewed this aspect of plant phenolics. Several classes of nonflavonoid phenolics (simple phenolics such as catechol, phenolic acids such as gallic acid, and cinnamic acid derivatives such as chlorogenic acid) and some naturally occurring flavonoids including quercetin have been reported to inhibit mutagenesis induced by direct-acting as well as S-9 requiring mutagens, inhibit the formation of mutagenic nitrosation products *in vivo,* and counteract benzo[*a*]pyrene-, and *β*-propiolactone-induced carcinogenesis in rodents. Polyphenols (tannins, etc.) have been implicated in oral, pharyngeal, and esophageal cancer associated with high consumption of high-tannin sorghums and/or dark beer prepared from them, tea, red wines, areca nuts, and coffee (224). Reports of negative association between tea drinking and stomach cancer (226) and coffee consumption and kidney cancer (102) also exist. Polyphenols, however, are not directly damaging to the DNA.

Other notable examples of phenolic toxicants include anthraquinone derivatives from senna leaf, *Cassia sp.,* aloe sap, and rhubarb root with severe purgative action, and the more than 20 yellow gossypol pigments from cottonseed (215). Despite the known toxicity of gossypol, which is the most studied of the gossypol pigments to monogastric animals such as swine and poultry, cottonseed meal has been successfully used in ruminant diets over the years and in human diets in developing countries in the recent years. The occurrence, chemistry, and nutritional and toxicologic aspects of gossypol have recently been reviewed (12).

As a result of its extreme reactivity, gossypol (1,1′,6,6′,7,7′-hexahydroxy-5,5′-diisopropyl-3,3′-dimethyl [2,2′-binaphthalene]-8,8′-dicarboxaldehyde) binds to cottonseed protein, thus reducing the biological availability of lysine. Toxicologically, bound gossypol is mostly inactive. Toxicity of gossypol is apparently related to its ability to inhibit oxidative phosphorylation, interference with prothrombin synthesis, binding to dietary and/or tissue iron, and its protein binding activity (215). Acute oral toxicity of gossypol is low (LD_{50} 550–3340 mg/kg), with pigs being the most sensitive (12). A dietary level of 0.01% gossypol is the safe recommended level for swine (215). Signs of gossypol toxicity include loss of appetite and body weight; reduced levels of plasma prothrombin and hemoglobin; reduced red blood cell count and serum protein; edematous fluid in body cavities, lungs, and heart giving rise to gasping; degenerative changes in liver and spleen, and hemorrhages in liver, stomach, and small intestines; diarrhea; hair discoloration; and olive discoloration of yolk and decreased egg hatchability in poultry.

Berardi and Goldblatt (12) reviewed the antifertility effects of gossypol following oral administration and observed reduced sperm production as well as motility during the late stages of spermatogenesis. Hematopoietic effects can be mostly reversed by supplemental iron and partially reversed by dietary vitamin K (Vit K; 215). A combination of iron and 1% calcium hydroxide prevented gossypol toxicity. At the present time, no reports of human toxicity from gossypol exist. There is a worldwide trend of increasing the use of cottonseed in bread and bakery goods. Incaparina (18–38% cottonseed flour) is used in Columbia, Guatemala, Honduras, Nicaragua, Panama, Salvador, and Venezuela. Cottonseed protein supplements and liquid cyclone processed flour products from glandless (gossypol-free) cottonseed are also produced. It is used as an antifertility pill in China. These increased uses may uncover undesirable and heretofore unknown effects following long-term gossypol exposure in humans.

As with gossypol, polyphenol (tannin) toxicity can be prevented by the addition of iron, supplemental protein, and alkalinizing agents such as sodium hydroxide. In addition, nonionic detergents such as Tween 80, methyl donors such as choline and methionine, and dehulling and peeling of grains and fruits have also been shown to prevent the toxic effects of tannins (47).

Lipids

Adverse effects from naturally occurring plant lipids are potential problems when factors are introduced such as the departure from established food use patterns, the use of new lipid materials in human diets, or inborn errors of metabolism. Erucic acid (*cis*-13-docosenoic acid) is predominantly a component of the seeds of the rape (*Brassica napus* and *B. campestris*) and the mustard (*B. hirta* and *B. juncea*). Canada, Argentina, Mexico, China, India, Pakistan, Japan, and several European countries are the major producers and users of these oils. Although no reported cases of erucic acid toxicosis have been reported in humans, growth suppression, myocardial fatty infiltration, mononuclear cell infiltration, and fibrosis were observed in weanling rats fed erucic acid supplying greater than 20% of the calories. In addition, ducklings showed hydropericardium and cirrhosis and guinea pigs developed spleenomegaly and hemolytic anemia (see review by Mattson, ref. 143). Organ specific inhibition of glutamate oxidation and adenosine triphosphate (ATP) synthesis in cardiac mitochondria (96) could be mechanistically involved in the pathogenesis of these lesions.

Refum's disease is characterized by a genetic inability of certain individuals to convert phytanic acid (3,7,11,15-tetramethylhexadecanoic acid, a product of chlorophyll metabolism in the rumen) from dairy products and ruminant fats to *α*-hydroxyphytanic acid in preparation for further *α*-oxidation. This results in accumulation of lipids containing phytanic acid in many tissues and a characteristic neurologic syndrome (143). Elimination of dairy and ruminant fats from the diet of these individuals results in partial remission.

Cyclopropene fatty acids such as sterculic acid (C_{19}) and malvalic acid (C_{18}) are natural components of oils from plants of the order *Malvales,* most important of which are cottonseed and kapok seed oils. Cyclopropene fatty acids have been incriminated in the pink discoloration of egg whites and reduced egg production in cottonseed-fed laying hens, growth suppression and impaired female reproduction in rats, and increased saturated fatty acids in the tissues of pigs and other animals (143).

The recent increase in consumption of polyunsaturated fatty acids in the diet in order to lower blood cholesterol, although beneficial in decreasing the incidence of coronary disease, has raised concern for adverse effects such as induction of Vit E deficiency (143). Carrol (33) demonstrated a strong correlation between dietary fat and age-adjusted mortality rate from breast and intestinal cancer. Pancreatic cancer was found to be enhanced by a diet containing 20% corn oil but not by one containing 18% hydrogenated coconut oil and 2% corn oil (194). Hayatsu et al. (88), however, demonstrated antimutagenic effects of oleic and linoleic acids. Fats seem to act mainly at the promotional stage of carcinogenesis involving alterations in composition of cell membranes and the hormonal environment. Inhibition of the immune responses, and enhanced formation of some of the known tumor promotors such as prostaglandins and bile acids also have been reported (33).

Saponins

The saponins are bitter tasting glycosides in various plant materials, composed of steroids (C_{27}) or triterpenoids (C_{30}) conjugated with sugars or sugar acids, capable of hemolyzing red blood cells and are extremely toxic to cold-blooded animals. Their toxic potential is related to their capacity to reduce surface tension (15). In addition, carboxylic-acid-type aglycones which can bind to cholesterol (e.g., medicagenic acid of alfalfa), appear to be quantitatively related to the hemolytic activity of the saponin fraction (15). Recent demonstration of antiatherosclerotic effects of alfalfa meal in monkeys (137), and the potential for alfalfa leaf protein concentrates in swine, poultry, and possibly human nutrition (129), are likely to encourage alfalfa utilization in foods and feeds. However, high saponin content in the alfalfa products is not only associated with lower growth rate in chicks, rats, and swine but also with anemia and other signs of systemic lupus erythematosus in nonhuman primates (129). Coagulation and washing at alkaline pH effectively reduces saponin contents of leaf protein concentrates.

Oxalates and Phytates

Certain plants including spinach, rhubarb, beet leaves, tea, and cocoa contain high (0.2–2.0% on fresh weight basis) levels of oxalic acid. Although consumption of 5 g or more of pure oxalic acid by human beings can be fatal, the likelihood that oxalates present in plant foods destined for human consumption (e.g., rhubarb) will cause problems appears remote (61). Cattle and sheep in the western states, however, have been poisoned following ingestion of large quantities of the plants *Halogeton* and *Sarcobatus* (grease wood). Most of the signs of oxalate intoxication are attributable to the ability of oxalic acid to bind to calcium ion and to the subsequent functional hypocalcemia and tetany or deposition of insoluble calcium oxalate crystals in the kidneys and vasculature causing degeneration and necrosis in these tissues. Death, however, appears to be due to oxalate-mediated inhibition of succinate dehydrogenase and carbohydrate metabolism (176).

Phytic acid (myoinositol hexdihydrogen phosphate) is a component of many plant foodstuffs, especially cereals, nuts and legumes, and is capable of binding di- and trivalent metals in the order $Cu^{++} > Zn^{++} > Co^{++} > Mn^{++} > Fe^{+++} > Ca^{++}$ (167). As a result, mineral deficiencies resulting from high phytates are of concern in countries such as Iran which are heavily reliant on cereal proteins.

Estrogens

Nonsteroidal estrogenic substances from plants, called phytoestrogens, although capable of causing infertility in animals grazing heavily on estrogen-containing forages, are rarely involved in human problems. However, signs of estrogen imbalance, such as uterine bleeding and abnormal menstrual cycle, have been reported under unusual circumstances, for example, the heavy consumption of tulip bulbs during food shortage in Holland. Hops, used in brewing beer, contain the estrogenic acids lupulon, colupulon, and adlupulon at high levels. However, no evidence of the estrogenic activity of beer is available to date in humans (225).

There are more than 50 plants containing one or more members of the isoflavone (e.g., genistein, genistin, daidzein), coumestan (e.g., coumestrol, 4-O-methylcoumestrol), and steroid (estrone and estriol) groups of estrogens (225). The isoflavone genistein from soybeans, and the coumestan coumestrol from alfalfa appear to be the most significant plant estrogens. Zearalenone and zearalenol, two major resorcylic acid lactone estrogens, are produced in corn in response to infection by toxigenic strains of the fungus *Fusarium roseum* and are discussed along with other mycotoxins. Phytoestrogens bind to the same intracellular receptors as those that bind estradiol, but at a much lower affinity, and produce similar physiologic responses including hypertrophy of the vulva, vagina, and uterus in the female and hypertrophy of the accessory glands in the male, and antigonadotropic effects at hypothalamic, anterior pituitary, and gonadal levels in mammals of both sexes (225).

Reports of growth stimulation in domestic animals and growth suppression in rodents (225) can be reconciled by higher dose levels of estrogens used in rodent studies which can cause inhibition of growth hormone secretion by the anterior pituitary. Phytoestrogens are not mutagenic in the Ames *Salmonella*/microsome assay (10) and appear to be noncarcinogenic when given orally (243). Stob (225) suggests that they may actually be anticarcinogenic owing to their antiestradiol effects.

Vitamins and Antivitamins

Vitamins are by far one of the world's most widely used pharmaceutical products, stemming primarily from the misconception that more is better (45). In general, toxicoses result from indiscriminate use of, as well as self-medication with, dietary supplements and not from the consumption of dietary vitamins. Omaye (171) has reviewed the safety issues related to megavitamin therapy.

Therapeutic uses of Vit A for deficiency states such as night blindness, steatorrhea, hyperkeratosis, and xerophthalmia, and potential therapy of acne vulgaris, certain immune disorders, and cancer, along with daily consumption of carotenoids and Vit A in plant and animal tissues, especially the liver, account for the total Vit A exposure in man (171). Doses of 75,000–300,000 IU and 2–5 million IU of Vit A can cause acute toxicosis, and 18,000–60,000 IU/day and 100,000 IU/day can cause chronic toxicity in infants and adults, respectively (171). Signs of acute intoxication include vomiting, drowsiness, and bulging of fontanelle in children, and headaches, vertigo, abdominal pain, vomiting, and diarrhea in adults. Following chronic exposure, children exhibit premature epiphyseal closure, cortical thickening, and retardation of long bone growth (45). In adults, signs include anorexia, headaches, blurred vision, postexercise muscle soreness, hair loss, drying and flaking of skin, pruritis, nose bleeds, anemia, and liver and spleen enlargement (171). Contrary to the membrane stabilization by smaller doses of Vit A, toxic doses are thought to alter cell membrane integrity and enhance the release and activity of lysosomal enzymes (181).

Vitamin D functions by facilitating the action of parathyroid hormone on the bone and promoting intestinal absorption of calcium and phosphate. A deficiency of this vitamin thus leads to rickets in children and to osteomalacia in adults. A plant steroid, ergosterol, converted to ergocalciferol (Vit D_2) by ultraviolet light, and endogenous dehydrocholesterol (in skin), converted to cholecalciferol (Vit D_3) by sunlight are two equally effective sources of Vit D for humans (171). Vitamin D_3 is converted to 25-OH cholecalciferol in the liver and then to the active 1,25-dihydroxy compound in the kidney. While the recommended dose is 400 IU/day, excessive exposure to supplemental Vit D from 1000 to 3000 IU/day in infants and 10,000 to 500,000 IU/day in adults has resulted in toxicosis. No recorded cases of Vit D toxicosis have resulted from excessive exposure to sunlight. Fish oils and animal tissues do not contain levels high enough to cause intoxication. Toxic signs of Vit D in humans, which are similar to those seen in laboratory animals, are a result of hypercalcemia leading to extraskeletal calcifications (171), especially blood vessel walls and kidneys, leading to hypertension, renal failure, and cardiac insufficiency. Other signs of hypervitaminosis D include anorexia, nausea, vomiting, diarrhea, headache, polyuria, polydypsia, and anemia (171).

Several unsupported claims of beneficial effects of Vit E (in muscular dystrophy, leg cramps, thrombophlebitis, burns, hypertension, rheumatic fever, immunologic conditions, and aging) together with some proven benefits (in anemia of premature or low-birth-weight infants, malabsorption syndrome, cystic fibrosis, and sickle cell anemia) are factors that enhance Vit E use. Severe weakness and fatigue associated with increased serum creatine kinase activity and urine creatine excretion in individuals given daily doses of 800 IU of α-tocopherol, skin sensitization in individuals following topical application, interference with normal clotting mechanism (increased Vit K requirement), and decreased response of anemics to iron dextran are the principal toxicologic effects (171). The major problem with rapidly administered therapeutic Vit K is the anaphylactoid reaction (8). Large doses of the synthetic Vit K_3 (menadione) can cause hemolytic anemia, skin irritation, polycythemia, and kidney and liver damage (171) resulting from damage by the quinone radical on RBC membrane.

Despite the lack of evidence of beneficial effects of ascorbic acid (Vit C) in conditions other than scurvy, it has been widely used in the treatment of dental caries, pyorrhea, gum infections, anemia, and various hemorrhagic conditions. Higher doses of Vit C (0.4–2.5 g/kg) may adversely influence β-carotene utilization, Vit B_{12} absorption and Vit B_6 metabolism in laboratory animals (171). In human beings, increased scorbutic tendencies during withdrawal of Vit C intake, abortions and failure of conception, increased oxalate excretion with possible kidney stones, increased incidence of thrombotic episodes, alteration of platelet function *in vitro*, reduced leukocyte counts, and hemolytic crisis in glucose-6-phosphate dehydrogenase-deficient individuals, have been reported (171). Ascorbic acid is mutagenic in human fibroblasts *in vitro* (221) and also in bacteria (190) but has not been reported to be carcinogenic. The genotoxic as well as some of the toxic effects could be mediated by free radicals generated by the autooxidation of ascorbic acid (171).

Limited human and animal data indicate that thiamin, folic acid, niacin, and other B-complex vitamins can cause toxic reactions only when large quantities are therapeutically administered, especially by the parenteral route, or as a result of genetic and biochemical variability in individuals. The reader is referred to the reviews of Omaye (171), Cumming et al. (45), and Hayes and Hagstead (91).

Antivitamin compounds include substances that diminish or abolish the effects of vitamins in a specific way, thus predominantly producing deficiency signs of the vitamin in question. Reviews of vitamin antagonists in plant and animals' foods are presented by Liener (126) and Somogyi (218). Vitamin A activity is antagonized by Vit E, the enzyme lipoxidase (an enzyme oxidizing and destroying carotene) in raw soybeans, and the orange oil component citral. In calves, inclusion of raw soybeans at 30% of the diet resulted in lower blood carotene and Vit A levels (126). Administration of citral in monkeys resulted in vascular endothelial damage that could be prevented by Vit A. The presence of citral in marmalade, orange drinks made from whole fruit, and products made from orange oil flavoring necessitates a close examination of possible increase in cardiovascular disease in individuals that consume these products heavily (126).

Several naturally occurring substances including a factor associated with soybean protein, β-carotene in green oats and other green feeds, a steroidal compound from the stems and leaves of fresh vegetables, and organic soluble factor from pig liver, have been shown to possess anti-Vit D activity.

A heat stable and alcohol soluble factor and a second relatively heat labile and alcohol insoluble factor, both from raw kidney beans (*Phaseolus vulgaris*), were able to prevent the protection offered by Vit E against development of nutritional muscular dystrophy in hens and liver necrosis in rats (126). The heat stable factor is thought to be linoleic acid. Similarly, elevated levels of polyunsaturated fatty acids in animal diets enhance Vit E requirement. The heat labile factor appears to be the enzyme α-tocopherol oxidase, which also occurs in other beans and alfalfa (126).

Dicoumarol, 3,3′-methylene-bis (4-hydroxycoumarin), is a component of moldy sweet clover (*Melilotus sp.*) hay known to cause a fatal hemorrhagic disease in cattle. During the process of activation (probably carboxylation) of the coagulation factors II, VII, IX, and X, the active hydroquinone form of Vit K is converted to inactive epoxide which needs to be reduced to Vit K (by epoxide reductase) to be reactivated again. Anti-Vit K coumarin compounds competitively inhibit the enzyme epoxide reductase and thus prevent its recycling (11). However, the occurrence of this compound in human food is insignificant. High doses of Vit A appear to interfere with absorption of Vit K causing similar effects (218).

The best known example of antithiamine factor is the heat labile enzyme thiaminase of the bracken fern (*Pteridium aquilinun*), which is consumed primarily by cattle and horses when other forage is unavailable. Antithiamine activity has been found, in addition, in many other plants including ragi, mung bean, rice bran, mustard seed, cottonseed, flaxseed, blackberries, blueberries, black currants, beets, brussels sprouts, and red cabbage (126), and also in fish and shellfish (218). The public health significance of these factors at the present time appears to be minor. Other anti-Vit B agents include the antiriboflavin agent hypoglycin A from ackee plum in Jamaica, which causes vomiting sickness; antiniacin compound (possibly high leucine) in millets and corn, which causes pallegra in certain regions of India where these cereals make up a major part of the diet; antibiotin factor avidin, in the white of bird eggs; antipyridoxin factor 1-amino-D-proline (linatine), in flaxseed; antipantothenic acid factor from pea seedlings; and anti-Vit-B_{12} factor from raw soybeans (126,218).

Flatus-Producing Factors

Many legumes and certain nonlegume foods such as wheat products and fruits (raisins, bananas) and fruit juices are known to produce intestinal gas composed largely of carbon dioxide, hydrogen, and methane (126). Signs of severe gas production include nausea, cramps, diarrhea, abdominal rumbling, and the social discomfort associated with ejection of rectal gas. The precursors for gas production in nonlegume products have not been identified. In legumes, however, the oligosaccharides raffinose and stachyose, which have α-1,6-galactosidic linkages, are clearly implicated. The absence of enzymes in the upper human intestinal mucosa that are capable of hydrolyzing this linkage results in anaerobic bacterial fermentation in the lower intestines. Cooking, preparation of protein isolates, fermentation, and treatment with microbial enzymes to hydrolyze the galactosidic linkage can all significantly reduce the flatulant activity of legumes (126).

Vaso- and Psychoactive Substances

Udenfriend et al. (235) found high levels of phenylalkylamines in plants such as pineapple, banana, plantain, and avocado. Subsequently, high levels of amines, predominantly tyramine and its methyl derivatives octopamine, synephrine. feruloylputrescine, dopamine, epinephrine, norepinephrine, histamine, serotonin, putrescine, and cadaverine, were demonstrated in cheese, yeast products, fermented foods, beer, wine, pickled herring, snails, chicken liver, large quantities of coffee, broad beans, chocolate, and cream products (132). Cheese and yeast products seem to be the most dangerous since they are likely to contain the needed dose of 10 mg of tyramine to cause a severe hypertensive crisis in individuals

treated with MAO inhibitors for disorders of mood (7). As a result of the inhibition of MAO, tyramine and other monoamines in food and those produced by the bacteria in the gut escape oxidative deamination in the liver and other organs and cause a release of catecholamines that are present in supranormal amounts (as a result of MAO inhibition) at the nerve endings and the adrenal medulla (7). Hypertensive crisis is associated with migraine headaches and in some instances intracranial bleeding and death. Other potential problems related to the consumption of bananas or plantains as a major part of the diet are the possible role of high levels of norepinephrine and serotonin in bananas whose metabolites in urine might yield false positive results for tests designed to detect pheochromocytoma, and carcinoid heart disease in Africans (132).

Psychoactive substances include CNS stimulants such as xanthines (caffeine, theophylline, and theobromine present in coffee, tea, and cocoa), depressants such as alcohol and high doses of atropine (from jimsonweed and henbane), and hallucinogens such as myristicin from nutmeg, psilocybin and psilocin from mushrooms, and nondietary consumption of cocaine and lysergic acid derivatives by drug cults (132). Chronic overindulgence in xanthine beverages may lead to restlessness, disturbed sleep, and myocardial stimulation reflected as premature systoles and tachycardia. The essential oils of coffee may cause gastrointestinal irritation (diarrhea) whereas the tannins in tea may cause constipation (186). Curatolo and Robertson (46) reviewed the toxic effects of caffeine and concluded that although caffeine inhibits DNA repair and is clastogenic and mutagenic in bacterial systems at high doses, it is neither mutagenic by itself nor enhances the mutagenic effects of other compounds in mammalian cells. Despite suggestions that caffeine consumption may be associated with cancer of the pancreas, kidney, and lower urinary tract, and methyl xanthene consumption with benign fibrocystic disease of the breast, clear evidence has yet to be presented. Based on the teratogenic effects of high doses of caffeine in animals, the Food and Drug Administration (FDA) has issued an advisory for pregnant women to limit their caffeine consumption.

Miscellaneous Plant Toxicants

Several plants contain toxic compounds that fall outside the chemical or physiological groupings discussed earlier. Creeping indigo (*Indigofera endecapylla*), which showed enormous promise as a tropical forage, contains a toxic amino acid indospicine. Indospicine causes liver damage in sheep, rats, and mice by inhibiting the incorporation of arginine, the amino acid it resembles, into protein (see ref. 126). 3-Nitropropionic acid is also present and is capable of inhibiting succinate dehydrogenase and thus cellular respiration (1).

A common human intoxication called *milk sickness* was one of the most dreaded diseases from colonial times to the early 19th century in an area extending from North Carolina to Virginia and to the midwestern United States (125). The disease is characterized by weakness, nausea and vomiting, constipation, tremors, prostration, delirium, and even death, and results from the consumption of dairy products made from milk derived from cows (even healthy ones) grazing on white snakeroot (*Eupatorium rugosum*). The causative agent appears to be an unsaturated alcohol trematol ($C_{16}H_{22}O_3$) in combination with a resin acid (125). Current processing methods have kept this condition in check for the most part. In cattle, consumption of 5–10 lbs of snakeroot causes weakness and trembling of various groups of muscles, labored respiration, and death.

Fool's parsley (*Aethusa cynapium*) and other members of *Umbelliferae* family contain highly toxic acetylene derivatives (e.g., aethusin) that are responsible for many human poisonings (see ref. 126). Carotatoxin, the acetylene compound in carrots, is less toxic and is not likely to cause problems.

Purple mint plant (*Perilla frustescens*) is widely distributed in the United States and Japan. In Japan, leaves as well as seeds are used as flavoring agents, volatile oil from seeds are used for medicinal purposes, and seed cake is used as animal feed. A ketone-substituted furan that is capable of causing acute pulmonary emphysema in cattle (208) and pulmonary lesions in rats, mice, and sheep was isolated from this plant, thus raising questions about the practice of using mint as a routine flavoring agent in human diets.

Cycads, the palm-like plants adapted for adverse climatic conditions of the tropical and subtropical areas of the world, are still occasionally used (seeds and stem) as a source of starch in Guam, Kenya, Amami Oshima, Miyako Island, and southern Japan by small groups of people (140). The starchy endosperm is cut into pieces, soaked in frequent changes of water over several days, dried in the sun, and ground into flour for use. Toxic effects result from incomplete extraction of toxicants during preparation of the flour.

In the mid 1900s, high morbidity and mortality from a paralytic neurologic disease amyotropic lateral sclerosis (ALS), among the native Chamorro in Guam suggested that cycad consumption may cause ALS. Also, older individuals suffer from parkinsonism and dementia (PD). Mice given cycasin and cattle grazing on cycads developed gait disturbances, motor weakness, and paralysis (140), and the aqueous extract of the seeds of cycads (*Encephalartos sp.*) has been shown to be neurotoxic in guinea pigs (131). Spencer et al. (219) recently produced corticomotoneuronal dysfunction, parkinsonian features, and behavioral anomalies with chromatolytic and degenerative changes of motor neurons in cerebral cortex and spinal cord, following repeated dosing of monkeys with the nonprotein amino acid β-*N*-methylamino-L-alanine (BMAA) from cycad flour. These are many of the same symptoms characteristic of human ALS-PD syndromes.

Further study has led to the discovery of the attenuation of this syndrome by AP7 and MK801, two selective antagonists of *N*-methyl-D-aspartate receptor and its associated ion channel, respectively (219). This may suggest a role for the excitatory neurotransmitters not only in the causation of ALS-PD syndrome and neurolathyrism, which is caused by another amino acid (ODAP) in *Lathyrus sativa* in India, but also in other motor-system diseases (Huntington's chorea, Parkinson's disease, and olivopontocerebellar atrophy) and Alzheimer's disease.

Other acute and chronic effects including hepatic necrosis, subserosal hemorrhages, accumulation of yellow fluid in serosal cavities, benign and malignant tumors in the liver, kidney, lungs, and gastrointestinal tract (mainly colon), and death have been reported in experimental animals (see ref.

140) either by feeding cycad flour or by administering cycacin, an azoxyglucoside isolated from toxic cycad flour. An interesting feature of cycacin toxicity and carcinogenicity is its inactivity when given parenterally to conventional rats and complete (both oral and parenteral) inactivity in germ-free rats, suggesting the essential role of intestinal flora in mediating cycacin toxicity. The aglycone methylazoxymethanol (MAM), formed as a result of enzymatic (bacterial β-glucosidase) hydrolysis of cycacin, was the active carcinogen producing hepatomas in rats. Organospecific action of MAM may be dependent on further activation of MAM by enzyme systems in various organs (68) in conjunction with the activities of repair enzymes. Cycacin, preincubated with β-glucosidase, and MAM are mutagenic in plant, bacterial, as well as animal test systems (see ref. 140). Malformations such as microcephalus, hydrocephalus, spina bifida, and cerebral and cerebellar abnormalities associated with cell loss were demonstrated in the offspring of hamsters, rats, and mice (140) exposed to MAM *in utero*.

The major biochemical effect of MAM appears to be the methylation of RNA, DNA, and proteins including enzymes involved in the synthesis of nucleic acids and proteins (see ref. 140). Nucleic acid methylation involves guanine resulting in the formation 7-methyl guanine, the RNA in liver being affected to a greater extent than that either in kidney or small intestines (212). The transient methylating intermediate formed by spontaneous breakdown of MAM appears to be methyldiazonium hydroxide (140). Inhibition of enzyme activity (e.g., catalase) also appears to be preferentially hepatic (140). Although the evidence for a role of cyacin in human cancer is not available, it appears that the increased mortality in Miyako Inlanders from cirrhosis of the liver could be related to consumption of hastily and improperly processed cycad flour containing cycasin (140).

Toxicants in Foods of Animal Origin

Phylogenetic closeness between man and animals whose products make up present-day human diets assures a wholesome diet unless human intervention introduces harmful agents into food supplies or agents into the human body that can interact with normal animal tissue constituents producing adverse reaction in the host. Examples of the former include residues of antibiotics or pesticides in the meat and milk of animals given diets or drugs containing these agents either for growth promotion or for prevention and treatment of animal disease, and contamination of foods with microorganisms or chemicals during growth, processing, storage, and preparation. A discussion of these agents will follow in a subsequent section. An example of the latter type is the treatment of human beings with MAO inhibitors to correct mood disorders, a situation that requires withholding foods such as cheese that contain high levels of pressor amines, as discussed above. The third group of toxic compounds are natural components of marine animals and eggs of fishes and amphibians, and have sometimes resulted in fatal toxic reactions. All foods derived from animals are likely to contain hormones such as estrogens and testosterone some of which are heat stable and can be consumed even in heat-processed foods. Although prolonged exposure to high doses of estrogens is carcinogenic in animals and likely to be so in humans (196), such exposures are unlikely by way of normal food consumption patterns.

Marine Toxins in Foods

Of the many marine organisms capable of producing toxins (up to 1200 species), only a few are involved in food poisoning. Problems of seafood (mainly fish) poisoning have spread to inland areas from the coastal fishing sites as a result of modern transportation and shipping of seafood products. Toxicants may be produced by the fish itself, by the marine plankton or algae consumed by the fish, or by the bacteria that contaminate fish products.

Shellfish poisoning is a paralytic disease resulting from the consumption of shellfish (clams, mussels, scallops, etc.) that have ingested toxic marine algae, especially the dinoflagellates *Gonyaulax catenella* and *G. tamarensis* (203). The shellfish are toxic during seasons of heavy algal bloom containing 200 organisms/ml or more. Toxicity increases proportionately to the concentration of algae and disappears within 2 weeks after the toxic plankton has disappeared from the waters (197). The phenomenon of *red tide* involves 20,000–50,000 organisms/ml of water containing a xanthophyll called peridinin. Saxitoxin (Fig. 3), one of several toxins present in the *paralytic shellfish poison,* was chemically identified by Schantz et al. (204). Subsequently, gonyautoxin II, gonyautoxin III, and neosaxitoxin, all of which differ from saxitoxin in their weak binding affinity to carboxylate resins, have been isolated from *G. tamarensis.* The LD$_{50}$ of saxitoxin in mice ranges between 3.4 μg/kg by the intravenous route and 263 μg/kg by the oral route. Man is four times more susceptible than mice (197). Although boiling at neutral pH does not destroy all of the toxin, inactivation is enhanced by acid and alkaline pH. Boiling in bicarbonate-treated water and discarding the broth is suggested as a means of preventing shellfish poisoning (86).

Consumption of 1 mg of the toxin (in 1–5 mussels or clams weighing 150 g each) can be mildly toxic whereas 4 mg can be fatal if not treated vigorously. Toxic symptoms begin as numbness of the lips, tongue, and fingertips within a few minutes after eating. Numbness then extends to the legs, arms, and neck, and is followed by general muscular incoordination, which progress to respiratory paralysis and death. Decreased heart rate and contractile force, headache, dizziness, increased sweating, and thirst may also be noted.

Saxitoxin blocks the action potential in nerves and muscles by preferential blockade of inward flow of sodium ions with no effect on the flow of potassium or chloride ions (110).

Halstead (86) describes three distinct syndromes of shellfish poisoning: paralytic, erythematous, and gastrointestinal. The latter two are characterized by typical allergic skin (erythema, urticaria, etc.) and digestive symptoms. In addition to *G. catenella* and *G. tamarensis* imparting toxicity to shellfish in the Pacific and Atlantic oceans off North America, respectively, *Gymnodium breve, Gym. veneficum,* and *Exuviaella mariae labouriae* (along with *G. catenella*) have caused toxicoses in humans consuming shellfish from the Gulf Coast, English Channel and sea of Japan, respectively (203).

Between 300 and 400 tropical reef and semipelagic species of edible marine animals, including barracudas, groupers, sea basses, snappers, surgeon fishes, parrot fishes, jacks, wrasses, eels as well as certain gastropods, are capable of causing *ciguatera poisoning,* a gastrointestinal–neurologic and occasionally cardiovascular syndrome. The intoxication, common in the South Pacific and the Caribbean, appears to follow the spacial and temporal pattern of the distribution of a photosynthetic dinoflagellate *Gambierdiscus toxicus,* which is consumed by the smaller herbivorous fish (197). Although the species incriminated in ciguatoxin poisoning are not direct plankton feeders, they acquire poisons by feeding on smaller plankton-feeding fish. Because of the large number of edible fish that potentially contain the toxin(s) from the dinoflagellate, ciguatera poisoning is the most significant public health problem involving seafood toxins.

Ciguatoxin is a colorless, lipid soluble and heat stable molecule (MW of 1100) that appears to be the major toxin with some contribution from maitotoxin and scaritoxin (197). Ciguatoxin increases membrane permeability to sodium ions causing depolarization of nerves. In addition, ciguatoxin possesses anticholinesterase activity and produces signs typical of cholinesterase inhibition in experimental animals (197). In humans, signs and symptoms include tingling of the lips, tongue, and throat followed by numbness, nausea, vomiting, abdominal pain, diarrhea, pruritis, bradycardia, dizziness, and muscle and joint pain. Severe cases exhibit paresis of the legs and infrequently death due to cardiovascular collapse (197,203). Prevention of ciguatera poisoning is difficult, although extensive evisceration in areas known to be affected should be a common sense approach, since viscera and liver seem to contain most of the toxin (203).

Pufferfish (fugu fish) poisoning has been known to occur as far back as 2000–3000 BC in China and Japan. In addition

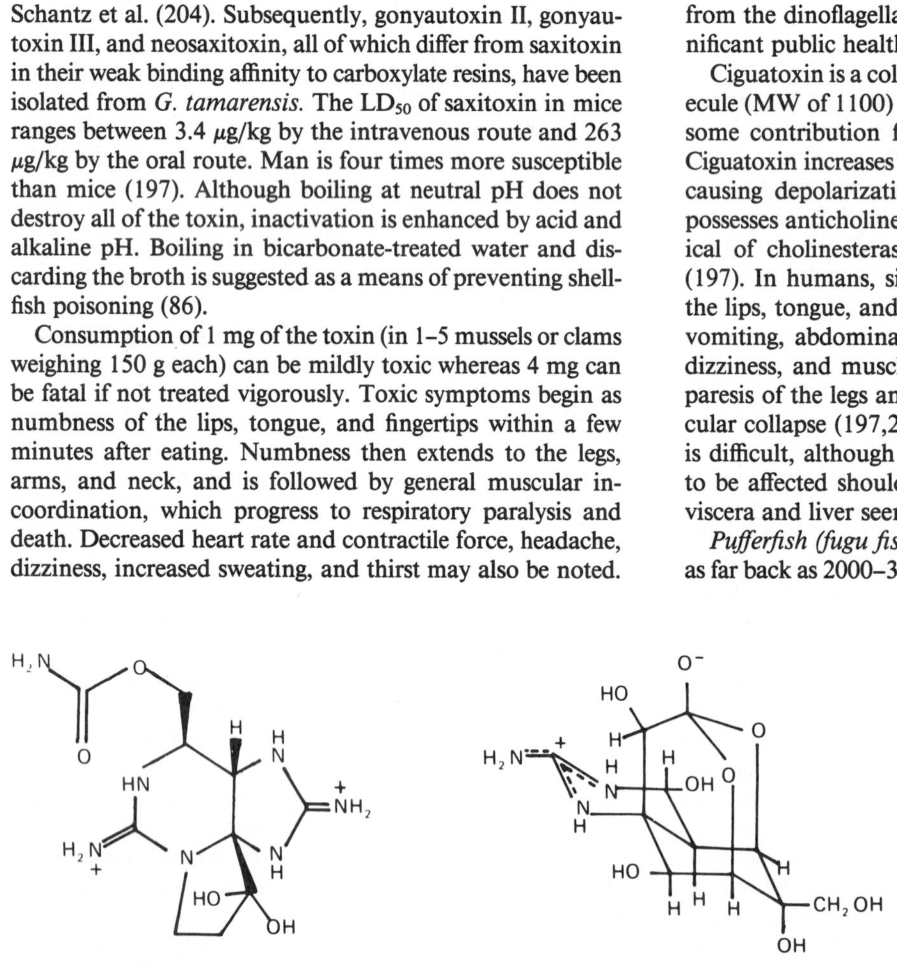

SAXITOXIN   TETRODOTOXIN

FIG. 3. Structure of two seafood toxins, saxitoxin and tetrodotoxin.

to puffers, the toxin (tetrodotoxin) is also found in ocean sunfishes, porcupine fishes, blue-ringed octopus, and certain amphibians of the family *Salamandridae* (197) concentrated mostly in liver and ovaries with lesser amounts in skin and intestines (109). The toxin accumulation is related to the reproductive cycle and is greater just prior to spawning in the spring. The choice edible species, considered a delicacy in China and Japan, are the ones that are most poisonous (203). Fuhrman (74) presented a list of fishes (mostly *Arothron spp., Fugu spp.,* and *Sphaeroides spp.*) and amphibia (*Taricha torosa* and *T. rivularis*) that contain tetrodotoxin and related substances in their eggs and ovaries.

The cyclic hemilactal structure of tetrodotoxin (Fig. 3) is unique in that only one other closely related natural toxin, chiriquitoxin, and no synthetic compound shares this structure. The toxin is active after boiling for 1 hr but is inactivated in acid and alkaline conditions, especially the latter (74). Tetrodotoxin is lethal to all vertebrates, except those that contain it, with a steep dose–response and an intraperitoneal LD$_{50}$ of about 10 μg/kg (74). Progressive paralysis of the voluntary muscles, hypotension, and respiratory paralysis are the predominant effects. In humans, numbness of the lips, tongue, fingers, and arms, muscular paralysis and ataxia, and respiratory paralysis leading to death progress rapidly beginning 30–60 min after consumption of 1–2 mg of tetrodotoxin (1–10 μg of roe or liver).

Tetrodotoxin prevents the increase in the early transient ionic permeability of neuronal membrane associated with the inward flow of sodium ions without affecting the later increase in outward flow of potassium ions, much like that of saxitoxin, despite structural dissimilarity (197). Both sensory and motor nerves are affected. Similar block also occurs at the skeletal muscle membrane. Treatment consists of oxygen, intravenous fluids, atropine, and, when appropriate, activated charcoal. Training of personnel in proper evisceration techniques and licensing of fugu restaurants in Japan have reduced the mortality in Japan to about 75 deaths per year. Only three known fatalities have occurred in the United States, all in Florida, from puffer fish poisoning since 1950.

Scombroid poisoning is an intoxication resulting from the consumption of inadequately preserved tuna, mackerel, shipjack, and bonito, in which histamine and saurine are produced as a result of bacterial action. Scombroid fish apparently has a sharp or peppery taste. Signs and symptoms of intoxication include nausea, vomiting, diarrhea, epigastric distress, flushing of the face, throbbing headache, and burning of the throat followed by numbness and urticaria. Severe cases may develop cyanosis and respiratory distress and, rarely, death may ensue. These signs and symptoms appear within 2 hr of the meal and disappear in 16 hr (197). The disease quickly responds to antihistamine treatment (86).

Other examples of seafood intoxication include eggs of stickelback (*Dinogunellus sp.*) in Japan and Cabezon or marbled sculpin (*Scorpaenichthys marmoratus*) on the Pacific Coast of North America, both containing the lipoprotein dinogunellin; fish-borne botulism (discussed in a subsequent section); and hepatotoxic shellfish poison in oysters in the region of the Hamana Bay in Japan. A number of other uncommon fish and nonfish marine food intoxications are described in reviews by Schantz (203), Halstead (86), Fuhrman (74), and Russell (197).

Although it is generally recognized that an overwhelming number of synthetic compounds have been introduced into our environment in the past century, this number pales in comparison with the number of naturally occurring chemicals. The unidentified natural chemicals may vastly outnumber those identified so far. The potential interactions among this vast array of chemicals, both beneficial and adverse, make safety evaluation extremely difficult, if not impossible, based solely on the toxicologic information derived from testing individual compounds. Further complications arise from vastly differing compositions of the diet in different regions of the world and also from genetic and environmental variations in individuals within and among various population groups.

FOOD CONTAMINANTS

In addition to the naturally occurring food components discussed above, several important groups of toxic biologic (bacterial, fungal, etc.) as well as man-made chemical contaminants enter the food chain at various stages of food manufacture and storage. Whereas some naturally occurring toxicants as well as man-made chemicals categorized as food additives serve the purpose of either imparting resistance to plants against pests or of the preservation and/or nutritional enhancement of the diet, respectively, the categories of biological contaminants and man-made chemicals, present as residues resulting from environmental contamination, serve only to increase food-borne toxicologic risk. For this reason, it is justified to use a much broader margin of safety in the control of contaminants compared with food additives. The FDA, in consultation with other federal agencies when needed, is responsible for establishing legal *action levels,* i.e., the maximal level of the contaminant allowed in foods and feeds, based on economic considerations, technologic feasibility, and toxicologic risk assessment (90).

Bacterial Toxins

Microbial contaminated food is a major source of human disease despite the severe underreporting both from patients and physicians. Organisms that produce intoxications are all normal environmental contaminants originating from the soil, animals, and processing equipment and even from the personnel involved in food processing and preparation (21). The major factors that contribute to bacterial contamination during food preparation include inadequate cooking, improper cooling of cooked foods, improper hot storage, cross-contamination between cooked and raw foods, inadequate reheating, inadequate cleaning of equipment, and preparation of food too far in advance of serving (139). As a result, the education of food handlers (both commercial and domestic) in proper food handling, preparation, and storage can go a long way in preventing food-borne bacterial illness (21).

Bacterial food-borne disease may result from the presence in food of bacteria that can cause disease either by multiplying in the intestinal mucosa or by toxins (enterotoxins) produced by microbes in the intestinal tract following multiplication, sporulation, and/or lysis. Such diseases are referred to as *food-borne infections* and are exemplified by *Salmonella sp.* and

Clostridium perfringens. Food-borne intoxication, on the other hand, results from the consumption of preformed microbial toxins in the food. Staphylococcal enterotoxins, which are not destroyed by heat, and botulinum toxin, one of the most potent neurotoxins known, are two examples of this group. In terms of the frequency of occurrence, although *Salmonella sp.* caused the most outbreaks in 1981 (26.4% of total), *Staphylococcus aureus* accounted for the most cases (33.9% of total). Bacterial illness accounted for a total of 74% of the confirmed outbreaks and 93.2% of the confirmed cases of food-borne illness (Table 1). *Clostridium perfringens* was the next most frequent agent involved.

S. aureus is probably the leading cause of food-borne disease worldwide. The organisms are gram positive, nonmotile and nonspore forming cocci, and occur ubiquitously in the environment. Although man is the leading source of food contamination by way of nasal discharge and infected cuts and wounds, the organism can be present in milk derived from mastitic cows and meat derived from arthritic poultry (13). Baked ham, poultry, meat and potato salads, cream-filled bakery goods, and high-protein leftover foods are frequently involved in such intoxication (23). Multiplication of *S. aureus* in raw food products is inhibited by other spoilage organisms present. As a result, only cooked products, subsequently contaminated by infected handlers and stored at warm temperature for several hours before consumption, are capable of causing intoxication (23).

The causative agent is one of six immunologically distinct heat stable proteins (MW 26,000–34,000) called enterotoxins A, B, C, D, E, and F (13,23). In addition, *S. aureus* also produces many other substances such as coagulase, DNase, hemolysins, lipases, fibrinolysin, and hyaluronidase, that are toxic to one or more animal species. Although all strains of *S. aureus* are potentially pathogenic, the enterotoxin production is closely related to coagulase and DNase production. Signs and symptoms begin 1–6 hr after consumption of contaminated food, and include nausea, salivation, vomiting,

retching, occasional diarrhea, abdominal cramps, sweating, dehydration, and weakness. Severe cases may show fever, chills, drop in blood pressure, and prostration. Recovery usually occurs in 1–3 days. Fatalities are rare (13).

Diagnosis of *S. aureus* intoxication involves phage typing and matching of isolated organism in food as well as vomitus from the patients and lesions or nasal swabs from food handlers. Demonstration of the enterotoxin in suspect food by gel diffusion technique is confirmatory. Major preventive measures in reducing the incidence of *S. aureus* food intoxication involve education of food handlers regarding hygienic practices to reduce postcooking contamination of high protein foods and eliminating practices promoting prolonged storage of cooked foods at room temperature before consumption.

Botulism is a neurotoxic syndrome caused by consumption of foods containing a neurotoxin produced by *Clostridium botulinum*. The organism is widely distributed in soil and in the intestinal tracts of animals. It is an anaerobic gram positive, motile rod capable of forming heat-resistant spores. Moisture, a pH above 4.6, and storage under anaerobic conditions for a period of time are required for *C. botulinum* contaminated foods to accumulate sufficient quantity of the toxin (200). If such a product is consumed without sufficient reheating, the likelihood of bolutism increases.

Seven distinct types of neurotoxins A through G, all of which are heat labile, have been isolated from various food products. Common foods involved are home canned vegetables such as beans, corn, leafy vegetables, and especially peppers, all of which contain toxins A and B. Canned fruits are also involved, though to a lesser extent (200). Type E is isolated mostly from fish products and type F from liver paste. All of these toxins can cause botulism in humans, whereas types C and D which cause botulism in animals and birds do not affect humans (23).

Boiling for 3 min or heating at 80°C for 30 min destroys preformed toxin. Another factor in the prevention of botu-

TABLE 1. *Confirmed bacterial food-borne disease outbreaks, cases, and deaths, by agent (United States, 1981)*

Agent	Outbreaks		Cases		Deaths	
	No.	%[a]	No.	%[a]	No.	%[a]
Bacillus cereus	8	3.2	74	0.9	0	0.0
Campylobacter jejuni	10	4.0	487	5.6	0	0.0
Clostridium botulinum	11	4.4	22	0.3	1	3.1
Clostridium perfringens	28	11.2	1,162	13.4	2	6.3
Salmonella	66	26.4	2,456	26.8	21	65.6
Shigella	9	3.6	351	4.1	0	0.0
Staphylococcus aureus	44	17.6	2,934	33.9	1	3.1
Streptococcus Group A	2	0.8	307	3.5	0	0.0
Streptococcus Group D	1	0.4	24	0.3	0	0.0
Vibrio cholerae non-01	1	0.4	4	<0.1	0	0.0
Vibrio parahaemolyticus	2	0.8	13	0.2	0	0.0
Yersinia enterocolitica	2	0.8	326	3.8	0	0.0
Other	1	0.4	48	0.6	0	0.0
Total:	185	74.0	8,208	93.2	25	78.1

[a] Percent of total confirmed food-borne disease outbreaks for 1981.
Data from ref. 35.

linum toxin formation in cured meats is the concentration of nitrite. An inverse relationship exists between the concentration of nitrite initially added to the food and the probability of toxin formation (see ref. 78). If the recent scientific and public pressure is successful in decreasing the nitrite content of foods as a means of decreasing the levels of carcinogenic nitrosamines, it is conceivable that the incidence of botulism from the consumption of cured meats and fish as well as fermented sausages will increase.

Studies with type E toxin (MW 350,000) indicated that the botulinum toxin is stable in the acid pH of the stomach where it is protected from the gastric juice and pepsin by a nontoxic component of the toxin molecule. Once in the duodenum, it is activated by trypsin with no change in molecular size (200) and subsequently absorbed into lymphatics. Botulinum toxin irreversibly binds to the myoneural junction and prevents the release of acetylcholine (ACh) at the peripheral cholinergic nerve endings with no effect on ACh synthesis or on the activity of cholinesterase. The toxin has no effect on the CNS (200).

Signs and symptoms of botulism usually appear 12–24 hr (range: 2 hr to 6 days) following consumption of botulinogenic food. Initial signs of nausea, vomiting, and diarrhea are followed later by predominantly neurologic signs including headache, dizziness, blurred vision, weakness of facial muscles, loss of light reflex, and pharyngeal paralysis (difficulty in speech and swallowing). Fever is absent. Sensory reflex and mental status are normal. Paralysis of the respiratory muscles leads to failure of respiration and death, usually in 3–10 days (217). In survivors, partial paralysis might persist 6–8 months and recovery is associated with growth of new fibrils outside the area of old fibrils. Food-borne botulism can be prevented by proper home as well as commercial canning, boiling vegetables for at least 3 min before serving, discarding all swollen and damaged canned products after boiling, and the use of a C. botulinum toxoid to protect individuals involved in research and testing. Control of cases of botulism involves the use of monovalent (E), bivalent (A and B), or polyvalent (A, B, and E) antitoxin, recall of all involved commercial products, and epidemiologic investigation and reporting of the extent of the problem.

Bacillus cereus, considered a harmless saprophyte, is a gram positive, spore-forming aerobe implicated in a number of non-food-borne infections including bronchopneumonia, meningitis, endocarditis, osteomyelitis, bovine mastitis, and wound infection. The majority of food-borne disease outbreaks have occurred in Northern and Eastern Europe. A diarrheal illness involving a wide variety of meats and vegetables, various desserts, fish, pasta, milk, and ice cream (similar to that of C. perfringens), and a vomiting illness involving cereals and fried rice served in Chinese restaurants (similar to that of S. aureus) are both apparently caused by B. cereus (80). A comparison between these three syndromes is presented in Table 2.

Two mouse lethal factors appear to be produced by the organism in food: One is unstable, possesses dermonecrotic, intestinonecrotic activity, and increases vascular permeability causing fluid accumulation and diarrhea; The other is a heat-stable emetic toxin (MW < 5,000). Toxin production occurs when foods are kept warm for several hours and/or cooled slowly.

C. perfringens, in addition to causing gangrene, appendicitis, puerperal fever, and enteritis in humans by non-food-borne routes, frequently causes food-borne infections which subsequently lead to sporulation of the organism in the large intestine. The enterotoxin (lecithinase), released during sporulation of the bacteria, is capable of causing fluid accumulation in the intestines. Lecithinase, also called α-toxin, possesses lethal, necrotizing as well as hemolytic activities, and is produced in greatest quantities by type A organisms. Among the five antigenically (toxicologically) distinct types of C. perfringens (type A through E), type A is almost always involved in food-borne gastroenteritis in humans in the United States. Type C produces two different (lethal-necrotizing and hemolytic) toxins and has caused only two outbreaks of sometimes fatal enteritis necroticans in Europe (92). Only meat and fish products are involved due to the availability of all the amino acids and growth factors required for growth of C. perfringens. Roast beef, beef stew, gravy, and meat pies for type A, and pork, other meats, and fish for type C are frequently involved (23). Typically, foods involved are cooked at <100°C for less than an hour and are subsequently kept warm or slowly cooled. Spores that survive the heat shock multiply faster in the food than those not subjected to heat treatment, and also are capable of elaborating greater quantities of enterotoxin in the gut.

Several mechanisms of action of the enterotoxin in the intestinal lumen have been proposed. The first suggests cholinergic action from phosphatidylcholine formed as a result of the action of lecithinase on lecithin in the diet. Alternately, or even at the same time, cholera toxin-like action involving active secretion of chloride ions into the lumen leading to retention of sodium and sequestration of water in the lumen has been proposed. The third mechanism suggests vascular endothelial effects leading to vasodilation in the gut with resultant increase in permeability (92).

TABLE 2. *Comparison of food poisoning caused by* Clostridium perfringens, Bacillus cereus, *and* Staphylococcus aureus

Variable	C. perfringens	B. cereus	B. cereus	S. aureus
Incubation period (hr)	8–22	8–16	1–5	2–6
Duration of illness (hr)	12–14	12–24	6–24	6–24
Diarrhea	Extremely common	Extremely common	Fairly common	Common
Vomiting	Rare	Occasional	Extremely common	Extremely common
Foods most frequently implicated	Cooked meat and poultry	Meat products, soups, vegetables, puddings, and sauces	Fried rice from Chinese restaurants and take-out shops	Cooked meat and poultry and dairy products

From ref. 80, with permission.

Signs of intoxication are mainly related to diarrhea with occasional fever, vomiting, shock, and rare death in the elderly. Outbreaks usually involve banquets, and meals served in hospitals, nursing homes, and schools. Due to the ubiquitous distribution of the organism in soil and in the gastrointestinal tract of man and animals, prevention of contamination is difficult. Multiplication and toxin production can be inhibited by heating food to proper temperatures (165–212°F), prompt and effective cooling, and avoiding prolonged reheating before consumption.

Salmonella sp. consists of over 1800 serotypes possessing somatic O, flagellar H, and capsular Vi antigens, of which 50 serotypes commonly occur. *S. typhi, S. paratyphi,* and *S. sendai* are adapted to human hosts which serve as sole carriers for those organisms. Feces of infected man, domestic and wild animals, and birds serve as sources of contamination of a variety of meat and milk products, causing severe gastrointestinal signs along with fever and septicemia. Mortality is rare and occurs in very young and very old patients. Although enteritis is a direct result of bacterial multiplication and penetration of the mucosa, the role of enterotoxins secreted by some serotypes cannot be ruled out. Fever is thought to result from the absorption of endotoxins (21). Thorough cooking of meats, pasteurization of milk and dairy and egg products; prevention of cross-contamination between cooked and raw products; and finally testing, isolation, and treatment of carrier animals and food handling personnel are all extremely important in controlling the incidence of this most common food-borne disease (21,23).

Recently, *Vibrio fetus,* an organism isolated originally in 1919 from bovine abortus and blood of some humans suffering from gastroenteritis, was found to differ from vibrios. The renamed organism *Campylobacter jejuni* and other species (*C. sputorum*) are frequently associated with food-borne disease similar to salmonellosis in many respects. Culture supernatant of *C. jejuni* was shown to induce a secretory response in jejunal segments of rats, suggesting the presence of toxins contributing to the loss of fluid through the gastrointestinal tract (67). Other bacterial species including *Vibrio cholerae* (cholera), certain strains of *Shigella dysenteriae* (bacillary dysentery), *Escherichia coli* (diarrhea), and *Pseudomonas cocovenenans* (Bangkrek poisoning) cause disease syndromes that result, at least in part, from toxins elaborated by the organisms. Alternately, there are organisms such as *Arizona hinshawii,* nonenterotoxigenic *Shigella spp., V. parahemolyticus,* and beta hemolytic *Streptococcus pyogenes* that cause enteric disease by way of multiplication and colonization of the gastrointestinal tract. The reader is referred to reviews by Bryan (22,23) for further information. Certain viral (e.g., hepatitis A) and parasitic (e.g., trichinosis) diseases are also transmitted through food, with no known involvement of toxic products. Problems arise mostly from consumption of infected seafood (shell fish) and meats (pork) without adequate cooking (23).

Mycotoxins

Mycotoxins are secondary fungal metabolites produced in animal feed and human food ingredients that cause adverse biological effects when consumed in sufficient quantities. Secondary metabolites perform minor or no obvious function in the metabolic scheme of the organism and are products of reactions that branch off at limited number of steps such as those involving acetate, pyruvate, melonate, mevalonate, shikimate, and amino acids (220). From the standpoint of human and animal health, molds belonging to the genera *Aspergillus, Fusarium,* and *Penicillium* have received most attention owing to their frequent occurrence in food and feed commodities. The storage fungi *Aspergillus sp.* and *Penicillium sp.* typically do not invade intact grain prior to harvest (234), whereas *Fusarium sp.* along with others such as *Alternaria sp.* are predominantly field (preharvest) fungi. Unfavorable conditions such as drought and damage of seeds by insects or during mechanical harvesting can enhance mycotoxin production during both growth and storage. Toxin production can take place over a wide range of moisture (10–33%), relative humidity (>70%), and temperature (4–35°C) depending on the fungal organism involved (39).

Following the discovery of aflatoxins and their potent carcinogenicity, the search for mycotoxins in the last three decades has led to the identification of more than a hundred toxigenic fungal organisms and mycotoxins throughout the world; the public health significance, however, of most of these remains unknown. A summary of experimental and domestic animal studies as well as some current epidemiologic associations of mycotoxins with human disease is pertinent.

Ergots

The history of human mycotoxicoses dates back to the Middle Ages when ergotism (St. Anthony's fire) was the scourge of Central Europe (9). Ergotism, which is now rare, was first associated with the consumption of scabrous (ergotized) grain in the mid-16th century (27). Subsequent studies led to the identification of *Claviceps purpurea* as the fungal agent invading rye, oats, wheat and Kentucky bluegrass and *C. paspali* invading Dallis grass. Lysergic acid derivatives, the amine and amino acid alkaloids of ergot, were identified as the causative agents of the gangrenous (*C. purpurea*) and nervous (*C. paspali*) forms of the disease. Gangrenous ergotism typically manifested as prickly and intense hot and cold sensations in the limbs, and swollen, inflamed, necrotic, and gangrenous extremities which eventually sloughed off. Convulsive ergotism was characterized by CNS signs, numbness, cramps, severe convulsions, and death. Both syndromes have been documented in the recent literature in domestic animals consuming ergotized grains (176) and in humans treated with ergotamine for migraine headaches (see ref. 211).

Ergot alkaloids are smooth muscle stimulants, promoting vasoconstriction (leading to gangrenous ergotism) and inducing uterine contractions (oxytocic effect). Van Rensburg and Altenkirk (242) reviewed evidence indicating that ergot alkaloids antagonize serotonin and block both the stimulatory and inhibitory CNS responses of epinephrine. The United States Department of Agriculture (USDA) grains division has set a tolerance limit of 0.3% (by weight) of contaminated grain in commercial trade.

Trichothecenes

In the first half of the 20th century, a large human mycotoxicosis was reported in Russia (106). The disease, termed alimentary toxic aleukia (ATA), was characterized by total atrophy of the bone marrow, agranulocytosis, necrotic angina, sepsis, hemorrhagic diathesis, and mortality ranging from 2 to 80%. It was later linked to the consumption of overwintered cereal grains and wheat or bread made from them. *Fusarium poae* and *F. sporotrichioides,* now considered synonymous with *F. tricinctum,* grow on these grains and have been shown to produce several trichothecene toxins including T-2 toxin (Fig. 4), neosolaniol, HT-2 toxin, and T-2 tetraol (154). Lutsky et al. (133) reproduced similar signs of ATA in cats given pure T-2 toxin orally.

Several outbreaks of a seasonal intoxication in horses and cattle caused by consumption of hay contaminated with *Stachybotys atra* (*S. alternans*) have been reported from Russia between 1930 and 1960 (27). Two forms, the atypical or typical, of intoxication reflecting acute or chronic exposure are characterized by sudden onset of neurological signs (loss of vision, poor control of movements, and tremors) or signs of dermonecrosis, leukopenia and gastrointestinal ulceration and hemorrhages, respectively. In these regions, humans may exhibit severe dermatitis following handling of or sleeping on contaminated hay. Inhalation of dust from the infected hay can result in rhinitis, fever, chest pain, and leukopenia (27). Eppley (57) reported the isolation of five trichothecene compounds of which three belonged to the group of macrocyclics, roridin-verrucarin, containing a conjugated butadiene system attached to the trichothecene structure.

A group of trichothecene toxins including nivalenol and fusarinon-X, containing carbonyl group at position 8 and different hydroxy and acetoxy substitution at the 3, 4, 6, and

AFLATOXINS

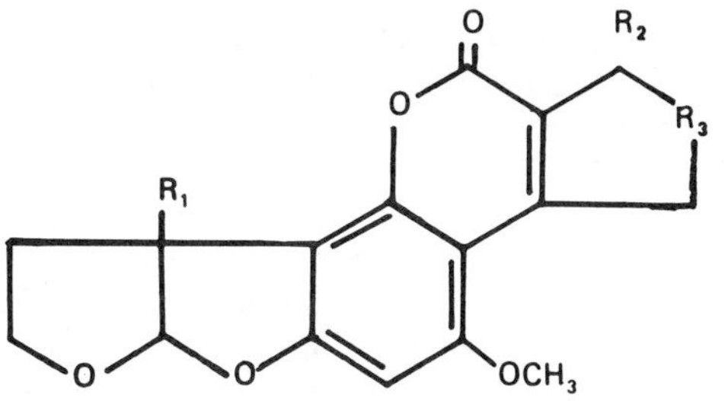

	R_1	R_2	R_3
Aflatoxin B_1	H	C	O
Aflatoxin G_1	H	O	O
Aflatoxin M_1	OH	C	O
Aflatoxicol	H	C	OH

TRICHOTHECENES

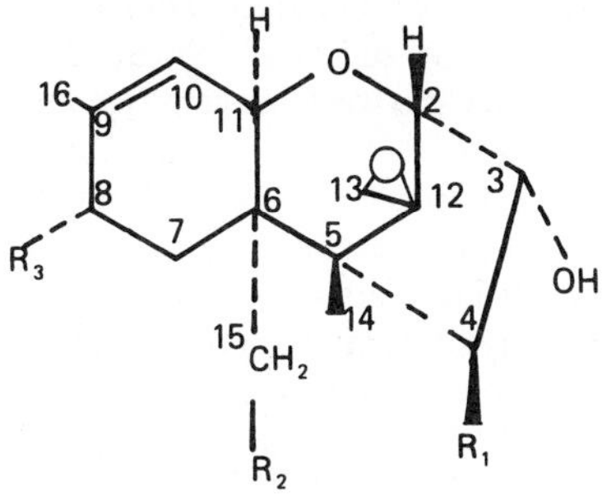

T-2 toxin $R_1=R_2=CH_3COO$-, $R_3=(CH_3)_2CHCH_2COO$-;
HT-2 toxin $R_1=OH$, $R_2=CH_3COO$-, $R_3=(CH_3)_2CHCH_2COO$-
Neosolaniol $R_1=CH_3COO$-, $R_3=OH$, $R_2=CH_3COO$-;
Diacetoxyscirpenol $R_1=R_2=CH_3COO$-, $R_3=H$;
Monoacetoxyscirpenol $R_1=OH$, $R_2=CH_3COO$-, $R_3=H$.

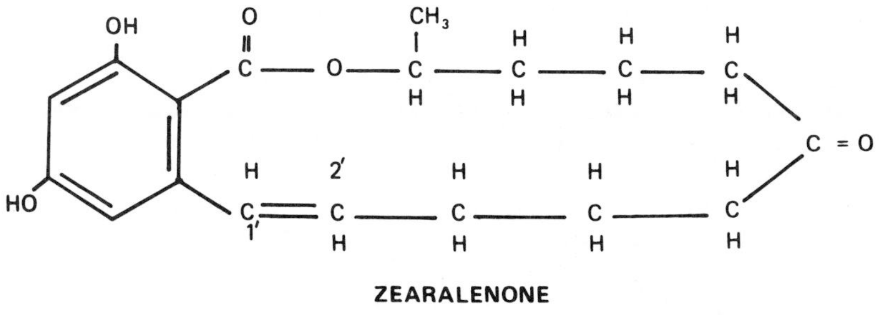

ZEARALENONE

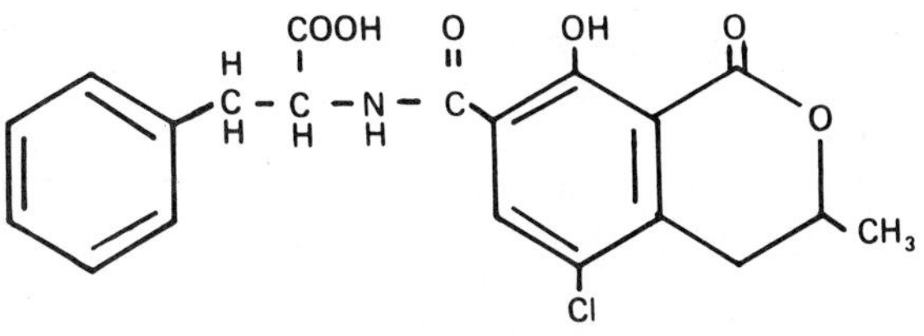

OCHRATOXIN A

FIG. 4. Structure of some common mycotoxins, aflatoxins, trichothecenes, ochratoxin A, and zearalenone.

7 positions, is produced by *F. nivale* in the flowering grain-head of wheat, barley, rice, corn, other cereals, and certain forage grasses. The disease in cereal grains called *red-mold disease* (akakabi-byo) or *black spot disease* (kokuten-byo) has been associated with intoxications in humans, horses, and sheep in Japan. Symptoms in humans include headaches, vomiting, and diarrhea, with no fatalities (27). *F. roseum,* capable of producing deoxynevalenol and its acetylated derivatives on rice and barley, was also isolated suggesting multiple causation.

F. solani, known to produce T-2 toxin and neosolaniol, has been isolated from bean hulls incriminated in a disease (bean hull poisoning) in horses characterized by retarded reflexes, decreased heart rate, disturbed respiration, cyclic movements, convulsions, and death in 10 to 15% of the affected horses (238).

Other diseases attributable to trichothecenes include dendrodochiotoxicosis in horses, sheep, and pigs in Russia that ingested feedstuffs contaminated with *Myrothecium roridum* (produces roridins and verrucarins); various syndromes reported in the United States and Canada involving corn (moldy corn toxicosis) and cereal grains consumed by farm animals (T-2 toxin and others); and finally the alleged use of trichothecene toxins as chemical warfare agent (yellow rain) in Southeast Asia (106,248).

Although many fungal genera such as *Fusarium, Myrothecium,* and *Stachybotrys* can produce these toxins, most trichothecenes of health significance are produced by *Fusarium spp.* Despite the diversity of human and animal diseases associated with this group of toxins, characteristic signs and symptoms of radiomimetic damage such as emesis, feed refusal, irritation and necrosis of skin and mucus membranes, hemorrhage, destruction of thymus and bone marrow, hematologic changes, nervous disturbances, and necrotic angina are common to all toxic syndromes (238). Feed-refusal and vomiting are common problems in farm animals, especially swine, in the midwestern United States and are associated predominantly with the presence of the trichothecene deoxynevalenol (vomitoxin) in wheat and corn. Although T-2 toxin and diacetoxyscirpenol (DAS) can also cause emesis and feed-refusal, their role in the swine feed-refusal syndrome appears negligible because of their rare presence in food and feed commodities in the United States (176). For a comprehensive review of the effects of environmental trichothecenes on domestic animals, the reader is referred to Osweiler et al. (176). Trichothecenes (T-2 toxin) can cause fetal death and abortions along with tail and limb abnormalities in rodent offspring (89). Although fusarinon-X and T-2 toxin are mutagenic at high doses in bacterial and yeast systems (169,205), trichothecenes exhibit no mutagenic effect in most other systems. Carcinogenic effects of trichothecenes still need to be addressed systematically, both in epidemiologic and experimental settings.

Metabolism of trichothecenes occurs rapidly through deacetylation and hydroxylation and subsequent glucuronidation in the liver and kidneys (77). Trichothecenes are generally recognized as potent inhibitors of protein synthesis in eukaryotic systems, inhibiting initiation, elongation as well as termination of protein synthesis by way of their inhibition of peptidyl transferase activity, and also their ability to cause disaggregation of polysomes (147). T-2 toxin, DAS, nivalenol, and fusarenon-X inhibit initiation whereas trichodermin, crotocin, and verrucarol inhibit elongation or termination. Many of the toxic effects of trichothecenes can be explained by this mechanism. Despite the severe toxic effects of trichothecenes, their low frequency of occurrence in nature, their rapid metabolism to apparently nontoxic metabolites in animals, and their low potential for residue transfer to humans reduce the risk of human disease to extremely low levels, if not completely. Farm animals, however, are at a higher risk of intoxication than humans because of the greater likelihood of consumption of trichothecenes in moldy feeds.

Aflatoxins

It was not until the early 1960s, that aflatoxins were discovered as the causative agents of *turkey X disease* in England, which resulted in the death of thousands of turkey poults, ducklings, and chicks that were fed diets containing *Aspergillus flavus*-contaminated peanut meal. This outbreak coupled with the reported carcinogenicity of the aflatoxins in experimental animals (4) helped fuel the scientific curiosity surrounding this group of food contaminants.

The aflatoxins are a group of highly substituted coumarins containing a fused dihydrofuran moiety (Fig. 4). Four major aflatoxins designated B_1, B_2, G_1, and G_2 (based on blue or green fluorescence under ultraviolet light) are produced in varying quantities in a variety of grains and nuts that have not been adequately dried at harvest and stored at relatively high temperatures (28). Commodities most often shown to contain aflatoxins are peanuts, various other nuts, cottonseed, corn, and figs. In addition to *A. flavus, A. parasiticus* and to a minor extent some species of *Penicillium* may be capable of producing aflatoxins (252). Human exposure can occur from consumption of aflatoxins from these sources and the products derived from them, as well as from tissues and the milk (aflatoxin M_1) of food animals consuming contaminated feeds.

Aflatoxin B_1 (AFB$_1$), the most potent and most commonly occurring aflatoxin has been shown to be acutely toxic (LD_{50} 0.3–9.0 mg/kg) to all species of animals, birds, and fishes tested. Sheep and mice are the most resistant whereas cats, dogs, and rabbits are the most sensitive species. Acute effects in animals include death without signs, or signs of anorexia, depression, ataxia, dyspnea, anemia, and hemorrhages from body orifices. In subchronic cases, icterus, hypoprothrombinemia, hematomas, and gastroenteritis are common (176). Chronic aflatoxicosis is more prevalent in domestic animals and is likely to occur in humans. Chronic aflatoxicosis is characterized by bile duct proliferation, periportal fibrosis, icterus, and cirrhosis of liver, and is associated with loss of weight, and reduced resistance to disease (176).

Dietary levels as low as 0.3 ppm can cause such effects. Prolonged exposure to low levels leads to hepatoma, cholangiocarcinoma, or hepatocellular carcinoma and other tumors (28). Osborne and Hamilton (173) described a lipid malabsorption syndrome in poultry characterized by decreased pancreatic lipase and steatorrhea. Reductions in serum triglycerides, cholesterol, phospholipids, and carotenoids were also seen following AFB$_1$ exposure. Mutagenicity of AFB$_1$ has been demonstrated in many systems including HeLa cells,

Bacillus subtilis, Neurospora crossa, and *Salmonella typhimurium* (reverse mutation). Metabolic activation of AFB$_1$ was required in most systems, (28). Aflatoxin B$_1$ is primarily metabolized by microsomal mixed function oxidase system in the liver and other organs forming, in addition to many hydroxylated detoxified products which subsequently are conjugated and excreted, a variety of reactive products that interact with various macromolecules such as DNA.

Swenson et al. (229) isolated 2,3-dihydro-2,3-dihydroxy AFB$_1$ as a product of mild acid hydrolysis of RNA-AFB$_1$ adduct. Aflatoxin B$_2$, which lacks unsaturation at the 2,3-position of the terminal furan ring, failed to form adducts. This led to the suggestion that AFB$_1$-2,3-epoxide was the reactive precursor. Essigman et al. (58) and Croy et al. (44) identified the N^7-guanyl residue of DNA as the major site of epoxide interaction. Hsieh (99) suggested subsequent formation of repair resistant adduct, apurination or error-prone DNA repair leading to single strand breaks, base-pair substitution, or frame shift mutations. Mispairing of the adduct could lead to transversion-type mutations. Involvement of oncogenes in such interactions may result in oncogene activation (99). In addition, AFB$_1$ inhibits DNA synthesis, DNA-dependent RNA polymerase activity, messenger RNA synthesis, and protein synthesis (97). Inhibition of protein synthesis may be related to several lesions and signs of aflatoxicosis including fatty liver (failure to mobilize fats from the liver), coagulopathy (inhibition of prothrombin synthesis), and reduced immune function.

In addition to aflatoxin contamination of foods such as peanuts and corn, aflatoxins and their metabolites can occur also in animal tissues. Especially important is the metabolite aflatoxin M$_1$, a ring hydroxylation product of AFB$_1$, present mainly in milk of AFB$_1$ exposed dairy animals. Hsieh (98) calculated the average daily *per capita* consumption of AFB$_1$ and AFM$_1$ in human populations in the United States as 25.73 ng/kg body weight (BW) and 0.3 ng/kg BW, respectively. Using the epidemiologic data generated from Asia and Africa by Carlborg (32) a lifetime risk of liver cancer was calculated to be 10 deaths/100,000/1 ng AFB$_1$/kg BW/day. McKay's (146) liver cancer statistics in United States males translate to a rate of 3.24/100,000, which corresponds to a lifetime risk of 227/100,000 (106/100,000 following background correction) and an AFB$_1$ exposure of 10.6 ng/kg BW/day. This suggests that United States males are twice as resistant to AFB$_1$ hepatocarcinogenicity as the males in Asia and Africa. Hsieh (98) considers the carcinogenicity of AFM$_1$ to be two orders of magnitude lower than that of AFB$_1$, which translates to a negligible lifetime risk for adult humans for liver cancer from AFM$_1$. However, in view of the higher susceptibility of young animals to AFB$_1$ carcinogenicity (244), the effect of AFM$_1$ on human infants needs to be evaluated separately. Evidence of the role of aflatoxins in human cancer and other diseases has been reviewed by Busby and Wogan (28) and Shank (211).

Other less widespread human clinical syndromes in which aflatoxins have been implicated include acute hepatitis (aflatoxicosis) in India; Taiwan, and certain countries in Africa; childhood cirrhosis in India, and possibly Reye's syndrome in many parts of the world (211). Reye's syndrome is a childhood neurologic disease that resembles viral encephalitis and actually involves a viral prodrome followed by rapid progression into coma and convulsions leading to death. Characteristic lesions include enlarged, pale, fatty liver and kidneys and severe cerebral edema. Evidence from Thailand and other countries including the United States (93,216) associates aflatoxin consumption or high levels of AFB$_1$ in victims' tissues with Reye's syndrome. Burgeois et al. (26) produced a syndrome strikingly similar to Reye's in monkeys given 4.5–13.5 mg/kg of AFB$_1$ orally. Epidemiologic evidence, however, also suggested a link between the use of aspirin and Reye's syndrome prompting the United States Surgeon General to advise against the use of salicylates in children with chickenpox or influenza (41).

Widespread concern regarding the toxic effects of aflatoxins in humans and animals and the possible transfer of residues from animal tissues and milk to humans has led to regulatory actions governing the interstate as well as global transport and consumption of aflatoxin-contaminated food and feed commodities. Action levels of aflatoxins in corn and other feed commodities used to feed mature nonlactating animals is 100 ppb, although temporary increases in limits are allowed on a case-by-case basis by the FDA in situations such as drought where availability of uncontaminated corn is extremely limited. For commodities destined for human consumption and interstate commerce, the action limit is 20 ppb. For milk, the action level of AFM$_1$ is 0.5 ppb. Among the many approaches tried to limit the aflatoxin contamination of grain, prevention of stress, the use of fungus-resistant varieties of grains, avoiding mechanical injury to grain during harvesting, drying of grains to contain less than 12% moisture, and strict control of humidity during storage are important to prevent AFB$_1$ production.

Ochratoxins

In 1957 and 1958, up to 75% of the households in several villages located in the valley floor in contiguous areas of Yugoslavia, Romania, and Bulgaria were found to be affected by chronic nephropathy (Balkan or endemic nephropathy). Although genetic factors appear to be partially involved, Krogh and co-workers (121) presented evidence implicating a mycotoxin, ochratoxin A (Fig. 4), produced in foodstuffs by *Aspergillus ochraceus* and a number of other aspergilli and penicillia, consumed at higher levels more frequently by people in these endemic areas compared with areas free from nephropathy. In addition, a remarkably similar nephropathy was identified in swine (porcine nephropathy) in Denmark (121) and in swine and bovine in the United States (130). Signs include lassitude, fatigue, anorexia, abdominal (epigastric or diffuse) pain, and severe anemia followed by signs of renal damage. Reduced concentrating ability, reduced renal plasma flow, and decreased glomerular filtration occur sequentially, accompanied by gross and microscopic renal changes including dystrophy, necrosis, fibrosis with some tubular regeneration, glomerular hyalinization, and interstitial sclerosis. Death results from uremia (211).

The ochratoxins, a group of seven isocoumarin derivatives linked with phenylalanine by an amide bond, are found in barley, corn, wheat, oats, rye, green coffee beans, and peanuts (29). In experimental animals, ochratoxin A produces renal lesions and liver degeneration. The acute LD$_{50}$ ranges between 2 ppm in birds and 59 ppm in mice. In poultry, ochratoxin A causes reduced weight gains and decreased egg shell quality and egg production in addition to the renal effects (176). Teratogenic effects of ochratoxin A in rodents include malformations of the head, jaws, tail, limbs, and heart (29,89). Ochratoxins are not mutagenic in several assay systems tested but appear to induce hepatomas and renal adenomas in 30% of the mice exposed to 40 ppm in the diet (108).

Ochratoxin A is hydrolyzed by carboxypeptidase A and α-chymotrypsin to nontoxic ochratoxin α. Absorbed ochratoxin A distributes mainly to the kidney and liver and is excreted in the urine and feces (50% and 20% of total in 24 hr). Ochratoxin A inhibits mitochondrial respiration and reduces ATP levels, these effects also being produced by nontoxic ochratoxin α. Depletion of glycogen, inhibition of gluconeogenesis, a pathway that accounts for 50–60% of the blood glucose in the starved or diabetic stage, and several key cyclic adenosine monophosphate (cAMP)-mediated enzymes in this pathway, including phosphoenolpyruvate carboxykinase by ochratoxin A, have received major attention in recent years. These effects seem to be mediated by a 50% decrease in multiple species of mRNA involved in the synthesis of these enzymes (148). However, whether any of these enzymatic steps is the critical target in the pathogenesis of ochratoxicosis and whether this response is limited to kidneys remain to be investigated.

Psoralens

Psoralens are furocoumarin compounds that have been used in repigmenting achromatic skin lesions in an acquired disease called vitiligo. Psoralens are in some suntan lotions and in drugs used to treat psoriasis (30). Abuse of such compounds can result in dermatitis following exposure to the sun as well as nausea, vomiting, vertigo, and mental excitation. A phototoxic dermatitis in celery pickers has also been linked to the presence of psoralens (8-methoxypsoralen, 5-methoxypsoralen, and trimethylpsoralen) in stalks infected with *Sclerotinia sclerotiorum* (pink rot), *S. rolfsii, Rhizoctonia solani* or *Erwinia aroideae,* or celery stalks soaked in 5% NaCl (211). In addition to celery, fig, parsley, parsnip, lime, and clove also contain psoralens. Unlike other photosensitizing agents, psoralens seem to act by photoreacting with DNA and to a lesser extent with RNA. Treatment with 8-methoxypsoralen and ultraviolet light induced squamous cell carcinomas of the ear in mice (30). Psoralens are rapidly excreted in the urine as fluorescent nontoxic metabolites, carboxypsoralen being one of the major metabolites. 8-Methoxypsoralen, however, appears to undergo epoxidation of the furan ring similar to aflatoxins and may thus react with DNA in a similar fashion.

The mechanism of psoralen photosensitivity appears to involve intercalation and crosslinking psoralen in the DNA which occurs in three steps: (a) reversible intercalation of psoralen between two pyrimidines on opposing sides of the helix; (b) formation of a monoadduct with the 5,6-double bond of the pyrimidine following absorption of 1 quantum of ultraviolet light; and (c) the crosslink formation by absorption of a second quantum of ultraviolet light and linking of the monoadduct to the 5,6-double bond of thymidine

(207). In general, there is an excellent correlation between photoadduct formation and photosensitization of psoralens.

Citreoviridin (Yellow Rice Toxin)

Acute cardiac beriberi (Shoshin-Kakke), characterized by palpitation, nausea, vomiting, rapid and difficult breathing, cold and cyanotic extremities, rapid pulse, abnormal heart sounds, low blood pressure, restlessness, and violent mania leading to respiratory failure and death, was observed in Japan in the late 1800s and early 1900s (239). The following pieces of evidence together eliminate avitaminosis as the cause of cardiac beriberi and suggest citreoviridin as the etiological agent: the growth of a variety of penicillia including *P. citreoviride* on polished rice consumed by this population; subsequent isolation of a number of toxic compounds such as anthraquinones, islandicin, catenarin, leuteoskyrin, rubroskyrin, iridoskyrin, skyrin, cyclochlorotine, islanditoxin, and erythroskyrin from *P. islandienum,* and the dark yellow toxic metabolite citreoviridin from *P. citreoviride;* experimental production of neurologic syndrome and respiratory failure in rats given crude extract of *P. citreoviride* contaminated rice; and recovery of animals suffering from avitaminosis following supplementation with livers from victims of acute cardiac beriberi. Other toxins identified failed to produce signs resembling cardiac beriberi (211). In 1921, the Japanese government passed the Rice Act to reduce the availability of moldy rice in markets. The act resulted in a sharp decrease in the disease during the same year (39), while maintaining rice as a prominent dietary ingredient. This provides additional support for the involvement of mycotoxins in the causation of cardiac beriberi.

Bishydroxycoumarin (Dicoumarol)

Dicoumarol is a Vit K antagonist which acts to inhibit epoxide reductase, an enzyme that plays a major role in the reactivation of Vit K that has been inactivated during its function in the synthesis of clotting factors II, VII, IX, and X (see ref. 176). Resulting effects lead to bleeding disorders and death from blood loss from undetectable bleeding sites. Naturally occurring coumarins in sweet clover (*Melilotus sp.*) hay are dimerized to dicoumarol as a result of fungal spoilage during curing. Cattle consuming such hay were poisoned in the 1920s in North Dakota and Alberta (211). Most human poisonings result from therapeutic accidents involving coumarin therapy of clotting disorders.

Zearalenone

In addition to zearalenone and zearalenol being contaminants in grains such as corn, wheat, sorghum, barley, and oats, zearalanol, a synthetic analog of zearalenol (Ralgro) is used as an anabolic agent in cattle. Under natural conditions, zearalenone and its derivatives are produced by *Fusarium roseum* mostly in ear corn stored in cribs. Zearalenone, despite its structural dissimilarity with estrogens (Fig. 4), induces effects consistent with those produced by excessive steroidal as well as synthetic estrogens, i.e., anabolic and uterotropic activities and regulation of serum gonadotropins. Among the domestic animals, swine appear to be the most sensitive, exhibiting signs of hyperestrogenic syndrome, i.e., swollen and edematous vulva, hypertrophic myometrium, vaginal cornification, and prolapse in extreme cases (176).

Gentry (79) summarized the mode of action of zearalenone as involving interaction with estrogen receptors, translocation of receptor–zearalenone complex to the nucleus, combination with chromatin receptors, selective RNA transcription leading to biochemical effects including increased water and lowered lipid content in muscle, increased permeability of uterus to glucose, RNA, and protein precursors. Zearalenone induces biphasic changes in luteinizing hormone but not follicle-stimulating hormone in serum (31). Available evidence indicates that rapid metabolism of zearalenone and zearalanol to conjugated metabolites to be excreted in urine and feces makes consumption of meat and milk from animals receiving Ralgro an insignificant risk to humans.

Recent evidence from Italy (60) and Puerto Rico (198), however, suggests that estrogenic substances (18), especially residues of zearalenone and zearanol (199) in red meats and poultry, may have caused premature thelarche (development of breasts before age 8) in Italy, and premature thelarche, pubarche, gynecomastia, and precocious pseudopuberty in Puerto Rico. Also, zearalenone has been shown to be mutagenic and carcinogenic in animals (99), suggesting the need to look at the residue issue much more closely.

Other Mycotoxins

A number of other mycotoxins (Table 3) have been identified either as contaminants in foods destined for human consumption, or as metabolites of fungi isolated from human foods (27). Although some of these have been associated with outbreaks of domestic animal diseases, no current link between human consumption and disease has been established. Others have been shown to induce toxic and lethal effects in laboratory animals with no association between consumption of these toxins by animals or humans and a disease syndrome. Several of these, for example, cytochalasins, and secalonic acid D (188), have been used to expand our understanding of normal as well as abnormal cellular responses to xenobiotics. For detailed information on the mycotoxins the reader is referred to reviews by several authors (27,39,176,193,252).

Although it is difficult to assess the total significance of consumption of mycotoxins in human foods, it is easy to conceive that such a task requires extensive research into hundreds of known and potentially at least thousands of as yet unknown mycotoxins. In spite of the vast number of toxic metabolites, prevention of mycotoxicoses in humans and animals can be achieved for the most part by avoiding stress, damage to seeds by pests and during harvesting, rapid postharvest drying, and finally by avoiding conditions conducive to mold growth during storage.

Metals

A high proportion of the total daily exposure to metals by the general population occurs from their natural presence in foods, beverages, water, and air; contact with metal-containing consumer products contributes the rest. Children consume more calories per unit body weight and have a higher absorption rate than adults, placing them at a higher risk than adults (82). Industrial and agricultural uses of metal products pose a hazard of food contamination associated with their use, storage, accidental spillage, and improper disposal. The recent decline in the use of heavy metal based pesticides, including herbicides, makes acute poisonings from dietary toxic metals less likely. A decline in the use of containers with metal coatings that dissolve during food manufacture, cooking, and storage has also contributed to the decline in acute toxicities associated with metals. Food-borne heavy metal intoxications are mostly limited to long-term consumption of water and food products from environments that contain naturally high levels of metals (e.g., selenium and fluoride) or that are contaminated by mining, smelting, and industrial discharge (e.g., methylmercury and Minamata disease). The reader is referred to ref. 237 for information on food and to several reviews on nonfood sources of metal exposure and toxicologic effects and mechanisms (82,95,245).

Arsenic

Most arsenic (As) intoxications in man are either accidental or deliberate (suicidal or homicidal). Occasional exposure to toxic levels of As can occur orally by way of contaminated water and beverages made from such water or by the ingestion of plant foods (fruits and vegetables) containing high levels of surface As applied as a pesticide (48,231). Examples of water-borne As intoxication include a mass poisoning in Chile in the early 1960s and another in Taiwan from artesian well-water in the late 1960s (48). Goiter and deaf-mutism are endemic in certain regions of Argentina where natural water supplies have levels of As as high as 1.4 mg/liter (231). Oregon and Nova Scotia are two regions in North America with high levels of As in natural water supplies. Although seafood such as molluscs, crustaceans, and fishes can accumulate organic forms of As, such foods are unlikely to induce a toxic reaction in the absence of other sources of exposure such as occupational exposure involving smelting and manufacture of pesticides and other agricultural products.

Acute oral arsenic intoxication is characterized by severe gastrointestinal signs including abdominal cramps, vomiting, watery diarrhea, hypotension, loss of urinary output, and cardiovascular collapse in both man and animals. Survivors may experience a reversible sensory loss of the peripheral nervous system after 1 or 2 weeks of exposure accompanied by Wallerian degeneration of axons (48,82). Chronic As toxicosis is characterized by liver injury progressing from hepatomegaly and jaundice to cirrhosis and ascites, peripheral vascular disease (acrocyanosis, Raynaud's phenomenon), loss of hair, loosening of nails with appearance of Mees' lines (transverse white bands across fingernails), skin rash, and hyperkeratosis of palms and soles. Conjunctivitis, bronchitis, laryngitis, and hematologic changes such as anemia, leukopenia, and thrombocytopenia have also been reported. A tragic case of chronic arsenicism was recorded in Japan in babies given formula prepared from contaminated powdered milk (48). Aside from many reversible signs and symptoms described above, concern was raised on possible incidence

TABLE 3. *Miscellaneous mycotoxins*

Mycotoxin	Major producing organisms	Source of fungi	Principal toxic effects
Alternariol and alternariol methyl ether	*Alternaria sp.*	Sorghum, peanuts, wheat	Highly teratogenic to mice; cytotoxic to HeLa cells; lethal to mice
Altenuene, altenuisol	*Alternaria sp.*	Peanuts	Cytotoxic to HeLa cells
Altertoxin I	*Alternaria sp.*	Sorghum, peanuts, wheat	Cytotoxic to HeLa cells; lethal to mice
Ascladiol	*Aspergillus clavatus*	Wheat flour	Lethal to mice
Austamide and congeners	*Aspergillus ustus*	Stored foodstuffs	Toxic to ducklings
Austdiol	*Aspergillus ustus*	Stored foodstuffs	Toxic to ducklings
Austin	*Aspergillus ustus*	Peas	Lethal to chicks
Austocystins	*Aspergillus ustus*	Stored foodstuffs	Toxic to ducklings; cytotoxic to monkey kidney epithelial cells
Chaetoglobosins	*Penicillium aurantiovirens, Chaetomium globosum*	Pecans	Toxic to chicks; cytotoxic to HeLa cells
Citreoviridin	*Penicillium citreoviride*	Rice	Neurotoxic, producing convulsions in mice
Citrinin	*Penicillium viridicatum, Penicillium citrinum*	Corn, barley	Nephrotoxic to swine
Cyclopiazonic acid	*Penicillium cyclopium*	Ground nuts, meat products	Nephrotoxic, enterotoxic
Cytochalasins	*Aspergillus clavatus, Phoma sp., Phomopsis sp.* *Hormiscium sp., Helminthosporium dematioideum, Metarrhizium anisopliae*	Rice, potatoes, Kodo millet, pecans, tomatoes	Cytotoxic to HeLa cells; teratogenic to mice and chickens
Diplodiatoxin	*Diplodia maydis*	Corn	Nephrotoxic and enterotoxic to cattle and sheep
Emodin	*Aspergillus wentii*	Chestnuts	Lethal to chicks
Fumigaclavines	*Aspergillus fumigatus*	Silage	Enterotoxic to chicks
Kojic acid	*Aspergillus flavus*	Squash, spices	Lethal to mice
Malformins	*Aspergillus niger*	Onions, rice	Lethal to rats
Maltoryzine	*Aspergillus oryzae*	Malted barley	Hepatotoxic and causes paralysis
Oosporein (Chaetomidin)	*Chaetomium trilaterale*	Peanuts	Lethal to chicks
Paspalamines	*Claviceps paspali*	Dallisgrass	Neurotoxic to cattle and horses, causes paspalum staggers
Patulin	*Penicillium urticae*	Apple juice	Lethal to mice; mutagenic; teratogenic to chicks; pulmonary effects in dogs; carcinogenic to rats
Penicillic acid	*Penicillium spp.*	Corn, dried beans	Lethal to mice; mutagenic; carcinogenic to rats
PR toxin	*Penicillium roqueforti*	Mixed grains	Hepatotoxic and nephrotoxic to rats; causes abortion in cattle
Roseotoxin B	*Trichothecium roseum*	Corn	Toxic to mice and ducklings
Rubratoxins	*Penicillium rubrum*	Corn	Causes hemorrhage in animals; hepatotoxic to cattle
Secalonic acids	*Aspergillus aculeatus, Penicillium oxalicum*	Rice, corn	Lethal, cardiotoxic, teratogenic, and causes lung irritation in mice
Slaframine	*Rhizoctonia leguminicola*	Red clover	Causes salivation and lacrimation in horses and cattle
Sporidesmins	*Pithomyces chartarum*	Pasture grasses	Hepatotoxic, causes photosensitization in ruminants
Sterigmatocystin	*Aspergillus flavus*	Mammals	Mutagenic carcinogenic, and hepatotoxic to mammals
Tenuazonic acid	*Alternaria sp.*	Grains, nuts	Lethal to mice
Terphenyllins	*Aspergillus candidus*	Wheat flour	Hepatotoxic to mice; cytotoxic to HeLa cells
Tremorgenic Mycotoxins			
Fumitremorgens A and B	*Aspergillus fumigatus*	Rice	Neurotoxic (prolonged tremors and convulsions)

TABLE 3. *Continued*

Mycotoxin	Major producing organisms	Source of fungi	Principal toxic effects
Paxilline	*Penicillium paxilli*	Pecans	Neurotoxic (prolonged tremors and convulsions)
Penitrems A, B, and C	*Penicillium cyclopium*	Peanuts, meat products, cheese	Penitrem A: Neurotoxic (prolonged tremors and convulsions) to cattle, sheep, dogs, and horses
Tryptoquivalines	*Aspergillus clavatus*	Rice	Neurotoxic (prolonged tremors and convulsions)
Verruculogen (TR-1)	*Penicillium verruculosum*	Peanuts	Neurotoxic (prolonged tremors and convulsions)
Unidentified toxin(s)	*Aspergillus terrus, Balansia epichloe, Epichloe typhina, Fusarium tricinctum,* and others	Fescue grass	Gangrene (fescue foot); summer slump syndrome; causes fat necrosis and agalactia in cattle
Xanthoascin	*Aspergillus candidus*	Wheat flour	Hepatotoxic and cardiotoxic to mice

Condensed and modified from ref. 27.

of mental retardation, epilepsy, and other forms of brain damage. Overexposure to certain organic arsenical growth promotants, approved for use in swine and poultry, result predominantly in demyelination and gliosis of peripheral and cranial nerves with no concurrent gastrointestinal or other signs (176).

The biologic half-life of As ranges between 10 and 30 hr. Although both forms of As are absorbed almost completely from the gastrointestinal tract, trivalent arsenicals (e.g., As trioxide, sodium arsenite) are more toxic than pentavalent ones (arsenates, arsanilic acid). Significant interconversion between the two forms *in vivo,* and also biomethylation of inorganic forms to rapidly excretable methylated As are known to occur (82). The key effects mediating As toxicity are its interaction with dihydrolipoic acid cofactor, necessary for substrate oxidation, its inhibition of the enzyme succinate dehydrogenase, and uncoupling of oxidative phosphorylation possibly by competing with phosphate (82), all of which are related to the interaction of As with —SH groups. Due to the abundance of —SH groups, skin, hair, and nails are the sites of accumulation for As. In addition to the characteristic hyperkeratosis, As causes skin cancer in humans in a dose-related manner. Cancer of the lung following occupational exposure and angiosarcoma of the liver following long-term As exposure in drinking water has also been reported. Interestingly, As has not been shown to be a carcinogen in animals following oral or dermal exposure (48). Arsenic can induce chromosomal breakage in human leukocyte cultures (48). In contrast to carcinogenicity, teratogenicity of As has been shown in animals (94) but not in humans. Current limits on exposure to As in the United States are 50 ppb in drinking water and 0.005 mg/cm^3 in the work environment.

Cadmium

Cadmium (Cd) is a biproduct of lead and zinc mining and is used in electroplating (45%), pigment (21%), plastics (15%), alloys (7.5%), batteries (3%), and other (8.5%) industries. In addition, it is also found in industrial sludges, phosphate fertilizers, and cigarettes (62). Human exposure to Cd occurs, in addition to direct exposure from occupations in Cd in-

dustries and to pollution, from plant and animal foods, water, and smoking (53). Food is by far the major source of Cd to the nonsmoking population, with total Cd intake ranging from 5 to 19 µg/day in the United States (187) to greater than 150 µg/day in some parts of Japan (53). Cereal grains, liver, and kidney from contaminated animals, and shellfish contain the highest amounts of Cd. Smoking of 20 cigarettes/day could result in inhalation of 2–4 µg of Cd of which 25–50% (0.5–2 µg) is absorbed via lungs (53). This exceeds the total Cd retention (5% absorption by the gastrointestinal tract) from the average Western diet (0.5–1.5 µg/day).

Absorbed Cd is transported in the blood, bound to RBC, albumin, and other large MW proteins and subsequently taken up by various organs (mainly liver and kidneys). Most Cd in food is bound to organic molecules such as cysteine and tends to accumulate preferentially in kidney whereas inorganic Cd is initially taken up by the liver. Once in the liver, Cd stimulates the synthesis of a low MW —SH-containing protein called metallothionein (MT), which strongly binds Cd. The half-life of Cd has been estimated at 10–30 years in humans. After repeated exposures to smaller doses or after a prolonged period following a single exposure to Cd, the Cd-MT enters the bloodstream and a major portion is filtered by the glomerulus and reabsorbed by proximal tubules, so that as much as half of the total Cd burden is in the kidneys (166).

In addition to the liver and kidneys, pancreas, spleen, and intestinal tissues seem to contain appreciable quantities of Cd, most of which is bound to MT. Cadmium is excreted via urine and feces. Urinary excretion closely parallels the body burden before renal damage. Following renal damage, a drastic increase in Cd excretion parallels a decline in Cd body (kidney) burden. Fecal Cd represents unabsorbed dietary Cd, biliary excretion (minor), and intestinal mucosal sloughing (166). Several nutritional deficiencies (calcium, iron, and protein) enhance Cd absorption, and excess zinc decreases Cd absorption (82).

Acute Cd intoxication is rare and usually results from consumption of contaminated beverages or excessive occupational exposure to Cd fumes or dust. The former type of exposure results in nausea, vomiting, and abdominal pain which regress without residual effects if exposure ceases, whereas the latter may produce acute chemical pneumonitis and pulmonary edema (82). Long-term inhalation exposure, on the other hand, leads to renal tubular disease in addition to obstructive and emphysematous pulmonary lesions. Lung lesions including chronic bronchitis, fibrosis of lower respiratory tract, alveolar damage, and interstitial fibrosis, result from necrosis of alveolar macrophages and subsequent enzyme release (82).

The kidney is the critical organ for long-term Cd exposure with renal tubular and glomerular disease resulting from either inhalational or oral exposure. Reports of chronic toxicosis following oral Cd exposure have come exclusively from Japan, whereas occupational intoxication has occurred in hundreds of workers in Europe, the United States, and Australia. After entering the kidney, Cd-MT accumulates preferentially in the cortex where the lysosomal enzymes break down the MT moiety. The released Cd stimulates MT synthesis and binds to new MT until renal Cd accumulation exceeds the capacity of the kidney to synthesize MT. When the level of non-MT-bound Cd exceeds a certain level (critical concentration), Cd is thought to interfere with the activities of critical biological molecules (e.g., zinc-requiring enzymes) in the kidney and thus cause renal tubular damage (116). Data from Ellis et al. (56) suggest that at a concentration of 190 mg Cd/kg renal cortex, 10% of the population would likely show renal damage. This agrees well with animal data suggesting a critical concentration of 200 mg/kg. Nomiyama and Nomiyama (165) concluded that the critical concentration of non-MT-bound Cd in the kidney cortex of rabbits was as low as 13 mg/kg. A WHO task force estimated that a daily dietary intake of 200–300 μg of Cd/day would be required to reach critical kidney Cd concentrations at the age of 50 for a 70-kg man.

Signs of Cd nephropathy include increased Cd in urine, proteinuria, aminoaciduria, glucosuria, and decreased renal tubular phosphate reabsorption as well as morphologic damage including tubular degeneration leading to interstitial nephritis and fibrosis (82). Proteinuria is predominantly tubular; low MW proteins such as β_2-microglobulin, retinol binding protein, ribonuclease, and light chains of immunoglobulins are excreted as a result of proximal tubular reabsorption failure. In later stages, glomerular disease is indicated by excretion of high MW proteins such as transferrin and albumin (124).

In addition, Cd also affects the skeletal system. These effects, reported predominantly from an endemic area of Japan (Fuchu prefecture), included osteomalacia and/or osteoporosis leading to multiple bone fractures and severe bone pain (*itai-itai* disease meaning "ouch-ouch"). Skeletal effects appear to be brought about by a combination of Cd-induced inhibition of calcium absorption, Vit D hydroxylation in the kidney, lysyl oxidase activity, and normal crosslinkage of collagen fibers (117).

Early associations of hypertension in humans in several parts of the world with increased urinary Cd concentrations, higher renal Cd concentrations, higher renal Cd/zinc ratio, and higher plasma Cd levels remain unconfirmed by more recent studies (see reviews in refs. 19 and 54). Hypertension is not a feature of itai-itai disease. However, people with Cd-induced proteinuria appear to have a mortality rate from cerebrovascular disease twice as high as those without proteinuria (164). Animal studies, however, indicate that low levels of Cd in drinking water could cause hypertension (181) by increasing sodium retention, direct vasoconstriction, increased plasma renin concentrations, and/or increased cardiac output (82).

Several other effects of Cd in experimental animals that await confirmation in human beings include acute testicular necrosis, liver necrosis, pancreatic dysfunction, teratogenic effects, and effects on the nervous and immune systems. Details of these effects are given in two recent reviews (72,150). Epidemiologic evidence, viewed collectively, suggests that Cd inhalation and/or ingestion may cause lung and prostatic cancer. Experimental studies, in general, have supported Cd carcinogenicity (sarcomas at injection sites, and Leydig cell tumors). Cadmium is mutagenic in mammalian cells *in vitro* and in animal systems (55).

In general, Cd effects on kidney are thought to be irreversible. Acute Cd intoxication can be treated with chelators such as dimercaprol (BAL) and penicillamine both of which enhance Cd elimination by biliary excretion, and ethylenediamine tetraacetic acid (EDTA) and diethylenetriamine pentaacetic acid (DTPA) which enhance urinary excretion (37). However, once MT induction has occurred such as in chronic Cd exposure, there appears to be little benefit from chelation therapy. Although dithiocarbamate (DTC) derivatives may effectively mobilize tissue levels of Cd following repeated doses, they are ineffective orally and may cause accumulation of mobilized Cd in some tissues while depleting others of essential metals (75,118). Zinc is known to protect animals from toxic effects of Cd in various organs. Data from Reddy et al. (189) indicate that oral doses of zinc not only mobilized Cd from a number of tissues in mice and reduced total Cd burden but also did not increase Cd in any tissues measured, and at the same time reversed some of the biochemical effects of Cd that could not be reversed by Cd withdrawal alone. Additional work on the possible therapeutic use of zinc in antagonizing chronic Cd toxicity is warranted.

Cobalt

Cobalt (Co) is an essential element (component of Vit B$_{12}$) produced mainly as a biproduct of copper, and is used in high temperature alloys, permanent magnets, paint driers, as catalysts, and in pigments (82). Leafy plants such as lettuce, cabbage, and spinach are relatively high in Co (up to 0.6 ppm). Animal tissues, ambient air, and drinking water are rarely sources of toxic levels of Co. Intoxication in man is usually a result of overzealous therapeutic administration or occupational exposure to various forms of Co. In humans, excessive oral intake has caused gastrointestinal signs and polycythemia; and parenteral Co exposure leads to deafness, palpitation, and hypertension. Cobalt is goitrogenic by both oral and parenteral routes (115). Industrial exposures have caused allergic manifestations (dermatitis, asthma, etc.) and a highly fatal hard metal disease (severe pulmonary fibrosis) in tungsten carbide workers. Addition of Co (1 ppm) to beer as a foam stabilizer and to prevent gushing has been associated with cardiomyopathy in heavy beer drinkers, causing signs of congestive heart failure (82). The FDA banned the use of Co salts in beers in 1966. The role of alcohol in enhancing toxicity of ordinarily nontoxic levels of Co, in this instance, needs further study. In experimental animals, toxicity of Co is moderate (LD$_{50}$ 100–500 mg/kg) causing, in addition to polycythemia, β-cell damage in pancreas and hyperglycemia which has not been reported in humans. Cobalt is carcinogenic in rats at the sites of injection; however, no evidence of carcinogenicity exists in humans (115).

Copper and Molybdenum

Copper (Cu) is an essential element required for iron utilization and for the activity of several enzymes including tyrosinase, cytochrome oxidase, superoxide dismutase, catalase, peroxidase, amine oxidases, and uricase. Despite its widespread use in the past in coloring and preserving of foods, in fungicides, insecticides, and anthelmintics, and its current uses in brass and Cu water pipes and domestic utensils, dietary contamination in the magnitude needed to cause toxic problems in man is rare. Leafy plant foods contain less than 25 ppm of Cu, cereal grains contain 4–6 ppm, and certain fruits and cocoa contain 20–40 ppm. Although organ meats (liver, kidney, etc.), crustacea, and shellfish contain up to 400 ppm of Cu on a dry weight basis, their consumption in human diets is too low to cause problems. Humans, similar to rats and other monogastrics, appear to be resistant to Cu toxicity as long as diets are adequate in iron, zinc, molybdenum (Mo), and sulfate (236). Sheep, however, are susceptible to dietary Cu levels (including normal 8–10 ppm) giving a Cu:Mo ratio of greater than 10:1 (176). Characteristic syndrome in sheep manifests as a severe hemolytic crisis apparently triggered by stress (starvation, shipping, shearing, even Cu withdrawal) following excessive Cu accumulation in liver. Such episodes have also been reported in burn patients treated with Cu compounds as well as following the use of Cu-containing dialysis equipment (82).

Once absorbed, albumin-bound Cu is slowly exchanged to ceruloplasmin (Cu-binding protein) which is subsequently taken up by the liver and stored as MT-bound Cu. Two genetic disorders in man, Wilson's disease and Menke's disease, and a genetic disorder similar to Wilson's disease in certain breeds of dogs, occur following the consumption of diets with normal Cu levels. Wilson's disease is characterized by abnormalities of, and excessive Cu accumulation in, the liver, brain, kidneys, and cornea, and by low serum ceruloplasmin and high serum Cu. In dogs, abnormalities of the liver are prominent. Penicillamine and trien (triethylene tetramine) are used to chelate Cu in both humans (247) and dogs. Patients with Menke's disease, on the other hand, show low Cu levels in the brain and liver with higher Cu levels in other organs, and lower Cu–enzyme activities in all organs. Symptoms of the disease include peculiar (kinky) hair, severe mental retardation, and death before 3 years of age. The basic defect appears to be in the regulation of MT synthesis (191).

Molybdenum is an essential component of xanthine oxidase and aldehyde oxidase. Its role in nitrogen fixation in plants by bacteria makes it ubiquitous in food. The average daily intake in humans is approximately 300 µg. Pastures containing a Cu:Mo ratio of less than 2:1 (high Mo or low Cu) produce molybdenosis (teart) in cattle and sheep char-

acterized by diarrhea, poor growth rate, anemia, achromatrichia (loss of hair color), demyelination of the CNS (neonatal ataxia), fibrosis and atrophy of the myocardium (falling disease), and deformities of joints (176). In rats, repeated oral administration resulted in degeneration of liver and kidneys (82). Underwood (236) suggested that Mo toxicosis in man is unlikely from naturally occurring dietary Mo.

Interactions of Cu and Mo occur at several levels. Copper may antagonize absorption of Mo and also prevents Mo accumulation in liver. Molybdenum and Cu form an *in vivo* complex with a 3:4 molar ratio and thus make Cu unavailable. It is likely that most signs of molybdenosis are a result of functional Cu deficiency. This is supported by the fact that molybdenosis can be effectively treated by oral or parenteral Cu (176).

Fluoride

Food is the major source of fluorine in individuals not exposed to industrial contamination (ceramics plants, aluminum refineries, mines, superphosphate manufacturing plants, etc.) or to naturally (artesian or other deep wells) or artificially fluoridated water supplies (236). Fluoride concentrations in deep well waters are usually 4–8 ppm, in some cases (India and South Africa) reaching toxic levels (up to 50 ppm). Sea fish, fish products, and tea leaves, and contaminated forages for cattle constitute the biggest sources of dietary fluorine (236). Protection against potentially toxic intakes of fluorine in all species is afforded by urinary excretion (saturable) and deposition in skeletal tissue. Levels in the bones can reach as high as 2500 ppm without any signs following a dietary level of 2 ppm for 50 years. Exposure to 8 ppm in the diet for 35 years or 10 ppm for several years is estimated to yield bone levels of fluoride of 6000 ppm at which time severe skeletal fluorosis results (236).

Exposure to fluoride during tooth development results in discoloration (mottling) and pitting of teeth that wear out much more rapidly. Bone changes include exostosis, lameness, pain, and stiffness of the spine which, in humans, may ultimately become one continuous column of bone. Secondary signs associated with teeth and skeletal changes include the inability to eat and drink and emaciation leading to death (176,236). The primary effect of fluoride is thought to be a delaying or alteration in the mineralization of matrix laid down by damaged ameloblasts, odontoblasts, and osteoblasts.

In bone, fluoride also replaces hydroxyl radicals of the hydroxyapatite crystals, thus decreasing their dimensions and leading to defective bone mineralization (176). Skeletal fluorosis has been reported in cryolite workers in several countries (95). Accidental acute fluoride ingestion results in gastroenteritis, muscular weakness, and respiratory and cardiac failure. Fluoride levels in urine can be used to monitor both suspected recent exposure or, in the absence of recent exposure, long-term exposure and body burden.

Iodine

Iodine is ubiquitous in occurrence and is present in toxicologically significant quantities in sea weeds, sea fish, and shellfish and in their oils. Iodine consumption in the United States is on an upward trend, the average consumption being four- to 13-fold greater than the required 100 μg/day. Fortuitous sources of iodine include bread (potassium iodate added as dough conditioner), salt, vitamin preparations, medications, and coloring agents (236). The use of iodophores as antiseptics in milking machines, storage vats, and bulk tanks, and the use of organic iodides (EDDI) in the prevention and treatment of footrot, lumpy jaw, and respiratory infections (176) can also contribute to the daily intake. Although iodine is generally regarded as safe (GRAS), endemic iodine goiter (myxedema) has been reported from the coastal regions of Hakkaido, a northern island of Japan where diets were high in seaweed which contains 4000–6000 ppm (0.4–0.6% of dry weight) of iodine. Experimental exposure to high (50 mg EDDI/day) iodine levels resulted in impaired humoral and cellular immune systems in young calves (84), suggesting the need to monitor human populations for such effects.

Iron

Dietary sources of iron (Fe) include organ meats (liver, kidney, heart), egg yolk, dried legumes, cocoa, cane molasses, shellfish, and various wines (236). Normal humans regulate Fe stores in the body mainly by regulating absorption of Fe from the intestines, since excretory mechanisms for Fe only eliminate 0.01% of body burden daily (82). Ingested Fe is absorbed (2–15%), bound to the β-globulin transferrin in plasma, taken up by the liver, and stored as a complex with ferritin. Following further intake Fe is bound to hemosiderin, a biproduct of lysosomal action on ferritin. When the Fe load increases to 20–40 g (normal: 3–5 g), the saturation of Fe binding capacity of the body leads to free Fe in tissues and serum. Free Fe at the cellular level induces membrane damage to mitochondria, microsomes, and other organelles by a mechanism involving free radical generation and subsequent lipid peroxidation (101).

Consequences of Fe-induced membrane damage include increased capillary permeability, fluid loss, and cardiovascular collapse (82,176) in man and animals. Other effects such as hepatic insufficiency and enlargement, pigmentation of skin, diabetes mellitus, and hemosiderosis of all organs, especially liver and pancreas, also may occur. Chronic Fe overload has been reported in humans in three situations: (a) idiopathic hemochromatosis due to an inherited abnormality of Fe absorption; (b) following prolonged intakes of medicinal Fe or repeated blood transfusions (transfusional siderosis); and (c) in alcoholics with high dietary Fe, such as the Bantus in South Africa (Bantu siderosis), who cook food and ferment beer in Fe vessels (236). Occupational exposure to Fe oxide fumes and dust in metal industries produced changes in lungs similar to silicosis. An increase in lung cancer, tuberculosis, and interstitial fibrosis was reported in hemalite (Fe ore) miners, although the role of other cocontaminants needs to be evaluated (82).

Lead

The principal source of lead (Pb) for the general human population is food, with the intake from uncontaminated sources of food (plant and animal) ranging from 220 to 400 μg/day for adults (236) and from 75 to 120 μg/day for small children (82). Although most municipal water supplies (at the tap) and air are insignificant sources of Pb, concern has recently been raised regarding the use of Pb pipes in domestic water supply systems in many areas of the United States. In highly urbanized communities, motor vehicle exhausts can increase human exposure both directly by inhalation of Pb-laden dust in air and indirectly through consumption of plant foods grown in the vicinity of highways where significant deposition of airborne Pb occurs. Other sources of Pb include Pb-based paints in old dwellings, industrial emissions, dust-laden clothes and shoes of workers, and the use of Pb-glazed earthenware.

The absorption of ingested inorganic Pb is about 10% whereas that of organolead compounds (tetraalkyl Pb in gasoline) may be up to 75%, with less than 5% of the absorbed Pb retained. In children, both absorption and retention are higher (82). In general, absorption is higher through the pulmonary route and lower by skin than via the gastrointestinal tract (82,246). Absorbed inorganic Pb is transported in blood mostly (90%) bound to RBC (membrane as well as hemoglobin) in equilibrium with that in plasma, which, in turn, is in equilibrium with that in soft tissues (246) but not with that in bone (half-life > 20 years) where major Pb accumulation takes place with time. Following organolead exposure, major accumulation takes place in the liver and kidney. Metabolism of tetraalkyl Pb to trialkyl and inorganic Pb, mainly by P-450-dependent oxidative dealkylation in the liver and subsequent transport of trialkyl Pb to the critical organ, the brain, seems to be responsible for the neurotoxic effects.

The neurotoxicity of organolead compounds appears to be brought about by a change in the chloride/hydroxide distribution across the nerve cell membrane, resulting from the induction of electrically silent anion exchange (16). Urine is the major excretory route for inorganic Pb whereas two-thirds of organic Pb is excreted via feces. The biologic half-life of organic Pb compounds appears to be only 1–7 days whereas half-lives as long as 1 year have been estimated in the brain following low level exposure (105). In addition to neurotoxic effects, Pb is known to affect the hematopoietic, renal, gastrointestinal, and reproductive systems.

Acute inorganic Pb poisoning in adults usually results from accidental ingestion or from drinking wine made and/or stored in poorly glazed earthenware, and manifests as abdominal pain, nausea, and vomiting. Occupational exposure has been reported to cause wrist drop and foot drop associated mainly with motor nerve dysfunction resulting from decreased nerve conduction velocities (even at subclinical Pb levels), Schwann cell degeneration (segmental demyelination), possibly axonal degeneration, and Wallerian degeneration of posterior roots of the tibial and sciatic nerves (82).

Encephalopathy, the common neurologic effect of Pb in children, is rare in adults and is characterized by stupor, ataxia, coma, convulsions, and even death. Pathologic changes associated with these signs include cerebral edema, increase in cerebrospinal fluid pressure, proliferation and swelling of capillary and arteriolar endothelial cells, proliferation of glial cells, neuronal degeneration, and areas of cortical necrosis. Subclinical effects of Pb exposure in children (blood Pb of 30–50 μg/dl) include hyperactivity, poor classroom behavior, and small decrements in I.Q. scores (161) which are associated with changes in electroencephalographic (EEG) patterns. In experimental animals, inhibition of cholinergic function, impairment of dopamine uptake, and altered function of GABA have been observed.

Renal effects of Pb can be divided into either an acute and reversible tubular dysfunction in children associated with CNS effects or a chronic irreversible interstitial nephropathy in occupational workers (82). Renal disease in early stages is characterized by accumulation of Pb as intranuclear inclusion bodies (Pb complexed with protein) in proximal tubular cells. The mechanism of tubular dysfunction may be related to the swelling of mitochondria and impaired oxidative phosphorylation leading to amino aciduria, glucosuria, hyperphosphaturia, and possible impairment of sodium transport. Interstitial nephropathy in occupational exposures is associated early with reduced glomerular filtration rate.

The effects of Pb on the hematopoietic system ultimately result in anemia from impaired heme synthesis and reduced erythrocyte life span (due to increased membrane fragility). Effects of Pb on heme synthesis result mainly from its inhibitory action on enzymes containing sulfhydril groups. Several enzymes in the pathway of heme synthesis are affected (Fig. 5). Delta-amino levulinic acid dehydrogenase (ALAD) appears to be the most sensitive enzyme, inhibition occurring even at blood Pb levels below 10 μg/dl (see ref. 246). This effect of Pb as well as the feedback stimulation of ALA synthetase (due to decreased heme synthesis) results in increased accumulation of ALA in the blood as well as in urine. Considerable evidence exists to support that Pb also inhibits ferrochelatase activity, resulting in depressed heme synthesis and a buildup of protoporphyrin which chelates zinc and takes the place of hemoglobin in circulating erythrocytes (82). Increased urinary coproporphyrin in Pb-exposed individuals suggests that coproporphyrin oxidase may also be affected (246). These changes in blood and urine biochemicals, i.e., blood ALAD, urinary ALA, and RBC zinc-protoporphyrin, correlate well with blood Pb levels and serve as early biochemical indices of Pb effects (82). Anemia, however, only occurs in very marked Pb toxicity.

Organic Pb appears to cause reduced sexual potency with decreased spermatogenesis in humans (168). Extremely high doses of Pb can cause increased fetal deaths (resorptions) and reduced fetal body weight. Organolead compounds seem to be less toxic to neonatal animals compared with adults due to the lack of enzyme systems necessary to metabolize organolead compounds to more active species. The human fetus, however, is capable of oxidizing several drugs and steroid hormones by 10–12 weeks of gestation (178), making it likely that the human unborn can adversely react to Pb exposure. Lead in cord blood, although slightly lower, correlates with lead in maternal blood from which there may be a transfer of Pb to the fetus as pregnancy progresses (see ref. 82). In addition, Pb-induced immunosuppression in animals (119), increased susceptibility of children to febrile illness (180), and mutagenic and carcinogenic effects in man and animals (see ref. 163) have been reported. Although carcinogenic effects in man (respiratory and digestive tract tumors) and animals (kidney) have not been correlated, it appears that Pb-induced inhibition of microsomal enzymes may enhance the carcinogenic potential of other chemicals (163).

Toxic effects of Pb are enhanced by dietary deficiencies of calcium, iron, and zinc, all of which enhance Pb absorption and tissue storage (136). Conversely, excess of these metals decreases toxic effects of Pb by mechanisms involving absorption as well as reversal of some calcium- and iron-dependent physiologic functions adversely altered by Pb (see ref. 246). Both chronic and acute cases of Pb intoxication can benefit from chelation therapy with calcium EDTA, BAL, or preferably a combination. Kidney function and blood calcium levels have to be carefully monitored during chelation therapy.

Standards have been developed for most environmental sources of Pb. The upper limit for ambient air is 2 μg/m^3 by the Environmental Protection Agency (EPA), and for industry the threshold limit value is 150 μg/m^3 (246). The maximum permissible Pb concentration in gasoline ranges from 0.15 g/liter for West Germany to 0.45 g/liter in the United Kingdom. The United States limit has been set at 0.10 g/gallon. The joint Food and Agriculture Organization–World Health Organization (FAO/WHO) expert committee on food additives suggested a tolerable weekly Pb intake from food and drinks of 3 mg/person, with lower limits (e.g., 0.5 mg/kg of food as in the U.K.) advisable for foods intended for infants and young children. The EPA recommends a limit of 0.05 mg/liter for all drinking water, whereas WHO recommends a level of 0.30 mg/liter. The Council of European Communities has set standards for blood Pb as 20 μg/dl or less in half the population, 30 μg/dl or less in 90% of the population, and 35 μg/dl or less in 98% of the population

MITOCHONDRION

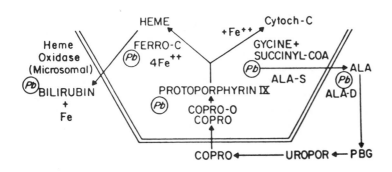

FIG. 5. Scheme of heme synthesis showing sites where lead has an effect. COA, coenzyme A; ALA-S, aminolevulinic acid synthetase; ALA, d-aminolevulinic acid; ALA-D, aminolevulinic acid dehydratase; PBG, porphobilinogen; UROPOR, uroporphyrinogen; COPRO, coproporphyrinogen; COPRO-O, coproporphyrinogen oxidase; FERRO-C, ferrochelatase; CYTOCH-C, cytochrome C; Pb, site for lead effect. (From ref. 82, with permission.)

when 100 or more persons in a population of 500,000 are sampled (246). In the absence of an understanding the significance of contamination in individual components of man's environment, the assessment of total exposure by biologic monitoring becomes extremely important in preventing overexposure to environmental hazards such as lead.

Manganese

Manganese (Mn) is an essential element that functions as a cofactor in a variety of enzymes including carboxylases, and is involved in phosphorylation and in the synthesis of cholesterol, fatty acids, and mucopolysaccharides (82,95). Deficiency of Mn can cause slipped tendon in poultry, ataxia in pallid mice, and reproductive disorders in adult animals. Uses of Mn include steel alloys, dry cell batteries, electrical coils, ceramics, glass, dyes, matches, fertilizers, welding rods as oxidizers, and animal feed additives. Although food is the major source of Mn for the general human population, and Mn at higher than recommended levels can lead to loss of appetite, growth depression, and anemia in domestic animals, toxicity in man from normal dietary levels of Mn alone is unlikely (236). Plant and animal foods generally contain levels of 20–30 ppm and 0.2–0.5 ppm, respectively, with the highest levels being consumed in tea and cloves. Shellfish seem to accumulate Mn 1100–13,500 times that in sea water (149). Since absorption of Mn is closely tied with that of iron, children and adults with iron deficiency anemia or cirrhosis appear to be highly sensitive to the toxic effects of industrial Mn. Except for one report from Japan of Mn poisoning in individuals drinking water from a well near which Mn-containing batteries had been buried, and another case of dementia and extrapyramidal involvement following consumption of mineral tablets (149), all reported Mn poisonings have come from occupational exposures.

Two principal syndromes of Mn toxicosis are (a) pneumonitis following acute exposure to high levels, and (b) a chronic CNS disorder characterized by psychosis (hallucinations and delusions) followed by a Parkinson-like syndrome (bradykinesia, loss of balance, impaired speech, and in some cases facial rigidity and loss of expression). Morphologic and biochemical lesions include damage to subthalamic nucleus and pallidum in humans and a marked decrease in dopamine and serotonin levels in the caudate nucleus of exposed squirrel monkeys (82). Manganese encephalopathy is only slowly reversible with effective symptomatic relief provided by the anti-Parkinson drug L-dopa. The United States Public Health Service recommends a drinking water limit for Mn of 0.05 mg/liter.

Mercury

Mercury (Hg) is a nonessential element that is used significantly as cathodes in the chloralkali and battery industries; as an antifungal agent in the paint, wood pulp, and paper industries; as seed dressing for antifungal activity in agriculture; in measuring and control equipment such as switches, vacuum pump seals, thermometers, and barometers which are used in industries, laboratories and medicine; as a catalyst

in organic synthesis of vinylchloride, acetaldehyde, etc.; and finally, in dentistry and medicine. Although the agricultural and medicinal uses of Hg are declining as a result of our understanding of the impact of mercurials on man and his environment, other uses still pose a significant health threat. In addition, up to 5000 tons of Hg/year may be released into the environment as a result of burning of coal, natural gas, and refining petroleum products (82). Mercury is used in inorganic as well as organic forms (e.g., phenylmercury) and significant interconversions between the two forms of Hg occur in the environment by bacterial action (112).

One of the most important reactions involves biomethylation of divalent Hg in water by a variety of bacteria and fungi resulting in the formation of mono- or dimethyl mercury in aquatic sediments. Mercury from the sediments is taken up by fauna and plankton which are fed upon by small fish which, in turn, are consumed by larger carnivorous fish. The Hg levels increase with each increase in the level of aquatic food chain. This phenomenon, called biomagnification, is aided by filtration of large quantities of sea water by larger fish and by their longer life cycle (112). Among the sources of Hg for man, i.e., air, water, and food, food is the largest source of Hg in unpolluted areas, the total dietary intake amounting to an average of 3.5 μg/day from nonfish diets and 9.0 μg/day from fish diets (236) with at least 80% of Hg in fish being methyl Hg. Heavy fish-eaters may consume 200 μg of Hg/day or more, which easily exceeds the Provisional Tolerable Weekly Intake of 0.3 mg/week (of which less than 0.2 mg should be methyl Hg) established by the Joint FAO/WHO Expert Committee on Food Additives (see ref. 112). In individuals consuming mercurial-treated grains or seafood from contaminated waters, the organic Hg levels far exceed these limits. In one incident in Iraq in 1971–1972, bread made from methyl Hg-treated wheat was consumed by a large number of farm families, resulting in 6530 admitted cases of Hg poisoning and 459 deaths. The flour samples were found to contain 4.8–14.6 μg/g of methyl Hg. Average daily consumption of methyl Hg was 130 μg/kg BW/day in the most severely affected group (6). Two incidents of alkyl mercurial intoxication in Japan, one in the area of Minamata Bay and the other at Niigata, resulted from consumption of fish contaminated with Hg from water polluted with industrial effluent. More than 1200 combined cases of alkyl Hg poisoning occurred from Hg levels as high as 36 mg/kg of fish (112).

Absorption of mercuric salts is 10–15% and that of alkyl- and arylmercurials is almost complete (95%). In the blood, inorganic Hg is distributed equally between plasma and RBC whereas 90% of organic Hg in blood is bound to RBC. Inorganic Hg rapidly accumulates in the kidney whereas organic Hg slowly accumulates in all organs. Subsequent demethylation of organic Hg in all tissues other than the brain results in a decline of Hg in other organs whereas Hg levels in brain remain relatively higher longer (112). Within cells, Hg binds to enzymes and other ligands containing —SH groups, thus affecting enzyme function, membrane integrity and active transport, and finally release of lysosomal enzymes. Methyl mercury also accumulates in hair with a hair/blood ratio of 250, making hair suitable to monitor environmental exposure. Methyl Hg also selectively accumulates in fetal blood and can be selectively toxic. Inorganic Hg is excreted in urine whereas organic Hg is excreted mostly in feces (152). Although biologic half-lives of mercurials range between 58 and 76 days, the half-life in the brain may be as long as 190 days in some individuals.

Accidental or suicidal ingestion of mercuric salts result in corrosive ulceration, bleeding, and necrosis of the gastrointestinal tract with shock and circulatory collapse. Survival during this phase leads to renal failure in 25 hr with tubular necrosis, oliguria or anuria, and uremia. Placement of victims on dialysis leads to tubular regeneration (82). Chronic exposure to mercuric salts in occupational settings leads to immunologic glomerular disease characterized by proteinuria which is reversible after removal of the source. Continued exposure may lead to interstitial immune-complex nephritis (233). Inhalation of Hg vapor in several occupational settings has led either to pneumonitis (acute) or to *mercurialism* (chronic) characterized by gingivitis (salivation), increased excitability, and tremors with a proportion of individuals showing nephropathy (112). Several historical accounts of mercurialism, summarized by Kazantzis (112), include syphilis patients who were made to inhale Hg vapor until their teeth loosened; syphilis patients who were treated by surgeons with mercurial ointments; craftsmen in Venice, particularly goldsmiths and mirror markers; and workers who used hot mercuric nitrate to convert rabbit fur into felt for hat making, and suffered from *mad hatter's* disease. The less toxic mercurous compounds (e.g., mercurous chloride), used in the recent past as a teething powder, have caused *pink disease* or acrodynia, a skin hypersensitivity characterized by vasodilation, pink-colored rash, hyperkeratosis, hypersecretion of sweat, fever, and swelling of spleen and lymph nodes (82). Phenyl and alkoxyalkyl mercurials produce effects similar to inorganic mercurials in most respects.

Among the organic Hg compounds, methyl Hg is the most important from the standpoint of food-borne Hg intoxication. In addition to the episodes of methyl Hg intoxication in Minamata Bay and Niigata, both of which were caused by industrial Hg contamination of waters followed by accumulation in edible fish, and the episode in Iraq of ingestion of bread made from methyl Hg-treated seed, several smaller scale episodes have occurred in Iraq in 1961, in Pakistan in 1963, and in Guatemala in 1966 (82). The major clinical features of methyl Hg poisoning involve the nervous system. The earliest and the most frequent sign was paresthesia with tingling and numbness involving the hands and feet, the circumoral region, and the chest, developing 6 weeks after the beginning of consumption. Disturbances in gait (ataxia), visual disturbances (tunnel vision and blindness), dysarthria, difficulty in speech, and deafness developed subsequently in that order (112). Degeneration and necrosis of neurons in the visual cortex, granular layer of the cerebellum, and other focal areas of the cerebral cortex accompanied the gross changes of atrophy of the convolutions of the cerebral cortex and folia and vermis of the cerebellum. The brainstem, spinal cord, and cranial nerves were not affected (112). Clarkson (40) found that recovery of protein synthesis inhibited by methyl Hg does not occur in granular cells of cerebellum as it does in other neuronal cells, possibly explaining the selective sensitivity of these cells to subsequent damage.

Kazantzis (112) summarized several reports of infants with features of cerebral palsy, generalized spasticity, increased reflexes, blindness, deafness, and abnormality of external ear, who were born to methyl Hg-exposed mothers in Minamata as well as in Iraq. Pathologic changes included microcephaly (reduced brain weight) and hypoplastic and dysplastic changes in the cerebellum and cerebrum. Similar changes have been reported in animals.

Treatment of inorganic Hg intoxication requires restoration of organ function (e.g., hemodialysis for renal failure) and removal of Hg from the critical organs. Agents such as cysteine, penicillamine, or BAL may be effective in such cases. Chelation, however, is ineffective in organomercurial intoxication. Surgical drainage of the gallbladder or oral administration of an insoluble polythiol ion-exchange resin to interrupt enterohepatic cycling of Hg may be helpful (112).

Control of environmental Hg contamination and prevention of human and animal intoxication from Hg can be achieved by appropriate surveillance of food, water, and ambient as well as industrial air and adherence to standards set by regulatory agencies. The reader is referred to reviews by Kazantzis (112) and Goyer (82) for pertinent information.

Selenium

Selenium (Se) is an essential element varying widely (in levels) in soils and thus in foods and feeds produced on these soils. Certain plant species such as *Astragalus, Oonopsis* (goldenweed), *Stanleya,* and *Xylorrhiza* (woody aster) require Se and accumulate high levels of Se from seleniferous soils, whereas others such as *Atriplex, Machaeronthera,* and *Sideranthus* accumulate Se although it is not needed for plant growth. Grazing on these plants, feeding forages grown on seleniferous soils, use of Se as a feed supplement (0.1–0.3 ppm of complete diets) as well as industrial contamination of forages are all factors that contribute to animal poisonings.

In humans, however, problems of food-borne Se toxicosis are rare owing to the wide geographical sources of components of modern diets and processing (e.g., dehulling, peeling) of plant foods before consumption. Although plants and forages consumed by animals may accumulate levels of Se in excess of 1000 ppm, normal human diets rarely exceed the recommended safe level of 3–4 ppm (236). Seafood (especially shrimp), meat (especially kidney), milk products, and whole grains constitute the major sources of Se in human diets.

Most Se from plant food sources is bound to nonprotein sulfur-containing amino acids such as methylselenocysteine and selenocystathionine, and protein amino acids such as selenocysteine and selenomethionine (126), although some uptake of selenates does occur. Organic Se and selenates are readily absorbed, distributed mainly to the liver and kidneys where they may be incorporated into proteins or methylated to trimethyl Se prior to urinary excretion (82). Sweat and exhaled air are two minor excretory pathways. Exhalation of highly volatile dimethyl Se gives rise to garlicky breath.

As a result of its role in the activity of glutathione peroxidase, which is involved in protecting membranes, proteins, and nucleic acids from organic hydroperoxides generated as a result of high oxidant stress, Se deficiency causes necrosis of liver and other organs in many animals. Some examples are muscular dystrophy, referred to as *stiff limb disease* in lambs and *white muscle disease* in calves, exudative diathesis in chicks, embryomortality in ewes, and cardiomyopathy in pigs and humans (82,95). Selenium protects against the toxic effects of cadmium, mercury, aflatoxin B_1, and a number of other toxins. Toxicity, on the other hand, appears to be related to displacement of sulfur in sulfur-containing amino acids in proteins and accumulation of Se in organs containing high —SH proteins such as skin, hair, hooves, and nails. Acute Se toxicosis in humans is restricted to industrial exposure to inorganic Se including hydrogen selenide gas, with signs of eye and nasal irritation, nausea, dizziness, lassitude, and garlic breath and CNS signs including drowsiness and convulsions. Chronic inhalation may lead to coated tongue, liver and spleen damage, and anemia (82).

Chronic dietary Se intoxication in man results mainly from consumption of locally produced foods grown on seleniferous soils. Signs include discolored or decayed teeth, skin eruptions, gastrointestinal distress, lassitude, and partial loss of hair and nails. One such case was reported following consumption of coco de mono (*Lecythis ollaria*) nuts containing high levels of selenocystathionine (5). Acute toxicosis in animals is characterized by muscle weakness, gait disturbances, bloody diarrhea, and respiratory failure whereas chronic consumption of high Se forages and feeds results in rough skin, loss of hair, deformation and sloughing off hooves, lameness, anemia, emaciation, and liver necrosis (176). Sterility, embryotoxicity, and teratogenicity of Se have been reported in laboratory animals (82). Although Se sulfide produced increased incidence of hepatocellular carcinomas and adenomas in mice (159), epidemiologic studies indicated an inverse relationship between Se levels in forages and human cancer rates (210). This correlates well with animal studies demonstrating anticlastogenic and anticarcinogenic effects of Se against clastogenic and carcinogenic effects of benzo[*a*]pyrene, benzanthracene, *N*-fluorenylacetamide, and dimethylaminoazobenzene in rodents, possibly by inhibiting the formation of the carcinogen melonaldehyde (82,210). Toxicity of Se is antagonized by high dietary protein, arsenic, and naphthalene. The latter two chemicals have been suggested as possible therapeutic agents in domestic animals (176).

Zinc

Zinc (Zn) is a ubiquitous essential element required for the activity of more than 70 metalloenzymes. Seafood, meats, dairy products, whole grains, nuts, and legumes are the predominant sources of Zn, contributing to a total intake of 12–15 mg/day (82). Zinc toxicity in humans from excessive dietary levels has not been reported. However, cases of intoxication from inhalation of Zn fumes (metal fume fever), consumption of beverages following prolonged storage in galvanized containers, cooking with galvanized utensils, and accidental ingestion of Zn salts, metallic toys, and other foreign objects have been reported in humans and animals (except metal fume fever). Zinc induces MT in the intestinal mucosal cells (as well as other organs) which, when saturated with metal, inhibit absorption (normally 20–30% of ingested) of Zn. Absorption of Zn is reduced by high, dietary calcium, phosphorus, copper, cadmium, and phytic acid (95,236) and by a deficiency of pyridoxine and tryptophan (82). Zinc is

distributed mainly to the liver, kidney, muscle, and pancreas and is eliminated in the urine.

Acute ingestion of toxic doses of Zn results mainly in gastrointestinal discomfort whereas inhalation of fumes leads to chills, fever, sweating, and weakness. As discussed by Brietschwerdt et al. (20), chronic therapeutic use of Zn in humans can lead to interference with iron and copper absorption, leading to hypochromic anemia. This has been demonstrated in dogs (20). Other consistent findings in dogs accidentally ingesting several forms of Zn included vomiting and renal tubular damage. In young horses grazing on pastures contaminated with industrial Zn, hypocuprosis in association with periarticular enlargement of long bones was the main feature (52). In birds, consumption of Zn from wire mesh cages (new wire disease) resulted mainly in nephritis and pancreatic degeneration.

Miscellaneous Toxic Metals

In addition to the food-borne toxic elements discussed above, a number of other elements occur in nature that can cause adverse effects in humans or animals following exposure in occupational settings, by the use of such elements in therapeutic or diagnostic modalities, or by being ingested occasionally in excessive quantities. These elements and their effects are summarized in Table 4. The reader is referred to reviews cited earlier for additional information and for references to the original articles. It should be pointed out, however, that the general population is exposed to most of these metals through food but at toxicologically insignificant levels.

FOOD ADDITIVES

The increasing demand for food by an ever-increasing world population, as well as by changes in life styles in developed societies, has invited the use of chemical additives to preserve foods as well as to process and fortify raw foods into nutritionally adequate ready-to-eat foods. Problems of adulteration of food (masking of low quality food by chemical additives) in the early 20th century coupled with the increasing awareness of toxic effects from chronic chemical exposure have led to the passage of the Food and Drug Act of 1906 followed by several expansions and amendments in 1938, 1958, and 1962 leading to the 1976 Federal Food Drug and Cosmetic Act (As Amended) (FFDCA; 63). The term *food additive* is defined in this Act as follows:

> . . . any substance the intended use of which results or may reasonably be expected to result, directly or indirectly, in its becoming a component or otherwise affecting the characteristic of any food (including any substance intended for use in producing, manufacturing, packing, processing, preparing, treating, packaging, transporting or holding food; and including any source of radiation intended for any such use), if such substance is not generally recognized, among experts qualified by scientific training and experience to evaluate its safety as having been adequately shown through scientific procedures (or, in the case of substances used in food prior to January 1, 1958, through either scientific procedures or experience based on common use in food) to be safe under the conditions of its intended use. . . .

TABLE 4. *Miscellaneous toxic metals—Their sources and effects*

Element	Essential	Source	Major effects	Treatment	Comments
Aluminum	No	Dialysis, occupational	Dementia, pulmonary fibrosis	Desferioxamine	No danger from oral antacids
Antimony	No	Occupational	Pneumoconiosis, emphysema	BAL (questionable)	Clastogenic
Barium	No	X-ray diagnosis, occupational	Digitalis-like (ventricular fibrillation), pneumoconiosis	Potassium (iv)	High level in Brazil nuts
Beryllium	No	Occupational	Contact dermatitis, acute chemical pneumonitis, chronic granulomatous disease (berylliosis)	Corticosteroids	Carcinogenic
Bismuth	No	Therapeutic use	Acute renal tubular degeneration, chronic rheumatic disease, encephalopathy in colostomy patients	BAL	—
Chromium	Yes	Occupational	Asthma and allergic dermatitis	Symptomatic	Carcinogenic
Gallium	No	Radiographic	Gastrointestinal disturbance, bone marrow depression	—	Rare
Gold	No	Therapeutic	Immune complex glomerulonephritis	—	—
Lithium	No	Therapy for depression	Neuromuscular, CNS, gastrointestinal, cardiovascular, and renal	Acetazolamide plus furosemide	—
Magnesium	Yes	Occupational	Metal fume fever	Symptomatic	—
Nickel	Maybe	Contact with coins and jewelry, occupational	Dermatitis, Pulmonary and CNS	Dithiocarb	Well-known carcinogen
Platinum	No	Jewelry, therapy, occupational	Dermatitis, nephrotoxic, platinosis (asthma)	—	Animal carcinogen
Silver	No	Jewelry, therapy, occupational	Dermal (patchy discoloration)	—	—
Tellurium	No	Diet (condiments, nuts, fish, garlic), accidental (man)	Teratogenic Cyanosis, stupor, loss of consciousness	—	Only in animals
Thallium	No	Food, therapy, occupational	Nervous system, alopecia, blindness	Diphenyl dithiocarbazone	—
Tin	No	Occupational	Pneumoconiosis, cerebral edema (organotin)	—	—
Titanium	No	Occupational	Mild pulmonary fibrosis	—	Titanocene is an animal carcinogen
Uranium	No	Nuclear industry (occupational)	Nephritis	—	—
Vanadium	No	Occupational	Bronchopneumonia	—	—

For regulatory purposes, the definition of food additive does not include substances generally recognized as safe (GRAS), substances used in accordance with sanction or approval granted prior to enactment of the 1958 amendment, pesticide residues in or on raw agricultural products, color additives, or new animal drugs. The latter three categories are covered under different sections of the Act. Frequently overlooked but included in this definition are those additives occurring through processing, such as pyrolysis or degradation products (carbonyls, peroxides, polycyclic aromatic hydrocarbons), proteolytic products, interactants between carbohydrates and proteins (browning) and radiolytic products (hydroxyhydroperoxides) from ionizing radiation, sterilization, and pasteurization of foods. A broad definition of food additive, however, includes any substance or mixture of substances, other than a basic foodstuff, that is present in a food as a result of any aspect of production, processing, storage, or packaging (158).

Food additives fall into two broad categories, i.e., direct and indirect. Direct additives are those that are intentionally added to foods to preserve or improve the quality of the product or to aid in the processing. Some examples of direct additives are antioxidants, inhibitors of bacterial and mold growth, vitamins and minerals, color, and antifoaming agents. Indirect additives are chemicals that may be incorporated into foods unintentionally or unavoidably during some phase of production, processing, storage, or packaging. Pesticide residues, animal feed additives and drug residues, and components of packaging materials that migrate into foods fall under this category. Direct additives are added in quantities established to be safe (e.g., <5.67 g of potassium iodide per 100 lbs of salt, or 5.5 g of synthetic color in estimated yearly consumption of 1420 lbs of food) whereas the indirect additives are allowed only if they are present below the levels considered safe (81).

Safety Assessment of Food Additives

The FFDCA of 1976 (63), together with the Meat Inspection Act of 1907 and Poultry Inspection Act of 1957 control the safety and quality of foods entering interstate commerce. The Food Additive Amendment (to FFDCA) of 1958 requires manufacturers to test all chemicals added to foods (except pesticides, GRAS substances, color additives, and animal drugs) and allows for an increase or an improvement in the quality of the food supply by the safe use of additives. The Pesticide Chemicals Amendment of 1954, the Color Additive Amendment of 1950, and the Animal Drug Amendment of 1968 regulate pesticide residues in or on raw agricultural commodities (including fruits, vegetables, grains, nuts, eggs, raw milk, meats, animal feed, and forage crops) under the authority of the EPA; color additive use in foods; and animal drugs and medicated feeds that may enter the human food chain as residues, respectively. Substances that qualify for GRAS status (553 direct and 154 indirect additives on the FDA-GRAS list in 1973) and those given prior sanction (prior to September 6, 1958; the list includes 150 substances) by FDA and USDA are currently undergoing FDA review to be finally classified as (a) reaffirmed as GRAS, (b) GRAS for a prescribed time while additional tests are ongoing, and (c) food additive status (non-GRAS status) requiring safety assessment before further use. The Food Additive, Color Additive, as well as the Animal Drug Amendments of the FFDCA contain anticancer clauses, including the Delaney Clause in the Food Additive Amendment. These clauses prohibit the use of these additives "if they are found to induce cancer when ingested by man or animal, or if found, after tests which are appropriate to the evaluation of safety of such substances, to induce cancer in man or animal" (63). New animal drugs and feed additives are exempt from this proviso, provided no residue of the additive is found in any edible portion of such animals after slaughter or in any food yielded by or derived from the living animals.

Safety evaluation of food additives involves establishment of a no observable adverse effect level (NOAEL) in experimental animals followed by establishment of *safe level* or *maximum acceptable daily intake* (ADI) in the total diet for man using a suitable *safety factor* (usually 2000). Due to the time and expense involved in testing the thousands of food additive chemicals, the Food Safety Council (71) developed a "decision-tree" approach to safety evaluation. This approach involves serial steps including (a) assessment of exposure in cases of high level intake (for additives already in use), (b) acute toxicity studies, (c) genetic and pharmacokinetic studies, (d) subchronic toxicity studies including reproduction and teratology studies, and (e) chronic toxicity study.

Following step a, risk analysis from the toxicity data at each subsequent step will determine if testing should proceed beyond that step. Testing is terminated at the step where excessive risk is encountered. If toxic metabolites are identified in step c, additional toxicology tests to uncover their effects may be needed. Pharmacokinetic studies also indicate the biologic half-life of the compound as well as the propensity for tissue accumulation (undesirable). The Food Safety Council recommends acceptance of the additive at step c if no mutagenicity and no toxic metabolites are detected at this point.

The FDA, however, proposed an alternative approach based on the concept of "level of concern" (25). Level of concern is based on the level of exposure, structural correlation with known compounds (if no toxicity data are available), and existing toxicologic data. Subjective categorization of additives into concern levels I, II, or III (level III being of highest concern) are made for compounds contributing <0.05 ppm, 0.05–1.0 ppm, and >1.0 ppm, respectively. Also, structural similarity to compounds with low, medium, or high toxicity would place them in concern levels I, II, or III, respectively. Furthermore, formation of active metabolites would place the compound in level III. Table 5 lists recommended toxicologic tests for each level of concern. This testing scheme allows compounds producing effects at high levels and those with lower levels of human exposure to be tested less extensively. Protocols for testing color additives and indirect food additives are similar to direct food additive testing. Testing animal drugs and feed additives, however, is much more complex not only because an additional animal species (target animal) is involved but also because of the necessity to understand the impact of target animal metabolism on the diversity and toxic potential of the metabolites to humans and the need for the development of residue detection methods and elimination strategies in the target animal species and to set maximum allowable residues (tolerance) of the parent compound and metabolites in tissues of the target animal.

Finally, a distinction between the ADI and *tolerance* should be made. Tolerance refers to the maximum allowable residue of the additive in or on a particular food (not the whole diet) and is determined following exposure to the additive at the *proposed use level* rather than *maximum tolerated* or *safe* level. As a result, tolerance levels are invariably lower than the levels calculated based on the ADI.

Safety of Food Additives

Food additives, although numbering in the thousands and at times used in large quantities, rank at the bottom of the list of food-borne hazards, behind pesticides, natural toxicants, environmental contaminants, and microbial toxins. Among the food additives subjected to regulatory action, only one direct food additive, i.e., cobaltous salts, has been strongly linked with an adverse effect in humans. The remaining additives were banned either on the basis of toxic responses in animals or on an association of therapeutic or other (including additive) use of the compound with human toxic reactions or cancer (e.g., diethylstilbestrol). The following sections summarize the use of various classes of food additives and currently available safety data on selected compounds.

TABLE 5. *Test schedule recommended by the FDA for additives at various concern levels*

Concern level I	Concern level II	Concern level III
1. Short-term (at least 28 days) feeding study in a rodent species	1. Subchronic feeding study in a rodent species	1. Chronic (at least 1 yr) feeding study in a rodent species
2. Short-term test for carcinogenic potential	2. Subchronic feeding study in a nonrodent species	2. Chronic (at least 1 yr) feeding study in a nonrodent species
	3. Multi- (at least two) generation reproduction study with teratology, in a rodent species	3. Multi- (at least two) generation reproduction study with teratology, in a rodent species
	4. Short-term test for carcinogenic potential	4. Short-term test for carcinogenic potential
		5. Carcinogenicity studies in two rodent species (test 1 can be a part of this)

Pesticides

Pesticides are essential in agriculture. The National Monitoring Program for Food and Feed, comprised of three federal surveillance programs (i.e., the Total Diet Study of market foods by the FDA, nationwide monitoring of unprocessed food and feed by the FDA, and analysis of meat and poultry by the USDA), detects residues of chlorinated hydrocarbon insecticides, organophosphates and carbamates, and very infrequently, herbicides and inorganic pesticides such as As and bromide in various agricultural products (51). Despite the ban of DDT in 1972, aldrin and dieldrin in 1975, a partial ban of heptachlor and chlordane in 1978, and a complete ban of heptachlor in 1983, residues of these and other chlorinated pesticides and metabolites continue to appear especially in dairy products, meat, fish, and poultry. In most cases, however, the daily intake of a pesticide did not exceed the ADI established by a Joint FAO/WHO Expert Committee on Pesticide Residues (107). Intoxication with a pesticide usually results from accidental or suicidal ingestion, careless storage, or improper use. Three reports of pesticide poisoning, summarized by Gilchrist (81), involved consumption of (a) collard greens sprayed with toxaphene three days before harvest, (b) mustard greens sprayed with nicotine sulfate on the day of harvest, and (c) meat from a hog fed alkyl mercury-treated seed. Details of the toxic effects of pesticides are presented in Chapter 5.

Food Colors

Color is a quality of foods that makes them visually acceptable and aids in their recognition. Foods containing added colors include candy and confections, bakery goods, soft drinks, cereals, dairy products such as butter, ice cream, and sherbet, margarine, snack foods, jams and jellies, and dessert powders. Following the passage of the Color Additive Amendment of 1960, 20 natural colors (comprising preparations such as dried algae meal, beet, powder, grape skin extract, fruit juice, paprika, caramel, carrot oil, cochineal extract, ferrous gluconate, and iron oxide) were exempted from certification, whereas all the synthetic colors including the ones approved prior to the Amendment were required to be retested if questions regarding their safety arose. A pro-

visional certification was given to those in use that required further testing. Currently, there are seven certified synthetic colors (FDC colors Blue No. 1, Red No. 3, Red No. 40, and Yellow No. 5 are permanently listed whereas FDC Blue No. 7, Green No. 3, and Yellow No. 6 are provisionally listed), with unlimited uses (according to good manufacturing practices) and one permanently listed color (Citrus Red No. 2) used only for coloring skins of oranges at 2 ppm. Several colors including Green 1, Green 2, Orange B, Red 2, Red 4, and Violet 1 were delisted due to concerns over carcinogenicity and other chronic toxic effects. Red No. 3 (disodium or dipotassium salt of 2,4,5,7-tetraiodofluorescein) was shown to cause thyroid hyperplasia and tumors in Sprague–Dawley rats (70), suggesting a likely delisting of this color in the near future.

A controversy exists regarding food colors and allergies and hyperkinesis in children (64). Recent evidence failed to establish a role for food colors in hyperkinesia and learning disabilities (43,128,138).

Animal Drugs

A *new animal drug* is defined as any drug intended for use in animals other than man. All new animal drugs and feeds containing them must receive premarket clearance from the Bureau of Veterinary Medicine of the FDA. Animal drugs used in the treatment of individual animal diseases are used sporadically and present few, if any, economic problems to producers resulting from withholding of residue-containing products. Feed additives and compounds used in feeds either in prevention of disease or for growth promotion, on the other hand, are widely used in animal production. Sixty to 100% of food-producing animals are raised on additive supplemented diets. Antibiotics and steroidal as well as nonsteroidal growth promotants are the predominant groups of feed additives currently used in the animal industry.

Two major concerns with the use of antibiotics in animal feeds are (a) the development of resistance in bacteria that could be transferred via plasmids to other bacteria in the gut of animals and thus transferred to humans (2), making antibiotics currently in use in humans ineffective, and (b) allergic reactions to residues of antibiotics present in milk and possibly other animal products, especially if the recommended waiting period following treatment is not allowed before using these products. Increasing pressure on the FDA has resulted in the exclusion of kanamycin, gentamycin, semisynthetic penicillins, and chloramphenicol from use in animal feeds. Total exclusion of penicillins and tetracyclines as feed additives is being considered.

Concerns about the use of growth promotants in feeds are related to possible chronic toxic effects, mainly carcinogenicity. A notable example is the synthetic estrogen diethylstilbestrol (DES), which has been shown to increase feed efficiency and the rate of weight gain in animals. A ban on DES use went into effect in 1979 when the FDA determined that the safety of DES had not been proven. This ban was based on the fact that a rare vaginal cancer developed in the daughters of a few of the pregnant women who, years ago, were given DES (up to 300 mg/day) in an attempt to prevent miscarriage. The applicability of the results of high dose therapy of DES to extremely low residues (<2 ppb) of DES in animals fed DES has to be questioned. At the maximum observed residue level, one would have to consume 26,666 lbs of beef liver (17,000 years) to equal one therapeutic dose of DES. A recent CAST report (34) summarized several studies and concluded that the cancer risk from DES residues in edible beef tissues is essentially zero. The second factor contributing to the ban on DES use was the lack of an acceptable method to demonstrate lack of residues in edible animal tissues. The FDA, prior to its ban, had withdrawn approval of an existing but less sensitive method.

Other steroids approved for use in one or more animal species include estradiol, progesterone, testosterone, melengestrol acetate, and zearanol. Although an excess of natural estrogens is considered to be carcinogenic, the residues resulting from feed additive use of steroids as well as other additives are negligible and pose little or no danger to humans.

Other additives commonly used in animal production include monensin, EDDI, phenothiazine, and thiabendazole. The Delaney Clause, as invoked in the ban of DES, although prohibiting the use of food additives if they "induce cancer when ingested by man or animal", also provides for approval of animal drugs by adding: "unless no residue of such drug will be found (by methods of examination prescribed or approved by the secretary . . .) in any edible portion of such animals after slaughter or in any food yielded by or derived from the living animals." Carcinogenic animal drugs can be approved for use by the FDA if an adequate period is recommended between the last dose of the additive and slaughter (withdrawal period) to allow residues to fall below detection limits.

Packaging Materials

Packaging is an essential part of food processing that aids in the preservation of the wholesomeness of foods by preventing (a) contamination or destruction by dirt, microorganisms, insects, and rodents, (b) loss or gain of moisture, odors, flavors, or aroma, and (c) deterioration from air, light, heat, and contaminating gases (81). Other functions served by packaging include assembling a variety of items, convenient handling, labeling, and finally sales promotion. A variety of materials ranging from metal foils to complex plastic films are in use. Examples of package modifications employing chemical additives are oleoresinous coating with or without suspended ZnO, which is used in the preservation of acid foods that do (e.g., sea food) or do not (e.g., cherries) produce sulfides; stabilizers to prevent degradation of plastic when exposed to heat and light; and hot-melt adhesives used to glue multilayered packages (tea, dehydrated soups, potato chips, etc.). A complete list of additives approved for use in packaging is given by Gilchrist (81).

In 1973, the National Science Foundation (NSF) estimated that as many as 3000 chemicals may enter foods indirectly from the process of packaging itself (90). A review of the safety of packaging ingredients by the FDA has resulted in banning the adhesive Flectol H, polyurethane resins and the polyurethane curing agent and component of food packaging adhesives, 4,4'-methylenebis (2-chloroanaline), and the synthetic chemicals mercaptoimidazoline and 2-mercaptoimidazoline, used in the production of rubber articles (90).

Direct Food Additives

Among the approximately 2800 chemicals added to foods, sucrose, corn syrup, dextrose, and salt make up 93% by weight. These additives serve a variety of purposes in foods including flavoring (natural and synthetic flavoring agents, nutritive and non-nutritive sweeteners), preservation (antioxidants, antibacterials, curing and pickling agents, gases, and sequestrants), and texturing (enzymes, firming agents, formulation aids, binders, thickeners, aerating agents, and texturizers), and also serve as processing aids (anticaking agents, dough conditioners, drying agents, emulsifiers, leavening agents, lubricants, surface-active agents, etc.) and as nutritional supplements (variety of macro- and micronutrients including amino acids, vitamins, and minerals). Colors, which are also direct additives have been discussed. For a detailed classification of food additives and a list of compounds in each class of additives, the reader is referred to reviews by Kraybill (120), Gilchrist (81), and Hayes and Campbell (90).

In spite of rigorous testing and requirements for the demonstration of safety of all food additives, absolute safety cannot be assured owing to species and individual differences in the composition of the diet, absorption, metabolism, and excretion of the additives. Toxic reactions associated with the use of selected additives that have been restricted, banned, or are currently being critically reviewed are presented below.

Monosodium glutamate

MSG was on the FDA GRAS list in 1958 and was used both as a seasoning agent and as a flavor enhancer. Its suspected role in the Chinese restaurant syndrome or Kwok's disease (described earlier) coupled with the demonstration of lesions in the retina and the lateral geniculate nucleus of neonatal rats and mice (170) led to the establishment of an ADI of up to 120 mg/kg in the general population (except for infants under 1 year of age) and voluntary discontinuation by United States manufacturers of MSG use in infant foods. Recent studies, however, cast doubt on the role of MSG in Chinese restaurant syndrome.

Cyclamate

Sodium and calcium cyclamates were introduced as non-nutritive sweeteners in 1950 following five years of testing showing no significant effects at a dose level as high as 5% of the diet in rats. Following FDA approval as a drug for use in obese and diabetic patients and establishment of safety in special purpose foods at 5 g/day by the National Academy of Sciences (NAS), cyclamates were included in the 1959 GRAS list. Significant consumption of cyclamates in low calorie foods and drinks followed. The FAO–WHO expert committee on food additives and the NAS established an ADI of 50 and 75 mg/kg, respectively, the former being adapted by the FDA. Subsequently, a study using implantation of cholesterol pellets containing cyclamate into the bladders of mice showed carcinogenic effects. Another study showed bladder tumors in 8 of the 60 rats given 2500 mg/kg of a mixture of cyclamate and saccharin (another non-nutritive sweetener) followed by cyclohexylamine, a metabolite of cyclamate.

Despite serious questions regarding the validity of these results in indicating carcinogenic potential of oral cyclamates, cyclamates were removed from the GRAS list and hence essentially banned. Several petitions following additional testing failed to bring cyclamates back on to the market. A more detailed account can be found in Kraybill (120) and Gilchrist (81).

Saccharin

After having been in use for more than 50 years with little indication of hazard, the above cyclamate/saccharin study of the FDA suggested the need to further study the carcinogenicity of saccharin. A review of saccharin carcinogenicity studies reveals problems with impurities of orthotoluene sulfonamide in the saccharin used as well as with bladder stones and parasites in test animals fed saccharin at 5 and 7.5% of the diet throughout gestation and lifetime of the first generation (242a). The effect was confirmed at the 5% dietary level in a later multigeneration study.

Following an extension of Interim Food Additive status for saccharin, the FDA proposed to ban food additive use of saccharin in 1977, drawing an enormous public outcry that led to a postponement of the ban by a congressional moratorium and pending results of additional studies (174). Saccharin is not considered to be a mutagen although it produces mitotic aneuploidy in the yeast *Saccharomyces cerevisiae*. It is known to promote the development of bladder cancer following exposure to a bladder carcinogen (160) apparently mediated by increased urinary indoles generated as a result of altered protein metabolism in the cecum (214). Several recent studies failed to detect urinary mutagens following chronic saccharin feeding in animals.

Nitrates, nitrites, and nitrosamines

Nitrates and nitrites are used to cure meats and contribute to (a) the development of the characteristic flavor and pink color, (b) the prevention of rancidity, and (c) the prevention of growth of *Clostridium botulinum* spores in or on meats.

Other sources of nitrates and nitrites as summarized by Newberne (162) include water (from soils, rocks, chemical fertilizers, and decomposing organic matter), vegetables (beets, radishes, lettuce, celery, and spinach), and endogenous secretion (saliva and bacterial action in the mouth and gut). Menzer and Nelson (151) quoted the total daily intake of nitrates in humans from all sources at 75 mg/person.

Nitrates can be reduced endogenously by microbial systems to nitrites which then oxidize the hemoglobin to methemoglobin (heme iron from ferrous to ferric state). Methemoglobin, being unable to combine with oxygen, following accumulation in sufficient quantities can lead to anoxia. The use of water with high nitrate content in making bottle formulae, baby foods, spinach with high nitrate content, and occasionally meats with high levels of added nitrates and nitrites have resulted in life-threatening methemoglobinemia in humans, especially children (162). The consumption of plants high in nitrates by animals has caused significant economic loss for owners (176).

Another aspect of nitrates and thus nitrites in foods is the reaction of nitrite with secondary amines to form a variety of nitrosamines including *N*-nitrosodimethylamine (DMN), *N*-nitrosodiethylamine (DEN), *N*-nitrosodibutylamine (DBN), *N*-nitrosodipropylamine (DPN), *N*-nitrosopyrolidine, *N*-nitrosopiperidine, and *N*-nitrososarcosine (195). In addition to their presence in foods, nitrosamines have been found in air, tobacco smoke, alcoholic beverages, and cow's milk. Nitrosamines are converted to active electrophilic species following α-hydroxylation, resulting in the formation of unstable hydroxyalkyl compounds which are subsequently converted to reactive alkyl carbonium ions. Biotransformation of nitrosamines is summarized by Williams and Weisburger (251).

Nitrosamines are acutely toxic causing centrilobular hepatic necrosis in animals and humans, fibrous occlusion of the central veins, and pleural and peritoneal hemorrhages in animals (see ref. 195). Chronic toxicity results in hepatic fibrosis, bile duct proliferation, hepatic hyperplasia, and focal abnormalities of hepatocyte structure. Nitrosamines are mutagenic and carcinogenic. Nitrosamines are potent carcinogens, producing cancer in a variety of organs including the liver, respiratory tract, kidney, urinary bladder, esophagus, stomach, lower gastrointestinal tract, and pancreas (see refs. 195 and 251). Although nitrosamines are carcinogenic, because they are not added to foods they are thus not subject to the restrictions of the Delaney Amendment. Newberne (162) has summarized the earlier work with nitrites which indicates carcinogenicity or at the least the promoting activity of nitrite itself in animals. Evaluation of these data by the FDA has resulted in a recent lowering of nitrite added to meats for curing 200 ppm to 120 ppm (34). Also, inhibition of nitrosamine formation in foods by ascorbate and sodium erythorbate prompted the FDA to suggest the addition of 550 ppm of one of these compounds to meats during curing. Because of the threat of *C. botulinum* growth in the complete absence of nitrite, a total ban of nitrite use is ill-advised in the absence of a safer substitute.

Safrole

Safrole and other alkenylbenzene compounds (β-asarone, methyleugenol, estragole, and isosafrole) are active components of many spice flavors. Sassafras, which contains high levels of safrole, has been used as a flavoring agent in sarsaparilla root beer. Safrole consumption also occurred in the form of sassafras oil and sassafras tea, the latter still occurring to a limited extent in the United States (see ref. 153). Hall (85) summarized the hepatotoxic effects of safrole at doses less than 40 mg/kg, and also the early FDA studies demonstrating hepatocarcinogenicity of safrole in rats at high doses. Later studies showed that a total dose of only 0.5–1.5 mg orally or intraperitoneally to infant male mice caused high liver tumor incidence. Dihydrosafrole, a synthetic safrole, caused esophageal tumors in rats, and some of the other natural alkenylbenzenes also are carcinogenic (see ref. 153). This finding resulted in the FDA banning the use of safrole, sassafras, and sassafras oil from commercial use in foods, including root beer, in 1960. Safrole appears to be activated to a 1-hydroxy metabolite which is then sulfated. The 1-hydroxy sulfate ester is apparently the ultimate carcinogen forming adducts with guanine and adenine (153). Although the role of 1-hydroxy sulfate ester is supported by lower DNA binding and liver cancer incidence in brachymorphic mice deficient in sulfate ester (66), the possibility of a role for additional active metabolites exists.

Several other chemical additives prohibited from use due to a potential risk or to lack of demonstration of safety include calamus and its derivatives in 1968 (containing alkenylbenzene flavoring agents); coumarin flavoring compounds in 1953; chlorofluorocarbon propellants in self-pressurized containers in 1978 (due to their role in the dissolution of the earth's ozone layer, which results in increased skin cancer risk from ultraviolet radiation from the sun); diethyl pyrocarbonate (DEPC), an antimicrobial agent in beers and juices (cold pasteurization) and a ferment inhibitor, in 1972 due to the presence of the carcinogen urethan in DEPC-treated products; and Dulcin, a sweetener, in 1950 due to liver and bladder cancer in rats. A summary of the toxicity of some food chemicals and restrictive actions are presented by Kraybill (120) and Gilchrist (81).

As exemplified by the above, only a few of the several thousand food additives have been subjected to regulatory action in the last three decades. This suggests that the trial and error pattern of introduction of chemical additives by our predecessors has left us with a virtually safe food supply. Unrecognized, however, are the low-level long-term effects such as carcinogenicity, idiosyncratic reactions due to poorly understood factors, and interactions between two or more chemical additives present simultaneously in foods. Our current understanding of the effect of various processing methods including simple ones such as frying, broiling, and baking, on the various chemicals in foods needs expansion. The effect of chemical additives on the natural constituents of foods also needs study. The role of the FDA and other regulatory agencies lies not only in recognizing food chemical hazards to man through epidemiologic reports and sensible extrapolations from existing animal data, but also weighing them against the total package of benefits (economic as well as human). Both areas are, at this time, somewhat subjective.

Toxic Factors Produced During Processing

Food processing is aimed at improving the quality of foodstuffs, ensuring safety, and finally enhancing the ease of preparation. This requires various chemical and physical treatments of food which may result in (a) partial or complete destruction or removal of nutrients, (b) inferior digestibility or utilization of nutrients, and (c) generation of new, potentially harmful chemicals (253). The first two effects can be overcome by nutritional supplementation. The latter represents a need for appropriate toxicologic investigation. In addition, similar products can form during storage due to continuous effects of heat, humidity, light, oxygen, and catalysts present in foods.

Formation of crosslinked amino acid side chains such as lysinoalanine, ornithinoalanine, and lanthionine, as well as racemization of amino acids to D-analogs appear to take place during alkali treatment, for example, of soybean protein for preparing imitation meat (73). These products, especially lysinoalanine, have been shown to cause nephrocytomegaly (enlarged nuclei and cytoplasm) of the pars recta cells. Nonenzymatic browning reactions (Maillard reactions) occurring during heating of foods (drying, frying, roasting, baking, and broiling) involve chemical interactions between amino acids and sugars (aldoses and ketoses) often forming mutagenic premelanoid secondary amine derivatives (Amadori and Heyns' products) which have been proposed to have a role in aging and the development of lens lesions in diabetes mellitus. Gruenwadel et al. (83) have shown that nitrosation of these products can result in the formation of mutagenic substances.

A further series of reactions during heating yields reductones, furans, aminocarbonyls, and pyrazines among others, all of which have been reported to be mutagenic (183). In general, high protein foods appear to possess more mutagenic activity compared with foods rich in carbohydrates and/or fats. Pyrolysis of proteins and amino acids at high temperatures (300°C or more) may also yield mutagenic substances. Sugimura (228) has reported a series of heterocyclic compounds which were positive in one or more rodent species for carcinogenicity (Table 6). Felton et al. (65) demonstrated that at least some of these are metabolized to N-hydroxy derivative involving P-448 IIa (a form of P-450), the derivative itself being mutagenic.

Cooked foods also contain a variety of polycyclic aromatic hydrocarbons (PAH) acquired by pyrolysis during cooking or by their prior contact with petroleum and/or coal tar products. Although the carcinogenic effects of PAH are known, the contribution of diet to the overall PAH exposure in humans and its significance in the absence of other substantial exposures has yet to be determined.

Fats undergo three basic changes during storage and/or heat treatments, i.e., auto-oxidation (oxidation below 100°C), thermal oxidation, and thermal polymerization. Auto-oxidation leads to generation of hydroperoxides via a free-radical mechanism and to rancidity. High levels of rancid fats (5% or more of the diet) caused decreased food consumption, diarrhea, weight loss, leukopenia, hair loss, and eventually death at higher doses. Lesions were mainly restricted to the intestinal tract (see ref. 253 for review). Hydroperoxides are also carcinogenic, inducing lymphosarcoma and tumors of the pituitary, mammary gland, cervix, and interstitial cells (of testes) in various animals. The question of the safety of heated and oxidized fats is still under debate. Those components of heated oils that fail to form adducts with urea (NAF, i.e., nonurea-adduct-forming) appear to be the toxic

TABLE 6. *Carcinogenicities of dietary heterocyclic amines isolated from cooked foods and pyrolysates of amino acids and proteins*

		Carcinogenicity	
Chemical name	Abbreviation	Mouse	Rat
2-Amino-3-methylimidazo[4,5-f]quinoline	IQ	Liver, forestomach, lung	Liver, intestine, Zymbal gland, clitoral gland, skin
2-Amino-3,4-dimethylimidazo[4,5-f]quinoline	MeIQ	Liver, forestomach	Ongoing
2-Amino-3,8-dimethylimidazo[4,5-f]quinoxaline	MeIQx	Liver	Liver, Zymbal gland, skin
3-Amino-1,4-dimethyl-5H-pyrido[4,3-b]indole	Trp-P-1	Liver	Liver
3-Amino-1,4-dimethyl-5H-pyrido[4,3-b]indole	Trp-P-2	Liver	Liver
2-Amino-6-methyldipyrido[1,2-a:3′,2′-d]imidazole	Glu-P-1	Liver, blood vessel	Liver, intestine, Zymbal gland, clitoral gland
2-Aminodipyrido[1,2-a:3′,2′-d]imidazole	Glu-P-1	Liver, blood vessel	Liver, intestine, Zymbal gland, clitoral gland
2-Amino-9H-pyrido[2,3-b]indole	AαC	Liver, blood vessel	Ongoing
2-Amino-3-methyl-9H-pyrido[2,3-b]indole	MeAαC	Liver, blood vessel	Ongoing

From ref. 228, with permission.

components. Most toxic among these appear to be the cyclic manomeric fatty acids followed by polymers of fatty acids. Toxic effects include, in addition to those described above, hepatomegaly and carcinogenic effects. The reader is referred to the review by Yannai (254) for further details.

CONCLUSION

Although this discussion on the variety of naturally occurring and man-made chemicals in food is by no means complete, it emphasizes the array of chemical toxicants present in food. Yet the incidence of known acute human disease is surprisingly small. In addition to our ability to learn from experience and avoid demonstrated or known hazards, this remarkable safety record seems to be complemented by a variety of antitoxic dietary compounds.

Long-term chemical effects, however, are harder to discern. A greater understanding of the balance between toxic and antitoxic compounds in our food is indispensible to the prevention and treatment of food-borne diseases. Our march toward this goal is highlighted by recent recommendations by Sugimura (228) aimed at preventing environmental mutagens/carcinogens and tumor promotors. These include consumption of a variety of foods and vitamins for a nutritionally balanced diet and avoidance of excess calories (especially as fats), fungal contaminated foods, excessive salt intake and eating charred parts of cooked foods.

REFERENCES

1. Alston, T. A., Mela, L., and Bright, H. G. (1977): 3-Nitropropionate, the toxic substance of Indigofera, is a suicide inactivator of succinate dehydrogenase, *Proc. Natl. Acad. Sci., USA,* 74:3767–3771.
2. Anderson, E. S. (1968): Middlesbrough outbreak of infantile enteritis and transferable drug resistance, *Br. Med. J.,* 1:293.
3. Arbeiter, H. I. (1967): How prevalent is allergy among United States school children? A survey of findings in the Munster (Indiana) school system. *Clin. Pediatr.,* 6:140–142.
4. Argus, M. F., and Hock-Ligeti, C. (1961): Comparative study of the carcinogenic activity of nitrosamines, *J. Natl. Cancer Inst.,* 27:695–703.
5. Aronow, L., and Kerdel-Vegas, F. (1965): Selino-cystathionine, a pharmacologically active factor in the seeds of *Lecythis ollaria:* Cytotoxic and depilatory effects, *Nature (Lond.),* 205:1185–86.
6. Bakir, F., Damluji, S. F., Amin-Zaki, L., Murtadha, M., Khalidi, A., Al-Rawi, N. Y., Tikritis, Dhahir, H. I., Clarkson, T. W., Smith, J. C., and Doherty, R. A. (1973): Methyl mercury poisoning in Iraq. *Science,* 181:230–241.
7. Baldessarini, R. J. (1985): Drugs and the treatment of psychiatric disorders. In: *Goodman and Gilman's The Pharmacological Basis of Therapeutics,* 7th ed., edited by A. G. Gilman, L. S. Goodman, T. W. Rall, and F. Murad, pp. 387–445, Macmillan, NY.
8. Barash, P. G. (1978): Nutrient toxicities of vitamin K. In: *Handbook of Nutrition and Food,* edited by M. Rechigl, Jr., pp. 97–100. CRC Press, Boca Raton, FL.
9. Barger, G. (1931): *Ergot and Ergotism.* Guerney and Jackson, London.
10. Bartholomew, R. M., and Ryan, D. A. (1980): Lack of mutagenicity of some phytoestrogens in the *Salmonella*/mammalian microsome assay, *Mut. Res.,* 78:317–321.
11. Bell, R. G. (1978): Metabolism of vitamin K and prothrombin synthesis: Anticoagulants and the vitamin K–epoxide cycle. *Proc. Soc. Exp. Biol. Med.,* 37:2599–2604.
12. Berardi, L. C., and Goldblatt, L. A. (1980): Gossypol. In: *Toxic Constituents of Plant Foodstuffs,* 2nd ed, edited by I. E. Liener, pp. 193–237. Academic Press, NY.
13. Bergdoll, M. S. (1979): Staphylococcal intoxications. In: *Foodborne Infections and Intoxications,* 2nd ed., edited by H. Riemann and F. L. Bryan, pp. 443–494. Academic Press, NY.
14. Bingham, S., Williams, D. R. R., Cole, T. J., and James, W. P. T. (1979): Dietary fibre and regional large bowel cancer mortality in Britain. *Br. J. Cancer,* 40:456–463.
15. Birk, Y., and Peri, I. (1980): Saponins. In: *Toxic Constituents of Plant Foodstuffs,* 2nd ed., edited by I. E. Liener, pp. 161–182. Academic Press, NY.
16. Bjerrum, P. J. (1984): Induction of anion transport in biological membranes. In: *Biological Effects of Organolead Compounds,* edited by P. Grandjean, pp. 125–136. CRC Press, Boca Raton, FL.
17. Bo-Linn, G., Santa Ana, C., Morawski, S., and Fordstran, J. (1982): Starch Blockers—Their effect on calorie absorption from a high starch meal. *N. Engl. J. Med.,* 307:1413–1416.
18. Bongiovanni, A. M. (1983): An epidemic of premature thelarche in Puerto Rico. *J. Pediatr.,* 103:245–246.
19. Bousquet, W. F. (1979): Cardiovascular and renal effects of cadmium. In: *Cadmium Toxicity,* edited by J. H. Mennear, pp. 133–157. Marcel Dekker, NY.
20. Brietschwerdt, E. B., Armstrong, P. J., Robinette, C. L., Dillman, R. C., and Karl, M. L. (1986): Three cases of acute zinc toxicosis in dogs. *Vet. Hum. Toxicol.,* 28:109–117.
21. Bryan, F. L. (1979): Epidemiology of food-borne diseases. In:

Foodborne Infections and Intoxications, 2nd ed., edited by H. Riemann and F. L. Bryan, pp. 3–69. Academic Press, NY.

22. Bryan, F. L. (1979): Infections and intoxications caused by other bacteria. In: *Foodborne Infections and Intoxications,* 2nd ed., edited by H. Riemann and F. L. Bryan, pp. 212–298. Academic Press, NY.

23. Bryan, F. L. (1982): *Diseases Transmitted by Foods* (a classification and summary), 2nd ed. HHA Publ. No. 83-8327.

24. Bryan, F. L., Fanelli, M. J., and Riemann, H. (1979): *Salmonella* infections. In: *Foodborne Infections and Intoxications,* 2nd ed., edited by H. Riemann and F. L. Bryan, pp. 74–130. Academic Press, NY.

25. Bureau of Foods (1982): *Toxicological Principles for the Safety Assessment of Direct Food Additives and Color Additives Used in Food.* U.S. Food and Drug Administration, Washington, DC.

26. Burgeois, C. H., Shank, R. C., Grossman, R. A., Johnson, D. O., Wooding, W. L., and Chandavomil, P. (1971): Acute aflatoxin B_1 toxicity in the macaque and its similarities to Reye's syndrome. *Lab. Invest.,* 24:206–216.

27. Busby, W. F., Jr., and Wogan, G. N. (1979): Foodborne mycotoxins and alimentary mycotoxicoses. In: *Foodborne Infections and Intoxications,* 2nd ed., edited by H. Riemann and F. L. Bryan, pp. 519–610. Academic Press, NY.

28. Busby, W. F., Jr., and Wogan, G. N. (1981): Aflatoxins. In: *Mycotoxins and N-Nitroso Compounds: Environmental Risks,* Vol. II., edited by R. C. Shank, pp. 3–28. CRC Press, Boca Raton, FL.

29. Busby, W. F., Jr., and Wogan, G. N. (1981): Ochratoxins. In: *Mycotoxins and N-Nitroso Compounds: Environmental Risks,* Vol. II., edited by R. C. Shank, pp. 129–136. CRC Press, Boca Raton, FL.

30. Busby, W. F., Jr., and Wogan, G. N. (1981): Psoralens. In: *Mycotoxins and N-Nitroso compounds: Environmental Risks,* Vol. II., edited by R. C. Shank, pp. 105–119. CRC Press, Boca Raton, FL.

31. Busby, W. F., Jr., and Wogan, G. N. (1981): Zearalenone and its derivatives. In: *Mycotoxins and N-Nitroso Compounds: Environmental Risks,* Vol. II, edited by R. C. Shank, pp. 145–154. CRC Press, Boca Raton, FL.

32. Carlborg, F. W. (1979): Cancer mathematical models and aflatoxin. *Food Cosmet. Toxicol.,* 17:159–166.

33. Carrol, K. K. (1982): Dietary fat and its relationship to human cancer. In: *Carcinogens and Mutagens in the Environment,* Vol. 1, edited by H. F. Stich, pp. 31–38, CRC Press, Boca Raton, FL.

34. CAST (1980): Foods From Animals: Quantity, Quality and Safety. Report No. 82, Council for Agricultural Science and Technology, Ames, IA.

35. CDC (1983): Foodborne Disease Outbreaks. Annual Summary, 1981. HHA Publ. No. 83-8185.

36. Chen, K. K., and Rose, C. L. (1952): Nitrite and thiosulfate therapy in cyanide poisoning. *JAMA,* 149:113–119.

37. Cherian, M. G., and Rodgers, K. (1982): Chelation of cadmium from metallothioneine *in vivo* and its excretion in rats repeatedly injected with cadmium chloride. *J. Pharmacol. Exp. Ther.,* 222: 699–704.

38. Chevion, M., Mager, J., and Glaser, G. (1983): Favism producing agents. In: *Handbook of Naturally Occurring Food Toxicants,* edited by M. Richcigl, Jr., pp. 63–79. CRC Press, Boca Raton, FL.

39. Ciegler, A., Burmeister, H. R., Vesonder, R. F., and Hesseltine, C. W. (1981): Mycotoxins: Occurrence in the environment. In: *Mycotoxins and N-Nitroso Compounds: Environmental Risks,* Vol. II., edited by R. C. Shank, pp. 1–50. CRC Press, Boca Raton, FL.

40. Clarkson, T. W. (1983): Methyl mercury toxicity to the mature and developing nervous system: Possible mechanisms. In: *Biological Aspects of Metals and Metal-Related Diseases,* edited by D. Sarkar, pp. 183–197. Raven Press, NY.

41. Committee on Infectious Diseases (1982): Aspirin and Reye's syndrome. *Pediatrics,* 69:810–812.

42. Conn, E. E. (1973): Cyanogenetic glycosides. In: *Toxicants Occurring Naturally in Foods,* pp. 299–308. National Academy of Science, Washington, DC.

43. Conners, C. K. (1980): *Food Additives and Hyperactive Children.* Plenum Press, NY.

44. Croy, R. G., Essigman, J. M., Reinhold, V. N., and Wogan, G. N. (1978): Identification of the principal aflatoxin B_1-DNA adduct formed *in vivo* in rat liver. *Proc. Natl. Acad. Sci. USA,* 75:1745–1749.

45. Cumming, F., Briggs, M., and Briggs, M. (1981): Clinical toxicology of vitamin supplements. In: *Vitamins in Human Biology and Medicine,* edited by M. H. Briggs, pp. 187–243. CRC Press, Boca Raton, FL.

46. Curatolo, P. W., and Robertson, D. (1983): The health consequences of caffeine. *Ann. Intern. Med.,* 98:641–653.

47. Deshpande, S. S., Sathe, S. K., and Salunkhe, D. K. (1984): Chemistry and safety of plant polyphenols. In: *Nutritional and Toxicological Aspects of Food Safety,* edited by M. Friedman, pp. 457–495. Plenum Press, NY.

48. Dickerson, O. B. (1980): Arsenic. In: *Metals in the Environment,* edited by H. A. Waldron, pp. 1–24. Academic Press, New York.

49. Doll, R., and Peto, R. (1981): The causes of cancer: Quantitative estimates of avoidable risks of cancer in the United States today. *J. Natl. Cancer Inst.,* 66:1193–1308.

50. Dorr, R. T., and Paxinos, J. (1978): The current status of laetrile. *Ann. Intern. Med.,* 89:389–397.

51. Duggan, R. E., and Corneliussen, P. E. (1972): Dietary intake of pesticide chemicals in the United States (III), June 1968–April 1970. *Pestic. Monit. J.,* 5:331–341.

52. Eamens, G. J., Macadam, J. F., and Laing, E. A. (1984): Skeletal abnormalities in young horses associated with zinc toxicity and hypocuprosis. *Aust. Vet. J.,* 61:205–207.

53. Elinder, C.-G. (1985): Cadmium uses, occurrence and intake. In: *Cadmium and Health: A Toxicological and Epidemiological Appraisal,* Vol. I, edited by L. Friberg, C.-G. Elinder, T. Kjellstrom, and G. F. Nordberg, pp. 23–64. CRC Press, Boca Raton, FL.

54. Elinder, C.-G. (1985): Other toxic effects. In: *Cadmium and Health: A Toxicological and Epidemiological Appraisal,* Vol. II., edited by L. Friberg, C.-G. Elinder, T. Kjellstrom, and G. F. Nordberg, pp. 159–204. CRC Press, Boca Raton, FL.

55. Elinder, C.-G., and Kjellstrom, T. (1985): Carcinogenic and genetic effects. In: *Cadmium and Health: A Toxicological and Epidemiological Appraisal,* Vol. II., edited by L. Friberg, C.-G. Elinder, T. Kjellstrom, and G. F. Nordberg, pp. 205–230. CRC Press, Boca Raton, FL.

56. Ellis, K. J., Yuen, K., Yasumura, S., and Cohn, S. H. (1984): Dose response analysis of Cd in man: Body burden vs. kidney dysfunction. *Environ. Res.,* 33:216–226.

57. Eppley, R. M. (1977): Chemistry of stachybotryotoxicosis. In: *Mycotoxins in Human and Animal Health,* edited by J. V. Rodricks, C. W. Hesseltine, and M. A. Mehlman, pp. 285–293. Pathotox, Park Forest South, IL.

58. Essigman, J. M., Croy, R. G., Nadzan, A. M., Busby, W. F. Jr., Reinhold, V. N., Buchi, G., and Wogan, G. N. (1977): Structural identification of the major DNA adduct formed by aflatoxin B_1 *in vitro. Proc. Natl. Acad. Sci. USA,* 74:1870–1874.

59. Evans, C. S. (1983): Toxic amino acids. In: *Handbook of Naturally Occurring Plant Toxicants,* edited by M. Richcigl, Jr., pp. 3–14. CRC Press, Boca Raton, FL.

60. Fara, D., Del Corvo, G., Bernuzzi, S., Bigatello, A., DiPietro, C., Scaglioni, S., and Chiumello, G. (1979): Epidemic of breast enlargement in an Italian school. *Lancet,* ii:295–297.

61. Fassett, D. W. (1973): Oxalates. In: *Toxicants Occurring Naturally in Foods,* 2nd ed., pp. 346–362. National Academy of Sciences, Washington, DC.

62. Fassett, D. W. (1980): Cadmium. In: *Metals in the Environment,* edited by H. A. Waldron, pp. 61–110. Academic Press, NY.

63. *Federal Food, Drug and Cosmetic Act, As Amended* (1976): U.S. Government Printing Office, Washington, DC.

64. Feingold, B. F. (1975): *Why Your Child is Hyperactive,* Random House, NY.

65. Felton, J. S., Bjeldanes, L. F., and Hatch, F. T. (1984): Mutagens in cooked foods: Metabolism and genetic toxicity. In: *Nutritional and Toxicological Aspects of Food Safety,* edited by M. Friedman, pp. 555–566. Plenum Press, NY.

66. Fennell, T. R., Eiseman, R. W., Miller, J. A., and Miller, E. C. (1985): Major role of hepatic sulfotransferase activity in the metabolic activation, DNA adduct formation, and carcinogenicity of 1′-hydroxy 2′,3′-dehydroestragole in infant male C57BL/6J X C3H/HeJF$_1$ mice. *Cancer Res.,* 45:5310–5320.

67. Fernandez, H., Ruzpala, G. M., and Wodstrom, T. (1983): Culture supernatants of *Campylobacter jejuni* induce secretory response in jejunal segments of adult rats. *Infect. Immunol.,* 40:429–431.

68. Fiala, E. S., Caswell, N., Sohn, O. S., Felder, M. R., McCoy,

G. D., and Weisburger, J. H. (1984): Non-alcohol dehydrogenase-mediated metabolism of methylazoxymethanol in the deer mouse *Peromyscus maniculatus. Cancer Res.,* 44:2885–2891.

69. Folsch, U., Grieb, N., Caspary, W., and Creutzfeldt, W. (1981): Influence of short- and long-term feeding of an α-amylase inhibitor (BAYe 4609) on the exocrine pancreas of the rat. *Digestion,* 21: 74–82.

70. Food Chemical News (1983): FD and C red 3 is carcinogenic in rats, NTP peer reviewers conclude, *Food Chem. News,* 25:50–51.

71. Food Safety Council Scientific Committee (1978): Proposed system for food safety assessment. *Food Cosmet. Toxicol.,* 16:1–136.

72. Friberg, L., Elinder, C.-G., Kjellstrom, T., and Nordberg, G. F. (1985): *Cadmium and Health: A Toxicological and Epidemiological Appraisal,* Vol. II. CRC Press, Boca Raton, FL.

73. Friedman, M., Gumbmann, M. R., and Masters, P. M. (1984): Protein-alkali reactions: Chemistry, toxicology and nutritional consequences. In: *Nutritional and Toxicological Aspects of Food Safety,* edited by M. Friedman, pp. 367–412. Plenum Press, NY.

74. Fuhrman, F. A. (1983): Toxic constituents of animal foodstuffs: Eggs of fishes and amphibians. In: *Handbook of Naturally Occurring Food Toxicants,* edited by M. Rechcigl, Jr., pp. 301–311. CRC Press, Boca Raton, FL.

75. Gale, G. R., Alkins, L. M., Smith, A. B., and Jones, M. M. (1986): Comparative effects of parenteral and oral administration of selected dithiocarbamates on body burden and organ distribution of cadmium. *Res. Commun. Chem. Pathol. Pharmacol.,* 53:129–132.

76. Gallaher, D., and Schneeman, B. O. (1984): Nutritional and metabolic response to plant inhibitors of digestive enzymes. *Adv. Exp. Med. Biol.,* 177:299–320.

77. Gareis, M., Hashem, A., Bauer, T., and Gadek, B. (1986): Glucuronide metabolites of T-2 toxin and diacetoxy-scirpenol in the bile of isolated perfused rat liver. *Toxicol. Appl. Pharmacol.,* 84: 168–172.

78. Genigeorgis, C., and Riemann, H. (1979): Food processing and hygiene. In: *Foodborne Infections and Intoxications,* 2nd ed., edited by H. Riemann and F. L. Bryan, pp. 613–714. Academic Press, NY.

79. Gentry, P. A. (1986): Comparative biochemical changes associated with mycotoxicosis other than aflatoxicosis and trichothecene toxicosis. In: *Diagnosis of Mycotoxicoses,* edited by J. R. Richard and J. R. Thurston, pp. 125–139. Martinus Nijhoff, Dordrecht, Netherlands.

80. Gilbert, R. J. (1979): *Bacillus cereus* gastroenteritis. In: *Foodborne Infections and Intoxications,* 2nd ed., edited by H. Riemann and F. L. Bryan, pp. 495–518. Academic Press, NY.

81. Gilchrist, A. (1981): *Foodborne Disease and Food Safety.* American Medical Association, Monroe, WI.

82. Goyer, R. A. (1986): Toxic effects of metals. In: *Casarette and Doull's Toxicology: The Basic Science of Poisons,* 3rd ed., edited by C. D. Klaassen, M. O. Amdor, J. Doull, pp. 582–635. MacMillan, NY.

83. Gruenwadel, D. W., Lynch, S. C., and Russell, G. F. (1984): The influence of 1-(N-L-tryptophan)-1-deoxy-D-fructose (FRU-TRP) and its N-nitrosated analogue (NO-FRU-TRP) on the viability and intracellular synthetic activity (DNA, RNA and protein) of HeLa S3-carcinoma cells. In: *Nutritional and Toxicological Aspects of Food Safety,* edited by M. Friedman, pp. 269–285. Plenum Press, NY.

84. Haggard, D. L., Stowe, H. D., Conner, G. H., and Johnson, D. W. (1980): Immunologic effects of experimental iodine toxicosis in young cattle. *Am. J. Vet. Res.,* 41:539–543.

85. Hall, R. L. (1973): Toxicants occurring naturally in spices and flavors. In: *Toxicants Occurring Naturally in Foods,* 2nd ed., pp. 448–463. National Academy of Sciences, Washington, DC.

86. Halstead, B. W. (1978): *Poisonous and Venomous Marine Animals of the World.* Darwin Press, Princeton, NJ.

87. Harper, A. E. (1973): Amino acids of nutritional importance. In: *Toxicants Occurring Naturally in Foods,* 2nd ed., edited by Committee on Food Protection, NRC, pp. 130–152. National Academy of Sciences, Washington, DC.

88. Hayatsu, S., Arimoto, K., Togawa, K., and Mokita, M. (1981): Inhibitory effects of the ether extract of human feces on activities of mutagens: Inhibition of oleic and linoleic acids. *Mutat. Res.,* 81:287–293.

89. Hayes, A. W. (1981): *Mycotoxin Teratogenicity and Mutagenicity.* CRC Press, Boca Raton, FL.

90. Hayes, J. R., and Campbell, T. C. (1986): Food additives and contaminants. In: *Casarett and Doull's Toxicology, The Basic Science of Poisons,* 3rd ed., edited by C. D. Klaassen, M. O. Amdur, and J. Doull, pp. 771–800. Macmillan, NY.

91. Hayes, K. C., and Haystead, D. M. (1973): Toxicity of the vitamins. In: *Toxicants Occurring Naturally in Foods,* 2nd ed., pp. 235–253. National Academy of Sciences, Washington, DC.

92. Hobbs, B. C. (1979): *Clostridium perfringens* gastroenteritis. In: *Foodborne Infections and Intoxications,* 2nd ed., edited by H. Riemann, and F. L. Bryan, pp. 131–173. Academic Press, NY.

93. Hogan, G. R., Ryan, N. J., and Hayes, A. W. (1978): Aflatoxin B$_1$ and Reye's syndrome. *Lancet,* i:561.

94. Hood, R. D., Bishop, S. L. (1972): Teratogenic effects of sodium arsenate in mice. *Arch. Environ. Health,* 24:62–65.

95. Horvath, D. J. (1976): Trace elements and health. In: *Trace Substances and Health: A Handbook,* Part 1, edited by P. M. Newberne, pp. 319–356. Marcel Dekker, New York.

96. Houtsmuller, U. M. T., Struijk, C. B., and Van Der Beek, A. (1970): Decrease in rate of ATP synthesis of isolated rat heart mitochondria induced by dietary erucic acid. *Biochim. Biophys. Acta,* 218:564–566.

97. Hsieh, D. P. H. (1979): Basic metabolic effects of mycotoxins. In: *Interactions of Mycotoxins in Animal Production,* pp. 43–55. National Academy of Sciences, Washington, DC.

98. Hsieh, D. P. H. (1985): An assessment of liver cancer risk posed by aflatoxin M$_1$ in the Western World. In: *Trichothecenes and Other Mycotoxins,* edited by J. Lacey, pp. 521–528. Wiley, NY.

99. Hsieh, D. P. H. (1986): Genotoxicity of mycotoxins. In: *New Concepts and Developments in Toxicology,* edited by P. L. Chambers, P. Gehring, and F. Sakai, pp. 251–259. Elsevier, NY.

100. Ikeguonu, F. I., and Bassir, O. (1977): Effects of phytohemagglutinins from immature legume seeds on the function and enzyme activities of the liver and on the organs of the rat. *Toxicol. Appl. Pharmacol.,* 40:217–226.

101. Jacobs, A. (1977): Iron overload—Clinical and pathological aspects. *Semin. Hematol.,* 14:89–113.

102. Jacobsen, B. K., and Bjelke, E. (1982): Coffee consumption and cancer: A prospective study. In: *Proceedings of the 13th International Cancer Congress.* Seattle, WA (abstr.).

103. Jaffe, W. G. (1980): Hemagglutinins (lectins). In: *Toxic Constituents of Plant Foodstuffs,* edited by I. E. Liener, 2nd ed., pp. 73–102. Academic Press, NY.

104. Jaffe, W. G. (1983): Nutritional significance of lectins. In: *Handbook of Naturally Occurring Food Toxicants,* edited by M. Rechcigl, Jr., pp. 31–38, CRC Press, Boca Raton, FL.

105. Jensen, A. A. (1984): Metabolism and toxicokinetics. In: *Biological Effects of Organolead Compounds,* edited by P. Grandjean, pp. 97–116. CRC Press, Boca Raton, FL.

106. Joffe, A. Z. (1986): *Fusarium species: Their biology and toxicology.* John Wiley, NY.

107. Joint FAO/WHO Expert Committee on Pesticide Residues (1973): Joint Meeting of the FAO Working Party of Experts on Pesticide Residues. WHO Tech Rep. Ser. No. 55, Washington, DC.

108. Kanisawa, M., and Suzuki, S. (1978): Induction of renal and hepatic tumors in mice by ochratoxin A, a mycotoxin. *Gann,* 69:599–600.

109. Kao, C. Y. (1966): Tetrodotoxin, saxitoxin and their significance in the study of excitation phenomena. *Pharmacol. Rev.,* 18:997–1049.

110. Kao, C. Y. (1967): Comparison of the biological actions of tetrodotoxin and saxitoxin. In: *Animal Toxins,* edited by F. E. Russell, and P. R. Saunders, pp. 109–114. Pergamon Press, Oxford.

111. Kassell, B. (1970): Inhibitors of proteolytic enzymes. *Methods Enzymol.,* 19:839–906.

112. Kazantzis, G. (1980): Mercury. In: *Metals in the Environment,* edited by H. A. Waldron, pp. 221–261. Academic Press, NY.

113. King, T. P., Pusztai, A., and Clarke, E. M. W. (1980): Kidney bean lectin-induced lesions in rat small intestine, I. Light microscopic studies. *J. Comp. Pathol.,* 90:585–593.

114. Kingsbury, J. M. (1980): Phytotoxicology. In: *Casarett and Doull's Toxicology, The basic Science of Poisons,* 2nd ed., edited by J. Doull, C. D. Klaassen, and M. O. Amdur, pp. 578–592. Macmillan, NY.

115. Kipling, M. D. (1980): Cobalt. In: *Metals in the Environment,* edited by H. A. Waldron, pp. 133–153. Academic Press, NY.

116. Kjellstrom, T. (1985): Renal effects. In: *Cadmium and Health: A Toxicological and Epidemiological Appraisal,* Vol. II, pp. 21–109. CRC Press, Boca Raton, FL.

117. Kjellstrom, T. (1985): Effects on bone on vitamin D and calcium metabolism. In: *Cadmium and Health: A Toxicological and Epidemiological Appraisal,* Vol. II, pp. 111–158. CRC Press, Boca Raton, FL.

118. Kojima, S., Kaminaka, K., Kiyozumi, M., and Honda, T. (1986): Comparative effects of three chelating agents on distribution and excretion of Cd in rats. *Toxicol. Appl. Pharmacol.,* 83:516–524.

119. Koller, L. D., Exon, J. H., Moore, S. A., and Watanabe, P. G. (1983): Evaluation of ELISA for detecting *in vivo* chemical immunomodulation. *J. Toxicol. Environ. Health,* 11:15–22.

120. Kraybill, H. F. (1976): Food chemicals and food additives. In: *Trace Substances and Health, A Handbook,* Part I, edited by P. M. Newberne, pp. 245–318. Marcel Dekker, NY.

121. Krogh, P., Hald, B., Plestina, R., and Ceovic, S. (1977): Balkan nephropathy and food-borne ochratoxin A: Preliminary results of a survey of foodstuffs. *Acta Pathol. Microbiol. Scand. (B),* 85:238–240.

122. Lampe, K. F. (1983): Mushroom poisoning. In: *Handbook of Naturally Occurring Food Toxicants,* edited by Rechcigl, Jr., M., pp. 193–212. CRC Press, Boca Raton, FL.

123. Lampe, K. F. (1986): Toxic effects of plant toxins. In: *Casarett and Doull's Toxicology, The Basic Science of Poisons,* 3rd ed., edited by C. D. Klaassen, M. O. Amdur, and J. Doull, pp. 757–770. Macmillan, New York.

124. Lauwerys, R. R., Bernard, A., Roels, H. A., Buchet, J.-P., and Viau, C. (1984): Characterization of Cd proteinuria in man and rat. *Environ. Health Perspect.,* 54:147–152.

125. Lewis, W. H., and Elvin-Lewis, M. P. F. (1977): *Medical Botany: Plants Affecting Human Health,* p. 57. John Wiley, NY.

126. Liener, I. E. (1980): Miscellaneous toxic factors. In: *Toxic Constituents of Plant Foodstuffs,* 2nd ed., edited by I. E. Liener, pp. 429–467. Academic Press, NY.

127. Liener, I. E., and Kakade, M. L. (1980): Protease inhibitors. In: *Toxic Constituents of Plant Foodstuffs,* 2nd ed., edited by I. E. Liener, pp. 7–71. Academic Press, NY.

128. Lipton, M. A., and Mayo, J. P. (1983): Diet and hyperkinesis—An update. *J. Am. Diet. Assoc.,* 83:132–134.

129. Livingston, A. L., Knuckles, B. E., Teuber, L. R., Hesterman, O. B., and Tsai, L. S. (1984): Minimizing the saponin content of alfalfa sprouts and leaf protein concentrates. In: *Nutritional and Toxicological Aspects of Food Safety,* edited by M. Friedman, pp. 253–268. Plenum Press, NY.

130. Lloyd, W. E., Daniels, G. N., and Stahr, H. M. (1985): Cases of nephrotoxic mycotoxicoses in cattle and swine in the United States. In: *Trichothecenes and Other Mycotoxins,* edited by J. Lacey, pp. 545–548. John Wiley, NY.

131. Louw, W. K. A., and Oelofsen, W. (1975): Carcinogenic and neurotoxic components in the cycad *Encephalartos alternsteinii* Leh. (family Zamiaceae). *Toxicology,* 13:447–452.

132. Lovenberg, W. (1973): Some vaso- and psychoactive substances in food. In: *Toxicants Occurring Naturally in Foods,* 2nd ed., pp. 170–188. National Academy of Sciences, Washington, DC.

133. Lutsky, I., Mor, N., Yagen, B., and Joffe, A. Z. (1978): The role of T-2 toxin in experimental alimentary toxic aleukia: A toxicity study of cats. *Toxicol. Appl. Pharmacol.,* 43:111–124.

134. MacGregor, J. T. (1984): Genetic and carcinogenic effects of plant flavonoids: An overview. In: *Nutritional and Toxicological Aspects of Food Safety,* edited by M. Friedman, pp. 497–526. Plenum Press, NY.

135. Mager, J., Chevion, M., and Glaser, G. (1980): Favism. In: *Toxic Constituents of Plant Foodstuffs,* 2nd ed., edited by I. E. Liener, pp. 266–294. Academic Press, NY.

136. Mahaffey, K. R., and Michaelson, J. A. (1980): Interaction between lead and nutrition. In: *Low Level Lead Exposure: Clinical Implications of Current Research,* edited by H. E. Needleman, pp. 159–200. Raven Press, NY.

137. Malinow, M. R., Bardana, E. J., Jr., Pirofsky, B., Craig, S., and McCluaghlin, P. (1982): Systemic lupus erythematosus-like syndrome in monkeys fed alfalfa sprouts: Role of a non-protein amino acid. *Science,* 216:415–417.

138. Maltes, J. A., and Giltelman, R. (1981): Effects of artificial food-colorings in children with hyperactive symptoms. A critical review and results of a controlled study. *Arch. Gen. Psychiatry,* 38:714–718.

139. Marth, E. H. (1981): Food-borne hazards of microbial origin. In: *Food Safety,* edited by H. R. Roberts, pp. 15–65. John Wiley, NY.

140. Matsumoto, H. (1983): Cycasin. In: *Handbook of Naturally Occurring Food Toxicants,* edited by M. Rechcigl, Jr., pp. 43–61. CRC Press, Boca Raton, FL.

141. Matsumoto, T., Itoh, H., and Akiba, Y. (1968): Goitrogenic effects of 5-vinyl-2-oxazolidinethione, a goitrogen in rapeseed, in growing chicks. *Poultry Sci.,* 47:1323–1330.

142. Mattocks, A. R. (1982): Plant toxins. In: *Trace Substances and Health: A handbook,* Part II, edited by P. M. Newberne, pp. 81–110. Marcel Dekker, NY.

143. Mattson, F. H. (1973): Potential toxicity of food lipids. In: *Toxicants Naturally Occurring in Foods,* pp. 189–209. National Academy of Sciences, Washington, DC.

144. Maurer, T. (1986): Skin as a target organ of immunotoxicity reactions. In: *New Concepts and Developments in Toxicology,* edited by P. L. Chambers, P. Gehring, and F. Sakai, pp. 147–157. Elsevier, NY.

145. McCawley, E. L., Brummet, R. E., and Dana, G. W. (1962): Convulsions from psylocybe mushroom poisoning. *Proc. West. Pharmacol. Soc.,* 5:27–33.

146. McKay, F. W. (1982): Biliary passages and liver. In: *Cancer Mortality in the United States, 1950–1977,* edited by M. R. Hanson, and R. W. Miller, p. 116, NCI Monograph No. 59. National Cancer Institute, Washington, DC.

147. McLaughlin, C. S., Vaughan, M. H., Campbell, I. M., Wei, C. M., Stafford, M. E., and Hansen, B. S. (1977): Inhibition of protein synthesis by trichothecenes. In: *Mycotoxins in Human and Animal Health,* edited by J. V. Rodricks, C. W. Hesseltine, and M. A. Mehlman, pp. 263–273. Pathotox, Park Forest South, IL.

148. Meisner, H., and Cimbala, M. (1985): Effect of ochratoxin A on gene expression in rat kidneys. In: *New Concepts and Developments in Toxicology,* edited by P. L. Chambers, P. Gehring, and F. Sakai, pp. 261–271. Elsevier, NY.

149. Mena, I. (1980): Manganese. In: *Metals in the Environment,* edited by H. A. Waldron, pp. 199–220. Academic Press, NY.

150. Mennear, J. H. (1979): *Cadmium Toxicity.* Marcel Dekker, NY.

151. Menzer, R. E., and Nelson, J. E. (1986): Water and soil pollutants. In: *Casarett and Doull's Toxicology: The Basic Science of Poisons,* 3rd ed., edited by C. D. Klaassen, M. O. Amdur, and J. Doull, pp. 825–853. Macmillan, New York.

152. Miettinen, J. K. (1973): Absorption and elimination of dietary mercury and methyl mercury in man. In: *Mercury, Mercurials and Mercaptans,* edited by M. W. Miller, and T. W. Clarkson, pp. 233–243. Charles C Thomas, Springfield, IL.

153. Miller, J. A., Miller, E. C., and Phillips, D. H. (1982): The metabolic activation and carcinogenicity of alkenylbenzenes that occur naturally in many spices. In: *Carcinogens and Mutagens in the Environment,* Vol. 1, edited by H. S. Stich, pp. 83–96. CRC Press, Boca Raton, FL.

154. Mirocha, C. J., and Pathre, S. (1973): Identification of toxic principle in a sample of Poaefusarin. *Appl. Microbiol.,* 26:719–724.

155. Montgomery, R. D. (1980): Cyanogens. In: *Toxic Constituents of Plant Foodstuffs,* edited by I. E. Liener, pp. 143–160. Academic Press, NY.

156. Morgan, R. G. H., Levinson, D. A., Hopwood, D., Saunders, J. H. B., and Wormsley, K. G. (1977): Potentiation of the action of azaserine on the rat pancreas by raw soybean flour. *Cancer Lett.,* 3:87–90.

157. NAS (1977): *Leucaena, Promising Forage and Tree Crop for the Tropics.* National Academy of Sciences, Washington, DC.

158. NAS (1979): *Food Safety Policy: Scientific and Societal Considerations.* National Academy of Sciences, Washington, DC.

159. NCI (1980): Bioassay of selenium sulfide (dermal study) for possible carcinogenicity. NCI Technical Report Service No. 197, NTP No. 80-18. National Cancer Institute, Washington, DC.

160. Nakanishi, K., Hagiwara, A., Shibata, M., Imaida, K., Tetematsu, M., and Ito, N. (1980): Dose response of saccharin in induction of urinary bladder hyperplasias in Fischer 344 rats pretreated with *N*-butyl-*n*-(4-hyroxybutyl) nitrosamine. *J. Natl. Cancer Inst.,* 65:1005–1010.

161. Needleman, H. L., Gunnoe, E. E., Leviton, A., Reed, R., Peresie, H., Maher, C., and Barrett, P. (1979): Deficits in psychologic and

classroom performance of children with elevated blood lead levels. *N. Engl. J. Med.,* 300:689–695.

162. Newberne, P. M. (1982): Nitrates and nitrites in foods and in biological systems. In: *Trace Substances and Health: A Handbook,* Part II, edited by P. M. Newberne, pp. 1–46. Marcel Dekker, New York.

163. Niebuhr, E., and Wulf, H. C. (1984): Genotoxic effects. In: *Biological Effects of Organolead Compounds,* edited by P. Grandjean, pp. 117–124. CRC Press, Boca Raton, FL.

164. Nogawa, K., Kobayashi, E., and Houda, R. (1979): A study of relationship between cadmium concentrations in urine and renal effects of cadmium. *Environ. Health Perspect.,* 28:161–168.

165. Nomiyama, K., and Nomiyama, H. (1986): Critical concentration of unbound cadmium in the rabbit renal cortex. *Experimentia,* 42: 149.

166. Nordberg, G. F., Kjellstrom, T., and Nordberg, M. (1985): Kinetics and Metabolism. In: *Cadmium and Health: A Toxicological and Environmental Appraisal,* edited by L. Friberg, C.-G. Elinder, T. Kjellstrom, and G. F. Nordberg, Vol. I, pp. 103–178. CRC Press, Boca Raton, FL.

167. Oberleas, D. (1973): Phytates. In: *Toxicants Occurring Naturally in Foods,* 2nd ed., pp. 363–371. National Academy of Sciences, Washington, DC.

168. Odenbro, A. (1984): Effects on reproduction and hormone metabolism. In: *Biological Effects of Organolead Compounds,* edited by P. Grandjean, pp. 161–176. CRC Press, Boca Raton, FL.

169. Ohtsubo, K., and Saito, M. (1977): Chronic effects of trichothecenes. In: *Mycotoxins in Human and Animal Health,* edited by J. V. Rodricks, C. W. Hesseltine, and M. A. Mehlman, pp. 255–262. Pathotox, Park Forest South, IL.

170. Olny, J. W. (1982): The toxic effects of glutamate and related compounds in the retina and the brain. *Retina,* 2:341–359.

171. Omaye, S. T. (1984): Safety of megavitamin therapy. In: *Nutritional and Toxicological Aspects of Food Safety,* edited by M. Friedman, pp. 169–203. Plenum Press, NY.

172. Osborne, T. B., and Mendel, L. S. (1917): The use of soybean as food. *J. Biol. Chem.,* 32:369–387.

173. Osborne, D. J., and Hamilton, P. B. (1981): Decreased pancreatic digestive enzymes during aflatoxicosis. *Poultry Sci.,* 60:1818–1821.

174. Oser, B. L. (1985): Highlights in the history of saccharin toxicology. *Food Chem. Toxicol.,* 23:535–542.

175. Osuntokun, B. O. (1973): Ataxic neuropathy associated with high cassava diets in West Africa. In: *Chronic Cassava Toxicity,* edited by B. Nestel and R. MacIntyre, pp. 127–138. International Development Research Center, Ottawa.

176. Osweiler, G. D., Carson, T. L., Buck, W. B., and Van Gelder, G. A. (1985): *Clinical and Diagnostic Veterinary Toxicology.* Kendall-Hunt, Dubuque, IA.

177. Padmanaban, G. (1980): Lathyrogens. In: *Toxic Constituents of Plant Foodstuffs,* 2nd ed., edited by I. E. Liener, pp. 239–263. Academic Press, NY.

178. Pelkonen, O. (1979): Prenatal and neonatal development of drug and carcinogen metabolism. In: *The Induction of Drug Metabolism,* edited by R. W. Estabrook and E. Lindenlaub, p. 407. Schattaur Verlag, Stuttgart.

179. Perlman, F. (1980): Allergens. In: *Toxic Constituents of Plant Foodstuffs,* 2nd ed., edited by I. E. Liener, pp. 295–327. Academic Press, NY.

180. Perlstein, M. A., and Attala, R. (1966): Neurologic sequela of plumbism in children. *Clin. Pediatr.,* 5:292–298.

181. Perry, A. M., and Erlanger, M. W. (1974): Metal-induced hypertension following chronic feeding of low doses of cadmium and mercury. *J. Lab. Clin. Med.,* 83:541–547.

182. Poulton, J. E. (1983): Cyanogenic compounds in higher plants and their toxic effects. In: *Handbook of Natural Toxins, Vol. 1, Plant and Fungal Toxins,* edited by R. F. Keeler and A. T. Tu, pp. 117–160. Marcel Dekker, NY.

183. Powrie, W. D., Wu, C. H., and Stich, H. F. (1982): Browning reaction systems as sources of mutagens and modulators. In: *Carcinogens and Mutagens in the Environment,* Vol. 1, edited by H. F. Stich, pp. 121–133. CRC Press, Boca Raton, FL.

184. Pressey, R. (1983): Naturally occurring inhibitors: Carbohydrase inhibitors. In: *Handbook of Naturally Occurring Food Toxicants,* edited by M. Rechcigl, Jr., pp. 39–42. CRC Press, Boca Raton, FL.

185. Puls, W., and Keup, U. (1974): Metabolic studies with an amylase inhibitor in acute starch loading tests in rats and men and its influence on the amylase content of the pancreas. In: *Recent Advances in Obesity Research,* edited by A. Howard. Newman, London.

186. Rall, T. W. (1985): Central nervous system stimulants: The methyl xanthenes. In: *Goodman and Gilman's The Pharmacological Basis of Therapeutics,* 7th ed., edited by A. G. Gilman, L. S. Goodman, T. W. Rall, and F. Murad, pp. 589–603. Macmillan, NY.

187. Reddy, C. S., and Dorn, C. R. (1985): Municipal sewage sludge application on Ohio farms: Estimation of cadmium intake. *Environ. Res.,* 38:377–388.

188. Reddy, C. S., Hanumaiah, B., Hayes, T. G., and Ehrlich, K. (1986): Developmental stage specificity and dose response of secalonic acid D-induced cleft palate and the absence of cytotoxicity in the developing mouse palate. *Toxicol. Appl. Pharmacol.,* 84:346–354.

189. Reddy, C. S., Mohammad, F. K., Ganjam, V. K., and Brown, E. M. (1987): Mobilization of tissue Cd in mice and calves and reversal of Cd induced tissue changes in calves by zinc. *Bull. Environ. Contam. Toxicol.,* 39:350–357.

190. Richter, H. E., and Loewen, P. C. (1982): Rapid inactivation of bacteriophage T7 by ascorbic acid is repairable. *Biochem. Biophys. Acta,* 697:25–30.

191. Riordan, J. R. (1983): Handling of heavy metals by cultured cells from patients with Menke's disease. In: *Biological Aspects of Metals and Metal Related Diseases,* edited by B. Sarkar, pp. 159–170. Raven Press, NY.

192. Rodricks, J. V., and Pohland, A. E. (1981): Food Hazards of Natural Origin. In: *Food Safety,* edited by H. R. Roberts, pp. 181–238. John Wiley, NY.

193. Rodricks, J. V., Hesseltine, C. W., and Mehlman, M. A. (1977): *Mycotoxins in Human and Animal Health.* Pathotox, Park Forest, IL.

194. Roebuck, B. D., Yeager, J. D., Jr., and Longnecker, D. S., Wilpone, S. A. (1981): Promotion by unsaturated fat of azaserine-induced pancreatic carcinogenesis in the rat. *Cancer Res.,* 41:3961–3966.

195. Rogers, A. E. (1982): Nitrosamines. In: *Trace Substances and Health: A Handbook,* Part II, edited by P. M. Newberne, pp. 47–80. Marcel Dekker, NY.

196. Rose, D. P. (1982): *Endocrinology of Cancer,* Vols. I–III. CRC Press, Boca Raton, FL.

197. Russell, F. E. (1986): Toxic effects of animal toxins. In: *Cararett and Doull's Toxicology: The Basic Science of Poisons.* 3rd ed., edited by C. D. Klaassen, M. O. Amdur, and J. Doull, pp. 706–756. Macmillan, NY.

198. Saenz de Rodriguez, C. A. (Letter) (1984): Environmental hormone contamination in Puerto Rico. *N. Engl. J. Med.,* 310:1741–1742.

199. Saenz de Rodriguez, C. A., and Toro-Sola, M. A. (1982): Anabolic steroids in meat and premature thelarche. *Lancet,* i:1300.

200. Sakaguchi, G. (1979): Botulism. In: *Foodborne Infections and Intoxications,* 2nd ed., edited by H. Riemann, and F. L. Bryan, pp. 389–442. Academic Press, NY.

201. Satouchi, K., and Matsushita, S. (1976): Purification and properties of a lipase inhibiting protein from soybean cotyledons. *Agric. Biol. Chem.,* 40:889–897.

202. Saunders, R. M. (1975): α-Amylase inhibitors in wheat and other cereals, *Cereal Foods World,* 20:282–285.

203. Schantz, E. J. (1973): Seafood toxicants. In: *Toxicants Occurring Naturally in Foods,* 2nd ed., pp. 424–447. National Academy of Sciences, Washington, DC.

204. Schantz, E. J., Ghazarossian, V. E., Schnoes, H. K., Strong, F. M., Springer, J. P., Pezzanie, J. D., and Clardy, J. (1975): The structure of saxitoxin. *J. Am. Chem. Soc.,* 97:1238.

205. Schappert, K. T., and Khachatourians, G. G. (1983): Effects of fusariotoxin T-2 on *Saccharomyces cerevisiae* and *Saccharomyces carlsbergensis. Appl. Environ. Microbiol.,* 45:862–867.

206. Schwarcz, E., and Coyle, J. T. (1977): Striatal lesions with kainic acid: Neurochemical characteristics. *Brain Res.,* 127:235–249.

207. Scott, B. R., Pathak, M. A., and Mohn, G. R. (1976): Molecular and genetic basis of furocoumarin reactions. *Mutat. Res.,* 39:29–74.

208. Selman, I. E., Wiseman, A., Breeze, R. G., and Pirie, H. M. (1976): Fod fever in cattle: Various theories on its etiology. *Vet. Rec.,* 99: 181–184.

209. Shamberger, R. J., Baughman, F. F., Kelchert, S. L., Willis, C. E., and Hoffman, G. C. (1973): Carcinogen-induced chromosomal breakage decreased by antioxidants. *Proc. Natl. Acad. Sci. USA,* 70:1461–1463.

210. Shamberger, R. J., Tytko, S. A., and Willis, C. E. (1976): Antiox-

idants and cancer, Part VI. Selenium and age-adjusted human cancer mortality. *Arch. Environ. Health,* 31:231–235.

211. Shank, R. C. (1981): Environmental toxicoses in humans. In: *Mycotoxins and N-Nitroso Compounds: Environmental Risks,* Vol. 1, edited by R. C. Shank, pp. 107–140. CRC Press, Boca Raton, FL.

212. Shank, R. C., and Magree, P. N. (1967): Similarities between biochemical actions of cycasin and dimethylnitrosamine. *Biochem. J.,* 105:521–527.

213. Sheff, D. (1982): Want to have your pasta and eat it too? *People Weekly,* June 28:30–32.

214. Sims, J., and Renwick, A. G. (1983): The effects of saccharin on the metabolism of dietary tryptophan to indole, a known dietary carcinogen for the urinary bladder of the rat. *Toxicol. Appl. Pharmacol.,* 67:132–151.

215. Singleton, V. L., and Kratzer, F. H. (1973): Plant phenolics. In: *Toxicants Occurring Naturally in Foods,* 2nd ed., pp. 309–345. National Academy of Sciences, Washington, DC.

216. Siraj, M. Y., Hayes, A. W., Unger, P. D., Hogan, G. R., Ryan, N. J., and Wray, B. B. (1981): Analysis of aflatoxin B_1 in human tissues with high pressure liquid chromatography. *Toxicol. Appl. Pharmacol.,* 58:422–430.

217. Smith, L. D. (1977): *Botulism: The Organism, Its Toxins, the Disease.* Charles C Thomas, Springfield, IL.

218. Somogyi, J. C. (1973): Antivitamins. In: *Toxicants Occurring Naturally in Foods,* 2nd ed., pp. 254–275. National Academy of Sciences, Washington, DC.

219. Spencer, P. D., Nunn, P. B., Hugon, J., Ludolph, A. C., Ross, S. M., Roy, D. N., and Robertson, R. C. (1987): Guam amyotrophic lateral sclerosis–parkinsonism–dementia linked to a plant excitant neurotoxin. *Science,* 237:517–522.

220. Steyn, P. S. (1977): Mycotoxins excluding aflatoxin, zearalenone, and the trichothecenes. In: *Mycotoxins in Human and Animal Health,* edited by J. V. Rodricks, C. W. Hesseltine, and M. A. Mehlman, pp. 419–467. Pathotox, Park Forest South, IL.

221. Stich, H. F., Karim, J., Koropatnik, J., and Lo, L. (1976): Mutagenic action of ascorbic acid. *Nature,* 260:722–724.

222. Stich, H. F., and Powrie, W. D. (1982): Plant phenolics as genotoxic agents and as modulators for the mutagenicity of other food components. In: *Carcinogens and Mutagens in the Environment,* Vol. I, edited by H. F. Stich, pp. 135–145. CRC Press, Boca Raton, FL.

223. Stich, H. F., Bohn, B., Chatterjee, K., and Sailo, J. (1983): The role of salvia-borne mutagens and carcinogens in the etiology of oral and esophageal carcinomas of betel nut and tobacco chewers. In: *Carcinogens and Mutagens in the Environment,* Vol. III, edited by H. F. Stich, pp. 43–58. CRC Press, Boca Raton, FL.

224. Stich, H. F., and Rosin, M. P. (1984): Naturally occurring phenolics as antimutagenic and anticarcinogenic agents. *Adv. Exp. Med. Biol.,* 177:1–29.

225. Stob, M. (1983): Estrogens. In: *Handbook of Naturally Occurring Food Toxicants,* edited by M. Rechcigl, Jr., pp. 81–100. CRC Press, Boca Raton, FL.

226. Stocks, P. (1970): Cancer mortality in relation to national consumption of cigarettes, solid fuel, tea and coffee. *Br. J. Cancer,* 24: 215–225.

227. Stults, V. J. (1981): Nutritional hazards. In: *Food Safety,* edited by H. R. Roberts, pp. 67–140. John Wiley, NY.

228. Sugimura, T. (1986): Historical background of studies on environmental carcinogenesis in Japan and recent progress in toxicology of carcinogens. In: *New Concepts and Developments in Toxicology,* edited by P. L. Chambers, P. Gehring, and F. Sakai, pp. 3–13. Elsevier, NY.

229. Swenson, D. H., Miller, J. A., and Miller, E. C. (1973): 2,3-Dihydro-2,3-dihydroxy-aflatoxin B_1: An acid hydrolysis product of an RNA-aflatoxin B_1 adduct formed by hamster and rat liver microsomes *in vitro. Biochem. Biophys. Res. Commun.,* 53:1260–1267.

230. Tani, N., Ohtsuru, M., and Hata, T. (1974): Purification and general characteristics of bacterial myrosinase produced by *Enterobacter cloacae. Agric. Biol. Chem.,* 38:1623–1630.

230a.Teratology Society (1987): Position paper: Recommendations for vitamin A use during pregnancy. *Teratology,* 35:269–275.

231. Tookey, H. L., Van Etten, C. H., and Daxenbichler, M. E. (1980): Glucosinolates. In: *Toxic Constituents of Plant Foodstuffs,* edited by I. E. Liener, pp. 103–142. Academic Press, NY.

232. Towill, L. E., Drury, J. S., Whitfield, B. L., Lewis, E. B., Gaylan, E. L., and Hammons, A. S. (1978): Review of the environmental

effects of pollutants. V. Cyanide, U. S. EPA Doc. EPA-600/1-78-027, USEPA. Cincinnati, OH.

233. Tubbs, R. R., Gephardt, G. N., McMahon, J. T., Phol, M. C., Vidt, D. G., Barenberg, S. A., and Valenzuela, R. (1982): Membranous glomerulonephritis associated with industrial mercury exposure. *Am. J. Clin. Pathol.,* 77:409–413.

234. Tuite, J. (1979): Field and storage conditions for the production of mycotoxins and geographic distribution of some mycotoxin problems in the United States. In: *Interactions of Mycotoxins in Animal Production,* pp. 19–42. National Academy of Sciences, Washington, DC.

235. Udenfriend, S., Lovenberg, W., and Sjoerdsma, A. (1959): Physiologically active amines in common fruits and vegetables. *Arch. Biochem. Biophys.,* 85:487–490.

236. Underwood, E. J. (1973): Trace elements. In: *Toxicants Occurring Naturally in Foods,* 2nd ed., pp. 43–87. National Academy of Sciences, Washington, DC.

237. Underwood, E. J. (1977): *Trace Elements in Human and Animal Nutrition,* 4th ed. Academic Press, NY.

238. Ueno, Y. (1977): Trichothecenes: Overview address. In: *Mycotoxins in Human and Animal Health,* edited by J. V. Rodricks, C. W. Hesseltine, and M. A. Mehlman, pp. 189–207. Pathotox, Park Forest South, IL.

239. Uraguchi, K. (1971): Yellowed rice toxins: Citreoviridin. In: *Microbiol Toxins,* Vol. 6, edited by A. Ciegler, S. Kadis, and S. J. Ajl, pp. 299–380. Academic Press, New York.

240. Vaisius, A. C., and Wieland, T. (1982): Formation of a single phosphodiester bond by RNA polymerase from calf thymus is not inhibited by alpha-amanitin. *Biochemistry,* 21:3097–3101.

241. Van Etten, C. H., and Tookey, H. L. (1983): Glucosinolates. In: *Handbook of Naturally Occurring Food Toxicants,* edited by M. Rechcigl, Jr., pp. 15–30. CRC Press, Boca Raton, FL.

242. van Rensburg, S. J., and Altenkirk, B. (1974): *Claviceps purpurea*—Ergotism. In: *Mycotoxins,* edited by I. F. H. Purchase, pp. 69–96. Elsevier, NY.

242a.Saccharin: Current status (1985): *Food Chem. Toxicol.,* 23:417–546.

243. Verdeal, K., Brown, R. R., Richardson, T., and Ryan, D. S. (1980): Affinity of phytoestrogens for the estradiol-binding proteins and effect of coumestrol on growth of 7,12-dimethylbenz[*a*]anthracene-induced rat mammary tumors. *J. Natl. Cancer Inst.,* 64:285–290.

244. Vesselinovitch, S. D., Mihailovich, N., Wogan, G. N., Lombard, L. S., and Rao, K. V. N. (1972): Aflatoxin B_1: A hepatocarcinogen in the infant mouse. *Cancer Res.,* 32:2289–2291.

245. Waldron, H. A. (1980): *Metals in the Environment.* Academic Press, NY.

246. Waldron, H. A. (1980): Lead. In: *Metals in the Environment,* edited by H. A. Waldron, pp. 155–197. Academic Press, NY.

247. Walshe, J. M. (1983): Assessment of treatment of Wilson's disease with triethylene tetramine HCl (trien HCl). In: *Biological Aspects of Metals and Metal Related Diseases,* edited by B. Sarkar, pp. 243–261. Raven Press, NY.

248. Watson, S. A., Mirocha, C. J., and Hayes, A. W. (1984): Analysis for trichothecenes in samples from Southeast Asia associated with "Yellow Rain." *Fund. Appl. Toxicol.,* 4:700–717.

249. Whitaker, J. R., and Feeney, R. E. (1983): Enzyme inhibitors in foods. In: *Toxicants Occurring Naturally in Foods,* 2nd ed., pp. 276–298, edited by National Academy of Sciences, Washington, DC.

250. Wieland, T., and Faulstich, H. (1983): Peptide Toxins from *Amanita.* In: *Handbook of Natural Toxins, Vol. 1, Plant and Fungal Toxins,* edited by R. F. Keeler and A. T. Tu, pp. 117–160. Marcel Dekker, NY.

251. Williams, G. M., and Weisburger, J. H. (1986): Chemical carcinogens. In: *Casarett and Doull's Toxicology: The Basic Science of Poisons,* 3rd ed., edited by C. D. Klaassen, M. O. Amdur, and J. Doull, pp. 99–173. Macmillan, NY.

252. Wilson, B. J., and Hayes, A. W. (1973): Microbial Toxins. In: *Toxicants Occurring Naturally in Foods,* 2nd ed., pp. 372–423. National Academy of Sciences, Washington, DC.

253. Wiseman, J. S., and Abeles, R. H. (1979): Mechanism of inhibition of aldehyde dehydrogenase by cyclopropamine hydrate and the mushroom toxin coprine. *Biochemistry,* 18:427.

254. Yannai, S. (1980): Toxic factors induced by processing. In: *Toxic Constituents of Plant Foodstuffs,* 2nd ed., edited by I. E. Liener, pp. 371–427. Academic Press, New York.

Principles and Methods of Toxicology, Second Edition, edited by A. Wallace Hayes, Raven Press, Ltd., New York © 1989.

CHAPTER 4

Solvents

Paul H. Ayres and *W. David Taylor

*Toxicology Research Division, R. J. Reynolds Tobacco Company, Bowman Gray Technical Center, Winston-Salem, North Carolina 27102, and *Center for Toxicology, RJR Nabisco Inc., Bowman Gray Technical Center, Winston-Salem, North Carolina 27102*

The nature and extent of health hazards related to the use of solvents are dependent on their physical, chemical, and toxicologic properties. Solvents encountered in industry for the most part are liquid; however, occasionally vapors are used because of their solvent properties. Organic solvents may be pure substances, such as toluene or xylene, and they may be complex mixtures of petroleum-based derivatives. Although solvents may be classified in various ways, it is usually beneficial for toxicologic assessments to group them by chemical class (aliphatic, aromatic, halogenated, etc.). In so doing, inhalation, dermal, and oral toxicologic properties can be compared.

A thorough knowledge and understanding of the basic physical and chemical properties associated with solvents is necessary for evaluating the toxicity of a specific solvent. A list of the physical properties of the most commonly encountered solvents in industry and research is presented in Table 1 (81,102). A brief review of these properties follows.

SOLVENT CHARACTERISTICS

Vapor Pressure

Vapor pressure is the measure of the amount of pressure exerted on the walls of a closed container by the vapors from a given solvent. Units are usually expressed as millimeters of mercury (mm Hg) or pounds per square inch (psi) at a given temperature. It is these vapors that produce potential toxic exposures and occupational health problems.

The vapor pressure of a solvent will be affected by mixing it with another solvent, if miscible. If a high vapor pressure liquid and a low vapor pressure liquid are mixed, the resulting vapor pressure will most probably lie between those for the pure materials. When such a mixture is exposed to the environment and vapors are continuously given off, the more volatile component evaporates first leaving the remaining mixture rich in the less volatile solvent. This phenomenon will continue until either the more volatile solvent is gone or an azeotropic (constant boiling) mixture is formed. If the azeotrope is formed, then both vapor constituents escape simultaneously (37). Examples of two commonly used solvents that form an azeotropic mixture are water and methanol. Vapor pressure is not only the quantitative term characterizing solvent volatility; it is also equivalent to the vapor concentration at the source and is the predominant chemical factor controlling the potential for vapor exposure in the workplace (74).

Boiling Point

The boiling point is the temperature at which the vapor pressure of the solvent reaches the external pressure. The

TABLE 1. *Solvent properties*

Name	BP	MP	Flash point	Vapor pressure	Vapor density	Density	LEL	UEL	TLV
Acetaldehyde	20.2C	−123.5C	−40F(OC)	740 mm @20C	—	0.783 @18C	—	—	100 ppm
Acetone	56.48C	−94.6C	0F(CC)	400 mm @39.5C	2.00	0.7972 @15C	2.6%	12.8%	750 ppm
2-Aminoethanol	170.5C	−78.5C	200F(OC)	6 mm @60C	2.11	1.0180 @20/4C	—	—	3 ppm
Amyl acetate	148C@737	5.5C	77F(CC)	—	4.5	0.879 @20/20C	1.1%	7.5%	125 ppm
Benzene	80.09C	5.5C	12F(CC)	100 mm @26.1C	2.77	0.8794 @20C	1.4%	8.0%	10 ppm
Bromoform	149.5C	7C	None	—	—	2.890 @20/4C	—	—	0.5 ppm (skin)
2-Butanone	79.57C	—	22F(TCC)	—	2.42	0.80615 @20/20C	1.8%	11.5%	200 ppm
Butyl acetates	120C	—	72F	15 mm @25C	4.00	0.86 @20/20C	1.4%	7.5%	150 ppm
n-Butyl alcohol	117.5C	—	95–100F	5.5 mm @20C	2.55	0.80978 @20/4C	1.4%	11.2%	50 ppm (skin)
Carbon disulfide	46.5C	−110.8C	−22F(CC)	400 mm @28C	2.64	1.261 @20/20C	1.3%	50%	10 ppm (skin)
Carbon tetrachloride	76.8C	−22.6C	None	100 mm @23C	—	1.597 @20C	—	—	5 ppm
Chlorobenzene	131.7C	−45C	85F(CC)	10 mm @22.2C	3.88	1.113 @15.5/15.5C	1.3% @150C	7.1% @150C	75 ppm
Chloroform	61.26C	−63.5C	None	100 mm @10.4C	4.12	1.49845 @15C	—	—	10 ppm
Cresol (all isomers)	191–203C	10.9–35.5C	178F	1 mm @38–53C	3.72	1.030–1.038 @25/25C	—	—	5 ppm (skin)
Crotonaldehyde	104C	—	55F	10 mm @38.3C	2.41	0.853 @20/20C	2.1%	15.5%	2 ppm
Cumene	152C	−96C	111F	100 mm @60.8C	4.1	0.864 @20/4C	0.9%	6.5%	50 ppm (skin)
Cyclohexane	80.7C	6.5C	1.4F	1 mm @21C	2.9	0.7791 @20/4C	1.3%	8.4%	300 ppm
Cyclohexanol	161.5C	24C	154F(CC)	10 mm @38.7C	3.45	0.9449 @25/4C	—	—	50 ppm
Cyclohexanone	115.6C	−45C	111F(147CC)	—	3.4	0.9478 @20/4C	1.1% @100C	—	25 ppm
Cyclohexylamine	134.5C	−17.7C	69.8F	—	3.42	0.865 @25/25C	—	—	10 ppm (skin)
1,2-Dichlorobenzene	180–183C	−17.5C	151F	10 mm @54.8C	5.05	1.307 @20/20C	2.2%	9.2%	50 ppm
1,4-Dichlorobenzene	173.4C	53C	150F(CC)	400 mm @38C	5.08	1.4581 @20.5/4C	—	—	75 ppm
Diethylamine	55.5C	−38.9C	−0.4F		2.53	0.7108 @20/20C	1.8%	10.1%	10 ppm
DEP diethyl-o-phthalate	302C	−40.5C	325F(OC)	1 mm @100.3C	7.66	1.110	—	—	5 mg/m³
Dimethyl phthalate	283.7C		295F(CC)		6.69	1.189 @25/25C	—	—	5 mg/m³
Dimethyl sulfate	188C	−31.8C	182F(OC)		4.35	1.3322 @20/4C	—	—	0.1 ppm (skin)
Ethanol	78.32C	—	55.6F	40 mm @19C	1.59	0.7893 @20/4C	3.3%	19% @60C	1000 ppm
Ethyl acetate	77.15C	−83.6C	24F	100 mm @27C	3.04	0.8946 @25C	2.2%	11%	400 ppm
Ethyl butyl ketone	148C	−36.7C	115F(OC)	—	3.93	0.8198 @20/20C	—	—	50 ppm
Ethylene glycol	197.5C	—	232F(OC)	0.05 mm @20C	2.14	1.113 @25/25C	3.2%	—	50 ppm
Ethylene glycol n-butyl ether	168.4–170.2C	—	160F(COC)	300 mm @140C	—	0.9012 @20/20C	—	—	50 ppm (skin)
Ethylene glycol monoethyl ether	135.1C	—	202F(CC)	3.8 mm @20C	3.10	0.9360 @15/15C	1.8%	14%	5 ppm (skin)
Ethylene glycol monoethyl ether acetate	156.4C	—	117F(COC)	1.2 mm @20C	4.72	0.9748 @20/20C	—	—	5 ppm (skin)

Compound	BP	MP	Flash point	Vapor pressure	Specific gravity	Vapor density	LEL	UEL	TLV
Ethyl glycol monomethyl ether	124 @757mm	—	115F	—	0.9663 @20/4C	—	—	—	5 ppm (skin)
Ethylene glycol monomethyl ether acetate	143C	—	111F(CC)	—	1.005 @20/20C	4.07	1.7%	8.2%	5 ppm (skin)
Ethyl ether	34.6C	—116.2C	—49F	442 mm @20C	0.7135 @20/4C	2.56	1.85%	36%	400 ppm
Formaldehyde	—3F	—	122F—185F	—	1	—	7%	73%	1 ppm
Formamide	210C	2.5C	310F(COC)	29.7 mm @129.4C	1.134 @20/40C 1.1292 @25/4C	—	—	—	20 ppm
Furfural	161.7C @764mm	—	140F(CC)	—	1.161 @20/20C	3.31	2.1%	19.3%	2 ppm
Furfural alcohol	171C @750mm	—31C	167F(OC)	1 mm @31.8C	1.129 @20/4C	3.37	1.8%	16.3%	10 ppm
Heptane	98.52C	—	25F(CC)	40 mm @22.3C	0.67 @20/4C	3.45	1.05%	6.7%	400 ppm
N-Hexane	69C	—	—9.4F	100 mm @15.8C	0.6603 @20/4C	2.97	1.2%	7.5%	50 ppm
Hexone	118	—	62.6F	16 mm @20C	0.803	3.45	1.4%	7.5%	50 ppm
Isoamyl acetate	142C	—73C	77F	—	0.876	4.49	1% @212F	7.5%	100 ppm
Isopropyl acetate	88C	—	39.2F	40 mm @17.0C	0.847 @20/20C	3.52	1.7%	7.8%	250 ppm
Isopropyl alcohol	82.5C	—88.5—89.5C	53F(CC)	—	0.7854 @20/4C	2.07	2.5%	12%	400 ppm
Isopropyl ether	68.5C	—60C	—18F(CC)	150 mm @25C	0.719 @25C	3.52	1.4%	7.9%	250 ppm
Methanol	64.8C	—97.8C	54F(CC)	100 mm @21.2C	0.7915 @20/4C	1.11	6%	36.5%	200 ppm
Nitroethane	114.0C	—90C	106F	15.6 mm @20C	1.052 @20/20C	2.58	4.0%	—	100 ppm
Nitromethane	101C	—	95F(CC)	27.8 mm @20C	1.1322 @25/4C	2.11	7.3%	—	100 ppm
1-Nitropropane	132C	—	93F(TCC)	7.5 mm @20C	1.003 @20/20C	3.06	2.2%	—	25 ppm
2-Nitropropane	120C	—	82F(TCC)	10 mm @15.8C	0.992 @20/20C	3.06	2.6%	—	10 ppm
N-Pentane	36.1C	—129.7C	—40F(CC)	—	0.64529 @0/4C	—	1.4%	8%	600 ppm
Propylene glycol monomethyl ether	120C	—96.7C	100F	—	0.919 @25/25C	—	—	—	100 ppm (skin)
Pyridine	115.3C	—	68F(CC)	10 mm @13.2C	0.982	2.73	1.8%	12.4%	5 ppm
Stoddard solvent	220—300C	—	100—110F	—	1.0	—	1.1%	6%	100 ppm
Styrene	146C	—31C	88F	—	0.9074 @20/4C	3.6	1.1%	6.1%	50 ppm
Tetrahydrofuran	65.4C	—	1.4(TCC)	114 mm @15C	0.888 @20/4C	2.5	1.8%	11.8%	200 ppm
Toluene	110.4C	—95—94.5C	40F(CC)	36.7 mm @30C	—	3.14	—	—	100 ppm
1,1,1-Trichloroethane	74.1C	—	None	100 mm @20.0C	1.3376 @20/4C	—	—	—	350 ppm (skin)
Trichloroethylene	86.7C	—73C	89.6F	100 mm @32C	1.4649 @20/4C	4.53	12.5% @ > 30C	90%	50 ppm
Turpentine	154—170C	—	95F(CC)	—	0.854—0.868 @25/25C	4.84	0.8%	—	100 ppm
Vinyl acetate	73C	—92.8C	18F	100 mm @21.5C	0.9335 @20C	3.0	2.6%	13.4%	10 ppm
VM&P Naphtha	80—130C	< —73C	<0F	—	0.730—0.750 @15.6/15.6C	2.50	1.1%	5.9%	300 ppm
Xylene	138.5C	—47.9C	77F(CC)	6.72 mm @21C	0.864 @20/4C	3.66	1.1%	7.0%	100 ppm

BP, boiling point; C, Centigrade; CC, closed cup; COC, Cleveland open cup; F, Fahrenheit; LEL, lower explosive limit; mm, mm Hg; MP, melting point; OC, open cup; ppm, parts per million; TLV, threshold limit value; TCC, Tagliabue closed cup; skin, potential exposure contribution due to cutaneous absorption; UEL, upper explosive limit. Constructed from refs. 2, 81, and 102.

boiling point is measured in degrees Centigrade (°C) or degrees Fahrenheit (°F), generally at one atmosphere (760 mm Hg or 14.7 psi). Generally, the solvent with the lower boiling point will have the higher vapor pressure.

Specific Gravity

Specific gravity is the ratio of the weight of a given volume of a substance to an equal volume of water at 4°C or some other specified temperature. A material having a specific gravity of less than 1.0 is lighter than water and, if not miscible, will float on it. A material with a specific gravity greater than 1.0 is heavier than water and, if not miscible, will sink. At 75°F, water has a specific weight of 8.31 pounds per gallon. The specific weight of a solvent such as ethyl alcohol at 75°F (specific gravity = 0.79) would be 0.79 times 8.31, or 6.56 pounds per gallon (102).

Evaporation Rate

The rate of evaporation is one of the most important properties to be considered when selecting a solvent for a particular process. The rate of evaporation of an organic solvent cannot be stated in absolute numbers because these rates are affected by a number of factors, many of which cannot be evaluated properly. Some of the factors that affect evaporation rate and consequently drying time are temperature of the fluid, temperature of the atmosphere above the liquid, surface tension, humidity, latent heat of evaporation, and vapor density (82). A simple relationship between the rate of evaporation and the boiling point of a solvent does not exist. A general rule to follow, however, when estimating the evaporation rate of a solvent is that the vapor pressure of liquids increases approximately three percent for every one-degree-Fahrenheit (1°F) rise in temperature. The evaporation rate of a solvent is frequently compared to the evaporation ratio of a standard solvent such as butyl acetate (considered as unity).

Vapor Density

Vapor density is the weight per unit volume of vapor at a given temperature and pressure (usually at 25°C and 1 psi). Generally, the vapor density of a solvent vapor is compared to air as unity (1.0). Dry air has a vapor density of 1.29 g per cubic meter at 0°C at 760 mm Hg (102). An important point to remember about solvent vapor is that if the density is greater than that of air, then the vapor tends to settle to lower points in the container. If there is little or no air movement, then a potentially hazardous situation exists.

Flash Point

The flash point of a solvent is the lowest temperature at which vapor is given off in sufficient quantities so that the air/vapor mixture above the surface of the solvent will propagate a flame away from the source of the ignition. In practical terms, it is the temperature below which a solvent may be used or stored in open containers without the formation of an explosive air/vapor mixture.

The flash point is determined by heating the solvent in a standard manner and measuring the temperature at which the flash will be obtained when a small flame is introduced into the vapor above the surface of the solvent. In Britain, the Abel and the Pensky–Martin apparatuses are commonly used; in the United States, either the Tag or the Cleveland is used. All four can be used to determine open or closed cup flash points (57).

When vapors of a flammable solvent are mixed with air in the proper proportions, ignition will produce an explosion. This proper proportion is called the flammable range and also is referred to as the explosive range.

Flash points are useful in defining combustibility and flammability (National Fire Protection Association). A solvent is classified as flammable if it has a flash point below 100°F (37.8°C) and a vapor pressure not exceeding 40 psia at 40°F (psia, absolute pressure measured in pounds per square inch). Combustible solvents are those solvents with flash points above 100°F. Figure 1 depicts the flammability characteristics of a vapor/air mixture as concentration and temperature vary (91).

CHEMICAL CLASSIFICATION FOR SOLVENTS

The majority of solvents fall into one of 11 chemical groups, with each group comprising one or more homologous series. Solvents from different groups differ markedly in their characteristics, even though the chemical and solvent properties of each group change only slightly with increases in molecular weight, and the differences between solvents belonging to different series within a group are relatively small.

Each group is characterized by a specific chemical radical which gives the individual members the properties typical of the group as a whole. The chemical configurations for these 11 groups are shown in Fig. 2. Common solvents from each of the classified groups are listed below the chemical configuration. Additionally, current American Conference of Governmental Industrial Hygienists (ACGIH) threshold limit values (TLV) in parts per million (ppm) are listed for selected solvents within the classes (64).

OCCUPATIONAL EXPOSURE LIMITS

Given the fact that almost all work environments involve some exposure to potentially hazardous materials and that the potential for exposure to these hazards cannot usually be eliminated completely, it becomes necessary to define exposure concentrations at which a worker's health and well-being will not be compromised. The most significant routes of chemical exposure in the industrial environment are by inhalation and through the skin. The most commonly accepted exposure limits in the United States are the TLVs and the biological exposure indices (BEI) published and updated yearly by the ACGIH; the maximum acceptable concentrations (MAC) of the American National Standards Institute (ANSI); the workplace environmental exposure level guide (WEEL) of the American Industrial Hygiene Associ-

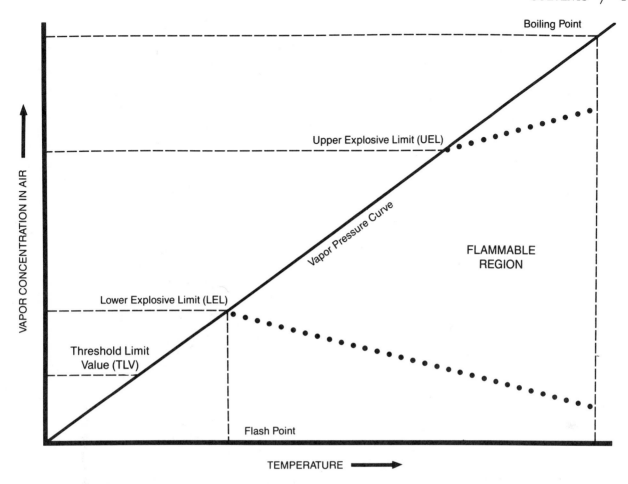

FIG. 1. Diagram of vapor pressure versus temperature showing relation between upper and lower flammable (explosive) limits, flammable and nonflammable regions, threshold limit value, boiling point, flash point, and vapor pressure curve. This diagram shows what happens to a vapor/air mixture as concentration and temperature vary.

ation (AIHA); the recommended exposure limits (REL) of the National Institute for Occupational Safety and Health (NIOSH); and the permissible exposure limits (PEL) promulgated by the Occupational Safety and Health Administration (OSHA). Only PELs have the force of law.

Fundamental to the development of an exposure limit is the concept that there is some concentration that does not produce adverse health effects. This threshold concept, however, is not applied to all health hazards, such as carcinogens.

Dr. Vernon Carter, Chairman of the ACGIH-TLV Committee, stated in 1983 that many compounds, because of their physical or toxic properties or small quantities manufactured, have not been given enough priority to warrant intensive investigations sufficient to establish an accurate TLV (70). However, the toxicity data on which TLVs are now set are much more rigorous and standardized (Table 2).

TLVs represent, with certain exceptions, time-weighted average concentrations (TWAs) of airborne substances associated with industrial operations. TLVs are designed as guides to protect the health and well-being of nearly all workers repeatedly exposed during a 7- or 8-hr workday and 40-hr workweek, not only for their working lifetime but after retirement. The concept of a TWA carries with it two important considerations. First, TWAs permit excursions above the limit, provided they are compensated by equivalent excursions below the limit during the workday. Secondly, the TWA method and its excursion limits merely represent guides in the control of occupational health hazards and are not to be considered as absolute figures differentiating precisely between hazardous and nonhazardous concentrations.

Other categories of TLVs are the short-term exposure limit (STEL) and ceilings. A STEL is defined as the maximum concentration to which workers can be exposed for a period up to 15 min continuously, provided that no more than four excursions per day are permitted with at least 60 min between exposure periods. The STEL allows short-term exposures during which workers will not suffer from irritation, chronic or irreversible tissue damage, or narcosis of sufficient degree to increase injury proneness, impair self-rescue, or materially reduce work efficiency. A ceiling is an airborne concentration that should not be exceeded even instantaneously. Examples of substances having ceilings are certain irritants whose short-term effects are so undesirable that they outweigh their long-term hazards.

Aliphatic Hydrocarbons

Straight or branched chains of carbon and hydrogen.

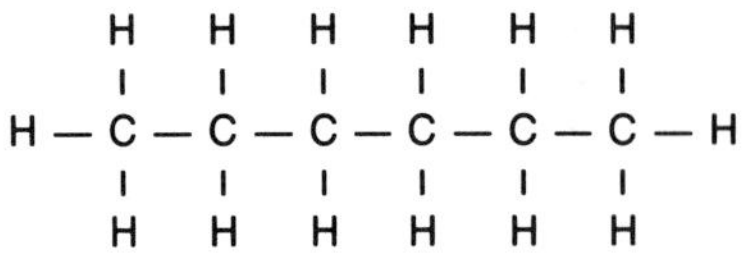

Aromatic Hydrocarbons

Contain a 6-carbon ring structure with one hydrogen per carbon bound by energy from several resonant forms.

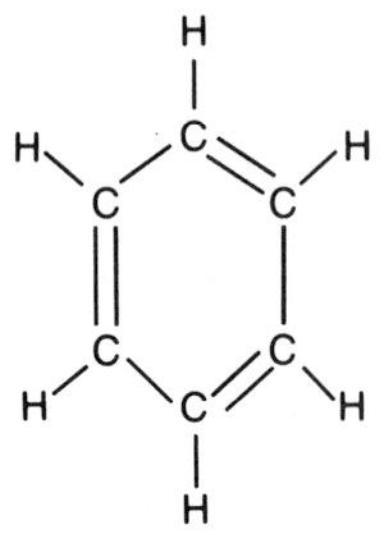

*Hexane   —   50 ppm
Heptane   — 400 ppm
VM+P Naptha — 300 ppm

Benzene   — 10 ppm
Toluene   — 100 ppm
Xylene   — 100 ppm

Cyclic Hydrocarbons

Ring stucture saturated and unsaturated with hydrogen.

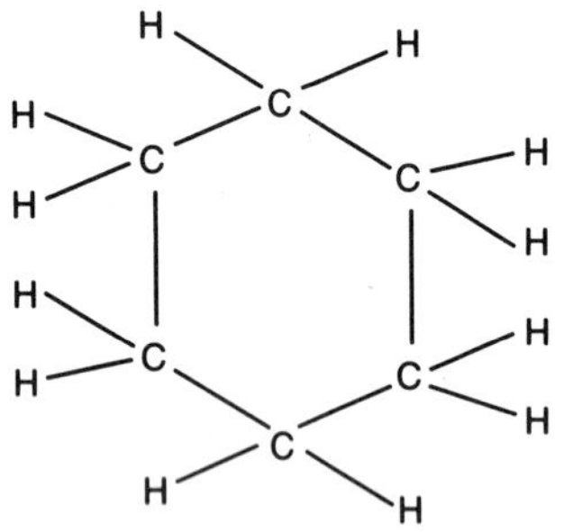

Alcohols

Contain a single hydroxyl group.

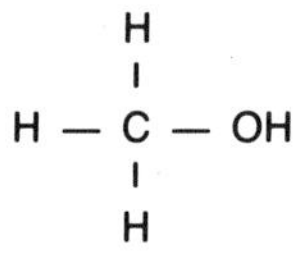

Cyclohexane — 300 ppm
Turpentine   — 100 ppm

Ethanol   — 1000 ppm
Methanol   — 200 ppm
Isopropanol — 400 ppm

Esters

Formed by interaction of an organic acid with an alcohol.

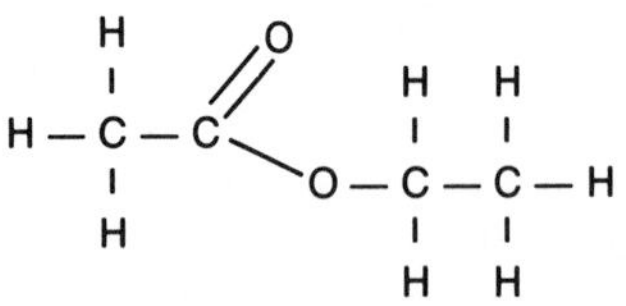

Ketones

Contain a double bonded carbonyl group, C=O, with two hydrocarbon groups on the carbon.

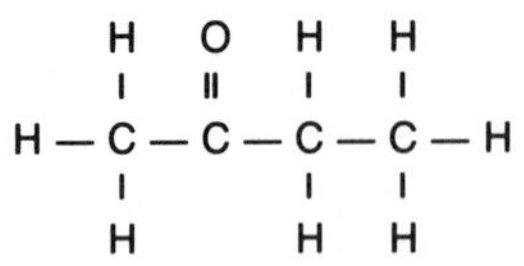

Ethyl Acetate   — 400 ppm
Isopropyl Acetate — 250 ppm

Methyl Ethyl Ketone   — 200 ppm
Acetone   — 750 ppm
Methyl Isobutyl Ketone — 50 ppm

*TLV – American Conference of Governmental Industrial Hygienists (ACGIH) Threshold Limit Value, 1986-1987.

FIG. 2. Classes of organic solvents. *ACGIH threshold limit value.

Halogenated Hydrocarbon

A halogen atom has replaced one or more hydrogen atoms on the hydrocarbon.

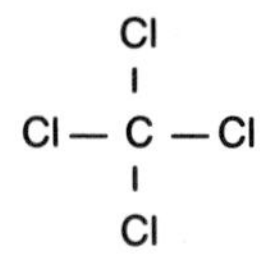

$$
\begin{array}{c}
Cl \\
| \\
Cl - C - Cl \\
| \\
Cl
\end{array}
$$

Carbon Tetrachloride	—	5 ppm
Methyl Chloroform	—	350 ppm
Chloroform	—	10 ppm

Glycols

Contains double hydroxyl groups.

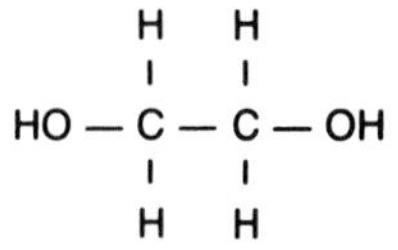

$$
\begin{array}{c}
H \quad H \\
| \quad | \\
HO - C - C - OH \\
| \quad | \\
H \quad H
\end{array}
$$

Ethylene Glycol	—	50 ppm
Hexylene Glycol	—	25 ppm

Aldehydes

Contain the double-bonded carbonyl group, C=O, with only one hydrocarbon group on the carbon.

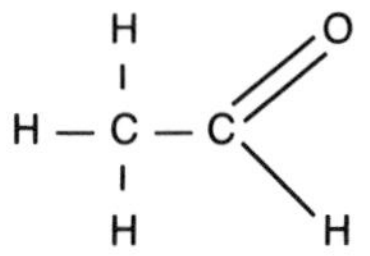

$$
\begin{array}{c}
H \quad\quad O \\
| \quad\quad \parallel \\
H - C - C \\
| \quad\quad \backslash \\
H \quad\quad H
\end{array}
$$

Acetaldehyde	—	100 ppm
Formaldehyde	—	1 ppm

Nitro-Hydrocarbons

Contain an NO_2 group.

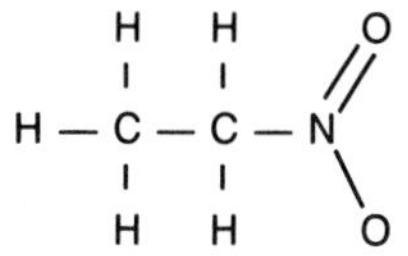

$$
\begin{array}{c}
H \quad H \quad\quad O \\
| \quad | \quad\quad \parallel \\
H - C - C - N \\
| \quad | \quad\quad \backslash \\
H \quad H \quad\quad O
\end{array}
$$

Nitroethane	—	100 ppm
Nitromethane	—	100 ppm

Ethers

Contain the C — O — C linkage.

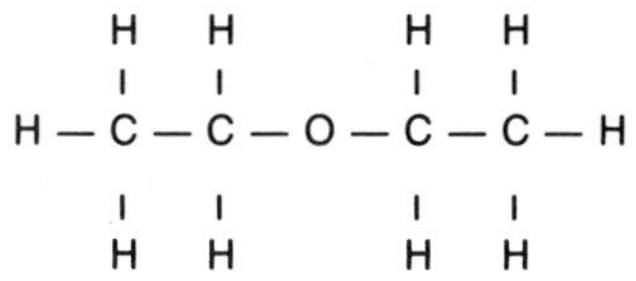

$$
\begin{array}{c}
H \quad H \quad\quad H \quad H \\
| \quad | \quad\quad | \quad | \\
H - C - C - O - C - C - H \\
| \quad | \quad\quad | \quad | \\
H \quad H \quad\quad H \quad H
\end{array}
$$

Diethyl Ether	—	400 ppm
Isopropyl Ether	—	250 ppm

FIG. 2. (*Continued.*)

The ACGIH-TLV Committee also has employed a *skin* notation for those substances where penetration of the worker's intact skin may make a significant contribution to the total body burden. The attention-calling designation is intended to suggest appropriate measures for the prevention of skin absorption so the TLV is not invalidated.

BEIs represent warning levels of biologic response to a specific chemical, or warning levels of specific chemicals or their metabolites in tissues, fluids, or exhaled air of exposed workers, regardless of whether the chemical was inhaled, ingested, or absorbed through the skin. The BEI is considered supplementary to an airborne TLV. TLVs are a measure of the composition of the external environment surrounding the worker. BEIs are a measure of the amount of chemical in the body. The concept of BEIs is extremely important when evaluating exposures to substances that are readily absorbed through the skin. Because elimination of chemicals and their metabolites, as well as biologic changes induced by chemical exposures, are kinetic events, the established BEIs are strictly related to 8-hr exposures and to the specified timing for the collection of biologic samples (2).

MACs are National Consensus Standards and have been established by the ANSI. These values are the highest airborne concentrations that can be justified consistent with the objective of maintaining unimpaired health or comfort of workers or both. The criteria on which the standard is established are the avoidance of (a) undesirable changes in body structures or biochemistry, (b) undesirable functional reac-

TABLE 2. *Data used in developing threshold limit values*

Physical properties
  Lipid solubility
  Water solubility
  Vapor pressure
  Odor threshold
Acute toxicity data
  Oral toxicity, LD_{50}
  Dermal toxicity, LD_{50}
  Dermal and eye irritation
  Inhalation toxicity, LC_{50}
Subchronic data (oral, dermal, or inhalation)
  14 day, NOEL[a]
  90 day, NOEL
  6 month, NOEL
Other data
  Developmental (teratology and embryotoxicity)
  Mutagenicity (Ames test, Drosophilia, etc.)
  Fertility
  Reproductive (3-generation)
  Reversibility study
  Dermal absorption tests
  Pharmacokinetics
  Cancer bioassay (2-year)
Epidemiologic data
  Morbidity
  Mortality
  Case reports
Industrial hygiene exposure data
  Area samples
  Personal samples

[a] NOEL, no observed effect level.

tions that may have no discernible effects on health, and (c) irritation or other adverse sensory effects (23,31).

WEELs are developed by the AIHA WEEL Committee for agents that have no current exposure guidelines established by other organizations. They represent the workplace exposure concentrations, to which, it is believed, nearly all employees could be repeatedly exposed without adverse effects. All WEELs are expressed as TWAs; however, different time periods are specified depending on the properties of the agent. A skin notation also is used in the same manner as the ACGIH TLV.

RELs, developed by NIOSH, are comprised of either a TWA or a ceiling or both. These recommended limits are published as criteria documents and are periodically revised. The recommended limits are established for up to a 10-hr workday and are intended to provide the maximum possible protection for all workers against acute and chronic effects of exposure. Skin notations are applied.

PELs refer to the legal allowable concentration of a contaminant in the air as established by OSHA. When the Occupational Safety and Health Act of 1970 was enacted, PELs were derived from existing standards. Thus, the TLVs from 1968 and ANSI values were adopted as legal limits. Although the ACGIH revises recommended TLVs each year, the PELs remain as created unless changes in the law are made. The PELs, in addition to TWA and ceiling values, contain values which were basically adopted from the ANSI standards. Skin notations are applied.

In addition to the conventional exposure limits such as TWAs, STELs, and ceilings, there are other specific limits or circumstances of concern. Immediately dangerous to life or health (IDLH) is a limit that addresses extremely hazardous conditions. It is meant to be an indication of the concentration which a worker can escape from within 30 min without losing his or her life or suffering permanent health impairment. Adjustments of worker exposure limits may be necessary under conditions of nontraditional work shifts (i.e., 12-hr days). Such adjustments may be predicated on a number of factors. For an extended workday, not only would a higher dose be accumulated, but the worker would have less time to recover before the next exposure. Exposures in confined spaces, for example, a submarine or space vehicle, present continuous exposures and require special consideration (17).

Occupational exposure limits are intended solely for the protection of the work force under the specific exposure conditions they may encounter. To apply such values to inhalation exposures unrelated to the occupational environment is a misapplication.

SAMPLING METHODOLOGY

Sampling methods used to evaluate the concentration of a solvent in the workplace environment are generally classified as follows: (a) direct reading; (b) those that remove the solvent from the environment via a measured quantity of air with subsequent laboratory analysis; (c) passive dosimetry; and (d) continuous area monitoring (39). No single method is available to assess the occupational environment; however, the trend is toward direct reading instruments and passive dosimetry.

To accurately reflect the concentration of an airborne solvent over a finite period of time in the workplace environment, the passive monitor is fast becoming the method of choice (25). These monitors utilize Brownian motion to control sampling into a collection medium. This technology is particularly well-suited for personal monitoring devices because these devices are (a) lightweight, (b) unobtrusive, (c) require no external power source, (d) require no calibration, and (e) can usually be used for up to 6 hr instead of the conventional 1 hr or less required for charcoal tubes (11). This binary diffusion concept was described first by Palmes and Gunnison (69) and Braun (16).

This type of sampling relies on a concentration gradient across a static or placid layer of air to induce mass transfer. The equation below, based on Fick's Law, gives the steady-state relationship for the rate of mass transfer.

$$W = D\left(\frac{A}{L}\right) \times (C_1 - C_0)$$

where W = mass transfer rate
  D = diffusional coefficient
  A = frontal area of static layer
  L = length or depth of static layer
  C_1 = ambient concentration
  C_0 = concentration at collection surface

It can be seen from the above equation that by choosing an effective collection surface, such that C_o is essentially zero, the mass transfer or collection rate is proportional to the ambient vapor concentration C_1. It also may be noted that the units of D(A/L) are volume per unit time, the same as for the volumetric flow in a battery-powered pump/solid sorbent monitoring system. The rate of sampling for the contaminant is then the product of the D(A/L) term and the average ambient concentration. A typical passive monitor is shown schematically in Fig. 3.

These devices are extremely useful for individuals exposed to low-concentration multiple-solvent vapors throughout a work shift. Meaningful data can thus be generated, allowing determination of appropriate controls and personnel protective measures (16,52,69).

EXPOSURE CONTROLS

Illnesses from exposure to solvents may be avoided by designing equipment in such a way that the employee is not subjected to vapor concentrations above the established safe limit during operations, does not become subjected to high concentrations of solvent vapor in occasional or intermittent operation, and does not have his or her skin wetted by a liquid solvent.

The OSHA Standard 29 Code of Federal Regulation (CFR) 1910.1000 states that compliance must be achieved by either engineering or administrative controls (Occupational Safety and Health Standards for General Industry). When such means are not available, personal protective equipment (PPE) should be used to minimize exposures to concentrations within the standard.

In general, potential deleterious health effects can be reduced by one or by a combination of the following methods:

1. Substitution of a less toxic material.
2. Isolation, either in space or time.
3. Process changes.
4. Engineering controls at the point of generation of the solvent (local exhaust).
5. Dilution of contaminant with uncontaminated air by general ventilation.
6. Use of personal protective devices (respirators, gloves, barrier creams) (20).

Substitution

Solvents, individually or mixed, often may be substituted by solvents of lower toxicity or higher flash points if the solvent's effectiveness and characteristics, such as boiling point, vapor pressure, and polarity, are acceptable. Substitutions may be made within a chemical series by retaining the active group. For example, substitution of butyl cellosolve for methyl cellosolve may be advantageous. The general group also may be retained such as in the substitution of aromatic naphtha for toluene, or toluene for benzene. Common solvents according to a chemical group classification are shown in Table 3.

Changing a solvent containing one chemical group for a solvent containing another chemical group of similar polar characteristics but of lower toxicity is possible. For example, changing from carbon tetrachloride to perchloroethylene or naphtha may work. Solvent-based adhesives or paints may be substituted with water-based products. Hot water detergent spray wash solutions followed by high temperature drying may be an alternative for trichloroethylene washes.

Isolation

The removal of an operation from one area to another and the complete structural containment of an operation where worker exposure to solvent vapors is eliminated are methods of isolation. Some operations may be run on the third shift of production where employee exposures are minimal.

Process Changes

A complete change of process or operation may effectively reduce or eliminate an exposure. Examples of such changes are paint dipping for spray painting and the use of electrostatic spraying instead of air pressurized spraying.

Engineering Controls (Local Exhaust)

One of the most common and effective ways to control exposures to solvent vapors is by the use of local exhaust

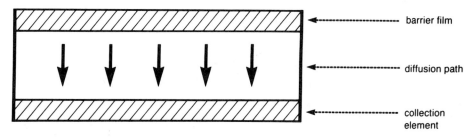

FIG. 3. Schematic of air being sampled by a passive monitoring system.

TABLE 3. *Common solvents classified by group*

Aliphatic Hydrocarbons

Gasoline	Petroleum benzene
High flash naphtha	Petroleum naphtha
Mineral spirits	VM&P naphtha

Aromatic Hydrocarbons

Benzene	Tetrahydronaphthalene
Decahydronaphthalene	Toluene
1-Methyl-4-isopropylbenzene	Xylene

Halogenated Aliphatic and Aromatic Hydrocarbons

Dichloroethylene	Monochlorobenzene
Ethylene dichloride	Tetrachloroethylene
Methylene chloride	Trichloroethylene

Alcohols

Amyl alcohol	2-Ethylbutyl alcohol
Benzyl alcohol	2-Ethylhexyl alcohol
Butyl alcohol	Isopropyl alcohol
Ethyl alcohol	Methyl alcohol

Ketones

Acetone	Diacetone alcohol
Cyclohexanone	Diisobutyl ketone

Esters

Acetates	Lactates
Alkyl formates	Propionates

Ethers

Butyl ether	Isopropyl ether
Ethyl ether	Diethyl cellosolve

ventilation. The solvent vapor is generally pulled into a one- or two-sided hood or booth, a slot, a canopy hood and exhausted externally, or a recirculation/purification system.

A properly designed exhaust hood is necessary to effectively control solvent vapors at their source with minimum air flow and power consumption. The reader is referred to a fundamental text for industrial ventilation published annually by the ACGIH, entitled *Industrial Ventilation, A Manual of Recommended Practice* (1). Figures 4–6 provide information basic to understanding proper ventilation design for local exhaust control.

Dilution Ventilation

Dilution ventilation refers to the dilution of contaminated air in a general area, room, etc., for the purpose of controlling exposures to solvents. It is usually accomplished by fans pulling or pushing clean fresh air past the employee's breathing zone. Dilution ventilation, which is not as effective as local or point source control, has at least four limiting factors:

1. The quantity of solvent generated must not be too great, because the air volume necessary for dilution will become impractical.
2. The worker must be far enough away from the source of

solvent vapor generation such that the TLV is not exceeded.
3. The toxicity of the solvent must be low.
4. The evaluation of contaminants must be uniform (1).

Figure 7 illustrates good fan location for dilution ventilation.

Personal Protection When Handling Solvents

The use of respiratory protective equipment and protective gloves or creams are necessary if appropriate control measures do not reduce the potential for overexposure to specific solvents. Typical operations and industries where respirators and gloves or creams are often found are (a) degreasing and cleaning, (b) painting, lacquering, and gluing, (c) reinforced plastics, (d) printing, and (e) repair and service (13).

Although personal protective devices are the last choice when designing control measures, often they are the only practical means. Therefore, qualified professional guidance is necessary when selecting both respiratory and skin/hand protection.

To provide adequate respiratory protection, the respirator must be effective enough to eliminate the exposure. When selecting and using a respirator, 29 CFR 1910.134 specifies (as a minimum) that certain requirements must be met (Occupational Safety and Health Standards for General Industry). Those that are most important are described below:

1. Identification and evaluation of the solvent.
2. Evaluation of the requirements of the task (mobility, physical demands, etc.).
3. Selection of appropriate respirator.
4. Instruction and training needs.
5. Maintenance of respirator (cleaning, inspecting, repair, and storage).
6. Medical surveillance (X-rays, pulmonary function, etc.).

An important factor to consider when selecting appropriate gloves for solvent handling is the protection afforded by the glove. Extensive research has been conducted on glove permeation through different kinds of materials (PVC, natural rubber, butyl rubber, neoprene, etc.) (67). The ACGIH have recently published a manual that has proven to be an excellent resource to aid in the selection of appropriate hand and skin protection (53).

Barrier creams are sometimes recommended as alternatives for protective gloves. However, the permeability of many barrier creams to organic solvents is high. Additionally, the thin film that is usually applied is easily worn away during the course of the day. Therefore, barrier cream is not a viable alternative for the protective glove.

ABSORPTION OF SOLVENTS AND INHALATION EXPOSURE

Probably the most important factor in the absorption of solvents by inhalation is the solubility of the compound in the blood and tissues. Uptake and tissue equilibrium con-

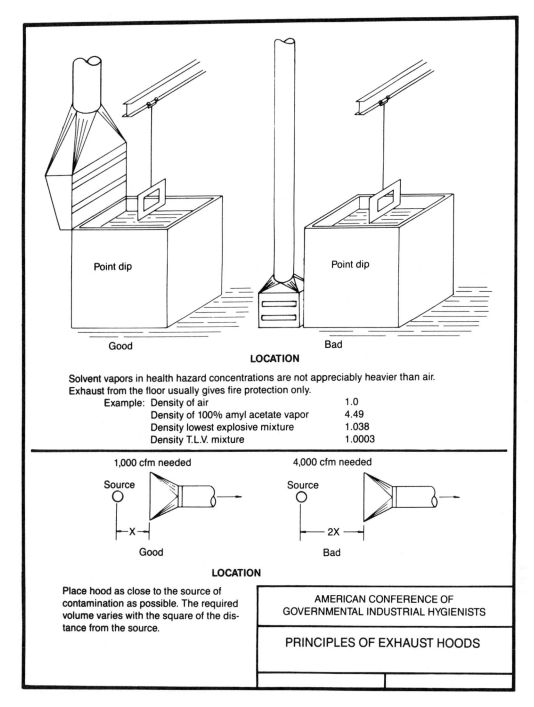

Point dip

Good

Point dip

Bad

LOCATION

Solvent vapors in health hazard concentrations are not appreciably heavier than air. Exhaust from the floor usually gives fire protection only.

Example: Density of air — 1.0
Density of 100% amyl acetate vapor — 4.49
Density lowest explosive mixture — 1.038
Density T.L.V. mixture — 1.0003

1,000 cfm needed

Source

X

Good

4,000 cfm needed

Source

2X

Bad

LOCATION

Place hood as close to the source of contamination as possible. The required volume varies with the square of the distance from the source.

AMERICAN CONFERENCE OF
GOVERNMENTAL INDUSTRIAL HYGIENISTS

PRINCIPLES OF EXHAUST HOODS

FIG. 4. Principles of exhaust hoods. (From ref. 1, with permission.)

centration of a solvent also are dependent on several different parameters. These factors are pulmonary ventilation, diffusibility through the alveolar–capillary membranes, solubility of the solvent in blood and in tissues, and blood flow through the tissue.

Solvents that are highly soluble in blood and tissues are absorbed very readily by inhalation, and blood concentrations can rise rapidly. The driving force is the difference in concentration between inspired air and blood. Concentration differences direct the diffusion of the inhaled solvent into the blood. The amount diffusing through the alveolar capillary membrane is dependent on the gas:blood partition coefficient. Tissue equilibrium concentrations with those solvents such as xylene, styrene, and acetone, which are highly soluble in blood and tissues, are not limited by pulmonary ventilation because the tissues act as a sink for the inhaled solvent. As pulmonary ventilation is increased, the blood and tissue concentrations continue to rise. The limiting factor in at-

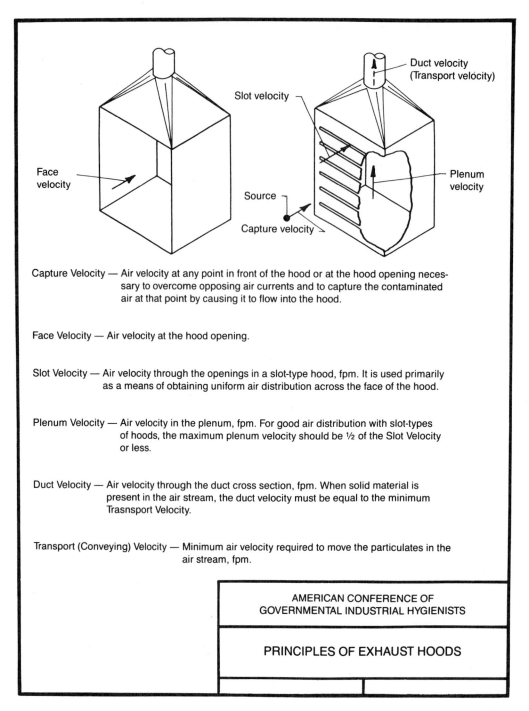

FIG. 5. Principles of exhaust hoods. (From ref. 1, with permission.)

taining the tissue equilibrium concentration is the blood flow through the tissues and the blood:tissue partition coefficient.

Solvents such as methyl chloroform, methylene chloride, trichloroethylene, and toluene, which have lower solubilities in blood and tissues, reach equilibrium rapidly because of low solubility or low blood:gas partition coefficient. Tissue concentrations also will reach equilibrium rapidly because of a low tissue:blood partition coefficient. Tissue concentration is limited then by tissue solubility and pulmonary ventilation. To achieve a higher concentration in tissues and blood, pulmonary ventilation must increase. When pulmonary ventilation is increased, more solvent can enter the blood and a new blood:tissue equilibrium can be obtained (6,7).

ELIMINATION OF SOLVENTS AFTER INHALATION EXPOSURE

Methylene chloride is widely used in industry and has a variety of applications (90). The volatile nature of methylene

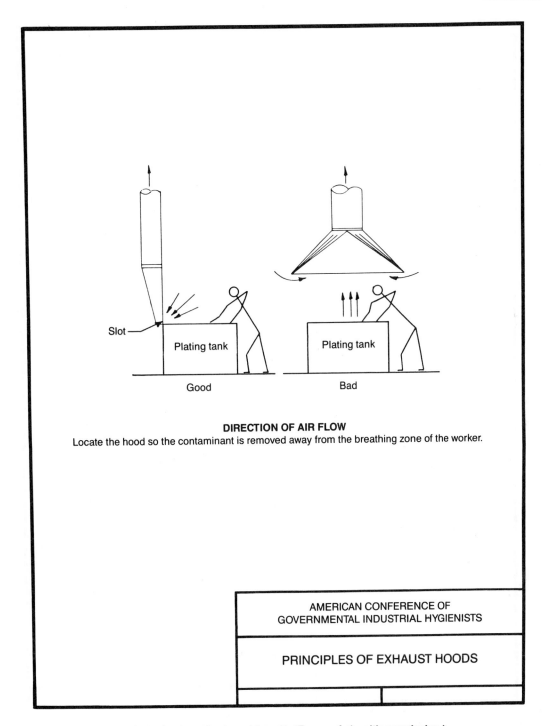

DIRECTION OF AIR FLOW
Locate the hood so the contaminant is removed away from the breathing zone of the worker.

AMERICAN CONFERENCE OF
GOVERNMENTAL INDUSTRIAL HYGIENISTS

PRINCIPLES OF EXHAUST HOODS

FIG. 6. Principles of exhaust hoods. (From ref. 1, with permission.)

chloride makes inhalation a predominant route of exposure. A study of the pharmacokinetics of ^{14}C-methylene chloride in rats at 50, 500, and 1500 ppm for 6 hr revealed that plasma concentrations of methylene chloride reached an apparent steady state after approximately 2 hr of exposure (62). However, it was found that steady-state plasma concentrations did not increase proportionally with exposure concentration. Investigation of the metabolism of inhaled methylene chlo-

ride indicated that metabolic processes were saturated above the 50-ppm exposure concentration which resulted in alterations in the metabolic profile. At 48 hr postexposure, approximately 95% of the body burden resulting from the 50-ppm exposure was metabolized in contrast to 69 and 45% at 500 and 1500 ppm, respectively.

Metabolism produced $^{14}CO_2$ and ^{14}CO and some radioactive components that remained in the carcass and were

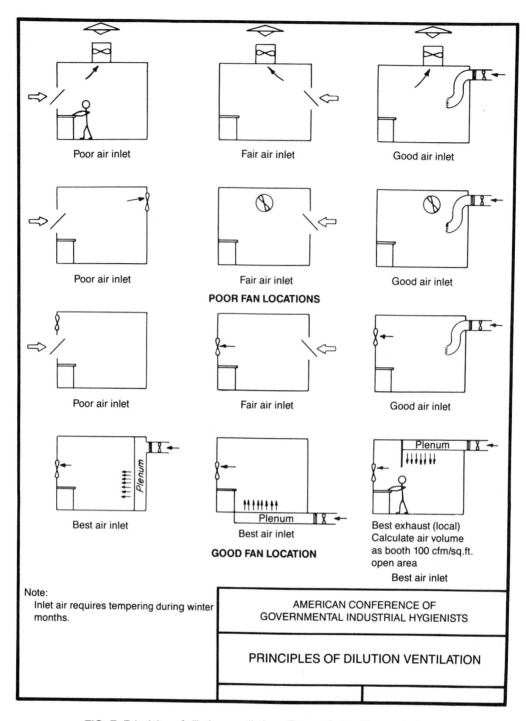

Poor air inlet

Fair air inlet

Good air inlet

Poor air inlet

Fair air inlet

Good air inlet

POOR FAN LOCATIONS

Poor air inlet

Fair air inlet

Good air inlet

Best air inlet

Best air inlet

Best exhaust (local)
Calculate air volume
as booth 100 cfm/sq.ft.
open area

Best air inlet

GOOD FAN LOCATION

Note:
Inlet air requires tempering during winter months.

AMERICAN CONFERENCE OF
GOVERNMENTAL INDUSTRIAL HYGIENISTS

PRINCIPLES OF DILUTION VENTILATION

FIG. 7. Principles of dilution ventilation. (From ref. 1, with permission.)

presumed to be nonvolatile metabolites. The highest concentrations of tissue radioactivity 48 hr postexposure were found in the liver, kidney, and lung. The fraction of the inhaled dose that remained in the carcass also decreased with increasing exposure concentration. Metabolism of methylene chloride to ^{14}CO led to the production of carboxyhemoglobin which reached a steady-state range of 10–13% irrespective of the exposure concentration, suggesting that a metabolic pathway that led to the production of CO was saturated.

Although disproportionately less compound was metabolized with increasing exposure concentration, the elimination rate of methylene chloride from the plasma was not affected. Elimination from the plasma was reported to be biphasic with a rapid component having a half-life of approximately 2 min and a slow component having a half-life of about 15 min.

Previous studies of the pharmacokinetics of methylene chloride after oral administration resulted in similar elimination patterns when compared with the inhalation route (61). The same phenomenon of saturation of metabolic pathways was observed when the administered dose was greater than 1 mg/kg.

These results with methylene chloride indicate that metabolic processes leading to the formation of metabolites that remain in tissues after the cessation of exposure can be saturated and that merely increasing the exposure concentration does not always increase the body burden in a linear manner. Such information can be valuable in safety evaluation to avoid overestimation of body burden.

Tetrachloroethylene represents another solvent in which elimination patterns are perturbed when metabolism is saturated (71). In a study comparing oral and inhalation exposure of rats to ^{14}C-tetrachloroethylene, it was found that with increasing dose, metabolism was saturated resulting in a greater percentage of the parent compound being eliminated unchanged (71) at 72 hr after exposure. A dose of 1 mg/kg by oral administration produced the same elimination patterns as did inhalation of 10 ppm for 6 hr. Radioactivity was found mainly in the liver, kidney, and fat and was not detectable in the brain. Approximately 70% of the body burden was eliminated in expired air as unchanged parent compound. Elimination in urine accounted for about 20% of the initial body burden. Radioactivity eliminated as $^{14}CO_2$ and nonvolatile metabolites in feces and carcass made up the remaining 10%. When the oral dose was increased to 500 mg/kg and the inhalation exposure was increased to 600 ppm for 6 hr, elimination patterns were altered with approximately 90% of the initial body burden being excreted in expired air as unchanged parent compound. Urinary excretion of radioactive nonvolatile metabolites decreased to approximately 5% of the body burden. Radioactivity eliminated as $^{14}CO_2$ and nonvolatile metabolites in feces and carcass represented about 5% of the body burden.

The elimination half-life from the blood of 7 hr was not affected by dose or route of administration. However, alteration of the proportion of parent compound metabolized due to saturation of metabolic pathways as a result of increasing dose was a phenomenon similar to that seen with methylene chloride. The effect of dose on the production of radioactivity bound to liver protein also was observed, in that although the oral dose differed by 500-fold, the amount of bound material differed by only 123-fold. When the inhalation dose was increased 60-fold from 10 to 600 ppm, the amount of bound material was increased by a factor of only 16. These results with tetrachloroethylene again point to the importance of pharmacokinetic and disposition studies when estimates of remaining body burden are to be extrapolated from low to high doses.

EFFECT OF SOLVENTS ON BIOLOGIC ACTIVITY

Selection of an appropriate solvent for dissolution of compounds for mutagenicity testing in bacterial mutagenicity assays is not always a simple task. Depending on the solvent selected, quantitative and qualitative differences in the results can occur with one compound but have little appreciable difference on other compounds. In experiments designed to evaluate solvent interaction, trichloroacetone dissolved in dimethylsulfoxide displayed a 1.6-fold higher mutagenic response than when dissolved in acetone, whereas, the mutagenic activity of tetrachloroacetone and pentachloroacetone showed no appreciable differences when dissolved in either solvent. Hexachloroacetone was inactive when acetone was used as a solvent but was positive in a time-dependent manner when dissolved in dimethyl sulfoxide (DMSO) (68). DMSO also modified the effects of the aromatic amine 2-aminoanthracene in the Salmonella/activation mutagenicity assay. The mutagenic activity of 2-aminoanthracene with S-9 could be decreased or enhanced in different strains depending on the amount of DMSO added to the plate (5).

Solvent selection can affect the comparative extraction of genotoxic components from filters used to collect air samples. Samples of rural air collected on glass fiber filters were evaluated in the TA100 strain of Salmonella typhimurium for estimation of mutagenic activity. The filters were extracted with water, benzene, or acetone alone and the extracts were dried before dissolving in DMSO for application on the plate. The use of water as a solvent produced the lowest yield of mutagenic activity with 6 revertants/mg extract. Extracts from the filters using benzene as a solvent produced 9.4 revertants/mg and acetone-extracted material produced 19 revertants/mg (95). These results indicate that the choice of solvent used to extract potentially mutagenic material can have a marked effect on resulting detected mutagenicity.

Bacterial mutagenicity assays are not alone in the confounding effects that solvents may produce. The use of DMSO in mutagenicity testing of the indirect mutagen dimethyl nitrosamine in Drosophila melanogaster resulted in a significant decrease in lethal mutations when compared with dimethyl nitrosamine alone (18).

In vitro metabolism of aniline, aminopyrine, 7-ethoxycoumarin, p-nitroanisole, and benzo[a]pyrene catalyzed by liver $9000 \times g$ supernatant fractions from Arochlor- and phenobarbital-treated rats was evaluated in the presence of a variety of solvents. Solvents used to dissolve compounds for these in vitro metabolism studies had a differential effect depending on the assay system and the substrate used. Additionally, the mutagenic potential of 2-aminoanthracene in the Ames assay with S-9 from Arochlor- or phenobarbital-treated rats was very dependent on the solvent used. Acetone, tetrahydrofuran, dioxane, and acetonitrile increased the mutagenic potential above that of other solvents when used with the S-9 from phenobarbital-treated rats, whereas, these same solvents reduced the mutagenic potential of 2-aminoanthracene with S-9 from Arochlor-treated rats with the exception of dioxane, which caused a stimulation of activity (44). These observations made by Kawalek and Andrews indicate the importance of testing for different effects of solvents on biochemical and bacterial mutagenesis assays.

Selection of a solvent as the vehicle of a potentially carcinogenic compound can influence the incidence and type of malignancy produced in whole animals. 3-Methylcholanthrene (MCA) was dissolved in either olive oil or benzene and administered subcutaneously to mice. Twenty weeks after the single administration of MCA the incidence of tumors in the group injected with MCA in benzene was 100% whereas the incidence of tumors in the MCA–olive oil group was only 50% without an alteration in the latency period. Control groups receiving olive oil or benzene alone had no appreciable incidence of tumors. The tumors found after administration of MCA in olive oil were predominantly fibrosarcomas whereas MCA in benzene yielded predominantly rhabdomyosarcomas. It was suggested that in the MCA–olive oil animals, MCA was slowly released from the injection site resulting in a lower tumor incidence. The difference in the type of tumors produced was hypothesized to occur because MCA in olive oil may remain longer in the subcutaneous tissues and produce fibrosarcomas. However, when MCA is dissolved in benzene, there may be rapid diffusion from the site of injection to the underlying muscle tissue resulting in the production of rhabdomyosarcoma (76).

These results from metabolism, mutagenicity, and carcinogenicity assays illustrate the importance of the choice of solvent. Care must be used to select a particular solvent vehicle for use in a study to avoid possible misinterpretation of potentially adverse effects.

DERMAL TOXICOLOGY OF SOLVENTS

It has been suggested that the barrier property of the epidermis is associated with filamentous proteins and lipids of the stratum corneum. The barrier may be composed of fibrous keratin in the stratum corneum which is surrounded by a lipid layer. The lipid is intercellular in location, and treatment of the skin with polar organic solvents, detergents, and some surfactants can remove lipids from the stratum corneum thereby increasing the permeability of the skin. Permeability is not always due to removal of lipids because permeability of the skin can increase as a result of hydration.

In a study of skin lipid removal by solvents, it was found that the ability of a solvent to penetrate the skin depends on the polarity of the solvent and the surface charge of the skin. In a study comparing penetration or removal of lipids by different solvents, it was found that of the solvents tested, ethanol extracted the most lipid followed by acetone and then ether (9). The solvent with the greatest polarity extracted the most intercellular lipid from the stratum corneum layer.

In consideration of the barrier the skin represents, the skin is one of our main areas of contact with solvents. Its surface area is approximately 18 sq. ft. and the main barrier of the skin is the stratum corneum. The intercellular spaces of the stratum corneum contain lipids which represent about 1% of the volume of the stratum corneum. Transfer or penetration of solvents across the stratum corneum is dependent on a number of factors. The thickness of the skin layer, difference in concentration of solvent on both sides of the epithelium, diffusion constant, partition coefficient, and the permeability constant all play a role in the ability of a solvent to penetrate the skin. Hair follicles and sweat glands, even though they comprise only a small proportion of the total surface area of the skin, are important pathways for dermal contact with solvents. The presence of hair follicles also increases absorption in localized areas. Even though hair follicles and sweat glands are important pathways for absorption, the magnitude of the effect is lessened because of the small surface area.

One of the main factors affecting skin penetration is the water content of the stratum corneum. Hydration of the stratum corneum can increase the permeability of the skin and increase the rate of diffusion of substances penetrating the skin. Movement of water soluble compounds may be impeded when the stratum corneum is highly hydrated. Intact skin has much better resistance to solvents than does injured skin.

The water/lipid solubility of a solvent is an important consideration for passage through the skin. The skin is composed of both hydrophilic and lipophilic regions. The lipophilic regions correspond to the intercellular spaces or membranes. The hydrophilic region is the proteinaceous portion of the cells. When compounds have near equality in the water/lipid partition coefficient their rate of skin absorption is increased. Molecular weight seems to have little importance on skin absorption and probably only affects absorption when a large molecule is considered (12). Low molecular weight solvents such as ethanol, ether, and acetone seem to enhance absorption and penetration of other compounds possibly through lipid depletion of the skin (12).

Uptake and elimination of solvents following percutaneous exposure have been investigated by several groups. Kinetics of percutaneous absorption and elimination of solvents was investigated by applying the solvent in a special depot fixed to the backs of guinea pigs (100). Solvents studied represented several chemical classes. Blood concentrations were somewhat related to the solubility of the solvent in water. The highest concentration obtained was with 1,2-dichloroethane which had the highest solubility in water, 870 mg/100 ml, of the solvents investigated. The solvent that had the lowest blood concentration was n-hexane, which also had the lowest water solubility (2.3 mg/100 ml).

Absorption of the organic solvents investigated followed three basic patterns. One pattern was seen in which the maximum blood concentration was reached after about 1 hr of exposure which was then followed by a rapid decline in concentration during the remainder of the exposure period. This pattern was observed with solvents that were relatively lipophilic, with water solubilities less than 100 mg/100 ml. Solvents that fit this kinetic profile were carbon tetrachloride, hexane, tetrachloroethylene, toluene, 1,1,1-trichloroethane, and trichloroethylene.

The second pattern of elimination observed was one in which the blood concentration reached an equilibrium after about 1 hr and maintained the equilibrium concentration throughout the remaining 5 hr of the exposure period. This pattern was seen with benzene and 1,2-dibromoethane.

The third pattern of absorption was observed with relatively hydrophilic solvents such as 1,2-dichloroethane and 1,1,2,2,-tetrachloroethane. With these solvents the blood concentration steadily increased with exposure duration. This steady increase in blood concentration was thought to be related to a local effect of the solvents on the barrier characteristics of the stratum corneum allowing more of the solvent to penetrate the skin with time. Elimination of solvents after percutaneous exposure generally fitted a biphasic pattern with the first phase having a short half-life of approximately 0.5–1 hr followed by a second phase with a longer half-life of several hours (42).

Solvents can cause damage to the skin by removing lipids and thus causing irritation, cellular hyperplasia, and swelling.

Treatment of the skin with solvents can cause an increase in penetration rate of other compounds. In a study (58) using excised human skin, the effect of several solvents including DMSO, dimethyl acetamide, formamide, and dimethyl formamide on the penetration rate of sarin was examined. After pretreatment with the solvents the rate of transport of sarin was increased 10–100 times that of sarin on control skin.

Penetration of solvents by the dermal route in humans was studied for toluene, xylene, and styrene. Volunteers were exposed to 300 or 600 ppm for 3.5 hr in a dynamic exposure situation in which the subjects wore full face respirators to prevent pulmonary absorption of the solvents. A 10-min exercise period was sufficient to make the subjects perspire and to raise the skin temperature about 0.5°C. Perspiration and warm skin temperature enhance the hydration of the skin and percutaneous absorption. These solvents had a biphasic elimination from blood into exhaled air after termination of exposure with a short half-life of about 1 hr and a longer half-life of approximately 10 hr for the second phase of excretion. Xylene and styrene had slightly delayed excretion in exhaled air after percutaneous exposure when compared with inhalation exposure. Delayed excretion after dermal exposure may be accounted for by a slow release from the skin after termination of exposure.

Overall percutaneous absorption of the compounds corresponded to only about 0.1% of the amount estimated to be absorbed by the pulmonary route, thus indicating a very small absorption potential by the percutaneous route for these compounds. When the percutaneous absorption of xylene vapor was compared with earlier work with xylene liquids, xylene vapor displayed an approximately 10-fold greater efficiency in penetration across the skin than xylene liquid. According to the authors, it was not uncommon to observe greater penetration with vapor exposure because liquid solvents removed the lipids from the stratum corneum and thus interfered with absorption. Additionally, exercise promoted the absorption of solvents because of the warm hydrated skin. In general, dermal absorption was on the order of 0.1–2% of the inhalation absorption, thereby indicating that at reasonable exposure conditions in the workplace, percutaneous absorption of solvent vapors would not contribute significantly to the blood concentrations of these solvents (78).

Even though dermal exposure to vapors of solvents appears to be an insignificant route of exposure, percutaneous exposure to liquid solvents is not without toxicological consequences. In a study investigating dermal toxicity, five industrial solvents, n-hexane, toluene, carbon tetrachloride, 2-chloroethanol, and n-butyl acetate, were evaluated on the skin of guinea pigs.

The solvents (1 ml) were administered percutaneously in a special well (100). Animals were killed at times ranging from 15 min to 16 hr after administration of the solvent. Skin as well as liver and kidney were examined. No gross changes were observed in the exposed skin. No changes were seen after administration of n-butyl acetate. With n-hexane, nuclear changes were seen in the layers of the epidermis even after only 15 min of exposure. These nuclei underwent a progressing degeneration with increasing length of exposure with pyknosis and karyolysis. Separation of the epidermis from the underlying basement membrane, called a junctional separation, occurred with slight progression with exposure period.

With toluene, morphologic changes in nuclei were observed after 15 min. There was a marked intercellular edema in the epidermal layers called spongiosis observed as early as 15 min of exposure and was more pronounced after 1 hr of exposure. Additionally, a junctional separation was seen after 1 hr of exposure.

Carbon tetrachloride produced nuclear changes as early as 15 min with the severity progressing with the length of exposure. As with toluene, there was a marked degree of spongiosis as early as 15 min of exposure which progressed up to the 4-hr time point with no increase in severity after that exposure time. A junctional separation was observed as early as 1 hr after exposure that was more pronounced at the 4-hr time point.

With 2-chloroethanol there were some nuclear changes as early as 15 min of exposure which progressed and became extremely severe to affect all epidermal layers. No spongiosis was observed; however, an almost complete junctional separation was observed after the 16-hr exposure.

Only carbon tetrachloride and 2-chloroethanol produced abnormalities in the livers examined. Hexane, toluene, and n-butyl acetate caused no histopathologic alterations in the liver. No morphologic alterations were seen in the kidney with any of the solvents tested. Even though 2-chloroethanol is acutely toxic by cutaneous exposure (101), there was only a slight histopathologic change in the skin which did not approach the severity of carbon tetrachloride-induced changes (48).

In a study designed to assess the percutaneous penetration of benzene, investigators studied the absorption of ^{14}C-benzene through the skin of the forearm or palm of the Rhesus monkey. Cutaneous administration of ^{14}C-benzene to the forearm of the monkeys resulted in an average of 0.13% of the dose penetrating the skin and being accounted for. When benzene was administered in a petroleum distillate mixture commonly used as a rubber solvent, only about half of the amount absorbed when pure benzene was applied was accounted for, indicating that the absorption of benzene was reduced when applied in this particular solvent mixture. When benzene was applied to the palmar surface in the rubber solvent mixture it was found that more of the benzene could be accounted for, indicating a greater potential penetration than in the forearm.

Mechanical damage to the stratum corneum of the skin resulted in five to six times greater absorption than penetration of intact skin. Even though the Rhesus monkey may not be the most appropriate model for the study of potential penetration of solvents through the skin, cutaneous exposure to benzene could account for only about 0.1–0.9% penetration of the applied dose. Due to the potentially toxic nature of benzene, safety concerns should be addressed even though the penetration may be less than 1% (56).

Investigation of the effects of solvents on the barrier characteristics of the stratum corneum was conducted with several compounds (14). Compounds with marked polar or nonpolar properties traverse the stratum corneum via different pathways. Using human skin in an *in vitro* preparation, the permeability constant of benzene (a nonpolar molecule) and water (a polar molecule) was investigated prior to and after exposure to several solvents. It was found that a 0.1% saline solution effected no change in the permeability constant of either benzene or tritiated water. However, it was found that butanol and hexane made the skin more permeable to both water and benzene. Gasoline treatment and benzene treatment both made the skin more permeable to water but did not alter the permeability to benzene. These studies indicate that treatment with solvents can alter the barrier characteristics of the stratum corneum (14).

TOXICOLOGY OF SELECTED SOLVENTS

This section deals with solvents of occupational concern that have reported reproductive, carcinogenic, or neurotoxic effects.

2-Ethoxyethanol

Ethylene glycol monoethyl ether (2-ethoxyethanol) is used as a solvent for epoxy coatings, paint, varnishes, inks, dyes, and cleaning fluids (79). Consumer products that may contain 2-ethoxyethanol are nail enamels, nail enamel removers, and hair conditioners. In an inhalation study, 2-ethoxyethanol was teratogenic and embryotoxic to rabbits and rats (35).

Dermal exposure to rats on gestational days 7–16 was accomplished by application of either 0.25 or 0.5 ml four times daily to the interscapular region with undiluted 2-ethoxyethanol. No signs of maternal toxicity were seen in the low or high dose group except some ataxia in the high dose group. There was a marked effect on embryotoxicity in the high dose group in that all of the fetuses died. The number of implants and the mean fetal body weight were reduced significantly when compared with controls. Visceral and skeletal examination of the live fetuses revealed significant increases in cardiovascular defects and skeletal malformations. An important point to consider with 2-ethoxyethanol exposure is that embryolethality was 100% at a dose that produced only mild signs of maternal toxicity. Dermal exposure of 2-ethoxyethanol to rats thus produced embryotoxic, fetotoxic, and teratogenic responses in a manner similar to inhalation exposure (36).

Other investigators have studied the potential interaction of ethanol and 2-ethoxyethanol because of similar metabolic pathways and the likelihood of concomitant exposure to ethanol in some individuals (65). 2-Ethoxyethanol, when presented alone or in combination with ethanol treatment, seemed to increase the duration of pregnancy. Exposure to 2-ethoxyethanol during gestational days 7–13 caused a decrease in certain behavioral tests such as rotorod performance. However, when 2-ethoxyethanol was exposed to animals that also consumed ethanol the behavioral deficit was diminished. When 2-ethoxyethanol was administered alone during late gestation, motor activity of pups was depressed and performance at avoidance conditioning trials was retarded. Combined administration to 2-ethoxyethanol and ethanol seemed to exaggerate the behavioral deficits induced by 2-ethoxyethanol and to depress both activity and learning.

Examination of neurotransmitters in 21-day-old pups that had been whelped by dams exposed to 2-ethoxyethanol alone on gestational days 7–13 revealed an increase in several neurotransmitters such as acetylcholine, dopamine, and nor-

epinephrine. Pups that were whelped by dams that had the combined treatment displayed a decrease in acetylcholine, dopamine, and 5-hydroxytryptamine. Thus, it was observed that ethanol during late gestation altered the neurochemical effects of 2-ethoxyethanol.

Concomitant exposure to ethanol therefore can have differential effects depending on the stage of gestation. Ethanol administration during the early period of gestation ameliorated both the behavioral and neurochemical effects of 2-ethoxyethanol to approximately 50% of the response produced by 2-ethoxyethanol alone. In the late stage of gestation the combination of ethanol with 2-ethoxyethanol exaggerates the effects of 2-ethoxyethanol alone. This indicates that the possibility exists for ethanol-induced exaggeration of the potential toxic effects of 2-ethoxyethanol exposure in pregnant workers.

Amides and Ureas

Because of significant potential dermal exposure to amide- and urea-type solvents in the workplace, studies were conducted to identify potential toxic effects of these solvent types in pregnant rats and rabbits. It was found that when these solvents were applied dermally to pregnant rats or rabbits during the period of fetal organogenesis, an array of toxic effects was observed. Ethylene thiourea resulted in teratogenic effects including skeletal malformations. n-Methyl formamide was found to be teratogenic (87) with no significant embryolethality. Formamide was a very weak embryotoxic agent. Dimethyl formamide (n-n-dimethyl formamide) was embryolethal in rats only at maternal lethal doses with no embryotoxic effects in rabbits. n-n-Di-n-butyl formamide and n-methyl acetamide caused slight embryolethal effects but were not teratogenic. n-n-d-Di-methyl acetamide caused a slight teratogenic effect (87) but only at exaggerated concentrations.

Tetramethylurea caused embryomortality in rats when administered on gestation day 9. Ethylene thiourea was found to be a potent teratogen at a dose of 100 mg/kg which was only about 5% of the dermal approximate lethal dose when applied on gestational days 12–13. Overall, among the amides and ureas, ethylene thiourea provided the greatest degree of teratogenic effects followed by n-methyl formamide. Those compounds with slight teratogenic effects were tetramethylurea, dimethyl acetamide, formamide, and n-methyl acetamide (87).

Glycol Ethers

Rats exposed to glycol ether solvents on gestational days 7–15 for 7 hr a day were killed and fetuses examined for terata (66). Methoxyethanol was administered at a concentration of 200 ppm and resulted in 100% resorption following exposure to 200 ppm of methoxyethanol. Heart abnormalities and skeletal malformations were seen. Inhalation of methoxyethanol at a concentration of only two to four times the OSHA 8-hr TWA has the potential for producing adverse effects in offspring of exposed mothers. Butoxyethanol was not teratogenic at the same dose.

2-Ethoxyethyl acetate was teratogenic with malformations of the heart as well as retardation in fetal weight.

Two solvents, 2-(2-ethoxyethoxy)ethanol and 2-methyl-aminoethanol, produced no maternal or fetal toxicity when administered by inhalation.

In the inhalation study of the glycol ethers and an amino derivative mentioned above, it appears that methoxyethanol produced the greatest embryotoxicity. Ethoxyethyl acetate displayed less potential to produce adverse effects than methoxyethanol. Butoxyethanol, 2-(2-ethoxyethoxy)ethanol, and 2-methylamino ethanol were not embryotoxic at the concentrations tested. These data suggest that the longer chain glycol ethers possess less potential to produce embryotoxic effects than the short chain compounds. The alarming fact that arises from the inhalation study of several glycol ethers is that these adverse effects were observed at concentrations that are near the permissible exposure limits.

Exposure to some of the glycol ethers produces adverse effects in male laboratory animals as well as offspring of pregnant animals. Early literature of male reproductive effects due to glycol ether exposure contains many instances of contradictory effects possibly because of contaminants in some of the solvents used. Experimental evidence on male reproductive effects after exposure to glycol ethers that has been confirmed by separate laboratories has been summarized in a recent review (34). On a molar comparison the methylated compounds produced more testicular toxicity than the ethyl derivatives. Expressed as a molar basis, the acetates of the ethers produced similar effects, suggesting that the acetate group is removed before a toxic compound is produced. Alongside a reduction in testicular weight, histopathologic evidence of tubular atrophy was observed in groups treated with ethylene glycol monomethyl ether and its corresponding acetate, ethylene glycol monomethyl ether acetate, as well as ethylene glycol monoethyl ether and its corresponding acetate, ethylene glycol monoethyl ether acetate.

Benzene

Benzene, used for many years as a solvent for paints, resins, rubber, inks and dyes, and many other products, has been implicated as a causative agent in the depression of bone marrow and production of aplastic anemia and leukemia. Because of its high lipid solubility, acute exposure to benzene can cause depression of the central nervous system to the point of narcosis. Headache, dizziness, nausea, and vomiting are all features of benzene exposure. Exposure to benzene at high concentrations can lead to blurring of vision, unconsciousness, convulsions, ventricular irregularities, and respiratory failure. Death as a result of exposure to extremely high concentrations of benzene may occur because of respiratory failure or cardiac arrhythmias (84,103). Concomitant exposure to benzene and high concentrations of catecholamines can sensitize the heart and lead to ventricular fibrillations.

Chronic exposure to benzene can result in headaches and a loss of appetite. Leukopenia and anemia may precede aplasia of the bone marrow. Epidemiologic evidence suggests that chronic exposure to high concentrations of industrial grades of benzene is responsible for the production of leukemia (84).

In exposed individuals, hematologic abnormalities were followed for several months to years. Improvement in the clinical aspects indicated a good prognosis for recovery from bone marrow disease. Seemingly, most exposures to benzene occurred before there was widespread concern about the toxicity (98). Clinical investigations reveal that benzene-induced leukemia can develop several years after the termination of exposure to the solvent (97).

The major metabolic pathway for benzene appears to be oxidation to a phenol which is then converted to a sulfate conjugate and excreted in urine. The sulfate conjugation reaction is an important facet of biologic monitoring of benzene exposure in that the ratio of inorganic to organic sulfate in the urine can be considered in determining the extent of benzene exposure. Normally, about 85% of the sulfate excreted in urine is in the inorganic form. With increasing benzene exposure, increasing amounts of organic sulfate are found in the urine (84).

The mechanism of benzene-induced leukemia is not known. Potential mechanisms for benzene-induced bone marrow disease include metabolism of the parent compound to phenols and other metabolites, in particular, quinone-type metabolites such as catechol, quinol, and pyrogallol which could react with chromosomes and interfere with mitosis. Another possibility could be the depletion of sulfur available for glutathione detoxification, thereby leading to interaction of toxic intermediates with critical elements of the bone marrow. Another suggested mechanism involves transfer of benzene metabolites from the liver to the bone marrow (84). Researchers have investigated the metabolism and binding of radiolabeled benzene in the isolated hindlimb of rats in which benzene was administered directly into the bone marrow space. Metabolites of benzene were found covalently bound to macromolecules in the bone marrow, indicating that the bone marrow has the potential of metabolizing benzene to reactive intermediates (41). The fact that benzene or benzene metabolites have been shown to inhibit the multiplication of erythrocyte precursor cells in the bone marrow may imply an additional mode of action (50).

The potential for benzene to induce leukemia in experimental animals has been difficult to demonstrate. In a study involving Sprague–Dawley rats and AKR mice, benzene vapor was administered for 6 hr a day, 5 days a week, for the lifetime of the animals. The rats showed signs of lymphocytopenia, mild anemia, and slightly decreased survival. The mice showed severe lymphocytopenia and anemia with significantly decreased weight gain and survival. However, no evidence of a leukemic or preleukemic response was observed in either species (83). Even though it has been shown that metabolism plays a role in benzene toxicity (54), and that benzene can interfere with erythrocyte development and binds to DNA, the exact mechanism of benzene-induced leukemia has not been elucidated.

Toluene

A cause-and-effect relationship has been difficult to establish even though solvents have been implicated in several central and peripheral nervous system symptoms. Toluene is an example of a solvent that has been implicated as a nervous system toxicant. Acute effects of toluene can resemble alcoholic intoxication by first stimulating and later depressing the central nervous system. In groups of volunteers exposed to 100 ppm of toluene vapor for 6 hr, complaints included fatigue, sleepiness, and the feeling of intoxication. Irritation of the eyes, nose, and throat was reported as well as decreased manual dexterity and accuracy in visual perception (8). High concentrations, as are seen when toluene is abused in cases such as glue sniffing, may cause death by sensitizing the myocardium (77,103). Chronic abuse of toluene may lead to hepatomegaly and nephrotoxic symptoms (88).

In humans, toluene is metabolized to benzoic acid, which is subsequently conjugated with glycine to form hippuric acid or with glucuronic acid to form benzoylglucuronates. Hippuric acid and benzoylglucuronic conjugates are excreted in the urine (49). Another metabolite that is excreted in urine is o-cresol. Efforts have been made to analyze for toluene in expired air and urinary metabolites of toluene to estimate the extent of toluene exposure. Examination of expired alveolar air in workers exposed to toluene revealed that toluene concentration in expired air was correlated to the exposure environment (19). The concentration of toluene in expired air represented approximately 15–20% of the environmental concentration.

In studies designed to investigate the effect of ethanol on the metabolism of toluene, ethanol inhibited the metabolism of toluene in humans when exposed to blood concentrations of ethanol of 21 mmol/liter (30). Alveolar air samples for analysis of expired toluene were collected before, during, and after the exposure period to determine the effect of ethanol on the rate of appearance, steady state, and elimination rate of toluene. Urine was collected before initiation of exposures and at 2-hr intervals during exposure and for 6 hr after termination of exposure to examine the elimination of the urinary metabolites of toluene, hippuric acid, and o-cresol. Following cessation of exposure, the concentration of toluene in alveolar air of volunteers exposed to toluene with concomitant ethanol treatment was significantly higher than in individuals exposed to toluene alone. During the exposure period, urinary excretion of hippuric acid in subjects who received the combined toluene/ethanol treatment accounted for only about 40% of that excreted by individuals who received toluene alone. During the 24 hr following the last exposure, excretion of both hippuric acid and o-cresol was reduced to about 40–50% of that excreted by subjects who received toluene alone. These results in human volunteers suggest that ethanol may alter the metabolism and time course of elimination of inhaled toluene. Prolongation of the elimination of toluene by ethanol may lead to an increase in the body burden of toluene and points out that ethanol consumption should be considered when biologically monitoring those individuals potentially exposed to toluene. Monitoring of individuals with concomitant ethanol intake could conceivably artifactually allow an underestimation of the exposure to toluene (30).

Experimental studies in the rat on the effect of phenobarbital pretreatment on the metabolism of toluene revealed that metabolism could be enhanced to form the intermediate metabolite benzoic acid, but did not have an appreciable effect on conjugation of benzoic acid with glycine to form hippuric acid. In the rats receiving toluene alone, the hippuric acid concentration in the urine was only about 33% of the phenobarbital-pretreated rats and blood toluene concentration was about twice that of pretreated rats. Not only did the phenobarbital pretreatment enhance metabolism of toluene to benzoic acid and subsequently to hippuric acid, but it also reduced the blood concentration of toluene and thus shortened the sleeping time induced by the narcotic effect of toluene.

Concentration of toluene in blood in phenobarbital-pretreated rats was reduced to about 50% of the group that received toluene alone. Benzoic acid in blood steadily increased in rats that received phenobarbital pretreatment, whereas benzoic acid was not detected in the group that received toluene alone. Administration of sodium benzoate to control and phenobarbital-pretreated rats resulted in no appreciable difference in conversion of benzoic acid to hippuric acid, thus leading to the conclusion that phenobarbital pretreatment had little effect on the conjugation reaction of glycine with benzoic acid to form hippuric acid (40).

From experimental studies it was seen that toluene metabolism may be altered by the pharmacologic status of the subject. It is important to take the pharmacologic status of the worker into account when monitoring either alveolar air or urine to avoid possible under- or overestimation of exposure to toluene.

When toluene is abused by individuals to produce the euphoric effect, a number of symptoms associated with exposure have been reported. Symptoms range from euphoria, mild tremors, and abnormality in walking, to behavioral changes (45). Encephalographic examination revealed abnormalities suggestive of cerebellar atrophy. Experimental evidence in rats subchronically exposed to 1000 ppm suggested that weaknesses of distal limbs and encephalographic alterations consistent with abnormalities of motor activity were associated with toluene exposure (59).

The mechanism of the neurotoxic effect of toluene is not well understood. Some experimental work with rats found that exposure of rats to very high concentrations of toluene at 30,000 ppm for a few minutes reduced the concentration of tryptophan and tyrosine in plasma by about 50 and 20%, respectively, when compared with controls. Tryptophan and tyrosine are known to be precursors of noradrenaline, dopamine, and 5-hydroxytryptamine. The reason for the decrease in neurotransmitter precursors was unknown, but it was speculated to be an alteration in the hepatic uptake or utilization of these amino acids (99). Occupational exposure to toluene has been associated with several neurophysiologic or neuropsychiatric abnormalities in workers that have a long history of environmental exposure to toluene. It is unusual to find instances of exposure to only a single solvent in the workplace and, after consideration of possible contributing influences such as drinking habits and exposure to solvent mixtures containing other known neurotoxicants such as n-hexane, it seems that the neurobehavioral deficits are not as closely associated with toluene exposure as once presumed (21).

Several solvents including n-hexane, methyl n-butyl ketone, and carbon disulfide exhibit characteristic histopathologic or neuropathologic disorders after exposure in humans or animals. Scientists have a reasonable understanding of the underlying mechanisms of toxicity in *n*-hexane, methyl *n*-butyl ketone, and carbon disulfide. These solvents affect the peripheral nervous system by producing a focal axonal swelling and distal axonal degeneration from the site of neurofilament protein accumulation (10). Solvents that are highly lipid soluble tend to seek tissue sites that have lipid concentrations and thus become deposited in organ systems such as the nervous system.

n-Hexane

Hexane is a highly toxic compound in the alkane class. It is generally used as a solvent for adhesives. Acute toxic responses after accidental ingestion include nausea, gastrointestinal irritation, and central nervous system effects. Inhalation exposure leads to a sense of dizziness, euphoria, and numbness of the extremities. Exposure to high concentrations yields vertigo and a marked anesthetic effect. Hexane is also an irritant to the skin upon dermal exposure.

Many cases of polyneuropathy in workers exposed to *n*-hexane have been noted, with the earliest occurring in Japan (104). Hexane is readily absorbed in laboratory animals and has an affinity for tissues high in lipid content (15). It is rapidly metabolized to hydroxylated compounds prior to being converted to a keto form (46,55). 2,5-Hexanedione and methyl *n*-butyl ketone are metabolites suspected of being responsible for the production of neurotoxicity. Inhalation of *n*-hexane in rats produced neurotoxicity with swelling of spinal tracts (86). Exposure to 2,5-hexanedione results in an accumulation of axonal neurofilaments in some central and peripheral myelinated nerve fibers (85).

The mechanism of 2,5-hexanedione-induced neuropathy is not known but several hypotheses have been suggested (26). These hypotheses include reduction in energy production in the axon resulting in disruption of axonal transport, alteration of protein structure, and inadequate proteolysis of neurofilaments in the nerve terminal. 2,5-Hexanedione has been shown to interact with glyceraldehyde-3,5-dehydrogenase and phosphofructokinase, inhibiting their glycolytic properties and resulting in decreased energy production and possible disruption of axonal flow. Reaction of 2,5-hexanedione with lysine amine moieties to form pyrrole adducts and modification of neurofilament or axonal skeletal proteins is also an attractive hypothesis (27). Modification of the proteins may lead to crosslinking of the neurofilaments, which could cause difficulty in passing through narrow regions of the axon such as the node of Ranvier, and therefore accumulate at the site of constriction. Possible biophysical membrane changes as a result of 2,5-hexanedione may influence the degeneration of the axon. 2,5-Hexanedione binding and inactivation of calcium-dependent proteases that are important for degradation of neurofilament proteins is the last mechanism mentioned that may lead to accumulation of neurofilaments. Although none of the mechanisms mentioned fully answers all of the questions concerning *n*-hexane-induced neurotoxicity, these hypotheses offer some suggestions to the understanding of the toxic interaction. It may

be that several mechanisms act in parallel to produce the neurotoxic effects.

The neurotoxic effect of *n*-hexane has characteristically been a progressive motor or sensorimotor neuropathy. Symptoms are first seen from several months to a year after the beginning of long-term hexane exposure (38). Symptoms in cases from occupational exposure have often been sensory in nature with numbness and paresthesias in the distal extremities, most notably in the feet or hands. Improvement of symptoms is noted after cessation of exposure, and mild cases can recover completely.

Methyl *n*-Butyl Ketone

Methyl *n*-butyl ketone and *n*-hexane share the same neurotoxic metabolite, 2,5-hexanedione. In fact, methyl *n*-butyl ketone is one of the metabolites of *n*-hexane. Methyl *n*-butyl ketone was implicated as a neurotoxic solvent in the 1970s after several instances of neurotoxicity were seen in the printing and painting industries (63). Exposure to methyl *n*-butyl ketone usually was by inhalation with the severity of the developed neuropathy related to the extent of exposure. The disorder caused by methyl *n*-butyl ketone begins several months after the beginning of chronic exposure. A frequent early symptom that occurs with methyl *n*-butyl ketone exposure is an unexplained weight loss. Generally, symptoms of a sensory distal neuropathy develop as a tingling paresthesia in the feet or hands. The muscular weakness that develops usually involves the hands and feet, but in severe cases may extend to the muscles of the legs and thighs. The sensory loss follows a similar symmetrical pattern with progression to the legs and thighs in severe cases. There is a moderate reduction of nerve conduction velocity in peripheral nerves associated with the methyl *n*-butyl ketone-induced neuropathy. It has been indicated that no central nervous system disorders have been linked to methyl *n*-butyl ketone exposure (3,4).

Termination of exposure in humans leads to an improvement in neurological signs, which generally show complete resolution in moderate cases. In severe cases improvement is seen, but sometimes a mild or moderate neuropathy persists that is characterized by a slight weakness and a distal sensory loss (3).

Histopathologic findings from experimentally induced methyl *n*-butyl ketone neuropathy have shown multiple swellings along individual nerve fibers at the node of Ranvier. In the area of axonal swelling, the myelin sheath becomes thin or denuded (86). When the areas of axonal enlargement were examined by transmission electron microscopy, increased accumulations of neurofilaments were noticed. Axonal degeneration began in the distal portion after the early changes in the nodal regions (85).

Rats were exposed to inhalation atmospheres of methyl *n*-butyl ketone vapor in order to investigate the development of the neuropathy seen in humans after exposure to the solvent. It was found that after exposure to methyl *n*-butyl ketone, the rats slowly developed a symmetrical weakness of the hindlimbs that progressed to the forelimbs after prolonged exposure. Examination of the peripheral nerves yielded a pattern of distal nerve fiber abnormalities that consisted of axonal swelling with demyelination around the affected nodes. Accumulation of neurofilaments at the affected nodes was noticed as well as abnormalities in regions of the central nervous system that supplied the motor nerves to the affected limbs (85).

Metabolism of methyl *n*-butyl ketone in rats after gavage led to about 40% of the administered dose being detected in urine. The radiolabeled compound was widely distributed in the tissues with the highest concentrations found in blood and liver. The principal metabolites of methyl *n*-butyl ketone detected in the serum were 2-hexanol, 5-hydroxy-2-hexanone, and 2,5-hexanedione. These major metabolites as well as some others were detected in urine. Elimination of 2-hexanol in the urine was found as the free compound, and suggestive evidence points to the possibility of a glucuronide conjugate. The 5-hydroxy-2-hexanone may be a key intermediate in the metabolic pathway of methyl *n*-butyl ketone. 5-Hydroxy-2-hexanone appears to be formed as a result of oxidation by the microsomal mixed function oxidase system. It is eliminated in the unchanged form and suggestive evidence indicates the possibility of glucuronide and sulfate conjugates. Further oxidation of the 5-hydroxy-2-hexanone leads to the toxic metabolite 2,5-hexanedione (28).

When volunteers were administered methyl *n*-butyl ketone by inhalation, orally, or by dermal application, 2,5-hexanedione appeared in the serum. It was found that radioactivity associated with the radiolabeled compound was excreted slowly, indicating that repeated exposures to high concentrations of methyl *n*-butyl ketone may lead to prolonged exposure to the potential neurotoxic metabolite 2,5-hexanedione (29).

The relative potency of the potentially neurotoxic compounds *n*-hexane and methyl *n*-butyl ketone and their metabolites was investigated in rats. Potency was estimated by determination of the length of time required to produce evidence of severe hindlimb weakness or paralysis. The compounds tested were *n*-hexane and methyl-*n*-butyl ketone and their metabolites 2-hexanol, 2,5-hexanediol, 5-hydroxy-2-hexanone, and 2,5-hexanedione. The relative neurotoxicity of these compounds in decreasing order was 2,5-hexanedione (the most toxic) followed by 5-hydroxy-2-hexanone, 2,5-hexanediol, methyl *n*-butyl ketone, 2-hexanol, and *n*-hexane. By measuring the serum concentration curves, the neurotoxic potency was found to be related to the amount of 2,5-hexanedione metabolically produced (47).

Carbon Disulfide

Carbon disulfide has had extensive use in the production of rayon. It has a characteristic rotten egg odor but adaptation to the odor occurs rapidly and the sense of smell cannot be used as a judge of exposure. Acute exposure to high concentrations of carbon disulfide can produce vomiting, headache, respiratory depression, loss of consciousness, a decrease in blood pressure, cyanosis, and death. Symptoms of nervous system involvement are exhibited by irritability, visual disturbances, bad dreams, psychoses, tremors, and convulsions (33,51,96). Improvement in the symptoms of acute carbon disulfide exposure occurs slowly over a period of 3–4 months and recovery may never be complete. Degenerative changes

in the brain and spinal cord have been seen after death due to carbon disulfide overexposure.

Prolonged exposure to carbon disulfide gas in the workplace results in a characteristic picture of the solvent-induced toxicity. The symptoms commonly seen with chronic exposure to carbon disulfide are polyneuritis with sensory loss in the extremities accompanied by muscular weakness, irritability, loss of memory, insomnia, mental depression, decreased visual acuity, loss of libido, and Parkinson-like tremors (51). Carbon disulfide exposure also produces some cerebrovascular changes and vascular changes in the retina. An increase in coronary heart disease has been reported in workers exposed to low concentrations of the solvent for prolonged periods (89,94). This increase in vascular disease may be related to increased atheroma formation (94).

The mechanism of carbon disulfide-induced toxicity is not known with certainty, but it appears to be related to an increase of neurofilament proteins in axons. An increase or accumulation of neurofilaments is seen in the axons of peripheral nerves and spinal cord with a concomitant decrease in nerve conduction velocity that may be causally related (22). Carbon disulfide does bind to neurofilament proteins (80) and may inhibit the action of dopamine beta hydroxylase by dithiocarbamate derivatives binding to enzymic copper necessary for normal dopamine beta hydroxylase function (60). Central nervous system involvement is seen with abnormal choreo and athetoid movements and evidence of lesions in the putamen, caudate nucleus, and globus pallidus (47).

The sequelae of morphologic alterations in the development of carbon disulfide-induced neuropathy in rats were studied after inhalation of the solvent for 5 hr a day, 5 days a week for 12 weeks, followed by a recovery period of 18 weeks. In the peripheral nervous system, examination of the sciatic nerve revealed swelling of axons proximal to the node of Ranvier and an increase of neurofilaments along with a decrease of neurotubules. The neuropathy that results after carbon disulfide exposure is termed distal axonopathy, because there is distal degeneration of the nerve distal to the site of axonal swelling. The axonopathy seen after carbon disulfide exposure is very similar to the type of neuropathy that develops after exposure to methyl *n*-butyl ketone, *n*-hexane, and acrylamide (22,85).

Exposure to carbon disulfide in the workplace is associated with several adverse health effects. These effects are cardiovascular such as vascular changes in the retina and coronary heart disease, psychoses, polyneuropathy, and reproductive effects as mentioned above. In a study of workers exposed to carbon disulfide at a concentration of approximately 3 ppm for at least 1 year, it was found that there was an increased frequency of retinal microaneurysms and hemorrhages and alterations in motor nerve conduction velocity (32). Workers exposed to carbon disulfide for an average of 22 years at concentrations up to seven times the TLV displayed definite signs of neuropathy consisting of distal sensory loss, altered tendon reflexes, reduced muscle power, and reduction in nerve conduction velocity. These abnormalities were present up to 10 years after cessation of exposure to carbon disulfide and were considered to be permanent alterations in nervous system physiology (24).

Additional studies were conducted of workers exposed to

carbon disulfide in the manufacture of rayon fibers for an average duration of 12 years at concentrations that had generally not exceeded 20 ppm. In contrast to the results obtained when exposure conditions to carbon disulfide were much higher, the group of workers that were exposed to low concentrations of less than 10 ppm displayed a reduction of motor nerve conduction velocity without the additional symptoms of peripheral nervous system damage.

These results suggest that exposure to concentrations of carbon disulfide less than 10 ppm do not produce the polyneuropathy that is associated with exposures at higher concentrations (43). In a companion study to investigate the potential behavioral deficits in the same workers, the investigators found that there were no behavioral changes of any major significance (75).

A convenient biologic index of carbon disulfide exposure is found in the urine of workers that correlates with magnitude of exposure during the workday. Metabolism of carbon disulfide leads to excretion of thio compounds into the urine. The metabolic pathway for degradation of carbon disulfide remains to be completely identified, but suggestive evidence exists that carbon disulfide combines with sulfur containing amino acids or glutathione which leads to the formation of thio compounds that are excreted into the urine. Several thio compounds have been identified in the urine that are quantitatively related to carbon disulfide exposure (72,73,91,92).

REFERENCES

1. ACGIH (1982): *Industrial Ventilation: A Manual of Recommended Practice,* Proceedings of the American Conference of Governmental Hygienists, Lansing, MI.
2. ACGIH (1987): *Threshold Limit Values and Biological Exposure Indices,* Proceedings of the American Conference of Governmental Hygienists, p. 111. Cincinnati, OH.
3. Allen, N. (1979): Solvents and other industrial organic compounds. In: *Handbook of Clinical Neurology Intoxications of the Nervous System,* Part 1(36), edited by P. J. Vinken and G. W. Bruyn, pp. 361–389. Elsevier/North Holland, NY.
4. Allen, N., Mendell, J. R., Billmaier, D. J., Fontaine, R. E., and O'Neill, J. (1975): Toxic polyneuropathy due to methyl *n*-butyl ketone. *Arch. Neurol.,* 32:209–218.
5. Anderson, D., and McGregor, D. B. (1980): The effect of solvents upon the yield of revertants in the *Salmonella*/activation mutagenicity assay. *Carcinogenesis,* 1:363–366.
6. Astrand, I. (1975): Uptake of solvents in the blood and tissues of man. *Scand. J. Work Environ. Health,* 1:199–218.
7. Astrand, I. (1985): Uptake of solvents from the lungs. *Br. J. Indust. Med.,* 42:217–218.
8. Baelum, J., Anderson, I., Lundqvist, G. R., Molhave, L., Pedersen, O. F., Vaeth, M., and Wyon, D. P. (1985): Response of solvent-exposed printers and unexposed controls to six-hour toluene exposure. *Scand. J. Work Environ. Health,* 11:271–280.
9. Bahl, M. K. (1985): ESCA studies on skin lipid removal by solvents and surfactants. *J. Soc. Cosmet. Chem.,* 36:287–296.
10. Baker, E. L., and Fine, L. J. (1986): Solvent neurotoxicity: The current evidence. *J. Occup. Med.,* 28:126–129.
11. Bamberger, R. L., Esposito, G. G., Jacobs, B. W., Podolak, G. E., and Mazur, J. F. (1978): A new personal sampler for organic vapors. *Am. Ind. Hyg. Assoc. J.,* 39:701–708.
12. Bird, M. G. (1981): Industrial solvents: Some factors affecting their passage into and through the skin. *Ann. Occup. Hyg.,* 24:235–244.
13. Birmingham, D. J. (1978): Occupational dermatoses. In: *Patty's Industrial Hygiene and Toxicology,* Vol. 1, edited by G. D. Clayton and F. E. Clayton, pp. 203–235. John Wiley, NY.
14. Blank, I. H., and McAuliffe, D. J. (1985): Penetration of benzene through human skin. *J. Invest. Dermatol.,* 85:522–526.
15. Bohlen, P., Schlunegger, U. P., and Lauppi, E. (1973): Uptake and distribution of hexane in rat tissues. *Toxicol. Appl. Pharmacol.,* 25:242–249.
16. Braun, D. L. (1972): Detection of mercury vapors as an adjunct to respiratory protective devices. Proceedings of the American Industrial Hygiene Association, San Francisco, CA.
17. Brief, R. S., and Scala, R. A. (1986): Occupational health aspects of unusual work schedules: A review of Exxon's experiences. *Am. Ind. Hyg. Assoc. J.,* 47:199–202.
18. Brodberg, R. K., and Woodruff, R. C. (1982): Dimethylsulfoxide reduces the mutagenicity of the indirect mutagen dimethylnitrosamine in *Drosophilia Melanogaster. Environ. Mutagen.,* 4:306–307.
19. Brugnone, F., Perbellini, L., Gaffuri, E., and Apostoli, P. (1980): Biomonitoring of industrial solvent exposures in workers' alveolar air. *Internat. Arch. Occup. Environ. Health,* 47:245–261.
20. Burson, J. L. (1985): Controls for industrial exposures. In: *Industrial Toxicology,* edited by P. L. Williams and J. L. Burson, pp. 433–450. Van Nostrand Reinhold, NY.
21. Cherry, N., Hutchins, H., Pace, T., and Waldron, H. A. (1985): Neurobehavioural effects of repeated occupational exposure to toluene and paint solvents. *Br. J. Indust. Med.,* 42:291–300.
22. Colombi, A., Maroni, M., Picchi, O., Rota, E., Castano, P., and Foa, V. (1981): Carbon disulfide neuropathy in rats. A morphological and ultrastructural study of degeneration and regeneration. *Clin. Toxicol.,* 18:1463–1474.
23. Cook, W. A. (1945): Maximum allowable concentrations of industrial atmospheric contaminants. *Indust. Med.,* 14:936–946.
24. Corsi, G., Maestrelli, P., Picotti, G., Manzoni, S., and Negrin, P. (1983): Chronic peripheral neuropathy in workers with previous exposure to carbon disulphide. *Br. J. Indust. Med.,* 40:209–211.
25. Cranmer, J. M., and Goldberg, L. (1987): Exposures issues in the evaluation of solvent effects. *Neurotoxicology,* 7:5–23.
26. DeCaprio, A. P. (1985): Molecular mechanisms of diketone neurotoxicity. *Chem. Biol. Interact.,* 54:257–270.
27. DeCaprio, A. P., and O'Neill, E. A. (1985): Alterations in rat axonal cytoskeletal proteins induced by *in vitro* and *in vivo* 2,5-hexanedione exposure. *Toxicol. Appl. Pharmacol.,* 78:235–247.
28. DiVincenzo, G. D., Hamilton, M. L., Kaplan, C. J., and Dedinas, J. (1977): Metabolic fate and disposition of 14C-labeled methyl *n*-butyl ketone in the rat. *Toxicol. Appl. Pharmacol.,* 41:547–560.
29. DiVincenzo, G. D., Hamilton, M. L., Kaplan, C. J., Krasavage, W. J., and O'Donoghue, J. L. (1978): Studies on the respiratory uptake and excretion and the skin absorption of methyl *n*-butyl ketone in humans and dogs. *Toxicol. Appl. Pharmacol.,* 44:593–604.
30. Dossing, M., Baelum, J., Hansen, S. H., and Lundqvist, G. R. (1984): Effect of ethanol, cimetidine and propranolol on toluene metabolism in man. *Internat. Arch. Occup. Environ. Health,* 54:309–315.
31. Elkins, H. B. (1948): The case for maximum allowable concentrations. *Am. Ind. Hyg. Assoc. J.,* 1:22–25.
32. Fajen, J., Albright, B., and Leffingwell, S. S. (1981): A cross-sectional medical and industrial hygiene survey of workers exposed to carbon disulfide. *Scand. J. Work Environ. Health,* 7:20–27.
33. Grasso, P., Sharratt, M., Davies, D. M., and Irvine, D. (1984): Neurophysiological and psychological disorders and occupational exposure to organic solvents. *Food Chem. Toxic.,* 22:819–852.
34. Hardin, B. D. (1983): Reproductive toxicity of the glycol ethers. *Toxicology,* 27:91–102.
35. Hardin, B. D., Bond, G. P., Sikov, M. R., Andrew, F. D., Beliles, R. P., and Niemeier, R. W. (1981): Testing of selected workplace chemicals for teratogenic potential. *Scand. J. Work Environ. Health,* 7:66–75.
36. Hardin, B. D., Niemeier, R. W., Smith, R. J., Kuczuk, M. H., Mathinos, P. R., and Weaver, T. F. (1982): Teratogenicity of 2-ethoxyethanol by dermal application. *Drug Chem. Toxicol.,* 5:277–294.
37. Hawley, G. G. (1981): *The Condensed Chemical Dictionary,* p. 1135. Van Nostrand Reinhold, NY.
38. Herskowitz, A., Ishii, N., and Schaumburg, H. (1971): *n*-Hexane neuropathy. *N. Engl. J. Med.,* 285:82–85.
39. Hosey, A. D. (1973): General principles in evaluating the occupational environment. In: *The Industrial Environment—Its Eval-*

uation and Control, edited by USDHEW, PHS, CDC, and NIOSH, pp. 95–100. United States Government Printing Office, Washington, D.C.

40. Ikeda, M., and Ohtsuji, H. (1971): Phenobarbital-induced protection against toxicity of toluene and benzene in the rat. *Toxicol. Appl. Pharmacol.,* 20:30–43.

41. Irons, R. D., Dent, J. G., Baker, T. S., and Rickert, D. E. (1980): Benzene is metabolized and covalently bound in bone marrow *in situ. Chem. Biol. Interact.,* 30:241–245.

42. Jakobson, I., Wahlberg, J. E., Holmberg, B., and Johansson, G. (1982): Uptake via the blood and elimination of 10 organic solvents following epicutaneous exposure of anesthetized guinea pigs. *Toxicol. Appl. Pharmacol.,* 63:181–187.

43. Johnson, B. L., Boyd, J., Burg, J. R., Lee, S. T., Xintaras, C., and Albright, B. E. (1983): Effects on the peripheral nervous system of workers' exposure to carbon disulfide. *Neurotoxicol.,* 4:53–66.

44. Kawalek, J. C., and Andrews, A. W. (1980): The effect of solvents on drug metabolism *in vitro. Drug Metab. Disposition,* 8:380–384.

45. Knox, J. W., and Nelson, J. R. (1966): Permanent encephalopathy from toluene inhalation. *N. Engl. J. Med.,* 273:1494–1496.

46. Kramer, A., Staudinger, H., and Ullrich, V. (1974): Effect of *n*-hexane inhalation on the monooxygenase system in mice liver microsomes. *Chem. Biol. Interact.,* 8:11–18.

47. Krasavage, W. J., O'Donoghue, J. L., DiVincenzo, G. D., and Terhaar, C. J. (1980): The relative neurotoxicity of methyl-*n*-butyl ketone, *n*-hexane and their metabolites. *Toxicol. Appl. Pharmacol.,* 52:433–441.

48. Kronevi, T., Wahlberg, J., and Holmberg, B. (1979): Histopathology of skin, liver, and kidney after epicutaneous administration of five industrial solvents to guinea pigs. *Environ. Res.,* 19:56–69.

49. Laham, S. (1970): Metabolism of industrial solvents. *Ind. Med.,* 39:61–64.

50. Lee, E. W., Kocsis, J. J., and Snyder, R. (1974): Acute effects of benzene on 59-Fe incorporation into circulating erythrocytes. *Toxicol. Appl. Pharmacol.,* 27:431–436.

51. Lewey, F. H. (1941): Neurological, medical, and biochemical signs and symptoms indicating chronic industrial carbon disulphide absorption. *Ann. Intern. Med.,* 15:869–883.

52. Linch, A. L. (1981): *Evaluation of Ambient Air Quality by Personnel Monitoring,* p. 363. CRC Press, Boca Raton, FL.

53. Little, A. D. (1983): *Guidelines for the Selection of Chemical Protective Clothing.* American Conference of Governmental Industrial Hygienists, Cincinnati, OH.

54. Longacre, S. L., Kocsis, J. J., and Snyder, R. (1981): Influence of strain differences in mice on the metabolism and toxicity of benzene. *Toxicol. Appl. Pharmacol.,* 60:398–409.

55. Lu, A. Y. H., Strobel, H. W., and Coon, M. J. (1970): Properties of a solubilized form of the cytochrome P-450-containing mixed-function oxidase of liver microsomes. *Mol. Pharmacol.,* 6:213–220.

56. Maibach, H. I., and Anjo, D. M. (1981): Percutaneous penetration of benzene and benzene contained in solvents used in the rubber industry. *Arch. Environ. Health,* 36:256–260.

57. Marsden, C., and Mann, S. (1963): *Solvents Guide,* p. 633. Interscience, NY.

58. Matheson, L. E., Jr., Wurster, D. E., and Ostrenga, J. A. (1979): Sarin transport across excised human skin. II: Effect of solvent pretreatment on permeability. *J. Pharm. Sci.,* 11:1410–1413.

59. Matsumoto, T. (1971): Experimental studies on the chronic toluene poisoning: 2. Electrophysiological changes of peripheral neuromuscular function in the rats exposed to toluene. *Jpn. J. Ind. Health,* 13:399–407.

60. McKenna, M. J., and DiStefano, V. (1977): Carbon disulfide. II. A proposed mechanism for the action of carbon disulfide on dopamine β-hydroxylase. *J. Pharmacol. Exp. Ther.,* 202:253–266.

61. McKenna, M. J., and Zempel, J. A. (1981): The dose-dependent metabolism of (14C)methylene chloride following oral administration to rats. *Food Cosmet. Toxicol.,* 19:73–78.

62. McKenna, M. J., Zempel, J. A., and Braun, W. H. (1982): The pharmacokinetics of inhaled methylene chloride in rats. *Toxicol. Appl. Pharmacol.,* 65:1–10.

63. Mendell, J. R., Saida, K., Ganansia, M. F., Jackson, D. B., Weiss, H., Gardier, R. W., Chrisman, C., Allen, N., Couri, D., O'Neill, J. J., Marks, B. H., and Hetland, L. B. (1974): Toxic polyneuropathy produced by methyl *n*-butyl ketone. *Science,* 185:787–789.

64. Menger, F. M., Goldsmith, D. J., and Mandell, L. (1972): *Organic Chemistry—A Concise Approach,* p. 450. W. A. Benjamin, Menlo Park, CA.

65. Nelson, B. K., Brightwell, W. S., Setzer, J. V., and O'Donohue, T. L. (1984): Reproductive toxicity of the industrial solvent 2-ethoxyethanol in rats and interactive effects of ethanol. *Environ. Health Perspect.,* 57:255–259.

66. Nelson, B. K., Setzer, J. V., Brightwell, W. S., Mathinos, P. R., Kuczuk, M. H., Weaver, T. E., and Goad, P. T. (1984): Comparative inhalation teratogenicity of four glycol ether solvents and an amino derivative in rats. *Environ. Health Perspect.,* 57:261–271.

67. Nelson, G. O., Lum, B. Y., Carlson, G. J., Wong, C. M., and Johnson, J. S. (1981): Glove permeation by organic solvents. *Am. Ind. Hyg. Assoc. J.,* 38:563–566.

68. Nestmann, E. R., Douglas, G. R., Kowbel, D. J., and Harrington, T. R. (1985): Solvent interactions with test compounds and recommendations for testing to avoid artifacts. *Environ. Mutagen.,* 7: 163–170.

69. Palmes, E. D., and Gunnison, A. F. (1973): Personal monitoring device for gaseous contaminants. *Am. Ind. Hyg. Assoc. J.,* 34:78.

70. Paustenbach, D., and Langer, R. (1986): Corporate occupational exposure limits: The current state of affairs. *Am. Ind. Hyg. Assoc. J.,* 47:809–818.

71. Pegg, D. G., Zempel, J. A., Braun, W. H., and Watanabe, P. G. (1979): Disposition of tetrachloro(14C)ethylene following oral and inhalation exposure in rats. *Toxicol. Appl. Pharmacol.,* 51:465–474.

72. Pergal, M., Vukojevic, N., Cirin-Popov, N., Djuric, D., and Bojovic, T. (1972): Carbon disulfide metabolites excreted in the urine of exposed workers. *Arch. Environ. Health,* 25:38–41.

73. Pergal, M., Vukojevic, N., and Djuric, D. (1972): Isolation and identification of thiocarbamide. *Arch. Environ. Health,* 25:42–44.

74. Popendorf, W. (1984): Vapor pressure and solvent vapor hazards. *Am. Ind. Hyg. Assoc. J.,* 45:719–726.

75. Putz-Anderson, V., Albright, B. E., Lee, S. T., Johnson, B. L., Chrislip, D. W., Taylor, B. J., Brightwell, W. S., Dickerson, N., Culver, M., Zentmeyer, D., and Smith, P. (1983): A behavioral examination of workers exposed to carbon disulfide. *Neurotoxicology,* 4:67–78.

76. Reddy, A. L., and Fialkow, P. J. (1981): Effect of solvents on methylcholanthrene-induced carcinogenesis in mice. *Int. J. Cancer,* 27: 501–504.

77. Reinhardt, C. F., Mullin, L. S., and Maxfield, M. E. (1973): Epinephrine-induced cardiac arrhythmia potential of some common industrial solvents. *J. Occup. Med.,* 15:953–955.

78. Riihimaki, V., and Pfaffli, P. (1978): Percutaneous absorption of solvent vapors in man. *Scand. J. Work Environ. Health,* 4:73–85.

79. Rowe, V. K., and Wolf, M. A. (1982): Derivatives of glycols. In: *Patty's Industrial Hygiene and Toxicology,* Vol. 3, edited by G. D. Clayton and F. E. Clayton, pp. 3909–4052. John Wiley, NY.

80. Savolainen, H., Lehtonen, E., and Vainio, H. (1977): CS2 binding to rat spinal neurofilaments. *Acta Neuropathol.,* 37:219–223.

81. Sax, N. I., and Lewis, R. J. (1986): *Rapid Guide to Hazardous Chemicals in the Workplace,* p. 236. Van Nostrand Reinhold, NY.

82. Scheflan, L., and Jacobs, M. B. (1953): *The Handbook of Solvents,* p. 728. Van Nostrand Reinhold, NY.

83. Snyder, C. A., Goldstein, B. D., Sellakumar, A., Wolman, S. R., Bromberg, I., Erlichman, M. N., and Laskin, S. (1978): Hematotoxicity of inhaled benzene to Sprague–Dawley Rats and AKR Mice at 300 ppm. *J. Toxicol. Environ. Health,* 4:605–618.

84. Snyder, R., and Kocsis, J. J. (1975): Current concepts of chronic benzene toxicity. *CRC Crit. Rev. Toxicol.,* 3:265–288.

85. Spencer, P. S., and Schaumburg, H. H. (1977): Ultrastructural Studies of the dying-back process, IV. Differential vulnerability of PNS and CNS fibers in experimental central-peripheral distal axonopathies. *J. Neuropathol. Exp. Neurol.,* 36:300–320.

86. Spencer, P. S., Schaumburg, H. H., Raleigh, R. L., and Terhaar, C. J. (1975): Nervous system degeneration produced by the industrial solvent methyl *n*-butyl ketone. *Arch. Neurol.,* 32:219–222.

87. Stula, E. F., and Krauss, W. C. (1977): Embryotoxicity in rats and rabbits from cutaneous application of amide-type solvents and substituted ureas. *Toxicol. Appl. Pharmacol.,* 41:35–55.

88. Taher, S. M., Anderson, R. J., McCartney, R., Popovtzer, M. M., and Schrier, R. W. (1974): Renal tubular acidosis associated with toluene "sniffing". *N. Engl. J. Med.,* 290:765–768.

89. Tiller, J. R., Schilling, R. S. F., and Morris, J. N. (1968): Occupational toxic factor in mortality from coronary heart disease. *Br. Med. J.,* 16:407–411.

90. Torkelson, T. R., and Rowe, V. K. (1982): Halogenated aliphatic hydrocarbons containing chlorine, bromine, and iodine. In: *Patty's Industrial Hygiene and Toxicology,* Vol. 2B, edited by G. D. Clayton and F. E. Clayton, pp. 3433–3601. John Wiley, NY.

91. Van Dolah, R. W. (1965): Flame propagation, extinguishment, and environmental effects on combustion. *Fire Technol.,* 2:138–145.

92. van Doorn, R., Delbressine, L. P. C., Leijdekkers, C. M., Vertin, P. G., and Henderson, P. H. (1981): Identification and determination of 2-thiothiazolidine-4-carboxylic acid in urine of workers exposed to carbon disulfide. *Arch. Toxicol.,* 47:51–58.

93. van Doorn, R., Leijdekkers, C. P. M. J. M., Henderson, P. T., Vanhoorne, M., and Vertin, P. G. (1981): Determination of thio compounds in urine of workers exposed to carbon disulfide. *Arch. Environ. Health,* 36:289–297.

94. Van Stee, E. W. (1982): Cardiovascular toxicology: Foundation and scope. In: *Cardiovascular Toxicology,* edited by E. W. Van Stee, pp. 1–35. Raven Press, NY.

95. Viau, C. J., Sherman, S. M., and Sabharwal, P. S. (1982): Comparative extraction of genotoxic components of air particulates with several solvent systems. *Mutat. Res.,* 105:133–137.

96. Vigliani, E. C. (1950): Clinical observations on carbon disulfide intoxication in Italy. *Ind. Med. Surg.,* 19:240–242.

97. Vigliani, E. C., and Forni, A. (1976): Benzene and leukemia. *Environ. Res.,* 11:122–127.

98. Vigliani, E. C., and Saita, G. (1964): Benzene and leukemia. *N. Engl. J. Med.,* 27:872–876.

99. Voog, L., and Eriksson, T. (1984): Toluene-induced decrease in rat plasma concentrations of tyrosine and tryptophan. *Acta Pharmacol. Toxicol.,* 54:151–153.

100. Wahlberg, J. E. (1976): Percutaneous toxicity of solvents. A comparative investigation in the guinea pig with benzene, toluene and 1,1,2-trichloroethane. *Ann. Occup. Hyg.,* 19:115–119.

101. Wahlberg, J. E., and Boman, A. (1978): 2-Chloroethanol—Percutaneous toxicity of a solvent. *Dermatologica.* 156:299–302.

102. Windholz, M. (1983): Monographs. In: *The Merck Index,* 10th ed., edited by M. Windholz, pp. 1–1463. Merck, Rahway, NJ.

103. Winek, C. L., and Collom, W. D. (1971): Benzene and toluene fatalities. *J. of Occup. Med.,* 13:259–261.

104. Yamada, S. (1964): An occurrence of polyneuritis by *n*-hexane in the polyethylene laminating plants. *Jpn. J. of Ind. Health,* 6:192–194.

Principles and Methods of Toxicology, Second Edition, edited by A. Wallace Hayes, Raven Press, Ltd., New York © 1989.

CHAPTER 5

Pesticides

Perry J. Kurtz, *Randy Deskin, and **Robert M. Harrington

*Health and Molecular Sciences Department, Battelle Columbus Division, Columbus, Ohio 43201; *Toxicology and Products Safety Department, American Cyanamid Company, Wayne, New Jersey 07470; and **R. J. Reynolds Tobacco Company, Bowman Gray Technical Center, Winston-Salem, North Carolina 27102*

Over the past forty years pesticides have become an indispensable part of world agriculture. It has been estimated that pesticide use has increased crop yield by a factor of greater than one-third (359). In the United States alone, annual commercial pesticide production is in the hundreds of millions of kilograms and represents a retail sales value of several billion dollars. The demand for pesticide products and the contributions that they make toward improved agricultural efficiency are clear, but the volume of production alone indicates that the potential for misapplication and accidental exposure is great. With the growth of the industry, therefore, the question of pesticide safety has become one of the most serious world public health concerns.

One of the factors underlying the increase in concern over the health hazards associated with the use of pesticides is a growing awareness of the hazards associated with long-term exposure to some of these chemicals among both health scientists and the public in general. The insidious nature of effects such as carcinogenicity and the potential for delayed manifestations of toxicity to the nervous and reproductive systems, in particular, has focused media and government attention on these problems. More comprehensive safety testing is required before a new pesticide is registered for use and a major effort to reexamine the safety data available for

chemicals already on the market is underway within the Environmental Protection Agency (EPA). Where there is special concern over a health or environmental problem, the pesticide may be placed under special review (formerly referred to as a rebuttable presumption against registration or RPAR). On the basis of the findings of the review, registration of the pesticide may be continued, restricted, or canceled.

The concern for long-term effects is reflected in the types of studies required for pesticide registration in the United States and abroad. While there is still a need to examine the hazards associated with high-level short-term (acute) exposure, there is also a need to understand the potential for effects resulting from lower levels during long-term (chronic) exposure. In general, it is the chronic exposure data which relate more directly to the safety of the general public, who may be exposed to low-level pesticide residues in food and drinking water. In contrast, acute and short-term exposure data are most relevant to those who may be exposed to high levels (particularly by the dermal and inhalation routes) during the formulation or application of the product. For those involved in the manufacturing of the chemical, both short- and long-term data are important.

It is important to recognize that while one pesticide may appear to represent a greater health hazard than another on the basis of acute toxicity data, it may actually be much less harmful in terms of its long-term effects. Furthermore, until the magnitude of exposure is known, which for chronic effects often means knowledge of the rate of pesticide application and other factors relating to residue in a specific crop, no valid judgment can be made about the relative hazards of the materials. Thus, it is not possible to evaluate the human health or environmental hazard associated with a given pesticide based on toxicity data alone.

At present, the typical acute toxicology data requirements for new pesticide registrations consist of the following: acute oral (rat), dermal (rabbit) and inhalation (for volatile materials) toxicity data, primary skin and eye irritation studies, dermal sensitization (guinea pig), and acute delayed neurotoxicity studies in the hen (for cholinesterase inhibitors). Subchronic (90-day) feeding studies in one rodent (rat) and nonrodent (dog) species may be supplemented by subchronic dermal, inhalation, and neurotoxicity studies depending on the chemical, the intended use, and the results of the other studies. Chronic (1- to 2-year) oral toxicity data must normally be submitted for one rodent (rat) and one nonrodent (dog) species as well as oncogenicity study data for rat and mouse. Reproductive effects are assessed from teratogenicity data in two species (rat and rabbit) and data from a multigeneration study (rats). *In vitro* mutagenicity tests are used to support information on reproductive toxicity and oncogenicity potential while general metabolism is examined in the rat. Data on dermal penetration and domestic animal safety may also be required.

Although this may appear to represent a formidable array of health safety studies, there are still many unanswered questions. For example, metabolism data are normally generated from studies employing a single or brief repeated exposure to the test materials. However, as discussed later in this chapter, many pesticides induce the production of metabolizing enzymes in the liver and elsewhere which may result in an altered metabolic state after long-term exposure. Thus, the data derived from such studies may not be helpful in understanding the disposition of the material in humans or animals subjected to chronic exposure. The problem is further complicated when attempting to apply the results of metabolism studies to long-term toxicity studies where dose levels necessary to elicit toxicity may have overloaded normal metabolic pathways.

Typically, long-term toxicity studies are conducted with a purified form of the active ingredient. Thus, interactions with other components of the pesticide formulation may not be examined in detail. As with all chemical substances, it is difficult to anticipate and test for all the possible combinations and uses for which a pesticide may be registered. Furthermore, the development and registration of new pesticides is already an extremely long and expensive process and the requirement of additional safety studies may discourage new product development. Thus, regulatory agencies must balance the need for adequate safety data with the cost of producing that data.

INSECTICIDES

The basic principle underlying the pesticidal activity of most traditional insecticides has been chemical interference with the function of the insect nervous system. Because of basic similarities between the neurophysiology of mammals and insects, the development of more effective insecticides often presents the dilemma of the double-edged sword in which increased insecticidal efficacy is accompanied by an increased hazard to animals and humans which may inadvertently be exposed as a result of insecticide application. Some of the most successful insecticides make use of differences in metabolic pathways available to mammals and insects, so that production of the actively neurotoxic chemical form is relatively greater in insects than it is in mammals. Unfortunately, with the use of such insecticides over time, more efficient detoxification mechanisms may evolve in the target insect and pesticide resistance develops.

CHLORINATED HYDROCARBON INSECTICIDES

There are three major categories of chlorinated hydrocarbon insecticides: DDT and its analogs, benzene hexachloride isomers, and cyclodiene compounds. DDT or dichlorodiphenyltrichloroethane (Fig. 1) is one of the oldest and most effective synthetic pesticides. Although it was synthesized in the 19th century, its insecticidal properties were not discovered until 1939. Its first important use was in the control of insects and the diseases carried by insects, notably typhus and malaria, during the Second World War. After the war, commercial production and use of DDT grew until the early 1960s when three factors contributed to its decline. First, there was evidence that some insect populations, particularly the housefly, were developing resistance to the effects of the chemical. Second, there was increasing concern that humans were being exposed through the environment and food residues and that this exposure was producing an accumulation of DDT in human adipose tissue. Third, there was developing concern about the effects of DDT in the ecosystem, a concern that was amplified by the publication of Rachel Carson's book, *Silent Spring*. These three factors have contributed to restrictions on the use of DDT and for other chlorinated hydrocarbons as well.

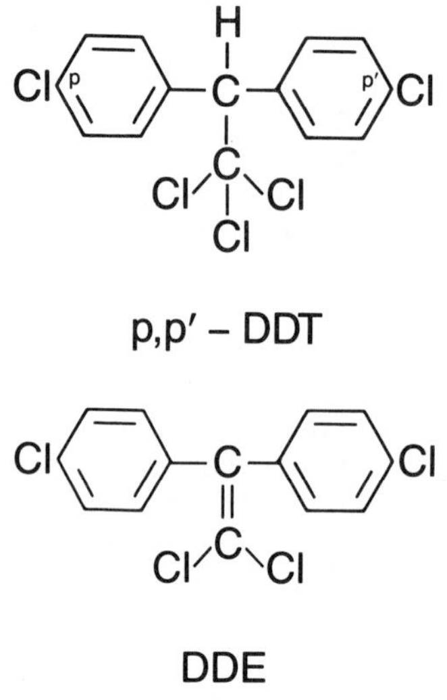

FIG. 1. Structures of DDT and DDE.

The principal site of DDT action is the nervous system. Acute poisoning results in repetitive neural discharges which are manifested outwardly as tremors, paralysis, and eventually, death, which is usually attributed to respiratory arrest. This abnormal neural activity appears to result from interference with the processes responsible for polarization of the nerve cell membrane and the lowering of normal neural excitation thresholds (207,227). Specifically, it acts by interfering with Na^+ and K^+ conductance gating. The normal cycle of increased followed by decreased Na^+ conductance during a nerve action potential is altered so that the inflow of Na^+ is not completely inactivated at the end of the cycle. This prevents the normal outflow of K^+ current from repolarizing the membrane to the resting (negative) level. Instead, the continuing Na^+ current depolarizes the cell membrane to the point where it triggers a new action potential, resulting in repetitive neural discharge (295a). DDT is stored in all body tissues, but the highest concentrations are found in adipose tissue (241) where it and a major lipophillic metabolite, dichlorodiphenyldichloroethylene (DDE) (Fig. 1), may be stored at very high concentrations. In wildlife, this leads to *biomagnification* or storage of increasing concentrations as animals higher in the food chain feed on and accumulate higher residues than their prey. DDE is interesting from another viewpoint because the development of resistance to the effects of DDT in some insect species appears to be related to the capacity to metabolize DDT to its less potent metabolite, DDE (320).

The rat acute oral LD_{50} for DDT administered in oil solution ranges from 100 to 500 mg/kg (130). Gaines (96) reported that the LD_{50} following 90 days of oral exposure to DDT was 46 mg/kg, which suggests moderate cumulative toxicity, probably attributable to increased body burden with storage of successive doses. In man, acute poisoning at a dose level of 10 mg/kg or higher may be expected to produce illness (132), although survival has been reported after dosages as high as 285 mg/kg (101). Muscle weakness, numbness, and eventually convulsions are observed at higher exposure concentrations, which is consistent with the notion that the nervous system is a primary target of DDT toxicity. In man as well as rat, toxicity through dermal exposure is much less than that associated with ingestion, mainly because dermal absorption of the technical powder is poor. Historically, this has facilitated the dermal application of DDT for treatment of human body lice and scabies (304).

In addition to its effects on the nervous system, DDT and numerous other chlorinated hydrocarbon insecticides cause histologic changes in the rodent liver consistent with the induction of microsomal enzymes. Chronic exposure to high dosages of DDT has been reported to produce hepatocarcinogenicity in mice but there is some dispute over the applicability of these findings to human hazard assessment (132). Epidemiologic evidence for carcinogenicity in humans has been negative (152,189).

Concerns about DDT residues in the adipose tissue of the general population has led to several epidemiologic and experimental studies in humans. Laws et al. (189) studied chemical workers who had been exposed to daily doses of DDT from 5 to 18 mg/day for an average of 15 years, an exposure several hundred times that of the general population. Routine clinical laboratory tests and chest radiographs indicated no abnormalities. Hayes et al. (131) administered DDT to human volunteers at doses up to 35 mg/day, also with no detectable effects. In these studies, DDT and DDE residues were much higher in fat than in blood serum, demonstrating the importance of adipose tissue biopsy in estimating the body burden of exposed populations.

The most important representative of the benzene hexachloride isomers is the gamma-isomer of hexachlorocyclohexane, often referred to as lindane (Fig. 2). The dose range and signs associated with acute lindane poisoning are similar to those of DDT except that the tremors and the more severe manifestations of central nervous system toxicity are frequently more obvious (48). The rat acute oral LD_{50} is in the range of 100–200 mg/kg. Chronic exposure has been reported to produce liver toxicity and carcinogenicity, particularly in mice (224,225). As with DDT, lindane exposure results in hepatic enzyme induction, which is manifested in the laboratory as a reduction in hexobarbital-induced sleeping time (179,223). In addition, effects on the immune system (361) and on reproduction have been reported (236).

One of the most interesting aspects of hexachlorocyclohexane toxicity is that different isomers have different pharmacologic effects. While the gamma isomer is a potent central nervous system stimulant, the beta- and delta-isomers produce depression (211). For this reason, the toxicity of the technical material, which is a mixture of the various isomeric forms, appears to represent the interaction of opposing pharmacologic actions. The antagonism of lindane by the other isomeric forms may be caused by competition for one or more common receptors (346) rather than a simple pharmacologic interaction. This is supported by evidence that the protective effects of the other isomers are enhanced if they are administered prior to lindane exposure (63,136).

Although worldwide use of lindane is probably decreasing, studies of its mechanism of action are providing new insights into insect and mammalian toxicology. Matsumura and Ghiasuddin (208) have discovered evidence to support the idea that the neuroexcitatory action of lindane is due to its ability to mimic picrotoxin, a convulsant pharmacologic agent which inhibits the action of gamma-aminobutyric acid (GABA). Since GABA normally suppresses transmission of nerve impulses, GABA antagonists produce excessive neural stimulation.

The chlorinated cyclodiene insecticides (Fig. 3) are among the most toxic and environmentally persistent pesticides. Among these are two pairs of stereoisomers, aldrin and

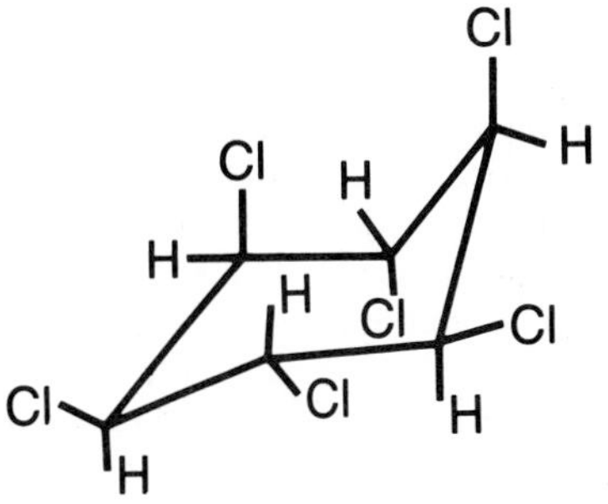

FIG. 2. Structure of lindane.

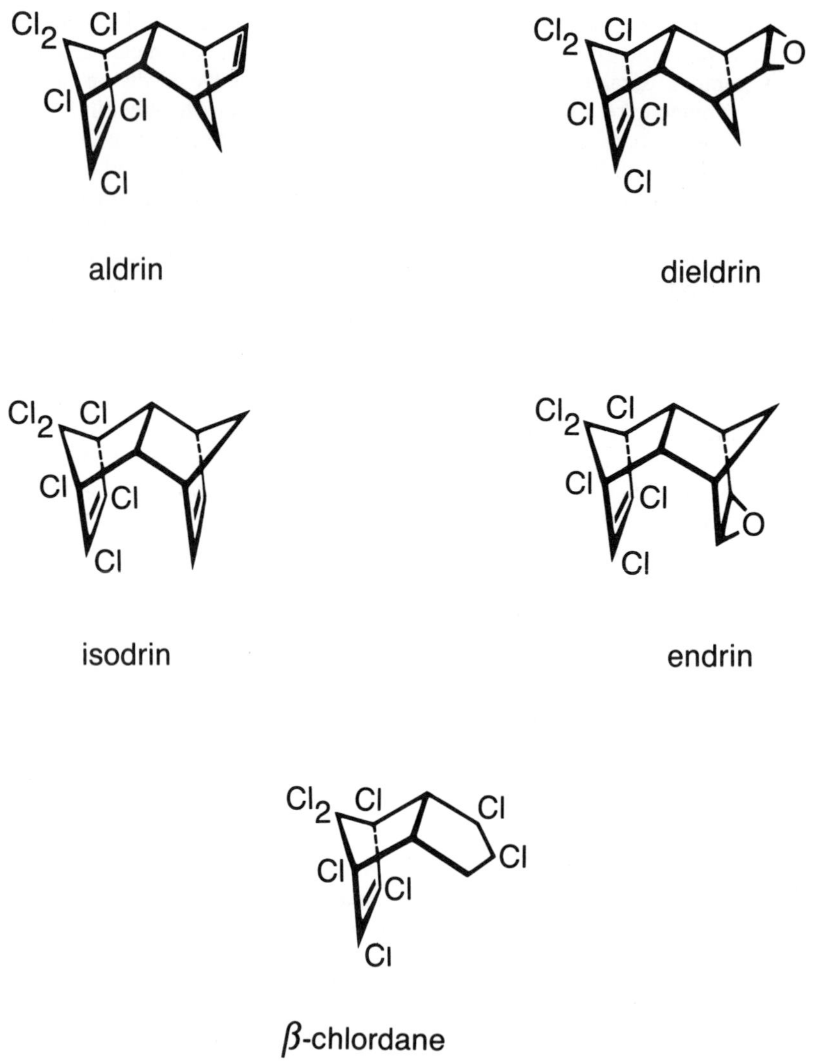

aldrin

dieldrin

isodrin

endrin

β-chlordane

FIG. 3. Chlorinated cyclodiene insecticides: aldrin, dieldrin, isodrin, endrin, and chlordane.

dieldrin, and isodrin and endrin. The first of each pair is rapidly metabolized to its companion stereoisomer so that the toxicity expressed is mainly produced by dieldrin or endrin, respectively. Other important representatives in this group are chlordane and toxaphene. The chlorinated cyclodienes produce similar neurotoxic signs as the other chlorinated hydrocarbon insecticides, although it appears that with many cyclodienes, convulsions are more likely to appear without preliminary indications of tremor or other milder signs of nervous system impairment. The rat acute oral LD_{50} for aldrin and dieldrin is typically well below 100 mg/kg (139) and, as with DDT, the mechanism of toxicity is believed to involve interference with the alteration in ion fluxes across the nerve axon membrane (44). Unlike DDT, the cyclodienes are well absorbed from the skin. Their oral and dermal LD_{50} values are generally within the same order of magnitude while for DDT these values may differ by two log units (96).

As with DDT, the chlorinated cyclodienes are capable of hepatic microsomal enzyme induction, and liver toxicity is a prominent feature in long-term studies. The evidence for carcinogenicity is equivocal; the conclusions of some reviews of the data for aldrin and dieldrin have been that there was sufficient evidence for carcinogenicity (338) while others (139) disagree.

Studies with aldrin and dieldrin have reported effects on reproduction. With aldrin, increased pup losses were reported in dogs (172) and rats (331). With dieldrin, for example, Treon and Cleveland (331) reported a reduction in fertility and an increase in pup mortality. Chernoff et al. (54) reported delayed ossification and an increase in supernumerary ribs in mice.

ORGANOPHOSPHORUS INSECTICIDES

The organophosphorus (OP) insecticides are esters of phosphoric acid or thiophosphoric acid. They were first studied in Germany at the time of the Second World War as possible substitutes for nicotine. In fact, the first important OP insecticide, tetraethylpyrophosphate (TEPP), was used as a substitute for nicotine against aphids. TEPP (Fig. 4) was

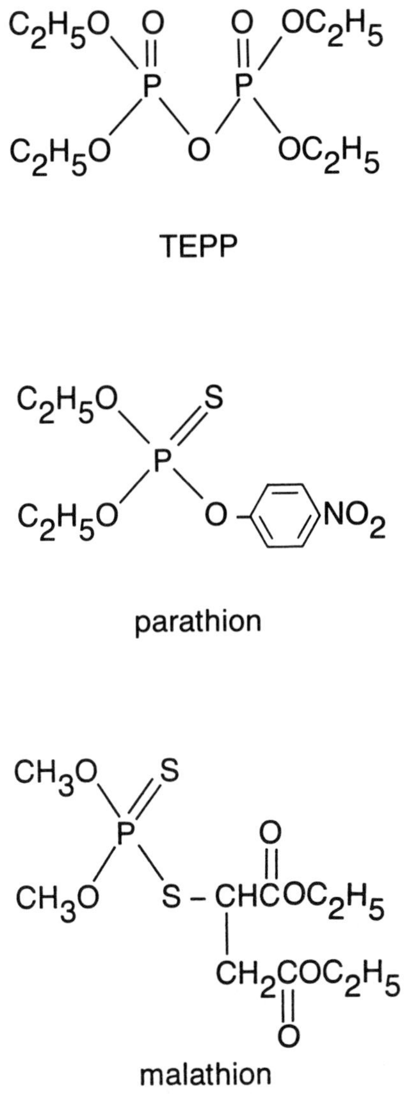

FIG. 4. Organophosphate insecticides TEPP, parathion, and malathion.

duced by binding with acetylcholine is terminated through hydrolysis of acetylcholine by acetylcholinesterase (AChE). Because of the similarities between the chemical structures of acetylcholine and OP compounds, AChE readily binds to OP agents. When this occurs, the esteratic bond formed is relatively stable, which prevents the enzyme from deactivating the normal substrate, acetylcholine. Thus, most of the acute signs associated with OP poisoning can be associated with the overstimulation of the cholinergic system due to excess acetylcholine.

Inhibition of AChE at the neuromuscular junction leads to muscular twitching, weakness, and later, paralysis. Paralysis of respiratory muscles eventually results in respiratory failure and death. Inhibition in the autonomic nervous system is also responsible for abdominal pain, diarrhea, involuntary urination and lacrimation, and pronounced pupillary construction (miosis). Effects on the central nervous system include confusion, slurred speech, poor coordination, and convulsions. The duration of these signs is generally a function of the time required for reactivation of the enzyme, and differs among OP agents. Treatment of OP poisoning typically consists of cholinergic antagonists (e.g., atropine) to block the excessive stimulation and oximes (e.g., 2-pyridine aldoxime methiodide (2-PAM)) to accelerate the hydrolysis of the phosphorylated enzyme.

Tolerance development after repeated or continuous exposure to OP agents has been studied since the early 1950s. Under certain conditions of exposure, animals and humans that survive acute poisoning may become functionally normal despite continued OP exposure and significantly lowered blood cholinesterase activity. As with the chlorinated hydrocarbons, drug metabolizing enzymes may be induced by exposure to OP agents (321), suggesting that accelerated metabolism might underlie the reduction in toxic response with repeated exposure. However, there is better evidence that at least part of the tolerance phenomenon is attributable to a decrease in the sensitivity of cholinergic receptors to acetylcholine (37,212,245,246).

Some of the more important OP insecticides require metabolic conversion to an active anticholinesterase form. For the phosphorothionates (e.g., parathion) and phosphorodithionates (e.g., malathion) this means substitution of $=O$ for the $=S$ on the phosphorous compound (producing paraoxon and malaoxon, respectively). In mammals, this step may not occur as readily as it does in insects because insects appear to possess a very active oxidative enzyme system. The difference between mammalian and insect toxicity is especially enhanced with malathion because a rich supply of carboxylesterase enables mammals to hydrolyze the carboxyester group on the malathion molecule, converting it to a form which does not inhibit cholinesterase. This reaction has been demonstrated in vivo and in vitro (76,333), but it is normally not a prominent feature of insect metabolism because insects possess relatively less hydrolytic enzyme (181). Thus, the differential toxicity of malathion to insects and mammals reflects different major pathways of metabolism dictated by the availability of metabolizing enzymes (Fig. 5). The development of insect resistance to the effects of malathion appears to be related to their ability to produce more carboxylesterase (330), in essence providing them with access to the same inactivation route as mammals.

soon replaced by more stable OP insecticides such as parathion (Fig. 4), and it, in turn, is now being replaced by OP insecticides with lower mammalian toxicity, such as malathion (Fig. 4). The rat oral LD_{50} of each of these three chemicals (TEPP, parathion, and malathion) is reduced from the preceding one by a factor of about 10 (96). In general, OP insecticides have significant advantages over the chlorinated hydrocarbons in agriculture because they are not persistent in the soil and do not accumulate in fat stores to the same extent.

The two most important aspects of OP insecticide toxicity are cholinesterase inhibition and delayed neurotoxicity. Cholinesterase inhibition is the basis for acute poisoning with these agents in both insects and mammals. In mammals, acetylcholine is responsible for transmission of nerve impulses across important synapses within both the peripheral and central nervous system. It also is responsible for the activation of skeletal muscle by motor neurons and the activation of certain effector organs within the autonomic nervous system. Normally, the stimulation of the postsynaptic receptor pro-

malathion

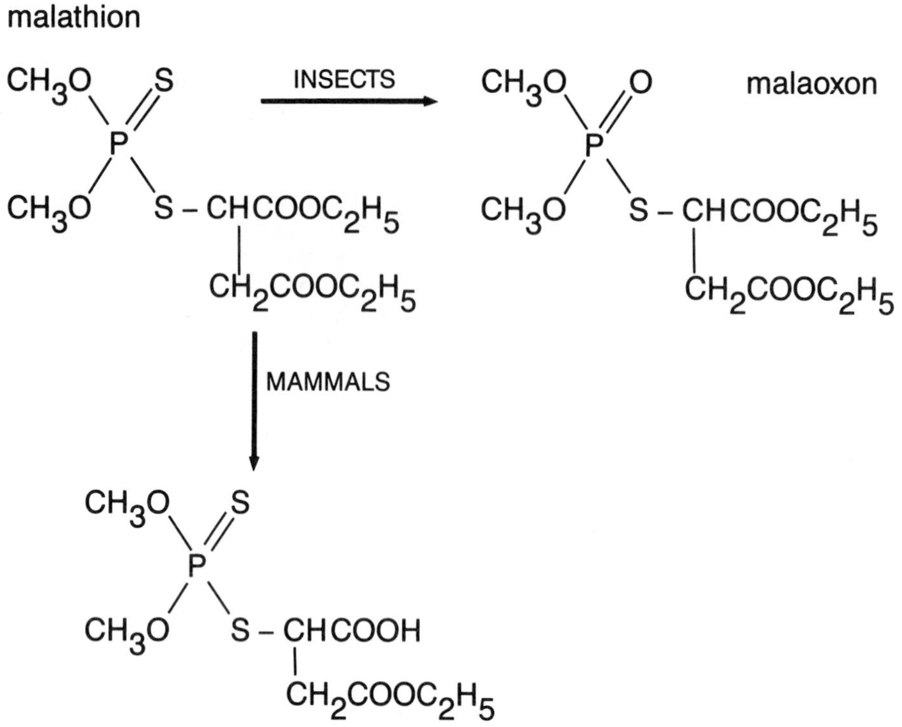

FIG. 5. Oxidation of malathion to the active metabolite malaoxon is relatively rapid in insects but slower in mammals. Hydrolysis to the inactive product is rapid in mammals but slower in insects.

Delayed neurotoxicity is a second major aspect of OP toxicity although it is not seen with all OP insecticides. The first major outbreak of OP-induced neurotoxicity occurred in the late 1920s when an alcoholic extract of Jamaican ginger was contaminated by triorthocresyl phosphate (Fig. 6) and caused a massive outbreak of neuropathy in the United States (312). The paresis of upper and lower extremities was known as *ginger jake paralysis*. Since that time similar human neuropathies have been associated with other OP compounds, mipafox and leptophos (Fig. 6), and testing for delayed neurotoxicity is now common practice as part of safety testing programs for OP pesticide registrations. Administration of a neurotoxic OP compound (in some cases, only a single dose is necessary) to a susceptible species produces clinical signs of weakness in about 1–3 weeks. Hens, a preferred species for OP-induced delayed neuropathy tests, develop a clumsy gait in about 8–10 days which progresses to weakness and paralysis (50). Recent research (247,351,352) has indicated that rats, long considered refractory to the neurotoxic effects of these agents, are susceptible to the structural damage produced by these agents, although perhaps not as likely to develop clinical signs. Histopathologic examination of the nervous system in typical cases of OP-induced neurotoxicity reveals "dying back" or Wallerian degeneration of peripheral nerve axons and their myelin covering. Usually, the distal portions of the nerve cell are affected first and large-diameter axons are affected more than small-diameter axons. Similar axonal degeneration may appear in the long spinal tracts of the spinal cord where it is most severe in the rostral ends of the ascending pathways and the distal ends of the descending pathways (50).

Johnson (153,154) has presented evidence that the manifestation of peripheral neuropathy by OP agents is mediated by phosphorylation of a specific protein receptor in the nerve axon referred to as *neurotoxic esterase* (NTE). However, not all NTE inhibitors are neurotoxic. In fact, some non-neurotoxic NTE inhibitors appear to protect animals against subsequent challenges with known OP neurotoxins. This protective effect now appears to derive from competitive blockade of the NTE binding site. The critical difference between the OP agents that are protective and those that produce delayed neurotoxicity is the ability of the neurotoxic compounds to undergo a second reaction called *aging* following phosphorylation at the active site. The aging process apparently results in a negatively charged phosphoryl moiety and prevents regeneration of the enzyme (155).

CARBAMATE INSECTICIDES

The carbamate insecticides are synthetic derivatives of carbamic acid (NH_2COOH), similar in chemical structure to the pharmaceutical agent physostigmine (eserine). As with the OP insecticides, the principal mechanism of toxicity of the carbamates is inhibition of cholinesterase activity, but the inhibition produced by the carbamates involves carbamylation of the esteratic site of AChE rather than phosphorylation. The resulting accumulation of acetylcholine at nerve synapses and myoneural junctions produces similar signs of toxicity as that produced by OP agents but with the carbamates, cholinesterase inhibition is apparently more labile and effects are typically shorter in duration. One con-

triortho cresyl phosphate

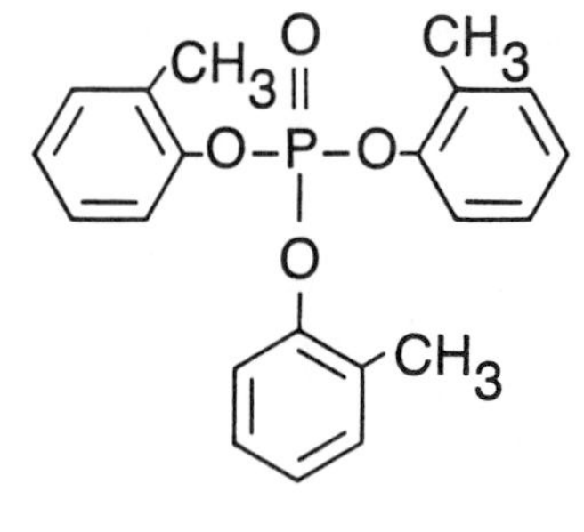

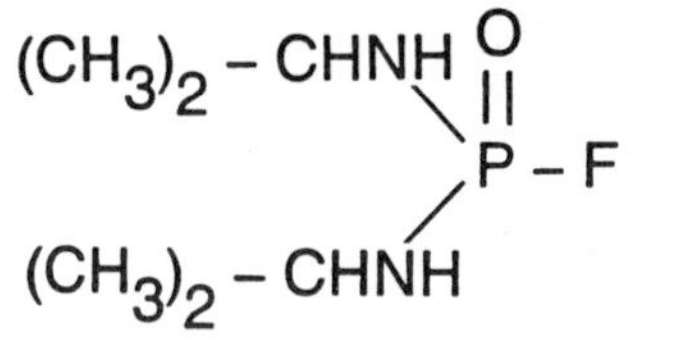

mipafox

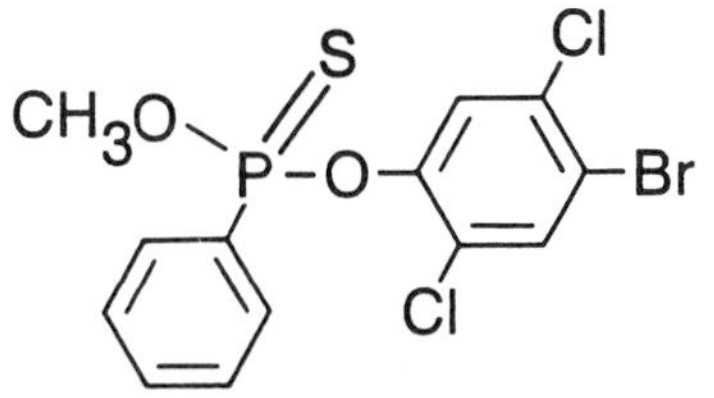

leptophos

FIG. 6. Structure of triorthocresyl phosphate, mipafox, and leptophos.

sequence of the reversibility of carbamate-induced cholinesterase inhibition is that the slope of the toxicity dose-response curve is reduced. That is, there is a wider dose range between a minimally toxic dose and a lethal dose with carbamates than typically exists with OP insecticides. From the point of view of hazard assessment, this property can be considered desirable since small increments in dosage are less likely to produce severe increases in toxic response.

Carbamates may inhibit two different enzymes with cholinesterase activity. Acetylcholinesterase (AChE) is considered "true" cholinesterase and is found in red blood cells and, most importantly, in the nervous system, as mentioned above. Butyrocholinesterase (or pseudocholinesterase) is found in the serum. A given agent may inhibit one, both, or neither. Furthermore, depending upon chemical structure, central nervous system function may be spared because of an agent's inability to pass the blood-brain barrier. The activity of quarternary carbamates, for example, is generally limited to the peripheral nervous system. However, this does not necessarily make them less toxic.

One of the most important carbamate insecticides is carbaryl or 1-naphthyl-*N*-methylcarbamate (Fig. 7). The rat oral LD_{50} is in the range of 500–850 mg/kg (132). High doses produce a reversible and short-duration (4–24 days) neurotoxicity in hens (96) but no evidence of nerve demyelination (49). Dogs were exposed to doses as high as 7 mg/kg for 5 days per week for 1 year without manifestation of significant clinical or anatomic pathology (49). Acute poisoning in humans is associated with abdominal pain, nausea, sweating, headache, and disturbed vision (132), but such incidents are rare despite the widespread use of this insecticide. Not all carbamates have the relatively benign toxicologic characteristics of carbaryl. The rat acute oral LD_{50} of aldicarb or 2-methyl - 2 - (methylthio)propylideneamino - *N* - methylcarbamate (Fig. 7), for example, is less than 1 mg/kg and the dermal LD_{50} is similarly low (2–3 mg/kg compared with >4000 mg/kg for carbaryl)(96). Acute poisoning with carbamate insecticides is usually treated with atropine sulfate and, unlike cases of OP poisoning, treatment with oximes may be of little benefit or even harmful (32,49).

FUMIGANTS

Methyl Bromide

Methyl bromide (monobromomethane) is a colorless gas at ordinary temperatures and is essentially odorless. One of the first references to a suitable use for methyl bromide was

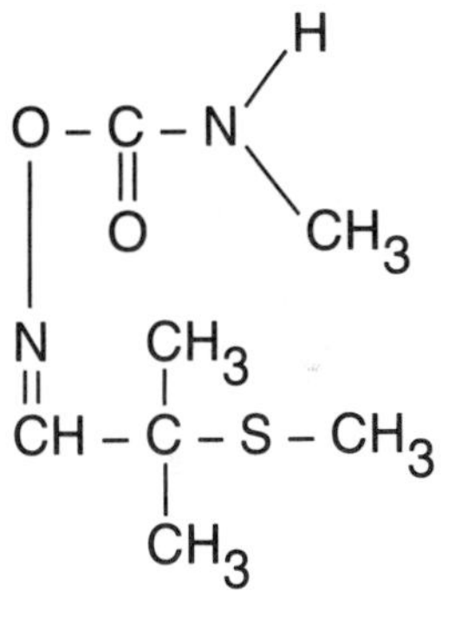

aldicarb

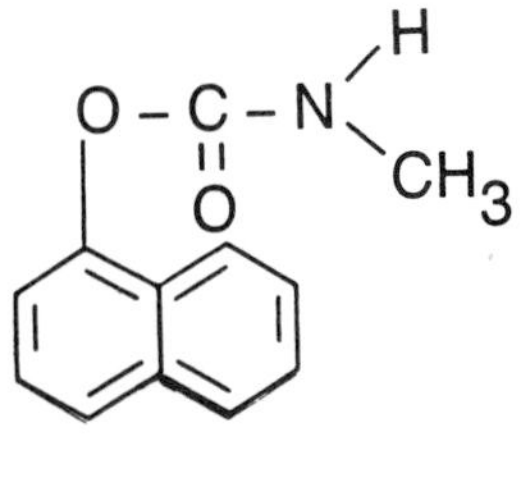

carbaryl

FIG. 7. Structure of carbaryl and aldicarb.

made by Richardson (276) who proposed its use as a chemical agent in medicine to destroy malignant tissue. Richardson (275) earlier condemned the existing practice of using methyl bromide as an anesthetic in dentistry, although effective as such, because it produced throat irritation, vomiting, and could be lethal. Methyl bromide is a direct alkylating agent and reacts via biomolecular nucleophilic substitution. It has been used as a methylating agent in the chemical industry, especially in the preparation of aniline dyes and antipyrine (135,240).

Because methyl bromide is nonflammable, considerably heavier than air, and vaporizes quickly, it was promoted as a fire extinguishing agent. The methyl bromide fire extinguisher was never accepted in the United States due to its toxic potential. The insecticidal properties of methyl bromide were first discovered by Le Goupil (192) when he added methyl bromide as a fire retardant to the fumigant ethylene oxide, and noticed the increased effectiveness of the mixture. Methyl bromide has subsequently been used to control a variety of pests including insects (31,85,201), nematodes (120), rodents (25), bacteria and viruses (200,287), fungi (215), mites (262), and weeds (365).

The annual production of methyl bromide in the United States is about 35 million pounds (335). The average amount of methyl bromide used annually in California in the last 11 years is approximately 7.9 million pounds (46), making methyl bromide one of the most widely used organic pesticides in California.

Methyl bromide (0.39–7.71 mg/liter) produced a dose-dependent increase in the number of mutants in *Salmonella typhimurium* without metabolic activation (303). The authors reported that the mutagenic potential increased with chemical reactivity, with the following order of mutagenicity: methyl iodide > methyl bromide > methyl chloride > bromochloromethane > methylene chloride. Mutagenicity studies conducted by Voogd and coworkers (355) revealed methyl bromide was mutagenic in four of five assays.

Perhaps the earliest investigation of methyl bromide toxicity was evaluated by Irish and co-workers (150). The authors exposed rats and rabbits to a single concentration of methyl bromide and repeatedly exposed rats, rabbits, guinea pigs, and monkeys to methyl bromide (0.065–0.85 mg/liter), 7.5–8 hr/day, 5 days/week, for 6 months or until the majority of the animals died or became moribund. Results obtained by the authors have been substantiated in subsequent studies. Rabbits were the most susceptible animals, showing severe nervous system responses (i.e., tremor and paralysis) after a few exposures. Animals tolerated a daily 8-hr exposure for an extended period of time at a concentration not far below that tolerated for a single 8-hr exposure. Irish and co-workers (150) also demonstrated that paralysis was reversible when exposures were discontinued. Recent work (125) has indicated no evidence of maternal toxicity, fetal toxicity, or teratogenicity in rats and rabbits in concentrations of methyl bromide up to 20 (rabbits) or 70 (rats) ppm.

A subchronic gavage study (74) resulted in the formation of squamous cell carcinomas in the forestomach of rats receiving methyl bromide (50 mg/kg) in oil. Whether the same results would be obtained using inhalation exposure is a matter of some question since Medinsky et al. (213,214) have shown that the patterns of excretion for ^{14}C-methyl bromide

given orally differs significantly from that seen with inhalation exposure.

Acute and chronic effects of methyl bromide can be broadly divided into two categories: neurologic and non-neurologic. The principal non-neurologic symptoms reported after acute inhalation of methyl bromide are effects on the respiratory system. Chest pain or difficulty in breathing have been reported in association with pulmonary edema (58,218). These symptoms are consistent with pathologic findings at autopsy, which have included pulmonary edema, bronchopneumonia, congestion, and hemorrhage (138,141). Acute neurologic and behavioral manifestations following inhalation or dermal methyl bromide exposure include headache, dizziness, fainting, drowsiness, apathy, lethargy, weakness, psychosis, loss of memory, anorexia, and vertigo (5). Acute exposure to methyl bromide has also been reported to cause specific effects such as slurred speech, limb weakness or numbness, tremors, epileptiform convulsions, ataxia, and clonic–tonic seizures (see ref. 5 for review). Toxic signs may develop immediately (250,372) or often a delay of more than 1 hr after exposure (138,141).

Toxic signs reported following subchronic and chronic exposure to methyl bromide are similar to those seen after acute poisoning with the addition of abnormalities of the digestive tract which are expressed as abdominal pain, nausea, and vomiting. If an acute exposure is preceded by a history of chronic exposure, there is a greater likelihood of severe neurologic signs, including convulsions and unconsciousness.

Ethylene Dibromide

Ethylene dibromide (EDB or 1,2-dibromoethane) is used as a soil fumigant to control nematodes and other soil organisms although its use as an agricultural chemical in the U.S. has been effectively eliminated by the USEPA (124,336,340). The halogenated nematocides such as ethylene dibromide in general are thought to act through chemical combination with an essential nucleophilic center in the nematode. One of the most important factors affecting toxicity of the nematocide is the reactivity of the leaving group. The toxicity decreases with increasing carbon chain length. Narcosis may also play a role in nematocidal action (171).

The toxicity of ethylene dibromide has been extensively reviewed (3,145,238,281,316). It is considered to be highly toxic to laboratory animals and humans by inhalation, ingestion, or skin absorption. The LD_{50} values for ethylene dibromide reported for various laboratory species (rats, mice, rabbits, and guinea pigs) range from 55 to 250 mg/kg. Reported inhalation LC_{50} values are 689 ppm (1 hr) in rats, 6425 ppm (1 hr) in rabbits, and 390 ppm (3 hr) in guinea pigs. The dermal LD_{50} in rabbits has been reported to be 300 mg/kg (282). A single exposure results in central nervous system depression, pulmonary irritation (after inhalation) and hepatic and renal damage, with death due to respiratory or cardiac failure.

Chronic and subchronic administration of ethylene dibromide to male rats has also been reported to adversely affect testicular function. Moderate-to-severe atrophy of reproductive tract tissues was seen in male rats exposed to ethylene dibromide concentrations sufficient to induce severe general toxicity over a 10-week period of exposure (302). In bulls dosed orally at doses which had no effect on general health however, sperm density was reduced, sperm motility was lowered, and sperm morphology was abnormal. At 2 years of age, examination of the testes revealed gross abnormalities (12,22). Further studies conducted in calves and bulls (10,11) suggest that ethylene dibromide does not act directly on spermatozoa but acts on spermiogenesis and epididymal maturation. Sperm morphology in calves returned to normal at about 3–4 weeks after cessation of dosing. The fact that it took 15 weeks for recovery of sperm morphology after cessation of treatment in adult bulls suggests that earlier stages of spermatogenesis may be affected.

Ethylene dibromide may also have adverse effects on female fertility which are reversible with cessation of exposure. Chickens exposed to 5–7.5 ppm ethylene dibromide in the feed produced eggs that were decreased in size and showed impaired ovarian follicular growth. Pituitary follicle-stimulating hormone (FSH) levels were unaffected at concentrations that would stop egglaying (10 mg/animal/day) (9,22). The estrus cycle of female rats exposed to 80 ppm ethylene dibromide by inhalation was disrupted; this dose also caused severe systemic toxicity. Lower doses had no effect on reproductive function (302).

In humans, ethylene dibromide is highly toxic following inhalation, ingestion, or skin absorption. Reported symptoms of intoxication include headache, prolonged vomiting, occasional diarrhea, and weak and rapid pulse. Brief exposures may produce severe conjunctival and respiratory irritation, anorexia, and headache. Prolonged inhalation may cause liver and renal damage and pulmonary lesions. Fatalities reported from case reports of exposure to ethylene dibromide appear to be due to respiratory or circulatory failure, complicated by pulmonary edema. In one case, ingestion of 4.5 ml ethylene dibromide caused death within 2 days (3). Fatalities after acute occupational exposure have also been reported; death was caused by metabolic acidosis, acute renal and hepatic failure, and necrosis of skeletal muscle and organs (193). Signs reported after chronic or subacute poisoning include conjunctivitis, pharyngeal and bronchial irritation, anorexia, headache, and depression (238).

Ethylene dibromide is a recognized animal carcinogen based on evidence from experiments in mice and rats by oral and inhalation administration (145,316). As with methyl bromide (74), gastric intubation of ethylene dibromide resulted in increased incidence of forestomach carcinomas in rodents (231). However, both oral and inhalation exposure of ethylene dibromide resulted in respiratory tract tumors (235). This pesticide has also been shown to produce evidence of mutagenicity in various in vitro assays (35,59,145,316,327). Epidemiologic evidence for the potential human carcinogenicity of ethylene dibromide is inconclusive (117,244). Ethylene dibromide has also been shown to cause an increase in the incidence of skin papillomas, skin carcinomas, and lung tumors in Ha:ICR mice after topical administration (348).

Sex-linked recessive lethal (SLRL) mutations are also consistently induced in male Drosophila melanogaster following inhalation exposure to ethylene dibromide vapor (145,316). In one study, SLRL mutations were induced following exposure to 0.2–2 ppm ethylene dibromide for 11–100 hr (159).

Unscheduled DNA synthesis (UDS) in vitro was induced in pachytene spermatocytes and F-344 primary rat hepatocytes when cultured with ethylene dibromide at concentrations of 10–100 mol. When ethylene dibromide was tested in the in vivo/in vitro UDS assay, only hepatocytes exhibited UDS when isolated from rats given ethylene dibromide 100 mg/kg intraperitoneally but not orally. UDS was not induced in spermatocytes or in hepatocytes when ethylene dibromide was administered at lower doses (370).

Results from available studies in laboratory animals (22,300,301) and a single epidemiologic study are inadequate to make a conclusive assessment of the teratogenic potential of ethylene dibromide.

Ethylene dibromide is readily absorbed by all routes of administration in experimental animals, where it is distributed to the liver, kidney, small intestine, adrenals, and finally eliminated via the kidney. There is also evidence from one study in guinea pigs that unchanged ethylene dibromide can be eliminated in expired air. After intraperitoneal administration of ^{14}C-ethylene dibromide to guinea pigs, the greatest concentration of ^{14}C was found in the kidneys, liver, and adrenals where pathologic changes were observed (257).

1,2-Dibromo-3-Chloropropane

1,2-Dibromo-3-chloropropane (DBCP) is a brominated organochlorine nematocide used as a fumigant primarily on citrus, grapes, peaches, pineapples, soybeans, and tomatoes. The use of DBCP expanded greatly during the two decades after its commercial production began in 1955, mainly due to its low acute toxicity, low vapor pressure, and prolonged half-life in soil (366). However, these apparent attributes could not outweigh the serious chronic reproductive toxicity and carcinogenicity hazard that became apparent with DBCP. In September, 1977, the EPA issued a notice of rebuttable presumption against renewal of registration or RPAR (now called special review) on all pesticide products containing DBCP based on reported carcinogenic and reproductive effects (339). Shortly thereafter, the EPA issued an order suspending registration of pesticide products containing DBCP as they were deemed to pose an "imminent hazard" to humans and/or to the environment (337).

Numerous reports have shown that DBCP is carcinogenic (146,230,235,271–273,348,363), mutagenic (29,263,279, 328,376), and a reproductive toxin (174,175,267,283) in animals. While there is no known association between human cancer and DBCP exposure, numerous reports link DBCP exposure to worker infertility (106,107,260,368). Following is an overview of the toxic potential of DBCP.

Oral administration of DBCP to rats (30 mg/kg) and mice (260 mg/kg), 5 days per week for 78 weeks produced increased incidences of squamous cell carcinomas of the forestomach in male and female rats and mice and adenocarcinomas of the mammary gland in female rats (233,363). Oral administration of DBCP (3.0 mg/kg/day) for 104 weeks resulted in significant instances in renal tubular adenomas and carcinomas and squamous cell carcinomas of the stomach in male and female rats. Dose-related increases in squamous cell papillomas and carcinomas of the stomach were observed in mice (92). Chronic inhalation exposure of rats and mice resulted in nasal cavity carcinomas, squamous cell carcinomas, and adenomas. Lung tumors, described as alveolar/bronchiolar adenomas or carcinomas, were significantly increased in both male and female mice. Squamous cell papillomas and carcinomas of the tongue were significantly increased in high-dose male and female rats. An increased incidence of squamous cell papillomas and carcinomas of the pharynx was observed in female rats exposed to 3.0 ppm DBCP (235,271–273). DBCP has also been shown to be active as an initiator of carcinogenesis following a single topical application in the mouse skin two-stage model system (348). Repeated dermal application (3 times per week for 440 days) of DBCP (11.7 and 35 mg per mouse) resulted in the presence of lung and stomach tumors (348). The latter results were ascribed to skin absorption and animal grooming.

Numerous reports in the literature demonstrate the mutagenic potential of DBCP (325). Rosenkrantz (279) reported that DBCP was mutagenic in *Salmonella typhimurium* strain TA1530 but not 1538, indicating that DBCP causes base-pair substitution but not a frame-shift type mutation. DBCP is reported to be mutagenic in strains TA100, TA1530, and TA1535, both in the presence and absence of a liver microsomal activation system (29,263,324).

Following a single, intraperitoneal dose of DBCP (100 mg/kg), a statistically significant increase in ^{3}H-thymidine incorporation was observed (191). Dose-dependent increases in sister chromatid exchanges (SCEs) and chromosomal aberrations were observed *in vitro* in CHO cells treated with DBCP. Cell cultures treated with DBCP (10^{-5}–10^{-3} M) exhibited an increase in the mean number of SCEs/cell. Chromosomal aberrations were induced in 92% of the cells scored (329). In the dominant lethal assay, DBCP was shown to be mutagenic in rats (284,328) but not in mice (102,328). Results obtained by Teramoto and co-workers (328) revealed an increased incidence (55.3%) of dead implants associated with a corresponding decrease in the number of live embryos when mating took place 5 weeks after treatment with 5 daily doses of 50 mg/kg/day DBCP.

Dibromochloropropane has been shown to be a reproductive toxin in rabbits and rats, but not in mice. Rao and co-workers evaluated reproductive effects of DBCP in rats (267) and rabbits (266). Semen analyses of exposed male rabbits revealed decreased sperm count, motility, and viability at 1 and 10 ppm. By the end of the exposure period, all male rabbits in the 10 ppm exposure group were infertile. Testicular atrophy and loss of spermatogenic cells occurred in male rabbits exposed to 10 ppm; these changes were partially reversible. Moderate, reversible testicular atrophy was observed at 1 ppm. In male rats fertility was not affected. Unexposed female rats mated to DBCP-exposed males (10 ppm) exhibited an increased incidence of fetal resorptions; this effect was reversible. Moderate testicular atrophy was seen in male rats exposed to 10 ppm DBCP; this effect also was partially reversible. The no observed effect level (NOEL) was 0.1 ppm in both rats and rabbits.

Results obtained by Warren and co-workers (360) demonstrated that DBCP and not allyl chloride, a contaminant of the technical formulation, is responsible for the male reproductive effects. Subcutaneous injection of 25 mg/kg DBCP produced elevations in serum leuteinizing hormone (LH) and FSH while reducing serum testosterone and reducing the weight of the testes, prostate gland, and seminal vesicles in male rats. These results demonstrate that the site of action of DBCP is on either androgen action or production and confirms the previous findings of Rao et al. (266,267), showing that DBCP acts at the interstitial compartment of the testes. Acute subantaneous injection of 100 mg/kg DBCP to adult male rats resulted in irreversible necrosis of epididymal epithelial cells, atrophy of testicular seminiferous tubules, and reduced sperm density (174). Irreversible fibrosis of the renal cortex and outer medulla was also seen.

Kluwe and co-workers (175) demonstrated that metabolism of DBCP to epichlorohydrin or 3-chloro-1,2-propanediol, or metabolism of DBCP, epichlorohydrin or 3-chloro-1,2-propanediol to oxalic acid, did not account for the toxic effects of DBCP on the male rat urogenital tract. Kluwe et al. (175) demonstrated that DBCP can cause immediate infertility by a direct action on post-testicular sperm by inhibiting glucose metabolism in ejaculated sperm. DBCP was not found to be teratogenic in rats at doses of up to 50 mg/kg DBCP administered on days 6 through 15 (283).

Effects on the reproductive system were not limited to animals. Whorton and co-workers (369) reported a dose-dependent decrease in sperm count and an increase in FSH and LH in 25 factory workers exposed to airborne DBCP concentrations of 0.4–0.6 ppm for 3 or more years. During subsequent years, numerous surveys were conducted to assess sperm counts in workers exposed to DBCP (106, 185,196,205,260,285). Results obtained from field applicators demonstrated that the sperm count depression was reversible (106). Several follow-up evaluations of factory workers have revealed an increase in sperm count over time (186,367).

Phosphine

Another widely used fumigant is phosphine (hydrogen phosphide, Phostoxin). Phosphine is effective against numerous insects and, more importantly, is effective against preadult or larval stages. These include fruit flies, assorted grain beetles, the bean weevil, and tobacco pests. Phostoxin has been approved by the United States EPA as a fumigant on processed foods including cereal flours and milled fractions, soybean flour and milled fractions, assorted chocolate, raisins, processed spices, almonds, and assorted nuts and coffee.

Upon exposure to atmospheric moisture or water in any form, phosphine tablets release hydrogen phosphide gas. Phosphine (molecular weight = 34; H_3P) is a colorless gas with an odor of decaying fish. The odor threshold for the pure gas is 2 ppm. Clinical signs in animals exposed to high concentrations of phosphine include lassitude, immobility, ataxia, pallor, epileptiform convulsions, apnea, and cardiac arrest. Exposure of rats, rabbits, guinea pigs, and cats via inhalation to phosphine indicated that at concentrations above 7.5 mg/m^3, the effects of phosphine were cumulative, but at concentrations of 3.7 mg/m^3 and below, there was no clinical evidence of cumulative effects. Rats tolerated a concentration of 3.75 mg/m^3 for 820 hr without apparent injury (173). Absorption and distribution studies indicate that phosphine is freely absorbed by the lungs and gastrointestinal mucosa and widely distributed in tissues. Regardless of the route of absorption, some phosphine is excreted by the lungs (132).

Phosphine has been shown to produce hypoxia by interfering with state 3 and state 4 respiratory activity, and by its interaction with cytochrome oxidase, with inhibition of electron transport in mouse liver mitochondria. The *in vitro* concentration of phosphine required to inhibit state 4 oxidation was reported as 3.74 ppm (52). Kashi and Chefurka (162) demonstrated that phosphine had little effect on the polypeptide chain of cytochrome oxidase but induced a valence change on the heme iron and a conformational change on the prosthetic group. The spectral change produced by phosphine was similar to that caused by sodium dithionite.

Numerous instances of accidental/intentional phosphine poisoning have been reported. Zipf et al. (377) reported on a 25-year-old man who swallowed six aluminum phosphide tablets dissolved in water (capable of releasing a total of 6000 mg phosphine). Clinical signs included abdominal pain, burning sensation, vomiting, unconsciousness, and loss of pulse. Hematuria, leukocyturia, proteinuria, and uremia were present. Cardiac effects included cardiac dilation, systolic murmur, atrial fibrillation, and ventricular arrhythmia. Electroencephalographic changes and hepatomegaly were also observed. Modrzejewski and Myslak (220) reported that concentrations ranging from 1 to 10 mg/m^3 produced vertigo, headache, nausea, vomiting, and psychomotor stimulation in five workers exposed to phosphine. Concentrations of 0.4 mg/m^3 for periods of 8 hr or more led to vertigo, headache, staggering gait, nausea, vomiting, diarrhea, epigastric pain, dyspnea, and palpitations. In half the cases, symptoms began almost immediately; in the remainder there was a delay of several hours to 2 days (157).

BOTANICAL INSECTICIDES

Nicotine

The three most important insecticide groups derived from natural products are nicotine, rotenone, and pyrethrum. Nicotine is one of the oldest known insecticidal chemicals. The rat acute oral LD$_{50}$ of nicotine sulfate is 83 mg/kg (96). The theoretical basis of nicotine toxicity is cholinergic hyperstimulation, which is achieved not by inhibition of cholinesterase activity but by direct action on the postsynaptic receptors normally occupied by acetylcholine in certain locations of the central and peripheral nervous system and in the neuromuscular junctions of skeletal muscles. The simultaneous activation of both the sympathetic and parasympathetic branches of the autonomic nervous system presents a complex toxicologic response which typically includes a rapid decrease in blood pressure and convulsions. The immediate cause of death is respiratory failure (104). Nicotine is readily absorbed from all mucosal surfaces and the alkaloid easily passes the skin barrier.

Rotenone

Rotenone is extracted from the root of the plant *Derris elliptica* which is native to Southeast Asia. Historically, it was used by island natives to poison fish. Its use as an insecticide was not common until the 20th century when it was employed for eradication of dermal parasites. Its acute oral toxicity is similar to DDT but it is much more irritating to the eye and mucous membranes. Acute poisoning in animals is characterized by initial respiratory stimulation followed by respiratory depression, ataxia, convulsions, and death from respiratory arrest (298). Dogs have survived exposure to 5 mg/kg/day for 1 month but this resulted in fatty changes to liver and kidneys (116). A dosage of 10 mg/kg/day was lethal to 3 of 5 dogs. Rotenone has an anesthetic effect on nerve axons and it is believed that the effects on respiration are attributable to the direct effects on respiratory control centers. Rotenone was reported to increase the incidence of mammary tumors in female rats treated for 6–12 months by intraperitoneal injection (109). However, Innes et al. (148) found no treatment-related increase in mouse tumors after daily exposure for 18 months.

Pyrethrum

Pyrethrum is an insecticide extracted from the dried flower heads of *Chrysanthemum cinerariaefolium*. The natural pyrethroids, believed to have been discovered initially by the Chinese in the first century A.D., are among the safest and most widely used insecticides. By 1982, one-third of worldwide insecticide usage consisted of pyrethroids (352c). Pyrethroids possess many of the most important characteristics desired in a pesticide. They are relatively safe to mammals and extremely toxic to arthropods. In addition, pyrethroids are much less persistent than the organochlorine insecticides, such as DDT and dieldrin, and do not accumulate in the environment (190,314). Naturally occurring pyrethroids are of limited value, however, due to their low photostability and high biodegradability (371).

Pyrethrum extract contains at least six closely related active components that occur in two fractions: pyrethrin I, which are esters of chrysanthemic acid (pyrethrin I, cinerin I, and jasmolin I), and pyrethrin II, which are esters of pyrethric acid (pyrethrin II, cinerin II, and jasmolin II). The first synthetic pyrethroids, allethrin and cycletrin were manufactured in 1949 (286a); they lacked photostability and were less effective as insecticides compared with the natural pyrethrins. Tetramethrin, the 3,4,5,6-tetrahydro derivative of *N*-hydroxymethylphthalimide, was found to have very high knockdown activity against houseflies (164a). Subsequent research has led to the synthesis of pyrethrum analogs which are photostable and efficacious synthetic pyrethroids including cypermethrin, permethrin, deltamethrin, and fernvalerate. The structures of these compounds are provided in Fig. 8.

Pyrethroids, like the organophosphate, organochlorine, and carbamate insecticides interfere with nervous system function. The symptomology of pyrethroid exposure is divided into two types and is the basis of classifying pyrethroids as type I or type II. Signs of type I exposure include tonic-like limb movements (tremor) and closely resemble the signs produced by DDT. Pyrethroids without a cyanosubstituent (e.g., cismethrin, permethrin, bromophenothrin) produce this type I or T syndrome. Cyanophenoxybenzyl pyrethroids (e.g., fenvalerate, deltamethrin, and cypermethrin) induce with-

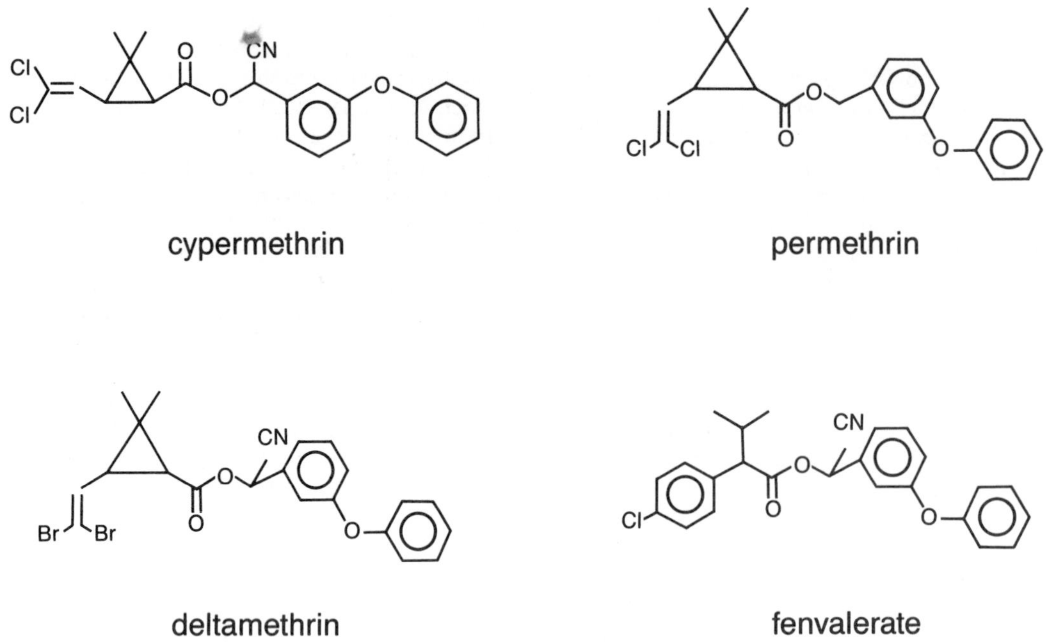

FIG. 8. Structure of pyrethroids.

ing, salivation, and clonic convulsions referred to as the CS (choreoathetosis and salivation) or type II syndrome (105a,98,111a,352a). Type I or T syndrome in rats is initially characterized by sparring and aggressive behavior (352a,364a); in rats and mice this is followed by the rapid onset of tremor, initially in the limbs and later extending over the entire body (364a). Body temperature can increase probably as a result of increased muscle activity (364a). Cis-methrin produces a large increase in oxygen consumption in association with elevated blood lactate levels. These effects probably result from increased motor activity (72). With progressing toxicity, mice exhibit periods of intense hyperactivity whereas rats become prostate and die. In mice, death is often associated with clonic seizures (111a) and respiratory failure (269). It is thought that type I pyrethroids produce signs mainly through actions on the peripheral nervous system (352a). The symptoms produced by type II or CS pyrethroids are characterized by profuse salivation, coarse whole body tremor, splayed hindlimb gait, tonic seizures, and death. In contrast to type I pyrethroids, type II compounds cause a decrease in body temperature in rats which has been attributed to evaporation of saliva (269a). Type II pyrethroids produce symptoms thought to be directed toward the central nervous system (318). Deltamethrin produces a marked increase in blood glucose levels; cardiovascular effects including increased pulse pressure and cardiac contractility have been reported both *in vivo* and *in vitro* (269). Fenpropathrin has been reported to produce both type I and II symptoms in mice (188).

The mechanism of action of pyrethroid insecticides has not been fully elucidated but their mode of action seems to involve alteration of sodium conductance. There is a similarity between symptoms of pyrethroid poisoning and a number of nonpyrethroids. DDT produces signs of toxicity similar to those characteristic of the type I syndrome described above while the plant alkaloid mixture, aconitine, produces effects similar to type II pyrethroids. The veratrine alkaloids, cevine and veratradine, produce a sequelae of events similar to type I and type II pyrethroids, respectively (352b). The similarity in signs of toxicity suggest that the pyrethroids produce both type I and II syndromes via an action on sodium channels. Type II pyrethroids depolarize nerves without repetitive firing whereas type I pyrethroids induce repetitive firing in sensory neurons (98). Research from numerous investigators has substantiated this assumption (98,199).

Lund and Narahasi (199) and Vijverberg (352c) demonstrated with *in vitro* preparations that pyrethroids prolong sodium influx by delaying the closing of a small percentage of sodium channels which reopen upon depolarization. Hence, at the end of the action potential sodium ions are still moving into the axon and the membrane potential difference becomes more positive. This leads to an increase in the negative after-potential. Where the after-potential exceeds the membrane threshold, another action potential is generated; the continuation of this process results in the repetitive firing observed (64).

Pyrethroids become more toxic to insects as the temperature is lowered; this effect is reversible (64). Blockage of axonal conduction induced by allethrin becomes enhanced as temperature is lowered (357). Further support for the importance of temperature-dependence is provided by Wouters and co-workers (371), who demonstrated an increase in repetitive nerve activity in allethrin-treated frog neuromuscular junction preparations as temperature was decreased. Two possible explanations have been proposed to explain this negative temperature correlation associated with pyrethroids. Holan (140) proposed the formation of a toxicant-receptor

TABLE 1. *Pyrethroid metabolism by esterases and oxidases and synergism by DEF and piperonyl butoxide*

| | Relative metabolism rate | | Synergism factor | | | |
| | | | DEF | | PB | |
Pyrethroid	Esterase	Oxidase	Mouse	Fly	Mouse	Fly
Tetramethrin						
Trans	32	79	1.6	2.1	0.8	2.9
Cis	4	95	1.4	3.0	1.4	2.1
Resmethrin						
Trans	100	25	—	2.3	—	3.2
Cis	<4	37	9.7	4.0	25	4.5
Permethrin						
Trans	98	38	—	1.1	—	—
Cis	<3	33	—	—	—	—
Cypermethrin						
Trans	22	5	>20	1.7	>10	—
Cis	<3	6	5	—	6	—

From ref. 105a, with permission.

complex for DDT that is more stable at lower temperatures. Due to apparent similarities in mode of action, this may apply to pyrethroids. An alternate possibility is that the reduction in temperature delays the closing of the sodium channels; the presence of the insecticide in the presence of reduced temperature may serve to enhance the sodium current (352c).

Although the primary site of action of pyrethroid insecticides appears to be nerve sodium channels, effects on other membrane components have been observed. Suppression of potassium current has been reported in squid axon preparations following allethrin perfusion (228,357). This effect is similar to suppressed potassium current induced by DDT in lobster axon preparations (229).

Cypermethrin (10^{-4} M) and permthrin (10^{-4}–10^{-3} M) inhibited calmodulin, a calcium-binding protein *in vitro* (268). Allethrin has been shown to inhibit Ca-ATPase activity *in vitro* whereas permethrin, cypermethrin, and deltamethrin inhibit Ca,Mg-ATPase (57). Inhibition of Ca,Mg-ATPase would serve to increase intracellular Ca. This effect is also considered to be inconsequential compared with sodium channel effects. Additional reported effects of pyrethroids on the nervous system include binding with GABA-receptors (99,188,318). Due to the excessive levels of pyrethroids required to attain these effects, the toxicologic significance of these findings is unclear. Finally, pyrethroids have been reported to interact with nicotinic cholinergic receptors *in vitro* (1,51,87,297).

The relative potency and species specificity of pyrethroids appears to be regulated, in part, by metabolism (49a,105a). Pyrethroids contain one or more ester groups potentially susceptible to esteratic hydrolysis. In addition, all pyrethroids are hydroxylated at methyl and aryl substituents or oxidized by the mixed function oxidase system. The fact that mammalian liver esterases and oxidases detoxify pyrethroids more rapidly than their counterparts in insects and fish liver may account for the high degree of species specificity (105a). The use of esterase and oxidase inhibitors (e.g., DEF (S,S,S,-tributyl phosphorotrithioate) and piperonyl butoxide, respec-

tively) has been shown to potentiate the toxicity of most pyrethroids (Table 1). For transpermethrin and transresmethrin, the limiting factor in their toxicity to mammals appears to be on intrinsic nerve insensitivity and not selective detoxification (105a).

HERBICIDES

Herbicides are chemicals specifically designed to destroy a specific type or types of plant. Ideally, a herbicide that kills one type of plant will not affect adjacent species. This property is commonly experienced by consumers who apply one of several commercial weed killers that kill many varieties of weeds but do not harm grass. As a class, herbicides exhibit less mammalian toxicity than insecticides since herbicides are designed specifically to effect the functions of a plant (e.g., inhibit a specific plant enzyme).

Chlorophenoxy Herbicides

2,4-Dichlorophenoxyacetic Acid

2,4-Dichlorophenoxyacetic acid (2,4-D) (Fig. 9) is used as a selective pre- and postemergence herbicide for broad-leaf weeds. At low concentrations it can be used to prevent an early fruit drop. It is commonly used along roadways and under power lines to control weed growth. 2,4-D mimics a plant auxin, specifically, indoleacetic acid. Auxins are plant hormones that normally cause elongation of the stem. Chlorophenoxy herbicides stimulate growth as do auxins, but are much more persistent. This abnormal stem elongation may alter the ability of the plant to adequately transport essential nutrients which results in death of the plant (350). The auxin-like activity of 2,4-D may cause a plant to increase its met-

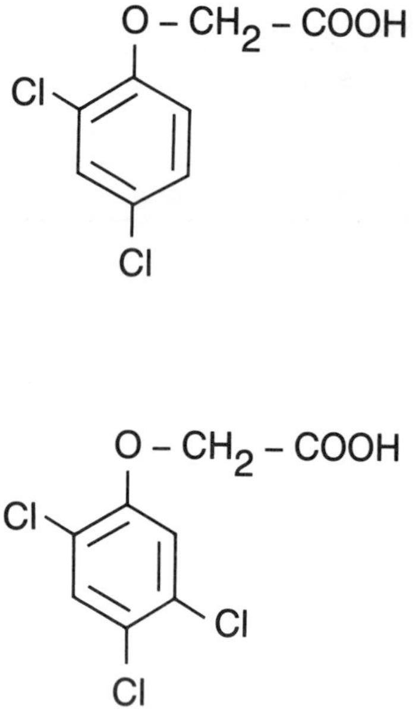

O – CH$_2$ – COOH

Cl

Cl

O – CH$_2$ – COOH

Cl

Cl

Cl

FIG. 9. Structure of 2,4-D and 2,4-5,-T.

abolic rate and "grow itself to death"; the exact mechanism of this process is not clearly understood. 2,4-D does not demonstrate hormonal activity in animals.

2,4-D is moderately toxic to most animals with a range of oral LD$_{50}$ values from 300 to 1200 mg/kg. There is no specific target organ for 2,4-D. Rather, toxicity is characterized by its effect on several organs. Congestion of all organs and degeneration of brain ganglia has been noted at autopsy following 2,4-D overdose (237). Acute fatal doses may result in ventricular fibrillation. If death is delayed, progressive ataxia, paralysis, muscular stiffness, followed by coma and death are observed. Disruption of the T-tubules in myocardial tissue may be seen. Myotonia (delayed relaxation of muscles following a contraction) is one of the most pronounced symptoms of 2,4-D poisoning in both man and animals (7).

Rats administered a diet containing 3000 ppm 2,4-D for 113 days did not demonstrate clinical or hematologic changes. At 1000 ppm there was depressed growth rate, increased liver weight, and increased mortality. A dietary level of 3000 ppm quickly resulted in death (280). Rats given a diet containing up to 1250 ppm 2,4-D for 2 years were not adversely affected (123). In a repeated dose study, rats receiving oral doses of 100–200 mg/kg 2,4-D showed reduced serum lipid levels, proliferation of hepatic microsomes, and increased utilization of lipids by the liver suggesting this compound may promote hypolipidemia (345).

2,4-D may be considered teratogenic and embryotoxic in rodents (168,292). In reproductive toxicity studies using rats, 2,4-D resulted in dose-dependent decreases in fetal weight and fetal viability, and various skeletal abnormalities. In a 3-generation reproductive toxicity study, rats consuming diets containing up to 1500 ppm 2,4-D (75 mg/kg/day) exhibited decreased survival of the pups and reduced weight of the survivors. There was no change in fertility or litter size (123).

Several reports have been published concerning accidental or intentional 2,4-D poisonings in man. In one case of accidental ingestion, toxic signs included profuse sweating, a burning sensation in the mouth, chest and abdomen, and sore, stiff muscles. Twenty-four hours after ingestion the patient had difficulty breathing and cyanosis (26). Another person voluntarily taking 3.6 g of 2,4-D intravenously lapsed into a coma and exhibited fibrillary twitching of muscles and urinary incontinence. He exhibited muscular weakness for 24 hr but by 48 hr the effects of 2,4-D had subsided (293).

2,4-D is rapidly excreted in urine. A dose of ^{14}C-labeled 2,4-D injected intravenously into volunteers was excreted unchanged (93); it was not stored extensively in body tissues. This rapid removal of 2,4-D may be partly responsible for its low toxicity. Treatment for 2,4-D poisoning is essentially symptomatic, but forced alkaline diureses and administration of quinidine sulfate to prevent cardiac arrhythmia may be beneficial (132).

2,4-D is not considered to be mutagenic or carcinogenic. When 2,4-D and its esters were evaluated in the Ames' *Salmonella* assay with and without a metabolic activation system, there was no increase in the frequency of revertants (14,123,148).

2,4,5-Trichlorophenoxyacetic Acid

2,4,5-Trichlorophenoxyacetic acid (2,4,5-T) (Fig. 9) is a herbicide with a mechanism of action very similar to 2,4-D but is much more effective against woody plants and weeds. It is sometimes used in conjunction with 2,4-D for increased effectiveness in elimination of unwanted vegetation. 2,4,5-T is moderately toxic with a range of LD$_{50}$ values from 100 to 500 mg/kg in laboratory animals. While 2,4,5-T is only of moderate toxicity, a common by-product of its synthesis is 2,3,7,8-tetrachlorodibenzo-*p*-dioxin (TCDD), one of the most toxic chemicals known. TCDD has an oral LD$_{50}$ in the rat of less than 50 μg/kg. Guinea pigs are one of the most sensitive species to TCDD with an oral LD$_{50}$ of 0.6 μg/kg (248). Levels of 30 ppm TCDD were commonly detected in 2,4,5-T formulations. Currently, the TCDD concentration in 2,4,5-T is regulated at 0.1 ppm. Clearly, TCDD contamination may play a significant role in the overall toxicity of 2,4,5-T.

The symptoms of acute toxicity of 2,4,5-T differ somewhat from that of 2,4-D. Dogs administered 2,4,5-T exhibited spastic muscle movement rather than myotonia. Death was not attributed to any single action. Upon gross examination, dogs exposed to excessive 2,4,5-T concentrations displayed mild necrosis of the intestinal mucosa. Tubular degeneration of the kidney and hepatic necrosis was also observed. Dogs did not survive past 5 days when given 20 mg/kg/day. At a dose of 10 mg/kg/day for 3 months, there was no alteration in organ weights, body weight, or blood count (84). There was no increase in the incidence of tumors (178) in rats receiving up to 30 mg/kg/day 2,4,5-T (<1 ppb TCDD) for 2 years.

The effects of 2,4,5-T on reproductive parameters have been evaluated in laboratory animals. It is necessary to consider the level of TCDD contamination in the 2,4,5-T formulation when interpreting the results of these studies, as TCDD itself is a potent teratogen. Mice treated orally or subcutaneously with 113 mg/kg 2,4,5-T (containing 30 ppm TCDD) during various stages of gestation exhibited a significant increase in the incidence of cleft pallets and cystic kidneys. Rats given 2,4,5-T (10 or 46 mg/kg) orally on days 10–15 of gestation demonstrated an increase in fetal mortality and cystic kidney but not cleft pallet (69). A follow-up study using 2,4,5-T (100 mg/kg containing up to 0.5 ppm TCDD) resulted in an increased incidence of cleft pallet and hydronephrosis in mice; no terata were noted in rats. It was concluded that 2,4,5-T was teratogenic in mice but not in rats (70). Similar results were noted in a study where rats received oral doses of up to 24 mg/kg 2,4,5-T (TCDD level of 0.5 ppm) on days 6–15 of gestation, and rabbits received up to 40 mg/kg 2,4,5-T on days 6–18 of gestation. This dosing regimen did not alter litter size, or number of resorptions and did not produce teratogenic or embryotoxic effects in either species (88). In another study, a dose of 100 mg/kg 2,4,5-T (0.5 ppm TCDD) given to rats on days 6–10 of gestation resulted in mortality to 21 of 25 dams. Only one litter of 13 fetuses survived; no terata were seen (315). A decrease in postnatal survival in the F_1, F_2, and F_3 litters was noted in a three-generation reproductive toxicity study in which rats were fed a diet containing 30 mg/kg/day of 2,4,5-T (<0.1 ppm TCDD). No evidence of teratogenesis was seen at any dosage (310).

There was no interference with normal development in the offspring or evidence of teratogenesis in rhesus monkeys given up to 10 mg/kg 2,4,5-T (0.05 ppm TCDD) on days 22–38 of gestation (83). In hamsters, 2,4,5-T (TCDD levels below the limit of detection) was teratogenic and fetotoxic. When 40 mg/kg was administered on days 6–10 of gestation, the litter size was slightly decreased. At 80 mg/kg the number of pups per litter and survival rate was reduced, and at 100 mg/kg, it was both fetotoxic and teratogenic. When 2,4,5-T contaminated with 45 ppm TCDD was administered, it was teratogenic to hamsters at only 20 mg/kg (61).

2,4,5-T is not considered to be carcinogenic in animals. Two strains of mice received the maximum tolerated dose (MTD) for 18 months without an increase in the incidence of tumors (148). This is consistent with the results later obtained by Kociba and co-workers (178). When 2,4,5-T and its esters were tested in the Ames' *Salmonella* assay with and without the presence of metabolic activation, no increase in revertants were noted (14,221).

2,4,5-T is excreted rather slowly by rats. The rate of excretion peaked on the first or second day after oral administration and declined thereafter. Almost 60% was excreted in the first 7 days, mostly unchanged (114). In a subsequent study in which 2,4,5-T (50 mg/kg) was administered to rats and mice, a majority of the chemical was excreted unchanged; taurine and glycerin conjugates of 2,4,5-T and 2,4,5 trichlorophenol were also excreted (113).

Radiolabeled 2,4,5-T administered to pregnant mice intravenously did not accumulate in the fetus during the early stages of gestation, but did at later stages. The kidney was the only organ with a higher concentration of 2,4,5-T than the blood (194). A rat study demonstrated that the half-life of 2,4,5-T after oral administration is inversely related to dose. The half-life for excretion from the body was 13.6 and 28.9 hr for doses of 5 and 20 mg/kg, respectively (254,255). In studies using isolated perfused rat kidneys, 2,4,5-T was readily excreted when present in the perfusate at low concentrations. At high concentrations it is nephrotoxic, resulting in the inhibition of its own excretion (179a).

In one human study, volunteers ingested 5 mg/kg 2,4,5-T without any clinically observable effects. The half-life for plasma clearance and excretion from the body was approximately 23 hr. Absorption from the gut was essentially complete. It was excreted in the urine unchanged following first order kinetics. In the bloodstream, 2,4,5-T is 98.7% bound to plasma proteins (103).

Much attention has been focused on the health effects of herbicides since the 1960s when the herbicide agent orange was used as a defoliant during the Vietnam War. Agent orange is a 1:1 mixture of 2,4-D and 2,4,5-T. TCDD levels in agent orange were as high as 47 ppm. It is believed that when large jungle areas were sprayed with this herbicide, soldiers in the area may have been inadvertently exposed to agent orange.

One of the most obvious effects of human TCDD exposure is the outbreak of chloracne (an acne-like condition usually the result of prolonged contact with chlorinated compounds). TCDD is hepatotoxic, teratogenic, immunotoxic, and a very potent microsomal enzyme inducer in animals. Workers exposed to 2,4,5-T have exhibited clearance, probably as a result of the TCDD content. Porphyria, liver disorders, neurologic, and psychological disturbances have also been reported (259).

Dicamba: A Benzoic Acid-Derived Herbicide

Dicamba (2-methoxy-3,6-dichlorobenzoic acid) (Fig. 10) is a pre- and postemergence herbicide used to control woody and broad-leaf weeds. It can be absorbed through the leaves and roots and acts as a plant growth regulator. Dicamba was first registered in the United States in 1967 and is approved by the EPA for use on soybeans, wheat, oats, barley, asparagus, and sugarcane. Residues of up to 3 ppm are allowed on asparagus. Dicamba, like most other herbicides, has a low acute toxicity in laboratory animals with oral LD_{50} values of 2629 mg/kg in rats, 2000 mg/kg in rabbits, 1190 mg/kg in mice, and 3000 mg/kg in guinea pigs (286). Dicamba is not acutely toxic following inhalation; the 4-hour LC_{50} is greater than 200 mg/liter (285a). The dermal LD_{50} in rabbits is greater than 2000 mg/kg. Rats acutely poisoned with dicamba exhibited myotonia, muscular spasms, dyspnea, and urinary incontinence. Some deaths occurred during spasms, with the muscles remaining contracted after death. Cyanosis, lung congestion, and occasional lung hemorrhages were noted. If death did not result, animals recovered in 2–3 days without pathologic effects. Repeated exposure to high levels of dicamba may result in mild-to-moderate skin irritation and

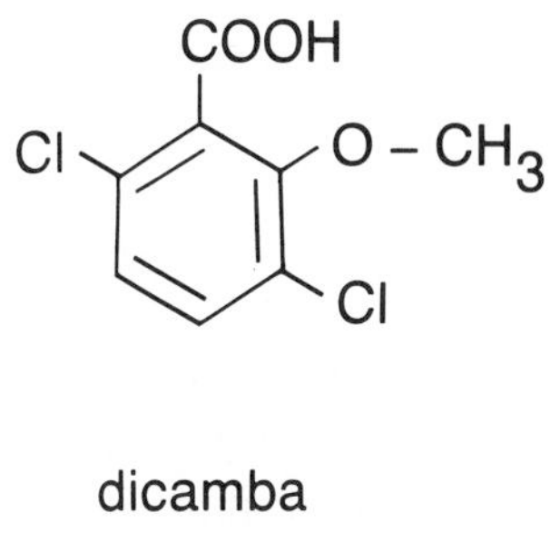

dicamba

FIG. 10. Structure of dicamba.

marked eye irritation in rabbits. In a 15-week study, rats ingesting 3162 ppm dicamba in their diets did not show toxic effects (86).

Dicamba is excreted rapidly in the urine. Rats given 100 mg/kg dicamba orally excreted 70–80% in the first 9 hr and 92–95% within 72 hr. When administered subcutaneously, approximately 90% of the dose was excreted in the urine within 11 hr.

Dicamba has been shown to be mutagenic in the Ames' assay without S9 activation but not with it (256). It was not reported to be carcinogenic (86).

Dicamba is not teratogenic and does not cause adverse effects on reproductive function. Dicamba administered to pregnant female rabbits at dosages up to 10 mg/kg/day did not result in an increased incidence of terata. The NOEL was 3 mg/kg/day. A teratology study in rats revealed a NOEL of 160 mg/kg/day. A three-generation reproductive toxicity study in rats showed no evidence of toxicity among rats from any of the generations utilized. The NOEL in this study was 25 mg/kg/day (285a).

Bipyridal Herbicides

Paraquat

Paraquat (1,1'-dimethyl-4,4'-bipyridinium ion) (Fig. 11) is a rapidly acting herbicide that kills green plants on contact. It may work by inhibiting photosynthesis or respiration in plants. Paraquat may also be reduced to toxic free radicals which, upon reoxidation, produce H_2O_2. Unsaturated lipids

paraquat
dichloride

diquat
dibromide

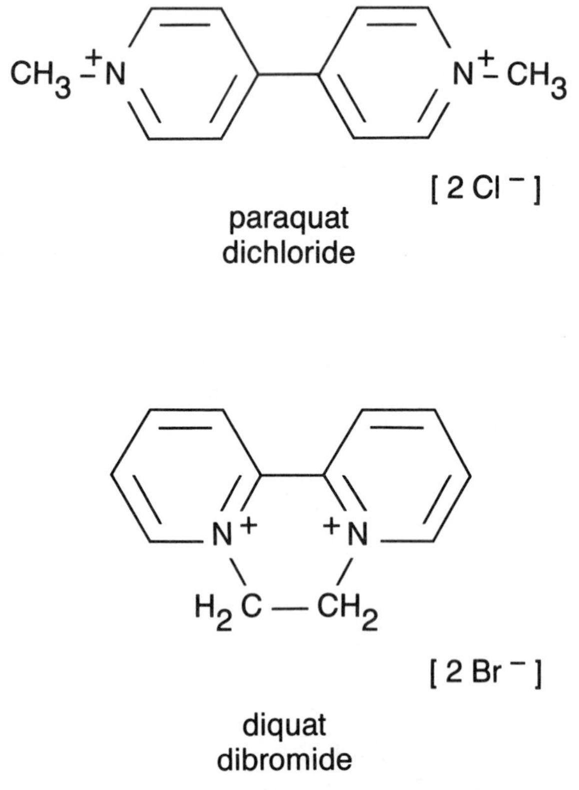

FIG. 11. Structure of bipyridal compounds.

in membranes may be oxidized by peroxides producing damage (121). Paraquat is rapidly inactivated in soil.

Paraquat is moderately toxic with a dermal LD_{50} in rats of 80 mg/kg and an oral LD_{50} of 100 mg/kg. Paraquat is considerably more toxic in man since doses above 14 mg/kg are likely to be fatal (28).

Paraquat is poorly absorbed from the gastrointestinal tract (96). When a dose of 126 mg/kg of paraquat was administered orally to rats, 52% of the dose was localized in the gastrointestinal tract 32 hr later, thus confirming its slow absorption rate (222). In an early experiment, 90% of a subcutaneous dose of ^{14}C-labeled paraquat was excreted in the urine within 24 hr. When paraquat was administered orally, 23% was excreted in the urine and most of the remainder in the feces. The entire dose was essentially cleared from the rat within 2–3 days (75). Later work failed to confirm these results and showed that rats given oral doses excreted it in the urine and feces for at least 3 weeks at measurable levels. A total of 45% of an orally administered dose was excreted in the urine and feces of monkeys within 48 hr. Measurable amounts were excreted for at least 21 days (222).

Rats consuming a diet of 500 ppm paraquat developed pulmonary lesions. No specific effects were observed until after 5–11 weeks of treatment, when animals began showing areas of consolidation in the lungs. Vacuolization and degeneration of the membranous pneumatocytes were the primary effects seen (170). Rats exposed to 3 μm aerosol particles of paraquat at 0.1 mg/m³ for 6 hr did not exhibit any health-related effects. At 1.3 mg/m³ rats did not show any immediate adverse effects during exposure. Later, respiration became impaired, shallow, and rapid. Death occurred within 11 days. Necropsy results showed congested lungs with edema around bronchi and blood vessels with an increase in polymorphonuclear lymphocytes around bronchi. Other organ systems were not significantly affected (95). Similar results were noted in rabbits where a single exposure to a high concentration of aerosol was fatal, whereas repeated exposures to lower concentrations were not harmful (295).

Death from paraquat exposure can occur in one of two ways. Animals receiving rapidly fatal doses of paraquat exhibit ataxia, hyperexcitability, and convulsions before death. Liver and kidney damage may be seen. If the animal survives beyond several days, respiratory problems may develop and death is due to respiratory failure (56). If death occurs 5 days after paraquat exposure, lungs are edematous and plum-colored. If death is delayed 10 or more days, the edema and hemorrhage are usually resolved but scarring, honeycombing, and fibrosis are present. Endothelial proliferation and squamous metaplasia are also observed (56,169). The development of intra-alveolar fibrosis during chronic paraquat exposure may be explained by the presence of a large number of infiltrating profibroblasts which are supported by the presence of oxygen and nutrients (311).

Mice injected intravenously with paraquat (27 mg/kg) had decreased pulmonary surfactant 3 days later. This would contribute to a decrease in respiratory function (94). Mice given 35 mg/kg paraquat subcutaneously had 75% less lecithin and four times as much protein in lung washings after only 24 hr. It was suggested that paraquat may alter lipid metabolism and thereby decrease pulmonary surfactant levels resulting in alveolar collapse (203).

When administered to rats orally at a dose of 126 mg/kg, the lung concentration of paraquat increased to 14 ppm at 32 hr while the serum concentration was only about 1 ppm. Kidney levels peaked at 27 ppm after 1 hr and then decreased rapidly. Serum values peaked at 4.8 ppm after only 30 min (222). Paraquat uptake by the lungs is believed to be carried out through an energy-dependent process by type I and II alveolar cells. This may explain the high concentration of paraquat in lung tissue following administration by all routes of exposure (278).

The mechanism of paraquat-induced pulmonary toxicity may be production of superoxide ions which leads to cellular membrane damage. NADPH-cytochrome c reductase can reduce paraquat. The reduced paraquat may in turn reduce O_2 to the superoxide anion (O_2^-) which can dismutate non-enzymatically to singlet O_2. Singlet O_2 can attack polyunsaturated lipids present in cell and organelle membranes producing lipid hydroperoxides. Lipid hydroperoxides spontaneously form lipid-free radicals which, in turn, react with other polyunsaturated molecules forming more lipid-free radicals which propagate this process. The end result is extensive lipid peroxidation, loss of membrane functional integrity, and death of the cell from membrane damage (40,326). The combination of active uptake by cells in the lung, and the generation of free radicals from paraquat may explain the selective toxicity of paraquat to the lung.

The toxicity of paraquat may be modulated by oxygen. Rats poisoned by paraquat kept in an atmosphere of only 10% oxygen had significantly less mortality than those exposed to normal air (274).

In a well-documented human case, a 30-year-old male attempted suicide by injecting 1 ml of a 20% solution of the dimethyl sulfate salt of paraquat subcutaneously. Gastrointestinal irritation was the first clinical sign noted. The patient vomited within the first several hours and passed bloody stools. After approximately 48 hr, right facial paralysis developed and lasted about 72 hr. On the third day he had a fever of 39°C (102°F) and experienced chest pain. After 14 days, tachycardia and dyspnea developed and opacity was noted in both lungs on a chest X-ray. The patient became oxygen-dependent and his condition deteriorated until the 18th day when he died from respiratory insufficiency (8). The pathogenesis is similar in paraquat poisoning regardless of the route of administration, except that when administered orally, necrosis of the mouth and pharynx is usually present.

Treatment of paraquat poisoning should include gastric lavage followed by administration of bentonite or Fuller's earth to absorb any paraquat not already absorbed by the gut. Purgatives should be given, but forced diuresis is not helpful (311). Hemodialysis or hemoperfusion may also be helpful. Hypoxia may also increase survival.

Diquat

Diquat (1,1'-ethylene-2,2'-bipyridylium ion) (Fig. 11) is a rapidly acting herbicide used for control of aquatic weeds and desiccation of seed crops prior to harvest. Its toxicity is similar to paraquat with oral LD_{50} values in the range of 100–200 mg/kg in laboratory animals. When administered subcutaneously in rats, the LD_{50} is 11–20 mg/kg (55). The higher oral LD_{50} is due to poor absorption of diquat from the gastrointestinal tract. Less than 6% of a dose of diquat is excreted in the urine following oral administration whereas 90–98% is excreted in the urine following subcutaneous administration. About 90% is excreted the first day following exposure and the balance on the next day (75).

A latency period of approximately 24 hr is commonly seen prior to the manifestation of toxic effects. Rats that received doses just above the threshold of lethality became lethargic, weak, and exhibited dyspnea and pupillary dilation the following day. Death usually occurred within 13 days. Animals that died 5 days after treatment had a grossly extended cecum. Doses five times the LD_{50} produced dyspnea within 1 hr. Muscular twitching progressed to convulsions, and death occurred within several hours. In cynomolgus monkeys, necrosis of the epithelial lining of the gastrointestinal tract and the epithelium of the proximal and distal convoluted tubules of the kidneys were observed after ingestion of 100–400 mg/kg diquat (60).

Chronic administration of diquat (4 mg/kg) to rats did not increase malignancies, mortality, or result in pathologic changes in the liver, kidneys, or heart; desquamation of the lung cells, thickening of intraalveolar septa and hyperplasia of the peribronchial lymph tissues were seen in the lungs (20). Rats consuming diets containing up to 1000 ppm diquat for 2 years had an increased incidence of cataracts. Similarly, dogs ingesting 15 mg/kg/day developed cataracts after 10–11 months of treatment (55). Diquat, like paraquat, can become a free radical and exert some of its toxic effects in this manner. There are differences in the biologic effects of these two compounds which are not clearly understood (319). Diquat is not as toxic to the lungs as paraquat, possibly because it is not actively accumulated by lung tissue to the same extent as paraquat.

Diquat is not mutagenic in mice (13) or in *Drosophila melanogaster* (24). It is not carcinogenic (20). In a three-generation reproductive toxicity study, rats consuming diets containing up to 500 ppm diquat did not exhibit behavioral or pathologic changes with the exception of an increase in cataracts (89).

Diquat toxicity in man is similar to that of paraquat. In one recorded case of diquat poisoning, gastrointestinal symptoms, ulceration of the mucous membranes, dyspnea, and liver and kidney damage were noted. Central nervous system involvement was more extensive. The cause of death was cardiac arrest on the sixth day following exposure. No fibrotic changes were noted in the lung (288). Treatment of diquat poisoning is the same as for paraquat poisoning.

RODENTICIDES

The toxicity of most rodenticides is much greater than that of herbicides since they are specifically designed to kill rodents at very low doses. Some rodenticides take advantage of certain physiologic differences between species (e.g., red squill) or rodent feeding habits (e.g., warfarin) in order to exert selective toxicity.

Sodium Fluoroacetate

Sodium fluoroacetate ($FCH_2\text{-}COONa$), also known as compound-1080 (Fig. 12), is especially toxic to rodents, with

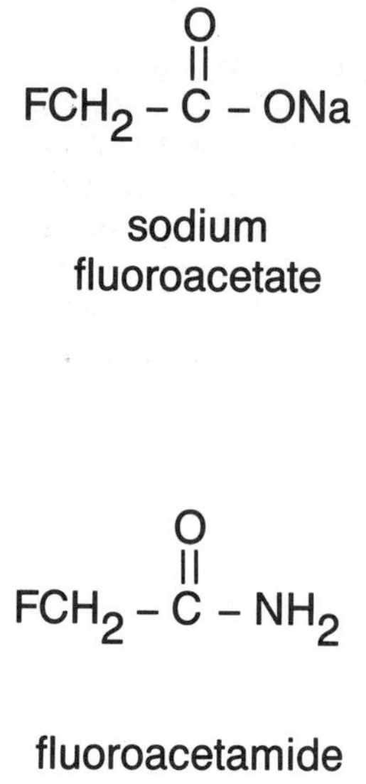

$$FCH_2 - \overset{\overset{\textstyle O}{\|}}{C} - ONa$$

sodium
fluoroacetate

$$FCH_2 - \overset{\overset{\textstyle O}{\|}}{C} - NH_2$$

fluoroacetamide

FIG. 12. Structure of rodenticides.

a rat oral LD_{50} of 0.22 mg/kg (81). The LD_{50} for several other species of rodents is also less than 5 mg/kg (358). However, sodium fluoroacetate is not selectively toxic to rodents. It is extremely toxic to humans with an LD_{50} ranging between 2 and 10 mg/kg (249).

The toxicity of fluoroacetate is due to its ability to inhibit the citric acid cycle (Krebs cycle) and thereby interfere with energy metabolism. *In vivo,* fluoroacetate links with coenzyme A (CoA) forming fluoroacetyl-CoA. Fluoroacetyl-CoA enters the citric acid cycle by condensing with oxaloacetate via the action of citrate synthetase. This results in the formation of fluorocitrate, an inhibitor of the enzyme, aconitase. Inhibition of aconitase blocks conversion of citrate to isocitrate, resulting in the accumulation of citrate (253). Mice injected with sodium fluoroacetate showed rapidly increasing levels of citrate in their tissues (209).

Sodium fluoroacetate is well absorbed from the gastrointestinal tract. It acts primarily on tissues that have a high energy requirement, specifically the central nervous system and the myocardium. Death in man and monkeys is usually the result of ventricular fibrillation or cardiac arrest. In one recorded case, a 17-year-old male ingested as much as 113 g of sodium fluoroacetate and vomited promptly. Upon admission to a hospital, gastric lavage was performed. Grand mal convulsions began within 3 hr. The patient displayed cardiac irregularities, hypertension, heart failure, infection with fever, and acute pulmonary edema. Autopsy findings revealed bronchopneumonia, septicemia, kidney damage, and mediastinal emphysema (36).

Currently no specific antidote is available for sodium fluoroacetate. Administration of glycerol monoacetate (competitive inhibitor to fluoroacetate), procainamide hydrochloride (to reduce the risk of cardiac arrhythmias), and supportive treatment may be of some benefit (53).

Fluoroacetamide

Fluoroacetamide (FCH_2CONH_2), also known as compound-1081 (Fig. 12), is a rodenticide that acts via a mechanism similar to fluoroacetate (209). Fluoroacetamide is not

as toxic as fluoroacetate. The oral LD_{50} of fluoroacetamide in rats is 15 mg/kg (253). Fluoroacetamide is slowly metabolized to fluoroacetate. Fluoroacetamide is toxic to the germinal epithelium in the testes. Rats consuming a diet of 50 ppm fluoroacetamide had a testes weight less than one-third that of controls. After 64 days of treatment, the germinal epithelium of the testes was almost devoid of seminal cells although some spermatogonia, sertoli cells, and interstitial cells did not appear to be damaged (210).

The mechanism of toxicity and clinical effects of fluoroacetamide poisoning are similar to that of fluoroacetate. Treatment of fluoroacetamide poisoning should be the same as fluoroacetate.

Strychnine

Strychnine (Fig. 13) is the principle alkaloid from the seeds of the *Strychnos nux-vomica* tree which has been used as a rodenticide for centuries. It is very toxic with intraperitoneal LD_{50} values of 2.3 and 1.4 mg/kg for male and female rats, respectively. Females and young rats are usually more susceptible than older males (258). A fatal dose in humans is estimated to be between 50 and 100 mg (104).

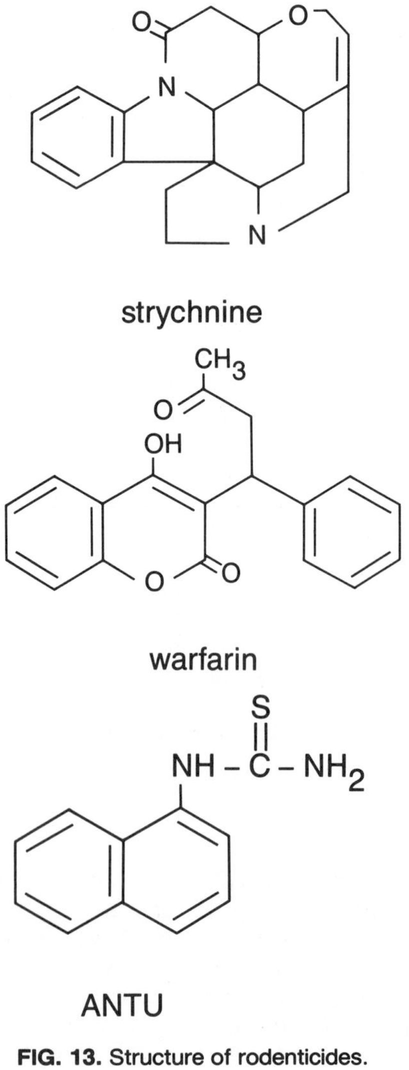

strychnine

warfarin

ANTU

FIG. 13. Structure of rodenticides.

Strychnine is rapidly absorbed from the intestine and acts by altering nerve impulses in the spinal cord. Strychnine interferes with postsynaptic inhibition of spinal and brain neurons. It acts specifically on Renshaw cells (inhibitory interneurons that lower the threshold for neural stimulation in postsynaptic spinal neurons). When Renshaw cell inhibition is blocked, the stimulation threshold for the postsynaptic spinal neurons is decreased, resulting in a hyperexcitable state. A sudden external stimulus coupled with the induced hyperexcitability of the spinal nerves may trigger fatal convulsions (104).

The most prominent response of strychnine poisoning is a violent startle response or seizures brought on by a sudden external stimulus such as touch, light, or noise. The responses of animals and man are strikingly similar. Initially, there is twitching of the muscles of the head and neck followed by clonic then tonic muscular contractions. During seizures the patient is conscious. Painful contraction of the muscles including the diaphragm inhibit breathing and may produce cyanosis. The seizures usually are short at first and tend to become longer with each episode. Death may be due to asphyxia during a seizure or from exhaustion (133). Pathologic findings at autopsy are nonspecific. Bone fractures and hematomas often result from violent convulsions (198).

Treatment involves intravenous administration of an anticonvulsant drug such as diazepam. Gastric lavage is contraindicated unless it is done almost immediately after ingestion. Strychnine is rapidly absorbed and gastric lavage may trigger convulsions. Charcoal may delay absorption. Succinylcholine or d-tubocurarine chloride, along with mechanical respiration, has also been used as a method to treat strychnine poisoning. Forced diuresis may also reduce the duration of poisoning (132).

Red Squill

Bulbs of red squill (*Urgimea martima*) contain scillaren glycosides. These glycosides, like digitalis glycosides, increase the force of myocardial contraction at therapeutic doses. At higher doses these glycosides cause cardiac irregularities, coma, and death due to ventricular fibrillation. Initial symptoms of red squill poisoning are gastrointestinal disturbances, abdominal pain, and blurred vision.

The selective toxicity of red squill is imparted by its ability to induce vomiting. When pets or children ingest it, the emetic action purges much of the dose from the gastrointestinal tract. Rats do not possess a gag reflex and thus are unable to vomit. Once the red squill is ingested by rats, it is absorbed and exerts its lethal effects. The treatment of red squill poisoning is similar to digitalis intoxication. Phenytoin, lidocaine, and potassium salts are the most effective treatments. Other antiarrhythmic drugs such as quinidine, procainamide, and propranolol may also be effective (104).

Warfarin

Warfarin (3(d-acetonylbenzyl)-4-hydroxycoumarin) (Fig. 13) is a rodenticide in the coumarin family. It is used clinically as an anticoagulant, which also serves as the basis for its rodenticidal property. Warfarin is moderately toxic with acute LD_{50} values in male and female rats of 61–102 and 21–33 mg/kg, respectively (264). Other studies have determined LD_{50} values of 323 mg/kg for male and 58 mg/kg for female rats (119). Gaines (96) reported the oral LD_{50} in male rats as only 3 mg/kg. Warfarin toxicity is enhanced following repeated exposure. The 90-dose LD_{50} in rats is only 0.77 mg/kg/day (133).

Warfarin acts as a vitamin K antagonist and inhibits the synthesis of prothrombin. It may block the reduction of vitamin K epoxide by NADH to the hydroquinone form. The hydroquinone form is needed for the synthesis of prothrombin (104). Warfarin is also capable of damaging capillaries. These two effects can combine to produce hematomas, severe blood loss, and death from shock or hemorrhage.

Animals repeatedly exposed to warfarin produce bloody stools and saliva, exhibit petechiae or hematomas, and display an overall pallor of the skin. Hemorrhage is common around the joints. Bleeding in the central nervous system can produce paralysis (134). Death is the result of hemorrhage throughout the body or hemorrhage into specific organs such as the brain.

Warfarin is detoxified by microsomal enzymes including cytochrome P-450 to the 6-, 7-, and 8-hydroxy derivatives (334). Rats excreted 4'-hydroxywarfarin, 6-hydroxywarfarin, 7-hydroxywarfarin, 8-hydroxywarfarin, 7-hydroxywarfarin glucuronide, and an intramolecular condensation product in the urine and feces (21). Rats excreted 90% of a warfarin dose within 14 days following intraperitoneal administration (195).

Warfarin is considered to be a human teratogen. Most of the teratogenic effects are seen in the nasal region of the fetus. The effects include nasal hypoplasia, stippling of bone, chondrodysplasia punctata, and mental retardation. Due to its low molecular weight, warfarin can cross the placenta in the early stages of pregnancy. The critical exposure period in humans is believed to be weeks 6–9 of gestation. These bony deformities may be caused by microhemorrhages into fetal cartilage which calcify and give the bone a stippled appearance (296,375).

In an instance of unintentional human poisoning, a Korean family ingested corn meal for 15 days contaminated with warfarin. Massive bruises and hematomas developed on the buttocks and at the knee and elbow joints after 7–10 days. Gum and nasal bleeding appeared later. Blood was noted in the urine and feces. The estimated exposure was less than 2 mg/kg/day. Of the 14 people exposed, 2 died; the others recovered following treatment (184).

Treatment for warfarin poisoning includes vitamin K_1 administration until the prothrombin time is restored to normal. Small transfusions of whole blood may be given regularly to a seriously ill patient.

Alpha-Naphthyl Thiourea

Alpha-naphthyl thiourea (ANTU) (Fig. 13) is a very potent rodenticide; the LD_{50} in rats is reported at 6.9 mg/kg (80). Dogs are also sensitive to ANTU; however, monkeys (and most likely humans) are essentially resistant to its lethal effects. ANTU and other monosubstituted thiourea derivatives produced pulmonary edema and plural effusion in the rat (79).

Radiolabeled ANTU was found covalently bound to macromolecules in the liver and lung after *in vivo* administration to rats. *In vitro* lung and liver microsomes catalyzed the covalent binding of ANTU to macromolecules in the presence of NADPH. Rats pretreated with 2 mg/kg ANTU for 5 days showed a decrease in microsomal enzyme activity. Pretreated rats survived a dose that was lethal to 60% of the untreated controls. Binding of ANTU to liver and especially lung microsomes was decreased. Depletion of glutathione by prior administration of dimethyl maleate increased the toxicity of ANTU. Thus, it appears that ANTU toxicity is dependent on metabolic activation by microsomal enzymes and the subsequent binding of a reactive intermediate to tissue macromolecules. Inhibition of microsomal enzymes by ANTU may explain the development of tolerance (33). This presents an interesting contrast with the hypothetical mechanism underlying tolerance development produced by agents mentioned earlier, in which tolerance is related to induction of detoxifying enzymes.

ANTU did not produce tumors in two strains of mice fed the maximum tolerated dosage for 18 months (148). ANTU transformed hamster embryo cells *in vitro* (165) and was mutagenic to *Salmonella* in the presence of a metabolic activation system from rats induced with phenobarbital (148). ANTU and other thioureas can induce hyperplasia of the thyroid gland by blocking thyroid hormone synthesis. They can also stop pigment production and impair hair growth.

FUNGICIDES

Nearly 90% of all agricultural fungicides are oncogenic. These oncogenic fungicides represent from 70 to 75 million of the 80 million pounds of all fungicides applied annually in the United States. A recent report by the National Research Council (232) concluded that fungicides contributed nearly 60% of all estimated oncogenic risk from pesticides (see Table 2). The committee evaluated 11 fungicides and concluded that while they represented only 10% of all acres treated with pesticides, they were responsible for about 60% of the total estimated dietary oncogenic risk. The committee went on to conclude that few nononcogenic new fungicides are being developed. The mode of action of fungicides makes it rather difficult to develop compounds that do not damage genetic material. Table 3 shows estimated oncogenic risk for fungicides in major food crops.

TABLE 2. *Distribution of estimated oncogenic risk by pesticide type*

Type of pesticide	Risk	Percentage
Fungicides	3.46×10^{-3}	59.2
Herbicides	1.58×10^{-3}	27.1
Insecticides	8.00×10^{-4}	13.7

From ref. 232, with permission.

TABLE 3. *Estimated oncogenic risk from fungicides in major foods*

Crop	Estimated risk no.	Percentage
Tomatoes	8.23×10^{-4}	14.1
Oranges	3.72×10^{-4}	6.3
Apples	3.18×10^{-4}	5.4
Peaches	2.86×10^{-4}	4.9
Lettuce	1.81×10^{-4}	0.1
Potatoes	1.29×10^{-4}	2.2
Beans	1.17×10^{-4}	2.0
Grapes	1.08×10^{-4}	1.8
Wheat	6.65×10^{-5}	1.1
Celery	6.04×10^{-5}	1.1
Percentage of total risk from herbicides, insecticides, and fungicides		42.0

From ref. 232, with permission.

Hexachlorobenzene

Hexachlorobenzene (Fig. 14) is not currently produced in the United States as a commercial product. It is generated as a waste byproduct from the manufacture of other products (i.e., chlorinated solvents). Because of its persistence and bioaccumulation, hexachlorobenzene is of toxicologic and environmental concern. The toxicity of hexachlorobenzene has been extensively reviewed (77,110,146,317). It is considered moderately toxic to humans following acute exposure,

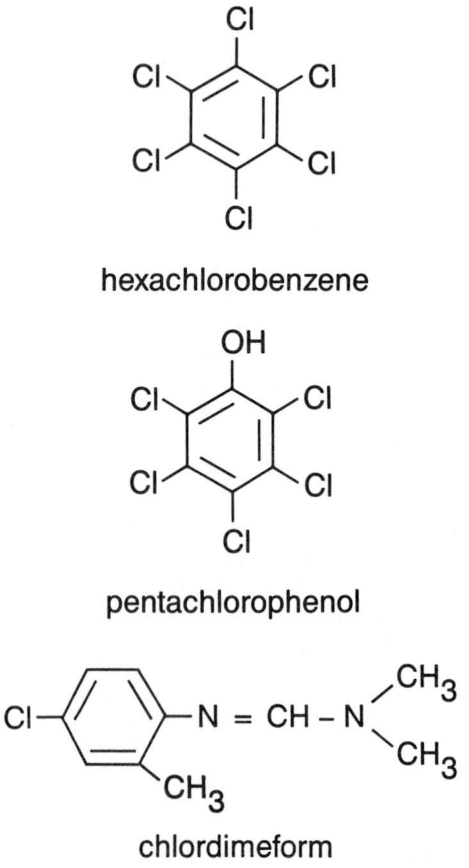

FIG. 14. Structure of fungicides.

with a probable human oral lethal dose ranging from 0.5 to 5 g/kg (or 1 ounce–1 pint for a 70-kg person) (110). Reported oral LD$_{50}$s in laboratory animals are 1700 mg/kg in cats, 2600 mg/kg in rabbits, 3500–10,000 mg/kg in rats, and 4000 mg/kg in mice (77,237a). Death is reportedly due to neurotoxic effects.

Symptoms following repeated exposure to hexachlorobenzene include neurologic effects such as excessive irritability, tremors, and in some cases, ataxia; focal alopecia; dermal changes such as itching and scabbing; and anorexia. Evidence in laboratory rats suggests that females are more susceptible than males to the toxic effects of hexachlorobenzene.

The immunotoxic potential of hexachlorobenzene has been investigated in experimental animals. Immunosuppression, as indicated by decreased resistance to infectious agents, decreased serum globulin levels, and decreased spleen lymphocyte response to sheep red blood cells was demonstrated in mice fed hexachlorobenzene up to 167 ppm in the diet for up to 4 months. Rats exposed pre- and postnatally to a diet containing up to 150 mg/kg showed two- to threefold decreased resistance to a lethal pathogen (77). The immunotoxicity of hexachlorobenzene may be related to its tendency to concentrate in the thymus and the spleen.

Porphyria has been observed in animals repeatedly exposed to hexachlorobenzene, suggesting an effect on the activity of uroporphyrinogen decarboxylase (UDC) (182).

Hexachlorobenzene appears to exert similar toxic effects in humans, according to the few case studies that have been reported (38,47,73). Porphyria cutanea tarda with photosensitivity, hyperpigmentation and hypertrichosis, osteoporosis, and enlargement of the liver, thyroid, and lymph nodes were among the symptoms reported in 4000 individuals in Turkey who unintentionally consumed hexachlorobenzene-treated seeds during the years 1955–1959. Daily consumption of hexachlorobenzene was estimated at 50–200 mg/day for several months before symptoms appeared (47,251). This episode illustrated the sensitivity of young children to the toxic effects of hexachlorobenzene since most of the patients were boys aged 4–14 years old. In addition, nursing infants of hexachlorobenzene-exposed mothers developed lesions on the skin termed *pink sore* and these were associated with 95% fatality. Placental transfer may have also contributed to exposure in these cases. A cohort study of 204 patients exhibited the following symptoms 20 years after exposure: abnormal porphyrin metabolism, hyperpigmentation, hirsutism, enlarged liver, weakness and paresthesis, sclerodermoid thickening, small hands, red urine, ascites, and jaundice. No effects on fertility were noted. In 10 patients, excretion of hexachlorobenzene in urine and feces was elevated, and the milk of 1 patient who was lactating was found to contain more than 0.7 ppm hexachlorobenzene (73). No evidence of carcinogenicity was observed in the 204 cohort patients.

Hexachlorobenzene found in the blood of occupationally exposed workers at levels averaging 3.6 µg/liter was not associated with porphyria; plasma coproporphyrin levels were elevated (38).

Hexachlorobenzene has been evaluated for carcinogenic potential in mice, rats, and hamsters by oral administration and has been found to be a carcinogen. Based on its activity in one bioassay, it may also be a cocarcinogen in rodents.

In an early study, groups of male and female Swiss mice were fed up to 24 mg/kg hexachlorobenzene in the diet, daily for up to 120 weeks. Concentrations of 12–24 mg/kg/day caused a significant increase in the incidence of hepatocellular tumors (44a).

Female Fischer 344/N rats were shown to be more sensitive to the effects of chronic oral administration of hexachlorobenzene than male rats. A diet containing 0.02% hexachlorobenzene fed to groups of 15 male and female rats for up to 90 weeks resulted in porphyria in female rats only. All 10 of the surviving females, but none of the males, developed neoplastic liver nodules or hepatocellular carcinomas (308).

Hexachlorobenzene induced liver tumors (hemangioendotheliomas) and thyroid adenomas in male and female Golden Syrian hamsters when administered in the diet at concentrations up to 16 mg/kg/day for up to 70 weeks. The frequency of tumor-bearing animals was dose-dependent; latency was 18 weeks in treated females (183).

Hexachlorobenzene has been shown to be a cocarcinogen in a single investigation. None of the 35 ICR mice fed up to 50 ppm hexachlorobenzene for 24 weeks developed tumors in the liver; 3 mice fed polychlorinated diterphenyl (PCT) developed tumors. Mice fed both compounds developed hepatocellular carcinomas (299).

Reports available in the published literature suggest that hexachlorobenzene is a nongenotoxic carcinogen. Hexachlorobenzene was nonmutagenic in the Ames' *Salmonella typhimurium* test in strains TA92, TA1535, TA100, TA1537, TA94, and TA98 both in the presence and absence of S-9 (129,219). Hexachlorobenzene was nonmutagenic when tested in three strains of *Saccharomyces cerevisiae* using reversion to methionine and histidine auxotrophy as measures of mutagenicity (115). Hexachlorobenzene has consistently failed to induce dominant lethal mutations in rats (167,237a,305).

The possible teratogenicity of hexachlorobenzene was originally suggested by a study in which cleft palate was observed in the offspring of adult C57BL6 and CD-1 mice treated with pentachloronitrobenzene (PCNB) (66). The deformation was linked to the hexachlorobenzene present as a contaminant at a concentration of 11%. Fewer cleft palates were observed with purified PCNB. Subsequently, hexachlorobenzene was administered alone to CD-1 mice, producing kidney and palate malformations. CD-rats tested by the same protocol were unaffected.

A study with Wistar rats has indicated that hexachlorobenzene is teratogenic. When hexachlorobenzene was administered in single daily doses of up to 120 µg/kg during days 6–9, 10–13, 6–16, or 6–21 of gestation, observations of a 14th rib increased over control levels. Depending on duration of treatment and dose, offspring of treated animals had incidences ranging from 12 to 55%, while controls ranged from 0 to 6%. No evidence of teratogenicity of hexachlorobenzene was found when Sprague–Dawley rats were dosed with up to 640 ppm in the diet during gestation; residues of hexachlorobenzene were present in weanlings in a dose-dependent manner. However, a high incidence of stillbirths was reported (111). Anecdotal evidence confirms the lack of sensitivity of Sprague–Dawley rats to the potential teratogenic effects of hexachlorobenzene. In a carcinogenesis study in rats, no excessive mortality was observed in offspring exposed *in utero* and during lactation and weaning to doses of up to 40 ppm hexachlorobenzene (18).

Dose-dependent, placental transfer has been demonstrated to occur in mice, rats, rabbits, hamsters, guinea pigs, and humans. As a lipophilic compound, hexachlorobenzene is readily transferred in the milk of lactating dams of mice, rats, and humans (15,43,67,68,354). The transfer of hexachlorobenzene in milk appears to play a more major role than placental transfer (67).

Hexachlorobenzene appears to be especially toxic to developing animals. Pre- and postnatal exposure to hexachlorobenzene resulted in renal malformations in CD-1 mice and CD rats in the form of enlarged kidneys and hydronephrosis (16). The developing immune system in rats may be susceptible to combined pre- and postnatal exposure to low levels of hexachlorobenzene. In the absence of other evidence of toxicity, hexachlorobenzene enhanced humoral and cell-mediated immunity and caused intraalveolar macrophage accumulation in rats (356).

Hexachlorobenzene is poorly absorbed via the lymphatic system after a single orally administered dose to rats, monkeys, and dogs. Once absorbed by the lymphatic system, hexachlorobenzene is rapidly distributed to all tissues, especially concentrating in lipid-rich tissues. It is excreted primarily through the intestines via the feces, but small amounts are excreted through the sebaceous, nasal, preputial, and Harderian glands in rats.

In rats, a single oral dose of radiolabeled hexachlorobenzene was distributed throughout the body within 2 hr. High concentrations of hexachlorobenzene were observed in the liver and brown fat within 4 hr, and in the abdominal and subcutaneous fat within 24 hr. High concentrations were found in adipose tissue, bone marrow, skin, Harderian gland, nasal mucosa, and preputial gland (147). A half-life of 20 days has been reported in rats following daily oral administration for 7 days (373).

The metabolic fate of hexachlorobenzene may be influenced by fat levels. Greater toxicity has been observed in food-deprived rats after administration of hexachlorobenzene (353).

The detoxication pathways for hexachlorobenzene have not been elucidated. It is thought that hexachlorobenzene initially reacts with glutathione in the liver, eliminating chlorine groups. The resulting conjugates, *S*-(pentachlorophenyl)glutathione, and *S,S'*-(tetrachlorophenyl)diglutathione may be further metabolized by cleavage of the glutamate and glycine residues, and acetylation of the amino groups of the cysteinyl moiety to yield mercapturic acid *N*-acetyl-*S*-*O*(pentachlorophenyl)cysteine, the major metabolite in rats. This is further metabolized in rats into pentachlorothiophenol and pentachlorothioanisole. The formation of phenol is thought to proceed either through the arene oxides or by direct oxygen insertion, although the mechanism by which this occurs is not completely understood.

Rats treated with hexachlorobenzene have excreted pentachlorobenzene, tetrachlorobenzene, pentachlorophenol, tetrachlorohydroquinone, pentachlorothiophenol, tetrachlorocatechol, pentachlorothiophenol, and trichlorophenol in urine (146,180). Tetrachlorohydroquinone, pentathioanisole, and pentachlorophenol have been found in the tissues of rats treated with hexachlorobenzene (270).

Hexachlorobenzene is an inducer of cytochrome P-450 enzymes in rat liver microsomes in *in vitro* studies (323). Hexachlorobenzene was metabolized to pentachlorophenol by the hepatic cytochrome P-450-mediated system; pentachlorophenol was subsequently converted to tetrachloro-1,2- or 1,4-benzenediols, but not to the 1,3-diol.

Differences between male and female rats in the metabolism and biotransformation of hexachlorobenzene have been demonstrated. When male and female rats were repeatedly fed hexachlorobenzene, significantly more pentachlorothiophenol was found in livers of females than male livers (277). This may relate to the propensity of females to develop porphyria more rapidly than males during long-term exposure (204,308,309).

The mechanism for the induction of porphyria by hexachlorobenzene has not been clearly determined. However, there is evidence that the presence of significant heme iron in susceptible individuals somehow potentiates the porphyrinogenic activity of hexachlorobenzene. Male mice with an iron overload fed a single 100 mg/kg dose of hexachlorobenzene developed porphyria, with no recovery by 14 weeks (314). In further studies by the same investigators, total microsomal P-450 content and activity of ethoxyphenoxazone, an enzymatic marker for the induction of P-450 isoenzymes induced by 3-methylchloroanthrene, peaked a few days after treatment then declined by the time of the inhibition of uroporphyrinogen decarboxylase (UDC). Addition of alpha-naphthoflavone, a P-450 inducer, enhanced inhibition of UDC; piperonyl butoxide, a P-450 inhibitor, partially protected against inhibition of UDC. Lipid peroxidation by a free radical metabolite of hexachlorobenzene may also play a role in its toxicity (6,309).

The registration of hexachlorobenzene and hexachlorobenzene-containing products for use as fungicides has been canceled by the EPA.

Pentachlorophenol

Pentachlorophenol or PCP (Fig. 14) has been used since the 1930s as a wood preservative. It is an effective fungicide, herbicide, and insecticide. It is also used to control termites and other wood-boring insects. It is moderately toxic with an oral LD_{50} in rats of approximately 150 mg/kg (291). The toxicity of PCP may be modified by some contaminants that are generated during its synthesis. Commercially available PCP may contain octa-, hepta-, and hexachlorodibenzo-*p*-dioxins although the levels of contaminants have been greatly reduced since the early 1970s. TCDD has not been shown to be a contaminant of this product. Other chlorinated phenols and polychlorinated dibenzofurans can also be found in commercial preparations. However, because of the varying levels and types of contaminants in samples of PCP, toxicity studies on this material may be difficult to compare.

In one subchronic study, rats fed a diet of technical grade PCP (30 mg/kg) exhibited a decrease in erythrocytes, hemoglobin, and serum albumin and an increase in serum alkaline phosphatase, liver, and kidney weights, and minimal hepatocellular degeneration. When a purified PCP formulation was tested, the only effect noted was an increase in liver and kidney weight (156). Rats ingesting a diet containing

50 or 200 ppm PCP (containing 200 and 82 ppm OCDD and pre-OCDD, respectively with no TCDD) demonstrated an increase in microsomal enzymes, and liver weights. The NOEL was determined to be 25 ppm (177). Female rats fed a diet containing 20, 100, or 500 ppm technical grade PCP for 8 months exhibited hepatic porphyria, increased cytochrome P-450 activity, and increased liver weight; rats fed purified PCP at the same dosages did not exhibit these changes. Both groups had decreased body weight at 500 ppm. The changes in the liver were considered to be due to the chlorinated dibenzodioxin and dibenzofuran contaminants (108). In a 2-year chronic study, 30 mg/kg/day PCP (approximately 22 ppm chlorinated dibenzodioxins) decreased growth and increased SGOT levels; at 3 mg/kg/day, no adverse effects were noted (291).

Following oral or intraperitoneal administration, PCP is primarily excreted unchanged in the urine. Rats also excreted tetrachloro-*p*-hydroquinone and a glucuronide conjugate in the urine. Over 90% of a 10 or 100 mg dose was excreted within 3 days of administration, primarily in the urine with some in the feces. A very small amount is lost as CO_2 in expired air (4,34).

PCP was not teratogenic in rats at dosages up to 50 mg/kg/day. It was fetotoxic at this dose level and resulted in an increase in resorptions and some bone abnormalities. When the dose was lowered to 5 mg/kg/day, no fetotoxicity or embryotoxicity was noted (289,290). PCP is not considered carcinogenic in mice (148) or in rats (291).

PCP is an uncoupler of oxidative phosphorylation at the level of Na^+-K^+ ATPase (78). Poisoning is characterized by muscular weakness, nausea, loss of appetite, dyspnea, profuse sweating, and loss of coordination. In fatal cases, chest pains, rapid pulse, dehydration, and a body temperature as high as 42°C (108°F) have been noted. There are no specific pathologic legions upon autopsy although congestion of organs and cerebral edema may be seen.

Treatment of acute PCP poisoning is generally supportive and nonspecific. It is readily absorbed through the skin. Gentle washing of the skin following direct contact helps remove some of PCP. Body temperature should be controlled by physical means since the use of antiseptic drugs will not be effective because the elevated temperature is due to altered body metabolism and is not controlled by the normal temperature regulatory system. Activated charcoal should be used for gastric lavage. Monitoring of electrolytes and forced diuresis may be beneficial (132).

Chlordimeform

Chlordimeform (*N'*-(4-chloro-*o*-tolyl)-*N'*,*N'*dimethylformamidine) (Fig. 14) is a formamidine pesticide used to control cattle ticks and mites. It is moderately toxic; reported oral LD_{50} values in male and female rats are 300 and 265 mg/kg, respectively (97). No specific pathologic legions were noted upon necropsy in rats following a lethal oral dose. In dogs, congestion of the liver, kidney, and lungs, and lung hemorrhage was observed (89).

Rats fed 80 mg/kg/day chlordimeform for 4 weeks did not show toxic effects. When 100 mg/kg/day was administered, growth rate was depressed, but no histologic changes were observed (118). In a chronic study, rats fed a diet containing 1000 ppm chlordimeform exhibited a retarded growth rate, and liver nodules with focal hyperplasia (89). When dogs ingested a diet containing 1000 ppm chlordimeform for 2 years, body weights were reduced and red blood cell indices were decreased. Bile duct hyperplasia, modular hyperplasia, and hypertrophy of hepatocytes were seen. No effects were detected at 250 ppm (89).

Chlordimeform possesses antiinflamatory and antipyretic properties very similar to aspirin. It acts as other nonsteroidal anti-inflammatory agents by inhibiting prostaglandin synthesis (374). Most other nonsteroidal anti-inflammatory agents cause gastric ulceration whereas chlordimeform does not (142). It is also a potent inhibitor of monamine oxidase. This property may contribute significantly to the overall toxicity of this compound (23). It also is a very potent uncoupler of oxidative phosphorylation (2).

Chlordimeform is primarily metabolized by the liver mixed function oxidase system to two principle metabolites, *N*-formyl-4-chloro-*o*-toluidine and 4-chloro-*o*-toluidine, and it is excreted rapidly. Approximately 96% of an oral dose of ^{14}C-labeled chlordimeform is excreted in the urine and the feces within 72 hr of administration (176).

Chlordimeform is not considered teratogenic. In a three-generation reproductive toxicity study, rats receiving a diet containing up to 500 ppm chlordimeform did not exhibit any changes in litter size, birth weight, sex ratio, or fertility index. No increase in terata was observed. When rabbits were given up to 30 mg/kg/day on days 8–16 of gestation, no changes in reproductive parameters or increases in teratogenesis were noted. Chlordimeform and both of its principle metabolites have been reported to be carcinogenic in mice, but not in rats (90,91).

In one case of accidental human poisoning, workers exposed to chlordimeform developed hematuria and other urologic symptoms accompanied by a fine eruption on the skin. Symptoms eventually resolved after exposure was discontinued. Treatment for overexposure is essentially supportive and symptomatic (132).

CONCLUSION

A principal goal in pesticide research and development is specificity of action. Only the target plant, animal, insect or fungus should be affected by the application of the product. This can be achieved in many different ways, including species-specific biochemistry, as with certain insecticides, or applications of antidotes to protect crops from herbicides. However, because pesticides are designed and selected for their biologic activity, toxicity to non-target species usually remains a significant potential problem.

Unintended exposure to pesticides can occur during their manufacturing, formulation, application, or from environmental residues after application. Each type of exposure has its own characteristics of magnitude and duration and may lead to different signs of toxicity. In some cases, the mechanisms underlying the observed toxicity are relatively well understood, while in others, our knowledge has not passed much beyond description of the symptomology. The pesticide studies reviewed in this chapter provide a good illustration of the variation in our knowledge of various pesticide groups. They also demonstrate that pesticides have the potential to disrupt virtually every major organ system. The further study of pesticide toxicology will contribute to a better understanding of the proper prevention and treatment of toxic effects after exposure to these substances. It will also facilitate the development of pesticides which are both safer and more effective.

REFERENCES

1. Abbassy, M. A., Eldefrawi, M. E., and Eldefrawi, A. T. (1983): Pyrethroid action on the nicotinic acetylcholine receptor channel. *Pest. Biochem. Physiol.*, 19:299–308.
2. Abo-khatwa, N., and Hollingworth, R. M. (1973): Chlordimeform: Uncoupling activity against liver mitochondria, *Pest. Biochem. Physiol.*, 3:358.
3. ACGIH (1986): *Documentation of the Threshold Limit Values and Biological Exposure Indices*, 5th ed. American Conference of Governmental Industrial Hygienists, Cincinnati, p. 250.
4. Ahlborg, V. G., Lindgren, J. E., and Mercier, M. (1974): Metabolism of pentachlorophenol. *Arch. Toxicol.*, 32:271.
5. Alexeeff, G. V., and Kilgore, W. W. (1983): Methyl bromide. *Residue Rev.*, 88:101.
6. Alleman, M. A., Koster, J. F., Wilson, J. H. P., et al. (1985): The involvement of iron and lipid peroxidation in the pathogenesis of HCB induced porphyria. *Biochem. Pharmacol.*, 34(2):161–166.
7. Allen, J. R., Hargraves, W. A., Hsia, M. T. S., and Lin, F. S. D. (1979): Comparative toxicology of chlorinated compounds on mammalian species. *Pharmacol. Ther.*, 7:513.
8. Almog, C., and Tal, E. (1967): Death from paraquat after subcutaneous injection. *Br. Med. J.*, 3:721.
9. Alumot, E., and Mandel, E. (1969): Gonadotropic hormones in hen treated with ethylene dibromide. *Poultry Sci.*, 48:957–960.
10. Amir, D. (1973): The sites of spermicidal action of ethylene dibromide in bulls. *J. Reprod. Fertil.*, 35:519–525.
11. Amir, D. (1975): Individual and age differences in the spermicidal effect of ethylene dibromide in bulls. *J. Reprod. Fertil.*, 44:561–565.
12. Amir, D., and Volcani, R. (1965): Effect of dietary ethylene dibromide on bull semen. *Nature*, 206:99–100.
13. Anderson, D., McGregor, D. B., and Purchase, I. F. H. (1976): Dominant lethal studies with paraquat and diquat in male CD-1 mice. *Mutat. Res.*, 40:349.
14. Anderson, K. J., Leighty, E. G., and Takahashi, M. J. (1972): Evaluation of herbicides for possible mutagenic properties. *J. Agric. Food Chem.*, 20:649.
15. Ando, M., Hirano, S., and Ito, H. (1984): Transfer of HCB (hexachlorobenzene) from mother to newborn baby through placenta and milk. *Kokuritsu Kogai Kenkyusho Kenkyu Hokoku*, 67:347–360.
16. Andrews, J. E., and Courtney, K. D. (1975): Hexachlorobenzene renal maldevelopment in CD-1 and CD rats. ISS Report; EPA/600/D-85/160. Order No. PB85-235976, p. 21.
17. Armstrong, J., Sommerville, O. R., Lovejoy, G., et al. (1975): Insecticide-induced acute hemorrhagic creptitis. *Tenn. Morbidity Mortality Weekly Rep.*, 24:374.
18. Arnold, D. L., Moodie, C. A., Charbonneau, S. M., et al. (1985): Long-term toxicity of hexachlorobenzene in the rat and the effect of dietary vitamin A. *Fed. Chem. Toxicol.*, 23:779–793.
19. Baage, G., Cekanova, E., and Larsson, K. (1973): Teratogenic and embryotoxic effects of the herbicides di- and trichlorophenoxyacetic acids (2,4-D and 2,4,5-T). *Acta Pharmacol. Toxicol.*, 32:408.
20. Bainova, A., and Vulcherla, V. S. (1978): Chronic action of diquat on the lungs. *Dokl. Bolg. Akad. Nauk.*, 31:1369–1372.
21. Barker, W. M., Hermodson, M. A., and Link, K. P. (1970): The metabolism of 4-^{14}C warfarin sodium by the rat. *J. Pharmacol. Exp. Ther.*, 171:307.
22. Barlow, S. M., and Sullivan, F. M. (1982): *Reproductive Hazards of Industrial Chemicals*. Academic Press, London, p. 296.
23. Beeman, R. W., and Matsumura, F. (1973): Chlordimeform: A pesticide acting upon regulatory mechanisms. *Nature*, 242:273.
24. Benes, V., and Sram, R. (1969): Mutagenic activity of some pesticides in *Drosophila melanogaster*. *Ind. Med. Surg.*, 38:441.
25. Berry, C. E. (1938): Methyl bromide as a rodenticide. *Calif. Dept. Agric. Bull.*, 27:173.
26. Berwick, P. (1970): 2,4-Dichlorophenoxyacetic acid poisoning in man: Some interesting clinical and laboratory findings. *JAMA*, 214:1114–1117.
27. Biles, R. W., Conner, T. H., Trieff, N. M., and Legator, M. S. (1978): The influence of contaminants on the mutagenic activity of dibromochloropropane (DBCP). *J. Environ. Pathol. Toxicol.*, 2:301–312.
28. Binnie, G. A. C. (1975): Paraquat. *Lancet*, 1:169.
29. Blum, A., and Ames, B. N. (1977): Flame-retardant additives as possible cancer hazards. The main flame retardant in children's pajamas is a mutagen and should not be used. *Science*, 195:17–23.
30. Bohm, G. M. (1973): Changes in lung arterioles in pulmonary oedema induced in rats by alpha-naphthyl-thiourea. *J. Pathol.*, 110:343–345.
31. Bond, E. J., and Buckland, C. T. (1978): Control of insects with fumigants at low temperatures: Toxicity of fumigants in atmospheres of carbon dioxide. *J. Econ. Entomol.*, 71:307.
32. Boskovic, B., Vojvodic, V., Maksimovic, M., et al. (1976): Effect of mono- and bis-quaternary pyridinium oximes on the acute toxicity and serum cholinesterase inhibiting activity of dioxacarb, carbaryl and carbofuran. *Arh. Hig. Rada Toksikol.*, 27:289–295.
33. Boyd, M. R., and Neal, R. A. (1976): Studies on the mechanism of toxicity and of development of tolerance to pulmonary toxin alpha-naphthylthiourea (ANTU). *Drug. Metab. Dispos.*, 4:314–322.
34. Braun, W. H., Young, J. D., Balu, G. E., and Gehring, P. J. (1977): Pharmacokinetics and metabolism of pentachlorophenol in rats. *Toxicol. Appl. Pharmacol.*, 41:395.
35. Brimer, P. A., Tan, E. L., and Hsie, A. W. (1982): Effect of metabolic activation on the cytotoxicity and mutagenicity of 1,2-dibromoethane in the CHO/HGPRT System. *Mutat. Res.*, 95:377–388.
36. Brockman, J. L., McDowell, A. V., and Leeds, W. G. (1955): Fatal poisoning with sodium fluoroacetate. Report of a case. *JAMA*, 159:1529.
37. Brodeur, J., and BuBois, K. P. (1964): Studies on the mechanism of acquired tolerance by rats to O,O-diethyl-S-2-(ethylthio)ethyl phosphonodithioate (Di-Syston). *Arch. Int. Pharmacodyn. Ther.*, 149:560–570.
38. Burns, J. E., and Miller, F. M. (1975): Hexachlorobenzene contamination: Its effects in a Louisiana population. *Arch. Environ. Health*, 30:44–48.
39. Bus, J. S., Aust, S. D., and Gibson, J. E. (1974): Superoxide and singlet oxygen-catalyzed lipid peroxidation as a possible mechanism for paraquat toxicity. *Biochem. Biophys. Res. Commun.*, 58:749.
40. Bus, J. S., Aust, S. D., and Gibson, J. E. (1975): Lipid peroxidation: A possible mechanism for paraquat toxicity. *Res. Commun. Chem. Pathol. Pharmacol.*, 11:31.
41. Bus, J. S., and Gibson, J. E. (1975): Postnatal toxicity of chemically administered paraquat in mice and interactions with oxygen and bromobenzene, *Toxicol. Appl. Pharmacol.*, 33:461.
42. Bus, J. S., Preache, M. M., Cagen, S. Z., et al. (1973): Fetal toxicity and distribution of paraquat and diquat in mice and rats. *Toxicol. Appl. Pharmacol.*, 33:450.
43. Bush, B., Snow, J., and Koblintz, R. (1984): Polychlorobiphenyl(PCB)congeners, p,p'-DDE, and hexachlorobenzene in maternal and fetal cord blood from mothers in upstate New York. *Arch. Environ. Contam. Toxicol.*, 13:517–527.
44. Butler, K. D., and Crowder, L. A. (1977): Increased cyclic nucleotides in several tissues of the cockroach and mouse following treatment with toxaphene. *Pestic. Biochem. Physiol.*, 7:474–480.
44a. Cabra, J. R. P., Mollimer, T., Kaitano, F., and Shubik, P. (1978): Carcinogenesis of hexachlorobenzene in mice. *Int. J. Cancer*, 23:47–51.
45. Cabrol-Telle, A. M., DeSaint Blanquat, G., Derache, R., et al. (1985): Nutritional and toxicological effects of long-term ingestion of phosphine-fumigated diet by the rat. *Food Chem. Toxicol.*, 23:1001–1009.
46. California Department of Food and Agriculture (1970–1981): Pesticide use report.
47. Cam, C., and Nigogosyan, G. (1963): Acquired toxic porphyria cutanea tarda due to hexachlorobenzene. *JAMA*, 183:88–91.

48. Cameron, G. R. (1945): Risks to man and animals from the use of 2,2-bis(*p*-chlorophenyl)-1,1,1-trichloroethane (DDT): With a note on the toxicology of gamma-benzene hexachloride. *Br. Med. Bull.*, 3:233–235.

49. Carpenter, C. P., Weil, C. S., Palm, P. E., et al. (1971): Mammalian toxicity of 1-naphthyl-*N*-methylcarbamate (Sevin insecticide). *J. Agric. Food Chem.*, 9:30–39.

49a.Casada, J. E., and Ruzo, L. U. (1980): Metabolic chemistry of pyrethroid insecticides. *Pest. Sci.*, 11:257–269.

50. Cavanagh, J. B. (1954): The toxic effect of triorthocresyl phosphate on the nervous system. *J. Neurol. Neurosurg. Psychiatry*, 17:163–172.

51. Chalmers, A. E., and Osborne, M. P. (1986): The crayfish receptor organ: A useful model system for investigating the effects of neuroactive substances. II. A pharmacological investigation of pyrethroid mode of action. *Pest. Biochem. Physiol.*, 26:139–149.

52. Chefurka, W., Kashi, K. P., and Bond, E. S. (1976): The effect of phosphine on electron transport. *Mitochondria, Pestic. Biochem. Physiol.*, 6:65–81.

53. Chenoweth, M. B., Kanoel, A., Johnson, L. B., and Bennett, D. R. (1951): Factors influencing fluoroacetate poisoning. Practical treatment with glycerol monoacetate. *Pharmacol. Exp. Ther.*, 102:31.

54. Chernoff, N., Kavlock, R. J., Kathrein, J. R., et al. (1975): Prenatal effects of dieldrin and photodieldrin in mice and rats. *Toxicol. Appl. Pharmacol.*, 31:302–308.

55. Clark, D. G., and Hurst, E. W. (1970): The toxicity of diquat. *Br. J. Ind. Med.*, 27:51.

56. Clark, D. G., McElligott, T. F., and Hurst, E. W. (1966): The toxicity of paraquat. *Br. J. Ind. Med.*, 23:126.

57. Clark, J. M., and Matsumura, F. (1982): Two different types of inhibitory effects of pyrethroids on nerve Ca and Ca$^+$Mg$^-$ ATPase activity in the squid, *Loligo pealei. Pestic. Biochem. Physiol.*, 18:180–190.

58. Clarke, C. A., Rowroth, C. G., and Holling, H. E. (1945): Methyl bromide poisoning. *Br. J. Ind. Med.*, 2:17.

59. Clive, D., Johnson, K. O., Spector, J. F. S., et al. (1979): Validation and characterization of the L5178Y/TK$^+$/$^-$ mouse lymphoma mutagen assay system. *Mutat. Res.*, 59:61–108.

60. Cobb, L. M., and Grimshaw, P. (1979): Acute toxicity of oral diquat (1,1-ethylene-2,2-bypyridenium) in cynomolgus monkeys. *Toxicol. Appl. Pharmacol.*, 51:277.

61. Collins, T. F. X., and Williams, C. H. (1971): Teratogenic studies with 2,4,5-T and 2,4-D in the hamster. *Bull. Environ. Contam. Toxicol.*, 6:559.

62. Conning, D. M., Fletcher, K., and Swan, A. A. (1969): Paraquat and related bipyridyls. *Br. Med. Bull.*, 25:245–259.

63. Coper, H., Herken, H., and Klempau (1951): I. Zur Pharmakologie und Toxikologie Chlorierter Cyclohexane. *Arch. Exp. Pathol. Pharmakol.*, 212:463–479.

64. Corbett, J. R., Wright, K., and Baillie, A. C. (1984): *The Biochemical Mode of Acton of Pesticides.* Academic Press, NY.

65. Corcos, A., Heuretematte, J., and Corcos, V. (1955): Intoxication Mortelle Par Le Bromure Ce Methyle. *Bull. Mem. Soc. Med. Hop. Paris.*, 71:1005.

66. Courtney, A., Copeland, M. F., and Robbins, A. (1976): The effects of pentachloronitrobenzene, hexachlorobenzene, and related compounds on fetal development. *Toxicol. Appl. Pharmacol.*, 35:239–256.

67. Courtney, K. D., and Andrews, J. E. (1985): Neonatal and maternal body burdens of hexachlorobenzene (HCB) in mice; gestational exposure and lactational transfer. *Fund. Appl. Toxicol.*, 5:265–277.

68. Courtney, K. D., Andrews, J. E., and Grady, M. A. (1985): Placental transfer and fetal deposition of hexachlorobenzene in the hamster and guinea pig. *Environ. Res.*, 37:239–249.

69. Courtney, K. D., Gaylor, D. W., and Falk, H. L. (1970): Teratogenic evaluation on 2,4,5-T. *Science*, 168:864.

70. Courtney, K. D., and Moore, J. A. (1971): Teratology studies with 2,4,5-T and TCDD. *Toxicol. Appl. Pharmacol.*, 20:396.

71. Crampton, M. A., and Rodgers (1983): Low doses of 2,4,5-trichlorophenoxyacetic acid are behaviorally teratogenic in rats. *Experientia*, 39:891.

72. Cremer, J. E., and Seville, M. P. (1985): Changes in regional cerebral blood flow and glucose metabolism associated with symptoms of pyrethroid toxicity. *Neurotoxicology*, 6:1–12.

73. Cripps, D. J., Peters, H. A., Gocmen, A., and Dogramici, I. (1984): Porphyria turcica due to hexachlorobenzene: A 20–30-year follow-up study of 204 patients. *Br. J. Dermatol.*, 111:413–422.

74. Danese, L. H. J. C., Van Velsen, F. L., and Van Der Heijden, C. A. (1984): Methyl bromide: Carcinogenic effects in the rat forestomach. *Toxicol. Appl. Pharmacol.*, 72:262.

75. Daniel, J. W., and Gage, J. C. (1966): Absorption and excretion of diquat and paraquat in rats. *Br. J. Ind. Med.*, 23:133.

76. Dauterman, W. C. (1971): Biological and nonbiological modifications of organophosphorous compounds. *Bull. WHO*, 44:133–150.

77. Deichman, W. B. (1981): Halogenated cyclic hydrocarbons. *Patty's Industrial Hygiene and Toxicology*, 3rd ed., edited by D. Clayton and F. E. Clayton, p. 3603. John Wiley, NY.

78. Desaiah, D. (1977): Effects of pentachlorophenol on the ATPases in rat tissue. In: *Pentachlorophenol*, edited by K. R. Rao, pp. 277–283. Plenum Press, NY.

79. Dieke, S. H., Allen, G. S., and Richter, C. P. (1947): Acute toxicity of thioureas and related compounds to wild and domestic Norway rats. *J. Pharmacol. Exp. Ther.*, 90:260–270.

80. Dieke, S. H., and Richter, C. P. (1945): Acute toxicity of thiourea to rats in relation to age, diet, strain and species variation. *J. Pharmacol. Exp. Ther.*, 83:195–202.

81. Dieke, S. H., and Richter, C. P. (1946): Comparative assays of rodenticides on wild Norway rats. *Public Health Rep.*, 61:672.

82. Dodge, A. D. (1972): The mode of action of the bipyridylium herbicides paraquat and diquat. *Endeavour*, 30:130–135.

83. Dougherty, W. J., Coulston, F., and Goldberg, L. (1973): Nonteratogenicity of 2,4,5-trichlorophenoxyacetic acid in monkeys (*Macaca mulatta*). *Toxicol. Appl. Pharmacol.*, 25:442.

84. Drill, V. A., and Hiratzka, T. (1953): Toxicity of 2,4-dichlorophenoxyacetic acid and 2,4,5-trichlorophenoxyacetic acid: A report on their acute and chronic toxicity in dogs. *Arch. Ind. Hyg. Occup. Med.*, 7:61.

85. Dudley, H. C., and Neal, P. (1942): Methyl bromide as a fumigant for food. *J. Food Sci.*, 7:421.

86. Edson, E. F., and Sanderson, D. M. (1965): Toxicity of the herbicides, 2-methoxy-3,6-dichlorobenzoic acid (dicamba) and 2-methoxy-3,5,6-trichlorobenzoic acid (tricamba). *Food Cosmet. Toxicol.*, 3:299.

87. Eldefrawi, M. E., Abbassy, M. A., and Eldefrawi, A. T. (1984): Effects of environmental toxicants on nicotinic acetylcholine receptors: Action of pyrethroids. In: *Cellular and Molecular Neurotoxicology*, edited by T. Narahasi, pp. 177–189. Raven Press, NY.

88. Emerson, S. L., and Thompson, D. J. (1971): Teratogenic studies of 2,4,5-trichlorophenoxyacetic acid in the rat and rabbit. *Food Cosmet. Toxicol.*, 9:395.

89. FAO/WHO (1973): 1972 Evaluation of some pesticide residues in food. WHO Pesticide Residue Series, No. 2, Geneva.

90. FAO (1980): FAO plant production and protection, Paper 20 (suppl.). Pesticide residues in food: 1979 Evaluations, p. 129. FAO of the U.N., Rome.

91. FAO (1979): FAO plant production and protection, Paper 15 (suppl.). Pesticide residues in food: 1978 Evaluations, p. 51. FAO of the U.N., Rome.

92. Federal Register (1979): Suspension order and notice of intent to cancel, 44:65135–65178.

93. Feldman, R. J., and Malibach, H. I. (1974): Percutaneous penetration of some pesticides and herbicides in man. *Toxicol. Appl. Pharmacol.*, 28:126.

94. Fisher, H. K., Clements, J. A., Tierney, D. F., and Wright, R. R. (1973): Enhancement of oxygen toxicity by the herbicide paraquat. *Am. Rev. Resp. Dis.*, 107:246.

95. Gage, J. E. (1968): Toxicity of paraquat and diquat aerosols generated by a size-selective cyclone: Effect of particle size distribution. *Br. J. Ind. Med.*, 25:304.

96. Gaines, T. B. (1969). Acute toxicology of pesticides. *Toxicol. Appl. Pharmacol.*, 14:515–534.

97. Gaines, T. B., and Linder, T. B. (1986): Acute toxicity of pesticides in adult and weanling rats. *Fund. Appl. Toxicol.*, 7:299.

98. Gammon, D. W., Brown, M. A., and Casida, J. E. (1981): Two classes of pyrethroid action in the cockroach. *Pestic. Biochem. Physiol.*, 15:181–91.

99. Gammon, D., and Casida, J. E. (1983): Pyrethroids of the most

potent class antagonize GABA action at the crayfish neuromuscular junction. *Neurosci. Lett.,* 40:163–168.

100. Gammon, D. W., Lawrence, L. J., and Casida, J. E. (1982): Pyrethroid toxicology: Protective effects of diazepam and phenobarbital in the mouse and the cockroach. *Toxicol. Appl. Pharmacol.,* 66:290–296.

101. Garrett, R. M. (1947): Toxicity of DDT for man. *J. Med. Assoc. State Ala.,* 17:74–76.

102. Generoso, W. M., Cain, K. T., and Hughes, L. A. (1985): Tests for dominant-lethal effects of 1,2-dibromo-3-chloropropane in male and female mice. *Mut. Res.,* 156:103–108.

103. Gerhing, P. J., Kramer, C. G., Schwetz, B. A., et al. (1973): The fate of 2,4,5-trichlorophenoxyacetic acid (2,4,5-T) following oral administration to man. *Toxicol. Appl. Pharmacol.,* 26:352–361.

104. Gilman, A. G., Goodman, L. D., and Gilman, A. (1980): *The Pharmacological Basis of Therapeutics,* 6th ed. McMillan, NY.

105. Glass, A. (1956): An account of suspected phosphine poisoning in a submarine. *J. R. Navy Med. Ser.,* pp. 42, 184.

105a. Glickman, A. H., and Casida, J. E. (1982): Species and structural variations affecting pyrethroid neurotoxicity. *Neurobehav. Toxicol. Teratol.,* 4:793–799.

106. Glass, R. I., Lyness, R. N., Mengle, D. C., et al. (1979): Sperm count depression in pesticide applicators exposed to dibromochloropropane. *Am. J. Epidemiol.,* 109:346–351.

107. Goldsmith, J. R., and Potashnik, G. (1984): Reproductive outcomes in families of DBCP-exposed men. *Arch. Environ. Health,* 39:85–89.

108. Goldstein, J. A., Fridsen, M., Linder, R. E., et al. (1977): Effects of pentachlorophenol on hepatic drug-metabolizing enzymes and porphyria related to contamination with chlorinated dibenzo-*p*-dioxins and dibenzofuran. *Biochem. Pharmacol.,* 26:1549.

109. Gosalvez, M., and Merchan, J. (1973): Induction of rat mammary adenomas with the respiratory inhibitor rotenone. *Cancer Res.,* 33:3047–3050.

110. Gosselin, R. E., Hodge, H. C., Smith, R. P., Gleason, M. N. (1976): *Clinical Toxicology of Commercial Products. Acute Poisoning,* p. 115. Williams and Wilkins, Baltimore.

111. Grant, D. L., Philips, W. E. J., and Hatina, G. V. (1977): Effect of hexachlorobenzene on reproduction in the rat. *Arch. Environ. Contam. Toxicol.,* 5:207–216.

111a. Gray, A. J. (1985): Pyrethroid structure-toxicity relationships in mammals. Neurotoxicology, 6:127–138.

112. Gray, A. J., and Rickard, J. (1982): Toxicity of pyrethroids to rats after direct injection into the central nervous system. *Neurotoxicology,* 3:25–35.

113. Grunow, W., and Boehme, C. (1974): Uber den Stoffwechsel von 2,4,5-T und 2,4-D bei ratten und mäusen. *Arch. Toxicol.,* 32:217–225.

114. Grunow, W., Boehme, C., and Budczies, B. (1971): Renale Avsscheidung von 2,4,5-T bei ratten. *Food Cosmet. Toxicol.,* 9:667.

115. Guerzoni, M. E., Del Cupolo, L., and Ponti, I. (1976): Mutagenic activity of pesticides. *Riv. Sci. Technol. Aliment. Nutr. Um.,* 6:161–165.

116. Haag, H. B. (1931): Toxicological studies of *Derris elliptica* and its constituents. I. Rotenone, *J. Pharmacol. Exp. Ther.,* 43:193–208.

117. Haar, G. T. (1980): An investigation of possible sterility and health effects from exposure to ethylene dibromide. In: *Banbury Report No. 5, Ethylene Dichloride: A Potential Health Risk?,* edited by B. Ames, P. Infante, and R. Reitz, pp. 167–176. Cold Spring Harbor Laboratory, Cold Spring Harbor, NY.

118. Haddow, B. C., and Shankland, B. A. (1969): C8514, *N*-(2-methyl-4-chloro-phenyl)-N′,N′-dimethylformamidine, a promising new acaricide. *Proceedings of the British Insecticide, Fungicide Conference,* Vol. 2, 5th ed., p. 538. Brighton, England.

119. Hagan, E. C., and Radomski, J. L. (1953): The toxicity of 3-(acetonylbenzyl)-4-hydroxycoumarin (warfarin) to laboratory animals. *J. Am. Pharm. Assoc.,* 42:379.

120. Hague, N. G., and Sood, U. (1963): Soil sterilization with methyl bromide to control soil nematodes. *Plant Pathol.,* 12:88.

121. Haley, T. J. (1979): Review of the toxicology of paraquat. *Clin. Toxicol.,* 14:1.

122. Hanify, J. A., Metcalf, P., Nobbs, C. L., and Worsley, K. J. (1981): Aerial spraying of 2,4,5-T and human birth malformations: An epidemiological investigation. *Science,* 212:349.

123. Hansen, W. H., Quaipe, M. L., Habermann, R. T., and Fitzhugh, O. G. (1971): Chronic toxicity of 2,4-dichlorophenoxyacetic acid in rats and dogs. *Toxicol. Appl. Pharmacol.,* 20:122–129.

124. Hanson, D. J. (1984): Agricultural uses of ethylene dibromide halted. *Chem. Engineer. News,* March 14:13–16.

125. Hardin, B. D., Bond, G. P., Sikon, M. R., et al. (1981): Testing of selected workplace chemicals for teratogenic potential. *Scand. J. Work Environ. Health,* 7(Suppl. 4):66.

126. Harger, R. N., and Spolyar, L. W. (1958): Toxicity of phosphine, with a possible fatality from this poison. *Arch. Ind. Health,* 18:497.

127. Harry, E. G., and Brown, W. B. (1974): Fumigation with methyl bromide: Applications in the poultry industry: A Review. *World Poultry Sci. J.,* 30:193.

128. Hatakeyama, H., and Shigel, T. (1971): Fine structured changes of alveolar walls in fibrin induced so-called neurogenic pulmonary edema of the rat: Comparative representation with adrenaline and ANTU-induced edema. *Jpn. J. Pharmacol.,* 21:673–675.

129. Haworth, S., Lawlor, T., Mortelmans, K., et al. (1983): *Salmonella* mutagenicity test results for 250 chemicals. *Environ. Mutagen. Suppl.,* 1:3–142.

130. Hayes, W. J., Jr. (1959): Pharmacology and toxicology of DDT. In *DDT, the Insecticide Dichlorodiphenyltrichloroethane and Its Significance, Vol. 2,* edited by P. Muller, pp. 9–247. Birkhauser Verlag, Basel.

131. Hayes, W. J., Jr., Dale, W. E., and Pirkle, C. I. (1971): Evidence of safety of long-term, high, oral doses of DDT for man. *Arch. Environ. Health,* 22:119–135.

132. Hayes, W. J., Jr. (1982): *Pesticides Studied in Man.* Williams and Wilkins, Baltimore.

133. Hayes, W. J., Jr. (1975): *Toxicology of Pesticides,* Williams and Wilkens, Baltimore.

134. Hayes, W. J., Jr., and Gaines, T. B. (1950): Control of Norway rats with residual rodenticide warfarin. *Public Health Rep.,* 65:1537.

135. Henning, C. H. (1933): Application of the halogen derivatives of the hydrocarbons with particular reference to methyl bromide. *Chem. Ind. (Lond.),* 52:462.

136. Herken, H., Kewitz, H., and Klempau, I. (1952): Wirkungsverluste von Krampfgiften durch Hexochlorcyclohexan. *Arch. Exp. Pharmacol.,* 215:217–230.

137. Hill, D. L., Shih, T. W., Johnston, T. P., and Struck, R. F. (1978): Macromolecular binding and metabolism of the carcinogen 1,2-dibromoethane. *Cancer Res.,* 38:2438–2442.

138. Hine, C. H. (1969): Methyl bromide poisoning: A review of ten cases. *J. Occup. Med.,* 11:1.

139. Hodge, H. C., Boyce, A. M., Deichmann, W. B., and Kraybill, H. F. (1967): Toxicology and no-effect levels of aldrin and dieldrin. *Toxicol. Appl. Pharmacol.,* 10:613–757.

140. Holan, G. (1969): New halocyclopropane insecticides and the mode of action of DDT. *Nature (Lond.),* 221:1025–1029.

141. Holling, H. E., and Clarke, C. A. (1944): Methyl bromide intoxication. *J. R. Navy Med. Ser.,* 30:218.

142. Holsapple, M. P., and Yim, G. K. W. (1981): Decreased gastrointestinal ulcerogenicity of chlordimeform, a basic anti-inflammatory agent. *Toxicol. Appl. Pharmacol.,* 59:107.

143. Hsu, L. L., Adams, P. M., Fanini, D., and Legator, M. S. (1985): Ethylene dibromide; effects of paternal exposure on the neurotransmitter enzymes in the developing brain of F_1 progeny. *Mutat. Res.,* 147:197–203.

144. Hughs, R. D., Milburn, P., and Williams, R. T. (1973): Biliary excretion of some dequaternary ammonium cations in the rat guinea pig and rabbit. *Biochem. J.,* 136:979–984.

145. IARC (1977): Ethylene dibromide. In: *IARC Monographs on the Evaluation of Carcinogenic Risk of Chemicals to Humans, Vol. 15: Some Fumigants, the Herbicides 2,4-D and 2,4,5-T, Chlorinated Dibenzodioxine, and Miscellaneous Industrial Chemicals.* pp. 195–204. International Agency for Research on Cancer, Lyon, France.

146. IARC (1979): Hexachlorobenzene. In: *IARC Monographs on the Evaluation of the Carcinogenic Risk of Chemicals to Humans, Vol. 20: Some Halogenated Hydrocarbons,* pp. 155 and 83–96. International Agency for Research on Cancer, Lyon, France.

147. Ingebrigtsen, K., and Nafstad, I. (1983): Distribution and elimination of ^{14}C-hexachlorobenzene after single oral exposure in the male rat. *Acta Pharmacol. Toxicol.,* 52:254–260.

148. Innes, J. R. M., Ulland, R. M., Valerio, M. G., et al. (1969): Bioassay

of pesticides and industrial chemicals for tumorogenicity in mice: A preliminary note. *J. Natl. Cancer Inst.*, 42:1101.

149. Inoue, T., Miyazawa, T., Tanahashi, N., et al. (1982): Induction of sex-linked recessive lethal mutations in *Drosophila melanogaster* males by gaseous 1,2-dibromo-3-chloropropane (DBCP). *Mutat. Res.*, 105:89.

150. Irish, D. D., Adams, E. M., Spencer, H. C., and Rowe, V. K., (1940): Response attending exposure of laboratory animals to vapors of methyl bromide. *J. Ind. Hyg. Toxicol.*, 22:218.

151. Jackson, D. A., and Gardner, D. R. (1978): *In vitro* effects of DDT analogs on trout brain M⁺⁺-ATPases. 1. Specificity and physiological significance. *Pestic. Biochem. Physiol.*, 8:113–122.

152. Jager, K. W. (1970): *Aldrin, Dieldrin, Endrin, and Telodrin.* Elsevier, NY.

153. Johnson, M. K. (1969): A phosphorylation site in brain and the delayed neurotoxic effect of some organophosphorus compounds. *Biochem. J.*, 111:487–495.

154. Johnson, M. K. (1970): Organophosphorus and other inhibitors of brain "neurotoxic esterase" and the development of delayed neuropathy in hens. *Biochem. J.*, 120:523–531.

155. Johnson, M. K. (1974): The primary biochemical lesion leading to the delayed neurotoxic effects of some organophosphorus esters. *J. Neurochem.*, 23:785–789.

156. Johnson, R. L., Gehring, P. J., Kociba, R. J., and Schwetz, B. A. (1973): Chlorinated dibenzodioxins and pentachlorophenol. *Environ. Health Perspect.*, 5:171.

157. Jones, A. T., Jones, R. C., and Longley, E. O. (1964): Environmental and clinical aspects of bulk wheat fumigation with aluminum phosphide. *Am. Ind. Hyg. Assoc. J.*, 25:376–379.

158. Jordi, A. U. (1953): Absorption of methyl bromide through the intact skin. A report of one fatal and two non-fatal cases. *J. Aviat. Med.*, 24:536–539.

159. Kale, P. G., and Baum, J. W. (1979): Sensitivity of *Drosophila melanogaster* to low concentrations of gaseous mutagens. II. Chronic exposures. *Mutat. Res.*, 68:59–68.

160. Kale, P. G., and Baum, J. W. (1981): Sensitivity of *Drosophila melanogaster* to low concentrations of gaseous mutagens. III. Dose-rate effects. *Environ. Mutagen.*, 3:65–70.

161. Kale, P. G., and Baum, J. W. (1982): Genetic effects of 1,2-dibromo-3-chloropropane (DBCP) in *Drosophila. Environ. Mutagen.*, 4:681–687.

162. Kashi, K. P., and Chefurka, W. (1976): The effect of phosphine on the absorption and circular dichronic spectra of cytochrome c and cytochrome oxidase. *Pestic. Biochem. Physiol.*, 6:350–362.

163. Kato, Y., Sato, K., Matano, O., and Goto, S. (1980): Alkylation of cellular macromolecules by reactive metabolic intermediate of DBCP. *J. Pestic. Sci.*, 5:45–53.

164. Kato, Y., Sato, K., Maki, S., et al. (1979): Metabolic fate of 1,2-dibromo-3-chloropropane (DBCP) in rats. *J. Pestic. Sci.*, 4:195–203.

164a. Kato, T., Ueda, K., Fujimoto, K. (1964): New insecticidally active chrysanthemates. *Agr. Biol. Chem.*, 28:914–915.

165. Kawalek, J. C., Andrews, A. W., and Pienta, R. J. (1979): 1-Naphthylthiourea: A mutagenic rodenticide that transforms hamster embryo cells. *Mol. Pharmacol.*, 15:678–684.

166. Kelso, G. L., Wilkinson, R. R., Ferguson, T. L., et al. (1976): Development of information on pesticides manufacturing for source assessment. EPA Contract No. 68-02-1324, Task 43, p. 75. Government Printing Office, Washington, D.C.

167. Khera, K. S. (1974): Teratogenicity and dominant lethal studies on hexachlorobenzene in rats. *Food Cosmet. Toxicol.*, 12:471–477.

168. Khera, K. S., and McKinley, W. P. (1972): Pre- and postnatal studies of 2,4,5-T and 2,4-D and their derivatives in rats. *Toxicol. Appl. Pharmacol.*, 22:14.

169. Kimbrough, R. D., and Gaines, T. B. (1970): Toxicity of paraquat to the rat and its effect on rat lungs. *Toxicol. Appl. Pharmacol.*, 17:679.

170. Kimbrough, R. D., and Linder, R. E. (1973): The ultrastructure of the paraquat lung legion in the rat. *Environ. Res.*, 6:265.

171. *Kirk-Othmer* (1982): *Encyclopedia of Chemical Technology, Vol. 18: Plant-Growth Substances to Potassium Compounds*, 3rd ed., p. 305. John Wiley, NY.

172. Kitselman, C. H. (1953): Long-term studies on dogs fed aldrin and dieldrin in sublethal dosages with reference to the histopathological findings and reproduction. *J. Am. Vet. Med. Assoc.*, 123:28.

173. Klimmer, O. R. (1969): Contribution to the study of the action of phosphine. On the question of so-called phosphine poisoning. *Arch. Toxicol.*, 24:164–187.

174. Kluwe, W. M. (1981): Acute toxicity of 1,2-dibromo-3-chloropropane in the F344 rat II. Development and repair of the renal, epididymal, testicular, and hepatic lesions. *Toxicol. Appl. Pharmacol.*, 59:84–95.

175. Kluwe, W. M., Lamb, J. C., Greenwell, A., and Harrington, F. W. (1983): 1,2-Dibromo-3-chloropropane (DBCP)-induced infertility in male rats mediated by a post-testicular effect. *Toxicol. Appl. Pharmacol.*, 71:294–298.

176. Knowles, C. O., and Sen Gupa, A. K. (1970): N′-(4-chloro-o-tolyl)-N,N-dimethylformamidine-¹⁴C (Galecron) and 4-chloro-o-toluidine-¹⁴C metabolism in the white rat. *J. Econ. Entomol.*, 63:856.

177. Knudsten, T., Verschuuren, H. G., Den Tonkelaar, E. M., and Kroes, R. (1974): Short-term toxicity of pentachlorophenol. *Toxicology*, 2:141.

178. Kociba, R. J., Keyes, D. J., Lisowe, R. W., et al. (1979): Results of a 2-year chronic toxicity and oncogenic study of rats ingesting diets containing 2,4,5-trichlorophenoxyacetic acid (2,4,5-T). *Food Cosmet. Toxicol.*, 17:205.

179. Kolmodin-Hedman, B., Alexanderson, B., and Sjoqvist, F. (1971): Effects of exposure to lindane on drug metabolism: Decreased hexobarbital sleeping times and increased antipyrine disappearance rate in rats. *Toxicol. Appl. Pharmacol.*, 20:299–307.

179a. Koschier, F. J., and Acara, M. (1978): Renal tubular transport of 2,4,5-trichlorophenoxyacetate (2,4,5-T). *Pharmacologist*, 20:222.

180. Koss, G., Seubert, S., Seubert, A., et al. (1980): Hexachlorobenzene and 2,4,5,2′,4′,5′-hexachlorobenzene—A comparison of their distribution, biotransformation and porphyrinogenic action in female rats. In: *Mechanisms of Toxicity and Hazard Evaluation*, edited by B. Holmstedt, R. Lauwerys, M. Mercier, and Roberfroids, pp. 517–520. Elsevier/North-Holland Bio-medical Press, NY.

181. Krueger, H. R., O'Brien, R. D., and Dauterman, W. C. (1960): Relationship between metabolism and differential toxicity in insects and mice of diazinon, dimethoate, parathion and acethion. *Econ. Entomol.*, 53:25–31.

182. Kuiper-Goodman, T., Grant, D. C., Moodie, C. A., et al. (1977): Subacute toxicity of hexachlorobenzene in the rat. *Toxicol. Appl. Pharmacol.*, 40:529–549.

183. Lambrecht, R. W., Erturk, E., Grunden, E., et al. (1982): Hepatoxicity and tumorigenicity of hexachlorobenzene (HCB) in Syrian golden hamsters (H) after subchronic administration. *Fed. Proc.*, 41:329.

184. Lange, P. F., and Terveer, J. (1954): Warfarin poisoning. *U. S. Armed Forces Med. J.*, 5:871–877.

185. Lanham, J. M. (1981): Effects of 1,2-dibromo-3-chloropropane (DBCP) on an exposed work population (abstract). *Annual Meeting of Society of Toxicology.*

186. Lantz, G. D., Cunningham, G. R., Huckins, C., and Lipshultz, L. I. (1981): Recovery from severe oligospermia after exposure to dibromochloropropane, *Fertil. Steril.*, 35:46–53.

187. Lawrence, L. J., and Casida, J. E. (1982): Pyrethroid toxicology: Mouse intracerebral structure–activity relationships. *Pestic. Biochem. Physiol.*, 18:9–14.

188. Lawrence, L. J., and Casida, J. E. (1983): Stereospecific action of pyrethroid insecticides in the gamma-aminobutyric acid receptor-ionophore complex. *Science*, 221:1399–1401.

189. Laws, E. R., Jr., Curley, A., and Biros, F. J. (1967): Men with intensive occupational exposure to DDT. A clinical and chemical study. *Arch. Environ. Health*, 15:766–775.

190. Leahy, J. P. (1985): The mode of action of pyrethroids on insects. In: *The Pyrethroid Insecticides*, edited by J. P. Leahy. Taylor and Francis, Philadelphia.

191. Lee, I. P., and Suzuki, K. (1979): Induction of unscheduled DNA synthesis in mouse germ cells following 1,2-dibromo-3-chloropropane (DBCP) exposure. *Mutat. Res.*, 68:169–173.

192. Le Goupil, M. (1932): Les Proprieties Insecticide du Bromure de methyle. *Rev. Pathol. Veg. Entomol. Agr. Fr.*, pp. 19, 169.

193. Letz, G. A., Pond, S. M., Osterloh, J. D., et al. (1984): Two fatalities after acute occupational exposure to ethylene dibromide. *JAMA*, 252:2428–2431.

194. Lindquest, N. G., and Ullberg, S. (1971): Distribution of the herbicides 2,4-D and 2,4,5-T in pregnant mice. Accumulation in the yoke sack epithelium. *Experientia*, 27:1439.

195. Link, K. P., Berg, D., and Barker, W. M. (1965): Partial fate of warfarin in the rat. *Science,* 150:378.
196. Lipschultz, L. I., Ross, E. C., Whorton, M. D., et al. (1980): Dibromochloropropane (DBCP) and its effects on testicular function in man. *J. Urol.,* 124:464–468.
197. Litchfield, M. H., Damel, J. W., and Longshaw, S. (1973): Tissue distribution of bipyridynium herbicides diquat and paraquat in rats and mice. *Toxicology,* 1:155.
198. Lovegrove, F. T. B. (1963): Three cases of strychnine poisoning. *Med. J. Aust.,* 1:783.
199. Lund, A. E., and Narahashi, T. (1981): Kinetics of sodium channel modification by the insecticide tetramethrin in squid axon membranes. *J. Pharmacol. Exp. Ther.,* 219:464–73.
200. Maag, T. A., and Schmittle, S. C. (1962): The effect of methyl bromide upon *Salmonella. Am. J. Vet. Res.,* 23:1289.
201. Mackie, D. B. (1938): Methyl bromide: Its expectancy as a fumigant. *J. Econ. Entomol.,* 31:70.
202. Maddy, K. T. (1976): Pesticides reported by physicians in California as causes of illness in employed persons in 1974. Pesticide Illness Report No. HS-171, p. 4. California Department of Food and Agriculture, Sacramento.
203. Malmqvist, E., Grossman, G., Ivenmark, B., and Robertson, B. (1973): Pulmonary phospholipids and surface properties of alveolar wash in experimental paraquat poisoning. *Scand. J. Respir. Dis.,* 54:206–214.
204. Manson, M. M., and Smith, A. G. (1984): Effect of hexachlorobenzene on male and female rat hepatic gamma-glutamyl transpeptidase levels. *Cancer Lett.,* 22:227–234.
205. Marquez, M. E. (1978): 1,2-Dibromo-3-chloropropane (DBCP), nematocide with sterilizing action in man. *S.P.M.,* 20:195–200.
206. Matsumura, F. (1985): *Toxicology of Insecticides.* Plenum Press, NY.
207. Matsumura, F., and Clark, J. M. (1982): ATP-utilizing systems in the squid axon: A review on the biochemical aspects of ion-transport. *Progr. Neurobiol.,* 18:231–255.
208. Matsumura, F., and Ghiasuddin, S. M. (1979): DDT-sensitive Ca-ATPase in the axonic membrane. In: *Neurotoxicology of Insecticides and Pheromones,* edited by T. Narahashi, pp. 245–257. Plenum Press, NY.
209. Matsumura, F., and O'Brien, R. D. (1963): A comparative study of the modes of action of fluoroacetamide and fluoroacetate in the mouse and American cockroach. *Biochem. Pharmacol.,* 12:1201.
210. Mazzanti, L., Lopez, M., and Berti, M. G. (1964): Selective destruction in testes induced by fluoroacetamide. *Experientia,* 20:492.
211. McNamara, B. P., and Krop, S. (1947): Pharmacological effects of lindane and isomers. Chemical Corps, U.S. Army Medical Division, Report 125.
212. McPhillips, J. J. (1969): Altered sensitivity to drugs following repeated injections of a cholinesterase inhibitor to rats. *Toxicol. Appl. Pharmacol.,* 14:67–73.
213. Medinsky, M. A., Bond, J. A., Dutcher, J. S., and Birnbaum, L. S. (1984): Disposition of [^{14}C] methyl bromide in Fischer 344 rats after oral and intraperitoneal administration. *Toxicology,* 32:187.
214. Medinsky, M. A., Dutcher, J. S., Bond, J. A., et al. (1985): Uptake and excretion of [^{14}C] methyl bromide as influenced by exposure concentration. *Toxicol. Appl. Pharmacol.,* 78:215.
215. Menge, J. A., Munnecke, D. E., Johnson, E. L., and Carnes, D. W. (1978): Dosage response of the vesicular-arbuscular aycorrhizal fungi glomus fasciuculatus and G. constrictus to methyl bromide. *Phytopathology,* 68(9):1368.
216. Meyrick, B., Miller, J., and Reid, L. (1972): Pulmonary oedema induced by ANTU or by high or low oxygen concentrations in rat—An electron microscopic study. *Br. J. Exp. Pathol.,* 45:347–358.
217. Millard, S. A., Hart, M. B., and Shimek, J. F. (1973): Enzymes controlling cerebral DNA synthesis: Response to 2,4,5-T and kerachlorophene. *Biochem. Biophys. Acta,* 308:270.
218. Miller, D. P., and Haggard, H. W. (1943): Intracellular penetration of bromide as a feature in the toxicity of alkyl bromides. *J. Ind. Hyg. Toxicol.,* 25:423.
219. Miyata, R., Nohmi, T., Yoshikawa, K., and Ishidate, M. (1981): Metabolic activation of *p*-nitrotoluene and trichloroethylene by rat-liver S9 or mouse-liver S-9 fractions in *Salmonella typhimurium* strains. *Bull. Natl. Inst. Hyg. Sci.,* 99:60–95 (abstr.).
220. Modrzejewski, J., and Myslak, Z. (1967): Phosphine poisoning during corn vermin fumigation in a port elevator. *J. Med. Pract.,* 18:78–82.
221. Mortelmans, K., Hayworth, S., Speck, W., and Zieger, E. (1984): Mutagenicity testing of agent orange components and related chemicals. *Toxicol. Appl. Pharmacol.,* 75:137.
222. Murray, R. E., and Gibson, J. E. (1974): Paraquat disposition in rats, guinea pigs, and monkeys. *Toxicol. Appl. Pharmacol.,* 27:283.
223. Nadzhimutdinov, K. N., Kamilov, I. K., and Muzrabekov, S. M. (1974): Influence of pesticides on the duration of hexobarbital induced sleep. *Farmakol. Toksikol.,* 37:533–537.
224. Nagasaki, H., Tomii, S., Mega, T., Marugami, M., and Ito, N. (1971): Development of hepatomas in mice treated with benzene hexachloride. *Gann,* 62:431.
225. Nagasaki, H., Tomii, S., Mega, T., et al. (1972): Hepatocarcinogenic effect of alpha-, beta-, gamma-, and delta-isomers of benzene hexachloride in mice. *Gann,* 63:393.
226. Narahashi, T. (1962): Nature of the negative afterpotential increased by the insecticide allethrin in cockroach giant axons. *J. Cell Comp. Physiol.,* 59:67–76.
227. Narahashi, T. (1963): Properties of insect axons. *Adv. Insect Physiol.,* 1:175–244.
228. Narahashi, T., and Anderson, N. C. (1967): Mechanism of excitation block by the insecticide allethrin applied externally and internally to squid giant axons. *Toxicol. Appl. Pharmacol.,* 10:529–547.
229. Narahashi, T., and Haas, H. G. (1968): Interaction of DDT with the components of lobster nerve membrane conductance. *J. Gen. Physiol.,* 51:177–198.
230. National Cancer Institute (1978): Bioassay of dibromochloropropane for possible carcinogenicity. Carcinogenesis Technical Report Series, No. 28, National Institutes of Health, U.S. Department of Health, Education and Welfare, DHEW Publication No. (NIH) 78-828, Washington, D.C.
231. National Cancer Institute (1978): Bioassay of 1,2-dibromoethane for possible carcinogenicity. Carcinogenesis Technical Report, No. 86, National Cancer Institute, NIH Publication No. 78-1336, Washington, D.C.
232. National Research Council (1987): *Regulating Pesticides in Food.* National Academy of Science Press, Washington, D.C.
233. National Toxicology Program (1987): Carcinogenesis bioassay of 1,2-dibromo-3-chloropropane. Technical Report No. 206, National Institutes of Health, U.S. Department of Health and Human Services, NIH Publication No. 87-1762, Washington, D.C.
234. National Toxicology Program (1985): Fourth annual report on carcinogens. National Toxicology Program, U.S. Department of Health and Human Services, NTP No. 85-002, Washington, D.C.
235. National Toxicology Program (1982): Carcinogenesis bioassay of 1,2-dibromoethane. Technical Report No. 210, National Toxicology Program, NIH Publication No. 82-1766, Washington, D.C.
236. Nayshteyn, S. Y., and Leybovich, D. L. (1971): Low doses of DDT, gamma-HCCH and mixtures of these: Effect on sexual function and embryogenesis in rats. *Gig. Sanit.,* 36:19–22.
237. Neilson, K., Kaempe, B., and Jensen-Holm, J. (1965): Fatal poisoning in man by 2,4-dichlorophenoxyacetic acid (2,4-D): Determination of the agent in forensic materials. *Acta Pharmacol. Toxicol.,* 22:224.
237a. NIOSH (1985): Registry of toxic effects of chemical substances, edited by R. C. Lewis and D. V. Sweet. U.S. Government Printing Office, Washington, D.C.
238. NIOSH (1977): NIOSH Criteria for a Recommended Standard Occupational Exposure to Ethylene Dibromide. National Institute for Occupational Safety and Health, U.S. Department of Health, Education, and Welfare, Washington, D.C.
239. Nishimura, M., Umeda, M., Ishizu, S., and Sato, M. (1980): Effect of methyl bromide on cultured mammalian cells. *J. Toxicol. Sci.,* 5:321.
240. Nuckolls, A. H. (1933): Report on the comparative life, fire and explosion hazards of common refrigerants. Underwriters' Laboratories Report on Miscellaneous Hazards, No. 2375.
241. Offner, R. R., and Cavery, H. O. (1945): Determination of DDT (2,2-bis(*p*-chlorophenyl)-1,1,1-trichloroethane) and its metabolite

in biological materials by use of the Schechter–Haller method. *J. Pharmacol. Exp. Ther.*, 85:363–370.

242. Olson, R. J., Trumble, T. E., and Gamble, W. (1974): Alterations in cholesterol and fatty acid synthesis in rat liver homogenates by aryloxy acids. *Biochem. J.*, 142:445–448.

243. Olson, W. A., Habermann, R. T., Weisburger, E. K., et al. (1973): Induction of stomach cancer in rats and mice by halogenated aliphatic fumigants. *J. Natl. Cancer Inst.*, 51:1993.

244. Ott, M. D., Scharnweber, H. C., and Langner, R. R. (1980): Mortality experience of 161 employees exposed to ethylene dibromide in two production units. *Br. J. Ind. Med.*, 37:163–168.

245. Overstreet, D. H. (1973): The effects of pilocarpine on the drinking behavior of rats following acute and chronic treatment with diisopropylfluorophosphate and during withdrawal. *Behav. Biol.*, 9:257–263.

246. Overstreet, D. H. (1974): Reduced behavioral effects of pilocarpine during chronic treatment with DFP. *Behav. Biol.*, 11:49–58.

247. Padilla, S., and Veronesi, B. (1985): The relationship between neurological damage and neurotoxic esterase inhibition in rats acutely exposed to triortho-cresyl phosphate. *Toxicol. Appl. Pharmacol.*, 78:78–87.

248. Panel on Herbicides (1971): Report on 2,4,5-T. A report of the panel on herbicides on the President's Science Advisory Committee. Executive Office of the President, Office of Science and Technology, U.S. Government Printing Office, Washington, D.C.

249. Pattison, F. L. M. (1959): *Toxic Aliphatic Fluorine Compounds.* Elsevier, NY.

250. Pernod, J., Tommasi, M., Damasio, R., and Magerand, J. (1961): Intoxication Aigue Collective Par Le Bromure De Methyle. *Bull. Soc. Med. (Paris)*, 7:235.

251. Peters, H. A. (1976): Hexachlorobenzene poisoning in Turkey. *Fed. Proc.*, 35:2400–2403.

252. Peters, R. A. (1963): *Biochemical Lesions and Lethal Synthesis.* Macmillan, NY.

253. Phillips, M. A., and Worden, A. N. (1956): Toxicity of fluoroacetamide. *Lancet*, ii:731.

254. Piper, W. N., Rose, J. Q., and Gehring, P. J. (1972): Metabolism of 2,4,5-trichlorophenoxyacetic acid (2,4,5-T) in rats. *Toxicol. Appl. Pharmacol.*, 22:317.

255. Piper, W. N., Rose, M. Q., Leng, M. L., and Gehring, P. J. (1973): The fate of 2,4,5-T following oral administration to rats and dogs. *Toxicol. Appl. Pharmacol.*, 26:399.

256. Plewa, M., Wagner, E. D., Gentile, G. J., and Gentile, J. M. (1984): An evaluation of the genotoxic properties of herbicides following plant and animal activation. *Mut. Res.*, 136:233.

257. Plotnick, H. B., and Conner, W. L. (1976): Tissue distribution of ^{14}C-labeled ethylene dibromide in the guinea pig. *Res. Commun. Chem. Pathol. Pharmacol.*, 13:251–258.

258. Poe, C. F., Suchy, J. E., and Sitt, N. E. (1936): Toxicity of strychnine for male and female rats of different ages. *J. Pharmacol. Exp. Ther.*, 58:239–242.

259. Poland, A. P., Smith, D., Metter, G., and Possick, P. (1971): A health survey of workers in a 2,4-D and 2,4,5-T plant with special attention to chloracne, porphyria cutanea tarda, and psychological parameters. *Arch. Environ. Health*, 22:316–327.

260. Potashnik, G. I., Ben-Aderet, N., Israeli, R., Yanai-Inbar, I., and Sober, I. (1978): Suppressive effect of DBCP on human spermatogenesis. *Fertil. Steril.*, 30:444–447.

261. Potashnik, G. I., Yanai-Inbar, I., and Sober, I. (1981): Recovery of human testicular function suppression caused by dibromochloropropane. Presented March 1981, Berlin.

262. Powell, D. F. (1978): The effects on Narcissus bulbs of methyl bromide fumigation used to control bulb scale mite. *Plant Pathol.*, 26(2):79.

263. Prival, M. J., McCoy, E. C., Gutter, B., and Rosenkranz, H. S. (1977): Tris-(2,3-dibromopropyl)phosphate: Mutagenicity of a widely used flame retardant. *Science*, 195:76–78.

264. Pyorala, K. (1968): Sex differences in the clotting factor response to warfarin and the rate of warfarin metabolism in the rat. *Ann. Med. Exp. Biol. Fenn.*, 46:35.

265. Rannug, U., Sundvall, A., and Ramel, C. (1978): The mutagenic effect of 1,2-dibromoethane on *Salmonella typhimurium*. I. Activation through conjugation with glutathione *in vitro*. *Chem. Biol. Interact.*, 20:1–16.

266. Rao, K. S., Burek, J. D., John, J. A., et al. (1983): Toxicologic and reproductive effects of inhaled 1,2-dibromo-3-chloropropane in rats. *Fund. Appl. Toxicol.*, 3:104–110.

267. Rao, K. S., Burek, J. D., Murray, F. J., et al. (1982): Toxicologic and reproductive effects of inhaled 1,2-dibromo-3-chloropropane in rabbits. *Fund. Appl. Toxicol.*, 2:41–251.

268. Rashatwar, S. S., and Matsumura, F. (1985): Interaction of DDT and pyrethroids with calmodulin and its significance in the expression of enzyme activities of phosphodiesterase. *Biochem. Pharmacol.*, 34:1689–1694.

269. Ray, D. E. (1982): The contrasting actions of two pyrethroids in the rat. *Neurobehav. Toxicol. Teratol.*, 4:801–804.

269a. Ray, D. E., and Crener, J. E. (1979): The action of decamethrin (a synthetic pyrethroid) on the rat. *Pestic. Biochem. Physiol.*, 10:330–340.

270. Renner, H. A. (1981): Biotransformation of the fungicides hexachlorobenzene and pentachloronitrobenzene. *Xenobiotica*, 11:435–446.

271. Reznik, G., Reznik-Schuller, H., Ward, J. M., and Stinson, S. F. (1980): Morphology of nasal-cavity tumours in rats after chronic inhalation of 1,2-dibromo-3-chloropropane. *Br. J. Cancer*, 42:772–781.

272. Reznik, G., Stinson, S. F., and Ward, J. M. (1980): Lung tumors induced by chronic inhalation of 1,2-dibromo-3-chloropropane in B6C3F$_1$ mice. *Cancer Lett.*, 10:339–342.

273. Reznik, G., Ulland, B., Stinson, S. F., and Ward, J. M. (1980): Morphology and sex-dependent manifestation of nasal tumors in B6C3F$_1$ mice after chronic inhalation of 1,2-dibromo-3-chloropropane. *J. Cancer Res. Clin. Oncol.*, 98:75–83.

274. Rhodes, M. L. (1974): Hypoxic protection in paraquat poisoning. A model for respiratory distress syndrome. *Chest.*, 66:341.

275. Richardson, B. W. (1891): Methyl bromide. *Asclepiad (Lond.)*, 8:239.

276. Richardson, B. W. (1897): Some further additions to therapeutics. *Practitioner*, 6:337.

277. Richter, E., Renner, G., Bayerl, J., and Wick, M. (1981): Differences in the biotransformation of hexachlorobenzene (HCB) in male and female rats. *Chemosphere*, 10:779–785.

278. Rose, M. S., and Smith, L. L. (1977): Tissue uptake of paraquat and diquat. *Gen. Pharmacol.*, 8:173–176.

279. Rosenkranz, H. S. (1975): Genetic activity of 1,2-dibromo-3-chloropropane, a widely used fumigant. *Bull. Environ. Contam. Toxicol.*, 14:8–12.

280. Rowe, U. K., and Hymas, T. A. (1954): Summary of toxicological information on 2,4-D and 2,4,5-T type herbicides and an evaluation of the hazards to livestock associated with their use. *Am. J. Vet. Res.*, 15:622.

281. Rowe, V. K., Spencer, H. C., McCollister, D. D., et al. (1952): Toxicity of ethylene dibromide determined in experimental animals. *Arch. Ind. Hyg.*, 6:158–173.

282. Rowe, V. K., Spencer, H. C., McCollister, D. D., et al. (1957): Toxicity of ethylene dibromide determined in experimental animals. *Am. Med. Assoc. Arch. Ind. Hyg. Occup. Med.*, 6:158–163.

283. Ruddick, J. A., and Newsome, W. H. (1979): A teratogenicity and tissue distribution study on dibromochloropropane in the rat. *Bull. Environ. Contam. Toxicol.*, 21:483–487.

284. Saito-Suzuki, R., Teramoto, S., and Shirasu, Y. (1982): Dominant lethal studies in rats with 1,2-dibromo-3-chloropropane and its structurally related compounds. *Mutat. Res.*, 101:321–327.

285. Sandifer, S. H., Wilkins, R. T., Loanholt, C. B., et al. (1979): Spermatogenesis in agricultural workers exposed to dibromochloropropane (DBCP). *Bull. Environ. Contam. Toxicol.*, 23:703–710.

285a. Sandoz Crop Protection Corporation (1986): Material safety data sheet for Banvel herbicide (dicamba) by Sandoz Crop Protection Corp., Chicago, IL.

286. Sax, N. I. (1984): *Dangerous Properties of Industrial Material*, 6th ed. Van Nostrand Reinhold, NY.

286a. Schechter, M. S., Green, N., and LaForge, F. B. (1949): Constituents of pyrethrum flowers. XXIII. Cinerolone and the synthesis of related cyclopentenolones. *J. Amer. Chem. Soc.*, 71:3165–3173.

287. Schmittle, S. C. (1955): Studies on methyl bromide. I. The efficacy of methyl bromide fumigation on Newcastle disease virus. *Poultry Sci.*, 34:1219.

288. Schonborn, H., Schuster, H. P., and Koessling, F. K. (1971): Klinik

und Morphologie der akuten peroralen diquatintoxikation (re-lone). *Arch. Toxicol.,* 27:204.

289. Schwetz, B. A., and Gehring, P. J. (1973): The effect of tetrachlorophenol and pentachlorophenol on rat embryonal and fetal development. *Toxicol. Appl. Pharmacol.,* 25:455.

290. Schwetz, B. A., Keeler, P. A., and Gehring, P. J. (1974): The effect of purified and commercial grade pentachlorophenol on rat embryonal and fetal development. *Toxicol. Appl. Pharmacol.,* 28:151.

291. Schwetz, B. A., Quast, J. F., Keeler, P. A., et al. (1977): Results of two-year toxicity and reproduction studies on pentachlorophenol in rats. In: *Pentachlorophenol,* edited by K. R. Rao, p. 301. Plenum Press, NY.

292. Schwetz, B. A., Sparchu, G. L., and Gehring, P. J. (1971): The effect of 2,4-D and esters of 2,4-D on rat embryonal, fetal and neonatal growth and development. *Food Cosmet. Toxicol.,* 9:801.

293. Seabury, J. H. (1963): Toxicity of 2,4-dichlorophenoxyacetic acid for man and dog. *Arch. Environ. Health,* 7:202.

294. Secretary's Commission on Pesticides (1969): Report of the Secretary's Commission on Pesticides and Their Relationship to Environmental Health. U.S. Department of Health, Education and Welfare, Government Printing Office, Washington, D.C.

295. Seidenfield, J., Wycoff, D., Zavala D., and Richardson, H. (1978): Paraquat lung injury in rabbits. *Br. J. Ind. Med.,* 35:245–257.

295a. Shankland, D. L. (1982): Neurotoxic action of chlorinated hydrocarbon insecticides. *Neurobehav. Toxicol. Teratol.,* 4:805–811.

296. Shaul, W. L., Emery, H., and Hall, J. G. (1975): Chrondrodesplasia punctata and maternal warfarin use during pregnancy. *Am. J. Dis. Child.,* 129:360–362.

297. Sherby, S. M., Eldefrawi, A. T., Deshpande, S. S., et al. (1986): Effects of pyrethroids on nicotinic acetylcholine receptor binding and function. *Pest. Biochem. Physiol.,* 26:107–115.

298. Shimkin, M. B., and Anderson, H. H. (1936): Acute toxicities of rotenone and mixed pyrethrins in mammals. *Proc. Soc. Exp. Biol. Med.,* 34:135–138.

299. Shirai, T., Miyata, Y., Nakanishi, K., et al. (1978): Hepatocarcinogenicity of polychlorinated diterphenyl (PCT) in ICR mice and its enhancement of hexachlorobenzene (HCB). *Cancer Lett.,* 4:271–275.

300. Short, R. D., Minor, J. L., Ferguson, B., et al. (1976): The developmental toxicity of ethylene dibromide inhaled by rats and mice during organogenesis. U.S. NTIS EPA 560/6-77-018 PB 256659.

301. Short, R. D., Minor, J. L., Winston, J. M., et al. (1978): Inhalation of ethylene dibromide during gestation by rats and mice. *Toxicol. Appl. Pharmacol.,* 46:173–182.

302. Short, R. D., Winston, J. M., Hong, C. B., et al. (1979): Effects of ethylene dibromide on reproduction in male and female rats. *Toxicol. Appl. Pharmacol.,* 49:79–105.

303. Simmon, V. F., and Tardiff, R. (1978): The mutagenic activity of halogenated compounds found in chlorinated drinking water. In: *Water Chlorination: Environmental Impact and Health Effects, Vol. 2,* edited by R. Jolley, p. 417. Ann Arbor Science Publishers, Ann Arbor.

304. Simmons, S. W. (1959): The use of DDT insecticides in human medicine. In: *DDT, The Insecticide Dichlorodiphenyltrichloroethane and Its Significance,* edited by P. Muller, pp. 251–502. Birkhauser Verlag, Basel.

305. Simon, G. S., Tardiff, R. G., and Borzelleca, J. F. (1979): Failure of hexachlorobenzene to induce dominant lethal mutations in the rat. *Toxicol. Appl. Pharmacol.,* 47:415–419.

306. Sjoden, P. O., and Soderberg, V. (1972): Sex dependent effects of prenatal 2,4,5-T on rats open-field behavior. *Physiol. Behav.,* 9:357.

307. Sjoden, P. O., and Soderberg, V. (1975): Long lasting effects of 2,4,5-T on open-field behavior in rats: Pre- and post-natal mediation. *Physiol. Psychol.,* 3:175.

308. Smith, A. G., Franscis, J. E., Dinsdale, D., et al. (1985): Hepatocarcinogenicity of hexachlorobenzene in rats and the sex difference in hepatic iron status and development of porphyria. *Carcinogenesis,* 6(4):631–636.

309. Smith, A. G., Franscis, J. E., Kay, S. J. E., et al. (1986): Mechanistic studies of the inhibition of hepatic uroporphyrinogen decarboxylase in C57BL/10 mice by iron-hexachlorobenzene synergism. *Biochem. J.,* 238:871–878.

310. Smith, F. A., Murray, F. J., John, K. D., et al. (1981): Three gen-

eration reproduction study of rats ingesting 2,4,5-trichlorophenoxyacetic acid in the diet. *Food Cosmet. Toxicol.,* 19:41.

311. Smith, L. L., Wright, A., Wyatt, I., and Rose, M. S. (1974): Effective treatment for paraquat poisoning in rats and its relevance to treatment of paraquat poisoning in man. *Br. Med. J.,* 4:469.

312. Smith, M. I., Elvove, E., Uglaer, P. J., Jr., et al. (1930): Pharmacological and chemical studies on the cause of so-called ginger paralysis. *Publ. Health Rep.,* 45:1703–1716.

313. Smith, P., Heath, D., and Kay, J. M. (1974): The pathogenesis and structure of paraquat-induced pulmonary fibroses in rats. *J. Pathol.,* 114:57–67.

314. Smith, T. M., and Stratton, G. W. (1986): Effects of pyrethroid insecticides on nontarget organisms. *Residue Rev.,* 97:93–120.

315. Sparschu, G. L., Dunn, F. L., Lisowe, R. W., and Rowe, U. K. (1971): Study on the effects of high levels of 2,4,5-trichlorophenoxyacetic acid on fetal development in the rat. *Food Cosmet. Toxicol.,* 9:527–530.

316. SRI (1983): Ethylene dibromide. In: *Monographs on Organic Air Pollutants.* Submitted to the National Cancer Institute under Contract No. NO1-CP-26004-02 by SRI International.

317. SRI (1983): Hexachlorobenzene. In: *Monographs on Organic Air Pollutants.* Submitted to NCI under Contract NO1-CP-26004-02 by SRI International, pp. 190, 1983.

318. Staatz, C. G., Bloom, A. S., and Lech, J. J. (1982): A pharmacological study of pyrethroid neurotoxicity in mice. *Pestic. Biochem. Physiol.,* 17:287–292.

319. Stancliffe, T. C., and Pirie, A. (1971): Production of superoxide radicals in reactions of the herbicide diquat. *Febs. Lett.,* 17:279–299.

320. Sternburg, J., Kearns, C. W., and Bruce, W. (1950): Absorption and metabolism of DDT by resistant and susceptible houseflies. *J. Econ. Entomol.,* 43:214–219.

321. Stevens, J. T., Stitzel, R. E., and McPhillips, J. J. (1972): Effects of anticholinesterase insecticides on hepatic microsomal metabolism. *J. Pharmacol. Exp. Ther.,* 181:576–583.

322. Stevens, K. M. (1981): Agent orange toxicity: A quantitative perspective. *Hum. Toxicol.,* 1:31.

323. Stewart, F. P., and Smith, A. G. (1986): Metabolism of the "mixed" cytochrome P-450 induced hexachlorobenzene by rat liver microsomes. *Biochem. Pharmacol.,* 35(13):2163–2170.

324. Stolzenberg, S. J., and Hine, C. H. (1979): Mutagenicity of halogenated and oxygenated 3-carbon compounds. *Toxicol. Appl. Pharmacol.,* 48:A47 (abstr.).

325. Stolzenberg, S. J., and Hine, C. H. (1980): Mutagenicity of 2- and 3-carbon halogenated compounds in the *Salmonella*/mammalian-microsome test. *Environ. Mutagen.,* 2:59–66.

326. Talcott, R. E., Shu, H., and Wei, E. T. (1977): Lipid peroxidation and paraquat toxicity. *Fed. Proc.,* 36:998.

327. Tan, E. L., and Hsie, A. W. (1981): Mutagenicity and cytotoxicity of haloethanes as studied in the CHO/HGPRT System. *Mutat. Res.,* 90:183–191.

328. Teramoto, S., Saito, R., Aoyama, H., and Shirasu, Y. (1980): Dominant lethal mutation induced in male rats by 1,2-dibromo-3-chloropropane. *Mutat. Res.,* 77:71–78.

329. Tezuka, H., Ando, N., Suzuki, R., et al. (1980): Sister-chromatid exchanges and chromosomal aberrations in cultured Chinese hamster cells treated with pesticides positive in microbial reversion assays. *Mutat. Res.,* 78:177–191.

330. Townsend, M. G., and Busvine, J. R. (1969): Mechanism of malathion resistance in the blowfly *Chrysomya putoria. Entomol. Exp. Appl.,* 12:243–267.

331. Treon, J. F., and Cleveland, F. P. (1955): Toxicity of certain chlorinated hydrocarbon insecticides for laboratory animals with special reference to aldrin and dieldrin. *Agric. Food Chem.,* 3:402–408.

332. Tye, R., and Engel, D. (1967): Distribution and excretion of dicamba by rats as determined by radiotracer technique. *J. Agric. Food Chem.,* 15:837–840.

333. Uchida, T., Dauterman, W. C., and O'Brien, R. D. (1964): The metabolism of dimethoate by vertebrate tissues. *J. Agric. Food Chem.,* 12:48–52.

334. Ullrich, V., and Staudinger, H. (1968): Metabolism in-vitro of warfarin by enzymatic and non-enzymatic systems. *Biochem. Pharmacol.,* 17:1662.

335. U.S. Department of Agriculture (1978): Agricultural stabilization and conservation service. *The Pesticide Review*, p. 32, Washington, D.C.

336. U.S. Environmental Protection Agency (1984): Ethylene dibromide; proposed revocation of exemption from the requirement of a tolerance. Proposed rule. *Fed. Register*, 49:6696–6703.

337. U.S. Environmental Protection Agency (1977): Intent to suspend any conditional registrations of pesticide products. *Fed. Register*, 42:48915–48922.

338. U.S. Environmental Protection Agency (1986): Pesticides; tolerances for ethylene dibromide on mangoes; extension of expiration date. Extension of rule, *Fed. Register*, 51:34469–34472.

339. U.S. Environmental Protection Agency (1977): Rebuttable presumption against registration and continued registration of pesticide products containing dibromochloropropane (DBCP). *Fed. Register*, 42:48026–48031.

340. U.S. Environmental Protection Agency (1984): Revocation of tolerances for ethylene dibromide. Final rule. *Fed. Register*, 49:22082–22085.

341. U.S. Environmental Protection Agency (1986): Tolerances and exemptions from tolerances for pesticide chemicals in or on raw agricultural commodities; revocation of exemption from tolerance for ethylene dibromide. Final rule, *Fed. Register*, 49:17144–17150.

342. U.S. Occupational Safety and Health Administration (1978): Occupational exposure to 1,2-dibromo-3-chloropropane (DBCP). Occupational safety and health standards, *Fed. Register*, 42:11514–11533.

343. U.S. Tariff Commission (1956): Synthetic organic chemicals. U.S. production and sales, 1955. Report No. 198, Second Series, p. 138. Government Printing Office, Washington, D.C. 1956.

344. U.S. Tariff Commission (1971): Synthetic organic chemicals. U.S. production and sales, 1969. TC Publication 412, pp. 191, 1971. Government Printing Office, Washington, D.C.

345. Vainio, H., Linnainmaa, K., Kahonon, M., et al. (1983): Hypolipidemia and peroxisome proliferation induced by phenoxyacetic acid herbicides in rats. *Biochem. Pharmacol.*, 32:2775.

346. van Asperen, K. (1954): Interaction of the isomers of benzenehexachloride in mice. *Arch. Int. Pharmacodyn. Ther.*, 99:368–377.

347. Van Bladeren, B. J., Breimer, D. D., Mohn, G. R., and Van der Gen, A. (1981): Metabolism and mutagenicity of dibromoethane and dibromomethane. *Mutat. Res.*, 85:270.

348. Van Duren, B. L., Goldschmidt, B. M., Loewengart, G., et al. (1979): Carcinogenicity of halogenated olefinic and aliphatic hydrocarbons in mice. *J. Natl. Cancer Inst.*, 63:1433–1439.

349. Van Gundy, S. D., and Van Gundy, R. L. (1971): Methyl bromide soil fumigation for continuous christmas tree (*Pinus radiata*) production. *Down to Earth*, 27:2.

350. Van Overbeek, J. (1964): Survey of mechanisms of herbicide action. In: *The Physiology and Biochemistry of Herbicides*, edited by L. J. Audus, pp. 387–400. Academic Press, London.

351. Veronisi, B. (1984): Effect of metabolic inhibition with piperonyl butoxide on rodent sensitivity to triortho-cresyl phosphate. *Exp. Neurol.*, 85:651–660.

352. Veronisi, B. (1984): A rodent model of organophosphorus-induced delayed neuropathy: Distribution of central (spinal cord) and peripheral nerve damage. *Neuropathol. Appl. Neurobiol.*, 110:357–368.

352a. Verschoyle, R. D., and Aldridge, W. N. (1980): Structure-activity relationships of some pyrethroids in rats. *Arch. Toxicol.*, 45:325–329.

352b. Verschoyle, R. D., and Barnes, J. M. (1972): Toxicity of natural and synthetic pyrethrins in rats. *Pestic. Biochem. Physiol.*, 2:308–311.

352c. Vijverberg, H. P. M., and van den Bercken, J. (1982): Structure related effects of pyrethroid insecticides on the lateral line sense organ and on peripheral nerves of the clawed frog, *Xenopus laerus*. *Pest. Biochem. Physiol.*, 18:315–324.

353. Villeneuve, D. C., van Logten, M. J., den Tonkelaar, E. M., et al. (1977): Combined effect of food deprivation and hexachlorobenzene feeding in rats. *Toxicol. Appl. Pharmacol.*, 41:202.

354. Villeneuve, D. C., and Hierlihy, S. L. (1975): Placental transfer of hexachlorobenzene. *Bull. Environ. Contam. Toxicol.*, 13:489–491.

355. Voogd, C. E., Knaap, A. G. A. C., Van Der Heijden, C. A., and Kramers, P. G. N. (1982): Gentoxicity of methyl bromide in short-term assay systems. *Mut. Res.*, 97:233.

356. Vos, J. G., Brouer, G. M. J., Van Leeuwen, F. X. R., and Wagenaar, S. (1983): Toxicity of hexachlorobenzene in the rat following combined pre- and post-natal exposure; comparison of effects on immune system, liver and lung. *Immunotoxicology (Proc. Int. Symp.)*, 1:219–235.

357. Wang, C. M., Narahashi, T., and Scuka, M. (1972): Mechanism of negative temperature coefficient of nerve blocking action of allethrin. *J. Pharmacol. Exp. Ther.*, 182:442–453.

358. Ward, J. C., and Spencer, D. A. (1947): Notes on the pharmacology of sodium fluoroacetate compound 1080. *J. Am. Pharm. Assoc. Sci. Ed.*, 36:59–62.

359. Ware, G. W. (1983): Pesticides: Chemical tools. In: *Pesticides: Theory and Application*, pp. 3–25. Freeman, NY.

360. Warren, D. W., Wisner, J. R., and Ahmad, N. (1984): Effects of 1,2-dibromo-3-chloropropane on male reproductive function in the rat. *Biol. Reprod.*, 31:454–463.

361. Wasserman, M., Wasserman, D., Kedar, E., et al. (1972): Effects of dieldrin and gamma BHC on serum proteins and PBI. *Bull. Environ. Contam. Toxicol.*, 8:177–185.

362. Weast, R. C. (1981): *Handbook of Chemistry and Physics*, 62nd ed., p. C-371. Chemical Rubber, Cleveland.

363. Weisburger, E. K. (1977): Carcinogenicity studies on halogenated hydrocarbons. *Environ. Health Perspect.*, 21:7–16.

364. Weisenberg, E., Arad, I., Grauer, F., and Sahm, Z. (1985): Polychlorinated biphenyls and organochlorine insecticides in human milk in Israel. *Arch. Environ. Contam. Toxicol.*, 14:517–521.

364a. White, I. N. H., Verschoyle, R. D., Moradian, M. H., and Barnes, J. M. (1976): The relationship between brain levels of cismethrin and bioresmethrin in female rats and neurotoxic effects. *Pestic. Biochem. Physiol.*, 6:491–500.

365. White, J. G. (1978): Weed control by soil partial sterilant chemicals: A Review. *Proc. Br. Crop Prot. Conf. Weeds*, 14:987.

366. Whorton, M. D., and Foliart, D. E. (1983): Mutagenicity, carcinogenicity and reproductive effects of dibromochloropropane (DBCP). *Mutat. Res.*, 123:13–30.

367. Whorton, M. D., and Milby, T. H. (1980): Recovery of testicular function among DBCP workers. *J. Occup. Med.*, 22:177–179.

368. Whorton, D., Milby, T. H., Krauss, R. M., and Stubbs, H. A. (1979): Testicular function in DBCP exposed pesticide workers. *J. Occup. Med.*, 21:161–166.

369. Whorton, M. D., Krauss, R. M., Marshall, S., and Milby, T. H. (1977): Infertility in male pesticide workers, *Lancet*, ii:1259–1261.

370. Working, P. K., Smith-Oliver, T., White, R. D., and Butterworth, B. E. (1986): Induction of DNA repair in rat spermatocytes and hepatocytes by 1,2-dibromoethane; the role of glutathione conjugation. *Carcinogenesis*, 7:467–472.

371. Wouters, W., van den Berckem, J., and van Ginneken, A. (1977): Presynaptic action of the pyrethroid insecticide allethrin in the frog. *Eur. J. Pharmacol.*, 43:163–171.

372. Wyers, H. (1934): Methyl bromide intoxication. *Br. J. Ind. Med.*, 2:24.

373. Yamaguchi, Y., Kawano, M., and Tatsukawa, R. (1986): Tissue distribution and excretion of hexabromobenzene (HBB) and hexachlorobenzene (HCB) administered to rats. *Chemosphere*, 15(4):453–459.

374. Yim, G. K. W., Holsapple, M. P., Pfister, W. R., and Hollingsworth, R. M. (1978): Prostaglandin synthesis inhibited by formamide pesticides. *Life Sci.*, 23:2509–2515.

375. Zakzouk, M. J. (1986): The congenital warfarin syndrome. *J. Laryngol. Otol.*, 100:215.

376. Zimmering, S. (1983): 1,2-Dibromo-3-chloropropane is positive for sex-linked recessive lethals, heritable translocations, and chromosome loss in *Drosophila. Mutat. Res.*, 119:287–288.

377. Zipf, K. E., Arndt, T., and Heintz, R. (1967): Clinical observations of a case of phostoxin poisoning. *Arch. Toxicol.*, 22:209–222.

Principles and Methods of Toxicology, Second Edition, edited by A. Wallace Hayes, Raven Press, Ltd., New York © 1989.

CHAPTER 6

Principles and Methods for Acute Toxicity and Eye Irritancy

Ping Kwong (Peter) Chan and *A. Wallace Hayes

*Toxicology Department, Rohm and Haas Company Research Laboratories, Spring House, Pennsylvania 19477; and *RJR Nabisco, Inc., Bowman Gray Technical Center, Winston-Salem, North Carolina 27102*

The methods and principles of identifying, evaluating, and extrapolating two categories of hazards, acute systemic toxicity and eye irritation, both of which result from a single or very short-term exposure, are described and discussed in this chapter. In recent years, economics and concerns over animal welfare have raised many issues on animal testings. Alternate methods for acute toxicity and eye irritation testings are being developed and the pros and cons of these issues are summarized. Laws and regulations controlling the risk of using chemicals are also reviewed.

GENERAL PRINCIPLES OF ACUTE TOXICOLOGY

Acute toxicity testing began nearly a century ago when physicians and pharmacologists were concerned with potent poisons and drugs. In 1927, Trevan (140) introduced the concept of a medium lethal dose (LD$_{50}$) for the standardization of digitalis extracts, insulin, and diphtheria toxin. He recognized that the precision of the LD$_{50}$ value was dependent on many factors such as seasonal variation and the number of animals used in a test. High precision of LD_{50} can only be established with a large number of animals.

The list of extraneous factors that affect the precision of LD_{50} has increased greatly since Trevan's work, and now includes, among other factors, sex, animal species, the strain of animal, age, diet, nutritional status, general health conditions, animal husbandry, experimental procedures, route of administration, stress, dosage formulation (vehicle), and intra- and interlaboratory variations. In spite of the many variables affecting LD_{50} determination, most governmental agencies have adopted the LD_{50} as the sole measurement of acute toxicity of all materials, but, a change in this attitude has emerged.

It is necessary and essential to obtain a precise measurement of the killing power of highly toxic substances, since a small difference in exposure can distinguish a safe from a lethal situation. However, a precise LD_{50} is not necessary for many less toxic materials such as pesticides and household products. For these substances, an approximate measurement of the killing ability is sufficient and still desirable, since overexposure to these products is possible and lethal cases are not uncommon. There are many errors inherent in the determination of LD_{50}, some of which cannot even be controlled by the experimenter, and it is therefore not scientifically sound to obtain a precise LD_{50} on these low-to-moderate toxic substances. Many methods have been developed over the years to calculate acceptably precise LD_{50}'s with a very small number of animals, and these methods are discussed in latter sections of this chapter.

Many scientists have advocated changes in the emphasis of acute toxicity testings. To date there is a general consensus among toxicologists in academia, industry, and government that a change in the emphasis of acute toxicity testing is needed (4,48,53,84,90,108,127,132,151). The value of a precise LD_{50}, except for highly toxic substances, is being de-emphasized and the focus is now on obtaining as much information as possible on the toxicity manifestation (symptomology) and mechanism (biochemical measurements). Undoubtedly, such information may be even more useful than the LD_{50} to physicians in treating overexposure to these products.

Even though the emphasis of acute toxicity testing is changing, the principles of dose–response and symptomology development remain the basis of today's science of toxicology and pharmacology. It is the objective of this section to refresh the experienced and introduce the novice to these general concepts.

Definition of Acute Toxicity

Toxicity is defined as any harmful effect of a chemical or a drug on a target organism. Acute and subchronic toxicities have been defined by various experts. The Organization for Economic Cooperation and Development (OECD) (112), defines acute toxicity as "the adverse effects occurring within a short time of (oral) administration of a single dose of a substance or multiple doses given within 24 hours." In terms of human exposure, this definition of acute toxicity refers to life-threatening crises such as accidental catastrophes, overdoses, and suicide attempts.

Dose–Response Relationship

Toxicologists often obtain two types of data, the quantal and the graded. The quantal response is called the "all or none" response; it either happens or it does not happen. On the other hand, the graded response can be quantitatively determined and it is continuous. Mortality and incidences of pharmacotoxic signs are examples of quantal data, whereas enzyme activity, protein concentration, body weight, food consumption, and electrolyte concentration are quantitative parameters. However, many apparently quantal responses are quantitative. If technical measurements permit, they may be graded. For example, the severity of a pharmacotoxic sign can be graded if detection methods are available.

At the molecular level, the graded dose–response relationship can often be explained by the *receptor,* a relatively old concept but still a valid one. Let S be a particular substance that is able to produce a specific response by interacting with a certain target protein molecule, the receptor R, in the body to form a substance–receptor complex, SR. Assuming the reaction is reversible and there is only one binding site on every target receptor molecule, this process can be described by the following expression:

$$S + R \underset{k_2}{\overset{k_1}{\rightleftharpoons}} SR$$

and the mass equation for this reversible process is

$$\frac{k_2}{k_1} = K_d = \frac{[S][R]}{[SR]} \qquad (1)$$

where [S], [R], and [SR] are the concentrations of the substance, the receptor, and the substance–receptor complex at any particular time, respectively, and K_d is the dissociation constant of the process. Let $[R]_0$ be the initial concentration of the receptor, which is usually very small and constant in number when compared with the concentration of the substance. Then

$$[R]_0 = [R] = [SR]$$

Thus

$$[R] = [R]_0 - [SR]$$

Substituting the above into the mass equation (Eq. 1) and rearranging:

$$[SR]K_d = [S]([R]_0 - [SR])$$

or

$$[SR](K_d + [S]) = [R]_0[S]$$

which can be rearranged to

$$\frac{[SR]}{[R]_0} = \frac{[S]}{K_d + [S]} \qquad (2)$$

$SR/[R]_0$ is the fraction of receptor that has reacted with the substance to form the substance–receptor complex. If we assume that the response (E) resulting from the interaction of the substance with the receptor is dependent on the fraction of total receptor concentration that has reacted with the substance, then

$$E = \frac{[S]}{K_d + [S]} \quad (3)$$

Equation 3 is a hyperbolic function; therefore, the response (*E*) is related to the concentration of the substance in a hyperbolic function relationship. If the concentration of the substance at the receptor site is dependent on the dose, then the response is dependent on the dose administered. This phenomenon is perhaps the simplest version of the receptor kinetic concept relating the dose of the chemical to a biologic response. The kinetics of the receptor–substrate interaction may be more complicated, and different dose–response relationships could be drawn based on these complicated kinetics. Readers who are interested in different receptor–substance kinetics are referred to a detailed discussion by Ferdinard (54).

The quantal dose–response relationship is often difficult to conceptualize based on the receptor theory. However, quantal response can also be viewed as a graded response if the whole population is considered as an individual. This relationship can best be explained in terms of a probability distribution. For a particular response, members of a population, for example, all the rats in the world, respond differently to a particular stimulus such as exposure to a chemical. Some rats will be highly sensitive whereas others will be very resistant. If these different responses are distributed normally within the population (i.e., with most members of the population being neither extremely sensitive nor resistant), the well-known bell-shaped population distribution curve results. If the probability of dose-response is expressed in terms of cumulative response, a sigmoidal curve can be obtained as shown in Fig. 1. However, most biologic response distributions are not exactly normal and tend to be skewed to the higher dose; i.e., extreme resistors have a larger *range of dose* to response than the extremely sensitive portion of the population. In general, a logarithmic dose transformation can normalize the distribution (i.e., convert the skewed distribution to a normal distribution) (Fig. 2). After this logarithmic dose transformation, if the probability of the log dose–response is expressed cumulatively, the sigmoidal response curve is obtained (Fig. 2). How is this log normal transfor-

mation related to a regular dose–response curve? Is there justification or basis for a log dose transformation? To answer these questions, let us again look at Eq. 3. This equation can be rearranged to

$$E = \frac{[S]}{(k_2/k_1) + [S]}$$

which also can be rearranged to

$$E = \frac{k_1[S]}{k_2 + k_1[S]} \quad (4)$$

Over a certain concentration range, Eq. 4 will produce a curve very similar to the logarithmic function $E = K_1\log(k_2[S] + 1)$ (27). Therefore, there may be justification for the log transformation besides simply a mathematical convenience.

Since a sigmoidal curve is more difficult to analyze than a straight line, many experts feel that further transformation of the log dose–response hyperbolic function is necessary to obtain a *straight-line* function curve. Perhaps the most widely used transformation is the normal equivalent deviate (NED) or the similar probit transformation (12,28,30,34,39,57,100). This technique involves the log dose transformation and the transformation of the cumulative response probability to the NED or probit. After both the probability and the dose are transformed, their transformed values are directly related to each other. A brief derivation of the straight-line direct function relationship between the log–dose and NED or probit will be presented later in this chapter.

LD$_{50}$ and Its Determination

Definition

The LD$_{50}$ in its simplest form is the dose of a compound that causes 50% mortality in a population. A more precise definition has been provided by the OECD panel of experts as the "statistically derived single dose of a substance that can be expected to cause death in 50% of the animals" (112).

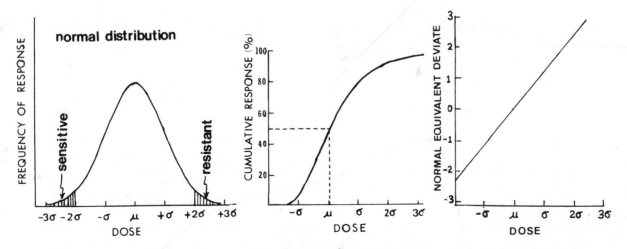

FIG. 1. Normal distribution of dose–response relationships: frequency of response, cumulative response, and cumulative response in terms of normal equivalent deviate.

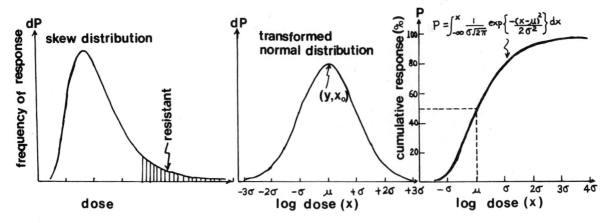

FIG. 2. Skew of dose–response can be normalized by log-dose transformation.

In other words, an LD_{50} of a compound is not a constant, as it has been treated by many; rather, it is a statistical term designed to describe the lethal response of a compound in a particular population under a discrete set of experimental conditions.

Significance of the LD₅₀ Value

The significance of LD_{50} values has been closely examined by many scientists (4,48,53,84,90,108,127,132,151) who have arrived at similar conclusions: the LD_{50} is an imprecise value; it is not a biologic constant and should be de-emphasised for most materials. They agree, furthermore, that approximate values of LD_{50} are often sufficient for all practical purposes and that more emphasis should be placed on symptomology, target organs, etc.

The numeric value of the LD_{50} has been used to classify and compare toxicity among chemicals. The extent of involvement of the LD_{50} in safety evaluation has almost reached a level of abuse. Although determining the LD_{50} under a set of experimental conditions can provide valuable information about the toxicity of a compound, the numeric LD_{50} per se is not equivalent to acute toxicity. One must always remember that lethality is only one of many reference points in defining acute toxicity. The slope (response/dose) of the dose–response curve, the time to death, pharmacotoxic signs, and pathologic findings are all vital or even more critical than the LD_{50} in the evaluation of acute toxicity. Therefore, defining acute toxicity based only on the numeric value of an LD_{50} is dangerous.

As pointed out in a previous paragraph, lethality is a quantal response, and the probability of a cumulative response is relative to dose in a hyperbolic (sigmoidal) function. The cumulative probability of response is directly related to the standard deviates of a log dose population (Fig. 1). Therefore, the slope of the log dose–response curve will indicate the relationship between the range of dose and the lethal response. This relationship is perhaps more important in risk assessment than the numeric value of LD_{50}, because more insight is available about the intrinsic toxic characteristics of a compound. Sometimes the slope can give a clue to the mechanism of toxicity. For example, a steep slope may indicate rapid

onset of action or faster absorption. A large margin of safety is predicted when a compound has a flat slope, i.e., only a small increase in response with a large increase in dose. With the slope, it is often possible to extrapolate the response to a low dose (e.g., LD_{10}, LD_1) or even to a no observed effect level. It is especially important to know the slope when comparing a set of compounds. Two compounds may have identical LD_{50} values but different slopes and thus have quite different toxicologic characteristics depending on the range of doses. Parallel dose–response curves may indicate a similar mechanism of toxicity, kinetic pattern, and probably similar prognosis. Neither the LD_{50} nor the slope can absolutely reveal a specific mechanism, but with pharmacokinetic and other biochemical studies elucidation of the mechanism of toxicity may be possible.

Determination of LD₅₀

Many methods are available for the determination of the LD_{50}. They can be grouped into two categories, the *normal population assumption* and the *normal population assumption-free* methods. The former usually can be analyzed by graphic procedures.

The normal population assumption-free methods are represented by the Thompson's moving average interpolation (138,144) and the "up-and-down" method (18,27,36). The former method is widely accepted, and convenient tables (39,144) are available for estimation of the value of the LD_{50} with confidence limits when either 0 or 100% mortality incidences are observed. However, there are some restrictions on the use of this method, i.e., four doses at equal log dose intervals and the number of animals per dose level must be equal. (The reader can find details of this method in Chapter 15.) The up-and-down or the pyramid method is designed to estimate the LD_{50} with a small number of samples. It has an economical advantage because fewer animals are needed, but the test may be time consuming and require excessive test material. Because of the advantage of using only a few animals, this method is popular when the test has to be conducted in large animals such as cows or sheep or expensive animals such as monkeys. A study comparing LD_{50}'s obtained by the up-and-down method and other methods revealed an excellent agreement (19). There are apparently two short-comings for this method, i.e., it is not adequate for estimating the incidence of delayed deaths, and a dose–response of mortality or signs of toxicity cannot easily be obtained. However, Weil (145) has adapted the up-and-down method to calculate the slope of acute toxicity response.

The normal population assumption method is represented by the probit analysis approach, which can be performed either by graphic means (89) or by mathematical calculations (57). Since the probit analysis is widely used in evaluating acute toxicity data, the principles will briefly be discussed. This method involves the transformation of both the cumulative response probability and the dose.

When the dose is transformed into a log dose (x), the frequency of response versus log doses follows a normal distribution (Fig. 2), which can be expressed mathematically as

$$dP = \frac{1}{\sigma\sqrt{2\pi}} \exp\left\{\frac{-(x - \mu)^2}{2\sigma^2}\right\} \tag{5}$$

where σ^2 and μ are the variance and the mean of the population, respectively, and P is the probability corresponding to each value of x (Fig. 2). The LD_{50} is defined as the log dose that can produce 50% mortality in a population (i.e., $P = 0.5$ or 50% cumulative response). Let x_0 be the log LD_{50}; then $P = 0.5$ will correspond to the area under the log normal distribution curve from $-\infty$ to x_0; or $P = 0.5$ will correspond to the integration of Eq. 5 from $-\infty$ to x_0: That is,

$$P = 0.5 = \int_{-\infty}^{x_0} \frac{1}{\sigma\sqrt{2\pi}} \exp\left\{\frac{-(x - \mu)^2}{2\sigma^2}\right\} dx \tag{6}$$

The solution of Eq. 6 is $x = \mu$, the true mean or the median of the log normal distribution. One way to solve this equation is by a graphic method. The integration of Eq. 5 from $x = -\infty$ to $+\infty$ can be graphically represented by a sigmoidal curve as illustrated in Fig. 2. Analysis of the sigmoidial curve is more difficult than a straight line. One way to transform the sigmoidal curve to a straight line is by NED analysis or similarly by probit analysis. For a detailed description of this analysis, the reader should consult Finney's test (57). A brief derivation of the straight-line function between log dose and the transformed probability of response is described below.

Probability (P) is normally expressed in terms of percentage or with values between 0 and 1; but Gaddum (62) has proposed to measure the probability of response on a transformed scale called the normal equivalent deviate (NED), or the standard deviation of a normal distribution, which can be described mathematically by Eq. 5. In a particular case, the normal distribution of response with mean equal to 0 and the standard deviation equal to 1, Eq. 5 can be written as

$$dP = \frac{1}{\sqrt{2\pi}} \exp\left\{\frac{-x^2}{2}\right\} dx$$

Similarly, if this distribution of response is plotted on the y axis (Fig. 3), then

$$dP = \frac{1}{\sqrt{2\pi}} \exp\left\{\frac{-y^2}{2}\right\} dx \tag{7}$$

The probability in such a case is defined by a value on the y axis of Fig. 3, i.e., the integration of Eq. 7 from $-\infty$ to y

$$P = \frac{1}{\sqrt{2\pi}} \int_{-\infty}^{y} \exp\left\{\frac{-y}{2}\right\} dy \tag{8}$$

In other words, for each value of y (from $-\infty$ to $+\infty$) expressed in terms of the standard deviation of a normal distribution with the mean equal to 0 and the standard deviation equal to 1, there is a corresponding value of probability (P) expressed in terms of percentage or having a value ranging from 0 to 1. Thus, equivalent values on the y axis can be used to define the value of P or vice versa; y and P define each other. This relationship is illustrated in Fig. 3.

The particular probability of response to a particular log dose value x, as described in Eq. 6, will be

$$P = \int_{-\infty}^{x} \frac{1}{\sigma\sqrt{2\pi}} \exp\left\{\frac{-(x - \mu)^2}{2\sigma^2}\right\} dx \tag{9}$$

where μ and σ are the mean and standard deviation of the log dose, respectively.

If P is expressed by a value of y on the y axis (standard deviations), then

$$P = \frac{1}{\sqrt{2\pi}} \int_{-\infty}^{y} \exp\left\{\frac{-y^2}{2}\right\} dy$$

$$= \int_{-\infty}^{x} \frac{1}{\sigma\sqrt{2\pi}} \exp\left\{\frac{-(x - \mu)^2}{2\sigma^2}\right\} dx$$

The solution of this equation is $x = \mu + \sigma y$ or

$$y = \frac{(x - \mu)}{\sigma} = \frac{1}{\sigma} x - \frac{\mu}{\sigma} \tag{10}$$

Therefore, the probability when expressed in terms of y (the NED scale) is linearly related to x, the log dose. If x is plotted against the corresponding y, a straight line with slope = $1/\sigma$ will be obtained. To further facilitate calculation, Bliss (11) suggested a slightly different NED unit called the probit, such that the new y value is equal to $[(x - \mu)/\sigma] + 5$. This procedure eliminates the negative values of NED when P has a value of less than 50%. Therefore, the probit is equal to the NED plus 5. The linear relationship between probits and log dose

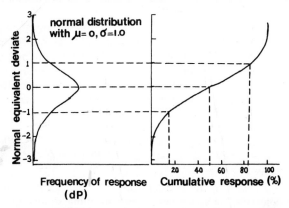

FIG. 3. Probability of response can be expressed in terms of percentage of the population or the NED of a normal distribution with mean = 0 and standard deviation = 1.

is similar to the relationship between NED and log dose. Thus, when $y = 5$, from Eq. 10,

$$5 = \frac{(x - \mu)}{\sigma} + 5$$

and $x = \mu$ (i.e., the median log dose which has a probability of response of 50%).

Logistic Transformation

Waud (143) has suggested a logistic approach to calculate the LD_{50}. Thus

$$P = \frac{D^E}{(D^E + K^E)}$$

where P is the probability of response, D is the dose, E and K are scale and location parameters, respectively, and K corresponds to the LD_{50}. With the procedure of iteration, K and E can be estimated with a range of confidence. The derivation of this equation is beyond the scope of this chapter, and interested readers are referred to the original article by Waud (143).

Nonlethal Parameters

Although the LD_{50} and the slope of the dose–response curve can provide valuable information on the toxicity of a compound, *the LD_{50} is not equivalent to toxicity.* Chemicals can induce damage to the physiologic, biochemical, immunologic, neurologic, or anatomical systems. Depending on the severity and the extent of the disturbance of the normal biologic functions, the animal may survive the toxic response but some irreversible damage may occur. These nonlethal, adverse effects are as undesirable as lethality and certainly should be taken into consideration in the risk assessment of a chemical.

The major problem in the analysis of nonlethal responses is that the data are not often quantal. For example, dermal toxicity ranges from slight to severe. This polychotomous data may be handled by *RIDIT analysis,* which was designed to analyze quantal responses with more than two outcomes (1,17,70).

While toxic effects may contribute to lethality, any attempt to correlate a particular nonlethal response to mortality may be irrational (133) unless that response is the only one responsible for the eventual death of the animal. Identification of the response or responses related to mortality is not often a straightforward matter. Nonlethal responses that affect the general well-being of an animal should be considered in the risk assessment of a compound.

If nonlethal responses can be viewed as true quantal data, the term called *median effective dose* (ED_{50}) and the corresponding dose–response curve may apply. The ED_{50}, which is often used in the standardization of biologically active compounds, such as a drug, has a meaning similar to the LD_{50} except that it is designated to examine nonlethal parameters such as pharmacologic responses and other nonlethal adverse effects. The ED_{50} is defined as a statistically derived single dose of a substance that can be expected to cause a particular effect to occur in 50% of the animal population. The therapeutic index (TI), defined by the ratio of LD_{50}/ED_{50} or LD_1/ED_{99}, has been applied to establish the safety margin of some biologically active drugs. The higher the index, the greater the margin of safety with the drug, i.e., a large difference exists between the amount of compound predicted to kill 50% of the animals and the amount of compound predicted to elicit a particular response in 50% of the animals. The TI gives an even greater estimate of safety when the LD_1 is compared with the ED_{99}.

Reversibility of Nonlethal Parameters

In general, reversible responses are those that diminish with elimination of the chemical from the body. A true reversible response will cause no residual effects when the chemical is completely eliminated from the body. Such responses are commonly seen in drugs used at therapeutic dose levels. As the amount of drug in the body increases, the magnitude of the effect also increases. If it is truly reversible, the effect will wear off when the drug is completely eliminated.

The reversibility of a particular response is dependent on the organ or system involved, the intrinsic toxicity of the chemical, the length of exposure, the total amount of the chemical in the body at a specific time, and the age and general health of the animal. If the amount of chemical in the body is high enough, the intensity of the response may overwhelm a particular organ. Effects indicated through hormonal imbalance such as thyroid effects are generally reversible unless the threshold is surpassed. Damage in rapidly regenerating organs such as the liver is usually more likely to be reversible than damage in nonregenerating tissues such as nerves. A good example is the delayed onset of neuropathy caused by many organophosphate insecticides. The chemical may be completely eliminated from the body before the effect manifests itself. Animals with renal or liver diseases are often more susceptible to damage (reversible or irreversible) by a chemical insult because of decreased ability to eliminate chemical. Exposure to a chemical at an early age in an animal may induce irreversible damage more easily than at an older age because of the limited development of the kidneys and/or functional capacity of other organs such as the liver.

In risk assessment, it is important to know whether a toxic effect is reversible. Irreversible effects seen in animals are obviously weighted more heavily in reaching a conclusion on the toxicity and hazard a chemical may pose for humans.

ACUTE TOXICITY TESTING

The objectives of acute toxicity testing are to define the intrinsic toxicity of the chemical, predict hazard to nontarget species or toxicity to target species, determine the most susceptible species, identify target organs, provide information for risk assessment of acute exposure to the chemical, provide information for the design and selection of dose levels for prolonged studies, and, most important and practical of all, provide valuable information for clinicians to predict, diagnose, and prescribe treatment for acute overexposure (poisoning) to chemicals. Acute studies are often called the "first line of defense" in the absence of data from long-term studies. These data help industrial, governmental, and academic institutions formulate safety measures for their researchers and for limited segments of their worker population during the early stage of the development of a chemical. From a regulatory standpoint, acute toxicity data are essential in the classification, labeling, and transportation of a chemical. From an academic standpoint, a carefully designed acute toxicity study can often provide important clues on the mechanism of toxicity and the structure–effect relationship for a particular class of chemicals.

Many acute toxicity studies have been conducted solely for the purpose of determining the LD_{50} of a chemical. However, the reader is reminded that acute toxicity is not equivalent to the LD_{50}, and that the LD_{50} is not an absolute biologic constant to be equated, as many investigators have, with such chemical constants as pH, pK_a, melting point, and solubility. The LD_{50} is only one of many indices used in defining acute toxicity. A well-designed acute toxicity study should include consideration of the dose–response relationship of both lethal and nonlethal parameters, as discussed above. Sometimes, biochemical measurements in an acute test can aid in elucidating the mechanism of toxic actions. Histopathology of organs may also be helpful in finding the cause of death and identifying the target organs.

Types of Acute Testing

Since acute toxicity data may provide the first line of defense, a battery of tests under different conditions and exposure routes should be conducted. In general, these tests should include oral, dermal, and inhalation toxicities, and skin and eye irritation studies. Other tests such as acute preneonatal and neonatal exposure, dermal contact sensitization, and phototoxicity should be considered. Depending on economical, practical, and sound scientific factors, which may vary from one chemical to another, the number and kind of acute tests needed to establish the initial toxicity data base may not be the same. For example, when inhalation exposure is not expected to occur because of the physical properties of the chemical, inhalation toxicity testing may not be needed. Such a case is not uncommon if respirable particles cannot be generated even under the most favorable laboratory conditions. Nonetheless, for all practical purposes, oral, dermal, skin, and eye tests should be considered in the initial acute investigation. These four tests are often sufficient for regulatory purposes, labeling, and classification of a chemical, although increasing concerns are also placed on the inhalation and skin sensitization studies. This chapter is concerned only with acute oral and dermal toxicity and eye irritation.

Acute Oral Toxicity Studies

Principles

The test substance, undiluted or diluted with appropriate solvents or suspending vehicles, is given to several groups of animals by gavage with a feeding needle or by gastric intu-

bation. A vehicle control group is included if needed, but generally this group is not necessary if the toxicity of the vehicle is known. Clinical signs, morbidity, and mortality are observed at specific intervals. Animals that die or become extremely moribund during the study are subjected to necropsies. Animals that survive the test period are killed and necropsied at the end of the observation period. Tissues may be saved for histopathologic examination to facilitate the understanding of the acute toxicity of the compound. In order to increase the reproducibility of the study, all experimental conditions and procedures should be standardized, and the study should be conducted according to "generally recognized good laboratory practices" (GLP) outlined by the Environmental Protection Agency (EPA) and the OECD (46, 47,114).

Animals

Species

The responses elicited by a compound often vary greatly among species. Ideally, toxicity tests should be conducted with an animal that will elicit compound-related toxic responses similar to those that occur in man, i.e., an animal that metabolizes the compound identically to man and which has the same susceptible organ system(s). Under ideal conditions, the animal data may then be extrapolated to man. Unfortunately, finding such an ideal animal is a difficult, if not impossible task.

A less ideal, but more manageable approach is to conduct acute toxicity studies in a variety of animal species under the assumption that if the toxicity of a compound is consistent in all the species tested, then a greater chance exists that such a response may also occur in man. Even though the response in different species is not consistent, it is generally considered better to err on the safe side with the risk assessment being based on the most sensitive species unless there is justification that such responses are less likely to occur in humans, for example, because of dissimilarity in metabolism between the less sensitive animal species and man. While these are logical assumptions and generally quite reliable, the danger of underestimating or overestimating the responses in humans still exists. Therefore, there is no absolute criterion for selecting a particular animal species. However, priority should be given to species with metabolism or other physiologic and biochemical parameters similar to man. Animal species should also be selected on the basis of convenience, economical factors, and the existing data base for the animal. Rats, mice, rabbits, and guinea pigs are most commonly chosen for acute toxicity studies.

Other animal variations

Acute toxicity, even within a particular species, can vary with health conditions, age, sex, genetic makeup, body weight, differences in absorption, distribution, metabolism and excretion of the compound, and the influence of hormones (37). A conscientious investigator should be aware of the possible interaction of chemical treatment with these parameters. For example, immature animals may lack an effective drug metabolizing enzyme system; this may contribute to higher toxicity of the compound in an immature animal if an enzyme is responsible for detoxification of the compound, or to decreased toxicity if an enzyme is responsible for activation of the compound. Obesity may affect the distribution and storage of a compound, especially when it is highly lipophilic. Sex hormones may be the target, or sex hormones may modify a particular toxic response, which then may account for different toxic responses between sexes. Liver and renal diseases associated with old age may contribute to a higher toxicity. Variations in genetic makeup among different strains may alter metabolism or other parameters, which may affect the toxicity of a particular compound. It is therefore important to document all data on animals: age, sex, body weight, strain, general health conditions, and source. In general, healthy, young adults should be used. For example, if rats are the test animal, then young adults weighing between 150 and 250 g should be used. The weight variation among animals should not exceed ±20% of the mean body weight.

Number and sex

The precision of the acute test is dependent to a large extent on the number of animals employed per dose level. Ten rats (5 male and 5 female) have been recommended in most regulatory guidelines (43,45,50,112,131). The degree of precision needed and, in turn, the number of animals per dose group needed depend on the purpose of the study. In screening tests or tests designed to define the range of toxicity, fewer animals per dose level or fewer numbers of dose levels may be considered. If a fairly precise LD_{50} is needed, the number of dose levels (at least three dose levels) and animals per dose group should be increased. The number of animals and dose levels should be based on sound scientific judgment as well as practical and economical factors.

In 1986, the OECD updating committee recommended that acute toxicity studies be conducted first in the male and then cross-checked if a marked sex difference appears when one dose level is used. This approach reduces the number of animals used in acute toxicity testings.

Housing and environment

Studies should be conducted in a controlled environment. The temperature (22 ± 3°C), relative humidity (30–70%), light and dark cycle (12 hr dark, 12 hr light), diet, and quality of drinking water should be standardized and maintained continuously. Animals may be caged in groups by sex or caged individually, depending on the species and size of the animal and on the needs of the particular study. Rodents can be caged in groups, usually not more than 3 per cage, but larger animals such as rabbits and dogs are generally housed individually.

Dose Levels

In general, the dose levels should be sufficient in number to allow a clear demonstration of a dose–response relationship and to permit an acceptable determination of the LD_{50}. Three dose levels are generally sufficient, although Japanese guidelines specifically recommend five doses (131). The selected dose levels should bracket the expected LD_{50} value with at least one dose level higher than the expected LD_{50} but not causing 100% mortality, and one dose level below the expected LD_{50} value but not causing 0% mortality, when the probit analysis method is applied to estimate the LD_{50}. However, with a method such as the moving average under some specific conditions (at least four dose levels with equal logarithmic intervals between each dose level, and with equal numbers of animals in each dose group), the LD_{50} can be estimated even with 0% mortality at the lower dose levels and 100% mortality at the two higher dose levels.

In any event, three or more dose levels with a wide range of toxicity responses are recommended if no other toxicity data are available. A pilot study may be needed for the selection of dose levels. Fewer animals per dose level and wider logarithmic intervals between dose levels are usually selected for the pilot study to ensure bracketing of the expected LD_{50} value. For example, if one desires an equal log interval of 0.6 between dose levels, and if the lowest dose is 1 mg/kg (log dose = 0), the next log doses would be 0 + 0.6, 0.6 + 0.6, 1.2 + 0.6, etc., corresponding to dose levels of antilogs 0.6, 1.2, 1.8 (i.e., the dose levels are: 1, 4, 16, 64, etc., in a geometric progression ratio of 4).

Dosages

If necessary, the test substance should be dissolved or suspended in a suitable vehicle, preferably in water, saline, or an aqueous suspension such as 0.5% methyl cellulose in water. If a test substance cannot be dissolved or suspended in an aqueous medium to form a homogeneous dosage preparation, corn oil or another solvent can be used. If the toxicity of the vehicle is not known, a vehicle control group should be included in the test. The animals in the vehicle control group should receive the same volume of vehicle given to animals in the highest dose group.

The test substance can be administered to animals at a constant concentration across all dose levels (i.e., varying the dose volume), or at a constant dose volume (i.e., varying the dose concentration). However, the investigator should be aware that the toxicity observed by administration in a constant concentration may be different from that observed when given in a constant dose volume. For instance, when a large volume of corn oil is given orally, the gastrointestinal motility is increased, causing diarrhea and decreasing the time for absorption of the test substance in the gastrointestinal tract. This situation arises when a highly lipid soluble chemical is tested. A large fraction of such a material may quickly pass through the gastrointestinal tract and remain unabsorbed. Local irritation of a test substance generally decreases when the material is diluted. If the objective of the study is to establish systemic toxicity, the test substance should be administered in a constant volume (diluted concentration) to minimize gastrointestinal irritation that may in turn affect the absorption of the test substance. On the other hand, the test substance should be administered undiluted to assess the irritation potential of the test substance. The choice of constant concentration versus constant dose volume should be based on sound scientific judgment. The OECD guideline suggests a constant dose volume approach (112). The maximum dose volume in rodents should not exceed 10 ml/kg body weight for nonaqueous vehicles or 20 ml/kg body weight for aqueous solution or suspension. In any event, the dose volume should be as small as possible.

Observation

As has been discussed previously, the emphasis in acute toxicity studies is on the determination of dose–response and the onset of symptoms and toxic signs. The observation period should be flexible depending on the purpose of the study. This period should be based on the onset of signs, the nature of the toxicity, time to death, and the rate of recovery. For most highly toxic substances, the onset of toxic signs and the time to death may be very short, and prolonged observation may not be necessary. The slope of the dose–response curve for such test substances is usually very steep, and the treated animals either die or survive within a very short time. For other substances, the onset of signs and the time to death may be delayed for a few days to a few weeks or longer. Obviously, a longer observation period is needed to detect these delayed acute effects. The observation period should also be long enough for the determination of reversibility or the recovery of an adverse effect. Under specific circumstances the observation period might be longer, but normally the observation period does not exceed 14 days.

Test Limit

All chemicals can produce toxicity under some experimental conditions, for instance, if a sufficiently large dose is given. It is therefore misleading to conduct acute toxicity studies at unreasonably high dose levels for the sake of demonstrating lethality and/or toxicity, which may be irrelevant to the compound itself. For example, an extremely high dose of a practically nontoxic compound can cause gastrointestinal blockage, which, in turn, can result in gastrointestinal tract dysfunction. Toxicity in this case is not related to the intrinsic characteristic of the test substance, since it is a direct result of the physical blockage caused by the biologically inert substance. There must be a point, however, at which an investigator can conclude that a test substance is practically nontoxic or nonlethal after an acute exposure. This test limit for acute oral toxicity is generally considered to be 5.0 g/kg body weight. If no mortality is observed at this dose level, a higher dose level is generally not necessary. A test limit of 2.0 g/kg body weight was recommended to the OECD Updating Committee in 1986, but has not been officially accepted as of publication of this volume.

Testing Methods and Procedures

While the purpose of this section is to describe practical experimentation in detail, it is not the authors' intention to list all technical procedures. A manual is available that de-

scribes technical procedures such as handling and dosing the animals (116). Since the Good Laboratory Practices Act has been implemented in both the United States and most OECD countries, all experimental procedures should be documented and the studies conducted by trained personnel. For more details on GLP guidelines, the reader may consult several recent EPA, OECD, and Japanese publications (46, 47,114,132). The Japanese guidelines contain some unique requirements that are not duplicated by other countries (132).

Grouping, Randomization, and Preparation of Animals

Animals not previously treated with test substances in other studies should be identified individually by coded marks, metal ear tags, or tatoos. The animals should then be quarantined for at least a week prior to dosing to acclimatize them to the conditions of the animal room.

The animals should be fasted prior to administration of the test substance if the route of administration is oral. Rats are usually fasted overnight. Because mice have a higher metabolic rate, withholding feed for 3–4 hr may be adequate. Overstarving small animals with a high metabolic rate may induce undesirable effects. The purpose of starving the animal is to eliminate feed in the gastrointestinal tract, which may complicate absorption of the test substance.

The animals should be randomly assigned to dose groups. Randomization, needed not only in acute toxicity studies but also in subchronic and chronic studies, ensures a homogeneous population and can minimize errors due to sampling bias. All animals with body weights and health conditions out of the normal range should be eliminated prior to the randomization procedure. With computer-generated random digit numbers or with tables of random digit numbers such as the one below, animals can be randomly assigned to groups by cage number or by individually assigned animal number.

Random Numbers

	00–04	05–09	10–14	15–19	20–24
00	01826	72696	67261	13748	57834
01	70731	12890	90395	45245	71282
02	46616	84522	17249	78172	14197
	25–29	30–34	35–39	40–44	45–49
00	27748	47492	43428	85524	19311
01	15960	02749	86763	80564	02631
02	84272	53226	96719	83462	05628

For example, by using a random number table, 50 rats from a total of 100 rats are assigned to 5 dose groups of 10 rats each. Assume that 20 rats will be excluded from the study because of overweight, underweight, or other health problems; this leaves 80 rats, from which 50 would be chosen. One method of randomization is to arbitrarily number the 80 rats from 1 to 80. The random number table gives the following series of random numbers (row 1): 01826, 72696, 67261, 13748, 57834, 27748. Since there are only 80 rats, the numbers should be 2-digit numbers. The first group of rats would be rat numbers 01, *82*, 67, 26, *96, 67,* 26, 11, 37, 48, 57, *83,* 42, and 77. The italicized numbers should be discarded because they are either repeated numbers or greater than 80. The second group of rats would be chosen similarly. The same procedure is repeated until 50 rats have been assigned to the 5 dose groups.

When the number of animals to be grouped is small, a large number of random numbers may be required to complete the grouping. Another way to use the random number table under such circumstances is by cycling. For example, 6 rabbits are assigned to 2 groups of 3 rabbits each from a total of 10 rabbits. From the second row of the same random digit number table, the first 3 two-digit numbers are 70, 73, and 11. Dividing these numbers by the total number of rabbits (i.e., 10), the remainders of these three numbers are 0, 3, and 1. If the remainder is zero, the denominator (in this case 10) will remain. Therefore the 3 rabbits in the first group would be rabbit numbers 10, 3, and 1. Again, if the remainder numbers are repeated, they would be discarded. Also, if the number is smaller than the total number of animals, the number would be used and no division is needed. For the second group, the next series of numbers from the table are 28, *90, 90,* 39, 54, 52, 45, 71, 28, *21,* 59, *60,* 02, 74, 98, 67, and the corresponding numbers are 8, 0, 0, 9, 4, 2, 5, 1, 8, 1, 9, 10, 2, 4, 8, 7. Therefore, the 3 rabbits in the second dose group would be rabbit numbers 8, 9, and 4. If a third group is needed, the 3 rabbits in this group would be rabbit numbers 2, 5, and 7. In general, the following rules apply when using the cycling method:

1. When the number from the random number table is less than the total number of animals to be chosen from, no division is needed.
2. When the number is greater than the total number of animals, the random number is divided by the total number of animals, and the remainder is used.
3. When the remainder is zero, the denominator is used.
4. No numbers or remainders should be allowed to repeat, i.e., any repeated numbers should be discarded.

The entry (the starting point) in the random number table should *not* be consistent. Thus the entry should be made at a different point each time the random number table is used (one can start along the rows or the columns).

Calculation and Preparation of Dosages

Dosages, in general, are based on the body weight of the animal (expressed as weight of the test substance per kilogram of body weight of the animal), although for larger animals, the surface area may be more appropriate. The weight (or dose) of the test substance is often expressed in milligrams or grams of active ingredient if the test substance is not 100% pure.

Ideally, only the 100% pure sample should be tested; however, impurity-free samples are difficult to obtain. While some toxicologists strongly advocate the use of pure samples in toxicity testings, others see the appropriateness of using technical samples, formulations, or crude products. It is accept-

able to study the test substance in its pure form or in its technical or product forms; however the toxicity of impurities should be examined separately if the investigator feels that the impurities may contribute significantly to the toxicity of the test substance.

Selection of dosages is often based on a pilot study, on existing toxicity data in other species, or on data obtained with a similar analog of the test substances. For example, if 0 of 3 and 3 of 3 rats died at dose levels of 500 and 1000 mg/kg, respectively, in the pilot study, the expected LD_{50} numeric value would be between these two dose levels. If the investigator decides to select five doses that will bracket the expected LD_{50}, the logical approach would be to select the LD_{50} of 750 mg/kg for the definitive study along with the following dose levels: 520, 625, 750, 900, and 1080 mg/kg. The dose levels progress by a value of the antilog 0.08 (i.e., multiplied or divided by 1.2 of the assumed LD_{50}).

If the test substance contains only 75% active ingredient and the investigator chooses a constant dose volume of 10 ml/kg body weight across all dose levels, it will be more convenient to prepare a stock solution such that when 10 ml/kg of this stock solution is given to the animal, the dose will be 1080 mg/kg (active ingredient). The concentration of this stock solution would be

$$(1080 \text{ mg/10 ml}) \div 0.75 = 144 \text{ mg of test substance/ml}$$

Aliquots of the test substance for other dose levels can then be prepared by dilution of the stock solution. For example, the solution concentration for the 900 mg/kg dose level is

$$(900 \text{ mg/10 ml}) \div 0.75 = 120 \text{ mg of test substance/ml}$$

This solution can be prepared by diluting the stock solution 1.2 times, i.e., for each milliliter of the 120 mg/ml solution to be prepared,

$$\frac{120 \text{ mg/ml} \times 1 \text{ ml}}{144 \text{ mg/ml}} = 0.833 \text{ ml of the stock solution}$$

should be diluted to a final volume in 1 ml with the vehicle.

The vehicle should be one with limited or no toxicity. In preparing dosage solutions or suspensions, the vehicle of choice is water; other choices include an aqueous suspending vehicle such as 0.5% (w/v) methyl cellulose (Methocel) in water; corn oil; or other solvents such as aqueous ethanol, propylene glycol, or diluted DMSO in 5.0% $NaHCO_3$ solution. Magnetic stirring bars, micromills, or homogenizers can be used in preparing suspensions. Sometimes a small amount of a surfactant such as Tween 80, Span 20, or Span 60 is helpful in obtaining a homogeneous suspension. If surfactants are used, one must be aware of the potential effects of these surfactants on the absorption of the test substance.

On many occasions, it is desirable to prepare dosage in an aqueous medium because of the undesirable effects of corn oil or other vehicles on the animals. In this case, one may try to prepare the dosage in a simple, water-suspensible, uniform formulation even though the test material is not soluble or cannot be suspended in aqueous medium. For example, a formulation can be prepared by dissolving a specific amount of the test material in an adequate amount of acetone followed by mixing the acetone solution with a known amount of small particle size and biologically inert dispensing agent such as HiSil, and evaporating to dryness under a hood. In the resulting formulation, the test material is uniformly coated on the small particles. Then, a dosage in a uniform suspension can be prepared from the formulated test substance. This dosage preparation procedure has been used successfully in many studies in our laboratory.

Administration of the Dose

The test substance can be administered as a solution or suspension as long as it is homogeneous. The solution or suspension is gavaged to the animal with a suitable stomach tube or feeding needle attached to a syringe. If the dose is too large to be administered at a single time, it can be divided into equal doses with 3 or 4 hr between each administration. Feed should be withheld until the last dose, which should be within 24 hr of the first dose.

Observations

Clinical examination, observation, and mortality check should be made shortly after dosing, at frequent intervals over the next 4 hr, and at least once daily thereafter. The intervals and frequency of observation should be flexible enough to determine the onset of signs, onset of recovery, and the time to death. The mortality checks should also be frequent enough to minimize unnecessary loss of animals due to autolysis or cannibalism. The cage side observation should include any changes in the skin, fur, eyes, mucus membranes, circulatory system, autonomic and central nervous systems, somatomotor activities, behavior, etc. Any pharmacotoxic signs such as tremor, convulsions, salivation, diarrhea, lethargy, sleepiness, morbidity, fasciculation, mydriasis, miosis, droppings, discharges, or hypotonia should be recorded. The most common pharmacotoxic signs that may provide valuable clues to the target organ or system of toxicity of a test substance are listed in Tables 1–3. Individual body weights should be determined just prior to dosing, once weekly, and at death or at termination. Body weight of animals found dead are generally not as useful as body weight of live animals. Necropsies should be performed on animals that are moribund, found dead, and killed at the conclusion of the study. All changes in the size, color, or texture of any organ should be recorded. Any observable gross change at necropsy should be described according to the size, color, and position of the lesion. Definitive pathologic diagnostic terms should be avoided. While a complete microscopic examination of tissues and organs is ideal and would be helpful in defining acute toxicity, economic and time factors may preclude such a study. If the investigator feels that microscopic examination of a lesion is essential, tissues from these lesions should be preserved in an appropriate fixative such as 10% buffered formalin.

Other Nonroutine Determinations

The cause of deaths in acute poisoning generally involved the nervous, cardiovascular, or respiratory systems. Effects on other organs such as the liver or kidney sometimes are masked by lethality or cannot be detected without some special determinations. Clinical laboratory studies (hematology, clinical chemistry, or specific functional tests) may be needed to identify these adverse effects. Since these laboratory tests are usually costly, they are only justifiable when there is evidence indicating that a particular laboratory test would be helpful in identifying the target organs or mechanism of toxic actions. For example, if the chemical structure of the test substance belongs to a class of hepatotoxins, a battery of clinical chemistry measurements may be conducted to verify its hepatotoxicity potential.

Histopathology can also be very valuable in aiding the identification of a target organ. As with clinical laboratory studies, histopathologic examination of organs could be expensive. However, the cost should not be the major limiting factor in deciding whether histopathologic examination is needed; rather the limiting factor should be whether there is evidence, such as by chemical structure or gross necropsy observation, that a particular organ is involved.

Data Processing

All signs of toxicity, onset of the signs, time to recovery, time to death, mortality, and necropsy findings can be summarized in tabular form. The LD_{50} may be determined by an acceptable method such as the graphic or nongraphic methods (89,138,144). While many laboratories are now equipped with calculators or computer programs to facilitate the estimation of LD_{50} values, fiducial limits, and the slopes of the dose–response curve, the reader is advised to review the manual estimation procedure for two widely adopted methods, the probit analysis and the moving average method. The latter method is detailed in another chapter and will not be discussed here. The graphic procedure of the probit analysis is rapid and is sufficient for most purposes. But for a more precise estimate of the LD_{50}, mathematical calculation may be necessary, and the reader is referred to the maximum likelihood estimation described in Finney's text (57).

Graphic Estimation of LD_{50} by Probit Analysis

The basic linear equation for the probit analysis as described in the previous section is

$$y = 5 + \frac{1}{\sigma}(x - \mu)$$

where y is the probit, σ is the standard deviation of a log normal distribution with mean μ, and x is the log dose. This equation is linear with respect to y and x and can often be expressed as a linear equation, e.g., $y = \alpha + \beta x$, where $\beta = 1/\sigma$ = slope, and $\alpha = 5 - (\mu/\sigma)$. When $y = 5$, $(x - \mu)/\sigma = 0$; thus $x = \mu$ (the median log dose). Further, y is related to P (the probability of response which has a value of 0 to 1) by the following equation:

$$P = \frac{1}{\sqrt{2\pi}} \int_{-\infty}^{y} \exp\left\{\frac{-y}{2}\right\} dy$$

TABLE 1. *Common signs and observation in acute toxicity test*

Clinical observation	Observed signs	Organs, tissues, or systems most likely to be involved
I. Respiratory: blockage in the nostrils, changes in rate and depth of breathing, changes in color of body surfaces	A. Dyspnea: difficult or labored breathing, essentially gasping for air, respiration rate usually slow	
	1. Abdominal breathing: breathing by diaphragm, greater deflection of abdomen upon inspiration	CNS respiratory center, paralysis of costal muscles, cholinergic inhibition
	2. Gasping: deep labored inspiration, accompanied by a wheezing sound	CNS respiratory center, pulmonary edema, secretion accumulation in airways (increase cholinergic)
	B. Apnea: a transient cessation of breathing following a forced respiration	CNS respiratory center, pulmonary cardiac insufficiency
	C. Cyanosis: bluish appearance of tail, mouth, foot pads	Pulmonary–cardiac insufficiency, pulmonary edema
	D. Tachypnea: quick and usually shallow respiration	Stimulation of respiratory center, pulmonary–cardiac insufficiency
	E. Nostril discharges: red or colorless	Pulmonary edema, hemorrhage
II. Motor activities: changes in frequency and nature of movements	A. Decrease or increase in spontaneous motor activities, curiosity, preening, or locomotions	Somatomotor, CNS
	B. Somnolence: animal appears drowsy, but can be aroused by prodding and resumes normal activities	CNS sleep center
	C. Loss of righting reflex: loss of reflex to maintain normal upright posture when placed on the back	CNS, sensory, neuromuscular
	D. Anesthesia: loss of righting reflex and pain response (animal will not respond to tail and toe pinch)	CNS, sensory
	E. Catalepsy: animal tends to remain in any position in which it is placed	CNS, sensory, neuromuscular, autonomic
	F. Ataxia: inability to control and coordinate movement while animal is walking with no spasticity, epraxia, paresis, or rigidity	CNS, sensory, autonomic
	G. Unusual locomotion: spastic, toe walking, pedaling, hopping, and low body posture	CNS, sensory, neuromuscular
	H. Prostration: immobile and rests on belly	CNS, sensory, neuromuscular
	I. Tremors: involving trembling and quivering of the limbs or entire body	Neuromuscular, CNS
	J. Fasciculation: involving movements of muscles, seen on the back, shoulders, hind limbs, and digits of the paws	Neuromuscular, CNS, autonomic
III. Convulsion (seizure): marked involuntary contraction or seizures of contraction of voluntary muscle	A. Clonic convulsion: convulsive alternating contraction and relaxation of muscles	CNS, respiratory failure, neuromuscular, autonomic
	B. Tonic convulsion: persistent contraction of muscles, attended by rigid extension of hind limbs	
	C. Tonic–clonic convulsion: both types may appear consecutively	
	D. Asphyxial convulsion: usually of clonic type, but accompanied by gasping and cyanosis	
	E. Opisthotonos: tetanic spasm in which the back is arched and the head is pulled towards the dorsal position	

TABLE 1. *Continued*

Clinical observation	Observed signs	Organs, tissues, or systems most likely to be involved
IV. Reflexes	A. Corneal (eyelid closure): touching of the cornea causes eye lids to close	Sensory, neuromuscular
	B. Pirmal: twitch of external ear elicited by light stroking of inside surface of ear	Sensory, neuromuscular, autonomic
	C. Righting	CNS, sensory, neuromuscular
	D. Myotact: ability of animal to retract its hind limb when limb is pulled down over the edge of a surface	Sensory, neuromuscular
	E. Light (pupillary): constriction of pupil in the presence of light	Sensory, neuromuscular, autonomic
	F. Startle reflex: response to external stimuli such as touch, noise	Sensory, neuromuscular
V. Ocular signs	A. Lacrimation: excessive tearing, clear or colored	Autonomic
	B. Miosis: constriction of pupil regardless of the presence or absence of light	Autonomic
	C. Mydriasis: dilation of pupils regardless of the presence or absence of light	Autonomic
	D. Exophthalmos: abnormal retraction of eye in orbit	Autonomic
	E. Ptosis: dropping of upper eyelids, not reversed by prodding animal	Autonomic
	F. Chromodacryorrhea (red lacrimation)	Autonomic, hemorrhage, infection
	G. Relaxation of nictitating membrane	Autonomic
	H. Corneal opacity, iritis, conjunctivitis	Irritation of the eye
VI. Cardiovascular signs	A. Bradycardia: decreased heart rate	Autonomic, pulmonary–cardiac insufficiency
	B. Tachycardia: increased heart rate	Autonomic, pulmonary–cardiac insufficiency
	C. Vasodilation: redness of skin, tail, tongue, ear, foot pad, conjunctivae sac, and warm body	Autonomic, CNS, increased cardiac output, hot environment
	D. Vasoconstriction: blanching or whitening of skin, cold body	Autonomic, CNS, cold environment, cardiac output decrease
	E. Arrhythmia: abnormal cardiac rhythm	CNS, autonomic, cardiac–pulmonary insufficiency, myocardiac infarction
VII. Salivation	A. Excessive secretion of saliva: hair around mouth becomes wet	Autonomic
VIII. Piloerection	A. Contraction of erectile tissue of hair follicles resulting in rough hair	Autonomic
IX. Analgesia	A. Decrease in reaction to induced pain (e.g., hot plate)	Sensory, CNS
X. Muscle tone	A. Hypotonia: generalized decrease in muscle tone	Autonomic
	B. Hypertonia: generalized increase in muscle tension	Autonomic
XI. Gastrointestinal signs: dropping (feces)	A. Solid, dried, and scant	Autonomic, constipation, GI motility
	B. Loss of fluid, watery stool	Autonomic, diarrhea, GI motility
Emesis	A. Vomiting and retching	Sensory, CNS, autonomic (in rat, emesis is absent)
Diuresis	A. Red urine (rhinorrhea)	Damage in kidney
	B. Involuntary urination	Autonomic, sensory
XII. Skin	A. Edema: swelling of tissue filled with fluid	Irritation, renal failure, tissue damage, long term immobility
	B. Erythema: redness of skin	Irritation, inflammation, sensitization

TABLE 2. *Autonomic signs*

Sympathomimetic	Piloerection
	Partial mydriasis
Sympathetic block	Ptosis
	Diagnostic if associated with sedation
Parasympathomimetic	Salivation (examined by holding blotting paper)
	Miosis
	Diarrhea
	Chromodacryorrhea in rats
Parasympathomimetic block	Mydriasis (maximal)
	Excessive dryness of mouth (detect with blotting paper)

The reader should bear in mind that both the μ and x are in log dose scale.

The following steps should be taken for graphic estimation of LD_{50} by probit analysis.

1. Convert response probabilities to probit units by a probit transformation table (see ref. 35, pp. 54–55).

2. Convert all doses into log dose units (e.g., $\log_{10}$ dose $= x$). (Steps 1 and 2 may be eliminated if probit–log graphic paper is available.)

3. Using the probit as the abscissa and $\log_{10}$ dose as the ordinate, plot the response probit units against the $\log_{10}$ dose.

4. Draw a straight line such that the vertical deviations of points (the probits) at each x value are as small as possible. Extreme probits, e.g., those outside the range of probit 7 and 1, carry little weight in the fitting of the probit–log dose–response line and thus should be excluded.

5. From the regression of the probit–log dose line, extrapolate the log dose corresponding to probit units of 5, which also correspond to the $P = 0.5$. Thus, this extrapolated dose should be the median lethal *log dose,* and the LD_{50} value would be the *antilog* of this log dose value.

6. Calculate the slope of the probit–log dose line. This slope, $\beta = 1/\sigma$, is defined as the number of increases in probit units for a unit increase in log dose. The slope defined by Litchfield and Wilcoxon (89) is equal to

$$\frac{1}{2}\left(\frac{LD_{84}}{LD_{50}} + \frac{LD_{50}}{LD_{16}}\right) = \sigma$$

This slope is different but related to the slope described here, thus the larger the slope value, the steeper the probit–log dose response. The opposite is true in the Litchfield and Wilcoxon definition.

7. A chi-square (χ^2) test should be conducted to determine if the fitted line is adequate. A small value of χ^2 statistic (within the limits of random variation) may indicate satisfactory agreement between the theoretically expected line and the fitted line. A significantly large χ^2 statistic may indicate either that the animals do not respond independently or that the fitted line (probit–log dose) does not adequately describe the dose–response relationship of the test substance. If the latter is true, forms of the dose–response curve other than the probit–log dose linearity may exist, and further transformation may be needed (57). If the former is the case, then precision of the line is reduced.

8. Determination of precision is by weighting the coefficient. The standard deviation of a binomial distribution is $\sqrt{PQ/n}$, where P and Q are the mean probabilities, P equals $(1 - Q)$, and n is the number of test subjects. Thus the variance is PQ/n, the square of the standard deviation. It is obvious that the variance (i.e., the spread of a distribution) is inversely related to n. This relationship means that the larger number of test subjects, the smaller the variance and the better the precision.

The reciprocal of the variance is invariance, which measures the weight, nW. Here W (weighting coefficient) $= Z^2/PQ$, where $Z = (1/\sqrt{2\pi}) \exp\{-y^2/2\}$ and is related to the normal frequency function corresponding to the NED. A table of weighting coefficients (see ref. 35, p. 53) corresponding to probits (y) is available (58). The standard error for the log LD_{50} is given by

$$\sigma/\sqrt{\Sigma nW}$$

if the estimated log LD_{50} does not greatly differ from the true mean log LD_{50}, because this estimation does not take into consideration the error in the estimation of σ for the probit–log dose–response line. A better equation for the estimation of the variance of the estimated log LD_{50} is given by

$$V(m) = \sigma^2 \left\{ \frac{1}{\Sigma nW} + \frac{(m - \bar{x})^2}{\Sigma nW(x - \bar{x})^2} \right\}$$

where $V(m)$ is the variance of LD_{50}, $\bar{x}$ is the weighted mean log dose, m is the median log dose, x is the log dose, and $1/\sigma = 1/\Sigma\, nW(x - \bar{x})$. If the χ^2 is large, indicating that the test subjects do not respond independently to the dose, the estimation of variance of log LD_{50} may not apply, and adjustment due to the sampling variation of the slope ($1/\sigma$) of the probit–log dose line may have to be made (57). For a quick estimation of the LD_{50}, this adjustment may be dropped, and the standard error would be the square root of the variance, i.e., $\sqrt{V(m)}$.

One must remember that the dose is expressed in log dose; therefore, the estimation of the standard error (SE) for the

TABLE 3. *Toxic signs of acetylcholinesterase inhibition*

Muscarinic effects[a]	Nicotinic effects[b]	CNS effects[c]
Bronchoconstriction	Muscular twitching	Giddiness
Increased bronchosecretion	Fasciculation	Anxiety
Nausea and vomiting (absent in rats)	Cramping	Insomnia
Diarrhea	Muscular weakness	Nightmares
Bradycardia		Headache
Hypotension		Apathy
Miosis		Depression
Urinary incontinence		Drowsiness
		Confusion
		Ataxia
		Coma
		Depressed reflex
		Seizure
		Respiratory depression

[a] Blocked by atropine.
[b] Not blocked by atropine.
[c] Atropine might block early signs.

LD_{50} in the original dose unit (e.g., mg/kg) is impossible. However, an approximation is given:

$$SE(LD_{50}) = (10^m) \cdot (\log_e (10) \cdot (S_m)$$

where S_m [which equals $\sigma/\sqrt{\Sigma \, nW}$ or $\sqrt{V(m)}$] is the estimated standard error for the median log dose m (i.e., $m = \log LD_{50}$ or $10^m = LD_{50}$).

A more rapid approximation of the standard error of log LD_{50} was given by Litchfield and Wilcoxon (89) as

$$S_m = \frac{S}{N'/2}$$

where S is the difference between two log doses of expected effects (as indicated by the probiting dose line) that differ by one unit of probit, and N' is the total number of animals between the log dose limits, corresponding to the expected probit 4.0–6.0 (i.e., the 16 and 80% responses).

9. Fiducial limits. The concept of fiducial limit is similar to the confidence limit. The value of the two may be the same, but they are not always identical. The fiducial probability F (e.g., 95%) can be defined as the situation when the true value of a parameter lies between the calculated upper and lower limits, which would not be contradicted by a significance test at the $\frac{1}{2}(1 - F)$ probability level. These higher

and lower limits are called the fiducial limits. For rapid analysis, the fiducial limits at the $F = 95\%$ level can be estimated by $\log LD_{50} \pm 1.96 \, (S_m)$. A more detailed estimation can be obtained by the *maximum likelihood estimation* (57).

Another simple approximation of the fiducial limits is given by Litchfield and Wilcoxon (89) as $LD_{50}/f \, LD_{50}$ or $LD_{50} \times f \, LD_{50}$ for the lower and upper limit, respectively, where LD_{50} is defined as the LD_{50} factor equal to $(s)(2.77/\sqrt{N'})$. Here s is the slope, which is defined as

$$\frac{1}{2}\left(\frac{LD_{84}}{LD_{50}} + \frac{LD_{50}}{LD_{16}}\right) = \frac{1}{2}(3.55 + 3.55) = 3.55$$

in this example, and N' is the total number of animals used between response probabilities 16 and 84% (i.e., probit 4 and 6, equal to 30 in this example). Then $f \, LD_{50}$ equals 1.896. Therefore, the lower fiducial limit is equal to 8.91/1.896 = 4.70, and the upper fiducial limit is equal to 8.96 × 1.896 = 16.90.

For all practical purposes, the graphic method should be sufficient to estimate the LD_{50} without using the detailed mathematical calculations of the maximum likelihood estimation (57). Nonetheless, since computer programs are available to handle the mathematics, the maximum likelihood estimation is used in many toxicology laboratories. An example of programming for the estimation of the LD_{50} with a small computer has been reported (88,124).

Various guidelines for acute oral toxicity testing are compared in Table 4.

■ *Example*

The following mortality data were obtained from an acute oral toxicity study. Calculate the LD_{50}, the SE of the LD_{50}, the fiducial limits, and the slope of the dose–response curve.

Dose (mg/kg)	1	2	4	8	16	32
Mortality	0/10	1/10	3/10	4/10	7/10	10/10
Procedure						
1. Log dose	0	0.30	0.6	0.9	1.2	1.5
2. Probits	—	3.72	4.48	4.75	5.52	—

3,4. Plot log dose versus probits (Fig. 4) and fit the best point(s) to a straight line.

5. From the log dose probits line, extrapolate the log $LD_{50} = 0.95$; then, LD_{50} = antilog 0.95 = 8.91 mg/kg body weight.

6. From the same line, calculate the slope as: (numbers of probit units)/unit log dose = 2/11 = 1.818. Thus, $\sigma = \frac{1}{\text{slope}} = 0.55$ (Fig. 4)

7. *Chi square (χ^2) test of goodness-of-fit.* Expected probability is converted from the expected probits. The test is conducted by converting each expected probit (y) back to the expected probability (P) and then to the number of expected responses (E) (i.e., multiply the expected probability P by n). The difference between expected and observed number of response will be used to calculate the χ^2 statistic, but instead of using $\Sigma[(E - O)^2/E]$, the weighted value will be used, i.e., $\Sigma[(E - O)^2/E(1 - P)]$. The degree of freedom (df) is $N - 2$, where N is the number of dose levels used in the calculation of χ^2. The critical χ^2 for $(4 - 2) = 2$ degrees of freedom is 6.0 at a $p = 0.05$, and the calculated $\chi^2 = 0.386$, which is less than the critical value, indicating that the fitted line is adequate.

Log dose (x)	n	Probits Observed	Probits Expected*	Probabilities expected (P)	Responses Observed (O)	Responses Expected (E)	χ^2
0.30	10	3.72	3.82	11.9	1	1.19	0.0344
0.60	10	4.48	4.36	26.1	3	2.61	0.0344
0.90	10	4.75	4.91	46.4	4	4.64	0.0789
1.20	10	5.52	5.45	67.4	7	6.74	0.1646
1.50	10	—	—	—	10	—	0.0307
						$\Sigma\chi^2 = 0.386$	
						$df = 2$	

* Expected probits = $y = \dfrac{(x - 0.95)}{\sigma} + 5$

8. *Determination of precision of LD_{50} by weighting.* The SE of log $LD_{50} = S_m = \sigma/\sqrt{\Sigma mW} = 0.55/\sqrt{18.5} = 0.129$. The approximation of the SE $(LD_{50}) = (10^m) \cdot (\log_e 10) \cdot (S_m) = 8.91 \times 2.302 \times 0.129 = 2.646$. The precision of $LD_{50} = 8.91 \pm 2.646$ mg/kg.

Dose (mg/g)	2	4	8	16
W	0.277	0.423	0.541	0.564
nW	2.77	4.23	5.41	5.64
nW		18.05		

9. *Fiducial limits.* Using the approximation formula, the fiducial limit calculated at the $F = 95\%$ level is given by $\log LD_{50} \pm 1.96 \cdot (S_m)$. Thus the lower log LD_{50} limit = 0.05 − 1.96 × 0.129 = 0.697, and the antilog 0.697 = 4.977. The upper log LD_{50} limit = 0.95 + 1.96 × 0.129 = 1.20, and the antilog 1.20 = 15.849. Antilogs of 0.697 and 1.20 give the fiducial LD_{50} limit 4.98 to 15.85 mg/kg.

TABLE 4. *Guidelines for acute oral toxicity testing*

Protocol provisions	EEC and OECD	U.K. USC notification scheme for toxic substances	U.S. EPA guideline under FIFRA (1982) or TSCA (1983)	Japan's MAFF guideline for pesticides (1985)
Animals	Rodents, rat preferred	Rat	Rat; other species need justification	2 Species required—rat and other mammal
Sex	M and F (F nulliparous and nonpregnant)	NS	Same as OECD	Same as OECD
Age and weight	Young adults and the weight variation within ±20% of group mean	NS	Same as OECD	Young adults
Number/dose	At least 10 (5/sex)	6 Animals	Same as OECD	For rodent at least 10 (5/sex)
Dose levels	Sufficient in number (min. 3) and spaced appropriately to produce a range of toxic effects and mortality rates for a dose–response curve and acceptable calculation of an LD_{50}	Precise LD_{50} not required; information needed on whether the test substance is of high, moderate, or low toxicity	Same as OECD	5 Doses usually required for rodents; other requirements same as OECD
Test limit	No compound-related mortality at 5000 mg/kg	Same as OECD	Same as OECD	Same as OECD
Controls	A vehicle control group if its toxicity is unknown	NS	Neither an untreated nor a vehicle control group is recommended except for vehicles of unknown toxicity	Toxicity of the vehicle used should be known
Fasting	Rat: overnight; shorter duration for rodent with higher metabolic rate	NS	Same as OECD duration for rodent with higher metabolic rate	Should be considered on the basis of species
Dosing	By gavage; single dose but if needed use divided doses over a 24-hr period. Withhold feed for 3–4 hr if divided doses are used. Dose volume not to exceed 10 ml/kg bw for nonaqueous vehicles and 20 ml/kg bw for aqueous vehicles. Variation in dose volume to be minimized by adjusting conc.	NS	Same as OECD	By gavage in a single dose; where necessary, the test substance should be dissolved or suspended in water or in a suitable vehicle
Observation period	At least 14 days. Extend if needed to establish the appearance/disappearance of the signs of toxicity	14 Days	Same as OECD	At least 14 days
Observation frequency	At leat once a day; more often if needed to minimize losing animals to cannibalism; necropsy animals found dead or refrigerate them; isolate or kill weak or moribund animals	NS	Same as OECD	Frequently on the first day; then at least once a day

Recording observations	Observations should include changes in the skin and fur, eyes, and mucus membranes; respiratory, circulatory, and autonomic and central nervous systems; and somatomotor activities and behavior pattern. Particular attentions to be directed to observations of tremors, convulsions, salivation, diarrhea, lethargy, sleep, and coma. Time of death should be recorded as precisely as possible	Any indications of general mode of toxic actions	Same as OECD	Types of visually observed signs of toxicity, the time at which the signs appear and disappear and the time of death should be recorded for each animal
Body weight	Record shortly before dosing and weekly thereafter and at death. Calculate changes in body weight for animals surviving longer than a day	NS	Same as OECD	Individual body weight should be determined shortly before dosing, weekly thereafter and at death
Necropsy/ pathology	Gross necropsy on all animals found dead or killed where indicated by the nature of toxic effects observed. Histologic examination of organs when evidence exists of gross pathologic changes in animals surviving longer than 24 hr	Histopathology not required if longer term studies are to be conducted with the test substance	Gross necropsy for all animals found dead or killed where indicated by the nature of toxic effects observed. Histopathologic examination not specified.	Same as OECD
Report	Should include species and strain; tables of responses with total number of animals exposed, number found dead and number showing signs of toxicity; time of death; and 14-day LD_{50} for each sex. 95% Confidence intervals, dose mortality curve and slope (where method of determination permits), body weights, and necropsy/pathology findings	NS	Basically the same as OECD	In order to be accepted by ACIS the report has to be in a specific format which includes: 1. Identification of the study, test facility, and purity of compound 2. Animals: specify strain, age in weeks, and number/sex/group 3. Duration of study 4. Method of dosing 5. Observation period; gross pathology of all tissues in all animals 6. Results: should be presented in a specific format including species and strain, route, dose, LD_{50}, time of first and last death, period of development and disappearance of symptoms 7. Conclusions/summary

NS, not specified.

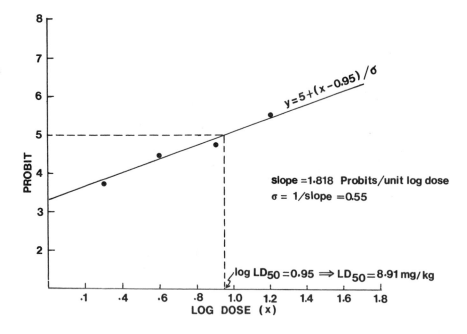

FIG. 4. Example of probit vs. log-dose plot.

Acute Dermal Toxicity Studies

Dermal exposure is an important route of exposure. The objective of conducting an acute dermal toxicity study is the same as an acute oral toxicity study. Such testing may provide information on the adverse effects resulting from a dermal application of a single dose of a test substance. The acute dermal test also provides the initial toxicity data for regulatory purposes, labeling, classification, transportation, and subsequent subchronic and chronic dermal toxicity studies. Comparison of acute toxicity by the oral and dermal routes may provide evidence of the relative penetration of a test material.

While the general experimental designs and principles of the acute dermal toxicity testing are similar to those of acute oral testing, there are differences. These differences include selection of the animal species, number of animals per dose level, preparation of animals, dosage, and administration of the test substance. Only differences in the acute dermal testing are described in this section.

Animals

The same concern about animal factors raised in conjunction with acute oral toxicity testing, such as species, age, health conditions, body weight, sex, and housing environment, can affect the outcome of an acute dermal test. The three most commonly used animal species are young, healthy adult rabbits (2–3 kg), rats (200–300 g), and guinea pigs (350–450 g). Other species can also be used. The animals should be housed individually in a controlled environment. Quarantine, acclimatization, and randomization are as described above for acute oral studies. The back of the animal or a band around the trunk should be clipped free of hair. When clipping the hair, care must be taken not to abrade the skin. If abraded skin is called for, a needle may be used, but care must be taken not to damage the dermis. Increasingly, investigators have come to question the value of conducting

tests on abraded skin and consider such tests to be irrevelant. To date, almost all testing guidelines call for conducting the dermal test only on intact skin (43,45,50,112,131). Starving the animals overnight is not necessary for the dermal test. Generally, 5 animals per dose level per sex are sufficient to allow for an acceptable estimation of the dermal LD$_{50}$. Smaller numbers of animals can be used.

Doses

Dose selection is similar to the acute oral test. It is generally believed that higher doses do not need to be tested when a test substance at a dose level of 2000 mg/kg has not produced test substance-related mortality.

While a control group is generally not needed, a vehicle control group should be included in the study if the toxicity of the vehicle is not known. Its influence on the dermal penetration of the test substance should be fully established prior to the study.

Preparation of Dosage and Dosing Procedure

The test substance should be applied uniformly to approximately 10% of the body surface of the animal (e.g., 4 cm × 5 cm for rats, 12 cm × 14 cm for rabbits, 7 cm × 10 cm for guinea pigs). This area may vary. For example, the area of application for highly toxic substances may be small because a smaller volume is applied. Liquid test substances are generally applied undiluted. If the test substance is a solid, it should be pulverized, weighed, placed on a plastic sheet or porous gauze dressing, moistened to a paste with normal saline (1 part test substance for 1 part saline) or with the appropriate solvent, and spread evenly on the closely clipped skin to ensure uniform contact with the skin. Grinding of the solid test substances may not be needed under some conditions. For example, when a granular formulation is tested, it may be more relevant to test the substance in its formulation state than to destroy the formulation by grinding.

Since rabbits are the most widely used animal for the acute dermal toxicity testing, the dosing procedure for the rabbit is detailed, especially for liquid test substances. Dermal application of the test substance ranges from occlusive to semiocclusive to unocclusive.

The choice of the application method depends on what the most likely exposure pattern is in humans. Skin irritation is usually the worst after occlusive exposure, followed by semiocclusive and unocclusive exposure. Skin irritation may not only cause stress to the animal but may also increase dermal penetration.

For unocclusive application, the application site remains uncovered, but the volume of liquid test substance that can be applied to the skin may be limited depending on the volatility of the liquid. Immobilizing the animal or using a device such as a collar is needed to prevent ingestion through licking of the application site. For occlusive or semiocclusive application, the application site is covered with an impervious material such as a plastic sheet, or with a porous gauze dressing, respectively, as described in the following paragraph. The volume that can be applied with the occlusive or semiocclusive patch is generally larger than that of the unocclusive method.

Dosing procedures for liquid test substances

Rabbits are clipped free of hair by using an electric animal hair clipper. The rabbit may have to be restrained by tightening the hind legs to a secured post and holding the nape of the neck during clipping. The area of skin to be clipped should be based on the need of the experiment and generally involves the entire band around the trunk between the flank and the shoulders if the dosage exceeds 5.0 ml/kg. If abraded skin is to be tested (generally not required), incisions on the stratum corneum may be made with a hypodermic needle ($20\frac{1}{2}$ G) 2–3 cm apart longitudinally over the application site. A plastic cuff in a cylindrical shape (approximately 12–15 inches long and 10 inches in diameter) open at both ends can be used. The cuff is put into the trunk of the rabbits, covering the application site. With the help of another investigator, the plastic cuff is folded around the trunk and secured at the thorax and flank of the rabbit with surgical adhesive tapes. Care should be exercised so that the cuff is sufficiently secured but not too tight to affect breathing. Using a long feeding needle, the correct amount of the liquid test substance is drawn into a syringe of appropriate size. The needle is then placed under the cuff and half of the dose is delivered evenly on each side of the vertebral column. After withdrawal of the needle, the test substance is then further evenly distributed over the application site by gently rubbing the top of the plastic cuff. A piece of cloth of appropriate size is then wrapped around the plastic cuff and taped in place to absorb any test substance that may spill off the cuff. After dosing, the investigator should observe the animal for a moment to see if breathing is affected, prior to putting the animal back into the cage. In the semiocclusive method, the plastic cuff is replaced by a porous gauze dressing. In unocclusive exposure, the test substance is simply applied uniformly over the skin; care must be taken to minimize run off from the skin, especially for aqueous dosing solutions. Applying the test substance in small amounts at a time may help.

Dosing procedure for solid test substances

If the test substance is a solid, it should be ground with a mortar and pestle unless there is justification not to pulverize. The correct dosage of the ground solid is weighed, placed in the center of a plastic sheet of appropriate size, and moistened with sufficient normal saline or another appropriate vehicle. If a vehicle other than saline or water is used, the effect of the vehicle on the skin penetration of the test substance should be considered, and its toxicity should be known. The type of vehicle selected should be based on the expected mode of exposure of the test substance and should be mixed into a paste. The paste is then spread evenly around the center of the plastic sheet. With one person holding the rabbit by grasping it at the back, another person moistens its belly and its back with paper towels soaked with saline. Then the rabbit is placed with its belly on the test substance paste on the plastic sheet, and another investigator wraps the sheet around the trunk of the rabbit. The plastic cuff is then secured in place with surgical tape at the thorax and the flank. A piece of cloth of appropriate size is then wrapped around the plastic cuff and secured in place in the same manner. In the semiocclusive method, the plastic sheet is replaced by a porous gauze dressing.

Dosing procedures for rats and guinea pigs

Similar dosing procedures can be applied to rats and guinea pigs. Liquid samples should be placed on the back instead of the belly or on the lateral trunk. If unocclusive exposure is called for in rats, the test substance should be applied to the skin as near to the head as possible to prevent ingestion by preening of the application site. In our experience, the plastic collars produce more stress in the rat, as indicated by chromodacryorrhea (red stain around the eyes), than in the rabbit. To minimize the stress in rats, we have successfully used small collars hand-made from light cardboard. The collar is lined with cut rubber tubing around the neck area and stapled in place. The cardboard collar is lighter and easier to place on small animals. It can readily be replaced if needed (the collar placed on the neck usually lasted about 3 days), and it is more economic than the commercially available plastic collars.

Exposure Period and Removal of Cuff

Almost all testing guidelines to date (43,45,50,112,131) call for 24-hr continuous exposure. After the 24-hr exposure, the cuff is removed and the application site is gently wiped with a paper towel soaked with saline, water, or any appropriate solvent to remove residual test substance remaining on the application site.

Observation Period

As in the acute oral toxicity test, the observation period and intervals should be flexible enough to establish onset of signs, time to death, and time to recovery, but should be frequent enough such that the loss of animals due to autolysis and cannibalizing is minimal. In addition, skin irritation should be assessed according to a scoring system such as the one described by Draize et al. (38).

Processing of Data

Data should be analyzed and handled as in the acute oral toxicity test. Since the exposure period in a dermal toxicity study is longer than in a skin irritancy test, the skin irritation resulting from the 24-hr exposure may not be relevant for assessing the skin irritancy potential of the test substance but may be considered as the worst case if the occlusive or semi-occlusive method is used.

Test Limit

If no test substance-related mortality is observed at 2,000 mg/kg, testing at higher doses may not be necessary because additional test substance may only be applied on top of the test substance layer already present. This layering may form a physical barrier to prevent further absorption of the test substance from the application site.

ASSESSMENT OF EYE IRRITATION INDUCED BY CHEMICALS

The eye captures visible energy and converts the energy into neurosignals which are transmitted to the intricated central nervous system in which they form neuroimages (vision). The importance of having this ability to perceive the external environment through vision is a giant step in the evolution process. In humans, vision along with hearing are vital for the development of speech, learning, and intelligence. Loss of vision can greatly curtail normal living.

There are three basic components of vision: optics, photoreceptors, and conducting nerves. All three components must function properly to form a clear and sharp neuroimage in the visual cortex. The optics of the eye (cornea, aqueous humor, iris, lens, and vitreous humor) must remain transparent and be able to refract and focus light on the right position on the photoreceptors. The photoreceptors (the cones and rods) of the retina must be able to undergo photolysis and convert light energy into neuropotential impulses. The optic nerves must be able to carry these neuroimpulses to the visual cortex.

Because the eye is constantly exposed to the external environment, its cornea must be protected from drying, dust, and microorganisms. The eyelids, the lacrimal system, and the somatosensory response of the cornea all work together to protect this outermost structure of the eye. Like other organs, the major portion of the eye is nourished by blood vessels. The retinal, circumcorneal, and uveal vessels also nourish and help maintain the eye. These vessels are so arranged and constructed that they normally do not alter the transparency of the ocular optics. Nutrients reach the transparent tissues of the eye via tears, the aqueous humor, and vitreous fluids.

Normal ocular functions are in delicate balance and are interdependent. Any traumatic insult, chemical or physical, can upset one or many of these ocular functions, thus creating a disturbance in vision. Depending on the extent of the traumatic injury (ranging from drying of the tear film to corneal ulceration or optic nerve damage), partial or complete loss of vision can result. Ocular injury not only can result from accidental physical trauma, but also radiation and chemicals.

Chemicals can cause ocular damage locally by accidental exposure to the eye, or systemically in ingestion of chemicals such as food contaminants and drugs. Because many chemicals can produce ocular damage either locally or systemically (65,72,99,123), it is important to test products for ocular effects before exposing workers during manufacturing and, ultimately, before subjecting consumers to products on the market. Ocular effects resulting from systemic exposure are beyond the scope of this chapter. This section focuses on eye irritation resulting from direct ocular contact.

Conducting ocular tests in humans is not only impractical but unethical. Consequently, many methods and techniques have been developed over the years for testing ocular effects in animals. This section describes the principles and methods for detecting potential eye irritants and discusses their limitations. In recent years, *in vitro* methods intended to replace eye irritancy tests in animals have evolved. The pros and cons of new alternative methods are discussed.

Testing for potential eye irritancy is required for the labeling and classification of chemicals by most regulatory agencies worldwide. The test protocol, interpretation of results, and classification scheme vary among countries. The differences among major industrial countries are also discussed.

Definition of Chemically Induced Eye Irritation and Corrosion

Eye irritation can be defined as reversible inflammatory changes in the eye and its surrounding mucus membranes following direct exposure to a material on the surface of the anterior portion of the eye. Eye corrosion is irreversible ocular tissue damage following exposure to a material. From a practical point of view, the distinction between reversible and irreversible changes sometimes is limited by the length of the observation period. Therefore, the term "eye corrosion" should be reserved for gross tissue destruction on the eye, which generally occurs rapidly following the exposure to a material. When interpreting results from an eye irritation study, one must take into consideration the biologic significance of ocular changes. For example, redness of the conjunctival is considered a mild ocular effect. Even if it does not completely disappear within a specific time period (e.g., 21 days) in a study, one can hardly justify classifying the material as corrosive.

Normal Physiology and Anatomy of the Eye

A brief description of normal physiology and anatomy is essential for understanding the development of eye irritation. Details can be found in some textbooks and reviews (56,97,120).

Functionally, the eye can be divided into three basic parts (Fig. 5). From posterior to anterior, they are as follows:

Photoreceptors (retina): the part of the eye that connects to the central nervous system via optic nerves;

Optics: structures that focus visible lights (images) onto the retina; they include (from anterior to posterior) the cornea, iris, aqueous humor in the anterior chamber, the lens, and its related organelles such as the zonules and ciliary body (muscles), and the vitreous in the posterior chamber;

Protective, lubricating, and nutritional structures: these include the anterior eyelids and conjunctiva and other associated secretory glands, the sclera and its outside layer (the fibrous tunic) and inside layer (uvea-vascular), and the ciliary body (secretory).

For chemically induced eye irritation, the main concern is generally on the direct exposed organelles such as the cornea, conjunctiva, and the iris. Effects on these structures can easily be detected by gross observation. If the chemical can penetrate deeper into the eye, other organelles also can be affected. Detection of the effects on these deeper ocular structures requires special aids.

Cornea

The cornea is composed of, from anterior to posterior, the epithelium, Bowman's membrane, stroma, Descemet's membrane, and endothelium. The epithelium is about five cells deep in the transitional zones at the periphery. The basal cells are columnar, the other cells are squamous, and the cells between the two layers are polygonal (wing cells). The Bowman's membrane (12 μm) is an acellular layer of collagen and ground substance which provides a functional interface between the stroma and epithelium. An intact Bowman's membrane and the epithelial basal cell layer are vital to the regeneration of damaged epithelium. Damage to the Bowman's membrane may predispose fibrosis. The stroma consists of lamellae of collagen fibrils and fibroblasts supported in ground substances. The stroma forms most (nine-tenths) of the cornea and it is limited on its inner surface by Descemet's membrane.

In addition to the organization of sheets of fibrils, other unique features such as proper hydration, also contribute to corneal transparency. The Descemet's membrane (5–10 μm), like the Bowman's membrane, is an acellular layer which is the basement membrane of the endothelium. The endothelium is a single layer of cells, which completely covers the posterior surface of the cornea. The cells are hexagonal with large nuclei. This layer of the cornea is particularly rich in the active transport enzyme adenine triphosphatase (ATPase). The maintenance of proper hydration of the cornea has been attributed to the activity of this enzyme, which catalyzes an active sodium–potassium pump (14,81,92). The

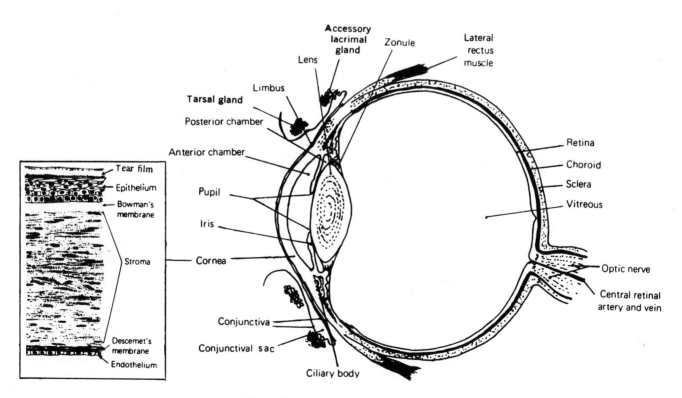

FIG. 5. Schematic illustration of the eye.

limbus is a transitional region between the cornea and the sclera. This region, rich in vascularization, is the source of fluid and infiltration cells during corneal injury.

The intrinsic protection for the cornea is provided by the epithelium and the overlying tear film. Other layers almost have no intrinsic resistance to injury. Penetration into the deeper layers of the cornea and other structure of the eye is limited by the chemicals' solubility and lipophilocity. Chemicals that are lipophilic and water soluble penetrate more rapidly and probably deeper into the eye than other chemicals.

The cornea is always covered with a film of tear, which consists of several oily and aqueous layers. Proper tear formation and drainage as well as as the stability of the precorneal tear film are important for a normal precorneal optical surface, proper lubrication, nutrition for the cornea, removal of bacteria and debris from the cornea, and antibacterial activity on the cornea. Reduction of tear formation can often lead to a dry eye, mechanical friction, irritation, or infection. A discussion on the assessment of tear film formation, stability, and drainage has been described (26).

The cornea is a powerful refractive biologic optic. Its refractive power is dependent on its being transparent and on proper hydration. Maintenance of proper transparency and hydration is dependent on many mechanisms, for example, proper tear flow, absence of deposits and blood vessels, proper arrangement of collagen fibrils, unimpaired nutritional supply for the metabolic active pump [(Na^+-K^+) pump], and proper intraocular pressure. Decreased transparency or hydration can be a result of corneal scars (decreased corneal thickness) or corneal edema (increased corneal thickness). Corneal edema can be caused by epithelial damage, endothelial damage, increased intraocular pressure, lack of oxygen, or inhibition of the electrolyte balance pump [(Na^+-K^+)-activated ATPase], which is located mainly in the endothelial membrane but is also found in the epithelium. The principles and methods for measuring the corneal curvature, corneal thickness, intraocular pressure, blood/aqueous humor barrier, and corneal endothelium damages have been reviewed (26).

Conjunctiva

The conjunctiva is part of the eyelid. It is the delicate membrane that lines the eyelid (palpebral conjunctiva) and covers the exposed surface of the eyeball (bulbar conjunctiva). Histologically, the conjunctiva is an aquamous, nonkeratinized epithelium with numerous mucus secreting cells. Accessory lacrimal glands are present in the conjunctiva, which contribute to the aqueous layer of a precorneal tear film. The Meibomian gland, a specialized sebaceous gland in the eyelid, secretes the outer oily layer of the tear film.

The main function of the eyelid is to protect the eye, especially the cornea, from external trauma through proper blinking reflexes and secretion of tears. Normal secretory and excretory functions of the tear is also important for normal optical functions of the eye. The precorneal tear film can form an optically uniform layer over the microscopically irregular surface of the corneal epithelial cells. The tear flow continuously flushes cellular debris or foreign bodies from the eye, lubricates the corneal surface from mechanical fric-

tion caused by blinking, provides nutrients to the cornea, and induces antibacterial activities by proteolytic enzymes and immunoglobulin. All of these functions are important to maintain an optically intact cornea surface. Substances that affect the stability of the precorneal tear film by interfering with the secretory/excretory functions or with the blinking mechanism can cause serious damage to the cornea, and may even cause corneal ulceration.

The nictitating membrane or the third eyelid is an important and prominent structure in many species of animals including the rabbit but is not as important in humans and nonhuman primates. It aids in protecting the conjunctiva and the cornea when the eyeball is retracted. The nictitating membrane, like the conjunctiva, also contains lacrimal glands and its secretion contributes to the aqueous layer of the precorneal tear film. In addition, the nictitating membrane helps to support the position of low eyelids and forms the lacrimal lake in the medial canthus. Vascularization in the conjunctiva generally consists of superficial and deep groups, mainly in the bulbar conjunctiva.

Three observation endpoints are generally associated with irritation in the conjunctiva: redness, chemosis, and discharge. In response to an irritant, the eyelids blink, the tear secretion increases, and the conjunctiva vessels dilate. Blinking and tearing (discharge) aid in removing the irritant from the eye, and tear flow also may reduce the acidity or basicity of the irritant. Vessel dilation may be triggered by histamine, prostaglandins, or other inflammatory mediators, resulting in an apparent increase in vascularity (redness) in the conjunctiva. If irritation is severe, the dilation of the vessel increases and vascular fluid and proteins leak into the conjunctiva resulting in edema (chemosis). If the edema is severe, the bulging may hinder normal functions of the eyelids.

Iris

The iris forms the pupil and functions in regulating the amount of light that may reach the retina. High intensity light causes constriction of the diameter of the pupil whereas low intensity light dilates it. It does so by two sets of muscles acting opposite to each other to control the diameter of the pupils. These muscles, circulatory and radiating, are innervated by both autonomic and sympathetic nervous systems. The set of muscles forms the distinct characteristic of iridic furrows of the iris.

The iris is anatomically located posterior to the cornea, and is a very vascular structure made of loose connective tissues, muscle, and pigmented cells. The amount of pigment in the iris varies. Heavily pigmented cells are found in most species except albino. Only a small amount of pigment is found in the albino rabbit eye. This is an advantage in ocular studies for it allows easier and better examination of the iridal vessels, lens, and retina.

The observation endpoints of local iridic injury are increased vascularity, edema (increased thickness of the stroma/swelling), reaction to light, aqueous flare, and gross destruction of tissue. These are the manifestations of an inflammatory process (iritis) responding to an irritant. Like the conjunctival vessels, the iridic vessels dilate and leak vascular fluid in response to irritants. Dilation of vessels and leakage cause edema and apparent changes in vascularity such as injection of iridic vessels (hyperemia). Aqueous flare is a result of protein leaking from the iridic vessels into the aqueous humor of the anterior chamber. Protein leakage into the anterior chamber alters the refractive index of the aqueous humors. Light beams entering the anterior chamber are scattered, giving the anterior chamber a cloudy appearance which contrasts with a clear appearance in normal eyes as a light beam passes through the pupil and the anterior chamber, for example, during examination with a slit lamp. This is called the aqueous flare or Tyndall phenomena which is usually not noted during routine gross examination of the eye. In a more severe form of iritis, tissue destruction may result and nerve innervation may be disrupted, causing the pupil to be unresponsive to light. Failure to react to light, from a practical standpoint, is the most reliable observation of severe iridic reaction since severe iritis is usually accompanied by severe opacity in the cornea, which may obscure the visible detection of changes on the iris.

THE DRAIZE TEST

The Draize test was developed in 1944 by Draize et al. to study eye irritation in rabbits (38). The test was based on the original work of Friedenwald et al. (61). For years, the Draize test has been used as the animal test to identify human eye irritants. It is a simple and generalized test. It is easy to conduct and requires no special instruments. While simplicity is probably the main reason for its popularity, it is also the limitation of the test per se. Undeniably, the Draize test can adequately identify most of the moderate-to-severe human eye irritants, but the test may fail to detect mild or subtle ocular irritation even with proper modification.

The result of the Draize test has been one of the key criteria for classifying and labeling chemicals in many countries. Although the test has been tailored by many regulatory agencies in terms of dosing procedure, numbers of animals, scoring of lesions, and interpretation of results, the basics remain constant (Table 8).

In the original Draize test, a standard 0.1-ml or 0.1-g of test substance is applied to the conjunctival sac of an albino rabbit's eye. The eyelid is held together for a few seconds and then released. The degree or extent of opacity on the cornea, the redness on the iris, and the chemosis and discharge on the conjunctiva are scored subjectively according to an arbitrary scale at preselected intervals (1, 24, 48, and 96 hr) after exposure. Scoring is based on the degree of effects caused by the testing substance. More emphasis is placed on the opacity of the cornea, which has a maximum score of 80, whereas emphasis is progressively less with other effects: conjunctival changes (maximum score of 20) and iritis (maximum score of 10) (20,64,94).

The Draize test has been a subject of controversy among animal-right groups (71,125) and even in the scientific community (8,20,64,67,73,94,122,146). This test has been widely criticized on the dose volume, use of animals as models, methods of exposure, irrigation, number of animals, observation and scoring including laboratory procedure variability, and interpretation of results, all of which are discussed below in detail.

Dose Volume

The 0.1-ml dose volume used in the original test was based on the volume used earlier by Friedenwald et al. (61) to study the mechanism of acid- and base-induced ocular damages. This dose volume was arbitrarily selected as a standard volume for intraocular injection. Draize et al. (38) adopted it solely for convenience which unfortunately has set a seemingly unchangeable doctrine for years even though the 0.1-ml dose volume absolutely lacks a scientific basis and, in conjunction with the conjunctival dosing method, often overpredicts the eye irritancy of a chemical.

Proponents of the 0.1-ml dose volume often argue that the dosage is a maximized test for the worst case, and that it can better predict human eye irritants. The Draize test is basically a safety test. Its main purpose is to predict what would happen to human eyes *within* the expected range of exposure. The 0.1-ml dose is far out of the range of any human exposure. The maximal volume the cul-de-sac of a rabbit's eye can hold is only 30–50 μl (101), thus even though one desires a maximal test, the dose volume should not be more than 50 μl. It has been our experience that any volume over this absolute maximum would simply fall from the eye. Furthermore, the worst case is not necessarily the best case. Constantly overrating eye irritation would have a desensitizing effect on consumers' and workers' awareness of potential eye irritation. This will defeat the purpose of testing for the eye irritancy to protect consumers and workers.

There are no data to substantiate the argument that the 0.1-ml dose can better predict human eye irritants. On the contrary, in at least one survey, there was little correlation between human accidental exposure experience and the rabbit data generated by the traditional 0.1-ml maximal dosage. The survey did not even support the general presumption that rabbit eyes are more sensitive than human eyes (24). Simply reducing the dose volume has produced data closer to eye irritation experienced in humans. For example, comparison of human eye irritation resulting from accidental exposure to many consumer products has revealed that lower dose volume predicts the eye irritancy potential much better than the 0.1-ml dose volume (60,67). In one of the studies, the time needed for full recovery from eye irritation in consumers or factory workers is compared with animal tests in monkeys and rabbits (60). This survey clearly demonstrated the modified Draize test [Federal Hazards Substances Act (FHSA) protocol] with a dose volume of 0.1 ml was the poorest predicting test, whereas the low dose volume and the monkey tests predicted better even though all three animal tests overpredicted the eye irritancy experienced in humans.

In 1977, a panel on eye irritancy test in the National Academy of Sciences (NAS), formed at the request of Consumer Product Safety Commission (CPSC), recommended lowering the dose volume (109). Subsequently, even smaller dose volumes ranging from 0.003 to 0.03 ml were proposed by others because they predict human eye irritants more accurately, cause less pain to animals, and can discriminate slight-to-moderate eye irritants (60,67,150). A recent study has shown that direct corneal application in a dose volume of 0.01 ml increased the response on the cornea when compared with the standard 0.1-ml dose, but did not change the response on the conjunctiva (150). The result, in the absence of compounding effects of a high dose volume, suggests that the lower dose volume is just as sensitive a method for eye irritancy testing. The lower dose volume protocol has been proposed to the revision committee of OECD; unfortunately, as of publication of this volume, the proposal had not been fully adopted. The reason given was "lack of an extensive data base." In the authors' opinion, there is sufficient evidence to date for lowering the dose volume.

Animal Models

As in other toxicologic tests in animals, the concerns of testing ocular irritancy in animals are similarity and predictability to humans. Recognizing that there are anatomic, physiologic, and biochemical differences between human and animal eyes, researchers are confronted with the difficult task of selecting the appropriate animal model and suitable test conditions to identify potential human eye irritants. The corneal thickness of dogs and rhesus monkeys is similar to that of humans (approximately 0.5 mm) (94,96,102), whereas rabbit corneal thickness is somewhat thinner (0.37 mm) (94). There is a lack of recognizable Bowman's membrane in rabbits, but they have a well-developed nictitating membrane (an additional target tissue), thick fur around the eye, loose eyelids susceptible to mild irritants, an ineffective tear drainage system, and a poorly developed blinking mechanism (109). There are also species differences in biochemistry, for example, variation in enzyme contents (86), and different penetration rates of various substances (93).

Even though there are shortcomings and exceptions in predictability, the rabbit has been selected for most eye irritancy studies. There are some obvious advantages for choosing the rabbit: a wide data base, economy, availability, ease of handling, and large, unpigmented eyes suitable for various ophthalmologic examinations. With some exceptions (66,122), the rabbit eye is generally more sensitive to irritating materials than human or monkey eyes (5,21). Thus, there are built-in safety factors for making extrapolation and assessment of hazards to humans.

In addition to rabbits, dogs and primates are sometime used for ocular testing. Eye irritancy in primates generally is more closely correlated with the exposure experience in humans, although dogs are also suitable under certain circumstances (9). Because they are much more expensive and less available, dogs and primates are only used occasionally to assess eye irritancy.

Regardless of which animal is used, the investigator should always have a good understanding of the animal eye being observed. Background ocular findings, if not observed prior to exposure, can be recorded falsely as chemically induced damage.

Methods of Exposure

Basically, there are two ways of applying a test substance to the eye: (a) applying the test material into the cul-de-sac of the conjunctiva or (b) applying it directly onto the cornea. The conjunctival exposure method has been adopted historically because of the ease of application. It has also been perceived as being accurate in dosing. However, it has been our experience and that of others (9,67) that conjunctival exposure is inappropriate under many circumstances, especially when the test material is a solid powder. The possibility exists of having the test material trapped in the conjunctival sac, thus producing some undesirable mechanical effects and making the interpretation of the results more difficult. It has also been our experience that a considerable amount of the standard 0.1-ml or 0.1-g dose (especially as a solid powder) either falls or is blinked from the eye once the animal's eyelids are released. Thus the claim that conjunctival dosing is more accurate is not valid.

The corneal exposure method, on the other hand, mimics more closely the actual accidental exposure experienced in humans. When assessing the hazard of most chemical accidents, this method should be considered except when such chemicals are intended for pharmaceutical use (109). Applicators developed for the corneal exposure method have been used in some studies (5,21). A more uniform corneal lesion was observed, resulting in less observation variability (5). For a study as specific as corneal wound healing, a corneal applicator is recommended (105). However, for hazard assessment, it is desirable to apply the test substance directly onto the cornea while the lids of the test eye are gently held open. The eyelids are closed for a second and then released to allow blinking; this action more closely mimics the actual exposure (67).

Irrigation

Washing the eye is a typical emergency remedy after accidental exposure to chemical substances. In experimental studies, the treated eye is usually irrigated 20–30 sec after exposure to the test substance. Water is rapidly but gently squeezed from a plastic bottle to produce a constant gentle stream of water irrigating the entire treated eye. Irrigation generally lasts for 1 min.

The effect of irrigation on the interpretation of test results has been the subject of many studies (5,7,9,13,31a, 59,66,68,115,128). While irrigation of the treated eye right after exposure can prevent or minimize eye irritation in rabbits, the effectiveness of irrigation is dependent on the chemical, the concentration, the time lag between exposure and initiation of the irrigation, and the volume of irrigation. Early washing (less than 1 min) is generally recommended to reduce irritation (31a,59,68,128). In other cases, ocular damage was almost instantaneous if irrigation did not begin after just a few seconds (5).

Number of Animals

It is generally true in experimental studies that the larger the group size the more precise the test results. Sometimes, the desired precision may be greatly offset by animal-to-animal variabilities. Economic considerations also are important factors in determining the number of animals used in a test group. The number of animals tested in a study should be determined by a balance between economic considerations and reliability of test results.

For eye irritation studies, a group size of 9 rabbits was recommended in the original Draize test, and group sizes of at least 6, 3, 3, and 4 rabbits have been recommended by the FHSA, Interagency Regulatory Liaison Group (IRLG), OECD, and NAS, respectively. The relationships of variability, classification, and group size are addressed throughout the literature (7,68,147). With a larger group size a smaller variability in results has been noted (147), whereas with decreased group size, lesser differentiation of irritancy has been suggested (7). Recognizing these facts, Guillot et al. (68) suggested a compromised approach. He suggested that with 3 rabbits in an initial study, there was a 96% chance that a positive or negative eye irritation result would be obtained. A similar conclusion was obtained in another study conducted with 67 petroleum products each with 6 rabbits (33). The eye irritation scores for the petroleum products based on all 6 rabbits were statistically compared with the scores from 2, 3, 4, or 5 animals. The comparison indicated that a subsample size of 2, 3, 4, and 5 rabbits correctly classified (compared with the original 6 rabbits/test classification) the chemicals at 88, 93, 95, and 96% accuracy, respectively.

Observation and Scoring

Reversibility and severity are the two major criteria used to measure eye irritancy in the Draize test. Reversibility refers to the time needed for all ocular effects to disappear and for the eye to return to its normal state. To determine this reference time, treated eyes are examined periodically at 24-hr intervals, on day 7 after exposure, or at longer intervals if needed to establish reversibility (38). The observation period varies for different guidelines. For example, the FHSA uses 24-, 48-, and 72-hr time spans (55); the OECD uses 1-, 24-, 48-, and 72-hr, and, if needed, extended observations (112); and the NAS uses 1, 3, 7, 14, and 21 days (109). In our opinion, the observation period should be flexible so that one can confidently assess the persistence of ocular effects and fully characterize the degree of involvement, since the onset and healing of ocular effects often are unpredictable (66).

The assessment of severity of different ocular effects is subjective. This subjective evaluation is the major source of error for intra- and interlaboratory variations (146). Therefore, to minimize at least the intralaboratory variability in scoring, uniformity in scoring techniques must exist among investigators regardless of which scoring system is followed. Pictorial references such as those prepared by the Food and Drug Administration (FDA; 52) and the CPSC (31) can be extremely helpful in the standardization of scoring eye irritation.

The types of ocular effects evaluated in the Draize test involve those on the cornea, iris, nectitating membrane, and conjunctiva. A grading system (Table 5) was originally proposed by Draize et al. (38), and subsequently a number of modifications were proposed (31,52,109). In the Draize system, the intensity and area of involvement on the cornea are graded separately on a scale of 0 to 4. The product of the two scores is multiplied by 5 to obtain a weighted corneal score. The congestion, swelling, circumcorneal injection, hemorrhage, and iridic failure of reactions to light are graded collectively on a scale of 0 to 2, and the score is multiplied

by 5 to obtain a weighted iridic score. The redness, chemosis, and discharge of the conjunctivae are graded on a scale of 0 to 3, 0 to 4, and 0 to 3, respectively. The sum of the conjunctival scores is then multiplied by 5 to obtain a weighted conjunctival score. Other lesions are also recorded, such as pannus (corneal neovascularization), phylctena, and rupture of the eyeball.

In the most recent guidelines set forth by the EPA, CPSC, FHSA, OECD, European Economic Community (EEC), and Japan's Ministry of Agriculture, Forestry and Food (MAFF) (31,43,45,55,112,131), only the degree [intensity of cornea damage, iritis, and redness and chemosis (swelling)] of the conjunctivitis is scored (Table 6). The area involved on the cornea as well as the discharge of the conjunctiva are not taken into consideration in scoring.

Various aids are used at times to facilitate or increase the resolution power of the observation. These aids include fluorescein staining and ophthalmoscopic or slit lamp microscopic examinations. A scoring system has been developed for the slit lamp and fluorescein staining examination (109) (Table 7). Other scoring systems have been proposed for lacrimation, blephamitis, chemosis, injection of conjunctival blood vessels, iritis, kerectasis, and corneal neovascularization (5).

Interpretation of Results

There are essentially four categories of data generated by the Draize test to be considered when interpreting the results of ocular testing: (a) the kind of ocular effects, (b) their severity, (c) their reversibility, and (d) their rate of incidence. Weighting the scores in the original Draize test has, to some extent, taken the first category into consideration, yet it biases toward the cornea—one of the most critical ocular tissues. Severity is measured according to a graded scoring system, whereas reversibility is expressed as the time needed for the affected ocular tissues to return to their normal state. Incidence is the number of animals that show some kind of ocular effect during the study. Interpretation of such data is a multiple and factorial undertaking. All four categories of data are somewhat interrelated; the individual scores do not represent an absolute standard for the irritancy of a material (113).

In one study, the interpretation of eye irritation was not considered to be the major factor contributing to interlaboratory variability (145). This finding is not surprising, if one assumes that everyone adheres to the same interpretation criteria. The question is, however, what are the appropriate criteria for interpreting eye irritation results that would have an impact on placing eye irritants into different categories. The individual scores do not represent an absolute standard for the irritancy of a material (113).

Many classification systems for eye irritants have been proposed. Some have been published in the literature (55,66,68,80,109) and in various testing guidelines (Table 8), yet there are many others that have been used in individual laboratories. There is general agreement among investigators on how to classify test substances when no irritation is observed or when severe irritation or corrosion is seen, but there is very little agreement on how to classify irritancy that

TABLE 5. *Scale of weighted scores for grading the severity of ocular lesions*

Lesion	Score
I. Cornea	
A. Opacity-degree of density (area which is most dense is taken for reading)	
Scattered or diffuse area—details of iris clearly visible	1
Easily discernible translucent areas, details of iris clearly visible	2
Opalescent areas, no details of iris visible, size of pupil barely discernible	3
Opaque, iris invisible	4
B. Area of cornea involved	
One-quarter (or less) but not zero	1
Greater than one-quarter—less than one-half	2
Greater than one-half—less than three-quarters	3
Greater than three-quarters—up to whole area	4
Score equals A × B × 5	
Total maximum = 80	
II. Iris	
A. Values	
Folds above normal, congestion, swelling, circumcorneal injection (any one or all of these or combination of any thereof), iris still reacting to light (sluggish reaction is positive)	1
No reaction to light, hemorrhage; gross destruction (any one or all of these)	2
Score equals A × 5	
Total possible maximum = 10	
III. Conjunctivae	
A. Redness (refers to palpebral conjunctivae only)	
Vessels definitely injected above normal	1
More diffuse, deeper crimson red, individual vessels not easily discernible	2
Diffuse beefy red	3
B. Chemosis	
Any swelling above normal (includes nictitating membrane)	1
Obvious swelling with partial eversion of the lids	2
Swelling with lids about half closed	3
Swelling with lids about half closed to completely closed	4
C. Discharge	
Any amount different from normal (does not include small amounts observed in inner canthus of normal animals)	1
Discharge with moistening of the lids and hairs just adjacent to the lids	2
Discharge with moistening of the lids and considerable area around the eye	3
Score (A + B + C) × 2	
Total maximum = 20	

The maximum total score is the sum of all scores obtained for the cornea, iris, and conjunctivae.

From ref. 38, with permission.

falls between these two extremes. The manner in which data are evaluated directly affects the conclusions that are reached.

Because of the complexity of eye irritancy data and their interdependence, some investigators chose to simplify the interpretation to a pass-or-fail approach. For example, in the FHSA guideline (55), if 4 or more of 6 test rabbits show ocular effects within 72 hr after a conjunctival sac exposure (0.1 ml or 100 mg of the test material), the test material is considered to be a positive eye irritant. The ocular effects in consideration are "ulceration of the cornea (other than a fine stippling), corneal opacity (other than a slight deepening of the normal luster), inflammation of the iris (other than deepening of folds), an obvious swelling with partial eversion of the lids, or a diffuse crimson-red with individual vessels but not easily discernible." If only 1 of the 6 tested animals shows the ocular effects within 72 hr, the test is considered negative. If 2 or 3 of the 6 tested animals show the ocular effects, the test should be repeated. The test substance is considered to be a positive irritant if 3 or more animals show ocular effects in the repeated test; otherwise, the test is repeated. Any positive ocular effect observed in the third test automatically classifies the test substance as an irritant. A similar approach has been adopted in the IRLG guideline (76), but in it an option is given to declare a test positive when 2 or 3 of 6 rabbits tested show a positive ocular effect and the test is not repeated. The pass-or-fail interpretation is too simplistic, however, and it does not separate eye irritants, especially those that fall between the two extreme irritancy categories (from nonirritating to severely irritating). Gradation of potential eye irritation is important to denote an anticipated hazard and to convey to the consumers or workers that a specific degree of precaution should be exercised whenever a potential of exposure to the substance exists.

Green et al. (66) used a different approach. Eye irritancy was classified into four easily recognizable categories based on the most severe responder in a group:

Nonirritation: Exposure of the eye to the material under the specified conditions causes no significant ocular changes. No tissue staining with fluorescein was observed. Any changes that did occur cleared within 24 hr and were no greater than those caused by normal saline under the same conditions.

Irritation: Exposure of the eye to the material under the specified conditions causes minor, superficial, and transient changes of the cornea, iris, or conjunctiva as determined by external or slit lamp examination with fluorescein staining. The appearance at any grading interval of any of the following changes was sufficient to characterize a response as an irritation: opacity of the cornea (other than a slight dulling of the normal luster), hyperemia of the iris, or swelling of the conjunctiva. Any changes that were seen cleared within 7 days.

Harmfulness: Exposure of the eye to the material under specified conditions causes significant injury to the eye, such as loss of the corneal epithelium, corneal opacity, iritis (other than a slight infection), conjunctivitis, pannus, or bullae. The effects healed or cleared within 21 days.

Corrosion: Exposure of the eye to the material under specified conditions results in the types of injury described in the previous category and also results in significant tissue de-

TABLE 6. *Grades for ocular lesions*

Lesion	Grades	Lesion	Grades
Cornea		**Conjunctivae**	
No ulceration or opacity	0	Redness (refers to palpebral and bulbar conjunctivae excluding cornea and iris)	
Scattered or diffuse areas of opacity (other than slight dulling of normal luster), details of iris clearly visible	1[a]	Vessels normal	0
		Some vessels definitely injected	1
Easily discernible translucent areas, details of iris slightly obscured	2	Diffuse, crimson red, individual vessels not easily discernible	2[a]
Nacreous areas, no details of iris visible, size of pupil barely discernible	3	Diffuse, beefy red	3
Complete corneal opacity, iris not discernible	4	Chemosis	
Iris		No swelling	0
Normal	0	Any swelling above normal (includes nictitating membrane)	1
Markedly deepened folds, congestion, swelling, moderate circumcorneal injection (any of these separately or combined); iris still reacting to light (sluggish reaction is positive)	1[a]	Obvious swelling with partial eversion of lids	2[a]
		Swelling of lids about half closed	3
No reaction to light, hemorrhage, gross destruction (any or all of these)	2	Swelling with lids more than half closed	4

[a] Lowest grade considered positive.

struction (necrosis) or injuries that adversely affect the visual process. Injuries persisted for 21 days or more.

The classification system has taken into consideration the kinds of ocular effects, the reversibility, and, to a certain extent, the qualitative severity, but not the incidence. The committee that revised NAS publication 1138 (109) put forward a system of classification similar to that of Green et al. (66). The categories are named differently: inconsequential or complete lack of irritation, moderate irritation, substantial irritation, and severe or corrosive irritation. The classification also is based on the most severe responder, and incidence is not considered. A provision for repeating the test is given as an option to increase the confidence level in making a judgment in some borderline cases. This eye irritancy classification system has been widely adopted in many laboratories.

One shortcoming of the NAS system is that too wide a spectrum is created for moderate irritancy, which may lead to overutilization of the cautionary term *moderate*. In order to fill the gap between the inconsequential or nonirritating and the moderate irritation categories, we have modified the classification system, taking into consideration the relative importance of ocular effects for visual function. Basically, the conjunctival effect is deemphasized and the nature of ocular effects is further qualified in our system. A slight irritation category is introduced to bridge the gap between inconsequential and moderate irritations. To be qualified for the *slight* category, the observed ocular effects must be conjunctival and all must disappear within a 72-hr period. Interpretation of neovascularization often proves to be frustrating. Neovascularization is generally considered part of the corneal healing process, but under some circumstances can interfere with the normal visual function by changing the transparency or hydration of the cornea. Recognizing this fact, we set up strict criteria for the interpretation of blood vessels seen on the cornea. Neovascularization is con-

sidered a corneal ocular effect, with some exceptions. Such exceptions are made because small vessels less than or equal to 1 mm in length, or a single vessel greater than 1 mm, are not considered to affect vision significantly (L. Rubin, *private communication*). Our system also is based on the most severe responder, but as in the NAS classification, the test can be repeated to increase confidence. In some borderline cases, judgments have to be made based on the investigator's experience.

Many investigators have at one time or the other experienced problems in interpreting results from fluorescein staining of the cornea when the NAS gradation system is used. The confusion arises mainly from the occasional artifacts inherent in fluorescein staining. Experience and sound scientific judgment are needed to properly interpret the fluorescein staining results (see also the following discussion on special aids and ophthalmologic techniques).

Griffith et al. (67) disagreed with using the most severe responder for classification of eye irritancy, claiming that there was no epidemiologic evidence to suggest that the most severe rabbit responder would correlate with the worst possible cases of human exposure experience. Instead, these investigators used the median time for recovery for classification according to the same temporal criteria as in the NAS system. The underlying logic is that the incidence of responders is being indirectly considered.

The classification systems of Green et al. (66), Griffith et al. (67), and the NAS (109) apparently have not taken into account the severity of irritancy. Although there is a perception of a direct relationship between severity and reversibility, we have examined the data of Griffith et al. (67) and found that a direct correlation of median time to recovery and the severity of irritancy did occur.

Kay and Colandra (80) proposed yet another rating system based on the Draize's scores, taking into account the extent and persistence of irritation and the overall consistency of

TABLE 7. *Scoring criteria for ocular effects observed in slit lamp microscopy*

Location of observations	Grades
Corneal observations	
Intensity	
Only epithelial edema (with only slight stromal edema or without stromal edema)	1
Corneal thickness 1.5 × normal	2
Corneal thickness 2 × normal	3
Cornea entirely opaque so that corneal thickness cannot be determined	4
Area involved	
≤25% of total corneal surface	1
>25% but ≤50%	2
>50% but ≤75%	3
>75%	4
Fluorescein staining	1
≤25% of total corneal surface	1
>25% but ≤50%	2
>50% but ≤75%	3
>75%	4
Neovascularization and pigment migration	
≤25% of total corneal surface	1
>25% but ≤50%	2
>50% but ≤75%	3
>75%	4
Perforation	4
Maximal corneal score	20
Iridal observations	
Iritis is quantitated by the cells and flare in the anterior chamber, iris, hyperemia, and capillary light reflex	
Cells in aqueous chamber	
A few	1
A moderate number	2
Many	3
Aqueous flare (Tyndall effect)	
Slight	1
Moderate	2
Marked	3
Iris hyperemia	
Slight	1
Moderate	2
Marked	3
Pupillary reflex	
Sluggish	1
Absent	2
Total maximal iridal score	11
Conjunctival observations	
Hyperemia	
Slight	1
Moderate	2
Marked	3
Chemosis	
Slight	1
Moderate	2
Marked	3
Fluorescein staining	
Slight	1
Moderate	2
Marked	3
Ulceration	
Slight	1
Moderate	2
Marked	3

the data. A similar system was proposed by Guillot et al. (68). Here, the greatest mean irritation score within an observation period is identified. On the basis of this score, the test substance is classified into six categories, ranging from nonirritating to maximum or extremely irritating. To maintain this initial rating, the data must also meet the arbitrary criteria for reversibility and frequency of occurrence, otherwise the rating is upgraded one category. The Kay and Colandra system has not been well verified for correlation to human exposure experience, nor has it been compared with other classification systems. Guillot et al. (68) made an attempt to compare the rating with the OECD protocol. They claimed that one-third of the 56 materials tested could be classified into a lower category by the OECD protocol.

OECD (113) basically has adopted the qualitative interpretation approach of Green et al. (66) and NAS (109), but the four gradations of irritancy was named slightly differently: nonirritation, irritation, substantial irritation, and corrosion. The OECD Committees stressed the importance of scientific judgement on severity, persistence, and the area of ocular involvement rather than reliance on a weighted scoring system for the interpretation of eye irritation. The most recent ECC Directives, on the contrary, have specified an average scores approach (Table 8) (43). The average scores of 6 animals at 24, 48, and 72 hr for each of the ocular effects (corneal opacity, iridal effects, conjunctival redness, and chemosis) are determined and a corresponding risk phrase (R-phrase) and safety phrase (S-phrase) then are assigned to the label of the chemical when the average scores fall within certain arbitrary numbers.

Despite such an elaborate scope of interpretation, fortunately there is little difference in the actual scoring system (basically adhering to the original Draizes) (38). Once the data are collected, the study should be acceptable to almost all regulatory agencies.

SPECIAL AIDS AND OPHTHALMOLOGIC TECHNIQUES

Draize's test, as stated previously, is a generalized gross test concentrating on the effects on the cornea, iris, and conjunctiva. Examination is usually performed grossly under a hand light. Accurate observations are limited by the experience and training of the investigator. Subtle ocular changes may be missed. If these subtle changes are to be detected and ambiguous gross observations resolved, or if internal tissues (e.g., the lens and the retina) are to be examined, the investigator must rely on special aids and techniques. Many such aids and techniques have been developed over the years, most of which are more objective than the gross examination itself. The principles and descriptions of these aids and techniques are beyond the scope of this chapter. A few comments on the most popular aids, the fluorescein staining techniques, and the slit lamp technique are presented below.

Fluorescein Staining for Corneal Damages

Fluorescein is a weak organic acid (Fig. 6) and is only slightly soluble in water, but its sodium salt is moderately soluble in water. It is very efficient in absorbing ultraviolet light and emitting fluorescent lights. The maximum absorption is 490 μm (excitation) in the violet region and its maximum emission is 520 μm in the green region of the spectrum. Its un-ionized form is less fluorescent than its ionized form. At a pH of 7.4, fluorescein does not seem to bind to tissue and is also nontoxic in animals, making it an ideal marker for an ocular fluid dynamics study. Because fluorescein is a deeply colored and highly fluorescent chemical, it can be detected at very low concentrations in biologic tissues or fluid; however, its detection sensitivity is often limited by the background fluorescence of biologic tissues.

Because sodium fluorescein is a polar molecule, it does not readily traverse lipophilic membranes, but easily diffuses into any aqueous medium. For example, if ulceration occurs on the cornea, the lipophilic membrane barrier is broken down and the fluorescein diffuses freely through the ulcerated area of the cornea and is either dissolved or suspended in the aqueous medium of the stroma. More detailed information on the chemical and biologic properties of fluorescein is provided in two excellent reviews (95,104).

Since its first use in studying the origin of aqueous humor secretion a century ago (44), fluorescein has become an important aid in ophthamology. It has been used as a marker in detecting obstructions in the nasolacrimal drainage systems, for studying changes in the flow dynamics of different ocular fluids, for demonstrating leakages of retinal vessels in angiography, for estimating permeability of the cornea and lens, and for identifying ulcerations on the cornea (95). Among these, the use in detecting subtle changes on the corneal epithelium (29,74) has been a routine procedure in animal eye irritation studies.

The corneal epithelium is a lipophilic barrier to sodium fluorescein, but such a barrier is broken when there is an ulceration or change in membrane structure. Some amount of fluorescein applied on the cornea will penetrate into the intercellular spaces of the stroma, which constitute a water-soluble layer of the stroma. When light is cast on the cornea, fluorescence is detected on the damaged area of the epithelium. Once the fluorescein enters the stroma, it will eventually pass through Descemet's membrane and the endothelium into the aqueous humor.

Fluorescein staining is usually accomplished either by solution or impregnated paper strips. Fluorescein solution is commercially available at several concentrations of 2, 1, or 0.25% sodium salt solutions. Preservatives are common in these commercially available solutions to minimize bacterial contamination (25). A drop of the solution is instilled onto the eye and excessive fluorescein is flushed immediately with a sufficient amount of water. The eye can then be examined grossly under a cobalt-filtered uv light for any epithelial defects.

Fluorescein is also available in impregnated paper strips (85). These strips are free of contamination and are easy to use. Moistened with collyria, a strip is lightly touched to the dorsal bulbar conjunctiva. The small amount of fluorescein should distribute uniformly on the cornea by either diffusion or blinking. Flushing is not usually necessary with the strips if applied properly. Nonetheless, if the strip touches the cornea, it then becomes necessary for the cornea to be flushed with water before examination. Better results are generally obtained with the fluorescein-impregnated strip when examination is by slit lamp microscopy.

The fluorescein staining has two valuable applications in a routine eye irritation test. It can be used for screening eyes prior to the study to ensure that healthy eyes are being used. The other application is for the determination of total recovery from grossly observed damages on the corneal. Slight epithelial effects still can be detected by fluorescein even though they are visible during gross observation. While most of these subtle effects on the cornea will disappear in a relatively short period of time, prolonged effects detected by fluorescein staining, but not by gross examination, should raise a concern over the healing process. However, when no gross lesions are detected at any time during a study (except for a few incidences of minor fluorescein staining on the cornea) one should not be overly concerned. If there are any effects on the cornea, they must be extremely minimal ones on the superficial epithelium, and eye irritation should be rated as nonirritating or inconsequential. If the staining is not an artifact, the minimal ocular effects detected under such circumstances should be readily reversible.

Although fluorescein staining can detect very subtle corneal epithelial changes, one can easily be misled by some very noticeable background staining. In addition, artifacts are quite common. For example, the apparent staining of the cornea can result from incomplete flushing of excessive fluorescein with water or even from reflected light. Mild damage to the cornea can be caused by a strong jet of water during irrigation. Damage can also occur if the eye is not handled properly during gross examination. These damages on the cornea are not related to the test compound but may be detected with fluorescein staining. Sometimes one may see haziness on the cornea after fluorescein staining even though a clear cornea is seen prior to fluorescein staining. Whether the hazy appearance of the cornea is a reflection of a mild change or artifact depends on several factors. If the hazy appearance is also visible under a cobalt filter and is preceded by grossly visible lesions, it is generally considered to be a residual effect of mild severity that will disappear within a short time. However, if the hazy appearance is seen intermittently or is not preceded by ocular effects, it is likely to be an artifact. Proper training and adequate experience are necessary for practitioners to recognize artifacts, and thus be able to obtain reliable, reproducible, and consistent results from fluorescein staining. In general, it is not necessary to stain lesions that are obvious and grossly evident. It is when lesions would otherwise go undetected by gross examination that fluorescein staining is of value.

Slit Lamp Microscopy

The slit lamp biomicroscope is an important instrument for studying many ocular tissues, especially the cornea. As its name suggests, a slit lamp biomicroscope consists of a microscope that views optical sections of different layers of the cornea made by an intense light beam acting as a surgical knife or microtome cutting through different layers of the eye. Many lesions can be observed with the slit lamp biomicroscope that would remain undetected by gross examination. Using recent models of slit lamp microscopes, one can not

TABLE 8. *Comparison of eye*

Protocol provisions	Draize et al. (1944, 1959)	FHSA (1972, 1979)	NAS (1977)
Animals (no./group)	9	6	At least 4
Sex	NS	NS	Male or female
Age	NS	NS	
Pretest eye examination	NS	NS	Gross examination and with fluorescein the day before test
Test substance	Acids/bases	Liquid, solids, or consumer products	Liquids, solids, consumer products, drugs, and others
Dose (solid/liquid)	0.1 ml/0.1 g for liquid	0.1 ml/0.1 g	2 Or more doses within range of human exposure. Suggested doses: 0.1–0.05 ml and the weight of these doses should be determined
Aerosol	NS	NS	Short burst from a distance similar to self-exposure by consumers
Dosing procedure for liquid/solid	Instill into the lower conjunctival sac of one eye, hold for 1 sec then release	Same as Draize, but one of the eyes serves as control	Manner of exposure should mimic human exposure conditions; for pharmaceuticals, conjunctival sac application can be justified, but for most other chemicals a direct corneal application more closely mimics accidental exposure in humans
Irrigation	3 Animals at 1 sec 4 Animals at 4 sec Washing with 20 ml tap water	Eyes may be washed at 24 hr after dosing with saline	Irrigation is not recommended for assessing inherent eye irritancy; the effects of washing should be assessed in separate study
Anesthetics	NS	NS	NS
Observation period	24, 48, 72 hr; 4 and 7 days	24, 48, 72 hr	1, 3, 7, 14, 21 days
Scoring system	See Table 5. The scores are weighed with a maximal corneal weighed score of 80 (severity × areas × 5), iridic score of 10 (severity × 5), and conjunctival scores of 20 (sum of redness, chemosis and discharge × 5)	See Table 6. Similar to Draize, except that corneal areas involved and conjunctival discharge are not scored. The scores are NOT weighed. (Based on CPSC, 1976)	Draize scoring system or a scoring system for using slit lamp

irritation test protocols in rabbits

IRLG (1981)	OECD (1981)	EPA (FIFRA/TSCA)	Japan (MAFF, 1985)
3 (Preliminary test) 6 (Definitive test) Young adult (2–3 kg)	At least 3 Healthy adult	At least 6 animals Male or female Young adult	At least 6 animals NS Young adult
Both eyes examined grossly, by instrument or with fluorescein at 24 hr before test	Both eyes examined 24 hr before test	All animals examined 24 hr before test	Both eyes examined 24 hr before test
General materials	No test needed for strongly acidic or basic materials (pH < 2 or >11.5) and materials cause severe irritation or corrosion to the skin	Same as OECD for manufacturing-use or end-use products	The end-use product should be tested, but no test is needed for strongly acidic or basic materials
Same as FHSA. If a vehicle is used its eye irritancy should be tested in a separate study	Liquid: 0.1 ml. Solid: amount equal to 0.1 ml which is not more than 0.1 g. The weight of 0.1 ml should be determined by slight tapping of the solid in a container.	Same as OECD	Same as OECD
1-Sec burst spray from approx. 4 in.; pump spray same as OECD	1-Sec burst from 10 cm directly in front of the eye. The dose can be estimated by weighing the container before and after the spray. Pump sprays should not be used but the contents expelled and tested as liquid or solid	Same as OECD	NS
Same as FHSA	Same as FHSA	Same as FHSA	Same as FHSA
Eyes may be washed at 24 hr after dosing with saline or tap water	May wash treated eyes at 24 hr after dosing if considered appropriate	Same as OECD	Similar to OECD; if irritation does not disappear at 72 hr after dosing, the effects of washing should be tested with 3 rabbits (washing at 2–3 min after dosing)
Should NOT be used unless extreme pain is expected and it should only be used once (prior to dosing) with the control eye also being anesthetized	May be used if extreme pain is expected; but the local anesthetics should not significantly affect the ocular reaction to the test substance; the control eye should also be anesthetized	Same as OECD	NS
24, 48, 72 hr	1, 24, 48, 72 hr. If no effects seen at 72 hr, the test may be ended. The period can be extended to establish reversibility or irreversibility of the effects observed, but the period normally does not have to exceed 21 days	Same as OECD	Same as OECD
Same as FHSA	Same as FHSA	Same as FHSA	Same as FHSA

TABLE 8.

Protocol provisions	Draize et al. (1944, 1959)	FHSA (1972, 1979)	NAS (1977)
Interpretation, evaluation, comments	NS	Positive: 4 of 6 rabbits responded Negative: 0 or 1 responded Repeat test if 2–3 responded; will be considered positive if >3 responded in the repeated test. If <2 responded, repeat test again and is positive if any rabbit responded in the 3rd test An animal is exhibiting positive reaction if corneal ulceration other than a fine stippling, corneal opacity other than a slight dulling of the normal luster, iritis other than a slight deepening of the folds (rugae or a slight circumcorneal injection of blood vessels), or conjunctival swelling (with partial eversion of lids) and diffused crimson redness with individual vessels not easily discernible	Reversibility is the major end point: Epithelial effects are considered reversible. Deep penetration may cause stromal necrosis which may result in scarring and vascularization. Persistent areas of peripheral corneal edema, especially after irrigation, may be due to residual inflammatory cells in the area of edema or an associated area of residual conjunctivitis in the same meridian. The precorneal and conjunctivitis are presumably reversible with time. Test may be repeated if results spurious.
Classification of irritants	NS	Pass/fail system (see interpretation)	Based on the most severe responder: Inconsequential/no irritation: no significant changes with 24 hr Moderate: minor superficial and transient changes detected by external, slit lamp or fluorescein staining at 24 hr, which include corneal opacity (other than a dulling of the normal luster), iridic hyperemia, or swelling, of the conjunctiva. Any changes clear within 7 days Substantial: significant injury, e.g., loss of corneal epiethelium, corneal opacity, iritis (other than slight injection) conjunctivitis, pannus, or bullae. The effects clear within 21 days Severe irritation or corrosion: significant injuries or necrosis that adversely affect vision. Injuries persist for 21 days

only observe the different layers of the cornea but can also examine other transparent parts of the eye such as the aqueous humor, lens, and vitreous body.

The slit lamp biomicroscope consists of an illuminating light source and a microscope. Both components are movable and adjustable, allowing the eye to be illuminated and observed from different angles and with different width and height adjustments of the slit light beam. An area on the cornea can simultaneously be illuminated and magnified by aligning the incidence of the light beam and the focus of the microscope. The light beam can also be directed at the area from different angles, providing several views of the same area.

Two types of slit images are used for illumination: parallelepiped and optical section (98). For the parallelepiped slit image, a rectangular light beam (approximately 1–2 mm wide and 5–10 mm high) is projected onto the cornea. The shape of the illuminated area is similar to a parallelepiped prism where the outer and inner surfaces are bent because of the shape of the cornea. For the optical section slit image, the width (20 μm) of the light beam is narrowed to its minimum and is projected onto the cornea, providing a sagittal view that is similar to a thin histologic section.

There are seven basic illumination techniques (Fig. 7): diffuse illumination, sclerotic scatter illumination, direct and indirect focal illumination, direct and indirect retroillumination, and specular reflection (98,135).

Diffuse Illumination

In diffuse illumination, a slightly out-of-focus wide beam is used to scan and localize any gross lesions of a large area

Continued

IRLG (1981)	OECD (1981)	EPA (FIFRA/TSCA)	Japan (MAFF, 1985)
Similar to FHSA; except that opacity grades of 2–4 and/or perforation of cornea are considered to be corrosive effects when opacities persist to 21 days.	OECD: Ocular irritation scores alone have only limited value and should be evaluated in conjunction with the nature of the effects and reversibility. EEC: NS	Same as OECD	NS
NS	OECD: same as NAS except that the classification terminology is changed to: No irritation Irritation Substantial irritation Corrosion EEC: a pass/fail system based on eye scores: Irritant: all ocular effects which occur within 72 hr and persist more than 24 hr have mean values of scores for each type of lesions calculated from 6 animals over 24, 48, and 72 hr to be: >2—corneal opacity >1—iridal lesions >2.5—conjunctival redness >2— chemosis or the above mean scores, when calculated separately, occur in 2 to 3 animals of a group of 3 animals	No irritation or inconsequential: effects clear within 24 hr Moderate: effects clear within 7 days Substantial: effects clear within 21 days Severe: effects not clear within 21 days Corrosion: irreversible tissue destruction	NS

of the eye. It is usually the first step in examining the eye under a microscope for gross lesions and their extent of change. This technique is similar to observing the eye with a hand light, except that the observation is made under a microscope (Fig. 7a).

Sclerotic Scatter Illumination

In sclerotic scatter illumination (Fig. 7b), a narrow light beam is directed at the temporal limbus, and the microscope is focused centrally on the area of the cornea to be examined. The light reflected from the sclera will transmit within the cornea by total reflection. Under normal conditions nothing will be seen, but if even minor changes are present the reflected light will be obstructed and the damaged area (e.g.,

mild corneal edema) will be illuminated. This technique is useful for detecting minimal changes in the cornea.

Direct Focal Illumination

In direct focal illumination, the light beam and the microscope are sharply focused at the same point of interest in the same plane (Fig. 7c). If a rectangular slit image is used for illumination and focused on the cornea, three general areas are seen when the parallelepiped is formed on the cornea: the epithelium (the anterior bright line), the stroma (the central clear marble-like area), and the endothelium (the posterior thin bright line). If an optical section slit image is used for illumination, the corneal layers seen from anterior to posterior are a thin bright layer, a thin dark layer, a granular

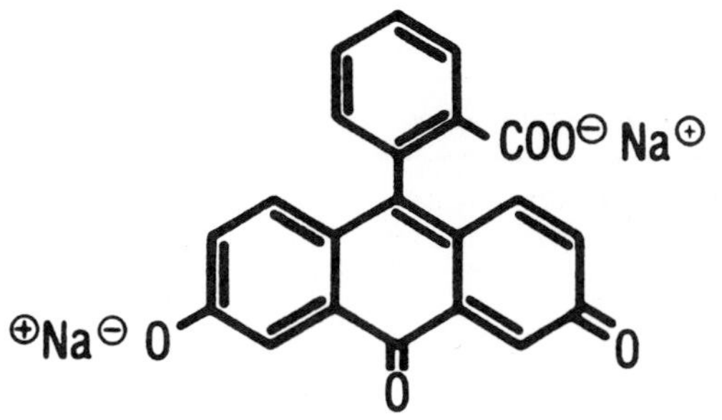

FIG. 6. Structural formula of fluorescein.

layer, and another thin bright layer. These correspond to the tear film, the epithelium, the stroma, and the endothelium, respectively. Altering the angle of incidence of the light beam decreases or increases the reflections. This allows for the detection of depth of the lesion. Opacities on the different layers can be easily detected as obstructions of the incident light beam.

Indirect Focal Illumination

Indirect focal illumination (Fig. 7d) is done by a narrow beam of light directed at an opaque area of the cornea. Changes, for example, in blood vessels at the cornea adjacent to the opaque area are illuminated and can be detected by focusing the microscope at these areas.

Direct and Indirect Retroillumination

In direct (Fig. 7e) and indirect (Fig. 7f) retroillumination, the light beam is directed at tissues behind the cornea, for example, the iris or the fundus. The reflected light illuminates the area of interest of the corneal tissue and can be focused under the microscope. The microscope can be directly located on the path of the reflected light (direct retroillumination), thus permitting subtle changes to be observed against a contrasting background. Any optical obstruction by lesions such as scars, pigment, or vessels located along the reflection light path will appear as darker areas on a brighter background. Lesions such as corneal edema and precipitates that can scatter the reflection light will show up as a brighter area against a darker background. When the microscope is located off the reflection light path (indirect retroillumination), the corneal structure is observed against a dark background such as the pupil or iris. Indirect retroillumination is better for observing opaque structures, whereas direct illumination is often used to detect corneal edema and precipitates.

Specular Reflection Illumination

Specular reflection (Fig. 7g) is most useful in studying the endothelium and precorneal tear film. This technique makes use of the difference in refractive properties between the cor-

neal surface and the adjacent medium of the posterior and anterior surfaces of the cornea. The microscope is focused on the cornea adjacent to the path of the incident slit light beam. By alternating the angle of incidence, a point can be reached such that a total reflection is obtained on the junction between the aqueous medium and the most posterior corneal surface, thus illuminating endothelial cell patterns and the Descemet's membrane. Similar techniques can be performed on the anterior corneal surface to visualize precorneal tear film.

Scoring System for Slit Lamp Examinations

By using slit lamp microscopic techniques, many subtle changes can be observed that would not otherwise be evident

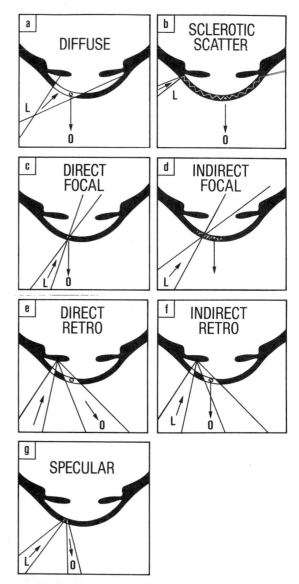

FIG. 7. Seven basic methods of illumination in slit lamp microscopy. (a) diffuse illumination; (b) sclerotic scatter illumination; (c) direct focal illumination; (d) indirect focal illumination; (e) direct retroillumination; (f) indirect retroillumination; (g) specular reflection illumination. O, observer; L, illuminator light. (Modified from ref. 135, with permission.)

from the Draize test. A different scoring system must be developed to reflect such subtle changes. Baldwin et al. (2) proposed a scoring system for the cornea, anterior chamber, iris, and lens. Subsequently, the NAS committee (109) developed a scoring system for slit lamp examinations that is similar to the Draize system in placing emphasis on the cornea, iris, and conjunctiva. Basically, in the NAS system the intensity and the area involved are the two main criteria for scoring. Using this scoring system, the investigator must have a good understanding of the physiology of a normal eye. Like the Draize score, the NAS system is also based on corneal effects; total maximal corneal score is 20 as compared with 11 and 15 for the iridic and conjunctival scores. A detailed scoring scale and criteria are listed in Table 7.

LOCAL ANESTHETICS

Primarily for humane reasons, guidelines such as those established by the IRLG and the OECD provide options for using local anesthetics in eye irritation studies. Tetracaine, lidocaine, butacaine, proparacaine, and cocaine have all been tested for their interaction with eye irritation, with the results being mixed and inconclusive. While most of these anesthetics can alleviate pain, they can also inhibit or reduce the somatosensory area of the eye and the blinking reflex. Tear flow is also reduced causing the test substance to be trapped and remain undiluted on the cornea instead of being blinked from the eye or diluted and flushed away by the tear flow. The blinking and tearing reflexes are important defense mechanisms, especially among higher primates, to accidental exposure to any substance (73). Some local anesthetics can cause delay in corneal epithelial regeneration and loss of surface cells from the cornea (69). Some local anesthetics such as procaine, lignocaine, piperocaine, amylocaine, amethocaine, and cinchocaine are cytotoxic to culture human cells including conjunctival cells (32). However, at least one study has shown that a 0.5% tetracaine solution apparently had no effect on corneal healing (118). Further research is needed to reveal the interaction of local anesthetics and chemically induced ocular effects. Local anesthesia is sometimes useful to induce akinesia of the eyelid during eye examination.

Local anesthetics are desirable to alleviate pain suffered by the animal, but one must always be aware of the potential physical, chemical, physiologic, and toxicologic incompatibilities before considering the use of any local anesthetics.

HISTOLOGIC APPROACHES

Histologic examination of the eyes has been routinely included in subchronic and chronic toxicity studies, but because it is time consuming and costly, it is performed only occasionally in eye irritation studies. Results may not be more informative than those from observations and measurements used in other techniques. However, histologic examination of ocular tissue under proper conditions can reveal the type of damage, tissues involved, and certain subtle changes in ocular tissue.

Both electron and light microscopic examinations have been used to evaluate local ocular injuries (22,66,78,79, 123,137,139,142; see ref. 73 for review). Although such methods can sometimes reveal morphologic changes of different parts of the cornea, conjunctiva, lens, and retina, as well as visual nerve degeneration, shortcomings are not uncommon. Among the many problems are sectioning the precise lesion, problems in slide preparation, and subjective interpretation of observations. A particularly important problem is that histologic examination is generally made on dehydrated tissue (22), which makes some lesions, such as corneal edema, difficult to detect. However, histologic examination of ocular tissues in local eye irritation studies has been considered an objective method because of its high sensitivity in detecting very mild ocular effects (73).

ALTERNATIVE METHODS FOR THE ASSESSMENT OF LOCAL EYE IRRITATION

Recent humane concerns with using animals in chemical-induced eye irritation tests have prompted many investigators to turn to alternative methods. Organizations such as the Johns Hopkins Center for Alternatives to Animal Testing, the Rockefeller Laboratory Animal Research Center, the Fund for Replacement of Animals in Medical Research (FRAME) of England, and many others have been very active in promoting alternatives. These attempts are successful in drawing the attention of many scientists. Consequently, the first generation of alternative methods for eye irritation testing has been emerging.

The development of alternatives is still in its infancy. Recent research has focused on validation of methods, most of which are *in vitro*. Basically, the current approaches for *in vitro* methods can be grouped into two categories: perfused organs (or tissues) and cell cultures. Many physiologic and biochemical markers of cellular function have been proposed. They include cytomorphology, enzyme leakage, corneal thickness and swelling, uptake of radioactive exogenous and endogenous chemicals, synthesis of tissue-specific proteins, and inflammatory parameters such as macrophage migration, and tetrahymena motility assay (10,15,16,51,82,83,106,107, 110,111,121,126,130,134,141). All of these are in one way or another indicators of the integrity of the cellular membrane and cytotoxicity. Some of these methods are briefly described below.

As early as 1956, Shapiro (129) used isolated corneas from rabbits to study the effect of sodium hydroxide solution on corneal swelling. Later, Mishima and Kudo (103), Hull (75), and Edelhauser et al. (40–42) used a perfused cornea to study the toxicity of selected chemicals on the corneal endothelium. In these studies, corneal thickness was the major end point measured. Besides specular microscopy, cytomorphologic examinations were also performed. Burton et al. (23) used similar end points to validate the *in vivo* and *in vitro* irritancy of a number of chemicals, and a broad correlation was noted.

The first successful corneal cell culture was achieved by Baum et al. in 1979 (6). The *in vitro* corneal culture technique was used later by Norton-Root et al. (111) to validate the irritancy of a series of surfactants. The end point measured was cytotoxicity. About 400 rabbit corneal cells were suspended in an incubating growth medium for 18 hr at 38°C. A solution of the surfactant or control medium was then added. The treated culture cells were incubated again for 7 to 8 days to allow the surviving cells to form colonies. The colonies were fixed with 10% formalin and stained with 0.1% crystal violet, and the number of colonies was counted. A fairly good rank correlation was observed between their *in vitro* results (cytotoxicity) and the repeated *in vivo* irritancy of surfactants by the Draize test modified by Griffith et al. (67). Using the same systems, Norton-Root et al. (111) evaluated six surfactant-based shampoo formulations and found good correlation between *in vivo* and *in vitro* ranking of eye irritation.

Borenfreund et al. (15) and Shopsis and Sathe (130) used HepG$_2$ cells (human epithelial hepatoma cell line) and Balb/c3T3 cells (murine fibroblast cell line) to validate the irritancy of different alcohols. Two end points were measured: cytotoxicity and membrane transport. Cytotoxicity was observed by phase microscopy for morphologic alterations such as changes in cell shape, vascularization and granularity, detachment and loss of viability as indicated by cell lysis, and trypan blue dye exclusion. Membrane transport was measured by ^{3}H-uridine uptake, which has been related to the status of membrane integrity and the metabolic phosphorylation process of cultured cells. A good rank correlation was noted between the *in vivo* irritancy by the Draize test and *in vitro* UI$_{50}$ values (concentration at which a 50% inhibition of uridine uptake was observed).

Stark et al. (134) used yet another approach: *in vitro* macrophage chemotaxis. The underlying principle of this method is that leukocytes migrate to the site of inflammation. Cultured Balb/c3T3 cells were treated with potential irritants for varying periods. The treated cells were washed with culture medium and re-fed with normal culture medium. The chemotactic factors in the re-fed cell culture media were detected by placing the media in the bottom wells of a microchemotaxis chamber, covering the wells with a polycarbonate membrane with 5 μm pores, placing about 10^5 cultured mouse peritoneal macrophages in the upper wells, and incubating the chamber for 4 hr at 37°C. After staining, the number of macrophages that migrated through the pores was counted on the membrane. Although preliminary results were encouraging, the method suffered from a number of technical problems.

Muir et al. (106) demonstrated that cytotoxicity, in terms of hemolytic potency *in vitro* of eight surfactants, did not correlate with *in vivo* eye irritation in rabbits. However, the ability of these surfactants to block spontaneous contractions of isolated mouse or rabbit ilea correlated better with the *in vivo* eye irritancy of these surfactants.

The chorioallantoic membrane (CAM) of chick embryo (hen's egg) method is a semi-*in vitro* technique which has been used to study irritation of mucus membrane (87,91). The method enjoys a key advantage of having a viable membrane with complete vasculature needed for an inflammatory response. A short exposure (91) and a longer exposure (87) have both been used. In the short exposure method, a fertilized hen's egg, incubated for 10 days was carefully opened around the air cell, exposing the CAM. Then, 0.2 ml of liquid or suspension was applied to the vascular chorioallantois, which was removed at 20 sec after dosing with 5 ml of warm water. The CAM, blood vessels, and albumin were examined and scored for irritation effects (hyperemia, hemorrhage, and

coagulation) according to an arbitrary scale with a maximal cumulative score of 21. A number of materials of several chemical classes have been tested using a cumulative index classification. A good correlation with the Draize results was noted.

In the longer exposure method (87), a false air space was created by withdrawing about 1.5–2 ml of albumin from the egg at 3 day of incubation. The CAM then formed the floor of the false air space, over the undisturbed fluid surface without focal artifact. The open shell was sealed with transparent adhesive tape and incubation was continued for another 11 days. The tape was then removed and the test substance applied onto an area of the CAM marked by a Teflon ring. The window was closed again and reopened at 17 days of incubation, whereupon the CAM was evaluated for contours and surface, color, retraction surrounding the CAM, spokewheel pattern of vessel, overall grade of severity, and necrosis (confirmed by microscopic examination). Preliminary results correlated well with the test results by the Draize test. However, using a method similar to that used by Leighton et al. (87) for acids, alkali, and surfactants, Parish (117) found that there was no reliable correlation between the CAM and the Draize results.

The survey of current *in vitro* eye irritation method development is by no means complete. Many unpublished reports of ongoing studies include histamine release from mast cells, plasminogen activator secretion, ^{51}Cr release from previously saturated corneal endothelium, contracellular ATP assay (83), and isolated eyes (119).

Eye irritation is a complex process involving multiple mechanisms (136). Although the idea of replacing *in vivo* testing in animals is admirable and the current thrust in method development and validation is encouraging, there are many problems with alternative *in vitro* methods. For example, most *in vitro* techniques are impeded by insolubility of certain chemicals. Testing extracts of these insoluble materials, however, may partially resolve this problem. A further problem is that the correlation between *in vitro* and *in vivo* data appears to be good only within certain classes of chemicals, requiring validation of different types and classes of chemicals. Most current *in vitro* techniques are not suitable to establish reversibility of eye irritation, which is extremely important in the classification of eye irritants. At the present time, none of the *in vitro* techniques appears to be able to replace *in vivo* testing in animals, but upon validation, some methods may be useful in screening ocular irritancy potential and aid in selection of a final product for further development.

It is generally agreed that *in vitro* techniques will not replace animal testing in the near future, so the immediate concern is to reduce the number of animals used and minimize the pain inflicted on animals during the study. As has been previously discussed, the precision of an eye irritancy test is a function of the number of animals used. The question then arises of whether it is justified to use a large number of animals to increase the precision. The answer is "no," for there is seldom an advantage to testing eye irritancy with more than 6 animals. The largest variability in an eye irritancy test is among animals, and the test itself is actually designed to be a gross bioassay. Therefore, to use a large number of animals in the hope of achieving a higher level of precision is neither realistic nor scientifically sound. As stated previously, a group of 3 rabbits can be sufficient for an initial attempt, which may be followed by more animals if the initial results indicate that clarification is needed.

Another proposal is to test for skin irritation instead of eye irritation. If the material causes severe skin irritation, it is presumed to be severely irritating to the eye as well. Thus, the argument concludes, an eye irritation test is not needed. There are two problems with this approach, however. First, pain and suffering inflicted to the skin of an animal are no less than to the eye. Second, the presumptive extrapolation from skin to eye is not always valid. In at least one study of 60 severe skin irritants, only 39 also caused severe eye irritation, 15 caused mild or no ocular effects, and the others caused moderate eye irritation (148,149). Nonetheless, this approach has been proposed as a criterion in a tier system to prevent conducting an eye irritancy test when intolerance in the skin irritancy test is noted (77).

Many test guidelines specifically indicate that there is no need to test materials that have an extremely high or low pH. This approach is fully justified, especially for compounds with high basicity. Alkali compounds generally can cause more severe eye irritation than acidic compounds.

A four-stage elaborated tier system, a gradual combination of the above approaches, has been proposed to reduce the number of animals used in eye irritation studies (77). Stage 1 involves physicochemical characterization of the test material: solubility, pH, shape, size of particle, and compatibility with local anesthetics. Conducting eye irritation tests may not be justified based on this information, particularly if the test material has a high or low pH or if certain unique physical properties of the test material prevent exposure under even the most likely conditions. In stage 2, the cytotoxicity of the test material is evaluated in cultured cells. If it is cytotoxic, further studies may not be needed. In Stage 3, a 6-hr exposure dermal irritancy test is performed and if any intolerance is noted, the assessment is terminated.

The final stage is to confirm the absence of eye irritancy. First, one rabbit, under local or general anesthesia, is dosed with a small quantity of the test material. A negative result is confirmed in yet another rabbit without anesthetics. Negative results will be confirmed with 6 rabbits with anesthetics. In theory, this is a logical approach, but in practice several questions arise: Should the test material be condemned as a severe eye irritant if it fails the *in vitro* cytotoxicity test or the dermal irritancy test? What are the criteria for cytotoxicity to be used at what concentrations? How is the cytotoxicity evaluated if the material is not soluble in the culture medium or if precipitation occurs at incubation temperature? Should the assessment be terminated if the material fails the first two phases of the final stage yet is only a slight or moderate eye irritant? As discussed above, extrapolation from skin irritation to eye irritation may not always be valid. Nonetheless, these questions can be properly addressed: The tier system may be a realistic approach that could potentially minimize pain and suffering to animals without significantly compromising the safety of consumers and workers. Undeniably, more research is necessary before the tier system can be adopted as a routine procedure.

The development of alternative *in vitro* tests for eye irritancy is extremely complex, partly because there are many physical and chemical mechanisms which can induce eye irritation. Most of the existing alternative tests cannot evaluate healing processes and some of them are not suitable for testing insoluble materials, or materials which can change the physiological pH of the test system.

Despite these problems, some trade organizations have launched programs to validate and evaluate some the first generation *in vitro* alternative tests. For example, the Cosmetic, Toiletries, and Fragrance Association are evaluating ten alternative tests: neutral red uptake assay, kenocid blue R protein determination, chorioallantoic membrane (CAM) assay, rabbit corneal cells (SIRC) colony-forming assay, EYTEX system, cell membrane permeability/dual dye-staining assay, mitochondrial activity (MIT) assay, tetrahymena motility assay, agarose diffusion method, and chromium-51 release assay. The Soap and Detergent Association has evaluated 14 alternative tests, and out of these, five tests (chorioallantoic membrane assay, corneal plasminogen activator assay, the SIRC cytotoxicity assay, a uridine uptake assay, and tetrahymena motility assay) were selected for validation.

LAWS AND REGULATIONS THAT GOVERN THE DESIGN, IMPLEMENTATION, AND INTERPRETATION OF TOXICITY STUDIES

To insure and safeguard the health and environment of their citizens, almost every country now has laws and regulations that govern the introduction and transportation of pesticides, food additives, human and animal drugs, and other chemicals. Many of these countries also have laws and regulations that govern medical devices, exposure to chemicals in the workplace, industrial chemicals introduced into commerce, and chemicals discharged into the environment. Within the last 10 years, the number of laws and regulations in various countries, especially in the developed and industrialized countries, has expanded exponentially. The development of these laws has involved politicians as well as special interest groups such as industrialists, lawyers, environmentalists, worker unions, and consumer advocates.

Increasingly, toxicologists are faced with difficult and conflicting situations in their attempt to comply or enforce these laws, for toxicologic and environmental sciences have not advanced as rapidly as the expanding laws and regulations. More often than not, a chemical may be regulated under many jurisdictions. For example, pesticides are not only regulated by pesticide laws at various levels of government but by antipollution laws, toxic substances control law, transportation laws, agricultural laws, occupational and consumer safety laws, worker right-to-know laws, etc.

The chemical and environmental laws to date are complex, imperfect, and often impregnated with political and emotional elements, but they have nevertheless met serious needs and have benefitted our well-being. Laws restricting chemical use have gradually brought about a cleaner environment worldwide; pesticides and drugs are being tested more thoroughly prior to marketing; and wildlife and endangered species are being preserved. However, behind this optimistic picture is an ever increasing bureaucratic situation in the regulatory arena. The promulgation of complex regulations under these laws often leads to conflicting requirements for toxicologic and other testings. There is too much duplicated effort. Efforts intended to increase agreement and uniformity in the regulation of chemicals are underway in the EEC and OECD countries as well as in the United States.

Chemical and environmental laws in all countries are still constantly changing. The enormous scope of these laws makes it almost impossible for one to comprehend them all, even to a modest degree. It is the intent of the authors to focus on the essential aspects of these laws.

UNITED STATES LAWS THAT REGULATE THE PRODUCTION, TRANSPORTATION, USE, AND DISPOSAL OF CHEMICALS

The United States leads the world in the number, sophistication, and, unfortunately, the confusion surrounding its laws and regulations for chemical use. Every year there are more new laws, amendments, guidelines, regulations, and policies. It is not our intention to interpret these laws or describe them in totality, but to review of a few important laws. Special emphasis is placed on FIFRA (Federal Insecticide Fungicide and Rodenticide Act) and the TSCA (Toxic Substances Control Act), since these are the most comprehensive laws and have had the greatest impact on the development and production of large-scale chemical use.

Food and Drugs, Pesticides, and Toxic Substances Laws

The Federal Food, Drug, and Cosmetic Act (FDCA)

The Federal Food, Drug, and Cosmetic Act (FDCA) is administered by the FDA and controls the introduction of new chemicals such as human and animal drugs, direct food additives, indirect food additives (such as packaging materials), and components of cosmetics. In the case of new human or animal drugs, *safety* and *efficacy* must be established for a particular therapeutic application before approval for marketing by the FDA. The approval process is lengthy. For the investigational new drug phase, industry is required to file with the FDA certain toxicity testing data at a stage when the investigation of the potential therapeutic usefulness of a chemical in limited numbers of humans or animals is desired. As the efficacy of the drug in the treatment of a particular disease is established through extensive clinical trials, these data, together with additional animal toxicity testing data, are filed as part of a New Drug Application or New Animal Drug Application for review of safety and efficacy by the FDA. Ultimately, as a consequence of the FDA review, the new drug application is either approved or deficiencies in the data are cited.

While informal guidelines do exist for what the FDA considers to be adequate toxicity testing for certain stages in human clinical investigation, it has not proposed guidelines for the conduct of particular animal toxicity studies. They have, however, issued regulations governing good laboratory practices (GLP) in the conduct of animal toxicity studies. The Pharmaceutical Manufacturers Association (PMA) felt

there should be guidelines for animal toxicity testing so that some agreement regarding basic methodology might be achieved.

Under the same act, industry must show that a chemical intended for direct addition to food such as a preservative or flavoring agent, or a new polymer having indirect contact with food such as in a packaging material or can-coating material, is safe for its intended use. Results of animal toxicity tests are submitted to the FDA for review as part of a Food Additive Petition. If the data demonstrate the safety of the chemical to the FDA, a regulation is published in the *Federal Register* allowing the chemical to be used for a particular purpose in food or in contact with food. The FDA has issued guidelines for the types of toxicity studies which should be conducted in support of a Food Additive Petition but has not given any guidelines in methodology.

At the present time, there are no requirements for the FDA to review cosmetic formulations for safety prior to marketing. While the FDCA only requires that cosmetics be free of any "poisonous and deleterious" substances, responsible suppliers of ingredients for use in cosmetics and manufacturers of the final product have been conducting relevant toxicity studies.

Medical Device Amendments of 1976 to the FDCA

Prior to 1976, the safety and efficacy of new medical devices was reviewed by the Division of Medical and Surgical Adjuncts of the FDA Bureau of Drugs. With congressional passage of the Medical Device Amendments, review of medical devices was placed in the Bureau of Medical Devices. This Bureau has classified existing medical devices into three categories and has been establishing standards for certain devices. The Bureau of Medical Devices has not issued guidelines for toxicity testing of plastic materials used in medical devices. Manufacturers of these devices and suppliers of plastic materials used in these devices have been conducting extensive toxicity tests to assure their safety in use.

Federal Insecticide, Fungicide and Rodenticide Act

FIFRA was originally passed by Congress in 1947 as a labeling statute that grouped all commercial poisons (insecticides, fungicides, rodenticides, herbicides, and preparations for pest control) under one law. The law was then administered by the United States Department of Agriculture (USDA). However, in 1954 and again in 1958, Congress amended the FDCA and required that tolerances be established for all agriculture commodities. Thus, registration of a pesticide also needed consent from the FDA. Two amendments were added to FIFRA before the creation of the EPA (Environmental Protection Agency):

The 1959 amendment added nematocides, plant regulators, defoliants, and desiccants to FIFRA jurisdiction;
The 1961 amendment authorized the Secretary of Agriculture to deny, suspend, or cancel pesticide registrations and assure the right of an appeal for the registrants.

Drastic overhaul of FIFRA took place in 1972 under the Federal Environmental Pesticide Control Act of 1972. The

EPA was not only charged with the authority to regulate labeling and the other original FIFRA provisions but was also given new powers to classify pesticides into general and restricted use, to require registration for interstate sales and production of pesticides, to require producers to keep records, and to inspect, seize, and order the suspension sales. Since then, FIFRA has been amended numerous times by Congress and further amendments are in progress as of publication of this volume. Some important provisions of the 1972 FIFRA, as amended in 1975, 1978, and 1980, are briefly described below:

Definitions

Section 2 of FIFRA defines all the terms in FIFRA.

Section 2(t) defines "pest" as any insect, rodent, nematode, fungus, weed, and others which the EPA declares as a pest.

Section 2(u) defines "pesticides" as any substance or mixtures intended for preventing, destroying, repelling, or mitigating any pest except those used as animal drugs and animal feed containing pesticides. The EPA also excludes deodorizers, bleaching agents, and cleaning agents with no pesticidal claim; and also excludes many products treated with pesticides but with no claim on pesticidal activity other than protecting the product itself (e.g., paint treated with a fungicide).

Section 2(bb) defines "unreasonable adverse effects on the environment" as any unreasonable risk to man or the environment, taking into account the economic, social, and environmental cost and benefit of the use of any pesticide.

Registration of pesticides

Section 3 empowers the EPA to register pesticides. The EPA has promulgated many regulations in registering pesticides. It has issued an extensive list of data requirements for pesticide registration (49), which includes testing guidelines and the GLP standards. The most recent toxicity testing guidelines for FIFRA were issued in 1982 (45).

Section 3(a) authorizes the EPA to register almost all pesticides for distribution, sales, delivery, etc. with two general exemptions under Section 3(b). One of the exemptions is the transfer of pesticides from one registered establishment to another registered establishment operated by the same producer solely for packaging or for use as a constituent part of another pesticide at the second establishment. The second exemption is the transfer of pesticides under the Experimental Use Permit (EUP) specified in Section 5 of FIFRA. In addition, pesticides intended solely for export, disposal, and use under Section 18 (emergency exemption) do not have to be registered; but all exemptions are still under the labeling and misbranding requirements of FIFRA.

Section 3(c) defines the procedure for registration and the criteria for granting a registration of a pesticide. Under Section 3(c)(1)(D), the applicant can submit data or, alternatively, a citation of data that appear in the public literature or which have previously been submitted to the EPA, to support the registration. The latter is often used in the so-called "me too registrations." Under Section 3(c)(1)(D)(i), the EPA permits 10 years of exclusive use of data of the initial registrant for active ingredient registered after September 30, 1978.

Under Section 3(c)(1)(D)(ii), if the data are originally submitted after December 31, 1969, the EPA can consider such data in support of an application without the permission of the original registrant provided that the new applicant has made an offer to compensate the original registrant. This provision only applies within 15 years of the original data submission. If the new applicant and the original registrant cannot agree on the amount of compensation, the matter will be decided by private binding arbitration. Section 3(c)(1)(D)(iii) permits the EPA to consider data in support of a new application without permission from the original registrant and without an offer for compensation, if the exclusive use period or the required compensation period has expired.

Section 3(c)(2)(A) requires the EPA to publish data guidelines specifying the kinds of information required to support the registration of a pesticide. Section 3(c)(2)(B) authorizes the EPA to require additional data from registrant(s) if the administrator determines such data are needed for maintaining an existing registration of a pesticide (also called the data-call-in provision). The EPA must allow sufficient time for the registrant(s) to generate such data. Each affected registrant must provide the EPA with evidence within 90 days after receipt of notification that the registrant is taking appropriate steps to secure the additional data. The cost may be shared by more than one registrant. If the EPA determines that a registrant, within the 90-day limit, has failed to take appropriate action, it may issue a notice of intent to suspend the registration. The suspension becomes final and effective after 30 days from the receipt of the notice by the registrant unless a request for a hearing is requested. The hearing deals only with the issue of whether the registrant has taken the appropriate action to secure the data. The hearing is held within 75 days after the receipt of the request for a hearing. At any time after suspension, the registration can be reinstated if the EPA determines that the registrant has complied fully with the requirements.

Section 3(c)(5) states the criteria for approval of pesticide registration. A pesticide can be approved if the following criteria are met:

1. Its composition warrants its proposed claims of efficacy.
2. Its labeling complies with FIFRA which requires certain precautionary statements and directions for use. A false or misleading label is considered misbranded under Section 2(g) of FIFRA.
3. It performs its intended function when used as directed by the label and causes no unreasonable risk to the environment.
4. It causes no unreasonable risk to the environment even though under generally misused conditions.

Under Section 2(bb), which defines "unreasonable adverse effect on health and environment," the EPA is required to consider the risks and benefits of a pesticide but cannot deny a registration simply because it determines that the pesticide is lacking essentiality (i.e., is not an important pesticide).

Section 3(c)(6) gives the EPA the authority to deny an application if it determines that the criteria for approval are not met.

Section 3(c)(7) allows the EPA to grant conditional registration in the absence of full supporting data under special circumstances, provided it has determined that there will be no unreasonable risk to health and environment. Conditional registration may be granted if the EPA determines that the pesticide is identical or substantially similar to a currently registered pesticide, or if it is an additional new use, or if the registration is only for a period sufficient for the generation of data.

Section 3(c)(8) gives the EPA the authority to initiate an interim administrative review (RPAR, or Special Review) if valid testing or other significant evidence raises prudent concerns of unreasonable risk.

Section 3(d) gives the EPA the power to classify pesticides into general and restricted use.

Certification of applicants

Section 4 of FIFRA requires the EPA to certify applicants for restricted use pesticides.

Experimental use permit

Section 5 of FIFRA empowers the EPA to issue an EUP allowing registrants to use unregistered pesticides solely for testing purposes in order to generate extensive data to support the registration application under Section 3. Small scale testing conducted under strictly limited conditions to determine the pesticide's efficacy, toxicity, and other properties are generally exempted from the EUP. This statute requires the EPA to complete the EUP application within 120 days. EUP's are valid for one year and are renewable upon request.

Administrative review and suspension

Section 6 of FIFRA lists the adverse effects reporting, and procedure and criteria for administrative review and suspension of a registration. All pesticide registrations shall be cancelled after 5 years unless the registrant requests, in accordance with the regulations prescribed by the EPA, that the registration be continued. If the EPA determines at any time after registration that the pesticide causes unreasonable adverse effects on the environment, the EPA may issue a notice of intent either to cancel or to hold a hearing to determine if the registration should be cancelled or its classification should be changed. The EPA is required to take into consideration the impact of its decision or intent on agriculture and must notify the Secretary of Agriculture. The EPA is also required to solicit comments from a Scientific Advisory Panel (SAP) on any proposed suspension actions. Before a hearing, the hearing examiner shall refer to a committee of the National Academy of Sciences (NAS) the relevant questions of scientific facts. The committee shall report in writing to the hearing examiner the scientific facts within 60 days. Section 6(a)(2) requires reporting any unreasonable adverse effects to the EPA after the pesticide is registered.

Confidentiality

Section 10 of FIFRA requires the EPA to protect trade secrets and other information and lists penalty for disclosure by a federal employee. Section 10 also prohibits the EPA to disclose trade secrets or other information to foreign or multinational companies.

Applicator standards

Section 11 of FIFRA sets the standard for commercial and general applicators of pesticides.

Unlawful acts, seizure, and penalties

Section 12 describes the unlawful acts of distributing, selling, holding, delivering, shipping, and receiving pesticides, and also lists the exemptions.

Section 13 empowers the EPA to stop the sale and use of pesticides and to remove and seize pesticides.

Section 14 describes the civil and criminal penalties for violating any provisions of FIFRA.

Reimbursement

Section 15 requires the EPA to make reimbursement (indemnities). If the EPA suspends or cancels the registration of a pesticide to prevent an imminent hazard, it must reimburse any person who owned any quantity of the pesticide, unless the EPA determines that the person knew the pesticide did not meet registration requirements under FIFRA Section 3(c)(5).

Right to appeal

Section 16 guarantees the registrant's right to jurisdictional appeals.

Import and exports

Section 17 describes the requirements and exemptions of import and exports of pesticides.

Emergency use exemption

Section 18 authorizes the EPA to grant emergency use of unregistered pesticides.

Research and monitoring

Section 20 requires the EPA to undertake research and monitoring pesticides.

Soliciting comments from the public and the USDA

Section 21 requires the EPA to solicit comments from the Secretary of Agriculture before publishing regulations, and from the public at the discretion of the EPA.

State regulations

Section 24 specifies the authority of individual states to regulate pesticides. States can regulate the sale and use of any federally registered pesticides but cannot permit any sale or use of pesticides prohibited by FIFRA (EPA). In other words, states should not be less strict than the federal government in regulating pesticides. A state may not impose additional labeling or packaging requirements but may provide registration for additional use of federally registered pesticides in that particular state. The state registration has certain restrictions and is still subject to the approval of the EPA.

Promulgation of regulations, the scientific advisory panel, and peer review

Section 25 specifies EPA's authority to promulgate regulations, to exempt pesticides, and to employ other authorities. One very important provision is **Section 25(d)** concerning the SAP. The EPA administrator is required to submit a notice of intent to an SAP advisory panel for comments on the impact of the EPA's proposed action to suspend or cancel registration under Section 6(b) or under any regulations on health and the environment (risk and benefit). The administrator can also solicit from the panel comments, evaluations, and recommendations for operating guidelines and must respond to the panel's report. The SAP may create temporary subpanels consisting of additional scientists for specific projects. The seven members of the SAP are selected by the EPA administrator from a list of twelve nominees who are chosen by the National Institute of Health (NIH, six nominees) and National Science Foundation (NSF, six nominees). **Section 25(e)** requires the administrator to specify procedures for peer review of the design, protocols, and conduct of major specific scientific studies performed or other agencies and studies that the EPA relies upon for initiating changes in classification, suspensions, or cancellation.

Authority of the state and the EPA

Section 26 specifies that the EPA may determine that a particular state has the primary responsibility to enforce violation of the uses of pesticides, but **Section 27** gives the EPA ultimate enforcement authority. The EPA may rescind the state's authority under specific emergency conditions or if the administrator determines that the state is unable or has failed to enforce the law.

Tolerances

FDCA Sections 408 and 409: Before the creation of the EPA, the FDA had the authority to set tolerances for pesticides in raw agricultural commodities (Section 408) and for food additives (Section 409). Section 3 of FIFRA (registration of pesticides) assigned to the EPA the responsibility of establishing safety levels for both pesticides and food additives. While the EPA also has the authority to monitor pesticide levels in foods, the FDA retains the basic responsibility of monitoring pesticide levels in food and of seizing food. The USDA continues to be responsible for monitoring meat and poultry for pesticides and other chemicals.

FDCA Section 409 contains a controversial clause, the Delaney clause (1958 amendment), which specifies that "no additive shall be deemed to be safe if it is found to induce cancer when ingested by man or animal, or if it is found, after tests which are appropriate for the evaluation of the safety of food additives, to induce cancer in man or animals." For chemicals that are found to be carcinogenic in laboratory animals, the EPA has two conflicting provisions. While Section 408 allows tolerances to be set on the basis of risk assessment, Section 409, the Delaney clause, prohibits tolerance setting. The Delaney clause was created more than two decades ago when the science of toxicology was still in its infancy. Advances in our understanding of carcinogens and the limitations of results generated in animal tests now permits safe levels to be set for some chemicals found to be carcinogenic in laboratory animals. Compounding the controversy is the fact that analytical equipment has advanced since 1958 to the point that extremely minute quantities of chemicals, often in parts per million (ppm), parts per billion (ppb), or even part per trillion (ppt), can now be detected in food. A solution to the Delaney controversy has not been found, although the FDA has used three approaches in avoiding the Delaney clause:

1. *Constituent approach.* When the food additive is not a carcinogen by itself but consists of a carcinogen as a constituent, the Delaney clause will not be applied.
2. *Sensitivity of the method approach.* If the carcinogen is not detected in food at the sensitivity of the method level, the Delaney clause will not be applied.
3. *Deminimus approach.* The risk of the carcinogen as a food additive is so trivial that the FDA does not have to act.

Toxic Substances Control Act (TSCA)

TSCA went into effect on January 1, 1977, and was enacted by Congress to fill the gaps among various statutes such as FIFRA and FDCA. TSCA is administered by the Office of Pesticides and Toxic Substances of the EPA. It is a complex and far reaching law which affects industrial chemicals existing in commerce in the United States as well as new chemicals. TSCA defines "new" chemicals as those that do not appear on the TSCA initial inventory list [TSCA **Section 8(b)** or any of its supplements]. One of the first tasks of TSCA was to inventory chemicals that were active in commerce between 1977 and 1979. In other words, all chemicals not exclusively under the jurisdiction of other statutes such as FIFRA are under the jurisdiction of TSCA. In 1980, the EPA determined that "significant-new-use-rule" chemicals would be treated as new chemicals, even though they were not on the original Section 8(b) inventory list; however, this ruling was withdrawn in 1983 by the EPA.

Under **Section 5** of TSCA, manufacturers or importers of industrial chemicals which meet the definition of being "new" under TSCA are required to notify the EPA at least 90 days prior to the manufacture or import of a new chemical. The act requires that certain information regarding the new chemical be submitted in a premanufacturer notification (PMN) to the EPA for review. While the act does not require that toxicity testing be conducted on a new chemical prior to manufacture, it does require that all existing health and safety data be submitted which demonstrate that the new chemical does not present an unreasonable risk to health or the environment. If the EPA determines that the new chemical presents an unreasonable risk or if there is insufficient evidence to make a risk assessment, the EPA can prevent or limit the manufacture or use of the new chemical.

The EPA may, for good cause, extend its normal review period of 90 days to 180 days. If the EPA determines in its review that the new chemical does present an unreasonable risk or that the chemical will be produced in substantial quantities to result in significant exposure to humans and the environment, one of several actions it may take is to require that the chemical be tested for specific toxic effects under Section 4 of the TSCA.

Under **Section 4** of the TSCA, the EPA may also issue a testing rule that would require a specified chemical or chemical mixture to be tested for certain toxic effects. Testing guidelines almost identical to the FIFRA guidelines were issued in 1983. The manufacturer(s) bear the costs which can be shared among affected manufacturers under TSCA **Section 4(c).** Before promulgating rules, certain criteria must be met under **Section 4(a).** The EPA must find that the chemicals may present an unreasonable risk to health or the environment or that they will be produced in substantial quantities resulting in substantial human or environmental exposure. In addition to these criteria, the EPA must show that available information is insufficient for evaluation of the chemical's health and environmental effects and that the testing is necessary to develop sufficient data concerning the effects. **Section 4(b)** authorizes the EPA to determine the time period within which the results must be submitted to the EPA, and to oversee the testing process to establish the identity of the test chemical, testing procedures, and methodology to the extent that is necessary to assure that data generated are reliable and adequate.

To aid the EPA in establishing priorities for testing, **Section 4(e)** of TSCA created an Interagency Testing Committee (ITC) composed of representatives from various federal agencies responsible for protecting health or the environment. The ITC is empowered to recommend a specific chemical for priority consideration by the EPA in the development of its testing rules (rule making). Within 12 months after a chemical has been recommended by the ITC, the EPA must either initiate a rule-making proceeding to require testing or publish in the *Federal Register* a notice explaining why this proceeding has not been initiated. The EPA can also designate chemicals even though they are not recommended by the ITC, or can propose more extensive testing than those recommended by the ITC.

Under TSCA **Section 6,** the administrator of the EPA is authorized to prohibit or limit production or impose labeling or other requirements, if the administrator determines, after taking into consideration risk and benefit, that a chemical presents an unreasonable risk of injury to health or the environment. Under TSCA **Section 7,** the EPA can seek an injunction or pursue other actions if the administrator recognizes an imminent and unreasonable risk of serious or widespread injury to health or the environment.

Section 8 of TSCA requires manufacturers and processors to collect, maintain, and submit chemical information [**Section 8(a)**], maintain records of significant adverse reactions to health or the environment [**Section 8(c)**], provide lists and copies of health and safety studies [**Section 8(d)**], and report information concerning substantial risk [**Section 8(e)**]. The EPA's interpretation of Section 8(e) is that the reporting obligation falls directly on any "officers and employees who are capable of appreciating the significance of pertinent information." The responsibility of the officers or employees can only be relieved if there is an official reporting procedure established within the employee's organization. The EPA requires reporting under **Section 8(e)** within 15 working days.

TSCA provides certain exemptions. For example, chemicals of small quantity produced or imported purely for research and development purposes are exempted from TSCA **Section 5** requiring premanufacture notification. However, the manufacturer or importer is required to evaluate data or information in its possession or control and notify all persons involved in research and development activities of any potential risk to health.

Submission of a premanufacture notification under TSCA

Manufacture or importation of a new chemical other than in limited quantities for research and development purposes is prohibited by the act. At the point when the developer of a new chemical foresees commercial application of the new chemical and wishes to produce or import it in commercial quantities, he should file a PMN. The information required by a PMN should be submitted to the extent that it is known or reasonably ascertainable. Obviously, in the early development of a chemical, data in all categories will not be fully developed. In such instances, the submitter should state that such information is not known and not reasonably ascertainable.

Under **Section 5** of TSCA, a manufacturer is required to submit the following information to the EPA as part of a PMN package.

1. Common or trade name, chemical identity, and molecular structure.
2. The categories or proposed categories of use.
3. The total amount of substance to be manufactured or processed.
4. The amount to be manufactured for each category of use.
5. A description of the by-products resulting from the manufacturing, process, use, or disposal of the product.
6. The number of persons exposed during manufacture and the duration of such exposure.
7. The manner or method of disposal (any change in the manner or method of disposal must be reported later).
8. Any test data, in the possession or control of the notifier, which "are related to the effect of any manufacture, processing, distribution in commerce, use, or disposal of such substance or any article containing such substance or, or,

any combination of such activities on health or the environment."

9. A description of any other data covering the environmental and health effects of the chemical.

While the act does not require that toxicity testing be conducted on a new chemical prior to manufacture or importation, it does require that all existing health and safety data which demonstrate that the new chemical does not present an unreasonable risk to health or the environment be submitted to the EPA.

The PMN procedure under TSCA is, in effect, a de facto registration system for new chemicals. While there is no requirement under TSCA to generate toxicity data on a new chemical, it seems rather unreasonable to expect the EPA to assess the potential risk of a new chemical in the absence of toxicity data. In practical terms, however, little or no toxicity information usually exists on a truly new chemical. While some estimates of its general toxicity might be approximated through categorization or the use of structure–activity relationships, a definition of chemical's toxicity must await actual testing in animals. For most new chemicals, the EPA may accept a minimal toxicology package of an acute toxicity profile (acute oral, dermal, and inhalation toxicity studies, eye and skin irritation tests), and possibly a skin sensitization study.

A PMN is submitted prior to any manufacture or importation of the new chemical. Following receipt, the EPA has 90 days to review the notification. The agency may, however, extend the review period another 90 days for good cause. If the 90 or 180 days pass without further action by the EPA, the notifier may begin to manufacture or import the new chemical. The PMN submitter should inform the EPA when manufacture or importation begins, and the EPA, in turn, should place the chemical on the TSCA inventory. If no patent problems exist, any other firm may manufacture or import that same chemical once it has been placed on the TSCA inventory.

During the EPA's review of a PMN, the agency may take one of two actions. If it finds that the data submitted in the PMN are insufficient to make a reasonable evaluation of the health or environmental effects of the chemical, it may issue a proposed order to prohibit or limit its manufacture, processing, and distribution in commerce, use, or disposal. These actions are regulated by **Section 5(e)** of TSCA, which is concerned with matters "pending development of information." The second action the EPA could take is specified in **Section 5(f)** of TSCA, entitled Protection Against Unreasonable Risks. If the EPA concludes from its review of a PMN that the manufacture, processing, and distribution in commerce, use, or disposal of the chemical (or combination of these activities) presents or will present an unreasonable risk to human health or the environment, it may issue a proposed rule to prohibit or limit the amount of the chemical that may be manufactured, processed, used, or distributed in commerce. The EPA may seek an injunction in a United States District Court to prohibit or limit the proposed activity with the new chemical.

The EPA may not place a PMN under continuing review, but must take a specific action under Sections 5(e) or 5(f) as noted. If the agency takes no action, the statutory time limits

for review will run out and the notifier is free to manufacture or import the new chemical.

If the EPA does propose to act against a chemical under Sections 5(e) or 5(f), the submitter of the PMN may file specific objections to such actions. The EPA may then seek an injunction or restraining order against the chemical through the U.S. District Court. The PMN submitter will then need to petition the Court to remove the injunction or restraining order.

The EPA takes a fairly practical approach to data deficiencies in a PMN or when suspicion exists of hazards associated with a PMN chemical. In the case of deficiencies of information, it may stop the clock on the review period until adequate information, including toxicity testing data, is furnished to the Agency. EPA may request further long-term testing based upon the similarity of the new chemical to others reported in the literature as having adverse findings.

The EPA has issued standards for the conduct of toxicity tests which might be required under a TSCA Section 4 test rule. It is implied, rather than stated, that all studies conducted as part of a PMN follow these test standards.

Hazardous Materials Transportation Act

The Hazardous Materials Transportation Act (HMTA) is administered by the Department of Transportation (DOT). HMTA defines a hazardous material as substance or material in a quantity and form which may pose an unreasonable risk to health and safety or property when transported in commerce. The designation of a material to be hazardous when transported in commerce is at the discretion of the Secretary of Transportation. Explosives, radioactive materials, etiologic agents, flammable liquids or solids, combustible liquid or solids, poisons, oxidizing or corrosive materials, and compressed gases may be included in the DOT list of hazardous materials.

DOT regulations require that materials shipped in interstate commerce be labeled and contained in a manner consistent with the degree of hazard they present. The DOT requires that acute toxicity studies be performed on Class B Poisons. These are chemicals that have not been classified as a Class A Poison ("extremely dangerous poison") or a Class C Poison ("tear gases or irritating substances"), but which are known or presumed to be toxic to humans. A Class B Poison is a substance that on oral administration, at a single dose of 50 mg or less per kilogram of body weight, produces death in 48 hr in half or more than half of a group of 10 or more white laboratory rats; or if when applied topically at a dose of 200 mg or less for 4 hr, produces death within 48 hr in half or more than half of a group of 10 or more rabbits. A substance may also be required to carry a Poison B label if it warrants testing by inhalation and meets the criteria of toxicity set forth by the DOT for this route of administration.

In other words, a Class B Poison label is required if the substance meets DOT toxicity criteria when tested by administration orally, dermally, or through inhalation. If a substance does meet these criteria through testing, but the physical characteristics or the probable hazards to humans, as shown by experience, indicate that the substance will not cause serious illness or death, then the Class B Poison label is not required.

Consumer Product Safety Act

Prior to the passage of the Consumer Product Safety Act (CPSA) in 1973, the classification and testing for acute toxicity of household products was conducted under regulations promulgated by the FDA which administered the FHSA. The function of administering FHSA and thus protecting the consumer from hazardous household substances has now fallen to the Consumer Product Safety Commission (CPSC) under the CPSA. If results obtained in acute oral or dermal toxicity tests, carried out according to the methods outlined in the Code of Federal Regulations for Hazardous Substances, meet prescribed criteria of toxicity, labeling and packaging as prescribed in the regulations must be used.

The Occupational Safety and Health Act

This law, enacted by Congress in 1970 and administered by the Occupational Safety and Health Administration (OSHA) of the Department of Labor, is designated "to assure so far as possible every man and woman safe and healthful working conditions." OSHA **Section 6(b)(5)** requires that the Secretary set the standard which must assure, to the extent feasible, on the basis of the best available evidence, that no employee will suffer from material impairment of health or functional capacity even if an employee has regular exposure to hazard during his or her working life. However, OSHA cannot duplicate the efforts of other agencies, such as the EPA, when exercising its statutory authority to prescribe or enforce standards or regulations affecting occupational safety.

OSHA **Section 3(8)** specifies that a new standard must be reasonably necessary and appropriate and must remedy a significant risk to health. Before setting an exposure standard (level), OSHA must first determine on the basis of sufficient evidence that there is significant risk by occupational exposure, and must also take into consideration other reasonable and appropriate factors such as economic impact and feasibility of the new standard.

No requirements exist in this law for manufacturers to test substances for toxicity prior to their use in the workplace. The impact of TSCA has an overlapping effect in that occupational exposure to new chemicals is considered in premanufacture notices. Specific test requirements under TSCA will affect new or existing chemicals that are manufactured or processed in the United States.

OSHA has been in the process of issuing exposure standards for commonly used chemicals. These standards are issued after consideration of the recommendations made by the National Institute of Occupational Safety and Health (NIOSH). Of interest, OSHA, in an effort to expedite the issuance of standards relative to potential carcinogens in the workplace, has prepared a generic approach. This proposed generic standard has been the subject of considerable controversy.

In 1980, OSHA published its generic cancer policy for the identification, classification, and regulation of toxic substances in the workplace. This policy, which has been challenged, provides the procedures and scientific principles for setting standards for carcinogenic chemicals in the workplace. The scientific principles may not be rebutted for an individual chemical unless the evidence presented meets certain criteria. In practice, a chemical listed by the National Toxicology Program (NTP) or even the International Agency for Research on Cancer (IARC) as carcinogenic automatically triggers OSHA's regulations. However, the NTP carcinogenicity classification system is only concerned with the evidence obtained from specific bioassay studies, showing that a chemical induces tumors in animals. Furthermore, the IARC system does not take into account the risk of an identified carcinogen, and its classification of carcinogens is established by a small panel of experts who receive very little or no public input. The IARC considers only published data, and many important data which are relevant to classification are often not considered. These limitations suggest that a chemical on the NTP or IARC lists may not necessarily pose unreasonable risk to the workplace and should not automatically trigger the OSHA regulation.

In 1980, OSHA promulgated a generic rule requiring employers to maintain employees' medical and exposure records for 30 years from the day of employment, or for the duration of their employment plus five years, in order to ensure that employees or their designated representatives or OSHA have access to these records. This rule has been challenged and modified by OSHA to reduce unnecessary burden to employers.

In 1982 OSHA issued yet another generic standard requiring employers to communicate hazard to employees. This provides employees with the information they need to protect themselves in the workplace through a simple performance-oriented standard. The procedure for hazard communication is at the discretion of the employers as long as they can demonstrate that they have adequately ascertained the scientifically well-established hazards of the chemicals. Labels to warn of a particular hazard, identify a chemical, and cross-reference to a Material Safety Data Sheet (MSDS) are required. Manufacturers are required to send the MSDS in the first shipment to users. These rules do not apply when there are other laws regulating the chemicals, such as pesticides under FIFRA.

ENVIRONMENTAL POLLUTION LAWS

To control pollution of the environment, Congress has enacted numerous laws governing the discharge of pollutants into the air and water and the disposal of solid waste. Among them, four important statutory laws have been enacted since 1970: the Clean Water Act, the Clean Air Act; the Resource Conservation and Recovery Act, and the Comprehensive Environmental Response, Compensation and Liability Act (Superfund or CERCLA).

The Clean Water Act and Its Amendment—The Federal Water Pollution Control Act

This law governs the discharges of waste water into the environment. The act provides the EPA with the authority to require facilities discharging waste water to install technological effluent controls to protect the quality of water. The Clean Water Act (CWA) also provides the EPA with the mechanism to regulate spills, leaks, and other unintentional discharges. Under the National Pollutant Discharge Elimination System (NPDES), all discharges of waste water must be permitted by the EPA or the states. Industry-by-industry effluent limitations reflecting the Best Practicable Technology currently available have been issued by the EPA.

Section 304(a) of the CWA requires the EPA to establish water quality standards for surface water. This gives the EPA the authority to develop the information or criteria for establishing the water quality standard. The information shall reflect the identifiable effects of each pollutant on the public health and welfare, aquatic life, and recreation. The EPA has published water quality criteria for a large number of organic and inorganic toxic compounds.

Under CWA **Section 307(a)(2),** the EPA is required to set effluent standards for toxic effluent based on health effects. The standard becomes effective one year after its promulgation unless the EPA determines that it is not technologically feasible.

Section 311 of the CWA prohibits the discharge of oil or hazardous substance into navigable water of the United States in quantity which may be harmful. The definition of harmful quantity of oil is defined as the quantity which exceeds the water quality standard or causes a sheen upon or discoloration of water or the shoreline. For hazardous substances, the EPA set a reportable quantity that may be harmful. There are only a few exemptions.

Clean Air Act

Under this act, the EPA is authorized to set national ambient air standards, emission standards for individual facilities, and standards for emission of hazardous air pollutants. However, enforcement of these standards is the responsibility of each state. The state is required to set up a implementation plan which specifies how it will limit emissions in order to comply with air quality standards.

Resource Conservation and Recovery Act

Decades of improper disposal of industrial and research wastes, particularly from the chemical and nuclear industries, have triggered public demand for the regulation of waste disposal. The Resource Conservation and Recovery Act (RCRA) of 1976 authorized the EPA to institute a national program to control hazardous waste. In 1980, the EPA put forward the final version of the RCRA regulations.

The main purpose of these regulations is to control the generation, storage, treatment, transportation, disposal, recordkeeping, and reporting of solid waste which is defined to include liquid, semisolid, and contained gaseous wastes. Solid waste is divided into hazardous and nonhazardous: non-hazardous wastes can be disposed of in sanitary landfills; open dumping is banned. A sanitary landfill must meet the criteria set under Subtitle D of the RCRA.

Hazardous wastes are regulated under RCRA subtitle C which is divided into six parts: (a) definition and scope; (b) standards for facilities that generate hazardous wastes; (c) standards for the transportation of hazardous wastes; (d) standards for facilities that treat, store, or dispose of hazardous wastes; (e) special standards for recycling and reclaiming hazardous wastes; and (f) the hazardous waste permit program.

RCRA defines a hazardous waste as "solid waste that may cause increased mortality or serious illness, or may cause substantial hazard to the health or the environment when improperly managed." There are listed wastes, characteristic wastes, and mixture wastes. The EPA has listed, periodically and specifically by names, those wastes including many commercial chemical products such as pesticides it considers hazardous. In addition, a waste material that exhibits any of the following characteristics set by EPA is considered hazardous:

1. *Ignitability*—posing a fire hazard during management.
2. *Corrosivity*—ability to corrode standard containers, or to dissolve toxic components of other wastes.
3. *Reactivity*—tendency to explode under normal management conditions, to react violently when mixed with water, or to generate toxic gases.
4. *EP toxicity* (as determined by a specific extraction procedure)—presence of certain toxic materials at levels greater than those specified in the regulations.

The fourth criterion permits the EPA to list waste materials that contain one or more substances known to cause toxicity in human or animals. In addition, the EPA may also consider the following factors in determining if a waste is hazardous: degree of toxicity, concentration, migration to the environment, persistence or degradation in the environment, bioaccumulation in the ecosystem, types of improper management, quantities of waste, and past human and environmental damage records.

If a listed hazardous waste is mixed with a nonhazardous waste, the waste is considered hazardous, with few exceptions. If a waste exhibiting one of the four characteristics is mixed with a nonhazardous waste, the mixture is considered hazardous only if the mixture exhibits any of the characteristics.

Certain solid wastes are exempted under the regulations. These include wastes already under the regulations of the Atomic Energy Act and Clean Water Act (e.g., domestic waste).

All facilities that generate hazardous solid wastes, except small quantity waste generators, must have an EPA identification number and must comply with the standards set for maintaining records, shipping hazardous wastes off-site, storing wastes on-site prior to shipment, and making annual reports and exception reports. Facilities that generate small quantities of waste, i.e., 1000 kg or less per month of an identified hazardous waste, are exempted from the initial waste controls. These facilities must be able to prove through recordkeeping that they are indeed generating small quantities of hazardous waste.

If a facility believes that the waste it generates should be exempted from the regulation even when it is listed, it must prove to the EPA that the waste does not meet the criteria which caused the EPA to list the specific waste as hazardous in the first place. This can be achieved either by conducting studies or by referring to test data that demonstrate that the criteria are not met.

Under the RCRA, transporters of hazardous wastes are required to keep records, take immediate action to contain a spill of hazardous waste during shipment, notify federal and state authorities of a spill, report a spill in writing to the DOT, clean up the spill, and obtain a waste generator identification number if the resultant wastes (contaminated soil and water) exceed the amount allowed for small quantity waste generators. Transporters also have to consider the requirements set by the DOT under the Hazard Material Transportation Act.

Facilities that treat, store, or dispose of hazardous wastes are subjected to an extensive standard and have to obtain a permit from the EPA. A generator of waste can store hazardous waste on-site up to 90 days provided that no treatment or disposal of the wastes are initiated by the generator.

Comprehensive Environmental Response Compensation and Liability Act

CERCA, enacted by the Congress in 1980, expands the authority of the federal (EPA) and the state government to investigate and respond to the release of materials into the environment. More importantly, the act permits the oil and chemical industries to be taxed in order to finance governmental action taken in response to the release of pollutants (Superfund), and also requires that all industries respond to releases immediately or reimburse the government for the costs it incurs in responding to the release of pollutants into the environment.

LAWS AND REGULATIONS THAT GOVERN TOXICITY EVALUATIONS IN OTHER COUNTRIES, AND INTERNATIONAL TOXICITY TESTING GUIDELINES

The United States has not been alone in developing laws to protect man and the environment from potentially dangerous effects of new industrial chemicals in the marketplace. Japan adopted regulations similar to an early version of what has become the TSCA in the United States. France has established a system for premarket notification of new chemicals. On June 19, 1979, the Council of Ministers of the EEC adopted the Sixth Amendment to the Council Directive 67/548/EEC of June 27, 1967. This Council Directive concerns the approximation of laws, regulations, and administrative procedures which relate to the classification, packaging, and labeling of dangerous substances. The Sixth Amendment is an effort to protect man and the environment from potential risks which might arise through the marketing of new chemicals. It requires that a new chemical be subjected to a "base set" of tests to define its physical and chemical properties, mammalian toxicity, and ecotoxicologic effects. When the Sixth Amendment takes effect in 1981, a manufacturer or importer will be required to furnish to the appropriate authorities in his EEC member state a notification containing, in part, the results of the tests on the new chemical. Notification will have to be filed 45 days prior to marketing in the member state.

The Sixth Amendment is the EEC counterpart of TSCA in the United States. There are, however, major differences, not the least of which is in the approach to toxicity testing. The EEC requires that notification be given prior to marketing of a new chemical whereas TSCA demands that notification, in the case of a domestic manufacturer, be given to the EPA at least 90 days prior to manufacture. Even test marketing of a new chemical in the United States requires that prior notification be given to the EPA. The "base set" consists of the following studies for acute toxicity: acute oral LD_{50}, acute dermal LD_{50}, acute inhalation LC_{50} (if applicable), skin and eye irritation, and dermal sensitization.

With many countries establishing their own regulations for safety assessment, it now becomes possible that manufacturers would have to perform several tests to satisfy the same objective in several different countries. In an attempt to avoid unnecessary duplication of work, the OECD, a group comprised of experts from a number of nations throughout the world, has produced a set of testing guidelines (109) which are sufficiently well defined to enable a test to be carried out in a similar manner in different countries and produce results that would be fully acceptable to various regulatory bodies.

Council Directives of the European Economic Community and Amendments

The EEC or Common Market has ten member countries: The Netherlands, Belgium, France, Luxembourg, Denmark, the United Kingdom, Ireland, Italy, Greece, and the Federal Republic of Germany. For several years, the Council of the EEC has been working on a system to identify and control toxic chemicals. The original EEC Council Directive 67/548/EEC of June 27, 1967 on the approximation of the laws, regulations, and administrative provisions of the member states relating to the classification, packaging, and labeling of dangerous substances has been amended a number of times. On September 18, 1979, the 1967 Council Directive was amended for the 6th time (79/831/EEC, or the 6th Amendment). The Council of the EEC felt that while Directive 67/548/EEC was adequate for the protection of workers through its system for classification, packaging, and labeling of dangerous substances, more extensive protection was needed to control the effects of dangerous substances on man and the environment. The adoption of the 6th Amendment by the EEC requires that an inventory of substances be compiled by the Common Market by September 18, 1981. New substances, defined as those not appearing on this inventory, will require notification by their manufacturer or importer at least 45 days prior to marketing. In contrast to the requirements of TSCA, which requires notification prior to manufacture, a new chemical may be introduced into the market in an EEC member country in quantities of less than one metric ton per year if the manufacturer notifies the authorities of his respective member country as to the identity, labeling, and quantity of the chemical to be marketed per year. No base-set data need be furnished.

If a manufacturer or importer wishes to initially market a new substance in yearly quantities of more than one metric ton but less than ten metric tons or a total marketing of less than 50 metric tons, he must submit a technical dossier containing base-set information on the new chemical to the authorities in one of the nine member countries at least 45 days prior to marketing. If a chemical has already been marketed in quantities of less than one metric ton per year, the dossier containing the base-set information must be presented at least 45 days before the marketing volume exceeds the one metric ton per year level.

The purpose of the technical dossier under the 6th Amendment is to supply information necessary for the authorities in a member country to evaluate the foreseeable, immediate, or delayed risks for man and the environment. One distinguishing concept of the 6th Amendment is that the toxicity and ecotoxicity studies required are tied into increments of marketing volumes per year or when total marketing reaches certain volumes.

At the base-set (marketing volume of 1–10 metric tons per year) the technical dossier must contain, in addition to such information as identity, composition, purity, impurities, spectral data, proposed uses, projected production volumes, methods, and precautions for handling, storage, and transport, physicochemical properties, and possibilities for rendering the substance harmless, the following toxicological studies as needed:

1. Acute oral LD_{50} (mg/kg) including the effects observed.
2. Acute inhalation LC_{50} (ppm) including the effects observed. Administration of the test substance must be for at least 4 hr.
3. Acute percutaneous LD_{50} (mg/kg) including the effects observed.

The 6th Amendment requires that substances other than gases must be administered via the oral route and at least one other route which will depend on their intended use and physical properties. In the acute toxicity studies, both male and female animals should be used. An observation period of at least 14 days is required. The rat is the preferred species for both the oral and inhalation studies unless there are overriding reasons. Skin and eye irritation studies are required, preferably using the rabbit. A dermal sensitization study using a recognized method in the guinea pig is also needed.

A subchronic study of at least 28 days' duration is required. The rat is again the preferred species for oral and inhalation studies. A 5- or 7-day per week schedule of administration may be used. The route of administration should be based on the intended use of the new chemical, its physical and chemical properties, and its acute toxicity. A no effect dose level should be established.

The new chemical's potential mutagenicity must be examined in two tests; a bacteriological test (with and without metabolic activation) and a nonbacteriological test.

Ecotoxicological studies including acute LD_{50} (ppm) for one or more species of fish and acute LD_{50} (ppm) for daphnia should be conducted.

With respect to degradation studies, determination of the (Biochemical Oxygen Demand) (BOD) and the BOC/COD (Chemical Oxygen Demand) ratio is considered a minimum requirement.

Level 1 is reached in the 6th Amendment when marketing of the new chemical reaches 10 metric tons per year or a total of 50 tons. At this point, authorities in the EEC member country may require further toxicologic studies after current

knowledge of the new substance is considered as well as its known or planned uses and the results obtained in the base-set of studies. At this level, in addition to possibly requiring a one-generation fertility study and/or a teratology study and/or additional mutagenesis studies, the authorities may require additional subchronic studies and/or a chronic study which may include special studies, depending on the results obtained in the 28-day subchronic study submitted as part of the technical dossier of base-set information. Any relevant information obtained from other sources may also be considered by the authorities in requesting these additional studies. Such additional studies may include exposure to the new chemical for 90 days or longer or more detailed examination for certain effects. Even a chronic study could be requested at this point.

Examples given in the 6th Amendment of effects that would indicate the need for additional subchronic studies include serious or irreversible lesions, a very low or lack of establishment of a no effect level, or a clear structural relationship of the new chemical to others that have been shown to be dangerous.

Additional ecotoxicology studies may also be required at level 1.

If the authorities have not required the above testing in the early stages of marketing, they will request that it be done when obligatory notification from the manufacturer is received that the quantity being marketed has reached a level of 100 metric tons per year or a total quantity of 500 metric tons.

The manufacturer is also required to notify the authorities when the marketing volume reaches 1000 metric tons per year or a total of 5000 metric tons. This is level 2 in the 6th Amendment incremental testing scheme.

The authorities, on receipt of notification, are obligated to design a testing program that covers chronic toxicity, carcinogenicity, fertility (only if an effect on fertility had been established in level 1 testing), teratology (nonrodent species), additional toxicokinetic studies as well as acute and subchronic studies in a second species if results of level 1 studies indicate a need. Results obtained in pharmacokinetic and biotransformation studies may also trigger a requirement to do these studies.

Additional ecotoxicology studies may also be required. These are noted in Annex VIII of the 6th Amendment.

On September 16, 1983, Annexes I, II, III, IV, and VI of the directives were amended again (83/467/EEC). The new directives specified that member states adopt and publish before January 1, 1985, the measures needed to comply with the new directive and immediately inform the EEC commission. The member states were required to apply these measures by January 1, 1986.

Annex I:	A list of dangerous substances.
Annex III:	The nature of the special risk of dangerous substances.
Annex IV:	Safety advice concerning dangerous substances.
Annex V:	Methods for determining physicochemical properties, toxicity, and ecotoxicity.
Annex VI:	General classification and labeling requirements for dangerous substances and the choice of risk and safety phrases.

Annex VII: Information required for the technical dossier (base set)

Annex VIII: Additional information and tests required at different levels

Specific Council directives have been issued for the classification, packaging, and labeling certain materials such as solvents (73/173/EEC and 80/781/EEC), pesticides (78/63/EEC), cosmetics (76/768/EEC), wastes (75/442/EEC), toxic and dangerous waste (78/319/EEC), and gaseous preparations (75/324/EEC).

Health and Safety Commission of the United Kingdom

As a result of recommendations made by a Committee of Inquiry chaired by Lord Robens and cited in its report "Safety and Health at Work," a comprehensive notification system for new chemicals or other potentially harmful substances being introduced for industrial or commercial use is currently being considered in the United Kingdom. There already exists a competent body, the Health and Safety Commission (HSC), for the receipt of such notifications. The HSC works with the Advisory Committee on Toxic Substances (ACTS) particularly on "methods of controlling the health hazards to persons at work and the related hazards to the public which may arise from toxic substances . . . with particular references to those requiring notification under regulations."

In 1977 a discussion document of the HSC presented proposals for a notification scheme covering new chemicals introduced into the United Kingdom by manufacturers or importers in quantities greater than one ton per year. Under this scheme, the manufacturer or importer will be required to furnish sufficient toxicologic and other information on the new chemical from which the likely hazards and the conditions of safe use may be inferred. The notification scheme, administered by the Health and Safety Executive (HSE) of the HSC, is intended principally to assess the potential of a chemical to cause harm to people in the workplace and also to people outside the workplace who might also be exposed from the work activity. This notification scheme does not include the requirement for data relating to environmental effects or waste disposal. However, some of the tests included in the scheme may provide basic information for these purposes also. Excluded from the notification scheme are those chemical substances already in use before the introduction of the scheme, those chemicals only available in small quantities, and chemical mixtures in which a new chemical is not present. Notification through this scheme is intended to assist the HSC in the early detection of substances likely to present more serious risks to safety and health and more adequately control them.

Included in the basic information to be provided by the notifier are details of the new substances' chemical and physical properties, biologic properties, recommendations for safe handling, proposed date of introduction to Great Britain, and scale of manufacturer or importation. Among the information requested for biologic properties are acute effects of ingestion, inhalation, or absorption through the skin and the effects of the new substance with respect to skin irritation or sensitization.

With regard to acute toxicity, the guidance given in Annex 1 to the notification scheme requests that while an acute LD_{50} must be provided, it need not be measured with precise accuracy but indicate whether the substance is of high, moderate, or low toxicity and show that careful observations have been made of the general mode of toxic action. Rats are suggested as the animals of choice, with groups of six animals used for each dose and observations continued for 14 days. This applies to studies of oral ingestion, dermal application, or inhalation exposure. Optionally, simultaneous assessment of dermal toxicity and skin irritation may be made. Rabbits may be used in studies of skin irritation. If the notifier also conducts studies of 30 days duration or longer on the substance, hematologic or histopathologic studies need not be conducted in an acute toxicity determination.

Due to the United Kingdom's treaty obligations to the EEC, the notification scheme of the HSC is being modified to conform with the proposals for the notification of the properties of dangerous substances.

Registration of Pesticides in the United Kingdom

Registration of pesticides in the United Kingdom is granted by the Ministry of Agriculture, Fisheries and Food (MAFF), which involves two schemes: the Pesticide Safety Precautions Scheme (PSPS) and the Agricultural Chemicals Approval Scheme (ACAS).

Before marketing a new pesticide or a new use for an existing pesticide, a manufacturer notifies MAFF under PSPS, a nonstatutory agreement between industry and government. The potential hazards of the pesticide are evaluated under PSPS through four levels of clearance. With each successful clearance, the pesticide is permitted more extensive marketing. The data requirements vary with each stage of clearance. At least as much data required in the United States is required for a complete clearance of a new pesticide in the United Kingdom. The evaluation under PSPS is handled by advisory committees with no industry representation, although the meetings are open to the industry.

Under the ACAS, the efficacy of the pesticide is evaluated and the labeling requirements are determined. The ACAS approves the registration of pesticides after they have obtained clearance under the PSPS. However, approval under the ACAS is not required for marketing.

Changes are underway in the United Kingdom. The voluntary approach of registering pesticides may eventually be replaced by more compulsory requirements.

Registration of Pesticides in Canada

Registration of pesticides in Canada is basically under two laws, the Pest Control Products Act and the Food and Drug Act. Agriculture Canada administers the Pest Control Products Acts and approves registrations of pesticides. The Food and Drug Act is administered by Health and Welfare Canada which sets the maximum residue limit of pesticides in food. Before granting registration of a pesticide, Agriculture Canada will consult various agencies such as Environment Canada, Fisheries and Oceans Canada, and Health and Welfare Canada. As in the United States and EEC countries, Canada has guidelines that outline the types of tests needed to fully evaluate the potential hazards of chemicals to humans. However, applicants are encouraged to discuss details and specific requirements with the Health Protection Branch of Health and Welfare Canada.

Agricultural Chemicals Laws of Japan

Japan is one of the most developed countries in the world and like the United States, Canada, and EEC countries has sophisticated chemical control laws. The major chemical control laws in Japan are The Poisonous and Deleterious Substances Control Law, The Food Sanitation Law, The Antipollution Law, and The Agricultural Regulation Law. Since the registration of agricultural chemicals often involves all of these laws, the registration process of agricultural chemicals is particularly involved and complicated.

The Agricultural Chemical Regulation Law was first enacted in 1948 and was amended in 1949, 1950, 1951, 1962, 1963, 1971, 1978, 1981, 1983, and 1984. This law governs the registration, labeling, recordkeeping, reporting, and inspection requirements for manufacturers, processors, dealers, and importers of pesticides. Only local registrants are allowed to manufacture pesticides in Japan. All importation of pesticides requires prior notification.

The Ministry of Agriculture, Forestry and Fisheries (MAFF) is charged with the responsibility of granting registrations of pesticides. The approval process basically involves two steps, the registration application and safety evaluation. The applicant makes a preliminary application to the Planning and Co-ordination Section of MAFF's Agricultural Chemicals Inspection Station (ACIS). The Planning Section will forward all data to various sections within ACIS including The Toxicology Section for reviews. Applicants can discuss the quality and adequacy of their data with ACIS officials. The ACIS is solely responsible for the quality of data and guideline compliance. If all data are deemed acceptable, the ACIS will forward the package to MAFF's Plant Protection Division which coordinates evaluations by Japan's Environmental Agency (EA) and the Ministry of Health and Welfare (MHW).

The acute toxicity data are submitted by MAFF's Plant Protection Division to the HMW's Pharmaceuticals and Chemicals Safety Division for the characterization and classification of chemicals which is authorized by the Poisonous and Deleterious Substances Control Law for all chemicals. Pesticides are classified as *common, poisonous,* or *deleterious.* For example, pesticides are classified as common if the LD_{50} in the mouse is greater than 300 mg/kg body weight, poisonous if the LD_{50} is less than 30 mg/kg, and deleterious if the LD_{50} is between 30 and 300 mg/kg.

Other toxicity data are submitted to the Food Chemistry Division of MHW to establish the Allowable Daily Intake (ADI) and tolerances as authorized by the Food Sanitation Law. The ADI is set by a Safety Evaluation Committee which is not accessible to the applicant. The tolerances are set jointly by the MAFF's Food Chemistry Division and Japan's EA.

As authorized by the Antipollution Law, all environment and residue data are submitted to EA by MAFF's Plant Pro-

tection Division for evaluation through the Agricultural Material Council, of effects on the environment. EA recommends the Maximum Residue Limit to MHW's Food Chemistry Division for setting tolerances, sets the standards for classifying pesticides with respect to potential effects on the environment, categorizes each pesticide with respect to (a) pesticides with high corp residue, (b) pesticides with high soil residue, (c) pesticides harmful to aquatic animals or plants, and (d) pesticides that can cause water pollution. EA is also responsible for monitoring the residues and setting standards for withholding the registration of pesticides. After obtaining the evaluations and recommendations from the MHW and EA, the MAFF's Plant Protection Division will grant the official approval for registration of a pesticide.

Japan is a member country of the OECD and theoretically should accept all data generated according to the OECD guidelines. However, there are some unique requirements. For example, certain data must be generated by Japanese Laboratories and certain portions of the data must be generated by independent laboratories not affiliated with the applicant. Another unique requirement in Japan is a set of pharmacologic studies, loosely defined by ACIS, with pesticides. As with the United States and EEC countries, Japan has its own toxicity testing guidelines (131), but unlike the United States, discussion between the applicant and the scientists in MHW and EA is not allowed in Japan. The only contact for the applicant is the ACIS. Since the ACIS is concerned only with quality of data and guideline compliance, applicants are often forced to comply with the Japanese guidelines regardless of what are specified in the OECD guideline. Registrants have encountered difficulty in registering pesticides in Japan. The most recently enforced GLP law has added to the already complicated situation in Japan. Under this new GLP law, all toxicity data generated after October of 1984 must be generated by a laboratory certified by the ACIS as a GLP laboratory. However laboratories in the United States and other countries have experienced difficulty with their applications for GLP certification in Japan.

REFERENCES

1. Ashford, J. R. (1959): An approach to the analysis of data for semiquantal responses in biological assay. *Biometrics,* 156:573–581.
2. Baldwin, H. Q., McDonald, T. D., and Beasley, C. H. (1973): Slit-lamp examination of experimental animal eyes. II. Grading scales and photographic evaluation of induced pathological conditions. *J. Soc. Cosmet. Chem.,* 24:181–195.
3. Ballantyne, B., and Swanston, D. W. (1974): The irritant effects of dilute solutions of dibenzoxyazepine (CR) on the eye and tongue. *Acta Pharmacol. Toxicol.,* 35:412–423.
4. Bass, R., Gunzel, P., Henschler, D., et al. (1982): LD_{50} versus acute toxicity. *Arch. Toxicol.,* 51:183–186.
5. Battista, S. P., and McSweeney, E. S. (1965): Approaches to a quantative method for testing eye irritation. *J. Soc. Cosmet. Chem.,* 16:199–301.
6. Baum, J. L., Niedra, R., Davis, C., and Yue, D. (1979): Mass culture of human corneal endothelial cells. *Arch. Ophthalmol.,* 97:1136–1140.
7. Bayard, S., and Hehir, R. M. (1976): Evaluation of proposed changes in the modified Draize rabbit irritation test. *Toxicol. Appl. Pharmacol.,* 37:186.
8. Beckley, J. H. (1965): Critique of the Draize eye test, now and then—Eighteen, nine or six rabbits. *Am. Perf. Cosmet.,* 80:51–54.

9. Beckley, J. H. (1965): Comparative eye testing: Man vs. animal. *Toxicol. Appl. Pharmacol.*, 7:93–101.

10. Bell, M., Holmes, P. M., Nisbet, T. M., Uttley, M., and Van Abbe, N. J. (1979): Evaluating the potential eye irritancy of shampoos. *Int. J. Cosmet. Sci.*, 1:123.

11. Bliss, C. I. (1934): The method of probits—A correction. *Science*, 79:409–410.

12. Bliss, C. I. (1964): *Insecticide Assays in Statistics and Mathematics in Biology*, edited by O. Kempthorne, T. A. Bancroft, J. W. Gowen, and J. L. Lush, pp. 345–360. Hofner, NY.

13. Bonfield, C. T., and Scala, R. A. (1965): The paradox in testing for eye irritation. A report on thirteen shampoos. *Proc. Sci. Sect. Toilet Goods Assoc.*, 43:34–43.

14. Bonting, S. L., Simon, K. A., and Hawkins, N. M. (1961): Studies on sodium-potassium-activated adenonsine triphosphatase. I. Quantitative distribution in several tissues of the rat. *Arch. Biochem.*, 95:416–423.

15. Borenfreund, E., Shopsis, C., Barrero, O., and Sathe, S. (1983): *In vitro* alternative irritancy assays: Comparison of cytotoxic and membrane transport effects of alcohols. *Ann. NY Acad. Sci.*, 407:416–419.

16. Borenfreund, E., and Borrero, O. (1984): *In vitro* cytotoxicity assays: Potential alternatives to the Draize ocular irritancy test. *Cell Biol. Toxicol.*, 1:33–39.

17. Bross, I. D. J. (1958): How to sue RIDIT analysis. *Biometrics*, 14:18–38.

18. Brownlee, K. A., Hodges, J. L., and Rosenblatt, M. (1953): The up-and-down method with small samples. *J. Am. Statist. Assoc.*, 48:262–277.

19. Bruce, R. D. (1984): An up-and-down procedure for acute toxicity testing. In: *Acute Toxicity Testing: Alternative Approaches*, edited by Alan M. Goldberg, p. 184. Mary Ann Liebert, NY.

20. Buehler, E. V. (1974): Testing to predict potential ocular hazards of household chemical. In: *Toxicology Annual*, edited by C. L. Winek, pp. 53–69. Marcel Dekker, NY.

21. Buehler, E. V., and Newman, E. A. (1964): A comparison of eye irritation in monkeys and rabbits. *Toxicol. Appl. Pharmacol.*, 6:701–710.

22. Burnstein, N. L. (1980): Corneal cytotoxicity of topically applied drugs, vehicles, and preservatives. *Surv. Ophthalmol.*, 25:15–30.

23. Burton, A. B. G., York, M., and Lawrence, R. S. (1981): The *in vitro* assessment of severe eye irritant. *Food Cosmet. Toxicol.*, 19:471–480.

24. Calabrese, E. J. (1983): Ocular toxicity. In: *Principles of Animal Extrapolation*, p. 400. John Wiley, NY.

25. Cello, R. M., and Lasmanis, J. (1958): *Pseudomonas* infection of the eye of the dog resulting from the use of contaminated fluorescein solution. *J. Am. Vet. Med. Assoc.*, 132:297.

26. Chan, P. K., and Hayes, A. W. (1985): Assessment of chemically induced ocular toxicity: A survey of methods. In: *Toxicology of the Eye, Ear and Other Special Senses*, edited by A. W. Hayes. Raven Press, NY.

27. Choi, S. C. (1971): An investigation of Wetherill's method of estimation for the up-and-down experiment. *Biometrics*, 27:961–970.

28. Clark, A. J. (1933): *Mode of Action of Drugs on Cells*. Williams and Wilkins, Baltimore.

29. Cohen, I. J. (1983): Use of fluorescein in eye injuries. *J. Occup. Med.*, 5:540.

30. Cornfield, J. (1964): Measurement and composition of toxicities: The quantal response. In: *Statistics and Mathematics in Biology*, edited by O. Kempthorne, T. A., Bancroft, J. W. Gowen, and J. L. Lush, pp. 327–344. Hofner, NY.

31. CPSC (1976): Illustrated guide for grading eye irritation by hazardous substances. Directorate for Engineering and Science, Consumer Product Safety Commission, Washington, D.C.

31a. Davies, R. G., Kynoch, S. R., and Liggett, M. P. (1976): Eye irritation tests—An assessment of the maximum delay time for remedial irrigation. *J. Soc. Cosmet. Chem.*, 27:301–306.

32. Dawson, M., and Mustafa, A. F. (1985): Use of cultured human conjunctival and other cells to assess the relative toxicity of six local anesthetics. *Food Chem. Toxicol.*, 23:305–308.

33. DeSousa, D. J., Rouse, A. A., and Smolon, W. J. (1984): Statistical consequences of reducing the number of rabbits utilized in eye irritation testing. Data on 67 petrochemicals. *Toxicol. Appl. Pharmacol.*, 76:234–242.

34. Dews, P. B., and Berkson, J. (1964): On the error of bioassay with quantal response. In: *Statistics and Mathematics in Biology*, edited by O. Kempthorne, T. A., Bancroft, J. W. Gowen, and J. L. Lush, pp. 361–370. Hofner, London.

35. Diem, K. (1968): Documenta Geigy Scientific Tables, 6th ed. Geigy Pharmaceutical Division of Geigy Chemical Corp., Ardsley, NY.

36. Dixon, W. J. (1965): The up-and-down method for small samples. *J. Am. Statist. Assoc.*, 60:967–978.

37. Doull, J. (1980): *Factors Influencing Toxicology in Cassarett and Doull's Toxicology: The Basic Science of Poisons*, edited by J. Doull, C. D. Klaassen, and M. O. Amdur, pp. 70–83. MacMillan, NY.

38. Draize, J. H., Woodward, G., and Calvery, H. O. (1944): Methods for the study of irritation and toxicity of substances applied topically to the skin and mucous membranes. *J. Pharmacol. Exp. Ther.*, 82:377–390.

39. Dunnett, C. W. (1968): Biostatistics in Pharmacological testing. In: *Selected Pharmacological Testing Methods*, edited by A. Burger, pp. 7–48. Edward Arnold, London.

40. Edelhauser, H. F., Gonnerings, R., and Van Horn, D. L. (1978): Intraocular irrigation solutions: A comparative study of BSS plus and lactated Ringer's solution. *Arch. Ophthalmol.*, 96:516.

41. Edelhauser, H. F., Van Horn, D. L., Hyndink, R. A., and Schultz, R. O. (1975): Intraocular irrigating solutions: Their effect on the corneal endothelium. *Arch. Ophthalmol.*, 93:648.

42. Edelhauser, H. F., Van Horn, D. L., Schultz, R. O., and Hundink, R. A. (1976): Comparative toxicity of intraocular irrigating solution on the corneal endothelium. *Am. J. Ophthalmol.*, 81:473–481.

43. EEC (1983): Methods for the determination of toxicity. EEC Directive 79/831 Annex V, Part B.

44. Ehrlich, P. (1882): Uber provocirte fluorescenzer—Scheinungen am Auge. *Dtsch. Med. Wochenschr.*, 2:21.

45. EPA/FIFRA (1982): Pesticide Assessment Guidelines, Subdivision F, Hazard Evaluation: Human and domestic animals, PB83-153916. Office of Pesticide Programs, U.S. EPA. Reproduced by the National Technical Information Service, U.S. Department of Commerce, Springfield, VA.

46. EPA (1983): Toxic substance control: Good laboratory practice standards; final rule. *Fed. Register*, 48(230):53921–53944, November 29.

47. EPA (1983): Pesticide programs: Good laboratory practice standards; final rule. *Fed. Register*, 48(230):53945–53969, November 29.

48. EPA (1984): EPA fact sheet: Background on acute toxicity testing for chemical safety, August, 1984.

49. EPA (1984): Data requirements for pesticide registration; final rule. 40 CFR Part 158. *Fed. Register*, Oct. 24:42855–42905.

50. EPA/TSCA (1984): Health effects test guidelines. PB84-233295. Office of Pesticides and Toxic Substances, U.S. EPA. Reproduced by NTIS, U.S. Department of Commerce, Springfield, VA.

51. Ernst, R., and Ardetti, J. (1980): Biological effects of surfactants IV. Effects of non-ionic and amphoterics on Hela Cells. *Toxicology*, 15:233.

52. FDA (1976): Illustrated guide for grading eye irritation by hazardous substances. FDA, Washington, D.C.

53. FDA (1983): Final report on acute studies workshop. Sponsored by the U.S. Food and Drug Administration on November 9, 1983.

53a. Federal Register (1980): 45:33063, May 19.

54. Ferdinard, W. (1976): The enzyme molecule. John Wiley, NY.

55. FHSA (1979): Regulations under the Federal Hazardous Substance Act. Chapter II. Title 16. Code of Federal Regulations.

56. Fine, B. S., and Yanoff, M. (1972): *Ocular Histology. A Text and Atlas*. Harper and Row, NY.

57. Finney, D. J. (1971): *Probit Analysis*, 3rd edition, Chapters 3 and 4 Cambridge University Press, Cambridge.

58. Fisher, R. A., and Yates, F. (1963): *Statistical Tables for Biological, Agricultural and Medical Research*, 6th ed., edited by Oliver and Boyd Ltd., Edinburgh, Scotland.

59. Floyd, E. P., and Stockinger, H. G. (1958): Toxicity studies of certain organic peroxides and hydroperoxides. *Am. Indust. Hyg. Asoc. J.*, 19:205–212.

60. Freeberg, F. E., Griffith, J. F., Bruce, R. D., and Bay, P. H. S. (1984): Correlation of animal test methods with human experience for household products. *J. Toxicol. Cutaneous and Ocular Toxicol.*, 1(3):53.

61. Friedenwald, J. S., Hughes, W. F., and Hermann, H. (1944): Acid-base tolerance of the cornea. *Arch. Ophthalmol.,* 31:279–283.

62. Gaddum, J. H. (1983): Reports on biological standards III. Methods of biological assay depending on a quantal response. *Spec. Rep. Ser. Med. Res.,* No. 813, London.

63. Gaunt, I. F., and Harper, K. H. (1964): The potential irritancy to rabbit eye mucosa of certain commercially available shampoos, *J. Soc. Cosmet. Chem.,* 15:209–230.

64. Giovacchini, R. P. (1972): Old and new issues in the safety evaluation of cosmetics and toiletries. *CRC Crit. Rev. Toxicol.,* 1:361–378.

65. Grant, W. M. (1974): *Toxicology of the Eye,* 2nd ed. Charles C Thomas, Springfield, IL.

66. Green, W. R., Sullivan, J. B., Hehir, R. M., et al. (1978): A chemically-induced eye injury in the albino rabbit and rhesus monkey. The Soap and Detergent Association, NY.

67. Griffith, J. F., Nixon, G. A., Bruce, R. D., et al. (1980): Dose-response studies with chemical irritants in the albino rabbit eye as a basis for selecting optimum testing conditions for predicting hazard to human eye. *Toxicol. Appl. Pharmacol.,* 55:501–513.

68. Guillot, J., Gonnet, J. F., and Clement, C. (1982): Evaluation of the ocular irritation potential of 56 compounds. *Food Chem. Toxicol.,* 20:573–582.

69. Gundersen, T., and Liebman, S. D. (1944): Effect of local anesthetics on regeneration of corneal epithelium. *Arch. Ophthalmol.,* 31:29–33.

70. Gurland, J., Lee, I., and Dahm, P. A. (1960): Polychotomous quantal response in biological assay. *Biometrics,* 16:382–398.

71. Harriton, L. (1981): Conversation with Henry Spira: Draize test activist. *Lab. Anim.,* 10:16–22.

72. Henkes, H., and Canta, L. R. (1973): Drug-induced disorders of the eye. In: *Excerpta Medica, Vol. 14: Proceedings of the European Society for the Study of Drug Toxicity,* edited by W. A. M. Duncan, pp. 146–153. Elsevier/North-Holland, NY.

73. Heywood, R., and James R. W. (1978): Towards objectivity in the assessment of eye irritation. *J. Soc. Cosmet. Chem.,* 29:25–29.

74. Holland, M. C. (1964): Fluorescein staining of the cornea. *JAMA,* 188:81.

75. Hull, D. S. (1979): Effects of epinephrine, benzalkonium chloride, and intraocular miotics on corneal endothelium. *S. Afr. Med. J.,* 2:1380–1381.

76. IRLG (Interagency Regulatory Liaison Group) (1981): Recommended guideline for acute eye irritation test.

77. Jackson, J., and Rutty, D. A. (1985): Ocular tolerance assessment—Integrated tier policy. *Food Chem. Toxicol.,* 23:309–310.

78. Jumblatt, M. M., Fogle, J. A., and Neufeld, A. H. (1980): Cholera toxin stimulates adenosine 3'5'-monophosphate synthesis and epithelial wound closure in the rabbit cornea. *Invest. Ophthalmol. Vis. Sci.,* 19:1321–1329.

79. Jumblatt, M. M., and Neufeld, A. H. (1981): Characterization of cyclic AMP-mediated wound closure of the rabbit corneal epithelium. *Curr. Eye Res.,* 1:189–195.

80. Kay, J. H., and Calandra, J. C. (1962): Interpretation of eye irritation tests. *J. Soc. Cosmet. Chem.,* 13:281–289.

81. Kaye, G. I., and Tice, L. W. (1966): Studies on the cornea. V. Electron microscopic localization of adenosine triphosphatase activity in the rabbit cornea in relation to transport. *Invest. Ophthalmol.,* 5:22–32.

82. Kemp, R. B., Meredith, R. W., Gamble, S., and Frost, M. (1983): A rapid cell culture technique for assessing the toxicity of detergent-based products *in vitro* as a possible screen for eye irritancy *in vivo.* *Cytobios,* 36:153.

83. Kemp, R. B., Meredith, R. W. J., and Gamble, S. H. (1985): Toxicity of commercial products on cells in suspension culture: A possible screen for the Draize eye irritation test. *Food Chem. Toxicol.,* 23:267–270.

84. Kennedy, G. L., Jr., Ferenz, R., and Burgess, B. A. (1986): Estimation of acute oral toxicity in rats by determination of the approximate lethal dose rather than the LD50. *J. Appl. Toxicol.,* 6:145–148.

85. Kimura, S. J. (1951): Fluorescein paper: Simple means of insuring use of sterile fluorescein. *Am. J. Ophthalmol.,* 34:466.

86. Kuhlman, R. E. (1959): Species variation in the enzyme content of corneal epithelium. *J. Cell. Comp. Physiol.,* 53:313–326.

87. Leighton, J., Nassaurer, J., and Tehoa, R. (1985): The chick embryo in toxicology: An alternative to the rabbit eye. *Food Chem. Toxicol.,* 23:293–298.

88. Lieberman, H. R. (1983): Estimating LD50 using the probit technique: A basic computer program. *Drug Chem. Toxicol.,* 6:111–116.

89. Litchfield, J. T., and Wilcoxon, F. (1949): A simplified method of evaluating dose-effect experiments. *J. Pharmacol. Exp. Ther.,* 96:99–115.

90. Lorke, D. (1983): A new approach to practical toxicity testing. *Arch. Toxicol.,* 54:275–287.

91. Luepke, N. P. (1985): Hen's egg chorioallantoic membrane test for irritation potential. *Food Chem. Toxicol.,* 23:287–291.

92. Maeda, K., and Sakagudin, K. (1965): Studies on sodium-potassium-activated adenosine triphosphatase in the cornea. Electron-microscopic observations on the rat cornea. *Jpn. J. Ophthalmol.,* 9:195–199.

93. Marzulli, F. N. (1965): New data on eye and skin tests. *Toxicol. Appl. Pharmacol.,* 7:79–85.

94. Marzulli, F. N., and Simmon, M. E. (1971): Eye irritation from topically applied drugs and cosmetics: Preclinical studies. *Am. J. Optom.,* 48:61–79.

95. Maurice, D. M. (1967): The use of fluorescein in ophthalmological research. *Invest. Ophthalmol.,* 6:465–477.

96. Maurice, D. M., and Giardini, A. A. (1951): A simple optical apparatus for measuring the corneal thickness, and the average thickness of the human cornea. *Br. J. Ophthalmol.,* 35:169–177.

97. McCaa, C. S. (1985): Anatomy, physiology and toxicology of the eye. In: *Toxicology of the Eye, Ear, and Other Special Senses,* edited by A. Wallace Hayes, pp. 1–15. Raven Press, NY.

98. McDonald, T. O., Baldwin, H. A., and Beasley, C. H. (1973): Slit-lamp examination of experimental animal eyes. I. Techniques of illumination and the normal eye. *J. Soc. Cosmet. Chem.,* 24:163–180.

99. Meier-Ruge, W. (1973): Eye toxicity. In: *Excerpta Medica, Vol. 14: Proceedings of the European Society for the Study of Drug Toxicity,* edited by W. A. M. Duncan, pp. 133–145. Elsevier/North-Holland, NY.

100. Miller, L. C. (1964): The quantal response in toxicity tests. In: *Statistics and Mathematics in Biology,* edited by O. Kempthorne, T. A. Bancroft, J. W. Gowen, and J. L. Lush, pp. 315–326. Hofner, NY.

101. Mishima, S. (1981): Clinical pharmacokinetics of the eye. *Invest. Ophthalmol. Vis. Sci.,* 21:504.

102. Mishima, S., and Hedbys, B. O. (1968): Measurement of corneal thickness with the Haag–Streit pachometer. *Arch. Ophthalmol.,* 80:710–713.

103. Mishima, S., and Kudo, T. (1967): *In vitro* incubation of rabbit cornea. *Invest. Ophthalmol. Vis. Sci.,* 6:329–339.

104. Mishimu, S., and Maurice, D. M. (1971): *In vivo* determination of the endothelial permeability to fluorescein. *Acta Soc. Ophthalmol. (Jpn.),* 75:236–243.

105. Moses, R. A., Parkinson, G., and Schuchardt, R. (1979): A standard large wound of the corneal epithelium in rabbits. *Invest. Ophthalmol. Vis. Sci.,* 18:103–106.

106. Muir, C. K. (1983): The toxic effect of some industrial chemicals on rabbit ileum *in vitro* compared with eye irritancy *in vivo.* *Toxicol. Lett.,* 19:309.

107. Muir, C. K., Flower, C., and Van Abbe, N. J. (1983): A novel approach to the search for *in vitro* alternatives to *in vivo* eye irritancy testing. *Toxicol. Lett.,* 18:1–5.

108. Muller, H., and Kley, H. P. (1982): Retrospective study on the reliability of an "approximate LD50" determined with a small number of animals. *Arch. Toxicol.,* 51:189–196.

109. NAS Committee for Revision of NAS publication 1138 (1977): Dermal and eye toxicity tests. In: *Principles and Procedures for Evaluating the Toxicity of Household Substances,* pp. 41–54. National Academy of Sciences, Washington, D.C.

110. Norton-Root, H., Yackovich, F., Demetrulias, J., et al. (1982): Evaluation of an *in vitro* cell toxicity test using rabbit corneal cells to predict the eye irritation potential of surfactants. *Toxicol. Lett.,* 14:207–212.

111. North-Root, H., Yackovich, F., Demetrullas, J., et al. (1985): Prediction of the eye irritation potential of shampoos using the *in vitro* SIRC cell toxicity test. *Food Chem. Toxicol.,* 23:271–273.

112. OECD (1981): OECD guidelines for testing of chemicals. OECD, Paris.

113. OECD (1984): Data interpretation guides for initial hazard assessment of chemicals. OECD, Paris.

114. OECD Test Guidelines (1981): Decision of the council concerning mutual acceptance of data in the assessment of chemicals. Annex 2. OECD Principles of Good Laboratory Practices. OECD, Paris.

115. Olson, K. J., Dupree, R. W., Plomer, E. T., and Rerve, V. (1962): Toxicological properties of several commercially available surfactants *J. Cos. Cosmet. Chem.*, 13:469–476.

116. Paget, G. E., and Thomson, R. (1979): *Standard Operation Procedures in Toxicology.* MTP Press, Lancaster, England.

117. Parish, W. E. (1985): Ability of *in vitro* (corneal injury-eye organ and chorioallantoic membrane) tests to represent histopathological features of acute eye inflammation. *Food Chem. Toxicol.*, 23:215–227.

118. Pfister, R. R., and Burstein, N. (1976): The effects of ophthalmic drugs, vehicles, and preservatives on corneal epithelium: A scanning electron microscope study. *Invest. Ophthalmol.*, 15:246–258.

119. Price, J. B., and Andrews, I. J. (1985): The *in vitro* assessment of eye irritancy using isolated eyes. *Food Chem. Toxicol.*, 23:313–315.

120. Prince, J. H., Diesem, C. D., Eglitis, I., and Ruskell, G. L. (1960): Anatomy and histology of the eye and orbit in domestic animals. Charles C Thomas, Springfield, IL.

121. Protty, C., and Ferguson, T. F. M. (1976): The effects of surfactants upon rat peritoneal mast cell *in vitro. Food Cosmet. Toxicol.*, 14:425.

122. Rieger, M. M., and Battista, G. W. (1964): Some experiences in the safety testing of cosmetics. *J. Soc. Cosmet. Chem.*, 15:161–172.

123. Roeig, D. L., Hasegawa, A. I., Harris, G. J., et al. (1980): Occurrence of corneal opacities in rats after acute administration of 1-alpha-acetylmethadol. *Toxicol. Appl. Pharmacol.*, 56:155–163.

124. Rosiello, A. P., Essigmann, J. M., and Wogan, G. N. (1977): Rapid and accurate determination of the median lethal dose (LD_{50}) and its error with a small computer. *J. Toxicol. Environ. Health*, 3:797–809.

125. Rowan, A. (1981): The Draize test: Political and scientific issues. *Cosmet. Tech.*, 3(7):32–48.

126. Scaife, M. C. (1982): An investigation of detergent action on cells *in vitro* and possible correlations with *in vivo* data. *Int. J. Cosmet. Sci.*, 4:179.

127. Schutz, E., and Fuchs, H. (1982): A new approach to minimizing the number of animals used in acute toxicity testing and optimizing the information of test results. *Arch. Toxicol.*, 51:197–220.

128. Seabrough, V. M., Osterberg, R. E., Hoheisel, C. A., et al. (1976): A comparative study of rabbit ocular reactions to various exposure times to chemicals. *Society of Toxicology, Fifteenth Annual Meeting.* Atlanta, Georgia.

129. Shapiro, H. (1956): Swetting and dissolution of the rabbit cornea in alkali. *Am. J. Ophthalmol.*, 42:292–298.

130. Shopsis, C., and Sathe, S. (1984): Uridine uptake inhibition as a cytotoxicity test: Correlation with the Draize test. *Toxicology*, 29:195–206.

131. Society of Agricultural Chemical Industry (1985): Agricultural Chemicals Laws and Regulations, Japan (II) (English translation).

132. Society of Toxicology of Canada (1985): Position paper on the LD_{50}. Adopted at the STC Annual meeting on December 3, 1985.

133. Sperling, F. (1976): Nonlethal parameters as indices of acute toxicity: Inadequacy of the acute LD_{50}. In: *New Concepts in Safety Evaluation*, edited by M. A. Mehlman, R. E. Shapiro, and H. Blumenthal, pp. 177–191. Hemisphere, Washington.

134. Stark, D. M., Shopsis, C., Borenfreund, E., and Walberg, J. (1983): *Alternative Approaches to the Draize Assay: Chemotoxic, Cytology, Differentiation and Membrane Transport Studies in Product Safety Evaluation*, edited by A. M. Goldberg, p. 179. Mary Ann Liebert, NY.

135. Sugar, J. (1980): Corneal examination. In: *Principles and Practice of Ophthalmology, Vol. 1*, edited by G. A. Peyman, D. R. Sanders, and M. F. Goldberg, pp. 393–395. Saunders, Philadelphia.

136. Swanston, D. W. (1983): Eye irritancy testing. In: *Animals and Alternatives in Toxicity Testing*, edited by M. Balls, R. J. Riddell, and A. N. Worden, p. 337. Academic Press, London.

137. Tanaka, N., Ohkawa, T., Hiyama, T., and Nakajima, A. (1982): Evaluation of ocular toxicity of two beta blocking drugs, cereteolol and practolol, in beagle dogs. *J. Pharmacol. Exp. Ther.*, 224:424–430.

138. Thompson, W. R. (1947): Use of moving averages and interpolation to estimate median effective dose. *Bacteriol. Rev.*, 11:115–145.

139. Tonjum, A. M. (1975): Effects of benzalkonium chloride upon the corneal epithelium: Studies with scanning electron microscopy. *Acta Ophthalmol.*, 53:358–366.

140. Trevan, J. W. (1927): The error of determination of toxicity. *Proc. R. Soc. Lond.*, 101B:483–514.

141. Walberg, J. (1983): Exfoliative cytology as a refinement of the Draize eye irritancy test. *Toxicol. Lett.*, 18:49.

142. Waltman, S. R., and Kaufman, H. E. (1970): *In vivo* studies of human corneal and endothelial permeability. *Am. J. Ophthalmol.*, 70:45–47.

143. Waud, D. R. (1972): On biological assays involving quantal responses. *J. Pharm. Exp. Ther.*, 183:577–607.

144. Weil, C. S. (1952): Tables for convenient calculation of median-effective dose (LD_{50} or EO_{50}) and instruction in their use. *Biometrics*, 8:249–263.

145. Weil, C. S. (1983): Economical LD_{50} and slope determinations. *Drug Chem. Toxicol.*, 6:595–603.

146. Weil, C. S., and Scala, R. A. (1971): Study of intra- and interlaboratory variability in the results of rabbit eye and skin irritation tests. *Toxicol. Appl. Pharmacol.*, 19:276–360.

147. Weltman, A. S., Sharber, S. B., and Jurtshuk, T. (1968): Comparative evaluation and influence of various factors on eye irritation scores. *Toxicol. Appl. Pharmacol.*, 7:308–319.

148. Williams, S. J. (1984): Prediction of ocular irritancy potential from dermal irritation test results. *Food Chem. Toxicol.*, 22:157–161.

149. Williams, S. J. (1985): Changing concepts of ocular irritation evaluation: Pitfalls and progress. *Food Chem. Toxicol.*, 23:189–193.

150. Williams, S. J., Grapel, G. J., and Kennedy, G. I. (1982): Evaluation of ocular irritancy: Potential intra-laboratory variability and effect of dosage volume. *Toxicol. Lett.*, 12:235–241.

151. Zbinden, G., and Flury-Roversi, M. (1981): Significance of the LD_{50}—Test for toxicological evaluation of chemical substances. *Arch. Toxicol.*, 47:77–99.

Principles and Methods of Toxicology, Second Edition, edited by A. Wallace Hayes, Raven Press, Ltd., New York © 1989.

CHAPTER **7**

Subchronic Toxicity Testing

A. T. Mosberg and A. W. Hayes

Center for Toxicology, R. J. R. Nabisco, Bowman Gray Technical Center, Winston-Salem, North Carolina 27102

Subchronic studies are designed to examine the adverse effects resulting from repeated exposure over a portion of the average life span of an experimental animal. Properly designed subchronic studies give valuable information on the cumulative toxicity of a substance on target organs and on physiologic and metabolic tolerance of a compound at low-dose (relative to acute toxicity testing doses) prolonged exposure. By monitoring many different parameters, including histopathologic evaluations, a wide variety of adverse effects can be detected. The results from such studies can provide information that will aid in selecting doses for chronic, reproductive, and carcinogenicity studies. Subchronic studies are also valuable in establishing doses at which no toxicologic effects are evident, a critical factor in risk assessment. It has been suggested that subchronic data may be sufficient to predict the hazard of long-term, low-dose exposure of a particular compound (47).

Although some experts have suggested that the long-term safety level of a compound can be predicted from acute or shorter than subchronic studies (47,49), one must bear in mind that these are only generalities and that exceptions are not at all uncommon. Even though acute data indicate that a compound is practically nontoxic, prolonged exposure studies cannot be automatically precluded from the process of safety evaluation. Acutely nontoxic compounds may be toxic after prolonged exposure, even at low doses, due to accumulation, changes in enzyme levels, and disruption of physiologic and biochemical homeostasis. Therefore, sub-chronic testing is considered essential for all new chemicals before their specific hazard can be assessed and legitimate safety assessment made.

The exposure period in subchronic studies may vary, depending on the objective of the study, the species selected for the study, and the route of administration employed. A generalization which is often made is that subchronic studies do not exceed 10% of the animal's lifespan. Oral and inhalation subchronic studies are generally carried out for 3 months in shorter lived animals (rodents) and 1 year in longer lived animals (dogs and monkeys). Subchronic dermal studies are usually performed for 1 month or less. The most common routes of administration employed in subchronic toxicity studies are oral, dermal, and inhalation. Subchronic toxicity studies should always attempt to expose the animals by the same route that man is most likely to be exposed.

The subsequent paragraphs will describe a classic 90-day oral subchronic toxicity study to illustrate the principles and methodologies employed in conducting subchronic toxicity studies.

THE 90-DAY SUBCHRONIC ORAL TOXICITY STUDY

Principles of Experimental Design

Oral administration of a test substance can be carried out by gavage, in capsules, or in the diet or drinking water. Dietary administration is the most common. Three to four doses of the substance should be employed. Numerous types of observations and evaluations are performed during and at the end of the dosing period. These may include daily observations, periodic physical examinations, monitoring of body weight and feed consumption, and analysis of hematology, biochemistry, and urinary parameters. When the animals have been killed at the end of the study, organ weights are recorded and histopathologic evaluation is performed. Prior to the initiation of the study, however, there are numerous factors to be considered and decisions to be made. Some of these factors will be discussed in the subsequent paragraphs.

Methods and Procedures

Animal Species

Any common laboratory animal may be selected, but it is recommended that subchronic studies be conducted in at least two species, one being a rodent and the other a non-rodent. Dogs are the most commonly used nonrodent species, mainly because of their availability and the large volume of background data available on these animals (17). Dogs and other larger animals have the advantage that blood samples can be collected at different time intervals during the study without killing the animals. One should not, however, confuse the size of the animal with its usefulness in toxicity testing. Bigger is not always better. Ideally, the animal of choice should be similar to humans in the pharmacokinetic handling of the test substance. However, this information is often missing or incomplete during the early stages of development of the chemical. Under such circumstances, it is a good practice to select the most sensitive species for evaluating the safety of a substance, a practice that can only be carried out after multiple species have been tested.

Age

Although immature or mature animals can be used, the decision should be based on the age population that is most likely to be exposed to the compound. Younger and still growing animals are preferred at the initiation of a subchronic study. When mice or rats are selected, initiation of treatment should be shortly after weaning (usually about 6 weeks old but not more than 8 weeks old). When the dog is chosen, initiation of treatment should begin at 4–6 months but not at more than 9 months of age.

Sex and Numbers

Variation in responses due to sex difference may be more important in a subchronic study than in an acute study. Subchronic studies should, therefore, be conducted employing both males and females to determine whether sex differences exist with regard to response to the test substance.

Each dose group should consist of equal numbers of males and females, usually 10–20 per sex per dose group for rodents and 6–8 per sex per dose group for dogs. The number of animals in a particular dose group may have to be increased

if interim kills (i.e., scheduled kill during the 90-day period) are scheduled. In general, not more than 10% of the animals in the high dose group should die during the study, and no deaths should occur in the intermediate and low dose groups. Obviously, the doses employed must be carefully selected. To examine the reversibility of adverse effects, the investigator may decide to include extra animals in each group. These animals are removed from the test compound after 90 days, fed standard lab chow for an additional 2–4-week period, and then subjected to the same analyses as those killed after the dosing period. The reversibility of adverse effects can be evaluated from these animals. This often produces valuable information in risk assessment of the compound.

Animal Husbandry and Randomization

As has been stated, subchronic toxicity studies are designed to determine responses produced by low-dose repeated exposure of a substance to a test animal. These responses are occasionally very low in incidence or severity, and it thus becomes essential that environmental conditions be tightly controlled to avoid unnecessary stress. These environmental stress-related responses may be interpreted as treatment-related effects. Such factors as room temperature, humidity, dark and light cycle, supply of quality drinking water, nutritionally balanced diet, and cleanliness of the environment, unless adequately controlled, can produce undue stress on, and unwanted responses in, the test animals. All things should be identical among the groups except for the dose of the test substance.

Each animal should be uniquely identified with a study. Ear tags, ear notching, or permanent markings such as tatoos may be employed. The animals should be housed in individual cages. To ensure a healthy and homogeneous animal population, the investigator should select only healthy animals, by weight, within a known age population. In a group of animals of the same age, animals whose weights are beyond two standard deviations of the group mean should be eliminated. The animals should be randomly assigned to test groups through the use of a random numbers table or a computer-generated randomization procedure. It is desirable and preferable to assign animals to groups on the basis of body weight so that no statistical difference exists in group mean body weights when the study is initiated. If the body weight means among groups are statistically different, the randomization procedure should be repeated.

Selection of Doses

Perhaps the most difficult task in designing a subchronic study is the selection of proper doses. Ideally, one should select doses that yield no toxicity at the low dose, none or only slight toxicity at the intermediate dose, and toxicity in the high dose. The high dose should produce frank toxicity but minimal mortality to allow meaningful evaluation of the data. Certain regulatory guidelines require that while toxicity should be observed in the high dose group, incidence of mortality should not exceed 10% in this group. These requirements, which are based more on ideal scientific logic than practical cases, sometimes compound the difficulty an investigator faces in selecting the proper doses. It is the authors' opinion that the arbitrary 10% mortality figure should only serve as a guideline and should not be mandatory. A more realistic target would be to establish toxicity in the high dose without producing excessive mortality. Whether three or four doses are selected, they should be spaced at concentrations or amounts such that graded responses can be observed. The low dose should be higher than the expected level of human exposure. With all these factors to consider, it should become apparent how difficult it can be to select appropriate doses for conducting a subchronic toxicity study.

It is a general practice that a range finding study be conducted (usually 2 weeks in duration) prior to initiating the subchronic study, to assist in the selection of doses. Toxicity in the pilot study is defined in the same manner and based on the same measurable parameters as those employed in the subchronic study, with the exception of histopathology. Remember that two of the primary goals of a subchronic study are to define a no observable effect dose and to determine the target organ or organs with greatest susceptibility. Unless a no observable effect dose has been established, it is difficult for one to do a risk assessment of the compound.

Many other factors must be taken into consideration in selecting proper dose levels. First, one has to consider the bioaccumulation potential of the test substance in the body. Determination of the half-life of the chemical in different tissues, organs, and biologic fluids may provide valuable information in determining the accumulation of the chemical in the body. For highly cumulative chemicals, the investigator may elect to decrease the daily dose; or toxic effects at all doses may be found after 90 days of exposure. Many investigators determine the half-life of a chemical by employing radioactively labeled chemicals.

Secondly, test-substance-related induction or inhibition of the enzyme systems that are normally responsible for the detoxification or bioactivation of the test substance may have an effect on the pharmacokinetics of the test substance. For example, the daily dose for a chemical that inhibits the enzymes responsible for its own metabolism and detoxification may have to be decreased.

Third, the stability of the test substance in the gastrointestinal tract should be considered. For test substances that have an affinity for the gastrointestinal content, the investigator may consider increasing the daily dose. Another consideration is that in such a case, the oral route may not be the proper route of administration. While all these factors may be more important in chronic studies, these factors must also be considered in subchronic studies, because subchronic toxicity data may be the only repeated animal exposure data available for a compound before it is presented to the public.

In addition to the group of animals treated with the test substance, a concurrent control group should also be included. This group should either be untreated animals or vehicle treated controls, if a vehicle is used in the formulation of the dosages. If the toxicity of the vehicle is not known, both an untreated and vehicle control group should be included in the study.

Preparation and Administration of Dosages

In a subchronic study, the test substance is often simply incorporated into the diet or added to the drinking water.

The test substance may also be given in a capsule or by gavage, although capsule administration is generally limited to larger animals. While the first two methods are more convenient, the latter two are more accurate because the amount of compound received by the animals is more closely controlled. When extremely accurate dosing is required, the administration method of choice should be one of the latter two. The doses may be expressed in terms of concentration of the test substance in the diet or drinking water (e.g., ppm) or it may be expressed in terms of the amount of the test substance received by the animal per kg of body weight per day (mg/kg/day) or per surface area per day (mg/cm^3/day).

If the test substance is given in the diet, the amount of feed consumed will be very important in determining the exact amount of test substance that an animal actually received in a day. For example, rabbits tend to spill feed when they eat and unless there is an acceptable method of determining the feed consumption, the total daily dose cannot be computed accurately. The investigator may consider dosing the animals by gavage or intubation. Rats and mice also spill feed. Drop sheets may be placed beneath the cages and checked daily for excessive spillage to assist in interpretation of feed consumption. Feed consumption varies from weaning to maturity, with younger animals consuming more feed on a per kilogram body weight basis. Under such circumstances it may be necessary to adjust the concentration of test substance in the diet on a weekly or biweekly basis. This dosage adjustment may have to be continuous until maturity or until the feed consumption rate has stabilized.

The same batch or lot of laboratory chow and test substance should be used in formulation of dosage throughout the study. This is true in any multiple dose study. If different lots of test substance are used at any time during the study, the physical and chemical properties and the composition of the new batch of test substance must be determined. The concentration of the test substance in the diet must be analytically determined periodically. Samples from freshly made diets are analyzed to insure adequate mixing. Samples from the top, middle, and bottom of each batch are analyzed to verify concentration. Residual samples which have been kept at room temperature for the same duration that the animals have been exposed to their feed are analyzed to assure stability. To achieve the goal of constant dosing throughout the study, the investigator should make predictions of changes in body weight and feed consumption and utilize such information for the adjustment of test substance concentrations. The example given below may help the reader to understand the procedures involved in such an adjustment.

The predicted body weight of the animals at the mid-2nd week will be equal to the group mean body weight at the beginning of the 2nd week plus the average (half) of the difference of the group mean body weight between the end of the first and the end of the 2nd week. Similarly, the predicted group mean feed consumption (g/animal/day) at the same time will be equal to the group mean feed consumption at the beginning of the 2nd week plus the average (half) of the difference of the group mean feed consumption at the beginning of the 2nd week plus the average (half) of the difference of the group mean feed consumption between the end of the first and the end of the 2nd week. Therefore, the predicted rate of diet intake at the middle of the 3rd week will be:

$$\frac{\text{Predicted group mean feed consumption}}{\text{Predicted group mean body weight}}$$

$$= \text{g of diet kg of body weight/animal/day}$$

And the concentration of the test substance at the middle of the 3rd week will be:

$$\frac{\text{Dose (mg/kg body weight/animal/day)}}{\text{Predicted diet intake (g of diet/kg body weight/animal/day)}}$$

$$= \text{mg/g of diet}$$

In a similar manner, these equations can be used to calculate the actual dose intake of the test substance if the diet concentration, the body weight, and the feed consumption are known.

Example

On Monday, an investigator wishes to know the concentration and the total quantity that must be prepared to feed at least 20 rats at a dose of 10 mg/kg/day on the coming Thursday and carry on until next Thursday. He has recorded the group mean body weight of the previous 2 weeks to be 150 and 250 g, and the group mean feed consumption to be 20 and 30 g/animal/day. The predicted group mean body weight on the coming Thursday would be $250 + \frac{1}{2}(250 - 150) = 300$ (g/animal), and the predicted group mean feed consumption would be $30 + \frac{1}{2}(30 - 20) = (30 + 5) = 35$ g diet/animal/day. Therefore, the average daily diet intake from the coming Thursday for the next 7 days would be:

$$\frac{35 \text{ (g diet/animal/day)}}{0.3 \text{ (kg/animal)}}$$

$$= 116.67 \text{ (g diet/day/kg of body weight)}$$

and the concentration of the diet would be

$$\frac{10 \text{ (mg test substance/kg body weight/day)}}{116.67 \text{ (g diet/day/kg of body weight)}}$$

$$= 0.086 \text{ (mg test substance/g diet)}$$

$$= 86 \text{ (mg test substance/kg diet)}$$

Since the average predicted feed consumption is 35 g diet/animal/day, the minimum quantity of diet needed for 20 rats for 7 days would be

$$(35 \text{ g diet/animal/day}) \times 20 \text{ animals} \times 7 \text{ days}$$

$$= 4,900 \text{ g diet or 4.9 kg diet}$$

Thus the investigator will need at least (86 mg test substance/kg diet) × 4.9 kg diet = 421.4 mg test substance, which has to be blended with the diet to obtain the 4.9-kg formulated diet. However, in practice, more diet mixture has to be blended to make up for the loss in transfer and weighing.

There are three generally accepted methods of mixing a test substance with the diet: direct dry mixing, serial addition, and premixing. The method selected will be determined to a large extent on the physical characteristics of the test substance. The first and simplest method is carried out by blending the required amount of the ground test substance directly with a corresponding amount of diet to achieve the required concentration. The second method is accomplished by sequentially adding a fraction of the total diet to the total amount of group test substance. The third method involves first blending the total amount of test substance with a portion of the diet and then blending this premix with the remainder of the diet for an additional period of time.

The choice among the three methods will depend on the nature of the compound, but the goal is to achieve a homogeneous diet and test substance mixture. A pilot diet mixing study may be necessary to find the most efficient method of mixing. In the premixing method, it is often desirable to dissolve the test substance in a volatile solvent prior to the premixing. The premixing is carried out in an open blender in a hood until all the volatile solvent has evaporated. If this is done, the same volatile solvent should be added in equal amount to all dose diets, including the control diet.

Samples from the top, middle, and bottom of the freshly prepared dietary mixture of each dose should be taken for test substance analysis to determine uniformity of mixing in the diet. If a vehicle other than water must be used to aid the diet mixing, the toxicity of the vehicle and its effects on the stability of the test substance should be determined.

If capsule administration is chosen, then inert diluents such as lactose, mannitol, milk solids, starch, kaolin, calcium carbonate, and dicalcium phosphate may be used to mix with the test substance. A predetermined amount of the mixture is weighed and packed into a gelatin capsule. The size of the capsule should be as small as possible but large enough to hold the entire dose without any spillage. For more accurate dosage, the dose mixture is weighed into the capsule until the desired amount of dose is obtained.

The test substance may also be given by gavage or intubation. In such cases, the test substance can be prepared as a solution or a suspension.

All dosing should be based on a 7-day per week basis. Five days a week is usually sufficient for inhalation or dermal exposure. Because all subchronic studies are relatively expensive, care must be exercised to minimize dosing errors. All calculations should be checked by two different people. Color-coded cage cards, color-coded feed cups, individual dosing schedule sheets, and double checking all procedures often decreases errors due to dosing. The investigator should check and verify the animal numbers, the feed cup color, and the cage card before changing feed cup or diet mixture to ensure that the animal receives the right dose.

In Vivo Observations and Measurements

The toxic effects of the test substance basically can be defined by physical examination, daily observations, ophthalmologic examination, determination of feed and water consumption, body and organ weights, hematology, urinalysis, biochemical organ function tests, and pathology studies. When possible, these parameters should be evaluated prior to initiation of the study to obtain baseline information on the animals. Detailed observations of each animal should be done at least once and preferably twice daily for the duration of the study. If the recovery groups are included in the study, these animals should be observed for a period of time after the termination of treatment. It is not usually necessary to exceed 28 days to determine reversibility of effects.

Daily observations should include close scrutiny for changes in fur texture, skin, eyes, mucus membranes, orifices, and clinical signs of the respiratory, circulatory, autonomic and central nervous systems, somatomotor activities, and behavioral changes. Special attention should be given to examine for any palpable mass which may be related to tumor incidence. All signs should be recorded. If deaths are found during the study, the animals should be necropsied within a short period of time and the tissues placed in 10% neutral buffered formalin or another appropriate fixative. If necropsies cannot be performed immediately, the dead animals should be refrigerated, but not frozen, until necropsies can be done. In any case, necropsies should be done within 16 hr of the death of the animal. Severely moribund animals should be killed and necropsied to prevent loss of valuable tissues due to autolysis. At the end of the 90-day test period, all animals except those in the recovery groups are killed. Animals in the satellite group should be observed during the recovery period and then bled and killed for hematology, clinical chemistry, and pathology studies.

Hematology

Hematologic analysis should include hematocrit and hemoglobin concentrations, red blood cell count, white blood cell count (total and differential count), morphology of the red blood cells, and a measure of clotting ability such as prothrombin and thromboplastin time or platelet count. These should be determined prior to treatment, once during the study and at the terminal sacrifice. The inclusion of an appropriately sized control group (up to double the number of animals in the treatment groups) can eliminate the need for pretest bleeding. For mice, additional groups of animals are usually added to the study for interim kill for hematologic analysis. Rats may be bled during dosing as well as at the end of the study; however, one must be cognizant of the fact that the interim retro-orbital bleeding can interfere with ophthalmologic examinations.

Biochemical Measurements

Part of the blood samples obtained for the hematologic analysis should also be subjected to biochemical analysis of the plasma or the serum. Such analysis should include, but not be limited to, electrolyte balance, carbohydrate and protein metabolism, and organ function tests. This information can be extremely important in the establishment of target organ toxicity. The animals should be fasted overnight prior to collecting blood samples. The period of time of fasting will depend on the species of animal; however, a 12–16 hr fast is adequate for most animals. For animals such as mice, with a high metabolism rate, 3–4 hr fasting may be sufficient.

Good clinical chemistry analyses will include most if not all of the following parameters in a subchronic study: Ca^{2+}, K^+, Na^+, Cl^-, PO_2^{4-}, fasting glucose, serum GOT (AST) and GPT (ALT), alkaline phosphatase, ornithine decarboxylase, γ-glutamyl transpeptidase, blood urea nitrogen (BUN), total protein, albumin, globulin, total bilirubin, blood creatinine, cholesterol, acid/base balance, lipids, cholinesterase (plasma, red blood cell, and/or brain), and any other biochemical parameters that may facilitate the definition of adverse effects. The list can be extensive. A good scientist selects an adequate battery of clinical chemistry tests. The number of biochemical parameters that should be examined are based on the class of chemicals and the expected toxicity. For example, cholinesterase activities should be considered if the test substance is an organophosphate or carbamate, which are expected to be inhibitors of the enzyme.

Urinalysis

Urinalysis is highly recommended if renal toxicity is suspected such as with organomercury compounds. The following should be determined: specific gravity and/or osmolarity, acidity, protein, glucose, ketones, bilirubin, epithelial cells, urobilinogen and stones, etc. Urinalysis is generally conducted at the same time as hematology and blood chemistry determination. Fresh urine should always be acquired for the analysis.

Other In-Vivo Tests

Other *in-vivo* tests may also be considered on a case-by-case basis. These include, but are not limited to, EKG, EEG, nerve conduction, and liver dye and kidney PAH functional tests.

Pathology Examination

All animals should be subjected to a gross pathology examination. All tissues from the high dose and control animals and any tissues with lesions in other groups should be further examined microscopically. When tissues from animals in the high dose group are detected as having microscopic lesions, those tissues should be examined from animals in lower dose groups. Because histopathology studies are generally expensive and time consuming, the numbers of tissues and organs to be examined should be based on sound scientific judgment. Certain regulatory guidelines have provided a list of tissues recommended for histopathology examination.

Analysis and Interpretation of Data

All quantitative and qualitative data, including histopathology findings, should be processed with appropriate statistics. Interpretation of *in-vivo* observations and measurements should be evaluated in conjunction with the histopathology findings in terms of incidence, severity, magnitude of deviation from normal range, and reversibility.

Feed consumption data along with body weight data may indicate changes in appetite or changes in the efficiency of feed utilization by the body. These two parameters are often very sensitive to chemical exposure, and occasionally they are the only significant toxicologic findings with compounds of low toxicity. However, the investigator should also be aware of the fact that feed consumption and body weight can be associated with other stresses such as diarrhea, dehydration, or decrease in water consumption. Elevated levels of serum or plasma enzymes which have a specific tissue origin are of great value in identifying target organs. For example, out of normal range levels and statistically significant increases in serum glutamic-pyruvic transaminase (SGPT) or sorbital dehydrogenase may suggest hepatotoxicity. While an increase in glutamic oxaloacetic transaminase and lactate dehydrogenase (LDH) activities indicates general tissue damage, increases in specific isoenzymes of LDH (LDH 1 and LDH 2) and α-hydroxybutyrate dehydrogenase may be related to myocardial damage. The level of serum alkaline phosphatase is elevated in certain osteologic diseases (e.g., osteogenic sarcoma, rickets) or biliary disorders such as obstructive jaundice and cirrhosis. Elevated acid phosphatase activity has been related to carcinoma of the prostate.

Electrolyte balance is essential for the normal function of all biologic systems and the general well-being of an animal; electrolytes are controlled and regulated by homeostatic mechanisms. Any significant deviation may indicate malfunction of these regulatory mechanisms, which may be related to the chemical exposure. Acid/base balance is regulated by renal and respiratory systems, and a significant deviation may indicate respiratory or renal problems. Renal damage may be substantiated by an increase in BUN level or by the appearance of stones, calculi, protein, or epithelial cells in the urine. Any changes in the morphology of blood cells may indicate blood dyscrasia. In such a case, bone marrow smears should be investigated. Pharmacotoxic signs can also often provide clues as to target organs. Autonomic or central signs may indicate the involvement of the nervous system, either primary or secondary to the exposure of the chemical.

In summary, the investigator should have a knowledge of physiology, pathology, biochemistry, and pharmacology to interpret the results of the study, to draw conclusions from the data, and to make a risk assessment of a chemical or drug. One must be able to distinguish chemically induced responses from normal biologic variations, especially since normal biologic variations will occasionally show up as statistically significant changes. Statistics can be a very useful tool in a toxicity decision, but it cannot be used as the only measure. The toxicologist may be able to assess the risk of a compound, but an acceptable risk level will be set by the public.

REGULATIONS THAT GOVERN THE DESIGN, IMPLEMENTATION, AND INTERPRETATION OF TOXICITY STUDIES

Following a strong demand from the public, governments are now more cautious in formulating their policies toward the use and development of chemicals. To insure and safeguard the health and the environment of their citizens, almost every industrialized country now has laws and regulations governing the introduction and transportation of new pesticides, food additives, human and animal drugs, and chemicals. Many of these countries also have, or will have in the near future, laws and regulations governing medical devices,

exposure to chemicals in the workplace, and the introduction of industrial chemicals into commerce.

While there is uniformity in the objectives of these laws, i.e., not to impede the beneficial use of chemicals but at the same time allow for a maximal safety in use, there have been considerable variations from country to country in approaches to evaluating the safety or setting safety standards for these chemicals. These variations are reflected in the numbers of tests, the methods, and experimentations required for generating toxicity data to support risk–benefit assessment. Considerable effort has been placed in harmonizing the many different approaches so that most testing guidelines are compatible both in the United States and worldwide. The World Health Organization (WHO) has long recognized the need for some uniformity in requirements for toxicity testing and evaluation. WHO has issued a number of technical reports and guidelines for testing and evaluating new chemicals having various applications as food additives and pesticides (50–66).

In the United States a number of laws have been passed with the intent that we might enjoy the benefits of innovations in chemistry with an acceptable degree of risk to health and environment. While the passage of these laws has served various real needs and basically has been to the benefit of our well-being, the promulgation of various regulations under these laws has led quite often to conflicting and confusing requirements for toxicologic testing. Guidelines for toxicity testing by the Environmental Protection Agency (EPA), for registration of pesticides under the Federal Insecticide, Fungicide and Rodenticide Act (FIFRA) (6) and for testing of new chemicals when required under the Toxic Substances Control Act (TSCA) (16), have set forth in great detail standards to be adhered to in the conduct of various toxicity studies from acute to chronic. Differences in guidelines that have been issued by the EPA have been almost eliminated. FIFRA guidelines now match TSCA guidelines as closely as possible (11,17).

Even though the agencies can agree on one framework of toxicity testing guidelines, the toxicologist, having a strong scientific background, must recognize the ramifications of particular guidelines to fulfill his role as a bridge between science and governmental affairs. These laws and regulations governing toxicity studies and safety evaluation are described briefly in the following paragraphs. Table 1 lists some of the differences in requirements of subacute toxicity testings under several United States and European guidelines, and Table 2 lists some differences in the subchronic testing guidelines.

UNITED STATES LAWS AND REGULATORY GUIDELINES

Federal Food, Drug and Cosmetic Act

The Federal Food, Drug and Cosmetic Act (FDCA; 24), administered by the Food and Drug Administration (FDA), controls the introduction of new chemicals such as human and animal drugs, direct food additives, indirect food additives (such as packaging materials), and components of cosmetics. In the case of new human or animal drugs, safety and efficacy must be established for a particular therapeutic

TABLE 1. *Guidelines for subacute toxicity testing*

	EPA TSCA FIFRA	OECD	FDA	UK	Japan	Japan
Age at start of study (wks)	NS	6	3–6	6	Adult	NS
Minimum duration of study (days)	NS	14–28	28	28	28	NS
No. of Tx Groups (no less than)	NS	3	3	3	3	NS
Control	NS	y	y	y	y	NS
Vehicle Control (if needed)	NS	y	y	y	y	NS
Route of administration (recommended or accepted)	NS					
Diet		y	y	y	y	NS
Gavage		y	y	y	y	NS
Capsule		y	y	y	y	NS
Water		y	y	y	y	NS
Dermal		y	NS	y	y	NS
Inhalation		y	NS	y	y	NS
No. of rats/sex/grp (not including interim sac. or clinical lab. testing #'s)	NS	5	10	5	10	NS
Record body wt. weekly	NS	y	y	y	y	NS
Record feed consumption wkly.	NS	y	y	y	y	NS
Daily observations	NS	y	y	y	y	NS
Minimum interval between obs.						
Acceptable mortality-high dose grp.	NS	NS	NS	NS	NS	NS
Ophthalmology	NS	NS	y	NS	y	NS
Pretest			y		y	
At termination			y		y	
All high dose and control (lower doses only if findings at high dose)			y		y	
Hematology and clinical chemistry (time periods for data collections)	NS	y	y	y	y	NS
Terminal		y	y	y	y	NS
Min. no. animals bled (no/sex/grp)	NS	All	5	All	All	NS
Urinalysis	NS	A	A	NS	y	NS
Organ weights recd. at termination						
Liver	NS	y	y	y	y	NS
Kidneys		y	y	y	y	
Heart					y	
Gonads		y	y	y	y	
Brain					y	
Adrenals		y	y	y	y	
Gross necropsy—all animals	NS	y	y	y	y	NS
Histopathology evaluation						
All tissues; high dose/control	NS	y	y	y	y	NS
Mid and low dose	NS	NS	NS	NS	y	NS
Gross lesions					y	
Target organs	NS	y	y	y	y	NS
Lungs	NS	y	NS	y	y	NS

A, urinalysis is not recommended on a routine basis, but only when there is an indication based on expected observed toxicity. NS, not specified; y, topic must be evaluated.

application before approval for marketing by the FDA. The approval process is lengthy. For the investigational new drug phase, industry is required to file with the FDA certain toxicity testing data at a stage when investigation of the potential therapeutic usefulness of a chemical in limited numbers of humans or animals is desired. As the efficacy of the drug in the treatment of a particular disease is established through extensive clinical trials, these data together with additional animal toxicity testing data are filed as part of a new drug application (NDA) or new animal drug applications for review of safety and efficacy by the FDA. Ultimately, as a con-sequence of the FDA review, the NDA is either approved or deficiencies in the data cited.

Regulations for investigational new drug (IND) applications were revised in 1987 regarding submission and review as well as defining the availability of such drugs for treatment and sale. These new regulations improved the methods of IND application and the responsiveness of the application evaluation. Patient safety evaluations by the FDA during clinical trials were also upgraded as a result of the 1987 changes (36,37). This was accomplished by limiting the FDA review of phase I studies to safety issues for human subjects.

TABLE 2. *Comparison of selected protocol provisions for subchronic oral toxicity studies in rats*

	EPA TSCA FIFRA	OECD	FDA	UK	Japan	Japan
Age at start of study (wks)	<6	<8	<6	<6	Adult	<8
Minimum duration of study (days)	90	90	90	90	30–90	
No. of Tx groups (no less than)	3	3	3	3	3	3
Control	y	y	y	y	y	y
Vehicle control (if needed)	y	y	y	y	y	y
Route of administration (recommended or accepted)						
Diet	y	y	y	y	y	y
Gavage	y	y	y	y	y	y
Capsule	y	y	y	y	y	y
Water	y	y	y	y	y	y
No. of rats/sex/group (not including interim sac. or clinical lab. testing #'s)	10	10	20	10	10	10
Record body wt. weekly	y	y	y	y	y	y
Record feed consumption wkly.	y	y	y	y	y	y
Daily observations						
Minimum interval between observations	12	12	12	12	24	24
Acceptable mortality—High D. Grp.	<10%	NS	NS	NS	NS	NS
Ophthalmology						
Pretest	y	y	y	y	n	y
At termination	y	y	y	y	y	y
All high dose and control (lower doses only if findings at high dose)	y	y	y	y	y	y
Hematology and clinical chemistry (time periods for data collection)						
Pretest	y	n	n	n	n	n
Monthly	y	n	n	n	n	n
Dosing midpoint	y	n	n	n	n	n
Terminal	y	y	y	y	y	y
Min. no. animals bled (no./sex/group)	NS	NS	10	NS	NS	NS
Urinalysis						
Pretest	n	n	n	n	n	y
Intermediate time	n	n	n	n	n	n
Terminal	n	n	n	n	y	y
Organ weights recd. at termination						
Liver	y	y	y	y	y	y
Kidneys	y	y	y	y	y	y
Heart	n	n	n	n	y	n
Gonads	y	y	y	y	y	y
Brain	y	n	n	n	y	y
Adrenals	n	y	y	y	y	y
Gross necropsy—all animals	y	n	n	y	y	y
All tissues; high dose/control	y	y	y	y	y	y
Mid and low dose						y
Liver	y	n	y	y	y	y
Kidney	y	n	y	y	y	y
Heart	y	n	y	y	y	n
Gross lesions	y	y	y	n	y	y
Target organs	y	y	NS	y	y	y
Lungs	y	y	NS	y	y	y

NS, not specified; y, topic must be evaluated; n, topic need not be evaluated.

The 1987 revisions to the Code of Federal Regulations (CFR) 312.21 (27) and 312.22 (28) provide a mechanism by which phase I study protocols may be modified by investigators without notifying the FDA beforehand. The adjustments to the study design must be based on information acquired during the conduct of the study. Another important aspect of the 1987 changes includes necessary feedback to define the degree of toxicology and chemistry information for the IND submission based on the anticipated chemical investigation study design.

Other important regulations regarding IND applications and the associated research include CFR 312.2 (26) in which it is stated that approved drug studies need not meet IND requirements if the studies are not intended for label changes or promotion of the drug.

Section 312.23 of the CFR (29) includes a format for IND submissions and requires a description of the suggested studies for the year and an indication of the number of human subjects needed. Protocols for each clinical trial must be included for those studies to be initiated first. Several other regulations associated with FDA IND applications were also approved as final rule in 1987. These were primarily associated with administration aspects of IND applications.

NDA and new antibiotic applications were addressed by 13 finalized guidelines by the FDA Center for Drugs and Biologics. Eight guidelines address the format of the applications and five are directed toward defining the supporting data necessary for controls, chemistry, and manufacturing. Packaging, stability, analytical data for methods validation, and manufacturing data requirements are specifically addressed. The summary of a New Drug and Antibiotic Application must address benefit/risk relationships, clinical data, nonclinical pharmacology and toxicology, human pharmacokinetics, and bioavailability and microbiology. It must also contain information on pharmacologic class, scientific rational and clinical benefits, as well as chemistry, controls, and manufacturing results (30).

The FDA has issued regulations governing good laboratory practices (GLP) (25) in the conduct of animal toxicity studies. The Pharmaceutical Manufacturers Association (PMA) felt there should be guidelines for animal toxicity testing so that some standardization of basic methodology might be achieved. Through the assistance of its member companies, these guidelines have now been finalized.

Under the FDC act, industry must also show that a chemical intended for direct addition to food, such as a preservative or flavoring agent, or a new polymer having indirect contact with food such as in a packaging material or can-coating material, is safe for its intended use. Results of animal toxicity tests are submitted to the FDA for review as part of a Food Additive Petition. If the data demonstrate the safety of the chemical to the FDA, a regulation is published allowing the chemical to be used for a particular purpose in food or in contact with food. In 1982, the FDA published *Toxicological Principles for the Safety Assessment of Direct Food Additives and Color Additives Used in Food* (46). This "Red Book" delineates the nature of evaluations that are necessary to determine food additive safety. This document provides a basic scheme for making scientifically sound decisions for the development of safety information. The FDA indicates that this new approach is built around a more cost-effective and flexible framework. The guidelines include a priority setting system that will increase the efficacy and timeliness of food additive evaluation. Importantly, food additive evaluations must now meet the guidelines of the Red Book and the FDA's GLP regulations.

The safety of carcinogenic studies in food-producing animals has now been addressed by a *sensitivity-of-method* approach (35) which was first proposed in 1973. These general principles are codified (31–34). Four steps are used to evaluate potentially carcinogenic residues. The first step is to ascertain if animal cancer bioassays are needed. The second phase is to conduct the cancer bioassays and determine the *de minimus* dose. The third stage is to develop and utilize an analytic method for monitoring the permitted residue concentrations in food-producing animals, and the last step is to conduct an elimination study with the chemical.

At the present time, there are no requirements for the FDA to review cosmetic formulations for safety prior to marketing. While the FDCA only requires that the cosmetics be free of any "poisonous and deleterious" substances, responsible suppliers of ingredients for use in cosmetics and manufacturers of the final product have been conducting relevant toxicity studies.

Medical Device Amendments of 1976

Prior to 1976, the safety and efficacy of new medical devices was reviewed by the Division of Medical and Surgical Adjuncts of the FDA Bureau of Drugs. With congressional passage of the Medical Device Amendment, review of medical devices became the responsibility of the newly created Bureau of Medical Devices. This bureau has classified existing medical devices into three categories and has been establishing standards for certain devices.

Class I devices under FDCA Section 513 are devices that have the lowest potential to be harmful. Manufacturers must comply with GLP regulations and must register the device with the FDA. Specified performance standards must be met for Class II devices prior to marketing. The construction and composition must meet specifications in order to operate in a safe and efficacious manner. Class III devices require premarket approval by the FDA.

Three use categories for medical devices are defined by the American Society of Testing and Materials (ASTM) Standard Practice F748-82. The categories are external use, implanted communicating devices, and externally communicating devices. The total series of recommended tests include cytotoxicity, systemic acute toxicity (mouse) (43), intracutaneous irritation (rabbit) (42), skin irritation (rabbit) (40), sensitization (rabbit) (41), hemolysis (44), short-term implantation (45), and long-term implantation (38,39).

Federal Insecticide, Fungicide and Rodenticide Act

FIFRA, which was passed by Congress in 1947 and amended in 1957, 1961, and 1964 (6), was administered initially by the Department of Agriculture and is now administered by the EPA. This act requires that extensive toxicity testing be conducted in mammalian, avian, and aquatic species to support the safety of a pesticide. Toxicity data submitted in an application for registration of a pesticide are reviewed by staff toxicologists in the Office of Pesticide Programs of the EPA. This agency proposed toxicity testing guidelines in 1975 (9), and revised and reproposed these guidelines again in 1978 (8), for the conduct of acute to chronic toxicity tests which are used to support pesticide registrations. In 1980 GLP regulations were proposed for pesticides and were published as a final rule in 1983 (11). The final rule which took effect in 1984 was almost completely harmonized with the FDA GLP regulations.

Also in 1984 regulations (10) were finalized. Specific topics of requirements included product chemistry, residue chemistry, environmental fate, toxicology, re-entry protection, spray drift, wildlife and aquatic organisms, plant protection, nontarget insects, product performance, biochemical pesticides, and microbial pesticides. A matrix of necessary tests and data are required for each of nine general pesticide use patterns and 14 pesticide use site groups.

In the area of toxicology, for example, 14 studies are required and five are conditionally required if the pesticide use group is assumed to be a terrestrial food crop. If the pesticide use group is assumed to be for aquatic nonfood use, then only seven toxicology studies are required and 11 are only conditionally required. This approach is applied for the appropriate combination of general use and use site groups and the required tests must be completed in each area of data requirement.

Toxic Substances Control Act

This act (16), which went into effect on January 1, 1977, and which is administered by the Office of Pesticides and Toxic Substances of the EPA, is a complex and far reaching law that affects industrial chemicals existing in commerce in the United States as well as new chemicals. TSCA defines *new* chemicals as those chemicals that do not appear on the TSCA initial inventory list or any of its supplements. One of the first requirements of TSCA was that an inventory be established of chemicals that were active in commerce in the years 1977–1979.

The EPA established an Interagency Testing Committee (ITC) to identify chemical classes or specific chemicals for evaluation under Section 4 of TSCA as existing chemicals. The ITC/EPA can choose to evaluate on either of two bases. If a chemical may be associated with untoward human health effects or adverse impact on the environment, or if the uses of a chemical may result in considerable exposure to humans or the environment, then the EPA may require that it be tested. Over 83 chemicals or classes of chemicals have been designated by the first 17 ITC reports to the EPA through the end of 1986.

Manufacturers or importers of industrial chemicals that are considered new under the TSCA definition are required to notify the EPA at least 90 days before the manufacture or import of a new chemical. The act requires that certain information regarding the new chemical be submitted in a premanufacture notification (PMN) to the EPA for review. While the act does not require that toxicity testing be conducted on a new chemical prior to manufacture, it does require that all existing health and safety data be submitted which demonstrate that the new chemical does not present an unreasonable risk to health or the environment.

The EPA may, for good cause, extend their normal review period of 90–180 days. If the EPA determines in their review that the new chemical does present an unreasonable risk, one of several actions it may take is to require that the chemicals be tested for specific toxic effects. The EPA, under Section 4 of TSCA, may also issue a testing rule which would require that a specified chemical or chemical mixture be tested for certain toxic effects. The EPA has finalized test standards for the conduct of toxicity studies on chemicals or chemical mixtures for which testing will be required under TSCA. These standards are similar to the guidelines proposed by the EPA for registering pesticides. GLP standards for toxic substances control were published as a final rule in late 1983 and became effective in mid-1984 (17).

Transportation Act

Regulations promulgated by the Department of Transportation (DOT) require that materials shipped in interstate commerce be labeled and containered in a manner consistent with the degree of hazard they present. The DOT requires that acute toxicity studies be performed on substances not already classified as a Class A poison ("extremely dangerous poison") or a Class C poison ("tear gas or irritating substances"), but which might be classified as a Class B poison. Substances require a Class B poison label in transportation if they are known to be so toxic to humans that they are hazardous to health or are presumed to be toxic to humans. A substance is also considered to be a Class B poison if, on oral administration, a single dose of 50 mg or less per kilogram of body weight produces death in 48 hr in half or more than half of a group of 10 or more white laboratory rats; or, if when applied topically at a dose of 200 mg or less for 4 hr, it produces death within 48 hr in half or more than half of a group of 10 or more rabbits.

A substance may also be required to carry a Class B poison label if it warrants testing by inhalation and meets the criteria of toxicity set forth by the DOT for this route. In other words, a Class B poison label is required if the substance meets criteria of toxicity when tested by administration orally, dermally, or through inhalation. If a substance does meet these criteria through testing, but the physical characteristics or the probable hazards to humans, as shown by experience, indicate that the substance will not cause serious illness or death, labeling as a Class B poison is not required.

The Coast Guard

Prior to importing a chemical into the United States, the Coast Guard requires a set of acute mammalian toxicity data of the chemical. This acute toxicity profile should minimally include the following: acute oral toxicity, acute dermal toxicity, and skin and eye irritation studies.

Consumer Product Safety Act

Prior to the passage of the Consumer Product Safety Act (CPSA;1) in 1973, the classification and testing for acute toxicity of household products was conducted under regulations promulgated by the FDA, which administered the Federal Hazardous Substances Act (FHSA). The function of administering FHSA and thus protecting the consumer from hazardous household substances now resides with the Consumer Product Safety Commission under responsibilities of the CPSA. If results obtained in acute oral or dermal toxicity tests, following methods outlined in the CFR for hazardous substances, meet prescribed criteria of toxicity, labeling and packaging as prescribed in the regulations must be used.

Occupational Safety and Health Act

This law (48), administered by the Occupational Safety and Health Administration (OSHA) of the Department of Labor, is designed to assure that safe and healthful conditions exist in the workplace. No requirements exist in this law for manufacturers to test substances for toxicity prior to their use in the workplace. The impact of the TSCA has an overlapping effect, in that occupational exposure to new chemicals is considered in premanufacture notices. Specific test requirements under TSCA affect new or existing chemicals which are manufactured or processed in the United States.

OSHA has been in the process of issuing exposure standards for commonly used chemicals. These standards are issued after consideration of the recommendations made by the National Institute of Occupational Safety and Health (NIOSH) of the Department of Health, Education and Welfare (DHEW). It is of interest that OSHA, in an effort to expedite the issuance of standards relative to potential carcinogens in the workplace, prepared a generic approach. This generic standard was the subject of considerable controversy from the time it was proposed in 1977 and adopted in 1980. This detailed description of methods for interpreting both animal and human data relative to cancer risk was delayed by the executive branch.

Resource Conservation and Recovery Act

Decades of improper disposal of industrial and research wastes, particularly from the chemical and nuclear industries, triggered public demand for regulating such waste disposal. The Resource Conservation and Recovery Act of 1976 (12) (RCRA) authorized the EPA to institute a national program to control hazardous waste. In 1980, the EPA put forward the final version of the RCRA regulations. (13–15).

The main purpose of these regulations is to control the generation, storage, treatment, transportation, disposal, record-keeping, and reporting of hazardous waste. RCRA places the primary responsibility of identifying and managing hazardous waste on the waste generators. Other persons or institutions involved in waste disposal and management also have an obligation to know if the waste is hazardous.

RCRA defines a hazardous waste as "solid, liquid, semisolid or gaseous waste that may cause increased mortality or serious illness, or may cause substantial hazard to the health or the environment when improperly managed." The EPA has listed specifically by names those wastes it considers hazardous. In addition, any waste material that exhibits any of the following criteria, set by the EPA, is considered as hazardous:

1. Ignitability: posing a fire hazard during management.
2. Corrosivity: ability to corrode standard containers, or to dissolve toxic components of other wastes.
3. Reactivity: Tendency to explode under normal management conditions, to react violently when mixed with water, or to generate toxic gases.
4. EP toxicity (as determined by a specific extraction procedure): Presence of certain toxic materials at levels greater than those specified in the regulation.

The fourth criterion permits the EPA to list waste material that contain one or more substances known to cause toxicity in humans or animals; however, the EPA may also consider other factors prior to determining if the waste is hazardous. The degree of toxicity, concentration, migration to the environment, persistence or degradation in the environment, bioaccumulation in the ecosystem, types of improper management, quantities of waste, past human and environmental damage records, and other factors are all taken into consideration.

Certain solid wastes are exempted under the regulations. These include wastes already under the regulations of the Atomic Energy Act and the Clean Water Act (e.g., domestic waste). Small waste generators which accumulate 1000 kg or less per month of an identifiable hazardous waste are exempted from the initial waste controls. These generators must be able to prove through record-keeping that they are indeed generating small quantities of hazardous waste.

If a waste generator believes that the waste should be exempted from the regulation even when it is listed, he should be able to prove to the EPA that the waste does not meet the criteria which caused the EPA to list the specific waste as hazardous. This can be achieved either by conducting one's own studies or by referring to test data that demonstrate that the criteria are not met.

LAWS AND REGULATIONS THAT GOVERN TOXICITY EVALUATIONS IN OTHER COUNTRIES AND INTERNATIONAL TOXICITY TESTING GUIDELINES

The United States has not been alone in developing laws to protect man and his environment from possibly dangerous effects of new industrial chemicals in the marketplace. Japan adopted regulations similar to an early version of what has become the TSCA in the United States. The Japanese Chemical Substances Controls Law was enacted in 1973 but was amended in 1987. France has a system established now for premarket notification of new chemicals.

On June 19, 1979, the Council of Ministers of the European Economic Community (EEC) adopted the Sixth Amendment to the Council Directive 67/548/EEC (2) of June 17, 1967. This Council Directive concerns laws, regulations, and administrative procedures which relate to the classification, packaging, and labeling of dangerous substances. The Sixth Amendment is an effort to protect man and his environment from potential risks which might arise through the marketing of new chemicals. It requires that a new chemical be subjected to a *base set* of tests to define its physical and chemical properties, mammalian toxicity, and ecotoxicologic effects. The Sixth Amendment requires a manufacturer or importer to furnish the appropriate authorities in his EEC member state with a notification containing, in part, the results of these tests on the new chemical. Such notification will be filed 45 days before marketing in the member state in which it is to occur.

The Sixth Amendment is the EEC counterpart of the U.S. TSCA. There are, however, some differences, not the least of which is in the approach to toxicity testing. The EEC requires premarket notification of a new chemical whereas TSCA demands that the notification, in the case of a domestic manufacturer, be given to the EPA at least 90 days prior to manufacture. Even test marketing of a new chemical in the United States requires that prior notification be given to the EPA. The base set consists of the following studies for acute toxicity: acute oral LD_{50}, acute dermal LD_{50}, acute inhalation LC_{50} (if applicable), skin and eye irritation, and dermal sensitization.

The EEC has also provided guidance on the evaluation of safety and efficacy of drugs. The EEC has now adopted guidance notes for efficacy testing of *pharmacokinetics in man* and *bioavailability of drugs for long term use,* as well as a number of more specific activity groups including cardiac glycosides, oral contraceptives, topical corticosteroids, nonsteroidal antiinflammatories, antimicrobials, anticonvulsants, antianginals, and chronic peripheral arterial disease agents. By the end of 1987, safety guidance notes were adopted for single-dose and repeated-dose toxicity, pharmacokinetic metabolism, mutagenic potential, carcinogenic potential, and reproduction studies (5).

With many countries establishing their own regulations for safety assessment, it now becomes possible that manufacturers would have to perform several tests to satisfy the same objective in several different countries. In an attempt to avoid unnecessary duplication of work, the Organization for Economic Cooperation and Development (OECD), a group comprised of experts from a number of nations throughout the world, has produced a set of testing guidelines that are sufficiently well defined to enable a test to be carried out in a similar manner in different countries and to produce results that would be fully acceptable to various regulatory bodies. The OECD package includes guidelines on acute oral, dermal, and inhalation studies; eye and skin irritation and skin sensitization studies; subchronic oral, dermal, and inhalation studies; and teratogenicity, carcinogenicity, and chronic and combined chronic/carcinogenicity studies. Some comparisons among FIFRA, TSCA, HSC, FDA, Japanese, and OECD guidelines can be seen in Tables 1 and 2.

Notification Schemes Under Different Guidelines

Health and Safety Commission of the United Kingdom

As a result of recommendations made by a committee of inquiry chaired by Lord Robens and cited in its report "Safety and Health at Work," a comprehensive notification system for new chemicals or other potentially harmful substances introduced for industrial or commercial use is currently employed in the United Kingdom. There is already in existence a competent body, the Health and Safety Commission (HSC), for the receipt of such notifications. The HSC is advised by the Advisory Committee on Toxic Substances (ACTS) on "methods of controlling the health hazards to persons at work and the related hazards to the public which may arise from toxic substances . . . with particular references to those requiring notification under regulations."

In 1977, a discussion document of the HSC presented proposals for a notification scheme covering new chemicals introduced into the United Kingdom by manufacture on importation in quantities greater than 1 ton per year. Under this scheme, the manufacturer or importer will be required to furnish sufficient toxicologic and other information on the new chemical from which the likely hazards and conditions of safe use may be inferred. The notification scheme, administered by the Health and Safety Executive of the HSC, is intended principally to assess the potential of a chemical to cause harm to people in the workplace and also to people outside the workplace who might also be exposed from the work activity. This notification scheme does not include the requirements for data relating to environmental effects or waste disposal. However, some of the tests included in the

scheme may provide basic information for these purposes. Excluded from the notification scheme are those chemical substances already in use before the introduction of the scheme, those chemicals only available in small quantities, and chemical mixtures where a new chemical is not present. Notification through this scheme is intended to assist substances likely to present the more serious risks to safety and health and consequently to more adequately control them.

Included in the basic information to be provided by the notifier are details as to the new substances' chemical and physical properties, biologic properties, recommendations for safe handling, proposed date of introduction to Great Britain, and scale of manufacture or importation. Among the information requested for biologic properties are acute effects of ingestion, inhalation, or absorption through the skin and the effects of the new substance with respect to skin irritation or sensitization.

With regard to acute toxicity, LD_{50} must be provided, but it is not so important that this be measured with precise accuracy. However, information is needed on whether the substance is of high, moderate, or low toxicity with careful observations having been made of general mode of toxic action. Rats are suggested as the animals of choice with groups of 6 animals being used for each dose and observations being continued for 14 days. This would apply for studies of oral ingestion, dermal application, or inhalation exposure. Optionally, simultaneous assessment of dermal toxicity and skin irritation may be made. Rabbits may be used in studies of skin irritation. If the notifier also conducts studies of 30 days or longer on the substance, hematologic or histopathology studies need not be conducted in an acute toxicity determination.

Japanese Chemical Substances Control Law

The 1973 implementation of this law was predicated on the determination of biodegradability, bioaccumulation, and toxic potential of specific chemicals. Two categories were used to classify chemicals. These were safe or specified. Specified chemicals were those that were identified as positive in all three evaluations above. Such chemicals required approval for manufacturing, use, or export. Safe chemicals possessed fewer than three positive responses to the determinations above and were not regulated.

In the amended law, new chemicals that will be manufactured or imported must adhere to chemical notification procedures if amounts are to exceed 1 ton per year. New chemicals in amounts of less than 1 ton must be verified for quantity but test data need not be submitted. Efforts have been made in the amended legislation to follow OECD testing guidelines where possible. The test data for notification of a new chemical must include a biodegradation test. If the chemical is found to be persistent in the environment, then it must also undergo evaluations of mutagenic activity, bioaccumulation, and subacute oral toxicity in the rat. Four classifications for chemical substances are possible and each chemical is assigned a class based on data from the above tests. These are *Class I, Class II, Designated,* and *Safe* (9).

Class I chemical substances demonstrate a lack of biodegradability, bioaccumulate, and are harmful to human health on chronic exposure. Importation of Class I substances or a product containing a Class I substance can be prohibited by MITI (Ministry of International Trade and Industry) Cabinet Order. Approval of manufacture or import must be given by MITI and must include specified allowable uses.

Substances in Class II as well as Class I are assigned by official Cabinet Order. Class II materials are also persistent in the environment and would be harmful to human health on chronic exposure. Manufacture and import figures must be provided before each year of operation and past estimates must be updated.

Designated chemical substances are also persistent in the environment and may be harmful to human health but are assessed to require less control than Class I or Class II materials. Reporting of chemical manufacture and importation is required.

Safe chemicals are not restricted and are defined as those chemicals not placed in any of the other three categories.

Toxic Substance Control Act

The main purpose of this act, administered by the EPA, is to require manufacturers to acquire adequate toxicity data on a chemical prior to its manufacture and marketing. Manufacture or importation of a new chemical other than in limited quantities for research and development purposes is prohibited by the act. At the time that the developer of a new chemical might foresee some commercial application of a new chemical and wishes to produce or import it in commercial quantities, one must file a PMN. The information required as part of a PMN should be submitted to the extent that it is known or reasonably ascertainable. Obviously, in the early development of a chemical, data in all categories will not be fully developed. In such instances, the submitter should state that such information is not known and not reasonably ascertainable.

Under this act, a manufacturer is required to have the following information submitted as part of a PMN package to EPA:

1. Common or trade name, chemical identity, and molecular structure;
2. Categories or proposed categories of use;
3. Total amount of substance to be manufactured or processed;
4. Amount to be manufactured for each category of use;
5. Description of the by-products resulting from the manufacturing, processing, use, or disposal of the product;
6. Number of persons exposed during manufacture and the duration of such exposure;
7. Manner or method of disposal (any change in the manner or method of disposal must be reported later);
8. Any test data, in the possession or control of the notifier, which "are related to the effect of any manufacture, processing, distribution in commerce, use or disposal of such substance or any article containing such substance, or, any combination of such activities on health or the environment";
9. Description of any other data covering the environmental and health effects of the chemical.

While the act does not require that toxicity testing be conducted on a new chemical prior to manufacture or importation, it does require that all existing health and safety data which demonstrate that the new chemical does not present an unreasonable risk to health or the environment be submitted to the EPA. The PMN procedure under TSCA is, in effect, a de facto registration system for new chemicals. While there is no requirement under TSCA to generate toxicity data on a new chemical, as a practical matter, it seems difficult to expect the EPA to assess the potential risk of a new chemical with no toxicity data available for review.

On May 9, 1979, the EPA proposed standards for the development of data on chronic health effects of chemicals which are the subject of a test rule under Section 4 of TSCA. Section 4 of TSCA gives the EPA the administrative authority to order that a chemical be tested in whatever parameters the EPA designates to determine if an unreasonable hazard exists to human health or the environment. The EPA later issued standards for the conduct of acute oral, dermal, and inhalation, and dermal sensitization as well as subchronic (up to 90 days) oral, dermal, and inhalation studies. These proposed standards, which follow very closely the August 22, 1978, proposed guidelines for registering pesticides under FIFRA in the United States, were very rigid protocols for the conduct of these various types of toxicity tests.

The EPA codified existing guidelines in the CFR Title 40, Parts 796–798 (18). Proposed test rules will include the references to appropriate test guidelines thus making them directly applicable only to those chemicals addressed in a given test rule.

Chemical selection rationale by the ITC was revised to include a fourth category of *intent-to-designate* (20). A single-phase method identifying tester responsibility, required tests, submission schedules, and representation substances was adopted for test rules in 1985 (21). This modified an earlier 1984 decision to utilize a two-phased approach (19). The short-lived two-phased test rule procedure was chosen in place of the proposed generic test standards of 1980. A continuing effort to harmonize testing guidelines is being made by the EPA. In 1985, the EPA codified 14 additional OECD testing guidelines as CFR Title 40, Part 796. These guidelines are specific to the chemical fate area (23).

In more practical terms, little or no toxicity information usually exists on a truly new chemical. While it is true that some estimate as to its general toxicity might be approximated through categorization or the use of structure–activity relationships, a definition of a chemical's toxicity must await actual testing in animals.

A PMN is submitted prior to any manufacture or importation of the new chemical. Following receipt, the EPA has 90 days to review the notification. The agency may, however, extend the review period another 90 days for good cause. If the 90 days passes, or 180 days if the review is extended, without further EPA actions, the notifier may then begin to manufacture or import the new chemical. Once such manufacture or importation begins, the PMN submitter informs the EPA of such activity. The EPA, in turn, places the chemical on the TSCA inventory. If no patent problems exist, any other firm may manufacture or import that same chemical once it has been placed on the TSCA inventory.

During the EPA's review of a PMN, the agency may take

one of two actions. It may, on finding that the data submitted in a PMN are insufficient to make a reasoned evaluation of the health or environmental effects of the subject chemical, issue a proposed order to prohibit or limit its manufacture, processing, distribution in commerce, and use or disposal. Such action would be under Section 5(e) of TSCA regulations pending development of information. The other action the EPA could take would be under Section 5(f) of TSCA–Protection Against Unreasonable Risks. The EPA may find, on review of the data in a PMN, that there is a reasonable basis to conclude that the manufacture, processing, distribution in commerce, and use or disposal of the chemical (or combination of these activities) presents or will present an unreasonable risk to human health or the environment. In such a case, the EPA may issue a proposed rule to prohibit or limit the amount of the chemical which may be manufactured, processed, used, or distributed in commerce. The EPA may also seek an injunction in a United States District Court to prohibit or limit the PMN notifier's proposed activity with the new chemical.

The EPA may not place a PMN under continuing review. They must take a specific action under Sections 5(e) or 5(f) as noted. If the Agency takes no action, the statutory time limits for review will run out and the notifier is free to manufacture or import the new chemical. If the EPA does propose orders under Sections 5(e) or 5(f) against a chemical that is the subject of a PMN, the submitter of the notification may file specific objections to such actions. The EPA may then seek an injunction or restraining order against the chemical through the United States District Court. The PMN submitter will then need to petition the Court to remove the injunction or restraining order.

The EPA has taken a fairly practical approach to data deficiencies in a PMN or suspicion of hazards associated with a PMN chemical. In the case of deficiencies of information, they have stopped the clock on the review period until adequate information, including toxicity testing data, has been furnished to the agency. In at least one instance, the agency has requested further long-term testing based on the similarity of the new chemical to others reported in the literature as having adverse findings.

The Sixth Amendment to Council Directive 67/548/EEC

The EEC, or Common Market, has 10 member countries: the Netherlands, Belgium, France, Luxembourg, Denmark, the United Kingdom, Ireland, Italy, Greece, and the Federal Republic of Germany. For several years, the Council of the EEC has been working on a system to identify and control toxic chemicals. The EEC Council Directive of September 18, 1979 (3), amended for the sixth time Directive 67/548/EEC on the laws, regulations, and administrative provisions relating to the classification, packaging, and labeling of dangerous substances. This amendment is commonly referred to as the Sixth Amendment. The Council of the EEC felt that, while Directive 67/548/EEC was adequate for the protection of workers through its system for classification, packaging, and labeling of dangerous substances, something more extensive was needed to control the effects of dangerous substances on man and the environment.

The adoption of the Sixth Amendment by the EEC required that an inventory of substances on the EEC or Common Market be compiled by September of 1981. The initial case inventory (ECOIN) was published in 1981 and contained about 35,000 substances. The European Inventory of Existing Chemicals (EINECS) represents all substances entered into the EEC commercial market from 1971 to 1981. New substances, defined as not appearing on this inventory, will require notification by their manufacturer or importer at least 45 days prior to marketing. In contrast to the requirements of TSCA, which requires notification prior to manufacture, a new chemical may be introduced onto the market in an EEC member country in quantities of less than 1 metric ton per year if the manufacturer notifies the authorities of his respective member country as to the identity, labeling, and quantity of the chemical to be marketed per year. No base-set data need be furnished.

If a manufacturer or importer wishes initially to market his new substance in yearly quantities of more than 1 metric ton but less than 10 metric tons or a total marketing of less than 50 metric tons, he must submit a technical dossier containing base-set information on the new chemical to the authorities in one of the 10 member countries at least 45 days prior to marketing. If a chemical has already been marketed in quantities of less than 1 metric ton per year, the dossier containing the base-set information must be presented at least 45 days before the marketing volume exceeds the 1 metric ton per year level.

The purpose of the technical dossier under the Sixth Amendment is to supply information necessary for the authorities in a member country to evaluate the foreseeable immediate or delayed risks for man and the environment. One distinguishing concept of the Sixth Amendment is that toxicity and ecotoxicity studies required are related to increments of marketing volumes per year or when total marketing reaches certain volumes.

The base-set methods were published under the Sixth Amendment in 1984 as Annex V (4). The three major parts of Annex V include:

Part A: Methods for the determination of physicochemical properties;
Part B: Methods for the determination of toxicity;
Part C: Methods for the determination of ecotoxicity.

The base-set is associated with a marketing volume of 1–10 metric tons per year. The technical dossier must contain, in addition to such information as identity, composition, purity, impurities, spectral data, proposed use, projected production volumes, methods and precautions for handling, storage, and transport, physicochemical properties, and possibilities for rendering the substance harmless, the following toxicologic studies as needed:

1. Acute oral LD_{50} (mg/kg), including the effects observed;
2. Acute inhalation LC_{50} (ppm), including the effects observed; (administration of the test substance must be for at least 4 hr);
3. Acute percutaneous LD_{50} (mg/kg), including the effects observed.

The Sixth Amendment requires that substances other than gases must be administered via the oral route and at least one other route, which will depend on the intended use and physical properties. In the acute toxicity studies, both male and female animals should be used. An observation period of at least 14 days is required. The rat is the preferred species for both the oral and inhalation studies unless there are overriding reasons why another test system must be chosen. Skin and eye irritation studies are required, preferably using the rabbit. A dermal sensitization study using a recognized method in the guinea pig is also needed.

A subchronic study of at least 28 days duration is required. The rat is again the preferred species for oral and inhalation studies. A 5- or 7-day per week schedule of administration may be used. Choosing the route of administration should be based on the intended use of the new chemical, its physical and chemical properties, and its acute toxicity. A no effect dose level should be established.

The new chemical's potential mutagenicity should be examined in two tests: a bacteriologic test, with and without metabolic activation, and a nonbacteriologic test. Ecotoxicologic studies, including an acute LC_{50} (ppm) for one or more species of fish and an acute LC_{50} (ppm) for daphnia should be conducted. With respect to degradation studies, determination of the biochemical oxygen demand and the ratio of biochemical oxygen demand/chemical oxygen demand are considered as a minimum requirement.

Level 1 is reached in the Sixth Amendment when marketing of the new chemical reaches 10 metric tons per year or a total of 50 tons. At this point, the authorities in the EEC member country may require further toxicologic studies after the current knowledge of the new substance is considered as well as its known or planned uses and the result obtained in the base-set studies. At this level, in addition to possibly requiring a one generation fertility study and/or a teratology study and/or additional mutagenesis studies, the authorities may require additional subchronic studies and/or a chronic study, which may include special studies, depending on the result obtained in the 28-day subchronic study submitted as part of the technical dossier of base-set information. Any relevant information obtained from other sources may also be considered by the authorities in requesting these additional studies. Such additional studies may include exposure to the new chemical for 90 days or longer or more detailed examination for certain effects. Even a chronic study could be requested at this point.

Examples given in the Sixth Amendment of effects that would indicate the need for additional subchronic studies include: serious or irreversible lesions, a very low or lack of establishment of a no effect level, or a clear structural relationship of the new chemical to others that have been shown to be dangerous. Additional ecotoxicology studies may also be required at level 1.

If the authorities have not required the above testing in the early stages of marketing, they will request that it be done when obligatory notification from the manufacturer is received that the quantity being marketed has reached a level of 100 metric tons per year or a total quantity of 500 metric tons. The manufacturer is also required to notify the authorities when the marketing volume reaches 1000 metric tons per year or a total of 5000 metric tons. This is level 2 in the Sixth Amendment incremental testing scheme.

The authorities, on receipt of such notification, are obligated to design a testing program that would cover chronic toxicity, carcinogenicity, fertility (only if an effect on fertility had been established in level 1 testing), teratology (nonrodent species), and additional toxicokinetic studies, as well as acute and subchronic studies in a second species if results of level 1 studies indicate a need. Results obtained in pharmacokinetic and biotransformation studies may also initiate a requirement to do these studies. Additional ecotoxicology studies may also be required. These are noted in Annex VIII of the Sixth Amendment.

Requirements of Acute Oral and Subchronic Oral Toxicity Testing Under Several United States and European Guidelines

Tables 1 and 2 present the requirements for conducting acute oral toxicity tests and subchronic oral toxicity tests, respectively, as set forth in the guidelines of the OECD for chemicals introduced into commerce by the member nations; the Notification Scheme for New Substances of the HSC of the United Kingdom; the EPA for registering pesticides in the United States under FIFRA and under the United States TSCA; the FDA Safety Assessment of Direct Food and Color Additives (Red Book); and the Japanese Drug and Agrichemical Requirements and Guidelines.

REFERENCES[a]

1. CPSC (1972): Consumer Product Safety Act, 15 U.S.C., 2051 et seq.
2. EEC (1967): Council Directive 67/548/EEC, Official Journal of the E.C.
3. EEC (1979): Council Directive 79/831/EEC, Official Journal of the E.C.
4. EEC (1984): Council Directive 84/449/EEC, Official Journal of the E.C.
5. EEC (1987): Council Recommendation 87/176/EEC, Official Journal of the E.C.
6. EPA (1976): Federal Insecticide, Fungicide and Rodenticide Act, 7 U.S.C., 135 et seq.
7. EPA (1978): FR, 48, Proposed Guidelines for Registering Pesticides in U.S. Hazard Evaluation: Human and Domestic Animals.
8. EPA FIFRA (1978): 40 CFR 153.
9. EPA FIFRA (1975): 40 CFR 162.
10. EPA FIFRA (1985): 40 CFR 158, Data Requirements for Proposed Pesticide Registration.
11. EPA FIFRA (1983): FR, 48, 53946, Pesticide Programs: Good Laboratory Practice Standards.
12. EPA Resource Conservation and Recovery Act (1976): 42 U.S.C.A., 6901.
13. EPA RCRA (1980): FR, 45, 12722.
14. EPA RCRA (1980): FR, 45, 33063.
15. EPA RCRA (1980): FR, 45, 34560.
16. EPA (1976): Toxic Substances Control Act, 15 U.S.C., 2601.
17. EPA TSCA (1983): FR, 48, 53922, Toxic Substances Control: Good Laboratory Practice Standards.
18. EPA TSCA (1985): 40 CFR 796–798.
19. EPA TSCA (1984): FR, 49, 39774.
20. EPA TSCA (1985): FR, 50, 13418.
21. EPA TSCA (1985): FR, 50, 20652.
22. EPA TSCA (1985): FR, 50, 39252.
23. EPA TSCA (1985): FR, 50, 39472.
24. FDA (1938): 21 U.S.C., 321 et seq. Federal Food, Drug and Cosmetic Act.
25. FDA (1983): 21 C.F.R. 58. Good Laboratory Practices for Nonclinical Laboratory Studies.

26. FDA (1987): 21 CFR 312.2.
27. FDA (1987): 21 CFR 312.21.
28. FDA (1987): 21 CFR 312.22.
29. FDA (1987): 21 CFR 312.23.
30. FDA (1987): 21 CFR 314.50.
31. FDA (1980): 21 CFR 70.
32. FDA (1985): 21 CFR 500.
33. FDA (1985): 21 CFR 514.
34. FDA (1985): 21 CFR 571.
35. FDA (1985): Federal Register, 50: 45530.
36. FDA (1987): Federal Register, 52: 8798.
37. FDA (1987): Federal Register, 52: 19466.
38. FDA MDA (1978): ASTM Practice F469, Practice for Assessment of Compatibility of Nonporous Polymeric Materials for Surgical Implants with Regard to Effect of Materials on Tissue. *J. ASTM*, Vol. 13.01.
39. FDA MDA (1980): ASTM Practice F361, Practice for Assessment of Compatibility of Metallic Materials for Surgical Implants with Respect to Effect of Material on Tissue. *J. ASTM*, Vol. 13.01.
40. FDA MDA (1981): ASTM Practice F719, Practice for Testing Biomaterials in Rabbits for Primary Skin Irritation. *J. ASTM*, Vol. 13.01.
41. FDA MDA (1981): ASTM Practice F720, Practice for Testing Guinea Pigs for Contact Allergens: Guinea Pig Maximization Test. *J. ASTM*, Vol. 13.01.
42. FDA MDA (1982): ASTM Practice F749, Practice for Evaluating Material Extracts by Intracutaneous Injection in the Rabbit. *J. ASTM*, Vol. 13.01.
43. FDA MDA (1982): ASTM Practice F750, Practice for Evaluating Material Extracts by Systemic Injection in the Mouse. *J. ASTM*, Vol. 13.01.
44. FDA MDA (1982): ASTM Practice F756, Practice for Assessment of the Hemolytic Properties of Materials. *J. ASTM*, Vol. 13.01.
45. FDA MDA (1982): ASTM Practice F763, Practice for Short-Term Screening of Implant Materials. *J. ASTM*, Vol. 13.01.
46. FDA (1982): Toxicological principles for the safety assessment of direct food additives and color additives used in food. Report by the U.S.F.D.A.
47. McNamara, B. P. (1976): Concepts in health evaluation of commercial and industrial chemicals. In: *New Concepts in Safety Evaluation,* edited by M. A. Mehlman, R. E. Shapiro, and H. Blumenthal. pp. 61–140. Hemisphere, Washington, D.C.
48. OSHA (1970): Occupational Safety and Health Act, 29 U.S.C., 651 et seq.
49. Weil, C. S., and McCallister, D. D. (1963): Safety evaluation of chemicals: Relationship between short- and long-term feeding studies in designing an effective toxicity test. *Agric. Food Chem.,* 11:486–491.
50. WHO (1957): WHO Technical Report Series No. 129 (General principles governing the use of food additives: First report of the Joint FAO/WHO Expert Committee on Food Additives), p. 22.
51. WHO (1958): WHO Technical Report Series No. 144 (Procedures for the testing of intentional food additives to establish their safety for use: Second report of the Joint FAO/WHO Expert Committee on Food Additives), p. 19.
52. WHO (1961): WHO Technical Report Series No. 220 (Evaluation of the carcinogenic hazards of food additives: Fifth report of the Joint FAO/WHO Expert Committee on Food Additives), p. 33.
53. WHO (1966): WHO Technical Report Series No. 341 (Principles for preclinical testing of drug safety: Report of a WHO Scientific Group), p. 22.
54. WHO (1967): WHO Technical Report Series No. 348 (Procedures for investigating intentional and unintentional food additives: Report of a WHO Scientific Group), p. 25.
55. WHO (1967): WHO Technical Report Series No. 364 (Principles for the testing of drugs for teratogenicity: Report of a WHO Scientific Group), p. 18.
56. WHO (1968): WHO Technical Report Series No. 403. (Principles for the clinical evaluation of drugs: Report of a WHO Scientific Group), p. 32.
57. WHO (1969): WHO Technical Report Series No. 426 (Principles for the testing and evaluation of drugs for carcinogenicity: Report of a WHO Scientific Group), p. 26.
58. WHO (1971): WHO Technical Report Series No. 482 (Evaluation and testing of drugs for mutagenicity: Principles and problems—Report of a WHO Scientific Group), p. 18.
59. WHO (1973): WHO Technical Report Series No. 535 (Environmental and health monitoring in occupational health: Report of a WHO Expert Committee), p. 48.
60. WHO (1974): WHO Technical Report Series No. 539 (Toxicological evaluation of certain food additives with a review of general principles and of specifications: Seventeenth report of the Joint FAO/WHO Expert Committee on Food Additives), p. 40.
61. WHO (1974): WHO Technical Report Series No. 546 (Assessment of the carcinogenicity and mutagenicity of chemicals: Report of a WHO Scientific Group), p. 19.
62. WHO (1975): WHO Technical Report Series No. 560 (Chemical and biochemical methodology for the assessment of hazards of pesticides for man), p. 26.
63. WHO (1975): WHO Technical Report Series No. 563 (Guidelines for evaluation of drugs for use in man: Report of a WHO Scientific Group), p. 59.
64. WHO (1975): WHO Technical Report Series No. 571 (Early detection of health impairment in occupational exposure to health hazards: report of a WHO Study Group), p. 80.
65. WHO (1976): Background and purpose of the WHO Environmental Health Criteria Program (Reprint from Environmental Health Criteria 1 Mercury). WHO, Geneva, p. 9.
66. WHO (1977): WHO Technical Report Series No. 601 (Methods used in establishing permissible levels in occupational exposure to harmful agents: Report of a WHO Expert Committee with the participation of ILO), p. 68.

---

a All CFR References pertain to Code of Federal Regulations. Office of the Federal Register, National Archives and Record Service, General Services Administration. U.S. Government Printing Office, Washington D.C.

All FR References pertain to Federal Register. Office of the Federal Register, National Archives and Record Service, General Services Administration. U.S. Government Printing Office, Washington D.C.

Principles and Methods of Toxicology, Second Edition, edited by A. Wallace Hayes, Raven Press, Ltd., New York © 1989.

CHAPTER 8

Practical Considerations in the Conduct of Chronic Toxicity Studies

Kent R. Stevens and *Michael A. Gallo

*Berlex Laboratories, Cedar Knolls, New Jersey 07927; and *Department of Environmental and Community Medicine, UMDNJ, Robert Wood Johnson Medical School, Piscataway, New Jersey 08854*

Long-term toxicity tests are usually defined as studies of longer than 3 months' duration, i.e., approximately 10% of the life span of the laboratory rat. These types of studies are conducted in all species of laboratory animals and in some economically important animals, wild and domestic. This class of tests encompasses the classic subchronic and chronic toxicity studies, multigeneration reproduction studies, and carcinogenicity studies.

This chapter deals primarily with the design, conduct, and interpretation of classic chronic toxicity study. Other chapters in this volume are concerned with the areas of reproductive toxicity and carcinogenicity. However, many of the basic tenets are the same for the several classes of nonacute toxicity studies.

The first step in assessing the toxicity of a test compound is to conduct one or more acute studies. Since single dose exposure is not generally sufficient to indicate the risk incurred with multiple dose, steady state exposure, it is therefore necessary to conduct the longer term chronic toxicity studies. There are two additional reasons for conducting chronic toxicity tests: (a) to induce a toxic effect through chronic exposure and (b) to determine an apparent no observable effect level

in the presence of such exposure. The chronic study is designed to elucidate any of a myriad of potential toxic effects of a xenobiotic on an organism's structural and functional entities. In contrast to the carcinogenicity studies, which are designed to assess tumor induction potential, the chronic toxicity study utilizes a holistic approach to detect the origin of an adverse response, and, parenthetically, to determine the safety margin between proposed use (exposure) levels and toxicity.

The results of a chronic toxicity study in animals should suggest signs and symptoms of adverse reactions to look for in man. With the exception of idiosyncratic reactions and hypersensitivity, many of the systemic and organismic responses are predictable from laboratory animal to man. To be useful as a tool in predicting human toxicity from animal data, the experimental design must be of such a power so as to eliminate false positive as well as false negative responses. False positives occur with a calculated probability, expressed statistically. However false negatives, while statistically unpredictable, can be avoided by establishing adequate control and treatment groups with sufficient representatives to make the conditions unlikely.

DESIGN OF CHRONIC TOXICITY STUDIES

All laboratory studies must be designed to test a working hypothesis. There are several basic principles that are invariably stated but at times not followed in conducting chronic toxicity studies.

First, the study should be conducted in a species whose metabolism is most similar to man. Since metabolic disposition in man can only be determined following exposure in man, this knowledge is not usually available because the metabolic disposition of xenobiotics in man is not usually known prior to initiating chronic studies. Such data are only available following cautious administration during phase I clinical trials on pharmaceuticals or, at times, following unplanned occupational exposure.

Second, the route of administration should be the same as the route of human exposure. In the laboratory, three modes of administration are most commonly used: diet, gavage, and inhalation. However, recent advances in drug delivery systems and consideration of occupational exposures has led many laboratories to examine chronic dermal administration. Multiple routes, such as might occur in the workplace, are generally not used in the experimental setting.

Third, the duration of exposure should be a reflection of the human situation. In practice, these studies are designed for daily (7 days a week) administration, with a duration of 6 months or greater in rodents and 1 year in nonrodents such as dogs or monkeys.

Fourth, the doses of the test article should span the range of the highest no effect level to the highest dose tolerated over the entire course of the study.

Species

A second nonrodent species is generally utilized, and the choice has usually been the purebred beagle because individuals of this species should respond more similarly than those of species that are genetically more variable. In addition, the larger animal permits more extensive clinical analyses, since more blood can be collected from each animal at frequent intervals than smaller species, i.e., rodents. There are several schools of thought on the use of the second species. The dog should be used with caution since it is a carnivore and often metabolizes compounds much differently than an omnivore or herbivore. The use of a primate, however, provides no greater assurance, a priori, that the model will be any more relevant to man.

In this regard, the nonhuman primates have been used as the nonrodent species with success. However, the question of compound bioavailability and metabolism as well as the difficulty of obtaining and handling these species must be considered. Nonhuman primates have not been shown to have metabolic systems any closer to man than those of other laboratory animals. In inhalation studies, the monkey is a preferred model since its respiratory anatomy and physiology are closer to man's than other laboratory animals.

An interesting alternative nonrodent species to consider in the future may be the ferret. This animal is a small carnivore that is readily available in a defined strain, has been used in several laboratories, and metabolizes many compounds similarly to man. It would be large enough to obtain multiple blood samples yet small enough to house easily and utilize a smaller quantity of test article over the course of the study. A much greater data base concerning normal behavior, clinical profile, and incidence of common diseases, pathology, and tumors will be necessary before this species can become a common subject for chronic studies. In this case, it is familiarity that will breed acceptance.

Duration of Study

Because of these constraints and the long-standing prejudice of practicing toxicologists, the classic chronic toxicity study in rats and mice usually consists of three treatment groups and a control group, all of equal number at the outset, in which the xenobiotic is administered 7 days per week for 6 months or 2 years. In nonrodents, studies are generally conducted for 1 year.

A consensus has not been reached as to whether exposures of 1 or 2 years are adequate for the chronic assessment of toxicity in laboratory animals. Reevaluation of data available to Canadian regulatory authorities found a number of compounds that developed toxicopathologic effects at periods beyond 1 year of exposure. Cataracts, renal toxicity, and other types of pathology arose following administration of several types of compounds for periods longer than 1 year.

For this reason, it is becoming more popular to conduct clinical assessments during the course of the longer term carcinogenicity studies in rodents. Some level of caution must be exercised here for two reasons: (a) the dose selection for carcinogenicity studies may not be optimal for chronic toxicity assessment, and (b) the influence of normally occurring geriatric pathology on the appearance of some specific finding cannot be determined. Such effects should be determined in separate, specifically designed studies if deemed important.

Dose of Test Article

The most difficult and intellectually stimulating task for the toxicologist preparing for a chronic toxicity study is selection of the dose levels to be tested. There are, as always, several approaches to the problem. One of these is the former approach of the National Toxicology Program's (NTP) Bioassay Program, which conducted a 3-month range-finding study with enough doses to find a level which suppressed body weight gain slightly, i.e., 10%. This dose, defined as the maximum tolerated dose (MTD), was selected as the highest dose. Two other levels, generally $\frac{1}{4}$ MTD and $\frac{1}{16}$ MTD, are then selected for testing. Currently, NTP and many other laboratories are following the more rigorous procedure of critically examining all the results of the 90-day studies (*in vivo*, post-morteus, chemistry, etc.) to determine the doses for the chronic bioassay.

The dose range finding study is a necessity in most cases, but the suppression of body weight is a scientifically questionable endpoint when dealing with establishment of safety factors. Physiologic or pharmacologic markers should generally be sought as better indicators of a systemic response than body weight. A series of well-defined acute and subchronic studies designed to determine the *chronicity factor* and to study the onset of pathology are more predictive for dose setting than body weight suppression. The chronicity factor is the ratio of the one-dose LD_{50} (mg/kg) divided by the 90-dose LD_{50} (mg/kg/day) for any particular compound. A comparison of day-1 with day-90 LD_{50}'s and the slopes of these curves can tell the toxicologist a great deal about the *in vivo* handling of the compounds. If the 90-day LD_{50} is far below that of the single-dose LD_{50}, it is probable that the compound is slowly metabolized and accumulates in the body. Recording organ weights (including brain weight), food consumption, body weight, behavior, and water consumption can go a long way in defining target organ toxicity.

Another excellent measure of the MTD in any one species is a qualitative and/or quantitative change in urinary metabolites of a given xenobiotic. This approach assumes some knowledge of the metabolites or at least methods to qualitatively determine metabolite patterns. The premise in this evaluation is that a change in profile of the urinary excretion pattern, as a function of dose, may indicate an overloading of the body's ability to handle the compound (13). Metabolite identification is not necessary for this evaluation, but rather only the ability to qualitatively evaluate the patterns by high performance liquid, thin-layer, or gas–liquid chromatography (HPLC, TLC, GLC). Knowledge of this type should be obtained during the initial acute and subchronic studies. Combining a metabolic assessment with acute and subchronic studies represents the most efficient use of laboratory animals.

The metabolism and pharmacokinetic profiles of a drug or other xenobiotics are major considerations in the assessment of toxicity. If a compound is metabolized, the toxic factor may be a metabolite and not the parent compound. Thus, nitrates are not normally considered chronic toxins until they are metabolized to nitrosamines. But, if the rat forms the toxic metabolite and the human does not, the compound will be erroneously considered toxic to the human on the basis of the rat studies. It is always best to evaluate the toxicity of a compound in an animal that metabolizes the compound in the same manner as the human. Of course, this information may only be available if the human has been deliberately or accidentally exposed to the material in question.

The half-life of the test material, its ability to bind to proteins or other macromolecules, the route of excretion and its clearance all have a potential influence on the rate of appearance and severity of pharmacologic and toxicologic manifestations following exposure. Many of the kinetic and metabolic considerations for chronic toxicology testing are presented in a recent review by Gillette et al. (4).

Dose setting also requires consideration of the end use of the xenobiotic in question. If the compound is to be a drug dispensed only by prescription or in a clinical setting, the dose levels may never approach an MTD but rather will be a function of the maximum therapeutic dose and thereby, a function of the therapeutic index (the ratio of therapeutic to toxic dose level). On the other hand, if the compound is an ubiquitous indirect food additive, the highest dose level should not be less than 100 times the maximum detectable residue in the prepared food. These examples are the extremes. For direct food additives, occupational hazards, household products, and environmental agents, other criteria such as use patterns, work habits, and routes of exposure should be considered when setting dose levels.

The major distinguishing factor in a chronic toxicity study, which separates it from an oncogenicity study is, as stated above, that the chronic toxicity study is designed to define no effect levels and potential systemic toxicity, whereas the oncogenicity study is designed to measure potential for induction of tumors. This difference in scope is one of the most important characteristics in determining dose levels for long-term testing. Some multiple (perhaps orders of magnitude) of the expected human exposure level might be used as the highest dose for a carcinogenicity study whereas subtle physiologic, pharmacologic, or biochemical markers should be used to determine dose levels for a chronic toxicity study.

Regardless of the purpose of the long-term toxicity study, certain laboratory practices must be followed dogmatically if the investigator is to rule out extraneous factors that may affect the interpretation of results. These practices are reviewed in the following sections on animal husbandry and laboratory considerations.

ANIMAL HUSBANDRY

Animal Requirements

Chronic and subchronic studies are commonly conducted using mice and rats (12–24 months) and dogs (12 months). The strains of these species are generally chosen to minimize, or select for, genetic characteristics and spontaneous appearances of lesions and/or tumors.

Feed

There are many types of animal feeds produced by major animal feed manufacturers. Semisynthetic feeds are formulated with chemically pure or refined ingredients. Vitamins, minerals, and carbohydrates of known purity are generally formulated with refined vegetable oils, starches, and casein to form a nutritious product capable of supporting all natural functions of the laboratory animal. Such diets may be designed and produced for any laboratory animal. The rationale for using semisynthetic diets includes constancy of ingredient mixture with low, controlled levels of contamination. Animal feeds formulated from vegetable products and fish and bone meals are not as likely to be of constant palatability or quality.

Laboratory animal feeds are formulated to achieve a minimum guaranteed nutrient analysis by combining the same quality of stipulated ingredients in each batch (closed formula) or by combining any of several commercially available ingredients in appropriate levels to achieve the guaranteed nutrient analysis (open formula). Feeds of the latter type are often produced even by the large feed manufacturers to allow use of the most readily available (and less costly) ingredients. The variable composition of open formula feeds leads to potential variation in quality of protein, carbohydrate, and lipids, as well as palatability and compatability with a test article. Even though the human diet is of the open formula type, this diet may give the investigator some problems in well-designed and controlled animal studies.

The type of diet used may affect not only palatability but also baseline plasma levels of liver enzymes. Glucose-6-phosphate dehydrogenase and alkaline phosphatase of the liver are reportedly lower in animals receiving semipurified diets than those receiving conventional commercial diets, and hepatic microsomal cytochromes P450 have been altered in rats fed diets ranging in alfalfa content. What effect this might have on the outcome of a toxicity study is not known. Regardless of the type of feed used, the diet is often used as a route of administration of the test material, as stated.

Housing

Rodents are generally housed in metal (stainless steel or galvanized steel) or plastic (polyethylene, polypropylene, or polycarbonate) cages. Metal caging or floor pens are used for dogs. Minimum cage sizes for all species are stipulated in the Guide for the Care and Use of Laboratory Animals (2) and compliance is monitored by federal and state health agencies. Since minimum sizes for cages are stipulated, only caging type remains to be decided. Two major types of caging are available: solid floor and grid or slatted floor cages. Following is a brief consideration of these housing types.

Solid floor cages

Solid bottom cages, often called shoebox cages, and pens require bedding to be added to the cage to absorb and contain waste materials. Such cages are usually used in reproduction studies but, for several reasons are not favored for chronic studies:

1. Additional effort is needed to clean the cages and change the bedding. In addition, the use of bedding may introduce dust, pesticides, or other contaminants. It has long been known that sawdusts and chips of some conifers induce liver mixed-function oxidase enzyme activity, which may affect the outcome of the study.

2. Animals have access to their waste.

3. It is difficult to calculate feed consumption because the quantity of spilled feed (if any) cannot be accounted for.

4. Clearance of the cage atmosphere is slower in this type of cage than in cages with wire mesh sides or bottoms, which may alter the outcome of the study.

5. Water from a malfunctioning automatic waterer can collect in the cage and drown the occupants.

6. Solid plastic cages can be fitted with filter tops to remove dust from the air. Added isolation is possible by HEPA filtration of the air flow passing over each cage.

Grid floor cages

Cages with metal, mesh floors are commonly suited for rodent and dog studies. However, these cages also have disadvantages:

1. They allow the extremities, especially of younger or smaller animals, to be caught in the mesh.

2. They also envelope the animal in room air on all sides so that there is no place for the animal to bed down. This means that the temperature control in the animal rooms must be rigorous so that animals are not exposed to the stress of extremes in temperature.

3. They permit animals to be exposed to dust particles suspended in the air. Thus, control animals may receive some exposure to test articles that are contained in the feed of other treated groups.

Cleaning cages at frequent intervals is a necessity in all toxicology studies. Failure to clean cages properly and frequently may result in skin lesions, alopecia, or appearance of signs and behavior that may be interpreted as an effect of the test article.

Animal Environment

Temperature

The temperature for housing laboratory animals is often dictated by the comfort of technicians working in the rooms or by the limitations of the heating and air conditioning systems. Temperatures of 70–72°F are common in rodent and large animal laboratories, but what temperatures do the animals prefer? Temperature recommendations for laboratory animals have been published by the National Academy of Sciences (6).

It is perhaps more important that the temperature remain fairly constant, wherever it may be set, rather than fluctuate around a given temperature. The fluctuations probably cause more stress than a constant temperature, even if it is slightly outside of the recommended range.

Ventilation

Airflow through the animal laboratory must be sufficient to prevent the air from becoming stale and must provide a low-odor environment. When more air is forced into a room than can be cleared completely by exhaust systems, air flows through the cracks and around the door, and the partial pressure of air in the room becomes positive with respect to the hallway or area outside the room. Establishing a positive room air pressure is an important method in reducing the possible exposure of animals to test substances being used in other animal rooms.

Ventilation must be homogeneous throughout the room; this is generally controlled by adjustable diffusers. The ventilation of all rooms in a facility must be balanced: All rooms should have the same relative air flow and positive pressure with regard to hallways. Balancing airflow in an entire facility should always be performed by airflow control specialists, who document their achievements with airflow meters. Balancing should be done only after changing all air filters in the system. Balancing is not a one-time task; it is affected by progressive filter clogging and is therefore an ongoing process.

Relative Humidity

Stringent control of humidity is probably not important; however, if moisture in the air is too low, the mucus membranes and eyes of the test animal will dry out. If humidity climbs too high, the growth of bacterial and fungal populations may permit respiratory distress and dermal involvement such as ringworm. In addition, urine and excreta do not dry, thereby increasing the room odor level.

Lighting

Common lighting schedules of 12-hr continuous light and 12-hr darkness are common. This schedule permits the animals to entrain upon the light cycle which, in turn, stimulates constant secretion of thyroid hormones, adrenocorticotropic hormone (ACTH), and growth hormone. Regulated lighting cycles are necessary in reproduction studies since rodents enter continuous estrus under conditions of constant light phases without darkness. The importance of stringently controlled light cycles has probably been underrated in toxicology.

Cleanliness

Freedom from filth and vermin should be an inalienable right of all laboratory animals. Insecticides should not be used in the rooms, if possible. However, if infestations are threatened, American Association for Accreditation of Laboratory Animal Care (AAALAC) permits the use of certain insecticides in animal rooms. Electric insect traps and electrocution devices may be used in laboratories to control flying insects. However, the best insect control is prevention of infestation by limiting the amount of materials brought into the lab from uncontrolled sources, i.e., food, bedding, and supplies. Dust and dirt will normally build up in a room and must be removed. Recirculated dust may be observed around incoming air vents, indicating a need for changing filters. Washing is the best method of removing such buildup. Technicians often like to carry portable radios into animal rooms as they work. This practice should be discouraged for reasons known to the parents of every teenager.

Floors should be mopped with a weak detergent solution with low volatility or known toxicity. Quaternary ammonium-based detergents are generally acceptable. Nonscented products would seem to be the best alternative, thereby avoiding volatile components in the test area. It should be noted that any gradients in lighting, temperature, or airborne products in an animal room will occur vertically. Thus, animals within groups should be distributed in cage racks in such a way as to be present equally at all vertical caging levels. This practice, and the practice of periodically changing the relative position of each animal within the room, avoids confounding treatment group with cage level in the room.

The preceding section has hopefully pointed out some methods that can be used to minimize exogenous factors which can affect the outcome of a long-term toxicity study.

LABORATORY CONSIDERATIONS

Animal Identification

Unique marking systems are necessary for conducting chronic toxicity studies, analyzing the results by animal and group, and retrieving data in the reconstruction of a study. Marking systems vary with species and type of study. Large animals can be tattooed, whereas smaller animals can be ear-tagged or leg-banded. Ear tags, which should be Monel metal rather than aluminum or steel to avoid irritation, have been and are being used in rodents, but tags may be lost during a study. The classic method for unique identification of rodents is the standard ear and toe clip system which allows for 999 animals without repetition. However, if rodents, particularly mice, are gang-housed, they will alter ear markings by chewing on each other's ears. Therefore, frequent checks and supplemental marking methods should be standard operating procedure.

Computerized systems for reading bar code implants have become available and may prove to be the best system for unique identification.

Cage Identification

Recent developments with computer "mark-sense" or bar code identification have proven to be a potential boon to the toxicologist with a computerized data-gathering system. As computers become more available (i.e., less expensive), the mark-sense identification systems should become more widespread. For those investigators who do not have a computerized system, color-coded cage cards are a good alternative. By using a systematic color coding (e.g., white for control, red for low dose, yellow for middose, blue for high dose), the chances of treatment level mixups are minimized. With the color code system, the cage, the container for the compound, and the page(s) in the notebooks should all be coded.

Administration of Test Material

The ideal situation is to be able to administer the test article by the same route and under the same conditions as those of human exposure. For example, if perchloroethylene is the chemical of interest and the exposure is in water, then drinking water would be the vehicle of choice. However, if we are concerned about perchloroethylene as an occupational hazard in the dry cleaning industry, then the routes of choice for one study should be dermal and/or inhalation. Lastly, when perchloroethylene was used as a drug to treat gastrointestinal parasites (see ref. 8), the route of administration in toxicology studies was again oral, but this time the delivery system was gavage in an oil base.

Parenteral routes of administration (intraperitoneal, intravenous, intramuscular, and subcutaneous) are also used in toxicology. These routes are of particular interest when the investigator is developing a drug for use by a parenteral route or when other routes are not useful in delivering a set dose to the animal.

The types of results may differ according to the means of introduction even though the doses are the same. Bioavailability is markedly affected by vehicle or delivery system. 2,3,7,8-Tetrachlorobenzo-p-dioxin was found to be considerably less toxic (about 100-fold) when given in soil rather than an oil vehicle (12) and several complex mixtures alleviated the toxicity of individual components of the mixture

(7). Differential bioavailability also changes the dynamics of a compound by altering the time to peak blood level. These findings are critical for all types of agents. General muscle weakness was seen in long-term feeding studies with zinc pyrithione in rats, but was not seen following daily intubation to rats in a shampoo base or when it was applied topically to the skin of rabbits (10).

Diet

Whenever possible, dosing should be accomplished by incorporating the test material in the diet. This lets the animal administer the test article to itself according to its size and metabolism. It is the easiest method for the laboratory personnel since the animals do not have to be handled to administer the compound. If feed is used as the route by which a test material is administered, it is important that the following procedures are observed:

1. The substance should be mixed uniformly throughout the feed at the specified level. The presence of "hot" and "cold" spots will contribute to the variation in response seen in the study.

2. The substance should be stable in the feed throughout the period of application. If the test material degrades in the oxidizing milieu of the feed, this route is clearly inappropriate. Establishing accurate and precise assays for test article in the complex medium of food is a prerequisite of conducting this stability evaluation.

3. The level of test material should be confirmed by acceptable analytical methods at stipulated intervals throughout the study. The extraction and assay of test materials from laboratory diets is a challenge to the analytical chemist. The establishment of adequate and appropriate analytical procedures is one of the first requirements for determining the uniformity and stability of the mixed feed.

4. The fortified feed is sufficiently palatable to permit normal intake of food for normal growth. If a loss of body weight and depressed food consumption is observed in treated groups during preliminary tests, a split-plate palatability test should be performed. In this test, treated and untreated (control) feeds are offered simultaneously for 4 days with the positions of the feed cups reversed daily. Preferential consumption of control feed indicates that the treated feed is not palatable, and either a paired-feeding study or another treatment route should be considered. Similarly, feed is not the preferred route when the test material must be administered as a bolus, when it is unstable in feed, or when it cannot be mixed properly.

Feed Mixing

Feed mixing is, at best, a messy operation, but it is also the foundation for many chronic studies. The techniques, equipment, and precautions used in feed mixing depend upon the properties of the feed and test material. It is obvious that no single statement can be made about the best method to use in all cases, but there are several principles that can be applied to all methods:

1. The test material, if solid, should be ground as finely as possible; the smaller the particle size the better. If the test material is liquid or can be dissolved in an innocuous liquid vehicle, the distribution in feed may be made more easily and more uniformly.

2. If mixing a diet that must provide 25 mg/kg to rats, one will want to calculate the total feed required and total test material required. The calculation can be performed as follows:

For feed	For test material
120 rats	120 rats (weight)
23 g feed/day/rat	0.25 kg/rat (avg)
2760 g total/day	30 kg total

Each day, 30 kg of rats will eat 2760 g of feed. At a dose of 25 mg test material per kilogram body weight, these rats must eat 750 mg of test material in their daily allotment of feed. If feed is mixed once weekly, 5.25 g of test material must be mixed into 19.32 kg of feed with no waste accounted for. Since losses always occur, one would make 25 kg of feed containing 6.8 g of test material mixed uniformly throughout. The very simplicity of these calculations could bore the dullest of students and is embarrassing to present except that it gives us a foundation to go on to a real-life situation.

In the laboratory, the situation is not always so simple. Feed is generally mixed a week before it is used so that the chemical analyses can be performed to confirm the intended test levels. A growing rat, depending on its sex, may grow 20–35 g in a week's time. Thus, the situation becomes more complex for the person calculating feed levels. What mean body weight will the rat achieve 2 weeks from now when the feed will be administered, and how much feed will the average rat be eating during that week? The answers that are selected for these questions will depend upon historical laboratory performance. It seems elementary that if dosing is calculated on a miligram test material per kilogram body weight basis, the feed will have to be mixed separately for each sex getting the same dose level. On the other hand, if the feed for both sexes contains the same quantity of test material per unit of feed, the females will receive higher doses per unit body weight than will the males during adulthood.

For example, 26-week-old male and female Fischer rats could weigh 313 and 193 g, respectively. They may eat 102 and 82 g of feed per week, respectively. If the diet for all animals contained 10 mg test material per kilogram, the males and females would have received daily doses of 47 and 61 mg/kg body weight, respectively.

Returning to our example above, we must add 6.8 g of test material to 25 kg of feed. It would be unreasonable to try to stir a teaspoon of test material into 25 kg of feed—we would be much more confident if we were mixing 2.5 kg of test material into 22.5 kg of basal feed. Therein lies the rationale for making a premix, which is then added to the commercial, untreated feed to achieve a final dosing level. Premixes often comprise approximately 10% of the final diet. In our example, we would mix the 6.8 g of test material into 2.5 kg of feed to make our premix, with the knowledge that any error created in making the premix will be magnified 10-fold in the final feed.

The premix is often mixed in an open bowl, stirring type mixer similar to a kitchen mixer. A powdered test material could be agitated into the air by mixing action or by electrostatic forces created by the mixing action in this system. Electrostatic forces can be overcome by adding a grounding wire to the mixer and adding 1% food grade oil to the feed to make it sticky.

Other techniques for achieving a uniform mix include the following. Layers of the feed and test material should be alternately added to the bowl. A bowl cover is recommended to prevent possible contamination or losses over the top, and, most importantly, the appropriate size mixer must be used. If one tries to use a 2-quart bowl to mix 2.5 kg of premix, one's efforts will be rewarded with spilled feed and a great sense of frustration. The 2.5 kg of premix should need no more than 5–10 min of mixing in the "kitchen mixer." So many labs use mixing times of 20–30 min that it is surprising that the feed can be mixed in a timely fashion. The bag and labels for the final feed should accompany the premix from this point forward.

The final feed is mixed using the premix in a similar way that the premix was developed from the test material. The 2.5 kg of premix is alternately layered into the mixing bowl with 22.0 kg of basal diet. One-half kilogram of basal diet is held back to "rinse" the premix container. The principles concerning adequate size of equipment, use of absolutely clean equipment, and appropriate mixing time apply to the development of the final feeds as well as to that of the premix. "Grab" several gloved handfuls of feed as it is poured into the final container. Save this sample of feed for analysis of the test material.

The open bowl, planetary mixer described above is only one of the types of mixers found in the laboratory. The other common type is the P-K or V blender. The V blender is named for its shape. The V rotates on an axis so that the feed flows back and forth between the tip and the legs of the V. Obviously, the feed is locked into this system so that spillage will not occur during the mixing process unless the ports are not properly tightened. This is an attractive feature when suspected carcinogenic or highly toxic materials are incorporated into feed. A premix is still important when mixing feed with a V blender, even though it is an efficient blender.

If the test material is a liquid with an aqueous base, too much test material can dampen the feed and encourage the growth of microflora, which make the feed unpalatable. If the test material is in a volatile vehicle, allow the vehicle to evaporate before adding the premix to the final feed. Failure to do so could result in treating the animals with an additional toxic component—namely the solvent.

Since many volatile vehicles are also explosive, one should provide sufficient ventilation to permit the evaporation of the solvents from the feed. Evaporation is most easily performed from shallow pans, not unlike cage waste pans. The air movement around these pans must be gentle so that the test material is not carried off to the air filters.

Drinking Water

Drinking water is also an acceptable vehicle for administering test substances. For soluble and stable compounds, this route may be preferred. This route is indicated when it simulates the route of human exposure. All of the caveats mentioned for feed are applicable to water. Close observation is essential because spillage is generally a more disastrous event when administering material by water. It cannot be recovered as easily as spilled feed. Losses of data because of this occurrence must be handled statistically.

Gavage

The French force-feed geese to fatten them sufficiently to obtain the enlarged, fatty livers to make paté de foie gras, which graces the tables of the gastronomically fortunate. While compensatory liver growth is an interesting toxicological phenomenon by itself, the subject is introduced here only because the French word for the process of forced feeding the geese is *gavage*. Thus, the word gavage has been adopted for "administer by stomach tube."

When the oral route is indicated, but feed and water are not appropriate vehicles, gavage may be the recommended method of administration. In this case, a test material is added to an appropriate vehicle and introduced into the esophagus with a tube attached to a graduated syringe. An appropriate vehicle is one that is compatible to both test material and animal. The most common gavage vehicles are water, water with suspending agents, and food grade oil—depending on the characteristics of the test material. When the test material is not soluble, a suspension is often formulated. Suspensions are made by increasing the viscosity of the vehicle with thickeners such as agar, carboxymethyl cellulose, or gum tragacanth. A wetting agent such as Tween 80 may also be used to increase the suspendability of the material. Stability assays will indicate the frequency with which the dosing formulation must be prepared during the test.

Dosing is commonly accomplished at a constant volume of 10 ml/kg body weight. In this way, a 260-g rat would receive a dose of 2.6 ml, and a 35-g mouse would receive 0.35 ml of material. Such ease of calculating the appropriate dose is important when many animals are treated daily for a long period of time. Errors arise if too much effort is required to determine the quantity of test material for each animal. Bioavailability and gastrointestinal uptake are also a function of gastric emptying time. Hence, there is a good scientific reason for a constant volume across groups. Body weights should be collected frequently during the growth phase of the animal, with dosing volume adjusted accordingly. Weekly adjustments are sufficient after the rapid growth phase.

Since rodents are nocturnal animals, they eat during the dark period. There is an increase in activity and eating just before lights on, at which time they become quiescent. Thought should be given to dosing animals after midmorning so that the food accumulation in the stomach will not interfere with dosing. For gavage delivery, it is not necessary to introduce the tip of the cannula into the stomach to obtain a good administration of the test material. Depositing the dose into the esophagus is quite sufficient in the rodent, which cannot regurgitate. The danger of course is intratracheal administration which is generally total. Proper holding of the animal and a skilled technician minimizes this possibility.

Other Methods of Administering Test Materials

Skin painting

The test material is applied by inunction of a specified dose onto an area from which the hair has been removed. Removal of hair by both shaving and depilatories alter skin permeability to applied materials. Also, a portion of the dosing material must be considered to be ingested since animals frequently lick the foreign material from their skin. It should be noted that oral ingestion from licking is also a major confounder in open-cage inhalation studies.

Subcutaneous injection

This method is a frequently used testing route for pharmaceutical preparations; the site of injection is altered daily so that a single site is not constantly punctured. The repeated irritation attributable to the method of administration may, by itself, induce fibrotic reactions and consequently tumors. The dosing vehicle when possible should be aqueous since the oil vehicles will track back along the needle path and be deposited on the skin and hair. If an oil vehicle must be used, "tracking" of the oil may be prevented by depositing the material under the skin of the inner thigh, having inserted the needle from the outer aspect of the thigh. An oil vehicle also functions as a delayed delivery system. Hence, it modifies the dynamics of the compound in the body.

Implantation

Subcutaneous or intramuscular implantation is common for evaluating biopolymers for medical devices or prostheses, and more recently for continuous delivery of drugs and other agents. A clean surgical technique is necessary to avoid the complication of infection or formation of fibrotic reactions. This route may prove to be an excellent way to test new biotechnology based agents such as growth hormones and insulin.

DATA COLLECTION IN CHRONIC TOXICITY STUDIES

Computer logging of data now permits an observation, for example, the death of an animal, to be accounted for in all future records. However, where handwritten records are kept, separate laboratory books are often made for weekly body weights, food consumption, daily observations, and clinical test results. If an animal dies, the event is dutifully and properly recorded in the daily observation book, but the entry lines are still available in the other laboratory books. At subsequent weighings or observations, an entry may mistakenly appear in the dead animal's space—and somehow the animal has reappeared. The more harried the technicians, the longer the reincarnation period. This is a serious problem which calls for appropriate care and vigilance.

The other aspect of manual data collection that promotes insomnia in Study Directors is transcription of data. Transferring data from a laboratory printout to a laboratory notebook is fraught with hazard, and, in the end, the laboratory notebook cannot be considered the "raw" data. The printout or machine output is, in fact, the raw data. Yet, how many times have "units of enzyme activity per milligram organ protein" been reported as raw data? Spectrophotometers speak in terms of optical density or percent transmission; scintillation counters report counts per minute, not microcuries per vial. The arithmetic gymnastics that must be performed to transform raw machine data to understandable toxicologic terms must be described fully and documented.

Daily Observations

It is an unavoidable fact that looking at animals huddled in the depths of cages is not exciting, and that it can turn even good technicians into poor observers. Every cage should be opened every day to assess the most gross state of the animal's well being, i.e., alive versus dead. The temptation to merely look into the cage each day without opening it is often irresistible, but in this case, if you've seen one you haven't seen them all. Rodents can die in the most lifelike poses, or they can get their appendages caught in the wire floor, and the technician will not know it if each animal is given only a glance.

If the technician does a good job of observing rats or mice, he or she will notice the amount, color, and consistency of feces, spilled feed beneath the cage, the water level in the bottle (if any), and evidence of urine on the paper or pan, and will then look at the rat for evidence of difficulty. Once the animal's condition is noted, the findings should be reported in descriptive terms rather than medical terms, which may be used inaccurately. A record stating that "winking, bloody nose, and bloody tears" were observed is more reliable than one which notes the presence of "blepharospasm, epistaxis, and chromodacryorrhea."

If, in the course of taking daily observations, an animal is found dead, it must undergo autopsy as soon as possible so that autolysis is minimized. If the autopsy cannot be performed right away, refrigerate the animal to retard autolysis. Since one of the major endpoints in a chronic study is histopathologic evaluation, every effort must be made to present the pathologist with the best samples of tissue from the experimental subject.

Routine Observations

Body Weights and Growth Rates

The true measure of growth rate of an experimental animal is the animal's response to the continued availability of food and water. Therefore, to evaluate growth, the investigator must record food consumption and body weight on a fixed schedule. Water consumption should be at least qualitatively compared between groups. This is particularly true when evaluating a diuretic or a salt of an acid.

Many protocols suggest that body weights can be recorded monthly after the rodent's weight plateaus at about 6 months. It is much better to weigh the animals weekly throughout the study. The weekly weighing assures the toxicologist that the animals will be examined closely and palpated at least once a week. Weekly weighings also give the investigator early warnings of the onset of disease or debilitation in aged animals. The latter consideration is a key factor in gathering data of toxicologic significance as the study winds down.

Food Consumption

Food consumption is often evaluated in chronic studies to assess the effect of a treatment on eating and food utilization, i.e., food consumed per unit weight gain. It is a widely collected and infrequently scrutinized item of data. Food consumption is measured by subtracting the average daily weight of feed remaining from the weight of feed introduced into an animal's cage and dividing by the number of days in the feeding period. It is not always obvious that there are three components to this value called "food consumption." It is comprised of food actually eaten plus food that is spilled minus fecal and urinary contributions to the feeder. Thus, whenever food consumption appears excessive, account should be taken of the spillage of feed attributable to different treatment groups.

Observations at Necropsy

Gross Observations

Post-morteus observations are some of the most important aspects of a toxicology study. Notations should be made of the animals general exterior condition, for example, haircoat thriftiness, color, and condition, position and size of external lesions, and muscle conditions.

Careful necropsy technique is critical to good histopathology. Prosection should be done with the supervision of an experienced laboratory animal pathologist. All organs and tissues should be examined for readily visible lesions or changes from normal. When possible, the lesions should be photographed (especially true for small neoplasms) and measured. Sectioning of organs should be done with scalpels using a drawing motion rather than a pushing or compressing. This type of sectioning avoids mechanical injury to tissues. All tissue should be quickly placed in buffered 10% formalin for fixation. Special fixatives may be required for some tissues. Good necropsy techniques will be rewarded with better fixed tissue and considerably less autolysis.

Organ Weights

Weighing the organs of treated animals may reveal a specific target-organ response. This is one of the first lessons taught in toxicology, yet there is an element of complexity in this lesson that is not always described. The major organs weighed in a chronic study include the liver, heart, kidneys, spleen, gonads, brain, adrenal, thyroid, pituitary, and thymus (at early interval sacrifices). The procedures for obtaining the weights of these organs include removal from the body, dissecting free of adhering tissue, and weighing. Removal from the body requires no major considerations except to place the organ on a moistened surface so that it will not dry out.

Dissecting the organ free of adhering tissues does require a few words of caution. The most easily dissected organs are the liver, spleen, kidney, testes, and perhaps pituitary. Very few decisions have to be made by the technician in preparing these discrete organs for weighing. The remaining organs have built-in hazards which are addressed below.

Heart. The atria of the rat or mouse heart are so thin that they are often removed with the major arteries; in addition, the heart may contain unexpelled blood in the ventricles, which will add weight to the organ. The ventricles should be incised to remove blood and inspect the valves and the endocardium.

Brain. While many organs are discrete, the brain continues posteriorly into the spinal column. In order to reduce variation in weights, necropsy, and dissection, procedures should be standardized. The spinal cord should be severed at the atlas joint before proceeding to the removal of the cranial cap. In this way, the brain will be cut in the same place each time. Similarly, the olfactory lobes, which extend forward into the snout, are often left in the animal, thereby increasing variability.

Adrenals. The adrenals of the rodent are similar in color to adhering fat. Without adequate training and care, the technicians may dissect the adrenals too closely, giving rise to excessive variation in the weights of adrenals. If one technician works on the control animals and another dissects the organs of a treated group, significant organ weight differences usually arise due to differences in procedures and not treatment. This is another reason to insist on randomization of animals at necropsy.

Thyroids. The thyroid is a small organ in rodents with a color similar to surrounding muscle. Like the adrenals, thyroid dissection requires care, training, and practice.

An indication of variability in organ weight, whether contributed by the animal or the technician, is the coefficient of variability (CV). The formula for CV is

$$\frac{100 \text{ (Standard deviation)}}{\text{Mean weight}}$$

A review of control groups of two mouse and four rat studies gives an approximation of the CV ranges of some organs (Table 1).

The contributions to variability are (a) animal variation, (b) technician dissecting variability, and (c) technician "balance reading" variability. It is interesting to compare the CV of the organs. The brain and testes have the least variability,

TABLE 1. *CV ranges in several organs*

Organ	Mouse	Rat
Liver	10–15	10–15
Heart	15–20	10–15
Kidney	10–15	10–15
Spleen	45–70	15–30
Testes	10–15	7–9
Brain	5–8	4–8
Adrenals	20–30	15–30

followed by the major organs, the liver, heart, and kidney. The greatest variability was seen with the spleen and adrenals (and thyroid weights, 20–30 in one mouse study).

When organ weights are compared statistically, they are often expressed as weight per gram of body weight, since animal size affects organ size. Peters found that intestinal content was rather constant in mature female rats and that no better correlation is obtained if organs were expressed relative to net body weight (total body weight minus weight of intestinal contents) rather than uncorrected weight. If body weights are greatly different between treatment groups, this expression of the relative size of the organ may not be valid. Calculation of relative organ weights may not be appropriate because depressed body weight due to treatment is frequently due to depressed deposition of fat, not depressed development of lean body mass. If it were possible, we would choose to express organ weights relative to lean body mass, but we have no way to determine this value for each animal. However, since the brain weight is measured with low variability and is not greatly influenced by nutritional factors, it is a good constant surrogate for lean body mass. Therefore, when significant treatment-related differences in a study are detected in many organ weights relative to body weight, organ to brain weight ratios should be analyzed.

CLINICAL DETERMINATIONS

General and Statistical Considerations

In the course of a chronic study, it is customary to monitor the state of the body fluids at several intervals, i.e., 3, 12, 18, and 24 months in rats. At these intervals, blood is collected from one of several sites (retroorbital sinus, tail tip, heart, or aorta, depending on the fate of the animal). Venipuncture is usual for large species, while blood is collected from the retroorbital sinus or the tail tip in rodents destined to continue treatment in the chronic study. Rodents may be bled from the abdominal aorta at the time of sacrifice. This permits greater amounts of blood to be collected for special purposes. Bleeding methods which require the technician to "milk" the blood out of the animal (such as cutting off the tip of the tail) run the risk of obtaining anomalous results on concentrations of microscopic or high molecular weight components. For routine hematologic and chemical determinations, no more than 1–2 ml of blood are required if newer microanalytical methods are used. This is important in mouse studies, in which it was once necessary to pool blood from several animals to provide enough blood to perform the desired analyses.

Clinical characteristics of blood are generally investigated in plasma obtained from blood mixed with an anticoagulant (heparin, EDTA, sodium citrate, sodium oxalate, etc.). The choice of anticoagulant depends on the analyses to be performed. For red blood cell (RBC) cholinesterase and serum alkaline phosphatase determinations, heparin is the anticoagulant of choice since chelating anticoagulants interfere with the assay.

Plasma to be used for clinical evaluation must be clear and straw-colored in appearance. Hemolysis, depending on extent, is associated with lower hematocrit and red blood cell concentration, elevated serum lactic dehydrogenase, alanine and aspartate aminotransferases, alkaline phosphatase, and creatinine. These are the RBC components released into the blood. The hemoglobin released by hemolysis interferes with photometric measurements of bilirubin and with chemical reactions needed to measure lipase activity.

When conducting clinical evaluations on a series of animals, it is a good policy to submit duplicate samples from 10 randomly selected animals to the clinical laboratory. The data from these samples may be analyzed to provide an estimate of the laboratory repeatability. The samples which are coded as duplicate would not be included in the statistical analysis of the results.

Statistical analyses for hematologic tests often reveal *statistically significant* results in pretest treatment groups. It is obvious that these results could not be *toxicologically significant* since treatment will not have been initiated. The "significant" results must be attributed to chance. The dilemma that this introduces is how to know which of the posttreatment significant results are due to chance and which are due to treatment.

Significant treatment differences can arise from systematic error. It is not unusual for technicians to bleed (in sequence) control, low-, mid-, and high-dose animals. This practice is dangerous since endogenous diurnal cycles of blood constituents may be rising or falling during the period of bleeding. This would introduce a *dose-related* rise or fall in concentration of the affected constituent. It is obvious that blood constituents from nutrient sources often decrease with time after eating (e.g., lipids), so animals are fasted to prevent this complication. But this does not eliminate the cycles of blood concentration found for glucose. For example, when control, young adult male rats were fasted and bled throughout the day, the glucose level was highest at 10 a.m. and 2 p.m. with troughs at 11:30 a.m. and 4 p.m. Thus, if control, low-, mid-, and high-dose groups were bled sequentially between 10 a.m. and noon (how often has that been done?), a dose-related depression of blood glucose would be obtained. To avoid the needless mess provided by this situation, one should randomly distribute animals to be bled from all treatment groups across the duration of the bleeding period of the day. Some investigators claim that animals that were randomly distributed at the beginning of the study need not be rerandomized later because, after all, random is random. However, animals become "ordered" merely by being housed in a specific cage at a specific position in the room and must be randomized to eliminate the effect of being ordered; systematic error can arise if this is not recognized. Randomization may not eliminate all of the "chance" treatment effects to be seen.

Some other precautions may be desirable. Often 5 animals per sex per treatment group are sampled for interim clinical evaluation. Using so few animals encourages the occurrence of inexplicable results, especially when the results are so often analyzed by a series of *t*-tests, each pitting a treatment group against its appropriate control. A better method of analysis would be an analysis of variance within each sex; better yet, one should employ a two-factor analysis and determine the effect of *sex* as well as *treatment* on the parameters being studied. If statistically significant differences occur using analyses of variance, the response should be dose-related before attributing toxicologic significance to the differences.

Care should be taken not to dismiss significant differences

because the values fall in the normal range. For instance, the range for serum alkaline phosphatase (SAP) values of the rat from several of our studies at the Food and Drug Research Laboratories is 56.8–128 IU/liter. This wide range is due to the ever-decreasing SAP values with age after weaning. A high value in an aged animal may be clearly significant, even though the value may fall within the normal range that was generated by including young and old control animals in the historical file. Average SAP values for male and female control rats evaluated at several intervals during a 2-year test decrease from approximately 150 IU/liter at 4 weeks to 85 IU/liter at 26 weeks and slowly decline to 70 IU/liter at 104 weeks. Paget (10) presents a lower range 40–95 IU/liter with a note "specifically lower in adult animals."

Rules for decreasing false significant differences are as follows:

1. Randomize animals.
2. Use sufficient numbers of animals.
3. Use appropriate statistical analysis.
4. Look for dose–response relationships.
5. Compare data with appropriate historical values from animals of similar age, sex, and physiologic state.
6. Never use plasma samples that are hemolyzed.

Hematology

The classic hematologic parameters are the erythrocyte count, leukocyte count, differential leukocyte count, and hemoglobin, hematocrit, platelets, and reticulocyte counts. From these data, the mean corpuscular hemoglobin (MCH) and mean corpuscular volume (MCV) can be calculated. With the added concern for blood dyscrasias, it behooves the investigator to examine red cell fragility, sedimentation rate, and coagulation factors, and to closely examine the bone marrow.

Generally, hematologic evaluations are carried out at several intervals throughout the study. These assays, along with the clinical chemistry assays, should be conducted on at least 10–15 animals per sex per group selected at random. It is critical that the blood be taken in the same manner for each sampling.

It is often desirable to perform pretreatment or time zero assays to establish baseline values. The value of zero time assays is underscored when one considers *early onset leukemia* in mice. This random phenomenon in some strains would be missed if initial hematologic evaluations were not conducted. Being unaware of the background leukocyte count could lead to a false positive finding of treatment-related leukemia.

Evaluation of bone marrow is a more tedious procedure. The most beneficial approach is to remove a section of a long bone at necropsy, allow the marrow to fix in the shaft, process the marrow, and examine its contents. The major variable in marrow examination is the site of sampling. In rodents, the epiphyseal plates of the femurs can be clipped, and the complete shaft fixed. In larger animals, the femur is a good site for sampling, but a standard distance from one of the epiphyseal plates should be selected.

A word of caution in handling long bones of dogs, monkeys, pigs, etc., must be offered. In general, the femur of the

adult animal is well developed and must be sampled using a Stryker saw or hand saw. Do not place the bone on the table when sawing. The vibration causes scrambling and movement of the marrow and, in some cases, complete loss of marrow from the shaft. Rather, score the shaft longitudinally and then sever the shaft in a 5–8-cm length. A rongers can then be positioned into the score marks and the bone split.

Differential White Cell Count

White cells are classed as neutrophils, basophils, lymphocytes, eosinophils, and monocytes. Occasionally, the relative quantity of one or more of these changes dramatically. Some specific changes are listed here with common interpretations:

1. *Neutrophils.* Elevated with acute infections (especially cocci), tissue necrosis (and hemolysis), strenuous exercise, convulsions, tachycardia, and acute hemorrhage.
2. *Lymphocytes.* Elevated with acute infection and chronic infection, e.g., hepatitis or malnutrition.
3. *Basophils.* Depressed in hyperthyroidism.
4. *Eosinophils.* Elevated with allergy, irradiation, pernicious anemia, parasitism, and some poisons, e.g., phosphorous or black widow spider venom.
5. *Monocytes.* Elevated with protozoal infection and some poisons, e.g., tetrachloroethane.

Nonspecific elevation of white blood cells, termed a *leukemia-like disorder,* may be due to acute hemolysis or hemorrhage, severe burns, mercury poisoning, or stress. Leukopenia, or nonspecific depression of white blood cells, may be associated with some infections, inanition and debilitation, splenic disorders, and intoxication with chemical agents, for example, sulphonamides or arsenicals. False leukopenia may also appear when automated cell counting is performed on white cells that have a tendency to clump or lyse. Unexpected occurrence of leukopenia is the obvious indication for manual counting to avoid errors in interpretation. It may be worth mentioning that mere shipment of animals is associated with leukocyte elevation in the blood. The elevated levels may persist for 3–8 weeks—the longer the transportation time, the longer the effect. Thus, one should be careful when placing animals on a test which have been received on different dates.

Clinical Chemistry

Clinical chemistry evaluations have been a major area of concern to the toxicologist for several reasons. The first concern is the variability of results. Standardized techniques have to be applied within any one laboratory, and an intralaboratory variance has to be established before the values have meaning. The second concern is the value of the change observed. It is assumed that intracellular damage in the laboratory rodent manifests itself in the same fashion as damage or physiologic alteration manifests itself in humans. A basic assumption in animal testing is that the results reflect what will occur in the exposed human.

The introduction of automated equipment in human clinical laboratories has channeled the toxicologist's approach to clinical chemistry by permitting almost effortless analysis of such classical serum enzymes as alkaline phosphatase (SAP), alanine aminotransferase, and aspartate aminotransferase (formerly known as SGPT and SGOT, respectively), and sorbitol dehydrogenase, which serve as indicators of liver toxicity. The electrolytes and blood urea nitrogen (BUN) along with creatinine are the major measures of renal function and remain major assays for the toxicologist. Several other enzyme systems have been suggested for aiding in diagnosis of organ damage, but the criteria of repeatability and interpretability in the laboratory animal must be followed.

Before selecting a battery of tests, it is better to evaluate organ specific activity during the early studies (acute and subchronic) and to focus on the areas of concern in the chronic study. A thumbnail sketch of common clinical chemistry evaluations is provided below.

Bilirubin

Arising from the breakdown of red blood cells, the major amount of bilirubin is bound to albumin in blood but is termed *free bilirubin*. Bilirubin is converted to the glucuronide form in the liver. In liver blockage, the yellowish cast to tissues is due to hyperbilirubinemia. Plasma bilirubin is also elevated with prolonged fasting and hemolysis.

Amylase

This enzyme hydrolyzes 1,4-glucosidic linkages of starch to form dextrins, maltotetrose, maltotriose, maltose, and glucose. Amylase is elevated in pancreatitis and renal insufficiency and depressed in hepatobiliary toxicity.

Creatine and creatinine

Known as methyl-guanacetic acid and its anhydride, respectively, these compounds are important in the physiology of muscle contraction. Normally, creatine is found in muscle, whereas creatinine is the waste product found in the circulation. Creatine is found in urine in some muscular disorders. Values for creatinine are elevated in younger and more active animals. There is an elevation of serum creatinine after eating meat; this could be an important consideration in dog studies. Pathologic elevation of serum creatinine occurs with renal failure.

Creatine phosphokinase

This enzyme is found in heart, skeletal muscle, brain, and testes, but not in liver. Elevated levels are found in muscular disorders, myocardial infarction, and pulmonary disorders.

Cholinesterase

True cholinesterase, found in red blood cells, can cleave only acetylcholine, whereas other esterases found in plasma, termed *pseudocholinesterases,* can cleave acetylcholine as well as other esters. Depressions of true and pseudocholinesterases accompany intoxication with some organophosphates and carbamates, as well as certain dietary restrictions.

Nonesterified fatty acids

These are also termed *free fatty acids* and are elevated during fasting and depressed following ingestion of food or glucose and following insulin injection.

Glucose

Glucose is a nutrient in blood that is utilized by all cells of the body, including erythrocytes. For this reason, analyses should be performed soon after blood withdrawal. Samples may be stored for 48 hr if refrigerated and preserved with potassium oxalate. If a glucose oxidase method of assay is used, contamination of samples or glassware with ascorbic acid (vitamin C) will cause false negatives, whereas peroxide and hypochlorite detergents will result in false positives.

Lactic dehydrogenase

This substance is found in all cells capable of glycolysis. Different tissues have different forms of this enzyme, called isoenzymes. Their activity in plasma rises in pernicious anemia, myocardial infarction, pulmonary embolism, renal toxicity, malignant neoplasms, and other disorders. The activity may be depressed following X-ray exposure.

Serum alkaline phosphatase

This substance is found in most tissues, including bone, liver, and kidney; isoenzymes characteristic of different tissues may also be found. These enzymes catalyze the transfer of phosphate to suitable acceptor alcohols. The plasma levels are generally higher in males and decrease with age in both sexes. Elevations are seen following eating and with osteoblastic activity, impairment of liver function, and obstruction of bile flow. Depressions are seen in malnutrition.

Total protein

Depressions are almost always due to a fall in albumin concentrations. This is complicated by compensatory increases in globulins. Thus, determination of total protein is generally not very useful. Measurement of specific proteins are more instructive, for instance:

Albumin: has colloidal osmotic function
Metal binding proteins: ceruloplasmin, lactoferrin, metalothionine
Hemoglobin binding proteins: haptoglobin
Globulins: antibodies
Clotting factors
Trace proteins: hormones, enzymes

Electrolytes

These are sodium, potassium, and chloride. Normally, they are very stable components of blood. However, depressions accompany vomiting and diarrhea, while elevations in concentration are found in renal disorders, dehydration, and cardiac failure.

Aminotransferases

Aspartate and alanine aminotransferases, formerly known as glutamic oxalacetic and glutamic pyruvic transaminases, respectively, are elevated following tissue damage in which the cellular enzymes are released from the cells into the bloodstream. Aspartate aminotransferase is found in high constitutive levels in heart and liver, whereas alanine aminotransferase is most active in liver. This latter enzyme increases dramatically in mice following bodily handling as opposed to picking up by the tail.

Uric acid

This end product of purine metabolism is classically elevated in humans with gout. It may also be elevated in renal toxicity and depressed with ACTH treatment.

Urobilinogen

This bacterial product of bilirubin metabolism in the intestines is partially reabsorbed and found in high levels in urine in liver toxicity or disease (cirrhosis and hepatitis).

Urea nitrogen

Generally termed BUN, it is elevated in renal toxicity or disease and with increased protein catabolism but is depressed with overhydration and severe liver damage.

Urinalysis

Urinalysis has been fraught with difficulty and clouded with controversy since the advent of routine analysis in toxicology studies. Generally, the crudest possible procedures are used in collection and analysis of urine. The results and their toxicologic meaning generally correspond with the primitive methods employed.

Analysis of body fluids, be it blood, urine, lymph, or other, is conducted to determine if the source organ(s) is functioning properly or is being taxed beyond its capacity. If the techniques for gathering the fluid are not consistent, the interpretation will not be consistent. Urine is generally collected from troughs or trays placed below the cages in which the animals are housed. The urine so collected is then evaluated for color and cloudiness, pH, and specific gravity; dipstick tests as well as microscopic inspection are employed for particulate matter.

Values of urinary pH may differ by treatment but will not reflect the normal physiologic situation since the dissolved CO_2 will have dissipated, resulting in an elevation of the pH. Hair, dander, and room dust often settle in the urine, to provide interesting viewing for the examiner and to contribute to the specific gravity of the urine. In addition, bacterial populations often develop in the urine collected in this manner. The addition of classic preservatives such as thymol or toluene is scarcely more than a symbolic gesture due to their lack of solubility. Other antibacterial or fungistatic agents would have to be evaluated for their interfering effects on clinical measurements before being used.

The results of urinalyses are generally so variable, especially with the current tendency to evaluate 5 animals per sex per group, as to be meaningless. If there is a real concern and reason to consider urinalysis important enough to characterize well, then it should be important enough to devote sufficient animals to the analyses so that the animals may be sacrificed with urine collected directly from the bladder and analyzed by sensitive means. Again, be sure to randomly select animals from different treatment groups throughout the day of collection, since the first urine of the day may be decidedly different from that collected at other times of the day. As an example, the clarity of urine of saccharin-treated male rats is reported to be visibly diminished in the first urine sample of the lights-on period, but clear at all other collection intervals during the day.

Finally, the clinical chemistry of urine may provide toxicologic information as follows:

1. *Ketonuria:* Elevated in starvation and low carbohydrate diets.
2. *Prophyrinuria:* Elevated in lead poisoning and hepatic disorders, e.g., cirrhosis and other liver damage.
3. *Hemoglobinuria/hematuria:* Elevated in direct toxicity, e.g., naphthalene, sulfonamides, ethylene glycol.
4. *Glucosuria:* Occurs in diabetes.
5. *Osmolality:* Usually crudely estimated by measuring specific gravity. Indicates degree to which kidney concentrates the urine. Osmolality decreases with some types of nephrotoxicity, e.g., high-output renal failure.
6. *pH:* Generally meaningless unless outside the range of 6.0–7.0. Urine in the bladder has lower pH than urine in the collection trough because dissolved CO_2 is liberated following urination.
7. *Crystalluria:* This occurs when urine becomes supersaturated in crystal forming molecule(s). May precede kidney stones or bladder stones.

Blood Levels of Test Material

The complex field of pharmacokinetics cannot be covered in this review, but one aspect should be mentioned. It is reasonable to check blood levels of the test material throughout the duration of the chronic test at a specified time after dosing or after lights on. It is normal, in such tests, to administer the test material on a dose per unit body weight basis. One must understand that body weight is the sum of weights of all tissues and that these tissues do not vary allometrically (in the same ratio to body weight) over the life of an animal. Rats put on weight primarily in the form of fat after they are 2–4 months old. Thus, increments in doses are largely in response to added fat. The dose of material thereby increases at a rate faster than the increase in lean body mass. If fat is not an active metabolizing or storage compartment for the test material, increases in blood concentration of the compound may be seen with age and increase in body weight. Such findings could easily be misinterpreted, for instance, as an inhibition of metabolizing enzyme activity. Thus, once again, body weight is seen as a poor indicator of the quantity that the investigator is really in search of—lean body mass.

Histopathology

This section is not written to present a histopathology primer. One of the best techniques for histopathology examination is now used by the NTP. The primary stains used in toxicopathology are hematoxylin and eosin (H&E). The pathologist's responsibility is to evaluate the normal and abnormal tissues and to account for all the lesions reported at necropsy. The quality control function of the pathology team is critical for the evaluation of a chemical (1).

STATISTICS

When a test is completed and the data have all been recorded, the interpretation of toxicity is often not obvious. That is to say, the toxicologic meaning must be derived from statistical analyses. But just as a researcher can use inappropriate toxicologic methods, so can also inappropriate statistical methods be used to support one's conclusions. If appropriate statistical tests reveal a significant effect on a measured parameter; the detected effect may not be meaningful (3). The results may lie within the normal range of variability seen historically for that parameter. Hence, it is not always enough to conduct an adequately designed study—one must also have historical data to give a proper perspective to the results (5).

The Task Force of Past Presidents of the Society of Toxicology was not pleased with the regulatory decision-making process that cited inappropriate scientific conclusions derived from biological and statistical findings of toxicology and epidemiological studies. The superficial and inappropriate application of statistics can have lasting and detrimental consequences depending on who believes the erroneous conclusions. Because we have computers that can perform complex statistical procedures does not mean that the results of their application are either correct or appropriate. The report of the Past Presidents should be required reading for all toxicologists (11).

REPORTS

Finally, it is worth stating that, like the tree that falls unattended in the forest, a toxicology study that is conducted,

but not reported, makes no impact. When the report is written, it should be clear and concise enough to convey the meaningful findings of the study with proper detail to permit the reader to introduce his or her own level of experience into the interpretation.

CONCLUSIONS

This chapter may seem to be a patchwork quilt of facts and fantasies in toxicity testing. If so, perhaps some of the unstated threads that are woven into this area can be connected. First, for any chronic evaluation, the experimental designs and setup should be logical and based on the background knowledge of the test material. There is no reason to adhere to a standard protocol if it is inappropriate for the specific test material. Second, be sure the statistical design is one that can be analyzed appropriately when the study is over. Third, the experiment should be run as though each day was the first day of the experiment. That is, the same care, caution, and enthusiasm should be maintained throughout the study as existed on the first day. Finally, enough information should be recorded, and reported, so that anyone else could duplicate the test exactly as conducted—"warts" and all.

REFERENCES

1. Boorman, G. A., et al. (1985): Quality assurance in pathology for rodent carcinogenicity studies. In: *Handbook of Carcinogen Testing,* edited by H. Milman and E. Weisburger, pp. 345–357. Noyes Publications, Park Ridge, NJ.
2. DHEW Publication (1977): Guide for Care and Use of Laboratory Animals. NIH 77-23.
3. Gart, J. J., Chu, K. C., and Tarone, R. E. (1979): Statistical issues in interpretation of chronic bioassay tests for carcinogenicity. *J. Natl. Cancer Inst.,* 62:957–974.
4. Gillette, J., Weisburger, E. K., Kraybill, H., and Kelsey, M. (1985): Strategies for determining the mechanisms of toxicity. *Clin. Toxicol.,* 23(1):1–78.
5. Haseman, J. K., Huff, J., and Boorman, G. A. (1984): Use of historical control data in carcinogenicity studies in rodents. *Toxicol. Pathol.,* 12:126–135.
6. National Academy of Sciences (1971): *Defining the Laboratory Animal.* National Academy of Sciences, Washington, D.C.
7. National Academy of Sciences (1987): *Complex Mixtures.* National Academy of Sciences/National Research Council, Washington, D.C.
8. Fingl, E. (1980): *The Pharmacologic Basis of Therapeutics,* 6th ed., edited by A. G. Gilman, L. S. Goodman, and A. Gilman. Macmillan, New York.
9. Paget, G. E. (1970): *Methods in Toxicology,* edited by G. E. Paget. F. A. Davis Company, Philadelphia.
10. Snyder, D. R., Gralla, E. J., Coleman, G. L., and Wedig, J. H. (1977): Preliminary Neurological Evaluation of Generalized Weakness in Zinc Pyrithione-treated Rats. *Food and Cosmetic Toxicol.,* 15:43–47.
11. Task Force of Past Presidents (1982): Animal data in hazard evaluation: Paths and pitfalls. *Fund. Appl. Toxicol.,* 2:101–107.
12. Umbreit, T. H., Hesse, E. J., and Gallo, M. A. (1986): Bioavailability of Dioxin in soil from a 2,4,5-T manufacturing site. *Science,* 232:497–499.
13. Wolf, F. J. (1980): Effect of overloading pathways on toxicity. *J. Environ. Pathol. Toxicol.,* 3:113–134.

Principles and Methods of Toxicology, Second Edition, edited by A. Wallace Hayes, Raven Press, Ltd., New York © 1989.

CHAPTER 9

Methods of Testing for Carcinogenicity

J. F. Robens, *W. W. Piegorsch, and **R. L. Schueler

*USDA/ARS, Beltsville Agricultural Research Center, Beltsville, Maryland 20705; *National Institute of Environmental Health Sciences, National Institutes of Health, Research Triangle Park, North Carolina 27709; and **6271 Old Washington Road, Sykesville, Maryland 21784*

Quality Control of the Test Chemicals
  Test Chemical • Dosage Mixture • Effect of Highly Toxic Impurities or Contaminants
Animals and Their Environment
  Species and Strain • Feed and Water • Caging • Ventilation, Temperature, Humidity, Emergency Power
Route of Administration
  Oral Gavage and Feed • Dermal Route • Inhalation Including Intratracheal Administration • Parenteral Administration

Clinical Examination and Health of Animals
Prechronic Studies for Dose Setting
  Type and Length of Studies • Repeated-Dose Study • Subchronic Study • Role of Pathology • Metabolism and Kinetic Studies • Dose Setting
Chronic Study
  Design • Pathology • Statistical Analyses
Transplacental Carcinogenesis
Health and Safety Procedures
Documents Considering Testing for Carcinogenicity
References

Testing for carcinogenicity has become a national priority in the United States and has taken a substantial share of both federal and industrial research dollars and resources. As of this writing there are 21 major federal laws related to exposures to toxic substances. These laws and their respective areas of concern are listed in Table 1 (111).

Testing for carcinogenicity has as many legal components as it has scientific. The implications of a positive finding that are greater than for any other toxic effect emanate from (a) the public concern of developing cancer from new and unknown substances and (b) uncertainty surrounding our evaluation of the relative hazards of small amounts of carcinogenic chemicals. Even with extensive investigation we do not generally understand the biological mechanisms of chemical toxicity sufficiently well to be able to extrapolate from a test species to humans accurately enough to quantify the hazard associated with exposure to specific chemicals. This concern has led to the philosophy of absolute exclusion embodied in some of the laws listed in Table 1, starting with that of the Food Additives Amendment to the Food, Drug, and Cosmetics Act in 1958. Thus the approval for use of a substance associated with significant increase in tumors has become difficult, time-consuming, and expensive. The testing process is subject to intense scrutiny by government, industry, and public interest groups. Both the state of the art of testing and

the action on any given chemical are continually examined by committees of Congress, the Executive branch of government, the industry seeking to market "new" chemicals or save "old" ones or the products containing them, and "environmental factions" wishing to protect the populace from potential harm.

Present methods for testing for carcinogenicity have evolved from the basic long-term studies in rodents first initiated on a large scale during the 1960s. We still use the same basic procedures today but in the context of a mature science utilizing, for instance, sufficient numbers of animals to yield statistically significant results and quality control procedures for all aspects of the studies. These improved controls have greatly increased public confidence in the results of testing.

Many sophisticated short-term tests for determining genotoxicity have been developed, but they are used primarily for screening for genetic toxicity. They have not replaced the classic carcinogenicity studies because the correlation between genotoxicity and carcinogenicity is not as direct as was originally hoped. The tests do not necessarily screen for all potential means of early detection of tumors and mimic only a part of the reactions that would occur *in vivo* (61).

Tumors can be induced by a number of agents including radiation, biological agents, and chemicals of diverse origin. They apparently originate as alterations in the genetic pro-

TABLE 1. *Federal laws related to exposures to toxic substances*

Legislation	Agency	Area of concern
Food, Drug and Cosmetics Act (1906, 1938, amended 1958, 1960, 1962, 1968, 1976)	FDA	Food, drugs, cosmetics, food additives, color additives, new drugs, animal and feed additives, medical devices
Federal Insecticide, Fungicide and Rodenticide Act (1948, amended 1972, 1975, 1978)	EPA	Pesticides
Dangerous Cargo Act (1952)	DOT, USCG	Water shipment of toxic materials
Atomic Energy Act (1954)	NRC	Radioactive substances
Federal Hazardous Substances Act (1960, amended 1981)	CPSC	Toxic household products
Federal Meat Inspection Act (1967) Poultry Products Inspection Act (1968) Egg Products Inspection Act (1970)	USDA	Food, feed, color additives, pesticide residues
Occupational Safety and Health Act (1970)	OSHA, NIOSH	Workplace toxic chemicals
Poison Prevention Packaging Act (1970, amended 1981)	CPSC	Packaging of hazardous household products
Clean Air Act (1970, amended, 1974, 1977)	EPA	Air pollutants
Hazardous Materials Transportation Act (1972)	DOT	Transport of hazardous materials
Clean Water Act (formerly Federal Water Control Act) (1972, amended 1977, 1978)	EPA	Water pollutants
Marine Protection, Research and Sanctuaries Act (1972)	EPA	Ocean dumping
Consumer Product Safety Act (1972, amended 1981)	CPSC	Hazardous consumer products
Lead-Based Paint Poison Prevention Act (1973, amended 1976)	CPSC, HHS, HUD	Use of lead paint in federally assisted housing
Safe Drinking Water Act (1974, amended 1977)	EPA	Drinking water contaminants
Resource Conservation and Recovery Act (1976)	EPA	Solid waste, including hazardous wastes
Toxic Substances Control Act (1976)	EPA	Hazardous chemicals not covered by other laws, includes premarket review
Federal Mine Safety and Health Act (1977)	DOL, NIOSH	Toxic substances in coal and other mines
Comprehensive Environmental Response, Compensation, and Liability Act (1981)	EPA	Hazardous substances, pollutants, contaminants

grams or information content of cells and in the subsequent fixation and replication of those alterations. The specific changes in DNA sequences associated with certain tumors are just now beginning to be delineated.

Carcinogenesis is believed to be a multistage phenomenon that may involve the genome both directly and indirectly through two operational stages, i.e., neoplastic conversion of the cell, often referred to as initiation, and neoplastic development (166). Neoplastic *conversion* is the process in which a normal cell is transformed to a neoplastic cell, and neoplastic *development* is the process of growth of the neoplastic cell into a tumor and the further acquisition of abnormal properties by that tumor (166). The testing addressed in this chapter does not differentiate between these two stages but is concerned primarily with the end result, i.e., the number and type of tumors present when the animal dies or at the termination of the study.

Carcinogenic agents, as with any xenobiotic, may be altered from the time they are ingested or otherwise enter the body until the time they reach the target site. These alterations include (a) interaction or coating with cellular secretions of the lungs (98), and (b) metabolic conversions by microorganisms in the gastrointestinal tract (147), which may occur before the substance has been absorbed. The latter is the most important for polar compounds that are not well ab-

sorbed from the gut and for those that are excreted in the bile. Once the xenobiotic has been absorbed, it may be deactivated, detoxified, and/or reactivated as it is transported throughout the body before finally being excreted or incorporated into cellular macromolecules (166). This metabolism does not take place just in the liver; it may occur in varying amounts in almost any tissue. For example, nasal epithelium can activate chemical carcinogens (27), and lung, kidney, and intestinal epithelium contain substantial amounts of metabolizing enzymes.

Miller and Miller (99) have proposed a generally accepted mechanism for the reaction of metabolically activated agents with cells: The ultimate carcinogenic forms of organic chemical carcinogens are electrophilic (electron-deficient), and they bind with intracellular nucleophilic (electron-rich) macromolecules such as DNA and protein. The reactive metabolites may also react with other nucleophiles, e.g., glutathione and water, to form polar and less biologically reactive metabolites that are easily excreted. This sequence of alterations, both parenteral and preparenteral, helps explain some of the reasons for species differences in the apparent potency of carcinogens. If sufficient reactive metabolite is not formed or is not available at the target site for the required reaction time, the substance is not carcinogenic in that species. Lesser quantitative alterations in the pattern of both activation and deactivation of a particular agent may also account for individual differences in tumor formation among individuals of a species.

Positive results from long-term carcinogenicity studies in laboratory animals demonstrate that a test chemical is carcinogenic to animals under the conditions of the test and indicate that exposure to the chemical has the potential for hazard to humans. However, these studies do not explain why the lesions occurred and provide only a general, albeit the best available, basis for extrapolation to humans. The relevance of laboratory animal studies is supported by the fact that known human carcinogens, with one possible exception, are carcinogenic in appropriately conducted studies in some animal systems (111). Also, many chemicals are known to have similar pharmacologic and pathologic effects on humans and test animals and frequently produce carcinogenic effects at the same target organ (164). Although laboratory animal studies are not infallible, most scientists working in the area agree with the principle set forth by the International Agency for Research on Cancer (77) and endorsed by the Office of Science and Technology Policy (OSTP) (111) that "in the absence of adequate data on humans, it is reasonable, for practical purposes, to regard chemicals for which there is sufficient evidence of carcinogenicity in animals as if they presented a carcinogenic risk to humans."

When an alleged carcinogenic chemical is considered highly important either to society or to its sponsor, an extensive sophisticated series of tests designed to elucidate the metabolic pathways, factors altering this pathway, ultimate carcinogenic forms, and pathogenesis of the lesions are necessary. The extensive scope of possible modulation of activity was outlined by Williams (166).

A closely associated area not covered in this chapter is the study of carcinogenic effects of nonionizing radiation. In this case the dosimetry must be carefully designed and controlled by persons having the appropriate scientific expertise. However, all other aspects of such studies, including such factors as the animals, length and types of studies, assessment of lesions, and statistical analysis of results, are no different than for studies using chemicals.

QUALITY CONTROL OF THE TEST CHEMICALS

Test Chemical

Quality control of the test chemical is necessary to determine that the chemical is actually what it is expected to be at all times during a study. It is particularly important with carcinogenicity and other long-term toxicity studies because of the funds and time invested. The first step in a quality control program is to obtain all relevant information on the test chemical, including synonyms and trade names, structural and molecular formulas and weight, and the methods of analysis, including chemical and physical properties of the pure substance. Also, the method of manufacture or route of synthesis, if known, may help determine what impurities are present. After the chemical is obtained, at least the following factors must be checked and controlled when nec-

essary: (a) identity of the major ingredient, with identification and quantification of impurities; (b) homogeneity of the product; (c) particle size; and (d) stability of the known or suspected active ingredients. All of these factors need to be considered for the test chemical both as obtained and in the vehicle used for administering the chemical. These points were considered more fully by Jameson (79).

An adequate method(s) for identification and quantification for the long-term storage of the test agent is necessary prior to initiating the first animal studies, and samples are analyzed periodically during the studies to determine if the test chemical has retained its original characteristics. When possible, the same batch of chemical is used throughout all test phases of a bioassay for carcinogenicity, and certainly the same batch is necessary for the entire chronic study. Accelerated stability studies may be conducted, but only periodic tests over the duration of the study can determine if in fact the compound is stable with time. Therefore initial analyses are vital to identify and quantify all impurities with some sort of "fingerprinting" technique (168). If more chemical is required, the new batch should be as close as possible to the old one.

Chemicals that are hydroscopic present special problems. When put in cold storage and warmed to room temperature, they tend to absorb water. Compounds that decompose or form addition products or polymerize in the presence of water need special handling. Toluene diisocyanate, for example, which is known to polymerize with water, can apparently absorb water from corn oil and form dimers, a white insoluble precipitate (38).

Dosage Mixture

Chemicals to be given by gavage, skin paint, or various routes of parenteral administration are ideally soluble and chemically stable in the vehicle used. When it is not possible, mixtures in a suspending agent can be used for gavage and skin painting. If corn oil is used, it must be periodically checked for rancidity (see also the section Oral Gavage and Feed, below).

The analytical methods for the active ingredients need to be modified for the vehicle being used, particularly the difficult and complex matrix afforded by animal feed. The precision and accuracy of the method, along with the limits of detection, must be known prior to sampling. Mixing protocols are developed before use to help ensure the stability of the test chemical in the feed. If stability is highly temperature-dependent, storage at low temperatures or more frequent mixing may be necessary.

All batches of dosage preparations are analyzed for accuracy in the mixing process, and the turn-around time for the analysis of dosage mixtures must be short enough to allow confirmation of accurate preparation prior to use. A misdosage could result in inadequate exposure to the test chemical, untoward toxicity, or even animal death.

At the beginning of the subchronic study, one sample of each dosage mixture for any route of administration is analyzed in duplicate to demonstrate the effectiveness of the mixing procedure and the analytical method. The length of time an insoluble chemical remains homogeneously suspended is checked to determine if either constant mixing or remixing at intervals is required even while dosing is in progress (38). In addition, for dosed-feed studies, three samples are taken from the blender (e.g., top left, top right, and bottom of twin shell blender with intensifier bar) at the highest and lowest concentrations and analyzed in duplicate to check the homogeneity of the mixture.

Quality control of the test material continues through its administration in the various control and dosage mixtures. This method prevents using a test mixture from an incorrect container and thus underdosing or, more critically, overdosing certain groups. Some suggestions include different-shaped bottles for the different species, color coding of various dosage concentrations, complete labeling indicating compound names, number, species, dosage group, different refrigerators for rat and mouse dosage mixtures or at the least individual racks on different shelves, and handling and removal of only one chemical at a time by any technician.

Effect of Highly Toxic Impurities or Contaminants

Three examples demonstrate the necessity of performing adequate chemical analysis. The first is that of 1,1,1-trichloroethane (methylchloroform). Assays of this chemical showed it to be present at an average of 95.5%; however, an additional component, p-dioxane, a protein-denaturing agent added to the commercial product as a stabilizer was found to be present at 3.7%. This compound is known to cause carcinomas of both the nasal cavity and the liver (5,6,72). In this case it is not clear whether an observed carcinogenic response could be attributed to methylchloroform treatment or to the presence of the stabilizing agent. The presence of p-dioxane illustrates the problem of using a commercial product rather than the pure chemical and raises the question of whether the product to be tested should be the one to which the public is exposed. Because exposure of humans usually involves a mixture of chemicals, often changing in relative amounts, the effects of testing technical grade versus highly purified substances must be carefully considered, although it is usually preferable to test analytical grade chemicals.

A second example is that of octachlorodibenzo-p-dioxin, a dioxin of lesser toxicity than others. A chemical analysis showed that the product was 99% pure, but the impurities included 0.4 to 0.6% heptachlorodibenzo-p-dioxin and 0.02 to 0.03% hexachlorodibenzo-p-dioxin. These impurities could not be removed by various attempted procedures. The toxicity of heptachlorodibenzo-p-dioxin has not been established; however, hexachlorodibenzo-p-dioxin is highly toxic (94). Because of the significant toxicity of the contaminants, a meaningful test of the toxicity of octochlorodibenzo-p-dioxin was not possible.

Another example of the possible "confounding" effects of impurities is the varying amounts of o-toluenesulfonamide (OTS) in different batches of saccharin that were used in the early carcinogenicity studies of this compound. Because the test animals in these early studies were exposed to the varying amounts of OTS present, tumors that appeared could not be attributed to saccharin itself (100).

ANIMALS AND THEIR ENVIRONMENT

Species and Strain

Animals used in carcinogenicity studies must (a) be reasonable in cost to allow for adequately large numbers of both test and control animals; (b) have a life-span within both the financial capabilities of the sponsor to maintain them and the public health and political time constraints for determining an answer, i.e., 2 to 3 years; and (c) be well adapted to the laboratory environment without serious interfering infectious disease. Thus the choice of species is practically limited at this time to mice (52), rats, and occasionally hamsters (1,139). Guinea pigs, rabbits, dogs (14), monkeys, or other species may be considered if the metabolism of the compound and its availability at the expected target site are similar to that in humans and if the value or extensive use of the test product warrants the extra cost. Strains of rodents with reasonable longevity are needed, i.e., 18 months to 2 years for mice, and 2.0 to 2.5 years for rats. Animal strains with shorter life-spans, e.g., the A-strain mouse, are used only in special test systems utilizing their particular sensitivities (137,138). When the information is available, the strains chosen are those most likely to be susceptible, but not hypersensitive, to cancer from the particular test chemical. For example, it is difficult to interpret the significance of the proliferative liver lesions in the widely used B6C3F1 hybrid mouse because of high background incidence in the male mice (67,116).

It is important for the testing laboratory to establish the background tumor incidence and other lesions of aging to help determine if the incidence of tumors among the controls in any specific test is representative of reported tumor incidences and remains stable through years of testing (11,18,21,34,49,51,67,96,132,136,156,157).

Use of at least two species to test any chemical helps compensate for genetic differences in tumor susceptibility and to reduce the incidence of false-negative results. Similarly, equal numbers of animals of both sexes help detect certain tumors more characteristic of one sex than of the other, e.g., mammary tumors in females and certain liver tumors in males. Inbred or hybrid strains are believed to produce more precise and more stable biological responses; however, inbred strains are subject to deterioration from genetic drift. When one or more histological or biochemical parameters measurable in the growing rodent (167) are known to be associated with the tumor, subchronic studies may be used to select the genetically defined inbred or F_1 hybrid animal stocks most appropriate for the chronic study.

Feed and Water

The composition of the laboratory animal feed including possible contaminants is established, held as constant as possible throughout the study, and checked by periodic analyses; these results are retained for inclusion in the final report. Naturally occurring toxic substances such as nitrosamines (35,107,109,110) and aflatoxins (108) may occur in animal feeds, although the latter was not found in a survey of the feeds of one major manufacturer (22). If diets for laboratory animals are subjected to heat during their manufacture or to a steam-sterilization process to decrease volatile nitrosamine concentrations, the effects of such procedures on the test substance and dietary constituents should be established (82). In Coleman and Tardiff's (22) survey, the levels of chlorinated hydrocarbon insecticides were too low to quantify despite constant occurrence. Limits for contaminants have been established in the National Toxicology Program's General Statement of Work for Conduct of Acute, 14-Day Repeated Dose, 90-Day Subchronic, and 2-Year Chronic Studies in Laboratory Animals.

It remains common practice to feed the same diet throughout the life-span of the test animals because of inadequate knowledge of nutrient requirements of different age rodents as well as for simplicity. However, a diet formulated for young, growing rodents may not be an optimum diet for longevity. Caloric intake has been shown to influence the life-span of rats (21,89,90,124,170) in conventional as well as barrier-maintained housing, to delay age-associated changes in kidney function (154), and to affect the incidence of spontaneous tumors (120,126). (See also the section on oral administration by gavage and feed.) An effect of the chemical on the range of individual body weights may indirectly alter survival and tumor incidence (155). Varying amounts of naturally occurring enzyme inducers and inhibitors from plant material in animal feeds may affect tumor incidence or other parameters following long-term feeding (58,88,119,146). Similarly, with dietary protein, Silverstone and Tannenbaum (141) showed that increases in sulfur-containing amino acids were associated with increases in spontaneous hepatomas in C3H mice, and Ross and Bras (125) demonstrated that chronic marginal protein undernutrition in rats led to earlier and more frequent tumors. In a comparison of caloric and protein restrictions with Wistar rats fed a synthetic diet, caloric restrictions decreased mature body weight and increased survival, whereas protein restriction had no effect on mature body weight but decreased survival (28). The effect of variations in components of the diet on carcinogenesis has been reviewed by Gilbert et al. (49), Newberne (107,108), Tannenbaum (150), and Kraft (85).

Purified and semipurified diets may be employed to reduce the incidence of contaminants, and they are less likely to vary in nutrient content; however, they are expensive and present problems of mixing, handling, and palatability. Furthermore, the incidence of tumors using these diets may vary from that observed with the usual laboratory diets and would have to be reestablished for any animal strain used.

Open-formula feeds are usually recommended, as both the individual ingredients of an open formula and their concentrations are known at all times. In contrast, the ingredients and amounts of a closed formula can be changed by the manufacturer at will, as dictated by availability and price. However, even with an open formula the nutritional profile of the diet may vary with changes in the source of the ingredients, a different year's crop, or different handling conditions for the ingredient. A comparison of open- and closed-formula diets in three strains of laboratory mice showed no differences in the reproduction parameters measured (83).

Caging

No adequate comparison of the effects of single versus group housing on the incidence of tumors is available, although Andervont (3) observed that female mice kept eight to a cage developed fewer mammary tumors more slowly than did mice housed singly. The choice depends on a balancing of many factors: (a) the aggressiveness of the species and strain (male B6C3F1 mice may fight, injure, and cannibalize one another when housed together, whereas the Fischer 344, Sprague-Dawley, and many other rat strains are placid); (b) the space and caging available for the number of animals needed to satisfy the requirements for statistical evaluation; and (c) the method of administration of the test chemical. Single housing is generally needed for (a) inhalation studies to prevent cannibalism because the animals are unavailable for several hours per day in the inhalation chambers, and (b) skin painting studies because the animals may lick and chew their own and their cagemates' irritated skin. This activity leads to ingestion of the test chemical or exacerbation of the lesion and occasionally cannibalization. There are also questions about the assumption of statistical independence of results for individual animals when animals are caged together.

Balancing of dosage groups over rows, columns, and racks allows control of potential location effects across dosage levels. Alternatively, rotation of cages or racks periodically can be used to balance potential confounding sources of variability. Eye lesions (retinal and lenticular degeneration) have been observed in animals kept in cages closest to light (86,122).

Shoebox-type cages are generally preferable to hanging wire cages for long-term holding of animals. Bedding materials and absorbent papers must be free of added antibiotics such as neomycin as well as naturally occurring enzyme inducers as may occur in soft woods (158). These cages allow bedding to be used and provide a more defined environment for the animals by affording greater protection from aerosolized microbial agents.

They are, of course, not feasible for inhalation studies utilizing whole body exposure. Cagetop filters are useful for preventing the spread of disease organisms and particulates in and out of the cages. They may increase the concentration of ammonia in a cage, but they should not be expected to keep volatile chemicals exhaled or eliminated by the animals confined to the cage area. If highly toxic chemicals such as the dioxins are being tested, sealed cages with individual intake and exhaust air systems comprise the most satisfactory method to protect both caretakers and other animals. Laminar flow cage systems provide an intermediate degree of protection. Decreased exposure to disease organisms in these improved housing systems may be associated with a lower incidence of tumors (142).

Each study with a different chemical is conducted in a separate room. More than one animal species can be housed in a room only if they are disease-free and from the same source, have similar microbiological flora, and are placed on test at approximately the same time with the same chemical. Also, it should be recognized that rodents, in particular mice, can be reservoirs of asymptomatic viral disease. Dedicated cages, water bottles, rubber stoppers, and sipper tubes should be considered in order to limit possible cross-contamination among test groups.

Ventilation, Temperature, Humidity, Emergency Power

Environmental stress to test animals must be minimized, particularly with mice, which are easily stressed even when maintained under conventional housing conditions and handled in the usual manner. The incidence of tumors carried by viruses in mice was increased by providing varying degrees of chronic stress (123,135).

Standards for care include: (a) 10 to 15 fresh air changes per hour in each animal room; (b) air pressure adjusted so that the animal rooms are slightly positive to the "dirty" corridor and negative to the "clean" one, with minimal crossovers between the corridors; (c) all air adequately filtered before it enters the animal facility and diluted or filtered after it leaves to prevent possibly toxic concentrations of the test chemical from entering the outside air (a process that is particularly important with inhalation studies because of the large amounts of chemical used); (d) temperature and humidity maintained within those ranges reported to be optimal, i.e., $74° \pm 2°F$ ($23.3° \pm 1.1°C$) and a relative humidity of $40 \pm 5\%$ in rat and mouse rooms (49,74); (e) automatic control systems that record both temperature and humidity at least three or four times per day. Variations of these factors in inhalation studies affect the distribution of the test chemical as well as the health of the animal; (f) control of cockroaches, field mice, and other vermin by adequate building design and sanitary procedures (pesticides are not allowed to contaminate the animal rooms, feed rooms, or cage washing areas and are dispensed only in closed traps in limited areas); (g) detergents and cleaning agents selected for the floors, cage washers, and other equipment to be nonvolatile or otherwise not leave a residue; and (h) emergency power, tested on a regular schedule and with the capacity to provide for the operation of storage freezers and refrigerators, lighting, autotechnicons, and some degree of air-conditioning, as well as air handling, as power failure can occur on extremely hot, humid days. Provision is also made for emergency heat sources and for when personnel are unable to get to work.

The relation of all of the above points regarding housing to the conduct of chronic studies has been reviewed by the Committee on Long Term Handling of Laboratory Rodents (23).

ROUTE OF ADMINISTRATION

Chemicals are generally administered to test animals by the route that most closely mimics the occupational or otherwise predominant method of human exposure unless it is not possible for technical reasons. Different routes of administration are tried in the prechronic studies if any question exists about which is the most appropriate or if there is more than one route of human exposure. Comparison of urinary excretion of radiolabeled compounds and of other qualitative and quantitative measures of chemical disposition and metabolism by each route assists when choosing the route of administration (143). These comparisons are mandatory for

bioassays utilizing gavage or other "atypical" routes of exposure. Significantly different results were obtained in the lung tumor bioassay when comparing intraperitoneal and oral administration (149).

With inhalation exposure, the test compound is absorbed directly from the alveoli into the parenteral circulation, thereby providing initial exposure of the tissues prior to any metabolism in the gastrointestinal tract or liver. However, production of uniform concentrations throughout the exposure chamber is an infinitely more sophisticated and expensive procedure than is obtaining uniformity of chemical in feed or gavage mixtures. It is particularly true with aerosols and dusts. In addition, inhalation facilities are more expensive, and the animals cannot be handled during the exposure period. Thus as a practical matter, oral administration may be considered to replace inhalation unless the effects of the gastrointestinal tract or the initial metabolism by the liver must be avoided or unless the breakdown products in the air would result in a substantially different exposure.

Oral Gavage and Feed

Addition of the test chemical to feed, when possible, is the most cost-efficient method of administration. However, it is difficult to measure feed consumption accurately, and concentrations of the chemical must be recalculated every week as the animals grow if the protocol calls for maintaining a constant milligram per kilogram dosage. It is particularly important for rats, which have large weight gains during the early part of the long-term test period but whose feed intake is not increased proportionally as they grow older. Thus test chemical intake as a factor of body weight is decreased if the chemical percentage in feed is not corrected, and the weanling animal can be markedly overdosed in comparison to the adult.

Dosing by gavage affords the most accurate intake of test chemical, but its suitability for chronic studies is being increasingly questioned. It may be useful where volatility, stability, or palatability are problems. This method does require handling and weighing of both treated and control animals at each dosing, but the additional handling and observation of the animals may be beneficial to the test. It is particularly important to search for a vehicle or dose delivery system that has little or no impact on the final carcinogenicity outcome. Even when it is believed that gavage of animals with the solvent or suspending agent has no effect on tumor incidence in the particular testing laboratory, a second control group of controls, which are not gavaged, are added.

Rats are administered the dose of test material in a volume of 3 to 5 ml/kg. Mice can be given approximately the same volume per unit of body weight, although up to 10 ml/kg has been given for extended periods of time without problems. It is sometimes advantageous to give mice doses in a larger volume on a weight basis to enable the dose to be measured more accurately. The dosing syringes are checked periodically to ensure accuracy in the volume of administration.

The dilution of the test chemical may affect its absorption and the degree of local irritating effect. Both dibromochloropropane and 1,2-dibromoethane produced squamous cell carcinomas of the forestomach, i.e., at the site of initial contact with the test animals (101,103). Unfortunately, because these chemicals are strong carcinogens, no studies were done to test the effects of various dilutions on the mucosa of the stomach and the degree of absorption. Borowitz et al. (17) reported that drugs that are weak acids or weak bases are absorbed more rapidly into the systemic circulation when given orally in dilute rather than in concentrated solution.

Technicians vary greatly in their ability to accurately gavage animals, particularly when pressed to dose large numbers of animals quickly. If unexpected deaths occur, the animals must be necropsied and the lungs and trachea checked closely for the presence of vehicle or test compound. Technician stress may result from handling large, active animals and fatigue from a large workload, and the stress is further increased by gavage dosing in a hood to reduce human exposure. If animals are always dosed in the same order, a large number of deaths in certain groups may be due to this order rather than to the test chemical itself.

It is increasingly recognized that corn oil used as a vehicle in chronic gavage studies may have its own effect on the test results. Recognized effects include (a) an increase in experimental animals' consumption of both calories and fat to amounts not consistent with known dietary requirements (12,85); (b) alteration of the pharmacokinetics of the test chemical; and (c) increased pancreatic tumors in some gavage studies in F344/n rats (15,62,67,120). Moreover, the maximum tolerated doses may have been exceeded in many gavage studies conducted by the National Toxicology Program (NTP) (65). Thus the use of this route of administration must be carefully considered.

The NTP has made considerable progress in evaluating microencapsulation as a means of providing for oral administration of chemicals that are volatile or unstable when included in the diet (97). Microencapsulation is a costly and time-consuming procedure that entails a significant research and development project for each chemical involved, but it should be considered for important chemicals. Other alternatives include (a) the use of powdered basal diets in combination with a small portion of the diet containing the test compound in nonscatter feed cups when the animals normally begin to eat (at night with rodents); and (b) the use of a dispensing agent, e.g., Tween 80, or a suspending agent, e.g., carboxymethylcellulose, for the test compound in an aqueous gavage solvent.

Dermal Route

Test compounds can be administered by skin painting either to study their effects as a skin carcinogen or to use the skin as a portal of entry for whole body exposure. Dermal administration is thus considered for compounds for which there is dermal human exposure, e.g., ethylene chlorohydrin, or in occasional instances for compounds poorly absorbed from the gastrointestinal tract or rapidly destroyed there. The potential of the skin to metabolize the agent to the ultimate carcinogen must be considered if metabolic activation is required. Dermal administration is often used for initiation and promotion studies, not because this method of tumor induction is unique to skin but because the tumors can be easily observed at all stages of development.

When choosing the skin painting route, it must be considered that the test material may (1) adhere or build up at the site of exposure; (2) be partly removed by scratching and licking; or (3) be ingested by the animals, particularly when they are group-housed. The remaining buildup may impede absorption and may even be chemically changed by exposure to air and light. Rats are large enough and vary in size sufficiently to make dosing on an individual milligram per kilogram basis worthwhile. Mice generally do not vary in size sufficiently to justify dosing by individual weight.

The extent of skin penetration in the various test species is variable and has been reviewed by Bock (13). Some strains of mice, e.g., Swiss, have been shown to be remarkably sensitive to the development of skin tumors from the polyaromatic hydrocarbons. However, these mice may be relatively short-lived and would not be the strain of choice when skin is used as a portal of entry for testing a potential carcinogen.

Administration is usually to the anterior dorsal area of the back where the skin is clipped weekly and at least 24 hours prior to skin painting. However, it was noted by Lavbelin et al. (87) that induction of skin tumors was more rapid when the test chemical was applied ventrally rather than dorsally. Usually, 0.25 to 1.00 ml of test material is allowed to flow over the clipped area, and a glass rod is used to rub the material into the skin. The test site must be clearly delineated and closely observed, and individual animal diagrams are used to show the location and size of the lesion. If the test material is irritating, administration is spaced at intervals that allow some recovery between treatments or the material is diluted sufficiently, as determined in subchronic studies. Administration intervals are usually less frequent than for gavage dosing. Too much inflammation results only in local lesions; the animals may also lose their conditioning, become bald, and be susceptible to infections and have compromised survival times. Mite infestations that are not apparent in untreated animals may become clinical problems.

Different compounds penetrate the skin at different rates in different solvents (134). However, the solvents and suspending agents available for skin painting are limited, as many of those formerly used may be either too drying (acetone) or irritating or are carcinogens themselves (benzene). Those with greater coefficients of lipoid solubility may enhance absorption. In addition, the use of a highly volatile and rapidly evaporating solvent as a vehicle may be associated with marked changes in the concentration of the test chemical. Corn oil, water, and possibly ethyl alcohol and carboxymethylcellulose are the best candidates.

Inhalation Including Intratracheal Administration

Whole body exposure is generally utilized for carcinogenicity or other long-term, chronic inhalation studies because the labor costs involved in the daily handling of individual animals for nose cone exposure would be prohibitive. Commonly, animals are exposed 6 hr/day during the usual working day but remain in the inhalation chambers throughout the entire 24-hr period. However, for the same exposure concentration, greater lung burdens may be obtained if rats are exposed at night (70). Some facilities provide space for housing the animals outside the chambers when they are not being exposed, but this method provides no particular advantage. Constant airflow through the chamber at a rate sufficient to avoid the buildup of expired fecal and urinary ammonia is necessary to help ensure animal health. If the estimated maximum tolerated dose (EMTD) for the chronic study is different for the two sexes within a species, planning must be done for a large number of exposure chambers.

It must be recognized that whole body inhalation exposure also includes both dermal and oral exposure because of grooming by the animals, even though feed is generally removed each day prior to initiation of exposure. If exposure is maintained 23 to 24 hr/day, the feed is exposed to the test compound and a greater proportion of the dose may be by oral exposure.

The concentrations achievable in inhalation studies may be limited by the physical properties of the test chemical, in particular its flammability and its explosive properties. With chemicals whose use concentration approaches the lower explosive limits (LEL), continuous monitoring with an automatic alarm system is employed during exposure periods. Continuous or frequent monitoring is also essential to verify (a) actual achievement and maintenance of the desired concentrations of test chemical and (b) the profile of the various particle sizes to ensure that most are in the respirable size range.

Initially, samples of each chemical must be taken from several areas from chambers containing a full animal load to test for layering (nonhomogeneity), but one location is sufficient for continued monitoring throughout the test period. Standard references must be consulted prior to initiation of such studies (60,71,91,106,153).

Intratracheal administration has been used to study the effects of specific chemicals in the respiratory tract and in initiation and promotion studies (127,128,142). Because the animals must be anesthetized with sodium pentobarbital, ketamine, or another suitable anesthetic for the procedure, another control group is needed. Even with technicians experienced with both anesthetization and intratracheal administration, the procedure cannot be repeated more often than at weekly intervals over a period of a few months. Some substances, e.g., low viscosity petroleum distillates, may initiate a chemical pneumonitis.

Parenteral Administration

Parenteral administration allows a test compound to be given in precise amounts that reach the general circulation without being changed by passage through the gastrointestinal tract and liver. However, many substances have been shown to produce local sarcomas at the sites of repeated subcutaneous injection, and the induction of both neoplastic and nonneoplastic lesions can be varied by modifying the surface activity of the injection solution or other physical chemical means (53). This method of administration is a valid measure of chemical carcinogenicity only when the tumors are produced at a site remote from the area of injection. If subcutaneous or intraperitoneal injection is used because of compound destruction in the gastrointestinal tract, it is essential to use separate clean needles for each animal to preclude transmission of any tumor-producing agents (102).

Such factors as volume, concentration, molecular size, and pH affect absorption from the injection site (9).

Intraperitoneal and intravenous injection are generally not well suited to repeated administration of test compounds. These methods are more suited for research using a single or limited number of doses than for studies to detect suspect carcinogens.

CLINICAL EXAMINATION AND HEALTH OF ANIMALS

Clinical monitoring is important to detect incipient disease unrelated to treatment in the test animals and becomes of greater importance with carcinogenicity studies because of the increased value of the animals held for extended periods of time. It is also useful for helping to interpret the significance of histopathologic lesions at the termination of the study. All clinical assessments of laboratory animals must consider that their immediate environment as well as the test agent may influence the biochemical, physiological, and behavioral status of the animals. Thus the daily records of the various environmental parameters, e.g., temperature and humidity, are vitally important when assessing the etiology of clinical signs (43).

Lesions of any system, organ, or tissue can result from infectious agents, parasites, dietary factors, fighting, trauma from cage parts, animal habits, heredity, residual amounts of chemicals remaining in animal care equipment, or any combination of these factors (43). The veterinarian supervising animal care must be able to recognize and correctly diagnose conditions resulting from each of these etiologies, and the animal care technicians performing the routine examinations must be intimately familiar with the normal appearance and behavior of the animals so they can recognize any deviation. Some of these lesions may predispose a particular organ to tumor formation such as the presence of the bladder parasite *Trichosomoides crassicauda* (19,20). If bladder tumors are suspected from the test chemical, urine is collected regularly, filtered, and examined for the ova and adult forms of the parasite.

Because of the numerous associations of viral infections with tumors in animals, recognized first by Bittner (10), the clinical and subclinical disease status of the test animals is assessed before they are placed on test and at regular intervals during the test period. The pretest examination while the animals are in quarantine includes clinical examination, necropsy, and parasite and microbiologic examination. Clinical examination of the actual test animals is necessary to detect overt disease conditions, whereas monitoring for subclinical infections in rodents can best be accomplished by laboratory examination of sentinel animals killed for this purpose (8). In one program, serum from five animals of each sex and species is tested at the termination of the subchronic study. Subsequently, 15 sentinel animals (additional untreated) of each sex and species are placed on the chronic study. Five of these animals are killed for testing at 6, 12, and 18 months as well as five control animals at the termination of the chronic study.

Serum collected at these various time periods is serologically tested for viruses in rats and mice by hemagglutination inhibition or complement fixation. The viruses in rats are pneumonitis virus of mice (PVM), Kilham rat virus (KRV), Toolan's H-1 virus, Sendai, and rat coronavirus-sialodacryoadenitis virus (RCV-SDA); in mice they are PVM, reovirus 3, Theiler's mouse encephalomyelitis (GD7), mouse polyoma, minute virus of mice (MVM), ectromelia, Sendai, mouse adenoma, mouse hepatitis (MHV), and lymphocytic choriomeningitis (LCM) virus. The precise significance of positive titers of these viruses regarding the incidence of specific tumors is not yet known (44,59).

The watchfulness and interest of animal technicians makes it possible to have animals remain on test as long as reasonably possible to develop latent lesions, yet be killed as they become moribund. Mediocre animal care results in a large proportion of unsupervised deaths. If animal technicians are assigned the major care of unique rooms, it should be recognized that there may be a personnel effect on the study. Animals found to have life-threatening tumors or lesions, or that are in poor health from undetermined causes, are isolated in separate cages to help prolong their lives. Persistent anorexia, advanced debilitation, and obvious pain indicate that the animal should be euthanized (8). Weekend observations should not be left to guards, and a person with senior scientific responsibility in the laboratory should be on call for emergencies 24 hr a day, 7 days a week.

All observations made during the twice-daily monitoring and weekly physical examinations can be entered in a daily log book maintained for each study. A computer-based system helps in recording the clinical signs in large studies; however, it is necessary to have some workable program of summarizing and analyzing the data on an animal, test group, and study basis so that the observations are helpful to the study director and to others assessing the results of the study. Too often the only sign that can be followed easily in detail in such reports is the presence and size of the easily palpable and finally highly visible mammary tumors whose presence is usually unrelated to the test compound.

PRECHRONIC STUDIES FOR DOSE SETTING

Type and Length of Studies

The studies performed prior to a carcinogenicity study depend on the amount of prior knowledge concerning the test chemical and the desire to have information relating to metabolism and target organ effects for use in a comprehensive evaluation of results. Under the NTP, carcinogenesis test procedures are evolving toward meeting the objective of broadened toxicologic characterization of the test chemicals. Certain chemicals may be referred to specific organ system groups for more detailed study of the functional, biochemical, and morphologic effects, including observations in the areas of reproduction, neurobehavior, immunotoxicity, and clinical pathology.

If a 2-year study has been performed previously with the same species and strain of animal with the same or similar route of administration, no prechronic studies are necessary. If less information is available, at least a 90-day study is necessary; and if delayed effects are suspected, a longer study, i.e., 6 months, may more accurately predict the maximum

dose tolerated over a 2-year period. With little available information, shorter studies are necessary to arrive at the correct doses for the 90-day subchronic study. Previous reports have tried to provide an estimate of the relation between doses in studies of different length (68,160,161); however, there is no substitute for a complete, well conducted 90-day or greater prechronic study in arriving at a defensible estimated maximum tolerated dose (EMTD). The NTP, in its carcinogenesis bioassay, currently employs two prechronic studies before proceeding to long-term testing of an untested chemical: a 14-day repeated-dose study and a 90-day subchronic study (74).

Repeated-Dose Study

In the repeated-dose study, it is advisable to administer the doses by the same route as anticipated in the chronic study to allow problems of administration to surface at this time and because inferences are made for the subchronic study. Five animals at each dose level are necessary, and ten are advisable. The endpoints of a repeated dose study, in addition to survival over a 10- to 14-day period, include other signs of toxicity such as failure to gain weight or dose-related pathology. The use of weight gain as an endpoint requires that each randomly constructed dose group be assigned animals as homogeneous in weight as possible. If the compound is to be administered in feed, it is given continuously over a 2-week period and the animals necropsied on the day following the last administration. If treatment is by gavage, skin paint, or inhalation, a five times per week administration schedule for 10 to 14 treatments is followed; scheduling must allow for necropsy the day following the last treatment. Histopathologic examination of all tissues is not required because the purpose of the study is generally limited to setting doses for the subchronic study. If gross lesions are found that need further identification, or if it is necessary to determine if they occurred in lower dose groups, the tissues are examined microscopically. Again, the highest dose resulting in few or no deaths is chosen as the high dose for the subchronic study. It is suggested that each of these studies employ four or five dosages with the high dosages chosen to produce toxicologic effects in the animals. This method precludes a study resulting in no significant effects, which must then be repeated using higher dosages.

Subchronic Study

The subchronic study was originally a straightforward 90-day study used to establish the estimated maximum tolerated dose for the chronic study. It is now evolving to a more complex study designed to examine, in depth, the toxicity in several organ systems. A well conducted subchronic study helps differentiate the many aging lesions found in the terminal histopathologic examination in the chronic study from lesions caused by the test chemical.

Ten and preferably 20 animals per sex per species are used in the 13-week subchronic study. Food intake is determined for rats at least; figures for mice are notoriously unreliable, as feed dishes may become filled with excreta or the feed may be dug out onto the cage floor and mixed with bedding, particularly if it is unpalatable. If a constant milligram per kilogram intake is specified by the test design, careful records of feed consumption must be kept and the concentration of the test chemical changed at regular intervals during the early part of the test period when the animals are growing rapidly. All of the effect parameters used in the chronic study are measured closely in the subchronic study, in addition to appropriate clinical chemistries, hematology tests, and organ weights. These tests include the 1978 suggestions by the Food Safety Council (42) (Table 2).

Species variation in serum chemical parameters is often great and needs further clarification, especially for rodents. Adequate technical methodology for serum chemistry determinations in small laboratory animals, in addition to selection of species-specific enzyme profiles, is critical for interpretation of toxicity in prechronic testing. The use and interpretation of specific enzyme studies has been discussed by Cornish (24), Grice et al. (54,57), Korsrud et al. (84), and Plaa (114) (see Chapter 20). In addition to these parameters, the NTP is routinely collecting information on sperm morphology and sperm counts as well as vaginal cytology and cyclicity of female rodents in all 13-week studies (NTP Board of Scientific Counselors, Summary Minutes of April 30 and May 1, 1985).

TABLE 2. *Food Safety Council recommendations for food safety assessment*

Physical observations
  Twice-daily cage check for appearance, morbidity, and mortality
  Daily examination for toxic signs or deviant activity, posture, or behavior
  Weekly record of body weight
  Weekly record of food consumption
  Periodic tests for neurologic response
  Periodic ophthalmologic examination (cornea and retina)
  Functional tests as indicated (e.g., cardiovascular, hepatic, renal, respiratory systems)
Hematologic examinations
  Hemoglobin, hematocrit, red and white blood cell and differential counts, platelets, reticulocytes, prothrombin and clotting times
Biochemical examinations
  Blood glucose, urea nitrogen, creatinine
  Serum albumin/globulin ratio
  Serum lipids (total and free cholesterol, glycerides, fatty acids)
  Serum electrolytes and osmolarity
  Serum enzymes (transaminases, phosphatases)
  Functional tests such as Bromsulphalein and urea clearance, especially in large animals
Urine analyses
  Semiquantitative for reducing sugar, albumin, ketones, pH, and specific gravity
  Microscopic examination of centrifuged sediment
Fecal analyses
  Occult blood
  Moisture content
Postmortem examinations
  Gross necropsy (note autolysis)
  Organ weights
  Histopathology

From ref. 42, with permission.

The decision to include specific functional tests, neurologic responses, ophthalmologic and biochemical examinations, and urine and fecal analyses in the subchronic study must be carefully considered. They may not all be needed to monitor the health of the test animals or to select the EMTD. Effects can often be detected at lower dosages by microscopic examination of the tissues. The low success rate of functional and other tests may originate from selection of inappropriate test(s), lack of correlation with microscopic changes, or both. Urinalyses have not proved to be generally useful in setting the EMTD. The toxicologic activity of the particular chemical being tested and other objectives of the study must be considered when choosing specific tests.

Weight Changes and Randomization

In the 2-week study and, more particularly, the 90-day study, the weight gained by the animals is considered to be an important endpoint. A useful randomization scheme in the assignment of animals to treatment and control groups stratifies the animals by initial body weight. Using this approach for d dosed groups, the animals are numbered and their weights recorded; then the $d + 1$ lowest-weight animals, are randomly assigned to the $d + 1$ dosed groups (d dosed groups and the control group). This process is repeated, ascending in weight, until the animals are all assigned. An alternative, which eliminates prenumbering the animals, consists in putting the animals in temporary cages marked with weight intervals covering the range of the initial weights. A random assignment to the treatment cages is then prepared. This assignment must be a partial randomization, in that for c = number of cages, the first c lowest-weight animals are randomly assigned to the c cages, the next c heavier animals are assigned to the c cages, and so on, ascending in weight. Starting with the cage at the lowest weight interval, the animals as obtained are placed in the cages indicated by the order of this prepared list. The cages are then randomly assigned to the study groups. In this way the cages have a mean and variance as homogeneous as possible, as each cage has a representative animal for each of the n/c weight classes (n is the number of animals to be randomized).

The endpoint of weight is best represented by the amount of weight gained by each dosed animal compared with the weight gained by the controls. A multiple comparison procedure (33,148,165) is that used to distinguish those groups statistically significantly different from the controls. The highest dose levels below these groups are taken to be the no-effect level. Weight differences are usually pronounced in a longer study unless the animals become acclimated to the taste or other effect of the test compound. Thus the 3-month study usually yields better results than the repeated-dose test, especially for mice that gain only a few grams in 2 weeks. Careful randomization by weight, taking weights to the tenth of a gram in mice, cleaning the scale between animals, and periodically recalibrating the scales against National Bureau of Standards (NBS) standards may help to produce interpretable results.

It should be emphasized that weight gain is only one endpoint in any study, and it must be appraised in conjunction with survival, toxicology, and pathology. In the assessment of weight gained, only those groups with good survival (approximately 80%) are used, and animals dying before the end of the study are censored (removed completely from consideration). When multiple comparisons are to be made with unequal numbers in the groups, an adjustment procedure such as that described by Gabriel (45) can be employed. Deaths in a dose group in the subchronic study preclude the use of that dose in the chronic study.

The cumulative effects of the compound are considered by those involved in the dose setting. In some instances it is helpful to apply the weight gain calculations to the first half of the subchronic study and similar calculations to the second half of the study to determine if the failure to gain weight is consistent over the 90 days or is mainly attributed to the first few weeks of the study. If weight gain stabilizes in the dosed groups relative to the controls, the EMTD may be higher than indicated by using the initial and final weights alone.

Data Analysis

Data collected from organ weight and hematologic and clinical chemistry analyses can provide useful information to help determine an EMTD (discussed earlier). Various organ weights can be calculated either in absolute form or as relative ratios, i.e., organ weight/body weight. Hematologic analyses include hemoglobin, hematocrit, and the various blood cell, platelet, and reticulocyte counts. Clinical chemistry analyses include alkaline phosphatase, bilirubin, triglycerides, blood urea nitrogen, and many others.

When examining relative organ weights, caution is advised. Scharer (133) contrasted the relative organ weight effects of outright toxicity to that of underfeeding. In his toxicity study dosed groups' relative liver weights increased substantively over the corresponding controls, whereas in his underfeeding study relative liver weights were lower than those in the corresponding controls. In contrast, relative brain weights increased in both the underfeeding and toxicity studies. Oishi et al. (112) also reported that relative organ weights were decreased by underfeeding.

Statistical analyses can determine if the dosed groups differ from the control group by employing multiple comparison procedures. Specific procedures for control-only comparisons were developed by Dunnett (33) and Williams (165). Williams' test is a specialized version of Dunnett's test; it is designed to detect dose-related differences when the response consistently increases (or decreases) as the dose increases. Although Williams' test employs a data-smoothing algorithm to adjust for dose-response inversions, Dunnett's test is more appropriate if the departure from monotonicity is severe. To assess this departure, Jonckheere's (80) test for a dose-related trend can be applied to the data. If the Jonckheere test indicates the presence of such a trend, Williams' test is used in place of Dunnett's test.

Role of Pathology

Emphasis is placed on both routine and special pathology methods when interpreting the early test phases. Careful attention to subtle lesions of toxicity and critical interpretation of their potential effects on the longevity of the host can enhance accuracy when forecasting "maximal tolerated doses" for chronic bioassay studies. Additionally, unless interim evaluations are made in the chronic study, the results of the subchronic study provide the only tissues for meaningful evaluation of nonneoplastic toxic lesions. In chronic studies toxic lesions are often masked by spontaneous aging lesions (56).

For the subchronic test, all control animals, all animals that die before group sacrifice, and all animals in the highest dose group with survivors at the time of group sacrifice are examined by the pathologist. If any lesion is found in a tissue of a subchronic animal that may be test-compound-related, this organ is examined at the next lower dose until a dose level can be found with no test-compound-related change. Clinical signs, particularly as they relate to the nervous, respiratory, or enteric systems, can be useful to the pathologist. When signs are evaluated prior to necropsy, the necropsy procedure might be modified to investigate possible target organs more thoroughly. Availability of clinical signs and clinical pathology data during microscopic evaluation can also influence the interpretation of lesions.

Toxic lesions in prechronic studies are often subtle and require careful microscopic evaluation. Cellular changes indicating cell death seldom present a problem to the experienced pathologist. However, the fine distinction between certain degenerative or atrophic changes and normal variation can be difficult. Experience with the species involved and awareness of the limits of normal are essential to the identification and interpretation of such changes. Microscopic evaluation of tissues in a "blind" fashion is one method employed to eliminate bias in borderline situations. More frequent use of special techniques can also be useful for elucidating controversial or uncertain results of the light microscopic examination of hematoxylin and eosin (H&E)-stained tissues.

Finally, the pathologist must correlate clinical observations and hematology, clinical chemistry, etc. results with the gross and microscopic pathologic changes observed. This correlation should lead to a reasonably well balanced, logical interpretation of the findings, which becomes a major factor when selecting the EMTD (or other type of dose selection). This evaluation helps preclude life-threatening toxic changes that might compromise the conduct of the chronic study.

Metabolism and Kinetic Studies

To learn why a chemical is carcinogenic and to provide an improved basis for estimation of human risk, it is necessary to perform metabolic absorption distribution, and excretion studies. These studies help determine the extent of absorption from the initially exposed tissue, which metabolites reach which tissue, and in what amount. Because the carcinogenic activity of many chemicals results from biotransformation products rather than the chemical per se, the response may be smaller with increasing dose or exposure when activation does not follow first-order kinetics (48). These studies are also important for more rational and selective spacing of doses below the MTD. Metabolic studies are usually open-ended, and limits must be set on the amount of information needed to help establish the EMTD lest initiation of the chronic study is delayed indefinitely. At the least, biological specimens are collected during the subchronic test phases to provide material for future investigation.

Dose Setting

The subchronic study is the most important study used to determine the doses for the chronic study. The EMTD may vary for the sexes of each species; therefore it should be viewed in context with the earlier, shorter studies to determine if the results are compatible. If the test compound appears to be more toxic in the 2-week study than in the 13-week study, it is imperative to review the conduct and results of each carefully. Did the animals come from the same source? Is the chemical stable? Are all of the technicians competent? Is the dose-response curve so steep that minor changes in conduct and material result in drastically altered patterns of death?

The EMTD is chosen to achieve a dose that, when given for the duration of the chronic study as the highest dose, does not shorten the treated animals' longevity because of any toxic effects other than the induction of neoplasms. It is not chosen to cause morphologic evidence of toxicity of a severity that would interfere with the interpretation of the study. For example, necrosis of a degree to be associated with a significant amount of regeneration may complicate the interpretation of a neoplastic response in that organ. The high dose for the chronic toxicity test generally lies between the dose level that produces a positive endpoint and the dose that produces a minimal effect in the 3-month subchronic test. The spread of doses below the MTD in chronic studies depends on the slope of the dose-response curve in the prechronic studies, the need for a no effect dose, the relevance to exposure guidelines such as a TLV, and the pharmacokinetics of the chemical, e.g., saturation and altered metabolism. For most of the chronic tests currently conducted by the NTP, the EMTD is supplemented by dose levels at one-half and one-fourth the EMTD (65). This is balanced modification of the optimal design(s) given by Portier and Hoel (118).

It goes without saying that all disciplines are involved in dose setting, particularly for the chronic study, as it is an extremely critical point. Political considerations all too often surface at this point, with those who believe the chemical to be carcinogenic or believe in the one-molecule theory opting for a higher dose and those who have a financial stake in the determination of noncarcinogenicity or who simply believe that results of doses far above human exposure are irrelevant opting for a lower dose. This case is particularly so when results of the subchronic test are equivocal or even conflicting, so the dose setting becomes not scientific but somewhat arbitrary and a reflection of one's "feeling about the situation." After all, we have no rapid method for determining if the dose selection for the chronic test was the best that could have been made. With results requiring 2.5 years for completion, there is seldom the opportunity to try again using exactly the same conditions so that an evaluation of the original selection can be made. Because of the extended time periods involved, it may be more practical to lean on the side of a high EMTD. If too many deaths occur during the early part of the study or the animals become debilitated, it

is obvious that an incorrect selection was made and the study can be terminated and started again using lower doses. However, if the initial selection was too low, all of the dosing, histopathologic examination, and statistical analysis must be completed before it is known.

CHRONIC STUDY

Design

Length and Frequency of Treatment

In most carcinogenicity studies, animals are placed on treatment at weaning so they can be exposed during the greater part of their life. This span is 18 to 24 months for mice and 24 months for rats. With Fischer rats the NTP considers that after 24 months the background incidence of some neoplasms increases rapidly, making the model less sensitive (144). There is some evidence that the neonatal animal is more susceptible than the adult, and transplacental carcinogenicity studies are considered separately in this chapter. Allowing all animals to live out their normal lifespan would not appreciably increase the sensitivity of the assay, as animals die at inconvenient times and more tissues may be lost for pathologic study because of cannibalism and autolysis of tissues. Also there is a higher background incidence of several types of neoplasm in lifetime studies, which could increase the chance of obtaining false-positive results (55).

Treatment groups are not allowed to live longer than control groups. Conversely, if the high-dose group dies prematurely from obvious toxicity, it does not trigger termination of the lower-dose groups or controls. A survival standard in the Pesticide Assessment Guidelines of the Environmental Protection Agency (EPA) (36) is that survival should not be less than (a) 50% for mice at 15 months and rats at 18 months and (b) 25% for mice at 18 months and rats at 24 months. Also, if there is more than 10 percent loss due to autolysis, cannibalism, or other management problems, the agency greatly discounts the value of the study.

For chemicals of particular importance, variations on the standard protocol yield valuable additional information for interpretation of results. The NTP has begun to include in some studies additional groups of animals for what are called "stop studies." Here a group or groups are given the chemical for a restricted period of time (usually 12 to 18 months); the animals are then held unexposed for the remainder of the study (usually up to 24 months) to determine if the toxicologic response, including tumor spectrum, is different from that in a group given the chemical similarly for the full 24 months. Also, additional groups of 10 to 20 animals per sex per dose may be killed at 15 months to evaluate chronic toxicity at an age where they are not compromised by aging lesions that appear with progressive severity after this time. Additionally, observation periods at the end of a predetermined treatment period may allow a higher dose to be used during treatment. Treatment is terminated early and the animals held on a control diet if it appears that it will significantly increase their life-span. Treatment may be stopped a few days prior to the end of the study so the prosectors are exposed to lesser amounts of potentially carcinogenic material. Because the lesions here are long-standing in contrast to those in the shorter prechronic studies, no regression is expected.

Administration of the test chemical in most toxicity studies is ideally carried out at the interval that maintains the desired minimum blood level in the animal that mimics the human exposure pattern without large variations or unduly high peak concentrations. It could be daily, twice a day, or even twice a week. Only pharmacokinetic studies during the prechronic phases yield the necessary information to make such a considered determination. It is not known if a relatively constant blood level of tumorigen is likely to lead to tumor formation. There is some information from a carbon tetrachloride study that an interrupted dosage schedule is more efficient; that is, lower doses can be used to produce the same tumor response (37). As a practical matter, most carcinogenicity studies, as with other toxicity studies, utilize an arbitrary treatment frequency built around a 5-day work week to accommodate the labor force unless the substance is added to the animal feed. If the test agent has a significant pharmacologic or toxic effect, as with some tumor suppressants, an interrupted dosage schedule resembling that used to treat human patients and allowing recovery between treatments may be preferable.

Number of Animals Necessary

The principal endpoint of the chronic test for carcinogenicity is whether the animals develop tumors as a result of exposure to the test chemical. Expressed in this way, it is apparent that the statistical analysis must be based on the proportion of animals with tumors in the various groups. The use of data comprising the total number of tumors, as opposed to the number of animals with a tumor of specific morphological site or tissue of origin, has many theoretical difficulties, among which are competing risks, the weighting provided by a high spontaneous tumor rate at some site, and the multiple contribution of a single animal to the total tumor count. The true carcinogenic potential of a compound is that proportion of the animals that incur tumors over and above the true spontaneous tumor rate. This potential may be any value between 0 and 1.00. The latter figure implies a zero spontaneous tumor rate. Because the determination of a true potential near zero is of lesser importance and would require a multitude of animals, the tradeoff between the determination of a potent carcinogen and the use of an unnecessarily large number of animals to determine a small potential must be made in the design of the chronic test. The degree of the ability of a statistical test to indicate correctly that a compound is carcinogenic is called its *power;* it is expressed as a number from 0 to 1, and it depends on the number of animals used in the experiment, the statistical significance level, and the true carcinogenic potential of the compound compared with the spontaneous tumor rate (46). For example, the power of a test is 0.80, with 55 animals each in a dosed group and a control group when the true carcinogenic potential in the dosed groups is 0.20, and the true spontaneous tumor proportion in the control groups is 0.05, assuming a 0.05 significance level in the statistical test. Table 3 gives the power of various experiments given assumed carcinogenic potentials. The number of animals are those that are uncensored in the sense that all had equal opportunity to present tumor development and all were examined in the same manner. Thus autolyzed animals or animals dying early in the experiment from causes extraneous to tumor are not included. Fifty animals per group, with possible additional animals for interim kills, is a sufficient number for most rodent studies unless the incidence of a particular tumor is at issue.

Positive Controls

Positive controls have been recommended and used for carcinogenicity studies ostensibly to demonstrate that the

TABLE 3. *Sample size required to obtain a specified power at 0.05 one-tailed significance level for various combinations of carcinogenic potential (P_1, P_2)*

P_2 (control)	P_1 (treatment)									
	0.95	0.90	0.80	0.70	0.60	0.50	0.40	0.30	0.20	0.10
0.30	10[a]	12	18	31	46	102	389			
	9	10	15	23	33	74	281			
	6	6	9	12	22	32	123			
0.20	8	10	12	18	30	42	88	320		
	6	8	10	15	23	30	64	230		
	5	5	6	9	12	19	28	101		
0.10	6	8	10	12	17	25	33	65	214	
	5	6	8	10	13	19	30	47	154	
	3	3	5	6	9	11	17	31	68	
0.05	5	6	8	10	13	18	25	35	76	464
	5	5	6	9	11	14	20	34	55	334
	3	3	5	6	7	9	12	19	24	147
0.01	5	5	7	8	10	13	19	27	46	114
	4	4	6	7	8	11	14	23	38	87
	3	3	5	5	6	8	10	13	25	56

[a] Power in descending order (0.90, 0.80, 0.50) for each P_1 and P_2.

test animals are sensitive to carcinogens (162). However, they yield little valuable information concerning the specific chemical in question. They may demonstrate that the laboratory can detect a carcinogen; or if a known carcinogen is chemically closely related to the test chemical, such a control group could be of possible value when assessing the results of the study. Similarly, the use of a positive control may help to verify that the products of a known carcinogen have lost their carcinogenic potential following chemical treatment or metabolism, as with aflatoxin B_1. Aside from the frequently dubious scientific value of a positive control group, the safety officer in the laboratory may be reluctant to introduce a known carcinogen into the laboratory. The chemical and its dosage form, the animals and their excreta, and the air are sources of possible contamination that may compromise the health of the staff and the results of other ongoing tests.

Pathology

Necropsy

The final outcome of long-term animal testing for carcinogenicity hinges on the quality of the postmortem examination, as the test results are contained in the tissues of the animal at the end of the study and recognition of gross lesions depends on a careful systematic necropsy technique. Adequate evaluation of lesions begins with a prenecropsy meeting so the pathologist becomes fully knowledgeable about the animal health background and environmental factors that existed during the study. Clinical findings can then be better correlated with pathologic changes. Organs should be examined *in situ* as well as after removal from the animal. Microscopic evaluation of these tissues is of little value unless the animals are carefully inspected to ensure that small tumors and lesions due to other toxic effects are detected and fixed. Adequate time is alloted for a brisk but unhurried postmortem examination of every animal. The necropsy facility is environmentally controlled for comfort, is well lighted, and has instrumentation available for special procedures or techniques. Improper necropsy examination can seriously influence the outcome of a carcinogenesis experiment.

When performing a necropsy, the prosector must handle the tissues with utmost care and respect. Instruments are used properly to avoid artifactual tissue damage from crushing, tearing, or excessive stretching of tissues, which interferes with their microscopic evaluation. For example, thumb forceps are used to grasp the connective tissue coverings at the edges of tissues and organs. Scissors and blades are kept sharp to prevent crushing. Tissues are cleansed of blood and excrement by rinsing in physiological saline. Use of tap water is not recommended because of the potential for cell damage owing to excessively low osmolarity.

The necropsy examination begins with the examination of body orifices (eyes, mouth, anus, ears, penis, vulva) and skin, and palpation for possible masses. A ventral midline incision through the skin, with extension of the incision along the medial aspects of the limbs, is made with a scalpel. The skin is reflected so that subcutaneous tissue, superficial lymph nodes, and the mammary line are readily examined for masses. The abdominal wall is incised along the midline and along the margins of the last rib, thereby exposing the abdominal viscera. The sternal plate, including the costochondral junction, is removed as a unit. Thoracic and abdominal organs, separated by the diaphragm, can now be examined *in situ.* Following such examination, each organ is removed and examined in detail before placing it in fixative. All abnormal findings are recorded. Lesions are accurately and concisely described using nonmedical terms with which the technicians have complete familiarity. Gross lesions are described according to location, size and number, shape, architecture, consistency, and color. Accurate description of lesions allows the pathologist to correlate gross and microscopic changes.

Examination of the gastrointestinal tract as one of the initial steps in the necropsy procedure is recommended because of the rapid rate of autolysis in this organ system. All hollow organs (e.g., esophagus, gastrointestinal tract, uterus, urinary bladder) are opened and the mucosal surfaces examined for lesions. Lungs are inflated by gently injecting formalin (approximately 2 ml in the mouse and 4 ml in the rat) into the trachea. The technician must use sound judgment with this procedure to avoid overinflation and artifact production. Inflation of the urinary bladder with formalin to detect small lesions can also be employed.

Multiple incisions are made in large organs (e.g., liver) and masses to promote proper fixation of their interior. To prevent curling, the flaccid organs and tissues (especially opened segments of gastrointestinal tract) can be placed on a dry piece of white blotter paper, labeled with pencil, and placed in fixative. Neoplasms are dissected to include a portion of surrounding normal tissue, which serves as a landmark for the pathologist.

Neutral, buffered formalin, which is inexpensive and reliable, is the fixative of choice. Millonig's phosphate-buffered formalin can also be used and results in better preservation of cell membranes for retrospective electron microscopy. Other techniques may be necessary when collecting tissue samples for chemical analysis. Table 4 lists the tissues that are taken for histopathologic examination under the most inclusive protocol of the NTP.

Because of the expense of harvesting and preparing this extensive list of tissues from each animal, attempts have been made to ascertain if it is in excess of what is required to determine if a given chemical causes cancer in the test species (92). McConnell (93) proposed an alternative protocol to answer this question which at the same time would give superior information on nonneoplastic chemical-related pathology. These alternative proposals include an "inverse pyramid" with the following steps: (a) "Complete" (31 to 33 tissues/organs) histopathologic examination of all animals from the highest-dose and control groups; (b) histopathologic examination of tissues/organs at lower doses where chemically related neoplastic or nonneoplastic effects were identified in the high-dose animals or in which there is a grossly visible lesion; and (c) "complete" histopathology on all of the animals in the next-high-dose group in addition to the high-dose group if survival in the latter group is reduced because of toxicity (unrelated to neoplasia). Target organs and gross lesions are examined in lower-dose group(s) if they are part of the study. Portier (117) has shown that there is only

TABLE 4. *Organs and tissues to be examined and fixed during necropsy*

Adrenals	Parathyroids
Brain	Pituitary
Cecum	Prostate
Colon	Rectum
Costochondral junction, rib	Salivary gland
Duodenum	Sciatic nerve
Esophagus	Seminal vesicles
Eyes	Skin
Gallbladder	Spinal cord
Gross lesions	Spleen
Heart	Sternebrae, vertebrae, or
Ileum	femur including marrow
Jejunum	Stomach
Kidneys	Testes
Larynx	Thigh muscle
Liver	Tissue masses or suspect
Lungs and bronchi	tumors and regional
Mammary gland	lymph nodes
Mandibular lymph node	Thyroid
Mesenteric lymph node	Thymus
Nasal cavity	Urinary bladder
Ovaries	Uterus
Pancreas	

a negligible loss in the probability of detecting significant results using this modified protocol. A second approach involves the "selected inverse pyramid," which focuses on a subset of 16 to 18 "core" tissues that have previously been associated with neoplasia or that are suspect target organs based on previous observations.

Any time the examination of tissues is deferred, it must be recognized that it will be more expensive to examine them later if examination is ultimately required. Also, if any protocol for reduction in the number of tissues to be examined is to succeed, a thorough postmortem examination becomes even more critical. If a given lesion is not recognized at necropsy and therefore not saved (fixed), it is lost forever. A pathologist has only one chance to perform the necropsy of a given animal and to recognize abnormalities, in contrast to stained sections, which can be reevaluated innumerable times.

Histology

Processing of tissues for preparation of glass microslides begins with proper tissue trimming techniques. Tissues selected for examination are taken from similar anatomic sites in each animal to ensure consistency of the sampling technique. For example, if the liver is to be sampled, the median and left lateral lobes are sectioned at the midportion of the lobes in each animal; the sites selected must not be left to the discretion of the tissue-trimming technician. It is preferable to section more than one site in multilobed (e.g., lung) or complex (e.g., brain) organs. Tissue trimmers must be alert for gross changes that might have been overlooked at necropsy. On occasion, a lesion is more easily recognized after fixation than before.

A variety of processing machines are available to prepare tissues for paraffin embedding. Whichever one is used, the technician must be on guard constantly to prevent overprocessing. A common cause of overprocessing is exposure of small rodent tissues to excessive heat in paraffin stations. Daily temperature checks entered in a log book help minimize this common error in tissue processing. Old and overused reagents (dehydrating and clearing agents) are also a frequent cause of poor tissue sections.

Depending on the preference of the pathologist, there are several schemes for embedding tissues, but the chosen system must be used routinely for each animal in the study. Some approach the tissue sequence from an anatomic viewpoint: e.g., slide 1 is nasal cavity; slide 2 is eyes, brain, and pituitary; slide 3 is salivary gland, mandibular lymph node. Another method is to embed those tissues of comparable cutting consistency in the same block, e.g., liver and kidney in one block, gastrointestinal organs in one block. A combination of the two methods is probably best.

Staining can be carried out either by hand or by automatic staining machines. The latter are probably best for large laboratories with a heavy histology workload; they also increase the consistency in staining quality.

To ensure consistency in the histology laboratory product (the glass microslide), all production procedures must be standardized to the greatest extent possible. Schematics or drawings depicting how tissues are to be handled, particularly for trimming and embedding, are helpful. Drawings that clearly show the specific anatomic site for tissue sampling and the position of the tissue in the proper block are displayed in the areas where the tasks are being done, so the proper procedures are readily available to the technician should a question arise.

Following the preparation of slides, a "slide/block checkout" station can be advantageous. Slides are matched with blocks to ensure that each block has been sectioned, labeling is accurate, all required tissues have been taken, and any artifacts that would preclude interpretation by the pathologist are corrected. The tissue section along with the necropsy record are now ready for the pathologist.

Special studies sometimes necessitate use of special histologic techniques. Inhalation studies usually require multiple sectioning of nasal structures, longitudinal sections of trachea, or coronal sections of lung. Sections of the middle and inner ear could be required if ototoxicity is encountered. Use of "thin" sections (1 μm), prepared on the ultramicrotome, are of value when thin, membranous structures, e.g., those found in the kidney and lung, must be examined. Electron microscopy is often of value when attempting to identify cell types, especially in neoplasms. Many special techniques can be utilized by the typical histology laboratory geared for light microscopy. Success, however, generally depends on the interest and willingness of the laboratory participants to learn and perfect the techniques.

Tissue Evaluation and Data Recording

The data are recorded and tabulated in a consistent manner, with the pathologist using a standardized dictionary of terms to provide for uniformity of reports. The dictionary can be generated *de novo* or modified from several already in existence (e.g., *Systematized Nomenclature of Pathology,* College of American Pathologists, 1965). It is imperative that one pathologist examine and report on all animals of one species from a bioassay study. If more than one pathologist is involved in the evaluation of a single species, the potential exists for enormous multiplicity of terms, often resulting in confusion and inaccuracy in data interpretation. This situation occurs particularly when nonpathologists interpret pathology data.

A standardized format, including all relevant identifiers, is commonly used to record gross and microscopic pathologic changes. The form includes columns for identifying the tissues examined grossly and microscopically (i.e., tissue count). Blocks for gross and microscopic description of lesions and diagnoses must be included in the format. A system for recording missing tissues, autolysis, artifacts, etc. by the pathologist is desirable; moreover, under certain circumstances, e.g., in prechronic studies, a method for recording the grading of lesions is a valuable addition to the format. A computerized system for recording all of the necropsy findings can speed the accurate generation of tables, perform tissue counts, and aid in general data retrieval.

Once the data have been properly recorded and entered into the computer, and an incidence table generated, the pathologist writes a narrative report of the findings. It includes a description of the important lesions or reference to such descriptions, interpretation of the results, and a conclusion as to their significance. A composite description of treatment-related neoplastic and nonneoplastic lesions is included. Other pertinent findings that could influence the outcome of the study, e.g., intercurrent disease, are also described and an assessment made of their influence on the study.

Certain neoplasms have similar origins that allow grouping for statistical analysis. For example, hemangioma and hemangiosarcoma that occur at multiple sites (i.e., skin, spleen, retroperitoneum) are often significant when tabulated together for a treatment group, whereas evaluation of either without grouping or on a system-by-system basis might fail to demonstrate statistical significance. Guidelines for such groupings have been proposed (95).

A question frequently arises about whether the microscopic evaluation of slides should be conducted in a "blind" fashion, i.e., without knowledge of the treatment of the animals. The American College of Veterinary Pathologists (2) does not believe that such an evaluation is appropriate for the routine evaluation of slides. They have stated that it may introduce such complications as (a) the probability of error in encoding and decoding, (b) increased time required to conduct studies, and (c) difficulty in tracking animals through an entire study, i.e., auditing a study. Blind reading is appropriate for second reviews of identified study endpoints, however, either by the original pathologist or by peer review.

Personnel Training

Doctoral level and technical support staff must have had training and experience sufficient to carry out the tasks outlined in the protocol. It is preferable for the pathologist to have a medical background (veterinary, medical, or dental).

Qualification in one of the medical disciplines provides some assurance that clinical signs, clinical chemistry, hematologic data, and other parameters are correctly interpreted. Interpretation of pathophysiological disturbances and correlation with anatomic pathologic changes requires an individual who has been formally trained in anatomy, physiology, biochemistry of metabolism, and other basic sciences commonly included in the "medical" curriculum.

It is essential that the pathologist have a broad background in general pathology, as a variety of organs must be examined from all animals. Evaluation by individuals with detailed experience in one organ or system and limited experience with others is undesirable. Extensive experience by the pathologist with the species being tested is of extreme importance to the success of the pathology program. There is no substitute for thorough familiarity with strain differences, intercurrent diseases, aging phenomena, and other idiosyncrasies that are unique to the species under test. Board certification is desirable but not essential if experience is judged to be comparable.

The technical staff, consisting of prosectors and histology technicians, must be thoroughly trained in their respective specialty areas. Often a "pathology laboratory technician" can be developed by cross-training in necropsy techniques, tissue trimming, and histologic technique, generally with an in-house training program. Such an individual often shows an appreciation for all tasks carried out in the laboratory. The histology section of the laboratory should be supervised by a registered histology technician (HT/ASCP).

Quality Assurance

Quality assurance ensures to the maximum extent possible the accuracy and integrity of the pathology laboratory results through the reduction or control of variables that might affect the outcome of the study. It is discussed in greater depth by Boorman et al. (16). Quality assurance (QA) is an ongoing process and must be accomplished while the study is in progress as well as at termination. Particularly during a large study, one must be concerned with proper identification of animals as they enter necropsy. Discrepancies in identification, e.g., torn ears, inability to read punches, and missing ear tags, are noted and every attempt made to correctly identify the animal. The necropsy technique of technicians must be assessed periodically (e.g., Is the protocol being followed? Are all required tissues being taken? Are all gross findings recorded and described accurately on the necropsy form?). A system of accounting can be employed to ensure completeness of tissue collections. Lesions noted clinically and at necropsy must be tracked through histology and microscopy (e.g., via numbered or coded cassettes or tags) to correlate clinical gross or microscopic findings. Tissues are trimmed in a standardized, uniform fashion and a procedure established to confirm that all lesions described are actually being trimmed. Random sampling of early-death necropsy forms and the companion microslides is useful for this purpose. In the histology laboratory, tissue processing is carefully monitored with use of log books; and such items as entry into the laboratory, temperature of paraffin pots, and so on are recorded. Individual animals are accounted for at each station in the histology laboratory (e.g., embedding, microtomy, staining, coverslipping, and check-out). All tasks, including those at the prosector, tissue trimmer, and histology stations, are initialed and dated by the technician performing the task. Standard operating procedures must be available in written form to the technician at the appropriate location. A specific method for making corrections of raw data that is compatible with good laboratory practices (39) (see below) is employed.

Once the study is completed and the data evaluated, a system of data verification or poststudy audits can be used to further confirm the integrity of the results. Neoplasms and any compound-related lesions (neoplastic or nonneoplastic) can be verified by an "impartial" pathologist. Differences of opinion, lesions that cannot be accounted for, and lesions that were not recorded are noted. Wet tissue checks help prevent discrepancies in untrimmed lesions and unverified animal identification.

A complete review of 10% of randomly selected animals in a chronic study (more than 10% for prechronic studies) can be included as part of the data verification procedure. Tissue counts and assessment of the quality of slide preparation can also be a part of the QA procedure. A QA report is generated in which the QA findings are compared with the original data. Differences of opinion or discrepancies of significant proportion can be resolved by a forum or roundtable discussion that includes the original pathologist, the QA pathologist, and one or more pathologists who have no association with the conduct of the study.

Good Laboratory Practices

Implementation of good laboratory practices (GLPs), those of either the Federal Drug Administration (FDA) or the EPA, increase assurance of the quality and integrity of the data. GLPs require that adequate numbers of personnel sufficiently trained and experienced to perform assigned tasks are available. Inspections of the laboratory by the study sponsor are unannounced and occur at least every 3 months in studies lasting more than 6 months.

Much controversy has arisen as to what constitutes "raw data." The term has been defined as any laboratory work sheets, records, memoranda, notes, or exact copies of such materials that result from original observations. Original tapes do not have to be retained if exact transcripts are prepared from the tapes. Copies of data must be dated and signed in order to be accepted as substitutes for the original. Photographs, computer printouts, and dictated observations are also viewed as raw data.

Good laboratory practices necessitate that standard operating procedures be written for all procedures in the laboratory and any changes from the protocol be made only with written authorization. Data entries must be dated and signed or initialed by the person responsible for the data; lists of data need be signed only once. All changes must indicate the reason for the change and be dated and signed, and the original entry must not be obscured by this change. Finally, an archive for storage and retrieval of material and reports is maintained.

Statistical Analyses

Testing Survival

Survival of the animals is an important endpoint of the chronic study. A test for homogeneity of survival in two or more groups is the "life table" analysis proposed by Cox (26); a test for the presence of a linear trend is also available (151). A significant trend toward increased mortality in the dosed groups, as indicated by these statistical tests, forms the basis for consideration that the EMTD has been reached or exceeded. If this situation occurs, a lack of tumor development in the dose groups is interpreted with great care, as the power of the test for detecting tumorigenic differences may be low. When survival is curtailed in some or all of the treated groups, the effective number of animals available for testing carcinogenicity becomes a matter of subjective interpretation, which can seriously impair acceptance of the results.

Testing Tumor Incidence

After the incidence of neoplasia of a particular morphology at a particular site has been determined, statistical testing can be employed to assess the differences in incidence among the control and treated groups. If survival differences among the groups are minimal, unadjusted tests such as the Fisher-Irwin exact test (25) may be used. This test compares tumor incidences between the controls and a specific dose group. It assumes that the number of observed tumors is spontaneous, so that any observed differences occur only because of the initial randomization of the experimental animals to these groups. The number of ways in which the disproportionality between groups could have been the same or greater than that observed, divided by the number of ways in which the total observed tumor load could have been distributed between the two groups, is the "p-value" of the test. Small p-values (<0.05) suggest more extreme disproportionality between the two groups and less chance that randomization alone influenced the outcome.

If more than one dose group is available, a test for linear trend in tumor incidence may be applied. Under the linearity hypothesis, the Cochran-Armitage test (7) assesses the degree of departure from zero of the slope of the dose-response curve. As with the Fisher-Irwin test, this procedure does not adjust for possible survival differences between the animal groups.

When the test compound does not affect the survival patterns of the animal groups, the Fisher-Irwin and Cochran-Armitage tests' results do not differ dramatically from those of more complex, survival-adjusted analyses. However, when there are suspected differences in the survival patterns of the animal groups, the power of the unadjusted statistical procedures to detect differences or trends among the dose groups can suffer. The ideal circumstances involve either (a) comparable and satisfactory survival in all groups or (b) early deaths in the dosed groups that can be clearly related to observation of the tumor. In many cases, however, neither of these instances occurs, and the use of statistical methods that compensate for differing patterns of survival among the groups of animals is advocated (113).

Different statistical methodologies exist for neoplasms with differing fatal effects. When it can be supposed that the tumor instantaneously (or nearly so) leads to the death of the animal, application of the life table test—including the test for trend (151)—is appropriate. It involves a simple substitution of "time to observation of tumor" for "death" (128). This generalization of survival testing implicitly assumes that the time to death closely approximates the time to tumor onset. Life table methods can therefore provide a comparison of the time-specific tumor incidences between control and treated groups (73).

When it is not reasonable to attribute animal mortality to a particular neoplasm, alternative survival-adjusted methods are available. These methods hinge primarily on the supposition that the tumors observed in animals that died before the end of the study are strictly nonlethal, or "incidental." Incidental tumor tests based on a statistical regression model, e.g., the logistic score test (32), have a number of desirable properties, including the ability to incorporate tests for trend and tests for differences from the control group as well as greater power to assess such differences (30). Logistic regression tests adjust for intercurrent mortality by directly incorporating the individual death times as covariables into the survival analysis. In fact, this framework can be extended to include information on any important covariables that might otherwise confound analyses that ignore these explanatory factors (31).

Use of Historical Control Data

The concurrent control group in any experiment is the most important source of information regarding the background effects of an endpoint of interest (e.g., survival, tumor incidence). However, in some cases (e.g., rare tumors or only-marginal increases in tumor incidence over the control rates) the use of historical control data can add valuable information when assessing the significance of the observed result (64). Historical control information can be misused, however, and care must be taken regarding its worth to the overall decision process. As noted by Haseman et al. (66), nomenclature conventions and diagnostic criteria must be carefully calibrated so as to allow meaningful comparisons among similar neoplastic effects. Also, outside sources of variability, e.g., laboratory differences or changes in tumorigenic susceptibility of a species over time, must be isolated. Once recognized, such extrabinomial factors, as they are called, must be properly accounted for in the statistical analysis (29,152).

Interpretation of Statistical Findings

Statistical tests can be applied to as many as 30 examined sites in two or more dose groups of both sexes in several species within a single bioassay. Such multiple application can lead to a larger-than-expected probability of falsely assessing some tumor incidence as significant (the "false-positive rate"). This situation is more true of the commonly occurring tumors, e.g., liver tumors in male B6C3F1 mice or anterior pituitary tumors in F344/N rats, because it is virtually impossible for rare tumors to occur in large enough numbers in a particular study to lead to spurious statistical

significance (64). Gart et al. (47) and Haseman (63) discussed the false-positive issue in greater detail.

To help protect against unaccounted-for growth in the false-positive rate, the nominal p-value required to conclude statistical significance can be lowered, but a number of more basic issues must also be considered. Most importantly, recognition that the interpretation of carcinogenicity data involves a complex, multidisciplinary process is vital. No one input should be given disproportionate weight in the evaluatory mechanism. In terms of the statistical decisions, it argues against the use of a formal, rigid, statistical rule. Factors such as (a) the relative survival of the control and dosed animals, (b) supporting evidence by related, nonneoplastic effects, (c) similar tumorigenic evidence across species or between sexes within a species, (d) target organ effects, and (e) any historical data must be taken into account during the evaluation of a compound's carcinogenic potential. Clearly, the wide range of possible outcomes emphasizes the need for all disciplines to apply their best efforts when assessing results from a carcinogenesis study.

TRANSPLACENTAL CARCINOGENESIS

Transplacental carcinogenicity studies are carried out because of the high susceptibility to chemical agents of the rapidly differentiating and dividing cells during organ and tissue formation. These studies are considered when the test agent has reproductive or teratogenic activity or when the nature and degree of exposure and the pharmacokinetics or metabolism suggest that it is an appropriate method of exposure. Although some highly potent carcinogens produce tumors within a few months when administered during these periods, delayed effects are more often expected. Specific periods of susceptibility to carcinogens have been identified for specific tissues and organs just as they have been for teratogens (159).

The discrete effect of a potential carcinogen on the developing fetus is tested by exposing animals to the agent only during fetal life followed by observation during the greater part of the life-span of the test animals. For an agent of particular concern or for strictly research purposes, this method is satisfactory. However, when the effect of the agent during postnatal life is also important, pre- and postnatal exposure is followed by lifetime administration to the F_1 generation. It is not possible to conclude from such a study whether (a) the neonate is more sensitive than the adult and tumors would occur after maternal exposure alone, or (b) exposure during both prenatal and postnatal periods of life is necessary.

A pilot study helps determine if the selected doses are fetotoxic. At weaning in the pilot study the maximal dose that does not depress weanling survival or body weight is defined as the maximum neonatal dose, which is used for the subsequent transplacental bioassay.

Dosing of the F_0 generation female animals begins anywhere from 4 weeks before breeding until day 6 of pregnancy, depending on the half-life of the compound. For test chemicals with short half-lives, the start of administration is delayed as long as possible to avoid secondary effects due to maternal toxicity. Dosing begins early enough for sufficient buildup of the test compound in maternal storage tissues to permit exposure of the developing fetus. Administration of the test chemical to the F_0 females is continued until the end of weaning. The levels of the test compound used to ensure that reproductive or teratogenic effects do not occur may be much lower than those selected for conventional carcinogenicity tests, and the validity of the test could be questioned.

Breeding and handling of the females and examination of the litters proceed as with a reproduction study. If methods are available, milk can be analyzed during the study to determine the contribution of this route of exposure. The F_1 animals then become the chronic test animals, and at weaning not more than two or three males and two or three females are randomly selected from each litter to obtain the total required for the lifetime study. No animal surviving to weaning is excluded from selection. Each animal and the litter of origin must be identified. The F_1 animals are fed the appropriate test diet at weaning and are continued on these diets until termination.

HEALTH AND SAFETY PROCEDURES

A comprehensive, rigidly followed Health and Safety Plan is necessary for the laboratory testing of substances for their carcinogenic activity. The fact that the substance is tested for such activity makes it, in effect, a suspect carcinogen at least during the test and makes necessary strict handling procedures for every step, from receipt of the chemical through disposal of animal waste and processing of tissues for histopathologic examination.

Such a plan (81,104) must address the responsibility within management for development and adherence of the plan; medical surveillance for employees; employee training; safe handling practices for the chemical; animal handling; general laboratory safety; safe personnel practices; safe work area practices, e.g., spill control and decontamination; handling of air, liquid, and solid wastes; monitoring of workers and physical equipment; emergency control; record keeping; the design of facilities; and the pollution potential. Applicable regulations of the Occupational Safety and Health Administration (OSHA) provide only a minimum structure from which to work, and lessening of the hazard within the particular facility must be addressed individually and with ingenuity. Laboratory directors must appreciate that chemicals may penetrate protective clothing and travel a considerable distance from their point of use (129–131).

There are no safety measures that are unique to a carcinogenicity study; it is the degree of adherence to them that distinguishes the conduct of these studies from all others. It is beyond the scope of this section to address each individually. A few examples of areas that are often overlooked include the following: (a) use of a properly ventilated cage dumping area or an enclosed animal bedding disposal cabinet to prevent inhalation of contaminated dust and aerosols by employees; (b) an air handling system that provides decreasing gradations of air pressure from clean corridor to the animal rooms to the dirty corridor and that is periodically tested under such stress as several doors being opened at one time or with all possible chemical hoods in operation; (c) maintenance personnel as well as scientific supervisors that follow the same rules as technicians for personal protection; (d) storage facilities that protect the integrity of the chemicals over the extended period of time during which unused material may be held and the immediate containers checked for deterioration; (e) a "breathable air" line available for use with an air-supplied respirator in the dosage preparation areas; and (f) workers, including weekend staff, who are familiar with emergency safety instructions within the laboratory and know whom to notify in the event of various types of potential emergency situations.

DOCUMENTS CONSIDERING TESTING FOR CARCINOGENICITY

Specific protocol suggestions and directions for carcinogenicity testing and monitoring continue to be the subject of numerous reviews by individuals, expert panels, and government agencies. The older reviews include those of Shubik and Sice (140), the National Academy of Sciences Subcommittee on Carcinogenesis (41), Weisburger and Weisburger (163), Arcos et al. (4), the International Union Against Cancer (78), the World Health Organization (169), and the Food and Drug Administration Advisory Committee (40). Later came such reviews as the Proceedings of the Conference on Carcinogenesis Testing in the Development of New Drugs (50) and the review of the Canadian Ministry of Health and Welfare (69), the guidelines of the National Cancer Institute (NCI) (145), the Food Safety Council (42), the Regulatory Council (121), the International Agency for Research on Cancer (76), and the NCI/NTP (105). More recent were the report of the NTP Ad Hoc Panel on Chemical Carcinogenesis and Evaluation (12) and the review of the Office of Science and Technology Policy (111).

REFERENCES

1. Adams, R. A., DiPaolo, J. A., and Homburger, F. (1978): The Syrian hamster in toxicology and carcinogenesis research. *Cancer Res.*, 38:2642–2645.
2. American College of Veterinary Pathologists (1986): Letter to the editor. *Toxicol. Appl. Pharmacol.*, 83:184–185.
3. Andervont, H. B. (1944): Influence of environment on mammary cancer in mice. *J. Natl. Cancer Inst.*, 4:579–581.
4. Arcos, J. F., Argus, M. F., and Wolf, G. (1968): Testing procedures. In: *Chemical Induction of Cancer*, Vol. I, pp. 340–463. Academic Press, New York.
5. Argus, M. F., Arcos, J. C., and Hoch-Ligeti, C. (1965): Studies on the carcinogenic activity of protein-denaturing agents: hepatocarcinogenicity of dioxane. *J. Natl. Cancer Inst.*, 35:949–958.
6. Argus, M. F., Sohal, R. S., Bryant, G. M., Hoch-Ligeti, C., and Arcos, J. C. (1973): Dose-response and ultrastructural alterations in dioxane carcinogenesis. *Eur. J. Cancer*, 9:237–243.
7. Armitage, P. (1971): *Statistical Methods in Medical Research*, pp. 362–365. Wiley, New York.
8. Arnold, D. L., Charbonneau, S. M., Zawidzka, Z. Z., and Grice, H. C. (1977): Monitoring animal health during chronic toxicity studies. *J. Environ. Pathol. Toxicity*, 1:227–239.
9. Ballard, B. E. (1968): Biopharmaceutical consideration in subcutaneous and intramuscular drug administration. *J. Pharm. Sci.*, 57:357–378.
10. Bittner, J. J. (1936): Some possible effects of nursing on the mammary gland tumor incidence in mice. *Science*, 84:162.
11. Blumenthal, H. T., and Rogers, J. B. (1967): Spontaneous and induced tumors in the guinea pig, with special reference to the factor of age. *Prog. Exp. Tumor Res.*, 9:261–285.
12. Board of Scientific Counselors National Toxicology Program (1984):

Report of the NTP Ad Hoc Panel on Chemical Carcinogenesis Testing and Evaluation. U.S. Dept. of Health and Human Services, Public Health Service, Washington, D. C.

13. Bock, F. G. (1963): Species differences in penetration and absorption of chemical carcinogens. *Natl. Cancer Inst. Monogr.,* 10:361–372.

14. Bonser, G. M. (1969): How valuable is the dog in the routine testing of suspected carcinogens? *J. Natl. Cancer Inst.,* 43:271–274.

15. Boorman, G. A., and Eustis, S. L. (1984): Proliferative lesions of the exocrine pancreas in male F344/N rats. *Environ. Health Perspect.,* 56:213–217.

16. Boorman, G. A., Montgomery, C. A., Eustis, S. L., Wolfe, M. J., McConnell, E. E., and Hardisty, J. F. (1985): Quality assurance in pathology for rodent toxicology and carcinogenicity testing. In: *Handbook of Carcinogen Testing,* edited by H. A. Milman and E. K. Weisburger. Noyes Publications, Park Ridge, New Jersey.

17. Borowitz, J. L., Moore, P. F., Yim, G. K. W., and Miya, T. S. (1971): Mechanism of enhanced drug effects produced by dilution of the oral dose. *Toxicol. Appl. Pharmacol.,* 19:164–168.

18. Burek, J. D., and Hollander, C. F. (1977): Incidence patterns of spontaneous tumors in BN/Bi rats. *J. Natl. Cancer Inst.,* 58:99–105.

19. Chapman, W. H. (1969): Infection with Trichosomoides crassicauda as a factor in the induction of bladder tumors in rats fed 2-acetylaminofluorine. *Invest. Urol.,* 7:154–159.

20. Clayson, D. B. (1974): Bladder carcinogenesis in rats and mice: possibility of artifacts. *J. Natl. Cancer Inst.,* 52:1685–1689.

21. Coleman, G. L., Barthold, S. W., Osbaldiston, G. W., Foster, S. J., and Jonas, A. M. (1977): Pathological changes during aging in barrier-reared Fischer 344 male rats. *J. Gerontol.,* 32:158–178.

22. Coleman, W. E., and Tardiff, R. G. (1979): Containment levels in animal feed used for toxicity studies. *Arch. Environ. Contam. Toxicol.,* 8:693–702.

23. Committee on Long-Term Holding of Laboratory Rodents (1976): *Long-Term Holding of Laboratory Rodents.* Institute of Laboratory Resources, National Academy of Sciences, National Research Council, Washington, D. C.

24. Cornish, H. H. (1971): Problems posed by observations of serum enzyme changes in toxicology. *CRC Crit. Rev. Toxicol.,* 1:1–32.

25. Cox, D. R. (1970): *Analysis of Bioassay Data,* pp. 48–52. Methuen, London.

26. Cox, D. R. (1972): Regression models and life tables. *J. R. Stat. Soc.,* 13,34:187–220.

27. Dahl, A. R., Hadley, W. M., Hahn, F. F., Benson, J. M., and McClelland, R. O. (1982): Cytochrome P-450 dependent monooxygenases in olfactory epithelium of dogs: possible role in tumorigenicity. *Science,* 216:57–59.

28. Davis, T. A., Bales, C. W., and Beauchene, R. E. (1983): Differential effects of dietary caloric and protein restriction in the aging rat. *Exp. Gerontol.,* 18:427–435.

29. Dempster, A. P., Selwyn, M. D., and Weeks, B. J. (1983): Combining historical and randomized controls for assessing trends in proportions. *J. Am. Statist. Assoc.,* 78:221–227.

30. Dinse, G. E. (1985): Testing for a trend in tumor prevalence. I. Nonlethal tumors. *Biometrics,* 41:751–770.

31. Dinse, G. E., and Haseman, J. K. (1986): Logistic regression analysis of incidental-tumor data from animal carcinogenicity experiments. *Fundam. Appl. Toxicol.,* 6:44–52.

32. Dinse, G. E., and Lagakos, S. W. (1983): Regression analysis of tumor prevalence data. *Appl. Statist.,* 32:236–248.

33. Dunnett, C. W. (1955): A multiple comparison procedure for comparing several treatments with a control. *J. Am. Statist. Assoc.,* 50:1096–1122.

34. Ediger, R. D., and Kovatch, R. M. (1976): Spontaneous tumors in the Dunkin-Hartley guinea pig. *J. Natl. Cancer Inst.,* 56:293–294.

35. Edwards, G. S., Policastro, P., Goff, U., Wolf, M. H., and Fine, D. H. (1979): Volatile nitrosamine contamination of laboratory animal diets. *Cancer Res.,* 39:1857–1858.

36. Environmental Protection Agency (1985): Pesticide assessment guidelines, subdivision F, hazard evaluation humans and domestic animals. In: *40 CFR,* Section 158.135, 83–1, p107 and 83–2, p117. EPA, Washington, D. C.

37. Eschenbrenner, A. D., and Miller, E. (1944): Studies on hepatomas. I. Size and spacing of multiple doses in the induction of carbon tetrachloride hepatomas. *J. Natl. Cancer Inst.,* 4:385–388.

38. Fitzgerald, J. M., Boyd, V. F., and Manus, A. G. (1984): Formulation of insoluble and inmiscible test agents in liquid vehicles for toxicity testing. In: *Chemistry for Toxicity Testing,* edited by C. W. Jameson and D. B. Walters. Butterworth, Stoneham, Massachusetts.

39. Food and Drug Administration (1978): Nonclinical laboratory studies, good laboratory practice recommendations. *Fed. Register,* 43:59986–60025.

40. Food and Drug Administration Advisory Committee on Protocols for Safety Evaluation (1971): Panel on carcinogenesis: report on cancer testing in the safety evaluation of food additives and pesticides. *Toxicol. Appl. Pharmacol.,* 20:419–438.

41. Food Protection Committee, Food and Nutrition Board (1961): Problems in the evaluation of carcinogenic hazard from the use of food additives: National Academy of Sciences, National Research Council, Publ. No. 749, p. 44, 1960. *Cancer Res.,* 21:429–456.

42. Food Safety Council—Scientific Committee (1978): Proposed system for food safety assessment. *Food Cosmet. Toxicol.,* 16, (Suppl. 2):1–136.

43. Fox, J. G. (1977): Clinical assessment of laboratory rodents on long term bioassay studies. *J. Environ. Pathol. Toxicol.,* 1:199–226.

44. Fox, J. G., Cohen, B. J., and Loew, F. M. (1984): *Laboratory Animal Medicine.* Academic Press, New York.

45. Gabriel, K. R. (1978): A simple method of multiple comparison of means. *J. Am. Statist. Assoc.,* 73:724–729.

46. Gail, M., and Gart, J. J. (1973): The determination of sample signs for use with the exact conditional test in 2×2 comparative trials. *Biometrics,* 29:441–448.

47. Gart, J. J., Chu, K. C., and Tarone, R. E. (1979): Statistical issues in the interpretation of chronic bioassay tess for carcinogenicity. *J. Natl. Cancer Inst.,* 62:957–974.

48. Gehring, P. J., Watanabe, P. G., and Park, C. N. (1978): Resolution of dose response toxicity data for chemicals requiring metabolic activation: example—vinyl chloride. *Toxicol. Appl. Pharmacol.,* 44:581–591.

49. Gilbert, C., Gillman, J., Loustalot, P., and Lutz, W. (1958): The modifying influence of diet and the physical environment on spontaneous tumor frequency in rats. *Br. J. Cancer,* 12:565–593.

50. Golberg, L., editor (1974): *Carcinogenesis Testing of Chemicals.* CRC Press, Cleveland.

51. Goodman, D. G., Ward, J. M., Squire, R. A., Chu, K. C., and Linhart, M. S. (1979): Neoplastic and nonneoplastic lesions in aging F344 rats. *Toxicol. Appl. Pharmacol.,* 48:237–248.

52. Grasso, P., and Crampton, R. F. (1972): The value of the mouse in carcinogenicity testing. *Food Cosmet. Toxicol.,* 10:418–426.

53. Grasso, P., Gangolli, S. D., Golberg, L., and Hooson, J. (1971): Physiochemical and other factors determining local sarcoma production by food additives. *Food Cosmet. Toxicol.,* 9:463–478.

54. Grice, H. C. (1972): The changing role of pathology in modern safety evaluation. *CRC Crit. Rev. Toxicol.,* 1:119–152.

55. Grice, H. C., and Burek, J. D. (1984): Age-associated (geriatric) pathology: its impact on long term toxicity studies. In: *Current Issues in Toxicity.* Springer-Verlag, New York.

56. Grice, H. C., Arnold, D. L., Blumenthal, D. L., Emmerson, J. L., and Krewski, D. (1984): *The Selection of Doses in Chronic Toxicity/ Carcinogenicity Studies in Current Issues in Toxicity.* Springer-Verlag, New York.

57. Grice, H. C., Barth, M. L., Cornish, H. H., Foster, G. V., and Gran, R. H. (1971): Correlation between serum enzymes, isozyme patterns and histologically detectable organ damage. *Food Cosmet. Toxicol.,* 9:847–855.

58. Gumbmann, M. R., Spangler, W. L., Dugan, G. M., Rackis, J. J., and Liener, I. E. (1985): The USDA trypsin inhibitor study. IV. The chronic effects of soy flour and soy protein isolate on the pancreas in rats after two years. *Qual. Plant Foods Hum. Nutr.,* 35:275–314.

59. Hamm, T. E., editor (1986): *Complications of Viral and Mycoplasmal Infections in Rodents to Toxicology Research and Testing.* Hemisphere, New York.

60. Hanna, M. G., Nettesheim, P., and Bilgert, J. R. (1970): Inhalation carcinogenesis. In: *Conference on the Morphology of Experimental Respiratory Carcinogenesis,* Gatlinburg, Tennessee. U.S. Atomic Energy Commission Series No. 18.

61. Harper, B. L., and Morris, D. L. (1984): Implications of multiple mechanisms of carcinogenesis for short-term testing. *Teratogenesis Carcinog. Mutagen.*, 4:483–503.

62. Haseman, J. K. (1983): Patterns of tumor incidence in two-year cancer bioassay: feeding studies in Fischer 344 rats. *Fundam. Appl. Toxicol.*, 3:1–9.

63. Haseman, J. K. (1983): A reexamination of false-positive rates for carcinogenesis studies. *Fundam. Appl. Toxicol.*, 3:334–339.

64. Haseman, J. K. (1984): Statistical issues in the design analysis and interpretation of animal carcinogenicity studies. *Environ. Health Perspect.*, 58:385–392.

65. Haseman, J. K. (1985): Issues in carcinogenicity testing: dose selection. *Fundam. Appl. Toxicol.*, 5:66–78.

66. Haseman, J. K., Huff, J., and Boorman, G. A. (1984): Use of historical control data in carcinogenicity studies in rodents. *Toxicol. Pathol.*, 12:126–135.

67. Haseman, J. K., Huff, J. E., Rao, G. N., Arnold, J. E., Boorman, G. A., and McConnell, E. E. (1985): Neoplasms observed in untreated and corn oil gavage control groups of F344/N rats and (C57BL/6N × C3H/HeN)F₁ (B6C3F₁) mice. *J. Natl. Cancer Inst.*, 75:975–984.

68. Hayes, W. J. (1972): Tests for detecting and measuring long term toxicity. In: *Essays in Toxicology,* Vol. 3. Academic Press, New York.

69. Health and Welfare, Canada (1973): *The Testing of Chemicals for Carcinogenicity, Mutagenicity and Teratogenicity.* Ministry of Health and Welfare, Ottawa, Canada.

70. Hesseltine, G. R., Wolff, R. K., Hanson, R. L., Mauderly, J. L., and McClellan, R. O. (1984): Effect of day vs. night inhalation exposure on lung burdens of gallium oxide in rats. In: *Inhalation Toxicology Research Institute Annual Report.* Albuquerque, New Mexico.

71. Hobbs, C. H., and McClellan, R. O. (1986): Deposition, retention and responses to inhaled materials. In: *Safety Evaluation of Drugs and Chemicals,* edited by W. E. Lloyd. Hemisphere, Washington, D. C.

72. Hoch-Ligeti, C., Argus, M. F., and Arcos, J. C. (1970): Induction of carcinomas in the nasal cavity of rats by dioxane. *Br. J. Cancer,* 24:164–167.

73. Hoel, D. G., and Walburg, H. E. (1972): Statistical analysis of survival experiments. *J. Natl. Cancer Inst.*, 49:361–372.

74. Huff, J. E., Haseman, J. K., McConnell, E. E., and Moore, J. A. (1986): The National Toxicology Program, toxicology data evaluation techniques and long-term carcinogenesis studies. In: *Safety Evaluation of Drugs and Chemicals,* edited by W. E. Lloyd, pp. 411–446. Hemisphere, Washington, D.C.

75. Institute of Laboratory Animal Resources (1974): *Guide for the Care and Use of Laboratory Animals.* DHEW Publ. No. (NIH) 74-23. Public Health Services, National Institutes of Health, Washington, D. C.

76. International Agency for Research on Cancer (1980): Long-term and short-term screening assays for carcinogens: a critical appraisal. *IARC Monogr. [Suppl.]* 2.

77. International Agency for Research on Cancer (1985): Polynuclear aromatic compounds. 4. Bitumens, coal-tars and derived products, shale-oils and soots. *IARC Monogr. Eval. Carcinog. Risk Chem. Hum.,* 35.

78. International Union Against Cancer (1969): *Panel on Carcinogenicity of Cancer Research Commission, Carcinogenicity Testing.* UICC Technical Report Series, Vol. 2, pp. 1–43.

79. Jameson, C. W. (1984): Analytical chemistry requirements for toxicity testing of environmental chemicals. In: *Chemistry for Toxicity Testing,* edited by C. W. Jameson and D. B. Walters. Butterworth, Stoneham, Massachusetts.

80. Jonckheere, A. (1954): A distribution-free k-sample test against ordered alternatives. *Biometrika,* 41:133–145.

81. Jurinski, N. (1977): *Carcinogenesis Bioassay Health and Safety Plan.* Tracor Jitco, Rockville, Maryland.

82. Knapka, J. J. (1979): Laboratory animal feed. *Science,* 204:1367.

83. Knapka, J. K., Smith, K. P., and Judge, F. J. (1974): Effect of open and closed formula rations on the performance of three strains of laboratory mice. *Lab. Anim. Sci.,* 24:480–487.

84. Korsrud, G. O., Grice, H. C., and McLaughlan, J. M. (1972): Sensitivity of several serum enzymes in detecting carbon tetrachloride-induced liver damage in rats. *Toxicol. Appl. Pharmacol.,* 22:474–483.

85. Kraft, P. L. (1983): The effect of dietary fat on tumor growth. *Regul. Toxicol. Pharmacol.,* 3:239–251.

86. Lai, Y. L., Jacoby, R., and Jonas, A. (1978): Age related and light associated retinal changes in Fischer rats. *Invest. Ophthalmol. Vis. Sci.,* 17:634–638.

87. Lavbelin, G., Roba, J., Roncucci, R., and Parmentier, R. (1975): Carcinogenicity of 6-aminochrysene in mice. *Eur. J. Cancer,* 11:327–334.

88. Liener, I. E., Nitsan, Z., Srisangnam, C., Rackis, J. J., and Gumbmann, M. R. (1985): The USDA trypsin inhibitor study. II. Time related biochemical changes in the pancreas of rats. *Qual. Plant Foods Hum. Nutr.,* 35:243–257.

89. McCay, C. M., Crowell, M. F., and Maynard, L. A. (1935): The effect of retarded growth upon the length of life span and the ultimate body size. *J. Nutr.,* 10:63–78.

90. McCay, C. M., Maynard, L. A., Sperling, G., and Barnes, L. L. (1939): Retarded growth, life span, ultimate body size and age changes in the albino rat after feeding diets restricted in calories. *J. Nutr.,* 18:1–13.

91. McClellan, R. O., and Hobbs, C. H. (1986): Generation, characterization and exposure systems for test atmospheres. In: *Safety Evaluation of Chemicals,* edited by W. E. Lloyd. Hemisphere, Washington, D. C.

92. McConnell, E. E. (1983): Pathology requirements for rodent two year studies. I. A review of current procedures. *Toxicol. Path.,* 11:60–64.

93. McConnell, E. E. (1983): Pathology requirements for rodent two year studies. II. Alternative approaches. *Toxicol. Pathol.,* 11:65–76.

94. McConnell, E. E., Moore, J., Haseman, J., and Harris, M. (1978): The comparative toxicity of chlorinated dibenzo-p-dioxins in mice and guinea pigs. *Toxicol. Appl. Pharmacol.,* 44:335–356.

95. McConnell, E. E., Solleveld, H. A., Swenberg, J. A., and Boorman, G. A. (1986): Guidelines for combining neoplasms for evaluation of rodent carcinogenesis studies. *J. Natl. Cancer Inst.,* 76:283–289.

96. Melby, E. D., and Altman, A. H. (1976): *Handbook of Laboratory Animal Science,* Vol. III, pp. 221–356. CRC Press, Cleveland.

97. Melnick, R. L., Jameson, C. W., Goehl, T. J., and Kuhn, G. O. (1987): Application of microencapsulation for toxicity studies: I. Principles and stabilization of trichlorethylene in geletin sorbitol microcapsules. *Fundam. Appl. Toxicol.,* 8:425–431.

98. Menzel, D. B., and McClellan, R. O. (1980): Toxic responses of the respiratory system. In: *Casarett and Doull's Toxicology, The Basic Science of Poisons,* edited by J. Doull, C. D. Klassen, and M. D. Anders. Macmillan, New York.

99. Miller, E. C., and Miller, J. A. (1976): The metabolism of chemical carcinogens to reactive electrophiles and their possible mechanisms of action in carcinogenesis. In: *Chemical Carcinogens,* edited by C. E. Searle, pp. 737–762. Monograph 173. American Chemical Society, Washington, D. C.

100. Munro, I. C. (1977): Considerations in chronic testing: the chemical, the dose, the design. *J. Environ. Pathol. Toxicol.,* 1:183–197.

101. National Cancer Institute (1978): *Bioassay of Dibromochloropropane for Possible Carcinogenicity.* Carcinogenesis Technical Report Series, No. 28.

102. National Cancer Institute (1978): *Bioassay of Acronycine for Possible Carcinogenicity.* Carcinogenesis Technical Report Series, No. 49.

103. National Cancer Institute (1978): *Bioassay of 1,2 Dibromoethane for Possible Carcinogenicity.* Carcinogenesis Technical Report Series, No. 86.

104. National Institutes of Health (1981): *NIH Guidelines for the Laboratory Use of Chemical Carcinogens.* NIH Publ. 81-2385.

105. National Toxicology Program (1981): *Monitoring Guidelines for the Conduct of Carcinogen Bioassays.* Technical Report Series, No. 218.

106. Nettesheim, P., Hanna, M. G., and Deatherage, J. W. (1970): *Morphology of Experimental Respiratory Carcinogenesis.* U.S. Atomic Energy Series, No. 21. U.S. AEC, Gatlinburg, Tennessee.

107. Newberne, P. M. (1974): Report of discussion group No. 2, diets. In: *Carcinogenesis Testing of Chemicals,* edited by L. Golberg. CRC Press, Cleveland.

108. Newberne, P. M. (1975): Influence on pharmacological experiments of chemicals and other factors in diets of laboratory animals. *Fed. Proc.*, 34:209–218.

109. Newberne, P. M. (1975): Diet: the neglected experimental variable. *Lab. Anim.*, 4:20–24.

110. Newberne, P. M. (1979): Nitrite promotes lymphoma incidence in rats. *Science*, 204:1079–1081.

111. Office of Science and Technology Policy (1985): Chemical carcinogens: a review of the science and its associated principles. *Fed. Register*, 50:10372–10418.

112. Oishi, S., Oishi, H., and Hiraga, K. (1979): The effect of food restriction for 4 weeks on common toxicity parameters in male rats. *Toxicol. Appl. Pharmacol.*, 47:15–22.

113. Peto, R., Pike, M., Day, N., Gray, R., Lee, P., Parish, S., Peto, J., Richards, S., and Wahrendorf, J. (1980): Guidelines for simple, sensitive significance tests for carcinogenic effects in long-term animal experiments. *IARC Monogr.* [*Suppl.*], 2:311–426.

114. Plaa, G. L. (1968): Evaluation of liver function methodology. In: *Selected Pharmacologic Testing Methods*, Vol. 3, edited by A. Burger, pp. 255–288. Dekker, New York.

115. Poiley, S. M. (1974): Housing requirements—general considerations. In: *Handbook of Laboratory Animal Science*, Vol. 1, edited by E. C. Melby Jr. and H. H. Altman. CRC Press, Cleveland.

116. Popp, J. A., editor (1984): *Mouse Liver Neoplasia.* Hemisphere, New York.

117. Portier, C. J. (1986): Type I error and power of the linear trend test in proportions under the National Toxicology Program's modified pathology protocol. *Fundam. Appl. Toxicol.*, 6:515–519.

118. Portier, C. J., and Hoel, D. G. (1983): Optimal design of the chronic animal bioassay. *J. Toxicol. Environ. Health*, 12:1–19.

119. Rackis, J. J., Gumbmann, M. R., and Liener, I. E. (1985): The USDA trypsin inhibitor study. I. Background, objectives, and procedural details. *Qual. Plant Foods Hum. Nutr.*, 35:213–242.

120. Rao, G. N., Piegorsch, W. W., and Haseman, J. K. (1987): Influence of body weight on the incidence of spontaneous tumors in rats and mice of long-term studies. *Am. J. Clin. Nutr.*, 45:252–260.

121. Regulatory Council (1979): Statement of regulation of chemical carcinogens. *Fed. Register*, 44:60038–60048.

122. Reuter, J., and Hobbelen, J. (1977): The effect of continuous light exposure on the retina in albino and pigmented rats. *Physiol. Behav.*, 18:939–944.

123. Riley, V. (1975): Mouse mammary tumors: alteration of incidence as apparent function of stress. *Science*, 189:465–467.

124. Ross, M. H., and Bras, G. (1976): Food preference and length of life. *Science*, 190:165–167.

125. Ross, M. H., and Bras, G. (1973): Influence of protein under and over nutrition on spontaneous tumor prevalence in the rat. *J. Nutr.*, 103:944–963.

126. Ross, M. H., Bras, G., and Ragbeer, M. S. (1970): Influence of protein and caloric intake upon spontaneous tumor incidence of the anterior pituitary gland of the rat. *J. Nutr.*, 100:177–189.

127. Saffiotti, U., Cefis, F., and Kolb, L. H. (1968): A method for the experimental induction of bronchogenic carcinoma. *Cancer Res.*, 28:104–124.

128. Saffiotti, U., Montesano, R., Sellakumar, A. R., Cefgis, F., and Kaufman, D. G. (1972): Respiratory tract carcinogenesis in hamsters induced by different numbers of administrations of benzo(a)pyrene and ferric oxide. *Cancer Res.*, 32:1073–1081.

129. Sansone, E. B., and Losikoff, A. M. (1978): Contamination from feeding volatile test chemicals. *Toxicol. Appl. Pharmacol.*, 46:703–708.

130. Sansone, E. B., and Tewari, Y. B. (1978): Penetration of protective clothing materials by 1,2-dibromo-3-chloropropane, ethylene dibromide, and acrylonitrile. *J. Am. Industr. Hyg. Assoc.*, 39:921–922.

131. Sansone, E. B., and Tewari, Y. B. (1978): The permeability of laboratory gloves to selected solvents. *J. Am. Industr. Hyg. Assoc.*, 39:169–174.

132. Sass, B., Rabstein, L. S., Madison, R., Nims, R. M., Peters, R. L., and Kelloff, G. J. (1975): Incidence of spontaneous neoplasms in F344 rats throughout the national lifespan. *J. Natl. Cancer Inst.*, 54:1449–1456.

133. Scharer, K. (1977): The effect of chronic underfeeding on organ weights in rats. *Toxicology*, 7:45–56.

134. Scheuplein, R. J., and Blank, I. H. (1971): Permeability of the skin. *Physiol. Rev.*, 51:702–743.

135. Seifter, E., Rettura, G., Zisblatt, M., Levenson, S. M., Levine, N., Davidson, A., and Seigter, J. (1973): Enhancement of tumor development of physically-stressed mice inoculated with an oncogenic virus. *Experientia*, 29:1379–1382.

136. Sher, S. P. (1974): Tumors in control mice: literature tabulation. *Toxicol. Appl. Pharmacol.*, 30:337–359.

137. Shimkin, M. B., and Stoner, G. D. (1975): Lung tumors in mice: application to carcinogenesis bioassay. *Adv. Cancer Res.*, 21:1–48.

138. Shimkin, M. B., Weisburger, J. H., Weisburger, E. K., Gubareff, N., and Suntzeff, V. (1966): Bioassay of 29 alkylating chemicals by the pulmonary tumor response in strain A. mice. *J. Natl. Cancer Inst.*, 36:915–935.

139. Shubik, P. (1972): The use of the Syrian golden hamster in chronic toxicity testing. *Prog. Exp. Tumor Res.*, 16:176–184.

140. Shubik, P., and Sice, J. (1956): Chemical carcinogenesis as a chronic toxicity test. *Cancer Res.*, 16:728–742.

141. Silverstone, H., and Tannenbaum, A. (1951): Proportion of dietary protein and the formation of spontaneous hepatomas in the mouse. *Cancer Res.*, 11:442–446.

142. Smith, D. M., Rogers, A. E., and Newberne, P. M. (1975): Vitamin A and benzo(a)pyrene carcinogenesis in the respiratory tract of hamsters fed a synthetic diet. *Cancer Res.*, 35:1485–1488.

143. Smyth, R. D., Gaver, R. C., Dandekar, K. A., Van Harken, D. R., and Hottendorf, G. H. (1979): Evaluation of the availability of drugs incorporated in rat laboratory diet. *Toxicol. Appl. Pharmacol.*, 50:493–499.

144. Solleveld, H. A., Haseman, J. K., and McConnell, E. E. (1984): Natural history of body weight gain, survival, and neoplasia in the F344 rat. *J. Natl. Cancer Inst.*, 72:929–940.

145. Sontag, J. M., Pae, N. P., and Saffiotti, U. (1976): *Guidelines for Carcinogen Bioassay in Small Rodents.* NCI Carcinogenesis Technical Report Series, No. 1. National Cancer Institute, Washington, D. C.

146. Spangler, W. L., Gumbmann, M. R., Liener, I. E., and Rackis, J. J. (1985): The USDA trypsin inhibitor study. III. Sequential development of pancreatic pathology in rats. *Qual. Plant Foods Hum. Nutr.*, 35:259–274.

147. Spatz, M., Smith, D. W. E., McDaniel, E. G., and Lacquer, G. L. (1967): Role of intestinal microorganisms in determining cycasin toxicity. *Proc. Soc. Exp. Biol. Med.*, 124:691–697.

148. Steel, R. G. D., and Torrie, H. H. (1960): *Principles and Procedures of Statistics*, pp. 111–112. McGraw-Hill, New York.

149. Stoner, G. D., Conran, P. B., Griesiger, E. A., Stober, J., Morgan, M., and Pereira, M. A. (1986): Comparison of two routes of chemical administration on the lung adenoma response in strain A/J mice. *Toxicol. Appl. Pharmacol.*, 82:19–31.

150. Tannenbaum, A. (1959): *Nutrition and Cancer in the Physiopathology of Cancer*, edited by F. Homberger, pp. 517–562. Phiebig, White Plains, New York.

151. Tarone, R. E. (1975): Tests for trend in life table analysis. *Biometrika*, 62:679–682.

152. Tarone, R. E. (1982): The use of historical control information in testing for a trend in proportion. *Biometrics*, 38:215–220.

153. Tillery, M. I., Wood, G. O., and Ettinger, H. T. (1976): Generation and characterization of aerosols and vapors for inhalation experiments. *Environ. Health Perspect.*, 16:25–40.

154. Tucker, S. M., Mason, R. L., and Beauchen, R. E. (1976): Influence of diet and feed restriction on kidney function of aging male rats. *J. Gerontol.*, 31:264–270.

155. Turnbull, G. J., Lee, P. N., and Roe, F. G. C. (1985): Relationship of body-weight gain to longevity and to risk of development of neuropathy and neoplasia in Sprague-Dawley rats. *Food Chem. Toxicol.*, 23:355–361.

156. Turusov, V. S., editor (1973): *Pathology of Tumors in Laboratory Animals, Vol. 1: Tumors of the Rat*, part 1. IARC, Lyon.

157. Turusov, V. S., editor (1976): *Pathology of Tumors in Laboratory Animals, Vol. 1: Tumors of the Rat*, part 2. IARC, Lyon.

158. Vessel, E. S. (1967): Induction of drug metabolizing enzymes in liver microsomes of mice and rats by softwood bedding. *Science*, 157:1057–1058.

159. Vesselinovitch, S. D., Kandala, V. N. R., and Mihailovich, N. (1979): Neoplastic response of mouse tissue during perinatal age

periods and its significance in chemical carcinogenesis. In: *Perinatal Carcinogenesis*. National Cancer Institute Monograph, No. 51.

160. Weil, C. S., and McCollister, D. M. (1963): Relationship between short- and long-term feeding studies in designing an effective toxicity test. *Agric. Food Chem.,* 11:486–491.

161. Weil, C. S., Woodside, M. D., Bernard, J. R., and Carpenter, C. P. (1969): Relationship between single-peroral, one-week, and ninety-day rat feeding studies. *Toxicol. Appl. Pharmacol.,* 14:426–431.

162. Weisburger, J. H. (1974): Report of discussion group No. 5. In: *Inclusion of Positive Control Compounds in Carcinogenesis Testing of Chemicals,* edited by L. Golberg. CRC Press, Cleveland.

163. Weisburger, J. H., and Weisburger, E. K. (1967): Tests for chemical carcinogens. In: *Methods in Cancer Research,* Vol. I, edited by H. Busch, pp. 307–387. Academic Press, New York.

164. Wilbourn, J. D., Haroun, L., Vainio, H., and Montesano, R. (1984): Identification of chemicals carcinogenic to man. *Toxicol. Pathol.,* 12:397–398.

165. Williams, D. (1972): The comparison of several dose levels with a control. *Biometrics,* 28:519–531.

166. Williams, G. M. (1984): Modulation of chemical carcinogenesis by xenobiotics. *Fundam. Appl. Toxicol.,* 4:325–344.

167. Wolff, G. L., Gaylor, D. W., Frith, C. H., and Suber, R. L. (1983): Controlled genetic variation in a subchronic toxicity assay: susceptibility to induction of bladder hyperplasia in mice by 2-acetyl-aminofluorene. *J. Toxicol. Environ. Health,* 12:255–265.

168. Woodhouse, E. J., Murrill, E. A., Stelting, K. M., Brown, R. R., and Jameson, C. W. (1984): Problems of testing commercial-grade chemicals. In: *Chemistry for Toxicity Testing,* edited by C. W. Jameson and D. B. Walters. Butterworth, Stoneham, Massachusetts.

169. World Health Organization (1969): *Principles for the Testing and Evaluation of Drugs for Carcinogenicity.* WHO Technical Report Series, No. 426.

170. Yu, B. P., Masoro, E. J., Murata, I., Bertrand, H. A., and Lynd, F. T. (1982): Life span study of SPF Fischer 344 male rats fed ad libitum or restricted diets: longevity, growth, lean body mass and disease. *J. Gerontol.,* 37:130–141.

Principles and Methods of Toxicology, Second Edition, edited by A. Wallace Hayes, Raven Press, Ltd., New York © 1989.

CHAPTER **10**

Assessment of Male Reproductive Toxicity: A Risk Assessment Approach[1]

Harold Zenick and Eric D. Clegg

Reproductive and Developmental Toxicology Branch, Office of Health and Environmental Assessment, Office of Research and Development, U.S. Environmental Protection Agency, Washington, DC 20460

OVERVIEW

Of the potential health risks associated with exposure to chemical or physical agents, a prominent concern is that these agents may interfere with the ability of individuals to produce normal, healthy children. Data suggest that the rate of infertility among couples in the United States may be as high as 10–15% (14). Also important is the estimate that as high as 80% of all conceptions fail to result in successful births (14). The male contribution to these reproductive failures, although unknown, is considered to be significant. Historically, efforts in the area of reproductive toxicology have focused on the effects of *in utero* exposures on embryo/fetal development (i.e., teratogenesis). However, evaluation of the reproductive hazards posed by an agent should also include assessment of the effects of exposure on the parental reproductive systems.

In the previous edition of this book, a combined overview of male and female reproductive toxicology was presented

(33). Separate coverage of these systems is provided in the current text. Female reproductive toxicity has been incorporated into the chapter on female reproductive and developmental toxicology (71), and male reproductive toxicity is covered in this chapter. Attention in this chapter primarily focuses on toxic effects that involve testicular and postspermatogenic processes that are essential for reproductive success. Male reproductive failure resulting from germ cell mutation (i.e., genotoxicity), and the role of the endocrine system in the support of reproductive function are discussed elsewhere in this volume.

BACKGROUND

Traditionally, data on agents affecting male reproduction were primarily derived from three sources: studies on potential male reproductive contraceptives, drugs to improve the fertility of subfertile men, or the spermatotoxic side effects of various therapeutic agents (e.g., chemotherapeutic drugs). In the mid 1970s, it was disclosed that male workers exposed to dibromochloropropane (DBCP) had impaired fertility in the absence of other clinical signs of toxicity. Those findings suggested that for certain agents the male reproductive system could be the first affected or the most sensitive target organ.

In the last 10 years, numerous reviews have classified a myriad of environmental agents as male reproductive toxicants (112). The outcomes of such exposures have included not only reduced fertility but also embryo/fetal loss, birth defects, childhood cancer, and other postnatal structural or functional deficits. However, the studies cited in support of such classification have often suffered from major flaws in experimental design and methodology. Thus the database remains limited, particularly for establishing safe exposure levels or for predicting the risk associated with a particular exposure level.

Compared with species routinely used in toxicity testing, the human male is particularly susceptible to agents that reduce the number or quality of sperm produced. Sperm production may have to be decreased by 80–90% in some strains of mice and rats to affect fertility with routine mating procedures (78,103). The human male produces substantially fewer sperm per gram of testis, and the epididymal sperm reserves are less in humans compared with other species (Table 1). Further, test species engage in multiple copulations during each estrus, ensuring delivery of increased numbers of sperm to participate in fertilization. It is unlikely that a similar copulatory pattern will occur in human couples. If such is the case, less dramatic decreases in normal sperm numbers in men could have serious consequences on their reproductive potential. In fact, many men (especially over the age of 30) have daily production rates of normal sperm that already place them close to or in the subfertile or infertile categories (4). It is reasonable to assume that insult to the human male reproductive system by a toxic agent may then decrease further the human reproductive potential compared with test species.

The remainder of this chapter will include the following: (a) a brief review of the systems and processes involved in spermatogenesis, maturation, and subsequent interaction with the female reproductive tract that result in fertilization, and (b) a critical analysis of the strategies and endpoints that are available for male reproductive risk assessment.

In addition to the chapter in the previous edition of this book, numerous reviews are available as background on the physiology and biochemistry of the male reproductive system (7,32,66,70,116,136).

THE SPERMATOGENIC PROCESS

Spermatogenesis

The testis is a multicompartmental organ with each compartment containing highly convoluted tubules called seminiferous tubules. These tubules, which account for approximately 80% of the normal adult testis weight, are the site of spermatogenesis. The intertubular tissue is called interstitial tissue and includes the Leydig cells, which are responsible for androgen production (Fig. 1). Spermatogenesis, for convenience of discussion, may be divided into three phases: spermatocytogenesis, meiosis, and spermiogenesis.

The seminiferous tubules contain two major cell types: Sertoli cells and spermatogenic (germinal) cells. The latter exist in several sequentially derived forms that may be labeled generally as spermatogonia, spermatocytes, spermatids, and spermatozoa (Fig. 2). The sperm are produced from mitotic divisions of spermatogonial stem cells that line the basement membrane of the tubule. They are gradually displaced toward the lumen during differentiation until, as immature spermatozoa, they are released into the lumen of the tubule (spermiation—Fig. 3). This matriculation of the germ cell occurs in close association with the Sertoli cells, suggesting important roles for the Sertoli cells in supporting and possibly coordinating spermatogenesis (see *Sertoli–Germ Cell Interrelationship*). The mitotic divisions of spermatogenesis differ from somatic cell mitoses in that the resulting cells remain connected by intercellular bridges, a configuration that persists throughout spermatogenesis (Fig. 4). Following spermiation, sperm are transported via the rete testis and vasa efferentia to the epididymis where they undergo further mat-

TABLE 1. *Approximate relationships among daily sperm production, number of sperm potentially available for ejaculation, and number of sperm in a typical ejaculate*

	Rabbit	Stallion	Bull	Human
At sexual rest[a]				
A. Daily sperm production (10^9)	0.16	5.3	7.5	0.12
B. Sperm available for ejaculation (10^9)[b]	0.85	28.7	23.5	0.24
C. Typical ejaculate (10^9) sperm[c]	0.25	13.5	12.0	0.33
Ratio B:A	5	5	3	2
Ratio B:C	3	2	2	1
With frequent ejaculation[d]				
D. Daily sperm production (10^9)	0.16	5.3	7.5	0.12
E. Sperm available for ejaculation (10^9)[b]	0.48	22.1	18.0	0.09
F. Typical ejaculate (10^9) sperm	0.15	5.3	7.3	0.08
Ratio E:D	3	4	2	1
Ratio E:F	3	4	2	1

[a] Assumes 7 or more days of sexual rest.
[b] Half the number of sperm in the cauda epididymidum, ductuli deferentia, and ampullae.
[c] Only the first ejaculate would contain this many sperm.
[d] One ejaculation every 1–2 days.
Calculated from published data plus data in referenced paper. (Modified from ref. 4.)

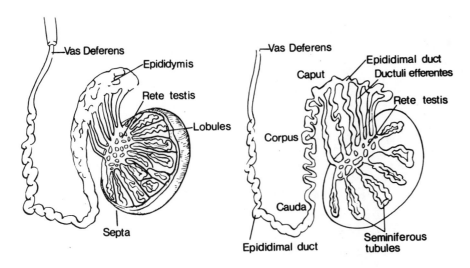

FIG. 1. Schematic representation of the testis and epididymis. (From ref. 135a, with permission.)

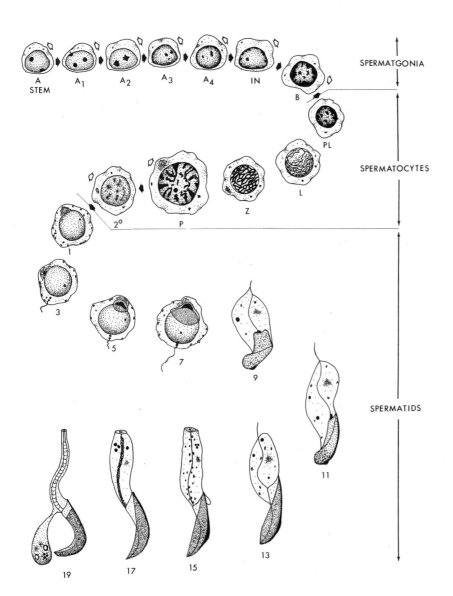

FIG. 2. Schematic representation of spermatogenesis in the rat. (From ref. 108, with permission.)

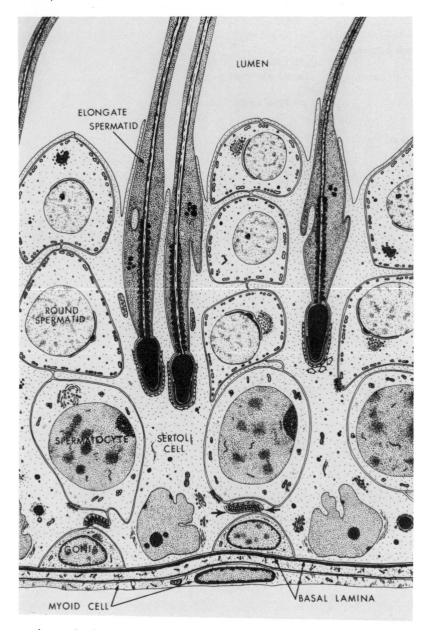

FIG. 3. Functional organization of the seminiferous tubule. (From ref. 108, with permission.)

uration and subsequent storage before ejaculation or elimination in urine.

The kinetics of spermatogenesis are highly synchronized and time locked. Although the timing of the sequence does not appear to be hormonally regulated, the maintenance of the various stages is dependent on the appropriate hormonal environment. Cells in the three developmental phases (spermatocytogenesis, meiosis, spermiogenesis) are arranged in defined associations (stages). Within the seminiferous tubules, a well-defined series of events occurs that follow each other in a precise, orderly sequence. The time interval between consecutive appearances of the same cell association at a given point of the tubule is constant and is called the cycle length of the seminiferous (germinal) epithelium. This concept is hypothetically presented in Fig. 5. The duration of the cycle for different species is presented in Table 2.

A precise description of the stages has been developed for the rat which uses primarily acrosomal and nuclear morphology of the spermatid (Fig. 6). Similar descriptions are

available for other species; however, the cellular associations do not appear to follow as regular a pattern in the human male (4).

Appreciation of the specific cellular associations at a given stage in normal testes is valuable in the histopathological evaluation of testicular tissue (see *Histopathological Evaluations*). Moreover, knowledge of the length of time required for a cell at a given point in the spermatogenic process to reach another point of maturity allows better coordination of the timing of the toxicity assessment relative to the timing of exposure and facilitates interpretation of test results (see *Dose Selection and Dosing Schedule*).

Spermatocytogenesis

This phase entails the maintenance of a population of spermatogenic stem cells as well as the production of sperm-

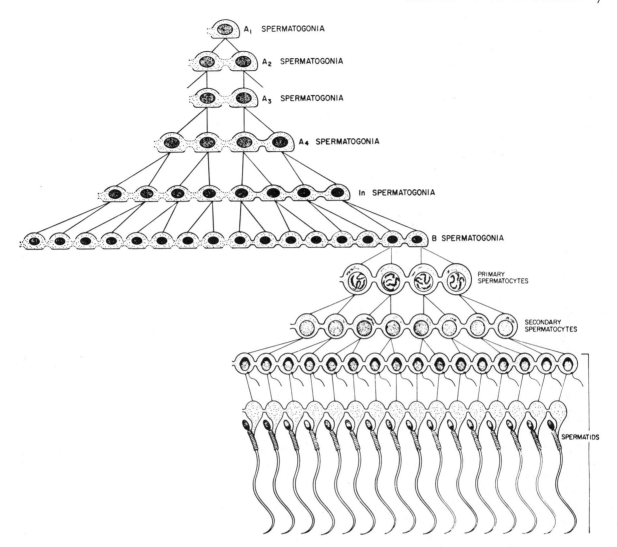

FIG. 4. Schematic representation of the development of mammalian male germ cells. Cytokinesis is incomplete in all but the earliest spermatogonial divisions, resulting in expanding clones of germ cells that remain joined by intercellular bridges. (From ref. 33a, with permission.)

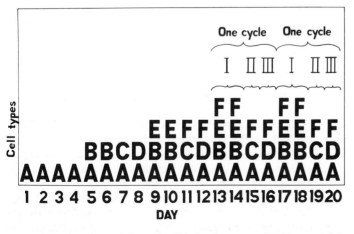

FIG. 5. A series of hypothetical cellular divisions representing spermatogenesis is depicted along a time axis. For this model, it is assumed that (1) A cells divide 4 days after their own formation to produce type A and B cells, (2) B cells divide every 2 days to form C cells, (3) C cells divide 1 day after their own formation to yield D cells, (4) D cells divide after 1 day to produce E cells, and (5) E cells divide after 2 days to form F cells that are released 4 days later as the final product of this process. Although two cells result from each division, only one member of each pair of identical daughter cells is shown. It can be seen that starting from a newly formed A cell shown on day 1, 14 days are required to produce a mature F cell, i.e., the duration of spermatogenesis in the example is 14 days. Once the first generation of F cells is released, distinct cellular associations are observed that reoccur at 4-day intervals. Thus, one cycle of the seminiferous epithelium lasts 4 days, and 3.5 cycles (14 days) are required to complete spermatogenesis. Three distinct cellular associations can be distinguished. These consist of cells ABEF, ACF, and ADF, respectively. These associations have been utilized as criteria for dividing the cycle of the seminiferous epithelium into three stages, designated by I, II, and III. (From ref. 9, with permission.)

TABLE 2. *Duration of various stages of spermatogenic cycle for different species*

	Mouse	Rat	Rabbit (New Zealand White)	Dog (beagle)	Monkey (rhesus)	Man
Duration of cycle of seminiferous epithelium (days)	8.6	12.9	10.7	13.6	9.5	16.0
Life span of						
B-type spermatogonia (days)	1.5	2.0	1.3	4.0	2.9	6.3
L + Z spermatocytes (days)	4.7	7.8	7.3	5.2	6.0	9.2
P + D spermatocytes (days)	8.3	12.2	10.7	13.5	9.5	15.6
Golgi spermatids (days)	1.7	2.9	2.1	6.9	1.8	7.9
Cap spermatids (days)	3.5	5.0	5.2	3.0	3.7	1.6
Fraction of lifespan as						
B-type spermatogonia	0.11	0.10	0.08	0.19	0.19	0.25
Primary spermatocyte	1.00	1.00	1.00	1.00	1.00	1.00
Round spermatid	0.41	0.40	0.43	0.48	0.35	0.38
Testes weight (g)	0.2	3.7	6.4	12.0	49	34
Daily sperm production						
Per gram testis (10^6/g)	28	24	25	20	23	4.4
Per male (10^6)	5	86	160	300	1100	125
Sperm reserves in cauda (at sexual rest: 10^6)	49	440	1600	?	5700	420
Transit time (days) through (at sexual rest)						
Caput + corpus epididymides	3.1	3.0	3.0	?	4.9	1.8
Cauda epididymides	5.6	5.1	9.7	?	5.6	3.7

From ref. 41, with permission.

atogonia that will become irreversibly committed to proceed to the meiotic stages that produce the haploid spermatid. It has been proposed that two populations of stem cells exist in the rodent (25): type A_1 cells that divide at fixed intervals to produce additional stem cells or differentiating spermatogonia; and type A_0 cells or reserve cells that are relatively dormant stem cells that exist in a negative feedback loop with type A_1. A decline in type A_1 may trigger type A_0 production of stem cells. The existence of such a reserve pool in humans is uncertain. The absence of such a compensatory reserve population or the presence of a somewhat different mechanism in the human male could contribute to an increased vulnerability of human males to longer-lasting and/or irreversible injury from exposure to spermatotoxic agents. Because potential for reversibility of toxic effects on stem cells depends on that compensation, a better understanding of the mechanism is important.

Meiosis

In early fetal life, there is proliferation of stem cells (known as gonocytes at this developmental stage), with mitotic arrest occurring at the prespermatogonial stage in late fetal/early postnatal life. At puberty, stem cell proliferation resumes to produce the succeeding types of spermatogonia. It has been proposed that the Sertoli cell may produce meiosis-preventing and meiosis-initiating substances, the ratio of which controls the resumption of spermatogenesis (96). In meiosis, the primary spermatocytes that are produced by the last spermatogonial division undergo a subsequent cellular division to produce secondary spermatocytes. The first meiotic prophase proceeds at a slow rate compared with mitotic prophase and consumes a substantial amount of the time required for the spermatogenic process. Meiotic prophase consists of five stages: preleptotene, leptotene, zygotene, pachytene, and diplotene. Pachytene is the longest phase and is characterized by high levels of RNA and protein synthesis and a unique reliance on lactate as its energy substrate. Genetic recombinations are also most likely to occur at this time. Cell atresia in normal animals also appears to be highest at this stage. The unique requirements of the pachytene stage suggest that this cell type may often be more sensitive to toxic insult than other stages. Knowledge of the requirements of the pachytene spermatocyte has proven valuable in guiding mechanism of action studies for several male reproductive toxicants (8,48,88).

Spermiogenesis

The transition from the secondary spermatocyte to the haploid spermatid is quite rapid. Subsequently, spermatids evolve morphologically in a process that includes formation of the acrosome, flagellum formation, and nuclear elongation and condensation. During nuclear elongation and condensation, there is a transition of the nucleus from a round structure with diffuse chromatin to a more compact mass wherein all detectable transcription of the spermatid nuclear genome ceases. Upon release of the spermatid into the lumen of the seminiferous tubule (spermiation), the spermatozoa are transported via the rete testis and vasa efferentia to the epi-

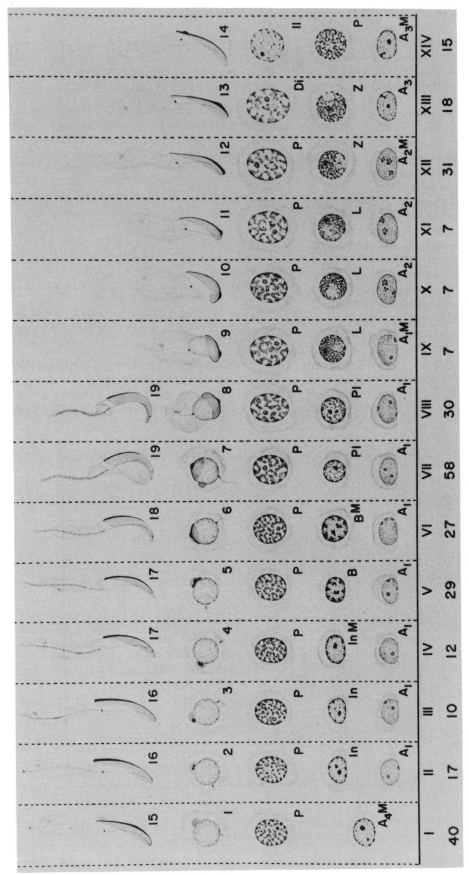

FIG. 6. This drawing shows the cellular composition in the 14 stages of the spermatogenesis cycle. Vertical columns are indicated by Roman numerals and represent associations of cells seen in cross sections of seminiferous tubules. The cells are designated similar to those in Fig. 2 and an M beside the designation indicates mitosis occurring as the cells progress in development to become part of the cell association in the next vertical column. Four and one-half cycles (horizontal rows) are necessary to complete spermatogenesis. The cells indicated by cross hatches are those seen degenerating in normal rats. Cross-hatched cells of stage VII degenerate with increased frequency in response to numerous treatments which influence the luteinizing hormone-testosterone stimulation of the testis. (Modified, by Y. Clermont, from ref. 8.)

didymis where the maturational process continues, including the acquisition of functional properties such as motility and potential to fertilize (see *Sperm Transport and Fertilization*).

The degree of germ cell degeneration can be substantial during the proliferation and differentiation phases described above. It has been proposed that the yield of spermatozoa is approximately 50% of that which could be theoretically produced based upon counts of the stem cell population (56). Three points have been emphasized as times at which cell loss may occur: the first is during the early mitotic divisions of spermatogonial development; the second, and highest level, during meiotic divisions (especially the pachytene stage); and the third during the early stages of spermiogenesis (stages 1–4). This background level of cell atresia must be considered in assessing and interpreting the effects of chemicals on sperm production. The mechanism(s) of this "normal" degeneration remains unknown. Elucidation of the mechanism(s) would improve understanding of the potential for toxicants to operate via similar or different pathways. Such knowledge would also help clarify the mechanisms that regulate regeneration and repopulation of the seminiferous tubules following injury. Recent investigations of chemotherapeutically induced azoospermia have suggested marked species differences between rodents and humans for the mechanisms that regulate these recovery processes (75).

The differentiation processes identified above represent some of the most highly complex cellular transformations that occur in the body. Insight into the mechanisms governing these processes has been slow to emerge. However, the uti-

lization of cell separation techniques in combination with cytochemical analyses of chromatin by flow cytometry has provided insight into the nucleoprotein transitions that occur during spermatogenesis. These changes are illustrated in Fig. 7. The description and possible functional significance of these changes have been discussed by Meistrich et al. (78) and are briefly summarized as follows:

1. The germ cells contain not only variants of the basic proteins (histones) that are found in somatic tissue but also at least five basic proteins that appear unique to the germ cells. Five are found in the testes and one of those—protamine—appears to be the major nucleoprotein of epididymal sperm.

2. Several roles have been proposed for these nucleoproteins during meiosis, including the facilitation of chromosomal pairings and genetic recombinations, and aiding in the mechanics of diploid to haploid reduction.

3. During spermiogenesis, these nucleoproteins may complex with the DNA in such a manner as to reduce its susceptibility to cleavage while forming cross-linking strands that promote nuclear condensation.

4. Further cross-linking during epididymal maturation may further stabilize the sperm for eventual transport in the female tract.

Although many of these roles are speculative, delineating these basic processes is important in delineating heretofore neglected mechanisms of spermatotoxicity. As an example, many of these basic proteins are rich in sulfhydryl-containing

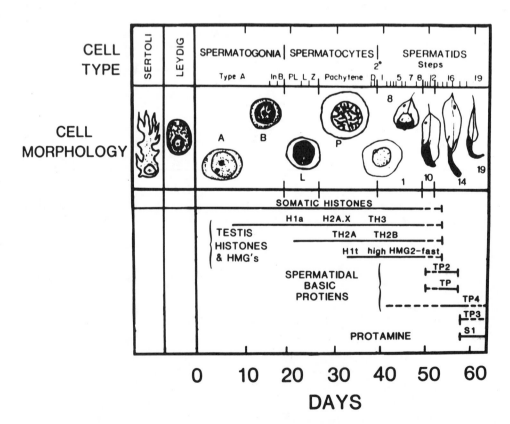

FIG. 7. Outline of the nucleoproteins present during the various stages of spermatogenesis correlated with the cell morphology and kinetics of spermatogenesis. (Provided by Dr. Marvin Meistrich.)

amino acids. A toxicant that would reduce the availability of sulfhydryl donors could interfere with the synthesis of these nucleoproteins. The subsequent failure in genomic inactivation or nuclear condensation during spermiogenesis could provide the opportunity for genetic damage in a manner different from that of "direct-acting" mutagens. Interestingly, a number of male reproductive toxicants are sulfhydryl scavengers (e.g., acrylamide, ethyl methane sulfonate). The potential for interference with sulfhydryl-containing detoxifying enzymes must also be accounted for in testing such hypotheses (see *Pharmacokinetic Considerations*).

Sertoli–Germ Cell Interrelationship

Sertoli cells are the other cellular component of the germinal epithelium. In the rat, Sertoli cells undergo rapid division after birth but cease dividing by 18–19 days of age. Numerous functions associated with coordination of the spermatogenic process have been ascribed to Sertoli cells.

The topographical relationship of germ cells to Sertoli cells is illustrated in Fig. 8. It has been proposed that Sertoli cells play a pivotal role in the cell-to-cell communication essential to coordinating the movement of germ cells through the seminiferous tubule while maintaining the precise pattern of cellular associations. This role includes involvement in spermiation (Fig. 9).

In addition to mechanical support for spermatogenesis, Sertoli cells may regulate the metabolic exchanges critical to meeting specific cellular needs at a given stage in the developmental process. They are also androgen targets and secrete specific proteins (e.g., androgen-binding protein) which may have important roles in development of meiotic and postmeiotic sperm. Another secretory product is inhibin, which may be involved in the negative feedback loop that regulates follicle-stimulating hormone.

Sertoli cells also appear to be primarily responsible for the formation of the blood–testis barrier. As seen in Fig. 8, adjacent Sertoli cells form occluding junctions interposed between the spermatogonia and early spermatocytes (basal

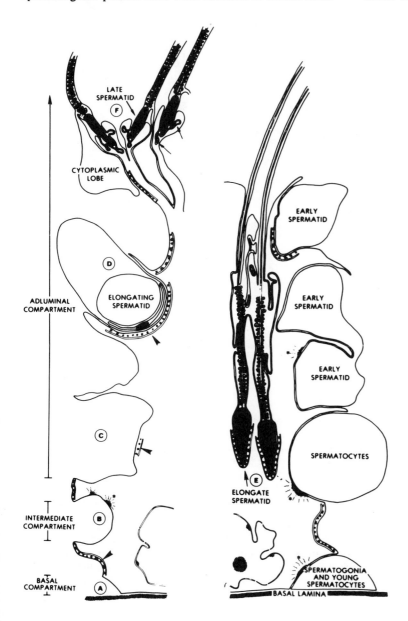

FIG. 8. Configurational relationships of Sertoli cell with germ cells: (**A**) Spermatogonia and young spermatocytes also share a position on the basal lamina and are covered on one surface by adjacent Sertoli cells that meet above them to form occluding junctions of the blood–testis barrier. These germ cells lie in free access to blood-borne nutrients and may be considered within the *basal compartment*; (**B**) Cells (leptotene-zygotene spermatocytes) leaving the basal compartment in their progressive translocation toward the lumen are removed from the basal lamina. Sertoli cells form junctional complexes both above and below them. This compartment, termed the *intermediate compartment*, is thought to allow passage of spermatocytes without interrupting the tight seal provided by the Sertoli cells (blood–testis barrier); (**C**) Once the Sertoli junctions above the spermatocyte dissociate, the germ cell is in the *adluminal compartment* and related to the lateral and apical processes of the Sertoli cell; (**D**) In the elongation phase of spermiogenesis, the nucleus of the spermatid is acentric within the cell. The cell becomes situated within a narrow recess of the trunk of the Sertoli cell; (**E**) This recess deepens as the germ cell elongates and the cell becomes deeply lodged within the body of the Sertoli cell. Numerous finger-like processes penetrate the spermatid cytoplasm that surrounds the flagellum; (**F**) In preparation for its release, the germ cell moves toward lumen where only its head region is related to the Sertoli cell. Specialized cell-to-cell contacts: *Asterisks*, desmosome-gap junction complex; *arrowheads*, ectoplasmic specialization; *isolated arrows*, tubulobulbar complexes. (From ref. 107a, with permission.)

compartment) and the subsequent spermatogenic cell types (adluminal compartment). Thus, a partial barrier is provided against the free access of certain lymphatic and blood-borne agents to cells in the adluminal compartment. Likewise, the blood–testis barrier protects these unique haploid cells from autoimmunological attack.

Sertoli cells have previously received little attention as a potential target for toxic agents. However, recent investigations have implicated these cells in the testicular pathophysiology associated with a variety of compounds including certain glycol ethers, dinitrobenzene, and phthalate esters (28,38,48). Disruption of their functions would have profound impact on the spermatogenic process. Also, important

is the fact that, in the adult, these cells are nonreplicating. Toxicity sufficient to produce Sertoli cell death is irreversible and would produce a permanent impairment in spermatogenic capability. This potential for irreparable damage makes the elucidation of Sertoli cell function and vulnerability an important research area in reproductive toxicology.

Spermiation

During spermiation, some of the plasma membrane in the midpiece region of the sperm remains associated with the Sertoli cell. As the sperm is released, a portion of the sperm

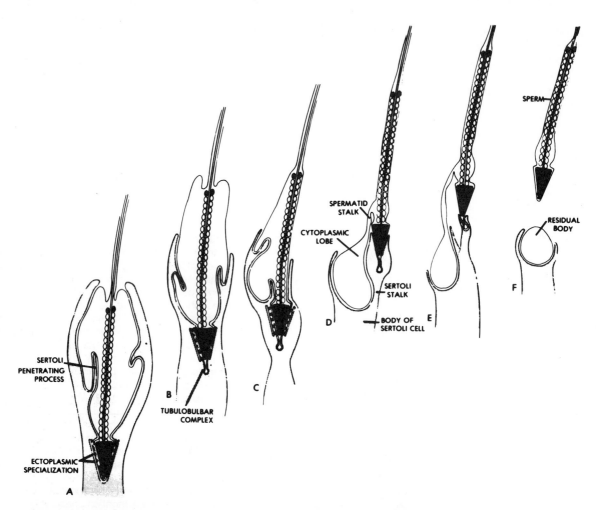

FIG. 9. Summary drawing depicting the general relationship of a spermatid to the Sertoli cells before, during, and after spermiation. **(A)** Prior to the beginning of spermiation, the spermatid is embedded in the deep crypts of a Sertoli cell. The Sertoli cell shows *ectoplasmic specializations* (EcSs) facing the spermatid head and Sertoli *penetrating processes* indenting the cytoplasm around the flagellum. **(B)** After rapid ascent to the lumen, the spermatids retain their configuration and are embedded in a shallower crypt of the Sertoli cell. **(C,D)** As the spermatid moves toward the lumen, the cytoplasm along the flagellum remains stationary with respect to the tubule and gathers into a *cytoplasmic lobe* that is attached to the *presumptive cytoplasmic droplet* by a *spermatid stalk*. The apical Sertoli cell constricts to form a *Sertoli stalk* that connects to an expanded extremity surrounding the heads termed the *apical Sertoli process*. Sertoli EcSs and penetrating processes are no longer present, although the timing of their disappearance is species-dependent. **(E)** The apical Sertoli process has withdrawn from most of the head, and the spermatid stalk has lengthened. **(F)** *Disengagement* occurs with the separation of the apical Sertoli process and the spermatid head and the severence of the spermatid stalk. The liberated spermatid cytoplasm is termed the *residual body*. The meager cytoplasm around the flagellum is termed the *cytoplasmic droplet*. (From ref. 109, with permission.)

plasma membrane plus a substantial amount of cytoplasm is removed from the sperm, forming a residual body. Residual bodies contain most of the Golgi and endoplasmic reticulum vesicles (residual organelles) from the sperm and are phagocytized by Sertoli cells.

The remainder of the residual subcellular organelles are localized in another structure called a cytoplasmic droplet at the top of the sperm midpiece. During normal sperm maturation in the epididymis, the cytoplasmic droplet migrates from the proximal portion of the midpiece to the distal end and then is released from the sperm by the time the sperm is ejaculated. Appearance of cytoplasmic droplets in ejaculated sperm or existence in an inappropriate position in epididymal sperm suggests that the process of sperm maturation has been compromised.

After spermiation, sperm are transported with fluid out of the seminiferous tubules, through the rete testis and vasa efferentia, and into the proximal caput epididymis (Fig. 1). In the vasa efferentia and proximal caput epididymis, a large amount of fluid is resorbed from the testicular product, leaving a substantially more concentrated sperm suspension. Maturation of sperm in the epididymis also begins in the caput, where at least one protein is added to the sperm that allows sperm to become capable of forward motility (55). Sperm acquire the potential to fertilize (see *Capacitation and Fertilization*) by the time they reach the distal corpus or proximal cauda epididymis. During passage through the epididymis, the fluid to which sperm are exposed undergoes substantial alteration in composition, including changes in osmolarity, ion ratios, energy sources, and protein types. The surface of the sperm is modified and chromatin condensation continues. These changes may influence survival of sperm after ejaculation and ensure competence for capacitation, the acrosome reaction, and fertilization. There is potential for toxic agents to affect adversely sperm survival and function at this level of sperm maturation.

During emission and ejaculation, spermatozoa plus the accompanying fluid from the distal cauda epididymis and the vas deferens are mixed with secretions from the accessory sex glands to comprise the ejaculate. Accessory sex gland secretions affect sperm metabolism and function, including motility (initially) and capacitation. Toxic agents in accessory sex gland secretions could affect sperm directly or produce effects in the female genital tract.

Sperm Transport and Fertilization

Deposition of semen by ejaculation or artificial insemination into the female reproductive tract initiates a sequence of events that may result in pregnancy. Although most aspects of those processes are similar across species, some details differ. Included in this discussion are the major components of that sequence: sperm transport and storage, capacitation, the acrosome reaction, and fertilization.

Sperm Transport

Important aspects of sperm transport in the female include the site of semen deposition, degree of stimulation or stress experienced by the female, timing of copulation or artificial insemination relative to time of ovulation, and site(s) of sperm storage and capacitation. Synchronization of these processes is essential for delivery of sperm to the site of fertilization (ampulla) that are capable of fertilizing when the oocyte(s) arrives. In most species, including rodents and humans, the normal site of semen deposition is the anterior vagina in the vicinity of the posterior cervical os. Stimulation of the female during copulation results in contractions of the female reproductive tract. Those contractions draw contents from the anterior vagina into the cervix and uterus, with some of the fluid propelled through the oviducts. This phase is called rapid sperm transport (89). Sperm reaching the ampulla during rapid sperm transport are considered to be incapable of fertilizing because of mechanical disruption. Subsequent contractions of the female reproductive tract during estrus are less violent and deliver sperm to the oviduct that have the potential to fertilize. Studies also indicate that the frequency and amplitude of those contractions increase as ovulation is approached (40). Contractile activity in different segments (uterus, isthmus, ampulla) as well as the diameter of the lumen of the uterotubal junction may differentially change. These contractions to move sperm toward the ampulla are a function of the estrogen-dominated reproductive tract. Contractions of the oviduct after fertilization are in the reverse direction.

Sperm Storage and Removal

In some species, a substantial proportion of the semen deposited in the vagina is lost because of backflow from the vulva. Deposition of semen in the posterior vagina potentiates increased loss by that mechanism. Vaginal plugs or semen coagulation reduces loss of semen by that route. Sperm in the uterus either gain access to the oviducts and ultimately the peritoneal cavity or are removed through the uterine endometrium after phagocytosis.

In some species, such as humans, the cervix appears to be an important site for sperm storage, with viable sperm moving from the cervix into the uterus for a substantial time after copulation. The uterus also may maintain a reservoir of viable sperm. Studies with rabbits indicate that the isthmus may serve as a reservoir for mammalian sperm, with sperm stored there until the time of ovulation is approached (89). At that time, the sperm appear to become activated and are released into the ampulla.

Capacitation and Fertilization

Even when mammalian sperm are produced by fertile males and have completed maturation, they must undergo the process of capacitation before they are capable of fertilizing oocytes (22,134). In capacitation, alterations in surface and other properties occur that prepare sperm to undergo the acrosome reaction if exposed to the proper conditions. Under normal conditions, the acrosome reaction is a vesiculation of the sperm plasma membrane and outer acrosomal membrane in the acrosomal region (Fig. 10) that occurs in capacitated sperm that are in close proximity to an oocyte

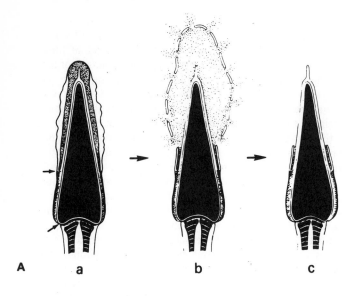

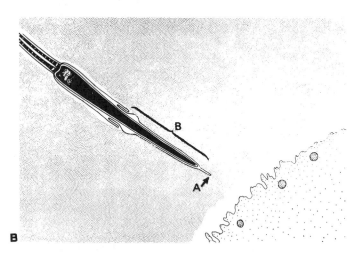

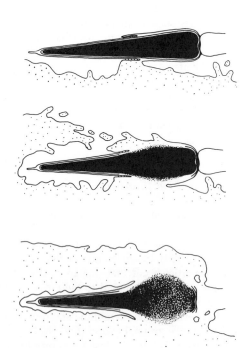

or cumulus cells in the ampulla (79,134). Sperm must undergo the acrosome reaction to fertilize intact ova. Agents that adversely alter surface properties of sperm either during maturation or while residing in the female reproductive tract could interfere with sperm survival, capacitation, and/or ability to undergo the acrosome reaction. As a result, fertility could be compromised. Also, if capacitation or the acrosome reaction is delayed, the potential exists for increased incidence of early embryo death caused by gamete aging. Fertilization that involves aged gametes can produce ova that are polyspermic or exhibit other disturbances of syngamy that are lethal or affect development (12).

During fertilization two acrosomal enzymes, hyaluronidase and acrosin, are released, which enable sperm to reach the plasma membrane (vitelline membrane) of the oocyte (134). Hyaluronidase disperses the cumulus cell mass, while acrosin facilitates penetration of the zona pellucida. Interference with acrosome formation during spermiogenesis or subsequent loss of acrosomal integrity would result in sperm that were incapable of fertilizing.

Following sperm penetration of the zona pellucida into the perivitelline space, the head of the fertilizing sperm comes into sufficiently close proximity to the plasma membrane of the oocyte for membrane fusion to occur (Fig. 10). The sperm

←

FIG. 10. A: Stages of the acrosome reaction in the eutherian spermatozoon, as seen in ultra-thin sections. **(a)** Intact acrosome in an unstimulated spermatozoon, showing the typical irregular contour of the plasma membrane over the acrosome. **(b)** As a first reaction response, multiple point fusions develop between the plasma membrane and outer acrosome membrane such that, in thin sections, these appear to constitute an array of vesicles. The acrosome content then swells and escapes through the ports that the fusion points create. This effectively completes the reaction. **(c)** The next step is acrosome loss which occurs in the fertilizing spermatozoon as it begins to penetrate the substance of the zona. (AC) acrosome; (OA) outer acrosome membrane; (PM) plasma membrane; (ES) equatorial segment whose limits are defined by arrowheads; (IA) inner acrosome membrane. (From ref. 8a, with permission.) **B:** Generalized diagram of a eutherian spermatozoon in the act of passing through the zona pellucida. Although the angle of approach to the oocyte may widely vary from sperm to sperm, the border (**A**) presents a relatively small area of inner acrosomal membrane to the zona substance opposing it. On the other hand, any lytic activity that persists on the lateral face of the sperm head (**B**) seems unlikely to be of major assistance in the penetration process. (See ref. 8a.) (From ref. 79, with permission.) **C:** Diagrammatic illustration of the successive stages of incorporation of a spermatozoon that has passed the zona pellucida. The fertilizing sperm approaches the oolemma. The sperm then fuses with the oolemma by way of the membrane overlying the equatorial segment of the sperm head (**a**). The zone of union then extends posteriorly into the postacrosomal region (**b**), the sperm nuclear envelope disappears, and the beginnings of nuclear decondensation may have become evident already. Finally, movement of the oocyte cortex anticipates the total engulfment of the acrosomal region of the head shown complete in (**c**).

plasma membrane becomes incorporated into the vitelline membrane and the remainder of the sperm becomes internalized into the oocyte (79). At the time of sperm–oocyte fusion, the oocyte is activated and initiates a block to polyspermy at the vitelline membrane or the inner portion of the zona pellucida (111). Penetration and activation of the oocyte are followed by decondensation of the sperm chromatin, formation of the male (and female) pronucleus, migration of the pronuclei toward the center of the ovum, and fusion of the pronuclei.

Fertilization provides a unique opportunity for sperm to deliver a toxic agent directly to an oocyte. Exposure of sperm to an agent during sperm development or in the female reproductive tract could result in binding of the agent to sperm plasma membrane, cytosolic components, or the nucleus. At fertilization, that agent could act directly on the oocyte, affecting the activation sequence or the genetic material.

RISK ASSESSMENT IN MALE REPRODUCTIVE TOXICOLOGY

The Risk Assessment Process

The risk assessment process has been described in detail for cancer in a publication by the National Academy of Sciences (83). Many of the components which are interdependent also apply to the assessment of noncancer health effects such as reproductive toxicity.

A risk assessment should begin with a thorough search and review of the literature and any other available information on that agent. A decision is then made concerning the potential of the agent to cause an effect on humans (hazard identification). In addition to identifying the potential effects, a statement should be developed on the weight of evidence supporting that decision. Included are consideration of the strength of the individual study(ies) and a description of the uncertainties that are associated with the hazard identification (see *Evaluating Reproductive Toxicity Data*).

When an agent has been identified as a potential hazard, it is appropriate to proceed with a quantitative risk assessment (see *Components of Quantitative Risk Assessment*). Included are the steps of dose-response assessment, exposure assessment, and risk characterization (83). The goals of those steps are to identify the lowest exposure level at which health effects occur in humans or in the most appropriate test species, and to combine that information with expected exposure levels for humans to arrive at an estimate of the risk for humans. The lowest dose at which an adverse effect is seen is called the lowest observed adverse effect level (LOAEL), whereas the highest dose at which no effect is observed is called the no observed adverse effect level (NOAEL).

When an appropriate NOAEL or LOAEL has been identified, uncertainty factors may be applied to that value to estimate a level of exposure that should be safe for humans. Alternatively, a margin of exposure may be calculated that is based on the ratio of the NOAEL for the most sensitive significant effect and the estimated exposure level for humans. The components of quantitative risk assessment are more fully discussed at the conclusion of this section.

Testing Protocols for Male Reproductive Toxicity Testing

Because of the range and complexity of the questions that should be answered in evaluating the potential toxicity of an agent to the male reproductive system, numerous test designs are possible. In this section, some of the factors that should be considered in designing protocols to test for male reproductive toxicity are examined. Subsequently, protocols that are routinely used for these tests are discussed.

Design Factors in Male Reproductive Toxicity Testing

Selection of species

When available, comparative pharmacokinetic data should be used to select a test species that appears similar to humans for the agent under consideration. In the absence of information on which to base selection of species, confidence in the results of testing for male reproductive toxicity is increased when multiple species have been examined. Under many circumstances, the rat or mouse is appropriate as one of the test species. Advantages for the rat are its widespread use and a resulting extensive data base on reproductive characteristics, convenient size of both the intact animal and its reproductive organs, uniformity within strains, and good reproductive performance. In addition, the basic mechanisms underlying male reproductive function in the rat are considered to reasonably represent those in human males.

For the second test species, the rabbit should be considered. The rabbit provides capabilities for assessment of male reproductive effects that are not as easily achieved with the smaller rodents. Ejaculated semen can be collected from bucks using an artificial vagina, allowing longitudinal sperm assessments. Alterations in the accessory sex gland secretions can be assessed. The influence of xenobiotics present in accessory sex gland secretions on sperm quality can also be examined. Ejaculated semen samples can also be used for artificial insemination. Use of artificial insemination with a limited number of sperm can be effective in detecting adverse effects on sperm fertilizing ability.

Number of animals

The number of animals per dose group that should be used in a toxicology study is determined by the number of animals expected to survive and to yield data, the expected variation between animals in the endpoints to be examined, the magnitude of effect that should be detected, and the level of probability selected for statistical significance. The number of animals needed per treatment should be calculated by standard statistical methods as part of the study design process. Estimates of the coefficients of variation for some parameters used for tests of the male reproductive system have been reported by several authors (13,113,127,139). (A more complete discussion is found below in the section on the evaluation of indices.) In general, when multiple end points will be used in a study of male reproductive toxicity, 20 males per treatment is often sufficient to detect effects. However, in tests designed to evaluate fertility, it is often necessary to start with 30 to 40 males per treatment group to obtain 20 pregnancies per treatment. There is no scientific justification for reducing the number of animals per treatment because a species (e.g., rabbit, dog) is more expensive to purchase or maintain.

Mating of two females per male at the same time or consecutively is frequently done. That practice does not double sample size for the statistical analysis of male-mediated reproductive outcomes. For statistical evaluation of effects on male fertility or of male-mediated effects on offspring, the male must be the unit of analysis. The use of the number of pregnant females as the unit of analysis artificially inflates sample size in the data analysis.

Dose selection and dosing schedule

Pharmacokinetic information is useful for selection of dose levels, as well as for determining the appropriate duration of dosing and timing of assessment relative to dosing. Such data would indicate the time course and degree of bioaccumulation. Initial range-finding studies are also useful in identifying the dose levels required to achieve the desired level(s) of toxicity. However, such data are often not available.

For hazard identification, it is important to use relatively high dose levels and a sufficient array of endpoints to be confident that a potential effect would not be missed. For such toxicity testing, the highest dose should produce systemic toxicity but not mortality. Dose–response assessment requires the generation of dose–response curves that adequately describe the increments in degree of effect as well as any changes in pattern of endpoints affected with increasing dose level. Dose–response data should also include sufficiently low dose levels that a low level of response or no effect is produced. Spacing between doses is especially critical in dose–response assessment. If the gaps between dose levels are too large, the estimate of the LOAEL could be too high and the NOAEL could be too conservative.

Adverse effects of an agent on the spermatogenic process may not be observed in semen evaluations or in fertility tests for a substantial time after initiation of treatment. Damage that is limited to spermatogonial stem cells would not appear in cauda epididymal sperm or in ejaculates for 8 to 14 weeks, depending on the species examined. To allow effects on spermatogonial stem cells to be expressed in all evaluations of cauda epididymal or ejaculated sperm in subchronic studies, treatment of adult males should be continued for a minimum of six cycles of the germinal epithelium (41) prior to sacrifice or mating. For the more commonly used species, one cycle of the germinal epithelium requires the following number of days: rat, 12.9; mouse, 8.6; rabbit, 10.7; rhesus monkey, 9.5; human, 16.0 (41). Therefore, treatment for six cycles of the seminiferous epithelium for the test species requires from 52 to 78 days to ensure that all possible adverse effects are expressed in each endpoint observed. This recommendation assumes that levels and cumulative effects of the agent at the site(s) of attack reach steady state within one cycle of the seminiferous epithelium after initiation of treatment. If that assumption is not valid for an agent, the treatment period may need to be extended accordingly.

Length of mating period

In fertility testing, pairs of rodents may be allowed to cohabit for periods of varying length. If prolonged cohabitation (i.e., 8–10 days or longer) is allowed, each nonpregnant female should be in estrus two or more times during that period. Under those conditions, reduced fertility in a male may be masked because of the multiple mating opportunities during each estrus and the multiple estrus periods.

During cohabitation, females should be examined daily for the presence of seminal plugs and/or by vaginal lavage for evidence of mating. Females are usually separated from the male on the day following mating. This practice limits mating to one estrus but still allows numerous copulations during that estrus. As a result, an adequate number of sperm may be ejaculated to ensure fertility even with males that have been severely compromised. The hypothesis that restricting the number of copulations would increase the sensitivity of fertility testing has been recently tested (24). Male rats were exposed to a well-documented spermatotoxicant, ethoxyethanol (EE) (0 or 450 mg/kg/day), by gavage for 7 weeks. That dose level produced severe depressions in sperm counts and testis weight (Table 3). Each control and EE-treated male was initially mated, in a counterbalanced design, to a female in estrus, with either a single mating or a minimum of three matings allowed. Three days later, each male was mated under the alternate condition. Despite the extreme reduction in sperm counts in EE males, no differences in fertility were observed relative to controls with multiple matings. However, a marked decrease in fertility was seen in the EE group when only a single mating was allowed (Table 3). These results suggest that the sensitivity of breeding protocols may be enhanced by limiting the number of mating copulations that are allowed. Such a model is also more analogous to the copulatory pattern of humans.

The observation and control of number of matings is facilitated by maintaining the animals on a reverse light–dark schedule so that estrus and matings occur during normal working hours. If sexually experienced rats are used, copulatory behavior can be rapidly and easily monitored, with several males simultaneously observed. Details of this mating procedure have been previously published (137,138,140).

Artificial insemination with a reduced number of sperm can also be used to reduce the number of sperm delivered to the female. This technique is primarily useful with rabbits. The interpretation of results is somewhat different when a

TABLE 3. *Reproductive toxicity data from restricted mating study*[a]

Dose (mg/kg/day)	Testis weight (g)	Spermatid count (10^6)	Cauda sperm count (10^6)	Fertility[b] 1× (%)	Fertility[b] >3× (%)
0	1.78	149.7	143.3	60	80
450	1.23	32.4	28.4	22	72

[a] Rats treated with ethylene glycol monoethyl ether for 7 weeks, given mating experience, then allowed either one copulation followed by separation or at least three copulations followed by overnight cohabitation with a female in estrus.
[b] Fertility index (number pregnant/number mated).

limited and fixed number of sperm is used. Under those conditions, the variable examined is quality of the sperm without regard to the number of sperm that the male is capable of ejaculating.

Protocols

There are several protocols that are routinely used to test for toxicity to the reproductive system. The basic types of "canned" protocols that can provide data on the male reproductive system include the single generation reproduction test, the multigeneration reproduction test, the Food and Drug Administration (FDA) Segment 1 protocol, and the dominant lethal test. The continuous breeding protocol, although not yet considered a standard protocol, is being routinely used by the National Toxicology Program and may assume increasing importance. In addition, the subchronic, and chronic toxicity test protocols can provide information on potential male reproductive effects from the histopathologic and organ weight observations.

The basic designs of the multigeneration reproduction, continuous breeding, and dominant lethal protocols are described elsewhere in this volume. In the following section, selected protocols are briefly described, along with discussions of their strengths and limitations. Modifications are identified that could be incorporated into some of the protocols to increase the information obtained on male reproductive effects.

Subchronic toxicity test

In a general subchronic toxicity test, dosing is usually initiated in young animals (often 35–56 days of age) and continued for 60 to 90 days. Dosing is often done orally but may be by inhalation or dermal application. Application of a test agent on the surface of or injection directly into a reproductive target organ is seldom appropriate for toxicologic testing and risk assessment, although those routes may be useful for studies of mechanism of action (110). Animals are monitored for clinical signs throughout the test and are necropsied at the end of dosing. The endpoints usually examined that are relevant to the male reproductive system include visual examination of the reproductive organs, testis weight, and testicular histology.

A substantial amount of additional, cost-effective information on effects on the male reproductive system could be obtained by expanding the male reproductive endpoints examined to include high quality evaluation of testicular histology (see *Histopathological Evaluations*), as well as measures of sperm production and quality. If properly done, such an array could serve as a screen for direct male reproductive effects. It could also provide information that would be useful to design any succeeding tests.

Chronic toxicity test

The chronic toxicity test provides the opportunity to obtain information on toxic effects of long-term dosing and effects on the aging male reproductive system. Although reproduction may be less important to aged individuals, maintenance of a normal hormonal pattern and sexual capability continue to be important (61).

In the chronic toxicity test, dosing is by oral, inhalation, or dermal routes, is initiated soon after weaning, and is continued for 12 to 24 months. Animals are usually observed daily. Body weights and food and water consumption should also be monitored. Because of the extended treatment period, some animals may be necropsied at 6-month intervals. The interim examinations can provide important insight into the progression of toxicity and its relationship to the normal changes associated with aging.

At necropsy, the reproductive organs are visually examined, testis weights obtained, and the testes subjected to gross histology. As suggested for the subchronic toxicity test, additional information could be obtained from high quality testicular histology, as well as from measures of sperm production and quality.

Single generation reproduction test

In a single generation reproduction test, both males and females are usually treated before and during mating. However, it is possible to mate treated with nonexposed animals to examine gender-specific effects. Dosing should be initiated at 10 weeks of age or older (see *Dose Selection and Dosing Schedule*). Following treatment of males for at least six cycles of the germinal epithelium, cohabitation is allowed for up to 3 weeks, during which time the females are monitored for evidence of mating. Males are necropsied at the end of the cohabitation period. Usually, females are allowed to complete gestation and nurse their litters to day 21. At necropsy, both the dam and the offspring are examined. Offspring are counted and weighed during the postnatal period, usually at days 1, 4, 7, 14, and 21.

This type of protocol can detect effects on the integrated reproductive process. Mating of exposed males with exposed females with continued treatment of the females through gestation and lactation is a "maximizing of effect" strategy. The results reflect the worst-case exposure situation for those animals at that dose level. However, as usually conducted, the single generation reproduction test is not usually adequate for comprehensive testing for male reproductive toxicity. A limited number of relatively insensitive endpoints such as fertility, organ weights, and routine histology are usually obtained.

This protocol is further limited in that it evaluates toxic reproductive effects on the young adult and provides only limited information on developmental toxicity. Because both males and females are usually treated, effects specific to the male may be detected only through the gross and histopathologic examinations of the males. Mating of treated males with untreated females and vice versa is the best way to delineate gender-specific effects on fertility.

Multigeneration reproduction test

Guidelines for the conduct of multigeneration reproduction tests have been published by the Office of Pesticide Programs and the Office of Toxic Substances (120,121), by the FDA (93), and by the Organization for Economic Cooperation and Development (OECD) (87). The test usually involves matings over two or three generations. The United States Environmental Protection Agency (EPA) recommends limiting the multigeneration reproduction test to reproduction by two generations because it is unlikely (but not impossible) that an adverse male reproductive effect caused by a nongenetic defect will be expressed in a third generation that is not also expressed in an earlier generation.

In evaluating results from a multigeneration reproduction test, it is important to recognize that the exposure history is different for each generation (Fig. 11). The initial parental (P) animals receive subchronic exposure during the early adult phase. F_1 animals are continuously exposed from the time of conception to early adulthood, allowing expression of effects on susceptible developmental stages in addition to the effects that would be expressed in the P generation. F_2 animals represent a third exposed generation. They are usually exposed only *in utero* and during the preweaning period. In cases of prolonged bioaccumulation or age-specific effects limited to the prenatal or prepubertal period, different effects or effects of increasing severity may be seen in the F_1 or F_2 generations that are not observed with the P animals. Moreover, many of the detoxifying enzyme systems and renal excretory mechanisms develop neonatally in the rodent, con-

tributing to the increased vulnerability of generations exposed during this critical period (95). Qualitative predictions of the increased risk of the filial generations could be strengthened by knowledge of the nature of the reproductive effects in the adult, the metabolic pathways and the likelihood of bioaccumulation of the agent, and the potential for increased sensitivity resulting from exposure during critical periods of development (46).

Increasing vulnerability of subsequent generations may not always be observed; effects may be static or possibly even of decreasing severity. The latter situation may be the result of the animals in the F_1 and/or F_2 generations representing "survivors" who are (become) more resistant to the agent than the average of the P generation. If such selection exists, subsequent generations may show a reduced toxic response. Also, the males and females are more experienced breeders for the second litter within a generation. Therefore, results between generations or between sequential litters within a generation should not necessarily be directly compared. Significant adverse effects in any generation should be considered cause for concern.

A recent review of 20 "positive" multigeneration reproduction studies has provided some preliminary observations on the relationship of male toxicity to effects on offspring within a given generation and the relationships of reproductive outcomes across generations (21):

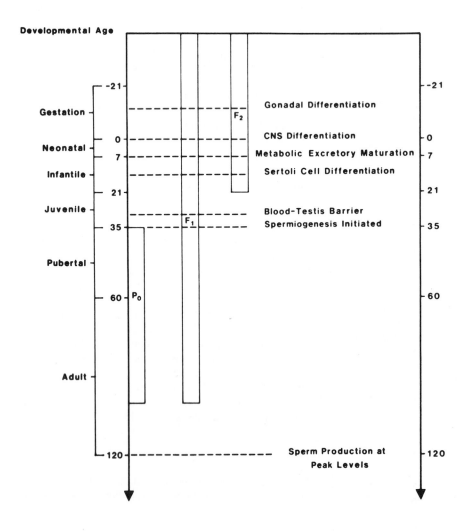

FIG. 11. The developmental stages and events encompassed by exposure of the P_0, F_1, or F_2 generations in a two-generation reproduction study.

1. The presence of toxicity in the adult male, reproductive or otherwise, was not a prerequisite for the occurrence of effects on offspring.

2. Approximately one-half of the studies were classified as "positive-increasing." In these cases, the second generation (F_1) animals exhibited effects that were more severe than those in the first generation and/or occurred at equivalent or lower doses.

3. The increasing toxicity across generations is consistent for chemicals that bioaccumulate. However, exposure of sequential generations that involve different developmental stages (P versus F_1 adults) might also contribute to differential effects across generations.

As noted for the single generation reproduction test, no distinction is usually made between male- and female-directed effects on fertility. Treated males can be mated with untreated females and vice versa to identify gender-specific effects on fertility.

As usually performed, the multigeneration reproduction test does not address the issue of reversibility. However, it is possible to produce more than one litter with either the F_1 or F_2 males. The additional offspring can provide animals for a developmental toxicity evaluation or a reversibility test. However, successive litters cannot be considered as replicates because of factors such as increased age, sexual experience, and parity of the parents.

Continuous breeding protocol

The continuous breeding protocol has been recently developed by the National Toxicology Program as a possible alternative to the multigeneration reproduction test. Validation of the protocol has been with the mouse (65). Its utility with rats is currently being tested. The distinctive feature is the use of continuous cohabitation of a male-female pair for 14 weeks with removal of each litter soon after birth. It is the only protocol currently in use that provides a measure of subfertility (increased time to mating) other than decreased litter size for mated pairs (see *Fertility and Pregnancy Outcomes*). Another feature is the inclusion of crossover matings of treated animals with untreated controls if effects on fertility are observed during the cohabitation of treated animals.

The continual production of litters from the same adults has the advantage of allowing observation of the timing of onset of an adverse effect on fertility. However, because treatment is continuous, a cumulative effect could increase severity of expression with subsequent litters. If offspring in the final litter are allowed to grow and reproduce, information can be produced on postnatal development or reproductive capability of a second generation. Because the animals used for the crossover matings are not treated during the matings with untreated animals, reversible effects may show a different pattern at necropsy than would have been observed had necropsy been done immediately after cessation of treatment.

As discussed for the multigeneration reproduction test, the increasing age, sexual experience, and multiparous state of the animals dictate caution in comparing results for different litters within each mated pair, between pairs within a dose level, and between dose levels.

Dominant lethal test

The dominant lethal test is intended to detect mutagenic effects in the spermatogenic process that are lethal to the embryo or fetus. A review of this test has been recently published as part of the EPA's Gene-Tox program (49). Dominant lethal protocols may use acute dosing (1–5 days) followed by serial matings with one or two females per male per week for the duration of the spermatogenic process. An alternative protocol may use subchronic dosing for the duration of the spermatogenic process followed by mating(s). Females are monitored for evidence of mating, sacrificed at approximately midgestation, and examined for incidence of pre- and postimplantation loss (see *Fertility and Pregnancy Outcomes*).

The acute exposure protocol of the standard dominant lethal test, combined with serial mating, allows identification of the spermatogenic cell type(s) that are adversely affected by treatment. Such information can be useful for identifying site and potential mechanism of action and thus facilitate design of subsequent studies.

Endpoints and Outcomes in Male Reproductive Toxicity Assessment

The following sections describe the various endpoints of male reproductive toxicity that can be obtained and their use in toxicity assessment. Three considerations are applicable throughout this discussion of measures of male reproductive toxicity. First, a comprehensive assessment requires information on a variety of endpoints. Ideally, the evaluation would include examination of data on the more sensitive endpoints (e.g., properly performed histopathology; see *Histopathological Evaluations*) to allow determination of the LOAEL. Positive effects on less sensitive, functional endpoints (e.g., fertility) are useful for hazard identification and in interpreting the biological significance of effects that are not as directly associated with function. The ability to form such associations between the more sensitive endpoints and those that measure function directly may provide a clearer picture of the risk to human reproduction.

A second issue is that alterations in these reproductive endpoints may be the result of direct or indirect toxicity to the male reproductive system. In either case, the agent should be considered a male reproductive hazard. Careful evaluation of the dose–response curves for the various target organs may provide insight into whether the reproductive effects are independent of these other toxicities. Estimating the dose levels at which these various target organ events occur has special significance in predicting the effects of anticipated human exposure. In addition, the likelihood that reproductive toxicity will be present in the absence of other systemic effects can be better characterized.

A third issue is that although the measures discussed in this section may reflect impairment to the various components of the reproductive process, they may not effectively discriminate nonmutagenic from mutagenic mechanisms. If the effects seen in evaluation of male reproductive endpoints are the result of mutagenic events (e.g., interaction with DNA), there is the potential for transmissible genetic damage.

(See Brusick, Chapter 14 *this Volume,* for a discussion of the approaches for evaluating potential germ cell mutagens.)

Data on the potential male reproductive toxicity of an agent may be obtained from a number of testing protocols. Some of the endpoints that can be readily evaluated in such studies are listed in Table 4.

Body and Organ Weights

Body and organ weights are usually obtained irrespective of the study protocol. Body weights should be recorded at a minimum of weekly intervals during the course of exposure and can provide a useful indicator of the general health status of the animal. Interpretation of reproductive effects in the presence of altered body weight may be uncertain. For at least the testes, organ weight and body weight are independent variables in the *normal* rat (104). Depression in body weight or reduction in weight gain may reflect a variety of responses including rejection of toxicant-adulterated food or water because of reduced palatability, treatment-induced anorexia, or systemic toxicity. Modest depressions in adult body weight as a result of decreased palatability or depressed appetite may have little effect on male reproductive function (e.g., 54,102). When body weight decline is produced by such factors, it may not be appropriate to dismiss the occurrence of male reproductive effects as simply secondary to the occurrence of a generalized toxicity. The factors underlying a decline in body weight or reduced weight gain often cannot be delineated. Also the impact of such weight changes may vary depending on the species and strain. Then the issue as to whether the observed reproductive effects are primary or secondary effects of exposure cannot be resolved. Additional data at other/lower exposure levels may further differentiate the toxic effects. In the absence of such data, alterations in a meaningful reproductive measure, irrespective of body weight change, are sufficient to identify an agent as a male reproductive hazard.

For the male, the reproductive organs that are often weighed include the testes, epididymides, pituitary gland, prostate, and seminal vesicles (the latter two are termed accessory sex glands in this chapter). Necropsy procedures for the reproductive organs other than the testes have not been standardized across laboratories. The development and application of uniform protocols might reduce some of the interstudy variability associated with these measurements as currently reflected across studies.

Organ weight data should be presented as both absolute weights and as relative weights (e.g., organ weight/body weight ratios). Organ weight data may also be reported relative to brain weight because, at maturity, brain weight remains quite stable. Evaluation of data on absolute organ weights is important because an organ weight/body weight ratio may show no significant difference if both body weight and organ weight change in the same direction. However, a change in the organ weight/body weight ratio is usually but not necessarily the result of a disproportionate change in the weight of that organ rather than a disproportionate change in body weight of exposed relative to nonexposed animals.

Testis weight demonstrates modest variation among normal members of a given test species (13,113). This low interanimal variability suggests that testis weight would be a sensitive early marker of gonadal injury. However, this is not always the case. Damage to the testes may often be detected as a weight change only at doses higher than those required to produce significant effects in other measures of gonadal status (9,36,37). This contradiction may arise from several factors including reactions to injury that may mask a decrease in testicular weight (e.g., edema and inflammation, cellular infiltration, and Leydig cell hyperplasia).

Pituitary and accessory sex gland weights can provide valuable insight into the androgen status of the animal. In fact, such measures may be more sensitive indicators of androgen status than testosterone values based upon single blood samples. However, the pituitary contains regions that are responsible for the regulation of a variety of physiologic functions separate from reproduction. Thus, changes in pituitary weight do not necessarily reflect reproductive impairment. If weight changes are observed, histopathological evaluations may be useful in identifying the regions of the pituitary that are altered.

Optimal evaluation of data on the pituitary and accessory sex glands requires information on the technique that was used in removal and dissection of extraneous tissue. Separation of the seminal vesicle and prostate is difficult in rodents. Moreover, published studies may report accessory sex gland weights with or without expression of the secreted fluids. Access to data on accessory sex gland weights, with and without the fluids, would facilitate comparisons across different data sets.

Changes in absolute or relative reproductive organ weights provide sufficient evidence for initially classifying an agent as a potential human male reproductive hazard and provide an important basis for obtaining additional information on the reproductive toxicity of that agent. Interpretation of the biological significance of such changes may be aided by examining data on other endpoints (e.g., histopathology, semen evaluations) as well as by comparison with historical control data. However, because changes in organ weights may only

TABLE 4. *Endpoints of male reproductive toxicity*

Body weight	
Organ weights	Testes, epididymides, seminal vesicles, prostate, pituitary
Histopathology	Testes, epididymides, seminal vesicles, prostate, pituitary
Semen evaluations	Sperm count (concentration), motility, morphology
Endocrine measures	Luteinizing hormone, follicle-stimulating hormone, testosterone
Sexual behavior	
Fertility	Mating ratio: number of confirmed matings/number mated
	Pregnancy ratio: number pregnant/number confirmed matings
Pregnancy outcomes	Litter size, number of live/dead pups, sex ratios, malformations, birth and postnatal weights, and survival

be apparent after substantial injury, reliance on more sensitive measures may be necessary to better define a LOAEL or NOAEL for an agent. Also, significant changes in other important endpoints may not always be reflected in organ weight data. Thus the absence of an organ weight effect does not provide a basis for assuming the absence of a reproductive effect (36,37).

Histopathological Evaluations

Histopathological evaluations have a prominent role in reproductive toxicity assessment. If properly conducted, histopathology is a sensitive tool not only for the detection of low dose effects but also for providing insight into the onset, site(s), and mechanism(s) of action. If similar mechanisms are known to exist in humans, the basis for interspecies extrapolation is strengthened. Depending upon the experimental design, information may also be obtained that will allow the prediction of the eventual extent of injury and the degree of recovery (108).

The histological analysis of spermatogenesis requires proper fixation and embedding of testicular tissue. Approaches that use formalin fixation combined with paraffin embedding of the testis result in artifacts in control as well as treated tissue (e.g., shrinkage, vacuoles, clumping of nuclear material) that can mask effects and confound interpretation. Detection and identification of degenerating cells may be difficult with such preparations. A description of the background level of lesions in control tissue, whether preparation-induced or otherwise, can facilitate the interpretation of the nature and extent of the lesions observed in tissues obtained from exposed animals. Reviews of fixation and embedding techniques for testes have been recently published (19,65), as well as comparisons of testes prepared in various fixation and embedding media (67).

Histological analysis of the testis may use a variety of approaches. Two prominent ones are those that involve "cell staging" and the use of morphometric techniques to count and size various elements in the testis. Both approaches require specialized training; however, once acquired, such expertise can be readily applied to the examination of various test species. Application of these techniques to properly prepared tissue can markedly enhance the ability to detect and interpret lesions.

Cell staging is based upon the examination of cross sections of the seminiferous tubules. As noted earlier, the proliferation and differentiation of germ cells is a highly ordered, time-locked process. Thus, for most species, the temporal and spatial relationships of the different spermatogenic cell types can be defined for the different stages of the spermatogenic cycle (Fig. 6). The photomicrographs shown in Figs. 12 and 13 provide examples of some of the various cell stages. Based on differences in light absorption of tubules containing different stages, transillumination has proven useful for isolating specific cell stages for subsequent biochemical analyses (97). Knowledge of the cytoarchitecture of the testis can allow delineation of specific lesions that have resulted from toxicity to the germ cell at a given stage of development. Quantification of cell staging may include analysis of frequency distributions of the cell stages present (17). The cell-staging ap-

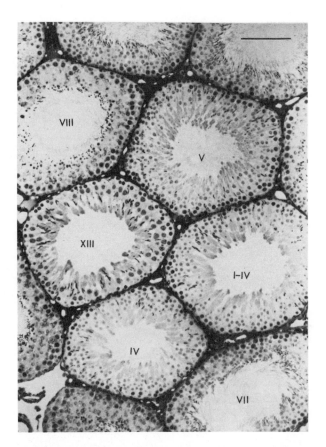

FIG. 12. Light micrograph of rat testis fixed by perfusion and embedded in Epon-Araldite. The seminiferous tubules and interstitial tissue are well maintained, providing favorable material for morphometric analysis. Stages of the cycle of the germinal epithelium are labeled. ×215. Bar = 100 μm. (From ref. 124, with permission.)

proach is being more frequently applied in the evaluation of environmental agents as witnessed by recent research on the glycol ethers (17,28), methyl chloride (20), and phthalate esters (27).

Morphometry is a broad category involving a variety of techniques to obtain quantitative data (9,80). The methods may be applied to measure diameters, areas, or volumes of testicular compartments (tubular versus interstitial); specific cell types; or subcellular structures (108). Cell counts may also be obtained as well as ratios of one cell type to another (e.g., pachytene spermatocytes/Sertoli cell).

Analysis of cell stages might be applied in standard histopathological evaluations to establish the presence of testicular damage. Morphometric analyses, which can be done with the same slides, could be delayed until tentative mechanisms of action had been identified. In the absence of information on mechanism, it would be difficult to state which of the many morphometric analyses should be pursued. The strength of this approach will be in providing additional support for hypotheses generated in earlier studies.

The degree to which histopathological effects are quantified is usually limited to classifying animals within dose groups

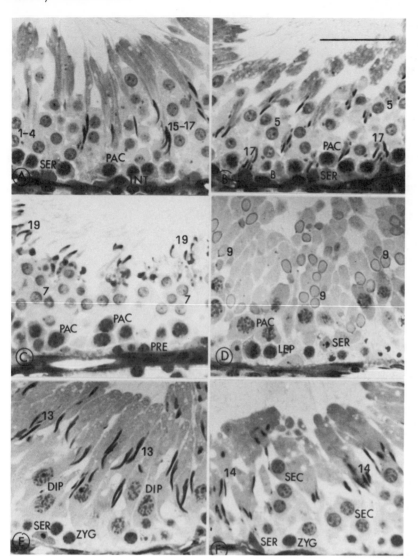

FIG. 13. Representative stages of the cycle of the seminiferous epithelium viewed at higher magnification, showing the level of preservation. Shown are (**A**) stages I–IV, which are pooled in the present study, (**B**) stage V, (**C**) stage VII, (**D**) stage IX, (**E**) stage XIII, and (**F**) stage XIV. Labeled in the figures are Sertoli cells (SER); type B (B) and intermediate (INT) spermatogonia; primary spermatocytes in preleptotene (PRE), leptotene (LEP), zygotene (ZYG), pachytene (PAC), and diplotene (DIP) phases; secondary spermatocytes (SEC); and spermatids at various steps (Arabic numerals) of spermatogenesis. ×575. Bar = 50 μm. (From ref. 124, with permission.)

as either affected or not affected. Little effort has been made to quantify the extent of injury, and standardized procedures for such classifications do not exist. The application of thorough evaluation procedures would be complemented by more uniform strategies for quantifying the extent of histopathological damage per individual. In the absence of a standardized scoring system, the evaluation of histopathological data would be facilitated by the presentation of the assessment criteria and the manner in which the level of lesions in exposed individuals would be judged to be in excess of controls.

The presence of histopathological damage in excess of the level seen in control tissue of test animals provides sufficient evidence for considering an agent to be a potential human male reproductive toxicant and can be used to establish a LOAEL/NOAEL. Thorough histopathological evaluations that fail to reveal any treatment-related effects may be equally convincing. However, in the presence of such "negative" data, consideration should be directed to the possible presence of reproductive effects that are not histologically detected (e.g., decreased sperm motility, increase in abnormal forms, germ cell mutation) but may influence reproductive function.

Fertility and Pregnancy Outcomes

Breeding studies are a major source of data on reproductive toxicants. Evaluations of fertility and the resulting pregnancy outcomes provide measures of the functional consequences of reproductive injury. A variety of measures can be obtained from fertility studies that may include the following: mating ratio (number with seminal plugs or sperm in a vaginal lavage/number cohabited), pregnancy ratio (number pregnant/number confirmed matings), pre- and postimplantation loss, litter size, the number of live and dead pups, sex ratio, malformations, birth weight and neonatal weight, and pup survival. Postnatal evaluations may be conducted on the surviving offspring to further assess growth and development, including an examination of functional endpoints such as behavior or reproductive capacity of the progeny.

As described in the protocols section, reproductive testing often entails the cohabitation of treated males with treated females. Therefore, the influences of the male and female parents on changes in fertility or other reproductive outcome (e.g., reduced survival) may not readily be discriminated.

Assignment to the male of at least some of the responsibility for a toxic effect on fertility may be possible from evaluation of data on other reproductive measures (organ weights, histopathology, sperm measures). Data on mating behavior could also clarify effects on fertility by indicating whether the males were behaviorally competent.

If evaluation of mating success is included, useful data would include confirmation of the day of insemination (i.e., sperm plugs or sperm-positive vaginal lavages), plus analysis of the length of time required for each animal to achieve successful mating (time to mating). The data routinely presented from the majority of breeding tests affirm the occurrence of matings but do not report the length of time required or any difficulties in achieving normal insemination. However, most laboratories conducting fertility studies obtain information on the number of days required for mating as part of their fertility record system. Although evidence of mating is not synonymous with successful impregnation and does not preclude undetected matings, such data could provide a more complete evaluation of reproductive competence.

Evaluations of time to mating might also help detect the presence of subfertility. Exposure to a reproductive toxicant may not produce a total absence of fertility (i.e., sterility) but rather a condition of subfertility seen as an increased time to conception. (Subfertility may also be reflected as a reduction in litter size in polytocous species.) The assessment of time to mating in reproductive studies might indicate the potential for increased time to conception in humans.

Data are available on the variability associated with some of these functional reproductive measures that allow evaluation of the power and group size requirements (113). Coefficients of variation range from approximately 10% for neonatal survival (to day 21) to 20% for fertility ratios. The background variability associated with rates of mating success may be markedly reduced if experienced males are mated to females that had been determined to be in proestrus by vaginal cytology.

Dominant lethal assays, in which the female is sacrificed in mid to late pregnancy, may also produce reproductive data. Endpoints examined from dominant lethal tests often include mating and fertility ratios and estimates of preimplantation loss (number of corpora lutea minus number of implantation sites/number of corpora lutea) and postimplantation loss (number of implantation sites minus number of fetuses/number of implantation sites). The occurrence of pre- and/or postimplantation loss is often considered to provide sufficient evidence that the agent has gained access to the reproductive organs and has induced mutagenic damage to the sperm.

A genotoxic basis for postimplantation loss is widely accepted. However, current methods of assessing preimplantation loss provide little distinction between contributions of mutagenic events that cause embryo/fetal death and nonmutagenic factors that result in failure of fertilization (e.g., inadequate numbers of normal and motile sperm, failure in sperm transport or ovum penetration). The interpretation of an increase in preimplantation loss may require additional data on the agent's mutagenic and/or spermatotoxic potential. Approaches are currently being developed that may prove useful in distinguishing these events. For example, *in vitro* techniques are available in the mouse that allow recovery of ova from females subsequent to mating (45). These ova can then be evaluated for the occurrence of fertilization and observed through several cellular divisions. Such data can discriminate between fertilization failure and early embryo mortality. This distinction is important because cytotoxicity does not imply the potential for transmissible genetic damage that is associated with mutagenic events.

Animal data on reproductive success (or the lack thereof) are difficult to verify in human populations. First, humans are characterized by low rates of conception. Thus, an insufficient number of pregnancies may occur in an exposed population to provide sufficient power to detect an effect. Moreover, both partners may be exposed to the toxicant(s), making it more difficult to ascribe reproductive failure solely to the male. Studies of gender-specific occupational work groups may provide some clarification as to the male's contribution. Such studies also provide the opportunity to study individuals with higher exposures than those encountered in the general population.

Data on fertility potential and other measures of reproductive outcome provide the most comprehensive and direct insight into reproductive capability. In studies with male-only exposure, substantial weight can be placed on results that demonstrate that an agent acted on the male to impair those outcomes. However, fertility assessments are limited by their insensitivity as measures of reproductive injury. Normal males of strains of most test species produce sperm in numbers that greatly exceed the minimum requirements for fertility as evaluated in current protocols that allow multiple matings (see *Length of Mating Period*). For example, in some strains of rats and mice, sperm production can be reduced by 90% without compromising fertility (74,103). However, less severe reductions can have dramatic consequences in human males who function nearer to the threshold for the number of sperm needed to ensure reproductive competence. This difference between test species and human means that data that fail to demonstrate an effect on fertility in a study using a test species should not be the basis for concluding that the test agent poses no reproductive hazard to fertility in humans. In such instances, data from additional reproductive endpoints may provide clarification and should be examined.

Sperm Evaluations

A major strength in conducting sperm evaluations in test animals is that similar data can be obtained from humans, enhancing the ability to confirm effects seen in test species and vice versa. A thorough assessment would include measures of sperm number, sperm motility, and sperm morphology.

The U.S. EPA Gene-Tox Program has published two reviews on sperm tests in test species and humans (130,131). The tests surveyed included sperm count, motility, and morphology. The most frequently reported sperm measure in laboratory studies was sperm morphology. This is a direct result of the use of sperm morphology as an *in vivo* screen for potential mutagens. The most frequently reported sperm measure in human studies was sperm count. A review of these reports emphasizes some of the major data gaps in this area. Aside from sperm morphology, limited animal data are available on other sperm changes associated with chemical exposures. More striking is the absence of sperm evaluations on human populations exposed to environmental agents. Of the 89 chemicals for which the panel reviewed human data, less than 10% were occupational or environmental agents. Research to expand these data bases is imperative if sperm evaluations are to be effectively used in male reproductive risk assessment.

Spermatogenic endpoints

Sperm production. Sperm counts may be derived from ejaculated, epididymal, or testicular samples. With ejaculates, both sperm concentration (number of sperm/milliliter of ejaculate) and total sperm per ejaculate (sperm concentration × volume) should be evaluated. Ejaculates provide the only source of semen readily obtained from the human male. However, ejaculated sperm counts from any species are influenced by several variables including the length of abstinence and the ability to obtain the entire ejaculate. Some of the intra- and interindividual variability may be reduced if repeated ejaculates are collected at regular, frequent intervals from the same male. Such a longitudinal study design may have greater detection sensitivity and require a smaller number of subjects (133). In addition, if a preexposure baseline can be obtained for each male (animal or human studies), changes during exposure and/or recovery can be better defined.

Historically, the only laboratory species in which it was convenient to obtain ejaculates were the rabbit and dog. However, recent strategies have been applied to evaluating serial ejaculates in the rat (100,137,138). These approaches entail recovering the ejaculate from the genital tract of a receptive female at a specified interval postcopulation. The use of ovariectomized, hormonally primed females can ensure availability of receptive females on demand (140).

Assessment of samples collected through electroejaculation is not recommended. It is uncertain that such a sample is representative of an ejaculate that would be delivered through normal copulation. Variation in factors such as electrode placement and intensity and duration of stimulation can cause substantial differences in the relative amounts of accessory sex gland secretions and effluent from the vas deferens. The possibility of contamination of the sample with urine is also increased. Therefore, both sperm concentration and sperm quality can be compromised in electroejaculated samples.

Epididymal sperm evaluations generally use sperm from only the caudal portion of the epididymis. The processing and evaluation of cauda epididymal samples are rapid and straightforward and can be readily incorporated into standard necropsy protocols. It has been customary to express sperm count on the basis of the weight of the cauda epididymis. However, because sperm contribute to epididymal weight, expression of the data as a ratio may actually mask true declines in sperm number. The inclusion of data on absolute sperm counts may provide further clarification. As was true for ejaculated sperm counts, epididymal sperm counts are also influenced by sexual activity (4,58).

Sperm production data may also be derived from the enumeration of elongated, condensed spermatid nuclei obtained by homogenization of the testis in a detergent-containing medium. The spermatid counts are a measure of sperm production by the stem cells and ensuing survival through the proliferative and differentiating stages of spermatogenesis (74). As with epididymal samples, the methods for sample procurement and evaluation are simple and straightforward. Spermatid enumerations provide an attractive alternative to the more laborious morphometric procedures for estimating sperm production such as counting the number of A_1 spermatogonia in histological sections (62). Moreover, the latter approach gives no insight into the survival of those cells through the course of spermatogenesis. However, the spermatid evaluation must be conducted at a time when the effect of the lesion would be reflected in the spermatid count.

The variability associated with spermatid counts across test animals is less than that seen with epididymal sperm count (13,127). This may, in part, be attributed to the fact that the cauda epididymides of most test species have large sperm reserves. This storage capacity may interfere with the ability to detect moderate changes in sperm production (58). Thus, the ability to detect a decrease in sperm production may be enhanced by use of spermatid counts. However, spermatid enumerations only reflect the integrity of spermatogenic processes within the testes and do not assess sperm that have been transported out of the testes. Posttesticular effects or toxicity expressed as alterations in motility, viability, fragility, and other properties of sperm other than count can be determined only from epididymal or ejaculated samples.

Sperm morphology. Sperm morphology refers to structural aspects of sperm. In the majority of studies with test species where sperm morphology is evaluated, only head shape is examined. Additional information may be gained from assessment of midpiece and tail morphology.

The traditional approach to characterizing morphology has relied on a subjective categorization of sperm shape from examination of stained slides at the light microscopic level. Such an approach may be adequate for mice and rats with their distinctly angular head shapes. However, the heterogeneity of structure in human sperm makes it difficult for the morphologist to define clearly the limits of normality (Fig. 14). The subjective assessment of sperm morphology can be markedly improved by employing reference slides and a systematic decision-tree process for categorization (Fig. 15) or utilizing a dimensionalized overlay with human sperm (Fig. 16). The process can be further quantified by employing image analysis using a variety of computer-linked digitizing systems to provide data on length, width, circumference, and area of the sperm head.

Flow cytometric techniques have also been developed to measure sperm morphology. When combined with cell-sorting technology, separation of large numbers of normal and abnormal sperm can be achieved. Those samples can then be subjected to further biochemical analyses (Fig. 17). Flow cytometry can also be used to quantify sperm DNA content, distinguish X- and Y-chromosome-bearing sperm (42), and sort different testicular cell types (34).

Sperm morphology profiles are quite stable and characteristic of a normal individual (and a strain within a species) over time. It has the least variability of the sperm measures

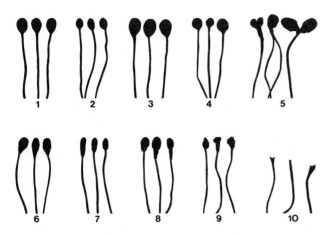

FIG. 14. Variations in shape of human sperm. The head shapes of the sperm in category 1 are oval and are considered by us to be normal. Those in categories 2–10 are scored as morphologically abnormal. The sperm in category 2 are small; 3, large; 4, round; 5, doubles; 6, narrow-at-base; 7, narrow; 8, pear-shaped; 9, irregular; and 10, ghost. Tail lengths are uniformly shortened. (From ref. 132, with permission.)

in normal individuals, which may enhance its utility in the detection of spermatotoxic events.

Several sources of morphological alterations need to be considered: mutagenic events (traditionally labeled teratospermia), nonmutagenic events during spermiogenesis, disruption of the maturational process during posttesticular development, or cellular degeneration. Mutagen-induced alterations in sperm morphology have received the greatest attention. However, the relationships between morphological changes and other sperm measures have not been thoroughly addressed.

As noted earlier, data on sperm morphology have been the most frequently reported sperm measure in animal studies. Its utility as a marker of mutagen exposure has been thoroughly evaluated (130). In spite of its extensive use, the ability to generalize these findings remains uncertain. The majority of studies has been conducted in one species (mouse), utilizing acute exposures (5 days), often administered parenterally, and assessed over a narrow window in the spermatogenic process (28–35 days postexposure). The ease with which this test can be conducted supports its application and validation using more environmentally and occupationally relevant exposure protocols and other test species.

The reproductive consequences of morphologically abnormal sperm are also uncertain. The majority of studies in test species and humans has suggested that abnormally shaped sperm may not reach the oviduct and/or participate in fertilization (85,101,106). This bias may be the result of an active selection process in the female tract against abnormal sperm and/or that the cells are incapable of reaching the site of fertilization [e.g., midpiece or tail defects (60,81); differences in flagellar beat frequency (63)]. Results from *in vitro* studies indicate that even if these abnormal cells gain access to the ova, fertilization and subsequent cellular divisions are unlikely. The implication is that the greater the number of abnormal sperm in the ejaculate, the greater the probability of reduced fertility.

Increase in abnormal sperm morphology has been considered supportive evidence that the agent has gained access to the reproductive organs (e.g., 122). Exposure of males to toxic agents may lead to sperm abnormalities in their progeny (57,129). However, transmissible germ cell mutations could also occur in the absence of any warning indicator such as abnormal sperm morphology. The relationship between these morphological alterations and other karyotypic changes remains uncertain (30).

Sperm motility. The biochemical environments in the testes and epididymides are highly regulated to assure the proper development and maturation of the sperm and the acquisition of critical functional characteristics. With chemical exposures, perturbations of this balance may occur, pro-

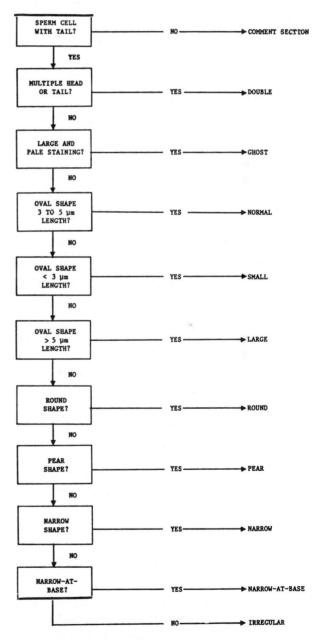

FIG. 15. Schematic of the decision process in assigning human sperm to shape categories. (From ref. 132, with permission.)

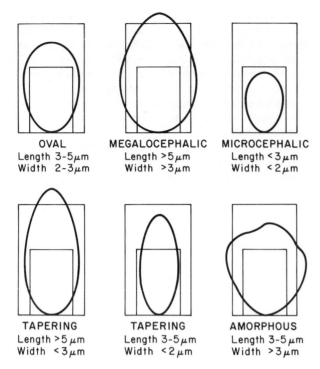

OVAL
Length 3-5 μm
Width 2-3 μm

MEGALOCEPHALIC
Length >5 μm
Width >3 μm

MICROCEPHALIC
Length <3 μm
Width <2 μm

TAPERING
Length >5 μm
Width <3 μm

TAPERING
Length 3-5 μm
Width <2 μm

AMORPHOUS
Length 3-5 μm
Width >3 μm

FIG. 16. Use of the morphology overlay. The base of the sperm head is aligned with the bottom of the overlay. If the length and the width lie between the two boxes, the classification is *oval*. If the length and the width lie outside the outer box, the classification is *megalocephalic*. If the length lies within the inner box, the classification is *microcephalic*. If the length lies outside the outer box and the width between the boxes, or if the length lies between the boxes and the width inside the inner box, the classification is *tapering*. If the length lies between the boxes and the width lies outside the outer box, the classification is *amorphous*. (From ref. 63, with permission.)

ducing alterations in sperm properties such as motility. Yet, few toxicologic studies have examined motility as an endpoint (130,131).

Motility estimates may be obtained on ejaculated, vas deferens, or cauda epididymal samples. Motility, like sperm count, is influenced by a number of variables including abstinence, the elapsed time between obtaining the sample and evaluation of motility, temperature, the medium utilized to dilute the sample, and the degree to which the sample is diluted.

Historically, motility has been measured using subjective microscopic evaluations. Estimates of percent motile sperm can be made and some rating of the quality of motility can be offered (i.e., the degree to which sperm show progressive linear motility). However, these techniques are subject to bias and may show a high intra- and interrater variability. Moreover, no opportunity is provided to obtain a permanent record for subsequent referral or validation.

Alternative methods of estimating motility calculate the degree of displacement or absorption of various energy sources as the sperm swim through a given medium (e.g., light or photon-scattering). Such approaches are accurate in deriving the relative percent motility for a population of cells; however, data on individual cells are not obtained. These

techniques also do not provide a permanent record for review or reevaluation.

Approaches have been introduced that use image analysis in conjunction with photomicrographic or videomicrographic techniques (e.g., 13,64,127). These strategies are far more objective, provide a permanent record, and allow additional data such as swimming speed and motility pattern to be obtained on the individual spermatozoa in a population. Several of these parameters are characterized by low variability among individuals, which suggests that they may be particularly sensitive indicators of reproductive toxicity (13,127).

In vitro measures of sperm function. Two tests of sperm function that can be clinically useful are the sperm-cervical mucus penetration test and the *in vitro* fertilization test (105). These tests may provide additional insight into the functional competence of the sperm. The diagnostic information obtained may identify subfertile men whose semen appears to be normal by other routine criteria. However, it is not feasible to implement these tests routinely for screening purposes in human populations or with test species. The techniques, which have not been standardized, are highly specialized and not readily established in every laboratory. Also an adequate normative data base does not exist for these tests (90,91). Their more appropriate application in toxicology may be in elucidating mechanisms of action of previously identified reproductive toxicants.

The extrapolation of *in vitro* data to predict the *in vivo* condition is also questionable. The ease with which *in vitro* fertilization can be achieved varies across species, being readily accomplished in the mouse but rather difficult in the rat. Such test systems do not reflect the dynamic role played by the female tract in sperm transport, survival, and capacitation before fertilization. The conditions required to achieve

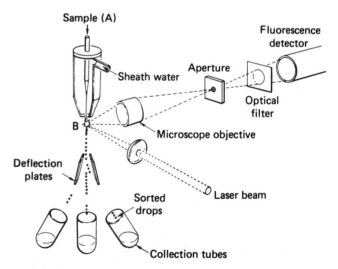

FIG. 17. Schematic of a fluorescence-activated flow sorter showing orthogonal axes of sample flow laser beam illumination, and fluorescent light detection. Fluorescently stained particles to be sorted are carried in a fast-moving jet of fluid past an optical detection system that responds to fluorescent light. The jet carrying the particles subsequently breaks up into individual droplets. Those droplets that contain desired particles can be electronically charged and deflected into a separate receptacle. (From ref. 42, with permission.)

TABLE 5. *Relative sensitivity of testicular and epididymal sperm parameters for the rat*

Parameter	Coefficient of variation	Percent difference detected		
		(N = 10)	(N = 15)	(N = 20)
Testis weight	4.65	6.08	4.96	4.31
Epididymal weight	9.40	12.30	10.03	8.70
Sperm production rate[a]	16.56	21.67	17.68	15.33
Sperm count/g epididymis	29.32	38.36	31.30	27.14
Percent motile	16.00	20.93	17.09	14.82
Swimming speed	7.24	9.47	7.73	6.70
Percent normal morphology[b]	2.70	3.53	2.88	2.49

[a] Sperm rate production = spermatid enumeration/rat.
[b] Derived from literature on Long–Evans and Sprague–Dawley rats.
Data from ref. 13.

successful fertilization *in vitro* may bear little resemblance to the state that exists *in vivo* (43,44,114). As routinely done, a far greater number of sperm is required at the site of fertilization for *in vitro* fertilization. A more straightforward approach to examining this functional component would be to recover ova from the mated female at the appropriate time postcopulation (species-dependent) and determine whether fertilization and normal initial development (timing of cleavage divisions) had occurred. In this approach, the test would utilize the natural environment, the female genital tract.

Evaluation of various indices of spermatotoxicity and their relationship to fertility

The relative sensitivity of a number of indices of spermatotoxicity in the rat is indicated in Table 5 (139). These data, for the most part, are in close agreement with values reported elsewhere in the literature (13,127) and reflect the percent difference that can be detected statistically for a change in a given measure as a function of sample size. Because sample size requirements under various federal testing guidelines vary (e.g., FDA Segment 1 test; EPA multigener-

ation reproduction study), the power of the studies that these agencies review varies accordingly.

Based on the data in Table 5, testis weight would appear to be a highly sensitive measure. However, as previously discussed, it may be a relatively insensitive marker of gonadal injury. Of the spermatogenic indices listed, percent normal morphology has the least variation and has been shown to be indicative of reproductive toxicity in both humans and test species for a variety of agents (130,131).

Similar data on endpoint sensitivity, including a variety of motility measures, are presented in Table 6. The motility measures were derived from computerized analyses of videomicrographic images (127) and are in agreement with previously published values (13). Although certain specific motility parameters exhibit low variability, research is needed that will help interpret the biological significance of changes in these measures.

Limited data are available that have examined the independent and interdependent relationships between these various spermatogenic indices. It is not clear how the expression of toxicity in one measure may influence the eventual expression of other markers.

Recent work has shown that spermatozoa with abnormal morphology exhibit poorer motility than normal sperm from

TABLE 6. *Variability in testicular and sperm motility parameters in Fischer 344 rats*

Indicator	n[a]	Range	Mean ± SD	CV[b] (%)
Testes weight (g)	30	2.3–2.9	2.6 ± 0.1	5.61
Sperm production rate ($\times 10^6$)				
Per testis/day	30	14.7–25.6	22.3 ± 2.7	12.09
Per g testis/day	30	14.6–21.1	17.8 ± 1.5	8.54
Cauda epididymal sperm no. ($\times 10^6$)				
Per cauda epididymis[c]	50	55.2–153.2	86.1 ± 20.8	24.16
Per g cauda epididymis	30	307.1–972.9	696.5 ± 151.9	21.81
Cauda epididymal sperm motility				
Motile cells (%)	50	39–82	61 ± 9	14.72
Curvilinear velocity (μm/sec)	50	98.3–156.5	128.3 ± 11.4	8.88
Straight-line velocity (μm/sec)	50	41.8–93.5	69.2 ± 10.2	14.68
Linearity	50	4.2–6.3	5.4 ± 0.5	9.45

[a] Number of animals examined for each indicator.
[b] Coefficient of variation = [(SD/mean) × 100].
[c] Regions 5, 6A, and 6B of the cauda epididymis.
From ref. 127, with permission.

TABLE 7. *Effects of methyl chloride exposure on various endpoints of male reproductive toxicity*

Endpoint	Dose (ppm)[a]	
	1,000	3,000
Fertility	–	D (wk 2, 3)
Fetal loss		
Preimplant	I (wk 3)	I (wk 2–4, 6, 8)
Postimplant	–	I (wk 1)
Histopathology		
Epididymis	–	+ (wk 2)
Testis	–	+ (wk 1–8)
Spermatid counts	–	D (wk 2–8)
Vas deferens sperm measures		
Sperm count	–	D (wk 3–8)
Percent motile	–	D (wk 1–8)
Percent abnormal forms	–	I (wk 1–3)
No. intact sperm	D (wk 3)	D (wk 2–8)

[a] 5-Day inhalation exposure. +, Effect observed; –, no effect; D, decrease; I, increase.
Modified from refs. 125 and 126.

the same ejaculate, whether the sample is from a fertile or infertile donor (63,92). However, the "normal-shaped" sperm from infertile men are also less likely to be motile and may swim more slowly than similarly shaped sperm from the semen of fertile men. These findings suggest that the normal sperm from these two populations differ in parameters not reflected in the standard evaluation.

Given that fertility tests are relatively insensitive, then reproductive risk assessment can benefit from the inclusion of data on additional variables such as sperm measures. Some support for using a more extensive protocol is provided by examining recent data on methyl chloride (125,126) and ethylene glycol monomethyl ether (16,18). Both of these investigations incorporated high quality histopathology (including cell staging), sperm measures, and fertility assessments. The results of these studies are summarized in Tables 7 and 8. For both agents, histopathological lesions and sperm alter-

ations were seen at either lower doses and/or earlier in time than were effects on fertility or fetal outcomes. Similar relationships can be observed in reviewing the effects of DBCP in rabbits (23,36,37).

Aside from the issue of relative sensitivity of these various measures, the quantitative relationships of these indices to fertility have not been well characterized for any species. Several investigators have attempted to define the critical correlates of sperm fertilizing ability by correlating various sperm properties with *in vitro* fertilizing capacity in fertile and infertile men. Yet, no sperm parameter or set of parameters has yielded consistently high, predictive results (e.g., 3,59).

Certain qualitative and quantitative sperm standards must be met to ensure fertility, but the lower limits that still allow fertility have not been delineated. For example, sperm counts in men that are lower than 20 million/ml have traditionally been taken as a sign of potential subfertility or infertility. However, there are men whose sperm counts fall below this level that have fathered children, whereas there are others whose sperm count exceeds the normal average (80–120 million/ml) but are infertile. Thus, the distributions of sperm counts for fertile and infertile men overlap (76). Additional animal and human research is needed to better understand the biological consequences of spermatogenic alterations. At this stage, spermatotoxicity observed in laboratory studies must be of concern in the extrapolation of the risk to man.

Paternally Mediated Postnatal Outcomes

Exposure of a female to toxic chemicals during gestation or lactation may produce death, structural abnormalities, altered growth, and functional deficits (e.g., behavioral changes) in her offspring. The probability of similar outcomes resulting from paternal-only exposure is less certain. Data for a variety of agents suggest that male-only exposure can produce deleterious effects in the offspring. Agents for which such adverse effects in test species have been reported include lead [behavioral deficits (15)], urethane [structural anomalies

TABLE 8. *Effects of ethylene glycol monomethyl ether on various endpoints of male reproductive toxicity*

Endpoint	Dose (mg/kg)[a]		
	50	100	200
Fertility	–	D (wk 5)	D (wk 4–16) Fetal loss
Preimplant	–	I (wk 5)	I (wk 3–16)
Live fetuses	–	D (wk 5)	D (wk 4–16)
Resorptions	–	–	I (wk 5–6)
Histopathology—Testis[b]	+ (wk 4–7)	+ (wk 1–8)	+ (wk 1–8)
Accessory sex organ weight	–	–	–
Epididymal sperm measures			
Sperm count	D (wk 5)	D (wk 2–16)	D (wk 2–16)
Percent motile	–	D (wk 4–7)	D (wk 3–16)
Percent abnormal forms	D (wk 5)	D (wk 5–16)	D (wk 3–16)
Percent headless forms	–	I (wk 5–?)	I (wk 5–?)

[a] 5-Day oral exposure (p.o.). +, Effect observed; –, no effect; D, decrease; I, increase.
[b] Assessed for only 8 weeks.
Modified from refs. 16 and 18.

and tumors (86)], cyclophosphamide [behavioral deficits (1); malformations and growth retardation (117–119); neonatal mortality and behavioral deficits (6)], marijuana [decreased reproductive performance in offspring (29)], and opiates [growth retardation (39)]. A number of studies has reported associations between a variety of paternal occupations and the occurrence of birth defects or childhood cancer (e.g., 35,52,98,99). However, others have failed to observe such relationships (e.g., 53,94,135).

These effects may be the result of direct damage to the sperm. However, xenobiotics present in seminal plasma or associated with the fertilizing sperm could also interfere with fertilization and/or early developmental events. With human exposures, the possibility also exists that the father could simply serve as a vehicle for transporting the toxic agent from the work environment to the home (e.g., on work clothes) wherein exposures to the mother or offspring could occur. Although the research findings in this area are intriguing, further work is needed to clarify the mechanisms by which paternal exposures may be associated with adverse effects on offspring.

Sexual Behavior

Sexual behavior is a very complicated process involving neural and endocrine components of the central and peripheral nervous systems and the reproductive system. For humans, complex interactions of personality, social, and experiential factors also influence the initiation and performance of these behaviors. Similar factors may exist in other species, but they are more controlled by standardized laboratory conditions. However, the perturbation of sexual behavior in animals suggests the potential for similar effects on humans. Consistent with this suggestion are data on CNS-active drugs that have been shown to disrupt sexual behavior in both animals and humans (107,123).

Although the functional components of sexual performance can be quantified in rats (31), no direct evaluation of this behavior is done in most breeding studies. Rather, the presence of copulatory plugs or sperm-positive vaginal lavages have been taken as indirect evidence of successful mating. These markers do not demonstrate that male performance necessarily resulted in adequate sexual stimulation of the female. In rats, the degree of sexual preparedness of the female partner can strongly influence the site of semen deposition and subsequent sperm transport in her genital tract (2). Failure of the female to achieve sufficient stimulation may adversely influence these processes, thereby reducing the probability of successful impregnation. Such a "mating failure" would be reflected in the fertility index as reduced fertility and could erroneously be attributed to a spermatotoxic effect. There are other aspects of current breeding protocols that also may serve to mask a decline in the fertility potential of a given male (see Length of Mating Period).

The need to directly evaluate sexual behavior routinely for all suspected reproductive toxicants is questionable. Likely candidates may be agents reported to exert neurotoxic effects because several neurotoxicants have also been shown to produce disruptions in copulatory behavior [trichloroethylene (84), carbon disulfide (137,138), acrylamide (141)]. Chemicals possessing or suspected to possess androgenic or estrogenic properties (or antagonistic properties) also are potential candidates for the evaluation of copulatory behavior, separate from effects on reproductive organs (e.g., chlorinated hydrocarbon pesticides).

Structure–Activity Relationships

Structure–activity relationships have not been well studied in reproductive toxicology. Data are available that suggest structure–activity relationships for certain classes of chemicals (e.g., glycol ethers, phthalate esters, heavy metals). Yet, for other agents, nothing in their structure would have identified them as male reproductive toxicants (e.g., chlordecone). Bernstein (10) reviewed the literature and offered a set of classifications relating structure to reported male reproductive activity. Although limited in scope and in need of rigorous validation, such schemes do provide hypotheses that can be tested.

Comparison of the chemical or physical properties of an agent with those of known male reproductive toxicants may provide some indication of a potential for reproductive toxicity. Such information may be helpful in setting priorities for testing of agents or for the evaluation of potential toxicity when only minimal data are available.

Pharmacokinetic Considerations

Pharmacokinetic data are most useful for risk assessment when the test agent has been administered by the route(s) expected for human exposure. Differences in metabolic fates at the site of entry, absorption rate into the blood, initial absorption into the portal versus the systemic blood, and lipophilic properties can markedly affect the amount, form, and time course in which a toxic agent is delivered to a target site.

Several major factors influence the pharmacokinetics of a given agent as related to gonadal toxicity, including (a) the existence of a blood–testis barrier that may restrict access of a compound to the adluminal compartment of the seminiferous tubules; and (b) the metabolic capability (including DNA repair) of the different compartments of the testes that determine the eventual disposition of the agent. The formation and role of the blood–testis barrier have been described earlier in this chapter.

The reproductive organs appear to have a wide range of metabolic capabilities directed at both steroid and xenobiotic metabolism. These properties have been best characterized for the testes. The distribution of these enzymes and cytochrome P-450 levels (multiple forms) in the testes differs between interstitial and germ cell compartments. Aryl hydrocarbon hydroxylase activity and cytochrome P-450 levels in interstitial tissue are approximately twice as high as those in the seminiferous tubules. On the other hand, activities of some of the detoxifying enzymes in the germ cells such as epoxide hydrase and glutathione transferase are nearly double those in the interstitial compartment (82). As seen in Fig. 18, high levels of glutathione transferase are seen in the neonatal rodent testis and rapidly approach adult levels (50), suggesting an early capacity to detoxify electrophilic agents.

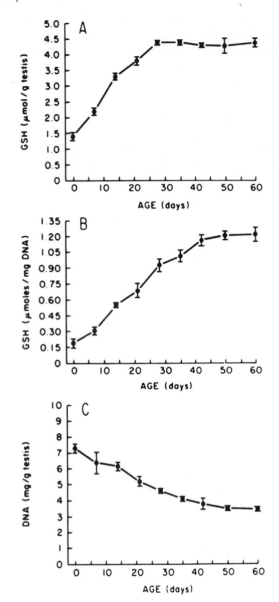

FIG. 18. Reduced glutathione (GSH) and DNA concentrations in mouse testis at 0, 7, 14, 21, 28, 35, 42, 50, and 60 days of age. Each point represents the mean ± SD of separate determinations on four to six individual mice (14–60 days of age) or pooled litter mates (0–7 days of age). Two aliquots of each testicular homogenate were removed for GSH assay and 4–5 aliquots for DNA assay. **(A)** GSH (μmol/g testis). **(B)** GSH (μmol/g DNA). **(C)** DNA (mg/g testis). (From ref. 50, with permission.)

The protective role of glutathione should not be underestimated because it may serve to prevent interactions between reactive electrophiles and critical cellular proteins and nucleic acids. For germ cell mutagens such as ethylene oxide, ethyl methane sulfonate, and acrylamide, the level of mutagenic response may be directly related to the rate of glutathione depletion (72,114a,115). Moreover, the concurrent exposure of an individual to a germ cell mutagen and a nonmutagenic glutathione depletor could significantly lower the dose–response threshold of the former. This has been demonstrated for the induction of dominant lethal mutations by ethyl methane sulfonate administered in combination with

the glutathione depletor, buthionine sulfoximine (11). The sensitivity of different species to germ cell mutagens may also, in part, be a function of the concentration of glutathione (72).

The majority of pharmacokinetic studies has incompletely characterized the distribution of toxic agents and their subsequent metabolic fate within the testis. Generalizations based on hepatic metabolism are inadequate because the metabolic profile for a given agent may differ between the liver and the testes (68). As an example, the isoenzyme patterns for glutathione transferase are markedly different for these two systems (51). Detailed interspecies comparisons of the metabolic capabilities of the testis also have not been conducted.

Attention also should be directed toward delineating the relationship between the pharmacokinetic fate of an agent in the testes and the occurrence of spermatotoxicity. Of primary importance is determining the relationships between different exposure conditions (acute, intermittent, subchronic, chronic), pharmacokinetic status (e.g., bioaccumulation, steady state) and the nature of the response (i.e., transient, static, or progressive) as a function of site or mechanism of action (e.g., stem cell, mature sperm). Understanding these interactions is critical to assessing more accurately the risk for different human exposure situations as well as for prediction of the degree of injury associated with prolonged exposures in humans. Such predictions must currently be based on test animal data from different exposure protocols.

Components of Quantitative Male Reproductive Risk Assessment

The quantitative component of reproductive risk assessment focuses on characterizing the relationship between dose and potential incidence of an adverse effect in humans. For most chemicals, human data are not available on which to base dose–response relationships, and data from test species must often be used to derive allowable exposure levels. Under those conditions, it is necessary to extrapolate to adjust for potential differences between species and possibly to predict effects at low doses from those observed at higher doses. The methodology to accomplish interspecies and high to low dose extrapolations has not been well developed. In this section, the methods currently used for such extrapolations are presented and approaches under development are discussed.

Threshold Assumption

For quantitative risk assessment of noncarcinogenic and nonmutagenic agents, the assumption is made that a finite level of exposure exists below which no effect would be observed. That level is termed the threshold. The threshold assumption is based on the concept that, at low dose levels, certain biological processes associated with the delivery and metabolism of a chemical, plus repair capabilities of affected tissues, result in too low a level of effect to be of significance. Using the threshold assumption, uncertainty factors are applied to a NOAEL or LOAEL to estimate an exposure level below which no adverse effect would occur in humans who are most sensitive to that chemical. Quantitative risk assessments involving male reproductive effects utilize the threshold approach.

Uncertainty Factors

Because the methodology for determination and application of quantitative extrapolation factors is inadequate, uncertainty factors are applied to a NOAEL or LOAEL. Such adjustments may be made for high to low dose and interspecies extrapolations as well as for intraspecies differences in sensitivity, for differences in expected exposure duration (e.g., subchronic to lifetime), and study quality.

Interspecies Extrapolation

Attempts to develop quantitative interspecies extrapolation factors have compared reductions in sperm count for humans and a test species that has been induced by the same agent. Male reproductive toxicants for which human as well as test species data exist include radiation, some chemotherapeutic drugs, and steroid hormones (see ref. 75 for review). Using these comparisons, Meistrich (75) has proposed the derivation of interspecies extrapolation factors (EF), which are expressions of relative potency, i.e., the ratio of the dose needed to produce a given effect in the test species to the dose needed to produce the same effect in humans. In the absence of adequate human data, that factor could then be applied to a NOAEL or LOAEL for a given agent from test animal data to predict the dose at which comparable effects would occur in humans. The relationship of that exposure level to actual human exposure could also be ascertained. For an effect such as a reduction in sperm count, the impact on fertility could potentially be calculated (76).

The only endpoints for which EFs have been calculated are measures of sperm production. For test species (usually mouse), frequently used measures have been counts of surviving stem cells, numbers of repopulated tubules, spermatid enumeration, and/or epididymal sperm counts. Measures of sperm production in humans are derived from ejaculated samples (sperm counts) or testicular biopsies (spermatid counts or numbers of affected or repopulated tubules). Spermatid counts from mice and ejaculated sperm counts from humans appear to be the most directly comparable for the agents tested. Such a relationship is anticipated because both endpoints are related to sperm production rate in the testes.

Initial findings (75) have shown that these EFs vary as a function of several variables including (a) the endpoints assayed; (b) degree to which the endpoints measured are comparable across species; (c) the manner in which the administered dose units are expressed (e.g., mg/kg body weight versus mg/m^3 surface area); and (d) the time of assessment relative to cessation of treatment. For example, interspecies differences may exist in the cell type that is most sensitive to a particular agent (e.g., stem cells versus differentiating spermatogonia). With that situation, an EF calculated from observations at the "time of minimal sperm counts" may be misleading because the survival of different cell types is being measured.

Assessment for determining EFs may also be done when cells that were stem cells at the time of exposure would be spermatozoa (56 days in mouse; 70–100 days in human). This approach would assure a comparison of effects on similar cell types. However, the resulting EF would be influenced by differences between species in the kinetics of stem cell regeneration and germinal epithelium repopulation. Whereas repopulation of the germinal epithelium may simultaneously occur with stem cell regeneration in the mouse, repopulation may be markedly delayed in humans.

An alternative approach is to derive EFs based on measurements made at the time at which maximum recovery occurs (i.e., no further increase in sperm count is obtained). Such a derivation is not influenced by differences between species in the kinetics of regeneration or repopulation. Moreover, this assay may be the most relevant if one is concerned primarily about permanent impairment of fertility (as opposed to temporary infertility). EFs based on assays obtained under the different conditions identified above are presented in Table 9 for radiation.

As noted earlier, the EF is influenced by the units in which dose is expressed (Table 10). To date, no consistent trend favoring one calculation over the other has emerged. Physiochemical properties and pharmacokinetics of a given agent must dictate the most appropriate method for expression of this relationship. Uniformity of approach will be important to assure maximum usefulness of such information.

The degree to which the EFs presented in Tables 9 and 10 can be generalized is unknown. The data have been primarily derived from acute exposures with a limited number of agents. Effects on only proliferating spermatogenic cell types (stem cells or differentiating spermatogonia) have been measured by a single outcome (reduction in sperm count). Moreover, the test animal data have been primarily derived from the mouse. Research that expands these dimensions is needed to develop and validate the use of EFs in predicting human risk from test species data.

Low Dose Extrapolation

Most current protocols are designed to generate data that are most useful for hazard identification. The need for inclusion of at least one high dose level, combined with use of a limited number of dose levels (often three plus control), may result in an insufficient range of dose levels. Guidelines for dose selection vary (see *Dose Selection and Dosing Schedule*). Recommendations from a recent EPA conference (41) include a second tier of testing that extends the dose range downward to the human exposure level (if known). The only study to date that has employed this approach utilized DBCP as the model agent with equivocal results (5). The absence of consistent dose-response trends across endpoints in that study limited the utility of these data in evaluating this dose-response strategy.

Many studies that must be used for quantitative risk as-

TABLE 9. *Summary of interspecies extrapolation factors*

Time of assay	Endpoint	EF[a]
Point of minimum counts	Sperm counts	2.6–7
Minute interval for stem cells to become sperm	Sperm counts	11–21
Time maximum recovery	Sperm counts	<1.7

[a] EF, dose needed to produce given effect in animal/dose needed to produce same effect in humans.

Modified from ref. 75.

TABLE 10. *Extrapolation factors for anticancer agents*

Agent	Endpoint	Extrapolation factor	Units of dose
Chlorambucil	Permanent	0.4	mg/m^2
	azoospermia	5	mg/kg
Procarbazine	Permanent	<2	mg/m^2
	azoospermia	<23	mg/kg
Adriamycin	Permanent	<0.05	mg/m^2
	azoospermia	<0.6	mg/kg

Modified from Meistrich (75).

sessments have an inadequate range of dose levels, with the result that substantial uncertainty exists as to the adequacy of a NOAEL or LOAEL. However, such values must often be used and uncertainty factors applied to estimate effects and to derive an allowable exposure level for humans. Research is needed on methods to predict effects at lower exposure levels for male reproductive toxicity. It is important that the effects of differences in mechanism of action on extrapolation models be included.

Linking Exposure and Reproductive Outcomes

Assessments of the human exposure patterns and levels are often not available for inclusion in the characterization of the reproductive risk for a given agent. Yet the confidence in a risk estimation should factor in the conditions under which the exposure occurred (e.g., route, duration, and concentration). Various combinations of these parameters of exposure will markedly influence the degree of risk that may be anticipated.

The nature of the exposure may be defined at a particular point in time or may reflect cumulative exposure. Each approach makes assumptions about the underlying relationship between exposure and outcome. For example, a cumulative exposure measure assumes that extended (lifetime) exposure is important and that the probability of effect increases with increasing total exposure (body burden). A dichotomous exposure measure (ever exposed versus never exposed) assumes an irreversible effect of exposure. Models that define exposure only at a specific time may assume that only the concurrent exposure is important (113a). The appropriate exposure model depends on the pharmacokinetic behavior of the agent and the biological processes affected. Thus, a cumulative or dichotomous exposure model may be appropriate if injury is to cells that cannot be replaced or repaired (e.g., Sertoli cells), whereas a concurrent exposure model may predict toxicity for cells that are continuously being generated or can be repaired (e.g., spermatids).

The relationship between time and/or duration of exposure and the observation of reproductive effects has particular significance for short-term exposures. Spermatogenesis is a temporally synchronized process. In humans, germ cells that were spermatozoa, spermatids, spermatocytes, or spermatogonia at the time of the acute exposure require 1–2, 3–5, 5–8, or 8–12 weeks, respectively, to appear in an ejaculate. That timing may vary somewhat depending on the degree of sexual activity because sexual activity affects rate of transport of sperm through the epididymis. It is possible that as-

sessments may be made too early or too late to detect an effect if only a particular cell type was affected during a relatively brief exposure to the agent. The absence of an effect when observations are made too late may result in the erroneous conclusion of either a reversible event or no effect. In addition, an effect that is reversible at lower exposures might become irreversible with higher or longer exposures or the exposure of a more susceptible individual. Thus, failure to detect transient effects because of improper timing of observations may have serious consequences for risk estimation. If information is available on the target/mechanism of action expected from that class of agents, it may be possible to predict the proper timing of the assessment or evaluate its appropriateness.

Compared to short-term exposures, the link between exposure and outcome may be more apparent with relatively constant, subchronic or longer exposures that are of sufficient duration to have covered all phases of spermatogenesis (in humans, approximately 70–100 days). Assessments may be made at any time after this point as long as exposure remains relatively constant. Time to attain steady-state levels should also be considered. Choice of exposure model (e.g., concurrent or cumulative) would still depend on the suspected target/mechanism of action.

Exposure at different stages of male development can also result in different outcomes. Such age-dependent variation has been well documented in both test animal and human studies. Prenatal and neonatal treatment can irreversibly alter reproductive function in a manner that may not be predicted from adult exposure. Chemicals that alter sexual differentiation in rodents during these periods may have similar effects in humans because some of the mechanisms underlying these developmental processes appear to be similar in all mammalian species.

The susceptibility of the aged male to chemical insult has not been well studied. Although reproductive competence may not be a pivotal health concern with older individuals, other biological functions maintained by the gonads (e.g., androgen production, sex drive) are of concern (61,122a).

An exposure assessment should characterize the probability of exposure of subgroups of different ages (embryo, fetus, neonate, juvenile, young adult, older adult). A risk characterization should then consider the susceptibility of these different age groups.

EVALUATING REPRODUCTIVE TOXICITY DATA—WEIGHT OF THE EVIDENCE

The weight of the evidence determination is the cumulative evaluation of the entire body of evidence to determine the degree of confidence that an agent could be a hazard to humans. The determination is qualitative in nature and does not approach issues related to severity of effect.

A recent EPA workshop (*manuscript in preparation*) has developed a weight of evidence approach that can be utilized with the male reproductive system. Although designed specifically for use with the male reproductive system, the overall outline is generic and could be adapted for use with other systems. One approach is presented in Fig. 19 and Table 11.

An agent may be categorized as having results that either implicate (positive results) or absolve (negative results) it as

MALE REPRODUCTIVE EFFECTS
WEIGHT OF EVIDENCE SCHEME

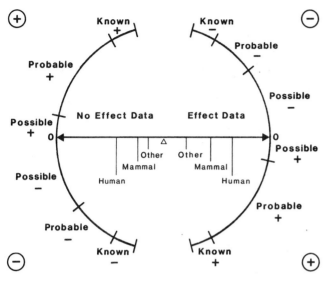

FIG. 19. A weight of evidence scheme for male reproductive effects.

a male reproductive toxicant. The criteria should be more stringent to place an agent in a particular negative category than in the equivalent positive category. For example, positive results from a *single* study based on a *single* endpoint may be sufficient to place an agent into a known positive or probable positive category. However, negative results from an adequate array of endpoints would be necessary to place an agent into the equivalent negative categories.

The description for each category allows flexibility by the user in assigning criteria. Data of equivalent quality from human exposures are given more weight than data from exposures of test species. Although a single study of high quality could be sufficient to achieve a relatively high level of confidence, replication increases the confidence that may be placed in the results.

The phrase "convincing body of evidence" allows the risk assessor to weigh the evidence from different studies and to arrive at an overall judgment as to the liklihood that the agent has toxic effects. The criteria for what constitutes a convincing body of evidence should be somewhat flexible. Some important considerations are presented below:

Data are available from *in vivo* study(ies) of acceptable quality with humans (known positive or negative) or other mammalian species (probable positive or negative) that are believed to be predictive of human responses.

When multiple studies are available, results are reproducible.

When multiple studies are available, the lines of evidence from independent study types are reinforcing.

Studies or other information are available that resolve discordant data.

Route(s), level, duration, and frequency of exposure are appropriate.

An adequate array of endpoints has been examined.

The resolving power and statistical treatment of the study(ies) are appropriate.

Data exhibit a dose–response relationship.

Results are statistically significant and biologically plausible.

Because many human males have sperm counts that place them near or in the subfertile or infertile categories (see *Overview*), a conservative stance should be taken with respect to the weight given to individual endpoints. Any statistically significant deviation from baseline levels for an *in vivo* effect warrants closer examination. To determine whether such a deviation constitutes an *adverse* effect requires an understanding of its role within a complex system and the determination of whether a "true effect" has been observed. Application of the above criteria can facilitate such determinations.

The greatest weight for male reproductive hazard identification should be placed on detection of effects on fertility and/or pregnancy outcomes or endpoints that are directly related to reproductive function such as sperm measures, reproductive histopathology, reproductive organ weight(s), and reproductive endocrinology. Positive results from those endpoints are assigned to known positive or probable positive

TABLE 11. *Weight of evidence categories for male reproductive risk assessment*

Known positive
A convincing body of evidence exists that an agent causes an adverse effect on the male reproductive system in humans.

Probable positive
A convincing body of evidence exists that an agent causes an adverse effect on the male reproductive system in nonhuman mammals.

Possible positive
Studies with acceptable quality produce inconsistent and conflicting results such that the possibility of adverse effects cannot be discounted.
Evidence from human or other mammalian studies shows statistically significant adverse effects, but the quality of the studies is questionable.
Other data, such as positive results from structure–activity relationships, *in vitro* testing or with nonmammalian species, exist from which biologically meaningful adverse effects are plausibly indicated.

Known negative
A convincing body of evidence that an agent does not cause an adverse effect on the male reproductive system in humans.

Probable negative
A convincing body of evidence that an agent does not cause an adverse effect on the male reproductive system in nonhuman mammals.

Possible negative
Studies with acceptable quality produce no adverse effects, but important aspects of the male reproductive system have not been evaluated.

No data or inadequate data
No data are available.
Results for which the predictive value of the test system or endpoint has not been established.
Negative data from studies for which the confidence in quality is questionable.

categories. Less confidence is placed in results from other measures such as *in vitro* tests or structure–activity relationship evaluation, but positive results could trigger follow-up studies to determine the likelihood and extent to which function might be affected. Positive results from these types of data are assigned to the possible positive category, whereas negative results are assigned to the inadequate data category.

The absence of effects on the endpoints routinely evaluated (i.e., fertility, histopathology, and organ weights) may constitute sufficient evidence to place low priority on the potential male reproductive toxicity of a chemical (i.e., possible or probable negative categories). However, in such cases, careful consideration should be given to the issues pertaining to the sensitivity of endpoint(s) and the quality of the data on these endpoints as previously detailed. Consideration should be given to the possibility of adverse effects that may not be reflected in these routine measures (e.g., germ cell mutation or alterations in sperm measures such as motility or morphology).

FACTORING REVERSIBILITY INTO MALE REPRODUCTIVE RISK ASSESSMENT

When an agent has been identified as a male reproductive hazard, it may be of interest to determine whether the effects are reversible. In the spermatogenic process, extensive damage to the spermatogonial stem cells is known to produce an irreversible effect. Even though an agent may affect only spermatocytes or spermatids at low dose levels, stem cells are often affected at higher doses. Damage to certain other cell types in the male reproductive system may also result in irreversible effects that are of concern.

When recovery from stem cell damage is possible, the duration of the recovery period is determined by the time for regeneration (for stem cells) and repopulation of the affected spermatogenic cell type(s). To that must be added the time required for appearance of those cells as sperm in the ejaculate. The time for these events to occur varies with species, pharmacokinetic properties of the agent, the extent to which the stem cell population has been destroyed, and the degree of sublethal toxicity inflicted on the stem cells and/or Sertoli cells. When the stem cell population has been partially destroyed, humans require longer to attain the same degree of recovery than mice (77).

The design of a protocol to study reversibility of effects on spermatogenesis requires assessment of degree of damage at intervals after cessation of treatment. In the absence of ability to monitor ejaculates in a longitudinal design, necropsy of satellite groups at intervals during the recovery phase is needed to specify the time required for recovery. Even with the ability to obtain ejaculates, data on testis parameters (e.g., histopathology and/or spermatid count) at the end of dosing and at intervals during recovery are useful in determining the potential for and progress of recovery.

Under some conditions, the level of concern associated with a reversible male reproductive effect might be less than with an irreversible effect. However, that stance is not necessarily justified for several reasons. First, reversibility assumes a discontinuation in exposure or a decrease in exposure below a critical (threshold) level. Thus, the assessment of reversibility must consider the exposure conditions. Second,

an agent that produces a reversible effect with a low exposure level may produce an irreversible effect at a higher exposure level. Third, the potential for reversibility may greatly vary between individuals. Individuals who border on subfertility may have a reduced capability to compensate for spermatotoxicity. Therefore, the extent of an effect on fertility may be greater in those individuals and the probability of full recovery less likely. Fourth, exposures that occur before puberty may produce effects that are not reversible, even if they would be reversible in adults. Finally, even if the effect is fully reversible, a period of infertility may be disruptive to family and career planning, as well as psychological health. Unless those factors described above have been carefully considered and judged to be insignificant relative to other considerations for that agent, the same level of concern should be given to an apparent reversible as to an irreversible male reproductive effect.

REFERENCES

1. Adams, P. M., Fabricant, J. D., and Legator, M. S. (1981): Cyclophosphamide-induced spermatogenic effects detected in the F_1 generation by behavioral testing. *Science,* 211:80–82.
2. Adler, N. T., and Toner, J. P. (1986): The effect of copulatory behavior on sperm transport and fertility in rats. *Ann. N.Y. Acad. Sci.,* 474:21–32.
3. Aitken, R. J., Best, F. S. M., Richardson, D. W., Djahanbakhch, O., and Lees, M. M. (1982): The correlates of fertilizing capacity in normal fertile men. *Fertil. Steril.,* 38:68–76.
4. Amann, R. P. (1981): A critical review of methods for evaluation of spermatogenesis from seminal characteristics. *J. Androl.,* 2:37–58.
5. Amann, R. P., and Berndtson, W. E. (1986): Assessment of procedures for screening agents for effects on male reproduction: effects of dibromochloropropane (DBCP) on the rat. *Fundam. Appl. Toxicol.,* 7:244–255.
6. Auroux, M. R., Dulioust, E. M., Nawar, N. Y., and Yacoub, S. G. (1986): Antimitotic drugs (cyclophosphamide and vinblastine) in the male rat. Deaths and behavioral abnormalities in the offspring. *J. Androl.,* 7:378–386.
7. Austin, C. R., and Short, R. V. (1982): *Reproduction in Mammals. Book 1. Germ Cells and Fertilization,* 2d ed. Cambridge University Press, New York.
8. Beattie, P. J., Welsh, M. J., and Brabec, M. J. (1984): The effect of 2-methoxyethanol and methoxyacetic acid on Sertoli cell lactate production and protein synthesis *in vitro. Toxicol. Appl. Pharmacol.,* 76:56–61.
8a. Bedford, J. M. (1982): *Germ Cells and Fertilization,* edited by C. R. Austin and R. V. Short. Cambridge University Press, New York.
9. Berndtson, W. E. (1977): Methods for quantifying mammalian spermatogenesis: a review. *J. Anim. Sci.,* 44:818–833.
10. Bernstein, M. E. (1984): Agents affecting the male reproductive system: effects of structure on activity. *Drug Metab. Rev.,* 15:941–996.
11. Bishop, J. B., and Teal, C. M. (1985): A dominant lethal mutation study in male F-344 rat: effects of ethyl methane sulfonate alone and in combination with agents perturbing the glutathione system in reproductive tissue. *NCTR Final Report.* Experiment 6298 and 6314.
12. Blandau, R. J. (1975): *Aging Gametes: Their Biology and Pathology.* S. Karger S. A., Basel.
13. Blazak, W. F., Ernst, T. L., and Stewart, B. E. (1985): Potential indicators of reproductive toxicity: testicular sperm production and epididymal sperm number, transit time, and motility in Fischer 344 rats. *Fundam. Appl. Toxicol.,* 5:1097–1103.
14. Bloom, A. D. (1981): *Guidelines for Studies of Human Populations Exposed to Mutagenic and Reproductive Hazards.* March of Dimes Birth Defects Foundation, White Plains, New York.
15. Brady, M., Herrera, Y., and Zenick, H. (1975): Influence of parental

lead exposure on subsequent learning ability in offspring. *Pharmacol. Biochem. Behav.*, 3:561–565.

16. Chapin, R. E., Dutton, S. L., Ross, M. D., and Lamb, J. C. (1985): Effects of ethylene glycol monomethyl ether (EGME) on mating performance and epididymal sperm parameters in F-344 rats. *Fundam. Appl. Toxicol.*, 5:182–189.

17. Chapin, R. E., Dutton, S. L., Ross, M. D., Sumrell, B. M., and Lamb, J. C. (1984): The effects of ethylene glycol monomethyl ether on testicular histology in F-344 rats. *J. Androl.*, 5:369–380.

18. Chapin, R. E., Dutton, S. L., Ross, M. D., Swaisgood, R. R., and Lamb, J. C. (1985): The recovery of the testes over eight weeks after short-term dosing with ethylene glycol monomethyl ether: histology, cell specific enzymes and rete testis fluid proteins. *Fundam. Appl. Toxicol.*, 5:515–525.

19. Chapin, R. E., Ross, M. D., and Lamb, J. C. (1984): Immersion fixation methods for glycol methacrylate-embedded testes. *Toxicol. Pathol.*, 12:221–225.

20. Chapin, R. E., White, R. D., Morgan, K. T., and Bus, J. S. (1984): Studies of lesions induced in the testis and epididymis of F-344 rats by inhaled methyl chloride. *Toxicol. Appl. Pharmacol.*, 76:328–343.

21. Christian, M. S. (1986): A critical review of multigeneration studies. *J. Am. Coll. Toxicol.*, 5:161–180.

22. Clegg, E. D. (1983): Mechanisms of mammalian sperm capacitation. In: *Mechanism and Control of Animal Fertilization*, edited by J. F. Hartmann, pp. 177–212. Academic Press, New York.

23. Clegg, E. D., Sakai, C. S., and Voytek, P. (1986): Assessment of reproductive risks. *Biol. Reprod.*, 34:5–16.

24. Clegg, E. D., and Zenick, H. (1988): Restricting mating trials enhanced the detection of ethoxyethanol-induced fertility impairment in rats. *Toxicologist* 8:119(A473).

25. Courot, M., Hochereau-de Reviers, M. T., and Ortavant, R. (1970): Spermatogenesis. In: *The Testis. Volume I. Development, Anatomy and Physiology*, edited by A. D. Johnson, W. R. Gomes, and N. L. Vandemark, pp. 339–432. Academic Press, New York.

26. Creasy, D. M., Flynn, J. C., Gray, T. J. B., and Butler, W. H. (1985): A quantitative study of stage specific spermatocyte damage following administration of ethylene glycol monomethyl ether in the rat. *Exp. Mol. Pathol.*, 43:321–336.

27. Creasy, D. M., Foster, J. R., and Foster, P. M. (1983): The morphological development of di-N-pentyl phthalate induced testicular atrophy in the rat. *J. Pathol.*, 139:309–321.

28. Creasy, D. M., Jones, H. B., Beech, L. M., and Gray, T. J. B. (1986): The effects of two testicular toxins on the ultrastructural morphology of mixed cultures of Sertoli and germ cells: a comparison with *in vivo* effects. *Fundam. Chem. Toxicol.*, 24:655–656.

29. Dalterio, S. L., Steger, R. W., and Bartke, A. (1984): Maternal or paternal exposure to cannabinoids affects central neurotransmitter levels and reproductive function in male offspring. In: *The Cannabinoids: Chemical, Pharmacologic and Therapeutic Aspects*, edited by S. Agurell, W. L. Dewey and R. E. Willette, pp. 411–425. Academic Press, Orlando.

30. De Boer, P., van der Hoeven, F. A., and Chardon, J. A. P. (1976): The production, morphology, karyotypes and transport of spermatozoa from tertiary trisomic mice and the consequences for egg fertilization. *J. Reprod. Fertil.*, 48:249–256.

31. Dewsbury, D. A. (1967): A quantitative description of the behavior of rats during copulation. *Behavior*, 29:154–178.

32. Dixon, R. L. (1985): *Reproductive Toxicology, Target Organ Toxicology Series.* Raven Press, New York.

33. Dixon, R. L., and Hall, J. L. (1984): Reproductive toxicology. In: *Principles and Methods of Toxicology*, edited by A. W. Hayes, pp. 107–140. Raven Press, New York.

33a. Dym, M., and Fawcett, D. W. (1971): Further observations on the number of spermatogonia, spermatocytes, and spermatids connected by intercellular bridges in the mammalian testis. *Biol. Reprod.*, 4:195–215.

34. Evenson, D. P. (1985): Male germ cell analysis by flow cytometry: effects of cancer, chemotherapy, and other factors on testicular function and sperm chromatin structure. *Ann. N.Y. Acad. Sci.*, 350:366.

35. Fedrick, J. (1976): Anencephalus in the Oxford record linkage study area. *Dev. Med. Child. Neurol.*, 18:643–656.

36. Foote, R. H., Berndtson, W. E., and Rounsaville, T. R. (1986): Use of quantitative testicular histology to assess the effect of di-bromochloropropane (DBCP) on reproduction in rabbits. *Fundam. Appl. Toxicol.*, 6:638–647.

37. Foote, R. H., Schermerhorn, E. C., and Simkin, M. E. (1986): Measurement of semen quality, fertility, and reproductive hormones to assess dibromochloropropane (DBCP) effects in live rabbits. *Fundam. Appl. Toxicol.*, 6:628–637.

38. Foster, P. M. D., Foster, J. R., Cook, M. W., Thomas, L. V., and Gangolli, S. D. (1982): Changes in ultrastructure and cytochemical localization of zinc in rat testis following administration of di-n-pentyl phthalate. *Toxicol. Appl. Pharmacol.*, 63:120–132.

39. Friedler, G., and Wheeling, H. S. (1979): Behavioral effects in offspring of males injected with opioids prior to mating. *Pharmacol. Biochem. Behav.*, 11 (Suppl.):23–28.

40. Fuchs, A. R. (1972): Uterine activity during and after mating in the rabbit. *Fertil. Steril.*, 23:915–923.

41. Galbraith, W. M., Voytek, P., and Ryon, M. S. (1983): Assessment of risks to human reproduction and development of the human conceptus from exposure to environmental substances. In: *Advances in Modern Environmental Toxicology, Vol. III. Assessment of Reproductive and Environmental Hazards*, edited by M. S. Christian, W. M. Galbraith, P. Voytek, and M. A. Mehlman, pp. 41–153. Princeton Scientific Publ., Princeton, NJ.

42. Gledhill, B. L. (1985): Cytometry of mammalian sperm. *Gamete Res.*, 12:423–438.

43. Goeden, H., and Zenick, H. (1985): Influence of the uterine environment on rat sperm motility and swimming speed. *J. Exp. Zool.*, 233:247–251.

44. Goeden, H., and Zenick, H. (1989): The effect of ethanol exposure on sperm residing in the female reproductive tract. *Biol. Reprod.* (in press).

45. Goldstein, L. S. (1984): Use of an *in vitro* technique to detect mutations induced by antineoplastic drugs in mouse germ cells. *Cancer Treat. Rep.*, 68:855–858.

46. Gray, L. E. (1989): Compound-induced developmental reproductive abnormalities in man and rodents: a review of effects in males. *J. Toxicol. Environ. Health* (in press).

47. Gray, T. J. B., and Beamand, J. A. (1984): Effect of some phthalate esters and other testicular toxins on primary cultures of testicular cells. *Fundam. Chem. Toxicol.*, 22:123–124.

48. Gray, T. J. B., Moss, E. J., Creasy, D. M., and Gangolli, S. D. (1985): Studies on the toxicity of some glycol ethers and alkoxyacetic acids in primary testicular cell cultures. *Toxicol. Appl. Pharmacol.*, 79:490–501.

49. Green, S., Auletta, A., Fabricant, J., Kapp, R., Manandhar, M., Sheu, C., Springer, J., and Whitfield, B. (1985): Current status of assays in genetic toxicology the dominant lethal test. *Mutat. Res.*, 54:49–67.

50. Grosshans, K., and Calvin, H. I. (1985): Estimation of glutathione in purified populations of mouse testis germ cells. *Biol. Reprod.*, 33:1197–1205.

51. Guthenberg, C., Astrand, I. M., Alin, P., and Mannervik, B. (1983): Glutathione transferase in rat testis. *Acta Scand.*, B37:261–262.

52. Hemminki, K., Saloniemi, I., and Salonen, T. (1981): Childhood cancer and paternal occupation in Finland. *J. Epidemiol. Community Health*, 35:11–15.

53. Hemminki, K. P., Mutanen, P., Luoma, K., and Saloniemi, I. (1980): Congenital malformations by the parental occupation in Finland. *Int. Arch. Environ. Health*, 46:93–98.

54. Heywood, R., and James, R. W. (1978): Assessment of testicular toxicity in laboratory animals. *Environ. Health Perspect.*, 24:73–80.

55. Hoskins, D. D., Johnson, D., Brandt, H., and Acott, T. S. (1979): Evidence for a role for a forward motility protein in the epididymal development of sperm motility. In: *The Spermatozoon*, edited by D. W. Fawcett and J. M. Bedford, pp. 43–53. Urban and Schwarzenberg, Baltimore.

56. Huckins, C. (1978): The morphology and kinetics of spermatogonial degeneration in normal adult rats: an analysis using a simplified classification of the germinal epithelium. *Anat. Rec.*, 4:905–926.

57. Hugenholtz, A. P., and Bruce, W. R. (1983): Radiation induction of mutations affecting sperm morphology in mice. *Mutat. Res.*, 107:177–185.

58. Hurtt, M. E., and Zenick, H. (1986): Decreasing epididymal sperm reserves enhance the detection of ethoxyethanol-induced spermatotoxicity. *Fundam. Appl. Toxicol.*, 7:348–353.

59. Jeulin, C., Feneux, D., Serres, C., Jouannet, P., Guillet-Rosso, F., Belaisch-Allart, J., Frydman, R., and Testart, J. (1986): Sperm factors related to failure of human *in vitro* fertilization. *J. Reprod. Fertil.*, 76:735–744.

60. Jeulin, C., Soumah, A., and Jouannet, P. (1985): Morphological factors influencing the penetration of human sperm into cervical mucus *in vitro*. *Int. J. Androl.*, 8:213–223.

61. Johnson, L. (1986): Spermatogenesis and aging in the human. *J. Androl.*, 7:331–354.

62. Johnson, L., Petty, C. S., and Neaves, W. B. (1980): A comparative study of daily sperm production and testicular composition in humans and rats. *Biol. Reprod.*, 22:1233–1243.

63. Katz, D. F., Diel, L., and Overstreet, J. W. (1982): Differences in the movement of morphologically normal and abnormal human seminal spermatozoa. *Biol. Reprod.*, 26:566–570.

64. Katz, D. F., and Overstreet, J. W. (1981): Sperm motility assessment by videomicrography. *Fertil. Steril.*, 35:188–193.

65. Lamb, J. C., and Chapin, R. E. (1985): Experimental models of male reproductive toxicology. In: *Endocrine Toxicology*, edited by J. A. Thomas, K. S. Korach, and J. A. McLachlan, pp. 85–115. Raven Press, New York.

66. Lamb, J. C., and Foster, P. M. D. (1988): *Physiology and Toxicology of Male Reproduction*. Academic Press, New York.

67. Lamb, J. C., Ross, M. D., and Chapin, R. E. (1986): Experimental methods for studying male reproductive function in standard toxicology studies. *J. Am. Coll. Toxicol.*, 5:225–234.

68. Lee, I. P., and Nagayama, J. (1980): Metabolism of benzo(a)pyrene by the isolated perfused rat testis. *Cancer Res.*, 40:3297–3303.

69. Macleod, J. (1971): Human male infertility. *Obstet. Gynecol. Surg.*, 26:335–351.

70. Mann, T., and Lutwak-Mann, C. (1981): *Male Reproductive Function and Semen: Themes and Trends in Physiology, Biochemistry and Investigative Andrology*. Springer-Verlag, New York.

71. Manson, J. M., and Kang, Y. J. (1988): Test methods for assessing female reproductive and developmental toxicology. In: *Principles and Methods of Toxicology, Second Edition*, edited by A. W. Hayes, pp. 311–359. Raven Press, New York.

72. McKelvey, J. A., and Zemaitis, M. A. (1986): The effects of ethylene oxide (EO) exposure on tissue glutathione levels in rats and mice. *Drug Chem. Toxicol.*, 9:51–66.

73. McRorie, R. A., and Williams, W. L. (1974): Biochemistry of mammalian fertilization. *Ann. Rev. Biochem.*, 43:777–803.

74. Meistrich, M. L. (1982): Quantitative correlation between testicular stem cell survival, sperm production, and fertility in the mouse after treatment with different cytotoxic agents. *J. Androl.*, 3:58–68.

75. Meistrich, M. L. (1986): Critical components of testicular function and sensitivity to disruption. *Biol. Reprod.*, 34:17–28.

76. Meistrich, M. L., and Brown, C. C. (1983): Estimation of the increased risk of human infertility from alterations in semen characteristics. *Fertil. Steril.*, 40:220–230.

77. Meistrich, M. L., and Samuels, R. C. (1985): Reduction in sperm levels after testicular irradiation of the mouse: a comparison with man. *Radiat. Res.*, 102:138–147.

78. Meistrich, M. L., Trostle, P. K., and Brock, W. A. (1981): Association of nucleo-protein transitions with chromatin changes during rat spermatogenesis. In: *Bioregulators of Reproduction*, edited by G. A. Jagiello and H. J. Vogel, pp. 151–167. Academic Press, New York.

79. Moore, H. D. M., and Bedford, J. M. (1983): The interaction of mammalian gametes in the female. In: *Mechanisms and Control of Animal Fertilization*, edited by J. F. Hartmann, pp. 453–497. Academic Press, New York.

80. Mori, H., and Christensen, A. K. (1980): Morphometric analysis of Leydig cells in the normal rat testis. *J. Cell Biol.*, 84:340–354.

81. Mortimer, D., Leslie, E. E., Kelly, R. W., and Templeton, A. A. (1982): Morphological selection of human spermatozoa *in vivo* and *in vitro*. *J. Reprod. Fertil.*, 64:391–399.

82. Mukhtar, H., Philpot, R. M., Lee, I. P., and Bend, J. R. (1978): Developmental aspects of epoxide-metabolizing enzyme activities in adrenals, ovaries, and testes of the rat. In: *Developmental Toxicology of Energy-related Pollutants*, edited by D. D. Mahlum, M. R. Sikov, P. L. Hackett, and F. D. Andrew, pp. 89–104. Technical Information Center, U. S. Department of Energy, Springfield, VA.

83. National Research Council (1983): *Risk Assessment in the Federal Government: Managing the Process*. National Academy Press, Washington, DC.

84. Nelson, J. L., and Zenick, H. (1986): The effect of trichloroethylene on male sexual behavior. Possible opioid role. *Neurobehav. Toxicol. Teratol.*, 8:441–445.

85. Nestor, A., and Handel, M. A. (1984): The transport of morphologically abnormal sperm in the female reproductive tract of mice. *Gamete Res.*, 10:119–125.

86. Nomura, T. (1982): Parental exposure to x-rays and chemicals induces heritable tumors and anomalies in mice. *Nature*, 296:575–577.

87. OECD Guideline for Testing of Chemicals. (1981): "One-generation reproduction toxicity study."

88. Oudiz, D., and Zenick, H. (1986): *In vivo* and *in vitro* evaluations of spermatotoxicity induced by 2-ethoxyethanol treatment. *Toxicol. Appl. Pharmacol.*, 84:576–583.

89. Overstreet, J. W. (1983): Transport of gametes in the reproductive tract of the female mammal. In: *Mechanisms and Control of Animal Fertilization*, edited by J. F. Hartmann, pp. 499–543. Academic Press, New York.

90. Overstreet, J. W. (1984): Laboratory tests for human male reproductive risk assessment. In: *Environmental Influences on Fertility, Pregnancy and Development. Strategies for Measurement and Evaluation*, edited by M. S. Legator, M. Rosenberg, and H. Zenick, pp. 67–82. Alan R. Liss, New York.

91. Overstreet, J. W. (1986): Sperm penetration of cervical mucus. *Fertil. Steril.*, 45:324–326.

92. Overstreet, J. W., Price, M. J., Blazak, W. F., Lewis, E. L., and Katz, D. F. (1981): Simultaneous assessment of human sperm motility and morphology by videomicrography. *J. Urol.*, 126:357–360.

93. Palmer, A. K. (1981): Regulatory requirements for reproductive toxicology: theory and practice. In: *Developmental Toxicology*, edited by C. A. Kimmel and J. Buelke-Sam, pp. 259–287. Raven Press, New York.

94. Papier, C. M. (1985): Parental occupation and congenital malformations in a series of 35,000 births in Israel. *Prog. Clin. Biol. Res.*, 163:291–294.

95. Parke, D. V. (1984): Development of detoxication mechanisms in the neonate. In: *Toxicology and the Newborn*, edited by S. Kacew and M. J. Reasor, pp. 1–32. Elsevier, New York.

96. Parvinen, M., Byskov, A. G., Andersen, C. Y., and Grinsted, J. (1982): Is the spermatogenic cycle regulated by MIS and MPS. *Ann. N.Y. Acad. Sci.*, 383:483–484.

97. Parvinen, M., and Vanha-Perttula, T. (1972): Identification and enzymatic quantification of the stages of the seminiferous epithelial wave in the rat. *Anat. Rec.*, 174:435–449.

98. Peters, J. M., Preston-Martin, S., and Yu, M. C. (1981): Brain tumors in children and occupational exposure of the parents. *Science*, 213:235–237.

99. Polednak, A. P., and Janerich, D. T. (1983): Use of available record systems in epidemiologic studies of reproductive toxicology. *Am. J. Ind. Med.*, 4:329–348.

100. Ratnasooriya, W. D. (1979): A simplified method for measuring ejaculated sperm content of male rats. *J. Pharmacol. Methods*, 2:379–381.

101. Redi, C. A., Garagna, S., Pellicciari, C., Manfredi-Romanini, M. G., Capanna, E., Winking, H., and Gropp, A. (1984): Spermatozoa of chromosomally heterozygous mice and their fate in male and female genital tracts. *Gamete Res.*, 9:273–286.

102. Ribelin, W. E. (1963): Atrophy of rat testis as index of chemical toxicity. *Arch. Pathol.*, 75:229–235.

103. Robaire, B., Smith, S., and Hales, B. F. (1984): Suppression of spermatogenesis by testosterone in adult male rats: effect on fertility, pregnancy outcome and progeny. *Biol. Reprod.*, 31:221–230.

104. Robb, G. W., Amann, R. P., and Killian, G. I. (1978): Daily sperm production and epididymal sperm reserves of pubertal and adult rat. *J. Reprod. Fertil.*, 54:103–107.

105. Rogers, B. J. (1985): The sperm penetration assay: its usefulness revisited. *Fertil. Steril.*, 43:821–840.

106. Rogers, B. J., Bentwood, B. J., Van Campen, H., Helmbrecht, G., Soderdahl, D., and Hale, R. W. (1983): Sperm morphology assessment as an indicator of human fertilizing capacity. *J. Androl.*, 4:119–125.

107. Rubin, H. B., and Henson, D. E. (1979): Effects of drugs on male

sexual function. In: *Advances in Behavioral Pharmacology, Volume 2*, pp. 65–86. Academic Press, New York.

107a. Russell, L. D. (1980): Sertoli-germ cell interrelations: A review. *Gamete Res., 3*:179–202.

108. Russell, L. D. (1983): Normal testicular structure and methods of evaluation under experimental and disruptive conditions. In: *Reproductive and Developmental Toxicity of Metals,* edited by T. W. Clarkson, G. F. Nordberg, and P. R. Sager, pp. 227–252. Plenum Publishing Co., New York.

109. Russell, L. D. (1984): Spermiation—the sperm release process: ultrastructural observations and unresolved problems. In: *Ultrastructure of Reproduction,* edited by J. Van Blerkom and P. M. Motta, pp. 46–66. Martinus Nijhoff, Boston.

110. Russell, L. D., Saxena, N. K., and Weber, J. E. (1987): Intratesticular injections as a method to assess the potential toxicity of various agents and to study mechanisms of normal spermatogenesis. *Gamete Res., 17*:43–56.

111. Schmell, E. D., Gulyas, B., and Hedrick, J. L. (1983): Egg surface changes during fertilization and the molecular mechanism of the block to polyspermy. In: *Mechanism and Control of Animal Fertilization,* edited by J. F. Hartmann, pp. 365–413. Academic Press, New York.

112. Schrag, S. D., and Dixon, R. L. (1985): Reproductive effects of chemicals. In: *Reproductive Toxicology,* edited by R. L. Dixon, pp. 301–320. Raven Press, New York.

113. Schwetz, B. A., Rao, K. S., and Park, C. N. (1980): Insensitivity of tests for reproductive problems. *J. Environ. Pathol. Toxicol., 3:* 81–98.

113a. Selevan and Lemasters (1987): The dose-response fallacy in human reproductive studies of toxic exposures. *J. Occup. Med., 29*:451–454.

114. Shalgi, R. (1984): Developmental capacity of rat embryos produced by *in vivo* or *in vitro* fertilization. *Gamete Res., 10*:77–82.

114a. Smith, M. K., Zenick, H., Preston, R. J. (1986): Dominant lethal effects of subchronic acrylamide administration in the male Long-Evans rat. *Mutat. Res., 173*:273–276.

115. Teal, C. M., Harbison, R. D., and Bishop, J. B. (1985): Germ cell mutagenesis and GSH depression in reproductive tissue of the F-344 rat induced by ethyl methanesulfonate. *Mutat. Res., 144*:93–98.

116. Thomas, J. A., Korach, K. S., and McLachlan, J. A. (1985): *Endocrine Toxicology. Target Organ Toxicology Series.* Raven Press, New York.

117. Trasler, J. M., Hales, B. F., and Robaire, B. (1985): Paternal cyclophosphamide treatment of rats causes fetal loss and malformations without affecting male fertility. *Nature, 316*:144–146.

118. Trasler, J. M., Hales, B. F., and Robaire, B. (1986): Chronic low dose cyclophosphamide treatment of adult male rats: effect on fertility, pregnancy outcome and progeny. *Biol. Reprod., 34*:275–283.

119. Trasler, J. M., Hales, B. F., and Robaire, B. (1987): A time-course study of chronic paternal cyclophosphamide treatment in rats: effects on pregnancy outcome and the male reproductive and hematologic systems. *Biol. Reprod., 37*:317–326.

120. U. S. Environmental Protection Agency (1982): *Pesticide assessment guidelines, subdivision F. Hazard Evaluation: human and domestic animals.* Office of Pesticides and Toxic Substances, Washington, DC. EPA report no. EPA-540/9-82-025.

121. U. S. Environmental Protection Agency (1985): Toxic substances control act test guidelines; final rules. *Fed. Reg.,* 50(188):39426–39436.

122. U. S. Environmental Protection Agency (1986): *Guidelines for mutagenicity assessment.* Office of Health and Environmental Assessment, Washington, DC.

122a. Walker (1986): Age factors potentiating drug toxicity in the reproductive axis. *Environ. Hlth. Perspect., 70*:185–191.

123. Waller, D. P., Killinger, J. M., and Zaneveld, L. J. D. (1985): Physiology and toxicology of the male reproductive tract. In: *Endocrine Toxicology,* edited by J. D. Thomas, pp. 269–333. Raven Press, New York.

124. Wing, T.-Y., and Christensen, A. K. (1982): Morphometric studies on rat seminiferous tubules. *Am. J. Anat., 165*:13–25.

125. Working, P. K., Bus, J. S., and Hamm, T. E. (1985): Reproductive effects of inhaled methyl chloride in the male Fischer 344 rat. I. *Toxicol. Appl. Pharmacol., 77*:133–143.

126. Working, P. K., Bus, J. S., and Hamm, T. E. (1985): Reproductive effects of inhaled methyl chloride in the male Fischer 344 rat. II. Spermatogonial toxicity and sperm quality. *Toxicol. Appl. Pharmacol., 77*:144–157.

127. Working, P. K., and Hurtt, M. E. (1987): Computerized videomicrographic analysis of rat sperm motility. *J. Androl., 8*:330–337.

128. Wyrobeck, A. J. (1984): Identifying agents that damage human spermatogenesis: abnormalities in sperm concentration and morphology. In: *Monitoring Human Exposure to Carcinogenic and Mutagenic Agents.* Proceedings of a joint symposium held in Espoo, Finland, International Agency for Research on Cancer, Lyon.

129. Wyrobek, A. J., and Bruce, W. R. (1978): The induction of sperm-shape abnormalities in mice and humans. In: *Chemical Mutagens, Principles and Methods for Their Detection, Vol. 5,* edited by A. Hollander and F. J. de Serres, pp. 257–285. Plenum Press, New York.

130. Wyrobek, A. J., Gordon, L. A., Burkhart, J. G., Francis, M. W., Kapp, R. W., Letz, G., Malling, H. V., Topham, J. C., and Whorton, M. D. (1983): An evaluation of human sperm as indicators of chemically-induced alterations of spermatogenic function. *Mutat. Res., 115*:73–148.

131. Wyrobek, A. J., Gordon, L. A., Burkhart, J. G., Francis, M. W., Kapp, R. W., Jr., Letz, G., Malling, H. V., Topham, J. C., and Whorton, M. D. (1983): An evaluation of the mouse sperm morphology test and other sperm tests in non-human mammals. *Mutat. Res., 115*:1–72.

132. Wyrobek, A. J., Gordon, L. A., Watchmaker, G., and Moore, D. H. (1982): Human sperm morphology. Description of a reliable method and its statistical power. In: *Banbury Report 13: Indicators of Genotoxic Exposure,* pp. 527–541. Cold Spring Harbor Laboratory, Cold Spring Harbor, New York.

133. Wyrobek, A. J., Watchmaker, G., and Gordon, L. (1984): An evaluation of sperm tests as indicators of germ-cell damage in men exposed to chemical or physical agents. In: *Reproduction: The New Frontier in Occupational and Environmental Health Research,* edited by J. E. Lockey, G. K. Lemasters, and W. R. Keye, Jr., pp. 385–407. Alan R. Liss, New York.

134. Yanagimachi, R. (1981): Mechanisms of fertilization in mammals. In: *Fertilization and Embryonic Development In Vitro,* edited by L. Mastroianni, Jr., and J. D. Biggers, pp. 81–188. Plenum Press, New York.

135. Zack, M., Cannon, S., Lloyd, D., Heath, C. W., Jr., Falletta, J. M., Jones, B., Housworth, J., and Crowley, S. (1980): Cancer in children of parents exposed to hydrocarbon-related industries and occupations. *Am. J. Epidemiol., 3*:329–336.

135a. Zaneveld, L. D. J. (1982): The epididymis. In: *Biochemistry of Mammalian Reproduction,* edited by L. D. J. Zaneveld and R. T. Chatterton, pp. 37–64. J. Wiley and Sons, New York.

136. Zaneveld, L. D. J., and Chatterton, R. T. (1982): *Biochemistry of Mammalian Reproduction.* J. Wiley and Sons, New York.

137. Zenick, H., Blackburn, K., Hope, E., and Baldwin, D. J. (1984): An assessment of the copulatory, endocrinologic, and spermatotoxic effects of carbon disulfide exposure in the rat. *Toxicol. Appl. Pharmacol., 73*:275–283.

138. Zenick, H., Blackburn, K., Hope, E., Oudiz, D., and Goeden, H. (1984): Evaluation of male reproductive toxicity: a new animal model. *Teratogenesis Carcinog. Mutagen., 4*:109–128.

139. Zenick, H., and Clegg, E. D. (1986): Issues in risk assessment in male reproductive toxicology. *J. Am. Coll. Toxicol., 5*:249–259.

140. Zenick, H., and Goeden, H. (1988): Evaluation of copulatory behavior and sperm in rats: role in reproductive risk assessment. In: *Physiology and Toxicology of Male Reproduction,* edited by J. C. Lamb and P. M. D. Foster, pp. 174–197. Academic Press, New York.

141. Zenick, H., Hope, E., and Smith, K. (1986): Reproductive toxicity associated with acrylamide treatment in male and female rats. *J. Toxicol. Environ. Health, 17*:457–472.

Principles and Methods of Toxicology, Second Edition, edited by A. Wallace Hayes, Raven Press, Ltd., New York © 1989.

CHAPTER 11

Test Methods for Assessing Female Reproductive and Developmental Toxicology

Jeanne M. Manson and Y. J. Kang

Reproductive and Developmental Toxicology, Smith Kline & French Laboratories, Philadelphia, Pennsylvania 19101

"Reproductive dysfunction" is broadly defined in this chapter to include all effects resulting from paternal or maternal exposure that interfere with the conception, development, birth, and maturation of offspring to healthy adult life. The relation between exposure and reproductive dysfunction is highly complex because exposure of the mother, the father, or both may influence reproductive outcome (89). In addition, exposures may have occurred at some time in the past, immediately prior to conception, or during gestation. For some specific dysfunctions, the relevant period of exposure can be identified, and for others it cannot. For example, chromosome abnormalities detected in the embryo can arise from mutations in the germ cells of either parent prior to conception or at fertilization, or from direct exposure of embryonic tissues during gestation. Major malformations, however, usually occur with exposure during a discrete period of pregnancy, extending from the third to the eighth week of human development.

Although extensive data are available on reproductive performance in human populations, most have been collected from routine surveillance and not from monitoring environmental exposures. Even though the effects of specific agents on reproductive function cannot be discerned from such data, useful information on trends and patterns in the frequency of various reproductive outcomes can be derived. An estimated 11 million married couples in the United States are infertile (i.e., not capable of having children), 3 million of whom have at least one partner who is noncontraceptively sterile (58). Although early spontaneous abortions often go unreported, particularly among pregnancies of less than 20 weeks' duration, their frequency has been estimated to be 15% of all recognized pregnancies (94). This figure is generally considered to be an underestimate of the true rate insofar as most spontaneous abortions occur early in gestation, often before the pregnancy is recognized. Of the approximately 3 million infants born alive each year, 13.1 per 1,000 die within the first year (59). Some 2 to 3% of infants born alive have major congenital malformations recognized within a year (14,29). When defects that become apparent later in life are included, the frequency of major and minor malformations increases to about 16% (10). Approximately 7% of babies are born prematurely (before the 37th week of gestation), and 7% of those born at full term have low birth weights (2.5 kg or less) (32,67).

The frequency of these adverse outcomes on a per-couple or per-pregnancy basis is given in Table 1. Exposure to an individual agent could be associated with the entire spectrum of effects or be linked to an individual outcome alone. The most frequent types of reproductive failure in the human population are infertility and spontaneous abortion, which occur in 10 to 15% of couples and 10 to 20% of pregnancies. These outcomes have received relatively little attention compared to the emotionally laden yet rarer outcomes of birth defects and functional disorders in infants.

In few cases has it been possible to separate the impact of a specific agent on human reproduction from the background rate of spontaneous genetic defects or from other causes such as radiation, infection, nutritional deficiencies, or maternal metabolic imbalance (34,65). There are also ethical limitations to conducting human studies, particularly regarding reproductive function. The enormous difficulty of conducting epidemiology studies, particularly in regard to obtaining adequate sample size, is illustrated in Table 2. To detect a 3.2-fold increase in all major malformations, which occur at a frequency of 3%, a sample of at least 300 live births would be needed (14). For more frequent outcomes such as spontaneous abortion (15% incidence), a smaller sample size of 50 pregnancies would be needed to detect a comparable threefold increase. Given the complexities of carrying out human clinical and epidemiologic studies, most information on agents that affect reproductive function is derived from animal studies.

The standard acute, subacute, and chronic toxicologic testing procedures are not sufficient to detect reproductive or developmental toxicity. A separate series of tests have been developed that specifically monitor these functions. The purpose of this chapter is to provide a rationale for and description of tests for monitoring effects on female fertility and pregnancy. A brief biologic description of these processes

TABLE 1. *Frequency of selected reproductive failures*

Event	Frequency	
	Per 100	Unit
Failure to conceive after 1 year	10–15	Couples
Spontaneous abortion 8–28 weeks	10–20	Pregnancies or women
Chromosome anomalies in spontaneous abortions, 8–28 weeks	30–40	Spontaneous abortion
Chromosome anomalies from amniocentesis, >35 years	2	Amniocentesis specimens
Stillbirths	2–4	Stillbirths and live births
Birth weight < 2,500 g	7	Live births
Birth defects	2–3	Live births
Chromosome anomalies, live births	0.2	Live births
Severe mental retardation	0.4	Children to age 15 years

Adapted from ref. 14.

TABLE 2. *Sample size calculations for epidemiologic studies of reproductive failure*

Frequency per 100[a]	Associated outcome	Sample size of comparison groups	Increase in frequency
3	Stillbirths, birth defects	50	7.7-fold
		100	5.3-fold
		250	3.3-fold
		300	3.2-fold
7	Low birth weight	50	4.6-fold
		100	3.4-fold
		250	2.3-fold
		300	2.3-fold
15	Infertility, spontaneous abortion	50	3.0-fold
		100	2.4-fold
		250	1.8-fold
		300	1.7-fold

[a] Detectable with 95% power.
Adapted from ref. 14.

is given to provide a background for the design of tests and selection of endpoints that are conventionally measured.

FEMALE REPRODUCTIVE TOXICOLOGY

Maturation of the Female Reproductive System

The ovarian follicle consists of three cell types: the germ cell (or oocyte), granulosa cells, and thecal endocrine cells. The growth, maturation, and differentiation of each cell type is required for successful ovulation of a fertilizable ovum and formation of a corpus luteum. Three major processes occurring during the life-span of a follicle that are susceptible to perturbation are *mitosis* of oogonia and granulosa cells occurring at specific stages of follicular growth, *meiosis* of oogonia to form oocytes, and *differentiation* of granulosa cells and theca cells, permitting them to respond to the luteinizing hormone (LH) surge and ovulate.

Formation of germ cells and follicles occurs during prenatal life. Early in embryonic development the progenitors of the germ cells, called primordial germ cells, are segregated from somatic cells. At 3 weeks of human development, the primordial germ cells are first detectable in the yolk sac, and thereafter they undergo mitotic divisions and migrate to the urogenital ridge, where they populate the "indifferent" gonad. Primordial germ cells then differentiate into oogonia or prespermatogonia. The oogonial stage is characterized by active mitotic divisions; the daughter cells do not separate but remain attached to each other by interconnecting cytoplasmic bridges in a syncytial mass. In the human embryo it has been estimated that approximately 1,700 germ cells are involved in migration to the gonads, with an increase to about 6×10^5 by 2 months of gestation. Mitotic activity peaks by the fifth month, with an increase to 7×10^6 cells. Oogonia first begin to enter meiosis at the third month, and by the end of the 5th month all the oogonia have entered early prophase I of meiosis and are called primary oocytes (27). The timing of gonadal sex differentiation and ovarian germ cell development in various mammalian species is presented in Table 3.

TABLE 3. *Ontogeny of ovarian germ cell development in mammalian species*

Species	Days of gestation	Gonadal sex differentiation	Initiation of meiosis	Completion of oogenesis	Arrest of meiosis
Mouse	19	12	13	16	*(5)*
Rat	21	13–14	17	19	*(5)*
Hamster	16	11–12	*(1)*	*(5)*	*(9)*
Rabbit	31	15–16	*(1)*	*(10)*	*(21)*
Monkey (rhesus)	165	38	56	165	Newborn
Human	270	40–42	84	150	Newborn

Numbers indicate days of gestation or postnatal age (italics). Completion of oogenesis refers to the time when all oogonia have been transformed to primary oocytes.
Adapted from ref. 27.

Each meiotic division has four stages: prophase, metaphase, anaphase, and telophase. The first meiotic division is initiated late in fetal life, with progression to early prophase during the fetal or neonatal period. By 8 weeks after birth, human oocytes have entered a resting phase of oocyte maturation, where meiosis remains blocked until the beginning of puberty (7). Given the long duration of prophase I, this stage has been subdivided into five subphases; leptotene, zygotene, pachytene, diplotene, and dictate (resting phase). Each substage is characterized by cytogenetic criteria of chromosome configuration.

Extensive physiological degeneration of germ cells occurs during the oogonial and primary oocyte stages of development. In humans it has been estimated that 60% of the germ cells present in a 5-month-old fetus are lost before birth. Three distinct waves of degeneration occur in the prenatal development of the human ovary, affecting oogonia in mitosis or in the final interphase, oocytes in pachytene, and oocytes in diplotene of prophase I. Oogonia connected by cytoplasmic bridges undergo atresia in synchrony, which accounts for most germ cell loss. After the completion of meiotic prophase, groups of oocytes no longer appear to undergo atresia simultaneously, but individual oocytes may degenerate at all stages of development. It is not understood why some oocytes degenerate whereas others mature (30).

After entering prophase, surviving oocytes are surrounded by granulosa cells to begin the process of folliculogenesis or the formation of follicles. In the "resting," or primordial (nongrowing), follicles, the granulosa cells are flat and unilayered. During the prepubertal and reproductive periods, most germ cells remain as primary oocytes enclosed within unilamellar follicles. These resting follicles comprise the pool from which a select number of oocytes are recruited for further maturation to preovulatory or graafian follicles. Progression of the ovulatory cycle in humans is diagramed in Fig. 1. Initiation of follicular growth occurs continuously on a daily basis and is characterized by three events: (a) oocyte enlargement; (b) transition of granulosa cells from a flattened to a rounded configuration; and (c) formation of the zona pellucida, a complex protein–carbohydrate extracellular matrix between granulosa cells and oocytes. This first stage of growth is characteristic of small, type 2 follicles (75), which have entered the pool of committed growing follicles. The factors that trigger the initiation of follicle growth are not known, but follicle-stimulating hormone (FSH) and LH are not involved (77).

Progression of follicle growth depends on FSH and LH and is associated with five events: (a) continued oocyte enlargement; (b) rapid proliferation and increase in layers of granulosa cells; (c) formation of the basal lamina, an extracellular matrix external to the outer layer of granulosa cells; (d) organization of the endocrine thecal cells around the basal lamina; and (e) formation of the antrum, a fluid-filled cavity within the follicle. Most of the type 2 follicles continue to grow until they reach the large, preantral stage (type 5–6). The few follicles that actually become antral, preovulatory follicles (type 7–8) are selected from the pool of the large preantral follicles by the surge of gonadotropins in the cycle preceding ovulation.

The preovulatory increase in LH stimulates the conversion of progesterone to androstenedione in theca cells (78). Androstenedione is then converted to estradiol in granulosa cells, and the estradiol is secreted by growing follicles. Estradiol, acting with FSH, is obligatory for differentiation of granulosa cells, which includes increased cellular content of FSH and LH receptors, and increased aromatose activity, cholesterol side chain cleavage, and prostaglandin synthetase activity (77,78). The latter regulates the synthesis of prostaglandins, which are necessary for ovulation to occur. Only those follicles capable of producing estradiol become preovulatory follicles. Thus any agent that inhibits either theca cell function (ability to synthesize androstenedione) or granulosa cell function (synthesis and action of estradiol) causes atresia. Furthermore, because FSH and LH act via cyclic adenosine monophosphate (AMP), agents that alter gonadotropin receptor content or the functional coupling of the receptor to adenylate cyclase also cause atresia.

Following the rise in FSH and LH levels, the primary oocytes in preovulatory follicles progress through the rest of the first meiotic division and form secondary oocytes that are blocked in metaphase of the second division. The first polar body, which contains half the chromosomes present in the primary oocyte, is extruded. As the time of ovulation nears, the follicle becomes more vascular and swells out from the ovarian surface; it is then macroscopically visible as a blister-like protuberance. The secondary oocyte is ovulated at metaphase II, and it stays in this stage preceding fertilization. At fertilization the second meiotic division is completed, the second polar body is extruded, and the female pronucleus is formed. The male and female pronucleus then combine to reestablish the diploid state (18).

In the absence of fertilization, the ovulated oocyte degen-

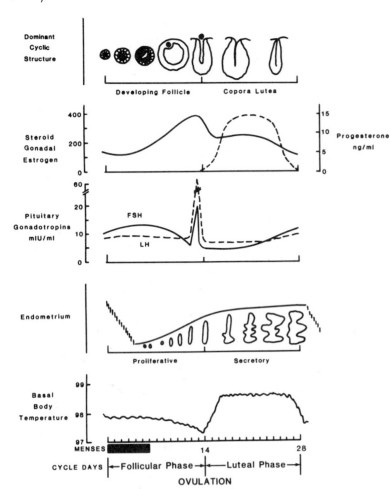

FIG. 1. Progression of ovulatory cycle in humans. Development of the dominant follicle, pattern of gonadal steroid production, levels of pituitary gonadotropins, endometrial proliferation, and basal body temperature are depicted. (Adapted from refs. 28 and 91.)

erates. Under continued LH stimulation, the emptied follicle luteinizes and develops into a corpus luteum, which secretes progesterone. This process continues throughout the reproductive life until the population of primordial follicles is depleted or menopause occurs.

Oocyte Toxicity

The ovary, as a repository of oocytes and as a source of steroid hormones that control the functional development of reproductive organs, plays a major role in fertility and initiation of pregnancy. As indicated in the preceding section, after mitotically active oogonia enter meiosis during fetal life, replacement of germ cells destroyed by toxins is no longer possible. Complete destruction of oocytes prepubertally results in primary amenorrhea and failure of pubertal onset (51).

If the preovulatory oocyte is destroyed, fertility is immediately interrupted. Growing follicles can repopulate the preovulatory pool, followed by a resumption in fertility. If a toxicant destroys growth-initiated, gonadotropin-independent follicles but spares preovulatory follicles, the delay in onset of infertility is proportional to the time required for growing follicles to reach the preovulatory stage. Destruction of resting or primordial follicles has the most delaying effect on fertility, and the results may not be evident until the end

of reproductive life. Partial destruction of the resting follicle pool is manifested as premature onset of menopause. Menopause generally occurs between 45 and 55 years of age, and premature onset is defined as occurrence before age 35 (53).

In a mathematical model of functional ovarian life-span, Mattison (53) estimated that menopause occurs when there are fewer than 3,500 oocytes per ovary. Calculations using this model indicated that the age of menopause was weakly dependent on the number of oocytes at birth. When 75, 50, or 25% of the normal complement of oocytes was present at birth, menopause was estimated to occur at 47, 44, or 37 years, respectively. The effect of varying the normal rate of atresia, or oocyte half-life (9.2 years), had a strong influence on age at menopause, however. If oocyte half-life was 75, 50, or 25% the normal rate, the age at menopause was 38, 25, or 12 years, respectively.

The results of this model are consistent with human data that suggest most forms of genetic or xenobiotic-induced premature ovarian failure are due to an increased rate of atresia. Surgical procedures, such as unilateral oophorectomy or bilateral wedge resection, that decrease resting oocyte number without altering the rate of atresia do not appear to influence the age of menopause (53).

In rodent species, female germ cells are extraordinarily sensitive to killing by exposure to ionizing radiation, especially during neonatal life. Primordial, or resting, follicles in juvenile mice have an LD_{50} of only 6 rad (13), whereas typical LD_{50} values for most other rapidly proliferating cell types range from 100 to 300 rad. The entire primordial follicle pool in female squirrel monkeys is destroyed by prenatal exposure to only 0.7 rad/day throughout pregnancy. Histopathological examination of other tissues failed to yield evidence of cytotoxic effects at any other site (13). High primordial follicle radiosensitivity has been demonstrated in relatively few species, most notably the neonatal mouse, prenatal pig, and prenatal squirrel monkey. In mice, primordial follicle radiosensitivity appears shortly after birth, increases rapidly to peak sensitivity from days 5 to 17 of life, and decreases moderately to adult levels. The rat displays a similar pattern but is considerably less radiosensitive.

The magnitude of prenatal germ cell loss in squirrel monkeys has led to examination of other nonhuman primates. Exposure of rhesus and bonnet monkeys to radiation during pregnancy has failed to yield evidence of primordial follicle radiosensitivity (13). Baker (4) emphasized that primordial follicles in humans are radioresistant, with x-ray LD_{50} values reaching 400 rad. X-ray exposures to the human ovary have most often been examined at prepubertal and adult stages, however, and a critical period during late fetal to early neonatal life would most likely have been missed.

In human adults the growing follicles appear to be most sensitive to ionizing radiation owing in part to the rapid rate of granulosa cell proliferation. Radiation effects on the ovary in women of reproductive age have been tabulated by Asch (3). Exposure to less than 60 centigrays had no deleterious effects at any age. At 150 centigrays, women over 40 were at risk of becoming sterile. From 250 to 500 centigrays, women under 40 had temporary amenorrhea, and 60% of the women were permanently sterile. All women over 40 had permanent sterility at this level of radiation.

With the onset of preovulatory maturation and resumption of meiosis, susceptibility to the lethal effects of radiation decreases, and sensitivity to genetic damage increases. Preovulatory oocytes in multilayered follicles are relatively resistant to cell killing, but they are sensitive to induction of both recessive and dominant mutations. Among irradiated preovulatory oocytes, the incidence of dominant lethal mutations is highest at metaphase I, slightly less at metaphase II, and low at other stages (4).

A number of xenobiotics and drugs have been associated with oocyte toxicity, the major classes of which are listed in Table 4. Several investigators have demonstrated that polycyclic aromatic hydrocarbons (PAHs) destroy resting or primordial follicles in mice and rats in a strain-, species-, age-, dose-, and metabolism-dependent manner (24,52). PAHs have also been demonstrated to cause ovarian tumors, chromosome aberrations in oocyte meiosis, and decreased fertility in laboratory animals (see ref. 52 for a review). Oocyte destruction by a PAH requires distribution of the parent hydrocarbon to the ovary, where ovarian enzymes metabolize it to reactive intermediates responsible for oocyte destruction. Although ovarian metabolism is necessary for oocyte destruction, inducibility at the *Ah* locus is not as highly correlated with this effect as is the rate of metabolism along the pathway leading to formation of dihydrodiol epoxides.

There are indications that cigarette smoking causes ovarian toxicity in humans, resulting in premature onset of menopause (93). The incidence of infertility, defined as a woman never being pregnant throughout her reproductive life, was about 12% among nonsmokers and 18% among smokers. There are more than 3,000 identifiable compounds in cigarette smoke, and the specific agents responsible for this effect are not known, although PAH and nicotine have been implicated.

A variety of antineoplastic agents have been associated with ovulatory dysfunction and destruction of oocytes (28). These agents destroy rapidly dividing granulosa cells in growing follicles and mutate preovulatory follicles. Dobson and Felton (13) reviewed data on the primordial follicle toxicity of 77 chemicals in 11 chemical classes. Of the 77 chemicals tested, 21 caused destruction of resting primordial follicles in mice. Positive compounds were found in 7 of the 11 classes, notably among the PAHs, alkylating agents, esters, epoxides and carbamates, fungal toxins and antibiotics, and nitrosamines. The four negative classes were the aromatic amines, aryl halides, metals, and steroids.

Antiestrogens such as *cis*-clomiphene have a selective effect on differentiating follicles insofar as estrogen acting with FSH (or cyclic AMP) is necessary for granulosa cell maturation. Only those follicles capable of producing estradiol survive to the preovulatory stage.

Because ovulation is considered to be an inflammatory process requiring prostaglandins and leukotrienes, drugs that block the synthesis of these products from arachidonic acid in the ovary can specifically inhibit ovulation (19). Under such conditions the ovary becomes macroscopically enlarged due to continued follicle growth as well as to swelling of preovulatory follicles that are blocked from expelling the oocyte. Microscopically, the preovulatory follicles begin to luteinize under uninterrupted LH stimulation but still contain an entrapped ovum (69). Female subjects maintain an estrous cycle, albeit irregular, in this state but are subfertile owing to blockade of ovulation.

Alterations in Reproductive Endocrinology

In addition to direct effects on survival of follicles, xenobiotic exposure can impair female fertility through alterations in the function of the hypothalamic-pituitary-uterine-ovarian axis. The central nervous system (CNS) component of the female reproductive system functions in a permissive/integrating role. Hypothalamic neurons synthesize and secrete gonadotropin-releasing hormone (GnRH). These hypotha-

TABLE 4. *Xenobiotics and drugs associated with oocyte toxicity*

Agent	Toxic actions
Polycyclic aromatic hydrocarbons	Destroy primordial follicles
Antineoplastic agents	Destroy growing follicles and mutate preovulatory follicles
Antiestrogens	Destroy growing and preovulatory follicles
Prostaglandin synthetase inhibitors	Block ovulation

lamic neurons adjoin a portal vascular system that transports GnRH, secreted in a pulsatile pattern, to the anterior pituitary. GnRH affects gonadotrophs of the anterior pituitary in a permissive capacity, allowing the release of FSH and LH. The pattern of gonadotropin release, although allowed by GnRH, is controlled by negative feedback from the circulating levels of sex hormones (46).

The hormones FSH and LH stimulate follicular maturation from the preantral to the preovulatory stage (Fig. 1). They influence the synthesis and secretion of estrogen by theca and granulosa cells in the follicle. With the surge in gonadotropins at midcycle, a series of events are set in motion that culminate in ovulation. These events include intrafollicular prostaglandin synthesis, terminal oocyte maturation, a shift in steroidogenesis from estrogen to progesterone production by granulosa cells, morphologic luteinization, and finally rupture of the follicle and release of the oocyte. Peripheral progesterone levels begin to rise with the initiation of the LH surge and continue to increase until the midpoint of the luteal phase, when they begin to gradually decrease, resulting in menses. In humans, chorionic gonadotropin (hCG) secreted by the embryo appears responsible for maintenance of the corpus luteum during early pregnancy.

There are a number of endocrine processes in which xenobiotics can interfere with ovarian function aside from direct injury of the follicle. It is difficult, however, to distinguish direct injury to the follicle from alterations in hypothalamic-pituitary-gonadal function. Interference with specific endocrine functions critical to follicular development yields the same endpoints as direct follicle toxicity, ovulatory dysfunction, and reproductive failure.

Endocrine Alterations During the Perinatal Period

Steroid hormones themselves have been the most thoroughly studied agents in female reproductive toxicology and have served as model agents for xenobiotic effects. It is well established that pharmacologic exposure of female rodents to androgens or estrogens during fetal and neonatal life results in disruption of the mechanisms that control cyclic secretion of gonadotropins. Although there are numerous functional and structural sex differences in the adult brain, they are imposed on an essentially feminine or bipotential brain by steroid hormones during a critical period of perinatal development in the rat.

The critical period for exposure to steroid hormones extends from day 18 of pregnancy to days 8 to 10 of neonatal life in the rat. During this time the hypothalamic centers believed to be involved in control of cyclic hormone secretion undergo neuronal maturation. Disruption or alteration of hypothalamic maturation in the female rat has a permanent effect that results in a male or acyclic (tonic) pattern of gonadotropin release and the persistent estrous syndrome that is characterized by infertility and a lack of estrous cyclicity (49).

In the rat and other rodent species, the persistent estrous syndrome appears to result from the action of estrogens on hypothalamic development during the neonatal period. Neonatal exposure to estrogenic substances stimulates uterine growth and early vaginal opening. These two responses are good indicators of estrogenic action, and when they occur during the neonatal period they can be predictive of persistent estrous and reproductive tract anomalies in the adult (84). Physiological estrogens (e.g., estradiol, estriol, and estrone), nonphysiological estrogens [e.g., diethylstilbestrol (DES), Kepone, o,p'-DDT, and methoxychlor], and triphenylethylene drugs (e.g., naloxidine, tamoxifen, and clomiphene) are known to cause these effects in the rat.

Endogenous estrogens are prevented from exerting these toxicities by their extensive binding to serum proteins. Consequently, the level of free hormone is low, leaving relatively little to bind to cellular estrogen receptors. This scenario has been well established in the rat, which has substantial quantities of α-fetoprotein (AFP) in the blood during fetal and neonatal development. AFP binds estradiol with high affinity and thus reduces the level of free hormone available for receptor binding in rodents. DES, however, is weakly bound by AFP, which permits more interaction of this estrogenic substance with cellular receptors. Those estrogens not extensively bound to AFP tend to be potent estrogenic toxins capable of disrupting normal reproduction in the rat (56).

Although these concepts have been validated in rodents, there is controversy about their applicability to humans. AFP does not bind physiological estrogens well in humans, and it cannot be equated with AFP in rodents. Other proteins, e.g., steroid hormone-binding globulin, along with the high levels of progesterone during human pregnancy may protect against estrogen action (11).

The mechanisms that control the development of the female reproductive system in primates, including humans, also appear to be different or less sensitive to toxic hormonal influences. In the rat it is generally accepted that androgens secreted by the testes during development are converted to estrogens in the hypothalamus (56). These estrogens act to defeminize the hypothalamus and to produce an acyclic, male pattern of gonadotropin secretion. However, these mechanisms do not appear to operate in primates; instead, testosterone is converted to dihydrotestosterone, which is the active agent. Insofar as aromatization of androgens to estrogens is not involved in masculinization of the primate hypothalamus, exposure to estrogenic toxins is not likely to lead to abnormal patterns of gonadotropin release or male infertility. The primate hypothalamus appears to be insensitive to androgens; pharmacological exposure of female fetuses to androgens can masculinize the external genitalia without influencing the periodicity of the adult menstrual cycle (11). Even though the evidence suggests that hormonal insult during human development does not influence hypothalamic maturation for cyclic gonadotropin release, it is clear the masculinized behavior patterns are produced in female primates with androgen exposure during pregnancy. Also, DES exposure during pregnancy has been associated with menstrual irregularity and subfertility, although the evidence for these effects is not as strong as for the structural and preneoplastic lesions in the reproductive tract. Steroid hormone exposure during the perinatal and adult periods is associated with reproductive tract abnormalities. Consequently, although there may be differences in the critical period and in the mechanism of action between rodent and primate species, in all mammalian species pharmacological exposure to sex steroids early in life predisposes the adult to subsequent reproductive abnormalities (11).

CNS-Mediated Endocrine Alterations in the Adult

Perinatal exposures that alter "sexual imprinting" in the CNS and that can cause permanent infertility and reproductive tract abnormalities in the adult have been discussed. In this section, exposures that can cause reversible disruption of hypothalamic pathways for gonadotropin release in the adult are covered. It is now well established that certain CNS-active drugs can cause reversible alterations in hypothalamic-pituitary function. In laboratory animals these effects are seen as suppression of the estrous cycle, ovulation, and fertility in females, and inhibition of androgen production and suppression of spermatogenesis in males.

The evidence now indicates that the major catecholamine pathways involved in hypothalamic control of gonadotropins are adrenergic and dopaminergic. There is profuse catecholaminergic innervation in the hypothalamus, and catecholamines play an important role in gonadotropin release. The surge-type gonadotropin release associated with the preovulatory rise in LH and FSH is under noradrenergic control and is stimulated by dopamine, norepinephrine, and epinephrine. These catecholamines stimulate the release of GnRH, which in turn controls the release of LH and to a lesser extent FSH. The stimulatory effect of these catecholamines, particularly norepinephrine, on GnRH release is mediated by α-adrenergic receptors. α-Receptor antagonists (e.g., phenoxybenzamine) block LH secretion, whereas agonists (e.g., clonidine) enhance LH secretion in most rat models. Reduction of norepinephrine or α-receptor blockade in the CNS has a greater effect on surge-type gonadotropin release associated with ovulation than basal gonadotropin release (55).

There is growing evidence that the endogenous opioid peptides may also be involved in GnRH release by reducing endogenous inhibitory tone at the time of the preovulatory surge in LH and FSH. Exogenous morphine or opioid peptides inhibit LH secretion, and naloxone injections, which block opioid receptors, augment the height of the preovulatory LH surge (54). The precise mechanism by which opioids modulate neuroendocrine function is unknown. Preliminary observations indicate that opioids may affect secretion of biogenic amines; i.e., they may decrease dopamine turnover and norepinephrine concentrations.

A wide variety of pharmacological agents can modify catecholamine levels by altering synthesis, release, receptor activation, and reuptake. Drugs that produce actions of this type are neuropharmacological agents that either inhibit CNS activities (anesthetics, analgesics, sedatives, and tranquilizers) or stimulate them (antidepressants, stimulants, and hallucinogens). In addition, drugs of abuse are increasingly implicated in the disruption of the hypothalamic-pituitary system, leading to reproductive dysfunction (87).

Marijuana and its principal psychoactive ingredient Δ-9-tetrahydrocannabinol (THC) inhibit secretion of FSH, LH, and prolactin in rodent and nonhuman primate models. In primates, acute administration of THC results in 50 to 80% reductions in serum FSH and LH for up to 24 hours. At blood THC levels comparable to those found in regular human marijuana users, nonhuman primates experienced disruption of the menstrual cycle and inhibition of ovulation. With an 18-day exposure to THC, continued disruption of the menstrual cycles persisted until 6 months after treatment. In both rodent and primate models, the antifertility effects of THC could be reversed by treatment with GnRH, suggesting that the primary lesion occurred at the hypothalamic level (reviewed in ref. 87).

Narcotic drugs have been found to cause reproductive dysfunction in human addicts: Clinical manifestations of decreased sexual desire and performance, menstrual irregularities, and infertility have been attributed to altered hypothalamic-pituitary function. Acute doses of morphine inhibit ovulation in rats and rabbits. Chronic doses of morphine or heroin abolish estrous cyclicity in rodents and the menstrual cycle in women. Evidence for a primary hypothalamic involvement has come from studies in men, where GnRH treatment prevented or reversed opioid-induced decrease in plasma testosterone levels (87).

The barbiturates are sedative-hypnotic agents that have been used as anesthetics in laboratory animals for many years. The general effect of barbiturates is an inhibition of both LH and FSH release, with subsequent depression in steroid hormone levels. Phenobarbital inhibits gonadotropin secretion and blocks the rise in serum gonadotropin levels that normally follows castration. LH secretion and ovulation can be restored in barbiturate-treated animals by treatment with GnRH, indicating a hypothalamic site of action (87).

Phencyclidine hydrochloride (PCP) was developed as an animal tranquilizer but has been used as a drug of abuse. Many areas of the CNS are affected by PCP, which alters several neurotransmitter systems. Acute administration of PCP at "recreational" dosage levels produced slight depressions in serum testosterone and LH levels in male rats. Marked depression occurred after nine daily treatments. After treatment, LH and testosterone levels were significantly elevated over controls, and they did not return to normal levels until 60 days after withdrawal of the drug. Juvenile male rats receiving an identical treatment regimen during sexual maturation had several-fold higher elevations in hormone levels after withdrawal than did adult male rats, and the period of elevation persisted for 80 days (87). Additional tranquilizers identified as causing alterations at the hypothalamic-GnRH level due to effects on endogenous catecholamines are reserpine, chlorpromazine, and perphenazine (57).

Most neuroactive drugs produce transient effects on CNS pathways necessary for normal gonadotropin secretion. The disruptive effects of these drugs on sexual and reproductive function are likely to be transient and reversible. Adults with compromised reproductive function and prepubertal adolescents may be at greater risk of long-term impairment due to lack of hypothalamic-pituitary-gonadal homeostasis.

Test Systems for Detection of Female Infertility

The study of female reproductive toxicology encompasses scientific approaches ranging from testing for toxicity to examination of mechanism of action. The first step of assessing the effect of an agent on the female reproductive function is to test the agent in the intact animal so the spectrum of physiological processes involved can be examined at one time. Such a test permits evaluation of the entire system regardless of the target organ, cell, or molecule. A comprehensive test

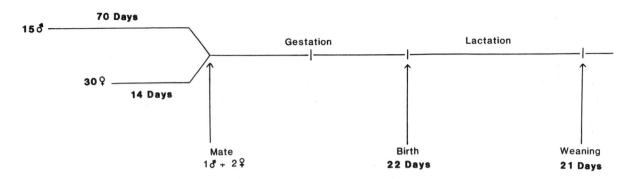

FIG. 2. Segment I: General Fertility and Reproductive Performance Study. See Appendix for details (50).

would encompass the varying susceptibilities of follicle growth and differentiation, the endocrine control of reproduction, the processes of ovulation and uterine migration of the fertilized ovum, and finally the ability of the conceptus to implant and successfully complete development through weaning. Disruption of female fertility can occur at a number of points during life and at a number of levels in the hypothalamic-pituitary-uterine-ovarian axis. Laboratory tests used in safety studies, however, tend to measure apical endpoints of estrous cyclicity and the ability to conceive and bear offspring.

Two basic designs have been developed for reproductive toxicity testing: one involving exposure during one generation and the other with exposure across several generations. These tests can include exposure of both male and female subjects or just one sex. The reproductive toxicity of therapeutic drugs is usually evaluated in single-generation, or segment I, studies, on the premise that most pharmaceuticals are taken for relatively short intervals and have comparatively short half-lives in the body. A typical design for a Segment I: General Fertility and Reproductive Performance Study is shown in Fig. 2. Multigeneration studies are used for compounds likely to concentrate in the body with long-term exposure, e.g., pesticides and food additives. Animals are continuously exposed to the test compound, usually in the food or drinking water, for three generations. A new test procedure being developed in the National Toxicology Program, entitled Fertility Assessment by Continuous Breeding (FACB), may provide a more accurate assessment of long-term, multigenerational effects on fertility (48). The basic designs of the multigeneration and FACB tests are shown in Figs. 3 and 4. These tests are designed to give an overview of the repro-

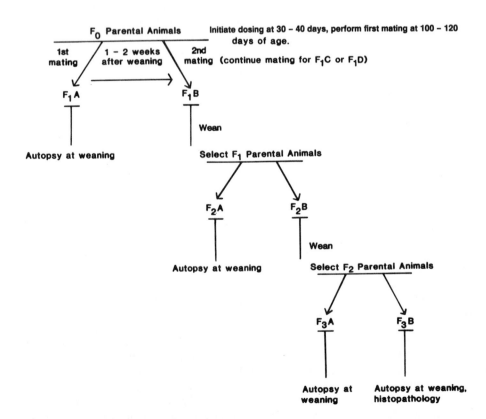

FIG. 3. Multigeneration study encompassing three generations (50).

ductive process. As such, a broad net is cast over a spectrum of reproductive endpoints to determine if any are impaired. Impairment often takes the form of inability to conceive and bear viable litters. If severe toxicity to parental animals is avoided, such impairments are indicative of specific effects on the reproductive system.

Details for conduct of the Segment I: Female Fertility Study, which is the definitive test for identifying adverse effects on the female reproductive system, are given in the Appendix. An overall view of the female reproductive process within one generation is obtained, and the effects of the test agent on estrous cyclicity, ovarian function, mating behavior, conception rates, development, natural delivery, and lactation are assessed. This test can also include exposure of both sexes, in which case males receive treatment for a minimum of 70 days and females for 14 days prior to mating, with the same endpoints measured as described for the female. Exposure of both sexes is not recommended. Identifying the critical period and process affected with exposure of both sexes is not possible, and positive results require the detailed examination of individual sexes as recommended here for the female.

Considerations for Risk Assessment

Various kinds of reproductive impairment occur frequently and are widespread. At least 15% of all recently married couples have difficulties conceiving a child. Approximately one-third of these infertility cases result from a pathologic condition in the man, one-third are attributed to the woman, and one-third are due to a combination of factors in the partners (71). It is surprising, therefore, that risk assessment is infrequently based on reproductive toxicity data and that safety testing programs do not always include measurements of adverse effects on reproduction. For example, the Toxic Substances Control Act (TSCA), P.L. 94-469, which regulates industrial chemicals, identifies four progressive levels of testing, depending on the extent, frequency, and nature of chemical use. Information on reproductive effects is not required until level IV, when the product is already on the market. At level II, the most comprehensive test is the subchronic (90-day) toxicity study designed to predict adverse effects on humans exposed during production or industrial use.

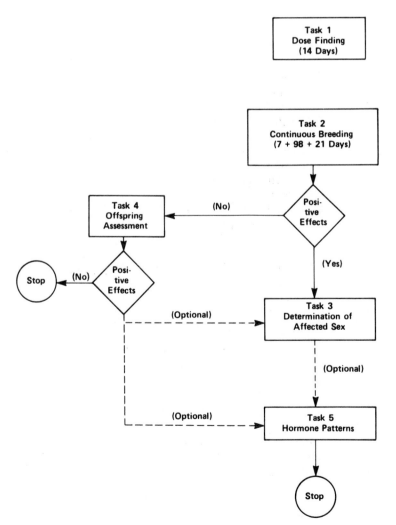

FIG. 4. Fertility assessment by the FACB protocol (48).

As demonstrated by Koeter (47), there is concern that the acceptable daily exposure level estimated from the subchronic toxicity study may be too high insofar as effects on reproductive function are not taken into consideration. Koeter evaluated toxicity data on 37 compounds tested in both subchronic studies and one or more reproductive toxicity studies to determine the impact of the latter in identifying the no-observed-effect level (NOEL) and the lowest-observed-effect level (LOEL). For the NOEL, reproductive toxicity studies were more sensitive than the subchronic studies for 35% of the compounds. For another 35% they were equally sensitive, and for 30% they were less sensitive. For the LOEL, reproductive toxicity studies were more sensitive for 21% of the compounds but were similar to the subchronic studies for 65% of the compounds. Koeter concluded that reproductive function is highly sensitive to impairment and should be examined at earlier stages in safety testing of industrial chemicals.

For therapeutic drugs, results from the Segment I: Female Fertility Study and Segment II: Developmental Toxicology Study must be available to the Federal Drug Administration (FDA) before women of child-bearing age can participate in clinical trials. Results from these and the Segment III: Perinatal/Postnatal Study must be available before the drug is marketed.

Even when data from reproductive toxicity studies are available for use in the assessment of a particular compound, there is much confusion about how to apply results from animal studies to humans. The confusion is due partly to the fact that considerably less is understood about the underlying events leading to reproductive toxicity than is known about other types of toxicity. There are currently no agree-on standard quantitative methods for cross-species extrapolation.

DEVELOPMENTAL TOXICOLOGY

The term *developmental toxicity* covers any detrimental effect produced by exposures to developing organisms during embryonic stages of development. Such lesions can be either irreversible or reversible. Embryolethal lesions are incompatible with survival of the conceptus and result in resorption, spontaneous abortion, or stillbirth. Irreversible lesions that are compatible with survival may result in structural or functional anomalies in live offspring and are referred to as *teratogenic*. Persistent lesions that cause overall growth retardation or delayed growth of specific organ systems are generally referred to as *embryotoxic*. For an agent to be labeled a *teratogen*, it must significantly increase the occurrence of structural or functional abnormalities in offspring after it is administered to either parent before conception, to the female during pregnancy, or directly to the developing organism.

Many developmental toxicologists believe that any agent administered under appropriate conditions of dosage and time of development can cause some disturbances in embryonic development in some laboratory species (20,38,88). For an agent to be classified as a developmental toxicant, it must produce adverse effects on the conceptus at exposure levels that do not induce severe toxicity in the mother (e.g., substantial reduction in weight gain, persistent emesis, hypo- or hyperactivity, convulsions). Adverse effects on develop-

ment under these conditions may be secondary to the stress on the maternal system. The main reason for conducting developmental toxicity studies is to ascertain if an agent causes specific or unique toxicity to pregnant animals or the conceptus. If these studies are conducted under extreme conditions of maternal toxicity, identification of exposures uniquely toxic to the conceptus or pregnant animal is not possible. Agents can be deliberately administered at maternally toxic doses to determine the threshold level for adverse effects on the offspring. In such cases conclusions can be qualified to indicate that adverse effects on the conceptus were obtained at maternally toxic exposure levels and may not be indicative of selective or unique developmental toxicity.

Developmental Considerations for Timing and Susceptibility

Compared to adults, developing organisms undergo rapid and complex changes within a relatively short period. Consequently, the susceptibility of the conceptus to chemical insult varies dramatically within each of the major developmental stages, i.e., preimplantation and embryonic, fetal, and neonatal stages. The relative timing of these stages in some mammalian species is given in Table 5. The preimplantation embryo appears to be more susceptible to lethality than to teratogenicity following chemical insult. Alterations in the hormonal milieu as well as direct secretion of chemicals into uterine fluids during this period can interfere with implantation and result in embryo lethality. In studies utilizing preimplantation embryo cultures, severe toxicity was manifested by rapid death of the embryo, whereas less severe effects were observed as decreased cleavage rates and arrested development (9). There have been few studies on the effects of sublethal exposures to preimplantation embryos, and the possibilities of persistent biochemical or morphologic alterations have not been adequately explored.

Following implantation, organogenesis takes place. The most characteristic susceptibility of the embryo during organogenesis is to the induction of structural birth defects. Individual organ systems possess highly specific periods of vulnerability to teratogenic insult during organogenesis. Figure 5 depicts the sensitive periods of the major embryonic organ systems in the rat to teratogenic insult. Administration of a teratogen on day 10 of rat gestation would likely result in a high level of brain and eye defects, intermediate levels of heart and skeletal defects, and a low level of urogenital defects. If the same agent were administered on day 11, a different spectrum of malformations would be anticipated, predominantly changes in the brain and palate. Figure 5 also illustrates that exposure to teratogens usually results in a spectrum of malformations involving a number of organ systems, reflecting the overlap of critical periods for individual organ systems. This pattern is most evident in species such as rodents, which have short gestation periods. Nonetheless, most human teratogens have been found to influence the development of several organ systems and cause clusters of malformations rather than single anomalies.

Histogenesis, functional maturation, and growth are the major processes occurring during the fetal and neonatal (i.e., perinatal) periods. Insult at these late developmental stages

TABLE 5. *Timing of early development in some mammalian species*

| Mammal | Times of early development (days from ovulation) | | | |
	Blastocyst formation	Implantation	Organogenesis period	Length of gestation
Mouse	3–4	4–5	6–15	19
Rat	3–4	5–6	6–15	22
Rabbit	3–4	7–8	6–18	33
Sheep	6–7	17–18	14–36	150
Monkey (rhesus)	5–7	9–11	20–45	164
Human	5–8	8–13	21–56	267

Adapted from ref. 9.

leads to a broad spectrum of effects that generally manifest as growth retardation or, more specifically, as functional disorders and transplacental carcinogenesis. The fetus is more resistant to lethal effects than is the embryo, but the incidence of stillbirths is measurable.

Dose-Response Patterns in Laboratory Animal Studies: Concordance with Humans

Functional deficits and perinatally induced cancers are often not manifested until adolescence or later. They are usually examined as endpoints in themselves without correlation to outcomes observable at the time of birth. The major effects from prenatal exposure measured at the time of birth in developmental toxicity studies are embryo lethality, malformations, and growth retardation. Three general dose-response patterns have been identified in animal studies for each of these outcomes (63) (Fig. 6). To clearly identify these patterns, exposure must be at levels below those causing frank maternal toxicity.

One pattern of response is seen with agents that cause malformations of the entire litter at exposure levels not causing embryo lethality. A depiction of the dose-response pattern for such agents is given in Fig. 6A. If the dose is increased beyond that which causes malformations of the entire litter, embryo lethality can occur but often in conjunction with maternal toxicity. Malformed fetuses are usually growth-re-

tarded, and the curve for growth retardation is often parallel to and slightly displaced from the curve for teratogenicity. Such a pattern of response is rare and indicates that the agents have high teratogenic potency (76). Generalities about the mode of action of these agents cannot be made except that they are likely to cause perturbations of processes unique or highly selective for developing/differentiating systems.

A more common dose-response pattern involves a combination of embryo lethality, malformation, and growth retardation, and apparently normal fetuses (Fig. 6B). Depending on the teratogenic potency of the agent, lower doses may cause predominantly lethality or malformations. As the dosage increases, however, embryo lethality predominates until the entire litter is resorbed or aborted. Growth retardation can precede both of the outcomes or parallel the malformation curve. This response pattern is typical of agents that are cytotoxic to replicating cells via alterations in replication, transcription, translation, or cell division (79). These substances include alkylating agents, antineoplastic agents, and many mutagenic agents. The susceptibility of the embryo to these substances derives from the high rate of cell division during organogenesis. Exposure to a cytotoxic agent during organogenesis can produce all three outcomes both within and among litters. Some litters may be totally resorbed, others may have only growth-retarded fetuses at term, and still others may have a mixture of malformed or growth-retarded fetuses and resorption sites.

A third dose-response pattern consists in growth retarda-

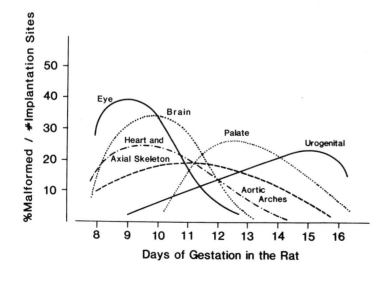

FIG. 5. Hypothetical pattern of susceptibility of embryonic organs to teratogenic insult. (Adapted from ref. 95.)

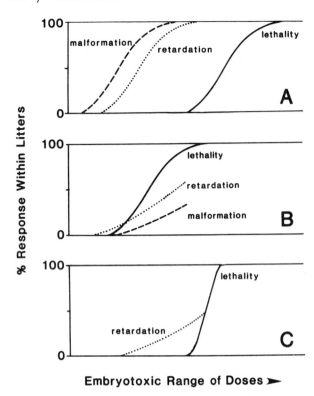

FIG. 6. Dose-response patterns (A–C) for different types of developmental toxicant. See text for explanation of the three patterns. (Adapted from ref. 63.)

tion and embryo lethality without malformations (Fig. 6C). The dose-response curve for embryo lethality in this case is usually steep, which may imply a dose threshold for survival of the embryo. Growth retardation of surviving fetuses usually precedes significant lethality. Developmental toxicants producing this pattern of response are considered embryotoxic or embryolethal but not teratogenic. When such a pattern is observed, it is necessary to conduct additional studies at doses within the range causing growth retardation and lethality. Results obtained at these intermediate doses can indicate if teratogenicity has been masked by embryo lethality. Agents inducing this response pattern typically affect fundamental cellular processes such as glycolysis, mitochondrial function, and membrane integrity (5). There is no basis for target-organ susceptibility in the early embryo to perturbation of such fundamental cellular processes. Consequently, all tissues appear to be equally affected. The early signs of perturbation are overall growth retardation, progressing to lethality of the entire litter once a threshold for cellular energy supply or survival is exceeded. These conditions are incompatible with teratogenicity, in which irreversible lesions are induced in some tissues while others are spared, permitting survival of abnormal embryos to term.

These dose-response patterns indicate that for some developmental toxicants, i.e., those cytotoxic to replicating cells (Fig. 6B), growth retardation, embryo lethality, and teratogenicity are different degrees of the manifestation of the same primary insult, cytotoxicity. For others there is a qualitative difference in response, and prenatal exposure leads primarily

to embryo lethality alone (Fig. 6C) or to malformations (Fig. 6A).

These dose-response patterns from animal studies have important implications in extrapolation of developmental toxicity data to humans. The major implication is that a spectrum of endpoints can be produced, even under the controlled conditions of timing and exposure that can be achieved in animal studies. When estimating the hazard to humans, all exposure-specific adverse outcomes identified in animal studies must be taken into consideration, not just malformations. A similar spectrum of growth retardation, embryo lethality, and malformations has been observed in humans after prenatal exposure to developmental toxicants, although clear dose-response patterns have rarely identified with individual agents (26). Consequently, manifestations of developmental toxicity cannot be presumed to be constant or specific across species. *Any* manifestation of exposure-related developmental toxicity in animal studies can be indicative of a variety of responses in humans (44).

An important factor to be considered in cross-species extrapolation is that the most common manifestation of developmental toxicity in humans is spontaneous abortion or early fetal loss (before the 28th week of pregnancy), occurring in at least 10 to 20% of all recognized pregnancies (Table 1). Estimates from prospective studies range even higher: 20 to 25% of all conceptions spontaneously abort (14). Approximately one-third of specimens obtained from spontaneous abortions occurring between 8 and 28 weeks of gestation contain chromosome aberrations. The frequency of such aberrations is at least 60-fold higher among spontaneous abortions than among term births. Among spontaneously aborted embryos and fetuses, the rate of structural malformation varies from 7 to 24%. The spectrum of abnormality found also varies with developmental age, and approximately 75% of structurally abnormal embryos and fetuses never reach the viable stage (85,86). The frequency of these malformations is not as well documented as for chromosome aberrations because they are difficult to observe in specimens that are often macerated or incomplete.

These observations suggest that most human conceptuses bearing chromosome aberrations or morphologic abnormalities are lost through early miscarriage (70). Epidemiological approaches to monitoring the frequency of early fetal loss and detecting such fetal abnormalities have been used only to a limited extent. Most studies of humans have focused on outcomes occurring at the time of birth or later, i.e., major malformations, stillbirths, low birth weight, and neonatal deaths. Underestimation of adverse pregnancy outcome, and thus true risk and pattern of response, is unavoidable in human studies whenever measurements are made only from the time of birth onward.

Developmental toxicants with dose-response patterns resembling those in Fig. 6A could be detected by monitoring malformations at the time of birth, especially if the malformations were rare (e.g., those resulting from thalidomide) or if the exposed populations were large (e.g., those with rubella infections). Agents with patterns B and C would probably be missed, because early fetal loss is not routinely monitored in human populations, even though it has been done successfully in isolated groups (45).

The sensitivity (ability to detect a true positive response

in humans) and specificity (ability to detect a true negative response in humans) of laboratory animal studies have been evaluated by the FDA (25) (Table 6). Of 38 compounds having demonstrated or suspected teratogenic activity in humans, all except one (tobramycin, which causes otological deficits in humans) tested positive in at least one animal species. Furthermore, more than 80% were positive in multiple species. A positive response was elicited 85% of the time in the mouse, 80% in the rat, 60% in the rabbit, 45% in the hamster, and only 30% in the monkey. Overall, these findings indicate that conventional animal species have high sensitivity for detecting human teratogens (64).

Evaluation of specificity (Table 6) has indicated that of 165 well-studied agents with no evidence of being human teratogens, 29% appeared negative in all animal species tested and 51% appeared negative in multiple species. However, 41% of these 165 compounds were positive in more than a single animal species. The nonhuman primate and the rabbit had the highest specificity of laboratory animal species, testing "negative" for substances reported to be negative in humans 80% and 70% of the time, respectively (25).

These findings indicate that laboratory animal species have high sensitivity but low specificity for predicting human teratogens. Schardein et al. (82,83) reviewed the literature on drugs and environmental chemicals and found that of the 2,800 agents now reported to have been tested in laboratory animals, approximately 1,000 demonstrated some measure of teratogenicity for which there is no evidence of positivity in humans. Consequently, the major concern in hazard assessment today is that far more agents have been shown to be positive in animal studies than have been identified in human studies. There are at least three possible explanations for this finding: No studies or inadequate studies have been conducted in humans with the animal teratogen; the animal

studies have yielded false-positive results because of test conditions and interpretation; and the true risk for adverse pregnancy outcome is underestimated in human studies that measure only outcomes from the time of birth onward. Human studies must be designed to measure developmental toxicity and not just teratogenicity before adequate cross-species comparisons can be made.

Relation Between Maternal and Developmental Toxicity

In developmental toxicity studies the usual sequence of testing begins with dose-range-finding studies using four to six treatment groups containing relatively small numbers of pregnant rodents. Details on study design and dose selection are given in the Appendix. The dose range study should be viewed as a toxicity study and designed to ensure that unequivocal toxic effects are obtained at the high dose. In the definitive study, diagrammed in Fig. 7, larger numbers of animals are exposed during organogenesis at three treatment levels. The highest dose level should cause measurable but modest maternal toxicity (e.g., significant depression in maternal weight gain), developmental toxicity (e.g., significant depression in fetal body weight), or both. The low dose should cause no observable effect. The definitive study is conducted to obtain information on the safety of the compound, although it is necessary to demonstrate a treatment effect in the high dose group.

If evidence of selective developmental toxicity is obtained from the definitive study (adverse effects on the conceptus at doses that are not maternally toxic), it may be necessary to conduct a third study exposing dams at nonmaternally toxic doses on single days during organogenesis (days 9, 10, 11, or 12) to obtain a clear definition of the dose-response pattern for developmental toxicity.

Despite the requirement for production of maternal toxicity in the dose-range and definitive studies, there is much controversy about what constitutes adequate demonstration of maternal toxicity. In some cases exhibition of frank clinical signs, e.g., sedation, hyperactivity, and convulsions, by the dam are considered sufficient. In other cases a marginal but statistically significant depression of maternal weight and weight gain throughout treatment during organogenesis or on individual days is considered adequate demonstration of maternal toxicity. The general definition for maximum tolerated dose in adult toxicity studies is one that causes a statistically significant weight loss and not more than 10% deaths.

The rationale for using a maternally toxic dose is to maximize the potential to detect adverse effects in the fetus (74). Effects observed in offspring at maternally toxic doses are used as landmarks to focus attention on outcomes at lower doses. If a statistically significant incidence of a particular adverse effect is found in the high dose group, the biological significance of a lesser and perhaps nonsignificant incidence at lower doses is magnified. It can be difficult, however, to interpret some effects observed only at maternally toxic dose levels. Are they indicative of unique and selective developmental toxicity, or are they a function of nonspecific alterations in maternal homeostasis (90)?

An initial factor to consider is that the state of pregnancy

TABLE 6. *Sensitivity and specificity of laboratory animal studies for predicting teratogenesis (FDA review)*

Parameter	No.	%
Sensitivity		
Compounds with positive teratologic findings in humans	38	100
Positive in at least one laboratory animal test species	37	97
Positive in more than one laboratory animal test species	29	76
Positive in all laboratory animal species tested	8	21
Specificity		
Compounds studied in humans with no teratologic findings	165	100
"Negative" in at least one laboratory animal test species	130	79
"Negative" in more than one laboratory animal test species	84	51
"Negative" in all laboratory animal species tested	47	29
Positive in more than a single laboratory animal test species	68	41

Adapted from ref. 25.

RATS OR MICE

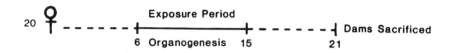

RABBITS

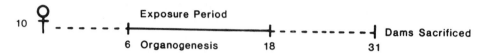

FIG. 7. Segment II: Developmental Toxicology Study. See Appendix for details. (Adapted from ref. 50.)

itself can confer increased susceptibility to xenobiotic insult. Table 7 details physiological changes in pregnancy related to drug handling. The general trend is that pregnancy-related physiological changes favor increased absorption of drugs. The one exception to this trend is the increase in renal function, which could result in elevated urinary excretion of free drug (33). Increased susceptibility due to these pregnancy-related changes can be addressed by comparing LOELs for adverse effects in the maternal system in pregnant versus nonpregnant animals. If this comparison is limited to those few measurements of maternal toxicity routinely made in developmental toxicity studies, i.e., clinical signs, food and water consumption, and body weight, it is unlikely that the LOEL for maternal toxicity would ever be lower than the LOEL for adult toxicity. It would be necessary to include a more complete assessment of health status (e.g., histology, hematology, and clinical chemistry studies), as routinely performed in adult toxicity studies, in those instances where increased susceptibility related to the state of pregnancy is suspected.

It is generally accepted that developmental toxicity in the form of increased embryo lethality and decreased fetal body weight can occur at maternally toxic dose levels. The role of maternal toxicity in the production of malformations is not clear, however. Khera (40,41) reviewed the published literature to examine the relation between maternal toxicity, em-

bryo toxicity, and malformations. He noted that doses of test agents that caused maternal toxicity, as indicated by reduced maternal body weight, clinical signs of toxicity, or death, commonly caused reduction in fetal body weight, increased resorptions, and rarely fetal death. The pattern of structural variants/malformations found to be associated with maternal toxicity in mice, rats, rabbits, and hamsters are listed in Table 8 (41). The severity and incidence of these defects could be directly related to the degree of maternal toxicity. They were absent or rare at doses that were nontoxic to the dam. Khera (40,41) concluded that these defects resulted from maternal toxicity and did not reflect the teratogenic potential of the compounds.

A number of other investigators (39,42,66,72) have addressed the association between maternal toxicity and the occurrence of retarded sternebral and vertebral ossification as well as supernumerary and wavy ribs in experimental animals. There is general agreement that these are variations and not malformations and that they are reversible and secondary to maternal toxicity. Those major malformations attributed to maternal toxicity in the Khera studies (exencephaly, open eyes, encephalocele, micro- or anophthalmia)

TABLE 7. Physiological changes in pregnancy related to drug handling

Parameter	Change
Absorption	Decreased gastric and intestinal motility
Distribution	40% Increase in blood and plasma volume
Protein binding	60% Reduction in plasma albumin levels; increase in proportion of free drug in pregnancy plasma
Metabolism	Decreased hepatic drug metabolism (?)
Excretion	Renal function increased; 50% elevation of renal plasma flow and glomerular filtration rate

Adapted from ref. 33.

TABLE 8. Structural variations/malformations associated with maternal toxicity

Mice
  Exencephaly
  Open eyes
  Hemivertebrae
  Fused arches or centrathoracic/lumbar vertebrae
  Missing or supernumerary ribs
  Fused or scrambled sternebrae
Rats and rabbits
  Fused, extra, missing, or wavy ribs
  Fused, retarded, missing, or split vertebrae
  Fused, missing, or nonaligned sternebrae
Hamsters
  Exencephaly
  Encephalocele (cranial blister)
  Micro- or anophthalmia
  Fused ribs

Adapted from refs. 40 and 41.

require more detailed examination to determine if they are representative of maternal toxicity or teratogenic activity.

As implied from this discussion, not all morphological variations observed in fetuses are of equal importance. Although there is little doubt that major effects such as irreversible and life-threatening malformations are deleterious, other effects are of considerably less consequence. Common skeletal variants, e.g., retarded ossification of the sternum and vertebrae, are reversible and indicative of slight developmental delays that invariably accompany modest depressions in fetal body weight. A clear understanding of the difference between structural malformations and variations, as provided by Palmer (73), is necessary for adequate interpretation of results. A low level of concern is attached to an increase in structural variations in animal studies, especially if they occur only in conjunction with maternal toxicity. Greater importance is given to variations that increase with dose and occur at nonmaternally toxic doses.

Considerations for Hazard and Risk Assessment

Regulatory agencies have developed a systematic scientific and administration framework to assess risks associated with exposure to chemical and physical agents (60). The process usually begins with the *identification of hazard,* which is defined as the potential of a given exposure to be toxic. Laboratory animal studies and occasionally human case reports are used to identify dose-response relations between exposure to a substance and associated adverse responses. The next step is the *identification of risk,* which is the likelihood of the adverse effect occurring under real conditions of exposure. Information is obtained on the range of dose levels to which human populations are likely to be exposed. Finally, the dose-response model from animal studies is applied to the expected human exposure levels to produce a quantitative estimate of risk. To date, quantitative risk assessment has been used largely for estimating the risk of developing or dying from cancer, and relatively little has been done in the area of developmental toxicity (see the next section). There are general guidelines for estimating hazard, however, that are concerned with the quality, quantity, and interpretation of data from laboratory animals.

Results from Segment II: Developmental Toxicology Studies in two species, preferably a rodent and a nonrodent, carried out according to prescribed guidelines (16,35) should be available. Treatment should be via the likely human route and the highest dose of sufficient magnitude to cause maternal toxicity. The minimum requirement is three treatment groups and a concurrent control group, each containing 20 pregnant rodents or 10 pregnant nonrodents (rabbits). Results should permit identification of the NOEL for maternal and developmental toxicity as well as the LOEL for maternal and/or developmental toxicity. Extrapolation to humans is from the most sensitive species (lowest LOEL) unless there is evidence this species is inappropriate because of major differences from humans in terms of pharmacokinetics or pharmacodynamics. These items represent minimal requirements for the quality of data necessary to carry out hazard assessment.

An important issue determining the quantity of data required involves the concept of statistical power. If an experimental result is found to be statistically significant, i.e., there is a statistically significant association ($p < 0.05$) between exposure and endpoint, the study had enough power to detect that difference at the chosen level of significance. If no statistically significant association is found, the reason may be that the study had insufficient power to detect a smaller but real effect, or that there was no effect.

Power is related to the number of subjects in a group, to the rarity of the endpoint, and to the variability of the frequency of the endpoint's occurrence. In general, the rarer the endpoint, the fewer the excess occurrences above background needed for detecting an effect. Thalidomide and DES, for example, induced lesions that rarely occur in control populations (1/10,000 to 1/100,000). Only several cases of phocomelia and vaginal adenocarcinoma were necessary to elevate the incidence of these lesions far above the background figure.

Most developmental toxicants tested in animal and human studies cause more common effects, e.g., intrauterine growth retardation and increases in the occurrence of minor anomalies and variants rather than major malformations. When evaluating these endpoints, it is necessary to consider their background incidence as well as their variance in order to estimate the sample sizes needed for their detection.

Historical control data on the frequency of major and minor fetal malformations in conventional laboratory animals are listed in Table 9. Major malformations are considered to be an insensitive indicator of developmental toxicity. Major malformations tend to occur within a relatively narrow range of doses; and unless the compound is a potent teratogen (pattern A, Fig. 6), large numbers of animals are required to detect a statistically significant increase in their occurrence. With 10 to 20 litters per treatment group, differences on the order of 40 to 50% between treatment and control means are required before statistical significance is achieved (74). When more common outcomes (e.g., embryonic death, intrauterine growth retardation, and elevated incidence of common variants and minor anomalies) are taken into consideration, a more sensitive appraisal of developmental toxicity can be obtained.

Table 10 contains information on the number of litters

TABLE 9. *Historical control data on major and minor fetal malformations*

Laboratory animal	No. of fetuses examined	Major malformations (%)	Minor malformations (%) Visceral	Minor malformations (%) Skeletal
New Zealand white rabbits	36,508	0.74	2.53	8.60
CD rats	51,349	0.41	2.02	2.35
CD1 mice	22,389	0.84	3.68	5.32

Adapted from ref. 74.

TABLE 10. *Litters per group required to detect designated changes in fetal weight and embryo lethality in rats and mice[a]*

Animal	Change in fetal weight		Change in embryo lethality	
	5%	10%	5%	10%
Mice				
A/J	84	22	1,176	324
C57BL/6	198	50	992	288
CD₁	84	22	805	235
Rats				
CD[b]	62	16	858	248
OM[c]	44	12	723	216

[a] Alpha = 0.05; beta = 0.10.
[b] Charles River Laboratories, Wilmington, Massachusetts.
[c] Osborne-Mendel, Charles River Laboratories, Wilmington, Massachusetts.
Adapted from ref. 61.

per group necessary to detect a 5 or 10% difference in embryo lethality or fetal body weight (alpha = 0.05; beta = 0.10). Twenty-two to fifty litters of mice are required to detect a 10% depression in fetal weight, whereas only 12 to 16 rat litters are required to detect the same magnitude of weight depression. For embryo lethality, 235 to 324 litters of mice are necessary to detect a 10% increase in resorptions, compared to 216 to 248 rat litters. Fewer litters are needed to detect a change in fetal weight, insofar as it is a continuously distributed parameter with relatively low variability. In contrast, embryo lethality is a highly variable, binomially distributed parameter, and more than 200 litters are required to detect even a 10% change in this response (61). Given the current testing requirements for 20 rats or mice per group, the most sensitive endpoint in developmental toxicology studies based on statistical power is fetal body weight. Within the range of normal variability for this response, a 10% change in fetal body weight would be statistically significant with 20 rodent litters in a group at the $p < 0.05$ level.

For accurate *biological* interpretation of depressed fetal weight and embryo lethality, however, the occurrence of maternal toxicity must be taken into consideration. Most experimental studies of developmental toxicity have been designed to provide information on the basic mechanisms of birth defects. Agents are administered under conditions that cause a high incidence of abnormal fetuses, without concern if they were secondary to toxic effects in the maternal system. In safety studies, however, failure to recognize that developmental toxicity will inevitably occur at exposure levels that cause severe maternal toxicity can lead to false-positive identification of many agents.

If the data are of sufficient quality and quantity, it should be possible to identify the NOEL or LOEL, the maternally toxic dose levels, and the specific types and incidences of adverse effects in the fetus. If these criteria are met, the next decision is whether to use the NOEL or LOEL for subsequent risk assessment. This decision depends largely on the value that can most accurately be identified from the data base. Greater experimental confidence can be placed on the LOEL insofar as this value is empirically derived, whereas the NOEL

can be orders of magnitude below the exposure level that would induce developmental toxicity.

Selection of the LOEL need not be restricted to responses that are statistically different. Trends in the data indicating biologically relevant elevations of adverse effects at low doses can be used if there are statistically significant elevations in these effects at higher doses. LOELs are most accurately selected when the response is at a threshold; i.e., it is slightly elevated above background and involves reversible developmental toxicity, which indicates that the NOEL is being approached. When statistical significance cannot be used as a guide to select the LOEL, which is often the case, minimal responses can be regarded as those that cause a doubling of the background rate (from concurrent or historical controls) for the particular response. To protect against the possibility that humans may have double the background rate of the response (which for major malformations would represent an unacceptable increase from approximately 60,000 malformed infants per year to 120,000), a large safety factor can be used for LOELs selected under these conditions.

There have been attempts to develop quantitative methodologies for comparing the developmental toxicity of individual agents across species. These attempts have been based on the perceived need to distinguish agents that are uniquely or selectively toxic to the conceptus from those that induce developmental toxicity at exposure levels that are also toxic to the mother. Agents in the latter category should be regulated based on their adult toxicity, whereas those in the former would be regulated based on their selective toxicity to the embryo.

Johnson (36) developed a testing system to quantitatively address this issue. He defined teratogenic hazard potential as the ratio of adult to developmental toxicity (A/D ratio):

$$\text{Log} \frac{\text{lowest adult toxic (lethal) dose}}{\text{lowest developmental toxic dose}}$$

Johnson and Gable calculated this ratio for more than 70 compounds using data from an *in vitro* system of *Hydra attenuata* adult and embryonic tissues. The A/D ratio from the *Hydra* assay has been within one-tenth to ten times greater than the mammalian A/D ratio. Most compounds had ratios near 1, several had ratios larger than 5, and a few had ratios larger than 10 (37). This system has been proposed for setting priorities for further testing of agents in mammalian developmental toxicity studies.

Fabro et al. (20) explored the quantitative characteristics of a similar type of index in mammalian studies. Dose-response data for adult lethality and fetal malformations were fitted (probit of response against log of dose) for eight structurally related compounds. The observed log-probit dose-response lines for lethality and teratogenicity were not parallel, and there was not a constant ratio between the slopes for the two lines. Consequently, a simple ratio between the median effective doses (i.e., LD_{50}/ED_{50}) could not be used. To calculate a relative teratogenic index (RTI), Fabro and colleagues established a ratio between one point on each dose-response line. The LD_{01} value was chosen to represent adult lethality, on the basis that a low LD value is necessary to guard against compounds that have a shallow dose-response curve for adult lethality. The tD_{05} value was chosen to represent teratogenicity, which is the dose causing a 5% elevation of the malformation rate above background. The investigators believed that the tD_{05} could be estimated with confidence for most teratogens because induced malformations often occur at a frequency between 1 and 20% in animal studies. This approach appeared to be satisfactory for ranking the candidate compounds according to teratogenic potency, provided the relation of dose to teratogenic response was not complicated by significant adult lethality.

This ranking system was developed to evaluate structure-teratogenicity relations between structurally related compounds. For this purpose, the RTI seemed adequate. The potential usefulness of this index for interspecies comparisons and risk estimation, however, has not been established. In their evaluation of the RTI, Hogan and Hoel (31) argued that because of the lack of parallelism between the probit lines for lethality and teratogenicity the index is not invariant in the selection of other LD and tD values; for example, if a ratio of LD_{10}/tD_{05} were chosen instead of LD_{01}/tD_{05}, a different ranking order for the RTI would be obtained. In addition, the index would be subject to the established deficiencies of the probit model, which tends to be insensitive in the low dose region near the origin of the dose-response curve.

Therefore until the RTI is more extensively applied and evaluated, it should not be used for risk assessment. It is apparent, however, that a uniform method for ranking agents according to their selective toxicity to the conceptus needs to be established. Such a method would provide a yardstick against which all agents could be compared, and it would standardize the selection of the numerator (NOEL or LOEL) for the risk assessment equation. Selection of the safety factor could then be based on the severity of the endpoint.

Existing models for quantitative risk assessment do not appear to be adequate for developmental toxicity data (22). Multistage models used for mutagenicity and carcinogenicity data are based on a no-threshold assumption (2), whereas it is generally accepted that thresholds do exist for developmental toxicity (96). The Environmental Protection Agency (EPA) (15) used a number of models to evaluate developmental toxicity data on PCBs and found that the safe dose varied by a factor of 7,000 for one set of data, depending on the model used. The EPA and Oak Ridge National Laboratory concluded that existing mathematical models are inappropriate for assessing developmental toxicity data and that the safety factor approach is appropriate for establishing exposure levels expected to yield acceptable levels of risk (17).

The FDA has also indicated that it will use the safety factor approach in developmental toxicity risk assessment but has not given specific details on how the safety factors will be chosen. It is likely that safety factors between 100 and 1,000 will be applied to NOELs identified in developmental toxicity studies of drug residues in human food. Smaller factors may be used when the prenatal effect can be ascribed to nonspecific maternal toxicity (68). Thus because of the absence of other widely accepted approaches, the use of safety factors seems to be the only available approach at present for quantitative assessment of developmental toxicity data.

Finally, criteria for what constitutes an acceptable risk must be developed (6). It involves defining what is meant by "ac-ceptable" and what is meant by "risk." What magnitude of risk is acceptable for a person or a given population? For example, is the doubling of a background rate for an adverse response of 1 in a 1,000 acceptable? To what extent should reversible effects and common variants be taken into consideration in risk assessment? These questions cannot be answered from a scientific point of view alone but require public policy decisions that take into account the benefit of the chemicals under consideration and priorities for protecting public health. Decisions at this level will greatly influence the requirements for safety testing and risk assessment.

APPENDIX: DETAILS OF TEST PROCEDURES

Methods for Developmental Toxicology Evaluation (Segment II)

This section describes methods for the collection, observation, and interpretation of developmental toxicology data. These methods have been developed from descriptions in the literature and personal experience in our laboratory. The reader is referred to references 8, 12, 21, 23, 92, and 95 for further descriptions of these methods. The species employed in our laboratory are the Sprague-Dawley rat, CD-1 mouse, and New Zealand white rabbit. These outbred strains are the usual choice for developmental toxicology studies because they have high fertility rates, low spontaneous malformation rates, a convenient size, genetic stability, large litters, a short gestation period, lack of seasonal breeding, and can be purchased free of common laboratory diseases such as murine pneumonia.

The day that sperm are found in the vagina (rats), a vaginal plug is seen (mice), or mating is observed (rabbits) is considered to be day 0 of pregnancy. Rats are sacrificed on day 21, mice on day 18, and rabbits on day 29 of pregnancy. For large experiments, a team approach is used for litter collections. One person performs the laparotomy, another the weighing of fetuses, and a third the corpora lutea counts and data recording. Throughout this section, the rat is used as the example, although the procedures are readily adaptable to other species (e.g., mouse, rabbit, ferret, hamster) (62).

Housing and Mating

Sexually mature male and female rats (10 to 11 weeks of age) are obtained; upon arrival the males are individually housed in metal cages with wire-grid floors. This type of housing unit permits observation of copulatory plugs in the underlying service pans. The females are individually housed in clear polycarbonate boxes containing bedding. They are kept in an air-conditioned room ($72° ± 4°F$; $50 ± 10\%$ relative humidity) with a 12-hr light/dark cycle. Food and drinking tap water are available *ad libitum* throughout the study. During the 2-week quarantine period, females are tattooed on the tail for permanent identification. The base of the tail is cleaned with AIMS Animal Tissue spray immediately before tattooing. Black Tattoo Pigment No. 242 (obtained from AIMS) is administered intradermally to the tail base by a vibrating tattoo machine using a three-point cluster stainless steel needle.

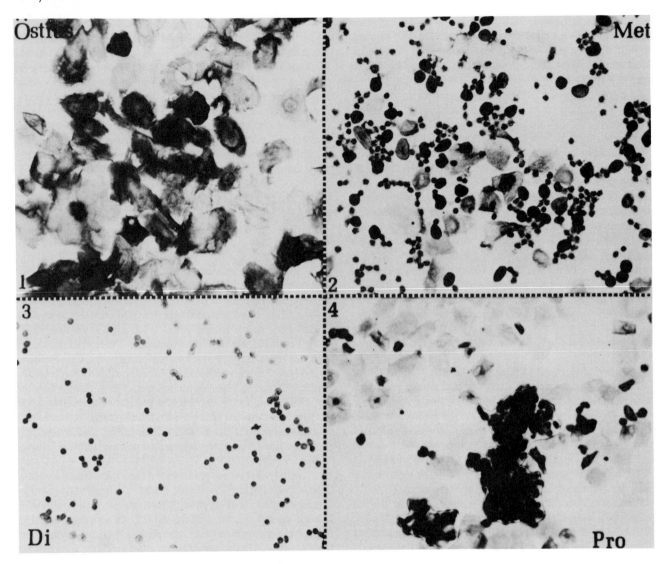

FIG. A-1. Phases of estrus in the rat. **1:** Estrus; masses of cornified cells with degenerating nuclei present. **2:** Metestrus; many leukocytes and epithelial cells. **3:** Diestrus; almost exclusively leukocytes. **4:** Proestrus; nucleated epithelial cells, singly or in sheets.

After the quarantine period, the females are introduced into the males' cages. The animals are paired on a one-to-one basis, usually in the early afternoon. The mating ratio is ideally one male to one female but can include up to one male to three females. The following morning and every subsequent morning of the mating period, the service pans are checked for copulatory plugs. Vaginal washings are then taken for each female. At this time the female is examined for signs of a retained intravaginal copulatory plug.

During vaginal lavage, a few drops of a saline solution are drawn into a pipette; the tip of the pipette is then inserted 1 to 2 mm into the rat's vagina, and the saline is gently flushed into the vagina and drawn back into the pipette. Insertion of the pipette too deeply into the vagina or excessive flushing can result in pseudopregnancy and disruption of the normal estrous cycle (Fig. A-1). A new, clean pipette is used for each female in order to prevent vaginal infection and carryover

of sperm from an inseminated female and thus incorrect identification of a nonmated female as inseminated. The saline solution with its cellular contents is smeared across a microslide and examined (wet and unstained) microscopically at 100× to 200× for the presence of sperm.

The female is considered mated if sperm are found in the vaginal washing or a vaginal plug is detected, and that day is designated day 0 of pregnancy. The copulatory plug in the service pan must be substantiated by the presence of sperm in the vaginal washing. When mated, the female is separated from the male, her body weight is recorded in the laboratory notebook, and she is returned to her original polycarbonate box. The mating date is recorded on the female's cage and in the laboratory notebook.

One would expect a maximum of 20 to 25% of randomly selected females to be in proestrus and to mate on a given day based on an estrous cycle length of 4 to 5 days. In practice, the first night of mating usually yields fewer matings than this number, and the second and third nights yield greater numbers. Within a 5-day mating period the entire cohort of females should be mated. Approximately 85 to 90% of mated females are actually pregnant.

Experimental Design

Dose-range study

The dose-range study is viewed as a toxicity study and is designed to ensure that unequivocal toxic effects are obtained at the high dose. It is of equal or greater importance than the definitive study and is designed with careful attention to dose levels and endpoints. We routinely include six treatment groups (eight mated females each), and a concurrent control and doses are selected based on the following projected outcomes:

Group 1: no effect
Group 2: no effect or minimal effect
Group 3: minimal effect
Group 4: moderate effect
Group 5: definitive toxicity
Group 6: definitive toxicity

Insofar as doses are usually selected based on minimal toxicity data in adult animals, it is necessary to build in redundancy for the projected no-effect and definitive-effect dose groups. With the high doses selected to produce unequivocal toxicity, it is particularly important to closely monitor animals for identification of distress or pain that would be incompatible with humane treatment. In developmental toxicity studies, the usual response in such an event is to immediately euthanize the animals rather than reduce or discontinue treatment. Alterations in maternal homeostasis generally accompanying severe distress can be sufficient to produce irreversible effects on the conceptus. The number of corpora lutea, implants, and live and dead fetuses are measured in dams removed or dying spontaneously during the study.

The route of administration must be similar to that used in normal human exposure. The vehicle should not exert systemic toxicity as evidenced by decrements in food and water consumption or maternal weight gain. If the vehicle does have some unavoidable effects on these parameters, inclusion of an untreated control group may be necessary. The treatment interval spans the period of organogenesis, which varies with species and length of gestation. Female body weights are recorded at mating, daily during dosing, and throughout the remainder of pregnancy as a whole number, in grams. Food consumption is recorded daily during days 7 to 21 of gestation to the nearest gram. During the treatment and posttreatment periods, clinical signs of toxicity are recorded. Each observation must have all relevant information including the date and time before or after dosing.

Rodent dams are weighed and killed on day 21 postcoitus by CO_2 asphyxiation. They are fastened to Plexiglas boards with spring clips, and an incision is made in the abdominal wall to expose the abdominal viscera. Maternal viscera are examined macroscopically, and major observations are recorded. The ovaries (Fig. A-2) are removed and placed in prelabeled containers; the corpora lutea are counted immediately or preserved in fixative and counted when time permits under a dissecting microscope. In some instances the periovarian sac and excess fat must be removed before the corpora lutea can be counted. This procedure is straightforward when performed on rat or rabbit ovaries at term but difficult with mice due to the small size of the ovaries.

The gravid uterus is removed (Fig. A-3) without confusing the left and right horns, trimmed of excess fat, blotted, and weighed. The isolated uterus is cut open with scissors along the side opposite the implantation sites, exposing the lining of the uterus (Fig. A-4) and the amniotic sacs. The sacs are ruptured one at a time, and the number and position of the implantations, early or late resorptions, and dead or live fetuses are counted. A resorption site resembling a dark brown blood clot and with no embryonic tissue visible is classified as an early postimplantation death (Fig. A-4); a resorption site with both placental and embryonic tissue visible is classified as a late postimplantation death. Fetuses that cannot be induced to respond or breathe are considered dead.

The umbilical cord of each fetus is cut, and fetuses are removed, blotted dry, and placed in specially designed trays that have slots corresponding to the positions within the uterus of each horn (from the ovary toward the cervix). The maternal identification number is placed on each tray, and neck tags are attached to the fetuses for identification of uterine position. The fetuses are then sexed by examining the location of the genital papilla, which is farther away from the base of the tail in males than in females. They are then individually weighed and the weights recorded to the second decimal place.

The uteri of apparently nonpregnant females are slit open and immersed in 0.5% ammonium sulfide solution for approximately 10 min under a chemical fume hood. The uteri are examined for implantation sites, which appear as dark residues (Fig. A-5) and are recorded as early resorptions.

The following data are recorded on the litter collection sheet, as illustrated in Fig. A-6: number of corpora lutea, number of implantation sites, number of resorption sites (early or late) and their location in the uterus, number and position of live or dead fetuses, fetal sex, weight and condition of the uterus, and general condition of other maternal viscera.

The last measurement made in a dose-range study is external examination of fetuses for morphological abnormalities. Under a dissecting microscope, the lips and palate are examined for cleft lip and palate by gently opening the mouth with forceps. The head (Fig. A-7) is examined in lateral profile for the presence of a dome-shaped cranium (Fig. A-8). From a face-on view, the eyes (closed), ears, jaw, and snout are examined for shape and size. External malformations of the head are pictured in Figs. A-8 through A-12.

External malformations of the trunk are easily discerned, and representative examples are shown in Figs. A-13 through A-16. They include craniorachischisis, gastroschisis, umbilical hernia, and thoracopagus twins. Various degrees of spina bifida are presented in Figs. A-17 through A-19, including a stained skeleton of a fetus with spina bifida (Fig. A-20).

Limbs are examined for shape, size, and position, and the digits for number and depth of the digital furrows. A normal forepaw is shown in Fig. A-21, and polydactyly (extra digits), ectrodactyly (missing digits), and syndactyly (fused digits) are shown in Figs. A-22 through A-26.

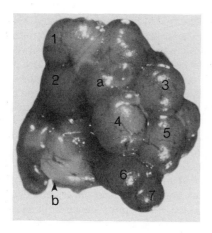

FIG. A-2. Normal rat ovary showing seven corpora lutea (1–7) and ovarian follicles; (a) of various sizes; (b) fimbriae fallopian tube.

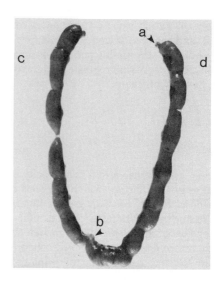

FIG. A-3. Normal rat gravid uterus at term; (a) left ovary; (b) cervix; (c) right uterine horn; (d) left uterine horn.

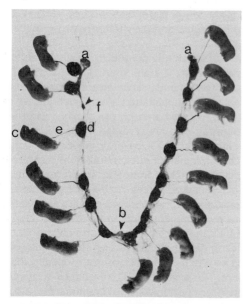

FIG. A-4. Normal rat gravid uterus at term, cut open with fetuses attached; (a) ovarian end; (b) cervical end; (c) fetus; (d) placenta; (e) umbilical cord; (f) early resorption site.

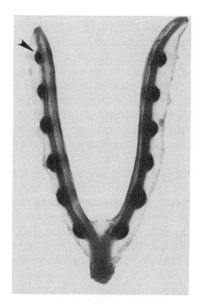

FIG. A-5. Normal rat uterine horn (day 10 postpartum) with stained implantation sites (arrowhead).

(SIDE A)

LITTER COLLECTION SHEET

Experiment _____ Female No. _____

Date Sperm Present _____ Male No. _____ Female Weight _____

Date	Day of Gest.	Weight and Comments

R   L

Autopsy Date _____ Body Wt. _____ Corpora Lutea

Comments: _____ Age _____ Days_____

Right   Left

Total implants   _____

No. early deaths (R)   _____

No. late deaths (X)   _____

No. living fetuses   _____

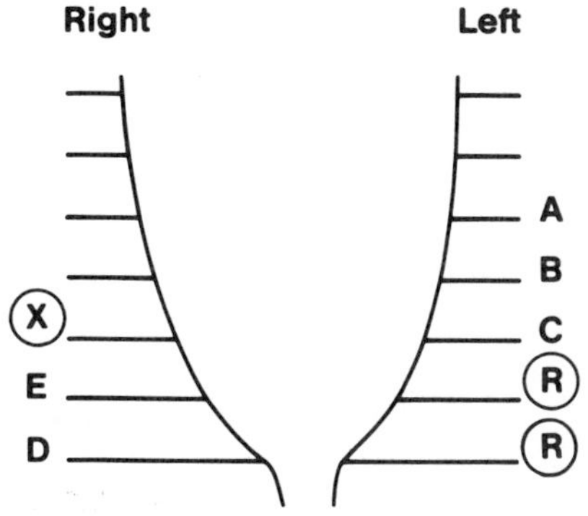

A
B
C
Ⓡ
Ⓡ

Ⓧ
E
D

Live fetuses are lettered alphabetically from left to right.

FIG. A-6. Data sheet for litter collection. **Side A:** Space is provided for the title of the experiment, identification of the dam and the sire, date of insemination, and weight of the female throughout gestation. The lower portion of the sheet is the record of the findings on the sacrifice dates.

(SIDE B)

GROSS EXTERNAL EXAMINATION

Fetus	Sex	Weight	FIX	Cranium	Eyes	Palate	Limbs	Tail	Genitals	Other

M/F Sex Ratio	X + S.D. Fetal Wt.	Corpora Lutea	Implants	Resorptions

Dead Fetuses	Live Fetuses	No. Fetuses w/ Abnormalities	Soft Tissue	Skeletal

Signed _____   Female No. _____

FIG. A-6. (*Continued.*) **Side B:** Space is provided to record the results of the gross examination of the fetuses as they are taken from the mother. A summary of all the data from the litter is recorded at the bottom.

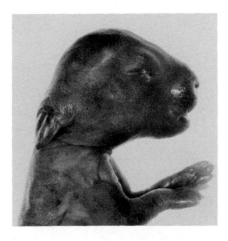

FIG. A-7. Normal head of rabbit fetus.

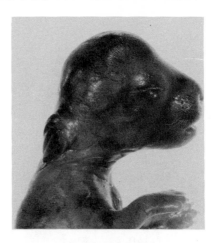

FIG. A-8. Malformed head of rabbit fetus: dome-shaped and hydrocephalic.

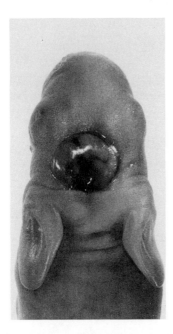

FIG. A-9. Malformed head of rabbit fetus: craniomeningocele.

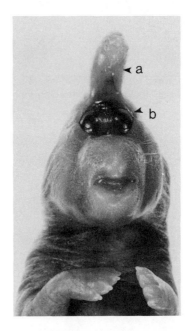

FIG. A-10. Malformed head of rabbit fetus: (*a*) rhinocephaly; (*b*) cyclopia.

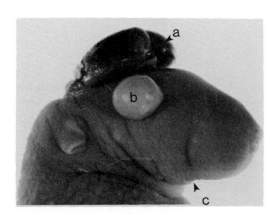

FIG. A-11. Malformed head of rat fetus: (*a*) excencephaly; (*b*) exophthalmia; (*c*) agnathia.

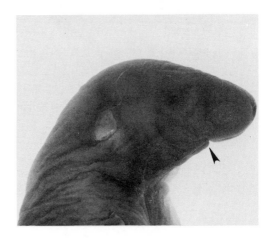

FIG. A-12. Malformed jaw of rat fetus: micrognathia (*arrowhead*).

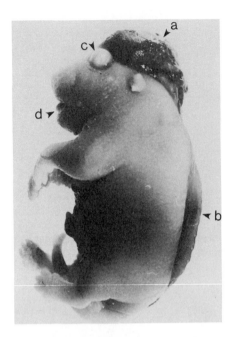

FIG. A-13. Malformed rat fetus: (*a*) excencephaly; (*b*) craniorachischisis; (*c*) exophthalmia; (*d*) protruding tongue.

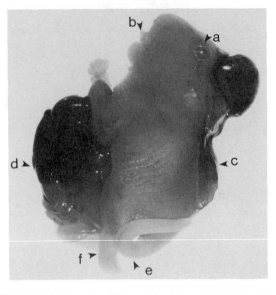

FIG. A-14. Malformed rat fetus: (*a*) open eyelids; (*b*) protruding tongue; (*c*) craniorachischisis; (*d*) gastroschisis; (*e*) bent tail; (*f*) club foot.

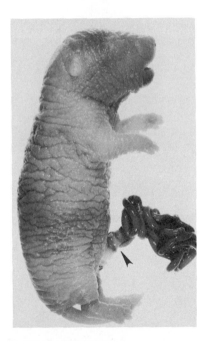

FIG. A-15. Malformed rat fetus: umbilical hernia.

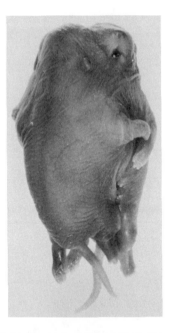

FIG. A-16. Malformed rat fetus: thoracopagus twins.

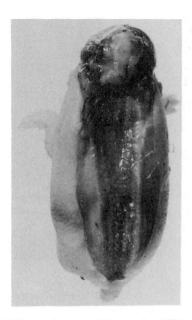

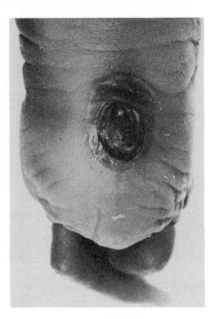

FIG. A-17. Malformed mouse fetus: spina bifida of total vertebral column.

FIG. A-18. Malformed rabbit fetus: spina bifida occulta.

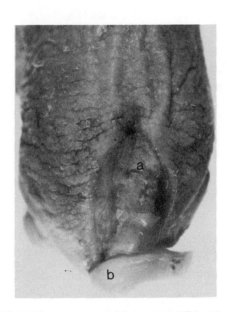

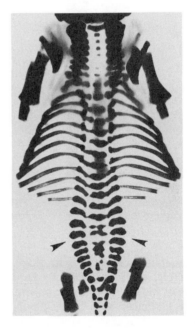

FIG. A-19. Malformed mouse fetus: spina bifida (*a*) with bent tail (*b*).

FIG. A-20. Spina bifida fetus: wide open lumbar vertebrae with irregularly shaped or fused lumbar centers (*arrowheads*).

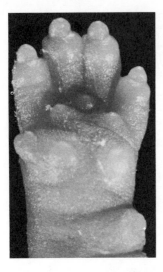

FIG. A-21. Normal left forepaw of mouse fetus.

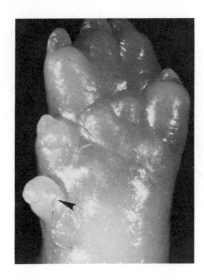

FIG. A-22. Malformed digits of mouse fetus: polydactyly (*arrowhead*).

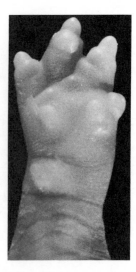

FIG. A-23. Malformed digits of mouse fetus: ectrodactyly, four digits.

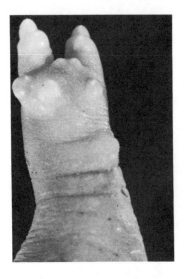

FIG. A-24. Malformed digits of mouse fetus: ectrodactyly, two digits.

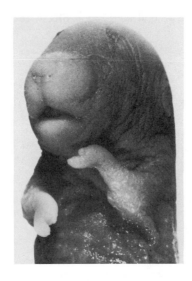

FIG. A-25. Malformed digits of mouse fetus: phocomelia and ectrodactyly.

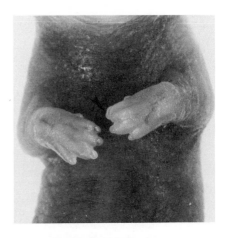

FIG. A-26. Malformed digits of mouse fetus: syndactyly.

The tail is examined for presence, size, shape, and position. A normal tail (Fig. A-27) is slightly curved and is 3 cm long. Kinky, vestigial, and missing tails are presented in Figs. A-28 through A-30. Fetuses with external malformations are photographed and then examined for skeletal and visceral malformations.

The following parameters are reported for a dose-range study:

1. Fate of females (survival, litters totally resorbed or aborted)
2. Clinical signs
3. Maternal food consumption
4. Maternal body weight (days 0 and 6–21) and weight gain (days 6–16, 6–21, or 16–21)
5. Gravid uterine weight and adjusted maternal weight (body weight day 21 − gravid uterus weight)
6. Maternal visceral changes

7. No. of corpora lutea per litter
8. No. of implantation sites per litter
9. Percent preimplantation loss

$$\left(\frac{\text{No. corpora lutea} - \text{No. implantations}}{\text{No. corpora lutea}}\right) \times 100$$

10. Number of resorption sites
    a. Early: no embryonic tissue visible at termination
    b. Late: placental and embryonic tissue visible at termination
11. Percent postimplantation death

$$\left(\frac{\text{No. implantations} - \text{No. live fetuses}}{\text{No. implantations}}\right) \times 100$$

12. No. of live fetuses per litter
13. Sex distribution
14. Fetal weight: male and female

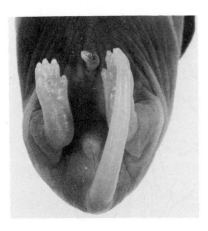

FIG. A-27. Normal tail of rat fetus.

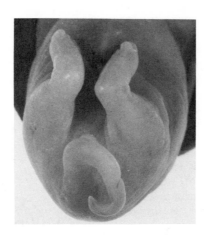

FIG. A-28. Malformed kinky tail.

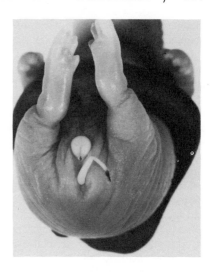

FIG. A-29. Malformed vestigial tail.

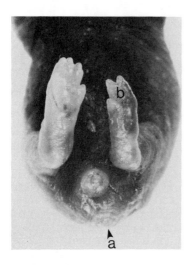

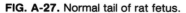

FIG. A-30. Malformed tail: anury (*a*) with ectrodactyly (*b*).

15. External malformations: total per treatment group and per litter

If a female is nonpregnant or has a totally resorbed or aborted litter, the food consumption and body weight data for this female are not included in the group mean. We routinely do not perform statistical analysis on results from dose-range studies given the small group size; rather, decisions are based on biologically significant trends in the data, such as:

1. Doses causing a 10% or more incidence of maternal death, abortion, or resorption of the entire litter, are generally too high for the definitive study.
2. If gravid uterine weight is depressed without a parallel decrease in adjusted maternal weight, the agent may be having a selective toxic effect on embryonic survival and growth.
3. In the absence of an indication of selective developmental toxicity (adverse effects on the conceptus at nonmaternally toxic doses), the most important parameter in the dose-range study to be used when selecting doses for the definitive study is usually fetal body weight.

By evaluating the conceptus at doses ranging from no effect to maternal toxic effects, an impression is gained as to whether the agent causes selective developmental toxicity. If it appears that the agent has this potential, the definitive study is designed for unambiguous identification of the effect, whether it is increased death, malformation, or growth retardation. The low dose is selected as the NOEL, the mid dose as the LOEL, and the high dose for full biological and statistical manifestation of the effect. If the agent causes adverse effects on the conceptus only at maternally toxic doses, a different strategy for dose selection is used. The most likely fetal effects encountered at maternally toxic doses are embryo lethality and growth retardation, although the rare occurrence of increased gross malformations cannot be discounted. Although many investigators select the high dose based on maternal toxic effects (e.g., significant reduction in maternal body weight), our practice has been to use fetal body weight as the criterion for dose selection. Selection of the high dose based on a 10% depression in fetal body weight ensures there will be a full cohort of fetuses surviving to term for detailed morphological analysis. This dimension of weight reduction in rat fetuses with a group size of 20 is statistically significant and is usually associated with a statistically significant reduction in maternal weight gain.

The dose-range study provides invaluable information for dose selection in the definitive study and for qualitative assessment of the potential developmental toxicity of the agent. With the limited group size and incomplete assessment of morphological alterations in the conceptus, however, a definitive study must be conducted before conclusions about the safety of the agent in pregnant animals can be drawn.

Definitive study

In the definitive study we start off with a group size of 24 mated females with the expectation there will be 20 dams bearing live litters at term per treatment group. The same procedures for housing, mating, and observations made in life and at cesarean section are followed as are described for the dose-range study. Following examination for external malformations, however, fetuses are processed for detailed skeletal and visceral examination.

Live fetuses are first placed on a Dry Ice bath for 2 to 3 min, which rapidly lowers body temperature and results in euthanasia. In our laboratory, half of the fetuses in each litter are randomly selected for fresh visceral examination by a modified Staples method and the other half for skeletal examination. This procedure is changed only when a fetus scheduled for skeletal examination is suspected of having an abnormality that can best be verified by visceral examination and vice versa.

The visceral examination takes place on the day of cesarean section. When complete (see below), the fetus is decapitated and the head placed in Bouin's fixative for 1 to 2 weeks for subsequent razorblade sectioning. The fetal carcass is stored in 70% ethanol. For the skeletal examination, fetuses are eviscerated, skinned, and placed in 70% ethanol on the day of cesarean section. They are then processed at a later date for skeletal staining and examination as described below.

Visceral examination of fetuses. Rodent fetuses are pinned to paraffin blocks, ventral side up (Fig. A-31). Visceral examination is then conducted under a dissecting microscope.

For examination of the abdominal viscera, the abdomen is cut horizontally at the level of the umbilicus and longitudinally from the pubis to below the level of the diaphragm. The abdominal cavity is then examined. A diagram of the abdominal viscera of a male rat fetus is presented in Fig. A-32 for reference. The *intestines, stomach, spleen,* and *pancreas* are examined for size and position. The *liver* has four distinguishable lobes: the right lobe, having an anterior and a posterior lobule; the left lobe, which is large; the median or cystic lobe, which bears a deep fissure for the ligamentum teres; and the caudate lobe, which is a small lobe on the caudal

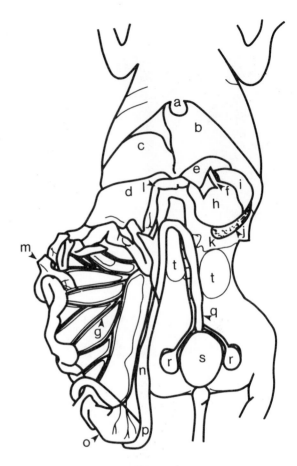

FIG. A-32. Normal abdominal viscera of male rat fetus: (*a*) xiphoid process; (*b*) left lobe of liver; (*c*) median lobe of liver; (*d*) right lobe of liver, anterior and posterior; (*e*) caudate lobe of liver; (*f*) esophagus; (*g*) mesentery; (*h*) pyloric region of stomach; (*i*) cardiac region of stomach; (*j*) spleen; (*k*) pancreas; (*l*) duodenum; (*m*) small intestines; (*n*) large intestines; (*o*) cecum; (*p*) ascending colon; (*q*) rectum; (*r*) testis (paired); (*s*) bladder; (*t*) kidney (paired).

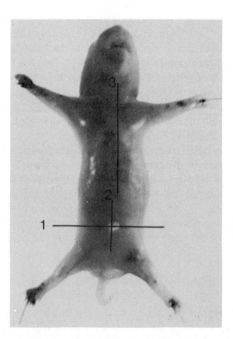

FIG. A-31. Rat fetus, ventral side, pinned to board in preparation for internal visceral examination; lines 1 and 2 show where cuts are made to examine abdominal viscera, and line 3 where to cut to expose thoracic viscera.

surface that fits around the esophagus. The rat does not have a gallbladder. The *reproductive organs* are exposed by raising the intestine and attached viscera from the dorsal wall with a cotton swab. In female fetuses (Fig. A-33), there is a bicornuate uterus; the two horns fuse at their cervical ends but have separate openings into the vagina. They extend from the vagina cranially almost to the caudal poles of the kidneys. Superiorly the uterine horns are related to the oviducts and ovaries. In male fetuses (Fig. A-34), testes have not fully descended and lie in the pelvic region on both sides of the bladder. In front of the testis and closely attached to it lies the caput, or head of the epididymis. The corpus, or body, of the epididymis lies along the surface of the testis and progresses to the cauda, or tail, of the epididymis. The ductus deferens is connected to the cauda epididymis and leads to the urethra. The seminal vesicles are relatively large and lobulated.

The *adrenals* and *kidneys* are examined for size and position. In the rat, the right kidney lies more cephalad than the left kidney, and on the superior pole of each is the adrenal. Transverse kidney cuts are made to expose the renal papillae.

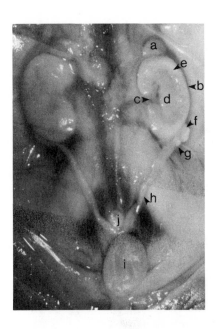

FIG. A-33. Normal female urogenital/reproductive organs of rat fetus: (*a*) adrenal; (*b*) normal horizontal kidney section; (*c*) renal pelvis; (*d*) medulla; (*e*) cortex; (*f*) ovary; (*g*) oviduct; (*h*) uterus; (*i*) bladder; (*j*) rectum.
←

FIG. A-34. Normal male urogenital/reproductive organs of rat fetus: (*a*) adrenal; (*b*) kidney; (*c*) ureter; (*d*) testis; (*e*) caput epididymis; (*f*) cauda epididymis; (*g*) vas deferens; (*h*) bladder.
→

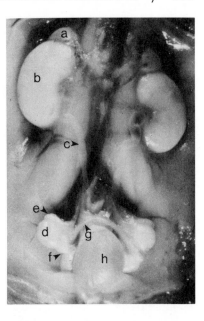

and pelvis. A distinction between "normal" delays in renal development and renal malformation (hydronephrosis) must be made. The varying degrees of renal distention and a rating scheme for these differences can be found in the work by Woo and Hoar (97). The *ureters* are traced from the kidney to the bladder to ensure that they are attached. A small amount of Bouin's solution can be applied to the ureters with a cotton swab to facilitate visibility. A moderate degree of tortuosity of the ureter is normal. Hydroureter and hydronephrosis are easily recognized (Figs. A-35 and A-36).

The liver is carefully lifted with a cotton swab to examine the diaphragm (Fig. A-37) for abnormal openings or herniation (Fig. A-38). Care is taken not to puncture the diaphragm in this process, as it would lead to incorrect identification of diaphragmatic hernia.

For examination of the thoracic cavity, a longitudinal cut is made extending anteriorly to the right of center so as not to disturb the integrity of the sternebrae. This cut is shallow in order to avoid damage to the underlying organs or blood vessels. Each side of the diaphragm is cut away to uncover the thoracic organs. The following features of the thoracic viscera are examined: The right and left auricular appendages of the heart are usually asymmetrical, their size and shape depending on the state of the organ at the time of death. The anterior portion of the heart is mainly occupied by the right ventricle, the left ventricle lying behind and to the left. The apex of the heart points to the left. The right lung has four lobes, and the left lung has one; the medial lobe of the right lung extends over to the left lobe and is dorsal and caudal to the heart. The lung lobes are counted and examined for size and maturity. The *thymus gland* (Figs. A-39 and A-40) is checked for size and position, and removed with sharp forceps. The *trachea* and *esophagus* are exposed for examination of fusion or tracheoesophageal fistula.

The pericardial sac is then opened and the pericardium cut away so the heart is fully exposed (Fig. A-41). On the right side are the right anterior (superior) vena cava (RSVC), right vagus nerve, and innominate artery; the latter arises from the aortic arch and divides into the right subclavian artery and right common carotid artery. On the left side of the aortic arch are the left common carotid artery and left subclavian artery. The left vagus nerve and the left anterior (superior) vena cava must be distinguished.

In the midline the *pulmonary artery,* arising from the base of the right ventricle ventral to the aorta, is relatively short and divides into right and left pulmonary branches, which extend to the right and left lung lobes. It is connected to the aorta by the *ductus arteriosus,* a fetal vessel that atrophies after birth. The *aorta* arises from the left ventricle, dorsal to the pulmonary artery, and extends anteriorly, then arches laterally to the left before extending posteriorly as the descending dorsal aorta. Malformed vessels of the rat fetal heart are shown in Figs. A-42 through A-44.

The heart consists of four muscle-walled chambers: the left and right atria and the left and right ventricles. The left and right sides of the heart are separated by the interatrial septum and the interventricular septum; atrioventricular septa separate the artria from the ventricles. To examine the internal anatomy of the heart, two cuts are made using microdissecting scissors.

The first cut (Fig. A-45) begins to the right of the ventral midline surface at the apex and extends anteriorly and ventrally into the pulmonary artery. This incision is opened with forceps; the tricuspid valve, between the right atrium and right ventricle, and the three cusps of the semilunar valve of the pulmonary artery are inspected. The interventricular septum is examined for the presence of ventricular septal defects. A membranous ventricular septal defect underneath the semilunar valve is shown in Fig. A-46.

The second cut (Fig. A-47) is made to the left of the ventral midline surface at the apex, extending through the left ventricle into the ascending aorta. The bicuspid valve between the left atrium and left ventricle and the three cusps of the semilunar valve of the aorta are observed. A fetal heart with both membranous and muscular ventricular septal defect is shown in Fig. A-48. Figure A-49 is a data collection sheet for recording visceral malformations and variations.

When this examination is complete, the fetus is decapitated

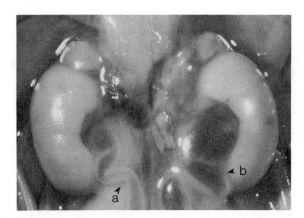

FIG. A-35. Malformed ureters: (*a*) slightly dilated ureter; (*b*) hydroureter (markedly dilated ureter).

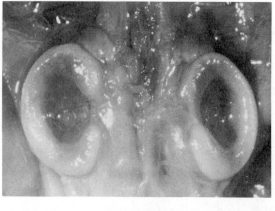

FIG. A-36. Malformed kidneys. Horizontal kidney sections showing bilateral hydronephrosis.

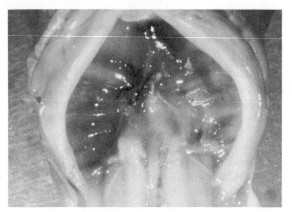

FIG. A-37. Normal diaphragm of rat fetus.

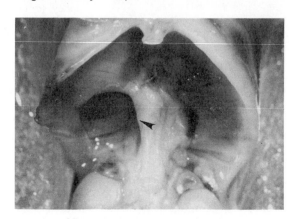

FIG. A-38. Diaphragmatic hernia.

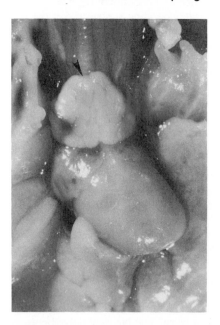

FIG. A-39. Normal thymus (*arrowhead*) of rat fetus.

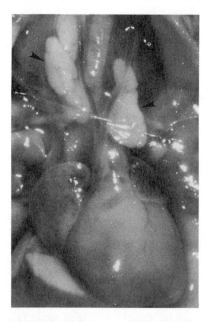

FIG. A-40. Malformed split thymus (*arrowheads*).

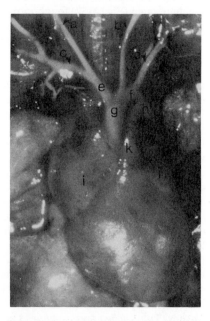

FIG. A-41. Normal heart vessels of rat fetus: (*a*) right carotid; (*b*) left carotid; (*c*) right subclavian; (*d*) left subclavian; (*e*) innominate; (*f*) aortic arch; (*g*) ascending aorta; (*h*) ductus arteriosus; (*i*) right atrium; (*j*) left atrium; (*k*) pulmonary artery.

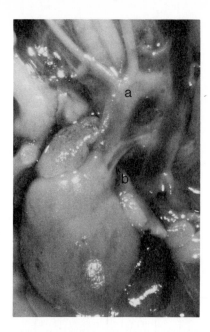

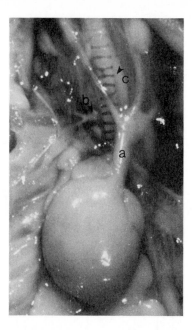

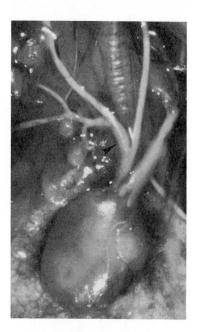

FIG. A-42. Malformed major vessels of rat fetus: (*a*) enlarged aortic arch; (*b*) hypoplastic pulmonary artery.

FIG. A-43. Malformed vessels of rat fetus: (*a*) persistent truncus arteriosus; (*b*) right subclavian under the trachea; (*c*) irregular tracheal cartilage.

FIG. A-44. Malformed vessels of rat fetus: right-sided aortic arch (*arrowhead*) and absent descending aorta.

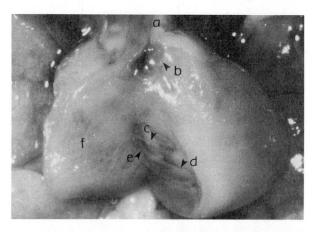

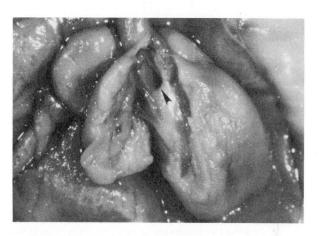

FIG. A-45. Normal heart of rat fetus, first cut from the right ventral surface into the pulmonary artery: (*a*) pulmonary artery; (*b*) semilunar valves; (*c*) chordae tendineae; (*d*) papillary muscles; (*e*) tricuspid valve; (*f*) right ventricle.

FIG. A-46. Malformed heart from the first cut: membranous ventricular septal defect (*arrowhead*) under the semilunar valve.

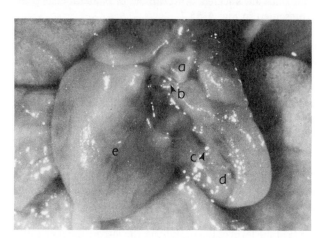

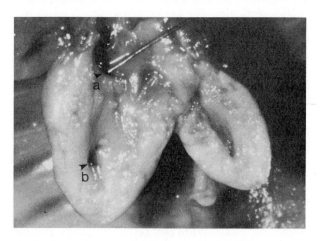

FIG. A-47. Normal heart of rat fetus, second cut from the left ventral surface into the ascending aorta: (*a*) ascending aorta; (*b*) semilunar valves; (*c*) bicuspid valve; (*d*) left ventricle; (*e*) interventricular septum.

FIG. A-48. Malformed heart from the second cut: (*a*) membranous ventricular septal defect (VSD) underneath aortic valve; (*b*) muscular VSD.

(SIDE A)

EXPERIMENT _____

SOFT TISSUE EXAMINATION

MATERNAL I.D. _____ SHEET ____ OF ____

TREATMENT _____

Fetus No.	External Sex	Head				Brain		Neck			Heart										Lung		
		Palate	Nares	Cornea	Lens	Ventricles	Other	Esophagus	Trachea	Thymus	Carotid Artery	Aortic Arch	Vena Cava Sup/Inf	Ductus Arteriosis	Pulmonary Valve	Aortic Valve	Atria	Ventricles	Septum	Other	Bronchi	Lungs	Diaphragm
1																							
2																							
3																							
4																							
5																							
6																							

FIG. A-49. Data sheet for visceral examination. **Side A:** Space is provided to record the observations made during this examination. A check (✓) is usually made if the organ is present and normal.

and the head placed in Bouin's fixative for subsequent razorblade sectioning. The head is first sectioned across from the opening of the mouth to the pinna, as illustrated in Fig. A-50. The top of the head is then detached, and the tongue is removed and examined for proper closure of the palate (Fig. A-51). An example of cleft palate is given in Fig. A-52. The top of the head is then flipped back to its original position, and five cuts are made, as illustrated in Fig. 53, to visualize internal structures. Each of these sections is placed in a well of a spotting plate with the anterior side facing up and then immersed in 70% ethanol.

The sections are examined under a dissecting microscope (×12.5), and both sides of each section are examined and compared with the preceding section and the following one. The first and second sections (Fig. A-54) of the head are examined for symmetry of external nares, conchae, nasal septum, and palate. When cleft palate occurs, it is classified as unilateral if only one side is affected and as bilateral if both sides are affected. An example of bilateral cleft palate is presented in Fig. A-55.

In the third section (Fig. A-56), the lenses and retinas of both eyes are examined for size, uniformity, and curvature, and the olfactory bulbs for development. Microphthalmia (small eye) and anophthalmia (missing eye) are shown in Fig. A-57. The fifth section (Fig. A-58) is examined for the lateral and third ventricles of the brain; the degree of enlargement is used for diagnosis of hydrocephalus. A brain section with hydrocephalus is shown in Fig. A-59. The remainder of the head, sectioned midsagittally, is examined for development of the cerebellum and brainstem.

Skeletal examination of fetuses. Fetuses scheduled for skeletal analyses are eviscerated and fixed in 70% ethanol until they are ready to be processed for the skeletal clearing procedure. To eviscerate the abdomen, a horizontal split is made at the level of the umbilicus; the viscera are then pulled away with forceps, starting at the level of the thorax. The

(SIDE B)

Fetus No.	Liver	Stomach	Intestines	Kidneys	Adrenals	Bladder	Ureter	INTERNAL SEX Ovaries	INTERNAL SEX Testes	Other and/or Comment
1										
2										
3										
4										
5										
6										

FIG. A-49. (*Continued.*) **Side B:** Remaining observations are recorded here along with any comments the examiner deems appropriate.

skin and the fat pad between the scapula is then removed. The skin need not be removed if a 2% KOH solution is used. Fixation in 70% ethanol is not necessary if fetuses are cleared immediately after being killed.

The unskinned fetuses (fresh or fixed) are placed in a 2% KOH solution with alizarin red S stain (1 mg/dl), and the skinned fetuses are placed in a 1% KOH solution with alizarin red S stain (1 mg/dl) for 1 day. They are transferred to fresh 1% KOH solution with alizarin red S stain (1 mg/dl) for 2 days more (each day specimens are transferred to fresh 1% KOH solution with stain) for tissue maceration and bone staining. The unskinned specimens may take longer to achieve favorable color or complete the maceration process in the 1% KOH solution. Specimens are then rinsed in cold tap water and cleared in a 1:1 mixture of glycerin and 70% ethanol for a minimum of 12 to 24 hours. Specimens are stored in pure glycerin.

A "double staining" procedure for visualization of cartilage

(alcian blue) and bone (alizarin red) can be used when detailed examination of the skeletal system is desirable. Fresh specimens are completely eviscerated and immersed for approximately 10 sec in hot water (70°–80°C) to remove skin from the hands, feet, and tail. Complete removal of the skin, especially around the digits, is necessary for alcian blue staining of cartilaginous elements. Adipose tissue between the scapula is removed. If skinning is not done immediately, the eviscerated specimens can be placed in 4% saltwater overnight and skinned the next day (43). The skinned specimens are fixed in 70% ethanol if staining is not done the same day.

Cartilage is stained in a alcian blue solution (10 mg alcian blue, 100 ml 70% ethanol, 5 ml acetic acid) for 3 days or until the optimum color is obtained. The specimens are rinsed in cold tap water and transferred to 1% fresh KOH solution with alizarin red S (1 mg/dl) each day for 2 days and then rinsed in cold tap water. The specimens are cleared and hardened in a 1:1 mixture of glycerin and 70% ethanol for

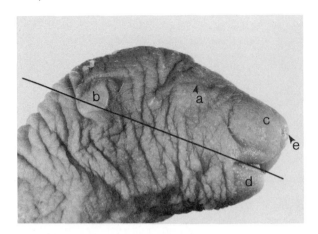

FIG. A-50. Normal head of rat fetus: (*a*) eyelids; (*b*) ear (pinna); (*c*) nares; (*d*) lower jaw; (*e*) nostrils. The line shows where section is made to examine the palatine shelf.

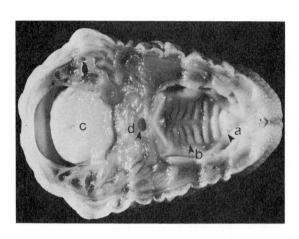

FIG. A-51. Normal palate from ventral aspect: (*a*) palatine shelves; (*b*) palatine ridges; (*c*) pons; (*d*) oral pharynx.

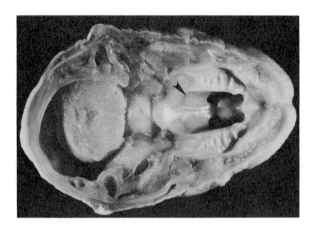

FIG. A-52. Malformed palate of rat fetus: cleft palate.

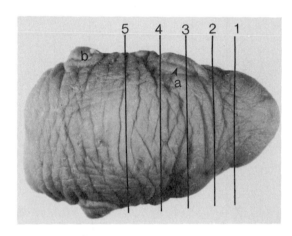

FIG. A-53. Normal head of rat fetus, coronal view: (*a*) eyelids; (*b*) ear (pinna). Lines 1 to 5 show where sections are made.

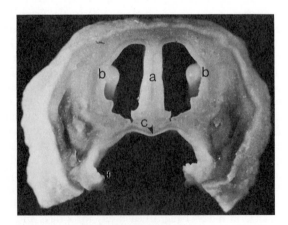

FIG. A-54. Normal head (section 2 in Fig. A-53): (*a*) nasal septum; (*b*) nasal conchae; (*c*) palatine shelf.

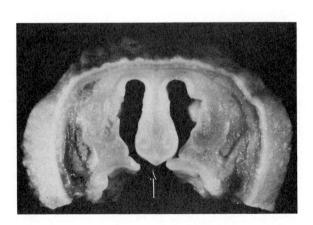

FIG. A-55. Malformed head section: cleft palate (*arrow*).

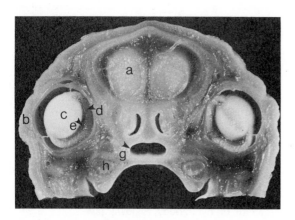

FIG. A-56. Normal head (section 3 in Fig. A-53): (a) olfactory bulbs; (b) eyelids; (c) lens; (d) retina; (e) vitreous body; (f) anterior chamber; (g) nasal tract (choana); (h) maxilla.

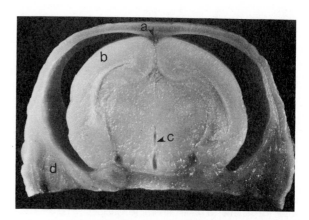

FIG. A-58. Normal head (section 5 in Fig. A-53): (a) superior sagittal sinus; (b) lateral ventricles; (c) third ventricle; (d) indication of internal ear.

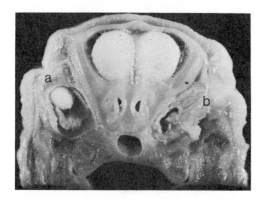

FIG. A-57. Section of malformed head: (a) microphthalmia; (b) anophthalmia.

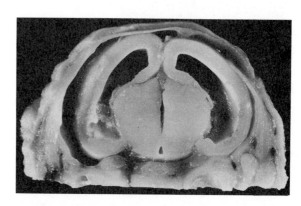

FIG. A-59. Malformed head section: hydrocephalic brain with marked dilation of lateral ventricles.

a minimum of 12 hr; they are stored in pure glycerin. The best results are obtained using the Varistain 24-3 (Shandon Inc., Pittsburgh, Pennsylvania) automatic stainer. The stainer can be programmed for constant agitation of specimens and for automatic transfer of specimens into fresh solutions.

Rat skeletons are examined under a dissection microscope at a magnification of 12.5×. The skull is examined for size, shape, and degree of ossification of the following bones: nasal, frontal, parietal, interparietal, occipital, lacrimal, zygomatic, squamosal, premaxillary, maxillary, mandible, basisphenoid, exoccipital, tympanic bullae (Figs. A-60 through A-62). A malformed skull with an extra sutural bone and large open fontanelle is pictured in Fig. A-63.

Vertebral arches and centers, ribs, and sternal centers are examined for size and shape, and counted for the number of ossification centers. The most frequently observed number of ossification centers at each site are as follows: cervical 7, thoracic 13 or 14, lumbar 7 or 6, sacral 5, caudal more than 5, sternal centers 6, and ribs 13 or 14 (Figs. A-64, A-68, and A-69). Figures A-65 through A-67 illustrate abnormally os-

sified ribs or vertebrae. Various degrees of abnormal sternal centers are presented in Figs. A-70 and A-71.

The thoracic and pelvic girdles and the forelimbs (Fig. A-72) and hindlimbs (Fig. A-73) are examined for development of the long bones; the number of phalanges are counted. The number of phalanges for the normal 21-day rat fetus are as follows: forelimb: metacarpals 4, proximal 4 (not shown in Fig. A-72), middle 4 (not ossified, stained in blue), distal 5; and hindlimb: metatarsals 5, proximal 5 (not shown in Fig. A-73), middle 4 (not ossified, stained in blue), distal 5. Examples of tibia and fibula long bone malformations are shown in Figs. A-74 and A-75. Any deviations from the normal development of the bone and cartilage are recorded in the data sheet shown in Fig. A-76.

Methods for Female Fertility Evaluation (Segment I)

Disruption of female fertility can occur at a number of stages in the life cycle and at many levels in the hypothalamic-pituitary-uterine-ovarian axis. The Segment I: General Re-

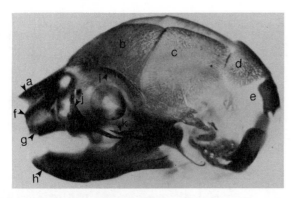

FIG. A-60. Normal skull of rat fetus, lateral view: (a) nasal; (b) frontal; (c) parietal; (d) interparietal; (e) occipital; (f) premaxillary; (g) maxillary; (h) mandible; (i) lacrimal; (j) zygomatic; (k) squamosa.

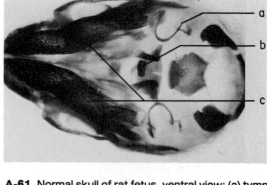

FIG. A-61. Normal skull of rat fetus, ventral view: (a) tympanic bulla (paired); (b) hyoid body; (c) lower jaw.

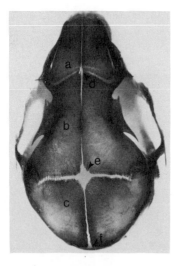

FIG. A-62. Normal skull of rabbit fetus, dorsal view: (a) nasal; (b) frontal; (c) parietal; (d) frontal suture; (e) anterior fontanelle; (f) posterior fontanelle.

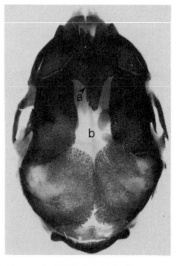

FIG. A-63. Malformed skull of rabbit fetus: (a) extra sutural bone; (b) large open fontanelle.

productive Performance Study in Female Rats is designed to detect potential adverse effects of an agent on estrous cycles and reproductive performance as well as on postnatal growth and survival of offspring throughout lactation. Female rats are treated for 2 weeks prior to mating, throughout mating and pregnancy to day 21 of lactation when offspring are weaned. Half the females are killed on day 21 of pregnancy for developmental toxicity assessment, as described in the previous section, and the other half go through natural deliveries with offspring maintained to weaning. The Segment I study measures a broad spectrum of apical endpoints related to fertility (estrous cycles, mating behavior, gonadal function, conception rates), reproductive performance (pregnancy outcome, natural delivery), and lactation (postnatal growth and viability). The usual procedure is to perform the Segment II: Developmental Toxicity Study first to obtain information on effects of the agent on prenatal development and to assist in dose selection for the Segment I: Female Fertility Study.

Even with availability of data from a Segment II study, a dose-range study for the Segment I: Female Fertility study

is recommended. Depending on the physiologic/pharmacologic mode of action of the agent, the Segment I study can provide the low-dose trigger for reproductive toxicity. This situation is particularly true for classes of drugs affecting smooth muscle contraction (antihypertensives), which can selectively impair uterine contractility at parturition, and those affecting prostaglandin synthesis (nonsteroidal antiinflammatory drugs), which can block ovulation and uterine contractility. It is also possible that *higher* doses of agents are needed in Segment I than in Segment II studies to "test to effect," given the longer prepregnancy treatment interval in Segment I studies, which permits detoxification and maternal homeostatic mechanisms to be established.

Dose-Range Study

For the dose-range study, we routinely include five treatment groups, each containing six females, and a concurrent

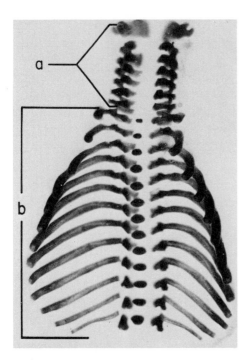

FIG. A-64. Normal vertebral column and ribs of rat fetus: (*a*) 7 cervical vertebrae; (*b*) 13 thoracic vertebrae with ribs (note centers in thoracic vertebrae).

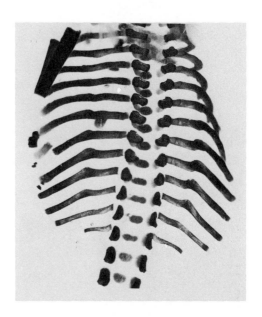

FIG. A-65. Malformed wavy ribs.

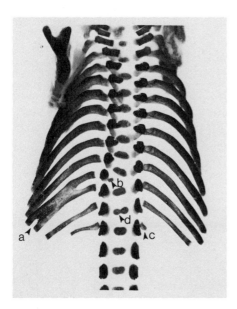

FIG. A-66. Malformed thoracic vertebrae and ribs: (*a*) fused ribs; (*b*) extra ossification center between 11th and 12th thoracic arches; (*c*) ossification center of 14th rib; (*d*) dumbbell-shaped thoracic center.

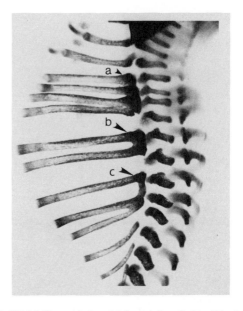

FIG. A-67. Malformed ribs: (*a*) fused ribs, 3rd to 5th; (*b*) fused ribs, 7th and 8th; (*c*) fused ribs, 9th to 11th.

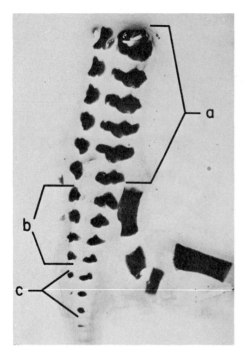

FIG. A-68. Normal lumbar, sacral, and caudal vertebrae of rat fetus: (a) 6 lumbar vertebrae; (b) 4 sacral vertebrae; (c) 2 to 3 caudal vertebrae.

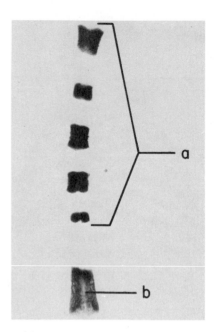

FIG. A-69. Normal sternum of rat fetus, detached from the torso: (a) five sternebrae; (b) xiphisternum.

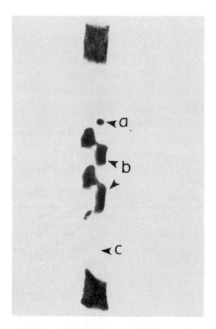

FIG. A-70. Malformed sternal centers: (a) hypoplastic, 2nd; (b) off center, 3rd and 4th; (c) missing, 5th.

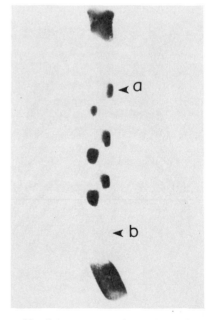

FIG. A-71. Malformed sternal centers: (a) split and off center, 2nd to 4th; (b) missing, 5th.

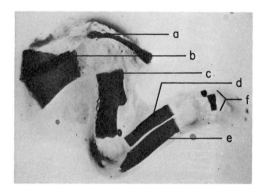

FIG. A-72. Normal long bones of fetal rat forelimb: (*a*) clavicle; (*b*) scapula; (*c*) humerus; (*d*) radius; (*e*) ulna; (*f*) three metacarpals.

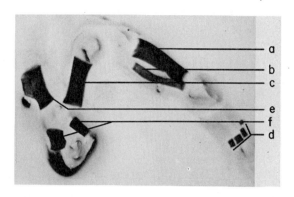

FIG. A-73. Normal long bones of fetal rat hindlimb: (*a*) tibia; (*b*) fibula; (*c*) femur; (*d*) four metatarsals; (*e*) ilium; (*f*) ischium.

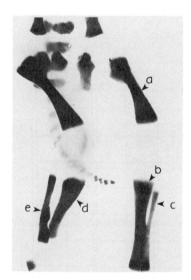

FIG. A-74. Long bones of fetal rabbit hindlimbs: (*a*) normal femur; (*b*) normal tibia; (*c*) normal fibula; (*d*) short tibia; (*e*) bent fibula.

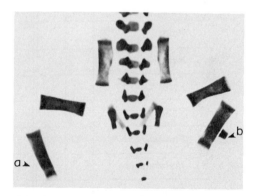

FIG. A-75. Malformed long bones of fetal mouse hindlimbs: (*a*) missing fibula; (*b*) hypoplastic fibula.

(SIDE A)

Experiment _____

Female No. _____

Treatment _____

Sheet _____ of _____

SKELETAL ANALYSIS

Abbreviations: ✓ – normal, A – absent, C – cleft (palate), I – irregular shape, M – misaligned, R – reduced, S – split, W – wavy

Fetus No.

Bone Description	1 L	1 R	2 L	2 R	3 L	3 R	4 L	4 R	5 L	5 R	6 L	6 R
Pectoral Girdle												
Clavicle												
Scapula												
Humerus												
Radius												
Ulna												
Metacarpals												
Phalanges												
TOTAL												
Pectoral Abnormalities												
Pelvic Girdle												
Ilium												
Ischium												
Femur												
Tibia												
Fibula												
Metatarsals												
Phalanges												
TOTAL												
Pelvic Abnormalities												
Pelvic & Pectoral Abnormalities												

FIG. A-76. Data sheet for skeletal examination. **Side A:** Space is provided for identification of the experiment, the dam, the treatment group(s), and the examination of pectoral and pelvic girdles. The abbreviations used to describe common abnormalities are indicated. They aid in consistency of recording and in data transcription to a computer file.

(SIDE B)

	Fetus No.					
	1	2	3	4	5	6
Skull						
Braincase						
Tympanic Bulla						
Body of Hyoid						
Palate						
Jaw						
TOTAL						
Skull Abnormalities						
Axial Skeleton						
Sternebrae						
Vertebrae						
Tail						
Ribs						
TOTAL						
Axial Abnormalities						
Axial & Skull Abnormalities						

Total # fetuses
with abnormalities   _____

fetuses examined
from this litter   _____

Total # anomalies   _____

Signed _____   Date_____

FIG. A-76. (*Continued.*) **Side B:** Space is provided for results of the examination of the skull and axial skeletons.

control with doses selected based on the following projected outcomes:

Group 1: no effect
Group 2: no effect or minimal effect
Group 3: minimal to moderate effect
Group 4: definitive toxicity
Group 5: definitive toxicity

After a 2-week quarantine period, females at approximately 70 days of age are monitored for two estrous cycles by taking vaginal smears for 10 days. Females not completing two cycles within this period are excluded from the study, and the remainder are randomized into treatment groups.

Treatment is then initiated and continued for all phases of the dose-range study, including a 10-day premating period, a mating period no longer than 10 days' duration, a pregnancy period of approximately 21 days, and a lactation period of 7 days. Food consumption, body weight, and clinical signs are monitored at intervals throughout the treatment period.

During the 2-week premating period, females are monitored for effects of the treatment on estrous cyclicity by daily vaginal smears. They are then placed in mating units with untreated males in a 1:1 (male/female) mating ratio. Females with sperm-positive vaginal smears are separated from the male and considered to be on day 0 of pregnancy. If a sperm-positive vaginal smear is not found during the first 5 mating days for a given female, she is transferred to a unit with a different male and allowed an additional 5-day mating period.

Treatment continues throughout pregnancy, and dams are permitted to deliver their litters naturally. The days of initiation and completion of delivery are recorded. Any female not delivering a litter by day 24 of presumed pregnancy is killed and the uterus stained with ammonium sulfide to visualize early implantation sites if products of conception are not evident.

At birth (day 1), pups are individually weighed, counted, sexed, examined for external malformations, and toe-clipped for permanent identification. Litters can be culled to a constant size of eight or ten pups whose body weights are closest to the litter mean. Pups are then counted and individually weighed daily or at intervals until day 7 of lactation, at which time they are killed. The decision can be made whether to perform gross internal examinations of pups on day 7 based on growth and viability data as well as previous results from a Segment II study. The dams are also killed on day 7, autopsied, and the uteri examined for number of implantation sites.

The following parameters are reported from a Segment I: Female Fertility Dose-Range Study:

1. Fate of females (percent mated, percent pregnant, survival, litters totally resorbed or aborted, litters surviving through lactation)
2. Clinical signs
3. Maternal food consumption and body weight
4. Number of estrous cycles completed during drug administration
5. Number of days needed for mating
6. Natural delivery data
   a. Length of pregnancy, days
   b. Number of pups at birth: litter size
   c. Sex distribution at birth and day 7
   d. Live birth index

   $$\left(\frac{\text{No. pups alive day 1}}{\text{No. pups born alive}}\right) \times 100$$

   e. Viability index

   $$\left(\frac{\text{No. pups alive day 7}}{\text{No. pups alive day 1}}\right) \times 100$$

   f. Growth rate of offspring during lactation
   g. Body weight of male and female pups during lactation
   h. Gross malformations and internal malformations
   i. Implantation sites at autopsy for determination of postimplantation death

In general, any female or entire litter lost from the study due to death, abortion, or resorption is accounted for under "fate of females," and the data for that female are not included in subsequent group mean determinations. We routinely do not perform statistical analysis on results from dose-range studies given the small group size; rather, decisions are made based on biologically significant trends in the data. Trends previously discussed for the Segment II dose-range studies are considered, in addition to the following:

1. Doses that cause a 25% or more decrease in mating or fertility indices, as well as live birth/viability indices, are generally too high for the definitive study.
2. In the absence of an indication of selective reproductive/developmental toxicity, the most important parameters in the dose-range study to be used when selecting doses for the definitive study are usually birth weight and the growth rate of offspring on days 1 to 7 of lactation.

By evaluating the spectrum of parameters measured in the study at treatment levels ranging up to those causing general systemic toxicity, an impression is gained as to whether the agent specifically impairs female fertility or pregnancy outcome. Perturbations in the ability to conceive or bear viable litters at treatment levels not causing systemic toxicity indicates specific impairment of the reproductive process. If it appears that the agent has this potential, the Definitive Study is designed for unambiguous identification of this effect, with the proviso that some viable litters must be produced in the high dose group for evaluation of postnatal viability. The low dose is selected as the NOEL, the middle dose as the LOEL, and the high dose for full biological and statistical manifestation of the effect.

If, on the other hand, the only adverse effects obtained at treatment levels causing frank systemic toxicity are depressions in birth weight and growth rates, a different strategy for dose selection is used. The most important consideration is to demonstrate that you have "tested to effect" in the high dose group for the definitive study. A 5–10% depression in birth weight will be statistically significant in the definitive study and will usually be associated with a statistically significant reduction in maternal weight gain during pregnancy and with the growth rate at intervals during lactation.

The dose-range study provides invaluable information for dose selection in the definitive study and for qualitative assessment of the potential reproductive and/or developmental toxicity of the agent. With the limited group size and incomplete characterization of pregnancy outcome, however, a definitive study must be carried out before conclusions about the safety of the agent can be drawn.

Definitive Study

For the definitive study, 30 females per treatment group are employed. This results in 15 females per group being available for cesarean delivery at term and 15 for natural deliveries. The same procedures for housing, mating, and observations made in life are followed as described for the dose-range study. Females are treated for 2 weeks prior to mating during which time estrous cycles are monitored, throughout a mating period with untreated males for 10 days' maximum duration, and throughout pregnancy. On day 21 of pregnancy, half the females per group are randomly selected for developmental toxicology assessment. A full cesarean delivery examination is made, as described for the definitive Segment II study. Fetuses are examined for external, skeletal, and visceral malformations. This protocol provides an additional assessment of the prenatal effects of the agent with treatment occurring throughout pregnancy rather than during the organogenesis period alone.

The remaining females go through natural delivery, and the times of initiation and completion of delivery are recorded. If there is an indication of delays in parturition from the dose-range study, evidenced by increased length of pregnancy or neonatal deaths on day 1, the actual delivery time per pup can be recorded in the definitive study. Offspring are maintained to day 21 of lactation, during which time survival and body weight are monitored. Dams are killed and autopsied for identification of gross lesions and the number of implantation sites in the uterus. The 21-day-old pups are also autopsied for identification of visceral malformations and morphological variations.

A frequent variation of the Segment I: Female Fertility Study is to perform behavioral testing of offspring during the preweaning and postweaning periods. Description of behavioral test methods is beyond the scope of this chapter, and the reader is referred to refs. 50 and 74 for additional information.

The same parameters are reported and analyzed for the definitive Segment I: Female Fertility Study as previously described for the Segment II study (cesarean delivery parameters) and the Segment I dose-range study.

Photography and Data Analysis

Photography is the most convenient way to produce permanent records of anomalies seen in these examinations. One method is macrophotography using a conventional 35-mm camera mounted on a stand with macrophotography lenses. This approach is reasonable for photographing external malformations and gross lesions in weanlings but may be inadequate for the degree of magnification needed for skeletal and visceral malformations. For this purpose a dissecting microscope with a camera attachment is necessary. With the dissecting microscope, several lighting modes are possible with a minimum of set-up time, greater magnifi-

cation can be achieved, and the operator can produce high quality, consistent results. The drawbacks are a loss of depth of field and a lack of versatility for other photographic applications. The unit we use is a dissecting microscope with an automatic camera equipped for substage and fiberoptic lighting.

A soft tissue section can be photographed wet or dry. For dry specimens the section is removed from the alcohol, carefully blotted dry, and placed on a nonabsorbent matte white background. A magnification is chosen that allows the specimen to fill the field (5–15×), the lighting angles adjusted to minimize the specular highlights, and the film exposed. These specimens photograph best when a combination of skim and fill lighting is used with a lighting ratio of 2:1 to 4:1, which can be achieved if fiberoptic lights are used to "pipe" the light where it is needed. Transillumination of specimens is also possible if a strong light source is available.

For black and white photographs, Tri-X Pan (400) or Plus-X films (Kodak), or their equivalent, have satisfactory accutance and contrast. Duraflo RT developer (Kodak) produces a good quality negative that prints well on grade 3 or 4 paper.

The use of filters to increase contrast in the negatives has been marginally successful in our hands. If lack of contrast is a serious problem, the sections can be counterstained with cresyl violet (62). We have found that we can produce adequate results without filtration or counterstaining. Color slides of soft tissue sections can be made with a tungsten balanced film (ET-135 Kodak) using the same photographic techniques stated above.

Photographs of skeletal anomalies are more difficult to take because of the jelly-like texture of the specimens and the specular highlights created by the glycerin solution that covers them. Transillumination of the specimens using substage lighting or off-axis illumination has produced the most satisfactory results. Diffusing the light reduces the specular problem in some instances, but it requires longer exposures and reduces contrast in the prints. An alternative is to totally immerse the specimens in glycerin, which eliminates spectral highlights but can lead to problems with maintaining the proper orientation. Records of the photographic procedure employed assists in the reproduction of any photograph and provides the laboratory with a permanent record of anomalies seen in any experiment.

The numerical data gathered in any reproductive and developmental toxicology study are extensive. There is an exponential increase in the amount of data generated compared to other toxicology studies because observations are made on approximately 10 to 15 fetuses per litter. All of these values are then entered into a final figure with the litter used as the basic unit of analysis, or the N for a given experiment. This situation is best handled by developing computer-assisted procedures for data analysis, where raw data need be entered into a file only once and then analyzed to suit the needs of the investigator. SAS Institute (80,81) statistical procedures are routinely used in our laboratory and are described below.

Body weight and food consumption data are tested using Bartlett's test or Levene's test for homogeneity of variance to determine if the groups have unequal variances at the 5% level of significance. If there is no evidence of inhomogeneity

TABLE A1. *Types and incidence of external malformations observed in 38,900 fetuses of control Sprague-Dawley rats*

Malformation	No. affected	Incidence (range)[a]	Malformation	No. affected	Incidence (range)[a]
Head (cranium)			**Tongue**		
Acephaly	0	0	Aglossia	2	0.005 (0.4–0.7)
Anencephaly	0	0	Macroglossia	0	0
Craniomeningocele	0	0	Protruding tongue	9	0.023 (0.4–1.8)
Craniorachischisis	4	0.010 (0.4–1.5)			
Exencephaly	5	0.013 (0.4–0.4)	**Trunk**		
Fonticulus open	0	0	Abdomen bloated	1	0.003 (1.6–1.6)
Hydrocephalus	13	0.033 (0.3–1.2)	Gastroschisis	2	0.005 (0.2–0.4)
Meningoencephalocele	0	0	Omphalocele	3	0.008 (0.1–0.4)
Microcephaly	0	0	Open peritoneum	2	0.005 (0.3–0.7)
Rhinocephaly	0	0	Rachischisis	0	0
Supraorbital meningocele	0	0	Short trunk	1	0.003 (0.4–0.4)
			Spina bifida	2	0.005 (0.4–0.4)
Ear			Umbilical hernia	6	0.015 (0.1–1.0)
Anotia	0	0			
Microtia	1	0.003 (0.7–0.7)	**Limb/digit**		
Low-set ear	0	0	Adactyly	0	0
			Amelia	1	0.003 (0.3–0.3)
Eye			Apodia	0	0
Anophthalmia	10	0.026 (0.3–1.5)	Brachydactyly	4	0.010 (0.7–2.2)
Buphthalmia	0	0	Club foot	1	0.003 (1.7–1.7)
Cataract	2	0.005 (0.5–0.5)	Ectrodactyly	8	0.021 (0.4–2.2)
Cyclopia	0	0	Limb flexure	0	0
Macrophthalmia/ exophthalmia	3	0.008 (0.4–1.5)	Nail absent/short	2	0.005 (1.5–1.5)
Microphthalmia	3	0.008 (0.3–1.7)	Phocomelia	4	0.010 (0.3–1.6)
Open eyelids	1	0.003 (0.7–0.7)	Pollex small	0	0
Synophthalmia	0	0	Polydactyly	7	0.018 (0.4–2.0)
			Postaxial polydactyly	0	0
Face/snout			Supernumerary limb	0	0
Facial cleft	0	0	Syndactyly	1	0.003 (0.4–0.4)
Pointed snout	3	0.008 (0.7–1.8)			
Short snout	1	0.003 (0.9–0.9)	**Tail**		
			Anury	7	0.018 (0.1–0.6)
Jaw			Brachyury	1	0.003 (0.7–0.7)
Agnathia	1	0.003 (0.7–0.7)	Kinky tail/bent tail	2	0.005 (0.7–1.7)
Micrognathia/brachygnathia	4	0.010 (0.4–1.5)	Vestigial tail	3	0.008 (0.4–1.7)
Short upper jaw	0	0			
			Anus		
Lip/mouth			Anal atresia	0	0
Asymmetrical lip	0	0	Imperforated anus	3	0.008 (0.3–1.6)
Astomia	0	0			
Harelip	1	0.003 (1.7–1.7)	**Twins**		
Microstomia	0	0	Conjoined twins	4	0.010 (0.06–0.5)
			Parasitic (thoracopagus) twins		
Nose					
Microstomia	0	0	**General**		
Dirhinia	0	0	Edema	10	0.026 (0.4–1.7)
Short nose	0	0	Hematoma	0	0
			Hemorrhagic	0	0
Palate			Lump	0	0
Cleft palate	7	0.018 (0.06–1.7)			
Cleft palate and harelip	0	0			

[a] The fetus was used as the basic unit of calculation. Incidence values were obtained by dividing the number of fetuses affected in the total population. Ranges were obtained from control groups in individual studies.

TABLE A2. *Types and incidence of visceral variations and malformations observed in 3,400 fetuses of control Sprague-Dawley rats*

Variation/malformation	No. affected	Incidence (range)[a]	Variation/malformation	No. affected	Incidence (range)[a]
Head			**Lung**		
Enlarged ventricles	8	0.24 (0.5–6.2)	Absent medial lobe	1	0.03 (0.7–0.7)
Eye			Hypoplastic	6	0.18 (1.6–5.2)
Folded retina	0	0	**Liver**		
Irregular vitreous chamber	0	0	Absent caudate	1	0.03 (0.7–0.7)
Irregular lens	0	0			
Nasal cavity asymmetrical	0	0	Diaphragmatic hernia	0	0
Olfactory bulbs underdeveloped	0	0			
			Stomach, right-sided	1	0.03 (0.7–0.7)
Heart					
Aorta			**Kidney**		
Absent descending arch	0	0	Absent	0	0
Hypoplastic	0	0	Dilated	260	7.65 (1.1–33.3)
Right-sided	0	0	Ectopic	0	0
Overriding	0	0	Fused	0	0
Fused with pulmonary artery	0	0	Small	0	0
Pulmonary artery					
Absent ductus arteriosus	0	0	**Ureter**		
Hypoplastic	0	0	Absent	0	0
Right-sided	0	0	Dilated	165	4.85 (0.7–26.7)
Fused with aorta	0	0			
Enlarged heart	0	0	**Testes**		
Levocardia	0	0	Absent	0	0
Minor vessels			Ectopic	3	0.09 (0.7–1.3)
Right subclavian under trachea	0	0			
Absent innominate	0	0	**Ovary**		
Double carotid	0	0	Absent	0	0
Tetralogy of fallot	0	0			
Ventricular septal defect	0	0			

[a] The fetus was used as the basic unit of calculation. Incidence values were obtained by dividing the number of fetuses affected in the total population. Ranges were obtained from control groups in individual studies.

of variance between groups, differences in group means are tested using a standard one-way analysis of variance (ANOVA) for each day. A repeated-measures model is used to analyze food consumption and body weight data across days. The repeated-measures ANOVA is a mixed model containing the parameters of GROUP, TIME, SUBJECT(GROUP), and GROUP*TIME, with SUBJECT(GROUP) being a random effect. If there is no significant interaction and if the data are balanced, the type III mean sum of squares for SUBJECT(GROUP) is used as the denominator of the F statistic for testing the GROUP effect and as the standard error for pairwise comparisons. When significant effects from the ANOVA are found, pairwise differences between two groups are evaluated with the Tukey's test.

If tests for homogeneity of variance indicate a lack of homogeneity, a Kruskal-Wallis (nonparametric) test is performed to determine if the treatment effects are equivalent.

When significant results are obtained from the nonparametric test, a rank sum comparison is used to determine which treatment groups differ from the control. Jonckheere's test for ordered response is performed in cases of unequal variances.

Developmental toxicity is assessed by evaluating the number of corpora lutea, implants, resorptions, dead and live fetuses, and fetal body weight. The average numbers of corpora lutea, implants, and live fetuses are calculated for each litter. The mean of litter means is then calculated within each treatment group. Percentages of preimplantation loss, postimplantation death, and dead fetuses are calculated for each litter and averaged for the total number of litters in a treatment group. The percent of litters with two or more resorptions/dead fetuses is ascertained to measure whether resorptions are spread over litters or concentrated in a few litters. Male and female weights are recorded separately in fetal body weight measurements. Weights of individual males

TABLE A3. *Types and incidence of skeletal variations and malformations observed in 5,500 fetuses of control Sprague-Dawley rats*

Variation/malformation	No. affected	Incidence (range)[a]	Variation/malformation	No. affected	Incidence (range)[a]
Skull			**Sacral-caudal vertebrae**		
Incomplete ossification	17	0.31 (0.6–5.5)	Fused/disorganized	0	0
Large open anterior			Hypoplastic	0	0
fontanelle	1	0.02 (0.4–0.4)			
Sutural bone	0	0	**Sternal centers**		
			>6	2	0.04 (0.5–1.7)
			<6	34	0.62 (0.5–3.1)
			Fused	5	0.09 (1.5–2.9)
Cervical vertebrae			Hypoplastic	450	8.18 (0.9–26.9)
Absent (<7) arch	0	0	**Ribs**		
Bifurcated arches	0	0	12 Ribs	0	0
Extra ossification on an arch	0	0	13th Rib, small	7	0.13 (0.6–4.3)
Fused arches/centers	0	0	14 Ribs	1,336	24.29 (3.4–61.3)
Hypoplastic arches/centers	2	0.04 (0.4–0.5)	Floating ribs	0	0
Variation in shape/size	0	0	Fused ribs	1	0.02 (0.5–0.5)
			Wavy and variation in shape	21	0.38 (0.4–1.7)
			Phalanges		
Thoracic-lumbar vertebrae			Metacarpals, <4	4	0.07 (0.2–1.0)
Absent arch	0	0	Metatarsals, <5	1,049	19.07 (7.2–44.3)
Bifurcated arches	0	0	Pubis hypoplastic	0	0
Fused arches/centers	1	0.02 (0.5–0.5)	Short/bent long bones	0	0

[a] The fetus was used as the basic unit of calculation. Incidence values were obtained by dividing the number of fetuses affected in the total population. Ranges were obtained from control groups in individual studies.

and females are averaged for a given litter, and then litter means are averaged within a treatment group.

Numbers of corpora lutea, implantations, fetuses, proportion of male fetuses, and length of pregnancy are analyzed with the one-way ANOVA model for GROUP effect, and Tukey's method is used for pairwise comparisons if the variances are equivalent as determined by Bartlett's test of homogeneity. Fetal weight, birth weight, and daily pup body weight are analyzed by a nested analysis of variance with fetuses or neonates nested within dams and with dams nested within groups. If differences in groups are identified, the Dunnett's test or Tukey's test is used to determine which test group(s) differ from the control group. Male and female fetuses and neonates are tested separately.

The nonparametric one-way procedure (NPAR1WAY) is used for analyzing the rates of preimplantation loss, postimplantation death, and incidence of external, skeletal, and visceral variations or malformations. The data are transformed for analysis using the Freeman-Tukey binomial arc sine-square root transformation. The data are then analyzed with the Kruskal-Wallis test for evaluation of the GROUP effect and the Wilcoxon rank sum test for pairwise comparisons. All tests are conducted at the 5% level using SAS (80,81). The mating index and fertility index are analyzed by chi-square followed by Fisher's exact one-tail test.

Teratogenicity is assessed by first determining the percent of abnormal fetuses in a litter. Abnormalities representing major malformations, minor malformations, and variations are considered separately. In each litter the number of abnormal fetuses is divided by the total number of fetuses examined for the particular anomaly (skeletal or soft tissue). Thus if four fetuses in a litter were subjected to soft tissue analysis, and one had a soft tissue anomaly, the figure $\frac{1}{4} \times 100$, or 25%, would be the percent of fetuses with soft tissue anomalies in that litter. Skeletal and soft tissue data are usually presented separately. The percentage of litters containing at least one abnormal fetus is then calculated to ascertain if abnormalities occur throughout the litters or are concentrated in a few litters.

Developmental toxicants cause embryonic death, reduced fetal weight, and increased incidence of morphological variants, minor and major malformations. Reduced fetal weight or birth weight can also occur as a result of decreased maternal body weight gains during pregnancy, or can be secondary to fetal immaturity due to a large litter. Evaluation of maternal and fetal effects in each treatment group is necessary to identify if the agent had a selective toxicity to the conceptus. Evaluation of fetal skeletal development can provide an additional index for retarded fetal development in developmental toxicology studies. However, delayed ossifications can occur sporadically in the absence of significant fetal weight reduction. Subtle structural changes due to delayed ossification are considered reversible, as indicated by the fact that the skeletons of day 21 rat fetuses are well advanced compared to those of day 19 and 20 fetuses (1).

Contributory roles of these factors must be clearly considered before relating retarded ossification directly to the drug treatment. Insofar as slight elevations in morphological variations, minor and major malformations are frequently not statistically significant, historical control background data are invaluable in the evaluation of sporadic cases of malformations and variations. Tables A-1, A-2, and A-3 show the incidence of external, visceral, and skeletal malformations and variations observed in control Sprague-Dawley rats in studies conducted in our laboratories. In cases where slight and sporadic elevations of these malformations occur in drug-treated groups, incidences are compared to the historical control data to gain an impression of their biological significance.

ACKNOWLEDGMENTS

The authors wish to thank Mr. Tom Covatta and Mr. Scott Wright for invaluable assistance in photography and Ms. Janet Koster for excellent secretarial support.

REFERENCES

1. Aliverti, V., Bonanomi, L., Giavini, E., Leone, V. G., and Mariani, L. (1979): The extent of fetal ossification as an index of delayed development in teratogenic studies on the rat. *Teratology,* 20:237–242.
2. Anderson, E. L., and CAG (Carcinogen Assessment Group of the U.S. Environmental Protection Agency) (1983): Quantitative approaches in use to assess cancer risk. *Risk Anal.,* 3:277–295.
3. Asch, P. (1980): The influence of radiation on fertility in man. *Br. J. Radiol.,* 53:271–278.
4. Baker, T. G. (1978): Effects of ionizing radiations on mammalian oogenesis: a model for chemical effects. *Environ. Health Perspect.,* 24:31–37.
5. Bass, R., Oerter, D., Krowke, R., and Speilmann, H. (1978): Embryonic development and mitochondrial function. III. Inhibition of respiration and ATP generation in rat embryos by thiamphenicol. *Teratology,* 18:93–102.
6. Bass, R., and Neubert, D. (1980): Testing for embryotoxicity. *Arch. Toxicol.* [*Suppl.*], 4:256–266.
7. Biggers, J. D. (1975): Oogenesis. In: *Gynecologic Endocrinology,* edited by J. J. Gold, pp. 612–620. Harper & Row, New York.
8. Brent, R. L. (1972): Drug testing for teratogenicity: its implications, limitations and application to man. In: *Drugs and Fetal Development,* edited by M. A. Klingberg, A. Abramovici, and J. Chemke, pp. 31–43. Plenum Press, New York.
9. Brinster, R. L. (1975): Teratogen testing using preimplantation mammalian embryos. In: *Methods for Detection of Environmental Agents That Produce Congenital Defects,* edited by T. H. Shepard, J. R. Miller, and M. Marois, pp. 113–124. American Elsevier, New York.
10. Chung, C. S., and Myrianthopoulos, N. C. (1975): Factors affecting risks of congenital malformations. In: *The National Foundation March of Dimes, Original Articles Series,* Vol. XI, No. 10.
11. Clark, J. H. (1982): Sex steroids and maturation in the female. In: *Environmental Factors in Human Growth and Development,* edited by V. Hunt, M. K. Smith, and D. Worth, pp. 315–328. Banbury Report 11. Cold Spring Harbor Laboratory, Cold Spring Harbor, New York.
12. Department of Health and Welfare, Canada (1973): *The Testing of Chemicals for Carcinogenicity, Mutagenicity and Teratogenicity.* DHW, Ottawa.
13. Dobson, R. L., and Felton, J. S. (1983): Female germ cell loss from radiation and chemical exposures. *Am. J. Industr. Med.,* 4:175–190.
14. Edmonds, L., Hatch, M., Holmes, L., Kline, J., Letz, G., Levin, B., Miller, R., Shrout, P., Stein, Z., Warburton, D., Weinstock, M., Whorton, R. D., and Wyrobek, A. (1981): Report of panel II: guidelines for reproductive studies in exposed human populations. In: *Guidelines for Studies of Human Populations Exposed to Mutagenic and Reproductive Hazards,* edited by A. D. Bloom, pp. 37–110. March of Dimes Birth Defects Foundation, White Plains, New York.
15. EPA (U.S. Environmental Protection Agency) (1983): *Quantitative Risk Assessment of Reproductive Risks Associated with Polychlorinated Biphenyl Exposure.* EPA, Office of Pesticides and Toxic Substances, Washington, D. C.
16. EPA (U.S. Environmental Protection Agency) (1986): Guidelines for the health assessment of suspect developmental toxicants. *Fed. Regul.,* 51:34028–34040.
17. EPA-ORNL (U.S. Environmental Protection Agency and Oak Ridge National Laboratory) (1982): *Assessment of Risks to Human Reproduction and to the Human Conceptus from Exposure to Environmental Substances,* pp. 99, 111. Report No. EPA–600/9–82–001. EPA, Washington, D.C.
18. Espey, L. L. (1978): Ovulation. In: *The Vertebrate Ovary,* edited by R. E. Jones, pp. 503–532. Plenum Press, New York.
19. Espey, L. L. (1980): Ovulation as an inflammatory reaction—a hypothesis. *Biol. Reprod.,* 22:1011–1020.
20. Fabro, S., Shull, G., and Brown, N. A. (1982): The relative teratogenic index and teratogenic potency: proposed components of developmental toxicity risk assessment. *Teratogenesis Carcinog. Mutagen.,* 2(1):61–76.
21. FDA (U.S. Food and Drug Administration) (1966): *Guidelines for Reproduction Studies for Safety Evaluation of Drugs for Human Use.* FDA, Washington, D.C.
22. FDA (U.S. Food and Drug Administration) (1980): Caffeine; deletion of GRAS status, proposed declaration that no prior sanction exists, and use on an interim basis pending additional study. *Fed. Regul.,* 45:69817–69838.
23. Food and Drug Administration (FDA) Advisory Committee on Protocols for Safety Evaluation, Panel on Reproduction (1970): Report on reproduction studies in the safety evaluation of food additives and pesticide residues. *Toxicol. Appl. Pharmacol.,* 16:264–296.
24. Felton, J. S., Kwan, T. C., Wuebbles, B. J., and Dobson, R. L. (1978): Genetic differences in polycyclic aromatic hydrocarbon metabolism and their effects on oocyte killing in developing mice. In: *Developmental Toxicity of Energy Related Pollutants,* edited by D. Mahlum, M. Skiov, P. Hackett, and F. Andrew, pp. 1526–1532. DOE Symposium Series 47. Technical Information Center, U.S. Department of Energy, Washington, D.C.
25. Frankos, V. H. (1985): FDA perspectives on the use of teratology data for human risk assessment. *Fundam. Appl. Toxicol.,* 5:615–625.
26. Fraser, F. C. (1977): Relation of animal studies to the problem in man. In: *Handbook of Teratology, General Principles and Etiology,* Vol. 1, edited by J. G. Wilson and F. C. Fraser, pp. 75–96. Plenum, New York.
27. Gondos, B. (1978): Oogonia and oocytes in mammals. In: *The Vertebrate Ovary,* edited by R. E. Jones, pp. 83–120. Plenum Press, New York.
28. Haney, A. F. (1985): Effects of toxic agents on ovarian function. In: *Endocrine Toxicology,* edited by J. A. Thomas, K. S. Korach, and J. M. McLachlin, pp. 181–210. Raven Press, New York.
29. Heinonen, O. P., Slone, D., and Shapiro, S. (1977): *Birth Defects and Drugs in Pregnancy,* pp. 127, 450. Publishing Sciences Group, Littleton, Massachusetts.
30. Hertig, A. T., and Barton, B. R. (1973): Fine structure of mammalian oocytes and ova. In: *Handbook of Physiology. Section 7: Endocrinology. Vol. II: Female Reproductive System,* part 1, edited by R. O. Greep and E. B. Astwood, pp. 317–348. American Physiological Society, Washington, D. C.
31. Hogan, M. D., and Hoel, D. G. (1982): Extrapolation to man. In: *Principles and Methods of Toxicology,* edited by A. W. Hayes, pp. 724–727. Raven Press, New York.
32. Hull, D., Dobbing, J., Miller, R. W., Naftolin, F., Ounsted, M., Rehder, H., Robinson, J. S., Tudge, C., and Usher, R. H. (1978): Definition, epidemiology, identification of abnormal fetal growth: group report. In: *Abnormal Fetal Growth: Biological Bases and Consequences,* edited by F. Naftolin, pp. 69–83. Dahlem Konferenzen, Berlin.
33. Hytten, F. E. (1984): Physiological changes in the mother related to drug handling. In: *Drugs and Pregnancy,* edited by B. Krauer, p. 7. Academic Press, New York.

34. IRLG (Interagency Regulatory Liaison Group), Epidemiology Work Group (1981): Guidelines for documentation of epidemiologic studies. *Am. J. Epidemiol.,* 114:609–613.

35. IRLG (Interagency Regulatory Liaison Group), Testing Standards and Guidelines Work Group (1981): *Recommended Guidelines for Teratogenicity Studies in the Rat, Mouse, Hamster or Rabbit.* Publication No. PB-82-119 488. National Technical Information Service, Springfield, Virginia.

36. Johnson, E. M. (1980): A subvertebrate system for rapid determination of potential teratogenic hazards. *J. Environ. Pathol. Toxicol.,* 4(5):153–156.

37. Johnson, E. M., and Gable, B. E. G. (1983): An artificial "embryo" for detection of abnormal developmental biology. *Fundam. Appl. Toxicol.,* 3:243–249.

38. Karnofsky, D. A. (1965): Mechanism of action of certain growth-inhibiting drugs. In: *Teratology: Principles and Techniques,* edited by J. G. Wilson and J. Warkany, pp. 185–194. University of Chicago Press, Chicago.

39. Kavlock, R. J., Chernoff, N., and Rogers, E. H. (1985): The effect of acute maternal toxicity on fetal development in the mouse. *Teratogenesis Carinog. Mutagen.,* 5:3.

40. Khera, K. S. (1984): Maternal toxicity—a possible factor in fetal malformations in mice. *Teratology,* 29:411–416.

41. Khera, K. S. (1985): Maternal toxicity: a possible etiologic factor in embryo-fetal deaths and fetal malformations of rodent-rabbit species. *Teratology,* 31:129–136.

42. Kimmel, C. A., and Wilson, J. G. (1973): Skeletal deviations in rats: malformations or variations? *Teratology,* 8:309.

43. Kimmel, C. A., and Trammell, C. (1981): A rapid procedure for routine double staining of cartilage and bone in fetal and adult animals. *Stain Technol.,* 56:271–273.

44. Kimmel, F. A., Holson, J. F., Hogue, C. J., and Carlo, G. L. (1984): *Reliability of Experimental Studies for Predicting Hazards to Human Development.* NCTR Technical Report for Experiment No. 6015.

45. Kline, J., Stein, Z., Strobino, B., Susser, M., and Warburton, D. (1977): Surveillance of spontaneous abortions: power in environmental monitoring. *Am. J. Epidemiol.,* 106:345–350.

46. Knobil, B. (1980): The neuroendocrine control of the menstrual cycle. *Recent Prog. Horm. Res.,* 36:53–88, 1980.

47. Koeter, H. B. (1983): Relevance of parameters related to fertility and reproduction in toxicity testing. *Am. J. Industr. Med.,* 4:81–86.

48. Lamb, J. C., IV, and Chapin, R. E. (1985): Experimental models of male reproductive toxicity. In: *Endocrine Toxicology,* edited by J. A. Thomas, K. S. Korach, and J. A. McLachlan, pp. 85–115. Raven Press, New York.

49. MacLusky, N. J., and Naftolin, F. (1981): Sexual differentiation of the central nervous system. *Science,* 211:1298–1306.

50. Manson, J. M., Zenick, H., and Costlow, R. D. (1982): Teratology test methods for laboratory animals. In: *Principles of Toxicology,* edited by A. W. Hayes, pp. 141–184. Raven Press, New York.

51. Mattison, D. R. (1983): Ovarian toxicity: effects on sexual maturation, reproduction and menopause. In: *Reproductive and Developmental Toxicity of Metals,* edited by T. Clarkson, G. Nordberg, and P. Sager, pp. 317–342. Plenum Press, New York.

52. Mattison, D. R., Shiromizu, K., and Nightingale, M. (1983): Oocyte destruction by polycyclic aromatic hydrocarbons. *Am. J. Industr. Med.,* 4:191–202.

53. Mattison, D. R. (1985): Clinical manifestations of ovarian toxicity. In: *Reproductive Toxicology,* edited by R. L. Dixon, pp. 109–130. Raven Press, New York.

54. McCann, S. M. (1982): Physiology, pharmacology and clinical application of LH-releasing hormone. In: *Recent Advances in Fertility Research, Part A: Developments in Reproductive Endocrinology,* edited by T. G. Muldoon, V. B. Mahesh, and B. P. Ballester, pp. 73–91. Alan R. Liss, New York.

55. McCann, S. M., Lumpkin, M. D., Mizunuma, H., Samson, W. K., Ojeda, S. R., and Negro-Vilar, A. (1982): Control of gonadotropin secretion by brain amines and peptides. In: *Recent Advances in Fertility Research, Part A: Developments in Reproductive Endocrinology,* edited by T. G. Muldoon, V. B. Mahesh, and B. P. Ballester, pp. 15–29. Alan R. Liss, New York.

56. McEwen, B. S. (1981): Neural gonadal steroid actions. *Science,* 211: 171–173.

57. McLachlin, J. A., Newbold, R. R., Korach, K. S., Lamb, J. C., and Suzuki, Y. (1981): Transplacental toxicology: prenatal factors influencing postnatal fertility. In: *Developmental Toxicology,* edited by C. Kimmel and J. Buelke-Sam, p. 213. Raven Press, New York.

58. Mosher, W. D. (1985): Reproductive impairments in the United States, 1965–1982. *Demography,* 22:415–430.

59. National Center for Health Statistics (NCHS) (1980): *Births, Marriages, Divorces and Deaths for 1979. Monthly Vital Statistics Report.* U.S. Department of Health, Education, and Welfare, Washington, D. C.

60. National Research Council (1983): *Risk Assessment in the Federal Government: Managing the Process.* National Academy Press, Washington, D. C.

61. Nelson, C. J., and Holson, J. F. (1978): Statistical analysis of teratologic data: problems and advancements. *J. Environ. Pathol. Toxicol.,* 2:187–199.

62. Neubert, D., Merker, H-J., and Kwasigroch, T. D., editors (1977): *Methods in Prenatal Toxicology.* PSG Publishing, Massachusetts.

63. Neubert, D., Barrach, H. J., and Merker, H. J. (1980): Drug-induced damage to the embryo or fetus: molecular and multilateral approach to prenatal toxicology. *Curr. Top. Pathol.,* 69:241–331.

64. Nisbet, I. C. T., and Karch, N. J., editors (1983): *Chemical Hazards to Human Reproduction.* Noyes Data Corp., Park Ridge, New Jersey.

65. Nishimura, H., and Tanimura, T. (1976): *Clinical Aspects of the Teratogenicity of Drugs.* American Elsevier, New York.

66. Nishimura, M. (1982): Repairability of drug-induced "wavy ribs" in rat offspring. *Drug Res.,* 32:1518.

67. Niswander, K. R., and Gordon, M., editors (1972): *The Women and Their Pregnancies: The Collaborative Perinatal Study of the National Institute of Neurological Diseases and Stroke.* Saunders, Philadelphia [originally: DHEW Publication No. (NIH) 73-379].

68. Norcross, M. A. (1983): Bureau of Veterinary Medicine to issue human food safety toxicology guidelines. *Food Chem. News,* 25(32): 3–6.

69. O'Grady, J. P., Caldwell, B. V., Auletta, F. J., and Speroff, L. (1972): The effects of an inhibitor of prostaglandin synthesis (indomethacin) on ovulation, pregnancy and pseudopregnancy in the rabbit. *Prostaglandins,* 1:97–105.

70. Ornoy, A., Salamon-Aron, J., Ben-Zur, B., and Kohn, G. (1981): Placental findings in spontaneous abortions and stillbirths. *Teratology,* 24:243–252.

71. Overstreet, J. W. (1984): Assessment of disorders in spermatogenesis. In: *Reproduction: The New Frontier in Occupational and Environmental Health Research,* edited by J. E. Lockey, G. K. Lemasters, and W. R. Keye, pp. 275–292. Alan R. Liss, New York.

72. Palmer, A. K. (1972): Specific malformations in laboratory animals and their influence on drug testing. In: *Drug and Fetal Development,* edited by M. A. Klingsbury et al., Vol. 7, p. 45. Plenum Press, New York.

73. Palmer, A. K. (1977): Incidence of sporadic malformations, anomalies and variations in random bred laboratory animals. In: *Methods in Prenatal Toxicology,* edited by D. Neubert, H. Merker, and T. Kwasigoch, pp. 52–71. PSG Publishing, Massachusetts.

74. Palmer, A. K. (1981): Regulatory requirements for reproductive toxicology: theory and practice. In: *Developmental Toxicology,* edited by C. A. Kimmel and J. Buelke-Sam, pp. 259–287. Raven Press, New York.

75. Pederson, T., and Peters, H. (1968): Proposal for a classification of oocytes and follicles in the mouse ovary. *J. Reprod. Fertil.,* 17:555–557.

76. Pratt, R. M., and Salomon, D. S. (1981): Biochemical basis for the teratogenic effects of glucocorticoids. In: *The Biochemical Basis of Chemical Teratogenesis,* edited by M. R. Juchau, pp. 179–199. Elsevier/North Holland, New York.

77. Richards, J. S. (1980): Maturation of ovarian follicles. *Physiol. Rev.,* 60:51–89.

78. Richards, J. S., and Bogvich, K. (1980): Development of gonadotropin receptors during follicular growth. In: *Functional Correlates of Hormone Receptors in Reproduction,* edited by Maresh, Muldoon, Saxena, and Sadler, pp. 223–244. Elsevier/North Holland, Amsterdam.

79. Ritter, E. J. (1977): Altered biosynthesis. In: *Handbook of Teratology, Vol. 2: Mechanisms and Pathogenesis,* edited by J. G. Wilson, and F. C. Fraser, pp. 99–116. Plenum Press, New York.

80. SAS Institute Inc. (1985): *SAS® User's Guide: Basics,* version 5 edition. SAS Institute, Cary, North Carolina.

81. SAS Institute Inc. (1985): *SAS® User's Guide: Statistics,* version 5 edition. SAS Institute, Cary, North Carolina.

82. Schardein, J. L. (1976): *Drugs as Teratogens.* CRC Press, Cleveland, Ohio.

83. Schardein, J. L., Schwartz, B. B., and Kenel, M. F. (1985): Species sensitivities and prediction of teratogenic potential. *Environ. Health Perspect.,* 61:55–62.

84. Sheehan, D. M., Branham, W. S., Medlock, K. L., Olson, M. E., and Zehr, D. (1980): Estrogen plasma binding and regulation of development in the neonatal rat. *Teratology,* 21:68A.

85. Shepard, T. H. (1980): *Catalog of Teratogenic Agents,* 3rd ed. Johns Hopkins University Press, Baltimore.

86. Shepard, T. H. (1986): Human teratogenicity. *Adv. Pediatr.,* 33: 225–268.

87. Smith, C. G., and Gilbeau, P. N. (1985): Drug abuse effects on reproductive hormones. In: *Endocrine Toxicology,* edited by J. A. Thomas et al., pp. 249–267. Raven Press, New York.

88. Staples, R. E. (1975): Definition of teratogenesis and teratogens. In: *Methods for Detection of Environmental Agents That Produce Con-genital Defects,* edited by T. H. Shepard, J. R. Miller, and M. Marois, pp. 25–26. American Elsevier, New York.

89. Strobino, B. R., Kline, J., and Stein, F. (1978): Chemical and physical exposure of parents: effects on human reproduction and offspring. *J. Early Hum. Dev.,* 1:371–399.

90. Szabo, K. T., and Brent, R. L. (1975): Reduction of drug-induced cleft palate in mice. *Lancet,* 1:1296–1297.

91. Takizawa, K., and Mattison, D. R. (1983): Female reproduction. *Am. J. Industr. Med.,* 4:17–30.

92. Taylor, P. (1986): *Practical Teratology.* Academic Press, London.

93. Tokuhata, G. (1968): Smoking in relation to infertility and fetal loss. *Arch. Environ. Health,* 17:353–359.

94. Warburton, D., and Fraser, F. C. (1964): Spontaneous abortion risks in man: data from reproductive histories collected in a medical genetics unit. *Hum. Genet.,* 16:1.

95. Wilson, J. G. (1965): *Teratology, Principles and Techniques.* University of Chicago Press, Chicago.

96. Wilson, J. G. (1973): *Environment and Birth Defects.* Academic Press, New York.

97. Woo, D. C., and Hoar, R. M. (1972): Apparent hydronephrosis as a normal aspect of renal development in late gestation of rats: the effects of methyl salicylate. *Teratology,* 6:191–196.

Principles and Methods of Toxicology, Second Edition, edited by A. Wallace Hayes, Raven Press, Ltd., New York © 1989.

CHAPTER 12

Inhalation Toxicology

Gerald L. Kennedy, Jr.

Haskell Laboratory for Toxicology and Internal Medicine, E. I. DuPont de Nemours and Company, Newark, Delaware 19711

The interactions between man and the materials that make up his environment occur continually with each having an influence on the other. With chemicals and physical agents, the response of the living organism comes after contact with the agent. There are three main routes by which man can come into contact with these agents: a material can land on his body surface (dermal exposure), it can be swallowed after contact with the mouth and oral cavity (oral exposure), and it can be breathed through the nose, mouth, and into the lungs (inhalation exposure). Through each route, an amount of the chemical or its converted form (metabolite) presents itself to the interior of the body and offers a chance for interaction with body cells, tissues, organs, and organ systems. Each route can and does contribute to the amount and form of chemical that gets into the system. Thus, the ultimate response of the organism will be to the integrated amount and form of the agent as it is received into the body from all three major entry points.

Because the lungs form a unique link between the blood supply of the body and the external environment, an understanding of the factors that can modify their function is of great importance to the toxicologist. Materials entering the lung have, by virtue of the rich vasculature of the organ, ready access to the internal milieu of the body. External influences that act to interfere with the operation of the respiratory system thus have profound effects on the organism which can be reflected by the full spectrum of unwanted responses ranging from minor irritation to death.

This chapter focuses on the methods used in measuring the effects of chemicals and physical agents on the respiratory system as the agents are presented through the air supply and inhaled into the lungs. The focus is not on describing the many types of physical and chemical changes that can be produced by agents, but selected examples of these interactions are presented that demonstrate applications of the experimental methodologies. Most of these examples are drawn from chemical agents, as these are the materials with which the author is most familiar, but the methods and principles apply to both chemical and physical agents. The chapter is intended to give the reader an overview of the principles and methods used in inhalation toxicology. A selected bibliography is provided at the end of the chapter for the reader who is interested in a more in-depth treatment of the material presented here.

ANATOMY AND FUNCTION OF THE RESPIRATORY TRACT

A brief discussion of the anatomy, function, and physiology of the mammalian respiratory system is presented here in order to clarify some of the complexities which face the inhalation toxicologist. The respiratory system can be simplified into three major components: (a) nasopharyngeal, (b) tracheobronchial, and (c) pulmonary. This is not the only system which can be used to compartmentalize the respiratory organs (for example, the physician might think in terms of large airways, small airways, the acinus, and the blood vessels), but it does serve to distinguish anatomically the various components of the system (Fig. 1).

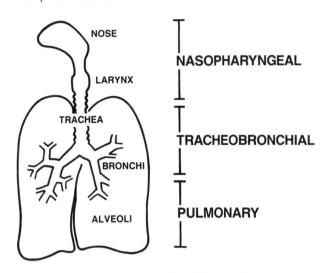

FIG. 1. Compartmental model of the respiratory tract.

The nasopharyngeal structure includes the turbinates, epiglottis, glottis, pharynx, and larynx. This is the entry port for inspired air. The region serves to remove the larger inhaled particles (through impaction in the turbinates and filtration by nasal hairs) and to condition the incoming air. The importance of this area is often overlooked but since it deals with the highest chemical concentrations, this oversight is inappropriate.

The tracheobronchial component delivers inspired air to the deeper portions of the lung, and includes branching ducts which begin at the trachea and end at the terminal bronchioles. Surfaces here are covered with mucus-secreting goblet cells and ciliated columnar cells which form a mucociliary blanket. This mucociliary blanket moves to the oral region (it is often referred to as the mucociliary "escalator"), and serves to move inspired particulate material from the bronchi and trachea to the back of the mouth where the material can be collected prior to swallowing or expectoration. These branching ducts continue to condition the inspired air by warming it to body temperature and saturating it with water vapor.

The pulmonary component is composed of respiratory bronchioles, alveolar ducts, and alveoli. The alveoli is the functional gas exchange unit of the lung and brings inspired air into direct contact with circulating blood and lymph. Oxygen diffuses from the inspired air in the lung through the alveolar-capillary membrane. After dissolution in plasma, oxygen then diffuses into the red blood cell where, bound to hemoglobin, it can be transported to tissues. The reverse diffusion of carbon dioxide occurs for presentation to and removal with the expired air.

A number of special cells and tissues of the respiratory tract deserve mention. The rear portions of the nose, the larynx, the trachea, the bronchi, and the bronchioles are lined by ciliated mucosa. Interspersed in these cells are columnar goblet cells which manufacture and secrete mucus. The alveolus itself has walls formed by very thin epithelial cells. Two such cell types have been described, the type I and type II cell. The type I cell is very thin, has a smooth surface, and covers the greatest part of the respiratory epithelium. The type II cell contains numerous microvilli, and manufactures and secretes surfactant(s) which serves to reduce the tendency for alveolar collapse.

Another major cell type found in the lung is the alveolar macrophage. This is a large, nucleated cell which functions to engulf foreign materials. These cells are very efficient particle removers and their location on the alveolar surfaces suggests an important function in preserving the sterility of the deep lung. The function of macrophages can be affected by airborne agents such as quartz and heavy metals and their lung-protective abilities compromised. Pulmonary instillation of 4 mg of carbon into the lung of a mouse induces a massive macrophage response within a few hours and by 24 hr the number of macrophages increases 10-fold (15). Alterations in macrophage numbers, viability, cell types, morphology, and changes in phagocytic capacity can be produced by chemical insult (41). The effects of inhaled gases and particulates on these defense cells are of major concern since the integrity and function of these pulmonary defense cells is important. Other mucus-secreting cells are found in the tracheobronchial tree which, along with goblet cells, functions to maintain the integrity of the mucociliary escalator.

A wide variation in the anatomy of the respiratory tract exists among the mammalian species that are often used as human surrogates for modeling purposes. One needs only to look around to see that there is also a wide variation within the human population starting from the most external part of the system. The nasal cavity of the dog, for example, can be many times longer than that of man and contains up to 25 turbinates (77). Species differences also exist in the tracheobronchial region where some species have a bronchus that branches off of the trachea near its midregion to enter a lobe of the lungs. This type of connection is seen in the goat, horse, and pig but not in man, laboratory rodents, or most other mammals. The branching patterns of the tracheobronchial tree are either monopodal or regular dichotomous. The monopodal type is characterized by long tapering airways with small lateral branches that leave the main tube at a 60° angle as seen in cats, dogs, hamsters, horses, mice, monkeys, pigs, rabbits, and rats. Regular dichotomous branching, typical of humans, involves division of a tube into nearly identical, equal-diameter smaller tubes with equal branching angles.

McLaughlin (76) classified mammalian lungs on the basis of pleural characteristics, the presence or absence of respiratory bronchioles, and the nature of the blood supply. Lung type I is characterized by a thick pleura, well-developed secondary lobulation, and marked interlobular septa and is found in the cow, pig, and sheep. Lung type II has a very thin pleura, no secondary lobulation, and poorly defined interlobular septa and is found in the cat, dog, and rhesus monkey. Lung type III, which is found in horses and man, is intermediate. When all of the anatomical features and classifications are taken into consideration, it becomes obvious that, although there are definable differences, the similarities in terms of tissues and functions between man and other mammals are remarkable.

The functional performance of the respiratory system can be estimated by measurement of lung volume and capabilities. A few definitions that are commonly encountered are presented in Table 1 (27). Measurement of breathing patterns,

TABLE 1. *Lung capacities*

Tidal volume	Volume of gas inspired or expired during each respiratory cycle
Inspiratory reserve volume	Maximum volume of gas that can be inspired from the end-inspiratory level
Expiratory reserve volume	Maximum volume of gas that can be expired from the end-expiration level
Total lung capacity	Volume of gas in the lungs at the end of maximum inspiration
Vital capacity	Maximum volume of gas that can be expelled from the lungs by forced effort following maximum inspiration
Functional residual capacity	Volume of gas remaining in the lungs upon resting

lung volumes, functional residual capacity, forced expirograms, and blood gas and pH are important in determining not only the functional ability of the lung but the actual dose of chemical received under experimental conditions (9). Obtaining reliable values for some of these parameters in many laboratory animal models is difficult because of size restrictions and the need for cooperation in maximal effort situations. The use of masks, mouthpieces, or anesthesia may alter the normal breathing patterns. Species such as the dog, horse, and sheep as well as some rodents have been trained to wear masks, or appropriate conversion factors have been employed to look at pulmonary function under normal conditions. A comparison of typical breathing patterns of a number of commonly studied species is shown in Table 2.

The relative sensitivity of pulmonary function studies to detect lung changes that would not be detected by standard toxicologic measures such as morphologic assessment has not been determined. Costa and Kutzman (29) found no functional abnormalities in rats exposed to silica dust whereas histopathologic assessment clearly differentiated exposed from background. However, rats exposed to 0.2 ppm ozone for 12 weeks showed significant flow–volume dysfunction in the absence of detectable morphologic change (30). The use of pulmonary function tests in experimental animals can serve as useful tools for the indication, identification, and quantification of chemically induced disease. These tests perform best as adjuncts to other bioassay techniques to provide a complete assessment of the potential for chemical-produced damage (28).

PULMONARY DEPOSITION AND CLEARANCE

Inspired air may contain toxic materials in many forms—gases, vapors, aerosols, and dusts. Gases and vapors dissolve throughout the respiratory tract with those of higher water solubility being removed predominantly by the upper respiratory tract. Less water-soluble materials may deposit in the deeper portions of the lung with the least soluble reaching the alveoli.

A large number of factors are involved in the deposition of particles. These mainly concern the nature of the aerosol,

the characteristics of the respiratory tract, and the breathing pattern. Characteristics of the breathing pattern which affect deposition include breathing rate and resulting air velocities, tidal volume and residual capacities, distribution within conducting channels, and breath-holding. The anatomy of the nasal, oral, and pharyngeal areas, nasal hairs, dimensions and geometry of the conducting airways from the nasal turbinates to the lower respiratory tract, size and shape of openings throughout the tract, and mucus distribution further define the characteristics of the respiratory tract that are major factors in particle deposition.

The predominant factor affecting deposition of airborne particulates is the size of the particle (Fig. 2). The motion of particles that results in their deposition is related to their size, density, and shape. Three independent mechanisms may be distinguished:

1. *Sedimentation.* Particles suspended in a gas slowly sediment under the influence of gravity. The speed at which the particle falls is proportional to the density of the particle and the square of its diameter.
2. *Diffusion.* Surrounding gas molecules bombard airborne particles, inducing random movement which results in the transfer of a gas volume from one region to another. This property is inversely proportional to particle diameter but is independent of its density.
3. *Inertia.* If the direction of air flow changes, then the inertia of any suspended particle will cause it to continue in the original direction for a certain distance, then respond to the change. This is dependent on the velocity and angle of change in airstream direction, which, in turn, is dependent on particle density and diameter squared. Impaction occurs when the inertial characteristics of the particles are such that they depart from the air line and impact on the surface. For a very long object such as a fiber, it is inevitable that one aspect or another of the fiber is going to come in contact with or be intercepted by the wall (Fig. 3).

The branching pattern of the bronchial area has two features that influence the nature of the air flow and resulting particle deposition. First, the diameter of the conducting airways becomes progressively smaller with each successive division. In man, major bronchi have diameters of 1 cm while bronchioles and alveolar ducts are 1 mm. Thus, the chances of a particle deposition in a given time due to diffusion or

TABLE 2. *Breathing patterns of commonly studied species*

Species	Size (g)	Frequency (breath/min)	Tidal volume (ml)	Minute ventilation (ml)
Man				
Rest	70,000	12	750	9000
Light exercise		17	1700	28,900
Dog	10,000	20	200	3600
Monkey	3000	40	21	840
Guinea pig	500	90	2.0	180
Rat	350	160	1.4	240
Mouse	30	180	0.25	45

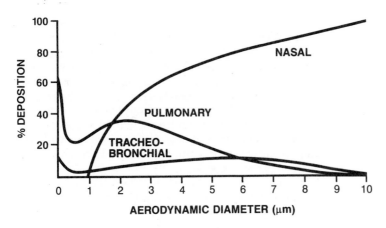

FIG. 2. Regional deposition of inhaled aerosols as a function of particle size.

sedimentation are much higher in a small airway, since it has a greater chance of contacting the boundary wall. The probability of deposition by these two mechanisms thus increases as the particle travels further into the lung. Second, since the total number of airways increases with each division, although the airway openings are small, the number of such airways is so great that the cross-sectional area is large. A given volume of air thus moves more and more slowly as it penetrates the deep lung (Table 3). Particles with a mass median diameter of 5–30 μm are deposited primarily in the nasopharyngeal region by inertial impaction; particles from 1 to 5 μm are deposited primarily in the trachea, bronchus, or bronchial regions by sedimentation; and particles less than 1 μm are deposited in the alveolar region by diffusion (21). Figure 4 shows the fractional deposition in the nose, ciliated airways, and alveoli in man.

The deposition of particulates by laboratory animals is, of course, not identical to that in man (81). Using polydisperse radioactive aerosols, total deposition in dogs, though slightly less, was in close agreement with that seen in humans (32). Nasal deposition was significantly less than that seen in man. Rats and hamsters showed deposition patterns that were similar, with particles of 1.5–2 μm being most easily deposited (87). The rodent nose was less effective at collecting particles

than the human nose. In general, the relative deposition efficiencies of various portions of the human and nonhuman respiratory tract are quite similar. When differences in lung, body size, and ventilation are considered, smaller animals inhaling the same atmospheric concentration will receive a greater dose (time constant) per unit of lung or body weight. For particles of approximately 1 μm in diameter, the rat can be expected to get a dose roughly 5–10 times and the dog about 3 times that of man on a per unit lung mass basis.

Particle clearance is related directly to the deposition site within the respiratory tract. The coarse nasal hairs filter out larger particles at the anterior of the nasopharyngeal region. Impaction and collection of particles in the nasal turbinate area results in further removal of materials from the inspired airstream. Sneezing is also an effective means of moving materials out of the respiratory system.

Irritation of the epithelial lining and other similar stimuli lead to the cough reflex which results in removal of particulate from the larger airways at the tracheobronchial level. A moving layer of mucus in the mucociliary escalator of this region continually moves deposited materials upward toward the oral cavity from which it is either expectorated or swallowed. This clearance rate may be faster in the larger rather than the smaller airways (80). Agents such as SO_2 can produce an

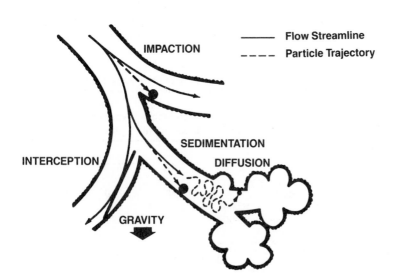

FIG. 3. Mechanisms of particle deposition.

TABLE 3. *Flow speeds in the human respiratory system*

Lung regions	No.	CS (m³)	Flow speed (cm/sec)
Main bronchi	2	1.1	180
Bronchi	770	14	14
Respiratory bronchioles	1.1×10^5	220	0.9
Alveolar sacs	5.2×10^7	1.47×10^5	0

CS, cross-section.

increase in mucus secretion which acts to slow down ciliary movement and subsequent clearance (94). Also, the mucus layer itself can dissolve substances allowing them to become absorbed into the system. The effects of inhaled materials on the nose can be classified as shown in Table 4.

Particles entering the alveolar region can be cleared by dissolution or direct passage and uptake by the vascular system, by movement into the lymphatic system, or by macrophage phagocytosis. Macrophages serve to bring the engulfed particle to the terminal bronchus to be cleared by the ciliary system or to the lymphatic drainage system. Particles may be sequestered within the alveoli as part of the condition known as pneumoconiosis.

The clearance rate for inhaled insoluble particles has been described to involve four phases (22). The first includes particles deposited in the nasopharyngeal region and reflects clearance from the upper respiratory tract. The clearance rate here is both constant and rapid with half-lives of 12–24 hr. The second phase reflects clearance of particles deposited in the lung parenchyma where clearance is primarily via the macrophage. These phagocytized particles migrate to the ciliated epithelium or to the lymphatic system at variable rates ranging from 2 to 6 weeks. A third phase can be demonstrated for some materials in which the clearance is still predominantly via the macrophage, but the time is protracted such that half-lives of many months are encountered. During this time, the action of body fluids leads to some solubilization of these stored materials. It may be that even the least soluble material shows gradual solubilization with this slow process explaining clearance phases which are measured in months to years.

The alveolar macrophage plays a significant role here (Table 5) and it has been clearly shown that certain chemicals have the ability to act directly on the macrophage to alter its clearance function. Clearly a cytotoxic material, when phagocytized, may be able to damage or destroy this cell. Silicon dioxide produces a cytotoxic response which results in the accumulation of particles in a given area. As the macrophage loses its activity these particles become less subject to removal, leading to the development of a mass which now includes dead cells and constitutes the beginning of the silicotic nodule (3).

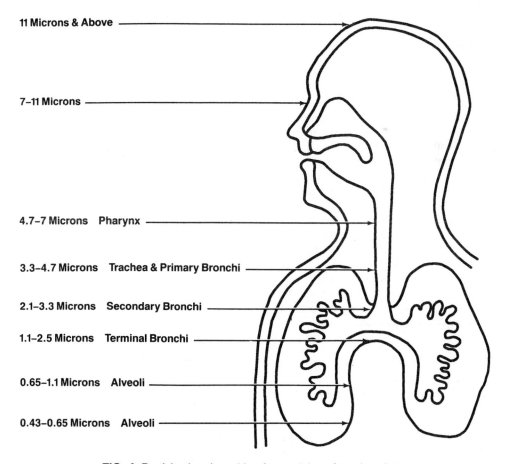

FIG. 4. Particle size deposition for particles of varying sizes.

TABLE 4. *Effects of inhaled materials on the nose*

Effect	Agent/Example
Restrict air flow	Temperature changes—cold air Irritants—acids, bases
Mucociliary flow	Slowing by SO_2, formaldehyde, methyl amines
Cellular changes/tumors	Irritants for lifetime periods (HCl, formaldehyde), organic dusts, radionuclides

Macrophages participate in pathologic processes that are classified as fibrogenic reactions (to inhaled dusts such as silica and asbestos), granulomatous reactions (to inhaled organic materials), or reactions of unknown etiology leading to emphysema. The phagocytic activity of the macrophage and its associated bactericidal activity is thus impaired by agents such as silica or cigarette smoke. The cytotoxic action of silica on the macrophage is produced by interaction with membrane phospholipids (24). Asbestos is less cytotoxic but induces secretion of hydrolytic enzymes which in part leads to a granulomatous response (33). This release of hydrolase is also encountered after exposure to beryllium which may contribute to the pathogenesis of emphysema (54).

An important, but often overlooked, principle in designing toxicology experiments to evaluate potential biologic sequelae of chemical exposure is that tolerated doses (exposures) be defined and incorporated. This is particularly important with particles that are relatively insoluble and have a low order of systemic and respiratory toxicity. It is important to determine the clearance of these particles from the lung for if clearance is impaired, particle burdens in the lung will far exceed those predicted based on data developed at lower exposure rates (36). Once the normal clearance mechanism(s) are destroyed, biologic effects could follow from the unusually high deposition rate. Recent experiments using titanium dioxide (68), antimony trioxide (37), gallium oxide (118), and diesel soot (75) point out the importance of not exceeding the lung clearance capability. This question was discussed by the National Toxicology Program and the need to determine particulate clearance was considered of prime importance (69).

To summarize, particle deposition and clearance is a complex series of interactions which depend on particle character, size, distribution within the respiratory tract, and the physiologic condition of the pulmonary tissues. Our understanding of these processes is far from complete, but the description and measurement of these processes is important in any toxicologic assessment of particulate materials.

EXPERIMENTAL INHALATION TOXICOLOGY

The potential toxic effects that need to be determined following inhalation exposure include irritation of the respiratory tract, changes in behavior, illness, pathologic change to vital organs or tissues within and distal to the respiratory tract, metabolic disturbances, carcinogenicity, and even death. Studies to measure the effects of chemical and physical agents as they enter the biological system through the respiratory tract must follow carefully designed protocols. The process of establishing exposure conditions is considerably more complex than that required for portals of entry such as oral or dermal. This is a result of the type of equipment needed to generate, maintain, and measure experimentally produced atmospheres. Further, there exists the inherent difficulty in measuring the applied dose; that is, relating the quantity of material inhaled to that absorbed or retained. The dose received depends on the physical and chemical properties of the material, the physiologic condition of the test animal, and the factors involved in deposition and clearance. One must also remember that inhalation exposures often result in simultaneous chemical exposure via the skin and the gastrointestinal tract.

Animal Models

The choice of an animal species selected for an inhalation study is an important one. It is apparent that there is no one ideal human surrogate but that each species presents its own advantages and disadvantages. Most commonly, rodents, including the rat, mouse, guinea pig, and hamster (probably in that order) are used. The extensive use of rodents in inhalation toxicology has provided a large body of background information for the investigator. Rodents have been used in toxicologic tests as models for particle deposition and clearance and as models for infectivity and immunologic function. The relative short lifespan of rodents certainly allows a reasonable approach to chronic toxicity evaluations and carcinogenesis bioassays. When extrapolating from experimental animal data to man, factors that need to be considered include the comparative anatomy of the respiratory tract, presence or absence of intercurrent diseases or infections, and similarities of the physical, biochemical, and physiologic responses.

In practice, however, selection of the test species is often based on criteria such as the size and availability of the test animals, the number of such animals needed to separate chemically induced change from background, and the expense involved in obtaining, using, and keeping these and larger numbers of animals for periods of time up to and including the total lifetime.

The guinea pig has been used in studies of the immune function and respiratory sensitization and has been particularly useful in determining the relative potencies of isocyanates (116,119). The unusually abundant bronchial smooth muscle makes this species a useful model to study bronchoconstriction.

TABLE 5. *Role of macrophages on particle clearance*

Insoluble particles	Soluble particles
Carry to mucociliary "escalator"	Dissolve
Dissolve slowly?	Engulf—to interstitium,
Carry to interstitium	lymphatics, "escalator"
Carry to lymphatics	in partial dissolution
Engulf; remain in alveoli	Little residual in alveoli

The hamster, having a relatively low spontaneous lung tumor rate and being highly resistant to pulmonary infection, has also been used in respiratory tract cancer studies. Some investigators feel that the hamster is the best animal model for the study of experimental lung cancer (91).

There are a number of major disadvantages in using the rodent to predict effects in man. The nasal/pharyngeal anatomy, with the tortuous anterior chambers, is unlike that of man and particle deposition may be quite different. These species are also obligate nose breathers, with superior nasal filtering efficiency. Assessment of pulmonary function in nonanesthetized rodents is difficult, although recent miniaturization of probes and detectors has allowed some success here (31). The most serious problems with rodents, especially rats, are those involving spontaneous respiratory infections and the sequelae.

There also exists a great deal of background data from inhalation toxicity studies on the dog, especially the beagle. The dog is a convenient size for a number of laboratory measurements including evaluation of pulmonary function. A great diversity of natural disease states exists in the dog making it a good model for evaluation of impact of the agent against such conditions as asthma. The cost and the facilities needed to properly care for the dog represent a minor disadvantage. The nasal anatomy of the dog is unlike that of humans and the subgross lung type is different. The dog may also be relatively insensitive to certain inhaled gases such as ozone (101).

The nasal anatomy of monkeys[1] is similar to humans and is sometimes used in inhalation experiments. Lung function can easily be determined. Considerable cost is involved in obtaining and maintaining monkey colonies and the lack of general availability is becoming a larger problem. The subgross pulmonary anatomy differs between types of monkeys and from that of humans (76). A potentially more serious limitation to the use of monkeys is the extreme care that must be taken to prevent the transmission of disease from monkey to man.

Other species such as the ferret, horse, donkey, sheep, cat, rabbit, and pig have been suggested for use in inhalation studies. Each of these species has been used for special applications which take advantage of a particular anatomical feature, chemical sensitivity, or research curiosity.

While the choice of animal model is seldom obvious, a compromise for general screening purposes is to use multiple species (45). This approach has been used in the testing of radionuclides (65,100), ozone (101), sulfur oxides (107), polychlorinated biphenyls (106), chlorinated hydrocarbons (86), and organofluorides (53). In the selection of an appropriate animal species, one must consider the background information available, the unique functional or structural characteristics, if any, of the species which make it a good (or bad) animal model, what the anticipated response might be that would enable the investigator to most accurately determine the number of animals needed and study duration, and finally, appropriate controls. The use of small rodents predominates because their smaller size allows testing of larger groups, their relatively short lifetime allows testing over the entire lifespan (a large body of data already exists on these species), and finally, the relatively low cost of their acquisition and upkeep.

STUDY TYPES

Evaluation of inhalation toxicity includes the determination of chemically induced changes following both short- and long-term exposures. Acute studies generally define both the amount of chemical needed to produce a given response (most often death) and the signs and symptoms associated with high exposure conditions. Longer term studies up to and including lifespan studies are conducted to determine the target organ or organ system for repeated exposures and carcinogenic potential (Table 6).

Acute studies generally involve single 4- or 6-hr exposure of small groups of rodents to the test chemical at a series of doses ranging from those producing little or no signs of response (clinical signs, body weight changes) to those producing death. The practice of using many groups and relatively many animals per group to define the LC_{50}[2] has been replaced to some extent by the determination of the approximate lethal concentration (the lowest concentration at which the first death is observed). This dramatically reduces the number of animals needed per study (from an average of 56 to 7 (58)). Another major purpose of the acute study is to help define exposure concentrations which can be used for further extended exposure studies.

A special application of the acute toxicity test relies on the fact that a large number of chemicals are sensory irritants and that animal models can be used to predict both the degree of irritancy and the relative potency. In this study animals are placed in whole-body cuffs and changes in respiration rate and pattern are recorded (1,4). Animals (usually rats or mice) are placed in small cylindrical tubes with the head protruding through a rubber dam. The neck fitting forms a relatively airtight seal which, with appropriate attachments, allows the unit to be used as a body plethysmograph. The animal in the tube is then placed with the head protruding into the exposure chamber. Following an acclimatization period, the animal is exposed to pre-equilibrated concentrations (Fig. 5) and the change in respiratory rate and pattern is determined. Each animal is exposed to a given concentration for approximately 10 min. This technique allows determination of the upper respiratory tract irritation potential in a simple and reproducible manner. The method is sensitive, appears to have a rather good correlation from animal to man, and detects irritating effects at concentrations in which pathologic changes at the light microscope level are not readily apparent.

Chemical irritants represent a very broad category of materials which are not always clearly defined. An irritant induces inflammation as a response to the noxious (irritating) stimulus. In our environment, there exist many different types

---

[1] Intraspecies differences exist so care must be taken when the species is identified as "monkey."

[2] Lethal concentration 50%, that concentration calculated to kill half of the exposed animals under the particular set of experimental conditions.

TABLE 6. *Study types for determination of inhalation toxicity*

To determine:	Duration (no. of exposures)	Examples
Acute response	Generally 1	LC_{50} (4–6 hr, sometimes shorter) ALC Sensory irritation (RD_{50})
Target organ	>1, <30	10 Doses repeated 28-Day study Increasing concentration study
Effects of chronic exposure (carcinogenic potential)	>1 month, to lifetime	2-Year rodent Lifetime rodent
Biochemical response	All of above	Lavage studies
Morphologic changes	All of above	Special microscopy; morphometrics, detailed staining
Functional capability	All of above	Pulmonary function parameters

ALC, approximate lethal concentration.

of respiratory tract irritants. Chlorine, for example, has been used as a war gas and methyl isocyanate was associated with massive accidental human exposures in India. Factors that influence the deposition of irritants in the respiratory tract include the physical and chemical characteristics of the irritant, the concentration of the irritant, regional airflow patterns and metabolism, and airway surface characteristics. The respiratory tract is a complex tube lined by protein-laden watery secretions which overlay a wide variety of epithelial cell types with variable metabolic activity. Lesions produced by irritants depend on regional deposition, exposure duration, and tissue susceptibility. Initial lesions include disturbances of mucociliary function, damage to lung surfactants, and epithelial and subepithelial damage.

Chemical irritants act on specific and different targets. For example, formaldehyde acts primarily on respiratory epithelial cells, chlorine acts on the nasal ciliae and the bronchial

functions, dimethylamine acts on olfactory sensory cells, and cigarette smoke affects the epiglottis epithelium. Furthermore, a number of disease states, including acute asphyxiations, chronic bronchitis, emphysema, pulmonary fibrosis, and pneumoconioses, can be induced or exacerbated by exposure to irritants.

Following acute studies, repeated exposure studies (subchronic—lasting 1 year or more, preferably for at least half the lifetime of the species studied) are conducted. The subchronic study precedes the chronic study and is used both to determine the target systems and to quantitate the exposure conditions associated with the changes. This also allows a preliminary estimation of the potential for cumulative toxicity. Our practice is to expose groups of animals, generally male rats, to concentrations of 1/5, 1/15, and 1/50 of the approximate lethal concentration, 6 hr per day, 5 days per week, for 2 weeks. The exposure level selection can also be based on the clinical observations seen in the acute study; for example, if it is seen that a large body weight loss follows a single 4-hr exposure at one-fifth the lethal dose, the range of exposures used in the study would be scaled downward. Animals are observed daily for signs of response; body weights are recorded weekly; clinical chemistry, hematology, and urine analysis are conducted at the end of the 10 exposures; and complete pathologic examinations including weights of selected key organs are conducted. Another group of rats is allowed a 14-day recovery period during which no additional test exposures are conducted and the above parameters are again measured to determine the reversibility of any test material-induced changes.

A variation of this approach to determine the target organ has been proposed by Calandra and Fancher (20). In their design, an increasing exposure concentration regimen is followed until severe biologic effects are observed. This provides information concerning minimal symptomatic and minimal toxic exposures, major symptoms of intoxication, duration of action, and major organs affected, but does not always allow correlating these changes with particular exposure conditions (the doses are changing).

Chronic studies add to the above information measurement of effects following extended exposures at concentra-

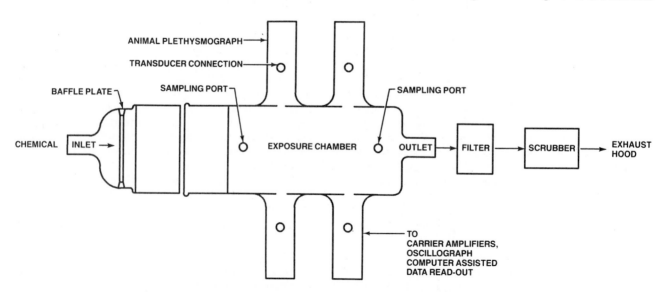

FIG. 5. Apparatus for determination of sensory irritation properties of a chemical.

tions where acute toxicity is not obvious. Here it needs to be noted that the investigator is trying to detect more subtle changes produced by chemical exposure and care must be taken to separate background noise from chemically induced effects. The need for appropriate parallel controls cannot be overemphasized. Chronic exposures usually mimic those encountered in the workplace with animals exposed 6 hr per day, 5 days per week for their lifetime. For environmental agents, exposures may be conducted around-the-clock. In both situations, the need to relate cause and effect uses fixed exposure concentrations, a situation that does not exist in either the environment or the workplace.

The end use of the data helps determine the exposure pattern. For example, investigators interested in the effects of chemicals in confined places such as a submarine would opt for continual 24-hr exposure conditions. This exposure pattern would also be preferred by those interested in setting guidelines for environmental air levels. Those needing to provide guidance for workplace situations would best be served by intermittent 6- or 8-hr per day exposure patterns.

Continuous 24-hr exposures of many species for extended periods of time to determine dose–response data for application to enclosed atmospheres has been conducted by Prendergast et al. (86) with carbon tetrachloride and by Weeks et al. (114) with ethanolamine. Changes in exposure times have been used to evaluate the effects of systemic toxicants for the purpose of setting exposure limits. The responses of rats to carbon tetrachloride following 11.5-hr exposures/day were different than those following 8 hr per day (84). Altering exposure schedules of rats from 8 hr per day for 5 days to 12 hr per day for 4 days produced both concentration- and time-dependent responses to aniline (60). Burgess (19) found that concentration was the primary determinant in a study where three aniline concentrations were tested in rats using three time periods, either 3, 6 or 12 hr per day.

Emergency releases of large volumes of biologically active materials, particularly gases or those that vaporize readily, may require more extensive testing to develop information relative to levels that can be used for evacuation purposes. These concentration profiles are designed to prevent both unwanted nonreversible injury and impairment of escape ability. To this end, we have studied the short-term lethality responses of rats to perfluoroisobutylene, a highly toxic gas, at time intervals ranging from 6 hr to 15 sec (97) and, from these data, have suggested both short- and long-term control limits (57).

The release of methyl isocyanate in Bhopal highlights the need for emergency planning measures to prevent escape of highly toxic chemicals into the community. Carefully conducted studies are needed to define exposure limits consistent with (a) survival, (b) production of irreversible damage, (c) production of reversible damage without impaired escape capability, and (d) production of no measurable damage. Short-term inhalation exposure studies are also recommended to define dose–response characteristics.

EXPOSURE TYPES

A variety of exposure types have been used to evaluate the effect of materials as they enter following respiration (Table 7). For inhalation studies where the entire animal is exposed

TABLE 7. *Exposure types used in evaluation of inhalation toxicity*

Class	Example
Common	Whole-body exposures
	Nose-only exposures
	Head-only exposures
Less common	Endotracheal intubation
	Tracheostomy
	Airway catheter
	Intratracheal instillation
	Insufflation

(whole-body exposures), the exposure chamber is essentially a jar or box containing an access for placing and removing the test animals and for introducing and removing the test chemical with provisions made to withdraw internal samples for chemical/physical analysis periodically throughout the test. This mode of operation reflects that usually encountered in the human situation; that is, the exposed individual may freely move about in an atmosphere containing the chemical such that absorption into the system only occurs through the lung following respiration, through the skin following contact with aerosols or vapors, and through the gastrointestinal tract after swallowing.

Whole-body inhalation exposures will result in the chemical being ingested regardless of physical form. Gases or vapors can dissolve in the mucus fluid lining the respiratory tract and, via the mucociliary escalator, reach the pharynx where they are swallowed. Droplets or solid particles also reach the gastrointestinal tract via this mechanism. Further contributions to total absorbed dose can be seen following dermal absorption of the test agent. The normal grooming and preening activities of rodents both during and after inhalation exposures can also deliver the chemical to the gastrointestinal tract. The quantitative aspects of both dermal and oral (preening) exposures have not been adequately studied but would be expected to vary greatly depending on the physical chemical properties of the material being studied. Rats exposed to respirable zinc chromate dust were housed either in conventional wire mesh cages or protected by fiberglass tubes so that the only exposure was through the external nares. Caged rats excreted 8.4 times as much fecal and 5.5 times as much urinary chromium as rats in the tubes, indicating that a significant amount of dust could be ingested or absorbed following whole-body exposures (63).

Conducting whole-body aerosol exposures in group-caged rodents would appear to reduce the actual amount of chemical to which each animal is exposed due to the filtering action of fur in groups of rodents huddled together. Ulrich and Marold (109) tested 3-μ aerosols of dodecyl alcohol and looked at lung and trachea concentrations in rats housed singly or in groups of 3 or 7. They found similar amounts of chemical in the lungs of each group and concluded that group housing does not appear to reduce the amount of aerosol inhaled by rats during a 6-hr whole-body exposure.

Head-only exposures are useful for repeated brief exposures, where the amount of test agent is somewhat limited, and for restricting the route of entry of the material into the animal to the respiratory tract. It is not possible for an animal to avoid inhalation exposure in this system. Disadvantages of this system include loss of material to the fur of the head, difficulty in obtaining a proper seal at the neck without impairing circulation, the possibility of restraint-induced stress to the animals, time and difficulty in handling the animals, and the limited number of animals that can be tested simultaneously. Further disadvantages are that exposures do not reflect those of workers and, to a lesser degree, the lack of standardized exposure systems.

All of the above disadvantages can be dealt with in a manner that does make this type of testing useful in safety evaluation programs. To ensure uniformity of exposure conditions on an animal-to-animal basis, a relatively large airflow is needed. This prevents animals from inhaling chemical-depleted atmospheres. For larger animals such as the dog and monkey, helmet exposures can be conducted which also require large airflows to prevent condensation, build-up of expiratory products, and chemical depletion. Pressure fluctuations in these systems may be great and records of breathing patterns during exposure may be needed to accurately measure the exposure doses. In addition, the fitting at the neck must be comfortable and easy to manipulate. Designs including both inflatable collars and thin rubber membranes have been successfully used.

Kirk et al. (61) describe a system for exposing guinea pigs to radioactive gases. The animals were placed in plethysmographs to record breathing patterns, a rubber seal isolated the head inside the exposure area, and the animals could also be immersed whole-body while breathing fresh air (if desired). Thomas and Lie (104) describe a similar system for aerosol testing in rats and mice. Dogs (103) and monkeys (93) have been tested using head-only techniques.

A typical exposure unit begins with an exposure cylinder, generally constructed from rigid plastic (or glass). This is placed inside a protective casing, the purpose of which is to allow introduction of equipment necessary to determine test concentrations, particle-size distributions, temperature/

humidity, etc. Both the cylinder and casing should be transparent to facilitate animal observations. Rodent holders consisting of Plexiglas or stainless steel cylinders (of varying sizes to accommodate rodents of differing sizes) fitted with conical head-pieces to project into holes drilled along the sides of the exposure cylinders. The holder needs to be supported carefully to minimize discomfort to the animal. This system was used successfully by Sachsse et al. (89) in their determination that the acute inhalation toxicity of five agricultural chemicals was essentially the same following head-only and whole body exposures (90).

Nose-only exposures are accomplished by attaching rodents to a dynamic chamber. Animals may breathe from chambers, large or small supply tubes, or directly from a generator such as a lighted cigarette or an exhaust pipe. Nose-only exposures limit entry of the materials to the respiratory tract, hence test material needs are reduced, the chemical can easily be contained, and test concentrations can be easily and quickly altered. Design considerations here are identical to those of head-only units. Mask designs represent a unique kind of nose-only exposure and are usually limited to relatively large animals. Masks for dogs (6), monkeys (43), ponies (74), donkeys (2), and chickens (8) have been successfully used.

It may be necessary to conduct brief or instantaneous exposure to airborne materials. This would be the case when developing data to deal with setting emergency exposure limits or when small sample quantities of materials must be pre-equilibrated prior to exposure. In our laboratory, we determined the lethal doses of perfluoroisobutylene in rats following exposure times of from 0.25 to 10 min (97). For this, we used a 1-liter cylindrical Plexiglas chamber (30" × 2" diameter) with 10 staggered animal ports and 3 sampling ports (Fig. 6). A high rate of airflow rapidly achieved chamber equilibrium. The rats were held in stainless-steel restraining tubes (Fig. 7) that were designed to facilitate loading and

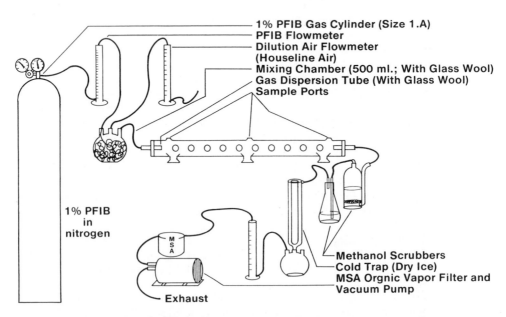

FIG. 6. PFIB generation apparatus uses for short-term responses to gases.

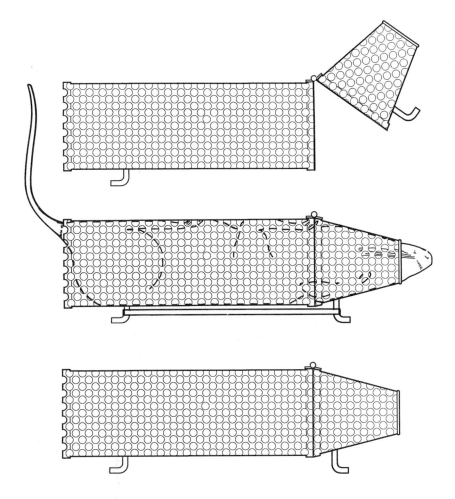

FIG. 7. Holder designed for rat head-only (or nose-only) exposures.

unloading. The front cone is hinged and, when open, allows the animal to walk out of the cylinder.

Sliding airlock mechanisms have been used to achieve essentially instantaneous exposures. One simple design is the drop-away headspace compartment shown in Fig. 8. Here animals are restrained and placed in slots which allow their heads to protrude into the exposure chamber. Prior to exposure, a headspace compartment is held in place over the head, allowing circulation of fresh air to the animals. Atmospheres are premixed to the desired concentration and the flap is dropped away to expose instantaneously. This design is inexpensive and easy to construct.

This apparatus was used to compare irritating and lethal concentrations of stannic chloride. Stannic chloride reacts with moisture in the air to form an irritant smoke which has been proposed to test for respirator fit in workers. In rats given a 1-min exposure (similar to the duration of an actual fit test), marked respiratory irritation and no mortalities were observed. With a 10-min exposure interval, respiratory irritation and mortality occurred—more importantly, in overlapping concentration ranges. On this basis, we decided that an insufficient safety margin existed for general use of stannic chloride irritant smoke to test respirator fit in workers (18).

Large-scale testing using head-only exposures has been conducted (99) in 0.5 m³ pyramidal vertical flow chambers which accommodated up to 60 rats per chamber. Rats were exposed to fibrous aerosols for 6 hr per day, 5 days per week for up to 24 months with relatively little test-condition-related stress as measured by growth, body temperature, and plasma corticosteroid levels. The amount of manpower needed to accomplish this, following training so that the tasks became routine, was not considered excessive.

Endotracheal intubation, tracheostomies, and airway catheters can be used to bypass the upper airway and expose only the lung to aerosols and gases. Endotracheal tubes are made of flexible rubber and are passed through the mouth to the trachea and are sealed by inflation of a balloon placed at the tip of the tube. A high degree of control of total dose delivered can be obtained, which is helpful when studying extremely toxic or expensive materials. Many disadvantages, including loss of natural upper respiratory tract defense mechanisms, mechanical complications, and interference with normal airflow characteristics, lead to a relatively nonphysiologic animal preparation that makes extrapolation from these data tenuous.

Tracheostomy generally has the same applications, advantages, and disadvantages. Airway catheters allow deep penetration into the lung and can be used to deliver very exact doses to specific localized sites. Examples of experiments involving endotracheal tubes include studies with exposure to radioactive metal fume aerosols (85), to fresh cigarette smoke (5), and to radioactive tantalum dust (14).

A comment on the use of intratracheal instillation as an alternative to exposure of animals by inhalation needs to be

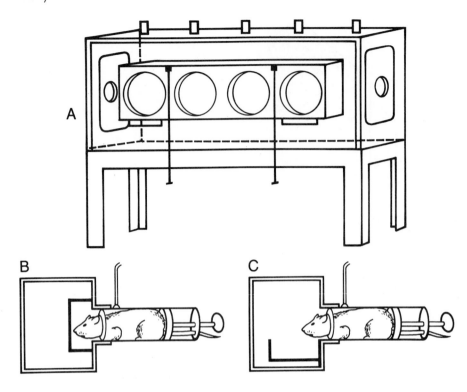

FIG. 8. Airlock exposure chamber for instantaneous exposures. **A:** Front view. **B:** End view, atmosphere preequilibrated while rats breathe fresh air. **C:** Airlock dropped for instantaneous exposure.

included here. This technique is extremely inexpensive in that small amounts of chemical are needed and expensive chambers, generating apparatus, and manpower support are avoided. High concentrations of test agent can be placed directly in contact with lung tissue and the delivered dose can be accurately controlled. The serious problem which limits its usefulness is that the distribution of dose to the respiratory tissue is highly artificial and does not accurately reflect lung distribution of chemical following inhalation exposures.

Deposition following inhalation is focal, i.e., inhaled particles deposit at selected sites in the distal lung. Subsequently, particles interact with complement proteins which are components of the surface lining layer of the distal lung generating chemotactic factors as a by-product of this reaction (112). These factors then serve to recruit pulmonary macrophages to the sites of particle deposition. Brain and co-workers (16) showed that intratracheal instillation of particles produced nonuniform deposition patterns which favored a greater dependence on gravitational settling. These investigators studied the distribution of particles labeled with ^{99m}Tc in both rats and hamsters following either intratracheal injection or aerosol inhalation. Particle distribution patterns in the lung following inhalation were evenly distributed and most of the dust deposited in apical lobes. Using electron microscopic techniques, Brody and Roe (17) have shown that inhaled particles and fibers, which are small enough to pass through the conducting airways, deposit at selective sites (i.e., alveolar duct bifurcations) in the distal lung. This preferential deposition pattern has been confirmed by Warheit et al. (113) in several rodent species, and substantiates the idea that the initial distribution patterns of inhaled particulates appear to be focal. Subsequently, particles may distribute throughout the alveolar regions during lung clearance.

As a consequence of these cellular and biochemical reac-

tions, it is clear that intratracheal instillations are relatively nonphysiologic with respect to the deposition patterns and create an artifactual series of cellular (macrophage) reactions which do not accurately reflect the events that occur following inhalation exposure to dusts.

CHAMBER OPERATION

Early inhalation experimentation utilized chambers that were made of glass walls in a wooden frame (52), or plywood and metal coated with a chemically resistant plastic (106), or were entirely of sheet metal (120). Acrylic chambers used by Gage (40), Montgomery et al. (78), and Laskin and Drew (64) were assembled from commercially available items. The Laskin and Drew chamber was portable, permitted food and water consumption determinations, and could accommodate up to 25 rats in a total volume of about 90 liters.

Larger units described by Fraser et al. (39) introduced solid aerosols through the bottom of the chamber and exhausted at the top. A plastic hexagonal prism of 2.7 m^3 was used (115) for dust studies and included a turntable allowing animals to be brought to the access windows for observation during the exposures. Wedge-shaped cages contained in plastic hemispheres were used to minimize loss of airborne agent through adsorption on the walls (102). This unit was about 3 m^3 and could expose 100 hamsters at a time.

Conventional chambers are constructed with stainless steel and have transparent observation ports of plastic or glass. Both stainless steel and glass are well-suited as chamber construction materials due to their excellent chemical resistance and their low adsorption characteristics. The Rochester chamber design described by Leach et al. (66) consists of a hexagonal prism fitted at the gases with hexagonal pyramids.

This design was shown to have two characteristics that are essential for accurate inhalation studies: good airflow pattern and uniform contaminant distribution. The chamber as originally designed also allows for good visibility of the test animals and could house simultaneously 8 dogs, 4 monkeys, and 40 rats. Hinners et al. (51) found the hexagonal construction to be unnecessary and obtained satisfactory performance using chambers with a square cross-section. This design provides a large access door for efficient animal loading, large windows for animal observations, appropriate sampling ports, control of air and contaminant flows, a slight negative pressure to prevent outward leaking, signal devices for equipment failure, temperature and humidity control, and has interior surfaces of stainless steel which prevent corrosion and facilitate cleaning.

Horizontal flow chambers can be constructed that seem to be comparable to vertical feed chambers in concentration gradient characteristics, but require higher flow rates to maintain test atmospheres. A system described by Hemenway and MacAskill (46) utilizes an inlet and outlet baffle/plenum configuration which, along with premixing of the test agent, allows achievement of a uniform exposure. Fecal catch pans do not interfere with the chamber concentrations, thus eliminating exposure of animals to fecal debris from above (82). The chambers also allow a higher packing density of animals for the volume occupied due to the lack of large inlet and outlet cones. These chambers can fit into most conventional animal rooms without major modification. The chambers are extremely sensitive to variations in chemical flow rates, hence the system could find application in experiments in which pulse dose/recovery responses are measured. Ferin and Leach (38) describe a horizontal flow unit comprised of four modules for air supply, contaminant addition, animal exposure, and exhaust. High air flow rates result in laminar flow entering the module becoming turbulent as it passes through the animal cages.

Most inhalation experiments utilize dynamic exposure conditions. Animals are placed in the exposure chamber and the generation apparatus is turned on. The concentration in the chamber rises rapidly to a theoretical equilibrium value which is the ratio of the flow of agent to the total flow in the chamber. The equation describing the concentration–time curve is:

$$Ct = f/F(1 - \exp{-F/V} \times t)$$

where Ct is concentration after t minutes, f is the flow of agent, F is total flow through the chamber, and V is the chamber volume. This is usually converted to an expression that defines the time required to attain a given percentage of the equilibrium concentration:

$$t_x = K \times V/F$$

where t_x is the time required to attain $x\%$ of the equilibrium concentration and K is a constant whose value depends on x. Most frequently the concentration–time relationship is described by $t(99)$, the time needed to attain 99% of the theoretical equilibrium concentration. For this, $K = 4.605$. At this point, the concentration in the chamber may be considered as constant. The concentration–time characteristics of a given chamber are described by the values of V and F, not by the outdated practice of giving air changes per hour (72,97).

The duration of exposure is defined as the interval from the start of flow of test agent to the point where delivery is discontinued. The exposure thus is terminated by stopping the flow of agent which leads to the decline in the chamber on an exponential curve that is the inverse of the rising curve (Fig. 9). Animals are not removed from the chamber (nor are the chamber doors opened to observe or treat the animals) until at least $t(99)$ min. For longer term exposures, the rising and falling curves can be neglected and the exposure is a square-wave form. For short exposures where t is less than $13 \times t(99)$, the system should include an airlock mechanism or some other instant expose/nonexpose mechanism (71).

Chambers should be operated at -2 cm H_2O pressure with respect to room pressure to protect personnel against leaks in the system. Pressure should be tested continually, especially in older units. The distribution of test agent within the chamber is determined carefully by using statistically valid sampling strategies to avoid the possibility of concentration gradients. After the proper distribution of test agent within the chamber has been established, the actual concentration should be measured several times during the exposure. For exposures of 4–6 hr, a common practice is to sample every 0.5 hr (or at least hourly). Continuous readout instruments are especially useful in long-term studies, for they are capable

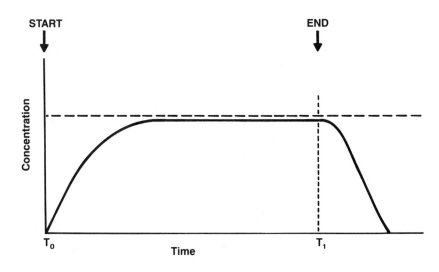

FIG. 9. Exponential concentration chamber build-up and decline.

of preventing anything greater than momentary excursions when appropriate alarms are integrated into the system. This single instrument can thus prevent many weeks or months of effort from being destroyed by sudden, prolonged upward concentration excursions.

Inhalation chambers operated in a dynamic mode should have a reasonably uniform distribution of test chemical throughout to avoid differential animal exposures. Variations exist in conventional chamber designs and also in the more unusual equipment involving modifications to improve distribution. It is generally felt that the concentration of gases and vapors shows less intrachamber variation than respirable aerosols. However, MacFarland (73) calculated the percentage differences and considers the deviations encountered under normal test conditions to be similar. Examples from the literature concerning the degree of variability encountered are presented in Table 8. Variations obviously do exist in all chamber types; hence the investigator is well advised to carefully characterize the distribution of test agent in the chamber under generating conditions to prevent concentration gradient errors from entering the experiment.

Actual concentrations measured in the chamber show variation within any single exposure or between exposure days. The control of vapor concentration is somewhat more readily obtained than that of aerosols and, after a few weeks of experience with most vapor generators, the standard deviation on a series of measurements through the day and from day to day should not vary by more than 10%. Variations of as much as 20% are commonly encountered with aerosols, particularly solid aerosols, and while this may be considered acceptable, greater control is usually possible.

The actual dose delivered to the target tissue depends on factors other than concentration. Breathing rates, respiratory volumes, and anatomic variations, for example, can be greater than the variation in concentration in terms of delivered dose. In long-term studies, if a chamber reached only 60–70% of the target value for one particular exposure day, this does not suggest that the study is invalid in terms of quantitative dose. The total accumulated exposure (concentration × time) should approach that specified in the experimental design,

but an occasional value of 40 or even 50% above or below the target value is not sufficient reason to terminate a study (35).

Air flow to a chamber can vary from approximately 10 to 60 changes per hour. This must be carefully defined as the addition and withdrawal of a volume of air equal to the volume of the chamber. Since added air mixes with that already present, a complete change of air has not occurred. The term "air change" is misleading, and the dynamics of mixing in inhalation chambers can be described by the statistical considerations first put forward by Silver (97).

Although used infrequently, the static method can generate useful comparative toxicity information. In this method, animals are exposed in a sealed chamber. Only materials that are gases or vapors at room temperature may be studied in this fashion. The substance is either injected through a sealable port or released from within the chamber (70) with the concentration rising to a rapid peak and slowly declining. The exposures of necessity can be at most 30–60 min, since CO_2 and internal temperatures rise rapidly depending on both the size of the jar and the number of animals contained therein. This method is also of some use when the availability of the test chemical is limited.

Control of the internal temperature of inhalation chambers is crucial to the proper conduct of animal inhalation studies. Elevated temperatures can alter animal physiology, affect metabolic rates, and increase chemical interactions. The volume of animals in a chamber should not exceed 5% of the chamber volume to avoid heat-induced problems. Even large chambers require that inlet air be cooled to maintain normal interior temperatures. Heat balance studies with rats in stainless steel and glass chambers of equal size and using a room air intake of 100 liters/min showed that the chamber walls were effective at removing approximately 90% of the animal body heat as compared with the airstream. With low flow rates, the heat transfer to the surrounding environment can be increased by painting the chambers, attaching cooling coils to the chamber walls, or by directing air conditioning ducts directly onto the chamber (12).

ADMINISTERED DOSE

Inhalation experiments present the investigator with the most difficulty in terms of expressing the dosage that is being tested. In this case, the dose needs to be expressed in terms of both concentration and time since the amount potentially inhalable depends heavily on these two factors. Dose is considered administered if the agent enters and remains in the respiratory tract regardless of absorption, since the lumina of the alveoli are, strictly speaking, outside the body, and transfer across the alveolar membrane would have to occur to bring the agent "into" the body. The actual dose the animal receives is related to the atmospheric concentration, individual respiratory physiology, and duration of the exposure. Dosage in inhalation studies is generally expressed as the concentration and time of exposure; for example, "rats were exposed to 'x' ppm of chemical 'y' for 6 hours a day, 5 days a week, for 13 weeks." For gases and vapors, the concentration may be expressed as percent, parts per million, or parts per billion. For dusts and aerosols (and gases and vapors)

TABLE 8. *Intrachamber variation reported in inhalation studies*

Test chemical	Physical form	% Difference from average concentration	Refs.
Ammonium fluorescein	Aerosol	3.0–7.6	102
Asbestos	Fiber	3.3–7.4	105
Carbon monoxide	Gas	0.7	50
Chlorine	Gas	2.1	97
Cobalt metal	Aerosol	11.7	39
Diesel exhaust	Aerosol	14.3–16.7	96
Formaldehyde	Gas	5.1	59
Methane	Gas	4.3	111
Nitrogen dioxide	Gas	4.3	110
Ozone	Gas	7.4	55
Sulfuric acid	Aerosol	3.4–18.0	11, 51
Sulfur colloid of technicium	Aerosol	9	11
Sulfur dioxide	Gas	14.9	50

concentrations are expressed in terms of milligrams per liter or per cubic meter.

Haber (44) determined that the response of an animal to a gas could be related to the product of the concentration and the time exposed. The equation known as Haber's law states that the product of the concentration and time of exposure required to produce a specific physiologic effect is equal to a constant, $CT = K$. The specific physiologic effect can be something other than death, but that is the most commonly applied endpoint. There are short (but finite) periods of time during which the physiologic endpoint may never be attained [mortality may not occur at attainable concentrations in short (0.1-, 1-, 10-min time periods)]. At the other end of the time scale are exposure levels (no-observed effect) at which no changes occur following continual, extended exposures. Rinehart and Hatch (88) and Kelly et al. (56) have shown that for the gas phosgene and the aerosol titanium tetrachloride, the equation holds when the endpoints of respiratory rate and death, respectively, were applied.

ATMOSPHERE GENERATION

Gases are the simplest atmosphere to generate. They can be metered by flowmeters, syringe drives, or some other suitable technique into a calibrated dilution air stream, allowed to mix, then introduced directly into the exposure chamber. A number of flow dilution devices are available. Saltzman (92) describes an asbestos-plugged capillary tube receiving a constant pressure of contaminant gas which ensures a constant flow. The pressure is regulated by the height of a dip tube immersed in either oil or water.

Vapors of either liquid or solid compounds can be heated by a furnace (care must be taken to prevent chemical conversion) or a flask equipped with a heating mantle, and the vapors generated can be passed into the exposure chamber in either nitrogen or houseline air. Another technique, depending on physical properties such as viscosity and chemical purity, is to use an infusion pump to syringe-drive the liquid test material onto a heated surface. The resulting vaporized components are then carried via nitrogen or air into the test chamber. Other liquid materials may be vaporized in a fitted-glass bubbler prior to being carried by air or nitrogen into the exposure chamber. In all of the above, the saturated airstream can be diluted with filtered air to the desired concentration.

The generation of particulate materials in a uniform manner is more difficult than vapor generation; these materials may be generated from a dry powder or from a liquid. The resultant particles range from being homogeneous to varying greatly in size. Dispersions of liquids in air possess a size between colloidal and macroscopic and are called aerosols. Examples that occur in industrial processes include dusts, fumes, smokes, mists, clouds, and fogs. These various forms are distinguished by their physical properties, particle-size range, and source.

The physiologic effect of airborne particles is closely related to their chemical and physical properties. Since these properties are related to particle size, the significance to inhalation toxicology is great. Small particles are generally more active than large particles, and the resulting biologic effects are greatly influenced by the particles of a given size retained by the test species. Models for the study of particle retention and elimination in the lung have been developed. Factors that influence deposition are indicated in general terms with no sharp demarcation between them. The term *aerodynamic diameter* describes the behavior of a unit density sphere in air. A particle exhibiting the same aerodynamic motion will be assigned that aerodynamic size regardless of actual size and shape. A detailed discussion of lung particle retention and deposition is given by Morrow (80).

The special need in toxicologic studies to express aerosol concentrations in terms of quantity as well as particle size should be stated. Size distribution should be given in terms of mass rather than size frequency for each size class. When particles are classified on the basis of their airborne behavior, the aerodynamic mass median diameter, which refers to the size of a unit density sphere having the same settling velocity as the particle in question, is used.

The generation of aerosols using dry dispersion techniques presents problems that are unique to each dust being studied. The need in toxicologic testing is for the particle size distribution to remain constant over long periods of time. The powder being tested must be dispersed into unitary particles rather than agglomerates. This requires a means of continuously metering a powder into the generator at a constant rate and a means of dispersing the powder. Most materials contain particles of irregular size and shape, which means that monodisperse conditions are rarely met and that in the generating system, the particle size distribution will differ from that in the original powder.

Simple dust metering systems use gravity feed of loose powder into an air stream, usually assisted by agitators or vibrators. Another method uses a turntable dust feed, where the powder is gently and continuously packed into grooves on a rotating disc. The material is removed from the groove at a constant rate by an air ejector. Systems such as volume feeders deliver specific amounts to a reservoir prior to generation. The Wright dust feed uses a scraping mechanism to remove a finely ground powder from the surface of a packed cylinder.

The dispersion of powder is accomplished by supplying sufficient energy, usually as a high velocity airstream, to a relatively small volume of the bulk powder to separate the particles by overcoming their own attraction forces. Hydrophobic materials such as talc are more easily dispersed than hydrophilic materials like limestone or quartz. Dry powders are considerably easier to disperse than humidified ones. The metered powder may be dispersed and agglomerates broken up directly by a turbulent air jet, or the dust-laden airstream can be passed through an impactor or fluidized bed. Elutriators, used to prevent escape of large agglomerates, are useful in dispersion. The importance of clean, dry air to generate particles should be stressed by noting that extremely dry air (relative humidity less than 5%) can cause strong electrostatic forces among particles, reducing their dispersibility.

Willeke et al. (117) describe fluidized-bed aerosol generators that are capable of a very stable output of particles from 0.5 to 30 μm. This generator uses a fluidized bed of glass or metallic beads (100–200 μm) into which the powder is directly added. The mechanism of dispersion involves the deposition of the particles onto the beads and their subsequent reentering into the airstream following the action of both impaction, as the beads collide with one another, and aerodynamic turbulence. The entire system also acts as an elutriator preventing large particles and agglomerates from leaving the system. This means of generation can only be used for dry, nonadhering powders, but does produce electrically charged aerosols, which need to be neutralized upon leaving the fluidized bed.

The NBS Dust Generator (34) is suitable for studies requiring high flow rates. In this system, the dust flows from a hopper (200–1200 cm²) with the aid of a vibrator into spaces of a metering gear. A spreader plate removes excess material as the gear turns at a given constant speed. Dust is pulled from the gears by a compressed air ejector, positioned to effectively remove the material from the gears. A plate can be fitted at the ejection output to remove large particles.

Lee et al. (67) used a high-pressure air-impingement device to separate fibrils from the larger Kevlar fiber matrix and directed to smaller fibers through a cyclone into the exposure chamber (Fig. 10). This system was used to generate fiber mass concentrations as high as 18 mg/m³ or as low as 2.5 fibers/cc for periods ranging from 2 weeks to 2 years.

Bernstein et al. (13) describe a brush feed micronizing jet mill which produces a relatively wide range of concentrations of respirable particles. Test concentrations from 0.22 to 7.48 mg/liter with particles less than 3 μ were attained and maintained. Only with higher concentrations of talc were these small particle sizes not attainable.

ATMOSPHERE ANALYSIS

The sampling system used in determining chamber concentrations should be designed to transmit a representative air sample (from the breathing zone of the animal) to the sensor or collection medium without significant losses. The sampling train should be designed to contain as few impaction locations (bends, reducers, turns) as possible. It is not necessary that the collection efficiency be 100%, but the efficiency should be known and consistent to be useful. For gases and vapors, lower efficiencies are acceptable, but with aerosols this is not the case. Aerosols are rarely monodisperse

and, since most particle entrapment mechanisms are size-dependent, the collection characteristics of a given sampler will change with particle size. Also, the efficiency will change in response to loading. A filter will be more efficient as dust collects on the surface. Electrostatic precipitator efficiency will drop as a resistive layer accumulates on the collecting electrode.

Sampling errors generally reflect the contribution of many small errors in the system rather than any single error source. Items that need to be carefully considered and examined in any such system include sampling train leakages and losses, flow rate and sample volumes, collection efficiency, sample stability, efficiency of recovery from the sampling substrate, and analytical background or interferences introduced by the sampling substrate.

Gases are fluids that occupy the entire space of the enclosure and can be liquified only by the combined effect of increased pressure and decreased temperature. Vapors (e.g., methanol and water) are the evaporation products of substances that are liquids at normal temperature. This distinction is made because in many instances they are collected by different devices, even though their thermodynamic behavior is identical.

Particulate matter (aerosol) is divided into solids and liquids. Solids are classified based on particle size and means of evaluation. Dusts are formed from solid inorganic or organic materials reduced in size by mechanical processing. Fumes are formed from solid materials by evaporation, condensation, and by gas phase molecular reactions. Smokes are products of incomplete combustion of organic materials and are characterized by optical density. Fibers are solids whose ratio of length to diameter (aspect ratio) exceeds 3.

Gases and vapors offer the least difficulty in sampling as they follow the normal laws of diffusion, mix freely with the general atmosphere, and equilibrate rapidly. Sampling can be conducted by direct reading instruments that have response times of seconds or less. Sensors in these instruments utilize infrared and ultraviolet radiation, flame and photoionization, and chemiluminescence

Direct samples may be instantaneous or continuous in nature. If grab sampling is conducted, samples should be taken frequently enough to reflect fluctuations in chamber

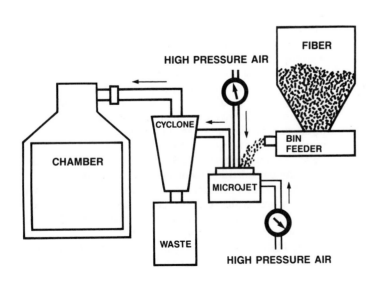

FIG. 10. Generation system used to produce airborne Kevlar fibrils.

concentration. Such samples may be collected in evacuated glass or metal containers, inflatable flexible polymer bags, or by gas-tight syringe. These samples may be taken remotely by directing the sample through sample lines and injecting aliquots of the stream directly into the analytical instrument. Continuous samples can be taken by pumping (or drawing) a constant stream of gas directly through a detector.

Extractive sampling involves removal of the chemical from air by scrubbing through a solvent or reagent, adsorption to a collection surface, or condensation on a cold surface. This type of collection involves use of a sample collector which may include sampling lines, a scrubbing device, an airflow rate or volume meter, a suction pump, or other specialty equipment.

Collection of particulate matter also may be performed by instantaneous or integrated sampling. Instantaneous sampling is unusual, and involves removing a small volume of the atmosphere and blasting it against a glass plate on which the particles are deposited and later characterized (counted and sized). For the more commonly conducted continuous sampling, physical forces such as gravity, impaction, electrophoresis, thermophoresis, and diffusion may be employed. Collectors for determination of mass of particulate matter in inhalation chambers include those listed in Table 9.

Filters represent the commonly used method of determining mass concentration in the chamber. All-glass filter papers made from superfine glass fibers having diameters well below 1 μ are available for collecting virtually all suspended particles. These have low airflow resistance and interfere negligibly with subsequent chemical analysis. Liquid particles such as sulfuric acid mist may be collected on glass filters with good results. Membrane filters with specific pore sizes are also available and have been used widely in characterizing atmospheres of mineral dusts by both optical and electron microscopy.

Complementary to monitoring by the filter method, rest-time aerosol monitors can be used to provide rapid input for *in vivo* concentration adjustments that are necessary to attain and maintain target exposure concentrations. Cheng and colleagues (23) describe the application of one such system to their research programs. The detector is a photometer which collects scattered light from the aerosol cloud within a 55–95° envelope prior to detection with a silicon photo detector. The system worked well at lower (<50 mg/m³) concentrations.

Impingers and impactors utilize inertial properties of particles to do the collecting. An impinger consists of a glass nozzle submerged in water (or alternative liquid media). For particle sizing, cascade impactors are used. These contain a number of impingement stages in series with graduated nozzle velocities and impaction distances to effect a progressive separation of smaller and smaller particles as the aerosol progresses through the unit. Particles deposited on each stage can be weighed and/or examined microscopically. The cascade impactor is calibrated to define the aerodynamic median size characteristics by calculating the percent by weight on each stage using weighings, radioactivity determinations, or chemical analysis to determine the amount of material deposited on each stage.

Electrostatic precipitators involve the use of an open tube with collection of the airborne particulate directly on the inside of the tube, on an inserted foil of transparent or opaque material, or on glass microscope slides placed between the collecting tube and a central ionizing wire. Thermal precipitators are limited in use since the dust-free zone around the hot body can be maintained only at very slow sampling rates. Settling chambers, centrifugal devices, and scrubbers are infrequently used but do have certain specialized applications.

PULMONARY FUNCTION STUDIES

Pulmonary function studies are frequently needed along with histomorphologic studies to adequately assess the inhalation toxicity of a material. The extra information over studies with histologic endpoints include greater assurance in the establishment of no or minimal effect levels, functional assessment of the magnitude of the injury, estimation of the time course of the lesion and its reversibility, correlation with physical changes, information of possible toxic mechanisms, identification of possible indicators to use for monitoring human populations, distinction between toxicologic and physiologic effects, and added sensitivity in being able at times to detect health changes not identifiable by histology.

Plethysmographic methods have been described to measure respiratory frequency and tidal volume and its product minute volume (25). Measurement of frequency alone has been shown to be misleading in that changes in rate can be counteracted by increased tidal volumes to yield no real change in minute volume. Landry (62) combined these determinations to evaluate metabolic rates and measured inhaled dose with both methyl and methylene chloride. Coggins (26) showed that the relationship between minute volume and dose of cigarette smoke is not linear but is described by a more complex set of functions.

Functional residual capacity is measured by placing an anesthetized animal in a plethysmograph. The animal breathes against a closed aperture and the pressure changes are recorded using a solenoid device operated by the computer and placed between the end of the tracheal cannula and a pneumotachograph. Forced expirograms generally require the cooperation of the subject but systems capable of measuring this in anaesthetized rats or hamsters have been described (8). Measurement of blood gases and pH is also needed to give complementary information to that obtained in the above battery.

Because most pulmonary function tests are nondestructive, they are useful for comparative studies in which the effects in laboratory animals can be compared with those in humans. The tests described above can be developed for essentially any species. Dogs (83), ponies (42), donkeys (95), as well as mice, guinea pigs, rats, and rabbits have been suc-

TABLE 9. Particulate matter collectors

Filters
Impingers and impactors
Electrostatic precipitators
Thermal precipitators
Settling chambers
Centrifugal devices
Scrubbers

cessfully studied. The tests used in measurement of pulmonary function are presented in Table 10. A detailed examination of the variety of methods used to obtain these measurements is beyond the scope of this chapter, but relevant references are suggested in *Further Readings* at the conclusion of this chapter.

BIOCHEMICAL STUDIES

Cytological analysis of bronchoalveolar lavage (BAL) fluid has been used in man for the diagnosis of lung disease for

TABLE 10. *Pulmonary function studies that can be used in evaluation of inhalation toxicity*

Parameter	Tests available
Blood gases	Several to determine O_2, CO_2, CO, pH, etc.
Diffusion	Several using blood–gas electrodes, tracer gases
Distribution of ventilation	Closing volume Single or multibreath nitrogen washout (or 133XE) regional pulmonary function, 133XE
Pulmonary circulation	Cardiovascular pressures Cardiovascular volumes, flow resistance, and work distribution of perfusion Edema determination (wet/dry weights, gas transfer, radioisotopes) Histamine, fibrinopeptide B, bradykinin analysis Matching of ventilation and perfusion Right-to-left pulmonary vascular shunt during O_2 breathing
Regional ventilation/perfusion matching	Several using arterial blood and alveolar gas measurements
Respiratory mechanics	Airway flow resistance Dynamic lung compliance Flow-volume inspiratory maximum inspiratory Flow-volume maximum expiratory flow volume curves Lung and thoracic cage flow resistance Small airways flow resistance Spirometry-forced expired volume vs. time Static lung and thoracic cage compliance Static volume pressure curves of saline-filled excised lungs Work of breathing
Static lung volumes	Expiratory reserve volume Functional residual capacity Inspiratory capacity Residual volume Total lung capacity Vital capacity
Ventilatory exchange	Minute ventilation Respiratory rate Tidal volume

many years. Not only the cellular but the enzymatic and soluble components of BAL have been used as indicators of pulmonary injury (10,47,79). Epithelial cell injury can result in release of cellular contents along the sites of damage in the respiratory tract. The lavage technique itself is easily performed both *in vivo* and *in vitro*. Physiologic saline or balanced salt solutions can be employed as the washing medium. The most effective practice is to wash the lungs twice, further washings generally only dilute the sample in terms of cells of interest. Total and differential cell counts are used to obtain the leukocyte profile. Cells are removed from BAL by centrifugation and the supernatent can be analyzed for markers of injury including the cytoplasmic enzymes lactic dehydrogenase, glutathione peroxidase, and glutathione reductase (glucose-6-phosphate dehydrogenase appears to be relatively insensitive) (49).

Increased phagocytic activity should be measured via the marker enzymes acid phosphatase, β-glucuronidase, β-N-acetylglucosaminidase, and peroxidase. Soluble protein or specific assays for albumin have been used as an indicator of increased permeability. Total sialic acid determinations can be used to reflect transudation of serum proteins. Increased protein or albumin in BAL plus the presence of neutrophils indicated an inflammatory process in this region.

The usefulness of this approach depends on the correlation between the biochemical marker and the cellular/tissue damage occurring. Correlations between lactic acid dehydrogenase (LDH) activity and injury from instilled surfactant have been demonstrated (48). Other agents in which biochemical changes have augmented morphologic studies in the determination and quantitation of lung effects include cadmium, nitrogen dioxide, oxygen, diesel exhaust soot, mineral dusts, and sulfuric acid (Table 11). These assays provide support information to the traditional histologic studies and may also find use in cytotoxicity screening assays where the question becomes one of relative potencies.

It is clear that detailed, nonartifactual structural analysis of the respiratory tract tissues at the most elemental level can be helpful in assessing the amount and degree of lung damage produced (or not produced) by chemical agents. Morphometric techniques are available to obtain quantitative data regarding changes in lung structure. These techniques allow the investigator to focus on specific regions of interest and to determine changes in lung tissue or in lung cellular population patterns (7). Clearly, structural evaluation of the respiratory system in toto needs to be conducted. Table 12 presents the recommendations of Tyler et al. (108) regarding structural evaluation of the respiratory system.

SAFETY

The safety of persons working in an experimental area dealing with the generation and maintenance of airborne chemicals must be carefully protected. The basic measures employed that prevent contact with chemicals or their spread within the laboratory must continually be reinforced. Specifically, to prevent the inhalation of test agents by those working on an experiment, a number of additional considerations apply. Dust masks provide only minimal protection, and only from larger dust particles such as animal dander

TABLE 11. *Biochemical indicators of lung damage*

Agent	Injury	Biochemical marker
Beryllium	Granuloma	Eosinophilia
Cadmium	Diffuse alveolitis	LDH, protein, PMN
Cyclophosphamide	Upper respiratory tract	Aniline hydroxylase
Diesel exhaust soot	Focal chronic alveolitis	LDH, protein, PMN, liposomal enzymes, glutathione reductase
Sulfuric acid	Upper respiratory tract	Not useful
Mineral dusts	Focal alveolitis	LDH, protein, PMN, liposomal enzymes
Nitrogen dioxide	Terminal bronchioles	Protein, PMN
Oxygen	Endothelial tissue	Protein, PMN
Silica	Alveolar proteinosis	Phospholipids, LDH

and hair. For chemical protection, half-face cartridge respirators can be used against certain organic vapors and dusts during times of potential exposure (e.g., transfer of test agents, removing animals from exposure chambers, observing animals following whole-body inhalation exposures). Air-supplied respirators should be used when handling open containers of highly toxic materials, and these transfers should additionally be made within a functional laboratory hood. Respirators should be test-fitted and personnel should be properly trained to use them. Air-supplied respirators should also be used when handling animals exposed to these agents.

Provisions to isolate animals following exposure to test agents should be made (walk-in storage areas for animal racks, portable hoods). The type of monitoring needed in any experimental situation must be geared to that particular chemical. Area monitoring should be conducted before, during, and after daily exposures to establish conditions that will avoid human exposure and to ensure that the conditions are being met.

The best practice to follow when conducting experimental inhalation tests is to remember that the subjects of the test must be isolated. The working area itself should be isolated so that only those directly involved with the experiment have access to the facility. Any potential for human contact should be removed prior to initiation of the experiment. This often is best accomplished by enclosing the entire generation and exposure system (including the exhaust) within a laboratory hood. The specific measures taken will follow from the type of test, the amount of chemical being handled during the test, and the toxicity of the chemical.

CONCLUSIONS

It is important to recognize that the evaluation of the toxicity of a material following inhalation is different from that following other routes of exposure. The effects of a given agent when inhaled must be understood so that appropriate control measures can be applied in the workplace and in the community to prevent the occurrence of adverse health effects. Both the qualitative and the quantitative aspects of these potential responses need to be properly considered. The tools for such evaluation exist even though the area of inhalation toxicology is continually making technical advances. The basic methodologies available to the investigator for studying the effects of chemicals as they enter the respiratory tract have been reviewed in this chapter, and these approaches remain constant in the face of technological advances. This chapter is not intended as a "cookbook," since the innovative and creative use of the materials discussed here is needed for the continual improvement of toxicology experiments. The information presented here should offer the reader some familiarity with the factors that must be considered when evaluating the toxicity of an agent following inhalation, and should give an understanding of the methods employed to accomplish that goal. It is important that information from several differing endpoints be integrated to ensure that the proper conclusions are reached. Inhalation toxicologists must continue to be receptive to new procedures and ideas so that the work of protecting the community at large from the adverse effects of inhaled agents can be conducted with appropriate, up-to-date tools.

TABLE 12. *Recommendations for structural evaluation of the respiratory system*

Procedure	Major value	Comment
Gross examination	Complete view	Comprehensive
Fixation *in vivo*	Lesser distortion	Tracheal infusion
Examination	With LM, SEM, TEM lung volumes[a]	Detail degrees Quantitation
Backscattered electrons and energy-dispersive X-rays	Localization elemental particle analysis	Includes autoradiography
Cytochemical	Characterize activities of specific cell types	With LM, SEM

[a] LM, light microscopy; SEM, scanning electron microscopy; TEM, transmission electron microscopy.

REFERENCES

1. Alarie, Y. (1973): Sensory irritation by airborne chemicals. *CRC Crit. Rev. Toxicol.*, 2:299–363.
2. Albert, R. E., Berger, J., Sanburn, K., and Lippmann, M. (1974): Effects of cigarette smoke components on bronchial clearance in the donkey. *Arch. Environ. Health*, 29:96–101.
3. Allison, A. C. (1976): Effects of silica, asbestos, and other pollutants on macrophages. In: *Air Pollution and the Lung*, edited by E. R. Aharonson, A. Ben-David, and M. A. Klingberg, pp. 114–134. John Wiley, NY.
4. Amdur, M. O. (1957): The influence of aerosols upon the respiratory response of guinea pigs to sulfur dioxide. *Am. Ind. Hyg. Assoc. Q.*, 18:149–155.
5. Auerbach, D., Hammond, E. C., Kirman, D., and Garfinkel, L. (1970): Effects of cigarette smoking in dogs. *Arch. Environ. Health*, 21:754–768.
6. Bair, W. J., Porter, N. S., Brown, D. P., and Wehner, A. P. (1969): Apparatus for direct inhalation of cigarette smoke by dogs. *J. Appl. Physiol.*, 26:847–850.
7. Barry, B. E., and Crapo, J. D. (1985): Application of morphometric methods to study diffuse and focal injury in the lung caused by toxic agents. *CRC Crit. Rev. Toxicol.*, 14:1–32.
8. Batista, S. P., Guerin, M. R., Gori, B. G., and Kensler, C. J. (1973): A new system for quantitatively exposing laboratory animals by direct inhalation. *Arch. Environ. Health*, 27:376–382.
9. Battelle Centre for Toxicology and Biosciences (1984): The assessment of pulmonary function in laboratory animals. Battelle Publ. 488:38.
10. Beck, B. D., Brain, J. D., and Bohannon, D. E. (1982): An *in vivo* hamster bioassay to assess the toxicity of particles for the lungs. *Toxicol. Appl. Pharmacol.*, 66:9–29.
11. Beethe, R. L., Wolff, R. K., Griffis, L. C., Hobbs, C. H., and McClellan, R. O. (1979): Evaluation of a recently designed multi-tiered exposure chamber. *Inhal. Toxicol. Res. Inst.*, LF-67.
12. Bernstein, D. M., and Drew, R. T. (1980): The major parameters affecting temperature inside inhalation chambers. *Am. Ind. Hyg. Assoc. J.*, 41:420–426.
13. Bernstein, D. M., Moss, O. R., Fleissner, H., and Bretz, R. (1984): A brush feed micronising jet mill powder aerosol generator for producing a wide range of concentrations of respirable particles, In *Aerosols: Science, Technology, and Industrial Application of Airborne Particles*, edited by B. Y. H. Liu, D. Y. H. Pui, and H. Fissan, pp. 721–724. Elsevier Sciences, NY.
14. Bianco, A., Gibb, F. R., Kilpper, R. W., et al. (1974): Studies of tantalum dust in the lungs. *Radiology*, 112:549–556.
15. Bowden, D. H., and Adamson, I. Y. R. (1978): Adaptive responses of the pulmonary macrophagic system to carbon. I. Kinetic studies. *Lab. Invest.*, 42:422–429.
16. Brain, J. D., Knudson, D. E., Sorokin, S. P., and Davis, M. A. (1976): Pulmonary distribution of particles given by intratracheal instillation or by aerosol inhalation. *Environ. Res.*, 11:13–33.
17. Brody, A. R., and Roe, M. W. (1983): Deposition pattern of inorganic particles at the alveolar level in the lungs of rats and mice. *Am. Rev. Respir. Dis.*, 128:724–729.
18. Burgess, B. A., and Brittelli, M. R. (1981): Acute inhalation toxicity of stannic chloride lethality and sensory irritation in rats. *Toxicologist*, 1:77.
19. Burgess, B. A., Pastoor, T. P., and Kennedy, G. L., Jr. (1984): Aniline-induced methemoglobinemia and hemolysis as a function of exposure concentration and duration. *Toxicologist*, 4:64.
20. Calandra, J. C., and Fancher, O. E. (1979): Target organ studies. In: *New Concepts in Safety Evaluation*, Part 2, edited by M. A. Mehlman, R. E. Shapiro, and H. Blumenthal, pp. 179–186. John Wiley, NY.
21. Casarett, L. J. (1972): The vital sacs: Alveolar clearance mechanisms in inhalation toxicology. In: *Essays in Toxicology*, Vol. 3, edited by W. J. Hayes, pp. 1–36. Academic Press, NY.
22. Casarett, L. J. (1975): Toxicology of the respiratory system. In: *Basic Science of Poisons*, edited by L. J. Casarett and J. Doull, pp. 212–214. Macmillan, NY.
23. Cheng, Y. S., Barr, E. B., Benson, J. M., et al. (1988): Evaluation of a real-time aerosol monitor (RAM-5) for inhalation studies. *Fund. Appl. Toxicol.*, 10:321–328.
24. Civil, G. W., and Heppleston, A. G. (1979): Replenishment of alveolar macrophages in silicosis: Implication of recruitment by lipid feed-back. *Br. J. Exp. Pathol.*, 60:537–547.
25. Coggins, C. R. E. (1981): Changes in the respiratory physiology of rats exposed to different phases of cigarette smoke. In: *Proceedings of the 19th Annual Hanford Life Sciences Symposium, Pulmonary Toxicology of Respirable Particles*. Department of Energy Symposium, 53(1979), pp. 420–430.
26. Coggins, C. R. E., Musy, C., and Ventrone, R. (1982): Changes in the minute ventilation of rats exposed to different concentrations of tobacco smoke. *Toxicol. Lett.*, 11:181–185.
27. Conroe, J. H., Forster, R. E., Dubois, A. B., et al. (1973): *The Lung*, 2nd ed. Year Book Medical, Chicago.
28. Costa, D. L. (1985): Interpretation of new techniques used in the determination of pulmonary function in rodents. *Fund. Appl. Toxicol.*, 5:423–434.
29. Costa, D. L., and Kutzman, R. S. (1983): Characterization of silicosis in the rat after subchronic inhalation of SiO_2 dust. *Am. Rev. Respir. Dis.*, 127:158.
30. Costa, D. L., Kutzman, R. S., Lehmann, J. R., et al. (1983): A subchronic multidose ozone study in rats. *Adv. Mod. Environ. Toxicol.*, 28:369–393.
31. Costa, D. L., Schafrank, S. N., Wehner, R. W., and Jellett, E. (1985): Alveolar permeability to protein in rats differentially susceptible to ozone. *J. Appl. Toxicol.*, 5:182–186.
32. Cuddihy, R. G., Brownstein, D. G., Raabe, O. G., and Kanapilly, G. M. (1973): Respiratory tract deposition of inhaled polydisperse aerosols in beagle dogs. *J. Aerosol Sci.*, 4:35–43.
33. Davies, P., Allison, A., Ackerman, J., et al. (1974): Asbestos induces selective release of lysosomal enzymes from mononuclear phagocytes. *Nature*, 251:423–425.
34. Dill, R. S. (1938): A test method for air filters. *Trans. Am. Sci. Heat. Vent. Eng.*, 44:379–393.
35. Drew, R. T. (1985): Design of inhalation exposure systems. Society of Toxicology Refresher Course, 24th Annual Meeting, San Diego, CA.
36. Drew, R. T. (1987): Inhalation toxicology—A status report. *Appl. Ind. Hyg.*, 2:213–217.
37. Drew, R. T., Terrill, J. B., Daly, I. W., and Sheldon, A. (1986): Dose-dependent clearance of antimony from rat lungs. *Toxicologist*, 6:141.
38. Ferin, J., and Leach, L. J. (1980): Horizontal air flow inhalation exposure chambers. In: *Generation of Aerosols and Facilities for Exposure Experiments*, edited by K. Willeke, pp. 517–523. Ann Arbor Science Publishers, Ann Arbor, MI.
39. Fraser, D. A., Bales, R. E., Lippmann, M., and Stockinger, H. E. (1959): Exposure chambers for research in animal inhalation. Public Health Monograph 357, U.S. Government Printing Office, Washington, D.C.
40. Gage, J. C. (1959): The toxicity of epichlorhydrin vapour. *Br. J. Ind. Med.*, 16:11–14.
41. Gardner, D. E. (1984): Alterations in macrophage functions by environmental chemicals. *Environ. Health Perspect.*, 55:343–358.
42. Garner, H. E., Rosborough, J. P., Amend, J. F., and Hoff, H. E. (1971): The grade pony as a new animal in cardiopulmonary physiology. *Cardiovas. Res. Cent. Bull.*, 9:91–94.
43. Greenberg, H. L., Avol, E. L., Bailey, R. M., and Bell, K. A. (1977): Effects of sulfate aerosols upon cardiopulmonary function in squirrel monkeys, PB. 279–393. National Technical Information Service, Springfield, VA.
44. Haber, F. (1924): *Funf vortrage aus den jahren 1920–1923*. Springer-Verlag, Berlin.
45. Hammond, P. B. (1970): The use of animals in toxicological research. National Library of Medicine, Bethesda, MD.
46. Hemenway, D. R., and MacAskill, S. M. (1982): Design, development and test results of a horizontal flow inhalation toxicology facility. *Am. Ind. Hyg. Assoc. J.*, 43:874–879.
47. Henderson, R. F., Benson, J. M., Hahn, F. F., et al. (1985): New approaches for the evaluation of pulmonary toxicity; bronchioalveolar lavage fluid analysis. *Fund. Appl. Toxicol.*, 5:451–458.
48. Henderson, R. F., Damon, E. G., and Henderson, T. R. (1978): Early damage indicators in the lungs. I. Lactate dehydrogenase activity in the airways. *Toxicol. Appl. Pharmacol.*, 44:291–297.
49. Henderson, R. F., Rebar, A. H., and DeNicola, D. B. (1979): Early

damage indicators in the lungs. IV. Biochemical and cytologic response of the lungs to lavage with metal salts. *Toxicol. Appl. Pharmacol.*, 51:129–135.

50. Hinners, R. G., Burkart, J. K., and Contner, G. L. (1966): Animal exposure chambers in air pollution studies. *Arch. Environ. Health*, 13:609–615.

51. Hinners, R. G., Burkart, J. K., and Punte, C. L. (1968): Animal inhalation exposure chambers. *Arch. Environ. Health*, 16:194–204.

52. Irish, D. D., and Adams, E. M. (1940): Apparatus and methods for testing the toxicity of vapors. *Am. Ind. Hyg. Assoc. Q.*, 1:1–5.

53. Jenkins, L. J., Jones, R. A., Coon, R. A., and Siegel, J. (1970): Repeated and continuous exposures of laboratory animals to trichlorofluoromethane. *Toxicol. Appl. Pharmacol.*, 16:133–142.

54. Kang, K. Y., and Salvaggio, J. (1976): Effects of asbestos and beryllium compounds on the alveolar macrophages. *Med. J. Osaka Univ.*, 27:47–52.

55. Kavlock, R. J., Meyer, E., and Grabowski, C. T. (1980): Studies on the developmental toxicity of ozone: Postnatal effects. *Toxicol. Lett.*, 5:3–9.

56. Kelly, D. P., Lee, K. P., and Burgess, B. A. (1981): Inhalation toxicity of titanium tetrachloride atmospheric hydrolysis products. *Toxicologist*, 1:76–77.

57. Kennedy, G. L., Jr., and Geisen, R. J. (1985): Setting occupational exposure limits for perfluoroisobutylene, a highly toxic chemical following acute exposure. *J. Occup. Med.*, 27:675.

58. Kennedy, G. L., Jr., Ferenz, R. L., and Burgess, B. A. (1986): Estimation of acute oral toxicity in rats by determination of the approximate lethal dose rather than the LD_{50}. *J. Appl. Toxicol.*, 6:145–148.

59. Kerns, W. D., Pavkov, K. L., Donofrio, D. J., Gralla, E., and Swenberg, J. A. (1983): Carcinogenicity of formaldehyde in rats and mice after long-term inhalation exposure. *Cancer Res.*, 43:4382–4392.

60. Kim, Y. C., and Carlson, G. P. (1986): The effect of an unusual workshift on chemical toxicity—II. Studies on the exposure of rats to aniline. *Fund. Appl. Toxicol.*, 7:144–152.

61. Kirk, W. P., Rennberg, B. F., and Morken, D. A. (1975): Acute lethality in guinea pigs following respiratory exposure to 85Kr. *Health Phys.*, 28:275–284.

62. Landry, T. D., Ramsey, J. C., and McKenna, M. J. (1983): Pulmonary physiology and inhalation dosimetry in rats: Development of a method and two examples. *Toxicol. Appl. Pharmacol.*, 71:72–83.

63. Langard, S., and Nordhagen, A. L. (1980): Small animal inhalation chambers and the significance of dust ingestion from the contaminated coat when exposing rats to zinc chromate. *Acta Pharmacol. Toxicol.*, 46:43–46.

64. Laskin, S., and Drew, R. T. (1970): An inexpensive portable inhalation chamber. *Lab. Anim. Sci.*, 26:645–646.

65. Leach, L. J., Maynard, E. A., Hodge, H. C., et al. (1970): A five-year inhalation study with natural uranium dioxide (UO_2) dust. I. Retention and biological effect in the monkey, dog, and rat. *Health Phys.*, 18:599–612.

66. Leach, L. J., Spiegl, C. J., Wilson, R. H., et al. (1959): A multiple chamber exposure unit designed for chronic inhalation studies. *Am. Ind. Hyg. Assoc. J.*, 20:13–22.

67. Lee, K. P., Kelly, D. P., and Kennedy, G. L., Jr. (1983): Pulmonary response to inhaled Kevlar aramid synthetic fibers in rats. *Toxicol. Appl. Pharmacol.*, 71:242–253.

68. Lee, K. P., Trochimowicz, H. J., and Reinhardt, C. F. (1985): Pulmonary response of rats exposed to titanium dioxide (TiO_2) by inhalation for two years. *Toxicol. Appl. Pharmacol.*, 79:179–192.

69. Lewis, T. R., Morrow, P. E., McClellan, et al. (1988): Establishing aerosol exposure concentrations for inhalation toxicity studies. *Fund. Appl. Toxicol.* (in press).

70. MacFarland, H. N. (1968): The pyrolysis products of plastics—Problems in defining their toxicity. *Am. Ind. Hyg. Assoc. J.*, 29:7–9.

71. MacFarland, H. N. (1976): Respiratory toxicology. In: *Essays in Toxicology*, Vol. 7, edited by W. J. Hayes, p. 136. Academic Press, NY.

72. MacFarland, H. N. (1981): A problem and a non-problem in chamber inhalation studies. In: *Inhalation Toxicology and Technology*, edited by B. K. J. Leong, pp. 11–18. Ann Arbor Science Publishers, Ann Arbor, MI.

73. MacFarland, H. N. (1983): Designs and operational characteristics of inhalation exposure equipment—A review. *Fund. Appl. Toxicol.*, 3:603–613.

74. Mauderly, J. L. (1974): Evaluation of the female pony as a pulmonary function model. *Am. J. Vet. Res.*, 35:1025–1029.

75. McClellan, R. O. (1985): Health effects of diesel exhaust—A case study in risk assessment. *Am. Gov. Ind. Hyg.*, 13:3–12.

76. McLaughlin, R. F., Jr., Tyler, W. S., and Canada, R. O. (1961): A study of the subgross pulmonary anatomy in various mammals. *Am. J. Anat.*, 108:149–166.

77. Miller, M. E. (1964): *Anatomy of the Dog*, Ch. 14. Saunders, Philadelphia.

78. Montgomery, M. R., Anderson, R. E., and Mortenson, G. A. (1976): A compact versatile inhalation exposure chamber for small animal studies. *Lab. Anim. Sci.*, 26:461–464.

79. Moores, S. R., Black, A., Evans, J. C., et al. (1981): The short-term cellular and biochemical response of the lung to toxic dusts: An *in vivo* cytotoxicity test. In: *The In Vitro Effect of Mineral Dusts*, edited by R. C. Brown, I. P. Gormley, M. Chamberlain, and R. Davies, pp. 297–303. Academic Press, NY.

80. Morrow, P. E. (1970): Models for the study of particle retention and elimination in the lung. In: *Inhalation Carcinogenesis*, edited by M. G. Hanna, Jr., P. Nettesheim, and J. R. Gilbert (CONF-691001), pp. 103–115. U. S. Atomic Energy Commission, Division of Technical Information, Oak Ridge, TN.

81. Morrow, P. E., Gibb, F. R., and Gazioglu, K. M. (1967): A study of particle clearance from the human lungs. *Am. Rev. Respir. Dis.*, 96:1209–1219.

82. Moss, O. R., Decker, J. R., and Cannon, W. C. (1982): Aerosol mixing in an animal exposure chamber having three levels of caging and excreta pans. *Am. Ind. Hyg. Assoc. J.*, 25:28–36.

83. Muggenburg, B. A., and Mauderly, J. L. (1974): Cardiopulmonary function of awake, sedated, and anesthetized beagle dogs. *J. Appl. Physiol.*, 37:152–162.

84. Paustenbach, D. J., Christian, J. E., Carlson, G. P., and Born, G. S. (1986): The effect of an 11.5-hr/day exposure schedule on the distribution and toxicity of inhaled carbon tetrachloride in the rat. *Fund. Appl. Toxicol.*, 6:472–483.

85. Phalen, R. F., and Morrow, P. E. (1973): Experimental inhalation of metallic silver. *Health Phys.*, 24:509–518.

86. Prendergast, J. A., Jones, R. A., Jenkins, L. J., and Siegel, J. (1967): Effects on experimental animals of long-term inhalation of trichloroethylene, carbon tetrachloride, 1,1,1-trichloroethane, dichlorodifluoromethane, and 1,1-dichloroethylene. *Toxicol. Appl. Pharmacol.*, 10:270–289.

87. Raabe, O. G., Yeh, H. C., Newton, C., Phalen, G. J., and Velasquez, D. J. (1977): Deposition of inhaled monodisperse aerosols in small rodents. In: *Inhaled Particles, IV*, edited by W. H. Walton, pp. 1–35. Pergamon Press, Oxford, England.

88. Rinehart, W. E., and Hatch, T. (1964): Concentration product (*Ct*) as an expression of dose in sublethal exposures to phosgene. *Am. Ind. Hyg. Assoc. J.*, 25:545–553.

89. Sachsse, K., Ullmann, L., Voss, G., and Hess, R. (1974): Measurement of inhalation toxicity of aerosols in small laboratory animals. In: *Experimental Model Systems in Toxicology and Their Significance in Man*. Proceedings of the European Society for the Study of Drug Toxicity. Vol. XV. pp. 239–251. Elsevier, NY.

90. Sachsse, K., Zbinden, K., and Ullmann, L. (1980): Significance of mode of exposure in aerosol inhalation toxicity studies—Head only versus whole body exposure. *Arch. Toxicol. Suppl.*, 4:305–311.

91. Saffiotti, U. (1970): Morphology of Experimental Respiratory Carcinogenesis, A.E.C. Symposium Series 21, U.S.A.E.C. Division of Technical Information. pp. 2, 45–250.

92. Saltzman, B. E. (1961): Preparation and analysis of calibrated low concentration of sixteen toxic gases. *Anal. Chem.*, 33:1100–1112.

93. Scheimberg, J., McShane, O. P., Carson, S., et al. (1973): Inhalation of a powdered aerosol medication by non-human primates in individual space-type exposure helmets. *Toxicol. Appl. Pharmacol.*, 25:478.

94. Schlesinger, R. B., Chen, L. C., and Driscoll, K. E. (1984): Exposure-response relationship of bronchial mucociliary clearance in rabbits following acute inhalations of sulfuric acid mist. *Toxicol. Lett.*, 22:249–254.

95. Schlesinger, R. B., Halpern, M., Albert, R. E., and Lippmann, M. (1979): Effect of chronic inhalation of sulfuric acid mist upon mu-

cociliary clearance from the lungs of donkeys. *J. Environ. Pathol. Toxicol.,* 2:1351–1367.

96. Schreck, R. M., Chan, T. L., and Soderholm, S. C. (1981): Design, operation and characterization of large volume exposure chambers. In: *Inhalation Toxicology and Technology,* edited by B. K. J. Leong, pp. 29–52. Ann Arbor Science Publishers, Ann Arbor, MI.

97. Silver, S. D. (1946): Constant flow gassing chambers: Principles influencing design and operation. *J. Lab. Clin. Med.,* 31:1153–1161.

98. Smith, L. W., Gardner, R. J., and Kennedy, G. L., Jr. (1982): Short-term inhalation toxicity of perfluoroisobutylene. *Drug Chem. Toxicol.,* 5:295–303.

99. Smith, D. M., Ortiz, L. W., Archuleta, R., et al. (1981): A method for chronic nose-only exposures of laboratory animals to inhaled fibrosis aerosols. In: *Inhalation Toxicology and Technology,* edited by B. K. J. Leong. Ann Arbor Science Publishers, Ann Arbor, MI.

100. Stockinger, H. E. (1949): Toxicity following inhalation. In: *Pharmacology and Toxicology of Uranium Compounds,* edited by C. Voegtlin and H. C. Hodge, p. 423. McGraw-Hill, NY.

101. Stockinger, H. E. (1957): Evaluation of the hazards of ozone and oxides of nitrogen-factors modifying toxicity. *Arch. Ind. Health,* 15:181–190.

102. Stuart, B. O., Willard, D. H., and Howard, E. B. (1970): In: *Inhalation Carcinogenesis,* edited by M. G. Hanna, P. Nettesheim, and J. R. Gilbert, pp. 131–135. Clearing-house for Federal Scientific and Technical Information, NBS, U.S. Dept. Commerce, Springfield, VA.

103. Stuart, B. O., Willard, D. H., and Howard, E. B. (1971): Studies of inhaled radon daughters, uranium ore dust, diesel exhaust and cigarette smoke in dogs and hamsters. In: *Inhaled Particles III,* edited by W. H. Walton, pp. 543–553. Unwin, Surrey, England.

104. Thomas, R. G., and Lie, R. (1963): Procedures and equipment used in inhalation studies on small animals. U.S. Atomic Energy Commission Research and Development Report, Lovelace Foundation Report No. LF-11, Albuquerque, NM.

105. Timbrell, V., Skidmore, J. W., Hyett, A. W., and Wagner, J. C. (1970): Exposure chambers for inhalation experiments with standard reference samples of asbestos of the International Union Against Cancer (UICC). *Aerosol Sci.,* 1:215–223.

106. Treon, J. F., Cleveland, F. P., Cappel, J. W., and Atchley, R. W. (1956): The toxicity of the vapors of Aroclor 1242 and Aroclor 1254. *Am. Ind. Hyg. Assoc. Q.,* 17:204–213.

107. Treon, J. F., Dutra, F. R., Cappel, J. W., Sigmon, H., and Younker, W. (1950): Toxicity of sulfuric acid mist. *Arch. Ind. Hyg. Occup. Med.,* 2:716–734.

108. Tyler, E. S., Dungworth, D. L., Plopper, C. G., et al. (1985): Structural evaluation of the respiratory system. *Fund. Appl. Toxicol.,* 5:405–422.

109. Ulrich, C. E., and Marold, B. W. (1979): Pulmonary deposition of aerosols in individual and group-caged rats. *Am. Ind. Hyg. Assoc. J.,* 40:633–636.

110. Wagner, W. D., Duncan, B. R., Wright, P. G., and Stokinger, H. E. (1965): Experimental study of threshold limit of nitrogen dioxide. *Arch. Environ. Health,* 10:455–466.

111. Wahrenbrock, E. A., Eger, E. I., Laravuso, R. G., and Maruschak, G. (1974): Anesthetic uptake of inert gases by mice and men. *Anesthesiology,* 40:19–23.

112. Warheit, D. B., George, G., Hill, L. H., et al. (1985): Inhaled asbestos activates a complement-dependent chemoattractant for macrophages. *Lab. Invest.,* 52:505–514.

113. Warheit, D. B., Hartsky, M. A., and Stefaniak, M. (1988): Comparative physiology of rodent pulmonary macrophages: *In vitro* functional responses. *J. Appl. Physiol.,* 64:1953–1959.

114. Weeks, M. W., Downing, T. O., Musselman, N. P., et al. (1960): The effects of continuous exposure of animals to ethanolamine vapor. *Am. Ind. Hyg. Assoc. J.,* 21:374–381.

115. Wehner, A. P., Craig, W. K., and Stuart, B. O. (1972): An aerosol exposure system for chronic inhalation studies with rodents. *Am. Ind. Hyg. Assoc. J.,* 33:483–487.

116. Weyel, D. A., and Schaeffer, R. B. (1985): Pulmonary and sensory irritation of diphenylmethane-4,4'- and dicyclohexylmethane-4,4'-diisocyanate. *Toxicol. Appl. Pharmacol.,* 77:427–433.

117. Willeke, K., Lo, C. S. K., and Whitby, K. J. (1974): Dispersion characteristics of a fluidized bed. *J. Aerosol Sci.,* 5:449–455.

118. Wilze, R. R., Henderson, R. F., Edison, A. F., and Hahn, F. F. (1987): Inhaled gallium oxide particles may be of comparable toxicity to quartz. American Industrial Hygiene Conference (abstr.), Montreal, Canada.

119. Wong, K. L., and Alarie, Y. (1982): A method for repeated evaluation of pulmonary performance in unanesthetized, unrestrained guinea pigs and its application to detect effects of sulfuric acid mist inhalation. *Toxicol. Appl. Pharmacol.,* 63:72–90.

120. Wright, B. M. (1957): Experimental studies on the relative importance of concentration and duration of exposure to dust inhalation. *Br. J. Ind. Med.,* 14:219–228.

Further Readings

Barrow, C. S. (1986): *Toxicology of the Nasal Passages.* Hemisphere, NY.

Brain, J. D., Proctor, D. F., and Reid, L. M. (1977): *Respiratory Defense Mechanisms,* Vols. I and II. Elsevier, NY.

Brown, S. S., and Davies, D. S. (1981): *Organ-directed Toxicity: Chemical Indices and Mechanisms.* Pergamon Press, NY.

Cralley, L. J., and Cralley, L. V. (1985): *Patty's Industrial Hygiene and Toxicology: Theory and Rationale of Industrial Hygiene Practice—Biological Responses.* Wiley, NY.

Fiserova-Bergerova, V. (1983): *Modeling of Inhalation Exposure to Vapors: Uptake, Distribution and Elimination.* CRC Press, Boca Raton, FL.

Hook, G. (1984): Monograph on pulmonary toxicology. *Environ. Health Perspect.,* 55:1–416.

Kennedy, G. L., Jr. (1988): Techniques for evaluating hazards of inhaled products. In: *Product Safety Evaluation Handbook,* edited by S. C. Gad, pp. 259–290. Marcel Dekker, NY.

Leong, B. K. J. (1981): *Inhalation Toxicology and Technology.* B. Herworth, London.

Menzel, D. B., and McClellan, R. O. (1980): Toxic response of the respiratory system. In: *Casarett and Doull's Toxicology,* edited by J. Doull, C. D. Klaassen, and M. O. Amdur, pp. 240–274. Macmillan, NY.

Phalen, R. F. (1984): *Inhalation Studies: Foundations and Techniques.* CRC Press, Boca Raton, FL.

Salem, H., (1986): *Inhalation Toxicology,* Marcel Dekker, NY.

Walton, W. H. (1982): *Inhaled Particles.* Proceedings of Symposium on Inhaled Particles and Vapours. Pergamon Press, NY.

Witschi, H. P., and Brain, J. D. (1985): *Toxicology of Inhaled Materials.* Springer-Verlag, NY.

Witschi, H. P., and Nettesheim, P. (1982): *Mechanisms in Respiratory Toxicology.* CRC Press, Boca Raton, FL.

Principles and Methods of Toxicology, Second Edition, edited by A. Wallace Hayes, Raven Press, Ltd., New York © 1989.

CHAPTER **13**

Dermatotoxicology

Esther Patrick and Howard I. Maibach

Department of Dermatology, University of California, San Francisco, California 94143-0989

Adult human skin constitutes approximately 10% of normal body weight. Its functions include regulation of body temperature and water loss, temporary storage of nutrients, vitamin synthesis, and its major function, protection (125,126,147,165). Resiliency and tensile strength protect against physical injury, pigmentation against ultraviolet light, barrier properties against environmental chemicals' entry into the body, and the growth pattern and surface characteristics against microbial colonization and invasion. The regenerative capacity following wounding and the number of processes by which skin can deal with environmental insults provide strong evidence of the importance of healthy skin to the organism. The psychological value of healthy skin has led in part to the development of multibillion dollar cosmetic and personal care industries.

The policies of agencies such as the Occupational Health and Safety Administration (OHSA), Department of Transportation (DOT), Consumer Product Safety Commission (CPSC), and Food and Drug Administration (FDA) in the United States and the Organization for Economic Cooperation and Development (OECD) and European Economic Community (EEC) internationally indicate that the identification of chemicals hazardous to the skin and the protection of society from exposure to those chemicals should be given high priority. These agencies mandate specific assays to evaluate the effects of skin exposure before registration, transport, or marketing of chemicals or formulated products.

The adverse skin responses associated with repetitive, low-dose exposure to industrial chemicals and consumer products all too often are not accurately predicted by the required assays. The need to market products with low risk of producing dermal and systemic injury to increase consumer satisfaction has led to the development of numerous assays to rank chemicals for their ability to injure the skin. Although these assays are not mandated by regulatory agencies, the frequency with which they are conducted and their utility warrant attention.

The field of dermatotoxicology includes measurement of absorption of materials as well as assays that evaluate the ability of topically applied chemicals to induce or promote the development of neoplasias, trigger an immune response in the skin, directly destroy the skin (corrosion), irritate the skin, produce urticaria (hives), and produce noninflammatory painful sensations. The inflammatory responses of skin are the most common chemically induced dermatoses in humans.

SKIN STRUCTURE AND PHYSIOLOGY

To understand the variety of adverse responses to skin and the basis for the predictive assays for skin injury, some understanding of skin anatomy and physiology is necessary. Approximately 2800 square inches of skin cover the body of an adult human. Skin is heterogeneous; the number of appendages, i.e., sweat glands, hair follicles, sebaceous glands, and the thickness of skin vary by body region. For example, thickness of skin of the eyelid is approximately 0.02 inch;

TABLE 1. *Comparative skin thicknesses of humans*[a]

Region	Thickness (μm)	Reference
Abdomen	46.6	Whitton and Ewell (179)
Stratum corneum of abdomen	8.2	Holbrook and Odland (67)
Forearm	60.9	Bergstressor et al. (8)
Stratum corneum of forearm	15.0	Holbrook and Odland (67)
Thigh	54.3	Bergstressor et al. (8)
Stratum corneum of thigh	10.9	Holbrook and Odland (67)
Back	43.2	Bergstressor et al. (8)
Stratum corneum of back	9.4	Holbrook and Odland (67)
Cheek	38.8	Whitton and Ewell (179)
Forehead	50.3	Whitton and Ewell (179)
Back of hand	84.5	Whitton and Ewell (179)
Fingertip	369.0	Whitton and Ewell (179)

[a] Values are for full thickness skin unless stratum corneum is specified.

the skin of the palm and sole are approximately 0.16 inch thick (Table 1).

A film composed of triglycerides, phospholipids, esterified cholesterol, and other materials released by holocrine sebaceous glands and salts and water released by eccrine sweat glands normally covers the outer surface (130). This surface film has been referred to as an acid mantle, pH of the skin normally varying between 4.2 and 5.6. *Micrococciae* and *Corynebacterium* species normally colonize the skin surface (125). Changes in surface film composition, for example, inflammatory conditions or occlusion, may result in a 1000-fold increase in absolute number of microorganisms colonizing the area and in a shift in flora present (11). The surface film penetrates the outermost cellular layers of the skin.

Based on structure and embryonic origin, the cellular layers of the skin are divided into two distinct regions (Fig. 1): the outer region, the epidermis, develops from embryonic ectoderm and covers the connective tissue; the dermis is derived from the mesoderm (68). The epidermis comprises approximately 5% of full thickness skin (104,126). For descriptive purposes, epidermis is subdivided into five to six layers based

on cellular characteristics (Fig. 2). Note that these layers of keratinocytes are formed by ordered differentiation of cells from one layer of mitotic basal cells. The number of distinguishable layers varies by anatomical site.

Basal layer keratinocytes are metabolically active cells with the capacity to divide. Some daughter cells of the basal layer move upward and differentiate. Cells adjacent to the basal layer contain large mitochondria; the golgi apparatus and rough endoplasmic reticulum (RER) are well developed. These cells produce lamellar granules, intracellular organelles, which later fuse to the cell membrane to release neutral lipids thought to form a barrier to penetration through the epidermis (32,33,162). Microscopically, the desmosomes and bridges connecting adjacent cells resemble spines and the three- to four-cell thick layer of cells above the basal layer is referred to as the stratum spinosum. The "spines" connecting adjacent cells are temporary structures; keratinocytes dissociate from neighboring cells and form new associations as they individually move upward in the epidermis (126). Cells of the third subdivision of the epidermis, the stratum granulosum, are characterized by the presence of keratohyalin granules, polyribosomes, large golgi apparatus, and RER. Cells of the granular layer are the uppermost viable cells of the epidermis. Here the lamellar granules are released at the cell surface. An intermediate zone of cells separates the cornified layers of the outer epidermis from the viable granulosum. In the palms and soles, the stratum lucidum, or "clear cell layer," lies above the stratum granulosum. This layer is indistinguishable in skin sections from other areas. Cells of the intermediate zone may contain enzymes capable of metabolizing exogenous chemicals, but have lost the ability to synthesize proteins. The outermost cornified layer, the stratum corneum, consists of cells that have lost their nucleus and all capacity for metabolic activity. The dominant constituent of these cells is keratin, a scleroprotein with chains linked by both disulfide and hydrogen bonds that were synthesized and stored in the deep epidermal layers. The intracellular attachments between these cells gradually break and the outermost cells are sloughed.

In addition to the visible intercellular and metabolic changes observed during keratinocyte differentiation, their size and shape have also changed. Cells derived from basal cuboidal cells approximately 5 μm in diameter have elongated and flattened to approximately 30 μm (104); four differen-

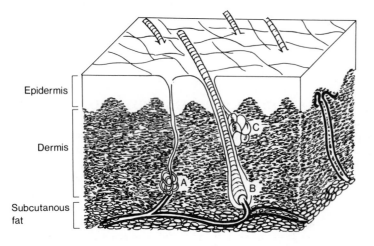

FIG. 1. Strata of the human skin. Eccrine sweat glands (**A**) are located in the dermis; a duct transports sweat through the epidermis to the surface. Hair follicles (**B**) are located deep in the dermis. Each hair extends through the skin via an epithelized channel. Contents of sebaceous glands (**C**) are released into the follicular channel as the sebocytes die. Each skin appendage has its own blood supply. Plexuses formed in the upper dermis (shown in the drawing to the far right) supply nutrients to the epidermis and upper dermis.

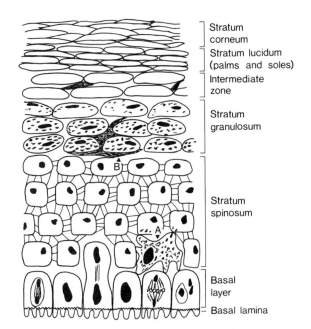

Stratum corneum
Stratum lucidum (palms and soles)
Intermediate zone
Stratum granulosum
Stratum spinosum
Basal layer
Basal lamina

FIG. 2. The epidermis. All possible cell layers and the locations of the two dendritic cell types, melanocytes (**A**) and Langerhans' cells (**B**), are shown.

tiated, cornified cells of the stratum corneum (2 × 2) would cover the same area as 100 basal keratinocytes (10 × 10). Each basal cell has the capacity to cover itself many times with modest mitotic rates. The pattern of papillae, ridges and grooves, of the basal layer formed by accessory structures from the dermis to the skin surface increases the area of germative layer relative to surface area, providing a large reserve in the capacity to cover the area. Normal turnover rate for keratinocytes has been estimated to be 28 days but varies considerably in disease states and somewhat by anatomical site, for example, 32 to 36 days for the human palm versus 58 days for the anterior surface of the forearm.

In addition to keratinocytes, the epidermis contains two dendritic cell types, melanocytes and Langerhans' cells. Between 460 and 1000 melanocytes and Langerhans' cells per square millimeter of glabrous nonspecified skin is normal (104). Melanocytes, derived from embryonic neural crest cells, lie directly adjacent to the basal layer. Melanocytes produce melanin, the principal pigment of human skin, which is then transferred to basal layer keratinocytes in granules. The dendrites of the melanocyte allow one cell to supply melanin to many basal cells. Langerhans' cells express immune recognition (Ia) antigen and receptors for IgG and C_3 on their surface. Like cells of the monocyte/macrophage lineage that bear these markers, they are believed to derive from the bone marrow mesenchyme. Presumably they process low molecular weight haptens during induction of immune responses (161). Although this function has been questioned, Langerhans' cells take up small molecules (nonlipid) and increase in number in areas that have developed allergic reactions (160). Note that Langerhans' cells lie in epidermal layers containing enzymes that can metabolize exogenous chemicals; in some cases, allergic contact dermatitis is due to metabolites of the agent applied to the skin.

The dermis and epidermis are separated by a basal lamina.

The dermis is attached to this membrane by fine fibers of connective tissue. Cells of the basal layer are anchored to the lamina by radicles. This area of attachment is called the marginal layer. Histologically, the area is identified by periodic acid-Schiff reaction. There are occasional breaks in the attachments. Large breaks are observed in exfoliative skin conditions (104). The dermal connective tissue enclosed by the epidermal papilla is referred to as papillary dermis; the area below the papilla is the stratum subpapillare, or reticular dermis. The fibers of the papillary dermis are finer than those of the reticular dermis. The reticular dermis contains thick collagen bundles, especially in areas adjacent to blood vessels and skin appendages. Connective tissue fibers are separated by the ground substance, an amorphous material consisting of proteins and glycosaminoglycans, such as chondroitin A sulfate and hyaluronic acid. The constituents of ground substance are derived from both fibrocytes and blood plasma. The physical behavior of the dermis, including elasticity, is determined by the fiber bundles and ground substance. Variations in plasma content of ground substance may alter physical properties substantially.

The dermis contains all tissue types except cartilage and bone. The skin appendages originate in the subpapillary dermis. Eccrine sweat glands, sebaceous glands, and hair follicles with their erector muscles are found in the skin of most anatomical sites. Sebaceous glands are normally adjacent to hair follicles, utilizing the hair shaft as an excretory duct. The axillae, anogenital region, eyelid, and external ear contain apocrine sweat glands. These glands develop at puberty and form odorless secretions that are decomposed by bacteria to produce characteristic odors. The dermis also contains nerve cells with highly specialized sensory endings in some areas, fat lobules, migratory white blood cells, and mast cells. Mast cells are indistinguishable from fibroblasts in size or appearance; however, they contain granules that stain metachromically with agents of a thiazine group. Mast cells are most numerous in areas adjacent to blood vessels, skin appendages, and nerves. The precise function of mast cells is unknown; however, they appear to be involved in the pathogenesis of some inflammatory conditions (172). Their granules contain histamine, heparin, and other vasoactive agents that may be released on stimulation of the cell surface by IgE crosslinking 48/80, activated serum compounds, and some enzymes. Release of these mediators is accompanied by formation of other agents that are inflammatory mediators in some conditions.

The dermis and fascia of muscles are separated by the subcutis, a layer of fatty tissue. The extent and development of subcutis depends on sex, age, diet, and body region. Blood vessels supplying the skin arise from the subcutis. Vascular plexuses are formed in the transition zone of the subcutis and dermis adjacent to coils of the eccrine sweat gland. Arteries extend upward to mid-dermis, forming anastomoses there. Similar but independent plexuses form at the base of the hair shaft and sebaceous glands. A third vascular network is formed from arteries branching off from vessels at the level of eccrine sweat glands that branch into finer vessels that form plexuses in the papillary dermis. Plexuses of the papillary dermis supply the upper dermis, including the upper hair shaft, and the epidermis with nutrients. The adjacent but separate vascular units in the dermis sometimes react differently in pathological processes, e.g., follicular rash.

A simple visual comparison allows the conclusion that the skin of humans and animals vary considerably. The most obvious difference is hair coat covering the skin. In lower mammals, each hair shaft may contain several follicles, a large follicle arising from the subpapillary dermis and several accessory follicles arising from the papillary dermis. In humans, sebaceous gland density varies from 100 to 900 glands/cm^2; in other mammals, sebaceous glands are more evenly distributed (158). Human sweat is produced by eccrine sweat glands. Apocrine sweat glands are the dominant sweat gland of animals. Eccrine sweat glands open directly to the skin surface, whereas apocrine glands empty into the hair shaft. Apocrine sweat is less acidic than eccrine sweat, and the pH of the skin surface of animals is usually somewhat higher than that of humans (93). The thickness of skin also varies extensively by species and body site. Differences in content of granules of mast cells from different species have been reported (172), as have differences in sensitivity to various inflammatory mediators applied to skin. These differences undoubtedly contribute to the lack of correlation between the results of some animal and human predictive assays and are ample justification for predictive skin testing in humans after preliminary screening in animals, if the risks to subjects are minimal.

PHARMACOKINETICS FOLLOWING APPLICATION OF CHEMICALS TO THE SKIN

Until the beginning of the twentieth century, skin was considered a relatively inert barrier to chemicals that might enter the body (148). We now know that this view is incorrect. Although the skin's barrier properties are impressive, many chemicals penetrate the skin, and the skin can metabolize exogenous compounds. Because of its large surface area, skin may be a major route of entry into the body for some exposure situations. Delivery of drugs through the skin to treat systemic conditions has become almost commonplace. Interest in cutaneous pharmacokinetics has increased as the skin has been reconsidered to be a route for systemic administration of drugs and chemicals, as well as a route of entry for toxins. A variety of assays, both *in vivo* and *in vitro,* for measuring absorption through the skin has been developed (4,5,139,178), and many factors that govern absorption through the skin have been determined (Table 2).

A major diffusion barrier of the skin is considered to be the stratum corneum. Removal of the stratum corneum by tape stripping increases the rate of absorption of some chemicals (10). Absorption of chemicals through shunts, openings of skin appendages, and gaps in the stratum corneum associated with these structures has been considered (157,164). Because of the relative surface area of these shunts, 0.1% to 1% of the total area, they do not play a decisive role in absorption. However, they may be important initially after application of the penetrant (149). The stratum corneum is nonviable and has no capacity for active transport processes. Therefore, absorption can be described as passive diffusion across this membrane by the equation, $J = (K_m C_v D_m) \div \delta$, or, rate of absorption = (vehicle/stratum corneum partition coefficient × concentration × diffusion constant of penetrant in stratum corneum) divided by thickness of stratum cor-

TABLE 2. *Ten factors determining percutaneous absorption*

Release from vehicle (varies by solubility in vehicle, concentration, pH)
Kinetics of skin penetration (varies by anatomical site, occlusion, skin condition, animal age, concentration, surface area dosed, frequency of dosing)
Tissue distribution
Excretion kinetics
Substantivity
Volatility
Wash-and-rub resistance
Binding
Cutaneous metabolism
Anatomic pathways

Adapted from ref. 178.

neum (31). It is obvious that skin from different animals or sites of different thicknesses from the same animal will vary in barrier properties to absorption. The concentration term is concentration at the skin surface. Application of suspensions of penetrant with slow dissolution rates, of emulsions, or of penetrants in vehicles in which diffusion rate is slow will alter surface concentration and may control the rate of penetration (15,19,23,66). This principle has been utilized in designing slow release transdermal delivery devices. Other factors that affect thermodynamic activity of the solution at the skin surface, e.g., pH and temperature, may vary the absorption rate (148,149). Vehicle influence cannot be overstated; for a specific concentration of drug, thermodynamic activity may vary by 1000-fold from one vehicle to another (30). Some vehicles may promote penetration by altering the characteristics of the stratum corneum (87). Other factors that affect percutaneous absorption include condition of the skin (42), age, surface area to which the material is applied (178), penetrant volatility, temperature and humidity (48), substantivity, and wash-and-rub resistance to removal from the skin and binding to the skin (137). Skin may become saturated by a penetrant and thus resist penetration from subsequent applications.

Once a chemical has gained access to the viable epidermal layers, it may initiate a local effect, be absorbed into the circulation and produce an effect, or produce no local or systemic effects. The viable epidermis contains many enzymes capable of metabolizing exogenous chemicals (132), including a cytochrome P-450 system, mixed function oxidases, and glucuronyltransferases. Early studies indicated that enzymatic activity in skin was only a fraction of the activity of the liver. Those studies were conducted *in vitro* using whole skin; the enzymatic activity is in the epidermis, which makes up <5% of whole skin. When enzymatic activities of the epidermis were calculated, activities ranged from 80% to 240% of those in liver. Comparison of metabolites formed after dermal and oral administration of [^{3}H]cortisol demonstrated that different metabolites were formed. The skin does not have the capacity to metabolize all chemicals. For example, topically applied hexachlorophene does not appear to be metabolized. At present, it is not possible to predict metabolic pathways or rates following topical application; these must be experimentally determined.

In Vivo Percutaneous Absorption Assays

Percutaneous absorption can be determined by applying a known amount of chemical to a specified surface area and then measuring levels of the chemical in the urine and/or feces. To correct for excretion of the material through the lungs, sweat, or retention in the body, levels measured following topical administration are usually expressed as a percentage of levels following parenteral administration of the chemical (179). Because the analytical techniques to measure the chemical are not always available and because some chemicals may be metabolized, radioactive-labeled chemicals, usually carbon 14 or tritium, are customarily used in these assays. Although studies with radiolabeled compounds accurately reflect absorption, they may not provide accurate estimates of bioavailability. For example, comparison of bioavailability from nitroglycerin (unmetabolized drug) levels and levels of radioactive tracer indicates that use of the tracer overestimates available drug by as much as 20%. This corresponds to the metabolism of the drug to an inactive form.

In vivo studies have been conducted in humans and in a number of species (5). Comparison of absorption rates of a number of compounds showed that absorption rates in the rat and rabbit tend to be higher than humans and that the skin permeability of monkeys and swine more closely resembles that of humans (Table 3). Although these differences are not predicted by any single factor, e.g., epidermal thickness, they are not unexpected in light of differences in skin characteristics. There are examples of differences in routes of excretion of some chemicals as well. This may be due in part to metabolism of the chemical, and the metabolic capabilities of the species should be considered when selecting an animal model and designing the experiment. Ingestion of the test material by the animal must be prevented, and this may require restraint of the animal or designing specialized protective apparatus for the site of application. Because urine and feces are collected for analysis, specialized cages are also required. Examples and descriptions of metabolic cage design and site-protective apparatus are available elsewhere. The difficulty of conducting these types of pharmacokinetic assays is obvious: collection of excrement requires a relatively long period of time (>24 hr), the use of specialized cages and specialized protective apparatus, and the increased space requirements for housing animals individually. Although there

is no question that pharmacokinetic studies of this type in humans or animals provide the best estimate of percutaneous absorption, the cost and difficulty in conducting well-controlled studies has led to the use of other in vivo assays that are poorer predictive tools and to the development of in vitro models.

Loss of radioactive material from the skin surface has been used to estimate in vivo percutaneous absorption (116). The difference in applied dose and residue on the skin is assumed to be absorbed. The characteristics of the radioisotope, penetrant, and vehicle may limit the usefulness of this procedure. Volatile materials leave the surface without penetration, and it is difficult to recover all material from the skin surface. In addition, skin may retain a reservoir of the penetrant that has not entered the circulation.

In vivo biological responses have been used to estimate the rate of penetration. Notable examples are the vasoconstriction assays estimating absorption of corticosteroids (122) and changes in blood flow to study penetration through various types of skin and under diverse conditions (62,63). These endpoints are complicated biological processes and may vary with the tissue's ability to produce the response. For example, application of histamine would be expected to produce increased blood flow; the degree of change would depend not only on the rate of penetration but on the reactivity of receptors at that time. Most exogenous chemicals produce their vascular effects by triggering formation or release of endogenous mediators. The usefulness of penetration studies utilizing biological endpoints is limited to comparisons between closely related chemical structures that can be assumed to trigger the same process.

In Vitro Percutaneous Penetration Assays

The excised skins of humans or animals can be used to measure penetration of chemicals. In vitro assays using excised skin utilize specially designed diffusion cells (4,46). The skin is stretched over the opening of a collecting receptacle, epidermal side up. The chemical to be studied is applied to the epidermis, and fluid from the receptacle is assayed to measure the penetration of the chemical. Chemicals are usually radioactively labeled. Although some investigators have used diffusion cells in which the epidermis was covered with

TABLE 3. Species differences in in vivo absorption

| | (% Dose absorbed) | | | | | | |
	Rat	Rabbit	Guinea pig	Pig	Squirrel monkey	Human	Reference
Haloprogin	95.8	113.0		19.7		11.0	Bartek et al. (5)
Acetylcysteine	3.5	2.0		6.0		2.4	Bartek et al. (5)
Cortisone	24.7	30.3		4.1		3.4	Bartek et al. (5)
Caffeine	53.1	69.2		32.4		47.6	Bartek et al. (5)
Butter yellow	48.2	100.0	34.9	41.9		21.6	Bartek et al. (5)
Testosterone	47.4	69.6		29.4		13.2	Bartek et al. (5)
Chlorophenathane	46.3			43.4	1.5	10.4	Bartek & LaBudde (4)
Lindane	51.2			37.6	16.0	9.3	Bartek & LaBudde (4)
Parathion	97.5			14.5	30.3	9.7	Bartek & LaBudde (4)
Malathion	64.6			15.5	19.3	8.2	Bartek & LaBudde (4)

fluid containing the chemical, the preferred method for toxicologic relevance is a one-chambered cell in which the stratum corneum is exposed to the air and the underside of the skin is bathed in saline or other receptacle fluid. Because diffusion through a membrane depends on relative concentrations on each side, some chambers have been designed to allow periodic replacement of the receptacle fluid. Fluid in the receptacle base is usually constantly stirred and maintained at a physiological temperature. Either full-thickness skin or epidermis alone may be used in *in vitro* assays. With relatively hairless skin, epidermis can be separated from the dermis by heat treatment.

This type of *in vitro* assay offers advantages over *in vivo* assays: highly toxic compounds can be studied in human skin; large numbers of cells can be run simultaneously; diffusion through the membrane, eliminating other pharmacokinetic factors, can be studied; and these assays may be cheaper and easier to conduct.

These assays do not mimic human exposure in some important areas. Because excised skin must often be stored before use, it cannot be assumed that the skin will retain full enzymatic activity. This may alter the metabolic profile of compounds entering the receptacle. In intact skin, chemicals penetrating the epidermis would enter the circulation through vessels and lymphatics located just below the epidermis. In excised full-thickness skin, the dermis is also involved in the absorptive process. The influence of the dermis can be minimized by using heat-separated epidermis or by removal of the skin with a dermatome at the level of the upper dermis. In the intact animal, the chemical enters the peripheral circulation in plasma; the collecting fluid of diffusion chambers is usually saline or water. The relative solubilities of hydrophobic and hydrophilic chemicals in these collecting fluids may alter the rate at which they leave the skin. Surface conditions of excised skin may vary from normal skin; changes in the surface emulsion occurring during storage have not been studied. Storage conditions and procedures for preparing the tissue may affect skin absorption and metabolism. It has been proposed that the suitability of each specimen of excised skin be verified by measurement of penetration of a standard, tritiated water through the tissue before its use to study penetration of other chemicals.

Comparisons of penetration rates obtained from *in vitro* and *in vivo* assays have been made (4). Often a good correlation between the two methods was obtained. However, with some compounds, correlation of the methods was poor. Differences in the methods for some compounds could be explained on the basis of solubilities in the receptacle fluid and blood; others could not be explained. *In vitro* penetration rates through skin of various species have also been compared. Skin of the weanling pig and miniature swine appears to be good *in vitro* models for most compounds (5). Although a limited number of studies have been reported, the skin of monkeys appears to be a good model as well (178). For most compounds, mouse and hairless mouse skin appears more permeable than skin of other species. Rat skin appears to be a good model for some compounds; however, when differences have been noted, they have been large.

A few investigators have estimated percutaneous absorption using "model" membranes, and physiochemical data have been used to predict absorption. Lipid:water partition coefficients have been correlated with skin permeability.

Smaller molecules (molecular weight <400) are more readily absorbed than large. Molecules with polar groups, in general, do not penetrate as well as nonpolar molecules (147). The addition of hydroxyl groups also lowers the permeability. Substitutions that increase lipid solubility may increase penetration, depending on the vehicle in which the chemicals are applied (148). Electrolytes do not penetrate the skin well (149); shunt diffusion for these molecules may be important.

NEOPLASTIC RESPONSE OF SKIN

The skin is the most common site of cancer in humans. Both benign and malignant tumors may be derived from viable keratinocytes and melanocytes of the epidermis and rarely from skin appendages, blood vessels, peripheral nerves, and lymphoid tissue of the dermis (104). Basal cell and squamous cell carcinomas, which develop from keratinocytes, account for 60 and 30%, respectively, of all skin cancer. The remaining 10% includes malignant melanoma and the rare tumors developing from other cell types. Malignant melanomas often metastasize, and prognosis for patients with this disease is poor. Only 4% to 5% of squamous cell carcinomas are metastatic, and basal cell tumors rarely metastasize. The relatively noninvasive nature of the common forms of skin cancer accounts for a high cure rate—>95%—and <0.01% of diagnosed patients die of the disease. Skin cancer accounts for <0.3% of all cancer deaths.

The association between exposure to environmental carcinogens and the development of basal cell and squamous cell carcinomas is strong. Epidemiologic studies have demonstrated a strong correlation between exposure to ultraviolet radiation and development of skin cancer (35). Clinical experience leaves little doubt that X-rays can also produce cancer of the skin. Both forms of radiation have induced tumors in experimental animals (14). The association between environmental chemicals and skin cancer was first demonstrated by Sir Percival Potts in 1775. Since Potts' association between skin cancer of the scrotum and soot exposure, experimental skin carcinogenesis studies with chemicals in animals have shown that the polycyclic aromatic hydrocarbons, e.g., benzo(a)pyrene, are the carcinogens in soot, coal tar, pitch, and various cutting oils (38) and that cancer development is a multistage process (13,14).

In spite of abundant experimental evidence that chemicals can produce skin cancer, few chemicals have been associated with increased incidences of skin cancer in humans. Epidemiologic studies have demonstrated associations between polycyclic aromatic hydrocarbons and arsenic and increased incidence of benign precancerous lesions and basal cell and squamous cell carcinomas (72). The ability to establish relationships between chemical exposure and the development of skin cancer by epidemiology is minimized by many confounding factors, e.g., exposure to ultraviolet light, high background incidence rates, long latency periods for development of cancer (38,39), and incomplete reporting caused by the nonlethal nature of the disease. The experimental evidence that chemical exposure of the skin can lead to development of tumors and the degree of exposure to chemicals in the workplace justify the practice of evaluating carcinogenic potential by the dermal route of exposure, in spite of few epidemiologic examples of its importance. Furthermore, it is likely that certain internal tumors (e.g., bladder cancer from aniline exposure) result from chemicals absorbed through the skin.

In vivo skin carcinogenesis studies are most often conducted in mice, although other species have been used. Differences in species sensitivity to various agents have been demonstrated (14,139). The design of carcinogenesis assays is described in Chapter 14 and reviewed in other texts (106,138). Two variations of standard skin exposure studies have been reported. The skin may be treated with the chemical of interest, then a promoting agent such as 12-o-tetradecanoyl phorbol 13-acetate (TPA) may be applied to reduce the latency period, or the skin may be treated with a single noncarcinogenic dose of a carcinogen such as dimethyl benzanthracene (DMBA), followed by repeated doses of the agent under study, to determine if that agent can promote the development of tumors initiated by other agents.

Numerous factors may influence the outcome of dermal carcinogenic assays, and the choice of what to test is crucial in such assays. Although it is tempting to evaluate pure chemicals, it should be remembered that other agents in mixtures can act as promoting agents. For example, coal tar and pitch may contain catechol and pyrogallol, which are promotors of the carcinogen benzo(*a*)pyrene found in these mixtures. Wounding increases the number of tumors that spontaneously develop, and severe inflammatory responses may cause tissue destruction. Care should be taken in selecting an appropriate nonirritant dose. The incidence of spontaneous skin tumors varies by strain and species (40) and should be considered in selecting test group size.

A number of *in vitro* assays for studying chemical carcinogenesis have been developed (71). Of particular interest for dermal carcinogenesis is the ability to cultivate epidermal keratinocytes of rats, mice, and, more recently, humans (94). Cultured human keratinocytes can metabolize polycyclic aromatic hydrocarbons, and chemical transformation using human fibroblasts has been achieved (94). The establishment of human epidermal lines for *in vitro* carcinogenesis testing will provide an important new predictive tool. Chapter 14 reviews the relationship of mutagenicity and carcinogenicity.

ALLERGIC CONTACT DERMATITIS

Since the turn of the century, certain forms of eczema have been recognized as allergic in nature. Joseph Jadassohn (73,74) demonstrated that in some patients dermatitis was due to increased sensitivity following repeated contact with a substance and not the toxic (irritant) properties of the material. By 1930, a procedure for producing this hypersensitivity to chemicals in guinea pigs had been developed (12). The pioneering work of Landsteiner and associates (100–102) demonstrated that low molecular weight chemicals conjugate with proteins to form an antigen that stimulates the immune system to form a hyperreactive state (102); that immunogenicity is related to chemical structure (101); and that two types of immunologic response exist, one transferable by serum and another transferred by suspensions of white blood cells (100). It is now known that most cases of allergic contact dermatitis are of the cell-mediated type, transferable by lymphocytes. This type of skin response is often referred to as delayed contact hypersensitivity because of the relatively

long period (~24 hr) required for the development of the inflammation following exposure.

Some understanding of the processes by which this hypersensitivity develops is helpful in selecting and interpreting results of predictive sensitization tests. During ontogenesis, stem cells from the yolk sac, fetal liver, and bone marrow migrate to the central lymphoid organs, i.e., the thymus and bone marrow in mammals. After birth, stem cells derive from bone marrow. In the central lymphoid organs, stem cells differentiate into immunocompetent lymphocytes. This results in two classes of lymphocytes: thymus-processed T-lymphocytes, and B-lymphocytes processed in bone marrow. B-lymphocytes are precursors of antibody-producing cells responsible for immune responses transferable by serum. T-lymphocytes are responsible for producing delayed-type hypersensitivity (DTH) and for regulation of the immune system. This regulation is accomplished by subsets of T cells, i.e., T-helper and T-suppressor cells. Lymphocytes leaving the lymphoid organs are "programmed" to recognize a specific chemical structure via a receptor molecule(s). If, during circulation through body tissues, a cell encounters the structure it is programmed to recognize, an immune response may be induced. The ability to develop and express a hypersensitivity response is determined by the relative activities of the T-helper and T-suppressor cell types (141).

To stimulate an immune response, a chemical must be presented to lymphocytes in an appropriate form (101,102). Chemicals are usually haptens, which must conjugate with proteins in the skin or in other tissues in order to be recognized by the immune system. Haptens conjugate with multiple proteins to form a number of different antigens that may stimulate an allergic response by stimulating T-lymphocytes with different recognition capabilities (142). Hapten-protein conjugates are processed by macrophages or other cells expressing Ia proteins on their surface. Although the exact nature of this processing is not completely understood, it is known that physical contact between macrophage and T cells is required (166), suggesting that receptor interactions are necessary. Physical interaction is accompanied by the release of interleukins, a family of soluble regulatory proteins that stimulate cell division, act as growth factors, and increase expression of immune proteins on the surface of some cells (41,70,124).

Following stimulation by antigen in the skin, lymphocytes enter the lymphatic system and migrate to the draining lymph nodes. Disruption of lymphatic drainage prevents sensitization of an animal (47). Stimulated T-lymphocytes settle in the paracortical regions of the lymph nodes and differentiate into immunoblasts. This differentiation involves interaction with other cell types. Immunoblasts eventually give rise to T-effector cells that enter the systemic circulation and, on encountering the antigen that they are programmed to recognize, release lymphokines that initiate a local inflammatory response. Immunoblasts also give rise to memory cells, which enter the systemic circulation. These memory cells are capable of similar activities as the T-processed lymphocytes; they recognize antigen and can be stimulated to divide. Memory cell production is essentially an expansion of the number of cells capable of recognizing a given antigen.

The lymphokines released by primed effector cells that encounter their stimulating antigen directly, and indirectly by stimulation of other white blood cells, produce a local inflammatory response. Actions of lymphokines include direct tissue damage, chemotactic factors, stimulation of mitosis, increased phagocytic activity of macrophages, and factors that inhibit migration of some cell types from the area (25). Only a small percentage of lymphocytes in an area of skin exhibiting a delayed hypersensitivity response is specifically stimulated by antigen (128). Most cells in the lesion are "recruited" by lymphokines. Histologically, the response has been described as a hyperproliferative epidermis with intracellular edema, spongiosis, intraepidermal vesiculation, and mononuclear cell infiltrate by 24 hr. The dermis shows perivenous accumulation of lymphocytes, monocytes, and edema. No reaction occurs if the local vascular supply is interrupted and the appearance of epidermal changes follows the invasion of monocytes. Vascular changes, e.g., increased blood flow, occur early—5 to 6 hr in the response. The histology of the response varies somewhat by species. For example, a higher proportion of polymorphonuclear cells in the cellular infiltrate has been observed in DTH reaction sites of mice than in guinea pigs or humans (75). These differences may be due in part to mixed immune responses. Mice develop both antibody and DTH responses to haptens applied to the skin (3). Exposure via the skin is thought to lead preferentially to DTH in guinea pigs and humans.

Many factors modulate development of DTH in experimental animals and in humans. The method of skin exposure may be important. Keratinocytes produce interleukin (25), an important regulatory protein for induction of DTH. Langerhans' cells express Ia antigen and may act as antigen-presenting cells (104,161). Intradermal injection in animals bypasses these processes but assures entry of the chemical into the skin. As one would expect, factors that govern rate of penetration also influence rate of sensitization. The effects of vehicle and occlusion are well documented (110). Application of haptens to damaged skin, e.g., irritated or tape-stripped, increases the sensitization rate. Increasing the dose per unit area increases the sensitization rate. Repeated applications to the same site are more effective for inducing sensitization than application to new sites each time (37,110). The incidence of sensitization increases with increased numbers of exposures (this applies through 10–15 exposures only) (110). An interval between exposures of 2 to 6 days increases the sensitization rate (110). This may be due to the "booster" effect of memory cells. Materials such as Freund's complete adjuvant nonspecifically enhance development of immune responses. Treatment of animals with adjuvant, either simultaneously or shortly after hapten exposure, increases sensitization rates (112,113). The development of DTH is under genetic control; all individuals do not have the capability to respond to a given hapten (110). The status of the immune system will determine if an immune response can be induced. For example, young animals may become tolerant to a hapten, and pregnancy may suppress expression of allergy (110). The intrinsic biological variables controlling sensitization can be influenced only by selection of animals likely to be capable of mounting an immune response to the hapten. The extrinsic variables of dose, vehicle, route of exposure, adjuvant, etc., can be manipulated to develop sensitive predictive assays.

Appropriate planning and execution of predictive sensitization assays is critical. All too often techniques are discredited when, in fact, the performance of the tests was inferior or study design, e.g., choice of dose, was inappropriate. The first priority is to choose an appropriate experimental design. Often the assay to be used is chosen on a *pro forma* basis, without realizing the inherent weaknesses and strengths of the method. A common error in choosing an animal assay is using Freund's complete adjuvant (FCA) when setting dose response relationships. The adjuvant provides such sensitivity that dose effect relationships are muted.

Choice of dose and vehicle appropriate to the assay and the study question is the second priority. Although dose must be high enough to ensure penetration, it must be below the irritation threshold at challenge to avoid misinterpretation of irritant inflammation as allergic. For instance, the quaternary ammonium compounds, e.g., benzalkonium chloride, rarely sensitize but have been identified as allergens in some guinea pig assays. Knowing the irritation potential of compounds will allow the investigator to design and execute these studies appropriately. Vehicle choice determines in part the absorption of the test material and can influence sensitization rate, ability to elicit response at challenge, and the irritation threshold. Inappropriate selections effectively invalidate studies.

Guinea Pig Sensitization Tests

Predictive animal tests to determine the potential of substances to induce delayed hypersensitivity in humans are conducted most often in guinea pigs. Several tests have been described. Each offers its own advantages and disadvantages; most have many features in common. All utilize young (1–3 months old or 250–550 g), randomly bred albino guinea pigs. To reduce the possibility of seasonal variability in reactivity, animals are maintained in facilities with temperature approximately $20 \pm 1°C$, 40% to 50% relative humidity, 12-hr automatic light cycle, a standard vitamin C-supplemented chow, and water available at all times. Test sites are clipped free of hair with electric clippers; some assays specify chemical depilation as well. Most visually evaluate the responses, using descriptive scales for erythema and edema. Because of genetic influences, sensitivity to a common chemical, e.g., dinitrochlorobenzene, is usually periodically confirmed for animals from each vendor. There is some disagreement about which sex, if either, is more susceptible to sensitization. Males are more aggressive and may damage the skin of cagemates. Some assays specify use of one sex or one-half of each sex. The tests differ significantly in route of exposure, use of adjuvants, induction interval, and number of exposures. The principal features of the most commonly used assays and assays acceptable to regulatory agencies (24,36,129,136) to predict sensitization are summarized in Table 4.

Even if proper assay, dose, and vehicles are chosen, improper conduct of the study may result in incorrect conclusions. Sensitization assays are often assigned to the novitiate, when they should be performed and read by the experienced. Experienced investigators will often recognize that marginal reactions should be further investigated or that positives may be irritant in nature. Working with laboratories and personnel with extensive experience greatly decreases errors and increases the reliability and relevance of all standard assays described below (69,80,83,146).

TABLE 4. *Principal features of guinea pig sensitization assays*

Feature	Draize test	Open epicutaneous test	Buehler test	Freund's complete adjuvant test	Optimization test	Split adjuvant test	Guinea pig maximization
Number in test group	20	6–8	10–20	8–10	20	10–20	20–25
Number in control group	20	6–8	10–20	8–10	20	10–20	20–25
Induction exposure route	i.d.	Open	Patch	i.d.	i.d.	—	i.d. and patch
Number of exposures	10	20 or 21	3	3	9	4	1 i.d., 1 dermal
Duration patches	—	Continuous open	6 hr each	—	—	48 hrs each	48 hrs
Concentration (%)	0.1	Nonirritating	Nonirritating	5–50	0.1	—	Max. tolerated
Test group(s)	TS	TS	TS	TS in FCA	TS in FCA	TS, FCA	TS, TS + FCA, FCA
Control group	—	V only	—	FCA only	—	—	FCA, FCA + V, V
Site	L. flank	R. flank	L. flank	Shoulder	Back	Midback	Shoulder
Frequency of exposure	Every 2nd day	Daily	Every 7 days	Every 4 days	Every other day	0, 2, 4, 7 days	0 (i.d.), 7 days (patch)
Duration (days)	1–18	0–20	0–14	0–9	0–21	0–9	0–7
Miscellaneous	—	—	—	—	—	Dry ice pretreatment	SLS pretreatment
Rest period (days)	19–34	21–34	15–27	9–21 22–34	22–34	10–21	9–20
Challenge exposure route	i.d.	Open	Patch	i.d., patch	i.d.	—	Patch
Number of exposures	1	2	1	2	2	1	1
Day(s)	35	21 and 35	28	22 and 35	14–28	22	21

FCA, Freund's complete adjuvant; SLS, sodium lauryl sulfate; V, vehicle; TS, test substance.

Draize Test

The Draize sensitization test (DT) (29,81,82) was the first predictive sensitization test accepted by regulatory agencies and is still widely used. One flank of 20 guinea pigs is shaved and 0.05 ml of a 0.1% solution of test material in saline, paraffin oil, or polyethylene glycol is injected into the anterior flank on day 0. The next day and every other day through day 20, 0.1 ml of the test solution is injected into a new site on the same flank. Challenge follows a 2-week rest period. The opposite untreated flank is shaved and 0.05 ml of test solution is injected into each animal. Twenty previously untreated controls are injected at the same time. The test site is visually evaluated 24 and 48 hr after injection. The intensity of the responses of test animals is compared with that of controls; a larger or more intensely erythematous response than that of controls is considered a positive response. Results are expressed as the percent of animals positive or as the ratio of positive animals to the number tested (actual numbers listed).

Open Epicutaneous Test

The open epicutaneous test (OET) (80–82) simulates the conditions of human use by utilizing topical application of the test material. As originally described, the procedure also determines the doses required to induce sensitization and to elicit a response in sensitized animals. The *irritancy* profile is determined by applying 0.025 ml of varying concentrations, typically undiluted, 30, 10, 3, and 1% in ethanol, acetone, water, polyethylene glycol, or petrolatum, to a 2-cm² area of the shaved flanks of six to eight guinea pigs. Vehicle solubility and use conditions, e.g., direct application to skin or dilution during normal use, is considered in selecting the concentration. Test sites are visually evaluated 24 hr after application of test solutions for the presence or absence of erythema. The dose not causing a reaction in any animal (maximal nonirritant concentration) and the dose causing a reaction in 25% of the animals (minimal irritant concentration) are determined. During induction, 0.10 ml of test solution is applied to an 8-cm² area of flank skin of six to eight guinea pigs for 3 weeks, or five times a week for 4 weeks. Up to six groups of animals are treated with different doses; a control group is treated with vehicle only. The highest dose tested is usually the minimal irritant concentration; lower doses are based on usage concentration or a stepwise reduction, e.g., 30–10–3–1. Solutions are applied to the same site each day unless a moderate inflammatory response develops. A new site on the same flank is treated when inflammation develops.

Twenty-four to 72 hr after the last induction treatment, each animal is challenged on the previously untreated flank. The minimal irritant concentration, the maximum nonirritant concentration (from irritancy screen), and five solutions of lower concentrations are applied, 0.025 ml to a 2-cm² area. Skin reactions are read on an all-or-none basis at 24, 48, and 72 hr after application of the solutions. The maximum nonirritating concentration in the vehicle-treated group is calculated. Animals in test groups that develop inflammatory responses to lower concentrations are considered sensitized. The dose required to sensitize is determined by comparing the number of positive animals in the test groups. The minimal concentration necessary to elicit a positive response in a sensitized animal is apparent from the challenge responses.

Buehler Test

The Buehler test (17,18,58,81,82) also employs topical application of the test material. However, the test site is covered with an occlusive patch to enhance penetration and prevent evaporation of the test material. An absorbent patch, 20 × 20 mm Webril, backed by Blenderm tape and saturated with 0.4 ml of the test material, is placed on the shaved flanks of 10 to 20 guinea pigs. Test concentration varies from undiluted to usage levels. A concentration that produces slight erythema is optimum and is selected based on an irritancy screen conducted in other animals. The patch is held in place by wrapping the animal with an occlusive wrapping, then placing the animal in a special restrainer fitted with a rubber dam to maintain even pressure over the patch for a 6-hr exposure period. This procedure is repeated 7 and 14 days after the initial exposure. A control group of 10 to 20 animals is patched with vehicle only. Two weeks after the last induction patch, animals are challenged with patches saturated with a nonirritating concentration of test material applied to both flanks and with the vehicle (if other than water or acetone). Wrapping and restraint are as during induction. After 6 hr, the patch is removed and the area depilated. Test sites are visually evaluated 24 and 48 hr after patch removal. Animals developing erythematous responses are considered sensitized (if irritant control animals do not respond). The incidence of positive reactions and the average intensity of the response are calculated.

Freund's Complete Adjuvant Test

Freund's complete adjuvant test (FCAT) is an intradermal technique incorporating test material in a 50/50 mixture of FCA and distilled water. The test has been significantly modified since originally described (81). The latest published description (82) is summarized here. A 6 × 2-cm area across the shoulders of two groups of 10 to 20 guinea pigs is shaved and used as the injection site. Animals of one group are injected with 0.1 ml of a 5% solution of the test material in FCA/water. Control animals are injected with FCA/water. Injections are repeated every 4 days until three injections are given. The minimal irritating and maximum nonirritating concentration following topical application of 0.025 ml solutions to a 2-cm² area of skin is determined on a minimum of four naive guinea pigs (See *OET procedure*). Twenty-one days after the first induction injection, 0.025 ml of the minimal irritant concentration, the maximum nonirritant concentration, and two lower concentrations are applied to 2-cm² areas of the shaved flank. Test sites are not covered and are evaluated for the presence of erythema at 24, 48, and 72 hr after application. The minimum nonirritating concentration in FCA/water-treated controls is determined. Animals injected with the test material during induction that respond to lower doses are considered sensitized. The incidence of

sensitization and the threshold concentration for elicitation of the response in these animals are calculated.

Optimization Test

The optimization test resembles the DT but incorporates the use of adjuvant for some induction injections and both intradermal and topical challenges (81,82,121). Injections during induction are 0.1 ml of 0.1% concentration of test material in 0.9% saline or in 50/50 FCA/saline. A total of 10 injections is given. On day 1 of the first week, one injection into the shaved flank and one into a shaved area of dorsal skin are given. Two and 4 days later, one injection into a new dorsal site is given. The test material is administered in saline during the first week. During the second and third weeks, test material is administered in FCA/saline every other day to a shaved area over the shoulders. Twenty test animals are treated; 20 controls are injected with saline during week 1 and FCA/saline during weeks 2 and 3. The intensity of the 24-hr responses during week 1 is calculated as reaction volume. Thickness of a skin fold over the injection site is measured with a caliper (mm), and the two largest diameters of the erythematous reaction are recorded (mm). The reaction volume is calculated by multiplying fold thickness times both diameters and is expressed as microliters. The mean reaction volume of each animal to the intradermal injections using saline as a vehicle (week 1) is calculated. Thirty-five days after the first injection, animals are challenged with 0.1 ml of 0.1% test material in saline. The challenge reaction volume for each animal is calculated and compared to the mean reaction volume for that animal. Any animal developing a reaction volume at challenge greater than the mean plus one standard deviation during induction is considered sensitized. Vehicle control animals are injected with saline at challenge. A second challenge is conducted 45 days after the first injection. A nonirritating concentration of the test material in a suitable vehicle is applied to the flank skin, away from injection sites; 0.05 ml is applied to approximately 1 cm². The area is covered with a 2 × 2-cm #2 filter paper backed by an occlusive dressing, which remains in place for 24 hr. Reactions are visually evaluated using the 4-point erythema scale of the Draize primary irritancy scale (See *Irritation Tests in Animals*). The control animals are patched with vehicle alone. The number of positive animals in the test group is statistically compared with the number of "pseudo-positive" animals in the control group using the exact Fisher test. Separate comparisons of intradermal and epicutaneous challenges are made; a *p* value of ≤0.01 is considered significant. To classify materials as strong/moderate/weak/nonsensitizer, a classification scheme has been devised using results of exact Fisher test and number of positives detected (Table 5).

Split Adjuvant Test

The split adjuvant test (82,112,113) utilizes skin damage and FCA as adjuvants; application of the test material is topical. An area of back skin just behind the scapulas of 10 to 20 guinea pigs is clipped, shaved to glistening, then treated with dry ice for 5 to 10 sec. A dressing of a layer of loose

TABLE 5. *Classification scheme based on results of the optimization test*

Intradermal positive animals (%)	Epidermal positive animals (%)	Classification
s, >75	And/or s, >50	Strong sensitizer
s, 50–75	And/or s, 30–50	Moderate sensitizer
s, 30–50	n.s., 0–30	Weak sensitizer
n.s., 0–30	n.s., 0	No sensitizer

s, significant; n.s., not significant (using exact Fisher test).

mesh gauze and stretch adhesive with a 2 × 2-cm² opening over the shaved area is placed around the animal and secured with adhesive tape. This dressing remains in place throughout induction. Approximately 0.2 ml of creams or solid test material, 0.1 ml if liquid, is spread over the test site and covered with two layers of #2 filter paper backed by occlusive tape and attached to the dressing by adhesive tape. The concentration tested varies by irritancy potential, use conditions, etc. Two days later, the filter paper is lifted from the test site, the test material reapplied, and the filter paper covering replaced. On day 4, the filter paper cover is removed, two injections of 0.075 cc FCA are given into the edges of the test site, the test material is reapplied, and the site is resealed. On day 7 the test material is reapplied, and on day 9 the dressing is removed. Twenty-two days after the initial treatment, animals are challenged by topical application of 0.5 ml of test material to a 2 × 2-cm area of the shaved midback. The test site is covered by filter paper backed with adhesive tape, held in place by wrapping the animal with an elastic adhesive bandage secured with adhesive tape. A group of naive controls, 10 to 20 animals, is treated by the same procedure at challenge. Twenty-four hr after application, the dressing is removed and the test site is visually evaluated at 24, 48, and 72 hr using a 7-point descriptive visual scale. Sensitization of individual animals is indicated by significantly stronger reactions than those of controls.

Guinea Pig Maximization Test

The guinea pig maximization test (GPMT) (81,82,110) combines FCA, irritancy, intradermal injection, and occlusive topical application during the induction period. The shoulder region of two groups of 20 to 25 guinea pigs is shaved. Two identical sets of 0.1 ml intradermal injections of 50/50 FCA/water, test material in water, paraffin oil, or propylene glycol, and the same dose of test material in FCA/vehicle are placed in a 2 × 4-cm filter paper, placed over the injection site, covered with approximately 4 × 8-cm occlusive surgical tape, and secured in place with an elastic bandage wrapped around the animal. If the test material is nonirritating, the test site is pretreated with 10% sodium lauryl sulfate in petrolatum on day 6 to provoke an irritant reaction. If a vehicle other than petrolatum is used for topical application of the test material, the filter is saturated with the solution. Control animals are patched with the vehicle alone. The dressing is removed from the animals 48 hr after application. Test and control animals are challenged on the shaved flank

with the highest nonirritating concentration, approximately one-half of the highest nonirritating concentration, and with the vehicle. Solutions are applied to 1 × 1-cm pieces of filter paper secured in place as during induction. Patches are removed 24 hr later. The challenge area is shaved, if needed, 21 hr after patch removal. Reactions are visually evaluated 24 and 48 hr after patch removal. The intensity of responses to test material and vehicle in the test group is compared to the responses in controls. Reactions are considered positive when they are more intense than the response to vehicle and the responses to the test material in controls. The test material is rated as a weak to extreme sensitizer, based on the incidence of positives in the test group (Table 6).

Human Sensitization Assays

Chemicals can be tested for their ability to induce contact hypersensitivity in panels of human volunteers from whom informed consent is obtained. Human studies should be undertaken only after the results of predictive tests in animals are available if the test material is a new compound or if it contains significantly increased levels of common ingredients. Testing higher doses in animals provides some margin of safety for potential human subjects. Generally, materials shown to be sensitizers in animals are not tested on humans. However, if the potential benefit of the material warrants it, a small group of human subjects may be tested with materials inducing sensitization in animals. Such situations should be reviewed by an Institutional Review Board, test subjects should be informed of the increased risks, and the number of subjects exposed should be limited (additional subjects can be exposed if members of a small group do not respond).

Subjects should be randomly selected; however, some precautions are indicated. Recurrence of skin conditions in remission, e.g., psoriasis or eczema, has been associated with patch testing, as well as other minor physical traumas. Subjects at risk should be informed of this possibility and encouraged to consult their dermatologist before testing. Allergic contact dermatitis to materials already in commerce is sometimes detected by early induction patches. This does not reflect the particular test material's ability to induce sensitization. It merely indicates that under patch conditions, the material may elicit a response in presensitized individuals. Although the incidence of preexisting sensitization to the material should be considered in risk assessment decisions regarding marketing, detection of preexisting sensitization is not helpful in evaluating a material's ability to induce sensitization. Subjects should not be tested with materials to which they are known to be allergic, i.e., demonstrated by

TABLE 6. *Classification of materials by maximization test*

Sensitization rate (%)	Grade	Class
0–8	I	Weak
9–28	II	Mild
29–64	III	Moderate
65–80	IV	Strong
81–100	V	Extreme

diagnostic patch test or in previous predictive assays. It is prudent to question potential subjects routinely concerning their history of dermatologic disease and allergies. Records of positive responses of individuals participating in multiple predictive assays should be reviewed before testing to eliminate presensitized subjects. Some investigators feel the presence of intact draining lymph nodes from the application site is necessary to induce sensitization, and patches should not be placed on areas adjacent to mastectomies. Persons with a unilateral mastectomy who wish to participate may be tested by applying patches to the opposite side of the body.

Although numerous variations have been reported, there are four basic predictive human sensitization tests in current use: (a) a single induction/single challenge patch test; (b) repeated insult patch test (RIPT); (c) RIPT with continuous exposure (modified Draize); and (d) the maximization test. Principal features of human sensitization assays are summarized in Table 7. As originally described, all used customized patches. Patch selection was governed by available adhesive systems. Description of customized patches would be of historical interest only; as currently conducted, all human assays use similar patches. Occlusive patches, consisting of a nonwoven pad, usually Webril, or four-ply gauze sponges, backed by a good occlusive surgical tape, e.g., Blenderm, are commercially available or may be custom-made in strips of four or five pads. Acceptable alternatives include the Hilltop Chamber (79), which contains a Webril pad inside an occlusive plastic disc backed by a porous tape; the Duhring Chamber (54), a stainless steel disc that contains a Webril pad; and the large Finn Chamber. Duhring and Finn chambers are usually secured in place by porous surgical tape. Occasionally, semiocclusive patches made of Webril backed by porous tape may be used; these are decidedly inferior to occlusive patches in inducing sensitization.

For assays other than maximization, 150 to 200 subjects are usually tested. Henderson and Riley (65) statistically showed that if no positive reactions are observed in 200 randomly selected subjects, as many as 15/1,000 of the general population *may* react (95% confidence). As sample size is reduced, the likelihood of unpredicted adverse reactions in the general population increases.

Schwartz–Peck Test (and Modifications)

A single application induction patch followed by a single application patch test was described by Schwartz (150,151) and Schwartz and Peck (152), with a usage test of 1 month after challenge to verify patch results. The test has been modified by some to eliminate the usage test (16), to eliminate patching altogether, and to place a usage period between induction and challenge patches (163). The term "complete Schwartz–Peck" refers to a single induction patch, usage period, single challenge patch test. This may also be referred to as the Traub–Tusing–Spoon method. Incomplete Schwartz–Peck tests do not incorporate a usage period.

A patch saturated with the test material, diluted if necessary, is applied to the outer upper arm of 200 test subjects and remains in place for 24 to 72 hr. The dose tested and duration of patch contact vary with intended use. Cosmetics may be tested without a covering (open application) or with

semiocclusive patches. The test site is visually evaluated at patch removal and at 24 and 48 hr after removal for erythema and edema. A 4-week normal usage period follows the induction patch in the complete Schwartz–Peck test. A challenge patch is applied to the same site on the upper arm at the conclusion of the usage period or 10 to 14 days after the induction patch of the incomplete Schwartz–Peck test. Duration of contact and evaluation of site are performed as during induction. The development of dermatitis at challenge, not present or much stronger than during induction, signifies sensitization. Schwartz originally described the incomplete Schwartz–Peck test. A usage test was to be conducted after the challenge patch, using 1,000 different subjects.

Although Schwartz and Peck referred to their assay as a "prophetic patch" test, experience has shown that only potent haptens will induce sensitization in this assay. In fairness, it should be noted that the test was originally designed to evaluate the effect of nylon garments on the skin. It was intended to detect adverse effects, irritation, and "secondary irritation" (sensitization). The mechanism of DTH was not understood by most scientists when the test was designed. Although the test was useful for its original purpose, its use was unfortunately expanded by its designers without considering new information generated by immunologists. Clearly, the assay is inferior to all other predictive human sensitization assays. However, a few groups continue to utilize the method.

Repeat Insult Patch Tests

Three major variations on the RIPT are in common use: (a) the Draize human sensitization test (27,28); (b) the Shelanski–Shelanski test (153–155); and (c) the Voss–Griffith test (18,57,58,171). Although the Shelanskis first published a description of a RIPT, they based its development on a verbal description of a method Draize was devising (154). Voss modified the Shelanski–Shelanski test (171), and his assay was later modified by Griffith (57). As one would expect, the three assays have much in common. There are, however, some significant differences in the assays as originally described.

In the Draize human sensitization test, an occlusive patch containing the test material is applied to the upper arm or upper back of 200 volunteers. The patch remains in place for 24 hr and is then removed. The test site is evaluated at patch removal for erythema and edema. A second patch test is applied to a *new* site 24 hr after the first patch is removed. This process is repeated until a total of 10 patches is applied. For convenience, the test may be run on a Monday-to-Friday schedule, with subjects removing their own patches Saturday (72 hr between Friday and Monday applications). Ten to 14 days after application of the last induction patches, subjects are challenged via a patch applied to a new site. Duration of contact is 24 hr; sites are visually evaluated at removal of the patch. The response at challenge is compared to the response to patches applied early in induction. The incidence of sensitization is reported.

Like the Draize RIPT, the Shelanski–Shelanski test employs occlusive patches that remain in contact with the skin of the upper arm for 24 hr. The patching cycle is the same;

TABLE 7. *Principal features of human sensitization tests*

	Complete Schwartz/Peck	Shelanski/ Shelanski	Draize	Griffith/Voss/ Stotts	Modified Draize	Human maximization
Number of subjects	200	200	200	200		25
Induction site	Upper arm	Upper arm; same site	Upper back; upper arm; new sites	Upper arm; same site	Upper arm; upper back; same site	Lower back; upper arm; same site
Number of exposures	1	15	10	9	10	5
Duration of exposures (hr)	24–72	24	24	24	48–72	48
Frequency of exposure	—	3/week	3/week	3/week	Continuous	24 hr rest periods
Evaluations at	Removal, 24, 48 hr	Patch removal	Patch removal	48–72 hr	30 min	
Miscellaneous	4-week usage period	Fatiguing index		Pilot group		Irritant dose or SLS[a] used
Rest period (days)		14–21	10–14	14	14	14
Challenge site	Upper arm	Upper arm	Upper back; upper arm; new site	Upper arms (2 patches)	Upper arm; upper back; new site	Lower back; upper arm; new site
Duration of challenge	24–72 hr	48 hr	24 hr	24 hr	72 hr	48 hr
Evaluations at	Removal, 24, 48 hr	Removal	Removal	48 & 96 hr	Removal, 24 hr	Removal, 24 & 48 hr
Miscellaneous				Challenge induct. and fresh site	May do 2 48-hr challenge patches	SLS provocative patch sensitization index

SLS, sodium lauryl sulfate.

however, patches are placed on the *same* test site each time, and a total of 15 patches is applied during induction. The test site is evaluated before application of a new patch to the site; if inflammation has developed, the patch is placed on an adjacent uninflamed site. Two to 3 weeks after the induction period, subjects are challenged by application of a patch that remains in place for 48 hr. Test sites are evaluated at patch removal for erythema and edema. The incidence of positive response is reported. Patch responses during induction were considered by Shelanski and Shelanski to be evidence of "skin fatigue" (cumulative irritation); the time to development, i.e., number of patches, was reported as a fatiguing index.

Voss (171) reduced the number of 24-hr patch exposures to nine over a 3-week period. At challenge 2 weeks after the last induction patch, duplicate patches applied to the original test site are worn for 24 hr. Patch sites are evaluated 48 and 96 hr after patch application. A pilot group of 10 to 12 subjects was tested before exposing the full panel of 60 to 70 subjects. Griffith later published more detailed accounts of the method (57,58). Up to four dissimilar materials were simultaneously tested, and duplicate challenges were applied to the sites of induction and to the opposite arm, thus testing on areas drained by different regional lymphatics. Griffith also described characteristics of allergic reactions at challenge, stronger reactions than during induction, persistence of the response through 96 hr, and reactions in a few subjects with no reactions in the rest of the panel. The concept of a rechallenge of subjects with reactions difficult to interpret was also introduced. The number of subjects was increased to 200 by conducting tests on multiple panels.

As currently conducted, the differences in Draize and Voss–Griffith RIPT are minimal. Many investigators apply patches to the same site during induction and refer to the procedure as a Draize RIPT. The value of multiple grades at challenge is widely recognized and utilized. Multiple test materials are simultaneously tested in all RIPT for reasons of efficiency and economy. Although the distinctions between Draize and Voss–Griffith procedures have blurred with common usage, the Shelanski–Shelanski test with five to six more induction applications remains distinct.

Human Maximization Test

Kligman (84) reviewed the common human predictive sensitization test methods in use in 1966 and found them to be unsatisfactory in inducing sensitization to nine clinical allergens. In panels of 200 subjects, the Shelanski–Shelanski method induced sensitization to four materials; the original Draize test and the complete Schwartz–Peck test induced sensitization to two allergens each; and the incomplete Schwartz–Peck test failed to induce sensitization to any allergen. He concluded that "emphasis must shift from prophecy to the more practical objective of identifying potential allergens. . . . Once the allergenic potential is known with reasonable certainty, a judgement of risk might be ventured after examining all the pertinent variables" (86). This represented a profound change in the intent of predictive sensitization assays. Based on his studies of factors affecting rates of sensitization in predictive assays (85,88), Kligman designed

the human maximization test (86). He later modified the procedure somewhat to reduce difficulties in performing the test and in interpreting the test (89).

The maximization test utilizes irritancy as an adjuvant. During induction, compounds that are irritating are tested at a concentration that produces a moderate erythema within 48 hr. For materials that are nonirritating, the test site is pretested with a 24-hr patch of 5% sodium lauryl sulfate (SLS); a second pretreatment SLS patch may be applied to produce a brisk erythema, and induction concentrations are at least five times higher than use levels. Petrolatum is the preferred vehicle. Often custom-made Webril/Blenderm patches or Duhring chambers are used. Patches are applied to either the outer aspect of the arm or lower back, and up to four dissimilar materials may be tested at one time. Wrapping with extra tape is often necessary to ensure occlusion. Bandage sprays may be used to ensure sealing of the test site. Five sets of patches are worn on the same site for 48 hr each, with a 24-hr rest period between removal and reapplication. Following a 2-week rest period after the last induction patch, an SLS provocative patch procedure is performed to prepare the skin for challenge. A patch saturated with a 2.5% to 5% solution of SLS is applied to previously untreated sites on the lower back. SLS concentration is based on the season and on individual subject response. The SLS patch is removed after 1 hr and a patch containing the test material applied. A control site is patched with SLS (1 hr) and petrolatum (48 hr) to aid in interpretation of the results. Forty-eight hours after application, the patch is removed and test sites are evaluated. Test sites are reexamined 24 and 48 hr after patch removal. The number of subjects developing a positive response is reported, and a sensitization index based on percent of subjects responding is assigned to the test material. Although it is clear that the maximization test is a sensitive tool for detection of allergenicity, the skin damage produced is dramatic and unacceptable to many subjects.

Modified Draize Human Sensitization Test

The RIPT procedure was modified to provide for continuous patch exposure to the test material during the 3-week induction period (117,118). Patches containing test material are applied to the outer upper arm each Monday, Wednesday, and Friday, until a total of 10 patches has been applied. Patches remain in place until about 30 min before application of a fresh patch. (This allows some clearing of responses to tape and facilitates grading.) Fresh patches are applied to the same site unless moderate inflammation has developed; the patches are placed on adjacent noninflamed skin if inflammation becomes pronounced. This produces a continuous exposure of 504 to 552 hr (some investigators apply only nine patches), compared to a total exposure period of 216 to 240 hr for RIPT of comparable induction periods. In addition, induction concentration was increased to levels above usage exposure. Two weeks after induction, subjects are challenged by exposure of a new site to a patch of 72-hr duration at a nonirritating concentration. Test sites are evaluated at patch removal and 24 hr after removal. Jordan and King (77) modified the challenge procedure to two consecutive 48-hr patch periods.

IRRITANT DERMATITIS

Historically, skin irritation has been described by exclusion as localized inflammation not mediated by either sensitized lymphocytes or by antibodies, e.g., that which develops by a process not involving the immune system. Application of some chemicals directly destroys tissue, producing skin necrosis at the site of application. Chemicals producing necrosis that results in formation of scar tissue are described as corrosive. Chemicals may disrupt cell functions and/or trigger the release, formation, or activation of autocoids that produce local increases in blood flow, increase vascular permeability, attract white blood cells in the area, or directly damage cells. The additive effects of the mediators result in local skin inflammation. A number of as yet poorly defined pathways involving different processes of mediator generation appear to exist. Although no agent has yet met all the criteria to establish it as a mediator of skin irritation, histamine, 5-hydrotryptamine, prostaglandins, leukotrienes, kinins, complement, reactive oxygen species, and products of white blood cells have been strongly implicated as mediators of some irritant reactions (144). Chemicals that produce inflammation as a result of a single exposure are termed acute irritants.

Some chemicals do not produce acute irritation from a single exposure but may produce inflammation following repeated application to the same area of skin. The cumulative irritation from repeated exposures has also been called skin fatigue (153). Because of the possibility of skin contact during transport and use of many chemicals, regulatory agencies have mandated screening chemicals for the ability to produce skin corrosion and acute irritation. These studies are conducted in animals, using standardized protocols. However, the protocols specified by some agencies vary somewhat. It is not appropriate to conduct screening studies for corrosion in humans, but acute irritation is sometimes evaluated in humans after animal studies have been completed. Tests for cumulative irritation in both animals and humans have been reported.

Irritation Tests in Animals

Draize-Type Tests

Primary irritation and corrosion are most often evaluated by modifications of the method described by John Draize and colleagues in 1944 (29). The Federal Hazardous Substance Act (FHSA) adopted one modification as a standard procedure (24). The backs of six albino rabbits are clipped free of hair. Each material is tested on two 1-inch-square sites on the same animal; one site is intact and one is abraded in such a way that the stratum corneum is opened but no bleeding produced. Abrasion can be performed using the tip of a hypoderm needle repeatedly drawn across the skin or commercial instruments such as the Berkeley Scarifier (64) or the Maryland Plastics skin abrader. Materials are tested undiluted; 0.5 ml liquid or 0.5 g solid or semisolid material is applied. In some cases the skin may be moistened to help solids adhere to the site, or an equal volume of solvent may be used to moisten the material. Each test site is covered with two layers of 1-inch-square surgical gauze secured in

place with tape. The entire trunk of the animal is then wrapped with rubberized cloth or other occlusive impervious material to retard evaporation of the substances and hold the patches in one position. Twenty-four hours after application, the wrappings are removed and the test sites are evaluated for erythema and edema, using a prescribed scale (Table 8). Evaluations of abraded and intact sites are separately recorded. Test sites are evaluated again 48 hr later (72 hr after application) by the same procedure. The reproducibility of the FHSA procedure (168,176) and the relevance of test results to human experience (26,69,105,120,131,143,159) have been questioned. Numerous modifications to the Draize procedure have been proposed to improve its prediction of human experience. Modifications that have been proposed include changing the species tested (127), reduction of exposure period, use of fewer animals, and testing on intact skin only (60). Several governmental bodies utilized their own modification of the Draize procedure for regulatory decisions. The FHSA, DOT, Environmental Protection Agency (EPA), Federal Insecticide, Fungicide, and Rodenticide Act (FIFRA), and OECD guidelines are contrasted to the original Draize methods in Table 9.

Summaries and evaluations of the scores vary somewhat. Draize reported values for individual animals at each time point, combined the erythema and edema values at each time point, and then averaged the 24- and 72-hr evaluations for intact and abraded sites separately. He also calculated a primary irritation index (PII), which was the average of the intact and abraded sites. Agents producing PII of <2 were considered only mildly irritating, 2 to 5 moderately irritating, and >5 severely irritating. The primary irritation calculated for the FHSA is essentially the PII of Draize. A minimum PII of 5 defines an irritant by Consumer Product Safety Commission (CPSC) standards. National Institute of Occupational Safety and Health (NIOSH) does not combine responses of abraded sites and includes probable effects on normal and damaged skin in their evaluation.

Although vesiculation, ulceration, and severe eschar formations are not included in the Draize scoring scales, all Draize-type tests are used to evaluate corrosion as well as irritation. When severe reactions that may not be reversible are noted, test sites are observed for a longer period. Delayed

TABLE 8. *Draize–FHSA scoring system*

Skin reaction	Score
Erythema and eschar formation	
No erythema	0
Very slight erythema (barely perceptible)	1
Well-defined erythema	2
Moderate to severe erythema	3
Severe erythema (beet redness) to slight eschar formations (injuries in depth)	4
Edema formation	
No edema	0
Very slight edema (barely perceptible)	1
Slight edema (edges of area well defined by definite raising)	2
Moderate edema (raised ~1 mm)	3
Severe edema (raised >1 mm and extending beyond the area of exposure)	4

TABLE 9. *Comparison of skin irritation tests based on the Draize method*

	Draize	FHSA	DOT	FIFRA	OECD[a]
No. of animals	3[b]	6	6	6	6
Abrasion	Abraded & intact	Abraded & intact	Intact	2 Abraded & 2 intact	Intact
Dose liquids	0.5 ml undiluted	0.5 ml undiluted	0.5 ml	0.5 ml undiluted	0.5 ml
Dose solids	0.5 g	0.5 g in solvent	0.5 g	0.5 g moistened	0.5 g moistened
Wrapping materials	Gauze and rubberized cloth	Impervious material			Semiocclusive
Exposure period (hr)	24	24	4	4	4
Examination (hr)	24, 72	24, 72	4, 48	0.5, 1, 24, 48, 72[c]	0.5, 1, 24, 48, 72[c]
Removal of test materials	Not specified	Not specified	Skin washed	Skin wiped—not washed	Skin washed
Excluded from testing	—	—	—	Toxic materials pH ≤ 2 or ≥11.5	Toxic materials pH ≤ 2 or ≥11.5

DOT, Department of Transportation; FHSA, Federal Hazardous Substance Act; FIFRA, Federal Insecticide, Fungicide, and Rodenticide Act; OECD, Organization for Economic Cooperation and Development.

[a] Although other species are acceptable, the albino rabbit is the preferred species.

[b] Draize tested four materials on six rabbits. Three abraded and three intact sites were tested with each material.

[c] Times listed are after patch removal for FIFRA and OECD. Times listed for Draize, FHSA, and DOT are after application.

evaluations are usually made on days 7 and 14. However, evaluations have been made as late as 35 days after application. EPA bases its interpretation on 7-day observations.

The basic exposure procedures for skin irritation/corrosion of OECD guidelines have been further modified to test for corrosion during shorter periods (136). Under a directive of the EEC, a 3-min exposure was added (with no wrapping procedure) and the United Nations recommendations for the Transport of Dangerous Goods are based on exposure times of 4 hr, 1 hr, and 3 min, with the recommendation that the 1-hr exposure be conducted first. Evaluations are made 1, 24, 48, 72 hr, and 7 days after dosing.

Non-Draize Animal Studies

Animal assays to evaluate the ability of chemicals to produce cumulative irritation have been developed (140). However, they are not required by any regulatory agency. The impetus for their use is largely development of products that are better tolerated by consumers. Although many such tests have been described, only a few are used extensively enough to summarize. Even those used more often are not as well standardized as Draize-type tests, and many variables have been introduced by multiple investigators.

Repeat application patch tests in which diluted materials are applied to the same site each day for 15 to 21 days have been reported using several species (140). The guinea pig or rabbit is most commonly used. Patches used vary considerably, with gauze Draize-type dressings and metal chambers being the extremes. Some authors recommend testing the materials with no covering, presumably with a restraining collar to prevent grooming of the area and ingestion of the material. Because the degree of occlusion is an important determinant of percutaneous penetration, the choice of covering materials may determine the sensitivity of a given test (107). A reference material of similar use or that produces a known effect in humans is included in almost all repeat application patch procedures. The degrees of inflammation produced by the materials in a single assay are compared.

Test sites are evaluated for erythema and edema, using either the scales of the Draize-type tests or more descriptive scales developed by the investigator. Although interpretation ratings such as "slight," "moderate," or "severe" irritant are not usually made, the data from cumulative irritancy assays in rabbits have been used to predict reactions in humans. Other investigators used multiple application with shorter periods of time to evaluate materials (78).

The guinea pig immersion assay has been used to evaluate the irritancy of aqueous detergent solutions (21,85,134,135). Ten guinea pigs are placed in restraining devices that are immersed in a 40°C test solution for 4 hr. The apparatus is designed to maintain the guinea pig's head above the solution. Immersion is repeated daily for three treatments. Twenty-four hours after the final immersion, the flank is shaved and skin is evaluated for erythema, edema, and fissures. Concentration of test materials varies somewhat but is usually <10% to limit systemic toxicity of the agents. Some materials are unsuitable for this assay because death may result from systemic absorption of toxic materials. A second group of animals is usually tested with a reference material for comparison to the material of interest.

Uttley and Van Abbe (167) developed a mouse ear test in which undiluted shampoos were applied to one ear daily for 4 days. The degree of inflammation was visually quantified as vessel dilation, erythema, and edema, using a visual scale. The degree of inflammation produced by materials of interest was compared to that produced by a reference material tested on another group of mice. Recently, others have used ear thickness to quantify degree of inflammation and have either pretreated the ear with a strong irritant to simulate damaged skin or have increased the frequency of application to increase the sensitivity of the assay.

Human Irritation Tests

Because only a small area of skin need be tested, it is possible to conduct predictive irritation assays in humans, provided systemic toxicity (from absorption) is low and informed consent is obtained. Although regulatory agencies do not routinely require testing in humans, human tests are preferred to animal tests in some cases because of the uncertainties of interspecies extrapolation. New materials, i.e., those of unknown or unfamiliar composition, should be tested on animal skin first to determine if application to humans is warranted (129).

Many forms of a single application patch test have been published. Duration of patch exposure has varied between 1 and 72 hr. Custom-made apparatus to hold the test material has been designed (79,107,154,156). A variety of adhesives no longer commercially available have been used (109). Although the individual assays provided important information to the investigators of the period, they were never standardized or gained wide acceptance.

The single application patch procedure outlined by the National Academy of Sciences (NAS) Publication 1138 (129) incorporates important aspects of assays used by many investigators. The procedure is similar to FHSA tests in rabbits. Commercial patches, chambers, gauze squares, or cotton bandage material, e.g., Webril, may be applied to either the intrascapular region of the back or to the dorsal surface of the upper arms (108). Patches are secured in place with surgical tape without wrapping the trunk or arm. For new materials or volatiles, a relatively nonocclusive tape, e.g., Micropore, Dermical, or Scanpore, should be used. Increasing the degree of occlusion with occlusive tapes, e.g., Blenderm, or chamber devices, e.g., the Duhring chamber or Hilltop chamber, generally increases the severity of responses.

A 4-hour exposure period was suggested by the NAS panel. However, it is desirable to test new materials and volatiles for shorter periods—30 min to 1 hr—and many investigators apply materials intended for skin contact for 24- to 48-hr periods. Subjects should routinely be instructed to remove patches immediately if any unusual discomfort develops. After the period of exposure, the patches should be removed, the area cleaned with water to remove any residue, and the test site marked by study personnel. Responses are evaluated 30 min to 1 hr after patch removal (to allow hydration and pressure effects to subside) and again 24 hr after the patch is removed. Persistent reactions may be evaluated for 3 to 4 days. The Draize scales for erythema and edema (Table 8) have been used for grading human skin responses. However, they have no provision for scoring papular, vesicular, or bullous responses. Integrated scales ranging from 4 to 16 points have been published and are generally preferred to the Draize scales (example, Table 10). Up to 10 materials can be si-

multaneously tested on each subject. The position that the materials are placed on the skin, e.g., upper right back or lower left back, should be systematically varied because skin reactivity differs by body region and some locations may receive more pressure from chairs, clothing, etc., than others. Each battery of patches should include at least one reference material. Scores from all subjects are averaged for each material, and comparisons between standards and other test materials are made. Some investigators have accepted an average difference of 1 unit on the grading scale as meaningful. Other investigators analyze the data by standard statistical tests. It is also possible to test multiple doses and calculate median irritant dose (ID_{50}) responses.

The development of inflammation after repeated application of patches containing a test material to the same area of skin was referred to as "skin fatigue" by Shelanski (153) to explain the development of inflammation late in the induction phase of sensitization tests without positive responses at challenge. The phenomenon was also referred to as secondary irritation and later as cumulative irritation. As with single application patch tests, many investigators developed their own version of a repeat application patch test. Most were patterned after human sensitization studies with 24-hr exposures, with or without a rest period between patches. Kligman and Wooding (90) applied the Litchfield and Wilcoxon probe analysis to cumulative irritation testing with calculation of IT_{50} and ID_{50} values and statistical comparison of those values for different materials. Their early work forms the basis for the 21-day cumulative irritation assay that currently is widely used.

The cumulative irritation assay as described by Lanman and co-workers (103) was used to compare antiperspirants, deodorants, and bath oils to provide guidance for product development. A 1-inch square of Webril was saturated with liquid or up to 0.5 g of viscous substances and applied to the surface of the pad to be applied to the skin. The patch was applied to the upper back and sealed in place with occlusive tape. After 24 hr the patch was removed, the area evaluated, and a fresh patch applied. The procedure was repeated daily for up to 21 days. The sensitivity of the assay was increased by increasing the number of test subjects from 10 to 24. The IT_{50} as described by Kligman and Wooding (90) was used to evaluate and compare test materials.

Modifications of the cumulative irritation assay have been reported. Data generated have been compared using other evaluation schemes (120), and the interval between application of fresh patches (145) has been varied. The newer chamber devices have replaced Webril with occlusive tape in some laboratories. Some investigators currently use cumulative scores to compare test materials and do not calculate an IT_{50}. The necessity of 21 applications has recently been questioned (7). Although the procedure came to be known as the 21-day cumulative irritation assay, the number of applications used was varied by Lanman et al. (103), depending on the types of materials to be tested. Twenty-one days was the *maximum* period of testing. Kligman and Wooding performed their studies on surfactants in 10 days. Lanman needed 21 applications to discriminate between baby lotions. The number of applications used to rank materials should be chosen based on the class of material being studied.

Repeated application patch tests as described above fail to

TABLE 10. *Simple integrated scale for irritant patch test*

0	No sign of inflammation; normal skin
±(1/2)	Glazed appearance of the sites, or barely perceptible erythema
1	Slight erythema
2	Moderate erythema, possibly with barely perceptible edema at the margin; papules may be present
3	Moderate erythema, with generalized edema
4	Severe erythema with severe edema, with or without vesicles
5	Severe reaction spread beyond the area of the patch

predict some adverse reactions because of repeated application of materials to damaged skin, e.g., acne, shaved underarms, or sensitive areas such as the face (6). The chamber scarification test (49–51,53) was developed to evaluate materials that would normally be applied to damaged skin. Light-skinned Caucasians who developed severe erythema with edema and vesicles following a 24-hr exposure to 5% SLS in Duhring chambers applied to the inner forearm are preselected as subjects. Six to eight 10-mm-square areas on the midvolar forearm are scarified with eight criss-cross scratches made with a 30-gauge needle. Four scratches are parallel, with another four at right angles. In scarifing the tissue, the bevel of the needle is to the side and is drawn across the tissue at a 45° angle with enough pressure to scratch the epidermis without drawing blood. Duhring chambers containing the test material, 0.1 g for ointments, creams, and powders or Webril saturated with 0.1 ml for liquids, are placed over the scarified areas and are secured in place with nonocclusive tape wrapped around the forearm. Fresh chambers containing the same materials are applied daily for 3 days. Thirty minutes after removal of the last set of chambers, the test sites are evaluated on a 0-to-4 scale (Table 11). The responses are averaged and materials are classified as low (0–0.4), slight (0.5–1.4), moderate (1.5–2.4), or severe irritants. In some cases, a scarification index (SI) is calculated by comparing responses on intact or scarified skin (scores from scarified sites divided by scores from intact skin). The SI is used to estimate the relative risk for damaged and normal tissue. It is not used to rank test materials.

Many variables of the chosen test procedure, e.g., vehicle, type of patch, concentration tested, may modify the intensity of the response (34,121). Selection of subjects tested may also influence the outcome. Differences in intensity of responses has been linked to differences in age (87), sex (87), and race (174,175). Some investigators select the test population based on proposed use of the test materials.

In addition to patch test procedures, exaggerated exposure tests simulating extreme usage and usage tests have been used to compare the irritation potential of a variety of consumer products. These tests include skin washing procedures (43), arm or hand immersion studies (44,59,78), and clinical usage tests in which subjects use exaggerated concentrations of test materials (22,76,92) or materials treated with the agent under investigation (173). The study designs vary significantly, and it is not possible to describe generally accepted procedures because of variabilities in design. Special emphasis should be placed on design in terms of statistical validity (1). Although some toxicologists specializing in the skin as a target organ are involved in tests of this type, they are more often conducted by groups specializing in clinical testing and claim support.

CONTACT URTICARIA

Contact urticaria has been defined as a wheal-and-flare response that develops within 30 to 60 min after exposure of the skin to certain agents (170). Symptoms of immediate contact reactions can be classified according to their morphology and severity:

Itching, tingling, and burning with erythema is the weakest type of immediate contact reaction.
Local wheal-and-flare with tingling and itching represents the prototype reaction of contact urticaria.
Generalized urticaria after local contact is rare but can occur from strong urticaria.
Symptoms in other organs can appear with the skin symptoms in cases of immunologic contact urticaria syndrome.

The strength of the reactions may greatly vary, and often the whole range of local symptoms—from slight erythema to strong edema and erythema—can be seen from the same substance if different concentrations are used in skin tests (95). Not only the concentration but also the site of the skin contact affects the reaction. A certain concentration of contact urticant may produce strong edema and erythema reactions on the skin of the upper back and face but only erythema on the volar surfaces of the lower arms or legs. In some cases, contact urticaria can be demonstrated only on damaged or previously eczematous skin, and it can be part of the mechanism responsible for maintenance of chronic eczemas (2,114,135). Some agents, such as formaldehyde, produce urticaria on healthy skin following repeated but not single applications to the skin. Diagnosis of immediate contact urticaria is based on a thorough history and skin testing with suspected substances. Skin tests for human diagnostic testing are summarized in a recent review (170). Because of the risk of systemic reactions, e.g., anaphylaxis, human diagnostic tests should only be performed by experienced personnel with facilities for resuscitation on hand. Contact urticaria has been divided into two main types on the basis of proposed pathophysiological mechanisms, nonimmunologic and immunologic (115). Recent reviews list agents suspected to cause each type of urticarial response (97). A few common urticants are listed in Table 12.

Nonimmunologic contact urticaria is the most common form and occurs without previous exposure in most individuals. The reaction remains localized and does not cause systemic symptoms or spread to become generalized urticaria. Typically, the strength of this type of contact urticaria reaction varies from erythema to a generalized urticarial response, depending on the concentration, skin site, and substance. The mechanism of nonimmunologic contact urticaria has not been delineated, but a direct influence on dermal vessel walls or a non-antibody-mediated release of histamine, prostaglandins, leukotrienes, substance P, or other inflammatory mediators represents possible mechanisms. Recent reports suggest that nonimmunologic urticaria produced by different agents may involve different combinations of mediators (97).

TABLE 11. *Grading scale for chamber scarification test*

0	Scratch marks barely visible
1	Erythema confined to scratches
2	Broader bands of increased erythema, with or without rows of vesicles, pustules, or erosions
3	Severe erythema with partial confluency, with or without other lesions
4	Confluent, severe erythema sometimes associated with edema, necrosis, or bulla

TABLE 12. *A few agents reported to cause urticaria in humans*

Immunologic mechanisms
  Bacitracin
  Ethyl and methyl paraben
  Seafood (high molecular weight protein extracts)
Nonimmunologic mechanisms
  Cinnamic aldehyde
  Balsam of Peru
  Benzoic acid
  Ethyl aminobenzoate
  Dimethyl sulfoxide
Unknown mechanisms
  Epoxy resin
  Lettuce/endive
  Cassia oil
  Formaldehyde
  Ammonium persulfate
  Neomycin

The most potent and best studied substances producing *nonimmunologic contact urticaria* are benzoic acid, cinnamic acid, cinnamic aldehyde, and nicotinic esters. Under optimal conditions, more than half of a random sample of individuals show local edema and erythema reactions within 45 min of application of these substances if the concentration is high enough. Benzoic acid and sodium benzoate are used as preservatives for cosmetics and other topical preparations at concentrations from 0.1% to 0.2% and are capable of producing immediate contact reactions at the same concentrations (118). Cinnamic aldehyde at a concentration of 0.01% may elicit an erythematous response associated with a burning or stinging feeling in the skin. Mouthwashes and chewing gums contain cinnamic aldehyde at concentrations high enough to produce a pleasant tingling or "lively" sensation in the mouth and enhance the sale of the product. Higher concentrations produce lip swelling or typical contact urticaria in normal skin. Eugenol in the mixture inhibits contact sensitization to cinnamic aldehyde and inhibits nonimmunologic contact urticaria from this same substance. The mechanism of the quenching effect is not certain, but a competitive inhibition at the receptor level may be the explanation (61).

Immunologic contact urticaria is an immediate Type 1 allergic reaction in people previously sensitized to the causative agent (170). The molecules of a contact urticant react with specific IgE molecules attached to mast cell membranes. The cutaneous symptoms are elicited by vasoactive substances, mainly histamine, released from mast cells. The role of histamine is conspicuous, but other mediators of inflammation, e.g., prostaglandins, leukotrienes, and kinins, may influence the degree of response. Immunologic contact urticaria reaction can extend beyond the contact site, and generalized urticaria may be accompanied by other symptoms, e.g., rhinitis, conjunctivitis, asthma, and even anaphylactic shock. The term "contact urticaria syndrome" was therefore suggested by Maibach and Johnson (115). The name generally has been accepted for a symptom complex in which local urticaria occurs at the contact site with symptoms in other parts of the skin or in target organs such as the nose and throat, lung, and gastrointestinal and cardiovascular sys-

tems. Fortunately, the appearance of systemic symptoms is rare, but it may be seen in cases of strong hypersensitivity or in a widespread exposure and abundant percutaneous absorption of an allergen.

Foodstuffs are the most common causes of *immunologic contact urticaria* (Table 12). The orolaryngeal area is a site where immediate contact reactions are frequently provoked by food allergens, most often among atopic individuals. The actual antigens are proteins or protein complexes. As a proof of immediate hypersensitivity, specific IgE antibodies against the causative agent can typically be found in the patient's serum using the RAST technique and skin test for immediate allergy. The passive transfer test (Prausnitz-Kustner test) also often gives a positive result.

Predictive assays for evaluating the ability of materials to produce nonimmunologic contact urticaria have been developed. No predictive assays for immunologic contact urticaria have been published. Lahti and Maibach (96) developed an assay in guinea pigs using materials known to produce urticaria in humans. One-tenth of a milliliter of the material is applied to one ear of the animal; an equal volume of the solvent in which the test material is dissolved or suspended is applied to the opposite ear as a control. Ear thickness is measured before application and then every 15 min for 1 or 2 hr after application. The swelling response is dependent on the concentration of the eliciting substance. The maximum response is about a 100% increase in ear thickness, and it appears within 50 min after application of a contact urticant. In histologic sections, marked dermal edema and intra- and perivascular infiltrate of heterophilic granulocytes appear 40 min after application of test substances.

This assay is the predictive test of choice for nonimmunologic contact urticaria if animals are to be tested. Guinea pig body skin reacts with quickly appearing erythema to cinnamic aldehyde, methyl nicotinate, and dimethyl sulfoxide but not benzoic acid, sorbic acid, or cinnamic acid. Analogous reactions can be elicited in the earlobes of other animal species. Cinnamic aldehyde and dimethyl sulfoxide produce a swelling reaction in guinea pig, rat, and mouse. Benzoic acid, sorbic acid, cinnamic acid, diethyl fumarate, and methyl nicotinate produce no response in the rat or mouse, but the guinea pig ear reacts to all of them (97). This suggests that either there are several mechanisms of nonimmunologic contact urticaria, or there are differences in the activation of sensitivity to mediators of inflammation among guinea pig, rat, and mouse.

Materials can also be screened for nonimmunologic contact urticaria in humans. A small amount of the test material is applied to a marked site on the forehead, and the vehicle is applied to a parallel site. The areas are evaluated at about 20 to 30 min after application for erythema and/or edema (170).

Differentiation between nonspecific irritant reactions and contact urticaria may be difficult. Strong irritants, e.g., hydrochloric acid, lactic acid, cobalt chloride, formaldehyde, and phenol, can cause clear-cut immediate whealing if the concentration is high enough, but the reactions do not usually fade away within a few hours. Instead, they are followed by signs of irritation; erythema, scaling, or crusting are seen 24 hr later. Some substances have only urticant properties (e.g., benzoic acid, nicotinic acid esters), some are pure irritants (e.g., SLS) and some have both these features (e.g., formaldehyde, dimethyl sulfoxide).

Contact urticaria reactions are much less frequently encountered than either skin irritation or skin allergy (98). However, increasing awareness of contact urticaria may expand the list of etiologic agents and hopefully will lead to the development of adequate predictive assays for detecting causative agents of other forms of urticaria.

SUBJECTIVE IRRITATION AND PARAESTHESIA

Cutaneous application of some chemicals elicits sensory discomfort, tingling, and burning without visible inflammation. This noninflammatory painful response has been termed subjective irritation (52,55). Materials reported to produce subjective irritation include dimethyl sulfoxide, some benzoyl peroxide preparations, and the chemicals salicylic acid, propylene glycol, amyl-dimethyl-p-amino benzoic acid, and 2-ethoxy ethyl-p-methoxy cinnamate, which are ingredients of cosmetics and over-the-counter (OTC) drugs. Pyrethnoids, a group of broad-spectrum insecticides, produce a similar condition that may lead to temporary numbness, which has been called paraesthesia (20,45,91). As in subjective irritation, the nasolabial folds, cheeks, and periorbital areas are frequently involved. The ear is also sensitive to the pyrethroids.

Only a portion of the human population seems to develop nonpyrethnoid subjective irritation. Frosh and Kligman found they needed to prescreen subjects to identify "stingers" for conducting predictive assays. Only 20% of subjects exposed to 5% aqueous lactic acid in a hot, humid environment developed stinging response (52). All stingers in their series reported a history of adverse reactions to facial cosmetics, soaps, etc. A similar screening procedure by Lammintausta et al. (99) identified 18% of their subjects as stingers. Prior skin damage, e.g., sunburn, pretreatment with surfactants, and tape stripping, increases the intensity of responses in stingers, and persons not normally experiencing a response report pain on exposure to lactic acid or other agents that produce subjective irritation (52). Attempts to identify reactive subjects by association with other skin descripters, e.g., atopy, skin type, or skin dryness, have not yet been fruitful. However, recent data show that stingers develop stronger reactions to materials causing nonimmunologic contact urticaria and some increase in transepidermal water loss and blood flow following application of irritants via patches than those of "nonstingers" (99).

The mechanisms by which materials produce subjective irritation have not been extensively investigated. Pyrethroids directly act on the axon by interfering with the channel gating mechanism and impulse firing (169). It has been suggested that agents causing subjective irritation act via a similar mechanism because no visible inflammation is present.

An animal model was developed to rate paraesthesia to pyrethroids and may be useful for other agents (20,123). The test site is the flank of 300–450-g guinea pigs. Both flanks are shaved, and animals are individually housed in observation cages. A volume of 100 μl of the test material is spread over approximately 30 mm^2 on one flank. The same amount of the vehicle is applied to the other flank. The animal's behavior is monitored by an unmanned video camera for 5 min at 0.5, 1, 2, 4, and 6 hr after application of the materials. Subsequently, the film is analyzed for the number of full turns of the head made to the control and pyrethroid-treated flank. Head turns were usually accompanied by attempted licking and biting of the application sites. Using this technique, it was possible to rank pyrethroids for their ability to produce paraesthesia. The ranking corresponded to the ranking available from human exposure.

As originally published, the human subjective irritation assay required the use of a 110°F environmental chamber with 80% relative humidity (52). Volunteers were seated in the chamber until a profuse facial sweating was observed. Sweat was removed from the nasolabial fold and cheek; then a 5% aqueous solution of lactic acid was briskly rubbed over the area. Those who reported stinging for 3 to 5 min within the first 15 min were designated as stingers and were used for subsequent tests. Subjects were asked to evaluate the degree of stinging as 0 = no stinging; 1 = slight stinging; 2 = moderate stinging; 3 = severe stinging. Stinging was evaluated 10 sec, 2.5, 5, and 8 min after application of the test material. Other investigators (99) used a 15-min treatment with a commercial facial sauna to produce facial sweating, had subjects turn away from the sauna for application of the test materials, and then turn back to face the sauna for the observation period. The facial sauna technique is less stressful to both subjects and investigators and produces similar results.

REFERENCES

1. Allen, A. M. (1978): Clinical trial design in dermatology: experimental design. Part I. *Int. J. Dermatol.*, 17:42–51.
2. Andersen, K. E., and Maibach, H. I. (1983): Multiple-application delayed-onset contact urticaria: possible relation to certain unusual formalin and textile reactions. *Contact Dermatitis*, 10:227–234.
3. Asherson, C. L., and Ptak, W. (1968): Contact and delayed hypersensitivity in the mouse. 1. Active sensitization and passive transfer. *Immunology*, 15:405–416.
4. Bartek, M. J., and LaBudde, J. A. (1975): Percutaneous absorption *in vitro*. In: *Animal Models in Dermatology*, edited by H. I. Maibach, pp. 103–120. Churchill-Livingstone, New York.
5. Bartek, M. J., LaBudde, J. A., and Maibach, H. I. (1972): Skin permeability *in vivo*: comparison in rat, rabbit, pig and man. *J. Invest. Dermatol.*, 58:114–123.
6. Battista, C. W., and Rieger, M. M. (1971): Some problems of predictive testing. *J. Soc. Cosmet. Chem.*, 22:349–359.
7. Berger, R. S., and Bowman, J. P. (1982): A reappraisal of the 21-day cumulative irritation test in man. *J. Toxicol. Cuta. Ocular Toxicol.*, 1:109–115.
8. Bergstressor, P. R., Paniser, R. J., and Taylor, J. R. (1978): Counting and sizing of epidermal cells in human skin. *J. Invest. Dermatol.*, 70:280–284.
9. Bjornberg, A. (1975): Skin reactions to primary irritants in men and women. *Acta Derm. Venereol.* (Stockh), 55:191–194.
10. Blank, H. I. (1953): Further observations on factors which influence the water content of the stratum corneum. *J. Invest. Dermatol.*, 21:259–269.
11. Blank, I. (1952): Water content of stratum corneum. *J. Invest. Dermatol.*, 18:433–440.
12. Bloch, B., and Steiner-Wourlisch, A. (1930): Die Sensibilisierung des Meerschweinchens gegen Primeln. *Arch. Dermatol. Syph.*, 162:349–378.
13. Boutwell, R. K. (1981): Chemical carcinogenesis. a. Biochemical role. In: *Biology of Skin Cancer (Excluding Melanomas)*, edited

by D. D. Laerum, and O. H. Iverson, pp. 134–150. International Union Against Cancer, Geneva.

14. Boutwell, R. K., Urbach, F., and Carpenter, G. (1981): Chemical carcinogenesis. b. Experimental models. In: *Biology of Skin Cancer (Excluding Melanomas)*, edited by D. D. Laerum, and O. H. Iverson, pp. 109–123. International Union Against Cancer, Geneva.

15. Bronaugh, R. L., Congolon, E. R., and Scheuplein, R. J. (1981): The effect of cosmetic vehicles on the penetration of *N*-nitro-diethanolamine through excised skin. *J. Invest. Dermatol.*, 76:94–96.

16. Brunner, M. J., and Smiljanic, A. (1952): Procedure for evaluation of skin sensitizing power of new materials. *Arch. Dermatol.*, 66:703–705.

17. Buehler, E. V. (1964): A new method for detecting potential sensitizers using the guinea pig. *Toxicol. Appl. Pharmacol.*, 6:341.

18. Buehler, E. V. (1965): Experimental skin sensitization in the guinea pig and man. *Arch. Dermatol.*, 91:171.

19. Busse, M. J., Hunt, P., Lees, K. A., Maggs, P. N. D., and McCarthy, T. M. (1969): Release of betamethasone derivatives from ointments—*in vivo* and *in vitro* studies. *Br. J. Dermatol.*, 81:103.

20. Cagen, S. Z., Malloy, L. A., Parker, C. M., Gardiner, T. H., Van Gelder, C. A., and Jud, V. A. (1984): Pyrethroid mediated skin sensory stimulation characterized by a new behavioral paradigm. *Toxicol. Appl. Pharmacol.*, 76:270–279.

21. Calandra, J. (1971): Comments on the guinea pig immersion test. *CTFA Cosmetic J.*, 3(3):47.

22. Carter, R. O., and Griffith, J. F. (1965): Experimental basis for the realistic assessment of safety of topical agents. *Toxicol. Appl. Pharmacol.*, 7:60–73.

23. Christie, G. A., and Moore-Robinson, M. (1970): Vehicle assessment—methodology and results. *Br. J. Dermatol.*, 82:93.

24. Code of Federal Regulations. (1985): Office of the Federal Registrar, National Archives of Records Service. General Services Administration Title 16, parts 1500.40–1500.42.

25. Cunningham-Rundles, S. (1981): Cell-mediated immunity. In: *Immunodermatology*, edited by B. Safai and R. A. Good, pp. 1–33. Plenum Medical Book Co., New York.

26. Davies, R. E., Harper, K. H., and Kynoch, S. R. (1972): Interspecies variation in dermal reactivity. *J. Soc. Cosmet. Chem.*, 23:371–381.

27. Draize, J. H. (1955): Procedures for the appraisal of the toxicity of chemicals in foods, drugs, and cosmetics. VIII. Dermal toxicity. *Food Drug Cosmetic Law J.*, 10:722–731.

28. Draize, J. H. (1959): *Dermal Toxicity*. Assoc. Food and Drug Officials, U.S. Appraisal of the Safety of Chemicals in Food, Drugs and Cosmetics, pp. 46–59. Texas State Dept. of Health, Austin, Texas.

29. Draize, J. H., Woodard, G., and Calvery, H. O. (1944): Methods for the study of irritation and toxicity of substances applied topically to the skin and mucous membrane. *J. Pharmacol. Exp. Ther.*, 82:377–390.

30. Drill, V. A., and Lazar, P. (1983): *Cutaneous Toxicity*. Raven Press, New York.

31. Dugard, P. J. (1983): Skin permeability theory in relation to measurements of percutaneous absorption. In: *Dermatotoxicology*, 2d ed., edited by F. N. Marzulli and H. I. Maibach. pp. 91–115. Hemisphere, New York.

32. Elias, P. M. (1987): Lipids and the epidermal permeability barriers. *Arch. Dermatol. Res.*, 270:95–117.

33. Elias, P. M., Cooper, E. R., Korc, A., and Brown, B. E. (1981): Percutaneous transport in relation to stratum corneum structure and lipid composition. *J. Invest. Dermatol.*, 76:297–301.

34. Emery, B. E., and Edwards, L. D. (1940): The pharmacology of soaps. II. The irritant action of soaps on human skin. *J. Am. Pharm. Assoc.*, 29:251–254.

35. Emmett, E. A. (1975): Occupational skin cancer: a review. *J. Occup. Med.*, 17:44–49.

36. Environmental Protection Agency (1982): Pesticides registrations: proposed data requirements. Sec. 158. 135: toxicology data requirements. *Fed. Reg.*, 47:53192.

37. Epstein, W. L., Kligman, A. M., and Senecal, I. P. (1963): Role of regional lymph nodes in contact sensitization. *Arch. Dermatol.*, 88:789.

38. Everall, J. D. (1981): Chemical carcinogenesis. A. Environmental carcinogens. In: *Biology of Skin Cancer (Excluding Melanomas)*, edited by D. D. Laerum, and D. H. Iverson, pp. 105–108. International Union Against Cancer, Geneva.

39. Everall, J. D., and Dowd, P. M. (1978): Influence of environmental factors excluding ultraviolet radiation on the incidence of skin cancer. *Bull. Cancer*, 65:241–248.

40. Fare, G. (1966): Rat skin carcinogenesis by topical applications of some azo dyes. *Cancer Res.*, 26:2466–2468.

41. Farrar, J. J., Benjamin, W. R., Hilficker, M. L., Howard, M., Farrar, W. L., and Fuller-Farrar, J. F. (1982): The biochemistry, biology, and role of interleukin in the induction of cytotoxic T-cell and antibody-forming B-cell responses. *Immunol. Rev.*, 63:129–166.

42. Feldman, R. J., and Maibach, H. I. (1967): Regional variation in percutaneous penetration of [^{14}C]cortisone in man. *J. Invest. Dermatol.*, 48:181–183.

43. Finkelstein, P., Laden, K., and Meichowski, W. (1963): New methods for evaluating cosmetic irritancy. *J. Invest. Dermatol.*, 40:11–14.

44. Finkelstein, P., Laden, K., and Meichowski, W. (1965): Laboratory methods for evaluating skin irritancy. *Toxicol. Appl. Pharmacol.*, 7:74–78.

45. Flannigan, S. A., and Tucker, S. B. (1986): Variation in cutaneous sensation between synthetic pyrethroic insecticides. *Contact Dermatitis*, 13:140–147.

46. Franz, T. J. (1975): Percutaneous absorption. On the relevance of *in vitro* data. *J. Invest. Dermatol.*, 64:190–195.

47. Frey, J. R., and Wenk, P. (1957): Experimental studies on the pathogenesis of contact eczema in the guinea pig. *Int. Arch. Allergy Appl. Immunol.*, 11:81–100.

48. Fritsch, W. C., and Stoughton, R. B. (1963): The effect of temperature and humidity on the penetration of [^{14}C]acetyl-salicylic acid in excised human skin. *J. Invest. Dermatol.*, 41:307.

49. Frosch, P. J. (1982): Irritancy of soap and detergent bars. In: *Principles of Cosmetics for the Dermatologist*, edited by P. Frost and S. N. Horwitz, pp. 5–12. C. V. Mosby, St. Louis.

50. Frosch, P. J., and Kligman, A. M. (1976): The chamber scarification test for irritancy. *Contact Dermatitis*, 2:314–324.

51. Frosch, P. J., and Kligman, A. M. (1977): The chamber scarification test for assessing irritancy of topically applied substances. In: *Cutaneous Toxicity*, edited by V. A. Drill and P. Lazar, pp. 127–144. Academic Press, New York.

52. Frosch, P. J., and Kligman, A. M. (1977): A method for appraising the stinging capacity of topically applied substances. *J. Soc. Cosmet. Chem.*, 28:197–207.

53. Frosch, P. J., and Kligman, A. M. (1979): The soap chamber test. A new method for assessing the irritancy of soaps. *J. Am. Acad. Dermatol.*, 1:35–41.

54. Frosch, P. J., and Kligman, A. M. (1979): The Duhring chamber: an improved technique for epicutaneous testing of irritant and allergic reactions. *Contact Dermatitis*, 5:73.

55. Frosch, P. J., and Kligman, A. M. (1982): Recognition of chemically vulnerable and delicate skin. In: *Principles of Cosmetics for the Dermatologist*, edited by P. Frost and S. N. Horwitz, pp. 287–296. Mosby, St. Louis.

56. Gilman, M. R., Evans, R. A., and DeSalva, S. J. (1978): The influence of concentration, exposure duration, and patch occlusivity upon rabbit primary dermal irritation indices. *Drug Chem. Toxicol.*, 1(4):391–400.

57. Griffith, J. F. (1969): Predictive and diagnostic test for contact sensitization. *Toxicol. Appl. Pharmacol. (Suppl.)*, 3:90–102.

58. Griffith, J. F., and Buehler, E. (1976): Prediction of skin irritancy and sensitization potential by testing with animals and man. In: *Cutaneous Toxicity*, edited by V. Drill and P. Lazar. Academic Press, New York.

59. Griffith, J. F., Weaver, J. E., Whitehouse, H. S., Poole, R. L., Newman, E. A., and Nixon, C. A. (1969): Safety evaluation of enzyme detergents. Oral and cutaneous toxicity, irritancy and skin sensitization studies. *Fd. Cosmet. Toxicol.*, 7:581–593.

60. Guillot, J. P., Gonnet, J. F., Clement, C., Caillard, L., and Truhaut, R. (1982): Evaluation of the cutaneous-irritation potential of 56 compounds. *Food Chem. Toxicol.*, 20:563–572.

61. Guin, J. D., Meyer, B. N., Drake, R. D., and Haffley, P. (1984): The effect of quenching agents on contact urticaria caused by cinnamic aldehyde. *J. Am. Acad. Dermatol.*, 10:45–51.

62. Guy, R. H., Tur, E., Bugatto, B., Gaebel, C., Sheiner, L., and Mai-

bach, H. I. (1984): Pharmacodynamic measurements of methyl nicotinate percutaneous absorption. *Pharmacol. Res.,* 1:76–81.

63. Guy, R. H., Wester, R. C., Tur, E., and Maibach, H. I. (1983): Noninvasive assessments of the percutaneous absorption of methyl nicotinate in humans. *J. Pharm. Sci.,* 72:1077–1079.

64. Haley, T., and Hunziger, J. (1974): Instrument for producing standardized skin abrasions. *J. Pharm. Sci.,* 63:106.

65. Henderson, C. R., and Riley, E. C. (1945): Certain statistical considerations in patch testing. *Invest. Dermatol.,* 6:227–230.

66. Higuchi, T. (1960): Physical chemical analysis of percutaneous absorption process from creams and ointments. *J. Soc. Cosmet. Chem.,* 11:85–97.

67. Holbrook, K. A., and Odland, G. F. (1974): Regional differences in the thickness (cell layers) of the human stratum corneum: an ultrastructural analysis. *J. Invest. Dermatol.,* 62:415–422.

68. Holbrook, K. A., and Smith, L. T. (1981): Ultrastructural aspects of human skin during the embryonic, fetal, premature, neonatal, and adult periods of life. In: *Morphogenesis and Malforming of the Skin,* edited by R. J. Blandau, pp. 9–38. Alan R. Liss, New York.

69. Hood, D. B., Neher, R. J., Reinke, R. E., and Zapp, J. A. (1965): Experience with the guinea pig in screening primary irritants and sensitizers. *Toxicol. Appl. Pharmacol.,* 7:485–486.

70. Ihle, J. N., Rebar, K., Keller, J., Lee, J. C., and Hapel, A. J. (1982): Interleukin 3: possible roles in the regulation of lymphocyte differentiation and visual assessment. *Br. J. Dermatol.,* 92:131–142.

71. Iverson, O. H. (1981): Chemical carcinogenesis. e. Short term tests for carcinogens. In: *Biology of Skin Cancer (Excluding Melanomas),* edited by D. D. Laerum, and O. H. Iverson, pp. 151–163. International Union Against Cancer, Geneva.

72. Jackson, R., and Grainge, J. W. (1975): Arsenic and cancer. *Can. Med. Assoc. J.,* 113:396–401.

73. Jadassohn, J. (1896): Zur Kenntniss der medicamentosen Dermatosen. *Verh. Dtsch. Dermatol. Ges. 5. Congress:* 103–129.

74. Jadassohn, J. (1896): A contribution to the study of dermatoses produced by drugs. *Verh. Dtsch. Dermatol. Ges.* In: *Selected essays and monographs,* transl. L. Elking, 1900: pp. 207–229. New Sydenham Society, London.

75. Jaffee, B. D., and Maguire, H. C., Jr. (1981): Delayed-type hypersensitivity and immunological tolerance to contact allergens in the rat. *Fed. Proc.,* 40:991 (abstract 4312).

76. Johnson, S. A. M., Kile, R. L., Kooyman, D. J., Whitehouse, H. S., and Brod, J. S. (1953): Comparison of effects of soaps and detergents on the hands of housewives. *Arch. Dermatol. Syph.,* 68:643–650.

77. Jordan, W. P., and King, S. E. (1977): Delayed hypersensitivity in females during the comparison of two predictive patch tests. *Contact Dermatitis,* 3:19–26.

78. Justice, J. D., Travers, J. J., and Vinson, L. J. (1961): The correlation between animal tests and human tests in assessing product mildness. *Proceedings of the Scientific Section of the Toilet Goods Association,* 35:12–17.

79. Kaminsky, M., Szivos, M. M., and Brown, K. R. (1986): Application of the Hill Top Patch Test Chamber to dermal irritancy testing in the albino rabbit. *J. Toxicol. Cuta. Ocular Toxicol.,* 5(2):81–87.

80. Kero, M., and Hannuksela, M. (1980): Guinea pig maximization test, open epicutaneous test and chamber test in induction of delayed contact hypersensitivity. *Contact Dermatitis,* 6:341–344.

81. Klecak, G. (1982): Identification of contact allergens: predictive tests in animals. In: *Dermatotoxicology,* 2d ed., edited by F. N. Marzulli and H. I. Maibach, pp. 200–219. Hemisphere, New York.

82. Klecak, G. (1985): The Freund's Complete Adjuvant test and the open epicutaneous test. In: *Contact Allergy, Predictive Tests in Guinea Pigs,* edited by H. I. Maibach and K. E. Anderson, pp. 152–171. Karger, Basel.

83. Kligman, A. (1964): Quantitative testing of chemical irritants. In: *Evaluation of Therapeutic Agents and Cosmetics,* edited by M. Steinberg, et al., pp. 186–192. McGraw-Hill, New York.

84. Kligman, A. M. (1966): The identification of contact allergens by human assay. I. A critique of standard methods. *J. Invest. Dermatol.,* 47:369–374.

85. Kligman, A. M. (1966): The identification of contact allergens by human assay. II. Factors influencing the induction and measurement of allergic contact dermatitis. *J. Invest. Dermatol.,* 47:375–392.

86. Kligman, A. M. (1966): The identification of contact allergens by human assay. III. The maximization test. A procedure for screening and rating contact sensitizers. *J. Invest. Dermatol.,* 47:393–409.

87. Kligman, A. M. (1983): A biological brief on percutaneous absorption. *Drug. Dev. Ind. Pharm.,* 521–560.

88. Kligman, A. M., and Epstein, W. (1959): Some factors affecting contact sensitization in man. In: *Mechanism of Hypersensitivity,* edited by J. H. Shaffer, G. A. LoGrippo, and M. W. Chase, pp. 713–722. Little, Brown, Boston.

89. Kligman, A. M., and Epstein, W. (1975): Updating the maximization test for identifying contact allergens. *Contact Dermatitis,* 1:231–239.

90. Kligman, A. M., and Wooding, W. M. (1967): A method for the measurement and evaluation of irritants on human skin. *J. Invest. Dermatol.,* 49:78–94.

91. Knox, J. M., Tucker, S. B., and Flannigan, S. A. (1984): Paresthesia from cutaneous exposure to synthetic pyrethroid insecticide. *Arch. Dermatol.,* 120:744–746.

92. Kooyman, D. J., and Snyder, F. H. (1942): Tests for the mildness of soaps. *Arch. Dermatol. Syph.,* 46:846–855.

93. Kral, F., and Schwartzman, R. M. (1964): *Veterinary and Comparative Dermatology.* J. B. Lippincott Co, Philadelphia.

94. Kuroki, T., Nemoto, N., and Kitano, Y. (1980): Use of human epidermal keratinocytes in studies on chemical carcinogenesis. In: *Carcinogenesis: Fundamental Mechanisms and Environmental Effects,* edited by B. Pullman, P. O. P. Ts'o, and H. Gelboin, pp. 417–426. Redel, Boston.

95. Lahti, A. (1980): Nonimmunologic contact urticaria. *Acta Derm. Venereol. (Suppl.) (Stockh),* 60(91):1–49.

96. Lahti, A., and Maibach, H. I. (1984): An animal model for nonimmunologic contact urticaria. *Toxicol. Appl. Pharmacol.,* 76:219–224.

97. Lahti, A., and Maibach, H. I. (1985): Species specificity of nonimmunologic contact urticaria: guinea pig, rat and mouse. *J. Am. Acad. Dermatol.,* 13:66–69.

98. Lahti, A., von Krogh, G., and Maibach, H. I. (1985): Contact urticaria syndrome. An expanding phenomenon. In: *Dermatologic Immunology and Allergy,* edited by J. Stone, pp. 379–390. Mosby, St. Louis.

99. Lammintausta, K., Maibach, H. I., and Wilson, D. (1988): Mechanisms of subjective (sensory) irritation: propensity of nonimmunologic contact urticaria and objective irritation in stingers. *Derm. Beruf Umwelt,* 36:45–49.

100. Landsteiner, K., and Chase, M. W. (1937): Studies on the sensitization of animals with simple chemical compounds. IV. Anaphylaxis induced by picryl chloride and 2:4 dinitrochlorobenzene. *J. Exp. Med.,* 66:337–351.

101. Landsteiner, K., and Jacobs, J. (1935): Studies on the sensitization of animals with simple chemical compounds. *J. Exp. Med.,* 61:643–648.

102. Landsteiner, K., and Jacobs, J. (1936): Studies on the sensitization of animals with simple chemical compounds. II. *J. Exp. Med.,* 64:625–629.

103. Lanman, B. M., Elvers, W. B., and Howard, C. S. (1968): The role of human patch testing in a product development program. In: *Proceedings of the Joint Conference on Cosmetic Sciences,* pp. 135–145. The Toilet Goods Association, Washington, DC.

104. Lever, W. F., and Schaumburg-Hevor (1983): *Histopathology of the Skin,* 6th ed. Lippincott, Philadelphia.

105. MacMillan, F. S. K., Rafft, R. R., and Elvers, W. B. (1975): A comparison of the skin irritation produced by cosmetic ingredients and formulations in the rabbit, guinea pig, beagle dog to that observed in the human. In: *Animal Models in Dermatology,* edited by H. I. Maibach, pp. 12–22. Churchill-Livingstone, Edinburgh.

106. Magee, P. N. (1970): Tests for carcinogenic potential. In: *Methods in Toxicology,* edited by G. E. Paget, pp. 158–196. Davis, Philadelphia.

107. Magnusson, B., and Hersle, K. (1965): Patch test methods. I. A comparative study of six different types of patch tests. *Acta Dermatol.,* 45:123–128.

108. Magnusson, B., and Hersle, K. (1965): Patch test methods. II. Regional variations of patch test responses. *Acta Dermatol.,* 45:257–261.

109. Magnusson, B., and Hersle, K. (1966): Patch test methods. III. Influence of adhesive tape on test response. *Acta Dermatol.*, 46:275–278.

110. Magnusson, B., and Kligman, A. M. (1969): The identification of contact allergens by animals assay. The guinea pig maximization test. *J. Invest. Dermatol.*, 52:268–276.

111. Magnusson, B., and Kligman, A. M. (1970): *Allergic Contact Dermatitis in the Guinea Pig.* Charles C Thomas, Springfield, IL.

112. Maguire, H. C. (1973): Mechanism of intensification by Freund's complete adjuvant of the acquisition of delayed hypersensitivity in the guinea pig. *Immunol. Commun.*, 1:239–246.

113. Maguire, H. C. (1974): Alteration in the acquisition of delayed hypersensitivity with adjuvant in the guinea pig. *Monogr. Allergy*, 8:13–26.

114. Maibach, H. I. (1976): Immediate hypersensitivity in hand dermatitis: role of food contact dermatitis. *Arch. Dermatol.*, 112:1289–1291.

115. Maibach, H. I., and Johnson, H. L. (1975): Contact urticaria syndrome. Contact urticaria to diethyltoluamide (immediate-type hypersensitivity). *Arch. Dermatol.*, 111:726–730.

116. Malkinson, F. D. (1958): Studies on the percutaneous absorption of C^{14} labeled steroids by use of the gas-flow cell. *J. Invest. Dermatol.*, 31:19.

117. Marzulli, F. N., and Maibach, H. I. (1973): Antimicrobials: experimental contact sensitization in man. *J. Soc. Cosmet. Chem.*, 24:399–421.

118. Marzulli, F. N., and Maibach, H. I. (1974): The use of graded concentration in studying skin sensitizers: experimental contact sensitization in man. *Food Cosmet. Toxicol.*, 12:219–227.

119. Mathias, C. G. T., Chappler, R. R., and Maibach, H. I. (1980): Contact urticaria from cinnamic aldehyde. *Arch. Dermatol.*, 116:74–76.

120. Mathias, C. G. T., and Maibach, H. I. (1978): Dermatoxicology monographs. I. Cutaneous irritation: factors influencing the response to irritants. *Clin. Toxicol.*, 13:333–346.

121. Maurer, T., Thomann, P., Weirich, E. G., and Hess, R. (1975): The optimization test in the guinea pig. A method for the predictive evaluation of the contact allergenicity of chemicals. *Agents Actions*, 5:174–179.

122. McKenzie, A. W., and Stoughton, R. M. (1962): Method for comparing percutaneous absorption of steroids. *Arch. Dermatol.*, 86:608–610.

123. McKillop, C. M., Brock, J. A. C., Oliver, C. J. A., and Rhodes, C. (1987): A quantitative assessment of pyrethroid-induced paresthesia in the guinea pig flank model. *Toxicol. Lett.*, 36:1–7.

124. Mizel, S. B. (1982): Interleukin 1 and T cell activation. *Immunol. Rev.*, 63:51–72.

125. Montagna, W. (1962): *The Structure and Function of Skin.* Academic Press, New York.

126. Montagna, W., and Lobitz, W. C. (1964): *The Epidermis.* Academic Press, New York.

127. Motoyoshi, K., Toyoshima, Y., Sato, M., and Yoshimura, M. (1979): Comparative studies on the irritancy of oils and synthetic perfumes to the skin of rabbit, guinea pig, rat, miniature swine, and man. *Cosmet. Toiletries*, 94:41–42.

128. Najarian, J. S., and Feldman, J. D. (1963): Specificity of passive transfer or delayed hypersensitivity. *J. Exp. Med.*, 118:341–352.

129. National Academy of Sciences, Committee for the Revision of NAS Publication 1138. (1977): *Principles and Procedures for Evaluating the Toxicity of Household Substances*, pp. 23–59. National Academy of Sciences, Washington, DC.

130. Nicolaides, N. (1963): Human skin surface lipids—origins, composition and possible function. In: *Advances in Biology of Skin*, Vol. IV, *The Sebaceous Glands*, edited by W. Montagna, R. A. Ellis, and A. F. Silver, pp. 167–187. Pergamon Press, Oxford.

131. Nixon, G. A., Tyson, C. A., and Wertz, W. C. (1975): Interspecies comparisons of skin irritancy. *Toxicol. Appl. Pharmacol.*, 31:481–490.

132. Noonan, P. K., and Wester, R. C. (1983): Cutaneous biotransformations and some pharmacological and toxicological implications. In: *Dermatotoxicology*, edited by F. N. Marzulli and H. I. Maibach, pp. 71–90. Hemisphere, New York.

133. Odom, R. B., and Maibach, H. I. (1976): Contact urticaria: a different contact dermatitis. *Cutis*, 18:672–676.

134. Opdyke, D. (1971): The guinea pig immersion test—a 20 year appraisal. *CTFA Cosmetic J.*, 3(3):46–47.

135. Opdyke, D. L., and Burnett, C. M. (1965): Practical problems in the evaluation of the safety of cosmetics. *Proceedings of the Scientific Section, Toilet Goods Association*, 44:3–4.

136. Organization for Economic Cooperation and Development. (1981): *OECD Guidelines for Testing of Chemicals, Section 4.* OECD, Paris, France.

137. Ostrenga, J., Steinmetz, C., Poulsen, B., and Yett, S. (1971): Significance of vehicle composition. II: Prediction of optimal vehicle composition. *J. Pharm. Sci.*, 60:1180–1183.

138. Page, N. P. (1977): Concepts of a bioassay program in environmental carcinogenesis. In: *Environmental Cancer*, Vol. 3, *Advances in Modern Toxicology*, edited by H. F. Kraybill and M. A. Mehlman, pp. 87–171. Hemisphere, New York.

139. Palotay, J. L., Adachi, K., Dobson, R. L., and Pinto, J. S. (1986): Carcinogen-induced cutaneous neoplasms in non-human primates. *J.N.C.I.*, 57:1269–1272.

140. Phillips, L., Steinberg, M., Maibach, H. I., and Akers, W. A. (1972): A comparison of rabbit and human skin response to certain irritants. *Toxicol. Appl. Pharmacol.*, 21:369–382.

141. Polak, L. (1977): Immunological aspects of contact sensitivity. In: *Dermatotoxicology and Pharmacology*, edited by F. N. Marzulli and H. I. Maibach, pp. 225–288. Hemisphere, New York.

142. Polak, L., Polak, A., and Frey, J. R. (1974): The development of contact sensitivity to DNFB in guinea pigs genetically differing in their response to DNP-skin protein conjugate. *Int. Arch. Allergy Appl. Immunol.*, 46:417–426.

143. Potokar, M. (1985): Studies on the design of animal tests for the corrosiveness of industrial chemicals. *Food Chem. Toxicol.*, 23:615–617.

144. Prottey, C. (1978): The molecular basis of skin irritation. In: *Cosmetic Science*, Vol. I, edited by M. M. Breuer, pp. 275–349. Academic Press, London.

145. Rapaport, M., Anderson, D., and Pierce, U. (1978): Performance of the 21 day patch test in civilian populations. *J. Toxicol. Cuta. Ocular Toxicol.*, 1:109–115.

146. Ritz, H. L., and Buehler, E. V. (1980): Planning conduct and interpretation of guinea pig sensitization patch tests. In: *Current Concepts in Cutaneous Toxicity*, edited by V. A. Drill and P. Lazar, p. 25. Academic Press, New York.

147. Rothman, S. (1954): *Physiology and Biochemistry of the Skin.* University of Chicago Press, Chicago.

148. Scheuplein, R. J. (1978): Permeability of skin: a review of major concepts. *Curr. Probl. Dermatol.*, 7:58–68.

149. Scheuplein, R. J., and Bronough, R. L. (1983): Percutaneous absorption. In: *Biochemistry and Physiology of the Skin*, edited by L. A. Goldsmith, pp. 1255–1295. Oxford Press, New York.

150. Schwartz, L. (1951): The skin testing of new cosmetics. *J. Soc. Cosmet. Chem.*, 2:321–324.

151. Schwartz, L. (1969): Twenty-two years' experience in the performance of 200,000 prophetic patch tests. *South. Med. J.*, 53:478–484.

152. Schwartz, L., and Peck, S. M. (1944): The patch test in contact dermatitis. *Public Health Rep.*, 59:546–557.

153. Shelanski, H. A. (1951): Experience with and considerations of the human patch test method. *J. Soc. Cosmet. Chem.*, 2:324–331.

154. Shelanski, H. A., and Shelanski, M. V. (1953): New technique of patch tests. *Drug Cosmet. Ind.*, 73:186.

155. Shelanski, H. A., and Shelanski, M. V. (1953): A new technique of human patch tests. *Proceedings of the Scientific Section of the Toilet Goods Association*, 19:46–49.

156. Shellow, W. V. R., and Rapaport, M. J. (1981): Comparison testing of soap irritancy using aluminum chamber and standard patch methods. *Contact Dermatitis*, 7:77–79.

157. Simpson, W. L., and Cramer, W. (1943): Fluorescence studies of carcinogens in skin. *Cancer Res.*, 3:362–369.

158. Sokolov, U. E. (1982): *Mammal Skin.* University of California Press, Berkeley, CA.

159. Steinberg, M., Akers, W. A., Weeks, M., McCreesh, A. H., and Maibach, H. I. (1975): I. A comparison of test techniques based on rabbit and human skin responses to irritants with recommendations regarding the evaluation of mildly or moderately irritating

compounds. In: *Animal Models in Dermatology,* edited by H. I. Maibach, pp. 1–11. Churchill-Livingstone, Edinburgh.

160. Stingl, G., and Abever, W. (1983): The Langerhans' cell. In: *Biochemistry and Physiology of the Skin,* edited by L. A. Goldsmith, pp. 907–921. Oxford University Press, New York.

161. Stingl, G., Katz, S. I., Clement, L., Green, I., and Shevach, E. (1978): Immunologic functions of Ia-bearing epidermal Langerhans' cells. *J. Immunol.,* 121:2005–2013.

162. Sweeney, T. M., and Downing, D. T. (1970): The role of lipids in the epidermal barrier to water diffusion. *J. Invest. Dermatol.,* 55:135–140.

163. Traub, E. F., Tusing, T. W., and Spoor, H. J. (1954): Evaluation of dermal sensitivity; animal and human tests compared. *Arch. Dermatol.,* 69:399–409.

164. Tregear, R. T. (1964): Relative penetrability of hair follicles and epidermis. *J. Physiol.* (Lond.), 156:303–313.

165. Tregear, R. T. (1966): *Physical Function of Skin.* Academic Press, New York.

166. Unanue, E. R. (1984): Antigen-presenting function of the macrophage. *Annu. Rev. Immunol.,* 2:395–428.

167. Uttley, M., and Van Abbe', N. J. (1973): Primary irritation of the skin: mouse ear test and human patch test procedures. *J. Soc. Cosmet. Chem.,* 24:217–227.

168. Vinegar, M. B. (1979): Regional variation in primary skin irritation and corrosivity potentials in rabbits. *Toxicol. Appl. Pharmacol.,* 49:63–69.

169. Vivjeberg, H. P., and VandenBercken, J. (1979): Frequency dependent effects of the pyrethroid insecticide decamethrin in frog myelinated nerve fibers. *Eur. J. Pharmacol.,* 58:501–504.

170. Von Krogh, C., and Maibach, H. I. (1982): The contact urticaria syndrome. *Semin. Dermatol.,* 1:59–66.

171. Voss, J. G. (1958): Skin sensitization by mercaptans of low molecular weight. *J. Invest. Dermatol.,* 31:273–279.

172. Wasserman, S. J. (1983): The mast cell and its mediators. In: *Biochemistry and Physiology of the Skin,* edited by L. A. Goldsmith, pp. 878–898. Oxford Press, New York.

173. Weaver, J. E. (1976): Dermatologic testing of household laundry products: a novel fabric softener. *Int. J. Dermatol.,* 15:297–300.

174. Weigand, D. A., and Gaylor, J. (1976): Irritant reaction in negro and caucasian skin. *South. Med. J.,* 67:548–551.

175. Weigand, D. A., Haygood, C., and Gaylor, J. R. (1974): Cell layer and density of negro and caucasian stratum corneum. *J. Invest. Dermatol.,* 62:563–568.

176. Weil, C. S., and Scala, R. A. (1971): Study of intra- and interlaboratory variability in the results of rabbit eye and skin irritation tests. *Toxicol. Appl. Pharmacol.,* 19:276–360.

177. Wester, R. C., and Maibach, H. I. (1975): Rhesus monkey as an animal model for percutaneous absorption. In: *Animal Models In Dermatology,* edited by H. I. Maibach, pp. 133–137. Churchill Livingstone, New York.

178. Wester, R. C., and Maibach, H. I. (1983): Cutaneous pharmacokinetics: 10 steps to percutaneous absorption. *Drug Metab. Rev.,* 14:169–205.

179. Whitton, J. T., and Ewell, J. D. (1973): The thickness of epidermis. *Br. J. Dermatol.,* 89:467–478.

180. Wooding, W. H., and Opdyke, D. L. (1967): A statistical approach to the evaluation of cutaneous responses to irritants. *J. Soc. Cosmet. Chem.,* 18:809–829.

Additional Resources

The field of dermatotoxicology has many subspecialties and is based on principles derived from other basic science disciplines and clinical medicine. It is impossible to cover adequately all topics that may be of interest. The following guide provides additional sources of information not cited in the references that provide greater detail than this text.

General:

Dermatotoxicology by Marzulli and Maibach; Hemisphere, 1987.

Clinical Aspects:

Contact Dermatitis by Fisher; Lea & Febiger, 1986.
Contact Dermatitis by Cronin; Churchill Livingstone, 1980.
Patch Test Guidelines by Malton, Nater, Van Ketel, & Nijmagen; Dekker & Van de Vogt, 1976.
Manual of Contact Dermatitis by Fregert; Muskgaard, 1976.

Percutaneous Penetration:

Dermatological Formulations by Barry; Marcel Dekker, 1983.
Percutaneous Absorption by Bronaugh & Maibach; Marcel Dekker, 1985.

Occupational Dermatology:

Occupational Contact Dermatitis by Foussereau, Benezra, & Maibach; Munksgaard, 1982.
Occupational and Industrial Dermatology by Maibach; Year Book Publishers, 1987.
Occupational Skin Diseases by Adams; Grune & Stratton, 1983.

Predictive Testing:

Contact and Photocontact Allergens by Maurer; Marcel Dekker, 1983.
Photochemical Toxicity Symposium Proceedings by Office of Health Affairs; FDA, 1981.
Contact Allergy Predictive Tests in Guinea Pigs by Anderson & Maibach; Karger, 1985.

Principles and Methods of Toxicology, Second
Edition, edited by A. Wallace Hayes,
Raven Press, Ltd., New York © 1989.

CHAPTER 14

Genetic Toxicology

David Brusick

Hazleton Laboratories America, Inc., Kensington, Maryland 20895

Genetic toxicology, as a subspecialty of toxicology, involves the identification and analysis of the action of agents with toxicity directed toward the hereditary components of living systems. Many agents damage genetic materials at concentrations that produce acute nonspecific cytotoxicity and death. The primary objective of genetic toxicologists, however, is to detect and analyze the hazard potential of agents highly specific for interactions with nucleic acids, thereby producing alterations in genetic elements at subtoxic concentrations.

Agents that produce alterations in the nucleic acids and associated components at subtoxic exposure levels, resulting in modified hereditary characteristics or DNA inactivation, are classified as *genotoxic*. Genotoxic substances usually have common chemical or physical properties that facilitate interaction with nucleic acids. Derivation of the term genotoxic is found in a publication by Ehrenberg et al. (33). A report of the International Commission for Protection Against Environmental Mutagens and Carcinogens (ICPEMC) provided

a more detailed definition of genotoxic and emphasized that categorization of a chemical as genotoxic is not an *a priori* indication of a health hazard (46). The term is a general descriptor meant to distinguish chemicals that have an affinity for direct DNA interactions from those that do not.

Genetic toxicology initially focused on the potential impact of mutagens on human germ cells; however, simultaneous with the concern over environmental mutagens were the reports from several independent groups of investigators showing a correlative relation between mammalian carcinogens and mutagens (2,12,17,64,95).

Thus genetic toxicology plays a dual role in safety evaluation programs. One is the implementation of testing and risk assessment methods to define the impact of genotoxic agents found in the environment and, more specifically, those whose presence may alter the integrity of the human gene pool. The second function is the application of genetic methodologies to the detection and mechanistic understanding of carcinogenic chemicals. In the latter regard, genetic toxicology has been applied as a front-line screen for potential carcinogens.

BASIC GENETIC MECHANISMS

Gene Structure

The informational molecules of all living systems, with the exception of some viruses that use RNA, are composed of DNA. Some of the characteristic features of DNA molecules are listed in Table 1. The mechanisms of information storage and gene expression are similar in all organisms.

The simplest complete functional unit in a DNA molecule is termed a *gene*. Most of what is known about the structure and operation of genes has been acquired from studies with bacteria or bacteriophages. The differences between the genes of prokaryotic (bacteria) and eukaryotic (plant and animal cells) organisms center primarily on their number, location on the respective chromosome entities, and mechanisms of gene regulation (Table 2). In prokaryotic cells there is a single chromosome entity with little or no differentiation along the DNA molecule so far as function is concerned. Eukaryotic cells, on the other hand, have DNA with nonfunctional, repeated sequences of some genes; these cells also have regions

TABLE 1. *Basic biochemical characteristics of all double-stranded DNA*

1. DNA consists of two purines (guanine, adenine) and two pyrimidines (thymine and cytosine).
2. A nucleotide pair consists of one purine and one pyrimidine [adenine/thymine (AT) or guanine/cytosine (GC)].
3. Nucleotide pairs are connected to a double helix molecule by sugar–phosphate backbone linkages and hydrogen bonding.
4. The AT base pair is held by two hydrogen bonds, and the GC is held by three.
5. The distance between each base pair in a molecule is 3.4 Å, producing 10 nucleotide pairs per turn of the DNA helix.
6. The number of adenine molecules must equal the number of thymine molecules in a DNA molecule. The same relation exists for guanine and cytosine molecules. The ratio of AT to GC base pairs, however, may vary in DNA from species to species.
7. The two strands of the double helix are complementary and antiparallel with respect to the polarity of the two sugar–phosphate backbones, one strand being 3′-5′ and the other 5′-3′ with respect to the terminal OH group on the ribose sugar.
8. DNA replicates by a semiconservative method in which the two strands separate and each is used as a template for the synthesis of a new complementary strand.
9. The rate of DNA nucleotide polymerization during replication is approximately 600 nucleotides per second. The helix must unwind to form templates at a rate of 3,600 rpm to accommodate this replication rate.
10. The DNA content of cells is variable (1.8×10^9 daltons for *Escherichia coli* to 1.9×10^{11} daltons for human cells).

TABLE 2. *Characteristics of DNA in prokaryotic and eukaryotic cell types*

Prokaryotic cells	Eukaryotic cells
Primarily haploid	Primarily diploid
DNA uncomplexed	DNA complexed with proteins forming chromosomes
DNA nonlocalized in the cell cytoplasm	DNA localized primarily within the nucleus of the cell
No morphologic stages in DNA replication	DNA replication described by mitotic cycle consisting of specific cytologic stages
DNA often found as a closed circle	DNA found in linear chromosomes
Replication not associated with cellular organelles	Replication and separation of chromosome associated with cellular organelles called centrioles
All genes encoded in the DNA are functional	Repetitive, nonfunctional gene sequences are common
Spacer sequences have not been identified	Noncoding spacer sequences identified as introns occur along the DNA molecule

of noncoding DNA, called *introns,* between coding sequences called *exons.* The function of repeated DNA sequences and intron regions is not known. The nucleotide composition and the mechanisms by which information encoded in a gene is transformed into gene products appear to be universal. This theory has been confirmed by recombinant DNA genetic engineering studies in which genes continue to function properly after having been transplanted from human cells to bacterial cells or from bacterial cells to plant cells (13,54).

In eukaryotic cells the process of gene expression follows the pattern shown in Fig. 1. Enzymes located in the nucleus of the cell excise intron regions and splice the coding sequence back together. The resulting mRNA is then transported to ribosomes outside the nucleus for translation. Intron regions are not present in prokaryotic cells, and the gene is read in one sequence.

Somatic Versus Germ Cells

Somatic cells constitute the major portion of the mammalian organism. The genomes of most somatic cells are diploid, and damage to somatic cells is not transmissible to subsequent generations. Virtually all *in vitro* assays measure damage in somatic cells. Germ cells are those cells that undergo meiotic division to haploid gametes. Damage to germ cells has the potential for transmission to the next generation.

DNA ALTERATIONS RESULTING IN GENOTOXIC EFFECTS IN CELLS

DNA replication and repair are not perfect processes, and in rare instances alterations in the genetic integrity of a cell

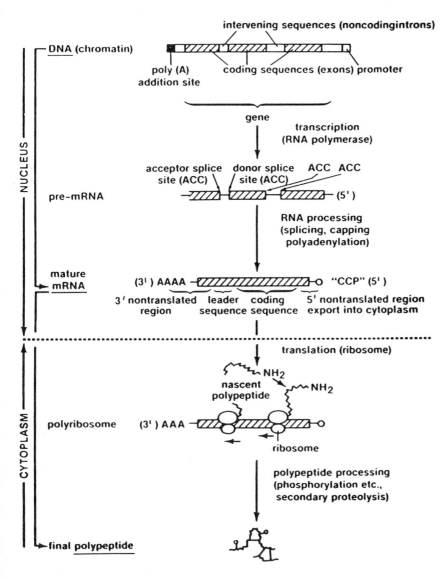

FIG. 1. Gene expression in eukaryotic cell types. Information is maintained in coding sequences (exons) in the DNA located in the nucleus. The information is transcribed into messenger RNA (mRNA) which is transported into the cytoplasm for translation into the gene product.

occur spontaneously. The occurrence of the changes follows a predictable rate per gene and forms the basis of "background" mutation frequencies. Spontaneous DNA changes occur at both the nucleotide and chromosome levels.

Classification Scheme for Genotoxic Effects

DNA damage falls into two broad categories: (a) visible effects detectable through cytologic analysis of chromosomes (*macrolesions*); and (b) nonvisible changes, which occur at the nucleotide level (*microlesions*). The specific types of DNA damage falling into these two categories are shown in Fig. 2.

The expected configurations of base pairs are shown in Fig. 3: Adenine and thymine form two hydrogen bonds, and guanine and cytosine form three. Hydrogen bonds are weak electrostatic forces involving oxygen and nitrogen atoms at specific sites on the purine and pyrimidine molecules. If electrophilic chemical species covalently bind to portions of the DNA bases involved in the formation of hydrogen bonds (Fig. 4), these covalently bound species (*adducts*) might result

in mispaired bases and, eventually, substitution of one base pair for another in the DNA molecule.

Base-pair addition–deletion mutations, also called *frameshift mutations,* result from the addition or deletion of one or a few nucleotide pairs from the nucleotide complement in a gene. Because the codon sequence of a gene is nonpunctuated, the loss or gain of a single base pair changes the reading frame of the gene—hence frameshift mutation. This type of change is illustrated in Fig. 5.

Macrolesions can be subdivided into changes in chromosome number (gain or loss of single chromosomes or sets of chromosomes) and changes in chromosome structure (breaks, deletions, rearrangements). Each specific type of chromosome change has a characteristic designation so that a reasonably high degree of uniformity can be maintained when scoring these changes. Variations in chromosome number can result from incomplete dissociation of single or entire sets of chromosomes at metaphase, producing serious effects in intact organisms. Some relatively common human disorders, e.g., mongolism (Down's syndrome), result from variations in chromosome number.

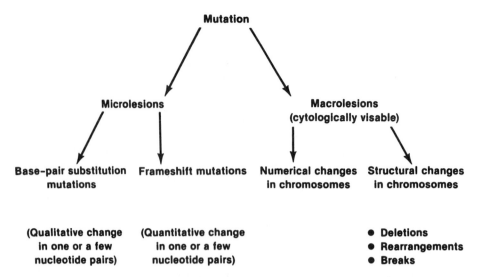

FIG. 2. Mutations can be classified by the extent of the DNA lesions. Microlesions are those mutations that result in the change of one or a few nucleotide pairs within a gene. These events do not extend beyond the altered gene. Macrolesions are generally visible using cytological analyses. They are represented by structural and/or numerical changes in chromosomes. Occasionally, changes will cover more than a single gene without producing visible chromosome alterations. These mutations are termed multilocus deletions and are not detected by most assays.

In addition to the tests that specifically measure nucleotide substitutions and chromosome alterations, a third, diverse group of ancillary tests have been identified that measure other indicators of genotoxicity. This mixed group of systems is generally grouped under the category of tests for primary DNA damage and includes tests measuring the DNA repair, mitotic recombination or mitotic gene conversion, and spermhead abnormalities (18).

Repair of DNA Damage

To maintain the fidelity and integrity of genetic information, several types of enzymatic DNA repair process developed during evolution. In lower eukaryotic organisms the number of genes already known to affect DNA repair is near 100. The number in humans is equal to or greater than that number and emphasizes how important the error recognition and correction processes have been during evaluation. DNA is the only molecule in living organisms with a capacity for self-repair. The common feature of repair processes is the ability to remove and replace damaged segments of DNA. Therefore if a DNA lesion induced by a mutagen can be repaired prior to fixation or stabilization, the net effect of the DNA insult may be nil. It is especially true following inter-mittent low level exposure where excision repair enzymes are not fully saturated by excessive numbers of damaged DNA sites. Systems measuring some parameter of DNA repair (87,92,102) have been used as measurements of primary DNA damage. Because all normal organisms are capable of some type of repair following chemical insult, a stimulation in the level of repair activity following chemical treatment at sublethal concentrations is a good general indicator that the test sample has experienced DNA-directed toxicity.

In the context of genetic toxicology, repair processes can play potentially critical roles at low exposure levels. Evidence from prokaryotic systems indicates that once premutational lesions have been induced in the DNA, both error-prone and error-free repair pathways are active, the results depending on the degree to which different pathways are used. The factors that determine whether error-prone or error-free pathways predominate include the target species, cell type, chemical mutagen, and the specific DNA lesion induced (32). Some data suggest that the error-free repair pathways predominate at low exposure levels, and error-prone pathways come into play only following saturation of the error-free enzymes. Thus repair processes can produce rather complex dose-response curves depending on many variables. Methods to incorporate these data into risk or threshold analyses are not available.

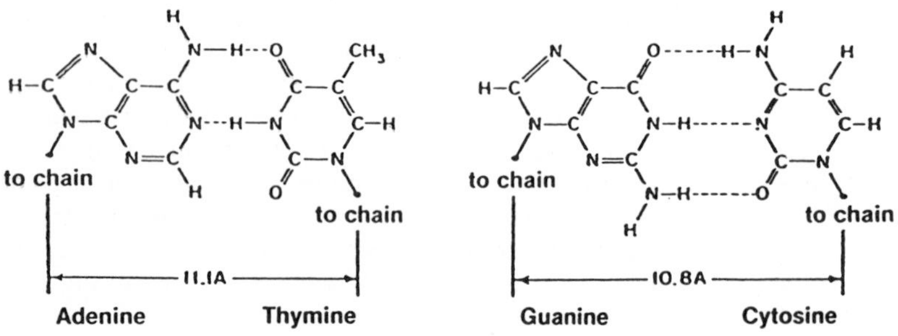

FIG. 3. Basic base-pairing configuration for adenine, cytosine, thymine, and guanine. Hydrogen bonds are relatively weak forces which hold the two strands of the DNA helix together except during replication or transcription.

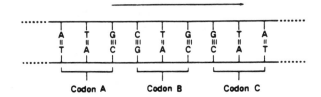

FIG. 4. Examples of two DNA adducts. **Top:** An aromatic amine adduct to guanine. **Bottom:** A benzo (α) pyrene metabolite bound to guanine.

Because of the influence that genetic background has on repair capacity, serious consideration should be given to determining the quantitative impact that DNA repair systems have in the assessment and extrapolation of genotoxic risk (75,89). An informative review of the evidence for thresholds from genotoxic agents addresses the potential for repair to modify dose-response curves at the low dose end (32). Theoretical assumptions and data from studies of repair mechanisms tend to support the belief that at low exposure levels an error-free removal of alkyl groups from DNA can be virtually 100% effective. Thus one observes survival shoulders and nonlinear kinetics for mutation induction in repair-pro-

ficient cells and the loss of apparent "no effect" regions in repair-deficient cells.

RELATION OF GENOTOXIC EFFECTS TO OTHER TOXICOLOGIC PHENOMENA

Because of the fundamental role genes play in all aspects of living organisms, the concept that altered genes lead to various disease states has considerable merit (99). Table 3 identifies examples of single gene and chromosome traits leading to genetic disease.

Other types of toxicologic endpoints appear to be under some type of genetic control, but the evidence is less direct. Among these endpoints are the following:

1. Oncogenesis (certain forms, e.g., retinoblastoma and familial polyposis, are clearly inherited) (55,80)
2. Teratogenesis (49)
3. Sterility or semisterility (22)
4. Heart disease (9)
5. Aging (21)

The primary emphasis placed on genetic testing, however, has been its ability to identify genotoxic carcinogens.

Carcinogens and Mutagens

A somatic mutation theory for the etiology of cancer was proposed by Bauer (8). The available database was insufficient to support such a theory through the 1950s (20) and even the late 1960s (66). The type of correlative database to support a mutation step in the induction of tumors was not available until the early 1970s, when microbial mutation assays were

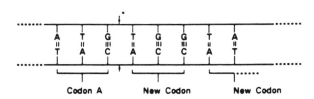

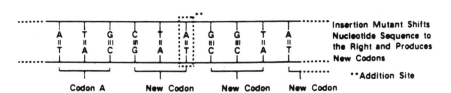

Direction of DNA Reading

Non Mutant DNA Showing 3 Codons

Deletion Mutant Shifts Nucleotide Sequence to the Left and Produces New Codons
*Deletion Site

Insertion Mutant Shifts Nucleotide Sequence to the Right and Produces New Codons
**Addition Site

FIG. 5. The induction of frameshift mutations occurs by the insertion and deletion of base pairs. Insertion or deletion will produce a shift in the transcription reading frame that results in genetic nonsense or missense.

TABLE 3. *Examples of genetic disorders in humans*

Category of genetic alteration	Estimated frequency/ 10^3 population[a]	Typical examples[b]
Chromosome abnormalities	6.86	Down's syndrome (trisomy)
		Klinefelter's syndrome (XXY)
		Turner's syndrome (XO)
		Cri du chat (deletion of chromosome)
		Numerous other trisomies XYY
Dominant mutations	1.85–2.64	Familial polyposis (AD)
		Neurofibromatosis (AD)
		Huntington's chorea (AD)
		Hepatic porphyria (AD)
		Crouzon's craniofacial dystosis (AD)
		Achondroplasia dwarfism (AD)
		Retinoblastoma (AD)
		Anitidia (AD)
		Chondrodystrophy (AD)
Recessive mutations	2.23–2.54 0.78–1.99	Xeroderma pigmentosa (AR)
		Duchenne muscular dystrophy (XR)
		Hemophilia (XR)
		Lesch-Nyhan syndrome (XR)
		Sickle cell disease (AR)
		Galactosemia (AR)
		Phenylketonuria (AR)
		Diabetes mellitus (AR)
		Fanconi's syndrome (AR)
		Albinism (AR)
		Cystic fibrosis (AR)
Polygenic (complex inheritance)	26.00–32.00	Cleft lip
		Anencephaly
		Spina bifida
		Clubfoot
		Idiopathic epilepsy
		Congenital heart defects

[a] *A Consultative Document on Guidelines for the Testing of Chemicals for Mutagenicity, Committee on Mutagenicity of Chemicals in Food, Consumer Products, and the Environment.* Department of Health and Social Security, Great Britain, March 1979.
[b] AD = autosomal dominant; AR = autosomal recessive; XR = X-linked recessive.

coupled with microsomal metabolic activation (S9 mix) systems (3). Many of the experimental animal carcinogens are biotransformed *in vivo* into biologically active agents and bacteria or *in vitro* mammalian cell assays cannot carry out such transformation without an exogenous metabolic source. Early analyses of animal carcinogens in S9 microsome enzyme-supplemented microbial tests produced highly suggestive evidence that most (85–90%) animal carcinogens were also mutagens (69). The degree of correlation between these

two phenomena appeared to be indicative of an intimate functional relation, and the probability that a genotoxic event was essential to the oncogenic process gained considerable support [reviewed by Brusick (16)].

Based on this relation, a generalized hypothesis associating mutagenic and carcinogenic mechanisms was proposed (Fig. 6). Chemicals that fit this scheme have been referred to as mutagenic carcinogens, genotoxic carcinogens, or initiating carcinogens, implying that their mechanism of action involves genotoxic events.

There were numerous problems associated with trying to use correlative evidence as a basis of proof. Although the correlation between animal carcinogens and their responses in *in vitro* assays is not trivial, the predictive values may range from 0.60 to 0.95, depending on the composition of the group of chemicals employed (16,78,96). Biasing the group with aromatic amines, polycyclic hydrocarbons, nitrosamines, and direct-acting alkylating agents has produced an exaggerated relation, whereas the inclusion of a high proportion of metal carcinogens, hormones, halogenated organic molecules, and aromatic solvents tends to reduce correlation coefficients. Thus concordance studies probably represent the least revealing strategy to understand the carcinogen–mutagen relationship.

The evidence linking carcinogens to genotoxic lesions might lead one to expect a better correlation between short-term mutagenicity test results and cancer in animals than is actually observed. Genetic tests are often viewed as too sensitive, producing unacceptable numbers of false-positive responses.

An argument to this assumption proposes that some false responses are not due to inadequacies of the short-term tests but rest with uncertainties regarding the resolving power and reproducibility of the animal cancer data used to "validate" the short-term bioassays. Conflicting responses between mouse and rat animal models tested with the same chemicals also tends to minimize the usefulness of animal data for an assessment of the reliability of mutagenicity tests (15).

Human carcinogenesis, which should be the true standard to determine the validity of a predictive test, consists in only confirmed positives; and by using the human carcinogens to validate tests one finds that a combination of one or two short-term bioassays is as predictive for positive results as are one or two rodent species (Table 4).

A discussion of false results is confusing at best, as the basis for it assumes that the truth can be clearly defined. Unfortunately, in the case of carcinogen prediction from short-term testing, false and true responses are only relative and tend to change with time and the accumulation of more knowledge of the processes leading to tumor development in mammals.

EFFECTS ON THE HUMAN GENE POOL

The human gene pool is the sum total of the genes at a given point in time that are available for transmission to the next generation. All of the human genes that formed the current population were acquired from the previous generation's gene pool. Obviously, deleterious genes are present in the gene pool as evidenced by the numerous genetic dis-

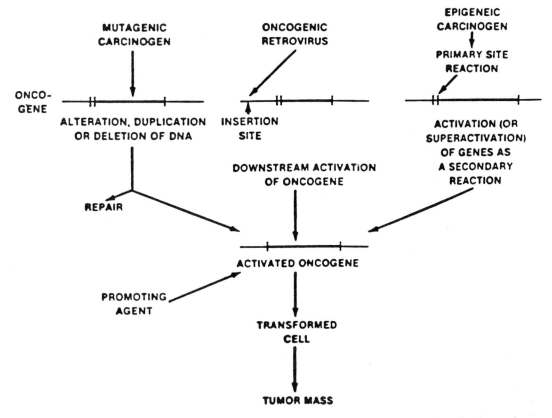

FIG. 6. A hypothetical model of cancer induction which harmonizes three proposed mechanisms of tumor inductions: mutation, retrovirus, and epigenetic.

eases observed in the human species. The specific origin of this disease burden (genetic load) is not known, but it is imperative that this generation transmit the pool to the next generation gene in no worse shape than it was received.

Genetic disease in humans is produced by various types of DNA alteration: (a) chromosome abnormalities resulting in stable changes in chromosome number or structure, per cell; (b) dominant gene mutations in which only a single mutant allele (of the normal gene pair) is required to produce the disease; (c) recessive gene mutations in which both alleles of the pair must be mutant for expression of the trait; and (d) polygenic mutations in which the trait is the result of the interaction of several genes.

Table 3 provides examples of human hereditary diseases as well as the frequency of these disorders per thousand individuals in the population. The examples given in the table represent only a small portion of the total human diseases and defects known to be of genetic origin (65).

The burden to the gene pool from each category of genetic alterations listed in Table 3 is not equivalent. Most of the chromosome abnormalities, for example, result in cell lethality and, if induced in either the ova or sperm, generally produce dominant lethal effects not transmitted to the next generation. Dominant mutations that are not lethal probably contribute moderately to the genetic load. These mutations are generally expressed in the generation immediately following their induction, as only one allele of the diploid pair must be mutant to express the trait. Reduced impact of these mutations is also expected because the affected individuals

can be informed that they are carrying the hereditary determinant and that there is a 50% probability of transmitting the trait to their children even if married to an unaffected individual. Thus depending on the severity of the effect, the parents may decide in advance if the risk associated with transmission is acceptable.

Recessive mutations are those that are not expressed unless both alleles of the pair are defective. This statement implies that both parents must carry at least one mutant gene in common. For example, two normal-appearing individuals could produce offspring (25% incidence) exhibiting a recessive disease, assuming the mutant allele is recessive to the normal allele. Recessive mutations pose the most serious threat to the gene pool, as they may accumulate in the heterozygous carrier state with no obvious effect on the individual.

New recessive mutations introduced into the gene pool are probably not expressed for several generations because of the requirement for homozygosity. Therefore expression of an environmentally induced mutation may have no apparent association with the exposure that induced it. This situation makes human epidemiological studies of mutagenic induction virtually impossible.

Intrinsic Differences Affecting Expression

Unlike the animal population used as human models in toxicology testing, the human population is heterogeneous and consists of subpopulations with a considerable range of

TABLE 4. *Responses of human carcinogens in rodent tumor models and* in vitro *short-term assays*

Group 1 chemicals	In vivo tumor assays				Ames	Mammalian cell mutation assays	Cell transformation	Cytogenetics		
	Human	Mouse	Rat	Other				ABS	SCE	UDS
4-Aminobiphenyl	+	+	+	+	+	ND	+	ND	ND	+
Analgesic mixtures containing phenacetin	+	−	+		+	ND	ND	+	+	ND
Arsenic and arsenic compounds	+	−	−		−	+	+	+	+	ND
Asbestos	+	+	+	+	−	(+)	+	+	ND	ND
Azathioprine	+	(+)	(+)		+	ND	ND	+	ND	ND
Benzene	+	−	−		−	−	−	+	ND	ND
Benzidine	+	ND	+	+	+	+	+	+	+	+
N,N-Bis(2-chloroethyl-2) naphthylamine (chlornaphazine)	+	+	+		+	ND	+	ND	ND	ND
Bis(chloromethyl)ether and chloromethyl methyl ether	+	+	+		+	ND	+	+	+	ND
Myleran	+	(+)	−		+	ND	+	+	+	ND
Certain combined lymphoma chemotherapy (MOPP)	+	ND	ND		ND	ND	ND	ND	ND	ND
Chlorambucil	+	+	+		+	ND	ND	+	ND	ND
Chromium and chromium compounds	+	−	+		+	+	+	+	+	+
Conjugated estrogens	+	ND	−		−	ND	ND	−	ND	ND
Cyclophosphamide	+	+	+		+	+	+	+	+	ND
Diethylstilbestrol	+	+	+	+	−	(+)	+	+	+	−
Melphalan	+	+	+		+	+	+	+	+	+
Methoxysalen plus UV light (PUVA)	+	+	ND		+	+	+	+	+	ND
Mustard gas	+	+	ND		+	+	ND	+	ND	ND
2-Naphthylamine	+	+	−	+	+	+	+	+	+	ND
Soots, tars, and oils	+	+	−		+	+	+	+	+	+
Treosulfan	+	ND	ND	ND	ND	ND	ND	ND	ND	ND
Vinyl chloride	+	+	+	+	+	+	ND	+	+	ND

ND = no data available; ( ) = limited data.
Data obtained from refs. 37 and 45.

susceptibilities to chemical-induced effects. Parameters such as metabolic variability, DNA repair capacity, and genetic predisposition influence the severity of a given exposure to a known genotoxic agent (32,90).

With respect to direct DNA damage, variability in DNA repair capacity affects both altered susceptibility to mutation induction and cancer induction. The test results shown in Fig. 7 clearly demonstrate the importance of the excision repair system in human cells to protect against mutation (68). The XP4BE cells were derived from an individual with xeroderma pigmentosum (XP). This genetic disease is produced by a mutation that affects the ability of the affected cells to repair most types of DNA lesions. Not only are these cells more susceptible to mutation, XP individuals as a group also show almost a 100-fold increase in cancer incidence compared to non-XP individuals. Other human syndromes associated with reduced repair capacity (e.g., ataxia telangiectasia and Fanconi's anemia) also result in increased cancer susceptibility (90). Thus it is clear that results from animal models may not produce data easily extrapolated to the human population because the variance of the response in humans is so broad. It is also clear from this illustration that generalizations regarding hazardous or safe limits of genotoxic chemicals may be rather meaningless.

A second study pointing out the importance of intrinsic factors was reported by Kopelovich et al. (56). This group exposed human cells from individuals known to be genetically susceptible to cancer to promoting agents. The assumption was that the genetic defect generated the initiating lesion and that individuals carrying this trait might even be at risk when exposed only to nongenotoxic promoting or enhancing agents. Their data seem to support this hypothesis and again emphasize the importance of intrinsic factors on the level of risk within the human species.

Life Style and Exposure

It is well documented that certain types of cancer and life expectancy correlate with life style. Tobacco smoke contains a broad range of mutagenic agents detectable in human lymphocytes and urine with the application of genetic assays. Whether mutagens or promoting and enhancing agents in the diet or tobacco smoke are involved in human genetic diseases remains controversial. Consumption of alcoholic beverages is associated with genetic alterations in humans (72a). The average human consumes about 10 tons (dry weight) of food by the age of 50 (94), and the list in Table 5

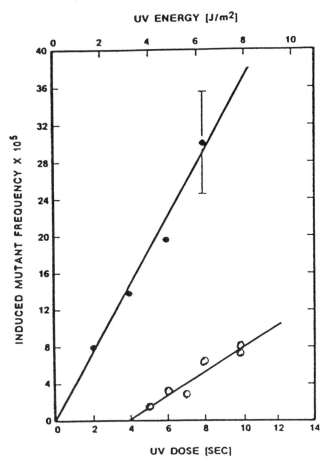

UV ENERGY [J/m²]

FIG. 7. Mutation induction data in human cell lines which are normal for DNA repair and deficient in some aspect of DNA repair. The repair normal cells suggest a threshold for mutation induction that is lacking in those cells incapable of repairing ultraviolet light-induced damage. *Open circles*, normal human diploid fibroblasts; *filled circles*, XP4BE repair deficient human diploid fibroblasts.

TABLE 5. *Foods with mutagenic activity in the Ames assay*

Coffee
Tea
Broiled beef and pork
Broiled fish
Pickled vegetables (Japanese)
Flavanoids in many edible plants
Mushrooms (*Agaricus bisporus*)
Salted fish (Chinese)
Caramelized sugars (glucose/fructose)
Pyrolysates of onion and garlic
Aflatoxin and other mycotoxins (food contamination)
Safrole

See Ames (1) and Nagao et al. (69–71) for general discussion.

peroxidation of fatty acids. The agents include aldehydes, peroxides, and other free radicals.

Considerable efforts are currently under way to evaluate the relative contributions of dietary, environmental, and endogenously formed mutagens to the human disease burden.

TESTING STRATEGIES AND DATA EVALUATION

Test batteries may consist of screening tests, risk assessment tests, or both. It is important at the outset of testing to carefully define the objectives desired in a testing program. A genotoxic material has been defined as "an agent that produces a positive response, e.g., mutation, unscheduled DNA synthesis (UDS), and chromosome breakage, in any bioassay measuring any genetic endpoint" (46). Although this definition considers virtually all forms of damage to DNA an expression of genotoxicity, it is not intended to confer an indication of hazard. This definition is, in fact, only a convenient method of classifying all chemicals into genotoxic or nongenotoxic groups. Additional evidence beyond this initial classification would be required to address concerns of increased genetic risk to somatic or germ cells. Figure 8 illustrates one method to develop additional information via a hypothetical genotoxic pathway leading from exposure and DNA interaction through the steps resulting in either cell death or induction of heritable genetic damage. The early events in the pathway are more likely to be reversed or repaired than those in later steps. Consequently, relative hazard gradient increasing from top to bottom can be proposed.

Screening Tests

Screening tests are those assays that measure the ability of the test substance to produce genotoxic effects. In screening tests, attempts are not generally made to relate the applied dose, route of administration, or type of metabolism to the human experience, and allegations of probable health hazards are difficult to justify if based solely on *in vitro* or submammalian test results.

illustrates that many food items normally consumed by humans contain substances found to be mutagenic in microbial assays. Other mutagenic components associated with modern life styles include cosmetic ingredients, drugs, food additives, and pesticide residues (2,4,5,91). At present, it is not possible to assess in quantitative terms the relevance, if any, of these agents on the mutational or cancer load in the human population.

In addition to tobacco smoke, alcoholic beverages, and consumption of preformed mutagens in or on food products, other life style factors that may be important are less subject to individual control. Ambient air, for example, contains carbonacious particles coated with agents producing mutagenic responses in a range of assays (60). The level of particle loading is location-dependent, and exposures encountered in urban areas or in certain occupations (e.g., coke oven workers) are considerably higher than exposures in more rural areas.

Ames hypothesized that endogenously formed mutagens are significant contributors to genotoxic risk (1). He reported the formation of numerous mutagens resulting from lipid

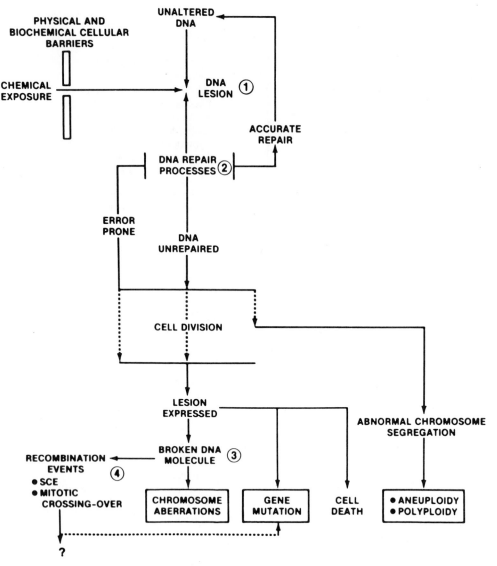

FIG. 8. A model for a genotoxicity pathway. This model indicates that only three types of DNA damage (*boxes*) are causally associated with human genetic disease. Other steps along the genotoxic pathway which are detected in various short term assays (e.g., DNA repair, DNA adducts, SCE) may or may not result in a mutation. Thus, measuring genotoxicity with one of these tests is not equivalent to detecting gene mutation, chromosome aberrations, or changes in chromosome number.

Hazard Assessment Tests

Tests that exceed the general characteristics of screening tests, yet are not adequate for quantitative risk assessment, are often classified as tests indicating possible human hazard. For the most part, these tests are somatic cell *in vivo* tests.

Risk Analysis Tests

Genetic risk analysis involves the development of quantitative estimates of transmissible mutation. Tests that qualify for this type of assessment usually measure either direct damage to the germ cells or heritable effects in the progeny of treated individuals.

Characteristics of Adequate Screening Tests

The following list provides several features of a bioassay that make it a candidate as a screening test.

1. It identifies agents with specific affinity for DNA, not agents with nonspecific toxicity for macromolecules. DNA interactions can be measured as primary DNA effects, point (gene) mutations, or chromosome alterations.
2. It has an adequate capacity for metabolic biotransformation.
3. It is reproducible. Study designs are prepared to ensure adequate sample sizes for definitive, reproducible determination of either positive or negative responses.
4. Test transferability among laboratories is documented.

Tests capable of being performed only in a single laboratory may not be suitable for routine screening.

STRATEGIES FOR BUILDING A TEST BATTERY

Test selection may be based on a variety of themes. For the most part, a test battery represents the experience and bias of the investigator as well as the financial resources available to conduct tests. Some batteries are constructed for carcinogenicity prediction; others encompass genetic risk, with emphasis on rodent germ cell mutagenesis. Accomplishing both objectives (detection of animal mutagens and carcinogens) with a single test battery is unlikely because the most suitable test battery for each type of toxic phenomenon is derived from an independent set of data.

Specific Approaches

The *concordance approach* was first recommended by Ray (79). The EPA-sponsored Gene-Tox program also has as one of its objectives the development of test batteries (100). Results of the working group reports are to be evaluated by an EPA steering committee for test performance with the intent of defining special test batteries optimal for detecting genotoxins in specific chemical classes. It is also presumed that analysis of the entire data set would facilitate emergence of a general test battery for carcinogenicity potential. A similar approach has been taken by Rosenkranz and colleagues at Case Western Reserve University (77). Using the Gene-Tox database and a computer analysis scheme, this group developed the carcinogen prediction and battery selection (CPBS) system, which uses the known performance of various test systems as predictors of animal carcinogenicity to estimate probable carcinogenicity and to suggest test batteries for specific chemical classes.

The *primary test plus complementary test* approach has been suggested primarily for carcinogen detection. The method rests on the use of a well established, routine assay, with extensive testing experience against carcinogens. This experience defines the strengths and weaknesses of the base test. A complementary test or set of tests known to compensate for the limitations of the base test are then recommended to complete the test battery. This approach has been suggested by Williams and Weisberger (101), by Ashby et al. (6), and by Shelby (90a). Williams and Weisberger combined the Ames assay and the rat hepatocyte UDS assay; Ashby recommended the use of the Ames test plus *in vitro* cytogenetic analysis or micronucleus assay; and Shelby proposed a battery of the Ames test coupled with an *in vivo* bone marrow test for chromosome aberrations.

The *endpoint/phylogenetic approach,* unlike the previous two methods, does not rely primarily on retrospective analysis of test performance in the selection of assays. It rests, instead, on the assumption that a reliable test battery covers the major genetic endpoints and contains a variety of organisms with diverse phylogenetic complexity. An example of this approach is the genetic toxicology requirements under EPA's pesticide registration program. These requirements call for at least three assays, including those for gene mutation, chromosome damage, and primary DNA damage. Some batteries also add cell transformation as a separate endpoint. The need for phylogenetic diversity is not explicitly stated, though encouraged.

The endpoint/phylogenetic approach is not tied to either carcinogenic or mutagenic prediction but, rather, addresses the broader view of genetic toxicity. Through the selection of individual tests one might focus the battery toward one or the other of those two toxic phenomena.

Considerations for Assay Selection

A final consideration relevant to all of the previously described approaches is how many assays to include in the battery. A general principle is that batteries with a few tests (e.g., two or three) are susceptible to false-negative outcomes, whereas a battery with more than five tests is more likely to have a false-positive result among the responses. Batteries skewed toward a single genetic endpoint or a single type of organism are also susceptible to false responses. Because this approach does not use test performance per se in test selection, an investigator may have several test options for each endpoint or phylogenetic level.

The selection and execution of protocols or study designs is as important to the genotoxic assessment of an agent as the selection of tests for the battery. Study designs should meet the Good Laboratory Practices requirements and be of sufficient size (power) to give good experimental resolution. Standard study designs for most of the routine genetic toxicology assays have been published by the EPA (34), OECD (73), and EEC (30).

The EPA (35) has also proposed guidelines for the interpretation of data, including *in vivo* tests, in the context of a weight-of-evidence approach to genetic risk. These guidelines provide a framework for evaluation but do not address when or how to select tests.

In Vivo Assay Use

Once a series of *in vitro* tests have been performed and evaluated, it may be necessary to extend the testing to *in vivo* assays. The following set of scenerios may be appropriate to trigger *in vivo* studies:

1. *In vitro* test battery responses are mixed with a key genetic endpoint (i.e., gene mutation or chromosome breakage) registering a clear positive response. The *in vivo* data are important to put this response into perspective.
2. *In vitro* test battery responses are mixed, and positive responses are found in more than one genotoxicity assay, e.g., DNA binding, UDS, sister chromatic exchange (SCE), cell transformation, but all mutation and chromosome aberration endpoints are negative. *In vivo* negative effects for mutation and clastogenesis would reduce concern for genetic hazard.
3. *In vitro* data are uniformly negative, but there is some

reason to believe that *in vivo* metabolism is not represented in activation systems used *in vitro*. Negative *in vivo* results support and provide additional evidence against a potential health risk.

4. *In vitro* responses are all negative, but the extent of compound use and human exposure levels necessitate extension of the database into those areas that involve germ cells in addition to somatic cells.

The following are other circumstances unrelated to *in vitro* responses that warrant *in vivo* analysis:

1. Cancer bioassay results from rodents are marginal or identified unusual target organ specificity. *In vivo* genotoxicity studies might assist in resolving the bioassay interpretation or aid in demonstrating activity in the target site through analysis of genotoxic damage in target organ explants.

2. Reproductive studies may have identified the gonads as target organs for toxicity, and *in vivo* germ cell mutagenicity data may be warranted to address concerns for heritable genetic risk.

In vivo genetic toxicology studies can be conducted as stand-alone assays or may be incorporated into planned acute or subchronic toxicology studies. There are advantages and limitations associated with both approaches.

Stand-Alone Techniques

The list of tests used as stand-alone assays is the most comprehensive and includes the most widely used assays. The tests can be applied as direct follow-up from their respective *in vitro* analogs. Direct follow-up of endpoints is the most reliable manner in which to apply this set of tests. Table 6 lists a set of *in vitro* tests and their follow-up *in vivo* models. The *in vivo* tests are listed in order of phylogenetic or methodologic preference.

The general interpretation applied to the use of *in vivo* data is that it may take precedence over *in vitro* results if (a) the design of the *in vivo* study is adequate to detect weak responses and (b) evidence can be provided that the test article or its metabolites have access to the target site.

Expansion of Standard Toxicology Assays

These *in vivo* models are particularly valuable for developing an *in vivo* database from planned toxicology studies. Most of the effort associated with dosage determination, compound administration, and animal care are incorporated into the toxicology study design. The genetic toxicology study requires (a) addition of a few animals or (b) removal of specific cells from existing treatment and control animals. Examples of expansion studies include analysis of genotoxic effects in isolated red blood cells, lymphocytes, hemoglobin, extracted DNA, and urine.

Data from these studies may be used to develop early hazard assessment for major products or to study target organ and metabolism questions that have arisen regarding the test material. The extent of these studies is similar to that of the

TABLE 6. In vitro *stand-alone techniques and their* in vivo *follow-up tests*

In vitro assays	Recommended in vivo follow-up models for in vitro tests
Gene mutation endpoint Ames (or other bacteria) Mouse lymphoma CHO (HGPRT) Yeast forward or reverse mutation	Gene mutation endpoint Mouse somatic cell coat color assay (spot test) *Drosophila* sex-linked recessive lethal test Mouse specific locus assay or suitable dominant mutation assay (germ cell)[a]
Chromosome aberration endpoint *In vitro* cytogenetic analysis in various cell lines	Chromosome aberration endpoint Rodent micronucleus Rodent bone marrow Dominant lethal assay (germ cell)[a] Heritable translocation (germ cell)[a] Germ cell chromosome aberrations[a]
UDS in primary hepatocytes	Rat *in vivo/in vitro* UDS in hepatocytes
Sister chromatid exchange (SCE)	*In vivo* SCE in bone marrow or other cell types
In vitro adduct formation (DNA binding)	DNA binding in selected target organs using radiolabeled chemical or ^{32}P-postlabeling[a]
In vitro cell transformation	Liver focus assay in rats

[a] Test or technique that may be applicable to the development of heritable genetic risk estimates.

previous group, as many of the same endpoints are included. The major limitations are that occasionally dose levels or routes of administration established for acute and subchronic toxicology studies might not be applicable for genetic evaluations. Occasionally, species selection prevents successful performance of genetic studies (e.g., peripheral blood cell micronuclei evaluations cannot be performed in rats).

Regulations Affecting Testing

Genetic toxicology studies submitted to U.S. or other international regulatory agencies must comply with certain regulations and testing guidelines. In the United States the Food and Drug Administration (FDA) and Environmental Protection Agency (EPA) Good Laboratory Practices regulations determine performance of tests and the documentation required for reporting the results. In addition, employee health and safety requirements and facility specifications are incumbent on most commercial testing operations (72).

Several government institutions and advisory bodies have published standard study designs for most genetic toxicology assays. Some regulatory agencies insist that all reports follow guideline protocols from one of these sources. Berry and Litchfield (10) have prepared a review of the regulatory re-

TABLE 7. *Minimal testing requirements of several countries*

Countries	Chemical category	Required testing[a]	Regulating agency
U.S.	Pesticides	Three tests minimum Gene mutation Chromosome aberration DNA repair	EPA
	Medical devices (implantable polymers)	Unofficial requirements Ames test Mammalian cell gene mutation *In vitro* cytogenetics Cell transformation	FDA
European community (EEC/OECD)	All industrial chemicals in commerce >1 but <10 tons of production per year	Two tests minimum Ames test *In vitro* cytogenetics	EEC 6th Amendment
	All industrial chemicals with ≥10 tons of production per year	Two tests above plus *in vivo* cytogenetics and mammalian cell test for gene mutation	EEC 6th Amendment
	All pharmaceuticals	Same as chemicals over 10-ton production[b]	EEC 6th Amendment
Japan	All chemicals in commerce not biodegradable	Two tests minimum Ames test (special version) *In vitro* cytogenetics	MOHW, MAFF, MITI[c]
Canada	Depends on exposure levels (levels of concern, LOC)	Two tests minimum (LOCI) Ames test *In vitro* cytogenetics	MOHW[c]

[a] Other testing may be requested after evaluation of the results from the required set.

[b] UDS possibly required for Italy as a fifth test.

[c] Respective Ministry of Health and Welfare, Ministry of Agriculture, Forestry and Fisheries, Ministry of International Trade and Industry.

quirements for mutagenicity testing. The general minimal requirements are similar in the United States, Japan, and Western Europe and are summarized in Table 7.

DATA ANALYSIS AND INTERPRETATION

Primary Evaluation of Individual Tests

Each type of test system is amenable to some form of data analysis. Most are evaluated mathematically to determine the statistical significance of the results. Criteria described in EPA, OECD, and EEC guidelines are not specific about the type of analysis to be used, although statistical methods are recommended. A careful review of published data such as those derived from the Gene-Tox program and other large collaborative studies is necessary for standardization of data analysis.

Evaluation Approaches for Batteries

The second level of data evaluation leads to a description or conclusion regarding the biological activity of a test substance. Is the compound a mutagen or a clastogen? Does exposure to the material constitute a health hazard? This level of data analysis is more elusive than the primary evaluation because it is based on a limited experience and requires intuitive processes. Therefore most interpretive evaluations are qualitative and define only hazard "potential."

The three most common methods for evaluating results from screening batteries are the following:

1. *Decision tree method,* in which results from one test direct the investigator to the next test or to an interpretation or categorization of the chemical.
2. *Critical mass approach,* in which a specified number of positive tests in a given category automatically defines the category of a test material, regardless of the spectrum of response or the concentration needed to achieve the response. Negative responses are not contributory unless the results are negative in all tests conducted.
3. *Weight-of-evidence approach,* in which each test has a specific weight proportional to its reliability in defining a true positive or negative effect. The overall evaluation is based on the trend of responses and is useful for mixed results, as both positive and negative data can be accommodated.

Interpretation of Results from Test Batteries

The ultimate application of test results is the assessment of hazard for humans exposed to the test agent. In this context, hazard assessment is defined as the most likely toxic outcome for humans exposed acutely or chronically to biologically significant levels of the agent. Hazard assessments are often expressed in degrees of concern rather than in expected increases in disease incidence as might be done for risk analysis.

TABLE 8. *Two-dimensional analysis of the relevance of test results*

MOST		
↑ *(Phylogenetic relevance)*	Tests that detect DNA alterations in somatic cells of humans exposed to genotoxic agents	Evidence from human studies for the induction of somatic and germ cell, gene, or chromosome mutations
	Tests that detect alterations in DNA synthesis and replication or tests that measure direct DNA damage and repair *in vivo* using mammalian models	Tests that detect gene or chromosome mutation *in vivo* using mammalian models
	Tests that detect alterations in DNA synthesis and replication or tests that measure direct DNA damage and repair *in vitro* using metabolically proficient mammalian cell systems	Tests that detect gene mutation or cell transformation *in vitro* using metabolically proficient mammalian cell systems
	Tests that detect alterations in DNA synthesis and replication or tests that measure direct DNA damage and repair using metabolically sufficient or exogenously supplemented nonmammalian cell systems	Tests that detect mutation or chromosome damage using metabolically sufficient or exogenously supplemented nonmammalian cell systems
LEAST ───→ MOST		

Relevance of the genotoxic endpoint detected

A generic method useful for genetic data assessment is a two-dimensional analysis of data that establishes estimates of hazard on the basis of positive test results (42a). Estimates are based on the assumption that tests measuring gene mutation or chromosome damage are directly responsible for, and therefore more relevant to, human disease than other genotoxic endpoints. Chemicals that induce only primary DNA damage, for example, are not accorded the same degree of concern because human diseases cannot be linked to non-mutational endpoints. Consequently, under the proposed approach to hazard assessment, test systems stratify into three classes indicating genotoxic hazard according to their position in the genotoxic pathway outlined in Fig. 8.

Class 3: assays that measure gene mutation or structural and numerical chromosome aberrations
Class 2: assays that measure SCE, recombination, DNA-repair synthesis, DNA-strand breakage, or DNA cross-linking
Class 1: assays that measure adduct formation or inhibition of DNA synthesis or replication

Class 1 represents the lowest degree of concern and class 3 the highest.

The second dimension of this analysis stratifies test organisms by their phylogenetic relatedness to humans. Data from a test battery that includes at least one test from each of the three end-point classes are analyzed using the scale in Table 8.

The information in Table 8 can be made semiquantitative by placing it in a two-way evaluation table (Table 9). In this table, there are five phylogenetic strata ranging from prokaryotic and plant cells to human *in vivo* responses.

A tested material may provide data from as few as three tests or as many as 10 or more. A proposed agent classification scheme is outlined in Table 10. An interpretation of the multitest is derived from combinations of numbers and letters from positive responses. The table uses combinations of the most relevant data acquired to classify the chemicals according to their potential hazard. In many cases, the data available on a chemical will not be sufficient to extend its classification of a chemical beyond *genotoxic* or *mutagenic;*

TABLE 9. *Data analysis table for categorizing hazard from positive test results*

Stratification of assays by complexity of bioassay system		Least relevant indicator of somatic mutation	→ Most relevant indicator of somatic mutation	
		Class 1	Class 2	Class 3
Least relevant assay	Plant prokaryotic systems (A)	1A	2A	3A
│	Lower eukaryotic microorganisms and insect systems (B)	1B	2B	3B
│	Mammalian *in vitro* systems (C)	1C	2C	3C
↓	Mammalian *in vivo* systems (D)	1D	2D	3D
Most relevant assay	Human *in vivo* data (E)	1E	2E	3E

TABLE 10. *Proposed scheme for classifying chemicals on the basis of test results*

Chemical classification	Responses required for classification of hazard potential	Implications for oncogenesis
Genotoxic agent	Positive response in at least one square	None, unless other conditions defined below are met.
Mutagenic agent	Positive response in at least one class 3 square	Carcinogenic potential is possible and the level of probability increases from 3A to 3D tests.
Animal cell somatic mutagen[a]	Positive responses in at least one test each from 1C and 2C and at least two tests from 3C	Relevance of test systems, correlation coefficients, and nature of the DNA lesions all point toward carcinogenic activity.
Probable animal (human) mutagen[b]	Positive responses in at least two tests each of 2C and 3C plus a positive response in 2D, 3D, or 2E	Relevance of test systems, correlation coefficients, nature of the DNA lesions, and *in vivo* chemical pharmacodynamics all point toward *in vivo* tumorigenicity.
Human mutagen	Positive results or evidence in 3E	Probable increase of risk of tumor induction if exposure persists.

[a] The test material has biological properties in common with materials known to produce cancer in experimental animals, but the pharmacodynamics of *in vivo* exposure are not known.

[b] The test material has relevant genotoxic activity in mammalian cells and has been shown to express that activity under *in vivo* test conditions.

in a few cases, a chemical may be defined as a human hazard. This approach is similar in many respects to the EPA (35) mutagenic risk assessment guidelines.

GENETIC HAZARD ASSESSMENTS

Assessing human risk to mutagenic substances represents a formidable task. There has been no conclusive evidence supporting chemical-induced mutation in human germ cells; however, mutagens are detected in rodent germ cells and quantitative estimates of mutagen-induced mutant rates per gene locus or the dose required to double a specific mutation rate can be calculated from results of the specific locus (84) or heritable translocation (41) assays. These estimates may be of limited value in calculating human risk or in setting safe exposure levels because they are based on male gametes

and, in the case of the specific locus assay, only on premeiotic stem cells (spermatogonia). The data do not reflect the risk to later cell stages in spermatogenesis or in female germ cells. Even if estimates were available from postmeiotic sperm or from female germ cells, other important biological variables would interfere with reliable risk estimates and extrapolation across species boundaries (Table 11).

DNA repair is probably the most confounding parameter when determining germ cell damage. Significant sex, age, and species differences would make extrapolation tenuous (39). In addition, postzygotic repair of damaged sperm is genotypically determined and varies widely (41).

Thus even under ideal testing situations it is virtually impossible to calculate accurate values for germ cell risk that address all aspects of human exposure. Most chemicals are handled using a form of hazard assessment that utilizes qualitative responses from an array of assays including *in vitro* and *in vivo* models.

Extrapolation of Somatic Cell Responses to Germ Cells

Two groups of investigators have attempted to examine *in vitro* and *in vivo* somatic cell assays to determine those that would most closely predict the germ cell effects of a mutagenic substance. The first group, Committee 1 of the International Commission for Protection Against Environmental Mutagens and Carcinogens (46), reviewed data on 53 chemicals that had been adequately tested in at least one of the following germ cell tests: mouse specific locus, heritable translocation, or dominant lethal.

Comparative data were obtained from 12 other tests including mammalian *in vivo* somatic cell tests, submammalian assays, and *in vitro* tests including bacteria and yeast organisms. Although the assays appear to stratify on the basis of common responses, none of the comparisons significantly exceeds overlapping responses due to chance. Thus it is difficult to conclude that non-germ-cell assays are predictive of effects in germ cells.

TABLE 11. *Biological barriers that protect gonads from mutagens*

Biological barrier	Function
Blood, testis	Limits access to male germ cells on the basis of molecular size, charge, and lipid solubility. Large, highly charged molecules or those with low lipid solubility are excluded from gonadal cells.
Hepatic biotransformation	Detoxifies highly reactive agents or promutagens prior to their access to other organs such as the gonads.
Gonadal biotransformation	Gonads contain low levels of mutagen-activating enzymes and high levels of detoxifying enzymes.
Germ cell DNA repair	DNA repair processes are active in premeiotic spermatogenic cells and throughout the meiotic process in female germ cells.

The second report was developed from phase II of the EPA GeneTox program. The report attempted to assess the relative value of various assays for genetic hazard identification (83). With this assessment the Specific Locus Test and the Heritable Translocation Test were matched separately against responses from the other assays. These results, like the ICPEMC comparison, stratified by concordance levels, but the effect of random assortment could not be excluded except in one case. Consequently, concordance between rodent germ cell results and results from tests among the other classes does not provide a reliable approach to definitive risk prediction.

At the present time the only acceptable method to define germ cell risk is to conduct *in vivo* studies that employ male and female germ cells as targets. Sensitive and reliable methods using sophisticated biochemical and biotechnology methods will probably be available for risk analysis purposes over the next several years.

Alternative Indirect Methods

Sobels (93) proposed an indirect approach to risk analysis that utilizes the ratio of somatic cell dosimetry and germ cell mutation in animals to predict germ cell mutation in exposed humans. The method, referred to as the *parallelogram approach,* makes direct measurements of germ cell mutation rates and somatic cell DNA dosimetry in animals. The measurements constitute an index of germ cell mutation/somatic cell genotoxicity. Mutagenic risk is calculated for humans by direct measurement of somatic cell (i.e., peripheral lymphocytes) genotoxicity combined with the assumption that the germ cell/somatic cell index for humans is similar to that for animals. The consequence is a calculated germ cell mutation rate for humans.

The second indirect method assesses somatic cell risk for cancer initiation using an index developed between cancer rates and *in vitro* test data potency for known human carcinogens (60). This ratio is used in a similar fashion to Sobel's parallelogram to calculate an index for an unknown agent using *in vitro* test data in combination with the risk ratio.

SELECTED STUDY DESIGNS FOR GENETIC TESTING

This section contains a set of seven protocols. These protocols include descriptions of assays designed to detect gene mutation, chromosome alterations, and primary DNA damage. The size of each study design is flexible and can be scaled up if so desired. The study designs as described are of sufficient diversity and size (power) to be used in most required testing programs (see Table 7).

Although not fully described in every protocol, it is recommended that each test article be examined for several chemical, physical, and biological parameters. Included in this preliminary assessment is an examination of the test article's solubility, volatility, and light sensitivity, as well as its stability in the recommended solvent. A preliminary toxicity study is performed to establish a maximum concentration or dose level. The protocols all contain specific criteria related to interpretation of toxicity, but it is often possible to save time and materials by knowing the approximate concentration range needed to achieve the desired toxicity.

This group of protocols does not represent the entire repertoire of methods available to genetic toxicologists. It provides, however, the essential tests needed for routine screening and gives a sufficient cross-section of the available tests that meet most general regulatory requirements outlined in Table 7.

Tests Measuring Gene Mutation

Protocol 1: Ames Salmonella/Microsome Plate Assay

The objective of the Ames *Salmonella*/microsome plate assay is to evaluate the test article for mutagenic activity in a bacterial reverse mutation system with and without a mammalian S9 activation component.

Materials

The strains of *Salmonella typhimurium* that are used routinely in the plate assay are described in Table 12. Other strains may be added or substituted (63).

An S9 homogenate is used as the activation system. The $9,000 \times g$ supernatant fluid is prepared from Sprague-Dawley adult male rat liver induced by Aroclor 1254 (4). The components of the S9 mix are described in Table 13.

Test procedures

An appropriate number of tubes of molten overlay agar (at least two per control or concentration level) are prepared. An equivalent number of Vogel Bonner plates also are prepared and properly labeled.

TABLE 12. Salmonella typhimurium *strains used in the plate assay*

| Strain designation | Gene affected | Additional mutations | | | Mutation type detected |
		Repair	LPS	R factor	
TA-1535	his G	Δ uvr B	rfa	—	Base-pair substitution
TA-1537	his C	Δ uvr B	rfa	—	Frameshift
TA-1538	his D	Δ uvr B	rfa	—	Frameshift
TA-98	his D	Δ uvr B	rfa	pKM101	Frameshift
TA-100	his G	Δ uvr B	rfa	pKM101	Base-pair substitution

TABLE 13. *Components of a standard S9 mix*

Components	Concentration (μmol/ml) S9 mix
NADP (sodium salt)	4
D-Glucose-6-phosphate	5
MgCl₂	8
KCl	33
Sodium phosphate buffer, pH 7.4	100
Organ homogenate from rat liver (S9 fraction)	100 μl

The test article is weighed or measured and diluted in a solvent to set up the stock solutions. The test article and other components are prepared fresh and added to the overlay. The contents then are mixed and poured on the surfaces of the Vogel Bonner plates. For activation studies, 0.5 ml of the S9 mix is added to each overlay tube. The entire test consists of nonactivation and activation (+S9 mix) test conditions, each with appropriate negative and positive controls.

The plates (once the overlay has solidified) are incubated at 37°C for 36 to 72 hr and scored for numbers of revertants per plate. Colonies are selected at random for verification of histidine independence by growth on minimal agar medium.

For the standard plate test, at least five dose levels of the test article, dissolved in a suitable solvent, are added to the test system. Duplicate or triplicate plates per dose per strain are used in the standard assay. The test concentrations can be based on preliminary toxicity dose selection test or selected from a set of standard test doses. When no toxicity is observed, concentrations of up to 50 μl or 5,000 to 10,000 μg per plate may be employed.

The chemicals that may be used as positive control agents are described in Table 14.

Evaluation criteria

Several methods for statistical analysis of the Ames test are suggested in the EPA GeneTox work group report for *Salmonella typhimurium* mutation assay (51).

Plate test data consist of direct revertant colony counts obtained from a set of selective agar plates seeded with populations of mutant cells suspended in a semisolid overlay. Because the test article and the cells are incubated in the overlay for 36 to 72 hr, and a few cell divisions occur during the incubation period, the test is semiquantitative in nature. Although these features of the assay reduce the quantitation of results, they provide certain advantages not contained in a quantitative suspension test:

1. The small number of cell divisions permits potential mutagens to act on replicating DNA, which is often more sensitive than nonreplicating DNA.
2. The combined incubation of the test article and the cells in the overlay permits constant exposure of the indicator cells for 36 to 72 hr.

Surviving populations. Plate test procedures do not permit exact quantitation of the number of cells surviving chemical treatment. At low concentrations of the test article, the surviving populations on the treatment plates are essentially the same as that on the negative control plate. At high concentrations, the surviving population is usually reduced by some unknown fraction. This protocol normally employs several doses ranging over two or three log concentrations; the highest of these doses is selected to show toxicity as determined by subjective criteria such as background clearing or a reduction in the number of spontaneous colonies on treated plates compared with the solvent control.

Dose-response phenomena. The demonstration of a dose-related increase in mutant counts is an important criterion for establishing mutagenicity. A factor that might modify dose-response results for a mutagen is the selection of doses that are too low (usually mutagenicity and toxicity are related). If the highest dose is far lower than a toxic concentration, no increase may be observed over the dose range selected. Conversely, if the lowest dose employed is highly cytotoxic, the test article may kill any mutants that are induced and thus does not appear to be mutagenic. Occasionally, high levels of toxicity produce microcolonies (not mutants), which can be confused for revertants by inexperienced investigators.

Control tests. Positive and negative control assays are conducted with each experiment and consist in direct-acting mutagens for nonactivation assays and mutagens that require metabolic biotransformation in activation assays. Negative controls consist of the test article solvent in the overlay agar together with the other essential components. The negative control plates for each strain give a reference point to which the test data can be compared. The positive control assay is conducted to demonstrate that the test systems are functional with known mutagens.

Replication. Each study is replicated with an independent test.

Evaluation criteria

Because the procedures used to evaluate the mutagenicity of the test article are semiquantitative, the criteria used to determine positive effects are inherently subjective and based

TABLE 14. *Positive control agents for the standard plate test*

Assay	Chemical	Solvent	Concentration per plate (μg)	Responding *Salmonella* strains
Nonactivation	Sodium azide	Water	1	TA-1535, TA-100
	2-Nitrofluorene	Dimethylsulfoxide	10	TA-1538, TA-98
	9-Aminoacridine	Ethanol	50	TA-1537
Activation	2-Anthramine	Dimethylsulfoxide	2.5	All strains

primarily on a historical database. Most data sets are evaluated using the following criteria:

1. *Strains TA-1535, TA-1537, and TA-1538.* If the solvent control value is within the typical range for the laboratory, a test article that produces a positive dose response over *three* concentrations, with the highest increase equal to three times the solvent control value, may be considered mutagenic.

2. *Strains TA-98 and TA-100.* If the solvent control value is within the normal range for the laboratory, a test article that produces a positive dose response over *three* concentrations, with the highest increase equal to twice the solvent control value, is considered mutagenic. Occasionally a doubling is not necessary for TA-100 if a clear dose-related pattern is observed over several concentrations.

3. *Pattern.* Because TA-1535 and TA-100 are derived from the parental strain (G-46) and because TA-1538 and TA-98 are derived from the same parental strain (D3052), to some extent there is a built-in redundancy in the microbial assay. In general, the two strains of a set respond to the same mutagen, and such a pattern is sought. Generally, if a strain responds to a mutagen in nonactivation tests, it does so in activation tests.

The preceding criteria are not absolute, and other extenuating factors may enter into a final evaluation decision. However, these criteria can be applied to most situations and are presented to aid individuals not familiar with this procedure. It must be emphasized that modifications of the procedure involving preincubation conditions or source of S9 mix are necessary for evaluation of specific chemicals or classes of chemicals.

Protocol 2: Forward Mutation at the TK Locus in L5178Y Mouse Lymphoma Cells

The objective of the mouse lymphoma assay is to evaluate a test article for its ability to induce forward mutation in the L5178Y TK+/− mouse lymphoma cell line, as assessed by colony growth in the presence of 5-trifluorothymidine (TFT).

Thymidine kinase (TK) is a cellular enzyme that allows cells to salvage thymidine from the surrounding medium for use in DNA synthesis. If a thymidine analog such as TFT is included in the growth medium, the analog is phosphorylated via the TK pathway and incorporated into DNA, eventually resulting in cellular death. Cells that are heterozygous at the TK locus (TK+/−) may undergo a single step forward mutation to the TK−/− genotype, in which little or no TK activity remains. Such mutants are as viable as the heterozygotes in normal medium because DNA synthesis proceeds by *de novo* synthetic pathways that do not involve thymidine as an intermediate. The basis for selection of the TK−/− mutants is the lack of any ability to utilize toxic analogs of thymidine, which enable only TK−/− mutants to grow in the presence of TFT. Cells that grow to form colonies in the presence of TFT are therefore assumed to have mutated either spontaneously or by the action of a test article to the TK−/− genotype.

Materials

Indicator cells. The mouse lymphoma cell line used in this assay, L5178Y TK+/−, is derived from the Fischer

L5178Y line. Stocks are maintained in liquid nitrogen and laboratory cultures periodically checked for the absence of *Mycoplasma* contamination. To reduce the negative control frequency (spontaneous frequency) of TK−/− mutants to as low a level as possible, cell cultures are exposed to conditions that select against the TK−/− phenotype and then returned to normal growth medium for 3 days or more before use.

Media. The cells are maintained in RPMI 1640 or Fischer's mouse leukemia medium supplemented with L-glutamine, sodium pyruvate, and horse serum (10% by volume). Cloning medium consists of the preceding growth medium with the addition of agar to a final concentration of 0.35% to achieve a semisolid state. Selection medium is cloning medium containing TFT 3 μg/ml.

Control articles. A negative control consisting in assay procedures performed on cells exposed to solvent in the medium is assayed as the solvent negative control article to determine any effects on survival or mutation caused by the solvent alone. For test articles assayed with activation, the solvent negative control articles include the activation mixture.

Ethylmethane sulfonate is highly mutagenic via alkylation of cellular DNA and may be used at 0.25 to 0.50 μl/ml as a positive control article for nonactivation studies.

3-Methylcholanthrene requires metabolic activation by microsomal enzymes to become mutagenic and may be used at 1.0 to 4.0 μg/ml as a positive control article for assays performed with activation.

Sample forms. All types of test article can be evaluated in the mouse lymphoma assay. Solid articles can be dissolved in water, if possible, or in dimethylsulfoxide (DMSO), ethanol, or acetone unless another solvent is requested. Liquids can be tested by direct addition to the test system at predetermined concentrations or following dilution in a suitable solvent.

Experimental design

Dose selection. The solubility of the test article in water or an organic solvent is determined first; then a wide range of test article concentrations are tested for cytotoxicity, starting with a maximum applied dose of 1 to 5 mg/ml for a solid test article or 1 to 5 μl/ml for a liquid test article and using twofold dilution steps. After an exposure time of 4 hr the cells are washed, and a viable cell count is obtained the next day. Relative cytotoxicities expressed as the reduction in growth compared to the growth of untreated cells are used to select seven to ten doses that cover the range from 0 to 50 to 80 to 90% reduction in 24-hr growth. These selected doses subsequently are applied to cell cultures prepared for mutagenicity testing, but only four or five of the doses are carried through the mutant selection process. This procedure compensates for daily variations in cellular cytotoxicity and ensures the choice of four or five doses spaced from 0 to 50 to 80 to 90% reduction in cell growth.

Mutagenicity testing. The procedure used for the nonactivation assay is based on that reported by Clive and Spector (25). Cultures exposed to the test article for 4 hr at the preselected doses are washed and placed in growth medium for 2 to 3 days to allow recovery, growth, and expression of the induced TK−/− phenotype. Cell counts are determined daily and appropriate dilutions made to allow optimal growth rates.

At the end of the expression period 3×10^4 cells for each selected dose are seeded in soft agar plates with selection medium, and resistant (mutant) colonies are counted after 10 to 14 days' incubation. To determine the number of cells capable of forming colonies, a portion of the cell suspension is also cloned in normal medium (nonselective). The ratio of resistant colonies to total vial cell number is the mutant frequency.

The activation assay can be run concurrently with the nonactivation assay. The only difference is the addition of the S9 fraction of rat liver homogenate and necessary cofactors (CORE) during the 4-hr treatment period. CORE consists of NADP (sodium salt) and isocitric acid. The final concentrations of the activation system components in the cell suspension should be 2.4 mg NADP (sodium salt)/ml, 4.5 mg isocitric acid/ml, and 10 to 50 μl S9/ml.

Preparation of 9,000 × g supernatant fluid (S9). Sprague-Dawley or Fischer 344 male rats are normally used as the source of hepatic microsomes. The S9 is obtained commercially. Briefly, induction with Aroclor 1254 or another agent is performed by injection 5 days prior to killing. After decapitation and bleeding, the liver is immediately dissected from the animal using aseptic technique and placed in ice-cold buffer at pH 7.4. When an adequate number of livers are obtained, the collection is washed twice with fresh buffer and completely homogenized. The homogenate is centrifuged for 10 min at $9,000 \times g$ in a refrigerated centrifuge, and the supernatant fluid (S9) from this centrifuged sample is retained and frozen at $-80°C$ until used in the activation system.

Assay acceptance criteria

An assay is considered acceptable for evaluation of test results only if all of the criteria in the following list are satisfied. The activation and nonactivation portions of the mutation assays usually are performed concurrently, but each portion is in fact an independent assay with its own positive and negative controls. The activation or nonactivation assays are repeated independently to satisfy general acceptance and evaluation criteria.

1. The average absolute cloning efficiency of the negative controls (average of the solvent and untreated controls) is 100 ± 30%. Assay variables can lead to artifically low cloning efficiencies in the range of 50 to 70% and still yield internally consistent and valid results. Assays with cloning efficiencies in this range are conditionally acceptable and dependent on the scientific judgment of the investigator. All assays below 50% cloning efficiency are unacceptable.

2. The average negative control suspension growth factor is not less than about 8. The optimal value is 25, which corresponds to fivefold increases in cell number for each of the 2 days following treatment of the experimental cultures.

3. The background mutant frequency (average of the solvent and untreated negative controls) is calculated separately for concurrent activation and nonactivation assays, even though the same population of cells is used for each assay. For both conditions the normal range of background frequencies for assays performed with different cell stocks is 10×10^{-6} to 100×10^{-6}. Assays with backgrounds outside this range are not necessarily invalid but are not used as primary evidence for evaluation of a test article. These assays can provide supporting evidence.

4. A positive control is included with each assay to provide confidence in the procedures used to detect mutagenic activity. The normal range of mutant frequencies induced by EMS 0.40 μl/ml (nonactivation assay) is 200×10^{-6} to 800×10^{-6}; for MCA 4.0 μg/ml (activation assay), the normal range is 200×10^{-6} to 800×10^{-6}. An assay is considered acceptable in the absence of a positive control (loss due to contamination or technical error) only if the test article clearly shows mutagenic activity as described in the evaluation criteria.

5. For test articles with little or no mutagenic activity, an assay must include applied concentrations that reduce the relative growth to between 10 and 20% of the average solvent control or reach the maximum applied concentrations given in the evaluation criteria. This requirement is waived if a dose increment of about 1.5 or less causes excessive toxicity.

6. An experimental treatment that results in fewer than 3.0×10^6 cells by the end of the 2-day growth period is not cloned for mutant analysis.

7. An experimental mutant frequency is considered acceptable for evaluation only if the relative cloning efficiency is 10% or greater and the total number of viable clones exceeds 20.

8. Mutant frequencies are derived normally from sets of three dishes for both the mutant and the viable colony count. To allow for contamination losses, an acceptable mutant frequency can be calculated from a minimum of two dishes per set.

9. The mutant frequencies for five treated cultures are normally determined in each assay. A required number of various concentrations cannot be explicitly stated, although a minimum of three analyzed cultures is considered necessary under the most favorable test conditions to accept a single assay for evaluation of the test article.

Assay evaluation criteria

The minimum condition considered necessary to demonstrate mutagenesis for any given treatment is a mutant frequency that is at least two times the concurrent background frequency. The *background frequency* is defined as the average mutant frequency of the solvent controls. The minimum increase is based on extensive experience that indicates that the calculated minimum increase is often a repeatable result.

The observation of a mutant frequency that meets the minimum criterion for a single treated culture within a range of assayed concentrations is not sufficient evidence to evaluate a test article as a mutagen. The following test results must be obtained to reach this conclusion for either activation or nonactivation conditions:

1. A dose-related or toxicity-related increase in mutant frequency is observed. It is desirable to obtain this relation for at least three doses, but it depends on the concentration steps chosen for the assay and the toxicity at which mutagenic activity appears.

2. An increase in mutant frequency may be followed by only small or no further increases at higher concentrations or toxicities. However, a decrease in mutant frequency to values below the minimum criterion is not acceptable in a single assay to classify the test article as a mutagen. If the mutagenic activity at lower concentrations or toxicities is large, a repeat assay is performed to confirm the mutagenic activity.

3. If an increase of about two times the minimum criterion or more is observed for a single dose near the highest testable toxicity, as defined in Assay Acceptance Criteria, the test article is considered mutagenic. Smaller increases at a single dose near the highest testable toxicity require confirmation by a repeat assay.

4. For some test articles the correlation between toxicity and applied concentration is poor. The proposition of the applied article that effectively interacts with the cells to cause genetic alterations is not always repeatable or under control. Conversely, measurable changes in the frequency of induced mutants may occur with concentration changes that cause only small changes in observable toxicity. Therefore either parameter—applied concentration or toxicity (percent relative growth)—can be used to establish if the mutagenic activity is related to an increase in effective treatment. A negative correlation with dose is acceptable only if a positive correlation with toxicity exists. An apparent increase in mutagenic activity as a function of decreasing toxicity is not acceptable evidence for mutagenicity.

A test article is evaluated as nonmutagenic in a single assay only if the minimum increase in mutant frequency is not observed for a range of applied concentrations that extends to toxicity causing 10 to 20% relative suspension growth. If the test article is relatively nontoxic, the maximum applied concentrations are normally 5 mg/ml (or 5 µl/ml) unless limited by solubility. If a repeat assay does not confirm an earlier, minimal response as discussed above, the test article is evaluated as nonmutagenic in this assay system.

Protocol 3: Sex-Linked Recessive Lethal Test in Drosophila melanogaster

The objective of the sex-linked recessive lethal test in *Drosophila melanogaster* is to provide a short-term *in vivo* mutagen screening system employing a eukaryotic organism. The test measures the frequency of lethal mutations in approximately one-fifth the total genome of the fly. Accumulated evidence has indicated that this test is the most sensitive among the various test systems available in *D. melanogaster*.

Materials

Several *Drosophila* strains are available for testing. Stocks can be obtained from the *Drosophila* stock culture center at Bowling Green State University, Bowling Green, Ohio. The stocks utilized for this test are chosen for their unique chromosome structure and visible markers. They may be maintained as permanent cultures and visually examined on a routine basis for any indication of genetic breakdown.

Ethylmethane sulfonate at 0.015 M in 1% sucrose solution given as a single, 24-hr exposure on the final day of the schedule is a suitable positive control. The males dosed are of the same age and stock as those used for the test article. The solvent or vehicle used for the test article is used as the negative control and is administered concurrently with the test article.

Drosophila cultures are maintained at 25°C. "Instant" culture medium may be purchased from Carolina Biological (Formula 4-24, without dyes) or the equivalent.

Experimental design

Solubility testing. Each test article is tested for solubility; the primary choice for a solvent is distilled water. If a test article is insoluble in water, it may be dissolved in DMSO, ethanol, acetic acid, or acetone and then diluted. The final concentration of solvent is 2% or below.

Palatability and toxicity testing. A test for palatability and toxicity is performed by preparing a test article in distilled water containing sucrose and any necessary solvents. The solution is then administered by the following method modified from Lewis and Bacher (59). A piece of chemically inert glass filter paper lining a shell vial is saturated with 1.5 ml of the test solution. Fifty adult males are then placed in each feeding vial and observed for feeding behavior and toxic effects. To ensure uptake, it may be necessary to use concentrations of sucrose varying between 1 and 5% and to vary the feeding time between 1 and 3 days. It may be useful at this point to include food coloring in the feeding solutions of certain vials, as the coloring is readily distinguishable in the gut and feces of *Drosophila*, and thus it can be easily determined that the flies have ingested the test article. Vials containing the coloring agent are not used for assessment of toxicity.

Fertility testing. Once the solution and toxicity have been established, a small pilot study is conducted to determine the fertility of the treated males at the selected concentrations of the test article. Dosed males are put through the same mating sequence as used in the actual test to ensure that sufficient numbers of progeny will be available for analysis.

Test size. The tests may be conducted at one, two, or three dose levels in conjunction with negative and positive controls. At least 200 treated males are used for each dose level of the test article and for the negative control. The suggested number of chromosomes to be tested for a two-dose study and a recommended brooding pattern are shown in Table 15.

TABLE 15. *Suggested number of chromosomes tested for a two-dose study*

| Tests | No. at 1 to 8 days posttreatment | | | |
	Brood I 1, 2	Brood II 3, 4, 5	Brood III 6, 7, 8	Total
Low concentration	2,000	2,000	2,000	6,000
High concentration	2,000	2,000	2,000	6,000
Negative control	2,000	2,000	2,000	6,000
Positive control	100	100	100	300

Procedure

Collection of males. To provide males of approximately uniform age for treatment, males from culture bottles under optimum conditions that are produced from timed (1-day) egg samples are collected and held for a 2-day maturation period. All males should then be between 2 and 3 days of age and have their full complement of sperm for treatment. Males are then randomized by the following unsystematized method. A sufficient number of healthy males for the test are transferred to a single empty bottle, mixed, parceled into groups of 50, and held in empty vials for several hours before exposure. This period of removal from a food supply ensures immediate uptake of the feeding solution.

Dosing. The males are dosed according to the methods described under Palatability and Toxicity Testing, using the concentration and duration of exposure determined in the preliminary studies. The high dose is normally set at one-half the LD_{50}. The maximum concentration administered, if the test article is nontoxic, is generally 5%.

Mating and scoring. The treated males are mated individually to sequential groups of three virgin *Basc* females. The brooding scheme consists in a 2–3–3-day sequence that samples spermatozoa, spermatids, and spermatocytes. Each treated male is assigned a unique identification number written on the vial that identifies the females inseminated by that male throughout the brooding sequence. In this way the progeny of each male can be kept separate and the data recorded in such a way that the origin of each tested chromosome is known. This method eliminates the possibility of false positives resulting from clusters of identical lethal mutations originating in one treated male.

The F_2 progeny of each culture are inspected to make certain the proper cross was made. The desired number of F_1 females are then pair-mated to their brothers. An approximately equal number of F_1 females per treated male are tested to avoid bias in the data.

In the F_1 generation, each culture vial (representing one treated X chromosome) is examined for the presence of males with yellow bodies. If this class of males is present, the culture is considered nonlethal and is discarded. If this class is absent, the vial is marked as a potential lethal and set aside for further examination. The following criteria are applied to cultures suspected of being lethal:

1. If 20 or more progeny are present and there are no yellow-bodied males, the culture is considered to carry a lethal mutation on the treated chromosome, and further testing

is not required. The chance of missing a male carrying the treated X chromosome in a population of this size is $(\frac{1}{2})^5$, or less than 0.05.

2. If there are fewer than 20 progeny, or if there is one yellow-bodied male, the culture is retested by mating three of the females heterozygous for the treated and *Basc* chromosomes to *Basc* males. The progeny of these crosses are scored for the presence of y males.

The *Basc* (*Muller-5*) mating scheme employed in this test is shown in Fig. 9. The treated X chromosome is marked with y (yellow body) for easy identification in the F_2 progeny, as the other three genotypes have normal black bodies. The X chromosome balancer, *Basc* (an acronym for Bar, apricot, scute), carries a dominant B (Bar-eyed) gene, which gives narrow eyes in a homozygous or hemizygous condition and kidney-shaped eyes in a heterozygous condition. The gene W^4 (white apricot) is recessive and gives an apricot-eyed phenotype in the homozygous condition. The visible expression of the recessive gene sc (scute) is a variable reduction in the length or number of the thoraxal bristles.

Data analysis

When the data are compiled, the total number of X chromosomes tested should equal the sum of the lethal and nonlethal cultures. The frequency of X-linked recessive lethals is calculated as:

$$\frac{\text{No. of lethals}}{\text{No. of lethals} + \text{No. of nonlethals}} \times 100 = \% \text{ lethal}$$

The Kastenbaum-Bowman test may be used to determine the significance of the results. An increase of twice the spontaneous frequency in conjunction with a dose-response relation is considered a positive response.

When evaluating the results, particular attention is given to multiple lethals occurring in progeny from a single treated male. In the positive control, where the mutation frequency is typically more than 20% sex-linked recessive lethals, several lethals occurring in a single brood from one parent male can be the result of individual mutational events and are counted as such when compiling the data. In the negative control, however, or in the test groups when the mutation frequency is low, such occurrences are generally interpreted as being in existence prior to treatment. The probability of a high number of independent events occurring by chance in one male is

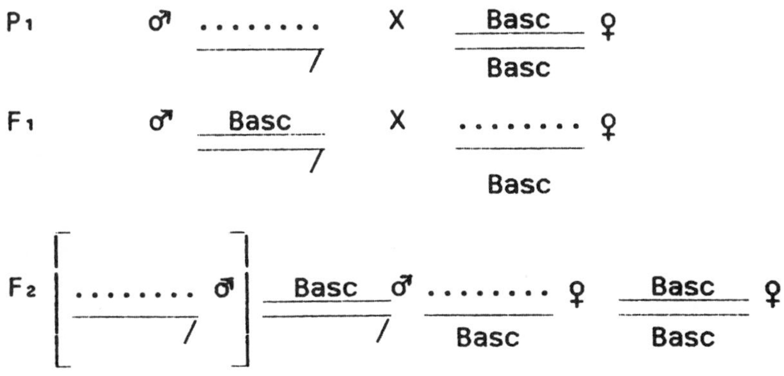

FIG. 9. The Basc (Muller-5) mating scheme. *Brackets* indicate the class of male absent if a lethal mutation occurred on its X chromosome. *Dotted line* indicates the exposed X chromosome.

calculated using a chi-square for goodness of fit. If it is determined that the unusual number of events, called a "cluster," cannot be attributed to handling or treatment, the cluster is determined to have arisen from a spontaneous mutation in a gonial cell that then replicated, and the cluster is counted as a single event to avoid bias in the interpretation of results. One-dose studies including an independent repeat are suitable for screening.

Tests Detecting Chromosome-Breaking (Clastogenic) Agents

Protocol 4: Chromosome Aberrations in Chinese Hamster Ovary Cells

The objective of the Chinese hamster *in vitro* assay is to evaluate the ability of a test article to induce chromosome aberrations in Chinese hamster ovary (CHO) cells.

Indicator cells

Cells to be used in this assay can be obtained from the American Type Culture Collection Repository No. CCL61, Rockville, Maryland. The original cells were obtained from an ovarian biopsy of a Chinese hamster. It is a permanent cell line with an average cycle time of 10 to 12 hr.

The CHO cells for this assay are grown in Ham's F12 medium supplemented with 10% fetal calf serum. The cells are split back to 3×10^5 per 75 cm^2 plastic flask and fed 24 hr prior to treatment with 10 ml of fresh medium.

Control articles

The solvent for the test article is used as the solvent vehicle for the control article.

Ethylmethane sulfonate, a known mutagen and chromosome-breaking (clastogenic) agent, may be dissolved in the culture medium and used as a positive control article for the nonactivation studies at a final concentration of 0.5 μl/ml.

Dimethylnitrosamine, a clastogen that requires metabolic transformation by microsomal enzymes, may be used as a positive control article for activation studies at a final concentration of 0.5 μl/ml.

Experimental design

Toxicity and dose determination. The solubility, toxicity, and doses for the test article are determined prior to screening. The effect of each test article on the survival of the indicator cells is determined by exposing the cells to a wide range of article concentrations in complete growth medium. Toxicity is measured as the loss in growth potential of the cells induced by a 4-hr exposure to the test article followed by a 24-hr expression period in growth medium. Doses are selected from the range of concentrations by bracketing the highest dose that shows no loss in growth potential with at least one higher and three lower doses. Otherwise, a half-log series of doses are employed, with the highest dose being perhaps limited by solubility, but in any case not

to exceed 5 mg/ml. The doses cover at least four orders of magnitude, and all doses that yield sufficient numbers of scorable metaphase cells are considered in the analysis. Alternatively, inhibition of cell cycling (BrdU staining, see below) can be used to set dose levels.

Cell treatment. For the nonactivation assay, approximately 10^6 cells are treated with the test article at predetermined doses for 2 hr at 37°C in growth medium. The exposure period is terminated by washing the cells twice with saline. Four replicate cultures per dose are employed in this assay. All receive fresh medium after washing, and 5-bromo-2'-deoxyuridine (BrdU) is added to two of the four replicates (10 μM final concentration). Incubation is continued in the dark for 20 hr. Colcemid is added for the last 3 hr of incubation (2×10^{-7} M final concentration), and metaphase cells are collected by mitotic shake-off. These cells are swollen with 0.075 M KCl hypotonic solution, washed three times in fixative (methanol/acetic acid, 3:1), dropped onto slides, and air-dried.

For the activation assay, the test article is tested in the presence of an S9 rat liver activation system. This assay differs from the nonactivation assay in that the S9 reaction mixture is added to the growth medium, together with the test article, for 2 hr. The S9 mix is the same as that used in the mouse lymphoma assay. The exposure period is terminated by washing the cells twice with saline. From this point, they are treated as described for the nonactivation assay.

Staining and scoring of slides. Slides are stained with 10% Giemsa at pH 6.8 for subsequent scoring of chromosome aberration frequencies. About 50 to 100 cells are scored from each of two replicate cultures per dose.

Standard forms are used to score and record gaps, breaks, fragments, and reunion figures, as well as numerical aberrations such as polypoid cells. The complete list of aberrations to be scored follows:

Chromatid gap	Pulverized chromosomes
Chromosome break	Pulverized chromosomes
Chromosome gap	Pulverized cells
Chromosome break	Complex rearrangement
Chromatid deletion	Ring chromosome
Fragment	Dicentric chromosome
Acentric fragment	Minute chromosome
Translocation	More than 10 aberrations
Triradial	Polypoid
Quadradial	Hyperdiploid

For control of bias, all slides are coded and scored blind.

Evaluation criteria

A number of general guidelines have been established to aid in determining the meaning of CHO chromosome aberrations. Basically, an attempt is made to establish if a test article or its metabolite(s) can interact with chromosomes to produce gross lesions or changes in chromosome numbers, and if these changes are of a type that can survive more than one mitotic cycle of the cell. All aberration figures detected by this assay result from breaks in the chromatin that either fail to repair or repair in atypical combinations.

It is anticipated that many of the cells bearing breaks or reunion figures would be eliminated (i.e., fail to divide again) after their first mitotic division and, as a corollary, that those cells that survive the first division would primarily bear balanced lesions. The detection of these lesions, and hence a complete risk evaluation, must usually rely on additional testing. In general, a cell bearing configurations such as small deletions or reciprocal translocations may be perpetuated and therefore constitutes a greater risk to an individual than one with large deletions or complex rearrangements.

Data are summarized in tabular form and evaluated. Gaps are not counted as significant aberrations unless they are present at a much higher than usual frequency. Open breaks are considered indicators of genetic damage, as are configurations resulting from the repair of breaks. The latter includes, for example, translocations, multiradials, rings, and multicenters. Reunion figures such as these are weighted higher than breaks, as they usually result from more than one break and may lead to stable configurations.

The number of aberrations per cell are also considered significant. Cells with more than one aberration indicate more genetic damage than those containing evidence of single events.

Frequently, one is unable to locate sufficient suitable metaphase spreads. Possible causes appear to be related to cytotoxic effects, which alter the duration of the cell cycle, kill the cell, or cause clumping of the chromosomes. Additional information can be gained from the mitotic index, which appears to reflect cytotoxic effects, as well as from the frequencies of M1, M2, and M3 cells.

Comparison with a concurrent negative control that shows an unusually low frequency of aberrations can suggest undue statistical significance. Therefore treatment data are considered against historical control data. In either event, the type of aberration, its frequency, and its correlation to dose trends within a given time period are all considered when evaluating a test article as being mutagenically positive or negative.

Statistical analysis employs a two-tailed t-test. This test can be performed on the number of breaks per chromosome in treated and control samples. Dose regression analysis also is useful.

Protocol 5: Mouse Micronucleus Assay

The objective of the mouse micronucleus assay is to evaluate a test article for clastogenic activity in polychromatic erythrocyte (PCE) stem cells in treated mice. The micronucleus test can serve as a rapid screen for clastogenic agents and test articles that interfere with normal mitotic cell division (43,88). Micronuclei are believed to be formed from chromosomes or chromosome fragments left behind during anaphase and scored during interphase because they persist. Thus, the time involved in searching for metaphase spreads in treated cell populations is eliminated. Test articles affecting spindle fiber function or formation, as well as clastogenic agents, can be detected through micronucleus induction.

Materials

Adult male and female mice, strain CD-1, from a randomly bred closed colony may be used as well as other strains or species. A healthy, random-bred strain is selected to maximize genetic heterogeneity and at the same time ensure access to a common source.

Triethylene melamine (TEM) at 1.0 mg/kg may be used as the positive control article and is administered via a split-dose intraperitoneal injection. The negative control article consists of the solvent or vehicle used for the test article and is administered by the same route as, and concurrently with, the test article in volumes equal to the maximum amount administered to the experimental animals.

Experimental design

Animal husbandry. Animals are group-housed up to 15 mice per cage. A commercial diet and water are available *ad libitum* unless contraindicated by the particular experimental design.

Five males and five females per dose level should be assigned to study groups at random. Prior to study initiation, animals are weighed to calculate dose levels. The volume of test article administered per animal is established using a mean weight unless there is significant variation among individuals; in this case individual calculations are made. Animals are uniquely identified by ear tag or ear punch, and dose or treatment groups are identified by cage card.

Sanitary cages and bedding are used. Personnel handling animals or working within the animal facilities are required to wear suitable protective garments. When appropriate, individuals with respiratory or other overt infections are excluded from the animal facilities.

Dose selection. If acute toxicity information (e.g., LD_{50}) is available, it can be used to determine dose levels. If it is not available, dose levels can be determined using five groups of six animals each in a toxicity study. The LD_{50} is determined statistically by probit analysis. In the event that an LD_{50} cannot be determined because the test article is nontoxic, the doses for the mutation studies are selected as high as possible in relation to conditions of human use.

Once the LD_{50} has been approximated, the high dose generally is selected as one-half the LD_{50}, with the low dose being one-tenth the high dose. An intermediate dose that is one-third the high dose is also commonly employed. An attempt is made in mutagenesis studies, as well as other toxicology work, to evaluate the extremes of dosage as well as values close to the use level.

Dosing schedule and route of administration. The test article is administered as an acute dose followed by micronuclei sampling at 12, 48, and 72 hr after the exposure. Oral gavage is employed as the route of administration. In the event that test article characteristics preclude oral gavage, intraperitoneal injection may be employed. These routes of administration are the ones most commonly used for this test procedure.

Extraction of bone marrow. Six hours after the last dose, animals are killed with CO_2 and the adhering soft tissue and epiphyses of both femurs removed. The marrow is aspirated from the bone and transferred to centrifuge tubes containing 5 ml fetal calf serum (one tube for each animal).

Preparation of slides. After centrifugation to pellet the tissue, the supernatant fluid is drawn off and portions of the pellet spread on slides and air-dried. The slides are then stained in May-Gruenwald solution and Giemsa, followed by clearing in distilled water.

Screening the slides. One thousand PCEs per animal are scored. The frequency of micronucleated cells is expressed as percent micronucleated cells based on the total PCEs present in the scored optic field. The frequencies of other bone marrow cell types are recorded for analysis of cytotoxic effects (reduced production of specific blood cell types).

Evaluation criteria

In tests performed for this evaluation, only PCEs are scored for micronuclei. Mature erythrocytes and other cells in the field are recorded but not scored. Loss of nucleated cells is an indication of cytotoxicity.

The dose levels are established to ensure that a nontoxic level of the test article is scored. Dose-response data are not necessary to define a test article as active. Responses considered active are assumed to reflect clastogenic and related activities of test articles. Agents that break chromosomes and induce nondisjunction, as well as other events that produce structural or numerical changes in chromosomes, can produce micronuclei.

The data generated in this study may be analyzed by a two-tailed t-test. Individual animal results are used as data points in the analysis. The set of micronuclei frequencies among the controls are compared to the set for each treatment level. Male and female animal data are combined unless there appears to be a sex difference, in which case the data are analyzed separately. Increases above the negative control frequency that are significant at $p < 0.01$ are considered indicative of an active agent.

For control of bias, all slides are coded prior to scoring and scored blind.

Protocol 6: Sister Chromatid Exchange in CHO Cells

The objective of the CHO *in vitro* assay is to evaluate the ability of a test article to induce sister chromatic exchange (SCE) in CHO cells, with and without metabolic activation.

Materials

Cells to be used in this assay can be obtained from the American Type Culture Collection Repository No. CCL61, Rockville, Maryland. The original cells were obtained from an ovarian biopsy of a Chinese hamster. This permanent cell line has an average cycle time of 10 to 12 hr.

The CHO cells for this assay are grown in Ham's F12 medium supplemented with 10% fetal calf serum. The cells are split back to 3×10^5 per 75 cm^2 plastic flask and fed 24 hr prior to treatment with 10 ml of fresh medium. The solvent for the test article is used as the solvent or vehicle control article.

Ethylmethane sulfonate, a chromosome-breaking agent that induces SCE, may be dissolved in culture medium and used as a positive control article for the nonactivation studies at a final concentration of 0.3 μl/ml.

Dimethylnitrosamine, an SCE inducer that requires metabolic biotransformation by microsomal enzymes, may be used as the positive control article for activation studies at a final concentration of 0.3 μl/ml.

Experimental design

Toxicity and dose determination. The solubility, toxicity, and doses for the test article are determined prior to screening. The effect of each test article on the survival of the indicator cells is determined by exposing the cells to a wide range of article concentrations in complete growth medium. Toxicity is measured as the loss in growth potential of the cells induced by 4-hr exposure to the test article followed by a 24-hr expression period in growth medium. Doses are selected from the range of concentrations by bracketing the highest dose that shows no loss in growth potential with at least one higher and three lower doses. Otherwise, a half-log series of doses are employed, with the highest dose being perhaps limited by solubility, but in any case not to exceed 5 mg/ml. The doses cover at least four orders of magnitude, and all doses that yield sufficient numbers of scorable metaphase cells are considered in the analysis.

Cell treatment. For the nonactivation assay, approximately 10^6 cells are treated in growth medium with the test article at predetermined doses and then incubated at 37°C for 2 hr on a rocker. The exposure period is terminated by washing the cells twice with saline. Then 5-bromo-2'-deoxyuridine (BrdU, 10 μM final concentration) is added to the culture tubes, and incubation is continued in the dark for 24 to 30 hr. Longer times are often necessary to permit cell passage through two DNA replication cycles in the presence of BrdU following treatments that cause mitotic delay. The timing can be determined experimentally. Colcemid is added for the last 3 hr of incubation (final concentration 2×10^{-7} M), and metaphase cells collected by mitotic shake-off. These cells are swollen with 0.75 M KCl hypotonic solution, then washed three times in fixative (methanol/acetic acid, 3:1), dropped onto slides, and air-dried.

For the activation assay, the test article is tested in the presence of an S9 rat liver activation system. This assay differs from the nonactivation assay in that the S9 reaction mixture is added to the growth medium, together with the test article, for 2 hr. The S9 mix is the same as used for the CHO cell aberration assay. The exposure period is terminated by washing the cells twice with saline. From this point they are treated as described for the nonactivation assay.

Staining and scoring of slides. Slides are stained for 10 min with Hoechst 33258 (5 μg/ml) in M/15 Sorensen's buffer (pH 6.8), mounted in the same buffer, and exposed to ultraviolet (UV) light from a mercury lamp for the amount of time required for sister chromatid differentiation (modification of the Perry and Wolff technique). Following UV exposure, the slides are stained with 10% Giemsa for 10 min and then mounted in Depex.

Second-division cells (M2 cells) are scored for the frequency of SCEs per cell and per chromosome. The proportions of cells in the first, second, and third divisions (i.e., M1, M2, and M3 cells) are also determined by scoring 50 cells. Typically, for SCE analysis, 40 M2 cells are scored.

For control of bias, all slides are coded prior to scoring and scored blind.

Evaluation criteria

Interpretation of data is based on the increase in SCE frequency as a function of dose or on the statistical significance of increases above the background or "spontaneous" level. The t-statistic is calculated, and an SCE frequency increase is considered positive if $p < 0.05$.

Tests Measuring Primary DNA Damage

Protocol 7: Unscheduled DNA Synthesis in Rat Liver Primary Cell Cultures

Protocol 7 assay is a highly sensitive test designed to measure unscheduled DNA synthesis (UDS) in primary rat liver cell cultures using the autoradiographic technique described by Williams. Primary hepatocytes have the advantage of having sufficient metabolic activity to eliminate the need for the addition of a microsomal activation system.

The existence and degree of DNA damage can be inferred from an increase in nuclear grain counts compared to untreated hepatocytes. The types of detectable DNA damage are unspecified but are recognizable by the cellular repair system and result in the incorporation of new bases (including ^{3}H-TdR) into the DNA.

Materials

The indicator cells for this assay are hepatocytes obtained from adult male Fischer 344 rats (weighing 150–300 g). The animals receive a commercial diet and water *ad libitum* prior to use.

The cells are cultured in William's Medium E (WME) supplemented with 5% fetal bovine serum, L-glutamine 2 mM, dexamethasone 2.4 μM, penicillin 90 U/ml, streptomycin sulfate 90 U/ml, and gentamicin 140 μg/ml. (This medium is referred to as complete WME; incomplete WME contains no serum or dexamethasone.)

A solvent control consisting of assay procedures performed on cells exposed to the solvent alone is included in all cases. If the test article is not soluble in medium, a stock solution in an organic solvent, normally DMSO, is prepared; the final concentration of solvent in the growth medium must be 1% or less in the treated cultures and the solvent control.

The positive control article should be known to induce UDS in rat hepatocyte primary cell cultures, e.g., 2-acetylaminofluorene (2-AAF) at 2.24×10^{-7} (0.05 μg/ml) or 4.48×10^{-7} (0.10 μg/ml). Aflatoxin B$_1$ (AFB$_1$) at 2×10^{-4} M (60 μg/ml) may be substituted for 2-AAF.

Dose selection

The preliminary cytotoxicity test is an integral part of the assay. The assay is initiated with a series of 15 applied concentrations of the test article, starting at a maximum concentration of 5,000 μg/ml (or 5 μg/ml). Cells are exposed for a period of 20 to 24 hr after initiation of the primary cultures. A viable cell count using trypan blue exclusion is obtained. At least five doses that span the range from *no apparent toxicity* to *complete loss of viable cells* in about 24 hr are chosen for the UDS assay.

UDS Assay Method

The assay described is based on the procedure reported by Williams. The hepatocytes are obtained by perfusion of livers *in situ* for about 4 min with Hank's balancing salts (Ca^{2+}- and Mg^{2+}-free) containing 0.5 mM ethyleneglycol-bis(β-aminoethyl ether)-N,N-tetraacetic acid (EGTA) and HEPES buffer at pH 7.2. Incomplete WME with type I collagenase (100 U/ml) is perfused through the liver for about 10 min. The hepatocytes are then dispersed by mechanical dispersion of excised liver in a culture dish containing incomplete WME and collagenase, and clumps are removed by allowing them to settle. The cells are then resuspended in complete WME and counted. A series of 35-mm culture dishes, each containing a 25-mm round plastic coverslip, are inoculated with approximately 0.5×10^{6} viable cells in 3 ml WME plus 5% serum per dish.

An attachment period of 1.5 hr at 37°C in a humidified atmosphere containing 5% CO$_2$ is allowed. Unattached cells are removed and the cultures refed with 2.5 ml complete WME.

The UDS assay is initiated by replacing the medium in the culture dishes with 2.5 ml WME containing only 1.0% fetal bovine serum, ^{3}H-thymidine 5 μCi/ml, and the test article at the desired concentration. Each treatment, including the positive and negative controls, is performed on five cultures. After treatment for 18 hr, the test article is removed and the cell monolayers washed twice with incomplete WME. Two of the cultures for each treatment are used to monitor the toxicity of treatment; these cultures are refed with complete WME and returned to the incubator. The other three cultures from each treatment are refed with 2.5 ml complete WME containing thymidine 1 mM and further processed as described below.

The nuclei in the labeled cells are swollen by placement of the coverslips in 1% sodium citrate for 10 min. The cells are then fixed in acetic acid/ethanol (1:3) and dried for at least 24 hr. The coverslips are mounted on glass slides (cells up), dipped in Kodak NTB2 emulsion, and dried. The coated slides are stored for 7 to 10 days at 4°C in light-tight boxes containing packets of Drierite. The emulsions then are developed in D19, fixed, and stained with William's modified hematoxylin and eosin.

The cells are examined microscopically at approximately 1,500× magnification under oil immersion and the field displayed on the video screen of an automatic counter. UDS is measured by counting nuclear grains and subtracting the average number of grains in three nuclear-sized areas adjacent to each nucleus (background count). This value is referred to as the *net nuclear gain count*. The coverslips are coded to prevent bias in grain counting.

Evaluation criteria

The net nuclear grain count is determined for 50 randomly selected cells on each coverslip, regardless of whether the nuclei contain grains. Only normal-appearing nuclei are scored, and occasional nuclei blackened by grains too numerous to count are excluded as cells in which replicative DNA synthesis occurred rather than repair synthesis. The mean net nuclear grain count is determined from the triplicate coverslips (150 total nuclei) for each treatment condition.

Several criteria have been established that, if met, provide a basis for evaluation of a test article as active in the UDS assay. These criteria are formulated on the basis of published results and laboratory experience and can be used in lieu of a statistical treatment to indicate a positive response.

The test article is considered active in the UDS assay at applied concentrations that cause any or all of the following:

1. An increase in the mean nuclear grain count to at least six grains per nucleus in excess of the concurrent negative control value
2. The percentage of nuclei with six or more grains to increase above 10% of the examined population, in excess of the concurrent negative control
3. The percentage of nuclei with 20 or more grains to reach or exceed 2% of the examined population

Generally, if the first condition is satisfied, the second and often the third condition are met. However, satisfaction of only the second or third condition indicates UDS activity. Various DNA-damaging agents give a variety of nuclear labeling patterns, and weak agents may strongly affect only a few cells. Therefore all three of the above conditions are considered in an evaluation.

A dose-related increase in UDS for at least two consecutive applied concentrations also is desirable to evaluate a test article as active in this assay. In some cases UDS increases with dose and then decreases to near zero with successively higher doses. If this behavior is associated with increased toxicity, the test article can be evaluated as active. If an isolated increase occurs for a treatment far removed from the toxic doses, the UDS must be considered spurious.

The test article is considered inactive in this assay if none of the above conditions is met and if the assay includes the maximum applied dose or other doses that are shown to be toxic by the survival measurements. If no toxicity is demonstrated for doses below the maximum applied dose, the assay is considered inconclusive and is repeated with higher doses.

The positive control values are not used as reference points to measure the UDS activity of the test article. UDS elicited by test agents in this assay is probably more dependent on the type of DNA damage inflicted and the available repair mechanisms than on the potency of the test agent as a mutagen or carcinogen. Some forms of DNA damage are repaired without incorporation of new nucleic acids. Thus the positive controls are used only to demonstrate that the cell population employed was responsive and that the methodology is adequate for the detection of UDS.

REFERENCES

1. Ames, B. N. (1984): Dietary carcinogens and anti-carcinogens. *Clin. Toxicol.*, 22:291–301.
2. Ames, B. N. (1979): Identifying environmental chemicals causing mutations and cancer. *Science*, 204:587–593.
3. Ames, B. N., Durston, W. E., Yamasaki, E., and Lee, F. D. (1973): Carcinogens are mutagens: a simple test system combining liver homogenates for activation and bacteria for detection. *Proc. Natl. Acad. Sci. USA*, 70:2281.
4. Ames, B. N., Kammen, H. L., and Yamasaki, E. (1975): Hair dyes are mutagenic: identification of a variety of mutagenic ingredients. *Proc. Natl. Acad. Sci. USA*, 72:2423–2427.
5. Ames, B. N., McCann, J., and Yamasaki, E. (1975): Methods for detecting carcinogens and mutagens with the Salmonella mammalian microsome mutagenicity test. *Mutat. Res.*, 31:347–364.
6. Ashby, J., de Serres, F. J., Draper, M., Ishidate, M., Margolin, B., Matter, B., and Shelby, M. D. (1985): *Short-Term Tests for Carcinogens: Results of the PICS Study.* Elsevier, Amsterdam.
7. Auerbach, C., Robson, J. M., and Carr, J. G. (1947): The chemical production of mutagens. *Science*, 105:243.
8. Bauer, K. H. (1928): *Mutationstheorie der Geschwulst-Entstehung. Ubergang von Körperzellen in Geschwulstzellen durch Gen-Anderung.* Springer, Berlin.
9. Benditt, E. P. (1977): The origins of atherosclerosis. *Sci. Am.*, 235:74.
10. Berry, D. J., and Litchfield, M. H. (1985): A review of the current regulatory requirements for mutagenicity testing. In: *Progress in Mutation Research*, Vol. 5, edited by J. Ashby and F. J. de Serres, pp. 727–740. Elsevier, Amsterdam.
11. Boutwell, R. K. (1974): The function and mechanism of promoters of carcinogenesis. *CRC Crit. Rev. Toxicol.*, 419–441.
12. Bridges, B. A. (1976): Short-term screening tests for carcinogens. *Nature*, 261:195–200.
13. Brousseau, R., Scarpulla, R., Sung, W., Hsing, H. M., Narang, S. A., and Ulu, R. (1982): Synthesis of a human insulin gene. V. Enzymatic assembly, cloning and characterization of the human proinsulin DNA. *Gene*, 17:279–289.
14. Brusick, D. J. (1979): Alterations of germ cells leading to mutagenesis and their detection. *Environ. Health Perspect.*, 24:105–112.
15. Brusick, D. J. (1983): Evaluation of chronic rodent bioassays and Ames assay tests as accurate models for predicting human carcinogens. In: *Application of Biological Markers to Carcinogen Testing*, edited by H. A. Milman and S. Sell, pp. 153–163. Plenum Press, New York.
16. Brusick, D. (1983): Mutagenicity and carcinogenicity correlations between bacteria and rodents. In: *Cellular Systems for Toxicity Testing 407*, reprinted from *Annals of the New York Academy of Sciences*, pp. 164–176.
17. Brusick, D. J. (1978): The role of short-term testing in carcinogen detection. *Chemosphere*, 5:403–417.
18. Brusick, D. J. (1980): *Principles of Genetic Toxicology.* Plenum Press, New York.
19. Brusick, D. J., and Mayer, V. W. (1973): New developments in mutagenicity screening techniques with yeast. *Environ. Health Perspect.*, 6:83–96.
20. Burdette, W. J. (1955): The significance of mutation in relation to the origin of tumors: a review. *Cancer Res.*, 15:201.
21. Burnet, F. M. (1974): *Intrinsic Mutagenesis: A Genetic Approach to Aging.* Medical & Technical Publishing, Lancaster, England.
22. Cacheiro, N. L. A., Russell, L. B., and Swartout, M. S. (1974): Translocations, the predominant cause of total sterility in sons of mice treated with mutagens. *Genetics*, 75:73–91.
23. Cattanach, B. M. (1966): Chemically induced mutations in mice. *Mutat. Res.*, 3:346–353.
24. Chromosome methodologies in mutagen testing (1972): Report of the Ad Hoc Committee of the Environmental Mutagen Society and the Institute for Medical Research. *Toxicol. Appl. Pharmacol.*, 22:269–275.
25. Clive, D., and Spector, J. F. S. (1975): Laboratory procedure for assessing specific locus mutations at the TK locus in cultured L5178Y mouse lymphoma cells. *Mutat. Res.*, 31:17–29.

26. Connor, T. H., Stoeckel, M., Evrard, J., and Legator, M. S. (1977): The contribution of metronidazole and two metabolites to the mutagenic activity detected in the urine of treated humans and mice. *Cancer Res.*, 37:629–633.

27. Dean, B. J. (1969): Chemically-induced chromosome damage. *Lab. Anim.*, 3:157–174.

28. Dean, B. J., and Senner, K. R. (1977): Detection of chemically-induced somatic mutation in Chinese hamsters. *Mutat. Res.*, 46:403–407.

29. De Serres, F., Fouts, J. R., Bend, J. R., and Philpot, editors (1976): *In Vitro Metabolic Activation in Mutagenesis Testing.* Elsevier/North-Holland, Amsterdam.

30. EEC (European Economic Community) Official Journal of the European Communities, 6th Amendment to Directive 67/548/EEC, Annex VII, 15.10.79, and Annex V, EEC Directive 79-831, part B, Toxicological Methods of Annex VIII, Draft, July 1983.

31. Ehling, U. H. (1978): Specific-locus metations in mice, In: *Chemical Mutagens: Principles and Methods for Their Detection,* Vol. 5, edited by A. Hollandaer and F. J. de Serres, pp. 233–256. Plenum Press, New York.

32. Ehling, U. H., Averbeck, D., Cerutti, P. A., Friedman, J., Greim, H., Kolbye, A. C., Jr., and Mendelsohn, M. L. (1983): Review of the evidence for the presence or absence of thresholds in the induction of genetic effects by genotoxic chemicals. *Mutat. Res.*, 123:281–341.

33. Ehrenberg, L., Brookes, P., Druckrey, H., Lagerlof, B., Litwin, J., and Williams, G. (1973): The relation of cancer induction and genetic damage. In: *Evaluation of Genetic Risks of Environmental Chemicals.* Report of Group 3, Ambio Special Report No. 3, Royal Swedish Academy of Sciences, Universitets forlaget.

34. EPA (Environmental Protection Agency) Office of Pesticides and Toxic Substances (1982): *Health Effects Test Guidelines.* EPA Publication 560/682-001. National Technical Information Service, Springfield, Virginia.

35. EPA (1986): EPA guidelines for mutagenicity risk assessment. *Fed. Register,* 51:34006–34012.

36. Finney, D. J. (1971): *Probit Analysis.* Cambridge University Press, Cambridge, England.

37. Garrett, N. E., Stack, H. F., Gross, M. R., and Waters, M. D. (1984): An analysis of the spectra of genetic activity produced by known or suspected human carcinogens. *Mutat. Res.*, 134:89–111.

38. Generoso, W. M., Bishop, J. B., Gosslee, D. G., Newell, G. W., Sheu, C., and von Halle, E. (1980): Heritable translocation in the male mouse. *Mutat. Res.*, 76:191–215.

39. Generoso, W. M., Cain, K. I., and Banby, A. J. (1983): Some factors affecting the mutagenic response of mouse germ cells to chemicals. In: *Utilization of Mammalian Specific Locus Studies in Hazard Evaluation and Estimation of Genetic Risk,* edited by F. J. de Serres and W. Sheridan, pp. 227–239. Plenum Press, New York.

40. Generoso, W. M., Cain, K. T., Huff, S. W., and Gosslee, D. G. (1978): Heritable translocation test in mice. In: *Chemical Mutagens: Principles and Methods for Their Detection,* Vol. 5, edited by A. Hollandaer and F. J. de Serres. Plenum Press, New York.

41. Generoso, W. M. (1980): Repair in fertilized eggs of mice and its role in the production of chromosomal aberrations. In: *DNA Repair and Mutagenesis in Eukaryotes,* edited by W. M. Generoso, M. D. Shelby, and F. J. de Serres, pp. 411–420. Plenum Press, New York.

42. Hardigree, A. A., and Epler, J. L. (1978): Comparative mutagenesis of plant flavonoids in microbial systems. *Mutat. Res.*, 58:231–239.

42a.Hart, R. W., and Brusick, D. (1988): Assessment of the hazard of genetic toxicology. In: *Toxic Substances and Human Risk,* edited by R. G. Tardiff and J. V. Rodricks, pp. 339–355. Plenum Press, New York.

43. Heddle, J. (1973): A rapid in vitro test for chromosomal damage. *Mutat. Res.*, 18:187–190.

44. Hollandaer, A., and de Serres, F. J., editors (1971–1979): *Chemical Mutagens: Principles and Methods for Their Detection,* Vols. 1–6. Plenum Press, New York.

45. *IARC Mongr.* [Suppl. 4], October 1982.

46. ICPEMC (1983): Committee 1 Final Report: screening strategy for chemicals that are potential germ-cell mutagens in mammals. *Mutat. Res.*, 114:117–177.

47. Jenssen, D., Ramel, C., and Gothe, R. (1974): The induction of micronuclei by frameshift mutagens at the time of nucleus expulsion in mouse erythroblasts. *Mutat. Res.*, 26:553–555.

48. Kakunaga, T. (1973): A quantitative system for assay of malignant transformation by chemical carcinogens using a clone derived from BALB/3T3. *Int. J. Cancer,* 12:463–473.

49. Kalter, H. (1977): Correlation between teratogenic and mutagenic effects of chemicals in mammals. In: *Chemical Mutagens: Principles and Methods for Their Detection,* Vol. 6, edited by A. Hollandaer. Plenum Press, New York.

50. Kastenbaum, M. A., and Bowman, K. O. (1970): Tables for determining the statistical significance of mutation frequencies. *Mutat. Res.*, 9:527–549.

51. Kier, L. D., Brusick, D. J., Auletta, A. E., Von Halle, E. S., Brown, M. M., Simmon, V. F., Dunkel, V., McCann, J., Mortelmans, K., Prival, M., Rao, T. K., and Ray, V. (1986): The Salmonella typhimurium/mammalian microsomal assay: a report of the U.S. EPA Gene-Tox Program. *Mutat. Res.*, 168:69–240.

52. Kier, L. D., Yamasaki, E., and Ames, B. N. (1974): Detection of mutagenic activity in cigarette smoke condensates. *Proc. Natl. Acad. Sci. USA,* 71:4159–4163.

53. Kilbey, B. J., Legator, M., Nichols, W., and Ramel, C., editors (1977): *Handbook of Mutagenicity Test Procedures.* Elsevier, Amsterdam.

54. Kleinhofs, A., and Behki, R. (1977): Prospects for plant genome modification by nonconventional methods. *Annu. Rev. Genet.,* 11:79–101.

55. Knudsen, A. G., Jr. (1973): Mutation and human cancer. *Adv. Cancer Res.,* 17:317–352.

56. Kopelovich, L., Bias, N. E., and Helson, L. (1979): Tumor promoter alone induces neoplastic transformation of fibroblasts from humans genetically predisposed to cancer. *Nature,* 282:619–621.

57. Lee, W. R. (1978): Dosimetry of chemical mutagens in eukaryote germ cells. In: *Chemical Mutagens: Principles and Methods for Their Detection,* Vol. 5, edited by A. Hollandaer and F. J. de Serres, pp. 177–202. Plenum Press, New York.

58. Legator, M. S., Palmer, K. A., Green, S., and Peterson, K. W. (1969): Cytogenetic studies in rats of cyclohexalamine, a metabolite of cyclamate. *Science,* 165:1139–1140.

59. Lewis, E. B., and Bacher, F. (1968): Method of feeding ethylmethane sulfonate (EMS) to Drosophila males. *Dros. Inf. Service,* 48:193.

60. Lewtas, J. (1986): A quantitative cancer risk assessment methodology using short-term genetic bioassays: the comparative potency method. In: *Risk and Reason: Risk Assessment in Relation to Environmental Mutagens and Carcinogens,* edited by P. Oftedal and A. Brogger, pp. 107–120. Alan R. Liss, New York.

61. Maier, R., and Schmid, W. (1976): Ten model mutagens evaluated by the micronucleus test. *Mutat. Res.*, 40:325–338.

62. Malling, H. V., and Valcovic, L. R. (1978): New approaches to detection of gene mutations in mammals. In: *Advances in Modern Toxicology,* Vol. 4, edited by G. Flamm and M. Mehlman, pp. 149–171. Hemisphere Press, New York.

63. Maron, D. M., and Ames, B. N. (1983): Revised methods for the Salmonella mutagenicity test. *Mutat. Res.*, 113:173–215.

64. McCann, J., Choi, E., Yamasaki, E., and Ames, B. N. (1975): Detection of carcinogens as mutagens in the Salmonella/microsome test: assay of 300 chemicals. *Proc. Natl. Acad. Sci. USA,* 72:5135–5139.

65. McKusick, V. A. (1978): *Mendelian Inheritance in Man: Catalogs of Autosomal Dominant, Autosomal Recessive and X-linked Phenotypes,* 5th ed. Johns Hopkins University Press, Baltimore.

66. Miller, J. A., and Miller, E. C. (1966): A survey of molecular aspects of chemical carcinogenesis. *Lab. Invest.,* 15:217.

67. Muller, H. J. (1927): Artificial transmutation of the gene. *Science,* 66:84–87.

68. Myhr, B. C., Turnbull, D., and DiPaolo, J. A. (1979): Ultraviolet mutagenesis of normal and xeroderma pigmentosum variant human fibroblasts. *Mutat. Res.*, 62:341–353.

69. Nagao, M., Sugimura, T., and Matsushima, T. (1978): Environmental mutagens and carcinogens. *Annu. Rev. Genet.,* 12:117–159.

70. Nagao, M., Takahashi, Y., Yamanaka, H., and Sugimura, T. (1979): Mutagens in coffee and tea. *Mutat. Res.*, 68:101–106.

71. Nagao, M., Yahagi, T., Kawachi, T., Seino, Y., Honda, M., Mat-

sukura, N., Sugimura, T., Wakabayashi, K. Tsuji, K., and Kosuge, T. (1977): Mutagens in foods, and especially pyrolysis products of protein. In: *Progress in Genetic Toxicology,* edited by D. Scott, B. A. Bridges, and F. H. Sobels, pp. 259–264. Elsevier/North-Holland, New York.

72. Nemchin, R. G., and Brusick, D. J. (1985): Basic principles of laboratory safety. *Environ. Mutagen.,* 7:947–971.

72a. Obe, G., and Anderson, D. (1987): Genetic effects of ethanol. *Mutation Res.,* 186:177–200.

73. OECD (Organization for Economic Co-operation and Development) (1981, revised May 1983): *Guidelines for Testing of Chemicals.*

74. OSHA (1980): Identification, classification and regulation of potential occupational carcinogens. *Fed. Register,* 45:5001–5296.

75. Pedersen, R. A., and Brandriff, B. (1980): Radiation- and drug-induced DNA repair in mammalian oocytes and embryos. In: *DNA Repair and Mutagenesis in Eukaryocytes,* edited by W. M. Generoso, M. D. Shelby, and F. J. de Serres, pp. 389–410. Plenum Press, New York.

76. Perry, P., and Wolff, S. (1974): New Giemsa method for the differential staining of sister chromatids. *Nature,* 251:156–158.

77. Pet-Edwards, J., Chankong, V., Rosenkranz, H. S., and Haimes, Y. Y. (1985): Applications of the carcinogenicity prediction and battery selection (CPBS) method to the Gene-Tox data base. *Mutat. Res.,* 153:187–200.

78. Pienta, R. J., Kushner, L. M., and Russell, L. S. (1984): The use of short-term tests and limited bioassays in carcinogenicity testing. *Regul. Toxicol. Pharmacol.,* 4:249–260.

79. Ray, V. A. (1979): Application of microbial and mammalian cells to the assessment of mutagenicity. *Pharmacol. Rev.,* 30:537–546.

80. Reedy, E. P., Reynolds, R. K., Santos, E., and Barbacid, M. (1982): A point mutation is responsible for the acquisition of transforming properties by the T24 human bladder carcinoma oncogene. *Nature,* 300:145–152.

81. Russell, L. B. (1976): Numerical sex-chromosome anomalies in mammals: their spontaneous occurrence and use in mutagenesis studies. In: *Chemical Mutagens: Principles and Methods for Their Detection,* Vol. 4, edited by A. Hollandaer, pp. 55–91. Plenum Press, New York.

82. Russell, L. B. (1977): Validation of the in vivo somatic mutation method in the mouse as a prescreen for germinal point mutations. *Arch. Toxicol.,* 38:7585.

83. Russell, L. B., Aaron, C. S., de Serres, F., Generoso, W. M., Kannan, K. L., Shelby, M., Springer, J., and Voytele, P. (1984): Evaluation of mutagenicity assays for purposes of genetic risk assessment. *Mutat. Res.,* 134:143–157.

84. Russell, L. B., Selby, P. B., van Halle, E., Sheridan, W., and Valcovic, L. (1981): The mouse specific locus test with agents other than radiation: interpretation of data and recommendations for future work. *Mutat. Res.,* 86:329–354.

85. Russell, W. L. (1951): X-ray induced mutations in mice. *Cold Spring Harbor Symp. Quant. Biol.,* 16:327–330.

86. Russell, W. L. (1977): The role of mammals in the future of chemical mutagenesis research. *Arch. Toxicol.,* 38:141–147.

87. San, R. H. C., and Stich, H. F. (1975): DNA repair synthesis of cultured human cells as a rapid bioassay for chemical carcinogens. *Int. J. Cancer,* 16:284–291.

88. Schmid, W. (1975): The micronucleus test. *Mutat. Res.,* 31:9–15.

89. Sega, G. A. (1982): DNA repair in spermatocytes and spermatids of the mouse. In: *Indicators of Genotoxic Exposure* (Banbury Report 13), edited by B. A. Bridges, B. E. Butterworth, and I. B. Weinstein, pp. 503–514. Cold Spring Harbor Laboratory, Cold Spring Harbor, New York.

90. Setlow, R. B. (1978): Repair deficient human disorders and cancer. *Nature,* 271:713–717.

90a. Shelby, M. D. (1988): The genetic toxicity of human carcinogens and its implications. *Mutation Res.,* 204:3–15.

91. Simmon, V. F., Mitchell, A. D., and Jorgenson, T. A.: Evaluation of selected pesticides as chemical mutagens, in vitro and in vivo studies. EPA-600/1-77-028. National Technical Information Center, Springfield, Virginia.

92. Slater, E. E., Anderson, M. D., and Rosenkranz, H. S. (1971): Rapid detection of mutagens and carcinogens. *Cancer Res.,* 31: 970–973.

93. Sobels, F. H. (1982): In: *Progress in Mutation Research,* Vol. 3, edited by K. C. Bora et al., pp. 323–327. Elsevier, Amsterdam.

94. Sugimura, T. (1978): Let's be scientific about the problem of mutagens in cooked food. *Mutat. Res.,* 55:149–152.

95. Sugimura, T., Sato, S., Nagao, M., Yahagi, T., Matsushima, T., Seino, Y., Takeuchi, M., and Kawachi, T. (1976): Overlapping of carcinogens and mutagens. In: *Fundamentals in Cancer Prevention,* edited by P. N. Magee, T. Matsushima, T. Sugimura, and S. Takayama, pp. 191–215. University of Tokyo Press, Tokyo, and University Park Press, Baltimore.

96. Tennant, R. W., Margolin, B. H., Shelby, M. D., Zeiger, E., Haseman, J. K., Spalding, J., Caspary, W., Resnick, M., Stasiewicz, S., Anderson, B., and Minor, R. (1987): Prediction of chemical carcinogenicity in rodents from in vitro genetic toxicity assays. *Science,* 236:933–941.

97. Teranishi, K., Hamada, K., and Watanabe, H. (1978): Mutagenicity in Salmonella typhimurium mutants of the benzene-soluble organic matter derived from airborne particulate matter and its five fractions. *Mutat. Res.,* 56:273–280.

98. Terasima, T., and Tolmach, L. J. (1961): Changes in x-ray sensitivity of HeLa cells during the division cycle. *Nature,* 190:1210–1211.

99. Turturro, A., and Hart, R. W. (1984): DNA repair mechanisms in aging. In: *Comparative Pathology of Major Age-Related Diseases,* edited by D. G. Scarpelli and G. Migaki, p. 1946. Mark R. Liss, New York.

100. Waters, M., and Auletta, A. (1981): The GeneTox program. *J. Chem. Inf. Comput. Sci.,* 21:35–38.

101. Weisburger, J. H., and Williams, G. M. (1981): The decision point approach for systematic carcinogen testing. *Food Cosmet. Toxicol.,* 19:561–566.

102. Williams, G. M. (1977): The detection of chemical carcinogens by unscheduled DNA synthesis in rat liver primary cell cultures. *Cancer Res.,* 37:1845–1851.

103. Wilson, J. G. (1973): *Environment and Birth Defects,* Chap. 8. Academic Press, New York.

104. Würgler, F. E., Graf, V., and Berchtold, W. (1975): Statistical problems connected with the sex-linked recessive lethal test in Drosophila melanogaster. I. The use of the Kastenbaum-Bowman test. *Arch. Genet.,* 48:158–178.

105. Yahagi, T., Nagao, M., Seino, Y., Matsushima, T., Sugimura, T., and Oleada, M. (1977): Mutagenicities of N-nitrosamines on Salmonella. *Mutat. Res.,* 48:121–130.

Principles and Methods of Toxicology, Second Edition, edited by A. Wallace Hayes, Raven Press, Ltd., New York © 1989.

CHAPTER 15

Statistics for Toxicologists

Shayne C. Gad and *Carrol S. Weil

*Director of Toxicology, G. D. Searle & Co., Skokie, Illinois 60077; and *Consultant, 4326 McCaslin Street, Pittsburgh, Pennsylvania 15217*

Philosophy and General Principles
   Functions of Statistics • Descriptive Statistics • Experimental Design • Outliers and Rounding of Numbers • Entry Devices • Computational Devices
Methods
Randomization • Bartlett's Test for Homogeneity of Variance • Student's *t*-Test (Unpaired *t*-Test) • Cochran *t*-Test • F Test • Scattergram • Analysis of Variance • *Post Hoc* Tests • Analysis of Covariance • Kruskal–Wallis Nonparametric ANOVA • Wilcoxon Rank-Sum Test • Distribution-Free Multiple Comparison • Fisher's Exact Test • R × C Chi-Square Test • Mann–Whitney *U* Test • Correlation Coefficient • Kendall's Coefficient of Rank Correlation • Life Tables
Transformations
   Linear Regression • Probit/Log Transforms and Re-
gression • Moving Averages • Nonlinear Regression • Trend Analysis • Exploratory Data Analysis • Multivariate Methods
Applications
   LD_{50} and LC_{50} • Body and Organ Weights • Clinical Chemistry • Hematology • Histopathologic Lesion Incidence • Reproduction • Teratology • Dominant Lethal Assay • Diet and Chamber Analysis • Mutagenesis • Behavioral Toxicology • Instrumentation and Technique Factors • Study Design Factors • Statistical Methodologies • Existing Versus Recommended Practice
References

Over the years that have passed since the writing of the first edition of this chapter, significant changes have come to pass in toxicology, in statistics, and in the interface of these two disciplines. The authors are hopeful that these changes are reflected in this complete revision of the original chapter.

PHILOSOPHY AND GENERAL PRINCIPLES

During the last 25 years, both the theory and practice that constitute the field of toxicology have become increasingly complex (or at least more detailed) and increasingly more controversial. Studies are designed to generate more data which must then be utilized to address escalating numbers of areas of concern. As our problem of data analysis has of its own nature become more complex, we have come to draw more deeply from the well of available statistical techniques to strengthen our understanding of the field.

One difficulty is that there are very few toxicologists who are also statisticians, or vice versa, and that there is a very real need to have an understanding of the biological realities and of the implications of a problem before a method of analysis is selected and employed. As a point of initiation, it is essential that any analysis of study results be interpreted by a professional who firmly understands both the difference between biological significance and statistical significance and the nature of different types of data. If we first consider the four possible combinations of the two types of significance, we find the relationship shown below.

		Statistical significance	
		No	Yes
Biological	No	Case I	Case III
significance	Yes	Case II	Case IV

Cases I and IV give us no problems, for the answers are the same statistically and biologically. But cases II and III present problems. In case II, we have a circumstance where there is a statistical significance in the measured difference between treated and control groups, but there is no true biological significance to the finding. This is not an uncommon happening, for example, in the case of clinical chemistry parameters. In case III, we have no statistical significance, but the differences between groups are biologically/toxicologically significant. An example of this second situation is when we see a few cases of a very rare tumor type in treated animals. In both of these latter instances, numerical analysis, no matter how well done, is no substitute for professional judgment. Here, perhaps, is the cutting edge of what really makes a practicing toxicologist. Along with this, however, must come a feeling for the different types of data and of the implications involved with them.

In all areas of biological research, optimal design and appropriate interpretation of experiments require that the researcher understand both the biological and technological underpinnings of the system being studied and of the data being generated. From the point of view of the statistician, it is vitally important that the experimenter both know and be able to communicate the nature of the data, as defined below in Table 1 (or in any of a number of similar schemes).

The nature of the data collected is determined by three considerations. These are the biological source of the data (the system being studied), the instrumentation and techniques being used to make measurements, and the design of the experiment. The researcher has some degree of control over each of these—the least over the biological system (he/she normally has a choice of one of several models to study) and the most over the design of the experiment or study. Such choices, in fact, dictate the type of data generated by a study.

This chapter has been assembled for toxicologists as a practical guide to the common statistical problems and procedures encountered in toxicology. It has been enriched by the addition of discussions of why (primarily for toxicologists) a particular procedure or interpretation is suggested, and by worked examples from toxicology. It is not intended as a complete course in statistics, but rather as a fundamental methods workbook.

TABLE 1. *Types of data and examples of each type*

Classification	Type	Example[a]
Scale		
Continuous	Scalar	Body weight
	Ranked	Severity of a lesion
Discontinuous	Scalar	Weeks until the first observation of a tumor in a carcinogenicity study
	Ranked	Clinical observations in animals
	Attribute	Eye colors in fruit flies
	Quantal	Dead/alive or present/absent
Distribution	Normal	Body weights
	Bimodal	Some clinical chemistry parameters
	Others	Measures of time to incapacitation

[a] It should be kept in mind that though these examples are most commonly of the data types assigned above, it is not always the case.

Statistical methods are each based on specific assumptions. Parametric statistics, which are most familiar to the majority of scientists, have more stringent sets of underlying assumptions than do nonparametric statistics. Among these underlying assumptions (for many parametric statistical methods, such as analysis of variance) is that the data are continuous. This means that, at least theoretically, the data can assume any of an infinite number of values between any two fixed points.

Limitations on our ability to measure constrain the extent to which the real-world situation approaches the theoretical here, but many of the variables studied in toxicology are in fact continuous. Examples of these are lengths, weights, concentrations, temperatures, periods of time, and percentages. For these continuous variables we may describe the character of a sample using measures of central tendency and dispersion with which we are most familiar—the mean, denoted by the symbol $\bar{X}$ and also called the arithmetic average (calculated by adding up all the values in a group then dividing by N), and the standard deviation (SD), which is denoted by the symbol σ and is calculated as being equal to

$$\sqrt{\frac{\sum X^2 - \frac{(\sum X)^2}{N}}{N - 1}}$$

where X is the individual datum and N is the total number of data in the group.

Contrasted with this continuous data, however, we have discontinuous (or discrete) data, which can only assume certain fixed numerical values. That is, no intermediate values are possible between the "fixed" points in discontinuous data. Examples of such data in toxicology have been detailed in Table 1. In these cases our selection of types of statistical tools or tests is, as will be explained later, more limited.

Functions of Statistics

Statistical methods may serve to do any combination of three possible tasks. The one we are most familiar with is hypothesis testing—that is, determining if two (or more) groups of data differ from each other at a predetermined level of confidence. A second function is the construction and use of models, which is most commonly seen as linear regression or as the derivation of some form of correlation coefficient. Model fitting allows us to relate one variable (typically a treatment or "independent" variable) with other variables (usually one or more effects or "dependent" variables). The third function, reduction of dimensionality, is still much less commonly utilized than the first two. In this final category are the methods for reducing the number of variables in a system while only minimally reducing the amount of information, therefore making a problem easier to visualize and to understand. Examples of such techniques are factor analysis and cluster analysis. A subset of this last function, discussed under descriptive statistics, is the reduction of raw data to single expressions of central tendency and variability (such as the mean and standard deviation).

There is also a special subset which is part of both the second and third functions of statistics. This is data transformation, which includes such things as the conversion of numbers to log or probit values.

As a matter of practicality, the contents of this chapter are primarily designed to address the first of the three functions of statistics that we presented. The second function, modeling—especially in the form of risk assessment—is becoming increasingly important as the science continues to evolve from the descriptive phase to a mechanistic phase (i.e., explaining of mechanisms), and as such is addressed in more detail here than in the first edition. Likewise, because the interrelation of multiple factors is becoming a real concern, the section on reduction of dimensionality has also been expanded.

Descriptive Statistics

Descriptive statistics are used to convey, in a summarized manner, the general nature of the data. As such, the parameters describing any single group of data have two components. One of these describes the location of the data, whereas the other gives a measure of the dispersion of the data in and about this location. Often overlooked is that the choice of what parameters are used to give these pieces of information implies a particular nature of distribution for the data.

Most commonly, location is described by giving the (arithmetic) mean and the dispersion by giving the SD or the standard error of measurement (SEM). The calculation of the first two of these has already been described. If we again denote the total number of data in a group as N, then the SEM would be calculated as

$$\text{SEM} = \frac{\text{SD}}{\sqrt{N}}$$

The use of these (the mean with either the SD or SEM) implies, however, that we have reason to believe that the data being summarized are from a population which is at least approximately normally distributed. If this is not the case, then we should rather use a set of terms which do not have such a rigid underpinning. These are the median, for location, and the semiquartile distance, for a measure of dispersion. These somewhat less commonly familiar parameters are characterized as follows.

Median When all the numbers in a group are arranged in a ranked order (that is, from smallest to largest), the median is the middle value. If there is an odd number of values in a group then the middle value is obvious (in the case of 13 values, for example, the seventh largest is the median). When the number of values in the sample is even, the median is calculated as the midpoint between the $[N/2]$th and the $([N/2] + 1)$th number. For example, in the series of numbers 7, 12, 13, 19, the median value would be the midpoint between 12 and 13, which is 12.5.

Semiquartile distance When all the data in a group are ranked, the values between any two quartiles contains one ordered quarter of the values. Typically, we are most interested in the borders (quartiles) of the middle two quarters of data, Q_1 and Q_3, which together bound the semiquartile distance and which contain the median as their center. Given that there are N values in an ordered group of data, the upper limit of any quarter of the data—that is, the jth quartile (Q_j) may be computed as being equal to the $[j(N + 1)/4th]$ value. Once we have used this formula to calculate the upper limits Q_1 and Q_3, we can then compute the semiquartile distance (which is also called the quartile deviation, and as such is abbreviated as the QD) with the formula $QD = (Q_3 - Q_1)/2$.

One final sample parameter which sees some use in toxicology (primarily in inhalation studies) is the geometric mean, denoted by the term $\bar{X}_g$. This is calculated as

$$\bar{X}_g = (X_1 \cdot X_2 \cdots X_N)1/N$$

and has the attractive feature that it does not give excessive weight to extreme values (or *outliers*), such as the mass of a single very large particle in a dust sample. In effect, it "folds" extreme values in toward the center of the distribution, decreasing the sensitivity of the parameter to the undue influence of the outlier.

Experimental Design

Both the cost to perform research and the value that society places upon the results of such efforts have continued to increase rapidly. Especially as this does not seem likely to become less the case in the foreseeable future, it is essential that every experiment and study yield as much information as possible, and that (more specifically) the results of each study have the greatest possible chance of answering the questions it was conducted to address. We have now become accustomed to developing exhaustively detailed protocols for an experiment or study prior to its conduct. But, typically, such protocols do not include or reflect a detailed plan for the statistical analysis of the data generated by the study. *A priori* selection of statistical methodology (as opposed to the *post hoc* approach) is as significant a portion of the process of protocol development and experimental design as any other and can measurably enhance the value of the study. Such prior selection of statistical methodologies is essential for effective detailing of such other portions of a protocol as the number of animals per group and the sampling intervals for body weight. Implied in such a selection is that the toxicologist has both an in-depth knowledge of the area of investigation and an understanding of the general principles of experimental design, for the analysis of any set of data is dictated to a large extent by the manner in which the data are obtained.

The four statistical principles of experimental design are replication, randomization, concurrent ("local") control and balance. In short form, these are summarized as follows.

Replication Any treatment must be applied to more than one experimental unit (animal, plate of cells, etc.). This provides more accuracy in the measurement of a response than can be obtained from a single observation, since underlying experimental errors tend to cancel each other out. It also supplies an estimate of the experimental error derived from the variability among all of the measurements taken (*replicates*).

Randomization This is practiced to ensure that every treatment will have its fair share of extreme high and extreme low values, and allows the toxicologist to proceed as if the assumption of "independence" is valid. That is, there is no avoidable/known systematic bias in how one obtains data.

Concurrent control Comparisons between treatments should be made, to the maximum extent possible, between experimental units from the same group. That is, animals used as a *control* group should come from the same source and lot as test group animals. And except for the treatment being evaluated, test and control animals should be maintained and handled in exactly the same manner.

Balance If the effect of several different factors is being evaluated simultaneously, the experiment should be laid out in such a way that the contributions of the different factors can be separately distinguished and estimated.

The goal of all of these principles is good statistical efficiency and the economizing of resources. An alternative way of looking at this in a step-wise logical manner is to do a logic flow analysis of the problem. Such an undertaking is conducted in three steps, and should be performed every time any major study or project is initiated. These steps are detailed below.

1. *Define the objective of the study—get a clear statement of what questions are being asked.*

Can the question, in fact, be broken down into a set of subquestions?

Are we asking one or more of these questions repeatedly? For example, does "*X*" develop at 30, 60, 90+ days and/or does it progress/regress or recover?

What is our model to be in answering this/these questions? Is it appropriate and acceptably sensitive?

2. *For each subquestion (i.e., separate major variable to be studied):*

How is the variable of interest to be measured?

What is the nature of the data generated by the measure? Are we getting an efficient set of data? Or are we buying (a) too little information, and would another technique improve the quality of the information generated to the point that it becomes a higher "class" of data? or (b) too much information, i.e., does some underlying aspect of the measure limit the class of data obtainable within the bounds of feasibility of effort?

Are there possible interactions between measurements? Can they be separated/identified?

Is our *N* (sample size) both sufficient and efficient?

What is the control—formal or informal? Is it appropriate?

Are we needlessly adding confounding variables (asking inadvertent or unwanted questions)?

Are there "lurking variables" present? These are undesired and not readily recognized differences which can affect results, such as different technicians observing different groups of animals?

How large an effect will be considered biologically significant? This is a question that can only be resolved by reference to experience or historical control data.

3. *What are the possible outcomes of the study—i.e., what answers are possible to both our subquestions and to our major question?*

How do we use these answers?

Do the possible answers offer a reasonable expectation of achieving the objectives that prompted us to initiate the study?

What new questions may these answers lead us to ask? Can the study be redesigned, before it is actually started, so that these "revealed" questions may be answered in the original study?

A practical example of the application of this approach can be demonstrated in the process of designing a chronic inhalation study. Although in such a situation the primary question being asked is usually "does the chemical result in cancer by this route?", even at the beginning there are a number of other questions that it is expected that the study will answer. Two such are (a) if cancer is produced, what is the relative risk associated with it and (b) are there other expressions of toxicity associated with chronic exposure? Several, if not all, of these three questions are actually to be asked repeatedly during the course of the study. Before the study starts, a plan and arrangements must be formed to make measurements to allow us to answer these questions.

When considering the last portion of our logic analysis, however, we must start by considering each of the things that may go wrong during the study. These include the occurrence of an infectious disease (Do we continue or stop exposures? Will we be able to separate the portions of observed effects that are due to the chemical under study and those that are due to the disease process?), finding that extreme nasal and respiratory irritation was occurring in test animals, or revealing the existence of some hidden variable. Can we preclude the possibility of a disease outbreak by doing a more extensive health surveillance and quarantine on our test animals prior to the start of the study? Could we select a better test model—one that is not as sensitive to upper respiratory or nasal irritation?

One last aspect of experimental design should be addressed here, however: determining sufficient test and control group sizes to allow us to have an adequate level of confidence in the results of an analysis. This number (*N*) can be calculated by using the formula (31)

$$N = \frac{(t_1 + t_2)^2}{\sigma^2} S^2$$

where t_1 is the one-tailed t value with $N-1$ degrees of freedom corresponding to the desired level of confidence, and t_2 is the one-tailed t value with $N-1$ degrees of freedom (*df*) corresponding to the probability that the sample size will be adequate to achieve the desired precision, and s is the sample standard deviation, derived typically from historical data and calculated as (with v being the variable of interest)

$$S = \sqrt{\frac{1}{N-1} \sum (v_1 - v_2)^2}$$

and σ is the acceptable range of variation in the variable of interest.

A good approximation can be generated by substituting t values for an infinite number of degrees of freedom. This entire process is demonstrated in the Example below.

Example

In a subchronic dermal study in rabbits, a key area of concern is the extent to which the compound results in oxidative damage to the circulating red blood cells. To quantitate this, we are measuring the levels of reticulocytes in the blood. What will be an adequate sample size to allow us to address the question at hand?

We use the one-tailed t value for an infinite number of degrees of freedom at a 95% confidence level (that is, $p \leq 0.05$). Going to a set of t tables, we find this number to be 1.645. From prior experience, we know that the usual values for reticulocytes in rabbit blood are from 0.5 to 1.9. The value of σ, therefore, is equal to the span of this range, or 1.4. Likewise, examining the control data from previous rabbit studies, we find our sample standard deviation (s) to be 0.825. When we place all of these numbers into the equation for sample size, we can calculate the required sample size (N) to be

$$= \frac{(1.645 + 1.645)^2}{(1.4)^2} 0.825$$

$$= \frac{10.824}{1.96} (0.825)$$

$$= 4.556$$

In other words, in this case where there is little natural variability, measuring the reticulocyte counts of groups of only 5 animals each should be sufficient to answer our question. More detailed texts are available to give guidance on the statistical aspects of experimental design (17, 24, 33, 57, 76).

Outliers and Rounding of Numbers

These two areas of consideration in the handling of numerical data can be, on occasion, of major concern to the toxicologist because of their pivotal nature in borderline cases. Outliers, at least, should also be of concern for other reasons. On the principle that one should always have a plan to deal with all reasonably likely contingencies in advance of their happening, early decisions should be made to select a policy for handling both outliers and the rounding of numbers.

Outliers are extreme (high or low) values that are widely divergent from the main body of a group of data and from what is our common experience. They may arise from an instrument (such as a balance) being faulty, the seeming natural urge of some animals to frustrate research, or they may be indicative of a "real" value. Outlying values can be detected by visual inspection of the data, use of a scattergram (as will be discussed later), or (if the data set is small enough, which is usually the case in toxicology) by a large increase in the parameter estimating the dispersion of data, such as the standard deviation.

When we can solidly tie one of the above error-producing processes (such as a balance being faulty) to an outlier, we can safely delete it from consideration. But if we cannot solidly tie such a cause to an outlier (even if we have strong suspicions), we have a much more complicated problem, for then such a value may be one of several other things. It could be a result of a particular cause that is the grounds for the entire study—that is, the very "effect" that we are looking for, or it could be because of the collection of legitimate effects which constitute sample error. As will be discussed later under exploratory data analysis, and as is now becoming more widely appreciated, in animal studies outliers can be

an indication of a biologically significant effect which is not yet statistically significant. Variance inflation can result from such outliers, and can be used to detect them. Outliers, in fact, by increasing the variability within a sample, decrease the sensitivity of our statistical tests and may actually preclude our having a statistically significant result (8).

Alternatively the outlier may be due to an unobserved technician error, etc. . . . In this last case we want to reject the data point—to exclude it from consideration with the rest of the data. But how can one identify these legitimate statistical rejection cases?

There are a wide variety of techniques for data rejection. Their proper use depends on one's having an understanding of the nature of the distribution of the data. For normally distributed data with a single extreme value, a simple method such as Chauvenet's criterion (73) may legitimately be employed. This states that if the probability of a value deviating from the mean is greater than $\frac{1}{2}N$, then we should consider that there are adequate grounds for its rejection. Another relatively straightforward approach, for when the data are normally distributed but contain several extreme values, is to winsorize the data. Though there are a number of variations on this approach, the simplest (also called $G = 1$) calls for replacing the highest and lowest values. For example, in a group of data consisting of the values 54, 22, 18, 15, 14, 13, 11, and 4, we would replace 54 with a second 22, and 4 with a replicate 11. This would give us a group consisting of 22, 22, 18, 15, 14, 14, 13, 11, and 11, which we would then treat as our original data. Winsorizing should not be performed, however, if the extreme values constitute more than a small minority of the entire data set.

If we have more information as to the nature of the data or the type of analysis to be performed, there are yet better ways to handle outliers. Extensive discussions of these may be found in Barnett and Lewis (6), Grubbs (50), or Beckman and Cook (8). Snedecor and Cochran (94) also give a nice short discussion.

When the number of digits in a number is to be reduced (due to the limitations of space or to reflect the extent of significance of a number) we must carry out the process of rounding off a number. Failure to have a rule for performing this operation can lead to both confusion and embarrassment for a facility (during such times as study audits). One common rule follows.

A digit to be rounded is not changed if it is followed by a digit less than 5—the digits following it are simply dropped off ("truncated"). If the number is followed by a digit greater than 5 or by a 5 followed by other nonzero digits, it is increased to the next highest number. When the digit to be rounded is followed by 5 alone or followed by zeros, it is unchanged if it is even but increased by one if it is odd. Examples of this rule in effect are (in a case where we must reduce to 3 digits)

1374	becomes	137
1376	becomes	138
13852	becomes	139
1375	becomes	138
1385	becomes	138

The rationale behind this procedure is that over a period of time the results should even out, for as many digits will be increased as are decreased.

Entry Devices

One approach for the selection of appropriate techniques to employ in a particular situation is to use a decision-tree method. Figure 1 is a decision tree that leads to the choice of one of three other trees to assist in technique selection, with each of the subsequent trees addressing one of the three functions of statistics that was defined earlier in this chapter. Figure 2 is for the selection of hypothesis-testing procedures, Fig. 3 for modeling procedures, and Fig. 4 for reduction of dimensionality procedures. For the vast majority of situations, these trees will guide the user into the choice of the proper technique.

Computational Devices

Both the range and availability of devices and software for the performance of the actual detailed calculation of most statistical techniques have continued to increase at a tremendous rate. Unlike when the first edition of this chapter was written, there are now four tiers of computational support available for statistical analysis. These range from programmable desktop calculators (such as the Texas Instruments and Hewlett–Packard models) to complete statistical packages available on mainframe computers. A brief review of some of the more common available supports is given in Table 2. As a general rule, as one goes from those systems listed under tier I to those listed under tier IV, both power and cost of the system decline while ease of use and flexibility increase. Everything described in this chapter can be performed by tier I through III systems, but only the univariate analysis procedures can be handled by tier IV items.

The difficulty with this wide availability of automated analysis systems is that it has become increasingly easy to perform the wrong tests on the wrong data and from there to proceed to the wrong conclusions. This serves to make at least a basic understanding of the procedures and discipline of statistics a vital necessity for the research toxicologist.

METHODS

In each of the subsequent sections, an example with detailed calculations is presented. These calculations can be performed rapidly by using a number of the programs previously discussed.

Randomization

Randomization is the act of assigning a number of items (e.g., plates of bacteria or test animals) to groups in such a manner that there is an equal chance for any one item to end up in any one group. This is a control against any possible unconscious bias in assignment of subjects to test groups. One variation on this is what is called a *censored randomization,* which insures that the groups are equivalent in some aspect after the assignment process is complete. The most common example of a censored randomization is one in which it is insured that the body weights of the test animals in each group are not significantly different from those in the other groups. This is done by analyzing weights by analysis of variance after animal assignment, then rerandomizing if there is a significant difference at some nominal level, such as $p \leq 0.10$. The process is repeated until there is no difference. A second valuation is stratified (or blocked) randomization, where members of subclasses (such as litter mates) are assigned to different groups.

There are several alternatives for actually performing the randomization process. The three most commonly used are card assignment, use of a random number table, and use of a computerized algorithm.

For the card-based method, individual identification numbers for items (e.g., plates or animals) are placed on separate index cards. These cards are then shuffled, and placed one at a time in succession into piles corresponding to the required number of test groups. The results are the random group assignment.

The random number table method requires only that one have unique numbers assigned to test subjects and access to

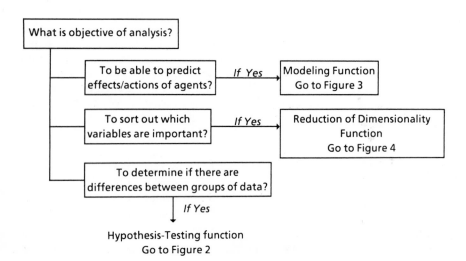

FIG. 1. Overall decision tree for selecting statistical procedures.

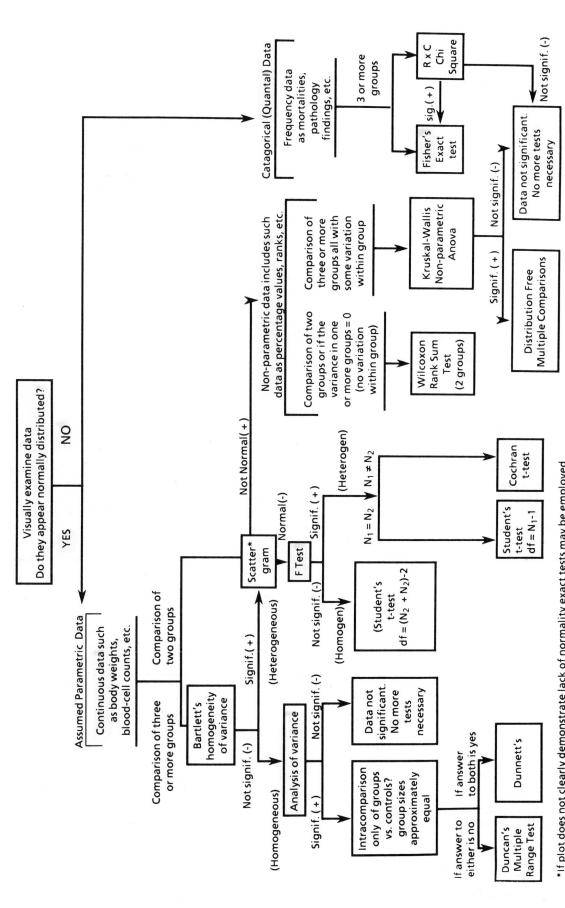

FIG. 2. Decision tree for selecting hypothesis-testing procedure. (∗) If plot does not clearly demonstrate lack of normality, exact tests may be employed. (+) If continuous data, Kolmongorox–Smirnov test may be used. (−) If discontinuous data, chi-square goodness-of-fit test may be used.

∗ If plot does not clearly demonstrate lack of normality exact tests may be employed.
–If continuous data, Kolmogorov Smirnov test.
–If discontinuous data, Chi-Square Goodness-of-Fit test may be used.

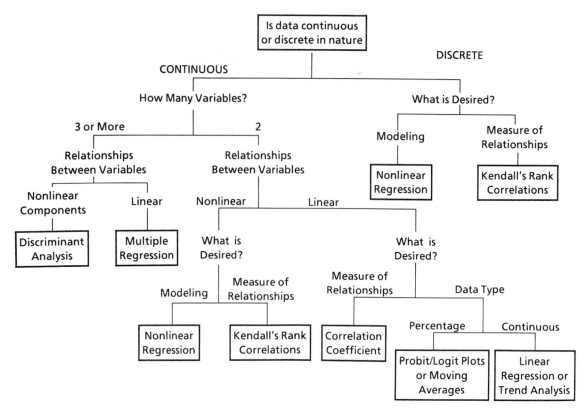

FIG. 3. Decision tree for selecting modeling procedures.

a random number table. One simply sets up a table with a column for each group to which subjects are to be assigned. We start from the head of any one column of numbers in the random number table (each time the table is used, a new starting point should be utilized). If our test subjects number less than 100, we utilize only the last two digits in each random number in the table. If they number more than 99 but less than 1000, we use only the last three digits. To generate group assignments, we read down a column, one number at a time. As we come across digits that correspond to a subject number, we assign that subject to a group (enter its identifying number in a column), proceeding from left to right and filling one row at a time. After an animal is assigned, any duplication of its unique number is ignored. We use as many successive

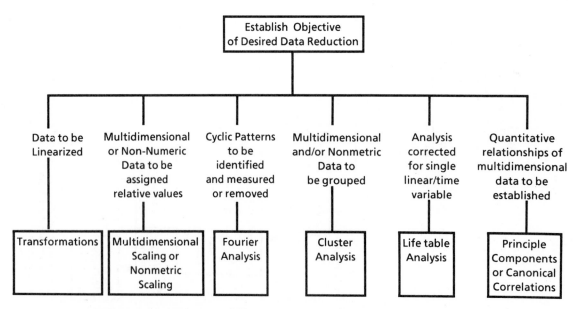

FIG. 4. Decision tree for selection of reduction of dimensionality procedures.

TABLE 2. *Selected available computational aids*

Tier/System	Description
I. Mainframe	
SPSS (78)	This commercial statistical software package is available in most university computer facilities. With manipulation it will perform almost all the procedures described in this chapter.
BMD (26)	Widely available, has greater capabilities than SPSS, and is more easily manipulated.
SAS (87)	Widely available, easier to format, better at summarizing data, and has its own higher level programming language.
Minitab (85)	Easiest to use of the mainframe packages and the least expensive of the four.
II. Minicomputer	
HP Stat	Available on the Hewlett–Packard 9836, 9826, and 9816. It can perform the full range of analysis except life-table analysis.
Stat Cat	SPSS on a made-to-order minicomputer.
III. Microcomputers[a]	
Statgraphics	For IBM PC or CP/M operating systems. Offers the full range of hypothesis-testing and modeling procedures, plus some multivariate and EDA procedures.
Statpro	For the IBM PC. Extensive coverage of the full range of procedures described in this chapter, though it is not complete on EDA.
HSD statistics series	This is a set of modules which, in combination, cover everything but EDA and multivariate functions.
IV. Programmable calculators	
Texas Instruments SR-59	Software, as described in the last edition of this chapter, is available to perform all the techniques described in Fig. 2 and most of the other univariate techniques.
Hewlett–Packard	This line of calculators also has a selection of statistical software available.

EDA, exploratory data analysis.

[a] At least 40 additional sets of statistical programs for microcomputers are known to the authors. The three specifically mentioned here currently seem to be the most powerful. Interested readers are referred to Woodward et al. (118) for more information.

columns of random numbers as we need to complete the process.

The third (and now most common) method is to use a random number generator that is built into a calculator or computer program. Procedures for generating these are documented in manuals that come with the machines and/or programs.

One is also occasionally required to evaluate whether or not a series of numbers (such as an assignment of animals to test groups) is random. This requires the use of a randomization test, of which there are a large variety. The chi-square test, as described later, can be used to evaluate the goodness-of-fit to a random assignment. If the result is not critical, a simple sign test will work. For the sign test, we first determine the middle value in the numbers being checked for randomness. We then go through a list of the numbers assigned to each group, scoring each as a "+" (greater than our middle number) or "−" (less than our middle number). The number of pluses and minuses in each group should be approximately equal. This is demonstrated in Example 1.

■ *Example 1*

In auditing a study performed at another lab, we wish to ensure that their assignment of animals to test groups was random. Thirty-three animals numbered 1–33 were assigned to groups of 11 animals each. Using the middle value in this series (17) as our check point, we assign signs as below.

Control		Test group A		Test group B	
Animal No.	Sign	Animal No.	Sign	Animal No.	Sign
17	0	18	−	11	−
14	−	1	−	2	−
7	−	12	−	22	+
26	+	9	−	28	+
21	+	5	−	19	+
15	−	20	+	3	−
16	−	33	+	29	+
6	−	27	+	10	−
25	+	8	−	23	+
32	+	24	+	30	+
4	−	31	+	13	−
Sums of signs	−2		+1		+1

Note that 17 was scored as a zero, insuring (as a check on results) that the sum of the sums of the three columns would be zero. The results in this case clearly demonstrate that there is not a systematic bias in animal number assignments. Tables for acceptance or rejection of sign test results can be found in most nonparametric texts (such as Hollander and Wolfe, ref. 58).

Bartlett's Test for Homogeneity of Variance

Bartlett's test (see ref. 95) is used to compare the variances (values reflecting the degree of variability in data sets) among three or more groups of data, where the data in the groups are continuous sets (such as body weights, organ weights, blood chemistry values, and diet consumptions). It is expected that such data will be suitable for parametric methods, and

Bartlett's is used as a check of the assumption of equivalent variances.

Bartlett's is based on the calculation of the corrected chi-square value by the formula:

$$\chi^2_{corr} = 2.3026 \frac{\sum df\left(\log_{10}\left[\frac{\sum [df(S^2)]}{\sum df}\right]\right) - \sum [df(\log_{10} S^2)]}{1 + \frac{1}{3(K-1)}\left[\sum \frac{1}{df} - \frac{1}{\sum df}\right]}$$

$$\text{where } S^2 = \text{variance} = \frac{\frac{N\sum X^2 - (\sum X)^2}{N}}{N-1}$$

X = individual datum within each group
N = number of data within each group
K = number of groups being compared
df = degrees of freedom for each group = $(N-1)$

The corrected chi-square value yielded by the above calculations is compared with the values listed in the chi-square table according to the numbers of degrees of freedom (such as found in Snedecor and Cochran, ref. 94).

If the calculated value is smaller than the table value at the selected p level (traditionally 0.05), the groups are accepted to be homogeneous and the use of ANOVA is assumed proper. If the calculated χ^2 is greater than the table value, the groups are heterogeneous and other tests (as indicated in Fig. 2, the decision tree) are necessary. This is demonstrated in Example 2.

■ **Example 2**

If monocytes in rat blood taken in the course of an inhalation study were counted, a possible set of results might be as follows:

	400 ppm		200 ppm		0 ppm	
	(X_1)	$(X_1)^2$	(X_2)	$(X_2)^2$	(X_3)	$(X_3)^2$
	9	81	5	25	7	49
	5	25	5	25	6	36
	5	25	4	16	5	25
	4	16	6	36	7	49
			7	49		
Sums	$\sum X_1 = 23$	$\sum X_1^2 = 147$	$\sum X_2 = 27$	$\sum X_2^2 = 151$	$\sum X_3 = 25$	$\sum X_3^2 = 159$

$$S_1^2 = \frac{\frac{4(147) - (23)^2}{4}}{4-1} = 4.9167 \qquad S_2^2 = \frac{\frac{5(151) - (27)^2}{5}}{5-1} = 1.3000$$

$$S_3^2 = \frac{\frac{4(159) - (25)^2}{4}}{4-1} = 0.9167$$

In continuing the calculations, it is helpful to set up a table such as follows:

Concentration	N	$df = (N-1)$	S^2	$(df)(S^2)$	$\log S^2$
400 ppm	4	3	4.9167	14.7501	0.6917
200 ppm	5	4	1.3000	5.2000	0.1139
0 ppm	4	3	0.9167	2.7501	-0.0378
Sums (Σ)	13	10		22.7002	

Concentration	$(df)(\log S^2)$	$\frac{1}{df}$
400 ppm	2.0751	0.3333
200 ppm	0.4556	0.2500
0 ppm	-0.1134	0.3333
Sums (Σ)	2.4173	0.9166

Now we substitute into our original formula and get corrected χ^2:

$$\chi^2 = 2.3026 \frac{10\left[\log_{10}\left(\frac{22.7002}{10}\right) - 2.4173\right]}{\frac{1}{3(3-1)}\left(0.9166 - \frac{1}{10}\right)}$$

$$= 2.3026 \frac{10(0.3560) - 2.4173}{1 + 0.1667(0.8166)}$$

$$= 2.32$$

The table value for 2 df at the 0.05 level is 5.99. As our calculated value is less than this, the corrected χ^2 is not significant and the variances are accepted as homogeneous. We may thus use parametric methods (such as ANOVA) for further comparisons.

Student's t-Test (Unpaired t-Test)

Pairs of groups of continuous, randomly distributed data are compared via this test. We can use this test to compare three or more groups of data, but they must be intercompared by examination of two groups taken at a time and are preferentially compared by ANOVA. Usually this means of comparison of a test group versus a control group, although two test groups may be compared as well. To determine which of the three types of t-tests described in this chapter should be employed, the F test is normally done first. This will tell us if the variances of the data are approximately equal, which is requirement for the use of a parametric method. If the F test indicates homogeneous variances and the numbers of data within the groups (N) are equal, then the Student's t-test is the appropriate procedure (Sokal and Rohlf, ref. 95, pp. 226–231). If the F is significant (the data are heterogeneous) and the two groups have equal numbers of data, the modified Student's t-test is applicable (25).

The value of t for the Student's t-test is calculated by the formula:

$$t = \frac{\bar{X}_1 - \bar{X}_2}{\sqrt{\sum D_1^2 + \sum D_2^2}} \sqrt{\frac{N_1 N_2}{N_1 + N_2}(N_1 + N_2 - 2)}$$

where the value of $\sum D^2 = \dfrac{N \sum X^2 - (\sum X)^2}{N}$

The value of t obtained from the above calculations is compared with the values in a t-distribution table (as may be found in any standard text) according to the appropriate number of degrees of freedom. If the F value was not significant (i.e., variances were homogeneous), $df = N_1 + N_2 - 2$. If the F was significant and $N_1 = N_2$, then $df = N - 1$. Although this case indicates a nonrandom distribution, the modified t-test is still valid. If the calculated value is larger than the table value at $p = 0.05$, it may then be compared with the appropriate other table values in order of decreasing probability to determine the degree of significance between the two groups. Example 3 demonstrates this methodology.

■ *Example 3*

Suppose we wish to compare two groups (a test and control group) of dog weights following inhalation of a vapor. First, we would test for homogeneity of variance using the F test. Assuming that this test gave negative (homogeneous) results, we would perform the t-test as follows:

Dog no.	Test weight (X_1 in kg)	X_1^2	Control weight (X_2 in kg)	X_2^2
1	8.3	68.89	8.4	70.56
2	8.8	77.44	10.2	104.04
3	9.3	86.49	9.6	92.16
4	9.3	86.49	9.4	88.36
Sums	$\sum X_1 = 35.7$	$\sum X_1^2 = 319.31$	$\sum X_2 = 37.6$	$\sum X_2^2 = 355.12$
Means	8.92		9.40	

The difference in means $= 9.40 - 8.92 = 0.48$

$$\sum D_1^2 = \frac{4(319.31) - (35.7)^2}{4} = \frac{2.75}{4} = 0.6875$$

$$\sum D_2^2 = \frac{4(355.12) - (37.6)^2}{4} = \frac{6.72}{4} = 1.6800$$

$$t = \frac{0.48}{\sqrt{0.6875 + 1.6800}} \sqrt{\frac{4(4)}{4+4}(4 + 4 - 2)}$$

$$= 1.08$$

The table value for t at the 0.05 probability level for $(4 + 4 - 2)$, or 6 df, is 2.447. Therefore, the dog weights are not significantly different at $p = 0.05$.

Cochran t-Test

The Cochran test should be used to compare two groups of continuous data when the variances (as indicated by the F test) are heterogeneous and the numbers of data within the groups are not equal ($N_1 \neq N_2$). This is a situation where the data, though expected to be randomly distributed, were found not to be (Cochran and Cox, ref. 17, pp. 100–102).

Two t values are calculated for this test, the "observed" t (t_{obs}) and the "expected" t (t'). The observed t is obtained by:

$$t_{obs} = \frac{\bar{X}_1 - \bar{X}_2}{\sqrt{W_1 + W_2}}$$

where $W = SEM^2 = S^2/N$

where S (variance) can be calculated from:

$$S = \frac{\dfrac{N \sum X^2 - (\sum X)^2}{N}}{N - 1}$$

The value for t' is obtained from:

$$t' = \frac{t_1' W_1 + t_2' W_2}{W_1 + W_2}$$

Where t_1' and t_2' are values for the two groups taken from the t-distribution table corresponding to $N - 1 df$ (for each group) at the 0.05 probability level (or such level as one may select).

The calculated t_{obs} is compared with the calculated t' value (or values, if t' values were prepared for more than one probability level). If t_{obs} is smaller than a t', the groups are not considered to be significantly different at that probability level. This procedure is shown in Example 4.

■ *Example 4*

Using the red blood cell count comparison from the F test (with $N_1 = 5$, $N_2 = 4$), the following results were determined:

$$X_1 = \frac{37.60}{5} = 7.52 \quad W_1 = \frac{0.804}{5} = 0.1608$$

$$X_2 = \frac{29.62}{4} = 7.40 \quad W_2 = \frac{0.025}{4} = 0.0062$$

(Note that the S^2 values of 0.804 and 0.025 are calculated in Example 5).

$$t_{obs} = \frac{7.52 - 7.40}{\sqrt{0.1608 + 0.0062}} = 0.29$$

From the t-distribution table we use $t_1 = 2.776$ ($df = 4$) and $t_2 = 3.182$ ($df = 3$) for the 0.05 level of probability.

$$t'_{05} = \frac{2.776(0.1608) + 3.182(0.0062)}{0.1608 + 0.0062}$$

$$= 2.79$$

Because t_{obs} is smaller than t' at the 0.05 level of significance, there is no statistical difference at $p = 0.05$ between the two groups.

F Test

This is a test of the homogeneity of variances between two groups of data (Sokal and Rohlf, ref. 95, pp. 187–188). It is used in two separate cases. The first is, if Bartlett's indicates heterogeneity of variances among three or more groups (i.e., it is used to determine which pairs of groups are heterogeneous). Second, the F test is the initial step in comparing two groups of continuous data that we would expect to be parametric (two groups not usually being compared using ANOVA), the results indicating whether the data are from the same population and whether subsequent parametric comparisons would be valid.

F is calculated by dividing the larger variance (S_1^2) by the smaller one (S_2^2). S^2 is calculated as

$$S^2 = \frac{\dfrac{N \sum X^2 - (\sum X)^2}{N}}{N - 1}$$

where N is the number of data in the group and X represents the individual values within the group. Frequently, S^2 values may be obtained from ANOVA calculations. Use of this is demonstrated in Example 5.

The calculated F value is compared with the appropriate number in F tables (as presented in Pearson and Hartley, ref. 82) for the appropriate degrees of freedom ($N - 1$) in the numerator (along the top of the table) and in the denominator (along the side of the table). If the calculated value is smaller, it is not significant and the variances are considered homogeneous (and the Student's t-test would be appropriate for further comparison). If the calculated F value is greater,

F is significant and the variances are heterogeneous (and the next test would be modified Student's t-test if $N_1 = N_2$ or the Cochran t-test if $N_1 \neq N_2$).

■ *Example 5*

If we wish to compare the red blood cell counts (RBC) of rats receiving a test material in their diet with the RBCs of control rats we might obtain the following results:

Test RBC (X_1)	X_1^2	Control RBC (X_2)	X_2^2
8.23	67.73	7.22	52.13
8.59	73.79	7.55	57.00
7.51	56.40	7.53	56.70
6.60	43.56	7.32	53.58
6.67	44.49	—	—
Sums $\sum X_1 = 37.60$	$\sum X_1^2 = 285.97$	$\sum X_2 = 29.62$	$\sum X_2^2 = 219.41$

$$\text{Variance for } X_1 = S_1^2 = \frac{\dfrac{5(285.97) - (37.60)^2}{5}}{5 - 1}$$

$$= 0.804$$

$$\text{Variance for } X_2 = S_2^2 = \frac{\dfrac{4(219.41) - (29.62)^2}{4}}{4 - 1}$$

$$= 0.025$$

$$F = \frac{0.804}{0.025} = 32.16$$

From the table for F values, for 4 (numerator) versus 3 (denominator) df, we read the limit of 15.1 at the 0.05 level. As our calculated value is larger (and, therefore, significant), the variances are heterogeneous and the Cochran t-test would be appropriate for comparison of the two groups of data.

Scattergram

Two of the major points to be made throughout this chapter are (a) the use of the appropriate statistical tests, and (b) the effects of small sample sizes (as is often the case in toxicology) on our selection of statistical techniques. It is these two points that cause us to include a section on scattergrams and their use.

We have shown that Bartlett's test may be used to determine if the values in groups of data are homogeneous. If they are, this (along with the knowledge that they are from a continuous distribution) is sufficient cause to trust that parametric methods are appropriate.

But, if the values in the (continuous data) groups fail Bartlett's (i.e., are heterogeneous), we cannot be secure in our belief that parametric methods are appropriate until we gain some confidence that the values are normally distributed. With large groups of data, we can compute parameters of the population (kurtosis and skewness, in particular) and from these parameters determine if the population is normal (with a certain level of confidence). If our concern is especially marked in these cases, we can use a chi-square goodness-of-fit test for normality. But when each group of data consists of 25 or fewer values, these tests (kurtosis, skewness, and chi-square goodness-of-fit) are not accurate determinants of normality. Instead, in these cases we should prepare a scattergram of the data, then evaluate the scattergram to estimate if the data are approximately normally distributed. This procedure consists of establishing a histogram of the data.

The abscissa (or horizontal scale) should be in the same scale as the values, and should be divided so that the entire range of our observed values is covered by the scale of our abscissa. Across such a scale we then simply enter symbols (stars, crosses, or dots) for each of our values. Example 6 shows such a plot.

■ *Example 6*

Suppose we have the two data sets below:

Group 1: 4.5, 5.4, 5.9, 6.0, 6.4, 6.5, 6.9, 7.0, 7.1, 7.0, 7.4, 7.5, 7.5, 7.5, 7.6, 8.0, 8.1, 8.4, 8,5, 8.6, 9.0, 9.4, 9.5 and 10.4.
Group 2: 4.0, 4.5, 5.0, 5.1, 5.4, 5.5, 5.6, 6.5, 6.5, 7.0, 7.4, 7.5, 7.5, 8.0, 8.1, 8.5, 8.5, 9.0, 9.1, 9.5, 9.5, 10.1, 10.0 and 10.4.

Both of these groups contain 24 values and cover the same range. From them we prepare the following scattergrams.

Group 1

Group 2

Group 1 can be seen to approximate a normal distribution (bell-shaped curve); we can proceed to perform the appropriate parametric tests with such data. But group 2 clearly does not appear to be normally distributed. In this case, the appropriate nonparametric technique must be used.

Analysis of Variance

ANOVA is used for the comparison of three or more groups of continuous data when the variances are homogeneous and the data are independent and normally distributed.

A series of calculations are required for ANOVA, starting with the values within each group being added ($\Sigma\ X$) and then these sums being added ($\Sigma\Sigma\ X$). Each figure within the groups is squared, and these squares are then summed ($\Sigma\ X^2$) and these sums added ($\Sigma\Sigma\ X^2$). Next the "correction factor" (CF) can be calculated from the following formula.

$$CF = \frac{(\overset{K}{\underset{1}{\Sigma}}\ \overset{N}{\underset{1}{\Sigma}}\ X)^2}{N_1 + N_2 + \cdots N_K}$$

where N is the number of values in each group and K is the number of groups. The total sum of squares (SS) is then determined as follows:

$$SS_{total} = \overset{K}{\underset{1}{\Sigma}}\ \overset{N}{\underset{1}{\Sigma}}\ X^2 - CF$$

In turn, the sum of squares between groups (bg) is found from

$$SS_{bg} = \frac{(\Sigma\ X_1)^2}{N_1} + \frac{(\Sigma\ X_2)^2}{N_2} + \cdots \frac{(\Sigma\ X_K)^2}{N_K} - CF$$

The sum of squares within group (wg) is then the difference between the last two figures, or

$$SS_{wg} = SS_{total} - SS_{bg}$$

Now, there are three types of degrees of freedom to determine. The first, total df, is the total number of data within all groups under analysis minus one ($N_1 + N_2 + \cdots N_K - 1$). The second figure ($df$ between groups) is the number of groups minus one ($K - 1$). The last figure (df within groups or "error df") is the difference between the first two figures ($df_{total} - df_{bg}$).

The next set of calculations requires determination of the two mean squares (MS_{bg} and MS_{wg}). These are the respective sum of square values divided by the corresponding df figures ($MS = SS/df$). The final calculation is that of the F ratio. For this, the MS between groups is divided by the MS within groups ($F = MS_{bg}/MS_{wg}$).

A table of the results of these calculations (using data from Example 7 at the end of this section) would appear as follows:

	df	SS	MS	F
bg	3	0.04075	0.01358	4.94
wg	12	0.03305	0.00275	
Total	15	0.07380		

For interpretation, the F ratio value obtained in the ANOVA is compared with a table of F values such as that found in Snedecor and Cochran (94, pp. 480–487) (If $F \leq 1.0$, the results are not significant and comparison with the table values is not necessary.) The df for the greater mean square (MS_{bg}) are indicated along the top of the table. Then read down the side of the table to the line corresponding to the df for the lesser mean square (MS_{wg}). The figure shown at the desired significance level (traditionally 0.05) is compared with the calculated F value. If the calculated number is smaller, there are no significant differences among the groups being compared. If the calculated value is larger, there is some difference, but further (*post hoc*) testing will be required before we know which groups differ significantly from which other groups. In such subsequent testing the groups are compared two at a time.

■ **Example 7**

Suppose we want to compare four groups of dog kidney weights, expressed as percentage of body weights, following an inhalation study. Assuming homogeneity of variance (from Bartlett's test), we could complete the following calculations:

400 ppm	200 ppm	100 ppm	0 ppm
0.43	0.49	0.34	0.34
0.52	0.48	0.40	0.32
0.43	0.40	0.42	0.33
0.55	0.34	0.40	0.39
ΣX 1.93	1.71	1.56	1.38

$$\Sigma\Sigma X = 1.93 + 1.71 + 1.56 + 1.38 = 6.58$$

Next, the preceding figures are squared:

400 ppm	200 ppm	100 ppm	0 ppm
0.1849	0.2401	0.1156	0.1156
0.2704	0.2304	0.1600	0.1024
0.1849	0.1600	0.1764	0.1089
0.3025	0.1156	0.1600	0.1521
ΣX^2 0.9427	0.7461	0.6120	0.4790

$$\Sigma\Sigma X^2 = 0.9427 + 0.7461 + 0.6120 + 0.4790 = 2.7798$$

$$CF = \frac{(6.58)^2}{4+4+4+4} = 2.7060$$

$$SS_{total} = 2.7798 - 2.7060 = 0.0738$$

$$SS_{bg} = \frac{(1.93)^2}{4} + \frac{(1.71)^2}{4} + \frac{(1.56)^2}{4} + \frac{(1.38)^2}{4} - 2.7060$$

$$= 0.04075$$

$$SS_{wg} = 0.07380 - 0.04075 = 0.03305$$

$$df_{total} = 4+4+4+4-1 = 15$$

$$df_{bg} = 4 - 1 = 3 \qquad df_{wg} = 15 - 3 = 12$$

$$MS_{bg} = \frac{0.4075}{3} = 0.01358$$

$$MS_{wg} = \frac{0.03305}{12} = 0.00275$$

$$F = \frac{0.01358}{0.00275} = 4.94$$

Going to an F value table we find that for 3 df_{bg} (greater mean square) and 12 df_{wg} (lesser mean square), the 0.05 value of F is 3.49. As our calculated value is greater, there is a difference among groups. To determine where the difference is, further comparisons by a *post hoc* test will be necessary.

Post Hoc Tests

There are a variety of *post hoc* tests available to analyze data after ANOVA. Each of these tests have proponents, advantages, and disadvantages. Four of these tests are used very commonly in toxicology: Duncan's multiple range test, Scheffe's test, Dunnett's t-test, and Williams' t-test.

Duncan's t-test [27,94 (pp. 233, 236)] is used to compare groups of continuous and randomly distributed data (such as body weights and organ weights). The test normally involves three or more groups, but the actual comparisons are made between pairs of groups taken one pair at a time. It should only follow observation of a significant F value in the ANOVA, when it can serve to determine which group (or groups) differs significantly from which other group (or groups).

There are two alternate methods of calculation here. The selection of the proper one is based on whether the number of data (N) are equal or unequal in the groups.

Groups with Equal Number of Data ($N_1 = N_2$)

Two sets of calculations must be carried out here: first, the determination of the difference between the means of pairs of groups; second, the preparation of a probability table against which each difference in means is compared (as shown in the first of the two examples in this section).

The means (averages) are determined (or taken from the ANOVA calculation) and ranked in either decreasing or increasing order. If two means are the same, they take up two equal positions (thus, for four means we could have ranks of 1, 2, 2, and 4 rather than 1, 2, 3, and 4). The groups are then taken in pairs and the differences between the means ($\bar{X}_1 - \bar{X}_2$), expressed as positive numbers, are calculated. Usually, each pair consists of a test group and the control group, though multiple test groups may be intracompared if so desired. The relative rank of the two groups being compared must be considered. If a test group is ranked "2" and the control group is ranked "1," then we say that there are two places between them, whereas if the test group were ranked "3," then there would be three places between it and the control.

To establish the probability table, the SEM must be calculated. This can be shown as:

$$SEM = \sqrt{\frac{\text{Error mean square}}{N}}$$

$$= \sqrt{\frac{\text{Mean square within group}}{N}}$$

where N is the number of animals or replications per dose level. The mean square within groups (MS_{wg}) can be calculated from the information given in the ANOVA procedure (refer to the ANOVA section). The SEM is then multiplied by a series of table values [as in Harter, ref. 54, or in Beyer, ref. 10 (pp. 369–378)] to set up a probability table. The table values used for the calculations are chosen according to the probability levels (note that the tables have sections for 0.05, 0.01, and 0.001 levels) and the number of means apart for the groups being compared and the number of "error" df. The "error" df is the number of df within the groups. This last figure is determined from the ANOVA calculation and can be taken from ANOVA output. For some values of df, the table values are not given and should thus be interpolated. Example 8 demonstrates this case.

■ *Example 8*

Using the kidney weight as percentage of body weight data described in Example 7 (4 groups of dogs, with 4 dogs in each group), we can make the following calculations:

	Ranks			
	1	2	3	4
Concentration	0 ppm	100 ppm	200 ppm	400 ppm
Mean kidney weight ($\bar{X}$)	0.345	0.390	0.428	0.483

Groups compared	$\bar{X}_1 - \bar{X}_2$	No. of means apart
2 vs. 1 (100 vs. 0 ppm)	0.045	2
3 vs. 1 (200 vs. 0 ppm)	0.083	3
4 vs. 1 (400 vs. 0 ppm)	0.138	4
4 vs. 2 (400 vs. 100 ppm)	0.093	3

The mean square within groups from the ANOVA example was 0.00275. Therefore, the SEM = $\sqrt{0.00275/4}$ = 0.02622. The "error" df (df_{wg}) was 12, so the following table values are used:

	Probability levels		
No. of means apart	0.05	0.01	0.001
2	3.082	4.320	6.106
3	3.225	4.504	6.340
4	3.313	4.622	6.494

When these are multiplied by the SEM we get the following probability table:

	Probability levels		
No. of means apart	0.05	0.01	0.001
2	0.0808	0.1133	0.1601
3	0.0846	0.1181	0.1662
4	0.0869	0.1212	0.1703

Groups with Unequal Number of Data ($N_1 \neq N_2$)

This procedure is very similar to that discussed above. As before, the means are ranked and the differences between the means are determined ($\bar{X}_1 - \bar{X}_2$). Next, weighting values ("a_{ij}" values) are calculated for the pairs of groups being compared in accordance with

$$a_{ij} = \sqrt{\frac{2N_iN_j}{(N_i + N_j)}} = \sqrt{\frac{2N_1N_2}{(N_1 + N_2)}}$$

This weighting value for each pair of groups is multiplied by $\bar{X}_1 - \bar{X}_2$ for each value to arrive at a "t" value. It is this "t" that will later be compared with a probability table.

The probability table is set up as above except that instead of multiplying the appropriate table values by SEM, SEM^2 is used. This is equal to $\sqrt{MS_{wg}}$.

For the desired comparison of two groups at a time, either the $\bar{X}_1 - \bar{X}_2$ value (if $N_1 = N_2$) or the "t" value (if $N_1 \neq N_2$) is compared with the appropriate probability table. Each comparison must be made according to the number of places between the means. If the table value is larger at the 0.05 level, the two groups are not considered to be statistically different. If the table value is smaller, the groups are different and the comparison is repeated at lower levels of significance. Thus, the degree of significance may be determined. We might have significant differences at 0.05 but not at 0.01, in which case the probability would be represented as 0.05 > p > 0.01. Example 9 demonstrates this case.

■ *Example 9*

Suppose that the 400 ppm level from the above example had only 3 dogs, but that the mean for the group and the mean square within groups were the same. To continue Duncan's we would calculate the weighing factors as follows:

100 ppm vs. 0 ppm

200 ppm vs. 0 ppm $N_1 = 4; N_2 = 4$ $a_{ij} = \sqrt{\dfrac{2(4)(4)}{4 + 4}} = 2.00$

400 ppm vs. 0 ppm $N_3 = 3; N_4 = 4$ $a_{ij} = \sqrt{\dfrac{2(3)(4)}{3 + 4}} = 1.852$

400 ppm vs. 100 ppm

Using the $\bar{X}_1 - \bar{X}_2$ from the above example we can set up the following tables:

Concentrations (ppm)	No. of means apart	$\bar{X}_1 - \bar{X}_2$	a_{ij}	$(\bar{X}_1 - \bar{X}_2)a_{ij}$
100 vs. 0	2	0.045	2.000	2.000(.045) = .090
200 vs. 0	3	0.083	2.000	2.000(.083) = .166
400 vs. 0	4	0.138	1.852	1.852(.138) = .256
400 vs. 100	3	0.093	1.852	1.852(.093) = .172

Next we calculate SEM$_2$ as being 0.00275 = 0.05244. This is multiplied by the appropriate table values chosen for 11 df (df_{wg} for this example). This gives the following probability table:

	Probability levels		
No. of means apart	0.05	0.01	0.001
2	0.1632	0.2303	0.3291
3	0.1707	0.2401	0.3417
4	0.1753	0.2463	0.3501

Comparing the t values with the probability table values we get the following:

Comparison	Probability
100 ppm vs. 0 ppm	$p > 0.05$
200 ppm vs. 0 ppm	$p > 0.05$
400 ppm vs. 0 ppm	$0.01 > p > 0.001$
400 ppm vs. 100 ppm	$0.05 > p > 0.01$

Scheffe's Test

Scheffe's test is another *post hoc* comparison method for groups of continuous and randomly distributed data. It also normally involves three or more groups (53,90). It is widely considered to be a more powerful significance test than Duncan's for the following reasons:

1. The Scheffe procedure is less sensitive to violations of normality and homogeneity of variance assumptions.
2. It is not formulated on the basis of groups with equal numbers (as is one of the Duncan procedures), and if $N_1 = N_2$ there are no separate weighting procedures.
3. It tests all linear contrasts among the population means (all alternative methods except the Bonferroni confine themselves to pairwise comparison).

Each *post hoc* comparison is tested by comparing an obtained test value (F_{contr}) with the appropriate critical F value at the selected level of significant (the table F value multiplied by $K - 1$ for an F with $K - 1$ and $N - K$ df[1]). F_{contr} is computed as follows:

a. Compute the mean for each sample (group).
b. Denote the residual mean square by MS_{wg}.
c. Compute the test statistic as

$$F_{contr} = \frac{(C_1\bar{X}_1 + C_2\bar{X}_2 + \cdots + C_K\bar{X}_K)^2}{(K - 1)MS_{wg}(C_1^2/n_1 + \cdots + C_K^2/n_K)}$$

where C_K is the comparison number such that the sum of $C_1, C_2 \cdots C_K = 0$. (See Example 10.)

■ *Example 10*

At the end of a short-term feeding study the following body weight changes were recorded:

	Group 1	Group 2	Group 3
	10.2	12.2	9.2
	8.2	10.6	10.5
	8.9	9.9	9.2
	8.0	13.0	8.7
	8.3	8.1	9.0
	8.0	10.8	
		11.5	
Totals	51.6	76.1	46.6
Means	8.60	10.87	9.32
$MS_{wg} = 1.395$			

To avoid logical inconsistencies with pair-wise comparisons, we compare the group having the largest sample mean (group 2) with that having the smallest sample mean (group 1), then with the group having the next smallest sample mean, and so on. As soon as we find a nonsignificant comparison in this process (or no group with a smaller sample mean remains), we replace the group having the largest sample mean with that having the second largest sample mean and repeat the comparison process.

Accordingly, our first comparison is between groups 2 and 1. We set $C_1 = -1$, $C_2 = 1$, and $C_3 = 0$, and calculate our test statistic

$$F_{contr} = \frac{(10.87 - 8.60)^2}{(3 - 1)1.395(1/6 + 1/7)}$$

$$= 5.97$$

---

[1] Where K = the number of groups and N = the total number of data.

The critical region for F at $p \le 0.05$ for 2 and 11 df is 3.98. Therefore, these groups are significantly different at this level. We next compare groups 2 and 3, using $C_1 = 0$, $C_2 = 1$, and $C_3 = -1$.

$$F_{contr} = \frac{(10.87 - 9.32)^2}{(3 - 1)1.395(1/7 + 1/5)} = 2.51$$

This is lower than the critical region value, so these groups are not significantly different.

Dunnett's t-Test

Dunnett's *t*-test (28,29) is based on the assumption that one wants to compare each of several means with one other mean and only one other mean—in other words, that one wishes to compare each and every treatment group with the control group, but not compare treatment groups with each other. The problem here is that, in toxicology, one is frequently interested in intercomparing treatment groups. However, if one does want only to compare treatment groups versus a control group, Dunnett's is a useful approach. In a study with K groups (one of them being the control) we will wish to make $K - 1$ comparisons. In such a situation, we want to have a level for the entire set of $K - 1$ decisions (not for each individual decision). The Dunnett's t distribution is predicated on this assumption. The parameters for utilizing a Dunnett's-t table, such as found in his original article, are K (as above) and the number of degrees of freedom for MS_{wg}. The test value is calculated as

$$t = \frac{|T_j - T_i|}{\sqrt{2MS_{wg}/n}}$$

where n is the number of observations in each of the groups. The mean square within group (MS_{wg}) is, as we have defined previously; T_j is the mean of control group observations and T_i is the mean of, in order, the successive test group observations. Note that one uses the absolute value of the number resulting from subtracting T_i from T_j. This is to ensure that we are dealing with a positive number of our final t.

Example 11 demonstrates this use with the data from Example 7.

■ *Example 11   Post Hoc* Tests (Dunnett's *t*-test)

The means, N's, and sums for the groups previously presented in Example 7 are:

	Control	100 ppm	200 ppm	400 ppm
Sum (ΣX)	1.38	1.56	1.71	1.93
N	4	4	4	4
Mean	0.345	0.39	0.4275	0.4825

MS_{wg} was 0.00275, and our test t for 4 groups and 12 df is 2.41. Substituting in the equation, we calculate our t for the control versus the 400 ppm to be

$$= \frac{|0.345 - 0.4825|}{\sqrt{2(0.00275)/4}}$$

$$= \frac{0.135}{\sqrt{0.001375}}$$

$$= \frac{0.1375}{0.03781} = 3.637$$

which exceeds our test value of 2.41, showing that these two groups are significantly different at $p \leq 0.05$. The values for the comparisons of the control versus the 200 and 100 ppm groups are then found to be, respectively, 2.182 and 1.190. Both of these are less than our test value, and therefore the groups are not significantly different.

Williams' t-Test

Williams' t-test (113,114) has also become popular for use in toxicology. It is designed to detect the highest level (in a set of dose/exposure levels) at which there is no significant effect. It assumes that the response of interest (such as change in body weights) occurs at higher levels, but not at lower levels, and that the responses are monotonically ordered so that $\bar{X}_0 \leq \bar{X}_1 \cdots \leq \bar{X}_K$. This is, however, frequently not the case. The Williams technique handles the occurrence of such discontinuities in a response series by replacing the offending value and the value immediately preceding it with weighted average values. The test also is adversely affected by any mortality at high dose levels. Such mortalities "impose a severe penalty, reducing the power of detecting an effect not only at level K but also at all lower doses" (114, p. 529). Accordingly, it is not generally applicable to use in the field.

Analysis of Covariance

Analysis of covariance (ANCOVA) is a method for comparing sets of data that consist of two variables (treatment and effect, with our effect variable being called the *variate*), when a third variable (called the *covariate*) exists that can be measured but not controlled and which has a definite effect on the variable of interest. In other words, it provides an indirect type of statistical control, allowing us to increase the precision of a study and to remove a potential source of bias. One common example of this is in the analysis of organ weights in toxicity studies. Our true interest here is the effect of our dose or exposure level on the specific organ weights, but most organ weights also increase (in the young, growing animals most commonly used in such studies) in proportion to increases in animal body weight. As we are not here interested in the effect of this covariate (body weight), we measure it to allow adjustment of the measurement of the variate which we are interested in (the organ weights). ANCOVA allows us to make this adjustment. We must be careful before using ANCOVA, however, to ensure that the underlying nature of the correspondence between the variate and covariate is such that we can rely on it as a tool for adjustments (3,69).

Calculation is performed in two steps. The first is a type of linear regression between the variate Y and the covariate X.

In a like manner, within-group sums of squares and cross products are calculated as

$$\sum xx = \sum_{k=1}^{k} \sum_{i} (X_{ik} - \bar{X}_k)^2$$

$$\sum yy = \sum_{k=1}^{k} \sum_{i} (Y_{ik} - \bar{Y}_k)^2$$

$$\sum xy = \sum_{k=1}^{k} \sum_{i} (X_{ik} - \bar{X}_k)(Y_{ik} - \bar{Y}_k)$$

where i indicates the sum from all the individuals within each group, and f equals the total number of subjects minus the number of groups

$$Sxx = Txx + \sum yy$$

$$Syy = Tyy + \sum yy$$

$$Sxy = Txy + \sum xy$$

With these in hand, we can then calculate the residual mean squares of treatments (St^2) and error (Se^2)

$$St^2 = \frac{\left(Tyy - \dfrac{S^2xy}{Sxx} + \dfrac{\sum^2 xy}{\sum xx}\right)}{K - 1}$$

$$Se^2 = \frac{\left(\sum yy - \dfrac{\sum^2 xy}{\sum xx}\right)}{F - 1}$$

These can be used to calculate an F statistic to test the null hypothesis that all treatment effects are equal:

$$F = \frac{S^2t}{S^2e}$$

The estimated regression coefficient of Y or X is

$$B = \frac{\sum xy}{\sum xx}$$

The estimated standard error for the adjusted difference between two groups is given by

$$Sd = Se \frac{1}{n_0} + \frac{1}{n_1} + \frac{(X_1 - X_0)^2}{\sum xx}$$

where n_0 and n_1 are the sample sizes of the two groups. A test of the null hypothesis that the adjusted difference between the groups is zero is provided by

$$t = \frac{Y_1 - Y_0 - B(X_1 - X_0)}{Sd}$$

The test value for the t is then looked up in the t-table with $f - 1$ df.

Computation is markedly simplified if all the groups are of equal size, as is demonstrated in Example 12.

The underlying assumptions for ANCOVA are fairly rigid and restrictive. These assumptions are as follows:

1. The regression slopes of Y and X are equal from group to group.
2. The relationship between X and Y is linear.
3. The covariate X is measured without error.
4. There are no unmeasured confounding variables.
5. The errors inherent in each variable are independent of each other.
6. The variances of the errors in groups are equal between groups.
7. The measured data which form the groups are normally distributed.

■ *Example 12*

As part of a program to characterize the mechanisms of action and biological effects of an ionophore, we measure the transport across an artificial membrane system of four different cations in the presence of different concentrations of our ionophore. As our real interest is the differential ability of our ionophore to facilitate transport of the cations in the presence of the ionophore, our measure of transport is our variate while the concentration of ionophore (which we cannot directly control) is our covariate. Our data appear as follows (X = concentration of ionophore; Y = measured transport factor of ion across membrane):

Cation	I		II		III		IV		V	
	X	Y	X	Y	X	Y	X	Y	X	Y
Sodium	0.47	1.40	0.57	1.75	0.42	1.34	0.63	1.85	0.55	1.61
Potassium	0.65	5.15	0.43	3.52	0.44	3.55	0.48	3.79	0.59	4.72
Calcium	0.54	10.77	0.64	12.36	0.41	8.31	0.59	11.18	0.53	10.37
Magnesium	0.59	0.27	0.68	0.36	0.53	0.28	0.48	0.22	0.43	0.19

	I		II		III		IV		V	
	X	Y	X	Y	X	Y	X	Y	X	Y
Sums X or Y	2.25	17.59	2.32	17.99	1.80	13.68	2.18	17.04	2.10	16.89
X^2 or Y^2	1.28	144.5	1.38	168.35	0.82	83.53	1.21	142.81	1.12	132.44
XY	9.981		10.666		5.680		9.687		9.248	
n	4		4		4		4		4	
Means	0.562	4.398	0.58	4.498	0.45	3.42	0.545	4.26	0.525	4.222

		X	Y
1. Grand totals			
Sums (X or Y)		10.65	83.19
Sum of squares (X^2 or Y^2)		5.81	671.68
2. Sum of squared group totals, divided by sample size $\dfrac{[\sum\limits^{n} (X \text{ or } Y)]^2}{n}$		5.7118	348.95608
3. Correction term $\dfrac{[\sum\limits^{a}\sum\limits^{n} (Y \text{ or } X)]^2}{\sum\limits^{a} n_i}$		5.6711	346.02881
4. SS total = 1–3		0.1389	325.65119
5. SS groups = 2–3		0.0407	2.92727
6. SS within = 4–5		0.0982	322.72392

ANOVA of the dependent variable

Sources of variation	df	SS	MS	F
Groups	4	2.92727	0.7318175	0.0340
Within	15	322.72392	21.514928	
Total	19	325.65119		

This preliminary ANOVA is not significant.

Analysis of Covariance

For each of the five groups we then compute SS_y, SP_{xy}, SS_x, $b_{y \cdot x}$, $SS_{\hat{y}}$, $SS_{y \cdot x}$, and $MS_{y \cdot x}$. This procedure is illustrated below for group I.

$$\sum^{n} y^2 = \sum^{n} Y_I^2 - \frac{(\sum^{n} Y_I)^2}{n_I} = 144.55 - \frac{(17.59)^2}{4} = 67.197975$$

$$\sum^{n} xy = \sum^{n} X_I Y_I - \frac{(\sum^{n} X_I)(\sum^{n} Y_I)}{n} = 9.981 - \frac{(17.59)(2.25)}{4} = 0.086625$$

$$\sum^{n} x^2 = \sum^{n} X_I^2 - \frac{(\sum^{n} X_I)^2}{n} = 1.28 - \frac{(2.25)^2}{4} = 0.014375$$

$$b_I = \frac{\sum^{n} xy}{\sum^{n} x^2} = \frac{0.086625}{0.014375} = 6.026087$$

$$\sum_{y}^{n} = \frac{(\sum^{n} xy)^2}{\sum^{n} x^2} = \frac{(.086625)^2}{0.014375} = 0.5220098$$

$$\sum d^2 y \cdot x = \sum^{n} y^2 - \sum^{n} \hat{y}^2 = 67.197975 - 0.5220098 = 66.675965$$

$$S_{y \cdot x}^2 = \frac{\sum^{n} d^2 y \cdot x}{(n_1 - 2)} = \frac{66.675965}{2} = 33.337982$$

$$F = \frac{\sum^{n} \hat{y}^2}{S^2 y \cdot x} = \frac{0.522098}{33.337982} = 0.0156608$$

Such an F ratio is not significant. The F ratios for the other groups are in like manner found to be

Group II = .0363761
Group III = 3.2168555
Group IV = .2325121
Group V = .3135638

Only the F for group III is significant.

$$\sum y_{within}^2 = \sum \sum^{n} y^2 = 67.197975 + 87.439975 + 36.7444 + 70.2196 + 61.121975 = 322.72393$$

$$\sum xy_{within} = \sum \sum^{n} xy = .086625 + .2318 + .476 + .4002 + .38075 = 1.57375$$

$$\sum x_{within}^2 = .014375 + .0344 + .01 + .0219 + .0175 = .098175$$

$$b_{within} = \frac{1.57375}{.098175} = 16.030048$$

$$\sum \hat{y}_{within}^2 = \frac{(1.57375)^2}{.098175} = 25.227289$$

$$\sum d^2 y \cdot x_{within} = 322.72393 - 25.227289 = 297.49664$$

$$S^2 y \cdot x_{within} = \frac{\sum d_{y \cdot x_{within}}^2}{\sum n - a - 1} = \frac{297.49664}{14} = 21.24976$$

$$F_s = \frac{\sum \hat{y}_{within}^2}{S_{y \cdot x_{within}}^2} = \frac{25.227289}{21.24976} = 1.1871799$$

This pooled regression is not significant.

$$\sum \sum^{n} d^2 y \cdot x = 0.5220098 + 85.87802 + 14.0868 + 62.906356 + 52.837943 = 216.23113$$

$$\sum n - 2a = 20 - 10 = 10$$

$$S_{y \cdot x}^2 = \frac{\sum \sum^{n} d_{y \cdot x}^2}{\sum n - 2a} = \frac{216.23113}{10} = 21.623113$$

$$SS_{among\,b's} = \sum d_{y \cdot x_{within}}^2 - \sum \sum^{n} d_{y \cdot x}^2 = 297.49664 - 21.6231113 = 275.87353$$

$$MS_{among\,b's} = \frac{SS_{among\,b's}}{a - 1} = \frac{275.87353}{4} = 68.968383$$

$$F = \frac{MS_{among\,b's}}{S_{y \cdot x}^2} = \frac{68.968383}{21.623113} = 3.1895677$$

This is significant at the $p \leq 0.05$ level.

Kruskal–Wallis Nonparametric ANOVA

The Kruskal–Wallis nonparametric one-way analysis of variance should be the initial analysis performed when we have three or more groups of data which are by nature nonparametric (either not a normally distributed population, or of a discontinuous nature, or all the groups being analyzed are not assumed to be from the same general underlying population) but are not of a categorical (or quantal) nature. Commonly, these will either be rank-type evaluation data (such as behavioral toxicity observation scores) or reproduction study data. The analysis is initiated (Pollard, ref. 83, pp. 170–173) by ranking all the observations from the combined groups to be analyzed. Ties (i.e., where two or more observations have the same value and are therefore "tied" in rank) are given the average rank of the tied values (i.e., if two values are tied for 12th rank—and would therefore be ranked 12th and 13th—both are assigned the average rank of 12.5).

The sum of ranks of each group ($r_1, r_2, \cdots r_k$) is computed by adding all the rank values for each group. The test value H is then computed as

$$H = \frac{12}{n(n+1)} (\sum r_1^2/n_1 + \sum r_2^2/n_2$$
$$+ \cdots + \sum r_k^2/n_k) - 3(n+1)$$

where $n_1, n_2, \cdots n_k$ are the number of observations in each group. The test statistic is then compared with a table of H values [such as in Beyer (10)]. If the calculated value of H is greater than the table value for the appropriate number of observations in each group, there is a significant difference between the groups, but further testing (using the distribution-free multiple comparisons method) is necessary to determine where the difference lies (as demonstrated in Example 13).

■ *Example 13*

As part of a neuro/behavioral toxicology study, righting reflex values (whole numbers ranging from 0 to 10) were determined for each of five rats in each of three groups. The values observed, and their ranks, are as follows:

	Control group		5 mg/kg group		10 mg/kg group	
	Reflex score	Rank	Reflex score	Rank	Reflex score	Rank
	0	2	1	5.5	4	10.5
	0	2	1	5.5	4	10.5
	1	5.5	2	8.5	8	14.5
	0	2	6	12.5	8	14.5
	1	5.5	2	8.5	6	12.5
Sums of ranks (Σr)		17.0		40.5		62.5

From these the H value is calculated as

$$H = \frac{12}{15(15+1)} \left(\frac{(17.0)^2}{5} + \frac{(40.5)^2}{5} + \frac{(62.5)^2}{5} \right) - 3(15+1)$$

$$= \frac{12}{240} \left(\frac{289 + 1640.25 + 3906.25}{5} \right) - 48$$

$$= \frac{1}{20} (1167.1) - 48$$

$$= 58.355 - 48$$

$$= 10.355$$

Consulting a table of values for H, we find that for the case where we have three groups of five observations each, the test values are 4.56 (for $p = 0.10$), 5.78 (for $p = 0.05$), and 7.98 (for $p = 0.01$). As our calculated H is greater than the $p = 0.01$ test value, we have determined that there is a significant difference between these groups at the level of $p < 0.01$, and would now have to continue to a multiple comparisons test to determine where the difference is.

Wilcoxon Rank-Sum Test

The Wilcoxon rank-sum test is commonly used for the comparison of two groups of nonparametric (interval or not normally distributed) data, such as those that are not measured exactly but rather as falling within certain limits (e.g., how many animals died during each hour of an acute study). The test is also used when there is no variability (variance =

0) within one or more of the groups we wish to compare (95, pp. 432–437).

The data in both groups being compared are initially arranged and listed in order of increasing value. Then each number in the two groups must receive a rank value. Beginning with the smallest number in both groups (which is given a rank of 1.0) each number is assigned a rank. If there are duplicate numbers (ties), then each value of equal size will receive the median rank for the entire identically sized group. Thus, if the lowest number appears twice, both figures receive the rank of 1.5. This, in turn, means that the ranks of 1.0 and 2.0 have been used and that the next highest number has a rank of 3.0. If the lowest number appears three times, then each is ranked as 2.0 and the next number has a rank of 4.0. Thus, each tied number gets a "median" rank. This process continues until all the numbers are ranked. Each of the two columns of ranks (one for each group) is totalled giving the "sum of ranks" for each group being compared. As a check, we can calculate the value:

$$\frac{(N)(N+1)}{2}$$

where N is the total number of data in both groups. The result should be equal to the sum of both sums of ranks.

The sums of rank values are compared with table values (10, pp. 409–413) to determine the degree of significant differences, if any. These tables include two limits (an upper and a lower) that are dependent upon the probability level. If the number of data is the same in both groups ($N_1 = N_2$), both of the calculated sums of ranks must fall within the two limit values. If this is the case, the two groups are not statistically different. If one or both of the sums of ranks is equal to or falls outside of the table limits, the groups are different at the probability level. If the numbers of data in the two groups are not equal ($N_1 \neq N_2$), then the lesser sum of ranks (smaller N) is compared with the table limits to find the degree of significance. Normally, the comparison of the two groups ends here and the degree of significant difference can be reported. This is demonstrated in Example 14.

■ *Example 14*

If we recorded the approximate times to death (in hours) of rats dosed with 5.0 g/kg (group A) or 2.5 g/kg (group B) of a given material, we might obtain the following results:

Hours to death (group A)	Hours to death (group B)	Group A ranks	Group B ranks
1	1	2.5	2.5
1	2	2.5	6.0
1	4	2.5	9.5
2	4	6.0	9.5
2	5	6.0	11.5
3	7	8.0	14.5
5	7	11.8	14.5
6	8	13.0	16.0
Sums		52.0	84.0

Sum of sums = 52.0 + 84.0 = 136

$$\text{Check} = \frac{16(17)}{2} = 136$$

From the probability table for $N_1 = 8$ we read the limit values (at 0.05) of 49 and 87. Since the calculated sums fall between these numbers, the two groups are not considered significantly different at $p = 0.05$.

Distribution-Free Multiple Comparison

The distribution-free multiple comparison test should be used to compare three or more groups of nonparametric data. These groups are analyzed two at a time for any significant differences (Hollander and Wolfe, ref. 58, pp. 124–129). The test can be used for data similar to those compared by the rank-sum test. We often employ this test for reproduction and mutagenicity studies (such as comparing survival rates of offspring of rats fed various amounts of test materials in the diet).

As shown in Example 15, we must calculate two values for each pair of groups: the difference in mean ranks and the probability level value against which the difference is compared. To determine the difference in mean ranks we must first rank the data within each of the groups in order of increasing values. Then we must assign rank values, beginning with the smallest figure. Note that this is done exactly like the ranking in the Wilcoxon test except that it applies to more than two groups.

The ranks are then added for each of the groups. As a check, the sum of these sums should equal

$$\frac{N_{total}(N_{total} + 1)}{2}$$

where N_{total} is the total number of figures from all groups. Next we can find the mean rank (R) for each group by dividing the sum of ranks by the number of data (N) in the group. These mean ranks are then taken in pairs according to which we want to compare (usually each test group versus the control) and the differences are found ($R_1 - R_2$). This value is expressed as an absolute figure; that is, it is always a positive number.

The second value for each pair of groups (the probability value) is calculated from the expression:

$$^z[a/K(K-1)] \sqrt{\frac{N_{total}(N_{total} + 1)}{12}} \sqrt{\frac{1}{N_1}\frac{1}{N_2}}$$

where a is the level of significance for the comparison (usually 0.05, 0.01, 0.001, etc.), K is the total number of groups, and Z is a figure obtained from a normal probability table. This last figure is found by reading the result of $a(K/K-1)$ within the table and determining the corresponding Z-score from the table.

The result of the probability value calculation for each pair of groups is compared with the corresponding mean difference $|R_1 - R_2|$. If $|R_1 - R_2|$ is smaller, there is not a significant difference between the groups. If it is larger, the groups are different and $|R_1 - R_2|$ must be compared with the calculated probability values for $a = 0.01$ and $a = 0.001$ to find the degree of significance.

■ *Example 15*

Consider the following set of data (ranked in increasing order), which could represent the proportion of rats surviving given periods of time during diet inclusion of test chemical at four dosage levels (survival index).

I (5.0 mg/kg)		II (2.5 mg/kg)		III (1.25 mg/kg)		IV (0.0 mg/kg)	
% Value	Rank	% Value	Rank	% Value	Rank	% Value	Rank
40	2.0	40	2.0	50	5.5	60	9.0
40	2.0	50	5.5	50	5.5	60	9.0
50	5.5	80	12.0	60	9.0	80	12.0
100	17.5	80	12.0	100	17.5	90	14.0
—		100	17.5	100	17.5	100	17.5
						100	17.5
Sum of ranks	27.0		49.0		55.0		79.0
N values	$N_I = 4$		$N_{II} = 5$		$N_{III} = 5$		$N_{IV} = 6$
$N_{total} = 20$							

Check: sum of sums = 210; $\frac{20(21)}{2} = 210$

Mean ranks (R): $R_1 = \frac{27.0}{4} = 6.75$

$$R_2 = \frac{49.0}{5} = 9.80$$

$$R_3 = \frac{55.0}{5} = 11.00$$

$$R_4 = \frac{79.0}{6} = 13.17$$

Comparison groups	$|R_1 - R_2|$	Probability test values
5.0 vs. 0.0	6.42	$(0.05/4(3)) = Z_{0.00417} = 2.637 \sqrt{\frac{(20)(21)}{12}} \sqrt{\frac{1}{4} + \frac{1}{6}} = 10.07$

| 2.5 vs. 0.0 | 3.37 | $(0.05/4(3)) = Z_{0.00417} = 2.637 \sqrt{\dfrac{(20)(21)}{12}} \sqrt{\dfrac{1}{5} + \dfrac{1}{6}} = 9.45$ |
| 1.25 vs. 0.0 | 2.17 | $(0.05/4(3)) = Z_{0.00417} = 2.637 \sqrt{\dfrac{(20)(21)}{12}} \sqrt{\dfrac{1}{5} + \dfrac{1}{6}} = 9.45$, |

Since each of the $|R_1 - R_2|$ values is smaller than the corresponding probability calculation, the pairs of groups compared are not different at the 0.05 level of significance.

Fisher's Exact Test

Fisher's exact test should be used to compare two sets of discontinuous, quantal (all or none) data. Small sets of such data can be checked by contingency data tables such as those of Finney et al. (36). Larger sets, however, require computation. These include frequency data such as incidences of mortality or certain histopathologic findings. Thus, the data can be expressed as ratios. These data do not fit on a continuous scale of measurement but usually involve numbers of responses classified as either negative or positive, i.e., a contingency table situation (95, pp. 738–743).

The analysis is started by setting up a 2 × 2 contingency table to summarize the numbers of positive and negative responses as well as the totals of these as follows:

	Positive	Negative	Total
Group I	A	B	$A + B$
Group II	C	D	$C + D$
Totals	$A + C$	$B + D$	$A + B + C + D = N_{total}$

Using the above set of symbols, the formula for the P appears as follows:[1]

$$P = \frac{(A + B)!(C + D)!(A + C)!(B + D)!}{N!\,A!\,B!\,C!\,D!}$$

The exact test produces a probability (p) which is the sum of the above calculation repeated for each possible arrangement of the numbers in the above cells showing an association equal to or stronger than that between the two variables.

The p resulting from these computations will be the exact one- or two-tailed probability depending on which of these two approaches is being employed. This value tells us if the groups differ significantly (with a probability, for example, less than 0.05) and the degree of significance. This is demonstrated in Example 16.

■ **Example 16**

The pathology reports from 22 control and 48 treated animals show that 1 control and 3 treated animals have tumors of the spleen. Setting this up as a contingency table we see:

	Tumor-bearing	No tumors	Total
Control	1	21	22
Treated	3	45	48
Total	4	66	70

[1] $A!$ is A factorial. For 4!, as an example, this would be $(4)(3)(2)(1) = 24$.

The probability for the worst case on this calculates as:

$$P = \frac{(1 + 21)!(3 + 45)!(1 + 3)!(21 + 45)!}{70!\,1!\,21!\,3!\,45!}$$

$$P = \frac{22!\,48!\,4!^2\,66!}{70!\,1!\,21!\,3!\,45!}$$

$$= 0.415002$$

All other possible stronger combinations must in turn be computed (in this case 0, 22, 4, 44 is the only other such combination and it computes as $P = 0.212216970$). The probabilities must be summed to give the total $P = 0.627$ (single-tailed probability, to be discussed later). Additionally, it should be kept in mind that Ghent proposed a good (though, by hand, laborious) method extending the calculation of exact probabilities to 2 × 3, 3 × 3, and R × C contingency tables (45).

R × C Chi-Square Test

The R × C chi-square test can be used to analyze discontinuous (frequency) data as in the Fisher's exact test. However, in the R × C test (R = row, C = column) we wish to compare three or more sets of data. An example would be comparison of the incidence of tumors among mice on three or more oral dosage levels. We can consider the data as positive (tumors) or negative (no tumors). One condition that should usually be met for this test is that none of the *expected* frequency values (assuming even distribution) should be less than 1.0 and that no more than 20% of the expected frequencies should be less than 5.0 (Zar, ref. 120, p. 50). The expected frequency for any box is equal to: (row total) (column total)/N_{total}.

As in the Fisher's exact test, the initial step is setting up a table (this time an R × C contingency table). This table would appear as follows:

	Positive	Negative	Total
Group I	A_1	B_1	$A_1 + B_1 = N_1$
Group II	A_2	B_2	$A_2 + B_2 = N_2$
	↓	↓	
Group R	A_R	B_R	$A_R + B_R = N_K$
Totals	N_A	N_B	N_{total}

Using these symbols, the formula for chi-square (χ^2) is

$$\chi^2 = \frac{N_{total}^2}{N_A N_B N_K}\left(\frac{A_1^2}{N_1} + \frac{A_2^2}{N_2} + \cdots \frac{A_K^2}{N_K} - \frac{N_A^2}{N_{total}}\right)$$

This resulting chi-square value is compared with table values (as in Snedecor and Cochran, ref. 94, pp. 470–471) according to the number of degrees of freedom, to which it is equal (R − 1) (C − 1). If chi square is smaller than the table value at the 0.05 probability level, the groups are not significantly different. If the calculated chi square is larger, there is some difference among the groups and $2 \times R$ chi-square or Fisher's exact tests will have to be completed to determine which group(s) differ from which other group(s). Example 17 demonstrates this.

■ *Example 17*

The R $\times$ C chi-square can be used to analyze tumor incidence data gathered during a mouse feeding study as follows:

Dosage (mg/kg)	No. of mice with tumors	No. of mice without tumors	Total no. of mice
2.00	19	16	35
1.00	13	24	37
0.50	17	20	37
0.25	22	12	34
0.00	20	23	43
Totals	91	95	186

$$\chi^2 = \frac{(186)^2}{91(95)}\left[\frac{19^2}{35} + \frac{13^2}{37} + \frac{17^2}{37} + \frac{22^2}{34} + \frac{20^2}{43} + \frac{91^2}{186}\right]$$

$$= (4.00)(1.71)$$

$$= 6.84$$

The smallest expected frequency would be $(91)(34)/186 = 16.6$; well above 5.0. The number of degrees of freedom is $(5 - 1)(2 - 1) = 4$. The chi-square table value for 4 df is 9.49 at the 0.05 probability level. Therefore, there is no significant association between tumor incidence and dose or concentration.

Mann–Whitney U Test

This is a nonparametric test in which the data in each group are first ordered from lowest to highest values, then the entire set (both control and treated values) is ranked, with the average rank being assigned to tied values. The ranks are then summed for each group. U is then determined according to

$$U_t = n_c n_t + \frac{n_t(n_t + 1)}{2} - R_t$$

and

$$U_c = n_c n_t + \frac{n_c(n_c + 1)}{2} - R_c$$

where n_c, n_t = sample size for control and treated groups; and R_c, R_t = sum of ranks for the control and treated groups.

For the level of significance for a comparison of the two groups, the larger value of U_c or U_t is used. This is compared with critical values as found in tables (93).

With the above discussion and methods in mind, we may now examine the actual variables that we encounter in teratology studies. These variables can be readily divided into two groups—measures of lethality and measures of teratogenic effect (44). Measures of lethality include (a) corpora lutea per pregnant female, (b) implants per pregnant female, (c) live fetuses per pregnant female, (d) percentage of preimplantation loss per pregnant female, (e) percentage of resorptions per pregnant female, and (f) percentage of dead

fetuses per pregnant female. Measure of teratogenic effect include (a) percentage of abnormal fetuses per litter, (b) percentage of litter with abnormal fetuses, and (c) fetal weight gain. As demonstrated in Example 18, the Mann–Whitney U test should be employed for the count data, but which test should be employed for the percentage variables should be decided on the same grounds as those described later in this chapter in the reproduction section.

■ *Example 18*

In a 2-week study, the levels of serum cholesterol in the treatment and control animals are successfully measured and assigned ranks as below:

Treatment		Control	
Value	Rank	Value	Rank
10	1	19	4
18	3	28	13
26	10.5	29	14.5
31	16	26	10.5
15	2	35	19
24	8	23	7
22	6	29	14.5
33	17	34	18
21	5	38	20
25	9	27	12
Sum of ranks	77.5		132.5

The critical value for a one-tailed $p \leq 0.05$ is $U \geq 73$. We then calculate

$$U_t = (10)(10) + \frac{10(10 + 1)}{2} - 77.5$$

$$= 100 + \frac{110}{2} - 77.5 = 77.5$$

$$U_c = (10)(10) + \frac{10(10 + 1)}{2} - 132.5 = 22.5$$

As 77.5 is greater than 73, these groups are significantly different at the 0.05 level.

Correlation Coefficient

The correlation coefficient procedure is used to determine the degree of linear correlation (direct relationship) between two groups of continuous (and normally distributed) variables; it will indicate whether there is any statistical relationship between the variables in the two groups. For example, we may wish to determine if the liver weights of dogs on a feeding study are correlated with their body weights. Thus, we will record the body and liver weights at the time of sacrifice and then calculate the correlation coefficient between these pairs of values to determine if there is some relationship.

The formula for calculating the linear correlation coefficient (r_{xy}) is as follows:

$$r_{xy} = \frac{N \sum XY - (\sum X)(\sum Y)}{\sqrt{N \sum X^2 - (\sum X)^2}\sqrt{N \sum Y^2 - (\sum Y)^2}}$$

where X is each value for one variable (such as the dog body weights in the above example), Y is the matching value for the second variable (the liver weights), and N is the number of pairs of X and Y. Once we have r_{xy} it is possible to calculate

t_r, which can be used for more precise examination of the degree of significant linear relationship between the two groups. This value is calculated as follows:

$$t_r = \frac{r_{xy}\sqrt{N - 2}}{\sqrt{1 - r_{xy}^2}}$$

The value obtained for r_{xy} can be compared with table values (94, p. 477) according to the number of pairs of data involved minus two. If the r_{xy} is smaller (at the selected test probability level, such as 0.05), the correlation is not significantly different from zero (no correlation). If r_{xy} is larger than the table value, there is a positive statistical relationship between the groups. Comparisons are then made at lower levels of probability to determine the degree of relationship (note that if r_{xy} equals either 1.0 or −1.0, there is complete correlation between the groups). If r_{xy} is a negative number and the absolute value is greater than the table value, there is an inverse relationship between the groups; that is, a change in one group is associated with a change in the opposite direction in the second group of variables. Both computations are demonstrated in Example 19.

Since the comparison of r_{xy} with the table values may be considered a somewhat weak test, it is perhaps more meaningful to compare the t_r value with values in a t-distribution table for $N - 2$ df, as is done for the Student's t-test. This will give a more exact determination of the degree of statistical correlation between the two groups.

It should be noted that this method examines only possible linear relationships between sets of continuous, normally distributed data. Other mathematical relationships (log, log/linear, exponential, etc.) between data sets exist which require either the use of another correlation testing method or that one or more of the data sets be transformed so that they are of linear nature. This second approach requires, of course, that one know the nature of the data so that an appropriate transform may be used. Some few transforms are discussed later in the sections on linear regression and probit/log analysis.

■ *Example 19*

If we computed the dog body weight versus dog liver weight for a study we could have the following results:

Dog no.	Body weight (kg) X	X^2	Liver weight (g) Y	Y^2	XY
1	8.4	70.56	243	59049	2041.2
2	8.5	72.25	225	50625	1912.5
3	9.3	86.49	241	58081	2241.3
4	9.5	90.25	263	69169	2498.5
5	10.5	110.25	256	65536	2688.0
6	8.6	73.96	266	70756	2287.6
Sums	$\Sigma X = 54.8$	$\Sigma X^2 = 503.76$	$\Sigma Y = 1494$	$\Sigma Y^2 = 373216$	$\Sigma XY = 13669.1$

$$r_{xy} = \frac{6(13669.1) - (54.8)(1494)}{\sqrt{6(503.76) - (54.8)^2}\ \sqrt{6(373216) - (1494)^2}}$$

$$= 0.381$$

The table value for six pairs of data (read beside the $N - 2$ value, or $6 - 2 = 4$) is 0.811 at a 0.05 probability level. Thus, there is a lack of statistical correlation (at $p = 0.05$) between the body weights and liver weights for this group of dogs.

The t_r value for these data would be calculated as follows:

$$t_r = \frac{0.381\sqrt{6 - 2}}{\sqrt{1 - (0.381)^2}} = 0.824$$

The value for the t-distribution table for 4 df at the 0.05 level is 2.776; therefore, this again suggests a lack of significant correlation at $p = 0.05$.

Kendall's Coefficient of Rank Correlation

Kendall's rank correlation, represented by τ (tau), should be used to evaluate the degree of association between two sets of data when the nature of the data is such that the relationship is not linear. Most commonly, this is when the data are not continuous. An example of such a case is when we are trying to determine if there is a relationship between length of hydra and their survival time in a test medium in hours, as is presented in Example 20. Both of our variables here are discontinuous, yet we suspect a relationship exists. Another common such use is in comparing the subjective scoring done by two different observers.

Tau is calculated as $\tau = N/n(n - 1)$ where n is the sample size and N is the count of ranks, calculated as $N = 4 \sum_{n}^{n} C_i - n(n - 1)$, with the computing of $\sum C_i$ being demonstrated in the example.

If a second variable Y_2 is exactly correlated with the first variable Y_1, then the variates Y_2 should be in the same order as the Y_1 variates. However, if the correlation is less than exact, the order of the variates Y_2 will not correspond entirely to that of Y. The quantity N measures how well the second variable corresponds to the order of the first. It has a maximum value of $n(n - 1)$ and a minimum value of $-n(n - 1)$.

A table of data is set up with each of the two variables being ranked separately. Tied ranks are assigned as demonstrated earlier under the Kruskall–Wallis test. From this point, disregard the original variates and deal only with the ranks. Place the ranks of one of the two variables in rank order (from lowest to highest), paired with the rank values assigned for the other variable. If one (but not the other) variable has tied ranks, order the pairs by the variable without ties (95, pp. 601–607).

The most common way to compute a sum of the counts is also demonstrated in Example 20.

The resulting value of tau will range from −1 to +1, as does the familiar parametric correlation coefficient, r.

■ *Example 20*

During the validation of an *in vitro* method, we notice that large hydra seem to last longer in test media than small individuals. To evaluate this, we take 15 hydra of random size, measure their length in millimeters, then place them all in a test media sample. Over the next day, we record how many hours each individual survives. These data are presented below, along with ranks for each variable.

Length	Rank (R_1)	Survival	Rank (B_2)
3	6.5	19	9
4	10	17	7
6	15	11	1
1	1.5	25	15
3	6.5	18	8
3	6.5	22	6
1	1.5	24	14
4	10	16	12
4	10	15	5
2	3.5	21	11
5	13	13	3
5	13	14	4
3	6.5	20	10
2	3.5	23	13
5	13	12	2

We then arrange this based on the order of the rank of survival time, as there are no ties here. We then proceed to calculate our count of ranks. The conventional method is to obtain a sum of the counts C_i, as follows. Examine the first value in the column of ranks paired with the ordered column. In the case below, this is rank 15. Count all ranks subsequent to it that are higher than the rank being considered. Thus, in this case, count all ranks greater than 15. There are 14 ranks following the 2 and all of them are less than 15. Therefore, we count a score of $C_i = 0$. We then repeat this process for each subsequent rank of R_1, giving us a final score of 1 (By this point it is obvious that our original hypothesis was in error).

R_2	R_1	Following (R_2) ranks greater than (R_1)	Counts (C_i)
1	15	—	$C_1 = 0$
2	13	—	$C_2 = 0$
3	13	—	$C_3 = 0$
4	13	—	$C_4 = 0$
5	10	—	$C_5 = 0$
6	6.5	10	$C_6 = 1$
7	10	—	$C_7 = 0$
8	6.5	—	$C_8 = 0$
9	6.5	—	$C_9 = 0$
10	6.5	—	$C_{10} = 0$
11	3.5	6.5	$C_{11} = 1$
12	6.5	—	$C_{12} = 0$
13	3.5	—	$C_{13} = 0$
14	1.5	—	$C_{14} = 0$
15	1.5	—	$C_{15} = 0$
			$\Sigma C_i = 1$

Our count of ranks, N, is then calculated as

$$N = 4(1) - 15(15 - 1)$$
$$= 4 - 15(14)$$
$$= -206$$

We can then calculate tau as

$$\text{tau} = \frac{-206}{15(15 - 1)}$$
$$= \frac{-206}{210}$$
$$= -0.9810$$

In other words, there is a strong negative correlation between our variables.

Life Tables

Chronic *in vivo* toxicity studies are generally the most complex and expensive studies conducted by a toxicologist. A number of answers to questions are sought in such a study—notably if a material results in a significant increase in mortality or in the incidence of tumors in those animals exposed to it. But we are also interested in the time course of these adverse effects (or risks).

It may readily be seen that during any selected period of time (t_i) we have a number of risks competing to affect an animal. There are the risks of (a) "natural death," (b) death induced by a direct or indirect action of the test compound, and (c) deaths due to such occurrences of interest as tumors (51). And we are indeed interested in determining if (and when) the last two of these risks become significantly different from the "natural" risks (defined as what is seen to happen in the control group). Life-table methods enable us to make such determinations as to the duration of survival (or time until tumors develop) and the probability of survival (or of developing a tumor) during any period of time.

We start by deciding the length of the intervals (t_i) we wish to examine within the study. The information we gain becomes more exact as the interval is shortened. But as interval length is decreased, the number of intervals increases and calculations become more cumbersome and less indicative of time-related trends because random fluctuations become more apparent. For a 2-year or lifetime rodent study, an interval length of a month is commonly employed.

Having established our interval length we can tabulate our data (21). We start by establishing the following columns in each table (a separate table being established for each group of animals—i.e., by sex and dose level):

1. Interval of time selected (t_i)
2. Number of animals in the group that entered that interval of the study alive (ℓ_i)
3. Number of animals withdrawn from study during the interval (such as those taken for an interim sacrifice or those that may have been killed by a technician's error) (ω_i)
4. Number of animals that died during the interval (d_i)
5. Number of animals at risk during the interval ($\ell_i = \ell_i - \frac{1}{2}\omega_i$) or the number on study at the start of the

interval minus one half of the number withdrawn during the interval

6. Proportion of animals that died ($D_i = d_i/\ell_i'$)
7. Cumulative probability of an animal surviving until the end of that interval of study ($P_i = 1 - D_i$, or one minus the number of animals that died during that interval divided by the number of animals at risk)
8. Number of animals dying until that interval (M_i)
9. Animals found to have died during the interval (m_i)
10. Probability of dying during the interval of the study [$c_i = 1 - (M_i + m_i/\ell_i)$, or the total number of animals dead until that interval plus the animals discovered to have died during that interval divided by the number of animals at risk through the end of that interval
11. Cumulative proportion surviving (P_i) is equivalent to the cumulative product of the interval probabilities of survival (i.e., $P_i = p_1 \cdot p_2 \cdot p_3 \cdot \cdot \cdot p_x$)
12. Cumulative probability of dying (C_i) is equal to the cumulative product of the interval probabilities to that point (i.e., $C_i = c_1 \cdot c_2 \cdot c_3 \cdot \cdot \cdot c_x$)

With such tables established for each group in a study (as shown in Example 21), we may now proceed to test the hypotheses that each of the treated groups has a significantly shorter duration of survival, or that each of the treated groups died more quickly (note that plots of total animals dead and total animals surviving will give one an appreciation of the data, but can lead to no statistical conclusions).

There are a multiplicity of methods for testing for significance in life tables, with (as often is the case) the power of the tests increasing as does the difficulty of computation (14,18,55,97).

We begin our method of statistical comparison of survival at any point in the study by determining the standard error of the K interval survival rate as (43):

$$S_K = P_K \sqrt{\sum_1^K \left(\frac{D_i}{\ell_x' - d_x} \right)}$$

We may also determine the effective sample size (ℓ_1) in accordance with

$$\ell_1 = \frac{P(1 - P)}{S^2}$$

We may now compute the standard error of difference for any two groups (1 and 2) as

$$S_D = \sqrt{S_1^2 + S_2^2}$$

The difference in survival probabilities for the two groups is then calculated as

$$P_D = P_1 - P_2$$

We can then calculate a test statistic as

$$\frac{P_D}{S_D} = t'$$

This is then compared to the z distribution table. If $t' > z$ at the desired probability level, it is significant at that level. Example 21 illustrates the life-table technique for mortality data.

■ *Example 21*

Interval (mos.) (t_i)	Alive at beginning of interval (ℓ_i)	Animals withdrawn (ω_i)	Died during interval (d_i)	Animals at risk (ℓ_i)	Proportion of animals dead (D_i)	Probability of survival (P_i)	Cumulative proportion surviving (P_i)	Standard error of survival (S_i)
Test level 1								
8–9	109	0	0	109	0	1.0000	1.0000	0.0000
9–10	109	0	2	109	0.0184	0.9816	0.9816	0.0129
10–11	107	0	0	107	0	1.0000	0.9816	0.0128
11–12	107	10	0	102	0	1.0000	0.9816	0.0128
12–13	97	0	1	97	0.0103	0.9897	0.9715	0.0162
13–14	96	0	1	96	0.0104	0.9896	0.9614	0.0190
14–15	95	0	12	95	0.1263	0.8737	0.8400	0.0367
15–16	83	0	2	83	0.0241	0.9759	0.8198	0.0385
16–17	81	0	3	81	0.0370	0.9630	0.7894	0.0409
17–18	78	20	1	68	0.0147	0.9853	0.7778	0.0419
18–19	57	0	2	57	0.0351	0.6949	0.7505	0.0446
Control level								
11–12	99	0	1	99	0.0101	0.9899	0.9899	0.0100
12–13	98	0	0	98	0	1.0000	0.9899	0.0100
13–14	98	0	0	98	0	1.0000	0.9899	0.0100
14–15	98	0	2	98	0.0204	0.9796	0.9697	0.0172
15–16	96	0	1	96	0.0104	0.9896	0.9596	0.0198
16–17	95	0	0	95	0	1.0000	0.9596	0.0198
17–18	95	20	2	85	0.0235	0.8765	0.9370	0.0249
18–19	73	0	2	73	0.0274	0.9726	0.9113	0.0302

Now, for these two groups, we wish to determine effective sample size and to compare survival probabilities in the interval months 14–15. For the exposure group we compute sample size as

$$\ell_{E14-15} = \frac{0.8400(1 - 0.8400)}{(0.0367)^2} = 99.7854$$

Likewise we get a sample size of 98.1720 for the control group.

The standard error of difference for the two groups here is

$$SD = \sqrt{0.0367^2 + 0.0173^2} = 0.040573$$

The probability of survival differences is $P_D = 0.9697 - 0.8400 = 0.1297$. Our test statistic is then $0.1297/0.040573 = 3.196$. From our z value table we see that the critical values are

$$p \leq 0.05 = 1.960$$
$$p \leq 0.01 = 2.575$$
$$p \leq 0.001 = 3.270$$

As our calculated value is larger than all but the last of these, we find our groups to be significantly different at the 0.01 level ($0.01 > p > 0.001$).

TRANSFORMATIONS

If our initial inspection of a data set reveals it to have an unusual or undesired set of characteristics (or to lack a desired set of characteristics), we have a choice of three courses of action. We may proceed to select a method or test appropriate to this new set of conditions, or abandon the entire exercise, or transform the variable(s) under consideration in such a manner that the resulting transformed variates (X' and Y', for example, as opposed to the original variates X and Y) meet the assumptions or have the characteristics that are desired.

The key to all this is that the scale of measurement of most (if not all) variables is arbitrary. That is, though we are most commonly familiar with a linear scale of measurement, there is nothing that makes this the "correct" scale on its own, as opposed to a logarithmic scale (a common logarithmic measurement is that of pH values). Transforming a set of data (converting X to X') is really only changing the scale of measurement.

There are at least four good reasons to transform data:

1. To normalize the data, making it suitable for analysis by our most common parametric techniques such as ANOVA. A simple test of whether a selected transformation will yield a distribution of data which satisfies the underlying assumptions for ANOVA is to plot the cumulative distribution of samples on probability paper. One can then alter the scale of the second axis (that is, the axis other than the one which is on a probability scale) from linear to any other (logarithmic, reciprocal, square root, etc.) and see if a previously curved line indicating a skewed distribution straightens out to indicate normality. The slope of the transformed line gives us an estimate of the standard deviation. And if the slopes of the lines of several samples or groups of data are similar, we accordingly know that the variances of the different groups are homogeneous.
2. To linearize the relationship between a paired set of data, such as dose and response. This is the most common use in toxicology for transforms and is demonstrated in the section under probit/logit plots.
3. To adjust data for the influence of another variable. This is an alternative in some situations to the more complicated process of analysis of covariance. A ready example of this usage is the calculation of organ weight to body weight ratios in *in vivo* toxicity studies, with the resulting ratios serving as the raw data from an analysis of variance performed to identify possible target organs. This use is discussed in detail later in this chapter.
4. Finally, to make the relationships between variables clearer by removing or adjusting for interactions with third, fourth, etc., uncontrolled variables which influence the pair of variables of interest. This case is discussed in detail under time series analysis.

Common transformations are presented in Table 3.

Linear Regression

The statistical methods described to this point, other than the correlation coefficient, have all been directed toward only one of the three functions of statistics that were initially discussed—hypothesis testing, or telling us if two or more groups of data are (or are not) significantly different from one another. But there are other things we would like to know from some sets of data including, given a known, but not yet tested

TABLE 3. *Common transformations of data*

Transformation	Calculation[a]	Example of use
Arithmetic	$x' = \dfrac{x}{y}$ or $x' = x + c$	Organ weight/body weight
Reciprocals	$x' = \dfrac{1}{x}$	Linearizing data, particularly rate phenomena[b]
Arcsine	$x' = 2 \text{ arcsine}$	Normalizing dominant lethal and mutation rate data
Logarithmic	$x' = \log x$	pH Values
Probability (probit)	$x' = \text{probability } X$	Percentage responding
Square roots	$x' = \sqrt{x}$	Surface area of animal

[a] x, y: original variables; x', y': transformed values; c: constant.

[b] Plotting a double reciprocal $\left(\text{i.e., } \dfrac{1}{x} \text{ vs. } \dfrac{1}{y}\right)$ will linearize almost any data set, as will plotting the log transforms of a set of variables.

(indeed, perhaps not possible to test) level of exposure, what will be the change in a response level? For example, having measured mortality at 100, 50, and 25 mg/kg, given a dose level of 10 mg/kg of material, how many of the 100 animals dosed will be expected to die? Foremost among the methods for interpolating within a known data relationship is regression—the fitting of a line or curve to a set of known points on a graph, and the extension ("estimation") of this line or curve to areas where we have no points. The simplest of these regression models is that of simple linear regression (valid when increasing the value of one variable changes the value of the related variable in a linear fashion, either positively or negatively). This is the case we will explore here, using the methods of least squares.

Given that we have two sets of variables, x (e.g., milligrams per kilogram of test material administered) and Y (e.g., percentage of animals so dosed that die), what is required is solving for a and b in the equation $Y_i = a + bx_i$ [where the uppercase Y_i is the fitted value of y_i at x_i, and we wish to minimize $(y_i - Y_i)^2$]. So we solve the equations

$$b = \frac{\sum x_i y_i - n\overline{xy}}{\sum x_i^2 - n\bar{x}^2}$$

$$a = \bar{y} - b\bar{x}$$

where n is the number of data points. Use of this is demonstrated in Example 22.

Note that in actuality, dose–response relationships are often not linear and instead we must use either a transform (to linearize the data) or a nonlinear regression method (a good discussion of which may be found in Gallant, ref. 42).

Note also that we can use the correlation test statistic described earlier (in the correlation coefficient section) to determine if the regression is significant (and, therefore, valid at a defined level of probability). A more specific test for significance would be the linear regression analysis of variance (83, pp. 260–262). To do so we start by developing the appropriate ANOVA table (see Table 4).

■ **Example 22**

From a short-term toxicity study we have the following results:

Dose administered (mg/kg)	% Animals dead		
x_i	x_i^2	y_i	$x_i y_i$
1	1	10	10
3	9	20	60
4	16	18	72
5	25	20	100
Sums $x_i = 13$	$x_i^2 = 51$	$y_i = 68$	$x_i y_i = 242$

$$\bar{x} = 3.25$$

$$\bar{y} = 17$$

$$b = \frac{242 - (4)(3.25)(17)}{51 - (4)(10.5625)} = \frac{21}{8.75} = 2.40$$

$$a = 17 - (2.4)(3.25) = 9.20$$

We therefore see that our fitted line is $Y = 9.2 + 2.4x$.

The ANOVA data in Table 4 are then used as shown in Example 23.

TABLE 4. *Linear regression analysis of variance*

Source of variation (1)	Sum of squares (2)	Degrees of freedom (3)	Mean square (4) $\left(\text{equal to } \frac{(2)}{(3)}\right)$
Regression	$b_1^2(\sum x_1^2 - n\bar{x}^2)$	1	By division
Residual	By difference	$n - 2$	By division
Total	$\sum y_1^2 - n\bar{y}^2$	$n - 1$	

We then calculate $F_{1,n-2} = \dfrac{\text{regression mean square}}{\text{residual mean square}}$

■ **Example 23**

We desire to test the significance of the regression line in Example 22.

$$\sum y_i^2 = 10^2 + 20^2 + 18^2 + 20^2 = 1224$$

$$\text{Regression } SS = (2.4)^2[51 - 4(3.25)^2] = 50.4$$

$$\text{Total } SS = 1224 - 4(17^2) = 68.0$$

$$\text{Residual } SS = 68.0 - 50.4 = 17.6$$

$$F_{1,2} = 50.4/8.8 = 5.73$$

This value is not significant at the 0.05 level; therefore, the regression is not significant. A significant F value (as found in an F distribution table for the appropriate degrees of freedom) indicates that the regression line is an accurate prediction of observed values at that confidence level. Note that the portion of the total sum of squares explained by the regression is called the coefficient of determination, denoted by R^2 (the square of the coefficient of correlation, which in the above example is equal to 0.86^2 or 0.74).

Finally, we might wish to determine the confidence intervals for our regression line—that is, given a regression line with calculated values for Y_i given x_i, what are the limits within which may we be certain (with say a 95% probability) of the real value of Y_i?

If we denote the residual mean square in the ANOVA by s^2, the 95% confidence limits for a (denoted by A, the notation for the true—as opposed to estimated—value for this parameter) are calculated as:

$$t_{n-2} = \frac{a - A}{\sqrt{\dfrac{s^2(\sum x_i^2)}{n\sum x_i^2 - n^2\bar{x}^2}}}$$

$$\frac{9.2 - A}{\sqrt{\dfrac{8.8(51)}{4(51) - (16)(10.562)}}} = \frac{9.2 - A}{\sqrt{\dfrac{448.8}{35.008}}}$$

$$= \frac{9.2 - A}{3.58} = \pm 4.303$$

$$9.2 - A = \pm 15.405$$

$$A = 9.2 \pm 15.405$$

with t_{n-2} being taken from a table of the upper and lower $2\frac{1}{2}\%$ points of the t distribution.

Probit/Log Transforms and Regression

As we noted in the previous section, dose–response problems (among the most common interpolation problems encountered in toxicology) rarely are such as to make a linear regression a valid operation. The most common valid interpolation methods are based upon probability (probit) and logarithmic (log) value scales, with percentage responses (death, tumor, incidence, etc.) being expressed on the probit scale while doses (Y_i) are expressed on the log scale. There are two strategies for such an approach. The first is based on transforming the data to these scales, then doing a weighted linear regression on the transformed data (if one does not have access to a computer or a high-powered programmable calculator, the only practical strategy is not to assign weights). The second requires the use of algorithms (approximate calculation techniques) for the probit value and regression process, and is extremely burdensome to perform manually.

Our approach to the first strategy requires that we construct a table with the pairs of values of x_i and y_i listed in order of increasing values of Y_i (percentage response). Beside each of these columns a set of blank columns should be left so that the transformed values may be listed. We then simply add the columns described in the linear regression procedure illustrated in Example 22. Log and probit values may be taken from any of a number of sets of tables (25) and the rest of the table is then developed from these transformed x_i and y_i values (denoted as x'_i and y'_i). A standard linear regression is then performed (see Example 24).

The second strategy we discussed has been approached by a number of authors (11,35,71,84). All of these methods are computationally cumbersome. It is possible to approximate the necessary iterative process using the algorithms developed by Abramowitz and Stegun (1), but even this merely reduces the complexity to the point that the procedure may be readily programmed on a small computer or programmable calculator.

■ *Example 24*

% Of animals killed (x_i)	Probit of $x_i = x'_i$	Dose of chemical (mg/kg) (y_i)	Log of $y_i = y'_i$	$(x'_i)^2$	$x'_i y'_i$
2	2.9463	3	0.4771	8.6806	1.40567
10	3.7184	5	0.6990	13.8264	2.59916
42	4.7981	10	1.0000	23.0217	4.79810
90	6.2816	20	1.3010	39.45724	8.17223
98	7.0537	30	1.4771	49.75468	10.4190
Sums	$\Sigma\, x'_i = 24.7981$		$\Sigma\, y'_i = 4.9542$	$\Sigma\, x'^2_i = 134.7461$	$\Sigma\, x'_i y'_i = 27.39416$
Means	$\bar{x}'_i = 4.95962$		$\bar{y}'_i = 0.99084$		

Calculating the regression values as before, we find

$$a = -0.200591$$

$$b = 0.240226$$

Our interpolated log of the LD_{50} (calculated by using 5.000—the probit of 50%—in the regression equation) is 1.000540338. When we convert this log value to its linear equivalent, we get an LD_{50} of 10.0 mg/kg.

Finally, our calculated correlation coefficient is $r = 0.997$.

Moving Averages

An obvious drawback to the interpolation procedures we have examined to date is that they do take a significant amount of time (though they are simple enough to be done manually), especially if the only result we desire is an LD_{50} or LC_{50}, or LT_{50}.

The method of moving averages (98,104) gives a rapid and reasonably accurate estimate of this median-effective dose and the estimated standard deviation of its logarithm.

Such methodology requires that the same number of animals be used per dosage level and that the spacing between successive dosage exposure levels be geometrically constant (i.e., levels of 1, 2, 4, and 8 mg/kg or 1, 3, 9, and 27 ppm). Given this and access to a table for the computation of moving averages (104), one can readily calculate the median effective dose with the following formula (illustrated for dose):

$$\log m = \log D + d(K-1)/2 + df$$

where m = median effective dose or exposure
D = the lowest dose tested
d = the log of the ratio of successive doses/exposures
f = a table value taken from Weil (104)

for the proper K (the total number of levels tested = $K + 1$)

Introduced here are additions to Weil's published tables (Tables 5–9), with coverage now added to include the full range of possibilities at N's of 4 and 5. Included are simplified formulas and calculated values useful if the factor between dosage levels is 2.0 (the logarithm of which is 0.30103 = d in this case).

Example 25 demonstrates the use of this method and the new tables.

■ *Example 25*

As part of an inhalation study we exposed groups of 5 rats each to levels of 20, 40, 80, and 160 ppm of a chemical vapor. These exposures killed 0, 1, 3, and 5 animals, respectively. From the $N = 5$, $K = 3$ tables on the r value 0, 1, 3, 5 line we get an f of 0.7 and $a\sigma_f$ of 0.31623 ($a\sigma_f$ is the constant the tables provide to calculate 95% confidence intervals). We can then calculate the LC_{50} to be:

$$\text{Log } LC_{50} = 1.30130 + 0.30103(2)/$$

$$2 + 0.30103(0.7)$$

$$= 1.30103 + 0.51175$$

$$= 1.81278$$

$$\therefore LC_{50} = 65.0 \text{ ppm with 95\% confidence}$$

$$\text{intervals of } \pm 2.179 \cdot d \cdot \sigma_f$$

$$\text{or } \pm 2.179(0.30103)(0.31623)$$

$$= \pm 0.20743$$

Therefore, the log confidence limits are $1.81278 \pm 0.20743 = 1.60535$ to 2.02021; on the linear scale, 40.3–104.8 ppm.

TABLE 5. *Tables for calculation of median-effective dose[a]*

r Values	f	σ_f	d = 0.30103 df	3.182 $d\sigma_f$
0, 4	0.5	(0)	0.15052	(0)
1, 4	0.33333	0.22222	0.10034	0.21286
2, 4	0.0	0.57735	0.0	0.55303
0, 3	0.66667	0.22222	0.20069	0.21286
1, 3	0.5	0.34355	0.15052	0.33866
2, 3	0.0	1.15470	0.0	1.10606
0, 2	1.0	0.57735	0.30103	0.55303
1, 2	1.0	1.15470	0.30103	1.1060
				2.776 $d\sigma_f$
0, 5	0.5	(0)	0.1505	(0)
1, 5	0.375	0.15625	0.11289	0.13057
2, 5	0.16667	0.34021	0.05017	0.28430
0, 4	0.625	0.15625	0.18814	0.13057
1, 4	0.5	0.23570	0.15052	0.19696
2, 4	0.25	0.47599	0.07526	0.39776
0, 3	0.83333	0.34021	0.25086	0.28430
1, 3	0.75	0.47599	0.22577	0.39776
2, 3	0.5	0.86603	0.15052	0.72371

[a] Calculation by moving average interpolation for $N = 4$ or 5, $K = 1$, $d = 0.30103$ from the formula: Log $m = \log D_a = \dfrac{d(K-1)}{2} + df = \log D_a + df$ in this case.

$N = 4$; upper section.
$N = 5$; lower section.

Nonlinear Regression

More often than not in toxicology (and, in fact, in the biological sciences in general) we find that our data demonstrate a relationship between two variables (such as age and body weight) which is not linear. That is, a change in one variable (e.g., age) is not coupled with a directly proportional change in the other (i.e., body weight). But some form of relationship between the variables is apparent. If understanding such a relationship and being able to predict unknown points from a limited set of measured data points is of value, we have a pair of options available to us. The first, which was discussed and reviewed above, is to use one or more transformations to linearize our data and then to make use of linear regression. This approach, though most commonly used, has a number of drawbacks. Not all data can be suitably transformed; sometimes the transformations necessary to linearize the data require cumbersome series of calculations; and the resulting linear regression is not always sufficient to account for the differences among sample val-

ues—there are significant deviations around the linear regression line (i.e., a line may still not give us a good fit to the data or do an adequate job of representing the relationships between the data). In such cases, we have available a second option—fitting the data to a nonlinear function such as some form of curve. This is, in the general form, nonlinear regression and may involve fitting data to an infinite number of possible functions. But most often we are interested in fitting curves to a polynomial function of the general form.

$$Y = a + bx + cx^2 + dx^3 + \cdots$$

where x is the independent variable. As the number of powers of x increases, the curve becomes increasingly complex and will be able to fit a given set of data increasingly well.

Generally in toxicology, if we plot the log of a response (such as body weight) versus a linear scale of our dose or stimulus, we get one of four types of nonlinear curves. These are as follows (Snedecor and Cochran, ref. 94, pp. 393–397):

1. Exponential growth

$$\text{where } \log Y = A(B^x)$$

TABLE 6. *Table for calculation of median-effective dose[a]*

r Values	f	σ_f	d = 0.30103 d(f + 0.5)	2.447 $d\sigma_f$
0, 0, 4	1.0	(0)	0.45154	(0)
0, 1, 4	0.75	0.25000	0.37629	0.18416
0, 2, 4	0.5	0.28868	0.30103	0.21265
0, 3, 4	0.25	0.25000	0.22577	0.18416
0, 4, 4	0.0	(0)	0.15052	(0)
1, 0, 4	1.0	(0)	0.45154	(0)
1, 1, 4	0.66667	0.35138	0.35120	0.25883
1, 2, 4	0.33333	0.44444	0.25086	0.32738
1, 3, 4	0.0	0.47140	0.15052	0.34724
2, 0, 4	1.0	(0)	0.45154	(0)
2, 1, 4	0.5	0.57735	0.30103	0.42529
2, 2, 4	0.0	0.81650	0.15052	0.60145
3, 0, 4	1.0	(0)	0.45154	(0)
3, 1, 4	0.0	1.41421	0.15052	1.04174
0, 1, 3	1.0	0.47140	0.45154	0.34724
0, 2, 3	0.66667	0.44444	0.35120	0.32738
0, 3, 3	0.33333	0.35138	0.25086	0.25883
0, 4, 3	0.0	(0)	0.15052	(0)
1, 1, 3	1.0	0.70711	0.45154	0.52087
1, 2, 3	0.5	0.6770	0.30103	0.49869
1, 3, 3	0.0	0.70711	0.15052	0.52087
2, 1, 3	1.0	1.41421	0.45154	1.04174
2, 2, 3	0.0	1.63299	0.15052	1.20289
0, 2, 2	1.0	0.81650	0.45154	0.60145
0, 3, 2	0.5	0.57735	0.30103	0.42529
0, 4, 2	0.0	(0)	0.15052	(0)
1, 2, 2	1.0	1.63299	0.45154	1.20289
1, 3, 2	0.0	1.41421	0.15052	1.04174
0, 3, 1	1.0	1.41421	0.45154	1.04174
0, 4, 1	0.0	(0)	0.15052	(0)

[a] Calculation by moving average interpolation for $N = 4$, $K = 2$, $d = 0.30103$ from the formula:

Log $m = \log D_a + \dfrac{d(K-1)}{2} + df = \log D_a + d(f + 0.5)$.

$2.447\ \sigma_{\log m} = 2.447\ \sigma_f (d)$.

TABLE 7. *Table for calculation of median-effective dose*[a]

| r Values | f | σ_f | d = 0.30103 | |
			d (f + 0.5)	2.306 $d\sigma_f$
0, 0, 5	1.0	(0)	0.45154	(0)
0, 1, 5	0.8	0.20000	0.39134	0.13884
0, 2, 5	0.6	0.24495	0.33113	0.17004
0, 3, 5	0.4	0.24495	0.27093	0.17004
0, 4, 5	0.2	0.20000	0.21072	0.13884
0, 5, 5	0.0	(0)	0.15052	(0)
1, 0, 5	1.0	(0)	0.45154	(0)
1, 1, 5	0.75	0.25769	0.37629	0.17888
1, 2, 5	0.5	0.33072	0.30103	0.22958
1, 3, 5	0.25	0.35904	0.22577	0.24924
1, 4, 5	0.0	0.35355	0.15052	0.24543
2, 0, 5	1.0	(0)	0.45154	(0)
2, 1, 5	0.66667	0.36004	0.35120	0.24993
2, 2, 5	0.33333	0.49065	0.25086	0.34060
2, 3, 5	0.0	0.57735	0.15052	0.40078
3, 0, 5	1.0	(0)	0.45154	(0)
3, 1, 5	0.5	0.58630	0.30103	0.40700
3, 2, 5	0.0	0.86603	0.15052	0.60118
4, 0, 5	1.0	(0)	0.45154	(0)
4, 1, 5	0.0	1.41421	0.15052	0.98171
0, 1, 4	1.0	0.35355	0.45154	0.24543
0, 2, 4	0.75	0.35904	0.37629	0.24924
0, 3, 4	0.5	0.33072	0.30103	0.22958
0, 4, 4	0.25	0.25769	0.22577	0.17888
0, 5, 4	0.0	(0)	0.15052	(0)
1, 1, 4	1.0	0.47140	0.45154	0.32723
1, 2, 4	0.66667	0.47791	0.35120	0.33175
1, 3, 4	0.33333	0.47791	0.25086	0.33175
1, 4, 4	0.0	0.47140	0.15052	0.32723
2, 1, 4	1.0	0.70711	0.45154	0.49086
2, 2, 4	0.5	0.72887	0.30103	0.50596
2, 3, 4	0.0	0.86603	0.15052	0.60118
3, 1, 4	1.0	1.41421	0.45154	0.98171
3, 2, 4	0.0	1.73205	0.15052	1.20235
0, 2, 3	1.0	0.57735	0.45154	0.40078
0, 3, 3	0.66667	0.49065	0.35120	0.35060
0, 4, 3	0.33333	0.36004	0.25086	0.24993
0, 5, 3	0.0	(0)	0.15052	(0)
1, 2, 3	1.0	0.86603	0.45154	0.60118
1, 3, 3	0.5	0.72887	0.30103	0.50596
1, 4, 3	0.0	0.70711	0.15052	0.49086
2, 2, 3	1.0	1.73205	0.45154	1.20235
2, 3, 3	0.0	1.73205	0.15052	1.20235
0, 3, 2	1.0	0.86603	0.45154	0.60118
0, 4, 2	0.5	0.58630	0.30103	0.40700
0, 5, 2	0.0	(0)	0.15052	(0)
1, 3, 2	1.0	1.73205	0.45154	1.20235
1, 4, 2	0.0	1.41421	0.15052	0.98171
0, 4, 1	1.0	1.41421	0.45154	0.98171
0, 5, 1	0.0	(0)	0.15052	(0)

[a] Calculation by moving average interpolation for $N = 5$, $K = 2$, $d = 0.30103$ from the formula: $\text{Log } m = \log D_a + \dfrac{d(K-1)}{2} + df = \log D_a + d(f + 0.5)$ in this case. $2.306 \, \sigma_{\log m} = 2.306 \, d\sigma_f$.

such as the growth curve for the log phase of a bacterial culture

2. Exponential decay

$$\log Y = A(B^{-x})$$

such as a radioactive decay curve

3. Asymptotic regression

$$\log Y = A - B(p^x)$$

such as a first order reaction curve

4. Logistic growth curve

$$\log Y = A/(1 + Bp^x)$$

such as a population growth curve

In all these cases, A and B are constants while p is a log transform. These curves are illustrated in Fig. 5.

All four types of these curves are fit by iterative processes—that is, best guess numbers are initially chosen for each of the constants. After a fit is attempted, the constants are modified to improve the fit. This process is repeated until an acceptable fit has been generated. Analysis of variance or covariance can be used to objectively evaluate the acceptability of the fit. Needless to say, the use of a computer generally accelerates such a curve-fitting process.

Trend Analysis

A variation on the theme of regression testing which has gained popularity in toxicology over the last 10 years is trend analysis. In the broadest sense, this is determining whether a sequence of observations taken over a period of time (e.g., the cumulative proportions of a group of animals which have tumors of a particular sort) exhibit some sort of pattern of change—either an increase (an upward trend) or a decrease (a downward trend). There are a number of tests that can be used to evaluate data to determine if a trend exists in data. The most popular test in toxicology is currently that presented by Tarone in 1975 (97) because it is that used by the National Cancer Institute (NCI) in the analysis of carcinogenicity data. A simple, but efficient alternative is the Cox and Stuart test (19) which is a modification of the sign test. For each point at which we have a measure (such as the incidence of animals observed with tumors) we form a pair of observations—one from each of the groups we wish to compare. In a traditional NCI bioassay this would mean pairing control with low dose and low dose with control (to explore a dose-related trend) or each time period observation in a dose group (except the first) with its predecessor (to evaluate time-related trend). When the second observation in a pair exceeds the earlier observation, we record a plus sign for that pair. When the first observation is greater than the later, we put a minus sign in place for that pair. A preponderance of plus signs suggests a downward trend while an excess of minus signs suggests an upward trend. A formal test of hypothesis at a preselected confidence level can then be performed.

Expressed more formally, we first (having defined what trend we want to test for) match pairs as $(X_1 + X_{1+c})$, (X_2, X_{2+c}), $\cdots (X_{n'-c}, X_{n'})$ where $c = n'/2$ when n' is even and $c = (n' + 1)/2$ when n' is odd (where n' is the number of observations in a set). The hypothesis is then tested by com-

TABLE 8. *Table for calculation of median-effective dose*[a]

r Values	f	σ_f	d (f + 1)	2.262 dσ_f	r Values	f	σ_f	d (f + 1)	2.262 dσ_f
			d = 0.30103					d = 0.30103	
0, 0, 2, 4	1.00000	0.28868	0.60206	0.19657	0, 1, 4, 3	0.33333	0.35136	0.40137	0.23925
0, 0, 3, 4	0.7500	0.2500	0.52680	0.17023	0, 2, 2, 3	0.66667	0.58794	0.50172	0.40035
0, 0, 4, 4	0.50000	0.0	0.45154	0.00	0, 2, 3, 3	0.33333	0.52116	0.40137	0.35487
0, 1, 1, 4	1.00000	0.35355	0.60206	0.24074	0, 2, 4, 3	0.00000	0.38490	0.30103	0.26209
0, 1, 2, 4	0.75000	0.38188	0.52680	0.26003	0, 3, 3, 3	0.00000	0.47140	0.30103	0.32099
0, 1, 3, 4	0.50000	0.35355	0.45154	0.24074	1, 0, 3, 3	1.00000	0.70711	0.60206	0.48149
0, 1, 4, 4	0.25000	0.25000	0.37629	0.17023	1, 0, 4, 3	0.50000	0.35355	0.45154	0.24074
0, 2, 2, 4	0.50000	0.40825	0.45154	0.27799	1, 1, 2, 3	1.00000	0.91287	0.60206	0.62160
0, 2, 3, 4	0.25000	0.38188	0.37629	0.26003	1, 1, 3, 3	0.50000	0.79057	0.45154	0.53832
0, 2, 4, 4	0.00000	0.28868	0.30103	0.19657	1, 1, 4, 3	0.00000	0.70711	0.30103	0.48149
0, 3, 3, 4	0.00000	0.35355	0.30103	0.24074	1, 2, 2, 3	0.50000	0.88976	0.45154	0.60586
1, 0, 2, 4	1.00000	0.38490	0.60206	0.26209	1, 2, 3, 3	0.00000	0.91287	0.30103	0.62160
1, 0, 3, 4	0.66667	0.35136	0.50172	0.23925	2, 0, 3, 3	1.00000	1.41421	0.60206	0.96298
1, 0, 4, 4	0.33333	0.22222	0.40137	0.15132	2, 0, 4, 3	0.00000	1.15470	0.30103	0.78627
1, 1, 1, 4	1.00000	0.47140	0.60206	0.32099	2, 1, 2, 3	1.00000	1.82574	0.60206	1.24320
1, 1, 2, 4	0.66667	0.52116	0.50172	0.35487	2, 1, 3, 3	0.00000	1.82574	0.30103	1.24320
1, 1, 3, 4	0.33333	0.52116	0.40137	0.35487	2, 2, 2, 3	0.00000	2.00000	0.30103	1.36186
1, 1, 4, 4	0.00000	0.47140	0.30103	0.32099	0, 0, 4, 2	1.00000	0.57735	0.60206	0.39313
1, 2, 2, 4	0.33333	0.58794	0.40137	0.40035	0, 1, 3, 2	1.00000	0.91287	0.60206	0.62160
1, 2, 3, 4	0.00000	0.60858	0.30103	0.41440	0, 1, 4, 2	0.50000	0.57735	0.45154	0.39313
2, 0, 2, 4	1.00000	0.57735	0.60206	0.39313	0, 2, 2, 2	1.00000	1.00000	0.60206	0.68093
2, 0, 3, 4	0.50000	0.57735	0.45154	0.39313	0, 2, 3, 2	0.50000	0.81650	0.45154	0.55598
2, 0, 4, 4	0.00000	0.57735	0.30103	0.39313	0, 2, 4, 2	0.00000	0.57735	0.30103	0.39313
2, 1, 1, 4	1.00000	0.70711	0.60206	0.48149	0, 3, 3, 2	0.00000	0.70711	0.30103	0.48149
2, 1, 2, 4	0.50000	0.81650	0.45154	0.55598	1, 0, 4, 2	1.00000	1.15470	0.60206	0.78627
2, 1, 3, 4	0.00000	0.91287	0.60206	0.62160	1, 1, 3, 2	1.00000	1.82574	0.60206	1.24320
2, 2, 2, 4	0.00000	1.00000	0.30103	0.68093	1, 1, 4, 2	0.00000	1.41421	0.30103	0.96298
3, 0, 2, 4	1.00000	1.15470	0.60206	0.78627	1, 2, 2, 2	1.00000	2.00000	0.60206	1.36186
3, 0, 3, 4	0.00000	1.41421	0.30103	0.96298	1, 2, 3, 2	0.00000	1.82574	0.30103	1.24320
3, 1, 1, 4	1.00000	1.41421	0.60206	0.96298	0, 2, 3, 1	1.00000	1.82574	0.60206	1.24320
3, 1, 2, 4	0.00000	1.82574	0.30103	1.24320	0, 2, 4, 1	0.00000	1.15470	0.80103	0.78627
0, 0, 3, 3	1.00000	0.47140	0.60206	0.32099	0, 3, 3, 1	0.00000	1.41421	0.30103	0.96298
0, 0, 4, 3	0.66667	0.22222	0.50172	0.15132	0, 1, 4, 1	1.00000	1.41421	0.60206	0.96298
0, 1, 2, 3	1.00000	0.60858	0.60206	0.41440					
0, 1, 3, 3	0.66667	0.52116	0.50172	0.35487					

[a] Calculation by moving average interpolation for N = 4, K = 3, d = 0.30103, from the formula: Log m = log D_a + d (K − 1)/2 + df = log D_a + d (f + 1) in this case. 2.262 $\sigma_{\log m}$ = 2.262 σ_f(d).

paring the resulting number of excess positive or negative signs against a sign test table such as are found in Beyer (10).

We can, of course, combine a number of observations to allow ourselves to actively test for a set of trends, such as the existence of a trend of increasing difference between two groups of animals over a period of time. This is demonstrated in Example 26.

■ *Example 26*

In a chronic feeding study in rats, we are interested in testing the hypothesis that, in the second year of the study, there was a dose responsive increase in tumor incidence over time associated with receiving the test compound. We utilize, below, a Cox–Stuart test for trend to address this question. All groups start the second year with an equal number of animals.

Month of study	Control Total X animals with tumors	Change [X_{A-B}]	Low dose Total Y animals with tumors	Change [Y_{A-B}]	Compared with control (Y − X)	High dose Total Z animals with tumors	Change [Z_{A-B}]	Compared with control (Z − X)
12 (A)	1	NA	0	NA	NA	5	NA	NA
13 (B)	1	0	0	0	0	7	2	(+)2
14 (C)	3	2	1	1	(−)1	11	4	(+)2
15 (D)	3	0	1	0	0	11	0	0
16 (E)	4	1	1	0	(−)1	13	2	(+)1
17 (F)	5	1	3	2	(+)1	14	1	0
18 (G)	5	0	3	0	0	15	1	(+)1
19 (H)	5	0	5	2	(+)2	18	3	(+)3

20 (I)	6	1	6	1	0	19	1	0
21 (J)	8	2	7	1	(−)1	22	3	(+)1
22 (K)	12	4	9	2	(−)2	26	4	0
23 (L)	14	2	12	3	(+)1	28	2	0
24 (M)	18	4	17	5	(+)1	31	3	(−)1
Sum of signs								
+					4+			6+
−					4−			1−
N = 12					Y − X = 0 (No trend)			Z − X = 5

Reference to a sign table is not necessary for the low dose comparison (where there is no trend) but clearly shows the high dose to be significant at the $p \leq 0.05$ level.

TABLE 9. *Table for calculation of median-effective dose*[a]

r Values	f	σ_f	d (f + 1)	2.179 dσ_f	r Values	f	σ_f	d (f + 1)	2.179 dσ_f
		d = 0.30103					d = 0.30103		
0, 0, 3, 5	0.9	0.24495	0.57196	0.16067	0, 2, 4, 4	0.375	0.40625	0.41392	0.26648
0, 0, 4, 5	0.7	0.20000	0.51175	0.13119	0, 2, 5, 4	0.125	0.30778	0.33866	0.20189
0, 0, 5, 5	0.5	0.0	0.45154	0.0	0, 3, 3, 4	0.375	0.44304	0.41392	0.29061
0, 1, 2, 5	0.9	0.31623	0.57196	0.20743	0, 3, 4, 4	0.125	0.39652	0.33866	0.26010
0, 1, 3, 5	0.7	0.31623	0.51175	0.20743	1, 0, 4, 4	0.83333	0.43744	0.55189	0.28694
0, 1, 4, 5	0.5	0.28284	0.45154	0.18553	1, 0, 5, 4	0.50	0.23570	0.45154	0.15461
0, 1, 5, 5	0.3	0.20000	0.39134	0.13119	1, 1, 3, 4	0.83333	0.59835	0.55189	0.39248
0, 2, 2, 5	0.7	0.34641	0.51175	0.22723	1, 1, 4, 4	0.50	0.52705	0.45154	0.34572
0, 2, 3, 5	0.5	0.34641	0.45154	0.22723	1, 1, 5, 4	0.16667	0.43744	0.35120	0.28694
0, 2, 4, 5	0.3	0.31623	0.39134	0.20743	1, 2, 2, 4	0.83333	0.64310	0.55189	0.42184
0, 2, 5, 5	0.1	0.24495	0.33113	0.16067	1, 2, 3, 4	0.50	0.62361	0.45154	0.40905
0, 3, 3, 5	0.3	0.34641	0.39134	0.22723	1, 2, 4, 4	0.16667	0.59835	0.35120	0.39248
0, 3, 4, 5	0.1	0.31623	0.33113	0.20743	1, 3, 3, 4	0.16667	0.64310	0.35120	0.42184
1, 0, 3, 5	0.875	0.30778	0.56443	0.20189	2, 0, 4, 4	0.75	0.64348	0.52680	0.42209
1, 0, 4, 5	0.625	0.26700	0.48917	0.17514	2, 0, 5, 4	0.25	0.47598	0.37629	0.31222
1, 0, 5, 5	0.375	0.15625	0.41392	0.10249	2, 1, 3, 4	0.75	0.88829	0.52680	0.58267
1, 1, 2, 5	0.875	0.39652	0.56443	0.26010	2, 1, 4, 4	0.25	0.85239	0.37629	0.55912
1, 1, 3, 5	0.625	0.40625	0.48917	0.26648	2, 2, 2, 4	0.75	0.95607	0.52680	0.62713
1, 1, 4, 5	0.375	0.38654	0.41392	0.25355	2, 2, 3, 4	0.25	0.98821	0.37629	0.64821
1, 1, 5, 5	0.125	0.33219	0.33866	0.21790	3, 0, 4, 4	0.5	1.27475	0.45154	0.83616
1, 2, 2, 5	0.625	0.44304	0.48917	0.29061	3, 1, 3, 4	0.5	1.76777	0.45154	1.15956
1, 2, 3, 5	0.375	0.46034	0.41392	0.30196	3, 2, 2, 4	0.5	1.90394	0.45154	1.24888
1, 2, 4, 5	0.125	0.45178	0.33866	0.29634	0, 0, 5, 3	0.83333	0.34021	0.55189	0.22316
1, 3, 3, 5	0.125	0.48513	0.33866	0.31822	0, 1, 4, 3	0.83333	0.58134	0.55189	0.38133
2, 0, 3, 5	0.83333	0.41388	0.55189	0.27148	0, 1, 5, 3	0.50000	0.39087	0.45154	0.25639
2, 0, 4, 5	0.50000	0.39087	0.45154	0.25639	0, 2, 3, 3	0.83333	0.67013	0.55189	0.43957
2, 0, 5, 5	0.16667	0.34021	0.35120	0.22316	0, 2, 4, 3	0.50000	0.56519	0.45154	0.37073
2, 1, 2, 5	0.83333	0.53142	0.55189	0.34858	0, 2, 5, 3	0.16667	0.41388	0.35120	0.27148
2, 1, 3, 5	0.50	0.56519	0.45154	0.37073	0, 3, 3, 3	0.50000	0.61237	0.45154	0.40168
2, 1, 4, 5	0.16667	0.58134	0.35120	0.38133	0, 3, 4, 3	0.16667	0.53142	0.35120	0.34858
2, 2, 2, 5	0.50	0.61237	0.45154	0.40168	1, 0, 5, 3	0.75	0.47598	0.52680	0.31222
2, 2, 3, 5	0.16667	0.67013	0.35120	0.43957	1, 1, 4, 3	0.75	0.85239	0.52680	0.55912
3, 0, 3, 5	0.75	0.63122	0.52680	0.41404	1, 1, 5, 3	0.25	0.64348	0.37629	0.42209
3, 0, 4, 5	0.25	0.67892	0.37629	0.44533	1, 2, 3, 3	0.75	0.98821	0.52680	0.64821
3, 1, 2, 5	0.75	0.80526	0.52680	0.52820	1, 2, 4, 3	0.25	0.88829	0.37629	0.58267
3, 1, 3, 5	0.25	0.91430	0.37629	0.59973	1, 3, 3, 3	0.25	0.95607	0.37629	0.62713
3, 2, 2, 5	0.25	0.98028	0.37629	0.64301	2, 0, 5, 3	0.5	0.86602	0.45154	0.56806
4, 0, 3, 5	0.5	1.32288	0.45154	0.86774	0, 1, 5, 2	0.75	0.67892	0.52680	0.44533
4, 1, 2, 5	0.5	1.64831	0.45154	1.08776	0, 2, 4, 2	0.25	0.91430	0.37629	0.59973
0, 0, 4, 4	0.875	0.33219	0.56443	0.21790	0, 2, 5, 2	0.25	0.63122	0.37629	0.41404
0, 0, 5, 4	0.625	0.15625	0.48917	0.10249	0, 3, 3, 2	0.75	0.98028	0.52680	0.64301
0, 1, 3, 4	0.875	0.45178	0.56443	0.29634	0, 3, 4, 2	0.25	0.80526	0.37625	0.52820
0, 1, 4, 4	0.625	0.38654	0.48917	0.25355	1, 1, 5, 2	0.5	1.27475	0.45154	0.83616
0, 1, 5, 4	0.375	0.26700	0.41392	0.17514	1, 2, 4, 2	0.5	1.76777	0.45154	1.15956
0, 2, 2, 4	0.875	0.48513	0.56443	0.31822	1, 3, 3, 2	0.5	1.90394	0.45154	1.24888
0, 2, 3, 4	0.625	0.46034	0.48917	0.30196	0, 2, 5, 1	0.5	1.32288	0.45154	0.86774
					0, 3, 4, 1	0.5	1.65831	0.45154	1.08776

[a] Calculation by moving average interpolation. For $N = 5$, $K = 3$, $d = 0.30103$ from the formula: $\text{Log } m = \log D_a + d (K - 1)/2 + df = \log D_a + d (f + 1)$ in this case. $2.179\ \sigma_{\log m} = 2.179\ \sigma_f(d)$.

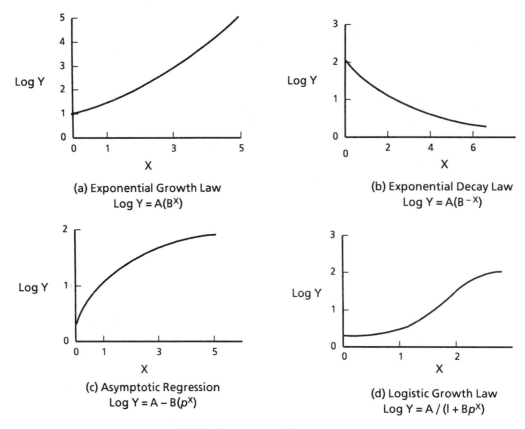

FIG. 5. Common curvilinear curves.

Exploratory Data Analysis

Over the past 10 years, an entirely new approach has been developed to get the most information out of the increasingly larger and more complex data sets that scientists are faced with. This approach involves the use of a very diverse set of fairly simple techniques which comprise exploratory data analysis (EDA). As expounded by Tukey (100), there are four major ingredients to EDA:

1. Displays, which visually reveal the behavior of the data and the structure of the analysis;
2. Residuals, which focus attention on what remains of data after some level of analysis;
3. Reexpressions, which use simple transformations such as the logarithm and square root to simplify data behavior (such as linearizing it) and clarify analysis; and
4. Resistance, which ensures that a few extreme outliers do not influence the results of analysis.

Further review of these techniques is beyond the scope of this text.

Velleman and Hoaglin (101) present a clear overview of the more important methods, along with code for their performance on the microcomputer (they have also now been incorporated into Minitab). A short examination of a single case of use, particularly relevant to toxicology, is in order.

Toxicology has long recognized that no population—animal or human—is completely uniform in its response to any particular toxicant. Rather, a population is composed of a (assumedly normal) distribution of individuals: some that are resistant to intoxication (hyporesponders), the majority responding close to an LD_{50} level, and some that are sensitive to intoxication (hyperresponders). This distribution of population can, in fact, result in a population that is less readily amenable to the detection of effects by traditional statistical techniques. The sensitivity of techniques such as ANOVA is markedly reduced by the occurrence of outliers (extreme high or low values, including hyper- and hyporesponders) which, in fact, serve to inflate markedly the variance (standard deviation) associated with a sample inflation. Such a variance inflation effect is particularly common in small groups that are exposed or dosed at just over or under a threshold level, causing a small number of individuals in the sample (who are more sensitive than the other members) to respond markedly. Such a situation is displayed in Fig. 6 which plots the mean and standard deviations of methemoglobin levels in a series of groups of animals exposed to successively higher levels of a hemolytic agent.

Though the mean level of methemoglobin in group C is more than double that of the control group (A), no hypothesis test will show this difference to be significant because it has such a large standard deviation associated with it. Yet this "inflated" variance exists because a single individual has such a marked response. The occurrence of the inflation is certainly an indicator that the data need to be examined closely. Indeed, all tabular data in toxicology should be visually inspected for both trend and variance inflation.

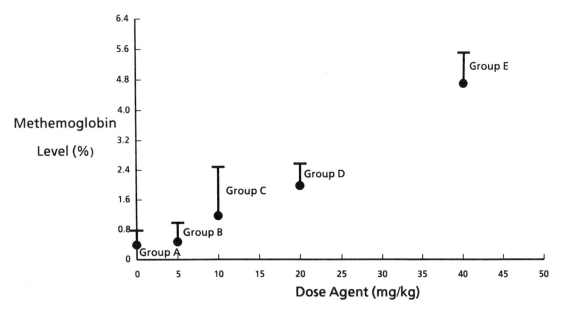

FIG. 6. Variance inflation. *Closed circles,* means; *error bars,* +1 standard deviation.

Multivariate Methods

In a chapter of this scope, any in-depth explanation of the available multivariate statistical techniques is an impossibility. However, with the increase of complexity of problems in toxicology, we can expect to be more frequently faced with data that are not univariate but rather multivariate (or multidimensional). For example, a multidimensional study might be one in which the animals are dosed with two materials that interact, and we are looking at body weight, tumor incidence, and two clinical chemistry values for effects and interaction. Our dimensions, or variables, are as follows: A = dose x, B = dose y, W = body weight, C = tumor incidence, D and E = levels of clinical chemistry parameters, and possibly also t (length of dosing).

These situations are more common in chronic studies (89). Though we can continue to use multiple sets of univariate techniques as we have in the past, there are significant losses of power, efficiency, and information when this is done, as well as an increased possibility of error (22).

Following is a brief examination of the most commonly employed multivariate techniques. Examples from the literature are also presented, illustrating their employment in toxicology and in other biological sciences. The techniques are categorized according to their primary function: *hypothesis testing* (are these significant or not?), *model fitting* (what is the relationship between these variables or what would happen if a population were exposed to x?), and *reduction of dimensionality* (which variables are most meaningful?). It should be noted, however, that most multivariate techniques perform several of these functions.

Hypothesis Testing

There are two significant multivariate techniques that have hypothesis testing as their primary function: MANOVA and factor analysis.

Multivariate analysis of variance

MANOVA is the multidimensional extension of the ANOVA process we explored before. It can be shown to have grown out of Hotelling's T^2 (59), which provides a means of testing the overall null hypothesis that two groups do not differ in their means on any of p measures. MANOVA accomplishes its comparison of two (or more) groups by reducing the set of p measures on each group to a simple number by applying the linear combining rule $W_i = w_j X_{ij}$ (where w_j is a weighting factor) and then computing a univariate F-ratio on the combined variables. New sets of weights (w_j) are selected in turn until the set that maximizes the F-ratio is found. The final resulting maximum F-ratio (based on the multiple discriminant functions) is then the basis of the significance test. As with ANOVA, MANOVA can be one-way or higher order.

Gray and Laskey (49) used MANOVA to analyze the reproductive effects of manganese on the mouse, allowing identification of significant effects at multiple sites. Witten et al. (117) utilized MANOVA to determine the significance of the effects of dose, time, and cell division in the action of abrin on the lymphocytes.

Factor analysis

Factor analysis is not purely a technique for hypothesis testing—it can also serve the reduction of dimensionality function. It seeks to separate the variance unique to particular sets of values from that common to all members in that variable system, and is based on the assumption that the intercorrelations among the n original variables are the result of there being some smaller number of variables ("factors") which explain the bulk of variation seen in the variables. There are several approaches to achieving the end results, but they all seek to determine the percentage of the variance of each variable that is explained by each factor (a factor

Group 1

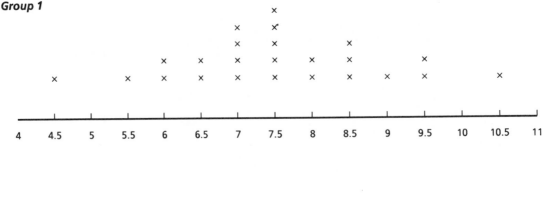

Group 2

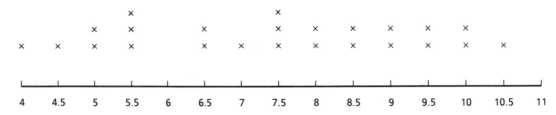

FIG. 7. **Group 1** can be seen to approximate a normal distribution (bell-shaped curve); we can proceed to perform the appropriate tests with such data. **Group 2** clearly does not appear to be normally distributed. In this case, the appropriate nonparametric technique must be used.

being one variable or a combination of variables). The model in factor analysis is $y = Af + z$, where

> y = n dimensional vector of observable responses
> A = factor loadings an $n \times q$ matrix
>   of unknown parameters
> f = q dimensional vector of common factors
> z = n dimensional vector of unique factors

Used for the reduction of dimensionality, factor analysis is said to be a linear technique because it does not change the linear relationships between the variables being examined.

Joung et al. (64) used factor analysis to develop a generalized water quality index that promises suitability across the United States, with appropriate weightings for 10 parameters.

Factor analysis promises great utility as a tool for developing models in risk analysis where a number of parameters act and interact.

Model fitting

Four multivariate modeling techniques are briefly discussed below: multiple regression, discriminant analysis, nonmetric scaling, and Fourier analysis (these last two not being purely multivariate techniques).

Multiple regression

Multiple regression and correlation seeks to predict one or more variables from many. It assumes that the available variables can be logically divided into two (or more) sets and

serves to establish maximal linear (or some other scale) relationships among the sets.

The linear model for the regression is simply

$$Y = b_0 + b_1 X_1 + b_2 X_2 + \cdots + b_p X_p$$

where Y = the predicted value,
   b = values set to maximize correlations
      between X and Y, and
X and Y = the actual observations

(with X's being independent of predictor variables and Y's being dependent variables or outcome measures). One of the outputs from the process will be the coefficient of multiple correlation, which is simply the multivariate equivalent of the correlation coefficient (r).

Schaeffer et al. (88) have neatly demonstrated the utilization of multiple regression in studying the contribution of two components of a mixture to its toxicologic action, using quantitative results from an Ames' test as an end point. Paintz et al. (81) similarly used multiple regression to model the quantitative structure–activity relationships of a series of 14 1-benzoyl-3-methyl-pyrazole derivatives.

Discriminant analysis

The main purpose of discriminant analysis is finding linear combinations of variables that maximize the differences between the populations being studied, with the objective of establishing a model to sort objects into their appropriate populations with minimal error. At least four major questions are asked of the data:

1. Are there significant differences among the K groups?
2. If the groups do exhibit statistical differences, in what directions do the central masses (or centroids, the multivariate equivalent of means) of the populations differ?
3. What are the relative distances among the K groups?
4. How are new (or at this point unknown) members allocated to established groups? How do you predict the set responses or characteristics of an as yet untried exposure case?

The discriminant functions used to produce the linear combinations are of the form:

$$D_i = d_{i1}Z_1 + d_{i2}Z_2 + \cdots + d_{ip}Z_p$$

where D_i = the score on the discriminant function i
  d's = weighting coefficients
  Z's = standardized values of the discriminating variables used in the analysis

It should be noted that discriminant analysis can also be used for the hypothesis testing function by the expedient of evaluating how well it correctly classifies members into proper groups (e.g., control, treatment 1, treatment 2, etc.). Taketomo et al. (96) used discriminant analysis in a retrospective study of gentamycin nephrotoxicity to identify patient risk factors (i.e., variables that contributed to a prediction of a patient being at risk).

Nonmetric scaling

Nonmetric or nondimensional scaling is not purely a technique for modeling (it also serves well to reduce the number of dimensions of the data). Its main purpose is to arrange the objects graphically in a few dimensions, while retaining the maximum possible fidelity to the original relationships between members. It is not a linear technique—it does not preserve the linear relationships (i.e., $A > B > C > D$). The spacings (interpoint distances) are kept such that if the distance of the original scale between members A and B is greater than that between C and D, the distances on the model scale shall likewise be greater between A and B than between C and D.

This technique functions by taking observed measures of similarity or dissimilarity between every pair of M objects, then finding a representation of the objects as points in Euclidean space such that the interpoint distances in some sense "match" the observed similarities or dissimilarities by means of weighting constants.

Fourier analysis

Fourier analysis (13) is not purely either a multivariate technique (it is more frequently univariate), or primarily for the modeling function (it can also be used to reduce dimensionality). In a sense, it is like trend analysis; it looks at the relationship of sets of data from a different perspective. In the case of the Fourier analysis, the approach is via resolving the time dimension variable in a data set. At the most simple level, it assumes that many events are periodic in nature,

and if we can remove the variation in other variables due to this periodicity (by using Fourier transforms), we can better analyze the remaining variation from other variables. The complications to this are (a) there may be several overlying cyclic-time-based periodicities, and (b) we may also be interested in the time-cycle events for their own sake.

Fourier analysis allows us to identify, quantitate, and (if we wish) remove the time-based cycles in data (with their amplitudes, phases, and frequencies) by use of the Fourier transform

$$nJ_i = x_i \exp(-iw_it)$$

where n = length
  J = the discrete Fourier transform for that case
  x = actual data
  i = increment in the series
  w = frequency
  t = time

Reduction of Dimensionality

Finally, we shall introduce four techniques whose primary function is the reduction of dimensionality—canonical correlation analysis, cluster analysis, principal components analysis, and biplot analysis.

Canonical correlation analysis

This technique provides the canonical R, an overall measure of the relationship between the two sets of variables we have (one set consisting of several outcome measures, the other of several predictor variables). The canonical R is calculated on two numbers for each subject:

$$W_i = \sum W_jX_{ij} \text{ and } V_i = \sum V_iY_{ij}$$

where X's = predictor variables
  Y's = outcome measures
  W_j and V_j = canonical coefficients

MANOVA can be considered a special case of canonical correlation analysis. Canonical can be used in hypothesis testing also—pairs of sets of weights, each with a corresponding coefficient of canonical correlation, each uncorrelated with any of the preceding sets of weights, and each accounting for successively less of the variation shared by the two sets of variables.

Young and Matthews (119) used canonical correlation analysis to evaluate the relationship between plant growth and environmental factors at 12 different sites.

Cluster analysis

Cluster analysis serves to sort a heterogeneous collection of objects into a series of sets, i.e., to identify sets and allocate objects to these sets simultaneously. It is a methodology almost entirely of an applied (as opposed to theoretical) nature and basis. The final result is a graphic display and a methodology for putting new members into the classification. The classification procedures are based on either density of population or distance between members. These methods can serve to generate a basis for classification of large numbers of dissimilar variables such as behavioral observations and compounds with distinct but related structures and mechanisms (40).

Principal components analysis

The main purpose of principal components analysis is to describe parsimoniously the total variance in a sample in a few dimensions; one wishes to reduce the dimensionality of the original data while minimizing the loss of information. It seeks to resolve the total variation of a set of variables into linearly independent composite variables which successively account for the maximum possible variability in the data. The fundamental equation is

$$Y = AZ$$

where A = matrix of scales eigenvectors
Z = original data matrix, and
Y = principal components

The concentration here, as in factor analysis, is on relationships within a single set of variables. Note that the results of principal components analysis are affected by linear transformations.

Cremer and Seville (20) used principal components to compare the difference in blood parameters resulting from each of two separate pyrethroids. Henry and Hidy (56), meanwhile, used principal components to identify the most significant contributors to air quality problems.

Biplot display

The biplot display (37) of multivariate data is a relatively new technique, but promises wide applicability to problems in toxicology. In a sense, it is a form of exploratory data analysis used for data summarization and description.

The biplot is a graphical display of a matrix Y_{nmx} of N rows and M columns by means of row and column marker. The display carries one marker for each row and each column. The "bi" in biplot refers to the joint display of rows and columns. The use of such plots is primarily for inspection of data and for data diagnostics when such data are in the form of matrices.

Shy-Modjeska et al. (92) illustrated this usage in the analysis of aminoglycoside renal data from beagle dogs, allowing the simultaneous clear display relationships among different observed variables and the exhibiting of the relationship of both individuals and treatment groups to these variables.

There are a number of good surveys of multivariate techniques available (5,15,91) which are not excessively mathematical in nature. More rigorous mathematical treatments on an introductory level are also readily available (47). It should be noted that most of the techniques we have described are computationally available in the better commercial computer statistical packages.

APPLICATIONS

LD$_{50}$ and LC$_{50}$

To calculate either of these figures, the data we have before us are, at each of several dosage (or exposure) levels, the number of animals dosed and the number that died. If we are seeking only to establish the median effective dose in a range-finding test, then 4 or 5 animals per dose level, using Thompson's method of moving averages is the most efficient methodology and will give a sufficiently accurate solution. With two dose levels, if the ratio between the high and low dose is two or less, even total and no mortality at these two dose levels will yield an acceptable accurate median lethal dose, although a partial mortality is desirable. If, however, we wish to estimate a number of toxicity levels (LD$_{10}$, LD$_{90}$) and are interested in more precisely establishing the slope of the dose/lethality curve, the use of at least 10 animals per dosage level with the log/probit regression technique described in the methods section is commonly used. Note that in the equation $Y_i = a + bx_i$, b is the slope of the regression line, and that our method already allows us to calculate 95% confidence intervals about any point on this line. Tests of significance between two or more such sets of data (i.e., slopes of mortality curves) may readily be done by the t-type test discussed earlier (at any one set of points, such as the LD$_{50}$'s of two curves). Note that the confidence interval at any one point will be different from the interval at other points, and must be calculated separately. Additionally, the nature of the probit transform is such that toward the extremes—LD$_{10}$ and LD$_{90}$, for example—the confidence intervals will "balloon," that is, they become very wide. Because the slope of the fitted line in these assays has a very large uncertainty, in relation to the uncertainty of the LD$_{50}$ itself (the midpoint of the distribution), much caution must be used with calculated LD$_x$'s other than LD$_{50}$'s. The imprecision of (a) the LD$_{35}$, a value close to the LD$_{50}$, is discussed by Weil (107), and (b) that of the slope of the log dose–probit line is also discussed by Weil (108).

Body and Organ Weights

Among the sets of data normally collected in studies where animals are repeatedly dosed with (or exposed to) a chemical, are body weight and the weights of selected organs. Body weight is frequently the most sensitive parameter to indicate an adverse effect. How to best analyze this and in what form to analyze the organ weight data (as absolute weights, weight changes, or percentages of body weight) have been the subject of a number of articles in the past (61,105,106,111). Our experience has been that the following procedures are appropriate if the sample sizes are sufficient (10 or more). With smaller sample sizes, the normality of the data becomes increasingly uncertain and nonparametric methods such as Kruskal–Wallis may be more appropriate (see ref. 120).

1. Organ weights as percentages of total body weights are calculated.

2. Body weights can be analyzed either as weights or changes in body weight. Even if the groups were randomized

properly at the beginning of a study (no group significantly different in mean body weight from any other group, and all animals in all groups within two standard deviations of the overall mean body weight), there is an advantage to using the computationally slightly more cumbersome changes in body weight.

3. Bartlett's test is performed on each set of data to ensure that the variances of the sets are homogeneous.

4. As appropriate, the sequence of analysis outlined in the decision trees, presented early in the chapter, is followed.

Clinical Chemistry

A number of clinical chemistry parameters are now determined on the blood and urine collected from the animals in chronic toxicity studies. In the past (and still, in some places), the accepted practice has been to evaluate these data using univariate–parametric methods (primarily *t*-tests and/ or ANOVA). However, this can be shown not to be the best approach on a number of grounds.

First, such biochemical parameters are rarely independent of each other. Neither is our interest often focused on just one of the parameters. Rather, there are batteries of the parameters associated with toxic actions at particular target organs. For example, increases in creatine phosphokinase (CPK), α-hydroxybutyrate dehydrogenase (α-HBDH), and lactate dehydrogenase (LDH) occurring together are strongly indicative of myocardial damage. In such cases, we are not just interested in a significant increase in one of these, but in all three. Table 10 gives a short summary of the association of various parameters with actions at particular target organs. Similarly, changes in serum electrolytes (sodium, potassium, and calcium) interact with each other; a decrease in one is frequently tied to an increase in one of the others. Furthermore, the nature of the data (in the case of some parameters), due either to the biological background of the parameter or the way in which it is measured, is frequently either not normally distributed (particularly because of being markedly skewed) or not continuous in nature. This can be seen in some of the reference data for experimental animals in Mitruka and Rawnsley (74) or Weil (110) in, for example, the cases of creatinine, sodium, potassium, chloride, calcium and blood urea nitrogen. Both normal distribution and continuous data are underlying assumptions in the parametric statistical techniques described in this chapter.

In subchronic and chronic studies that we have recently been involved with, clinical chemistry statistical test methodologies were selected according to the decision-tree approach presented at the beginning of this chapter. The methods that this approach most frequently led to are outlined in Table 11.

This may serve as a guide to what to expect. A more detailed discussion may be found in Martin et al. (72) or Harris (52).

Hematology

Much of what we said about clinical chemistry parameters is also true for the hematologic measurements made in chronic studies. The pragmatic approach of evaluating which test to utilize by use of a decision tree should be used until one becomes confident as to which are the most appropriate methods. Keeping in mind that both values and (in some cases) population distribution vary not only between species, but also between the commonly used strains of species (and that the "control" or "standard" values will "drift" over the course of only a few years), familiarity should not be taken for granted.

The majority of these parameters are, again, interrelated and highly dependent on the method used to determine them. RBC count, platelet counts, and mean corpuscular volume (MCV) may be determined by a device such as a Coulter counter taking direct measurements, and the resulting data are usually suitable for parametric methods. The hematocrit, however, may be actually a value calculated from the RBC and MCV values and, if so, is dependent on them. If the hematocrit is measured directly, instead of being calculated from the RBC and MCV, it may be compared by parametric methods.

Hemoglobin is directly measured and is an independent and continuous value. However, probably because at one time a number of forms and conformations (oxyhemoglobin, deoxyhemoglobin, methemoglobin, etc.) of hemoglobin are actually present, the distribution seen is not typically a normal one, but rather may be a multimodal one. Here, a nonparametric technique is called for such as the Wilcoxon or multiple rank-sum test.

Consideration of the white blood cell (WBC) and differential counts leads to another problem. The total WBC is typically a normal population amenable to parametric analysis, but differential counts are normally determined by manually counting one or more sets of 100 cells each. The resulting relative percentages of neutrophils are then reported as either percentages or are multiplied by the total WBC count with the resulting count being reported (as the "absolute" differential WBC). Such data, particularly in the case of eosinophils (where the distribution do not approach normality and should usually be analyzed by nonparametric methods. It is widely believed that "relative" (%) differential data should not be reported because it is so prone to being misleading.

Lastly, it should always be kept in mind that it is rare for a change in any single parameter to be biologically significant. Rather, because these parameters are so interrelated, patterns of changes in parameters should be expected and analyzed for.

Histopathologic Lesion Incidence

In recent years, there has been an increasing emphasis on histopathologic examination of many tissues collected from animals in subchronic and chronic toxicity studies. While it is not true that only those lesions which occur at a statistically significantly increased rate in treated/exposed animals are of concern (for there are the cases where a lesion may be of such a rare type that the occurrence of only one or a few such in treated animals "raises a flag"), it is true that, in most cases, a statistical evaluation is the only way to determine if what we are seeing in treated animals is significantly worse

TABLE 10. *Association of changes in biochemical parameters with actions at particular target organs*

Parameter				Organ system					Comments
	Blood	Heart	Lung	Kidney	Liver	Bone	Intestine	Pancreas	
Albumin				↓	↓				Produced by liver. Very significant reductions require extensive liver damage.
ALP					↑	↑	↑		Elevations usually associated with cholestasis. Bone alkaline phosphatase tends to be higher in young animals.
Total bilirubin	↑				↑				Elevations usually associated with cholestasis due to obstruction or hepatopathy.
BUN				↑	↓				Estimates blood filtering capacity of the kidneys. Doesn't become significantly elevated until kidney function is reduced 60–75%.
Calcium				↑					Can be life-threatening and result in acute death.
Cholinesterase				↑	↓				Found in plasma, brain and RBC.
CPK		↑			↑				Most often elevated due to skeletal muscle damage but can also be produced by cardiac muscle damage. Can be more sensitive than histopathology.
Creatinine				↑					Also estimates blood filtering capacity of kidney as does BUN, but is more specific.
Glucose								↑	Alterations other than those associated with stress are uncommon and reflect an effect on the pancreatic islets or anorexia.
GGT					↑				Elevated in cholestasis. This is a microsomal enzyme and levels often increase in response to microsomal enzyme induction.
HBDH		↑		↑	↑				Increases usually due to skeletal muscle, cardiac muscle, and liver damage. Not very specific.
LDH		↑	↑	↑	↑				
Total protein				↓	↓				Absolute alterations are usually associated with decreased production (liver) or increased loss (kidney). Can see increases in cases of muscle "wasting" (catabolism).
SGOT		↑		↑	↑			↑	Present in skeletal muscle and heart and most commonly associated with damage to these.
SGPT					↑				Elevations usually associated with hepatic damage or disease.
SDH					↑ or ↓				Liver enzyme. Can be quite sensitive but is fairly unstable. Samples should be processed as soon as possible.

↑, Increase of chemistry values; ↓ decrease in chemistry values.
ALP, alkaline phosphatase; BUN, blood urea nitrogen; CPK, creatinine phosphokinase; GGT, gamma glutamyl transferase; HBDH, hydroxybutyric dehydrogenase; LDH, lactic dehydrogenase; RBC, red blood cells; SDH, sorbitol dehydrogenase; SGOT, serum glutamic oxaloacetic transaminase [also called AST (asparate aminotransferase)]; SGPT, serum glutamic pyruvic transaminase [also called ALT (alanine amino transferase)].

TABLE 11. *Tests used in analysis of clinical chemistry data*

Clinical chemistry parameters	Statistical tests
Calcium	ANOVA, Bartlett's and/or F test, t-Test
Glucose	ANOVA, Bartlett's and/or F test, t-Test
BUN	ANOVA, Bartlett's and/or F test, t-Test
Creatinine	ANOVA, Bartlett's and/or F test, t-Test
Cholinesterase	ANOVA, Bartlett's and/or F test, t-Test
Total bilirubin	Kruskal-Wallis nonparametric ANOVA
Total protein	ANOVA, Bartlett's and/or F test, t-Test
Albumin	ANOVA, Bartlett's and/or F test, t-Test
GGT	Kruskal-Wallis nonparametric ANOVA
HBDH	ANOVA, Bartlett's and/or F test, t-Test
ALP	ANOVA, Bartlett's and/or F test, t-Test
CPK	ANOVA, Bartlett's and/or F test, t-Test
LDH	ANOVA, Bartlett's and/or F test, t-Test
SGOT	ANOVA, Bartlett's and/or F test, t-Test
SGPT	ANOVA, Bartlett's and/or F test, t-Test
Hemoglobin	ANOVA, Bartlett's and/or F test, t-Test

than what has been seen in control animals. And although cancer is not our only concern, it is the class of lesions that is of the greatest interest.

Typically, comparison of incidences of any one type of lesion between controls and treated animals are made using chi-square or Fisher's exact test with a modification of the numbers as the denominators. Too often, experimenters exclude from the consideration all those animals (in both groups) that died prior to the first animals being found with a tumor at that site.

Two major controversial questions are involved in such comparisons: (a) Should they be based on one-tailed or two-tailed distribution, and (b) what are the effects and implications of multiple comparisons?

The one- or two-tailed controversy revolves around the question of which hypothesis are we properly testing in a study such as a chronic carcinogenicity study. Is the tumor incidence different between the control and treated groups? In such cases, it is a bidirectional hypothesis and, therefore, a two-tailed distribution we are testing against. Or are we asking if the tumor incidence is greater in the treated group than in the control group? In the latter case, it is an undirectional hypothesis and we are contemplating only the right-hand tail of the distribution. The implications of the answer to this question are more than theoretical; significance is much greater (exactly double, in fact) in the one-tailed case than in the two-tailed. For example, a set of data analyzed by Fisher's exact test, which would have a two-tailed p level of 0.098 and a one-tailed level of 0.049, would therefore be flagged as significantly different.

Feinstein (34) provides an excellent discussion of the background in a nonmathematical way. Determination of the correct approach must rest on a clear definition by the researcher, beforehand, of the objective of his study and of the possible outcomes (if a bidirectional outcome is possible, are we justified in using a one-tailed test statistic?).

The multiple comparisons problem is a much more lively one. In chronic studies, we test lesion/tumor incidence on each of a number of tissues, for each sex and species, with each result being flagged if it exceeds the fiducial limit of $p \leq 0.05$.

The point we must ponder here is the meaning of "$p \leq 0.05$." This is the level of the probability of our making a type I error (incorrectly concluding we have an effect when, in fact, we do not). So we have accepted the fact that there is a 5% chance of our producing a false positive from this study. Our trade-off is a much lower chance (typically 1%) of a type II error, that is, of our passing as safe a compound that is not safe. These two error levels are connected; to achieve a lower type II level inflates our type I level. The problem in this case is that if we make a large number of such comparisons, we are repeatedly taking the chance that we will "find" a false positive result. The set of lesions and/or tumor comparisons described above may number more than 70 tests for significance in a single study, which will result in a large inflation of our false positive level.

The extent of this inflated false positive rate (and how to reduce its effects) has been discussed and estimated with a great degree of variability. Salsburg (86) has estimated that the typical NCI type cancer bioassay has a probability of type I error ranging between 20 and 50%. Fears and colleagues (31,32), however, have estimated it as being between 6 and 24%. Without some form of correction factor, the "false positive" rate of a series of multiple tests can be calculated as being equal to $1 - 0.95^N$ where N is the number of tests and the selected alpha level is 0.05.

Salsburg (86) expressed the concern that such an exaggerated false positive result may result in a good compound being banned. Though Haseman (55) challenged this on the point that a much more mature decision process than this is used by the regulatory agencies, Salsburg has pointed out at least two cases where the decision to ban was based purely on such a single statistical significance.

What, then, is a proper use of such results? Or, conversely, how can we control for such an inflated error rate?

There are statistical methods available for dealing with this multiple comparisons problem. One such is the use of Bonferroni inequalities to correct for successive multiple comparisons (112). These methods have the drawback that there is some accompanying loss of power expressed as an inability to identify true positives properly.

A second approach is to use the information in a more mature decision-making process. First, the historical control incidence rates [such as are given for the B6C3F1 mouse and the Fischer-344 rats in Fears et al. (32)] should be considered; some background incidences are so high that these tissues are "null and void" for making decisions. Second, we should look not just for a single significant incidence in a tissue but rather for a trend. For example, we might have the following percentages of a liver tumor incidence in the female rats of a study: (a) control—3%, (b) 10 mg/kg—6%, (c) 50 mg/kg—17%, and (d) 250 mg/kg—54%. In this study only the incidence at the 250 mg/kg level might be statistically significant. However, the trend through each of the levels is suggestive of a dose-response. Looking for such a trend is an essential step in a scientific assessment of the results, and one of the available trend analysis techniques, such as presented earlier in this chapter, should be utilized.

Another method for determining whether statistically significant incidences are merely random occurrences is to compare the results of the quantitative variables with two or more concurrently run control groups. Often the mean of one variable will differ from only one of these controls and be numerically within the range of this same variable of the two control means. If so, the statistical significance compared to that one control must be seriously questioned as to its being correlated with a biological significance.

Also enjoying current wide acceptance is risk assessment based on data from carcinogenicity bioassays. The results of test chemicals at high concentrations, including a certain incidence level of tumors in experimental animals, are used to project the risk of inducing cancer in humans at much lower real-life concentrations. There are a large number of models of projecting or extrapolating such data sets. None of these is universally accepted, and there are several orders of magnitude of uncertainty in such estimates. This area is an extremely complex one, and would require significantly more space than is available here to adequately explore and develop. A number of overviews are available to the interested reader, such as Gaylor and Shapiro (45) or Jayjock and Gad (62).

Reproduction

Reproductive implications of the toxic effects of chemicals have become increasingly important. Along with other types of studies that are closely related (such as teratogenesis and dominant lethal mutagenesis, which is discussed later in this chapter), reproduction studies are now common companions to chronic toxicity studies.

One point that must be kept in mind with all the reproduction-related studies is the nature of the appropriate sampling unit. Put another way: What is the appropriate N in such a study: the number of individual pups or the number of litters (or pregnant females)? Fortunately, it is now fairly well accepted that the first case (using the number of offspring as the N) is inappropriate (103). The real effects in such studies are actually occurring in the female that receives the dosage or exposure to the chemical, or that is mated to a male which received a dosage or exposure. What happens to her, and to the development of the litter she is carrying, is biologically independent of what happens to every other female/litter in the study. This cannot be said for each offspring in each litter; the death of, or other change in, one member of a litter can and will be related to what happens to every other member in numerous fashions. Or the effect on all of the offspring might be similar for all of those from one female and different or lacking in another.

As defined by Oser and Oser (80), there are four primary variables of interest in a reproduction study. First, there is the fertility index (FI), which may be defined as the percentage of attempted matings (i.e., each female housed with a male) that resulted in pregnancy, with pregnancy being determined by a method such as the presence of implantation sites in the female. Second, there is the gestation index (GI), which is defined as the percentage of mated females, as evidenced by a vaginal plug being dropped or a positive vaginal smear, that deliver viable litters (i.e., litters with at least one live pup). Two related variables which may also be studied are the mean number of pups born per litter and the percentage of total pups per litter that are stillborn. Third, there is the viability index (VI), which is defined as the percentage of offspring born that survives at least 4 days after birth. Finally (in this four-variable system) there is the lactation index (LI), which is the percentage of those animals per litter alive at 4 days that survive to weaning. In rats and mice, this is classically taken to be until 21 days after birth. An additional variable which may reasonably be included in such a study is the mean weight gain per pup per litter.

Given that our N is at least 10 (we will further explore proper sample size under the topic of teratology), we may test each of these variables for significance using a method such as the Wilcoxon–Mann–Whitney U test, or the Kruskal–Wallis nonparametric ANOVA. If N is less than 10, then we cannot expect the central limit theorem to be operative and should use the Wilcoxon sum of ranks (for two groups) or the Kruskal–Wallis nonparametric ANOVA (for three or more groups) to compare groups.

Teratology

When the primary concern of a reproductive/developmental study is the occurrence of birth defects or deformations (terata, either structural or functional) in the offspring of exposed animals, the study is one of teratology. In the analysis of the data from such a study, we must consider several points.

First is sample size. Earlier in this chapter we reviewed the general concerns with this topic, and presented a method to estimate a sufficient sample size. The difficulties with applying these methods here revolve around two points: (a) selecting a sufficient level of sensitivity for detecting an effect and (b) factoring in how many animals will be removed from study (without contributing a datum) by either not becoming pregnant or not surviving to a sufficiently late stage of pregnancy. Experience generally dictates that one should attempt to have 20 pregnant animals per study group if a pilot study has provided some confidence that the pregnant test animals will survive the dose levels selected. Again, it is essential to recognize that the litter, not the fetus, is the basic independent variable.

A more basic consideration, as we alluded to in the section on reproduction, is that as we use more animals, the mean of means (each variable will be such in a mathematical sense) will approach normality in its distribution. This is one of the implications of the Central Limit Theorem; even when the individual data are not normally distributed, their means will approach normality in their distribution. At sample size of 10 or greater, the approximation of normality is such that we may use a parametric test (such as a t-test or ANOVA) to evaluate results. At sample sizes less than 10, a nonparametric test (Wilcoxon rank-sum or Kruskal–Wallis nonparametric ANOVA) is more appropriate. Other methodologies have been suggested (70,77), but do not offer any widespread acceptance of usage. One nonparametric method that is widely used is the Wilcoxon–Mann–Whitney U test, which was described earlier. Williams and Buschbom (115) further discuss some of the available statistical options and their consequences.

Dominant Lethal Assay

The dominant lethal study is essentially a reproduction study which seeks to study the end point of lethality to the fetuses after implantation and before delivery. The prime statistical considerations of concern are (a) the proper identification of the sampling unit (the pregnant female), and (b) the design of the experiment so that a sufficiently large sample is available for analysis. The question of sampling unit has been adequately addressed in earlier sections. Sample size is of concern here because the hypothesis-testing techniques which are appropriate with small samples are of relatively low power, as the variability about the mean in such cases is relatively large. With sufficient sample size [e.g., from 30 to 50 pregnant females per dose level per week (7)], the variability about the mean and the nature of the distribution allow sensitive statistical techniques to be employed.

The variables of concern that are typically recorded and included in analysis are (for each level per week): (a) the number of pregnant females, (b) live fetuses per pregnancy, (c) total implants per pregnancy, (d) early fetal deaths (early resorptions) per pregnancy, and (e) late fetal deaths per pregnancy.

A wide variety of techniques for analysis of these data have been (and are) used. Most common is the use of ANOVA after the data have been transformed by the arc sine transform (75).

Beta binomial (2,103) and Poisson distributions (23) have also been attributed to these data, and transforms and appropriate tests have been proposed for use in each of these cases (in each case with the note that the transforms serve to "stabilize the variance" of the data). With sufficient sample size, as defined earlier in this section, the Mann–Whitney U test is to be recommended for use here. Smaller sample sizes should necessitate the use of the Wilcoxon rank-sum test.

Diet and Chamber Analysis

In feeding studies, we seek to deliver desired doses of a material to animals by mixing the material with their diet. Similarly, in an inhalation study we mix a material with the air the test animals breathe.

In both cases, we must then sample the medium (food or atmosphere) and analyze these samples to determine what levels or concentrations of material were actually present and to assure ourselves that the test material is homogeneously distributed. Having an accurate picture of these delivered concentrations, and how they varied over the course of time, is essential on a number of grounds:

1. The regulatory agencies and sound scientific practice require that analyzed diet and atmosphere levels be ±10% of the target level.

2. Marked peak concentrations could, due to the overloading of metabolic and repair systems, result in extreme acute effects that would lead to apparent results in a chronic study which are not truly indicative of the chronic low level effects of the compound, but rather of periods of metabolic and physiologic overload. Such results could be misinterpreted if the true exposure/diet levels were not known.

Sample strategies are not just a matter of numbers (for the statistical aspects) but of geometry, so that the contents of a container or the entire atmosphere in a chamber is truly sampled; and of time, in accordance with the stability of the test compound. The samples must be both randomly collected and *representative* of the entire mass of what one is trying to characterize. In the special case of sampling and characterizing the physical properties of aerosols in an inhalation study, some special considerations and terminology apply. Because of the physiologic characteristics of the respiration of humans and of test animals, our concern is very largely limited to those particles or droplets which are of a respirable size. Unfortunately, "respirable size" is a somewhat complexly defined characteristic based on aerodynamic diameter, density, and physiological characteristics. A second misfortune is that while those particles with an aerodynamic diameter of less than 10 μ are generally agreed to be respirable in humans (that is, they can be drawn down to the deep portions of the lungs), in the rat this characteristic is more realistically limited to those particles below 3 μ in aerodynamic diameter. The one favorable factor is that there are now available a selection of instruments that accurately (and relatively easily) collect and measure aerodynamically sized particles or droplets. These measurements result in concentrations in a defined volume of gas, and can be expressed as either a number concentration or a mass concentration (the latter being more common). Such measurements generate categorical data—concentrations are measured in each of a series of aerodynamic size groups (such as >100 μ, 100–25 μ, 25–10 μ, 10–3 μ). The appropriate descriptive statistics for this class of data are the geometric mean and its standard deviation. These aspects and the statistical interpretation of the data that are finally collected should be considered after sufficient interaction with the appropriate professionals. Typically, it then becomes a matter of the calculation of measures of central tendency and dispersion statistics, with the identification of those values which are beyond acceptable limits (12).

Mutagenesis

In the last 15 years a wide variety of tests (see ref. 68 for an overview of available tests) for mutagenicity have been developed and brought into use. These tests give us a quicker and cheaper (though not as conclusive) way of predicting whether a material of interest is a mutagen, and possibly a carcinogen, than do longer term whole-animal studies.

How to analyze the results of this multitude of tests (Ames, DNA repair, micronucleus, host-mediated, cell transformation, sister chromatid exchange, and *Drosophila*, just to name a few) is a new and extremely important question. Some workers in the field hold that it is not possible (or necessary) to perform statistical analysis, that the tests can simply be judged to be positive or not positive on the basis of whether or not they achieve a particular degree of increase in the incidence of mutations in the test organism. This is plainly not an acceptable response, when societal needs are not limited to yes-or-no answers but rather include at least relative quantitation of potencies (particularly in mutagenesis, where we have come to recognize the existence of a nonzero background level of activity from naturally occurring factors and agents). Such quantitations of potency are complicated by the fact that we are dealing with a nonlinear phenomenon. For though low doses of most mutagens produce a linear response curve, with increasing doses the curve will flatten out (and even turn into a declining curve) as higher doses take the target systems into levels of acute toxicity to the test system.

Several concepts that differ from those we have previously discussed need to be examined, for our concern has now shifted from how a multicellular organism acts in response to one of a number of complex actions to how a mutational event is expressed, most frequently by a single cell. Given that we can handle much larger numbers of experimental units in these systems that use smaller test organisms, we can seek to detect both weak and strong mutagens.

Conducting the appropriate statistical analysis, and utilizing the results of such an analysis properly, must start with understanding the biological system involved and, from this understanding developing the correct model and hypothesis. We start such a process by considering each of five interacting factors (48,102):

1. α: The probability of our committing a type I error (saying an agent is mutagenic when it is not, equivalent to our P in such earlier considered designs as the Fisher's exact test); false positive;

2. β: The probability of our committing a type II error (saying an agent is not mutagenic when it is); false negative;

3. Δ: Our desired sensitivity in an assay system (such as being able to detect an increase of 10% in mutations in a population);

4. σ: The variability of the biological system and the effects of chance errors; and

5. n: The necessary sample size to achieve each of these (as we can only, by our actions, change this one portion of the equation) as n is proportional to:

$$\frac{\sigma}{\alpha, \beta, \text{ and } \Delta}$$

The implications of this are, therefore, that (a) the greater σ is, the larger n must be to achieve the desired levels of α, β, and Δ, (b) the smaller the desired levels of α, β and/or Δ, if n is constant the larger our σ is.

What is the background mutation level and the variability in our technique? As any good genetic or general toxicologist will acknowledge, matched concurrent control groups are essential. Fortunately, with these test systems large n's are readily attainable, though there are other complications to this problem, which we shall consider later. An example of the confusion that would otherwise result is illustrated in the intralaboratory comparisons on some of these methods done to date, such as that reviewed by Weil (109).

New statistical tests based on these assumptions and upon the underlying population distributions have been proposed, along with the necessary computational background to allow one to alter one of the input variables (α, β, or Δ). A set that shows particular promise is that proposed by Katz (66,67) in his two articles. He described two separate test statistics: ϕ for when we can accurately estimate the number of individuals in both the experimental and control groups, and θ,

for when we do not actually estimate the number of surviving individuals in each group, and we can assume that the test material is only mildly toxic in terms of killing the test organisms. Each of these two test statistics is also formulated on the basis of only a single exposure of the organisms to the test chemicals. Given this, then we may compute

$$\phi = \frac{\alpha(M_E - 0.5) - Kb(M_C + 0.5)}{\sqrt{Kab(M_E + M_C)}}$$

where a and b are the number of groups of control (c) and experimental (e) organisms, respectively.

N_C and N_E are the numbers of surviving microorganisms.

$$K = N_E/N_C$$

M_E and M_C are the numbers of mutations in experimental and control groups.

μ_e and μ_c are the true (but unknown) mutation rates (as μ_c gets smaller, N's must increase).

We may compute the second case as

$$\theta = \frac{\alpha(M_E - 0.5) + (M_C + 0.5)}{ab(M_E + M_C)}$$

with the same constituents.

In both cases, at a confidence level for α of 0.05, we accept that μ_e equals μ_e if the test statistic (either ϕ or θ) is less than 1.64. If it is equal to or greater than 1.64, we may conclude that we have a mutagenic effect (at $\alpha = 0.05$).

In the second case (θ, where we do not have separate estimates of population sizes for the control and experimental groups) if K deviates widely from 1.0 (if the material is markedly toxic), we should use more containers of control organisms (tables for the proportions of each to use given different survival frequencies may be found in ref. 67). If different levels are desired, tables for θ and ϕ may be found in ref. 65.

An outgrowth of this is that the mutation rate per surviving cells (μ_c and μ_e) can be determined. It must be remembered that if the control mutation rate is high enough that a reduction in mutation rates can be achieved by the test compound, these test statistics must be adjusted to allow for a two-sided hypothesis (30). The β levels may likewise be adjusted in each case, or tested for, if what we want to do is assure ourselves that we do have a mutagenic effect at a certain level of confidence (note that this is different from disproving the null hypothesis).

It should be noted that there are numerous specific recommendations for statistical methods designed for individual mutagenicity techniques, such as that of Bernstein et al. (9) for the Ames test. Exploring them is beyond the scope of this chapter, however.

Behavioral Toxicology

A brief review of the types of studies and experiments conducted in the area of behavioral toxicology, and a classification of these into groups is in order. Although there are a small number of studies that do not fit into the following classification, the great majority may be fitted into one of the following four groups. Many of these points were first covered by one of the authors in an earlier article (39).

1. Observational score-type studies are based on observing and grading the response of an animal to its normal environment or to a stimulus which is imprecisely controlled. This type of result is generated by one of two major sorts of studies. Open-field studies involve placing an animal in the center of a flat, open area and counting each occurrence of several types of activities (grooming, moving outside a designated central area, rearing, etc.) or timing until the first occurrence of each type of activity. The data generated are scalar of either a continuous or discontinuous nature, but frequently are not of a normal distribution. Tilson et al. (99) have presented some examples of this sort. Observational screen studies involve a combination of observing behavior or evoking a response to a simple stimulus, the resulting observation being graded as normal or as deviating from normal on a graded scale. Most of the data so generated are of a rank nature, with some portions being quantal or interval in nature. Irwin (60) and Gad (38) have presented schemes for the conduct of such studies. Table 12 below gives an example of the nature (and of one form of statistical analysis) of such data generated after exposure to one material.

2. The second type of study is one that generates rates of response as data. The studies are based on the number of responses to a discrete controlled stimulus or are free of direct connection to a stimulus. The three most frequently measured parameters are (a) licking of a liquid (milk, sugar water, ethanol, or a psychoactive agent in water), (b) gross locomotor activity (measured by a photocell or electro-magnetic device), or (c) lever-pulling. Work presenting examples of such studies has been published by Annau (4) and Norton (79). The data generated are most often of a discontinuous or continuous scalar nature, and are often complicated by underlying patterns of biological rhythm (to be discussed more fully later).

3. The third type of study generates a variety of data which are classified as error rates. These are studies based on animals learning a response to a stimulus or memorizing a simple task (such as running a maze or a Skinner box-type shock avoidance system). These tests or trials are structured so that animals can pass or fail on each of a number of successive trials. The resulting data are quantal, though frequently expressed as a percentage.

4. The final major type of study is that which results in data which are measures of the time to an endpoint. They are based on animals being exposed to or dosed with a tox-

icant; then the time until an effect is observed is measured. Usually, the endpoint is failure to continue to be able to perform a task. The endpoints can, therefore, be death, incapacitation, or the learning of a response to a discrete stimulus. Burt (16) and Johnson et al. (63) present data of this form. The data are always of a censored nature—that is, the period of observation is always artificially limited on one end, such as in measuring time-to-incapacitation in combustion toxicology data, where animals are exposed to the thermal decomposition gases of plastics for a period of 30 min. If incapacitation is not observed during these 30 min, it is judged not to occur. The data generated by these studies (continuous or discontinuous because the researcher may check, or may be restricted to checking only, for the occurrence of the endpoint at certain discrete points in time) or rank (if the periods to check for occurrence of the endpoint are far enough apart, one may actually only know that the endpoint occurred during a broad period of time—but not where in that period) in nature.

5. There is a special class of test which should also be considered at this point: the behavioral teratology or reproduction study. These studies are based on dosing or exposing either parental animals during selected periods in the mating and gestation process or pregnant females at selected periods during gestation. The resulting offspring are then tested for developmental defects of a neurological and behavioral nature. Analysis is complicated by a number of facts: (a) The parental animals are the actual targets for toxic effects, but observations are made on offspring; (b) the toxic effects in the parental generation may alter the performance of the mother in rearing its offspring, which, in turn, can lead to a confusion of prenatal and postnatal effects; and (c) different capabilities and behaviors develop at different times (which will be discussed further below). Zero means no observed occurrence at those points (i.e., defining start of a regression from development) forcing one to develop a strong baseline data set before initiating such studies so that results may be analyzed in the proper context.

A researcher can, by varying the selection of the animal model (species, strain, sex), modify the nature of the data generated and the degree of dispersion of these data. Particularly in behavioral studies, limiting the within-group variability of data is a significant problem and generally should be a highly desirable goal.

TABLE 12. *Irwin screen parameters showing significant differences between treated and control groups*

Parameter[a]	Rats (18-crown-6 animals given 40 mg/kg i.p.)				Observed difference in treated animals (as compared with controls)
	Control (sum of ranks)	N_C	18-crown-6 (treated sum of ranks)	N_T	
Twitches	55.0	10	270.0	15	Involuntary muscle twitches
Visual placing	55.0	10	270.0	15	Less aware of visual stimuli
Grip strength	120.0	10	205.0	15	Considerable loss of strength, especially in hind limbs
Respiration	55.0	10	270.0	15	Increased rate of respiration
Tremors	55.0	10	270.0	15	Marked tremors

[a] All parameters significant at $p < 0.05$.

Instrumentation and Technique Factors

Most if not all behavioral toxicology studies depend on at least some instrumentation. Very frequently overlooked here (and, indeed, in most research) is that instrumentation, by its operating characteristics and limitations, goes a long way toward determining the nature of the data generated by it. An activity monitor measures motor activity in discrete segments. If it is a jiggle-cage type monitor, these segments are constricted so that only a distinctly limited number of counts can be achieved in a given period of time and then only if they are of the appropriate magnitude. Likewise, technique can also readily determine the nature of data. In measuring response to pain, for example, one could record it as a quantal measure (present or absent), a rank score (on a scale of 1–5 from decreased to increased responsiveness, with 3 being normal) or as scalar data (by using an analgesia meter which determines either how much pressure or heat is required to evoke a response).

Study Design Factors

These are probably the most widely recognized of the factors which influence the type of data resulting from a study. Number of animals used, frequency of measures, and length of period of observation are three obvious design factors that are readily under the control of the researcher and which directly help to determine the nature of the data.

Statistical Methodologies

A complete discussion of all the considerations entering into the selection of the "best" and most appropriate statistical tests has already been presented. However, certain basic considerations can be pointed out. These basic statistical considerations should include the following five points.

1. Before designing a study, consider all the factors which serve to determine the nature and power of the data to be generated. After establishing these, if at all possible, consult a statistician to assist in the study design.
2. The first step in analyzing a set of data should always be to identify its nature in terms of a classification like that presented at the beginning of this chapter. Is it continuous or discontinuous? Is it scalar, rank, quantal, or an attribute? Is it normally distributed, or does it fit some other known distribution?
3. Don't assume normality without at least some inspection of the distribution of the data.
4. Use the information in the data. That is, if you have data which you have gone to a great degree of effort to collect as scalar data as opposed to ranked data (which could have been collected with much less effort), utilize tests which make use of the extra information in scalar as opposed to rank data. The most frequent case for this is when one finds that the scalar data are markedly non-Gaussian, and do not lend themselves to be normalized by a transformation. In this case one should investigate using one of a number of tests which are robust as to the effects of normality yet use the detail of location information inherent in scalar data (a modification of a chi-square type test, for example, with the intervals of the cells delimited appropriately).
5. The first test should be the highest order test possible. That is, if one wishes to compare a multiple of sets of data, for example, a control group and four treatment groups, one should first use a test that makes this global comparison and not make a series of pairwise comparisons. Unfortunately, it is still common in behavioral work for a series, sometimes seemingly infinite, of Student's t-tests to be used as opposed to ANOVA. Likewise, it should be kept in mind that there are global comparison tests analogous to ANOVA for rank type data (the Kruskal–Wallis test, for example).

One should keep in mind that statistics can serve other purposes besides acting as tools to highlight points for concern. There are methods, especially among the multivariate techniques such as factor analysis, which can serve to help determine relationships and better understand the interactions between masses of observations which are commonly the result of behavior studies, especially in the observational score type studies.

Existing Versus Recommended Practice

Finally, it is appropriate to review each of the types of studies currently seen in behavioral toxicology, according to the classification presented at the beginning of this section,

TABLE 13. *Overview of statistical testing for behavioral toxicology: Those tests commonly used as opposed to those most frequently appropriate*

Type of observation	Most commonly used procedures[a]	Suggested procedures
Observational scores	Student's t-test or one-way ANOVA	Kruskal–Wallis nonparametric ANOVA or Wilcoxon rank sum
Response rates	Student's t-test or one-way ANOVA	Kruskal–Wallis ANOVA or one-way ANOVA
Error rates	ANOVA followed by a post-hoc test	Fisher's exact, or RXC chi-square, or Mann–Whitney U-test
Times to endpoint	Student's t-test or one-way ANOVA	ANOVA, then a post-hoc test or Kruskal–Wallis ANOVA
Teratology and reproduction	ANOVA followed by a post-hoc test	Fisher's exact test, Kruskal–Wallis ANOVA, or Mann–Whitney U-test

[a] That these are the most commonly used procedures was established by an extensive review of the literature. The reader is referred to the example articles cited in the text for verification of the scope of this review.

in terms of which statistical methods are used now and what procedures should be recommended for use. The recommendations, of course, should be viewed with a critical eye.

They are intended with current experimental design and technique in mind and can only claim to be the best when one is limited to addressing the most common problems from a "library" of readily and commonly available and understood tests.

Table 13 summarizes this review and recommendation process into a straightforward form. A more detailed examination of the topics in this chapter can be found in Gad and Weil (41).

REFERENCES

1. Abramowitz, M., and Stegun, I. A. (1964): *Handbook of Mathematical Functions,* pp. 925–964. National Bureau of Standards, Washington, D.C.
2. Aeschbacher, H. U., Vuataz, L., Sotek, J., and Stalder, R. (1977): Use of the beta binomial distribution in dominant-lethal testing for "weak mutagenic activity," Part 1. *Mutat. Res,* 44:369–390.
3. Anderson, S., Auquier, A., Hauck, W. W., et al. (1980): *Statistical Methods for Comparative Studies.* John Wiley, NY.
4. Annau, Z. (1972) The comparative effects of hypoxia and carbon monoxide hypoxia on behavior. In: *Behavioral Toxicology,* edited by B. Weiss and V. G. Laties, pp. 105–127. Plenum Press, NY.
5. Atchely, W. R., and Bryant, E. H. (1975): *Multivariate Statistical Methods: Among-Groups Covariation.* Dowden, Hutchinson and Ross, Stroudsburg, PA.
6. Barnett, V., and Lewis, T. (1978): *Outliers in Statistical Data.* John Wiley, NY.
7. Bateman, A. T. (1977): The dominant lethal assay in the male mouse. In: *Handbook of Mutagenicity Test Procedures,* edited by B. J. Kilbey, M. Legator, W. Nichols, and C. Ramel, pp. 325–334. Elsevier, NY.
8. Beckman, R. J., and Cook, R. D. (1983). *Outliers Technometrics* 25:119–163.
9. Bernstein, L., Kaldor, J., McCann, J., and Pike, M. C. (1982): An empirical approach to the statistical analysis of mutagenesis data from the *Salmonella* test. *Mutation Res.,* 97:267–281.
10. Beyer, W. H. (1976): *Handbook of Tables for Probability and Statistics,* pp. 269–378, 409–413. Chemical Rubber, Cleveland.
11. Bliss, C. I. (1935): The calculation of the dosage–mortality curve. *Ann. Appl. Biol.,* 22:134–167.
12. Bliss, C. I. (1965): Statistical relations in fertilizer inspection. *Bulletin,* p. 674. Connecticut Agricultural Experiment Station, New Haven, CT.
13. Bloomfield, P. (1976): *Fourier Analysis of Time Series: An Introduction.* John Wiley, NY.
14. Breslow, N. E. (1975): Analysis of survival data under the proportional hazards model. *Int. Stat. Rev.,* 43:45–58.
15. Bryant, F. H., and Atchley, W. R. (1975): *Multivariate Statistical Methods: Within-Groups Covariation.* Dowden, Hutchinson and Ross, Stroudsburg, PA.
16. Burt, G. S. (1972): Use of behavioral techniques in the assessment of environmental contaminants. In: *Behavioral Toxicology,* edited by B. Weiss and V. G. Laties, pp. 241–263. Plenum Press, NY.
17. Cochran, W. G., and Cox, G. M. (1975): *Experimental Designs,* pp. 100–102. John Wiley, NY.
18. Cox, D. R. (1972): Regression models and life-tables. *J. R. Stat. Soc.,* 34B:187–220.
19. Cox, D. R., and Stuart, A. (1955): Some quick tests for trend in location and dispersion. *Biometrics,* 42:80–95.
20. Cremer, J. E., and Seville, M. P. (1982): Comparative effects of two pyrethroids dietamethrin and cismethrin, on plasma catecholamines and on blood glucose and lactate. *Toxicol. Appl. Pharmacol.,* 66:124–133.
21. Cutler, S. J., and Ederer, F. (1958): Maximum utilization of the life table method in analyzing survival. *J. Chronic Dis.,* 8:699–712.
22. Davidson, M. L. (1972): Univariate versus multivariate tests in repeated-measures experiments. *Psych. Bull.,* 77:446–452.
23. Dean, B. J., and Johnston, A. (1977): Dominant lethal assays in the male mice: Evaluation of experimental design, statistical methods and the sensitivity of Charles River (CD1) mice. *Mutat. Res.,* 42:269–278.
24. Diamond, W. J. (1981): *Practical Experimental Designs.* Lifetime Learning Publications, Belmont, CA.
25. Diem, K., and Lentner, C. (1975): *Documenta Geigy Scientific Tables,* pp. 158–159. Geigy, NY.
26. Dixon, W. J. (1974): *BMD-Biomedical Computer Programs.* University of California Press, Berkeley, CA.
27. Duncan, D. B. (1955): Multiple range and multiple F tests. *Biometrics,* 11:1–42.
28. Dunnett, C. W. (1955): A multiple comparison procedure for comparing several treatments with a control. *J. Am. Stat. Assoc.,* 50: 1096–1121.
29. Dunnett, C. W. (1964): New tables for multiple comparison with a control. *Biometrics,* 20:482–492.
30. Ehrenberg, L. (1977): Aspects of statistical inference in testing for genetic toxicity. In: *Handbook of Mutagenicity Test Procedures,* edited by B. J. Kilbey, M. Legator, W. Nichols, and C. Ramel, pp. 419–459. Elsevier, NY.
31. Fears, T. R., and Tarone, R. E. (1977): Response to "use of statistics when examining life time studies in rodents to detect carcinogenicity." *J. Toxicol. Environ. Health,* 3:629–632.
32. Fears, T. R., Tarone, R. E., and Chu, K. C. (1977): False-positive and false-negative rates for carcinogenicity screens. *Cancer Res.,* 27:1941–1945.
33. Federer, W. T. (1955): *Experimental Design.* Macmillan, NY.
34. Feinstein, A. R. (1975): Clinical biostatistics, XXII: Biologic dependency, hypothesis testing, unilateral probabilities, and other issues in scientific direction vs. statistical duplexity. *Clin. Pharmacol. Ther.,* 17:499–513.
35. Finney, D. K. (1977): *Probit Analysis,* 3rd ed. Cambridge University Press, Cambridge, England.
36. Finney, D. J., Latscha, R., Bennet, B. M., and Hsu, P. (1963): *Tables for Testing Significance in a 2 × 2 Contingency Table.* Cambridge University Press, Cambridge, England.
37. Gabriel, K. R. (1981): Biplot display of multivariate matrices for inspection of data and diagnosis. In: *Interpreting Multivariate Data,* edited by V. Barnett, pp. 147–173. J. Wiley, NY.
38. Gad, S. C. (1982): A neuromuscular screen for use in industrial toxicology. *J. Toxicol. Environ. Health,* 9:691–704.
39. Gad, S. C. (1982): Statistical analysis of behavioral toxicology data and studies. *Arch. Toxicol. Suppl.,* 5:256–266.
40. Gad, S. C., Gavigan, F. A., Siino, K. M., and Reilly, C. (1984): The toxicology of eight ionophores: Neurobehavioral, membrane and acute effects and their structure activity relationships (SAR's). *Toxicologist,* 4:702.
41. Gad, S. C., and Weil, C. S. (1988): *Statistics and Experimental Design for Toxicologists.* Telford Press, Caldwell.
42. Gallant, A. R. (1975): Nonlinear regression. *Am. Stat.,* 29:73–81.
43. Garrett, H. E. (1947): *Statistics in Psychology and Education,* pp. 215–218. Longmans, Green, NY.
44. Gaylor, D. W. (1978): Methods and concepts of biometrics applied to teratology. In: *Handbook of Teratology,* Vol. 4, edited by J. G. Wilson and F. C. Fraser, pp. 429–444. Plenum Press, NY.
45. Gaylor, D. W., and Shapiro, R. E. (1979): Extrapolation and risk estimating for carcinogenesis. In: *New Concepts in Safety Evaluation,* edited by M. A. Mehlman, R. E. Shapiro, and H. Blumenthal, pp. 65–87. John Wiley, NY.
46. Ghent, A. W. (1972): A method for exact testing of 2 × 2, 2 × 3, 3 × 3 and other contingency tables, employing binomial coefficients. *Am. Midland Naturalist,* 88:15–27.
47. Gnanadesikan, R. (1977): *Methods for Statistical Data Analysis of Multivariate Observations.* John Wiley, NY.
48. Grafe, A., and Vollmar, J. (1977): Small numbers in mutagenicity tests. *Arch. Toxicol.,* 38:27–34.
49. Gray, L. E., and Laskey, J. W. (1980): Multivariate analysis of the effects of manganese on the reproductive physiology and behavior of the male house mouse. *J. Toxicol. Environ. Health,* 6:861–868.
50. Grubbs, F. E. (1969): Procedure for detecting outlying observations in samples. *Technometrics,* 11:1–21.

51. Hammond, E. C., Garfinkel, L., and Lew, E. A. (1978): Longevity, selective mortality, and competitive risks in relation to chemical carcinogenesis. *Environ. Res.*, 16:153–173.
52. Harris, E. K. (1978): Review of statistical methods of analysis of series of biochemical test results. *Ann. Biol. Clin.*, 36:194–197.
53. Harris, R. J. (1975): *A Primer of Multivariate Statistics*, pp. 96–101. Academic Press, NY.
54. Harter, A. L. (1960): Critical values for Duncan's new multiple range test. *Biometrics*, 16:671–685.
55. Haseman, J. K. (1977): Response to use of statistics when examining life time studies in rodents to detect carcinogenicity. *J. Toxicol. Environ. Health*, 3:633–636.
56. Henry, R. D., and Hidy G. M. (1979): Multivariate analysis of particulate sulfate and other air quality variables by principal components. *Atmos. Environ.*, 13:1581–1596.
57. Hicks, C. R. (1982): *Fundamental Concepts in the Design of Experiments.* Holt, Rinehart and Winston, NY.
58. Hollander, M., and Wolfe, D. A. (1973): *Nonparametric Statistical Methods*, pp. 124–129. John Wiley, NY.
59. Hotelling, H. (1931): The generalization of Student's ratio. *Ann. Math. Stat.*, 2:360–378.
60. Irwin, S. (1968): Comprehensive observational assessment. In: Systematic, quantitative procedure for assessing the behavioral and physiologic state of the mouse. *Psychopharmacologia*, 13:222–257.
61. Jackson, B. (1962): Statistical analysis of body weight data. *Toxicol. Appl. Pharmacol.*, 4:432–443.
62. Jayjock, M. A., and Gad, S. C. (1988): Hazard and risk assessment. In: *Handbook of Product Safety Evaluation*, edited by S. C. Gad, pp. 558–628. Marcel Dekker, NY.
63. Johnson, B. L., Anger, W. K., Setzer, J. V., and Xinytaras, C. (1972): The application of a computer controlled time discrimination performance to problems. In: Weiss, B. Laties, V. G. (eds) *Behavioral Toxicology*, edited by B. Weiss and V. G. Laties, pp. 129–153. Plenum Press, NY.
64. Joung, H. M., Miller, W. W., Mahannah, C. N., and Guitjens, J. C. (1979): A generalized water quality index based on multivariate factor analysis. *J. Environ. Qual.*, 8:95–100.
65. Kastenbaum, M. A., and Bowman, K. O. (1970): Tables for determining the statistical significance of mutation frequencies. *Mutat. Res.*, 9:527–549.
66. Katz, A. J. (1978): Design and analysis of experiments on mutagenicity. I. Minimal sample sizes. *Mutat. Res.*, 50:301–307.
67. Katz, A. J. (1979): Design and analysis of experiments on mutagenicity. II. Assays involving micro-organisms. *Mutat. Res.*, 64:61–77.
68. Kilbey, B. J., Legator, M., Nicholas, W., and Ramel, C. (1977): *Handbook of Mutagenicity Test Procedures*, pp. 425–433. Elsevier, NY.
69. Kotz, S., and Johnson, N. L. (1982): *Encyclopedia of Statistical Sciences, Vol 1*, pp. 61–69. John Wiley, NY.
70. Kupper, L. L., and Haseman, J. K. (1978): The use of a correlated binomial model for the analysis of certain toxicological experiments. *Biometrics*, 34:69–76.
71. Litchfield, J. T., and Wilcoxon, F. (1949): A simplified method of evaluating dose effect experiments. *J. Pharmacol. Exp. Ther.*, 96:99–113.
72. Martin, H. F., Gudzinowicz, B. J., and Fanger, H. (1975): *Normal Values in Clinical Chemistry.* Marcel Dekker, NY.
73. Meyer, S. L. (1975): *Data Analysis for Scientists and Engineers*, pp. 17–18. John Wiley, NY.
74. Mitruka, B. M., and Rawnsley, H. M. (1977): *Clinical Biochemical and Hematological Reference Values in Normal Experimental Animals.* Masson, NY.
75. Mosteller, F., and Youtz, C. (1961): Tables for the Freeman–Tukey transformations for the binomial and Poisson distributions. *Biometrika*, 48:433–440.
76. Myers, J. L. (1972): *Fundamentals of Experimental Design.* Allyn and Bacon, Boston, MA.
77. Nelson, C. J., and Holson, J. F. (1978): Statistical analysis of teratologic data: Problems and advancements. *J. Environ. Pathol. Toxicol.*, 2:187–199.
78. Nie, N. H., Hall, C. H., Jenkins, J. G., Steinbrenner, K., and Bent, D. H. (1975): *Statistical Package for the Social Sciences.* McGraw-Hill, NY.

79. Norton, S. (1973): Amphetamine as a model for hyperactivity in the rat. *Physiol. Behav.*, 11:181–186.
80. Oser, B. L., and Oser, M. (1956): Nutritional studies on rats on diets containing high levels of partial ester emulsifiers. II. Reproduction and lactation. *J. Nutr.*, 60:429.
81. Paintz, M., Bekemeier, H., Metzner, J., and Wenzel, U. (1982): Pharmacological activities of a homologous series of pyrazole derivatives including quantitative structure–activity relationships (QSAR). *Agents Actions (Suppl.)*, 10:47–58.
82. Pearson, E. S., and Hartley, H. O. (1958): *Biometrika Tables for Statisticians*, Vol. I, Table 18. Cambridge University Press, Cambridge, England.
83. Pollard, J. H. (1977): *Numerical and Statistical Techniques.* Cambridge University Press, NY.
84. Prentice, R. L. (1976): A generalization of the probit and logit methods for dose response curves. *Biometrics*, 32:761–768.
85. Ryan, T. A., Joiner, B. L., and Ryan, B. F. (1982): *Minitab Reference Manual.* Duxbury Press, Boston.
86. Salsburg, D. S. (1977): Use of statistics when examining life time studies in rodents to detect carcinogenicity. *J. Toxicol. Environ. Health*, 3:611–628.
87. SAS Institute (1979): *SAS Users Guide 1979 Edition.* SAS Institute, Raleigh, NC.
88. Schaeffer, D. J., Glave, W. R., and Janardan, K. G. (1982): Multivariate statistical methods in toxicology. III. Specifying joint toxic interaction using multiple regression analysis. *J. Toxicol. Environ. Health*, 9:705–718.
89. Schaffer, J. W., Forbes, J. A., and Defelice, E. A. (1967): Some suggested approaches to the analysis of chronic toxicity and chronic drug administration data. *Toxicol. Appl. Pharmacol.*, 10:514–522.
90. Scheffe, H. (1959): *The Analysis of Variance.* Wiley, NY.
91. Seal, H. L. (1964): *Multivariate Statistical Analysis for Biologists.* Methuen, London.
92. Shy-Modjeska, J. S., Riviere, J. E., and Rawldings, J. O. (1984): Application of biplot methods to the multivariate analysis of toxicological and pharmacokinetic data. *Toxicol. Appl. Pharmacol.*, 72:91–101.
93. Siegel, S. (1956): *Nonparametric Statistics for the Behavioral Sciences.* McGraw-Hill, NY.
94. Snedecor, G. W., and Cochran, W. G. (1980): *Statistical Methods*, 7th ed. Iowa State University Press, Ames, IA.
95. Sokal, R. R., and Rohlf, F. J. (1981): *Biometry.* Freeman, San Francisco.
96. Taketomo, R. T., McGhan, W. F., Fushiki, M. R., Shimada, A., and Gumpert, N. F. (1982): Gentamicin nephrotoxicity application of multivariate analysis. *Clin. Pharmacol.*, 1:544–549.
97. Tarone, R. E. (1975): Tests for trend in life table analysis. *Biometrika*, 62:679–682.
98. Thompson, W. R., and Weil, C. S. (1952): On the construction of tables for moving average interpolation. *Biometrics*, 8:51–54.
99. Tilson, H. A., Cabe, P. A., and Burne, T. A. (1980): Behavioral procedures for the assessment of neurotoxicity. In: *Experimental and Clinical Neurotoxicology*, edited by P. S. Spencer and N. H. Schaumburg, pp. 758–766. Williams & Wilkins, Baltimore.
100. Tukey, J. W. (1977) *Exploratory Data Analysis.* Addison-Wesley, Reading, MA.
101. Velleman, P. F., and Hoaglin, D. C. (1981): *Applications, Basics and Computing of Exploratory Data Analysis.* Duxbury Press, Boston.
102. Vollmar, J. (1977): Statistical problems in mutagenicity tests. *Arch. Toxicol.*, 38:13–25.
103. Vuataz, L., and Sotek, J. (1978): Use of the beta-binomial distribution in dominant-lethal testing for "weak mutagenic activity," Part 2. *Mutat. Res.*, 52:211–230.
104. Weil, C. S. (1952): Tables for convenient calculation of median-effective dose (LD_{50} or ED_{50}) and instructions in their use. *Biometrics*, 8:249–263.
105. Weil, C. S. (1962): Applications of methods of statistical analysis to efficient repeated-dose toxicological tests. I. General considerations and problems involved. Sex differences in rat liver and kidney weights. *Toxicol. Appl. Pharmacol.*, 4:561–571.
106. Weil, C. S. (1970): Selection of the valid number of sampling units and a consideration of their combination in toxicological studies

involving reproduction, teratogenesis or carcinogenesis. *Food Cosmet. Toxicol.,* 8:177–182.

107. Weil, C. S. (1972): Statistics vs. safety factors and scientific judgment in the evaluation of safety for man. *Toxicol. Appl. Pharmacol.,* 21: 459.

108. Weil, C. S. (1975): Toxicology experimental design and conduct as measured by interlaboratory collaboration studies. *J. Assoc. Anal. Chem.,* 58:687–688.

109. Weil, C. S. (1978): A critique of the collaborative cytogenetics study to measure and minimize interlaboratory variation. *Mutat. Res.,* 50:285–291.

110. Weil, C. S. (1982): Statistical analysis and normality of selected hematologic and clinical chemistry measurements used in toxicologic studies. *Arch. Toxicol. (Suppl.),* 5:237–253.

111. Weil, C. S., and Gad, S. C. (1980): Applications of methods of statistical analysis to efficient repeated-dose toxicologic tests. 2. Methods for analysis of body, liver, and kidney weight data. *Toxicol. Appl. Pharmacol.,* 52:214–226.

112. Wilks, S. S. (1962): *Mathematical Statistics,* pp. 290–291. John Wiley, NY.

113. Williams, D. A. (1971): A test for differences between treatment means when several dose levels are compared with a zero dose control. *Biometrics,* 27:103–117.

114. Williams, D. A. (1972): The comparison of several dose levels with a zero dose control. *Biometrics,* 28:519–531.

115. Williams, R., and Buschbom, R. L. (1982): Statistical Analysis of Litter Experiments in Teratology. Battelle PNL-4425.

116. Winer, B. J. (1971): *Statistical Principles in Experimental Design.* McGraw-Hill, NY.

117. Witten, M., Bennet, C. E., and Glassman, A. (1981): Studies on the toxicity and binding kinetics of abrin in normal and Epstein Barr virus–transformed lymphocyte culture—I: Experimental results. *Exp. Cell Biol.,* 49:306–318.

118. Woodward, W. A., Elliot, A. C., Gray, H. L., and Matlock, D. C. (1988): *Directory of Statistical Microcomputer Software.* Marcel Dekker, NY.

119. Young, J. E., and Matthews, P. (1981): Pollution injury in Southeast Northumberland, England UK: The analysis of field data using economical correlation analysis. *Environ. Pollut. Sen. B. Chem. Phys.,* 2:353–366.

120. Zar, J. H. (1974): *Biostatistical Analysis,* p. 50. Prentice-Hall, Englewood, NJ.

Principles and Methods of Toxicology, Second Edition, edited by A. Wallace Hayes, Raven Press, Ltd., New York © 1989.

CHAPTER 16

Clinical Pathology for Toxicologists

Robert L. Suber

Center for Toxicology, RJR Nabisco Inc., Bowman Gray Technical Center, Winston-Salem, North Carolina 27102

Clinical pathological parameters have been extensively studied and used in human clinical medicine for decades. The precision and accuracy of these data in diagnosing animal diseases, physiological state, and pathological condition have been adapted from the human to the animal diagnostician. With the onset of technology, we have adapted various laboratory equipment and technologies to the differences in hematological and biochemical parameters between humans and animals. The clinical pathologist must use this technology to increase the accuracy and precision of the diagnostic methodologies in defining the mechanisms and reasons for toxicity in animal models.

Clinical pathology should be used in the same manner as genetic toxicology, histopathology, body and organ weights, clinical signs, feed consumption, and metabolism in establishing a cause-and-effect relationship in toxicology. Clinical pathology parameters will not usually define carcinogenicity, but selected parameters may be developed to do so. Carcinogenicity is currently better diagnosed by the histopathologist as to the organ and cell type affected. The ease in evaluating animal tissues has prevented the effective use of the subtle changes in clinical pathological parameters. In humans, it has been easier to take body fluid samples, e.g., blood or urine, than tissue samples. This difference has allowed human medicine to develop specific methodologies to better assess the health status of humans. In toxicology, we must learn to understand these subtle differences in analyses of body fluids to apply this knowledge to animal models.

The incidence of chemical toxicities in the human population is relatively rare when compared with other maladies such as diseases, infections, and the effects of age. This has prevented the development of a large data base to assimilate the cause-and-effect mechanisms of toxic agents in animal models via clinical pathological parameters. The use of total tumor number and/or site specific carcinogenicity by regulatory agencies also has reduced the use of clinical pathology in defining toxicity. The current regulatory mind-set on the preoccupation of carcinogenicity will continue to slow the understanding of mechanisms of toxicity, inhibit the extrapolation of these data to human situations, and prevent the use of other forms of data in assessing appropriate ways to use agents safely, extrapolating threshold dose levels, and defining a virtually safe dose.

The scientist must optimize each clinical pathology parameter to the animal to have a parameter that is specific, accurate, and precise. It is only through diligent efforts and application of the scientific method that we will learn to use clinical pathology to assess the effects of compounds administered in toxicological protocols.

PHLEBOTOMY TECHNIQUES

The major prerequisite for an accurate hematology or clinical chemistry assay is the proper collection and processing of the sample. The methods of sample collection are varied depending on the species, the need for samples at frequent intervals, the volume of sample needed, the ease of sample collection, and the physiological state of the animal.

The usual collection sites in animals used in toxicology studies are noted in Table 1. Laboratories must perfect several routes of collection for each species in order to generate the most accurate data and reduce the trauma to the animal while on study or at termination. A procedure may also affect the number of technicians needed to collect and process the samples. In the dog, the jugular and cephalic veins provide the best collection sites, and the size of the dog allows for repetitive sample collection. The collection site should be clipped to allow the technician to see the vein, but it is better to occlude the area via a tourniquet for the cephalic vein or via pressure from the technician's finger for the cephalic or jugular veins. The better collection method is determined by feeling the collection area with the index finger of the right hand. This allows the technician to find a strong, large vessel instead of a small surface vessel. The area is then rubbed with a gauze pad or cotton ball soaked with isopropyl alcohol. Blood collection systems are available (Vacutainer, Becton-Dickinson) that allow single or multiple samples to be drawn directly into blood collection tubes. It is preferable to use such systems on large animals because the vacuum in the tube may collapse the blood vessel when withdrawal of blood is faster than the normal flow through that vessel. The better method is via the use of a syringe (usually 5–10 cc) and needle (20–22 gauge) held in the right hand while the vein is gently pressed against the thumb or finger of the left hand. The use of the left hand prevents the vein from moving and the technician from forcing the needle through both sides of the cephalic vein. When blood is collected from veins or arteries, the needle should be inserted parallel to the vessel instead of perpendicular to it.

The ear is the best collection site in the rabbit because anesthesia is not required. The color of the blood vessels in the rabbit's ear provides visual confirmation of arterial (red) or venous (blue) blood. The technician should be aware of

this difference and take samples from either the artery or vein for each animal on the study. Mixing arterial and venous blood samples will result in additional experimental error in a study. A major problem with the rabbit is the proper restraint because the hindlegs have nails that can scratch the technician. A wooden box or cloth towel is often used to restrain a rabbit and protect the technician.

Primates are usually bled from any of the arteries or veins listed on Table 1. The ease of collection and the need for arterial or venous blood should be the deciding factors when selecting the sampling site. If the animal is properly restrained, an anesthetic may not be required.

Rodents are the most often used laboratory animal in toxicology studies, and the sampling techniques are quite varied. The orbital sinus allows the most ease in collection of blood samples for both the technician and the animal, allows collection of many samples in a short time period, does not require chemicals for anesthesia, allows the use of hypoxic agents (e.g., carbon dioxide) to simplify sample collection, does not require surgical incisions (3), allows repetitive collection of blood samples, and reduces variance in clinical pathology parameters (101). For sample collection, the animal is restrained with one hand while a glass capillary tube (0.5–0.9 mm inside diameter) is inserted into the corner of the eye. To reduce clotting, the capillary tube may contain an anticoagulant and should be short (usually 2–3 mm long). The capillary tube should be rotated as it enters the retro-orbital sinus. This 90 to 180° rotation destroys the plexus and allows collection of more sample in a shorter time frame. The tail vein may be used for blood collection by insertion of a small needle (23–25 gauge) into the vein near the base of the tail and withdrawal of the sample into a small syringe (2–5 cc). The ease in collection of a sample from the tail may be increased by warming the tail via immersion in warm water, bathing with a warm towel, exposure to a sun lamp or light bulb, or placing the tail on a heating pad. The exposure of the tail to external heat causes vasodilation and increased blood flow to the tail. The technician must be care-

TABLE 1. *Species, sites, and collection techniques in animals often used in toxicology studies*

Species	Site	Collection technique/apparatus	Anesthesia required
Dog	Cephalic vein (foreleg)		No
	Jugular vein (neck)	18–20 gauge, 1-inch needle	No
	Saphenous vein (rear leg)		No
Rabbit	Heart	18–20 gauge, 2-inch needle	Yes
	Ear vein or artery	23–25 gauge, 3/4-inch needle	No
	Jugular vein	20–22 gauge, 1-inch needle	No
Pig	Anterior vena cava	16–18 gauge, 4-inch needle	No
Rat or mouse or other rodents	Orbital sinus (eye)	Capillary tube	Optional
	Jugular vein	20–23 gauge, 3/4- to 1-inch needle	Yes
	Femoral artery	20–23 gauge, 3/4- to 1-inch needle	Yes
	Tail vein	Excision or 23 gauge, 3/4-inch needle	Optional
	Abdominal (inferior) vena cava	20–22 gauge, 1-inch needle	Yes
	Cardiac puncture	20–22 gauge, 1-inch needle	Yes
Primate	Jugular vein (neck)		Optional
	Femoral artery (leg)	20–22 gauge, 1-inch needle	Optional
	Cubital vein (elbow/forearm)		Optional
	Saphenous vein (leg)		Optional

ful not to use too much heat for too long a time period because tissue damage will occur. Another collection method from the tail requires excision of the distal portions of the tail with a scalpel or razor blade and collection of the sample into an open vial. This method allows the technician to stop the blood flow by application of a clotting agent, e.g., styptic powder or a gauze pad, to the tail. However, this method increases contamination because scales from the tail or hair from the animal can fall into the open container. The other routes (Table 1) of bleeding laboratory rodents require anesthesia and have been reported to cause excessive variation in clinical pathology parameters (68,106).

Anesthesia

Various anesthetic agents have been used to allow rapid, safe collection of blood samples. Pentobarbital, xylazine, ketamine, methoxyflurane, carbon dioxide, and other chemical agents have been used to anesthetize laboratory rodents. At times, each has a benefit but also a risk caused by irritancy, technician safety, and induction of endogenous enzymes. If the anesthetic is inhaled, it may be an irritant that adds to the stress level of the animal. Stress has been reported to affect clinical pathological parameters (11,44). Some of the anesthetic agents may be explosive, require special storage conditions, or may be abused by the laboratory's staff. Many of the anesthetic agents are microsomal protein inducers and may cause effects on clinical pathological parameters that are not treatment related.

The best agent for laboratory rodents is carbon dioxide. This agent has few if any of the problems mentioned above. It is safe in the work environment, relatively nontoxic, does not induce microsomal enzymes, is a nonirritant, is readily available, does not require a controlled substance license, does not distort cellular architecture, is inexpensive, and has been recommended by the American Veterinary Medical Association as an acceptable euthanasia agent (80). It is preferable to use 70% carbon dioxide because pure carbon dioxide causes petechial hemorrhages in the lung, which may interfere with histopathological evaluation. Carbon dioxide may be provided as commercial bottled-gas or as dry ice. For 70% carbon dioxide exposure, the animal may be fitted with a nose cone made from a syringe casing or placed in a bell jar. If bottled carbon dioxide is used, a two-stage regulator is required for accurate flow control of the gas. The animal should be placed on a raised stainless steel grid in the bell jar. This allows collection of voided urine when the animal becomes hypoxic. Practice by the technician is required to ensure the least amount of hypoxia required to allow ease in sample collection without killing the animal. For rats and mice, this time varies from 15 to 45 sec, depending on the size and physiological state of the animal. If additional hypoxia is needed, the animal is simply returned to the bell jar. Proper depth of hypoxia may be judged by the color of the mucous membranes or ears, which change from a bright pink to a pale pink color. Recovery from exposure is rapid, does not require an antidote, and is accomplished by placing the animal back in its cage. Other chemical agents require from 30 min to several hours for complete recovery and may depress respiratory rate to the point of unwanted or ill-timed euthanasia.

Anticoagulants

A variety of anticoagulants are available to coat blood collection tubes. Several commercial blood collection tubes are available with anticoagulants coated to the tube as a powder or in the tube as a liquid. With larger animals and large blood volumes, the use of liquid anticoagulants may be acceptable in the tube. Because of the effects on blood volume of liquid anticoagulants, liquids are not preferred for collection of small volume samples from rodents. When coating syringes or other

TABLE 2. *The effects and use of anticoagulants*

Anticoagulants	Use	Advantages/disadvantages
Ethylenediaminetetraacetic acid (EDTA)	Hematology Platelet counts	Effective for several days No cell distortion Available as powder Allows cellular staining Complexes calcium to prevent clotting Excess shrinks erythrocytes
Heparin	Hematology Osmotic fragility tests	Effective for 10–12 hr Not suitable for coagulation tests Distorts cellular architecture Causes poor staining of cells Inhibits certain biochemical procedures Expensive
Sodium fluoride	Serum glucose	Inhibits glycolysis
Sodium citrate	Coagulation tests	Large amount required Causes blood volume dilution Useful for platelet count and function
Ammonium or potassium oxalate	Hematology Coagulation tests	Interferes with nitrogen determinations Minimal cell distortion if analyzed within 1 hr Leukocyte degeneration after 1 hr

items, the liquid may be used but the item should be allowed to dry to minimize volume effects.

A list of anticoagulants, their use, and their advantages and disadvantages are noted in Table 2. The anticoagulant of choice is ethylenediaminetetraacetic acid (EDTA). The potassium salt is more soluble and is preferred to the sodium salt. As little as one drop of a 10% solution will prevent coagulation of 5 ml of blood. EDTA also is available as a powder, which prevents blood volume distortion; is commercially available already coated to small (2–3 ml) blood collection tubes; allows proper cellular staining; maintains stable cell counts for up to 24 hr (60); and prevents distortion of cellular architecture (73). Excessive EDTA may shrink erythrocytes and cause artifacts in the measured hematocrit or packed cell volume (PCV), the calculated mean corpuscular volume (MCV), and the calculated mean corpuscular hemoglobin concentration (MCHC) (60). Animals with hypercalcemia may require additional EDTA to prevent clotting because EDTA complexes with calcium to prevent clotting.

Heparin has been used as an anticoagulant (Table 2), but its major disadvantages of causing autolysis of cell nuclei, inhibiting the clarity of cell morphology, and reducing stainability of leukocytes have limited its use. Heparin also is more expensive than EDTA because of the commercial need to extract it from the pig's pancreas.

Other anticoagulants and their uses also are noted in Table 2. Several of these anticoagulants have special uses that should be exploited in toxicological studies. With the advent of new clinical chemistry instruments, many serum or blood samples can be rapidly analyzed so there may be little need for specialized anticoagulants, e.g., sodium fluoride.

Sample Preparation

Proper sample preparation is also critical to accurate and precise analyses. Hematological profiles are conducted on whole, uncoagulated blood samples. Plasma is the extracellular fluid that contains the clotting factors found in blood. Plasma is separated from uncoagulated blood containing an anticoagulant. Serum is defined as the extracellular blood fluid that is separated from the blood after the blood is allowed to clot. Plasma and serum are normally clear to straw-colored.

Hematological profiles should be conducted on fresh blood samples. After the sample is drawn from the animal, the blood should be gently rotated for 30 sec with the anticoagulants. The sample should then be placed on a commercially available mechanical rotator to mix the sample thoroughly before analyses are conducted. If the sample remains stationary for any time, the sample must be thoroughly mixed for 2 to 5 min before taking an aliquot for analysis. If clots are observed, this sample should not be used for constructing a hematological profile because erroneous results would be reported.

Serum samples are prepared by allowing the blood sample to clot at room temperature for 15 to 30 min. The sample is then centrifuged in a refrigerated or unrefrigerated centrifuge at $2,000 \times g$ for 10 to 15 min. The tube is removed and the serum withdrawn by pipette. Changes in serum glucose, lactic acid, alanine aminotransferase (ALT), aspartate aminotransferase (AST), potassium, and alkaline phosphatase

(ALP) have been reported when serum was not removed within 48 hr (66). Care must be taken not to disturb the interface between the red cells and the serum. The sample may be recentrifuged to reestablish this interface. The removed serum may be recentrifuged to remove any cellular debris or any red cells. The serum sample may then be analyzed, refrigerated, or frozen. If frozen, proper tubes must be used to withstand the cold temperature. Polypropylene tubes are often used.

A silicone-based material has been developed that comes in the blood tube or may be added to the tube during centrifugation. This material forms a physical barrier between the erythrocytes and serum or plasma by acting as a molecular sieve, thus forcing or allowing the less dense extracellular fluid to rise to the surface and the more dense erythrocytes to settle to the bottom of the tube. This material does not interfere with the chemical assays and may save time in processing serum or plasma samples.

Blood is usually collected in glass tubes. Plastic tubes also are available. The larger tubes (>1 ml) are usually glass. The smaller tubes (100–500 ml) are usually plastic. The blood sample volume should be matched to an appropriate tube size with the proper amount of anticoagulant. The smaller tubes usually fit special tube holders that slide into specially designed centrifuges. These smaller centrifuges rotate at higher revolutions per minute so the separation time may be reduced to 2 to 3 min. Care must be taken to ensure that the smaller plastic tube diameter does not increase friction during separation. This increased resistance may lyse erythrocytes and result in hemolyzed samples.

The stability of the sample and the effect on cell types or blood constitution must be considered when determining how many samples are collected per day, the order in which the assays are conducted, and the relative importance of the assay. The stability of hematological parameters is listed in Table 3 (73), whereas the stability of selected clinical chemistry constitutents is listed in Table 4 (73). Stability of each constituent must be considered in order to produce accurate data that will be used to determine the toxicity of a selected agent.

QUALITY CONTROL

The quality control system for clinical pathology laboratories is to ensure the reliability of the data. The quality control system should include steps to reduce variability in sample analysis caused by instrumentation, reagents, methodologies, handling, sample collection and preparation, and

TABLE 3. *Stability of hematological parameters*

Parameter	Time
Erythrocyte count	2 Days
Leukocyte count	3 Days
Reticulocyte count	1 Day
Platelet count	2–4 Hr
Hemoglobin	7 Days
Hematocrit	2–4 Hr

TABLE 4. *Stability of specimens for clinical chemistry assays*

Parameter	Stability time/temperature		
	Room (37°C)	Refrigerated (4°C)	Frozen (−20°C)
Albumin	4 Days	30 Days	Stable
Alkaline phosphatase	2 Days	7 Days	Stable
Aspartate aminotransferase	4 Days	14 Days	Stable
Bilirubin (protect from light)	2 Days	4–7 Days	90 Days
Calcium	7 Days	Stable	Stable
Chloride	7 Days	7 Days	Stable
Cholesterol	7 Days	7+ Days	Stable
Creatine phosphokinase	48 Hr	7 Days	Stable
Creatinine	1 Day	1 Day	Stable
Globulin	4 Days	30 Days	Stable
Glucose	1 Hr	2 Days	Stable
Lactate dehydrogenase	7 Days	Not stable	Not stable
Potassium	14 Days	30 Days	Stable
Protein	7 Days	30 Days	Stable
Sodium	14 Days	30 Days	Stable
Triglycerides	4 Days	7+ Days	Stable
Urea nitrogen	3–5 Days	7 Days	Stable
Uric acid	3 Days	3–5 Days	Stable

other extraneous sources of variation. Many sources other than instrumentation and reagents have been discussed in other areas of this chapter.

Quality control is best evaluated in two parts: accuracy and precision. Accuracy as applied to clinical pathology is the ability to measure the real, "true" parameter. An example is the measurement of all the serum creatinine and only that creatinine, not the quantification of other chromogens. Accuracy must account for the specific activity of clinical pathological parameters in the model system. In toxicology this requires the modification of assay systems to animal characteristics instead of the optimized methods that are normally designed and sold for diagnosis of human pathological conditions. This requires optimization of buffering agents, reaction times, substrate concentrations, cross-reactivity with chemicals (including those administered to the animal), and reaction temperatures. One major portion of accuracy is to ensure that the chemical, i.e., toxin or its metabolite, does not absorb light or fluoresce in the same region as the desired reaction product.

Precision is the ability to reproduce a measurement with a reduction in errors. Precision is often reported as the standard deviation or variance: the smaller the variance, or standard deviation, the greater the precision. The reliability of assays in clinical laboratories is enhanced if the accuracy of the assay is maximized and the precision is enhanced, i.e., errors reduced. In the establishing of a particular assay, the accuracy should be determined before the method is accepted. Laboratory personnel must verify precision on a constant basis. Precision is established by documentation of instrument repair, preventative maintenance, and the use of biological controls that verify the reproducibility of the assay in day-to-day analyses or repetitive analyses of the same parameter.

Precision is determined by establishing the Gaussian distribution about the mean. There are many commercial programs that will calculate and prepare summaries of precision for a laboratory. Whether prepared by a commercial vendor or by the laboratory's personnel, a Levey–Jennings plot (16) is the best way to observe changes in precision. The mean is plotted as the center line, with the outer limits being plus or minus two standard deviations (solid lines, Fig. 1). An action line (dotted line, Fig. 1) also is drawn, which establishes the limits at which the laboratory will correct the loss of precision. This action line is usually set at 1.5 standard deviations and serves as a warning to laboratory personnel of analytical changes. Examples of various trends and shifts seen in clinical pathological parameters are noted in Fig. 1. A trend is a progressive drift or change away from the mean. A shift is an abrupt change away from the mean (16). A downward trend (Fig. 1, graph A) is often caused by contaminants in the system (instruments) or reagents, standards or controls that are too diluted, leaks in reagent lines, improper calibration of automatic diluters to deliver too little sample or too much reagent, deterioration of light sensitive reagents or controls, and weak spectrophotometer photocells or lamps. An upward systematic trend (Fig. 1, graph B) is often due to deteriorating or instability of standards or reagents, especially light sensitive materials, contamination of the system or reagents, and increased concentration of control or reagent caused by improper dilution. A systematic downward shift (Fig. 1, graph C) is often due to decreased concentration of reagents or controls caused by improper dilutions, contamination of reagents or systems, inaccurate timer, low reaction or incubation temperature, and contaminated glassware. A systematic upward shift (Fig. 1, graph D) is often associated with partial electrical failure in the instrument, unstable line voltage, undiluted control or reagent, deteriorated but stable reagent, contaminated reagent or water supply, dirty glassware, inaccurate timer, and excessive reaction or incubation temperature. Outliers are defined as spurious results caused by contamination of a single specimen or control lot, a faulty line that may be clogged with serum protein or fibrinogen, incorrect dilution of control or reagent, contamination of the system, and fluctuation in electrical voltage to the instrument (Fig. 1, graph E).

A good quality control program also incorporates good laboratory practices (46). Such concepts include scheduling and recording of preventative maintenance on instruments including refrigerators, cell counters, and spectrophotometers; proper grounding and suppression of line voltage peaks to instruments; calibration of all instruments including incubators and refrigerators; maintaining clean glassware; rotation of technicians to ensure abilities; use of controls or standards; labeling of all reagents as to contents, date prepared, and person who prepared it; and use of proper diluents, usually distilled water with conductivity of 5 to 10 MΩ. Laboratory directors also must prepare standard operating procedures so each technician can conduct the assay in the same manner. The hiring of properly qualified personnel, e.g., a registered medical technologist, and continuing education and training

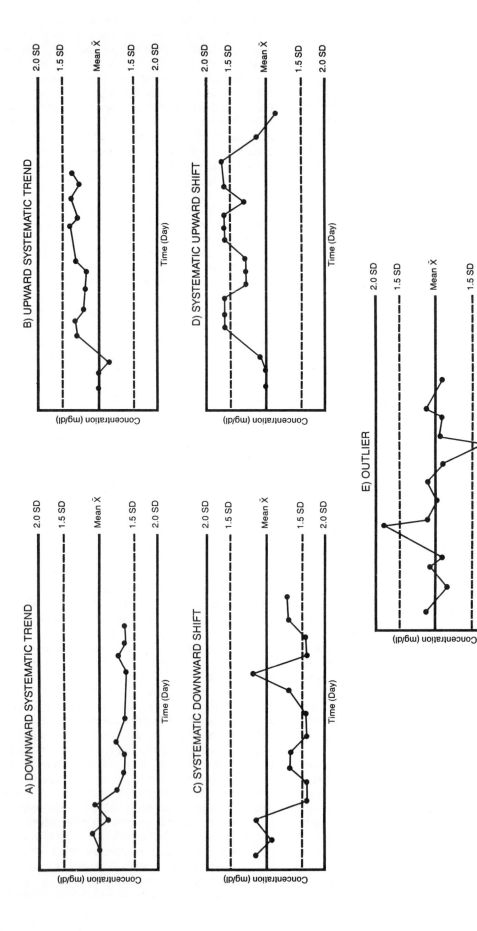

FIG. 1. Systematic trends and abrupt shifts in analytical results diagrammed by Levey–Jennings plots. **A:** Systematic downward trend; **B:** systematic upward trend; **C:** systematic downward shift; **D:** systematic upward shift; **E:** outliers or spurious analytical results.

are required to maintain consistent quality in the clinical pathology laboratory.

Many quality control systems involve standards or controls. Standards are compounds of exact chemical composition, e.g., serum protein. Standards are made by adding a known, precise concentration of the agent to a known medium. Controls are ranges of chemicals with known composition. Standards are most often used in establishing the accuracy of a procedure, whereas controls are usually cheaper and easier to use in assessing the day-to-day variability (precision) in an analytical procedure. Controls are usually based on human sera and therefore cannot be used as standards to ensure the accuracy of the procedure in animal clinical pathology laboratories. Controls can be used to verify the precision of the assay on a monitoring basis if the same control is used in each batch of analyses and on a day-to-day basis to show reproducibility of the procedure. In a good quality control program, controls are placed at selected intervals between biological samples. When analyses are conducted in groups, as with centrifugal analyzers, controls should be included in each group, as well as sera from animals from each group and sex. A statistical randomization of animals at termination permits the collection of random samples, which can then be assayed in the same order as the animals were killed. Controls that are within and above the physiological normal range of the analyte are used to verify that the reaction did not suffer from substrate depletion when sera with unknown concentration of analyte from treated animals are analyzed.

Instruments have become more precise but more complicated, often leading to instrument variance or failure. Therefore, a good quality control program must include a record of instrument repair and preventative maintenance and corroboration that the instrument is properly functioning. Its function must also be verified and not just accepted because a light is on or a display function provides the desired value. Instruments must be calibrated on a scheduled basis. The actual voltage delivered to an electrophoretic chamber must be verified with a voltmeter. Commercially available solutions must be placed in spectrophotometers to ensure proper light absorption and generation. Temperatures must be verified with quality thermometers instead of accepting the displayed value.

The major goal of any quality control program is to ensure that the analytical results are reliable. Programs should be developed that ensure this reliability for the laboratory's management and instill confidence in the laboratory staff. A modest quality control program that is adhered to and supported is superior to any exotic program that is not supported or maintained by the laboratory staff.

EXPERIMENTAL DESIGN

Proper experimental design is critical to accurate analyses. This requires a thorough understanding of normal animal physiology and an awareness of pathological processes that may occur in toxicological studies.

Stress is the major cause of inaccuracies and increased variation in clinical pathology parameters. Stress may be due to housing conditions, sex, handling, anesthetic agent, environmental conditions, light cycles, and euthanasia technique. It has been reported that peripheral leukocyte counts are reduced in BALB/Wm mice housed alone or in small groups of four animals versus groups of 20 mice (77). Excessive movement of cages, lack of fresh water or feed, improper bedding (e.g., dusty bedding material), and movement of animals between animal rooms and the necropsy area may induce stress (44). Stress can be reduced by movement of animals to an area next to the necropsy area, waiting to weigh the animal immediately before bleeding, and bleeding a single animal under a negative pressure hood so pheromones are not released to other animals in the room.

Improper application of anesthetic and sensing of euthanasia also have been reported to cause a stress response in rats (11), as noted by a decrease in serum lactate and glucose and a decrease in hematocrit, hemoglobin, and total leukocyte count. Serum glucose, pyruvate, and lactate increased by 20% to 100% after exposure to ether or cage movement, whereas serum potassium and glycerol decreased (44). No reported effects were reported on serum urea nitrogen, calcium, phosphate, ALT, AST, or ALP (44).

Diurnal variations may also affect proper interpretation of clinical pathological parameters. Plasma protein has been reported to be affected by time of day when the sample is drawn (11). Serum glucose and lactate have been reported to vary by 10% to 30% between 6 sampling days (11). The length of the light cycle also has been reported to reduce the hematocrit, eosinophil count, and plasma protein in rats on a 2-hr light to 3-hr dark cycle as compared to the normal 12-hr light to 12-hr dark cycle (11).

Phlebotomy also has been reported to affect clinical pathology parameters. Lower values for plasma lactate dehydrogenase (LDH), malate dehydrogenase (MDH), AST, creatine kinase, and ALP have been reported following the taking of samples from the carotid artery via a catheter than by cardiac puncture (68). There were no significant differences in plasma ALT, protein, urea, sodium, potassium, calcium, or phosphate (68).

This trend has been verified by the lower mean concentrations of erythrocytes, leukocytes, hemoglobin, hematoid, serum ALT, and serum urea nitrogen in female Sprague-Dawley rats bled via cardiac puncture than those bled from the retro-orbital sinus or excision of the tail (106).

It also has been reported that a greater coefficient of variation occurs in plasma samples taken by cardiac puncture than by catheterization of the carotid artery (68). A larger standard deviation in erythrocyte counts, hemoglobin, hematocrit, serum LDH, serum AST, serum ALT, serum gamma-glutamyltransferase (GGT), serum creatinine, and serum urea nitrogen has been reported in female Sprague-Dawley rats bled via cardiac puncture than animals bled via excision of the tail or via the retro-orbital sinus (106). There was also a larger deviation in the leukocyte count and serum ALP for Sprague-Dawley rats bled from the orbital sinus (106). Hematological and serum chemistries obtained from incision of the tail vein were similar to results from rats bled from the orbital sinus (106).

Hemolysis often results in erroneous serum chemistries and hematological values. It also is helpful to grade the level of hemolysis. Hemolysis may be a toxicological endpoint but is more often the result of mechanical injury to erythrocytes caused by phlebotomy route, technique or processing of the sample (e.g., excessive centrifugation), low temperatures, or improper pipetting of the serum. Cardiac puncture has been reported to cause a greater incidence of hemolysis in female Sprague-Dawley rats (106). The incidence of hemolysis varied from 50% to 80% in samples taken via cardiac puncture, 24% to 29% when taken via excision of the tail, and no hemolysis in samples taken via the retro-orbital sinus. This incidence of hemolysis leads to excessive amounts of serum LDH, AST, and ALT. The mean serum LDH was increased 300%, AST increased 200%, and ALT increased 300% in rats following cardiac puncture when compared to those bled via the retro-orbital sinus (106). An earlier study also had reported a 30% increase in serum AST and a fivefold increase in serum LDH, serum alpha-hydroxybutyrate dehydrogenase, and serum bilirubin, in male Fischer 344 (F344) rats bled via the orbital sinus with 0 to 1500 mg/L of hemoglobin added to the sample (26). There were minor changes in serum creatine phosphokinase (CPK), serum glucose, serum ALT, serum cholinesterase, serum ALP, serum albumin, serum protein, serum calcium, or serum urea nitrogen. Serum creatinine was reported to decrease twofold (26).

Age and sex also have been reported to affect clinical pathological parameters (42). Therefore, the experimental design should include both sexes for all treatment groups and ages. Age differences may prevent clear dose response. In BALB/C and C57BL/6 mice bled via the retro-orbital sinus, the leukocyte count was highest at 1 to 3 months of age and decreased until the mice were 18 months old. Erythrocyte count, hematocrit, and hemoglobin levels were similar between 1 and 12 months but decreased at 12 to 18 months and after 18 months of age for both strains. Serum phosphorus, calcium, ALP, and urea nitrogen decreased in both strains after 3 months of age, then increased after 12 months of age. Serum glucose and ALP decreased with age. Differences in hemoglobin, serum phosphorus, serum cholesterol, serum AST, serum glucose, serum protein, serum albumin, and serum ALP were also reported between sexes of one or both mouse strains.

Diet can affect clinical pathological parameters even when fed for a short time period, e.g., 3 weeks (50). The use of a semipurified diet (AIN-76) significantly increased the serum cholesterol by 36% to 43% in BALB/C and B6C3F1 female mice when compared with mice fed a cereal-based diet (NIH-07). Both mouse strains had higher (20–22%) serum urea, higher (2–3.5%) erythrocyte count, and higher hematocrit and hemoglobin when consuming the cereal-based diet than the semipurified, sucrose-based diet. There were no significant differences in serum creatinine, ALT, AST, or GGT. Storage of autoclaved, cereal-based diets for up to 130 days had no adverse effects on serum protein, body weight, or histopathology of BALB/C or B6C3F1 mice fed these diets for 13 weeks (76).

Fasting with *ad libitum* access to water is often used with laboratory animals to reduce interference in assays caused by excessive chylomicrons and lipids in the circulation. Excessive chylomicrons are a result of rodents being nocturnal animals. Therefore, their feeding habits do not coincide with the normal human workday or the usual light schedule. Fasting has been reported to decrease serum glucose (24) and increase serum bilirubin (101). Because of the smaller body and organ size, mice should not be fasted for the usual 12 to 18 hr. This period has not been reported to affect rat serum chemistries. The advent of improved assays that are specific for individual serum enzymes or components and the use of methodologies that detect serum component activities in spectrophotometers at ultraviolet wavelengths have reduced the interference of chylomicrons in these assays.

HEMATOLOGY

Methodology

The onset of technology has allowed a rapid advance in electronics, especially as it applies to biomedical instrumentation. These advances and the need to process large numbers of blood samples in hospitals and clinical practices have led to the development of semiautomated and automated instruments that allow accurate, rapid evaluation of hematological parameters. Advances in human medicine have provided reliable, cost-effective methods to evaluate the effects of chemicals and disease in research animals. These procedures also increase the reliability of the hematological data as compared to the earlier manual methods that required large dilutions between 1:20 to 1:200 of the blood sample and manual counting of erythrocytes (red blood cells) or leukocytes (white blood cells) on a hemocytometer. The hemocytometer method required the technologist to count the number of cells per grid, average the count from about five squares on the grid, and calculate the number of cells per volume of blood. The formula used is

Number of blood cells/mm^3 of blood

$$= \frac{\text{Total number of cells counted in five squares on the hemocytomer}}{\text{Surface area counted} \times \text{height of counting chamber} \times \text{dilution volume}}$$

There are several automated and semiautomated methods that reduce the variability caused by human error and that improve the validity of the data. Two methods count cells electronically by (a) aperture impedance and (b) laser light scatter. These systems provide a variety of cell parameters that can be counted or calculated (73). Ease of operation, maintenance or service, number of samples, and technologist's time should be considered.

The aperture impedance method employs the suspension of a blood sample (usually 10–20 μl) into isotonic saline. This sample is passed through an aperture (usually 100 μm in size for animal blood cells) at the same time as an electrical current. The cell's size is proportional to the impedance change generated when the cell passed through the aperture (90).

In the laser light scatter method, a cell suspension is hydrodynamically focused into a narrow stream of cells. As cells pass through the laser sensing zone in single file, the resulting angle light scatter is detected. During this time, the cell volume, cell refractive index, and time of passage are recorded (90).

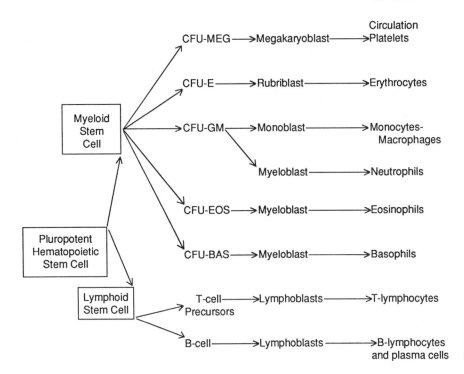

FIG. 2. Schematic origin of circulating blood cells. CFU, colony forming unit. (From ref. 60, with permission.)

By either method, the cell counts are determined by the number of electrical pulses. The cell volume is determined by the size of the electrical pulse for the impedance method, and the hematocrit determination is calculated from the volume. In the laser scatter method, the hematocrit is the sum of the red cell pulse integrals, and the cell volume is mathematically calculated by the machine from the hematocrit (90). For counting nucleated cells or leukocytes, a lysing agent, e.g., water, saponin, or dilute acid, is used. The lysed erythrocytes then do not interfere with counting of cells by either automated method or by the manual method. However, certain lytic agents may cause the leukocytes to shrink, which may interfere with automated methods and cause increased discrepancies between automated and manual methods (37,116).

Bone Marrow

Erythrocytes, leukocytes, monocytes, platelets, granulocytes (basophils and eosinophils), plasma cells, and megakaryocytes are produced in the bone marrow after birth (Fig. 2) and in the spleen, liver, and bone marrow in fetal life and in early postnatal life (60). Hematopoiesis is usually restricted to the bone marrow after birth, but the spleen and liver retain the hematopoietic potential, which may be reexpressed in times of stress (60). Hypoplasia and aplasia have been reported after exposure to viruses, bacteria, radiation, benzene, chloramphenicol, and certain alkylating agents (93).

As erythrocytes mature in the bone marrow, they are delivered into the circulation (4,30,111). The terminal stage of erythrocyte maturation is reported to occur next to the sinus wall. As the metarubricytes, leukocyte precursors, and platelet precursors press against the sinus wall, the nucleus is extruded and phagocytized (60). If any nuclear material is retained in the metarubricyte, it is referred to as a reticulocyte when found in the systemic circulation. The presence of systemic reticulocytes may suggest problems in cellular transport, effects on membrane dynamics, general anemia, or increased hematopoiesis.

In mammals, lymphoblasts (Fig. 2) are transported to the thymus from the bone marrow. After differentiation in the thymus (T), precursor cells are formed that localize in the spleen, lymph nodes, or other lymphoid tissue where T-lymphocytes are produced when the appropriate antigenic stimulation occurs.

Erythrocytes

Erythrocyte production is controlled by the production of erythropoietin. Renal hypoxia stimulates the production and release of erythropoietin from the kidney. In the absence of hypoxia, which may be the result of anemia or lack of the circulating erythrocytes to carry oxygen, basal stem cell turnover or extrarenal erythropoietic stimuli may induce erythropoietin production. Erythropoietin increases circulating erythrocyte numbers by inducing stem cells to differentiate into rubriblasts, increasing the stem cell numbers, increasing the rate of erythroid precursor maturation, and decreasing the marrow transit time by decreasing the cell cycle time or causing early denucleation and release into the systemic circulation (21).

The erythrocyte is a biconcave disk that transports oxygen, carbon dioxide, nutrients, and waste products. The bone marrow maturation time is normally 5 days. The erythrocyte life span (Table 5) in the peripheral circulation varies from 20 days in the mouse to 120 days in the dog (21,60).

Reduced erythrocyte counts as quantified by the automated, semiautomated, or manual methods previously discussed are a sign of anemia. This loss of erythrocytes results in a decreased oxygen carrying capacity, which may result in clinical signs of weakness or palor, fainting after stress or exercise, or a systolic heart murmur. In order to compensate, tachycardia, tachypnea, or lower temperature in the extremities may occur. The tachycardia and tachypneas are reflex mechanisms to increase the delivery rate of oxygen to the tissues. The shunting of blood from the extremities to maintain essential organ functions or to deliver oxygen results in a lowered body temperature in peripheral areas, e.g., limbs or ears.

Polycythemia or abnormally elevated levels of erythrocytes may also occur. Excess cobalt (from the addition of cobalt to stabilize beer foam) has been reported to cause polycythemia (100).

The only anemias that can be based on erythrocyte count alone are anemias caused by underproduction of erythrocytes, hemolysis (hemolytic anemia), or blood loss (hemorrhagic anemia). Diagnosis (Fig. 3) of these anemias requires a decrease in hematocrit also called packed red blood cell volume (PCV), which is the ratio of total erythrocyte volume to total blood volume, and a decrease in hemoglobin concentration in grams of hemoglobin per deciliter of blood sample. Anemia induced by underproduction of erythrocytes may be due to reduced or defective erythropoiesis. Reduced erythropoiesis has been reported because of the lack of erythropoietin following chronic renal disease and humeral disorders, e.g., hypopituitarism, hypoadrenocorticism, hypothyroidism, or hypoandrogenism (35). Chronic disease, e.g., chronic inflammation or neoplasia, also causes reduced erythropoiesis. Radiation, estrogen, phenylbutazone, cytotoxic cancer drugs, and bracken fern are reported to reduce erythropoiesis by cytotoxic bone marrow damage (47). Immune mediated diseases, myelophthisis, viral or bacterial infections, or infestation with selected parasites may be responsible for reduced erythropoiesis. Defective erythropoiesis may be induced by defects in nucleic acid synthesis, vitamin B-12 deficiency, folic acid deficiency, and disorders of heme synthesis caused by deficiencies of iron, pyridoxine, or copper or by excessive concentrations of lead, molybdenum, or chloramphenicol (35).

Hemolytic anemias are the result of increased erythrocyte destruction caused by intravascular effects or phagocytosis. Intravascular hemolysis may occur because of bacterial infections (*Leptospira* or *Clostridium*), parasitic infections (*Babesia*), immune mediated disease caused by autoimmune disease, hyposmolarity caused by injection of hypotonic fluids, or hypophosphatemia. Plant, animal, and chemical toxins may also be responsible for increased erythrocyte destruction. Ricin from the castor bean and snake venoms, particularly from pit vipers (e.g., rattlesnakes or moccasins in the United States), also cause erythrocyte destruction. Onions, rye grass, red maple, phenothiazine benzocaine, acetaminophen, phenazopyridine, copper, and members of *Brassiccae* family also have been reported to cause intravascular hemolysis with resulting Heinz-body formation. Phagocytic hemolysis may result because of erythrocytic parasites such as *Anaplasma, Eperythrozoon, Hemobartonella,* or *Cytauxzoon,* immune mediated diseases, erythrocytic defects, e.g., pyruvate kinase deficiencies or porphyria, or cellular fragmentation caused by intravascular coagulation, vasculitis, or hemangiosarcoma (35).

Hemorrhagic anemias are the result of acute blood loss caused by trauma, gastrointestinal ulcers, reduced intravascular coagulation, warfarin poisoning, sweet clover poisoning, and bracken fern poisoning. Acute blood loss may become a chronic problem caused by internal or external parasites, e.g., hookworms or mosquitoes, vascular neoplasia, hemophilia, or thrombocytopenia (35).

Polycythemia is an increase in the numbers of erythrocytes with a resulting increase in hematocrit and hemoglobin concentration. Polycythemia may occur from vascular shock, which depletes the serum (extracellular fluid) or shifts the extracellular fluid to an intracellular fluid compartment, water lost to excessive diuresis, splenic contraction to deliver more erythrocytes to the circulation, and increased erythropoiesis caused by chronic hypoxia, which may occur at high altitudes or with chronic pulmonary disease, neoplasia, hydronephrosis, or certain endocrine diseases, e.g., hyperadrenocorticism.

Hemoglobin

Hemoglobin is the combination of the metal iron conjugated to a protein. Each hemoglobin molecule is composed of four heme units, with each unit associated with a polypeptide chain. The synthesis of heme is outlined in Fig. 4. The hemoglobin molecule is a sphere with dimensions of $65 \times 55 \times 50$ Å and a molecular weight of 64,458.

Hemoglobin can be measured by a variety of methods. The preferred method employs the conversion of hemoglobin to cyanomethemoglobin following addition of potassium ferricyanide to the blood sample. The resulting cyanomethemoglobin concentration is proportional to its absorption at 540 nm in a spectrophotometer. Methemoglobin has oxidized the iron to the ferric state (+3), whereas hemoglobin's iron is in the ferrous state (+2).

Hemoglobin concentration is calculated by comparison to a standard solution of hemoglobin. The absorption spectra of the standard solution then is compared to the absorption spectra in the unknown solution. The resulting concentration is then expressed in grams of hemoglobin per deciliter of whole blood.

TABLE 5. *Life span of peripheral erythrocytes*

Species	Days
Mouse	20–45
Guinea pig	80–90
Hamster	60–70
Rat	50–65
Rabbit	45–70
Cat	75–90
Dog	100–120
Humans	130

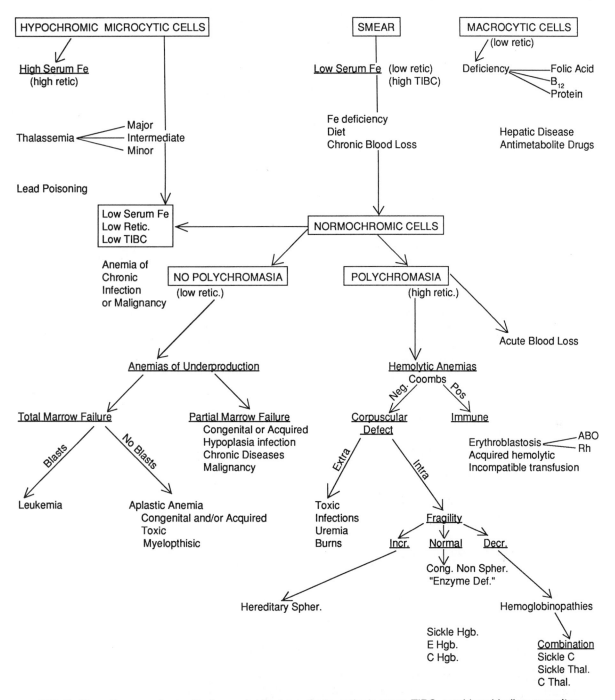

FIG. 3. Flow diagram of anemia diagnosis. Fe, iron; Retic, reticulocytes; TIBC, total iron binding capacity; Neg, negative; Pos, positive; Hgb, hemoglobin; Thal, thalassemia; Def, deficiency; ABO and RH, blood antigens; Decr, decrease; Incr, increase; Spher, spherocytes; Cong, congenital. (Modified from ref. 115.)

Hemoglobin deficiencies have been reported in lead poisoning (47) and occur in the anemias discussed above. In the hemorrhagic, hemolytic, and reduced erythropoiesis anemias, the hematocrit and erythrocyte count also are reduced. A unique diagnostic use of hemoglobin concentration is in the calculation of mean corpuscular hemoglobin (MCH), which is used to define the types of anemia as related to cellular hemoglobin concentrations.

In polycythemia, the measured hemoglobin is increased along with an increase in the hematocrit and erythrocyte count.

Hematocrits

The hematocrit, also referred to as PCV, is the proportion of the erythrocyte's mass to total blood volume, usually noted

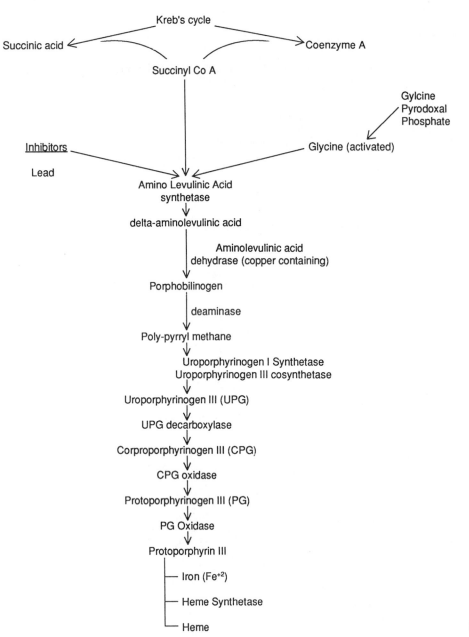

FIG. 4. Heme synthesis.

as plasma, in the peripheral circulation and is expressed as a percent. Centrifugation of whole blood samples containing an anticoagulant is the preferred method for determining the hematocrit. The Wintrobe macrohematocrit method requires a 3-mm diameter tube to which blood was added and centrifuged for 20 to 30 min at 3,000 rpm. The microhematocrit method uses a capillary tube of 1.0-nm diameter and 6 to 8 nm long. The tube is filled by capillary action, whereas the Wintrobe method requires pipetting of the sample into the tube. The capillary tube may contain an anticoagulant, which facilitates the direct filling of the capillary tube from the phlebotomy site. These tubes then are sealed with a silicone-based material and placed in a special high speed centrifuge equipped with grooves or notches that separate the capillary tubes and prevent breakage. The sealed end of the capillary tube is placed toward the outside rim of the centrifuge. The

tube is centrifuged for a short period (2–5 min) at 10,000 to 15,000 rpm. The hematocrit is read from a scale. The bottom of the erythrocyte line or the top of the silicone-based sealant is placed on the baseline of the scale. The demarcation line on the scale between the red-colored erythrocytes and the clear or straw-colored plasma is recorded in percent as the hematocrit. Errors caused by trapping of leukocytes or plasma in the erythrocyte volume need to be avoided. The layer of leukocytes, platelets, and other cellular material is usually called the "buffy coat" and is located on top of the erythrocyte mass and below the plasma component. An accurate hematocrit measures the erythrocyte mass below the buffy coat. The Wintrobe method is considered the more accurate, but the type and amount of anticoagulant are critical. Both methods require consistency in the centrifugal force generated and in the time that the force is exerted. The microhematocrit method requires less blood volume, which is important for rodents and for collecting samples directly from the phlebotomy site. It also requires less time for sample preparation and centrifugation and is less expensive in terms of equipment needed, e.g., tubes, and in terms of technician time. The major disadvantages of the microhematocrit method is the requirement of a special scale built into the centrifuge or held against the tube by hand. The hematocrit can be directly read from the Wintrobe tube because a scale is etched into the tube. Another disadvantage of the microhematocrit method is the difficulty in evaluating the depth or volume of the buffy coat.

On automated instruments, the hematocrit is calculated by multiplying the erythrocyte count and the MCV. The reproducibility of the hematocrit from automated instruments is better because technician error and trapping of plasma between cells are eliminated.

The plasma saved from either of these methods can be retained for analysis of biochemical markers or chemical metabolites. Because the normal plasma color is clear or slightly yellow (straw-colored), the color of the plasma may suggest pathological changes. For example, a red-colored or pink-colored plasma is a sign of hemolysis caused by improper sample preparation including phlebotomy technique or caused by cell lysis. Samples that are icteric (orange-yellow colored) because of the presence of bile acids or bilirubin metabolites in the plasma are indications of abnormal physiological states, e.g., hemolytic anemia, hepatic disease, or bile duct obstruction. White or opaque plasma is usually the result of lipemia (the presence of chylomicrons or other lipids) caused by metabolic disorders, liver disease, or recent feeding. Leukemia (the presence of excessive white blood cells) may also cause the serum or plasma to appear opaque.

The hematocrit is used to calculate the MCV and the MCHC and to verify the erythrocyte count. A decrease in the hematocrit value suggests anemia. However, the differential diagnosis requires evaluation of the erythrocyte count and the hemoglobin value. Hemoconcentration, i.e., increased numbers of erythrocytes, leads to an increased hematocrit. Hemoconcentration occurs in shock, which may be associated with stress (e.g., trauma or surgery), when extracellular fluid (plasma) is removed from the peripheral circulation. Hematocrit also is increased with primary polycythemia caused by increased erythropoiesis after chronic hypoxia, pulmonary disease, hydronephrosis, and certain endocrine diseases. Secondary or transitory polycythemia also can increase the hematocrit because of splenic contraction, which introduces more erythrocytes into the peripheral circulation, or excessive diuresis, which reduces extracellular fluid via excretion. The hematocrit is decreased with the hemolytic, hemorrhagic, and defective erythropoiesis anemias discussed earlier. Excessive hydration caused by administration of fluids, pregnancy, or cardiomyopathy also can reduce the hematocrit. Excessive concentrations of EDTA in blood samples (60) and venoms from snakes and spiders (34) have been reported to decrease the hematocrit.

Mean Corpuscular Volume (MCV)

The MCV is the calculated volume of the average erythrocyte. The MCV is calculated from the erythrocyte count and hematocrit and expressed in cubic micrometers via the following formula:

$$MCV\ (\mu m^3) = \frac{Hematocrit \times 10}{Erythrocyte\ count\ (10^6/\mu l)}$$

Most hematology instruments are programmed to calculate this value.

The cell volume is used to classify the cell size for descriptive hematology. If the cells have normal volume, they are called normocytes. Microcytosis refers to cells of less than normal volume, and macrocytes describe cells that have a volume larger than normal cells. The normal MCV is 58 to 64 μm^3 in young (3 weeks old) rats, 50 to 55 μm^3 in adult rats, 52 to 59 μm^3 in young (4 weeks old) rats, 43 to 52 μm^3 in adult mice, 74 to 86 μm^3 in young (5 weeks old) guinea pigs, and 78 to 85 μm^3 in adult guinea pigs (85). MCV also has been reported for most domestic and laboratory animals including Syrian and Chinese hamsters, rabbits, pigs, and dogs (60,85). Generally younger animals have higher MCVs because of the immaturity of the erythrocyte, because newly released erythrocytes may not have assumed the biconcave disc pattern, the presence of fetal or other types of hemoglobin in the cell, and borderline hypoxic often present in young animals or humans. In cases of anemia, newly generated and released erythrocytes result in an increased MCV in adults. Infectious agents, e.g., *Anaplasma* or *Hemobartonella*, osmotic fragility, and autoimmune diseases also increase the MCV (85). Interference with nucleic acid synthesis and deficiencies of vitamin B-12 or folic acid also cause an increased MCV (35). Transitory reticulocytosis (immature erythrocytes) may temporarily increase the MCV (85). A normal MCV can be presented if there are significant numbers of macrocytic and microcytic erythrocytes. A decreased MCV is normally symptomatic of an iron deficiency.

Mean Corpuscular Hemoglobin (MCH)

Mean corpuscular hemoglobin is a calculated erythrocytic index of the concentration of hemoglobin by weight in the average erythrocyte. This value is expressed in micromicrograms or picograms. The formula used is

$$MCH\ (pg) = \frac{Hemoglobin\ concentration\ (g/dl) \times 10}{Erythrocyte\ count\ (10^6\ cells/\mu l)}$$

In newborn babies and infants and in macrocytic anemias, the MCH is higher than normal (73). *In vivo* and *in vitro* hemolysis (35) and infection with *Anaplasma* (60) also have been reported to increase MCH. Reticulocytosis may present normal or slightly increased MCH values (35). MCH is decreased with iron deficiencies (35) and when excessive EDTA is used as an anticoagulant (60).

MCH also is higher in young mice and rats than in older animals (85). Values for other laboratory and domestic animals have been reported (73,85).

Mean Corpuscular Hemoglobin Concentration (MCHC)

Mean corpuscular hemoglobin concentration is a calculated erythrocytic index that expresses the ratio hemoglobin to hematocrit. This value (MCHC) is expressed in percentage or grams per deciliter of concentrated red cells. The formula used is

$$MCHC (\%) = \frac{Hemoglobin (g/dl) \times 100}{Hematocrit (\%)}$$

The MCHC is the best index in relation to MCV or MCH because the erythrocyte count is not used. In descriptive hematology, lower than normal values of MCHC are referred to as hypochromasia. Hyperchromasia cannot exist as a pathological condition because the normal erythrocyte contains the maximal hemoglobin concentration. Reticulocytosis (85), iron deficiency (85), and methemoglobinemia (60) are reported to cause decreased MCHC values.

Hemolysis causes increased MCHC values because of the inherent fault of the calculation that uses the hematocrit as a factor without correcting the total hemoglobin levels (2,35). Also increased numbers of spherocytes (35) or excessive levels of the anticoagulant EDTA (60) will increase the MCHC value.

Reticulocytes

A reticulocyte is a nonnucleated, immature erythrocyte that may contain some ribosomal or mitochondrial material and appears polychromatic. It occurs in the peripheral circulation because of defective or early release from the bone marrow. Following stimulation of the erythropoietic stem cell by erythropoietin, 5 days are normally required before reticulocytes are released from the bone marrow (60). Reticulocytes remain in the bone marrow 2 to 3 days before release into the peripheral circulation. When released, the reticulocyte is larger than the erythrocyte because the reticulocyte has not assumed the biconcave shape. It is able to synthesize hemoglobin and may have a sticky cell membrane that appears as a rouleaux formation on a blood smear under microscopic examination.

Qualitative and quantitative evaluation of reticulocytes requires a vital stain, i.e., the staining of fresh, live, unfixed cells. Vital stains such as brilliant cersyl green, brilliant cersyl blue using a 1% solution, or methylene blue are mixed with an equal aliquot of fresh blood sample in a test tube. The aliquots are allowed to interact at room temperature for 5 to 15 min. The cells then are smeared on a clean glass slide, allowed to air dry, and fixed in methanol. The smear may then be counterstained with Wright's or Giemsa stain, which differentiates leukocytes and other blood cells (60). The reticulocytes then are counted under oil immersion objective. The relative reticulocyte count is expressed as a percent and is based on the number of reticulocytes per 100 erythrocytes. Increased precision occurs when up to 1,000 erythrocytes are examined.

Reticulocytes appear as large, polychromatic cells without the lighter center normally characteristic of erythrocytes. The identifying character is the blue-colored (basophilic) clumps, dots, or strings of cellular material referred to as reticulum. Aggregate reticulocytes contain the clumps or strings of ribosomal or mitochondrial material, and punctate reticulocytes contain the dots of ribosomal or mitochondrial material.

To reduce variance in reticulocyte counts resulting from the subjective nature of the identifying characteristics of the reticulocytes, an absolute reticulocyte value can be calculated by multiplying the reticulocyte percentage times the total erythrocyte count. The corrected reticulocyte count attempts to reduce this variance by standardizing the hematocrit times the relative reticulocyte count. The formula is

Corrected reticulocyte count

$$= \frac{Observed\ hematocrit \times relative\ reticulocyte\ count}{Normal\ hematocrit}$$

The best method to correct for fewer erythrocytes in anemic animals and the persistence of reticulocytes in the circulation at an earlier stage following anemia is to calculate the reticulocyte production index:

Reticulocyte production index

$$= \frac{Corrected\ reticulocyte\ count}{Maturation\ factor\ (days)}$$

The maturation factor in days is a function of the hematocrit and increases as the hematocrit decreases. At 45% hematocrit, the maturation factor is 1.0 day; at 35% it is 1.5 days; at 25% it is 2.0 days; and at 15% it is 2.5 days (35). To calculate other maturation factors, the factor increases by 0.5 for each 10% decrease in hematocrit. Without contrary data, the maturation factor is considered the same for all mammals.

The normal reticulocyte concentration or count for adult rat reticulocytes is 2% but may be much higher (10–15%) in young rats (85). In very old rats, the reticulocyte count may decrease to 1% (85). The normal reticulocyte count in the young mouse is 7–8% and 3–4% in the adult mouse, 1.5–11.5% in the adult (38 weeks old) male Chinese hamster, 1.5–10.0% in the older (65 weeks old) male Chinese hamster, 2.5–9.0% in the female adult (38 weeks old) Chinese hamster, which is reduced to 2.5–5.0% by 65 weeks of age, and 2–5% in adult rabbits (85). The dog has been reported to have very small numbers of reticulocytes up to 1% (35) or 0.5–2.0% (85). Reticulocytes are virtually absent in ruminants and horses (85) but are 6–8% in young piglets (85), which decreases to <1.0% by adulthood (35).

Reticulocytes are the result of erythropoietin stimulation of bone marrow usually caused by hemorrhagic or hemolytic anemia. Hemolytic anemias usually result in more reticulocytes because of the increased availability of iron for erythropoiesis from the ruptured cells. If iron must be released from stored areas, the reticulocyte response is much slower. With regenerative responses to anemia, the reticulocyte production index is ≤1.5. In hemolytic anemias, the reticulocyte production index is >3.0 because the regeneration response is intense with the continued presence of the affecting agent. With hemorrhagic anemia caused by acute blood loss, the index is between 1.5 and 3.0.

Differential Erythrocyte Evaluation

Evaluation of a peripheral blood smear after staining with methylene blue, Wright–Giemsa stain, or other stains (see

Leukocytes) often reveals the presence of abnormal or unusual erythrocytes. These cells or cellular material include the following:

1. Howell–Jolly bodies contain nuclear material because of the lack of complete nucleus extrusion from the reticulocyte. Howell–Jolly bodies can be seen with nonvital stains, but differentiation is determined by a vital stain such as methylene blue. Usually <1.0% of erythrocytes in mice or rats contain Howell-Jolly bodies (85). Howell–Jolly bodies may increase during responsive anemia (60) or reduced splenic function (60).

2. Basophilic stippling of erythrocytes is note as bluish granular material following staining with a nonvital stain, e.g., Wright stain. A vital stain such as methylene blue is used to differentiate reticulocytes. Basophilic stippling may occur after arsenic or lead poisoning (18,34) and with vigorous erythrogenesis (60).

3. Nucleated erythrocytes are mature erythrocytes that exhibit the biconcave shape as noted by a lighter cellular center following a nonvital stain such as Wright's. Nucleated red blood cells may be present following splenectomy, reduced splenic function, 5' nucleotidase deficiency, or lead poisoning (60). Nucleated erythrocytes are occasionally found in young rats, young guinea pigs, or puppies but are not common in adult rats or mice, Syrian hamsters, adult guinea pigs, adult dogs, or rabbits (85). Increased total leukocyte counts may be reported with automated cell counters because of the methodology used to differentiate leukocyte and erythrocyte cell counts. When large numbers of nucleated erythrocytes are in the circulation, a corrected leukocyte count can then be calculated by the following formula:

Corrected leukocyte count

$$= \frac{\text{Observed leukocyte count} \times 100}{100 + \text{number (\%) of nucleated erythrocytes/}}$$
$$100 \text{ leukocytes}$$

4. Rouleaux formation is a stack of erythrocytes that appear as "stacks of coins." This formation is prominent in the horse, often seen in the dog and cat, but generally is not seen in laboratory rodents. The presence of excessive serum protein or "sticky" material on the reticulocyte membrane may account for some rouleaux formation.

5. Heinz bodies are erythrocytes that contain denatured hemoglobin, usually evident as extruded cellular hemoglobin, on the erythrocyte's surface. With the Wright stain, it appears like normal hemoglobin but stains blue with methylene blue. Heinz bodies are common in cats. Heinz bodies have been reported following administration of aniline, nitrobenzene, phenols, ascorbic acid, arsine, and dichromate (93). The cat, dog, mouse, and human are particularly susceptible, whereas the rabbit, monkey, chicken, and guinea pig are resistant to Heinz body formation (93). Heinz bodies also are often formed in response to anemias (35).

6. Leptocytes are thin cells with a decreased volume-to-surface ratio. Leptocytes can be seen in conjunction with hypercholesterolemia, iron deficiencies (60), and liver disease (60).

7. Spherocytes are spherically shaped cells that appear to contain increased hemoglobin. These cells stain more intensely than normal erythrocytes and appear hyperchromic without the pale center of normal erythrocytes. These cells may be caused by immune mediated diseases, membrane loss, or hereditary factors (60).

8. Acanthocytes are erythrocytes with thick, club-like projections from the cellular membrane. The cell surface appears knobby. The cells may be an artifact caused by the presence of EDTA as the anticoagulant, liver disease, pneumonia, abetalipoproteinemia (60), heparin therapy (60), or hemangiosarcoma in dogs (60).

Anemias

Anemias are classified as a loss of erythrocytes or hemoglobin or a reduction in hematocrit. The morphological classification of anemia requires calculated erythropoietic parameters, e.g., MCH, MCHC, or MCV. The MCH is often not used to classify anemia because it varies proportionally with MCV. It is impossible to have a hyperchromic anemia because excessive hemoglobin would precipitate in the cell. Morphological classification of anemia should always be confirmed by microscopic evaluation of a blood smear, keeping in mind the descriptions of erythrocytes and reticulocytes described earlier. Numerical classification of anemia may not be evident on microscopic examination of a blood smear unless the reduction in erythrocytes is overtly evident. Anemias may be attributed to chemicals; however, the administered chemical may have affected one or more organ systems, which leads to anemia after acute or chronic exposure.

Anemias and their known causes are outlined in Fig. 5. These anemias are based on the MCV and the MCHC.

Leukocytes

Leukocytes can be counted by methods similar to those described for erythrocytes. The manual method requires mixing blood in a special white cell diluting pipette, followed by lysis and dilution of the erythrocytes with water or a dilute acid (0.5–1.0% acetic or hydrochloric acid) solution containing Gentian violet. The cells then are placed on a hemocytometer with grids and counted under a 100× magnification.

Automated electronic cell counters employ either the aperture impedance (116) or laser light scatter (2) methods described earlier. The difference between counting erythrocytes and leukocytes is based on the diameter of the cell and lysing of the erythrocytes. Erythrocytes are smaller than leukocytes in rats, where the diameter is 5.9 μm for erythrocytes and 10 to 12 μm for neutrophils (85). Young rats have slightly larger, immature erythrocytes with a diameter of 6.2 to 6.4 μm (85). Mice have erythrocytes with a mean diameter of approximately 5.5 μm, whereas the neutrophil is 10 to 12 μm.

Extreme care must be exercised in using either the automated method or the manual method to prevent erroneous total leukocyte counts caused by clotted blood samples. Incomplete mixing of anticoagulant, which causes clumping of cells, may also introduce error. A third source of error is with increased numbers of nucleated erythrocytes.

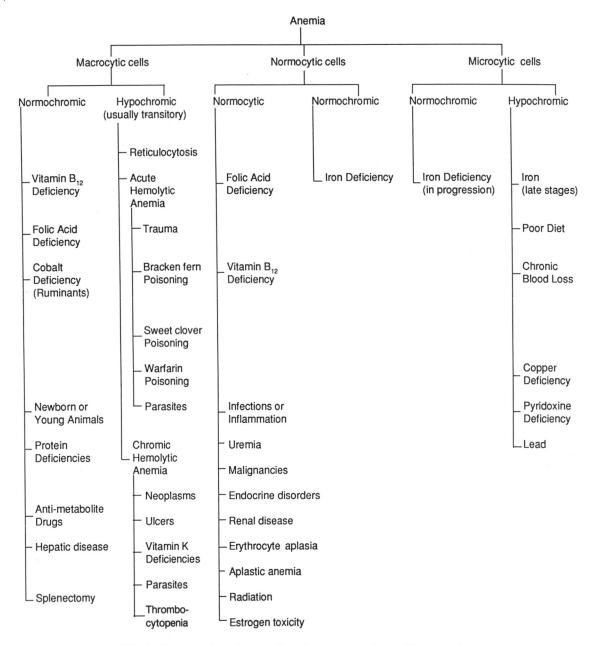

FIG. 5. Morphological classification of anemias and possible causations.

Leukocytes are identified by structure and function. A textbook on veterinary hematology (85) containing color photographs of the different cell types for rats, mice, dogs, guinea pigs, hamsters, rabbits, marmosets, sheep, cattle, and pigs should be consulted. Leukocytes are classified by function into neutrophils, eosinophils, basophils, lymphocytes, and monocytes.

Identification of these cells requires microscopic evaluation of a blood smear. A blood smear approximately one cell layer thick is prepared on a glass slide, allowed to air dry at room temperature, and fixed in methanol. Romanowsky-type stains with anionic and cationic type dyes (eosin and methylene blue) are most often used to stain leukocytes. Wright's stain is a combination of eosin and methylene blue in a basic solution, and Giemsa stain is a neutral stain composed of eosin and oxidized methylene blue. Methylene blue is basic and stains the acidic nuclei. Eosin dyes are acidic and stain the alkaline cytoplasmic components of the leukocyte. A phosphate buffered solution (pH 6.6–6.8) is used to bring the stains into solution. If the solution is too acid, e.g., distilled water, the cellular components will be stained by the eosin. If the solution is too alkaline, e.g., tap water, the staining emphasis is on the methylene blue dye.

The manual method of staining uses the following procedures:

1. The blood smear is fixed by immersing the entire slide in methanol for 5 min.
2. The fixed smear is placed in a solution of Wright's stain (0.1 g powdered stain/60 ml acetone-free methanol) for 3 to 5 min.
3. The cells then are counterstained with Giemsa stain (~4 ml stain/500 ml methanol diluted 1:10 with water or in

a 1% bicarbonate solution) for 10 to 15 min. An alkaline solution will intensify the stain.

4. The cells are washed in a phosphate buffer solution (pH 6.6–6.8) for 3 to 5 min, followed by a wash in distilled water for 3 to 5 min.
5. The cells then are allowed to air dry.

A commercial automatic stainer is available from Gam-Rad. The stains are premixed and should be made fresh daily or replaced after staining 400 slides. About 6 to 12 slides can be stained at once, depending on the tray size. The phosphate buffer should be replaced after three to four staining cycles. The automatic stainer allows many more slides per time period to be stained and requires less time than the manual method.

The staining procedure is enhanced if staining times are varied depending on the concentration of the stain, if only acetone-free, absolute methanol is used, if overstaining is corrected by washing the smear in methanol and restaining, and if only clean, methanol-washed, dry slides are used when preparing the blood smear.

The blood smear should be examined for proper preparation and staining, i.e., clean of debris or clumping under the lower power microscope objective. The high-dry objective and preferably the oil immersion objective should be used when conducting the differential count and classification of leukocytes.

Stains other than the Romanovsky type can be used for differentiation of cell type or cell content (60). The periodic acid–Schiff (PAS) stain colors granulocytic cells a magenta color and denotes cellular glycogen. Acid phosphatase stain will color leukocytes a dark blue color because of cellular acid phosphatase. Peroxidase stains the neutrophils and eosinophils (except in the cat) a greenish-blue color because of the peroxidase activity in the cell. ALP will color neutrophils of most animals a red color because of the presence of the enzyme in the cell. Dog, cat, and mouse neutrophils do not normally contain ALP and will not accept this stain.

The manual differential leukocyte count should be based on the identification of 100 to 200 leukocytes. An automated differential leukocyte counter has been developed for use on canine and murine blood smears (53). The automated methods use a Wright stained smear to differentiate six classes of leukocytes and will flag abnormal or unusual cells for further evaluation. The methodology requires the examination of three color images and extracts various morphological and statistical measurements from previously established identification guidelines. The differential leukocyte cell types are normally expressed as a percentage of total leukocytes. An absolute cell type count may be calculated by multiplying the total leukocyte count times this percentage.

Neutrophils

The neutrophil contains a dark blue-purple colored nuclear band or ring structure within a clear to pale pink-colored cytoplasm. At times the nucleus may appear as a lobulated structure or a "figure eight." In rats and mice, the ring shape is most often seen (85). In humans, neutrophilic nuclei are usually band-shaped. In the dog, the nuclei are lobulated and stain a much darker blue-purple (85). In young rats the neu-

trophil percentage is very small but increases with age and is predominant by 15 to 18 months of age (85).

Neutrophils are the first line of cellular defense that respond to infectious agents, tissue injury, parasites, and inflammatory or foreign materials. A colony stimulating factor is responsible for stimulating production and is controlled by a positive and negative feedback mechanism. Neutrophils migrate to the site because of chemotactic processes that include complement fractions, antibodies, and other proteinaceous materials. Neutrophils exert their activity by eliminating foreign material via phagocytosis and may also have a functional role in coagulation, fibrinolysis, lymphocyte stimulation, iron absorption, and cytotoxicity of other body cells (60). Phagocytosis may be enhanced by fever. Certain components of neutrophils, e.g., proteases, may cause tissue inflammation.

Increased total leukocyte counts (leukocytosis) are most often the result of an increase in neutrophils. An increase in neutrophils usually occurs from uremia, diabetes, lead or mercury poisoning, animal or arthropod venoms, and tissue necrosis. A decrease in neutrophils (neutropenia) often occurs following corticosteroid administration, acute hemorrhage, endotoxemia, *Salmonella* infections, bracken fern poisoning, cancer chemotherapy, irradiation, diphenylhydantoin administration, and leukemias (125).

Lymphocytes

Lymphocytes usually appear as spherical or oval cells with a blue-purple colored round nucleus that comprises 75–90% of the pale blue cytoplasmic area. The diameter of the rat lymphocyte varies from 5 to 10 μm but may be as large as 15 μm (85). The lymphocyte is the predominant leukocytic cell in the mouse and the young rat's peripheral circulation (85). Lymphocytes also are found in lymph nodes.

Tissue rejection and antibody production are major functions of lymphocytes. Cell mediated immunity, e.g., tissue rejection, is governed by the functional T cell or thymus-derived cell, whereas humeral immunity, e.g., antibody production, is mostly mediated in the lymph node by the B cell derived from the bursa of Fabricius in birds and bone marrow in mammals (60). Approximately 20% of the circulating lymphocytes are B cells, with the remainder being T cells (60). Differentiation of T and B cells cannot be determined under the microscope but are separated by cell membrane surface markers. A third class called null cells may be present but their function is unknown (41,51).

The plasma cell is a specialized B-lymphocyte recognized on the blood smear by an irregularly shaped nucleus with a small clear area near the nucleus and a basophilic (blue-colored) cytoplasm that is often mottled or stippled in appearance. The function of the plasma cell is to synthesize, store, and release immunoglobin (60). This cell type is not often seen in the circulation unless an antigenic challenge has been issued.

Eosinophils

The eosinophil is a relatively large (10–15 μ diameter in the rat or mouse) cell with bright pink to red stained cytoplasmic granules and a pale blue-colored polymorphic nucleus. The eosinophil's nucleus is less lobulated or segmented than the neutrophil and may be ring-shaped in the mouse and rat (85). The cellular cytoplasm when differentiated from the colored granules is usually clear or colorless.

Eosinophils contain high amounts of lysozymal enzymes and cationic proteins (60). These enzymes are predominately peroxidases, glucuronidases, and phospholipases with low concentrations of alkaline phosphatase (ALP) and hexokinase (HK). Eosinophils are produced mainly in the bone marrow but may be produced in the spleen, thymus, or cervical lymph node (57). In rats, eosinophils may be generated in 30 hr, with a marrow transit time of 5.5 days, and emerge into the circulation in 41 hr (98,99). Once in the circulation, rat eosinophils migrate into the spleen for additional maturation, where they may remain for 40 hr (28).

The actual function of eosinophils has not been clearly determined. Eosinophils may be important in controlling parasitic infections caused by the presence of surface IgE receptors, in regulating allergic or inflammatory reactions, in phagocytosis of bacteria with less activity than neutrophils, and in restructuring collagen formation in the later stages of inflammation. An increase in eosinophils may be seen in local areas after release of histamine from mast cells, in guinea pigs following hypoxia (49), or in rats with a magnesium deficiency (58). Eosinophilia may also occur in allergic conditions such as asthma or hay fever. Because the level of eosinophils is normally <1.0% of the total leukocytes, an eosinophil deficiency is difficult to assess. However, eosinopenia (fewer eosinophils) may occur with stress (9), corticosteroids or catecholamine release, uremia, acute infection or inflammation (60).

Basophils

Basophils are seldom found in the peripheral circulation of rats, mice, or dogs. The cytoplasm of basophils normally contains blue-colored granules and sometimes pink granules with an indented nucleus.

Basophils store and produce histamine, serotonin, and heparin. These cells are found in connective tissue and around blood vessels and may play a role in systemic allergic reactions (73). Basophils exist in the circulation for a few days, whereas the basophil's tissue corollary cell is the mast cell, which may exist for several months (60).

Monocytes

Monocytes (phagocytic cells found in the peripheral circulation) are related to similar cells found in tissues (macrophages), and monocytes may form macrophages when they migrate to the tissue. The rat and mouse monocyte has a vacuolated, blue-colored cytoplasm with a 12 to 16 μ cell diameter. When challenged, these cells may form giant cells (30–40 μ) or granulomas. The monocyte's nucleus may comprise 50% of the cell, is irregular, kidney or lobular in shape, and may stain blue or pink. The circulatory monocyte may exist for 1 to 4 days, whereas the macrophage may remain for up to 75 days (73).

The monocyte not only responds to infection but also functions in the destruction of damaged tissue and processes antigens in order to provoke a lymphocyte response.

Platelets

The platelet is a relatively small cell (1.0 μ diameter), approximately one-fourth the size of an erythrocyte, with an irregular shape and a delicate cellular membrane. The cell stains a pale blue-pink color (85). Platelets may exhibit as clumps if the blood sample was not adequately mixed with the anticoagulant or when samples are taken from the tail vein or heart.

Special instruments dedicated to platelet counting are available. A direct counting method can be performed with a special diluent and a hematocytometer (60). An indirect method for absolute platelet count can be calculated by counting the number of platelets in the same area as 100 leukocytes and using the following formula:

Platelet count/microliter

$$= \frac{\text{Platelet count} \times \text{leukocyte count}}{100}$$

A semiquantitative or qualitative assessment of absent, moderate, or excessive platelets is generally given. This determination can be made from a blood smear while determining the leukocyte differential count.

Leukocytosis, Leukopenia, and Leukemia

Leukocytosis is defined as an increase in the number of leukocytes above the normal, circulating level. Release of epinephrine or corticosteroids is responsible for a physiological leukocytosis. Disease processes, e.g., pyelonephritis or bacterial infections and hematopoietic or hepatic neoplasia, are responsible for pathological leukocytosis. The terms "right shift" and "left shift" have been used to describe the shift in circulating leukocyte differential counts. The right shift denotes increased numbers of neutrophils with a lobulated or segmented nucleus. The left shift denotes a regenerative response caused by a stimulus, e.g., inflammation, by induction of granulopoiesis or an inhibitory response to delay or prevent production and maturation of banded neutrophils. If the left shift is slight, it refers to an increase in banded neutrophils only. A moderate left shift includes both neutrophils and metamyelocytes (leukocytes with kidney-shaped nuclei). A marked left shift is demonstrated by the presence of myelocytes (leukocytes with rounded nuclei) and programulocytes (large, rounded leukocytes with rounded nuclei).

Leukopenia is defined as a reduction in peripheral, circulating leukocytes from the normal numbers. The reduction is usually limited to neutrophils in laboratory animals. Leukopenia is a pathological condition because no known physiological response causes a reduction in leukocyte numbers. Leukopenia may occur because of decreased leukocyte production, necrosis of lymphoid tissues, inhibited release into the circulation, or increased destruction of circulating leukocyte levels. Common causes of leukopenia are viral diseases, anaphylaxis, irradiation, endotoxins (bacterial), bracken fern poisoning, sulfonamides, and deficiencies of vitamin B-12, niacin, or folic acid (125).

Leukemia is a neoplastic disease that may involve one or more cell types of the hematopoietic systems. Diagnosis of leukemia must include histopathological confirmation including organ systems involvement, e.g., spleen, bone marrow, or lymph nodes. The descriptive classification of leukemia is conveyed by notation of cell type. In myeloproliferative disorders, the cell types are the granulocytic cells, e.g., eosinophils, basophils, myeloblasts, and promyeloblasts. The monocytes, megakaryocytes, and mast cells may also be used to differentiate types of myeloproliferative malignancies. In certain situations, myeloproliferative leukemias may be of mixed cell types, e.g., myelomonocytic leukemia. Lymphoproliferative leukemias are classified by the presence of lymphocytes or plasma cells.

The most often observed leukemia in laboratory animals occurs in the F344 rat (70,102). A review of the published literature also shows the confusion that occurs when determining cell type by appearance, biochemical markers, and function. The usual classification of F344 leukemia is a mononuclear cell leukemia that occurs in 20% to 50% of the rats in a colony with a time of onset of about 18 months. The incidence appears to vary by laboratory and by sex, with female rats usually having a higher incidence. The mononuclear cell nucleus may be round to kidney bean-shaped (semiform) that may be indented and located off-center (eccentric) of the cell. Many cells have cytoplasmic vacuoles with distinct eosinophilic (red to pink) granules. The total white cell count may vary from 5 to 370×10^3 cells/ml blood with signs of hemolytic anemia, left shift neutrophilia, reticulocytosis, polychromasia, lymphopenia, and thrombocytopenia (103). It is thought that the disease originates in the spleen and appears later in the bone marrow. Serum biochemical analyses, e.g., bilirubin, ALT, AST, LDH, and ALP, are elevated (104). Serum alpha globulins are decreased (104). These parameters suggest involvement of the liver. It has been reported that tetramethylthiuram disulfide may reduce the incidence of F344 leukemia (109). This leukemia should be considered when evaluating experiments with F344 rats. It is important to segregate individual animals within each treatment group to differentiate toxicological effects from spontaneous disease.

CLINICAL CHEMISTRY

Many of the diseases diagnosed by clinical chemistry parameters in animals are based on the correlation of organ systems and clinical chemistry parameters in humans. This is often insufficient for a proper understanding of the many varied and often slight changes associated with biochemical parameters caused by chemicals. The frequency of chemical toxicity in humans is very small in relation to the other disease states/disorders suffered by the general human population. Therefore minor changes in animal clinical chemistry parameters are often difficult to interpret.

The protein alignment and matching base pair differ in each animal species and between individual members of a species. This genetic variation increases the difficulty in interpretation of the effects of chemicals on biological systems. Therefore each animal per treatment group must be evaluated and these findings evaluated along with the histopathology to interpret the results properly. In most cases, the mean and standard deviation of each parameter is reported for all animals in a treatment group. This reduces the biological effects of the chemical to a mathematical calculation that averages most effects of the toxic agent across all members of the treatment group. Therefore, any mathematical calculation by the clinical pathologist must also evaluate tissue function and not just serum concentrations. The data may be more interpretable if an incidence table was generated. This might prevent the rationalization that a chemical's effect was due to toxicity when an enzyme's activity increased from 400 to 500 units between the medium and high dose groups while the control group's enzyme level was 300 units. Both the medium and high dose may be significantly different but not biologically different.

Many other factors, e.g., stress, sampling time caused by handling of the animals (to account for diurnal variation), stability at various times and temperature, biochemical applicability to that species or disease state, and optimization of the chemical reaction, must be considered. Handling stress and diurnal variation were discussed earlier. Biochemical stability is addressed in Table 6 for selected enzymes. Certain species may have individual variances that should be verified (22). For example, the half-life of ALP is 72 hr in the dog (55) but only 6 hr in the cat (56). Uric acid is species dependent and is a measure of renal function in reptiles and avian species but not in mammals where the corollary renal function test is urea nitrogen. In subprimate mammals, hepatic uricase coupled with ureosuric nitrogen excretion is a better indication of hepatic function than is uric acid. In primates, uric acid is quite variable because of the instability of hepatic uricase, rendering the diagnostic value of uric acid suspect as a measure of purine metabolism (69).

The optimization of biochemical reactions provides a challenge. There are many packaged, ready-to-use reagent kits available. A major disadvantage, however, is that these kits have been optimized for human serum volume and human parameters. Therefore biochemical tests must be optimized according to species, volume, reaction time, and spectral absorbency. An example is with the chemical ascorbic acid, which is normally higher in dogs and mice (69) and inhibits the glucose oxidase reaction often used in human medicine to determine serum glucose concentrations. The use of a glucose oxidase method would result in false serum glucose levels for dogs and mice as compared to human values. It would be better to use another methodology such as the glucose hexokinase method when analyzing dog and mouse serum.

An advantage in conducting multiple clinical chemistry assays is to perform a differential diagnosis. Certain enzymes are located within specific cellular organelles (Table 6). The presence of an enzyme (61) is often measured in the circulating blood serum or plasma to indicate the organ and cellular component affected.

Those clinical chemistry parameters that are most often associated with a particular mammalian target organ are listed

TABLE 6. *Cellular location of common enzymes*

Cytosol
    Lactate dehydrogenase
    Alanine aminotransferase
    Aspartate aminotransferase
Lysozymes
    Acid phosphatase
    β-Glucuronidase
Mitochondria
    Aspartate aminotransferase
    Cytochrome oxidase
    Isocitrate dehydrogenase (NADH-dependent)
    Succinic dehydrogenase
    Sorbitol dehydrogenase (NADPH-dependent)
Peroxisomes
    Catalase
    Amino oxidases
Membrane border
    Alkaline phosphatase
    Maltase
Golgi bodies
    Amylase
    Trypsinogen
Endoplasmic reticulum
    Cholesterol esterase
    Cholinesterase
    Glucose-6-phosphatase
    Glutathione reductase

in Table 7. An increase is most often attributed to an effect on that organ or organ system (22). Decreases in many of these parameters have been reported without a clear understanding of the biological consequences of such reduced concentrations. Decreases are most often associated with enzymes and not electrolytes.

Equipment

Improvements in the clinical pathology laboratory for human medicine with its concurrent reduction in sample size, assay time, and reagent costs have provided a cost effective means to extract more data from fewer animals. Laboratory automation also has increased efficiency, number of assays conducted, and types of assays available.

The earliest developments employed the continuous flow principle (124). For example, the Technicon Instrument Corporation used this principle in their Sequential Multiple Analyzer (SMA), which simultaneously performed a number of tests. Continuous flexible tubing of various diameters and peristaltic pumps to meter reagents and samples precisely were integral components of the system. A second unique principle employed air bubbles to separate samples and reagents and to prevent cross-contamination. When these bubbles were removed, reagents and samples were allowed to react. This technology allowed stepwise chemical reactions by removing air bubbles at set times. The third principle involves the use of semi-impermeable membranes to separate biochemical parameters from the biological fluid because selected proteins often interfere with the reaction of interest. In the past, preparation of a protein-free filtrate by manual methodologies was required. Finally, the concept of modular

equipment construction allowed rapid, convenient replacement of faulty components or substitution of components for different assays.

The second major group of instruments is known as discrete or "dedicated" instruments (124). These instruments are dedicated to conducting only one or two assays. This system usually adapts a manual method. The instrument manufacturer has adapted some form of technology, e.g., a smaller spectrophotometer, use of ion specific electrodes, automatic pipetting of a reduced sample/reagent volume, or the automatic transfer of reaction mixture into a cuvette, to conduct the assay. Discrete analyzers may be automated to deliver sample and reagent but most often require a technician to place the sample in the instrument while the reagent is drawn from a reservoir. Examples of such analyzers include the measurement of carboxyhemoglobin by spectrophotometric differentiation or sodium and potassium by flame photometry.

The third major type of clinical chemistry instrumentation involves the use of centrifugal force to mix sample and reagents (124). Microelectronics have allowed development of

TABLE 7. *Clinical chemistry parameters associated with organs and organ systems*

Heart
    Creatine kinase and isoenzymes
    Lactate dehydrogenase and isoenzymes
Liver
    Alanine aminotransferase
    Albumin
    Alkaline phosphatase
    Aspartate aminotransferase
    Bilirubin
    Gamma-glutamyl transferase
    Lactate dehydrogenase and isoenzymes
    Sorbitol dehydrogenase
    Total protein
Kidney
    Albumin
    Chloride
    Creatinine (urine and serum)
    Glucose
    Potassium
    Protein (urine and serum)
    Sodium
    Urea nitrogen
Pancreas
    Amylase
    Glucose
    Lipase
    Calcium
Bone
    Alkaline phosphatase and isoenzymes
    Calcium
    Phosphorus
    Uric acid
Miscellaneous
    Cholesterol (diet and liver)
    Triglycerides (diet and liver)
    High density lipoprotein cholesterol
    Lipoproteins
    Glucose
    Cholinesterase

such centrifugal analyzers equipped with computers to be more adaptable to many assays, sample/reagent volumes, reaction times, and/or collection of kinetic data. The centrifugal analyzer gives the clinical pathologist the most versatility in adaptation of reagent kits marketed for humans to modification for animal biological fluids. The methodology involves the transfer and mixing of reagents, solutions, and samples from discrete portions of a preloaded transfer disc into a peripheral cuvette with optically transparent materials. Spectrophotometers with filters or gradients or fluorometers are then used to determine the change in absorbance over time of the mixture in the peripheral cuvette. The application of a minicomputer allows the individual absorbance points to be collected at designated time periods. Collection of these kinetic data allows the technician to verify the optimization of the reaction and note interference in the reaction that may occur because of excess or inadequate sample or reagent volumes, interference caused by the administered chemical or its metabolite, or monitoring of individual peripheral cuvettes, e.g., scratched or dirty cuvettes. As with the flow-through analyzers, the centrifugal analyzers are self-cleaning, require less time, and employ modular component technology for replacement of mechanical parts. The only disadvantage of the centrifugal analyzer is the current inability to perform certain preparatory functions, e.g., the preparation of protein free filtrates within the reaction chamber.

Alkaline Phosphatase (ALP)

Alkaline phosphatase is composed of a group of enzymes with a wide substrate specificity to catalyze the hydrolysis of monophosphate esters (35). The actual substrates *in vivo* are not known but are postulated to be either ethanolamine phosphate or phosphatidylethanolamine because inborn genetic absence of ALP in humans results in increased excretion of these two substrates (61). The enzyme is inhibited by phosphate, borate, oxalate, and cyanide ions but activated by magnesium, cobalt, and manganese substrates (61). The enzymes are bound to intracellular microsomal membranes but do not leak out with increased permeability of the cell membranes. This has led to a postulate that only newly synthesized ALP is released because of cellular damage (35). Isoenzymes of ALP are found in every tissue (35), with the highest concentrations being in liver, bone, intestine, kidney, placenta, and leukocytes. The individual isoenzymes have been reported to be inhibited to different extents by L-phenylalanine, urea, zinc, or arsenic tetraoxide (61).

The preferred method for analysis of serum ALP is the Bessey-Lowry-Block method, which measures the rate of production of *p*-nitrophenol, a yellow chromogen, at 405 nm.

$$p\text{-Nitrophenylphosphate} \xrightarrow{\text{ALP}} p\text{-nitrophenol} + \text{phosphate}$$

The type of buffer used is critical because carbonate or barbital buffers are inert and glycine and propylamine buffers are inhibitors. Diethanolamine, tris-hydroxymethyl-amino-methane (Tris), and 2-methyl-2-aminopropanol-1 buffers are activators (35). In the above reaction, the diethanolamine has produced the highest reaction rates with an optimum pH 9.8 (12). The enzyme is reportedly stable for 5 days when stored at 2 to 8°C (12). If an anticoagulant is used, sodium fluoride is preferred, but oxalate and heparin will not interfere with the assay. EDTA and citrate should not be used (12) because these anticoagulants may inhibit the magnesium ion that acts as a cofactor.

The isoenzymes of ALP have been differentiated by a variety of analytical techniques. These techniques include differences in reaction rates with various substrates, use of selected inhibitors, stability differences caused by protein denaturation by heat or urea, differences in immunochemical characteristics, and differences in electrophoretic mobility. Starch, agar, polyacrylamide, and cellulose acetate have been used to electrophoretically separate ALP isoenzymes (35). Electrophoresis using cellulose acetate has been optimized with the following general methods in a commercial kit (48):

1. Apply serum to a cellulose acetate plate that has been soaked in a commercial buffer.
2. Electrophoresis for 25 min at 180 V.
3. Stain with alpha naphthol ASMX and Fast Blue RR in a sandwich manner with another cellulose acetate pad.
4. Incubate for color development for 30 min at 37°C. Let dry.
5. Read color development at 610 nm on a scanning densitometer.

The different isoenzyme bands from the anode end of the electrophoresized plate are from the liver, bone, intestine, and kidney, respectively. The placental isoenzyme may have the same migration pattern as the bone fraction. To differentiate this pattern, the serum is incubated at 65°C for 30 min (61). The intestinal isoenzyme can be clearly differentiated by treating the serum sample with neuraminidase, which removes negatively charged sialic acid groups from all the other isoenzymes to reduce the anodal mobility of all remaining isoenzymes (61). The bone isoenzyme is more sensitive to urea denaturation, and L-phenylalanine inhibits intestinal and placental isoenzymes (61). Because of differences in DNA base pairs, different species may have different protein molecular weights and charges. Therefore, a scanning densitometer, which allows the operator to adjust chart speed, slit width, and wavelengths, is better than a densitometer preset to human isoenzyme characteristics.

Alkaline phosphatase has been reported to be elevated in those diseases that affect the organs/tissues previously mentioned. With diseases of the bone, ALP is increased in rickets, osteomalacia, hyperparathyroidism, healing fractures, and bone tumors (128). The young person and pregnant women in the third trimester also have elevated ALP, probably because of skeletal development (128). ALP also has been reported to be elevated in liver diseases such as biliary cirrhosis and in primary or metastatic carcinoma where ALP is elevated more than the transaminases ALT and AST (127). Intrahepatic cholestasis causes a progressive increase in ALP, whereas extrahepatic obstructions of bile ducts may show a plateau or decline in ALP activity if recanalization of the duct occurs (127). Administration/exposure to acetaminophen, acetohexamide, allopurinol, aminosalicylic acid, ampherotericin, antifungal agents, aspirin, carbamazepine, chloramphenicol, chlortetracycline, clofibrate, diphenylhydantoin, halothane, gentamicin, and a multitude of other chemicals/pharmaceuticals have been reported to increase

ALP (125). Decreased ALP has been reported in hypophosphatasia and in malnourished patients (128). It is because of this multitude of diseases, chemicals, or pharmaceuticals that the isoenzyme pattern is most useful in differentiating the target tissue/organ in arriving at a differential diagnosis.

The ALP in dogs, cats, and horses is primarily of hepatic origin, with the bone isoenzymes being elevated in young animals. The serum half-life (indicative of stability) of ALP is 3 days in the dog and 5.8 hr in the cat. The intestinal, renal, and placental ALP half-life is <6 min in canine plasma, whereas the intestinal ALP isoenzyme has a 2-min half-life in the cat (35). The liver ALP isoenzyme half-life is reported to be 66 to 74 hr in the dog, 40 hr for the bone isoenzyme in the human, 21 hr for the placental isoenzyme in the human as compared to 6 min in the dog, and 24 min for the intestinal isoenzyme in the rat (22). In addition, a glucocorticoid-induced isoenzyme has been reported in the dog that moves more toward the anode than the liver isoenzyme (35).

Species differences as to isoenzyme concentrations have also been reported (22). In humans, the kidney contains 1.29 IU/g tissue, 3.09 IU/g is from the intestine, and the other organs contain <1.0 IU/g tissue. A similar pattern is seen in the dog, with 220.0 IU/g from the intestine, 6.4 IU/g from the kidney, and less from the other tissues, and in the rabbit, with 8.25 IU/g from the intestine and 2.82 IU/g from the kidney. In the rat, 300 IU/g comes from the kidney and 4.8 IU/g from the spleen.

Plasma ALP has been reported to increase two- to threefold after 15 days, five- to sevenfold after 20 days, 15-fold after 25 days, and 20- to 30-fold between 30 and 43 days in C_3H/HeJ mice with subcutaneous implantation of osteosarcoma cells (45).

Amylase

Amylases are a group of hydrolases that hydrolyze carbohydrates such as amylopectin, amylose, starches, and glycogen (61,123). The enzyme splits the alpha-, D-glucose bonds at the 1,4 carbon atoms of adjacent glucose units. Amylases exist as the alpha-isomer that functions as an endoamylase to cleave any 1,4 linkages along a polyglucan chain and the beta-isomer that cleaves two glucose units (maltose) at a time beginning at the terminal reducing end of a polyglucan chain (61). Both isomers exist in humans and animals, but the alpha-isomer is the one measured in diagnostic medicine. The greatest concentration of amylase is in the pancreas of mammals (22) and humans (61). The enzyme is synthesized by the pancreatic acinar cells and secreted into the small intestine for digestion of starches. The salivary glands also secrete an amylase called ptyalin, which hydrolyzes starches in the upper gastrointestinal tract, the mouth, and the esophagus. Both sites favor the hydrolysis of starches in an alkaline medium. The enzymes are destroyed by the acidity of the stomach and by the acidity or the presence of trypsin in the lower intestine.

The preferred analytical method for amylase requires measuring the increase in nicotinamide adenine dinucleotide (NADH) at 340 nm after a series of reactions where amylase hydrolyzes maltotetraose to maltose:

$$\text{Maltotetraose} \xrightarrow{\text{amylase}} 2 \text{ maltose}$$

$$\text{Maltose} + \text{phosphate} \xrightarrow[\text{phosphorylase}]{\text{maltose}} \text{glucose} + \beta\text{-glucose-1-phosphate}$$

$$\beta\text{-glucose-1-phosphate} \xrightarrow{\text{phosphoglucomutase}} \text{glucose-6-phosphate}$$

$$\text{Glucose-6-phosphate} + \text{NAD}^+ \xrightarrow[\text{dehydrogenase}]{\text{glucose-6-phosphate}}$$

$$\text{6-phosphogluconate} + \text{NADH}$$

Urine amylase can also be determined by diluting urine with 19 parts of distilled water (1:20 dilution). The production of NADH is directly proportional to enzyme activity. Serum amylase has been reported as stable for 1 week at 20 to 25°C and several months at 2 to 8°C (123). Amylase activity has been reported to be decreased with citrates and oxalates as anticoagulants (125). Several other methods employ the production of a chromogen that lacks specificity because of reactions with unknown components in serum and urine (61).

The clinical usefulness of amylase is based on its location in the pancreas. Pancreatic amylase has been reported to be approximately 100 times greater in the rat than in humans, and the serum level is approximately 30 times greater in the rat (22). Reported levels in the dog have been 100 times greater than in humans in the pancreas and 200 times greater in the serum (22). The rat also has 100 to 10,000 times greater concentration in the salivary gland than most other mammals. The rabbit is most similar to humans with 40 times more amylase in the rabbit's pancreas and four times more amylase in the serum (22).

Amylase is elevated within 8 to 72 hr of acute pancreatitis, with a peak at 24 to 30 hr. Increased levels in the urine may persist for several days while serum amylase has returned to normal (61). Serum amylase has also been reported to increase after administration/exposure to aminosalicylic acid, benthanechol, copper, dexamethasone, hydrochlorothiazide, sulfonamides, and other thiazides (125).

Creatinine

Creatinine is a waste product of creatine and is also excreted by the kidneys. Creatine is synthesized from the amino acids glycine, arginine, and methionine by the liver and pancreas. The increase in serum creatinine usually does not occur until renal function is substantially impaired. Glomerular filtration is responsible for removing creatinine from the extracellular fluid, e.g., serum, and serum creatinine is usually equated with glomerular filtration rate. Creatinine is not usually reabsorbed from renal tubules, but creatinine can be excreted through these tubules if the serum creatinine is above normal. Creatinine's major advantage over urea nitrogen is that creatinine is not affected by dietary protein levels (38). Creatinine clearance tests are also more accurate than serum creatinine in the same manner as nitrogen and its clearance test. This clearance test also suffers from the same disadvantage, i.e., the requirement for a simultaneously timed blood sample and timed urine sample.

The preferred method of determining serum or urine creatinine is the Jaffé reaction (97):

Creatinine + NaOH + picric acid → creatinine-picric acid

The production rate of the orange-red colored creatinine-picric acid solution is proportional to the serum creatinine concentration at 510 nm in a spectrophotometer. A commercial kit requires 20 μl of serum or urine reacted with 350 μl of reagent (95) to produce a linear reaction for animal fluids, with the first reading taken after 10 sec, with four consecutive readings being conducted 10 sec apart. This spectrophotometric reading is much shorter than for humans because of the presence of more chromogens in animal fluids. The same reaction can be used to determine urine creatinine if the specimen is diluted by 20- to 30-fold. The urine creatinine level can be correlated with serum creatinine for the creatine clearance assay.

As an endpoint reaction, this assay is subject to interference by glucose, proteins, temperature, pH, and other chromogens (121). The chromogens may be removed from the sample by addition of Lloyd's reagent (aluminum silicate) (121). Other endpoint reactions measure the colorimetric of complexes with 3,5 dinitrobenzoic acid or ortho-nitrobenzaldehyde, which are superior in terms of linearity, precision, and interference to the picrate method (121). However, the advantage offered by technological development of computers allows one to convert the Jaffe reaction to a kinetic-rate procedure that is relatively free of interfering chromogens. When commercial kits made for determination of human creatinine levels are modified, species differences in endogenous chromogens require the optimization of the method to locate the linear portion of the reaction curve. This eliminates the interference of fast- and slow-reacting chromogens. This reaction modification for creatinine determination in rats and mice usually requires the reduction of the incubation period to 10 sec before the first spectrophotometric reading is collected. The total reaction is usually completed in 30 to 40 sec.

Creatinine is usually increased in young or pregnant humans or after loss of skeletal muscle caused by trauma, atrophy, necrosis, or starvation (121). Destruction of muscle mass because of strenuous exercise may also increase urine creatine with the resulting increase in serum creatinine. Human muscle diseases (121), e.g., myasthenia gravis, poliomyelitis, or muscular dystrophia, and aging (125) will also increase serum creatinine. Hyperthyroidism and diabetic acidosis in humans also increase serum creatinine (121).

Increased serum creatinine has also been reported in humans after administration of acetaminophen, arsenic, gentamicin, neomycin, tetracyclines, and thiazides (125). Significantly increased serum creatinine has also been reported in spontaneously hypertensive male rats orally administered 20 mg/kg cyclosporin/day for 4 weeks (84).

Serum creatinine has been reported to increase significantly within 24 hr after subcutaneous injection of mercuric chloride into rats (114). Injection of dithiothreitol did not affect serum creatinine nor did it protect against an increase in serum creatinine when administered after mercuric chloride injection.

Significant increases in serum creatinine have also been reported within 6 hr after intramuscular injection of glycerol (113). The creatinine was also elevated after 48 hr. Significant changes were also reported within 24 hr and persisted at the 48-hr period if 1% saline was administered in the drinking water 4 weeks before glycerol injection. Injection of fructose resulted in increased serum creatinine 1 hr after injection but was not elevated at 6, 24, or 48 hr.

A transient postischemic increase in serum creatinine has been reported in young (3–4 months) rats that persisted through 96 hr post ischemia in older (3 years) rats (74).

Bilirubin

Bilirubin is the bile pigment in which hemoglobin from damaged or aged erythrocytes is metabolized through a series of biochemical reactions. Bilirubin is the reduced form of biliverdin, which has been reduced from the heme molecule. The globulin fraction and iron are then passed back into the body's amino acid and storage pools, respectively. Figure 6 illustrates the complex mechanism and organ function for metabolism of bilirubin. Bilirubin is transported to the liver via the blood stream via a saturable and probably active transport process. The bilirubin is "conjugated" or glucuronidated in the liver, transported in the serum, and excreted mainly into the bile. Bilirubin is further reduced to a class of compounds known as urobilinogens in the intestines and excreted in the feces. Because of enterohepatic recirculation, a majority of urobilinogen is removed by the liver and transported via the blood stream to the kidney. There, urobilinogen and bilirubin are excreted in the urine (83,127).

The preferred method for bilirubin analysis is to analyze total bilirubin by differential spectrophotometry at 454 nm. The direct or conjugated (glucuronidated) bilirubin is determined by adding diazotized sulfanilic acid in an acid media to the serum sample (Evelyn–Malloy reaction). The formation of azobilirubin (purple-colored) is then determined by absorbance at 540 nm. There are many instruments and methods for determining total and direct bilirubin, but the dedicated bilirubinometers offer the advantage of low sample size and ease of operation. One instrument (Advanced Instruments, Newton Highlands, MA) requires 30 μl to determine both direct and total bilirubin concentrations.

Another method, the Jendrassik and Grof method, uses sodium acetate and caffeine-sodium benzoate to buffer and accelerate the reaction. Ascorbic acid is used to inhibit this reaction, which may inhibit the reaction in animal serum caused by reported elevated levels of ascorbic acid (69).

Bilirubin is used to differentiate intrahepatic jaundice, extrahepatic obstructive jaundice, and hemolytic jaundice. Intrahepatic jaundice usually occurs because of hepatic conjugation failures, e.g., neonatal physiologic jaundice, transport disorders, hepatocellular damage by viral hepatitis, toxic hepatitis, and cirrhosis, and intrahepatic obstruction such as edema. Extrahepatic or posthepatic jaundice usually occurs because of bile duct obstructions by stones, neoplasms, or stricture. Hemolytic jaundice occurs because of acute or chronic hemolytic anemia and neonatal physiologic jaundice (83).

Serum bilirubin has been reported to increase with administration of acetaminophen, acetyl phenylhydrazine, aminopyrene, arsenic, cadmium, chloroform, and sorbitol (125). The increase in bilirubin with chemicals is dependent

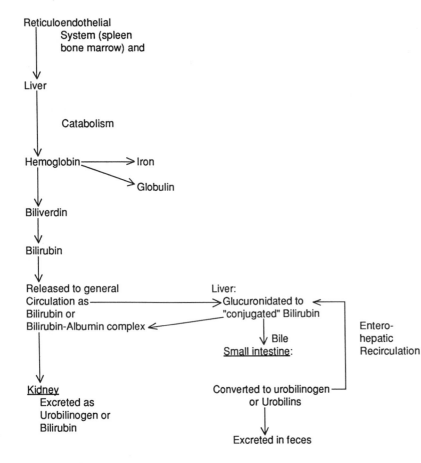

FIG. 6. Normal metabolism and excretion of bilirubin.

on the chemical's site of action, e.g., hemolytic anemia or intrahepatic jaundice.

Total plasma bilirubin has been reported to increase in male Sprague–Dawley rats pretreated with acetone followed by exposure to carbon tetrachloride (46). Whether the carbon tetrachloride was administered via inhalation or by gavage with corn oil or water, the plasma bilirubin paralleled plasma ALT and blood acetone levels. Total plasma bilirubin has also been reported to increase when male Sprague-Dawley rats were challenged via gavage of acetone, 2-butanone, 2-hexanone, Mirex, or Chlordecone and subsequently exposed to chloroform via gavage in corn oil (54). The 2-hexanone caused the greatest increase in plasma bilirubin from 18 to 72 hr. The 2-butanone exposure created the next highest plasma bilirubin levels from 18 to 48 hr. Acetone demonstrated a lesser effect than 2-butanone during the same time period. In each case, the plasma bilirubin was greatest at 24 hr after the subsequent chloroform exposure.

Total serum bilirubin has also been reported to increase twofold in F344 rats with leukemia at sacrifice and 20-fold in early-death animals with leukemia (64). The deviation in total bilirubin was also greater in rats with leukemia. The direct bilirubin was sevenfold greater in scheduled sacrifice animals with leukemia and 90- to 100-fold greater in early-death animals. The standard deviations of direct bilirubin were also increased in a pattern similar to total plasma bilirubin.

Cholesterol

Cholesterol is the most abundant unsaturated steroid alcohol in human tissues and fluids. It is a precursor to steroid hormones and bile acids, is a structural component of cellular membranes, and is transported by low density, very low density (VLDL), and high density lipoproteins. The majority of cholesterol is transported as the ester. Therefore the preferred method employs the use of cholesterol esterase to hydrolyze the ester to cholesterol. The cholesterol is oxidized with the generation of hydrogen peroxide (H_2O_2), which is coupled to form a quinonemine dye. The total change in absorbance after 8 min is proportional to the serum cholesterol as measured at 510 nm (15). The complete reaction is

$$\text{Cholesterol esters} \underset{\text{esterase}}{\overset{\text{cholesterol}}{\rightleftharpoons}} \text{Cholesterol + fatty acids}$$

$$\text{Cholesterol + oxygen} \underset{\text{esterase}}{\overset{\text{cholesterol}}{\rightleftharpoons}} \text{Cholest-4-en-3-one} + H_2O_2$$

$$2\ H_2O_2 + \text{4-aminoantipyrene + phenol} \overset{\text{peroxidase}}{\rightleftharpoons}$$

$$\text{Quinonemine dye + water}$$

Serum cholesterol may be affected by recent dietary intake of liquids or cholesterol. For consistent, comparable results in animal studies, the animals should be fasted 6 to 12 hr.

Hypercholesterolemia has been reported in renal disease, liver disease, hypothyroidism, and diabetes mellitus (36). Hypercholesterolemia has also been reported with administration of acetophenazine, acetohexamide, arsenicals, chlorpromazine, diphenylhydantoin, ether, and sulfonamides (125).

Hypocholesterolemia has been reported in hyperthyroidism (36), severe or chronic hepatitis (36), heart disease (36), arteriosclerosis (36), and high carbohydrate diets (125). Chemical agents that have been reported to cause hypocholesterolemia are androgens, ascorbic acid, chlortetracycline, ethanol, monoamine oxidase inhibitors, niacin, and thiouracil (125).

Hypercholesterolemia of dietary origin has been reported to enhance mammary carcinogenesis initiated with 7,12-dimethylbenz(a)anthracene in female Sprague-Dawley rats (62). Hypercholesterolemia has also been reported in young marmosets with vitamin C deficiency (71) caused by dietary influences in several animal species (27,71,112) and administration of streptozocin to diabetic rats (40), Chinese hamsters (39), and mice (39).

Cholinesterase

Cholinesterase refers to a group of related enzymes found in serum and erythrocytes that hydrolyze acetylcholine. In addition, the enzyme may act on substrates such as butyryl and other acyl thiocholine and choline esters. The enzyme found in serum is often referred to as "pseudocholinesterase" and is also found in the liver, pancreas, heart, and white matter of the brain. The other enzyme is referred to as "true" or red cell cholinesterase because of its presence in erythrocytes, nerve cells, spleen, lungs, and gray matter in the brain (61).

The serum cholinesterase rapidly hydrolyzes acetylcholine and other choline esters as well as benzoylcholine (128) but cannot hydrolyze acetyl-beta-methylcholine (61). The erythrocyte cholinesterase can hydrolyze the acetyl-beta-methylcholine but not benzoylcholine. Acetylcholine may also inhibit erythrocyte cholinesterase (61).

A commercial method is available that exploits the common acetylcholine substrate for both serum and erythrocytes (13). The enzyme activity is proportional to the increased production of the yellow chromogen thionitrobenzoic acid, also called 5-mercapto-2-nitrobenzoic acid, at 405 nm. This chromogen is developed from 5,5'-dithiobis (2-nitrobenzoic) acid (DTNB), also called Ellman's reagent.

$$\text{Acetylcholine} \xrightarrow{\text{cholinesterase}} \text{Thiocholine} + \text{acetate}$$

$$\text{Thiocholine} + \text{DTNB} \rightarrow \text{Thionitrobenzoic acid}$$

Cholinesterase is reportedly stable for several days at 4°C and in plasma when EDTA is used as an anticoagulant (13). On a GEMSAEC centrifugal analyzer (Electro-nucleonics), the enzyme is measured using 10 μl of sample and 310 μl of reagent and incubated for 5 sec, with six readings taken every 30 sec for 3 min (20). The same reaction can be used to measure serum and erythrocyte cholinesterase. Erythrocytes are washed three times with isotonic saline at the ratio of 0.2 ml whole blood to 2.0 ml saline. Between each wash, the centrifuged supernatant (saline) is removed. The erythrocytes are then lysed with 2.0 ml distilled water. The lysed solution is then used as outlined above, with 10 μl being used as the sample size.

Cholinesterase is most often decreased in humans after pesticide exposure, especially organophosphates (61,128). Serum levels are also decreased in hepatic disease, acute infections, muscular dystrophy, renal disease, pulmonary emboli, and myocardial infarctions (61).

The decrease in serum cholinesterase varied when rats or dogs were administered organophosphate pesticides (120). This decrease varied from 25% to 82% of normal in the dog and 0% to 80% in the rat administered several different pesticides. Carbaryl has been reported (75) to decrease erythrocyte and plasma cholinesterase to 30% of normal in rats after 450 to 1,200 mg of carbaryl/kg body weight was administered by gavage in polyethylene glycol. Plasma cholinesterase levels but not erythrocyte cholinesterase levels have been reported to decrease in rats following gavage of isopropyl methyl phosphonofluoridate (an organophosphate nerve gas) (126).

Creatine Phosphokinase (CP)

Creatine phosphokinase, also referred to as creatine kinase, catalyzes the reversible oxidation of creatine by adenosine triphosphate (ATP) (61). The enzyme concentration is highest in skeletal muscle, brain, and heart tissue, but unlike many other enzymes, very little is found in the liver or kidney (128). The rat and human have similar CPK activities in the heart and skeletal muscle, but the rat has twice the activity in the brain as compared to the human (22). The rabbit has similar CPK levels as humans and rats in the skeletal muscle, two- to threefold more in the heart, and an intermediate level in the brain (22). The CPK activity in the dog is more similar to the rabbit than to the rat or human (22).

The preferred method of analysis in animals is to measure the kinetic increase in production of nicotinamide adenine dinucleotide phosphate (NADPH) at 340 nm. The principle involves the dephosphorylation of creatine phosphate by CPK, which is coupled to phosphorylate glucose to glucose-6-phosphate with its subsequent oxidation to 6-phosphogluconate. The total enzyme activity is directly proportional to the increased NADPH production over a 3-min period at 340 nm:

$$\text{Creatine phosphate} + \text{ADP} \overset{\text{CPK}}{\leftrightarrow} \text{Creatine} + \text{ATP}$$

$$\text{ATP} + \text{glucose} \overset{\text{HK}}{\leftrightarrow} \text{Glucose-6-phosphate} + \text{ADP}$$

$$\text{Glucose-6-phosphate} + \text{NADP}^+ \xrightarrow{\text{glucose-6-phosphate dehydrogenase}}$$

$$\text{6-Phosphogluconate} + \text{NADPH}$$

The enzyme is reportedly stable in unhemolyzed serum or plasma for 4 hr at 20 to 25°C or 1 week at 2 to 8°C (18). Heparin and EDTA as anticoagulants are not reported to interfere with the assay (18). The reaction of creatine phosphate to creatine is favored at pH 6.7, whereas the reverse reaction occurs when the solution pH is 9.0 (61). Magnesium is an obligatory enzyme cofactor as with all kinases but excess magnesium is inhibitory (61). Other heavy metals, e.g., zinc or copper, iodoacetate, sulfhydryl binding reagents, excess adenosine diphosphate (ADP), citrate, fluoride, and L-thyroxine will inhibit CPK activity (61). The enzyme's activity may be restored by incubation with cysteine, glutathione, mercaptoethanol, thioglycolic acid, and dithiothreitol (61).

Isoenzymes of CPK are composed of two subunits, often referred to as muscle-derived (M) or brain-derived (B). Three isoenzymes are found in humans and most mammals. The CPK-1 (BB) predominates in nervous tissue such as the central nervous system. The CPK-2 (MB) predominates in the heart muscle. The CPK-3 (MM) is found most in the skeletal muscle with lesser levels in the heart. The isoenzymes may be separated by precipitation with antibodies, selective elution from a chromatographic column, differences in isoenzyme reaction rates, and electrophoresis (61). Electrophoresis on agarose, polyacrylamide, and cellulose acetate gels is the preferred method. One commercial method uses separation of CPK isoenzymes from serum on cellulose acetate plates at 300 volts for 10 min (52). A fluorescent color is developed from NADH after incubation with oxidized nicotinamide dinucleotide (NAD) for 25 min at 37°C. The colored isoenzymes' relative concentration is scanned at 570 nm. The actual concentration is calculated as the percentage of each isoenzyme multiplied by the total CPK activity. The CPK-1 moves more rapidly toward the anode and the CPK-3 moves the slowest.

Serum CPK is a very sensitive indicator, becoming rapidly elevated in 4 to 6 hr after the target tissue is affected. If the injury is not progressive, the serum CPK levels will return to normal in 24 to 48 hr (35). Total CPK is elevated in humans with muscle diseases such as muscular dystrophy, viral myositis, and polymyositis (61). Serum CPK activity may also be increased with cerebral diseases, e.g., ischemia, cerebrovascular diseases (61), and cardiovascular diseases, e.g., infarcts, coronary insufficiency, and angina (128). Total serum CPK has been reported to increase after administration/exposure to barbiturates, carbromal, clindamycin, ethanol, halothane, and intramuscular injections of many pharmaceutical agents (125). Decreases in serum CPK activity have been reported when phenothiazines are administered (125). The individual isoenzymes are increased in relation to the target organ. Activity of CPK-3 is related to the muscle diseases and muscular damage caused by injections of pharmaceuticals previously noted. The CPK-2 activity is elevated in diseases of myocardial origin and CPK-1 is elevated when nervous tissue is affected. Elevations in CPK-1 have also been reported in metastatic carcinoma of many organs, e.g., lung, prostate, breast, pancreas, blood cells, and nervous system (43).

In animals, serum CPK has been reported to increase following shipment of animals and during periods of strenuous exercise especially by dogs and horses (35). Total serum CPK has been reported to increase significantly ($p < 0.05$) in C3H mice after intraperitoneal injection of brown recluse spider venom (6). The fivefold increase in serum CPK occurred within 6 hr of injection but was only increased by twofold after 54 hr. Both CPK-1 and CPK-2 were increased approximately 20-fold greater than control after 6 hr but only two- to fourfold after 54 hr. The CPK-3 was slightly elevated at 6 hr and increased by fourfold after 54 hr. The sudden increase in CPK-1 and CPK-2 was postulated to be the result of rapid effects of the venom on the nervous system and the myocardium. The later increases in CPK-3 were postulated to be the result of muscular necrosis in the mice. When humans are bitten by the spider, the usual sign is muscular necrosis that may continue for months.

Gamma-Glutamyltransferase (GGT)

Gamma-glutamyltransferase specifically transfers the gamma-glutamyl group from peptides to another acceptor compound, usually another peptide or amino acid. The enzyme was first isolated from the kidney, but its diagnostic use is usually associated with the liver (Table 7). The renal GGT is thought to be excreted into the urine (35). A small amount is also present in the pancreas of certain species (22). The larger amount of the enzyme is found in the cellular membrane but some remains in the cytosol (61) (usually <5%) (35). As a component of the cell membrane, its function is postulated to transport proteins and amino acids across the cellular membrane as a gamma-glutamyl peptide (81), to play a role in glutathione metabolism (61), and to increase with microsomal induction (127).

The preferred assay technique for animal clinical chemistry is the transfer of a gamma-glutamyl from nitroanilide to glycylglycine with the increase in absorbance of the nitrobenzoate (yellow-colored) at 405 nm being proportional to the enzyme's activity. The reaction is often referred to as the SZASZ method (108):

L-gamma-glutamyl-3-carboxy 4-nitroanilide

$$+ \text{ glycylglycine} \xrightarrow{\text{GGT}} \text{5-Amino-2-nitrobenzoate}$$

$$+ \text{ gamma-glutamyl-glycylglycine}$$

The reaction requires unhemolyzed serum or plasma with EDTA as the anticoagulant. The enzyme is stable for seven days at 2 to 8°C or one day at 20 to 25°C.

The clinical value of GGT is in the diagnosis of liver diseases. The highest levels of GGT in humans are reported in intra- or posthepatic biliary obstruction when the enzyme may be 5 to 30 times normal (61). It is also considered to be a more sensitive enzyme than transaminases or ALP in detection of obstructive jaundice, cholangitis, and cholecystitis because GGT increases earlier and the increase persists longer than the other enzymes (7). With infectious hepatitis, the enzyme only increases by two- to fivefold, whereas the transaminases show a greater increase (61). These same increased levels may occur with fatty livers, pancreatitis, and drug intoxication (61).

Acetaminophen, barbiturates, ethanol, and phenytoin have been reported to induce or cause increased levels of serum GGT (125). When this is applied to animals, it is an additional reason not to use barbiturates as an anesthetic if animals are serially bled or if the induction period has not been identified for each species and sex.

It has been reported that GGT was markedly increased in rats after administration of N-2-fluorenylacetamide, a hepatic carcinogen, or phenobarbital (79). It has also been reported that serum circulating levels of GGT are lower in the rat than in the dog, humans, horses, or pigs (22).

Glucose

Glucose is the major circulating carbohydrate, which may be derived from the diet or metabolism of glycogen, fructose, or other sugars. The carbohydrate metabolic cycle, which is responsible for glucose anabolism and catabolism, is referred to as the glycolytic cycle. Glucose is the major energy source in mammals. Serum glucose levels may be abnormal in many diseases, e.g., those that affect the insulin (pancreas, Beta cells), growth hormone and adrenocorticotrophic hormone (anterior pituitary), thyroxine (thyroid gland), glucagon (pancreas, alpha cells), hydrocortisone (adrenal cortex), or epinephrine (adrenal medulla). Serum glucose levels may also be used to monitor the animal's physiological state, e.g., adequate nutrition or caloric intake (glucagon storage).

The preferred method to analyze serum or urine glucose in animals is to phosphorylate glucose via ATP and hexokinase to glucose-6-phosphate, which is then oxidized to 6-phosphogluconate by glucose-6-phosphate dehydrogenase (G6PD) with the reduction of NADPH. The increased absorbance of NADPH at 340 nm is proportional to the serum glucose concentration (86). This is an endpoint reaction with the change in absorbance being measured after 3 min:

$$\text{D-glucose} + \text{ATP} \overset{HK}{\rightleftarrows} \text{glucose-6-phosphate} + \text{ADP}$$

$$\text{Glucose-6-phosphate} + \text{NADP}^+ \overset{GPD}{\rightleftarrows}$$

$$\text{6-phosphogluconate} + \text{NADPH} + \text{H}^+$$

This method is also preferred in determining urinary glucose. Interference with anticoagulants that inhibit glycolysis, e.g., fluoride, heparin, or oxalate, has not been reported. EDTA may also be used as an anticoagulant. Other sugars such as fructose and mannose do not interfere with this assay. The major advantage with the hexokinase (HK) method is the lack of interference by uric acid or ascorbic acid (24). Dogs and mice have been reported to have high concentrations of urinary ascorbic acid (69), and it has been postulated that elevated levels are present in the serum of many animals. This is the major advantage of the HK method over other methods that use glucose oxidase (24,35). Other methods that employ alkaline ferricyanide or ortho-toluidine give falsely elevated results with uremia (the presence of urine constituents, e.g., creatinine or uric acid, in the blood) (24).

Serum should be separated from whole blood within 30 min. The use of automated instruments to analyze serum rapidly for glucose does not require the blood to contain an anticoagulant, e.g., fluoride or oxalate, to inhibit glycolysis. Without prompt separation, glucose levels have been reported to decrease 10% per hour at room temperature.

Hyperglycemia (increased serum glucose) has been reported to occur because of pancreatitis, diabetes mellitus, pancreatic tumors, pheochromocytomas of the adrenal gland, thyrotoxicosis, infection, chronic renal disease, and chronic liver disease (36). Drugs such as oral contraceptives, steroids, thiazide diuretics, phenytoin, and streptozocin have also been reported to cause hyperglycemia (36). In animals, hyperglycemia has been reported with administration of ketamine, morphine, xylazine, and phenothiazine and in moribund animals (35), as well as those conditions previously mentioned.

Hypoglycemia (reduced serum glucose) occurs with fasting, ethanol, sulfonylurea, salicylates, liver diseases, extrapancreatic lesions, adrenocortical insufficiency, and hypopituitarism (36). In animals, aflatoxicosis, extreme exercise, septicemia caused by gram-negative bacteria, and ketosis also cause hypoglycemia (35).

Lactate Dehydrogenase (LDH)

Lactate dehydrogenase catalyzes the oxidation of L-lactate to pyruvate with a transfer of a hydrogen ion to NADH. The reaction is reversible with the equilibrium favoring the conversion of pyruvate to lactate at physiological pH of 7.4–7.8. At pH 8.8–9.8, the lactate to pyruvate reaction is preferred (61). In mammalian tissues, LDH is widely distributed with the greatest concentration being found in the cytoplasm of myocardium, kidney, liver, and muscle cells (61,128). In specific tissue injury, maximal LDH activity is not reached until 48–72 hr and returns slowly, i.e., over several days, to normal levels if the injury is not progressive (35). Isoenzymes of LDH also exist with each isoenzyme being attributed to a particular organ. In humans the serum levels are similar to enzyme levels in the liver, heart, muscle, and kidney according to some reports on an enzyme unit per milligram tissue or per milliliter of serum (22) but are higher in tissues according to other reports (61). The level in rat serum has been reported to be 12-fold higher than levels in humans (22). The levels in the rat's liver, heart, and muscle have also been reported to be twofold, threefold, and threefold higher, respectively, than comparable levels in humans (22). This exceedingly high level of 1,370 IU/L in rat serum may be the reason for the reported large variability and the reduced diagnostic value of this enzyme in rats (33). A large variability has also been reported in monkeys (33). The dog's LDH level is approximately twice the value of humans for serum, heart, and kidney but similar to humans in the liver and muscle (33). The level is fourfold higher in the rabbit's heart, twofold in the liver, threefold in the muscle, and similar in the kidney, as compared to values in humans (33). These species differences may be indicative of different metabolic pathways or caused by differences in genetic function as animals evolved.

The preferred method to determine total serum LDH is to measure the reduction of L-lactate to pyruvate at 340 nm with the production of reduced NADH (117):

$$\text{L-Lactate} + \text{NAD}^+ \overset{LDH}{\longrightarrow} \text{Pyruvate} + \text{NADH} + \text{H}^+$$

The increasing intensity of NADH production in a kinetic reaction is proportional to the total LDH concentration at 340 nm. By using a buffer that maintains the reaction pH at ≥ 8.6, the production of pyruvate is favored. Because LDH is also found in erythrocytes, the serum should be free of hemolysis. The enzyme is reported to not be stable if frozen or refrigerated, so analyses should be conducted as soon as possible (31). The enzyme is inhibited by sulfhydryl reagents, e.g., mercuric acids or para-chloromercuricbenzoate, which can be reversed by addition of glutathione or cysteine. Borate and oxalate compete for lactate with the enzyme, and EDTA binds zinc to inhibit the enzyme. These compounds should not be used as anticoagulants. If plasma must be used, heparin is the anticoagulant of choice (61).

Isoenzymes of LDH may be measured by selective adsorption on DEAE cellulose, heat denaturation, solvent pre-cipitation, substrate-product inhibition, or coenzyme affinity (128). The preferred method is the electrophoretic separation of isoenzymes based on protein charge caused by amino acid composition and molecular weight. Cellulose acetate, agar, and polyacrylamide gels are most often used (61). One method employs separation on cellulose acetate and quan-titation on a scanning densitometer at 525 nm after color development with a tetrazolium salt to form the colored for-magen (52). Serum is applied to the cellulose acetate plate followed by electrophoresis at 300 volts for 10 min. A sand-wich technique is used to develop color with the cellulose acetate plate for 20 min at 37°C. The fraction with the greatest anodic mobility is often referred to as LDH-1, with the slow-est-moving enzyme being designated LDH-5. The individual isoenzyme concentration is mathematically determined by multiplying the total LDH times the percentage of that iso-enzyme. The LDH-1 and LDH-2 are usually attributed to be of myocardial origin in humans, with LDH-4 and LDH-5 being attributed to liver and skeletal muscle (128). These isoenzymes are also attributed to similar origins in animals but often one or two isoenzymes may be combined if the electrophoresis time, voltage, and medium (e.g., cellulose ac-etate) have not been optimized for each species.

Total lactate dehydrogenase is reported to be increased in a number of diseases such as myocardial infarction, pul-monary infarction, megaloblastic anemia, leukemia, meta-static carcinoma, and hepatic disease (61,128). The LDH is most useful in diagnosis of pulmonary and myocardial in-farction (128). Increased serum LDH levels are also reported with administration/exposure to copper, dicumarol, clofi-brate, quinidine, fluorides, sulfonamides, and xylitol (125).

The differentiation of particular isoenzymes allows the clinical pathologist to define the target organ. In acute myo-cardial infarction, LDH-1 and LDH-2 are usually elevated, with the LDH-1 level being greater than LDH-2. In normal situations LDH-1 is usually less than LDH-2. With liver dis-ease, LDH-4 and LDH-5 are elevated; usually LDH-5 is el-evated more than LDH-4. In pulmonary infarcts, LDH-3 is usually elevated, almost equal to LDH-2, whereas LDH-1 is decreased (61,128).

Total serum LDH has been reported to be increased in NMRI mice with Ehrlich ascites tumors 2 days after tumor implantation (10). The muscle LDH level significantly de-creased after implantation, liver LDH increased by 170%, and heart and brain LDH remained the same over a 12-day period, with a slight increase in heart LDH on day 12. Muscle LDH and the LDH-5 fraction increased when mammary carcinoma cells were implanted in C3H mice (59).

Carbon tetrachloride has been reported to increase serum total LDH in male Wistar rats (64). At gavaged doses between 0.075 ml/kg and 2.5 ml/kg, total LDH was significantly ($p < 0.05$) increased. The total serum activity of LDH has been reported to be fourfold higher after 72 hr in male Sprague-Dawley rats administered O,O,S trimethyl phos-phorothioate, a contaminant in organophosphate insecti-cides, via oral ingestion at 40 mg/kg (63). Carbon tetrachlo-ride at 1.0 mg/kg via intraperitoneal injection increased the total serum LDH by ninefold after 24 hr. Paraquat at 25 mg/kg by intraperitoneal injection did not affect total serum LDH at 48 hr. The trimethyl phosphorothioate administration also

increased the LDH-1 and LDH-2 isoenzymes as did paraquat administration. Carbon tetrachloride increased the LDH-5 isoenzyme. The authors postulated similar organ damage, i.e., lung and kidney, in paraquat- and trimethyl phospho-rothioate-treated animals based on the similarity of the elec-trophoretic LDH pattern.

Total serum LDH has also been reported to increase in F344 rats with leukemia (96). Serum LDH increased two- to threefold ($p < 0.05$) in scheduled sacrifice rats after 24 months of age. Early-death rats had levels that were 15-fold above normal ($p < 0.05$). However, the standard deviation was also increased significantly in the early-death rats. The range of serum LDH was 83 to 470 IU/L in the normal rats, 302 to 666 IU/L in the scheduled sacrifice leukemic rats, and 78 to 11,140 IU/L in the early-death leukemic rats. Scheduled sacrifice leukemic rats had significant ($p < 0.05$) elevations of LDH-2, LDH-3, LDH-4, and LDH-5 but not LDH-1 as compared to controls. The LDH-4 isoenzyme in-creased eight- to ninefold, whereas LDH-5 had the highest concentration.

Total serum LDH has been reported to increase two- to fourfold 6 hr after C3H mice were administered brown recluse spider venom by intraperitoneal injection (6). The simulta-neous increase in LDH-1, LDH-2, and LDH-3 was indicative of a pulmonary infarction, along with increases in LDH-4 and LDH-5, which represent damage to the liver and muscle.

The activity of LDH-1 and LDH-2 has been reported to be significantly ($p < 0.05$) decreased in B6C3F1 mice ad-ministered PRO-ven by intramuscular injection (105). PRO-ven is a mixture of snake venom components from cobras (*Naja*), pit vipers (*Agkistrodon*), and krait (*Bungarus*). These components are neurotoxic, hemolytic and nephrotoxic, and cardiotoxic and neurotoxic, respectively.

Protein

Plasma or serum proteins serve many functions, e.g., fac-tors in blood coagulation, transport characters, antibodies, and nutrients, because they are composed of amino acids. The major function is a physiochemical one that serves to maintain the normal blood volume by exerting colloidal os-motic pressure. Albumin (one component of plasma proteins) most often transports or binds drugs/chemicals and fatty ac-ids. Albumin also maintains the normal oncotic pressure in blood. If serum albumin levels fall, extracellular water leaves the blood stream and accumulates in the tissues or interstitial fluid to produce edema (48).

The remainder of plasma proteins often determined in clinical pathology laboratories are the alpha, beta, and gamma fractions (48). The alpha-1 fraction is composed of a pro-teinase inhibitor (antitrypsin); a lipoprotein (apoprotein A), which transports lipids, hormones, and fat-soluble vitamins; and an acid glycoprotein whose function is unknown. The alpha-2 fraction is composed of a macroglobulin, which is a plasmin inhibitor; haptoglobin, which binds hemoglobin and preserves the body's iron; and the pre-beta lipoprotein often referred to as VLDL (very low density lipoprotein), which transports triglycerides and lipids. The beta fraction is com-posed of beta-1, which contains transferrin, an iron transport protein; hemopexin, a heme binding protein; and the beta lipoprotein, which transports cholesterol, fat-soluble vitamins, and hormones. A beta-2 fraction is composed of complement C3 factors. The last serum protein fraction is the gamma-globulins, which are composed of all the immunoglobulin classes, e.g., IgA, IgG, and IgE.

Total plasma protein is best determined by the biuret method. In the biuret method, copper ions react with the protein in an alkaline solution to form a colored chelate of unknown structure. The color intensity is proportional to the number of peptide bonds undergoing reaction. The reaction is an endpoint reaction with the change in color being determined after 5 min. In one commercial kit for centrifugal analyzers, 10 μl of sample are reacted with 500 μl of reagent (122). Amino acids and dipeptides do not react but tri- and polypeptides form a pink to red-violet color. After 5 min the difference in absorbance at 540 nm before and after the reaction is compared to determine the color intensity, and the serum protein concentration is expressed in grams per deciliter. A simpler but less accurate method is to determine visually the refractive index of serum or plasma with a handheld refractometer.

The different serum protein fractions are usually determined by electrophoresis, which is the most accurate method. This procedure requires the following steps (91):

1. Presoaking cellulose acetate plates in a buffer solution.
2. Imprinting small volumes of serum onto the plate with a mechanical apparatus.
3. Placing the plates in an electrophoretic chamber, which separates the protein fractions by electrical charge and molecular weight. Plates are electrophoresized at 180 V for 15 min.
4. Staining strips for 6 to 8 min with Ponceau S, washing three times in 5% concentrated acetic acid for 2 min each, and air-drying.
5. Determining the density of each section of the plate in a scanning densitometer at 525 nm.
6. Multiplying the relative percent protein fraction times the total protein value from the biuret method to report each fraction in grams per deciliter.

Individual animal species or strains may require modification of electrophoretic charge, time, or staining because of differences in amino acid content and molecular weight.

Albumin may also be determined by the bromcresol green dye method. This method may give inaccurate results with low serum albumin because of the dye binding to other proteins. Serum bilirubin, anticonvulsants, and certain antibiotics may give a low value because of competitive binding to the dye (35).

Albumin and most alpha and beta proteins are synthesized by the liver, whereas the gamma globulins are synthesized by the plasma cells, or B lymphocytes, in the spleen, bone marrow, and lymph nodes (35,72). Therefore, the target organs or disease states in animals are postulated to correlate with similar results in humans.

In humans, serum proteins have been reported to be decreased because of benzene, carbon tetrachloride, phosgene, and estrogen exposure (125), reduced dietary protein (48), liver disease (48) and chronic intake of laxatives (48). Serum proteins are increased with corticosteroids, digitalis, dehydration caused by vomiting or diarrhea, exercise, or epinephrine (72,125). Albumin has been reported to be decreased with cirrhosis, nephrotic diseases, and malnutrition (48,72). Alpha-1 proteins are decreased because of congenital deficiencies, neonatal liver necrosis, and hepatic diseases but increased with chronic inflammation and arthritis (48,72). Alpha-2 proteins are increased in diabetes, liver diseases, nephrosis, chronic inflammation, and hyperlipoproteinemia or iron deficiencies but decreased in nephrotic syndrome, hemolytic anemia, and autoimmune diseases (48,72). Abnormal electrophoretic patterns are reported by Grant and Kachman (48) and McPherson (72) for humans and by Duncan and Prasse (35) for dogs and cats.

Elevated serum alpha-2 proteins have been reported in rats with dimethylnitrosamine and 3'-methyl-4-dimethyl aminozobenzene (32). In each case the serum alpha-2-macroglobulin was increased 25-fold above control levels in animals bearing hepatic tumors. There were no significant differences in animals not exhibiting hepatic carcinoma.

Sorbitol Dehydrogenase

Sorbitol dehydrogenase (SDH) catalyzes the reversible oxidation of D-sorbitol to D-fructose with NADH. The cytosolic SDH utilizes NADH, whereas the mitochondrial SDH activity is specific for NADPH as a cofactor (61). The majority of SDH activity is found in the liver, with very small quantities found in the prostate and kidney (61). A smaller increase in serum SDH has been reported for certain liver disorders than corresponding increases in serum transaminase levels (5,88,119). However, SDH remains elevated for shorter periods of time than ALT or AST (119) and therefore can be used to evaluate acute hepatic injury caused by chemical exposure.

The preferred method of determining SDH is to measure the increase in absorbance of NADH at 340 nm when sorbitol is oxidized to fructose:

$$\text{D-sorbitol} + \text{NAD}^+ \xrightarrow{\text{SDH}} \text{D-Fructose} + \text{NADH} + \text{H}^+$$

The oxidation to fructose is favored in an alkaline medium (pH 8.5–9.5), whereas the reduction of fructose to sorbitol is favored near a neutral (pH 6.0–7.5) medium (61). The enzyme is nonspecific and may oxidize other sugar alcohols, e.g., xylitol, iditol, or ribitol (61). Because erythrocytes are devoid of SDH, hemolysis does not affect the kinetic analysis method (96). Rat erythrocytes contain very little SDH and less than the mouse, dog, or man (1). At room temperature, SDH decreases approximately 8% after 8 hr but only 6.5% after 7 days if the serum is stored at 4°C (33).

In humans, SDH has been reported to increase 10- to 30-fold with acute hepatitis or other liver damage as a result of hypoxia or shock (61). Greater elevations are seen with intoxication following inhalation of organic solvents (61). In chronic hepatic injury, e.g., obstructive jaundice, cirrhosis, or chronic hepatitis, the initial rise in SDH activity is followed by a return to normal or marginally elevated level (61).

It has also been reported that experimental lead poisoning in guinea pigs causes an approximate threefold increase in SDH activity (87). As little as a single dose of 0.025 ml/kg of carbon tetrachloride has been reported to increase SDH significantly in male Wistar rats after 18 hr when fed a semipurified diet (65). Serum transaminase (ALT and AST) levels were not significantly affected at 18 hr in rats fed the semi-purified diet. SDH levels were increased approximately two-fold when the dose was increased to 1.0 ml/kg. In male Wistar rats fed a commercial cube diet, SDH, ALT, and AST were increased after 18 hr when 0.025 ml of carbon tetrachloride/kg was administered. SDH has also been reported (65) as elevated in rats administered acetaminophen (23) and vinyl chloride (29).

Transaminases

Alanine Aminotransferase (ALT)

Alanine aminotransferase was once referred to as serum glutamate pyruvate transaminase (SGPT) and catalyzes the transfer of an amino group from the amino acid alanine to oxoglutarate to produce glutamate. Pyridoxal-5′-phosphate and pyridoxamine-5′-phosphate function as coenzymes of the reaction that favors the production of alanine in the body.

The preferred assay procedure is the conversion of alanine to pyruvate, which is coupled to NAD$^+$. The oxidation rate of NADH to NAD$^+$ is catalyzed by LDH and measured in the ultraviolet light range at 340 nm. Several of the commercial reagent kits use this preferred coupled reaction:

$$\text{L-Alanine} + \alpha\text{-ketoglutarate} \underset{}{\overset{\text{ALT}}{\rightleftharpoons}} \text{L-Glutamate} + \text{pyruvate}$$

$$\text{Pyruvate} + \text{NADH} + \text{H} \underset{}{\overset{\text{LDH}}{\rightleftharpoons}} \text{L-Lactate} + \text{NAD}^+$$

Aspartate Aminotransferase (AST)

Aspartate aminotransferase was once referred to as serum glutamate oxaloacetate transaminase (SGOT). This enzyme catalyzes the transfer of an amino group from the amino acid aspartate to oxoglutarate to form L-glutamate. As with ALT, pyridoxal and pyridoxamine-5′-phosphate function as coenzymes, which favors the production of aspartate *in vivo*.

The preferred assay procedure is the conversion of aspartate to oxaloacetate, which is coupled to NAD$^+$. The oxidation of NADH to NAD$^+$ is catalyzed by malate dehydrogenase (MDH) and proportional to AST activity at 340 nm. Several of the commercial reagent kits are available that use the preferred coupled reaction:

$$\text{L-aspartate} + \alpha\text{-ketoglutarate} \underset{}{\overset{\text{AST}}{\rightleftharpoons}}$$

$$\text{L-Glutamate} + \text{oxaloacetate}$$

$$\text{Oxaloacetate} + \text{NADH} + \text{H} \underset{}{\overset{\text{MDH}}{\rightleftharpoons}} \text{Malate} + \text{NAD}^+$$

The diagnostic value of AST and ALT is manifested in the enzyme's location. The cellular cytosol contains both AST and ALT, whereas the cellular mitochondria contain only AST (61). The majority of AST is found in the cytosol but excessive serum levels of AST with minor or no changes in ALT will allow differentiation of the chemical's target site. Elevated levels of AST have been reported in humans with hepatic disease, myocardial necrosis, skeletal muscle necrosis, and often, metastatic carcinoma (127). Serum AST has also been reported to increase with ingestion of arsenicals, bar-

biturates, methotrexate, mushrooms, heptachlor, oral contraceptives, quinacrine, sulfonamides, and urethane (125). Serum ALT levels are increased in humans with hepatic disease (127). The low ALT concentrations in other tissues make any increase indicative of hepatic disease, and the increased serum levels persist for longer time periods than AST (61). Humans with posthepatic jaundice, intrahepatic cholestasis, and acute hepatitis caused by viral infections or toxic agents have increased ALT levels of 10 to 200 times normal and are equal to or higher than AST levels (127).

Humans with metastatic carcinoma, cirrhosis, or alcoholic hepatitis have AST levels that are much higher than ALT levels, which may not be elevated (127). Human serum ALT and AST levels are usually equally elevated in cases of acute hepatic necrosis, extrahepatic obstruction, congestive hepatomegalia, and infectious mononucleosis (127).

Increased levels of ALT have been reported in acetone potentiated carbon tetrachloride-induced hepatic injury (25). Linear correlations of ALT with blood acetone concentrations were significant when male Sprague–Dawley rats were administered acetone via inhalation or gavage before intraperitoneal injection of carbon tetrachloride. Plasma ALT levels increased by 70 times the control value when acetone was administered by inhalation and by 20 times when acetone was administered via gavage with corn oil or water.

Serum AST and ALT levels have also been reported to increase by 120% to 150%, respectively, when guinea pigs were administered ethanol with a low (0.025–0.050 mg/ml drinking water) ascorbic acid intake (107). When the ascorbic acid was increased to 2.0 mg/ml drinking water, the ALT levels were not significantly changed but AST levels were increased by 50%. The authors also reported hepatic necrosis and steatosis in the guinea pigs receiving the lower ascorbic acid water.

Consistent increases in serum ALT and AST have been reported in albino Wistar rats administered p-aminodiphenylamine, an azo reduction metabolite of metanil yellow (Acid Yellow 36) (92). When administered in a powdered diet, a significant dose-related increase (two- to threefold) in both serum AST and ALT was observed as dietary levels increased to 0.75% p-aminodiphenylamine in the diet.

In F344 rats, the ALT and AST levels have been reported to be increased by three- to fourfold, respectively, in control animals used in 2-year chronic toxicity and carcinogenicity studies (104). When F344 rats that died early were evaluated, the increase was more dramatic. The AST levels increased by approximately 25-fold and the ALT levels increased by approximately 15-fold. The authors attributed the increased ALT and AST levels to hepatocellular disease secondary to leukemic infiltration or hypoxia induced by the concomitant anemia. It should also be noted that the standard deviations also increased as the enzyme levels increased (104). This difference in standard deviations is indicative of the genetic biochemical variation between animals and enforces the need to diagnose each animal as an individual instead of a mathematical determination.

Triglycerides

Triglycerides are esters of glycerol, constitute up to 95% of the adipose tissue, and are the major form of lipid storage

(89). Triglycerides are transported in the extracellular fluid, e.g., serum, in the form of chylomicrons and VLDL. After eating, fatty acids are absorbed by intestinal mucosal cells and incorporated into triglycerides, which are then released into the intestinal lymph and transported to the adipose tissue (36). For several hours after dietary intake, triglycerides as chylomicrons (triglycerides combined with a protein) will appear in the systemic circulation. These chylomicrons interfere with many assays, especially those that depend on a colorimetric method that is measured in the visible light range, e.g., 360 to 600 nm.

The preferred method to determine triglycerides in animals is the hydrolysis of triglycerides to glycerol, which is then phosphorylated by ATP, dephosphorylated, and reduced to lactate by a series of coupled enzymatic reactions (94) via a bichromatic blanking method.

$$\text{Triglycerides} \underset{}{\overset{\text{lipase}}{\rightleftharpoons}} \text{Glycerol} + \text{Free Fatty acids}$$

$$\text{Glycerol} + \text{ATP} \underset{}{\overset{\text{glycerol kinase}}{\rightleftharpoons}} \text{Glycerol-1-Phosphate} + \text{ADP}$$

$$\text{Phosphophenol pyruvate} + \text{ADP} \underset{\text{kinase}}{\overset{\text{phosphophenol}}{\rightleftharpoons}}$$

$$\text{Pyruvate} + \text{ATP}$$

$$\text{Pyruvate} + \text{NADH} \underset{\text{dehydrogenase}}{\overset{\text{lactic}}{\rightleftharpoons}} \text{Lactate} + \text{NAD}^+$$

The change in ultraviolet light absorbance at 340 nm by the oxidation (NAD^+) of NADH is proportional to the serum triglyceride concentration. This kinetic reaction reduces the interference of chylomicrons in the serum, but the assay should use unhemolyzed serum/plasma and serum from fasted animals for less variation in the results. Increased chylomicrons can remain in the serum for 4 to 6 hr regardless of the diet (35). Slightly higher levels of triglycerides are reported in plasma than in serum, probably because of entrapment of chylomicrons or lipoproteins during clotting.

Hyperglyceridemia may be linked to inherited genetic disorders or caused by diseases such as diabetes mellitus, nephrosis, biliary obstruction, and metabolic disorders caused by endocrine dysfunctions (36). Triglycerides have been reported to increase after administration of ethanol, ethynodiol, glucocorticoids, oral contraceptives, or sucrose (125). Triglycerides have also been reported to decrease with administration of ascorbic acid, cholestyramine, clofibrate, glucagon, heparin, niacin, and sulfonylureas (125).

Male rats have been reported to have significantly ($p < 0.01$) reduced serum triglycerides following a portacaval shunt operation when compared with sham-operated, pair-fed, or *ad libitum* fed rats (82). Intravenous administration of 100 mg/g body weight of tetracycline has been reported to reduce serum triglycerides in male and female NMRI mice and lower doses of tetracycline (25 and 50 mg/g) also reduced the serum level in female mice (19). Butanol (25 nmol/kg body weight) administered by stomach tube has been reported to decrease significantly ($p < 0.01$) serum triglycerides in female Wistar rats (8). Intraperitoneal injection of sodium pentobarbital has been reported to increase serum triglycerides by twofold as compared to decapitated or ether-administered male Long Evans rats (67). The standard deviations of the mean serum triglycerides were also higher in the pentobarbital adminis-

tered rats. Intraperitoneal injection of propylene glycol was reported to interfere with a fluorometric method for determining serum triglycerides (67).

Urea Nitrogen

Urea nitrogen, also mistakenly referred to as blood urea nitrogen (BUN), is really the quantitative analysis of serum urea nitrogen. Urea is synthesized from two molecules of nitrogen by the liver. The source of ammonia (NH_3) is the catabolism of amino acids and absorption from the large intestine (35). In simple-stomached animals, the ammonia-urea cycle is closed because intestinal bacteria degrade urea to ammonia, which is then resynthesized by the liver to form urea. In ruminants, amino acids may be synthesized from the ammonia by rumen bacteria (35). Serum urea nitrogen is used to determine renal function but is much less sensitive than urea clearance tests (38). However, the urea clearance test requires collection of both blood (serum) and urine over a timed period, which is difficult to conduct in experimental animals. This extra handling and sampling induces additional animal stress and is inconvenient to conduct during a toxicological study. The serum urea nitrogen levels may not change significantly until 50% of renal function is impaired.

The preferred technique to determine urea nitrogen in animals is to measure the oxidation of NADH after catalysis of urea to ammonia by the enzyme urease:

$$\text{Urea} + H_2O \xrightarrow{\text{urease}} CO_2 + NH_3$$

$$\text{2-Alpha-ketoglutarate} + 2\text{NADH} + 2NH_4 \xrightarrow{\text{GLDH}}$$

$$\text{2 L-Glutamate} + 2\text{NAD}^+ + 2H_2O$$

Glutamate dehydrogenase (GLDH) then catalyzes the oxidation of NADH, which is measured as a reduction in absorbance at 340 nm in a spectrophotometer (17). The only interference in this assay is due to the presence of ammonia when ammonium heparinate or ammonium oxalate is used as an anticoagulant (17).

One other often used method also links the formation of ammonia after catalysis of urea by urease to phenol. The intensity of the resulting blue-colored indophenol is proportional to the urea nitrogen concentration (38). Hemolysis, icterus, and lipemia may interfere with this colorimetric method (38). Excessive levels of room ammonia, e.g., cleaning solutions, and sodium fluoride inhibit both reactions caused by the competition for ammonia in the reaction and inhibition of urease, respectively (38). Bacterial decomposition of urea in a contaminated specimen may cause inaccurate results. Refrigeration and the addition of thymol crystals will inhibit this bacterial action (38).

Serum urea nitrogen in humans has been reported to be affected by the degree of hydration, shock, reduced blood volume (e.g., hemorrhage), and dietary intake of protein. Glucocorticoids and thyroid hormones have also been reported to cause increased urea nitrogen (121). Acetaminophen, alkaline antacids, amyl nitrite, arsenic, cadmium, carbon tetrachloride, chloroform, copper, ethylene glycol, lead, phenacetin, phenylbutazone, and tetracyclines have also been reported to increase serum urea nitrogen (125).

Increased serum urea nitrogen has also been reported in spontaneously hypertensive male rats administered cyclosporin orally for 4 weeks at 20 mg/kg/day (84). Male Sprague–Dawley rats have also been reported to have increased urea nitrogen 48 hr after a single intraperitoneal injection of 0.8 mmol/kg of 3,5-dichloroaniline (78).

Renal ischemia has also been reported to increase serum urea nitrogen in rats (74), with the effects being more pronounced in older (3 years) rats than in younger rats (3–4 months).

Uric Acid

Uric acid is the major waste product of purine catabolism in man (121), the anthropoid apes (121), and in the Dalmatian dog (38). In other mammals, uric acid is further oxidized by uricase to allantoin. Birds and reptiles synthesize uric acid as the endproduct of purine and protein catabolism (121). Uric acid is usually formed from catabolism of endogenous and ingested nucleoproteins and transformation of endogenous purine nucleotides by xanthine oxidase in the liver and intestinal mucosa (121).

The preferred method to determine uric acid is the production of allantoin by uricase with a series of coupled reactions that produce a yellow-colored lutidine dye. The rate of the yellow color formed at 405 nm over a 10-min period is proportional to the uric acid concentration (14).

$$\text{Uric acid} + \text{water} + \text{oxygen} \underset{\text{uricase}}{\rightleftarrows}$$

$$\text{Allantoin} + \text{carbon dioxide} + \text{hydrogen peroxide}$$

$$\text{Hydrogen peroxide} + \text{methanol} \underset{\text{catalase}}{\rightleftarrows}$$

$$\text{Formaldehyde} + \text{water}$$

$$\text{Formaldehyde} \rightleftarrows \text{3,5-Diacetyl-1,4-dihydrolutidine}$$

Acetylacetone and ammonia are present in the buffer to transform the formaldehyde to the yellow lutidine derivative (14).

Uric acid is stable in serum or urine for 3 days at room temperature but can be stabilized for longer periods by the addition of thymol or fluoride (121). The anticoagulants, sodium heparin, fluoride, EDTA, and sodium citrate will not interfere with this assay (121). Lithium heparinate may decrease levels up to 8% (14). Bilirubin (up to 18 mg/dl) and hemoglobin (up to 350 mg) have not been reported to interfere with this assay (14).

Other reactions using phosphotungstic acid to form a tungsten blue chromogen and the decrease in absorbance at 290 nm when a specimen is incubated with uricase to form allantoin are also available (38). The presence of potassium caused by potassium salts in the anticoagulant or buffer will form insoluble phosphotungstates, which cause turbidity in the method that uses phosphotungstic acid. Ascorbic acid or sulfhydryl groups will also interfere with this phosphotungstic reaction. Pretreatment of the specimen with sodium hydroxide will inhibit this destructive oxidation and allow an accurate determination with uric acid. The first reaction is preferred because of these problems with the phosphotungstic reaction.

Uric acid has been used in the diagnosis of gout (38), which is a painful disease with crystallization of uric acid in the joints. Uric acid can also be increased with increased metabolism of nucleoproteins caused by leukemia, polycythemia, or diets rich in organ tissues such as liver, kidney, or sweetbreads (38). Decreased renal function may also result in increased serum uric acid (38). Serum uric acid has been reported to increase following exposure/administration of aspirin, beryllium, chloroform, ethacrynic acid, ethanol, lead, methanol, and anticancer drugs such as methotrexate or vincristine (125), as well as barbiturates and carbon monoxide (121). A decrease in serum uric acid is also reported with exposure/administration of cadmium, clofibrate, steroids, estrogens, lithium, oxyphenylbutazone, phenylbutazone, and sulfonamides (121).

SUMMARY

The adaptation of clinical diagnostic procedures to animal systems requires the development of the proper methodologies that are both precise and accurate. This requires an understanding of technology, biochemistry, physiology, and pathology of many species. The many differences between species require that we reduce the variability of each parameter, e.g., handling, anticoagulant, anesthesia, buffer, pH, enzyme specificity, and temperature, and optimize these parameters to generate accurate data. It is only by reducing these factors and enhancing our knowledge of the experimental animal's physiology that the toxicologist can determine the effects of chemicals and extrapolate those data to meaningful exposure conditions.

REFERENCES

1. Agar, N. S. (1979): The activity of sorbitol dehydrogenase in some mammalian erythrocytes. *Experientia*, 35:790–791.
2. Alpert, N. L. (1980): *Clinical Instrument Systems*, 1:1–8.
3. Annis, R., and Dorsheimer, W. T. (1975): *Blood Sampling Techniques in Small Laboratory Animals*. Technicon Industrial Systems, Tarrytown, NY.
4. Aoki, M., and Tavassoli, M. (1981): Dynamics of red cell egress from the bone marrow after blood letting. *Br. J. Haematol.*, 49:337.
5. Asada, M., and Galambos, J. T. (1963): Sorbitol dehydrogenase and hepatocellular injury: an experimental and clinical study. *Gastroenterology*, 44:578.
6. Babcock, J. L., Suber, R. L., Frith, C. H., and Geren, C. R. (1981): Systemic effect in mice of venom apparatus extract and toxin from the brown recluse spider (*Loxosceles reclusa*). *Toxicology*, 19:463–471.
7. Batsakis, J. G. (1974): Enzymes of the hepatobiliary tract. Biochemical and clinical comparison. *Ann. Clin. Lab. Sci.*, 4:255–266.
8. Beauge, F., Clement, M., Nordmann, J., and Nordmann, R. (1981): Liver lipid disposal following *t*-butanol administration to rats. *Chem. Biol. Interact.*, 38:45–51.
9. Beeson, P. B., and Bass, D. A. (1977): The eosinophil. In: *Major Problems in Internal Medicine*, Vol. 14, edited by L. H. Smith. W. B. Saunders, PA.
10. Bengtsson, G., and Andersson, G. (1981): The effect of Erelich ascites tumour growth on lactate dehydrogenase activities in tissues and physiological fluoride of tumour bearing mice. *Int. J. Biochem.*, 13:53–61.
11. Bickhardt, K., Buttner, D., Muschen, U., and Plonait, H. (1983):

Influence of bleeding procedures and some experimental conditions on stress-dependent blood constituents of laboratory rats. *Lab. Anim.*, 17:161–165.

12. Biodynamics (1977): Product circular 123846, Division of Boehringer Mannheim Corporation, Indianapolis, IN.

13. Biodynamics (1977): Product circular 124117, Division of Boehringer Mannheim Corporation, Indianapolis, IN.

14. Biodynamics (1977): Product circular 124753, Division of Boehringer Mannheim Corporation, Indianapolis, IN.

15. Biodynamics (1977): Product circular 204340, Division of Boehringer Mannheim Corporation, Indianapolis, IN.

16. Biodynamics (1978): Product circular 145006, Division of Boehringer Mannheim Corporation, Indianapolis, IN.

17. Biodynamics (1978): Product circular 166421, Division of Boehringer Mannheim Corporation, Indianapolis, IN.

18. Biodynamics (1978): Product circular 181188, Division of Boehringer Mannheim Corporation, Indianapolis, IN.

19. Bocker, R., Estler, C. J., Maywald, M., and Weber, D. (1981): Comparative evaluation of the effects of tetracycline and doxycycline on blood and liver lipids of male and female mice. *Arzneimittel-Helforschung*, 31:2118–2120.

20. Boehringer Mannheim Diagnostics (1981): Cholinesterase product 124117, Houston, TX.

21. Boon, G. D. (1986): *Hematology of Laboratory Animals: The Erythron*. Society of Toxicology, March, New Orleans, LA.

22. Boyd, J. W. (1983): The mechanisms relating to increases in plasma enzymes and isoenzymes in diseases of animals. *Vet. Clin. Pathol.*, 12(2):9–24.

23. Buttar, M. S., Nera, E. A., and Downie, R. H. (1976): Serum enzyme activities and hepatic triglyceride levels in acute and subacute acetaminophen treated rats. *Toxicology*, 6:9–20.

24. Caraway, W. T. (1976): Carbohydrates. In: *Fundamentals in Clinical Chemistry*, edited by N. Tietz, pp. 234–263. W. B. Saunders, Philadelphia.

25. Charbonneau, M., Brodeur, J., duSouich, P., and Plaa, G. L. (1986): Correlation between acetone potentiated CCl_4-induced liver injury and blood concentrations after inhalation or oral administration. *Toxicol. Appl. Pharmacol.*, 84:286–294.

26. Chin, B. H., Tyler, T. R., and Kozbelt, S. J. (1979): The interfering effects of hemolyzed blood on rat serum chemistry. *Toxicol. Pathol.*, 7(1):19–22.

27. Cho, B. H. S., Erdman, J. R. W., and Corbin, J. E. (1984): Effects of feeding raw eggs on levels of plasma and lipoprotein cholesterol in dogs. *Nutr. Rep. Int.*, 30(1):163–170.

28. Clark, R. A. F., and Kaplan, A. P. (1975): Eosinophil leukocytes: structure and function. *Clin. Haematol.*, 4:635–649.

29. Conolly, R. B., and Jaeger, R. J. (1979): Acute hepatoxicity of vinyl chloride. *Toxicol. Appl. Pharmacol.*, 50:523–531.

30. DeBruyn, P. H. (1981): Structural substrates of bone marrow function. *Semin. Hematol.*, 18:179.

31. Demetriou, J. A., Drewes, P. A., and Ginn, J. B., (1974): Enzymes. In: *Clinical Chemistry: Principles and Techniques*, 2d ed., edited by R. J. Henry, pp. 815–1001. Harper and Row, NY.

32. Dolezalova, V., Stratil, P., Simickova, M., et al. (1983): α-Fetoproteins and macroglobulin as the markers of distinct response of hepatocytes to carcinogens in the rat: carcinogenesis. *Ann. N.Y. Acad. Sci.*, 417:294–306.

33. Dooley, J. (1984): Sorbitol dehydrogenase and its use in toxicology testing in lab animals. *Lab. Anim.*, May/June: 20–21.

34. Doull, J., Klaassen, C. D., and Amdur, M. O. (1980): *Casarett and Doull's Toxicology: The Basic Science of Poisons*. Macmillan, NY.

35. Duncan, J. R., and Prasse, K. W. (1986): *Veterinary Clinical Medicine—Clinical Pathology*. 2d ed., pp. 1–285. Iowa State University Press, Ames, IA.

36. Ellefson, R. D., and Caraway, W. T. (1976): Lipids and lipoproteins. In: *Fundamentals in Clinical Chemistry*, edited by N. Tietz, pp. 474–541. W. B. Saunders, Philadelphia.

37. Faulkner, M., Dixon, J., and Green, J. (1982): *Veterinary Record*, Feb 27, 110(9):202.

38. Faulkner, W. R., and King, J. W. (1976): Renal function. In: *Fundamentals of Clinical Chemistry*, edited by Norbert Tietz, pp. 975–1014. W. B. Saunders, Philadelphia.

39. Feingold, K. R., Lear, S. R., and Moser, A. W. (1984): De novo cholesterol synthesis in three different animal models of diabetes. *Diabetologia*, 26:234–239.

40. Feingold, K. R., Wiley, M. H., MacRae, G., et al. (1982): The effect of diabetes mellitus on sterol synthesis in the diabetic rat. *Diabetes*, 31:388–395.

41. Ferrarin, M., Cadoni, A., Franzi, A. T., et al. (1980): Ultrastructure and cytochemistry of human peripheral blood lymphocytes: similarities between the cells of the third population and T6 lymphocytes. *Eur. J. Immunol.*, 10:562.

42. Frith, C. A., Suber, R. L., and Umboltz, R. (1980): Hematologic and clinical chemistry findings in control BALB/C and C57 BL/6 mice. *Lab. Anim. Sci.*, 30(5):835–840.

43. Ganz, P. A., Potter, D., Figlin, R., and Shell, W. E. (1981): Creatine kinase-BB (CK-BB): a tumor for active metastatic cancer. *Clin. Res.*, 29:435.

44. Gartner, K., Buttner, D., Dohler, K., et al. (1980): Stress response of rats to handling and experimental procedures. *Lab. Anim.*, 14:267–274.

45. Ghanta, V. K., Soong, S. J., Hurst, D. C., and Hiramoto, R. N. (1980): Osteosarcoma associated alkaline phosphatase and *in vivo* growth and development. *Proc. Soc. Exp. Biol. Med.*, 164:229–233.

46. Good Laboratory Practices (1978): Department of Health and Human Services. Nonclinical Laboratory Studies. *Fed. Reg.*, 43:59986–60025.

47. Gosselin, R. E., Hodge, A. C., Smith, R. P., and Gleason, M. N. (1960): *Clinical Toxicology of Commercial Products. Acute Poisoning*, 4th ed. Williams and Wilkins, Baltimore.

48. Grant, G. H., and Kachman, J. F. (1976): The proteins of body fluids. In: *Fundamentals of Clinical Chemistry*, edited by N. Tietz, pp. 298–400. W. B. Saunders, Philadelphia.

49. Grant, J. B. F., and Hudson, G. (1969): A quantitative study of blood and bone marrow eosinophils in severe hypoxia. *Br. J. Haematol.*, 17:121–127.

50. Greenman, D. L., Fullerton, F., Gough, B., and Suber, R. (1982): Clinical chemistry and hematology of mice: a comparison of cereal-based and semipurified diets. *33rd Annual Session of the American Association of Laboratory Animal Science*. Abstract No. 11.

51. Grossi, C. E., and Greaves, M. F. (1981): Normal lymphocytes. In: *Atlas of Blood Cells: Function and Pathology*. Vol. 2, edited by Zucker-Franklin et al., p 347. Lea & Febiger, Philadelphia.

52. Helena Laboratories (1983): *Electrophoresis Manual*. Beaumont, TX.

53. Hematrak Automated Differential System Operator's Manual. (1986): Geometric data. Wayne, PA.

54. Hewitt, L. A., Ayotte, P., and Plaa, G. L. (1986): Modifications in rat hepatobiliary function following treatment with acetone, 2-butanone, 2-hexanone, mirex, or chlordecone and subsequently exposed to chloroform. *Toxicol. Appl. Pharmacol.*, 83:465–473.

55. Hoffman, W. E., and Dorner, J. L. (1977): Disappearance rates of intravenously injected canine alkaline phosphatase isoenzymes. *Am. J. Vet. Res.*, 38:1553–1556.

56. Hoffman, W. E., and Dorner, J. L. (1977): Serum half-life of intravenously injected intestinal and hepatic alkaline phosphatase isoenzymes in the cat. *Am. J. Vet. Res.*, 38:1637.

57. Hudson, G. (1968): Quantitative study of eosinophilic granulocytes. *Semin. Hematol.*, 5(2):166–186.

58. Hungerford, G. F. (1964): Role of histamine in producing the eosinophilia of magnesium deficiency. *Blood*, 16:1642.

59. Ibratiim, G. A., Abbasnezhad, M., Hawmineh, W. G., and Thelogides, A. (1980): Changes in lactate dehydrogenase isoenzyme pattern in muscle of tumor bearing mice. *Experimentia*, 36:1415–1416.

60. Jain, N. C. (1986): *Schalm's Veterinary Hematology*, 4th ed. Lea & Febiger, Philadelphia.

61. Kachman, J. F., and Moss, D. W. (1976): Enzymes. In: *Fundamentals of Clinical Chemistry*, edited by N. Tietz, pp. 565–698. W. B. Saunders, Philadelphia.

62. Klurfeld, D. M., and Kritchevsky, D. (1981): Serum cholesterol and 7,12-dimethyl-benz(a)anthracene-induced mammary carcinogenesis. *Cancer Lett.*, 14(3):273–278.

63. Koizumi, A., Tada, V., and Imamura, T. (1986): Similarity of isozyme pattern of serum lactate dehydrogenase following treatments with *O,O,S*-trimethyl phosphorothioate and paraquat. *Toxicol. Lett.*, 31:85–90.

64. Korsrud, G. O., and Grice, H. C. (1972): Sensitivity of several

serum enzymes in detecting carbon tetrachloride-induced liver damage in rats. *Toxicol Appl. Pharmacol.,* 22:474–483.

65. Korsrud, G. O., Grice, H. C., and McLaughlin, J. M. (1972): Sensitivity of several serum enzymes in detecting carbon tetrachloride-induced liver damage in rats. *Toxicol. Appl. Pharmacol.,* 22:474–483.

66. Laessig, R. H., Indriksons, A. A., Hassemer, D. J., et al. (1976): Changes in serum chemical values as a result of prolonged contacts with the clot. *Am. J. Clin. Pathol.,* 6:598–604.

67. Lenz, P., Cargill, D. I., and Fleischman, A. I. (1973): Propylene glycol interference in determination of serum and lipid triglycerides. *Clin. Chem.,* 19:1071–1074.

68. Lindena, J., Buttner, D., and Trautschold, I. (1984): Biological, analytical and experimental components of variance in a long term study of plasma constituents in rat. *J. Clin. Chem. Clin. Biochem.,* 22:97–104.

69. Loeb, W. (1983): A review of species differences in clinical chemistry. *Vet. Clin. Pathol.,* 12(1):24.

70. Losco, P. E., and Ward, J. E. (1984): The early stage of large granular lymphocyte leukemia in the F344 rat. *Vet. Pathol.,* 21:286–291.

71. McIntosh, G. H., Bulman, F. H., Illman, R. J., and Topping, D. L. (1984): The influence of age, dietary cholesterol and vitamin C deficiency on plasma cholesterol concentration in the marmoset. *Nutr. Rep. Int.,* 29(3):673–682.

72. McPherson, R. A. (1984): Specific protein. In: *Clinical Diagnosis and Management by Laboratory Methods,* edited by J. B. Henry, pp. 204–216. W. B. Saunders, Philadelphia.

73. Mitruka, B. M., and Rawnsley, H. M. (1981): *Clinical Biochemical and Hematological Reference Values in Normal Experimental Animals and Normal Humans,* 2d ed. Year Book Medical Publishers, Chicago.

74. Miura, K., Goldstein, R. S., Morgan, D. G., et al. (1987): Age related differences in susceptibility to renal ischemia in rats. *Toxicol. Appl. Pharmacol.,* 87:284–296.

75. Mount, M. E., Dayton, A. D., and Aehme, F. W. (1981): Carbaryl residues in tissues and cholinesterase activities in brain and blood of rats receiving carbaryl. *Toxicol. Appl. Pharmacol.,* 58:282–296.

76. Oller, W. L., Greenman, D. L., and Suber, R. L. (1985): Quality changes in animal feed resulting from extended storage. *Lab. Anim. Sci.,* 35(6):646–650.

77. Plata, E. J., and Murphy, W. H. (1972): Growth and hematologic properties of the BALB/WM strain of inbred mice. *Lab. Anim. Sci.,* 22:712–720.

78. Rankin, G. O., Yang, D. J., Teets, V. J., et al. (1986): 3,5-Dichloroaniline induced nephrotoxicity in the Sprague–Dawley rat. *Toxicol. Lett.,* 30:173–179.

79. Remandet, B., Gouy, D., Berthe, J., et al. (1984): Lack of initiating or promoting activity of six benzodiazepine tranquilizers in rat liver limited bioassays monitored by histopathology and assay of liver and plasma enzymes. *Fundam. Appl. Toxicol.,* 4:152–163.

80. Report of the AUMA Panel on Euthanasia (1986). *J. Am. Vet. Med. Assoc.,* 188:252–268.

81. Rosalki, S. (1975): Gamma-glutamyl transpeptidase. In: *Advances in Clinical Chemistry,* Vol. 17, edited by O. Bodansky and A. L. Latner, p. 53. Academic Press, NY.

82. Rossouw, J. E., Labadarios, D., and de Villiers, A. S. (1978): Plasma lipids and hepatic lipid synthesis following portacaval shunt in the rat. *S. Afr. Med. J.,* 53:1024–1026.

83. Routh, J. I. (1976): Liver function. In: *Fundamentals of Clinical Chemistry,* edited by N. Tietz, pp. 1026–1062. W. B. Saunders, Philadelphia.

84. Ryffel, B. (1986): Toxicology—experimental studies. *Prog. Allergy,* 38:181–197.

85. Sanderson, J. H., and Phillips, C. E. (1981): *An Atlas of Laboratory Animal Haematology.* Clarendon Press, Oxford.

86. Schmidt, F. H. (1974): D-Glucose. In: *Methods of Enzymatic Analysis,* edited by H. U. Bergmeyer, p. 1196–1201. Academic Press, NY.

87. Secchi, G. C., Alessio, L., and Spreafico, F. (1971): Serum enzymatic activities in experimental lead poisoning. *Enzyme,* 12:63–69.

88. Secchi, G. C., and Ghidoni, A. (1962): Interesse clinico della determinazione dell' attivita sorbitoldeidrogenasica plasmatica in patologia epatica. *Enzymol. Biol. Clin.,* 2:99.

89. Segal, P., Bachorik, P. S., Rifkind, B. M., and Levy, R. I. (1984): Lipids and dyslipoproteinemia. In: *Clinical Diagnosis and Man-*

agement by *Laboratory Methods,* edited by J. B. Henry, pp. 180–203. W. B. Saunders, Philadelphia.

90. Sellers, T. S., and Bloom, J. C. (1982): Hematologic evaluation of laboratory animals. *Lab. Anim.,* 11(6):43–51.

91. Serum Protein Electrophoresis (1983): Helena Laboratory Electrophoresis Manual, Beaumont, TX.

92. Singh, R. L., Khana, S. K., Shanker, R., and Singh, G. B. (1986): Acute and short term toxicity studies on *p*-aminodiphenylamine. *Vet. Hum. Toxicol.,* 28(3):219–223.

93. Smith, R. P. (1980): Toxic responses of the blood. In: *Cassarett and Doull's Toxicology: The Science of Poisons,* edited by J. Doull, C. D. Klaassen, and M. O. Amdur, pp. 311–331. MacMillian, NY.

94. Smith Kline Beckman (1980): Eskalab adaptation of triglyceride method products 89804, 89808, 89802. Sunnyvale, CA.

95. Smith Kline Instruments (1979): Creatinine no. 89420, Sunnyvale, CA.

96. Sorbitol dehydrogenase (1983): Sigma Bulletin 50-UV, Sigma Chemical Company, St. Louis, MO.

97. Smith Kline Instruments (1979): *Spin Chem Reagents for Creatinine,* Circular 89420, Sunnyvale, CA.

98. Spry, C. J. F. (1971): Mechanism of eosinophila. V. Kinetics of normal and accelerated eosinoporesis. *Cell Tissue Kinetics,* 4:351–364.

99. Spry, C. J. F. (1971): Mechanism of eosinophilia. VI. Eosinophil mobilization. *Cell Tissue Kinet.,* 4:365–374.

100. Statland, B. E., and Westgard, J. O. (1984): Quality control: theory and practice. In: *Clinical Diagnosis and Management by Laboratory Methods,* edited by J. B. Henry, pp. 74–93. W. B. Saunders, Philadelphia.

101. Statland, B. E., and Winkel, P. (1984): Pre-instrumental sources of variation. In: *Clinical Diagnosis and Management of Laboratory Methods,* edited by J. B. Henry, pp. 61–73. W. B. Saunders, Philadelphia.

102. Stromberg, P. C., and Vogtsberger, L. M. (1983): Pathology of the mononuclear cell, leukemia of Fischer rats. I. Morphologic studies. *Vet. Pathol.,* 20:698–708.

103. Stromberg, P. C., and Vogtsberger, L. M. (1983): Pathology of the mononuclear cell, leukemia of Fischer rats. II. Hematology. *Vet. Pathol.,* 20:709–717.

104. Stromberg, P. C., and Vogtsberger, L. M. (1983): Pathology of the mononuclear cell, leukemia of Fischer rats. III. Clinical chemistry. *Vet. Pathol.,* 20:718–726.

105. Suber, R. L., and Frith, C. H. (1983): Biochemical, hematological and histological changes in B6C3F1 mice after intramuscular administration of PROven. *J. Toxicol. Environ. Health,* 12:641–651.

106. Suber, R. L., and Kodell, R. L. (1985): The effect of three phlebotomy techniques on hematological and clinical chemical evaluation in Sprague Dawley rats. *Vet. Clin. Pathol.* 14(1):23–30.

107. Susick, R. L., Abrams, G. D., Zurawski, C. A., and Zannoni, V. G. (1969): Ascorbic acid and chronic alcohol consumption in the guinea pig. *Toxicol. Appl. Pharmacol.,* 84:329–335.

108. Szasz, G., Weimann, G., Staehler, F., and Wahlefeld, A.-W. (1974): New substrates for measuring gamma glutamyl transpeptidase activity. *Klin. Chem. Klin. Biochem.,* 12(5):228.

109. Takahashi, M., Kokubo, T., Furukawa, F., et al. (1983): Inhibition of spontaneous leukemia in F344 rats by tetramethylthiuram disulfide (Thiram). *Gann.,* 74:810–813.

110. Taketa, F., Smits, M. R., DiBona, F., and Lessard, J. L. (1967): Studies on cat hemoglobin and hybrids with human hemoglobin A. *Biochemistry,* 6:3809–3816.

111. Tavassoli, M. (1981): Structure and function of sinusoidal endothelium of bone marrow. *Prog. Clin. Biol. Res.,* 59B:249.

112. Terpstra, A. H. M., and Beynen, A. C. (1984): Density profile and cholesterol concentration of serum lipoproteins in experimental animals and human subjects on hypercholesterolaemic diets. *Comp. Biochem. Physiol.,* 778(3):523–528.

113. Trifillis, A. L., Kahng, M. W., and Trump, B. F. (1981): Metabolic studies of glycerol induced acute renal failure in the rat. *Exp. Mol. Pathol.* 35:1–13.

114. Trifillis, A. L., Kahng, M. W., and Trump, B. F. (1981): Metabolic studies of mercuric chloride-induced acute renal failure in the rat. *Exp. Mol. Pathol.,* 35:14–24.

115. University of Arkansas Medical School (1980–81): *Hematology Manual.* Department of Pathology, Little Rock, AR.

116. Veterinary Applications for Coulter S Series Instruments (1982): Coulter Electronics, Inc., Hialeah, FL.

117. Wacker, W. E. C., Ulmer, D. D., and Vallee, B. L. (1956): Metalloenzymes and myocardial infarction. *N. Engl. J. Med.*, 225:449.

118. Ward, J. M., and Reynolds, C. W. (1983): Large granular lymphocytes leukemia: a heterogeneous lymphocytic leukemia in Fischer 344 rats. *Am. J. Pathol.*, 3(1):1–10.

119. Wiesner, I. S., Rawnsley, H. M., Brooks, F., and Senior J. R. (1965): Sorbitol dehydrogenase in the diagnosis of liver disease. *Am. J. Dig. Dis.*, 10:147.

120. Willis, J. H. (1972): The measurement and significance of changes in the cholinesterase activities of erythrocytes and plasma in man and animals. *CRC Crit. Rev. Toxicol.*, 3:153–202.

121. Woo, J., and Cannon, D. C. (1984): Metabolic intermediates and inorganic ions. In: *Clinical Diagnosis and Management by Laboratory Methods*, edited by J. B. Henry, pp. 133–164. W. B. Saunders, Philadelphia.

122. Worthington Diagnostics (1980): Total Protein, Catalog No. 27934.

123. Wu, W. T., and Kao, Y. S. (1984): Exocrine pancreatic function. In: *Clinical Diagnosis and Management by Laboratory Methods*, edited by J. B. Henry, pp. 537–575. W. B. Saunders, Philadelphia.

124. Young, D. S. (1976): Automation. In: *Fundamentals of Clinical Chemistry*, edited by N. Tietz, pp. 187–211. W. B. Saunders, Philadelphia.

125. Young, D. S., Pestaner, L. C., and Gibberman, V. (1975): Effects of drugs on clinical laboratory tests. *Clin. Chem.*, 21(5):1–431.

126. Young, J. F., Gough, B. J., and Suber, R. L. (1985): Correlation of blood cholinesterase levels with toxicity of agent GB in CD rats. *Toxicologist*, 5:274.

127. Zimmerman, H. J. (1984): Function and integrity of the liver. In: *Clinical Diagnosis and Management by Laboratory Methods*, edited by J. H. Henry, pp. 217–250. W. B. Saunders, Philadelphia.

128. Zimmerman, H. J., and Henry, J. B. (1984): Clinical enzymology. In: *Clinical Diagnosis and Management by Laboratory Methods*, edited by J. B. Henry, pp. 251–282. W. B. Saunders, Philadelphia.

Principles and Methods of Toxicology, Second Edition, edited by A. Wallace Hayes, Raven Press, Ltd., New York © 1989.

CHAPTER **17**

Animal Care and Facilities

Gary T. Burger and *L. Cheryl Miller

*R. J. Reynolds Tobacco Company, Bowman Gray Technical Center, Winston-Salem, North Carolina 27102; and *Sandoz, Ltd., Clinical Immunology, CH-4002, Basel, Switzerland*

This chapter provides a general guide and overview of the basic principles of laboratory animal care and the design and maintenance of laboratory animal facilities for toxicologists. Hopefully, other scientists engaged in basic research as well as the testing of chemicals and materials for the determination of their potential for toxicity will find this review helpful. It is not intended that this chapter be an in-depth treatise of laboratory animal care, nor is it intended to be an exhaustive review of the environmental factors and husbandry practices that may affect the results of toxicology research and testing. However, this chapter does provide scientists with an overview of these areas emphasizing appropriate laboratory animal care and maintenance practices and procedures.

An introduction and a discussion of selected government regulations and guidelines concerning the use and care of laboratory animals is presented to make scientists aware of pertinent public law, regulations, and guidelines. A brief discussion of environmental factors such as diet, drinking water, caging, temperature, humidity, lighting, noise, and room ventilation is also presented. A section on the physical plant and husbandry practices presents scientists with a discussion of the importance of providing quality care and facilities in

toxicology experimentation. This is followed by a discussion of factors to be considered in infectious disease control in a vivarium. Later in the chapter, a brief discussion of training and safety considerations for animal care personnel is presented. At the end of the chapter, the social and cultural climate that the scientist must face in using laboratory animals, as well as the philosophy of animal use, is discussed.

For more detail on each of the areas discussed, the reader is referred to review articles included in the references (66,96,109,183,192). The importance of proper and humane laboratory animal care cannot be overemphasized. Recent external social and political influences have stimulated concerned scientists to search diligently for *in vitro* bioassays to replace animal studies, as well as to seek ways to reduce the number of animals used in toxicology studies. These developments are to be applauded and encouraged. However, it is not probable that *in vitro* bioassays, computer simulated experiments, or the determination of structure activity relationships will provide a complete substitute of intact living organisms in the laboratory for the foreseeable future. Obviously, this is due to the complex interaction of different organ systems, as well as the variables of cell biology, that determines the reaction of organisms to exogenous xeno-biotics. Also, the field of toxicology is not yet at a "state-of-art" whereby biological phenomena and assessment of risk to humans and animals can be predicted with absolute certainty. Until toxicology reaches an era in which *in vitro* bioassays and the computer meet the requirements of safety assessment, the laboratory animal will be an irreplaceable resource. Therefore, it behooves toxicologists to understand the necessity for minimizing environmental influences, such as stress in the laboratory environment, that detract from producing objective, high quality research.

Many of the major advances in toxicology and medical research have depended on studies that have utilized animals as research subjects in one way or another. Viewed in this perspective, the use of laboratory animals constitutes a foundation for all other methodologies that are utilized in toxicological research. Although the care and use of laboratory animals have not usually been a part of the formal training of graduate students interested in toxicology, recent federal policies now make such training important, if not mandatory, for all investigators who plan to use animals for research. The principles and methods that are specific to the use of laboratory animals are aimed at accomplishing two major goals: (a) control of the animals' health and environment to ensure the validity of scientific results, and (b) compliance with federal regulations reflecting the public concern that animals be treated humanely. The first goal, the validity of scientific results, depends on methodologies that adequately control animal health and environmental factors. Scientific data are only as "good" as the system in which they are collected. The second goal, the humane treatment of animals, addresses the obligation of the biomedical research community as a whole to use research animals in a humane and responsible manner. Beyond scientists' ethical and moral obligations, federal regulations mandate that certain minimum standards be followed to ensure the humane care and use of laboratory animals.

GOVERNMENT REGULATIONS, LAWS, AND POLICIES

A major focus of this chapter is to introduce the basic principles governing the care and use of laboratory animals for toxicology research. It is essential for every investigator to become familiar with the laws, regulations, and policies relating to the use of animals in research and also to adopt a generally responsible attitude toward the use of laboratory animals. The current and increasingly stringent federal laws reflect the public's concern regarding the use of animals in research. These laws and regulations are designed to ensure that laboratory animals receive humane treatment and care. Compliance with the federal laws and a concerned, responsible, and humane policy of animal use by all research facilities will help alleviate the growing public concern regarding the use of laboratory animals and may prevent federal policies from becoming so stringent as to prohibit the use of animals for research.

National Laws and Policies

The Animal Welfare Act

Historical perspective

The United States Congress passed the first Laboratory Animal Welfare Act in 1966, Public Law (P.L.) 89-544. The Act, administered by the United States Department of Agriculture (USDA), established the first legal requirement for research facilities to provide the specified minimum standards of care for research animals and to provide the care of an attending veterinarian. In 1970, the Act was amended (P.L. 91-579) and renamed "The Animal Welfare Act." The scope of the law was broadened to include protection for additional animal species and to require research facilities to register with the USDA and provide an annual report of animal utilization and assurances of compliance with the standards for care. The Act was again amended in 1976 by P.L. 94-279 to include more stringent standards for transportation of animals. Each time the Animal Welfare Act is amended, the relevant federal regulations are also rewritten to include the new provisions of the law. The detailed rules and regulations for the Animal Welfare Act are published in the Code of Federal Regulations (CFR), Title 9, Chapter A, Parts 1, 2, and 3. These regulations are the guidelines that must be followed to assure compliance with the "intent" of the law (13).

Current law

The Animal Welfare Act was amended to its current status by the 1985 Food Security Act (P.L. 99-198), which became effective December 1, 1986 (13). The revised regulations are not yet complete and may add further restrictions of the use of animals in research. However, the following list is offered as an abbreviated reference for some of the basic components of the current law that are especially relevant to research facilities and investigators.

1. The purpose of the Act is to ensure that animals intended for use in research facilities are provided humane care and treatment and to regulate persons or organizations using animals for research or experimental purposes (Section 1, subpart b).
2. A "research facility" is defined as any school, institution, organization, or person that uses or intends to use live animals in research; such facilities fall under the jurisdiction of the law and must register with the USDA, unless specifically exempted by the Secretary of the USDA (Section 1, subpart b, and Section 6).
3. Animals that are protected by the law include any live or dead dog, cat, nonhuman primate, guinea pig, hamster, rabbit, or such other warm-blooded animal (Section 2, subpart g).
4. Standards to ensure the humane care of animals being transported (to and from research facilities) include minimum requirements for containers, food, water, ventilation, temperature, and handling (Section 18, subpart 4).

5. Standards for care of animals in research facilities include minimum requirements for housing (shelter, space allotment, ventilation, temperature control, etc.), feeding, watering, sanitation, handling, adequate veterinary care, and the appropriate use of anesthetic, analgesic, and tranquilizing drugs to ensure the minimization of pain and distress (Section 1, subpart b, and Section 13, subpart 3A).

6. In addition to minimum housing and care requirements, research animal environments must provide for (a) the separation of species, (b) adequate exercise for dogs, and (c) the "psychological well-being" of primates (Section 13, subparts 2A, 2B).

7. Experimental procedures must be designed to ensure that animal pain and distress are minimized, including the provisions that (a) the principal investigator considers alternatives to any procedures that may cause pain, and (b) a veterinarian be consulted during the planning of such procedures so that the appropriate use of tranquilizers, anesthetics, and analgesics are included in the study protocol (Section 13, subparts 3B, 3C).

8. The use of paralytics without anesthesia is prohibited, appropriate presurgical and postsurgical care procedures are mandatory, and no animal may be used in more than one major operative experiment from which it is allowed to recover except in cases of justified scientific necessity, which must be explained in writing and filed with the Institutional Animal Care and Use Committee (IACUC) (Section 13, subparts 3C, 3D, 3E).

9. Research facilities must be open for inspection by USDA representatives and be able to show that the provisions of the act are being followed. Each facility will be inspected once a year and follow-up inspections will be conducted as often as necessary until deficiencies are corrected (Section 13, subpart 7A, and Section 16, subpart A).

10. Research facilities must submit an annual report showing that professionally acceptable standards for the humane care and use of animals are in effect. The report must be comprehensive and include proof of compliance with all aspects of the Act. The USDA provides forms and guidelines for making the report. It is due on December 1 of each year and must cover the previous year ending September 30 (Section 13, subparts 7A, 7B).

11. An IACUC must be established at every research facility. The committee must be appointed by the chief executive officer of the research facility and must consist of at least three members who have sufficient expertise to assess animal care and use practices. One veterinarian and one person not in any way affiliated with the research facility must be appointed as members to the committee. The IACUC is assigned a variety of responsibilities including conducting semiannual inspection of all animal facilities and study areas in the research facility and assuring that pain and distress are minimized in all aspects of the care and use of laboratory animals. (For an example of how the IACUC may fit within an organization, see Fig. 1.)

12. Each research facility must conduct training for all personnel involved in the care and/or use of laboratory animals. The training must include instruction on the humane use of animals and methods that minimize pain and distress (e.g., the use of pain- or stress-reducing medication).

The above reference list provides only an abbreviated account of the issues covered by the Animal Welfare Act. All research facilities and investigators are legally obligated to comply with these laws. At the present, facilities using only rats, mice, and poultry are exempted. However, for institutions using only rats and mice, it behooves scientists to abide by the intent of the law so that at a future date, if other species are used, the institution could readily obtain registration and obtain successful approval upon inspection. Furthermore, there is the possibility that the law could be amended to include rats, mice, and poultry. Failure to comply could result in fines, jail sentences, and the revocation of licensing to conduct research with animals. For more complete infor-

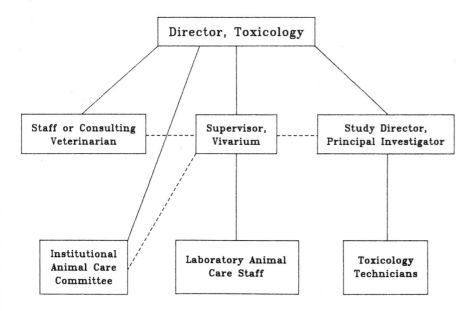

FIG. 1. Suggested scheme of institutional organizational chart for laboratory animal care.

mation, refer to the Act and the relevant parts of the CFR cited above.

Good Laboratory Practices

The Good Laboratory Practice (GLP) Regulations of the Food and Drug Administration (FDA) are guidelines that must be followed in nonclinical (nonhuman) studies for research results to be valid evidence of product safety (106). Such evidence is needed to obtain permits for research in or marketing for humans. These regulations, which are published in the CFR, Title 21, Chapter 1, Part 58, contain provisions for the care and use of laboratory animals. The minimum standards include requirements for housing, separation of species, quarantine of new and sick animals, and separation of projects. In addition, the health of research animals must be closely monitored and documented. Rigorous standard operating procedures must be developed and implemented for all aspects of such studies (including animal care and use), and documentation that procedures were followed is required.

Public Health Service Policy

The policy of the Public Health Service (PHS) requires that research institutions "establish and maintain proper measures to ensure the appropriate care and use of all animals involved in research, research training, and biological testing activities . . . conducted or supported by the PHS" (233). No individual may receive PHS funds (awarded grants) unless affiliated with or sponsored by an institution that assumes responsibility for complying with PHS policy. All the provisions of the Animal Welfare Act (P.L. 99-198) and the associated regulations are included in the PHS policy, along with further requirements relating to documentation and assurance of the status of the research institution with regard to the care and use of laboratory animals and associated increased responsibilities of the IACUC. Research organizations and institutes are required to have IACUCs and thorough records of the activities of the committee as well as records on animal care and husbandry practices. The administration and coordination of the PHS policy is the responsibility of the Office for Protection from Research Risks (OPRR). Each research facility must ensure that its procedures and facilities meet all the requirements of the policy by one of two ways:

Category 1—Accreditation by the American Association for Accreditation of Laboratory Animal Care (AAALAC).
Category 2—Evaluated by the Institution. This evaluation is conducted by the IACUC every 6 months.

In addition to stipulating requirements for establishing procedures to ensure appropriate care and use of animals, the policy provides guidelines for the operation and function of the IACUCs, general recordkeeping in animal facilities, review of research projects for proper and humane use of animals, and reporting requirements of research institutions to the PHS through the OPRR. Throughout the PHS policy is referral to the National Institutes of Health (NIH) Guide for the Care and Use of Laboratory Animals (70,71).

Guide for the Care and Use of Laboratory Animals

The Guide for the Care and Use of Laboratory Animals is published by the PHS and the NIH. It was first published in 1963 and has been revised five times (70,71). The purpose of the guide is to provide recommendations to research institutions to ensure appropriate and humane animal care in the laboratory setting. This guide should be read and referred to repeatedly by everyone involved with the use of laboratory animals in testing and research. It is discussed in other sections of this chapter and recommended as supplemental reading for toxicologists. The guide is an excellent document for scientists to use to ascertain the degree of compliance with standards required for accreditation by the AAALAC. This organization will be discussed later in this chapter.

STRUCTURE OF FACILITIES

Other than the husbandry practices of the animal care technicians and scientists working in the vivarium, the design and maintenance of facilities is the most important factor in controlling disease and minimizing stress in laboratory animals. Husbandry practices and safety will be discussed later in this chapter. Each aspect of the facility (e.g., walls, floors, hallways) will be discussed in this section. For more detailed information, the reader is referred to the reference section (14,21,51,67,71,74,151,157,182,201,248).

Floors

Floors should have smooth surfaces with as few crevices and cracks as possible. Surfaces should be resistant to water damage, nonabsorbent, skidproof, resistant to wear, and able to withstand detergents, solvents, and chemicals used for cleaning. The floor should be able to withstand friction from traffic of personnel and wheels of cages and cage racks, as well as resistant to stains from urine and feces. Where the walls and floors join, there should be sealants or special molding that prevents the presence of dead space or crevices that would collect dirt and materials or in which insects could hide. Materials satisfactory for floors include smooth surface concrete, epoxy aggregates, rubber base aggregates, and commercial specially designed flooring for a laboratory animal facility. In hallways and animal rooms with drains, floors should be designed to slant gradually toward drains. In facilities housing small rodents, drains are not necessary because correct use of wet vacuuming, sponge mopping, and rinsing will sufficiently clean such rooms.

Drains

Drains are often included in animal rooms, especially those designed for larger animals such as primates and dogs. Drains should be designed to allow adequate draining from rooms, as well as from pipes immediately below the floors. This draining will help curtail the buildup of humidity in rooms. Drainpipes should be at least 4 inches in diameter, and 6 inches are recommended in high use areas such as dog kennels (71). Drains should be periodically flushed and when not in use they should be capped. Drains can be equipped with trap buckets to trap solid wastes. Water with waste material or dirt should not be allowed to sit and stagnate.

Walls and Ceilings

Walls and ceilings should be as free from cracks and crevices and as smooth as possible. Epoxy paint over cinder blocks or cement plaster can work satisfactorily. In the event walls are equipped with guards or rails to prevent damage from cages or racks, they should be able to be easily sanitized. Curbs or rails should be smooth and have surfaces that withstand cleansing with detergents and/or disinfecting agents. Junctions of walls with ceilings should be tight and, if necessary, sealed. Walls and ceilings should be resistant to high pressure, high temperature water. In the event specialized ceilings are used with laminar flow rooms, they should be designed so that disassembly and cleaning can take place and filters above or around rooms can be easily changed.

Doors

Ideally, doors should be metal or metal covered with windows whereby viewing into the rooms is possible. Doors should be at least 42 inches wide to allow easy passage of racks and cages. Kick plates and recessed or shielded handles are advisable. The doors should fit tightly on frames and, where necessary, sealed. Self-sealing sweep strips are recommended (70,71). A strip or pad is advisable along the bottom if clearance is more than $\frac{1}{8}$ inch. Doors should open into animal rooms or open into specially designed vestibule areas.

Corridors (Hallways)

Corridors require the same type of surfaces on floors, walls, and ceilings as in the animal rooms. These should be smooth and resistant to stains, wear, and cleansing agents. Curbs or rails should be installed to prevent damage to walls from moving racks or cages. Likewise, exposed corners should be covered with steel or other durable surface. Corridors may have room monitors for temperature, humidity, and if possible, air flow. These monitors and service panels should be in corridors as opposed to animal rooms. If necessary, drains can be in hallways; however, covers should be utilized when drains are not in use. Corridors should be minimum of 7 feet wide and, if possible, 8 feet wide or more (51,71,151).

Miscellaneous Support Areas

Special areas for various functions that are separate from animal rooms are recommended. For example, separate rooms for surgery, diagnostic procedures, and treatment should be provided. Bathroom facilities including showers should be provided for personnel. Areas for breakroom activities such as drinking, eating, and smoking should be outside the vivarium or in special isolated areas. A storage area for feed and bedding should be provided. Specialized separate areas with separate ventilation should be provided for diet mixing and preparation of dosing solution. Areas for receiving shipment of supplies and animals are also suggested. An area should be set aside to store waste until it is incinerated or packed for disposal. A refrigerator unit for the storage of carcasses until disposal is highly recommended. The cage wash area should be separated from animal rooms but easily accessible to corridors. Ideally, automatic cage washers should divide a dirty cage area from a clean cage area. If possible, different personnel can operate each area on a given day. A special area for quarantine is also necessary to prevent potential spread of disease. A discussion on quarantine procedures is provided later in this chapter.

SPECIAL FACILITY CONSIDERATIONS

In any general consideration of facilities, a discussion of barrier and corridor systems is warranted. The use of single versus double corridor is a decision the scientists and engineers must consider in the design or modification of facilities. Other considerations regarding barriers and corridors include traffic flow, use of designated or disposable clothing, and the intended practices of laboratory animal husbandry.

Many toxicology laboratories were built before emphasis was placed on corridor and barrier systems. However, it is possible to maintain a conventional facility without double corridors and barrier systems that is at minimum risk of disease outbreak and stress for laboratory animals. Even the spread of disease or infections can be controlled by careful husbandry practices (29). Practices such as "dedicated" laboratory coats (or disposable laboratory coats); shoe and head covers; strict control of traffic into animal facility; use of disposable gloves for bleeding animals or handling serum or urine; cleaning equipment and supplies for each room; control of temperature, humidity, and noise in each room; procurement of animals from high quality suppliers; separation of species and studies; and strict quarantine procedures are some of the procedures that can help any facility maintain healthy, unstressed animals.

If an institution is building or modifying a vivarium, a decision must be made on corridor design and whether a double corridor system will be utilized (see Figs. 2, 3, 4). Many facilities with rooms that exit onto two hallways use a clean and dirty corridor system. The "clean" corridor is used to bring in sterilized material and feed, as well as used by personnel entering to work with animals and/or to clean and service rooms, whereas people exit the room into the "dirty" corridor with dirty cages, litter, and carcasses. The concept is for humans, animals, and material to flow from areas of least contamination to areas where contamination is the most probable. The use of a double corridor system requires more space, construction, and maintenance costs (151,157,201). Obviously, this type of system requires the flow of traffic and, ideally, the flow of air from the clean side to the dirty side (161). Toxicologists should be aware of a

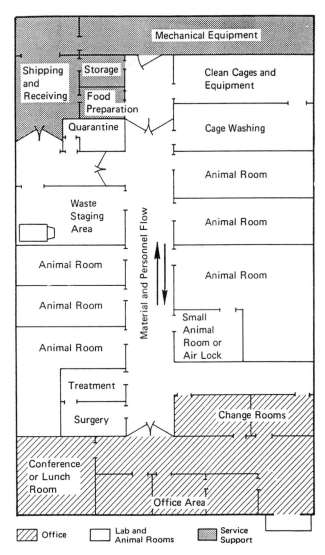

FIG. 2. A single-corridor design for an animal facility. (From ref. 157, with permission.)

barriers is based on the degree of containment necessary, which is based on potential risk. The reader is referred to the reference section for a more in-depth discussion (67,157). It is interesting to note that for most purposes in toxicology, conventional rooms in the vivarium will suffice. Even in the case of cesarian-derived rats, the lungs show evidence of disease essentially no different in goblet cell change and respiratory mechanics in rats under conventional conditions as compared to rats in a barrier system (36). Investigators will probably want to consider barrier systems if nude mice, immunosuppressive drugs, irradiation, or germfree animals are being used.

Another concern of toxicologists, engineers, and veterinarians is the monitoring of the air flow, levels of adequate ventilation, temperature and humidity, and flow of water in automatic water systems. The use of transducers to measure temperature and humidity pressure, as well as alarms, helps the scientist keep environmental control of experiments (300,337). The use of recorders and monitors for each room

study using sodium fluorescein in the diet of rats whereby the double corridor system was significantly less contaminated with the tracer chemical than a single corridor system (286). However, close monitoring of traffic flow and secure containment of contaminated items, as well as the use of disposable gowns, head covers, and shoe covers, can cut down on the chances for contamination. When potentially hazardous chemicals are being used in a study, widespread contamination of corridors, rooms, clothing, and equipment is possible (284,288). If known hazardous chemicals and microbes are being used, the reader is referred to the bibliography for requirements in design, traffic flow, and husbandry (67,71,74,151,157,239). For further discussion, see the section discussing ventilation.

Another consideration for the toxicologists and/or engineers building new facilities or modifying old facilities is the establishment of a barrier system. The purpose of a barrier system is to keep out infectious agents and chemical contamination (74,151) (see Table 1 and Fig. 5). Classification of

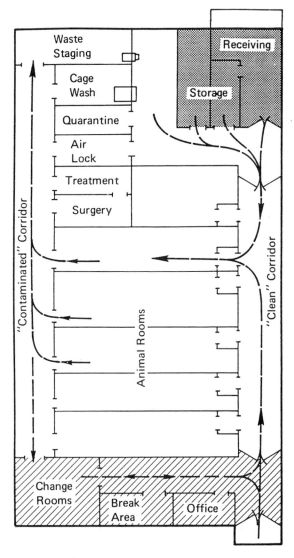

FIG. 3. A two-corridor design for an animal facility. (From ref. 157, with permission.)

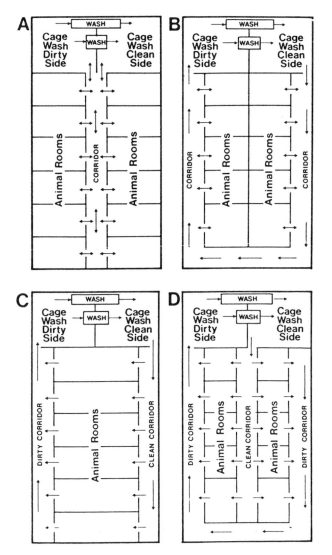

FIG. 4. Four types of traffic flow patterns are illustrated relative to the cage wash area. The *arrows* indicate the direction of cage traffic. All are drawn within the identical space to the same scale in order to demonstrate the relative "cost" in terms of animal housing space, both square footage and number of spaces. **A:** "To and fro" traffic pattern; **B:** unidirectional; **C:** clean–dirty with two corridors; **D:** clean–dirty with three corridors. (From ref. 116, with permission.)

helps investigators keep detailed records and monitor rooms while an experiment is ongoing.

Laminar flow circulation in rooms in conjunction with ventilation filtration systems should be continuously monitored for air flow and room ventilation. An alternative to expensive laminar flow rooms is the use of portable or self-contained laminar flow systems. These systems can help curtail the spread of microbes such as bacterial pathogens (27,198).

Before concluding any discussion on special facility considerations, the scientists using laboratory animals must consider providing comfortable housing or caging just as important as providing for the adequate prevention of the spread of disease. Stress-related disorders can cause as many com-

plications in experimental results as can infections. The reader is referred to references cited that deal with space and space requirements for laboratory animal species (14,51,67,71) (See Table 2).

LIGHTING

Lighting is an important factor in determining potential effects of the environment. Obviously, adequate illumination in animal rooms and adjacent auxiliary rooms provides easier observation of the clinical condition of animals as well as the status of their feed, water, and bedding. The sanitation of the walls, floors, drains, and animal equipment can also be evaluated easier with good lighting. High quality illumination might also provide animal care personnel with added incentive to maintain a clean, uncluttered work environment in order to provide pleasant surroundings.

Although exact lighting requirements for health and physiological stability of animals are unknown, it is known that past illumination standards of 75 to 100 footcandles can be a source of retinal damage in laboratory rodents (132). Even lower levels can be a problem (347). Consequently, these levels have to be used with caution and the position of cages in relation to lights should be carefully evaluated. In the case of lighting systems using timer controls, the performance of timers should be periodically checked (71). The light-dark cycle of animal rooms should be automatically controlled for each room. Windows in animal rooms are not recommended because they may affect light-dark cycles and the ability to control constant light cycles. They also provide extra surfaces, seams, and crevices for cleaning.

TABLE 1. *Chemical substances commonly found in the animal facility*

Source of contaminant	Type of contaminant
Organic solvents	Ethers, alcohols, chloroform, carbon tetrachloride, acetone
Air	Dust and bedding particles, irradiation, trace volatile anesthetics, animal room deodorants (volatile hydrocarbons), disinfectant sprays (eucalyptol), pheromones, vinyl chloride, ammonia, insecticides, piperonyl butoxide
Diet	Nitrates, cadmium, arsenic, lead, aluminum, mercury, nickel, insecticides, mycotoxins, herbicides, chloroform, food additives, estrogenic compounds, polycyclic hydrocarbons, phenothiazines, phenylthiazoles, flavones, antibiotics
Bedding, caging, and equipment	Detergents, disinfectants, soaps, acids, ethylene oxide, wood alkaloids, cedrene, cedrol, ammonia, lignin aldehydes, antibiotics, microbiocides
Dosing and treatment of animals	Mutagens, teratogens, carcinogens, toxic agents, drugs, vaccines

From ref. 157, with permission.

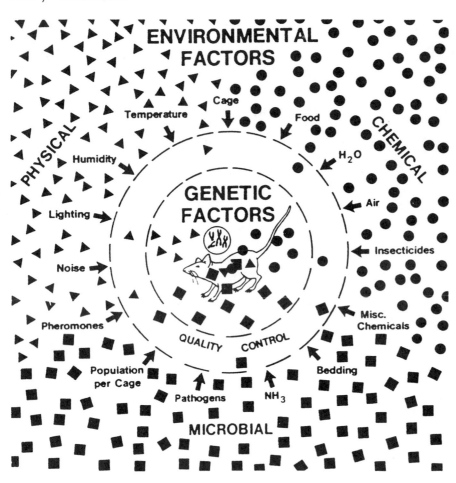

FIG. 5. Conceptual view of the modern laboratory animal. In terms of biologic response, every experimental animal is a composite of genetic and environmental effects—at each point in time from zygote to ultimate death. Many physical (▲), chemical (●), and microbial (■) factors of the environment contribute along with genetic factors (of the genome) toward each animal's responsiveness to experimental stimuli. Quality control has the important role of maintaining genetic purity while preventing, minimizing, or maintaining as nearly constant as possible the effects of various environmental factors. (From ref. 157, with permission.)

Intensity of lighting recommendations at cage level vary from 50 to 100 footcandles or lower (114) to 75 to 125 footcandles (75). In order to decide on a lighting intensity value, the toxicologist should be aware of several reports in the literature. High levels of lighting (75–100 footcandles) can cause retinal degeneration in rodents (132,266). Even low levels of lighting intensity (~30 footcandles) can cause lesions in albino rats (347). Continuous lighting (24 hr) at levels of 50 to 100 footcandles has been reported to cause retinal photoreceptor degeneration in both albino and pigmented rats (229,344). Continuous lighting can cause permanent vaginal cornification in mice and rats as well as ovarian follicle development without formation of corpora lutea (344,345). Exposure of albino rats and pigmented rats to 50 to 90 footcandles continuously produced regression of ovaries, Harderian glands, and pineal glands. In this same study, severe retinal degeneration occurred in albino rats, whereas only minimal change was seen in pigmented rats (260).

When considering effects of lighting, the scientists should be aware that the position of the rack and cage is also important in calculating light intensity reaching the animal (227,345). The level of cage level in a chronic study can be an important factor. Mice in cages on the high level can have an incidence of retinal atrophy as high as 30.2% and for lower shelves as low as 0.7% at 33 months (132). Cage rotation or random shelf assignment across treatment groups in chronic studies might aid the toxicologist in coping with light intensity retinal problems. This might also help avoid inci-

dence of neoplasia in mice as a consequence of cage position (133).

In determining length of light cycle, the toxicologist should be aware that changes or biological parameters can be affected by light–dark cycles. The light–dark cycle can affect the estrous cycle and breeding of laboratory rodents (136,210,260,345). Recommendations for life cycles range from 10 hr light/14 hr dark (75) to 14 hr light/10 hr dark (114). Whether an investigator goes with either extreme or a 12 hr light/12 hr dark cycle is less important than ensuring that the same cycle is maintained throughout an experiment.

Light intensity in the 50 to 100 footcandle range with a 12 hr/12 hr light–dark cycle with cage rotation or random assignment of cages across groups on different shelves appears to be a good compromise for the toxicologist concerned with retinal lesions in albino rodents.

VENTILATION

Ventilation is one of the most important aspects of the vivarium for the toxicologist to consider when controlling disease and minimizing stress. Ventilation supplies oxygen, removes heat buildup from animals, lights, and equipment, and dilutes and/or removes contaminants (particles and gases) (71). Ventilation is also an important factor for controlling humidity and temperature. Proper ventilation can

TABLE 2. *Minimum space recommendations for laboratory animals*

Animals	Weight	Housing	Floor area/animal		Height [a]	
Mice	<10 g	Cage	6.0 in.²	38.71 cm²	5 in.	12.70 cm
	10–15 g	Cage	8.0 in.²	51.62 cm²	5 in.	12.70 cm
	15–25 g	Cage	12.0 in.²	77.42 cm²	5 in.	12.70 cm
	>25 g	Cage	15.0 in.²	96.78 cm²	5 in.	12.70 cm
Rats	<100 g	Cage	17.0 in.²	109.68 cm²	7 in.	17.78 cm
	100–200 g	Cage	23.0 in.²	148.40 cm²	7 in.	17.78 cm
	200–300 g	Cage	29.0 in.²	187.11 cm²	7 in.	17.78 cm
	300–400 g	Cage	40.0 in.²	258.08 cm²	7 in.	17.78 cm
	400–500 g	Cage	60.0 in.²	387.12 cm²	7 in.	17.78 cm
	>500 g	Cage	70.0 in.²	451.64 cm²	7 in.	17.78 cm
Hamsters	<60 g	Cage	10.0 in.²	64.52 cm²	6 in.	15.24 cm
	60–80 g	Cage	13.0 in.²	83.88 cm²	6 in.	15.24 cm
	80–100 g	Cage	16.0 in.²	103.23 cm²	6 in.	15.24 cm
	>100 g	Cage	19.0 in.²	122.59 cm²	6 in.	15.24 cm
Guinea pigs	≤350 g	Cage	60.0 in.²	387.12 cm²	7 in.	17.78 cm
	>350 g	Cage	101.0 in.²	651.65 cm²	7 in.	17.78 cm
Rabbits	<2 kg	Cage	1.5 ft.²	0.14 m²	14 in.	35.56 cm
	2–4 kg	Cage	3.0 ft.²	0.28 m²	14 in.	35.56 cm
	4–5.4 kg	Cage	4.0 ft.²	0.37 m²	14 in.	35.56 cm
	>5.4 kg	Cage	5.0 ft.²	0.46 m²	14 in.	35.56 cm
Dogs[b]	<15 kg	Pen/run	8.0 ft.²	0.74 m²	—	—
	15–30 kg	Pen/run	12.1 ft.²	1.12 m²	—	—
	>30 kg	Pen/run	24.0 ft.²	2.23 m²	—	—
	<15 kg	Cage	8.0 ft.²	0.74 m²	32 in.	81.28 cm
	15–30 kg	Cage	12.1 ft.²	1.12 m²	36 in.	91.44 cm
	>30 kg	Cage	b	b	—	—
Nonhuman primates[c]						
Group 1	<1 kg	Cage	1.6 ft.²	0.15 m²	20 in.	50.80 cm
Group 2	1–3 kg	Cage	3.0 ft.²	0.28 m²	30 in.	76.20 cm
Group 3	3–10 kg	Cage	4.3 ft.²	0.40 m²	30 in.	76.20 cm
Group 4	10–15 kg	Cage	6.0 ft.²	0.56 m²	32 in.	81.28 cm
Group 5	15–25 kg	Cage	8.0 ft.²	0.74 m²	36 in.	91.44 cm
Group 6	>25 kg	Cage	25.1 ft.²	2.33 m²	84 in.	213.36 cm

Modified from ref. 71.

[a] Height measured from the floor to top of cage.

[b] These recommendations may vary according to breed and conformation of dogs.

[c] Primates vary in size and are divided into groups as follows:

Group 1—Marmosets, tamarins, and infants of various species
Group 2—Capuchins, squirrel monkeys, and similar species
Group 3—Macaques and African species
Group 4—Male macaques and large African species
Group 5—Baboons and nonbrachiating species > 15 kg
Group 6—Great apes and brachiating species

minimize biological changes induced by atmospheric contaminants (154).

Most guidelines and requirements call for a minimum of 10 to 15 air exchanges an hour for the animal room (51,71,75,304). This should control and help eliminate odors. If possible, air should be filtered entering the room. HEPA filters are recommended for room ventilation systems (78,151,201). Incoming air should be 100% fresh or recirculated only if adequate filtration is available (114). In controlling ventilation, the investigator should take into account the effect of structures in the room that might create uneven flow and dead spaces. Placement of cages and equipment

can affect effectiveness of ventilation (74). If filters in ventilation systems are not changed and maintained on a regular basis, the effectiveness of clean air on prevention of disease spread is lost. If air is being recirculated, it should be kept in mind that air exhausted from spaces where chemical carcinogens are present should not be recirculated to any other air supply in the facility. Room exhaust air should be passed through filtration systems including HEPA filters in animal rooms where hazardous or infectious agents are located (74).

Another consideration for disease and contamination control is the direction of air flow from animal rooms to corridors and service areas. In double or multiple corridor systems, air flow should go from clean corridors to animals' rooms to dirty corridors. In conventional, one-corridor systems, uninfected or unexposed animals should be in rooms slightly positive in pressure to hallways (unless infectious agents or hazardous agents are being used, in which case rooms with negative pressure may want to be considered). However, negative pressure should be present in rooms used for quarantine. Negative pressure should also be utilized in rooms in long-term studies in which known toxic agents are incorporated in the diet (71,75,114,284,288).

For added efficiency of ventilation and filtration, laminar flow units for small laboratory animals that can be placed inside animal rooms are available (27). Other systems make the whole room a "laminar-flow" room. These rooms provide 100+ air exchanges per hour of HEPA filtered air. Usually these systems use 100% fresh air. The HEPA filters can use recirculation with 10% outside air. These filters are 99.97% effective at 0.3 μm particle retention (74). This clean room concept works on the concept of mass air displacement. Air exchanges may range as high as 200 to 600 air exchanges per hour. Drafts are not created because of perforated ceiling air supplies and uniform air exits around the floor or walls (151).

TEMPERATURE AND HUMIDITY

Because the requirements for each room may vary by species on test and because, for energy conservation reasons, the number of animals per room and the weather may alter the internal energy requirements for each room, it is recommended that each room be independently monitored. Accordingly, each room should have its own temperature and humidity monitors. Each room should be able to be controlled to within 1°C (2°F) for any temperature in a range of 18 to 29°C (65–85°F) (151). A range of humidity control from 30% to 70% is also advisable (70). Humidity can be a special problem in rooms where flush racks are being used. Balance between the microenvironment and the macroenvironment can make determination of the proper setting of temperature and humidity difficult. Factors that determine the outcome of the interaction of the inner cage environment with the room environment include cage design, use of filter-top cages, number of animals in rooms, as well as number of animals in a cage, and the amount and velocity of air coming into rooms. All of these factors determine the temperature and humidity in the cage, which is typically slightly higher than the room (157). It should be noted that use of filter tops raise the humidity of ammonia levels in the cage but increases the control of contamination (34,75,176,296,298,359). To monitor the room environment diligently, managers of animal facilities should keep daily records or logs that include temperature and humidity records.

Overall, at lower temperatures and relative humidity, animals consume more food and achieve higher body weights, whereas at higher temperatures animals eat less, resulting in lower body weights (344). Another factor for consideration is that placement of racks and cages in a stagnant zone can lead to the cage environment deriving very little benefit from air movement. Consequently, placement of cages, exhausts, and air inlets must provide proper temperatures, humidity,

and air velocity gradients in the room (217). One point discussed in the section on cages is that plastic or polycarbonate cages are not as heat conductive as metal cages. Therefore, animals in metal cages will usually experience temperatures closer to that of the room than those animals in plastic cages (227).

Room or cage temperature may affect the action of drugs in animals. One investigator (343) reviewed the effects of temperature on drug action. He described an increase in the toxicity of amphetamines caused by increased temperature and group housing. One study (170) studied 58 different drugs given intraperitoneally to rats. Most CNS stimulants and depressants were more toxic at lower temperatures (e.g., chlorpromazine and promazine) than higher temperatures. Strychnine was more toxic at 8°C and 36°C than at 26°C. DBA female mice kept at 41 to 55°F had far fewer mammary tumors than mice kept at 80°F (10% versus 74%) (318). According to one investigator, many effects on the action of drugs will not be well recognized between 15 and 30°C (343). In many cases, when drugs were given at temperatures in the thermoneutral zone, minimal toxicity was seen, whereas toxicity was increased when temperatures were lowered or raised. Temperature and humidity can affect the susceptibility of chicks to Newcastle disease and mice to influenza (20). In lactating rats, high temperature resulted in a drop in milk production (361). In another study, rats exposed to a high temperature (80–89°F) as a result of a mechanical failure died. Many of the young male rats in this study that survived were sterile and had bilateral atrophied testes (254). Humidity can also be a problem. Low humidity was seen to cause ringtail in newborn Norway rats (325) and in albino rats (103,228). If investigators are interested in determining humidity and temperature in a cage and the factors of animal physiology that may affect temperature and humidity including basic physiology and basal metabolism rate, several review articles are available for more in-depth studies (6,42,143,342).

Toxicologists should be aware that there is a range of temperature and relative humidity whereby an animal's oxygen consumption is minimal and therefore physical activity or biochemical mechanisms for maintenance of body temperature or control of body heat is not required. Temperatures above that zone cause metabolism to increase. In those conditions, animals avoid overheating by evaporative heat loss (34,71,344). The range of recommended temperature and humidity (see Table 3) is below reported thermoneutral zones because experience with these numbers show them to be optimum settings. Animals adapt to changing temperatures by different behavior, such as increased physical activity, alteration of body position, huddling, increase in grooming, and use of more or less bedding. Toxicologists should also keep in mind that animals housed singly may eat significantly more than animals housed together (253), and this may be due to temperature as well as behavioral factors.

In summary, most laboratory animals can be kept comfortable in a range of 65 to 75°F and 45% to 55% relative humidity. Cages and racks should not be placed to block inlet or exhaust vents or to create dead space. Daily logs on humidity and temperature should be kept for each room, and each room should have individual controls for humidity and temperature. Toxicologists should refer to tables listing

TABLE 3. *Summary of ranges of temperature and relative humidity (thermoneutral zone)*

Species	Temperature		Relative humidity (%)
	°F	°C	
Rat	65–73	18–23	45–55
Mouse	68–75	20–24	50–60
Guinea pig	65–75	18–24	45–55
Rabbit	60–75	16–24	40–45
Hamster	68–75	20–24	40–55
Dog	65–75	18–24	45–55
Cat	70–75	21–24	40–45
Monkey	62–85	17–29	40–75

From ref. 114, with permission.

the thermoneutral zones of laboratory animal species when setting the temperature and humidity of a room.

CAGING

There are two general types of cages in laboratory settings. These are fixed and portable types of cages. Fixed cages are generally used for larger species (dogs and primates). In general, fixed cages are on the floor or on slightly raised floors. Fixed cages may be used in conjunction with kennels or runs. Portable cages are usually suspended from or set on racks that are equipped with casters. This type of system facilitates the sanitation as well as flexibility in use of the animal room. There are two basic kinds of portable cages. One type has solid sides and bottoms with a portable top (shoebox type), and the other has floors that are slotted or perforated with metal slats or mesh slats that allow urine and feces to drop into pans or trays beneath the cage. Some racks have trays or pans that are flushed automatically and periodically. Racks and trays are generally made of stainless steel, although aluminum and galvanized metal are also available; however, galvanized metal should not be used if it comes in contact with urine or cleansing agents because corrosion is apt to take place (151).

The shoebox cage is primarily used for rodents. It is recommended for breeding purposes. Typically, it is made of plastic (e.g., polycarbonate) with a metal perforated or rod lid that holds the feeder. In the event the toxicologist does not want the rodents in contact with their own bedding, removable wire mesh floors are available to separate animals from bedding. If the cage is made of polycarbonate, it can be autoclaved. Transparent plastic cages permit observation of animals. Opaque plastic cages or metal type shoebox cages can be used for animals that prefer a darker environment. It should be borne in mind that plastic cages do not last as long as metal cages, can scratch or stain, and usually are used with bedding that has to be frequently changed. Metal suspended cages have floors that are mesh or perforated above a tray or pan that can be lined with paper for excreta collection. These cages can be plastic or aluminum, but stainless steel is more durable and easy to sanitize. Metal cages transmit heat more readily than plastic cages. In general, these cages are not used for breeding purposes. The last type of cage is a front opening

cage, which is widely used for dogs, primates, rabbits, and occasionally, guinea pigs. In general, these are made of stainless steel or fiberglass. The floor is solid but may have an elevated second floor of grids or slats (51). The toxicologist should be aware that grids or bars on elevated floors and doors can break loose and be a potential source of injury for the animal. Frequent inspections and repairs can help prohibit the problem.

The choice of cages should be determined on the type of species and the kind of study being conducted. For example, in the case of rodents in inhalation studies where cages are placed in chambers, a suspended well-ventilated metal suspended cage is preferred. Breeding studies might dictate the use of opaque plastic or metal shoebox-type cages. Toxicology studies requiring frequent observation of animals might best be conducted in transparent plastic cages.

In selecting types of cages, several things should be considered. The dissipation of an animal's body heat into the room is determined by type of cages, population density, species of laboratory, and activity of the animals (152,213,227,360). In rodent cages open at the top, 90% of the heat generated by an animal is lost to the room environment by radiation and conduction through the sides of the cage (6). Toxicologists should remember animals in metal cages will have a cage temperature more like the room environment than animals kept in plastic cages. The physiology of the animal(s) in the cage can contribute to air movement from a cage because of convection from the heat of animals, as well as the activity of the animal(s) and the animal care technicians handling the animals. These factors along with type and volume of air from the ventilation of the room determine the internal cage environment (212,322).

Open-top cages tend to bring the cage conditions more in line with the environment of the room. However, open-top cages can serve as a source of distribution of dust, particles, and fomites (227). The use of filter tops for cages can help control the spread of dust, dander, and fomites and therefore disease from cage to cage (177,296). However, several points should be kept in mind. Filter tops have a disadvantage in that they potentially allow build-up of heat, humidity, CO_2, and ammonia (296). Because of these buildups, more frequent litter changes may be necessary (151,296). The higher levels of ammonia could lead to respiratory lesions or increased incidence and severity of infectious agents (44,121,188). Activity of hepatic microsomal enzymes is decreased in rodents housed in cages with filter tops (332). In the case of suspended steel cages, the toxicologist should be aware of several potential problems. Wire mesh floors can cause decubitus ulcers on the plantar surface of feet of rodents. Another problem is animals may break their mandibles when trying to free teeth from wire grids.

The decision to house singly or in groups in a study should be determined by considering the communal nature of the species and the type of protocol of a given study. The use of single versus group housing for rodents is controversial. If the decision is made to group house, efforts should be made to prevent overcrowding. The potential for single housing and group housing to affect animals will be discussed under the section on stress.

Proper sanitation of cages is one of the most important aspects of disease control in the vivarium. In the case of shoebox cages with bedding, bedding for rodents should be changed one to three times a week. Litter should not be emptied into litter containers in the same room to minimize dust or aerosolization of waste. Perforated metal or wire bottom cages should be washed at least once every 2 weeks. Shoebox cages should be washed once or twice a week and racks at least once every 2 weeks to once a month. Cages can be cleaned with detergents or chemicals but should be thoroughly rinsed. If sterilization depends on heat sterilization, rinse water should be at least 180°F for a sufficient period to destroy pathogenic microorganisms (71). Feeders should be changed at least once weekly, and water bottles should be removed at least twice weekly. Water bottles can be sterilized by heat or by chemicals (e.g., hyperchloride) (304). It is interesting to note that in addition to increasing the potential for spread of disease, a dirty environment can cause hepatic microsomal enzyme activity to decrease (332).

In addition to requirements of caging listed above, scientists should mandate that size of caging meet space requirements to minimize stress caused by crowding. An example of selected species space requirements is provided in Table 2 (71).

BEDDING

Although bedding and solid wall cages (polycarbonate or plastic) would not be practical in inhalation chambers, metabolism studies, or other special procedures, other toxicology studies can use bedding quite successfully. Transparent cages allow easy clinical observation of animals as well as allow animals to observe animals in the adjacent cages on a rack. However, if such cages are used, bedding should be used so that rodents are not always in direct contact with a substantial amount of urine and feces on the cage floor. Bedding also allows rodents to exhibit nesting behavior and may be a more natural environment. In general, small rodents' longevity is increased when kept in cages with bedding (51). Bedding provides thermal insulation and absorption of fecal and urinary wastes and spilled water. Abrasive, toxic, or edible material should not be used for bedding coming in contact with animals (75). Because of sanitation problems, use of bedding may not be warranted with certain larger animals such as dogs, nonhuman primates, and rabbits in the toxicology laboratory setting. However, in teratology and reproduction studies it is advisable to use bedding for most species before parturition (51).

The type of contact bedding to be used is very important. Cedar and other softwoods are not recommended. Cedar bedding has been reported to increase rate of mammary tumors in C_3H-A^{ry} mice (282), decrease threshold for chronic seizures induced in mice by pentylenetetrazol (244), and increase pup mortality in rats (46). One investigator speculates that the carcinogenicity of shavings may be due to alpha and beta unsaturated carbonyl compounds present in wood lignins. Other investigators have reported potential effects of softwood bedding on carcinogenic effects (290,291,334). Bedding made from softwood shavings has been reported to increase respiratory infection rates. Softwoods contain volatile hydrocarbons, which may be the cause of hepatic microsomal enzyme stimulation (63,81,97,251,330–332,336). Red cedar chips decreased "sleep time" in male albino mice given hex-obarbital and pentobarbitol (97) and decreased the threshold to pentylenetetrazol convulsions in mice.

The type of bedding can have a significant effect on fertility, parturition, and lactation. Corncob bedding may decrease reproductive productivity (250). Sawdust should not be used for bedding in reproduction studies. Guinea pigs used in breeding experiments on sawdust bedding had a significant decrease in deliveries (245). Overall, hardwood bedding, preferably sterilized, is preferred over softwood and corncob bedding (51,71,304). Sterilization of bedding is preferred over nontreated shavings.

Nesting material provided along with bedding can be an asset in breeding and reproductive studies. Shredded paper for nesting increased lactation in rats (230). Shredded material such as woodwool was superior to paper tissue for nesting material in rats (231). However, the problems of softwood shavings discussed above could present problems that should be considered while selecting nesting material.

Overall, bedding material should be able to absorb moisture without crumbling excessively, should be nonedible, nonabrasive, and relatively dust-free, and should be free of pathogens, pesticides, toxic chemicals, droppings from other animals, insects and parasites as well as their droppings, and natural volatile chemicals that may alter enzyme systems of the animals (341). For these reasons, bedding from hardwood shavings or cellulose (paper) chips may be the best choice (116). Bags or containers of bedding should be stored off the floor on pallets, racks, or carts (71).

WATER

In many animal experiments, the quality of drinking water is not often considered as a major factor impacting laboratory animal research. However, there are several reports in the literature whereby contamination of drinking water was incriminated as a source of disease or changes in laboratory animals. These include biological variation in male mice (137) and variation in immune response in mice (150). Drinking water and water containers can be a source of bacteria that can compromise the resistance of laboratory animals to effects of toxicology studies. An example of this phenomena is the cause of early death in mice receiving X-irradiation as the result of *Pseudomonas aeruginosa* bacterium infestation (197).

Contamination of drinking water can be reduced with treatment utilizing hydrochloric acid or chlorine (200). However, the toxicologist should consider whether such treatment would compromise the outcome of their studies. Even the transmission of metazoan parasites, such as the pinworm of the rat, *Syphacia muris,* can occur through ingestion of contaminated water (105).

Chemical contamination of public drinking water is often reported in the news media. Also, various water processing and distribution systems are used by a wide variety of laboratories. These methods may include acidification, chlorination, activated carbon, microinfiltration, deionization, and reverse osmosis. Toxicologists should be aware that chlorination techniques could lead to formation of carcinogenic chlorinated hydrocarbons because of chlorination of organic chemicals in drinking water (226).

The investigator using drinking water as the vehicle of exposure for toxicants or carcinogens could inadvertently cause contamination of the laboratory environment with test chemicals through husbandry and water bottle cleaning practices. However, such contamination is not apt to be nearly as marked as with dosed feed (287). Thorough and frequent cleaning of water bottles will minimize chemical contamination and spread of pathogens in the vivarium. In the case of automated watering systems, selection of systems with in-line filtration and automatic or manual flushing systems should be encouraged.

According to the 1985 *Guide for the Care and Use of Laboratory Animals* (71), to ensure continuous access to fresh potable uncontaminated water, periodic monitoring for pH, hardness, and microbial and chemical contamination should take place. Toxicologists should determine if local public testing of public water as well as any testing of water that may take place at their institution is adequate or if more testing is required to ensure high quality water free of contaminants. The guide recommends that investigators routinely check bottles or automatic watering devices to ensure their proper operation. In the case of water bottles, they should be replaced with clean bottles, but if refilled, care should be taken to put bottles back in the same cage from which they were retrieved. In the case of automatic watering systems, bacterial contaminants can be controlled by circulating or recirculating water through filtration systems or ultraviolet (UV) systems (259). Flushing the lines is also a practice that helps diminish bacterial contamination (151). Bacterial contamination can also be controlled by chlorine or hydrochlorine acid (28). However, the use of chemicals can affect research data (99,137,150) and obscure the interpretation of that data for the investigator.

In addition to consideration of potential contamination of water, scientists should be familiar with the drinking habits and appropriate water distribution systems for each species of laboratory animal being used in their studies (324). The appropriate volumes and water distribution systems will help minimize stress in laboratory animals.

DIET

An entire text or chapter could be dedicated to diet and its impact on toxicology studies. Obviously, it is not the intent of this section to give toxicologists a treatise on nutrition, factors affecting quality of diet, interaction of dietary factors on health of laboratory animals, complications of feed contamination on animal studies, or dietary factors influencing drug metabolizing enzymes, immunity, and neoplasia. Even though each of these areas will be briefly discussed in this section, interested scientists should refer to the cited references for more in-depth discussions. Other areas that will be discussed include the effect of quantity of diet on toxicology studies and a general discussion of husbandry practices regarding diet and feed storage.

All laboratory animals should receive palatable, nutritionally complete, and uncontaminated diets unless the aim of a particular study is to evaluate the effect of deprivation of a nutrient or addition of a known contaminant. The quality and quantity of a diet should be sufficient to ensure normal growth and health in an animal as well as to maintain normal reproduction and lactation in breeding or reproduction studies (51,71). All too frequently, toxicologists and other scientists assume that laboratory animals receiving commercial feed *ad lib* will have no problems related to diet in a toxicology study. Hopefully, this section will convince the toxicologist that a number of factors have to be considered when choosing and storing a diet for a given study. Depending on the nature of a study, scientists may want to conduct chemical analysis of the diet to ensure nutritional quality and lack of contamination.

Because there are 50 or more nutrients to consider, as well as required concentration of these nutrients for each species, it behooves a scientist to refer to the literature. There are several excellent references that can be consulted for a particular species or a specific ingredient (8,52,65,171,219,222,223,271,308,309). In considering the selection of a diet for a given study, there are a number of terms or classifications with which a scientist should be familiar.

Closed formula diets are those manufactured or marketed by feed companies that consider the exact quantities of ingredients proprietary and therefore would not list this information on a label. Usually one can get the ingredients and a "guaranteed" analysis on these products from the companies if requested (21,74,75,171). These diets are generally made up of natural ingredients (crops and animal products) and therefore are subject to variables such as weather, shipping, and storage conditions of crops, as well as the processing and storage practices of the feed manufacturer. In spite of this variability, these closed formulations are usually more than adequate to provide required nutrition of laboratory animals. In the event that nutritional quality of the closed formula diet is suspect or if particular nutrients or contaminants are of concern, the toxicologist should obtain a chemical or ingredient analysis from the manufacturer and/or an independent test laboratory. Should the study involve interactions between particular ingredients, chemicals, or toxicants, the investigator might consider an open formula diet. These are diets manufactured to obtain specified quantities of ingredients. In many cases, they are manufactured to meet the specifications on quantities of ingredients listed by the researcher. The quantitative and qualitative ingredient composition is readily available from the manufacturer (21,74,75,171,271). Although these diets are usually made from natural products and therefore subject to variability, the researcher has the advantage of specifying particular ingredients and a specific analysis of components with which he or she can be aware of potential problems. One study in three strains of mice demonstrated no difference in effect on reproductive performance and weight of pups weaned between open and closed rations (172). The disadvantage of open diets is cost and availability compared to closed formula diets. The choice between open and closed formula diet should be based on the design of a given experiment.

Other classifications of diets include natural ingredient diets, chemically defined diets, and purified diets (also referred to as semipurified diets). These are based on the type of ingredients used to formulate the ration (8,21,171,227,271,309). Natural product (cereal-based) diets consist of natural ingredients such as grains and fish meal.

Purified diets (some investigators use the terms "synthetic," "semisynthetic," and "semipurified") consist only of refined ingredients such as caesin, carbohydrates, fats, cellulose, and isolated soy protein (355). The third type of diet is the chemically defined diet that is composed of chemically pure compounds such as amino acids, triglycerides, sugars, fatty acids, minerals, vitamins, and inorganic salts.

Laboratory animal feed may come in several physical forms such as pellets, meal, baked, gel, and liquid. As stated above, the type and form of diets should be selected by an investigator on the basis of type of study, availability, and limitation of equipment and resources.

Regardless of the formulation of feed or physical form of the diet, laboratory animals should receive a palatable nutritional uncontaminated feed. Feed should be available in enough quantities to ensure normal growth in younger animals and maintenance of normal body weight, reproduction, and lactation in adult animals. Again, the selection of the diet will depend on the nutritional requirements of the species being studied as well as on the experimental objectives (51,71,72).

Invariably when discussing animal feed, the subject of autoclaving is eventually introduced. Autoclavable diets may require adjustments in nutrients. Also the dates of sterilization should be recorded and diets used as soon as is reasonably possible (71). One study (107) demonstrated no deleterious effects from autoclaving on reproduction or growth rate in mice. However, intervals between litters were increased in mice on an autoclaved diet. Another study (236) did not demonstrate any adverse effects of autoclaving on feed stored up to 130 days in hybrid mice ($B_6C_3F_1$) or Balb/C mice. There are diets available with heat-labile constituents that can be autoclaved (75).

Unless the objectives of a test or study (e.g., an immunology experiment) or the type of animals on a study (e.g., germfree rodents, nude mice) require sterilized feed, the use of autoclaves for diet is probably not warranted.

Another decision that scientists and animal care supervisors have to decide is what physical form of feed will be used. Feed may be in the form of a powder or meal, pelleted, or expanded. In one study, reproduction and weight gain were not affected in mice by pelleted versus expanded food; however, food utilization was poorer and food consumption higher for pelleted food. Increasing pellet hardness reduced food wastage in mice (108). Obviously, pelleted food can be too hard for rodents; therefore, pelleted feed should be hard enough not to crumble but not so hard that rodents have trouble chewing it (75).

Feeders or feed containers can also cause problems. For example, one study (144) reported weight loss and impaired reproduction when the hamsters could not pull pellets through slots in a feeder. Another problem can be with a powder- or meal-type feed sticking in the upper part of feeders and therefore not shaking down to the bottom half of the feeder. Frequent shaking or agitation of feeders by animal care technicians can avoid this problem.

In spite of the fact that most commercial products from well-established feed companies are more than adequate, problems can arise from diets stored for very long periods or those stored at high temperatures or if the diet is contaminated (72). The date of manufacture should be on feed, and lots delivered more than 90 days after formulation should not be accepted. Broken or torn bags of feed should not be accepted and feed should be stored off the floor (pallets, racks, or carts) in controlled environments. If feed is to be stored a long time, it should be stored in a cold environment. Open bags or unpacked feed should be stored in vermin-proof containers. If feed is stored for a long-term period, it should be analyzed for nutrients in accordance with the Association of Official Analytical Chemists (AOAC) methods of analysis. Feed should be marked for storage so that older shipments may be fed first. Bulk feed should not be stored in animal rooms. Small quantities stored in animal rooms should be in containers that can be sealed and can be easily disinfected. If cold storage is used, temperatures should be less than 15.5°C (60°F) (51,71,74,221). In choosing a commercial product and considering storage conditions and time from shipment to use, a scientist has to decide whether analysis for nutrients or contaminants is necessary. Assays for ingredients sensitive to environmental conditions such as thiamin or Vitamin A or for contaminants such as mycotoxins may be required (272).

Although commercial diets from reputable companies and dealers are usually more than adequate, toxicologists need to be aware of the variability that may be encountered in diets. As discussed earlier, the feed made from natural ingredients is going to be subject to the soil, climate conditions, and time of harvest of the grain and plants from which a diet is made (227). Additionally, the shipment and storage conditions of that grain will also impact the nutrient balance of a diet.

Several investigators have examined laboratory animal diets and found a wide range of variability for minerals, vitamins, and proteins, and these values do not always closely match the manufacturer's composition (64,134,221,356,357). Variation and/or difference in quality of natural ingredient products can have biological consequences. One study (37) examined two commercial diets and three special formulated diets from natural ingredients fed to hamsters. There were no significant differences for growth rates, litter size, and body weights of offspring. However, body weights were different in sexually mature adults (one of the commercial diets had the least mean weights), death rates (hamsters died earlier on one of the commercial diets), and total number of offspring weaned. The number of offspring weaned was greatest with a diet containing corn, soy, and alfalfa. The percentage of stillborn litters was lowest with the corn, soy, and alfalfa diet and one of the cornmeal diets.

In another study, six different commercial diets were examined in laboratory rats (64). In this experiment, all diets acceptably supported reproduction. However, one of the diets had a decreased body weight gain (−30%) and an increased plasma alanine transaminase activity. Nephrocalcinosis was seen in female rats fed diets with a calcium: phosphorus ratio of <1 (three of the diets). One interesting finding was that the levels of protein in the diet was positively correlated with the incidence of renal pelvic dilatation in offspring rats at 7 weeks of age.

It should be noted that guinea pigs, like rabbits, are sensitive to "acid" diets and that excess phosphorus can cause a decreased rate of growth, metastatic calcification, and death (232). Another point to be considered is the interaction of nutrients or dietary components with other factors. For example, one study (230) showed a "protective" effect of high dietary fat toward environmental stress in lactating guinea pigs using softwood shavings as nesting material. More pups were weaned from mothers using softwood shavings for nesting that are on a high fat diet as compared to mothers on a low fat diet using the same nesting material. However, as discussed later in this section, high fat diets may present problems. Fiber can be an important part of the diet and also vary considerably from one commercial diet to another. If there is concern regarding dietary fiber, investigators should know that rodents and lagomorphs can obtain fiber if kept on edible bedding.

One area that can be a significant problem in dietary considerations is feed contamination. Because of the limitations of space, this chapter will limit discussion to selected literature citations to acquaint toxicologists with general concepts. Obviously, major contaminants may consist of pesticides, herbicides, metals, polycyclic aromatic hydrocarbons, nitrosamines, and mycotoxins, as well as other classes of potentially toxic compounds (218,350) (see Figs. 5 and 6). These contaminants can potentially affect drug metabolizing enzymes, hematology values, clinical chemistry, and background of pathology lesions, as well as induction of tumors. One example is the effects high levels of selenium could have on a study evaluating mercury toxicity or the interaction of mercury, vitamin E, and selenium. Another example would be studies evaluating P-450 enzymes in rats that happen to receive a diet contaminated with polycyclic hydrocarbons. Even necessary constituents of the diet, depending on their level (excess or inadequate amounts) can affect the pharmacological and physiological variables of a biological system. Levels of vitamins, minerals, nitrates, fats, and lipotropes are also very important (218). Therefore, the discussion will emphasize common contaminants and issues that toxicologists may encounter.

Diet can be a major source of chemical contaminants in the laboratory environment (112,220,285). Contaminants that may be seen as constituents of the diet include metals such as cadmium, high levels of selenium, mercury, arsenic, and lead; mycotoxins; insecticides such as PDT, deldrin, malthion, lindane, and heptachlor; and other compounds such as polychlorinated biphenyls and nitrosamines (112,115,220–223,256,271).

Metals found in feed or other parts of the laboratory animal environment can lead to problems. Effects of selected metals are discussed to give the toxicologists insight to problems metals can cause. Swiss Webster mice orally given lead (1, 375, 137.5, or 13.75 ppm) showed a decreased antibody formation (174). A study using 5 ppm of chromium, cadmium, or lead in drinking water given to Long-Evans rats reported the following results: decreased life span in rats fed lead and cadmium, increased life span in rats fed chromium, fewer tumors in rats fed lead, arteriolar sclerosis in kidneys and ventricular hypertrophy in cadmium-fed animals, and cirrhoses of the liver in all groups (293). In another study, rabbits given lead acetate, cadmium chloride, or mercuric chloride in their drinking water all showed significantly lower levels of neutralizing antibodies to pseudorabies virus than did the control group rabbits (173). Lead can affect the resistance of mice to *Salmonella typhimurium* (149).

Even clinical signs and death can result from dietary contaminants. One case reported a fatal diarrhea in rabbits fed a diet contaminated with antibiotics (323).

Even carcinogens such as nitrosamines have been reported in diets (89,297). Other animal carcinogens that can be detected in commercial animal feed include aflatoxin, metals such as cadmium, PCBs, chlorinated hydrocarbons, and other pesticides (218,257). Obviously, trace amounts of carcinogens and other toxicants can be in animal feed, as well as the food supply that is part of our everyday diet, and therefore the discussion in this section should not surprise anyone. However, it is recommended that depending on the design and intent of the study that investigators conducting chronic studies on laboratory animals may want to consider monitoring pesticides, mycotoxins, selected trace minerals, and selected chemicals such as nitrosamines in the diets used on the study (see Tables 4 and 5).

Not only feed contamination can be an issue, but the amount of diet given animals may affect the results of a toxicology study. As discussed earlier, over the past 10 years much attention has been given by scientists to diet given *ad libitum* and the effects of dietary fat, protein, and total caloric content of the diet. Some toxicologists are considering the use of restricted diets for chronic studies. Another related area of interest is the effects of exercise and diet on chronic studies.

Even short-term acute studies may be affected by fasting. One investigator reported that fasting overnight showed a

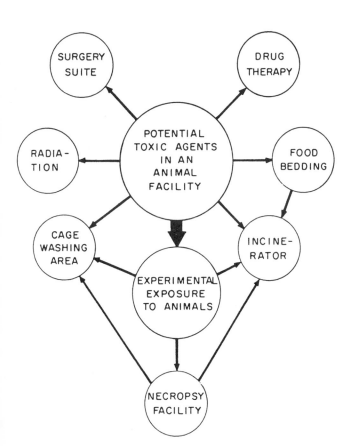

FIG. 6. Sources of potential exposure to chemicals and toxins in the animal facility. (From ref. 157, with permission.)

TABLE 4. *Maximum concentrations of feed contaminants considered acceptable for natural ingredient rations manufactured for use at the National Center for Toxicological Research at Jefferson, Arkansas[a]*

Agents	Maximum concentration
Cadmium	0.05 μg/g
Selenium	0.50 μg/g
Polychlorinated biphenyls	0.50 μg/g
Total DDT (DDE, DDT, TDE)	0.05 μg/g
Mercury	0.05 μg/g
Arsenic	0.25 μg/g
Lead	1.00 μg/g
Dieldrin	0.01 μg/g
Lindane	0.01 μg/g
Heplachlor	0.01 μg/g
Malathion	0.50 μg/g
Estrogenic activity	2.00 μg/kg
Total aflatoxins (B_1, B_2, G_1, G_2)	1.00 μg/kg

From ref. 74.

marked effect on diurnal rhythm with serum triglycerides in rats (57). Another study showed that concentrations or doses required to produce a median lethal dose (LD_{50}) were generally higher in nonfasted rats than in fasted rats (83). The feeding of pregnant female guinea pigs such that obesity ensues can predispose to pregnancy toxemia (122).

The practice of overfeeding or "over nutrition" in laboratory rats and mice on chronic studies can cause early deaths, increased incidences of neoplasms, and lesions of the kidneys and endocrine system (267,268,278,280). The effects of diet in laboratory animals have been reported in the literature for more than 40 years (313–317). Specific studies of interest with dietary restriction include the following:

- A study in rats and mice whereby a 20% restriction in diet decreased liver tumors in specific-pathogen free (SPF) Swiss albino mice and a decrease in pituitary, mammary, and skin tumors in SPF Wistar rats (326);
- An increase in longevity and a decrease in incidence of lymphoma in C57BL/6J mice (58) by dietary restrictions;
- An overall average of a 25% decrease in body weight and a 42% decrease in tumor incidence is reported in a summary reviewing 82 studies in mice in the scientific literature (4);
- An early occurrence (decreased latency period) of lymphoreticular tumors, hematopoietic tissues, and urinary papillary tumors in Charles River cesarian-obtained barrier-sustained Sprague-Dawley (COBS-SD) male rats given unrestricted diet as compared to rats on restricted diets (277);
- A study whereby C_3H mice reared in Australia, fed U.S. feed, and kept on cedar shavings from the United States had a much higher incidence of mammary and liver tumors (282); and
- A study that reported an inhibitory effect of low dietary protein on aflatoxin-induced tumors in rats (194).

In addition to the amount of overall diet affecting neoplasia, dietary fat can affect neoplasia incidence. A significant increase of tumors was seen in mice with a diet consisting of a 10% fat level as compared to diets with 3% or less (327). Another study showed that high fat and high calorie diets will cause an increased yield of neoplasms in female Sprague-Dawley rats given carcinogens; however, high calories appeared to have a stronger effect (178).

The effect of diet may be related to the overall body weight increase that is caused by unrestricted diet. One study demonstrated a decrease of pituitary and mammary tumors as the result of a 10% to 20% decrease in body weight in female rats (258). Another study reported an increase in mortality, nephropathy, and incidence of endocrine and mammary tumors with increased weight gain in Sprague-Dawley rats (328).

Another study in mice reported a slight increase in survival and a significant decrease of neoplasms of all types in outbred Swiss mice with restricted diets (76).

In several studies, lipotrope deficiencies have been shown to increase tumor incidence in rats given various carcinogens (77,225,269,270,275). It is also interesting to note that lipotrope deficiency can also increase the rats' susceptibility to acute toxicity of aflatoxin B_1 (274). Marginal levels of Vitamin A increased the incidence of rat colon carcinomas in rats exposed to aflatoxin (224) and slightly increased colon tumors in rats exposed to 1,2-dimethylhydrazine (273). Excess or added Vitamin A has been reported to increase the incidence of benign respiratory tract tumors in hamsters conventionally housed and decrease the incidence in hamsters housed in laminar flow units (302).

Nonneoplastic lesions can be affected by the levels of feed intake, as well as fat, protein, and calorie intake. Food restriction in rats may slow the progress of such lesions as nephropathy, cardiomyopathy, periarteritis, and muscular degeneration (32,33,196). In laboratory mice, dietary restriction can lessen age-related decline T-cell-dependent immunological function, enhance immune response, and increase longevity (59).

TABLE 5. *Proposed Environmental Protection Agency limits of contaminants in laboratory animal feeds and vehicles*

Parameter	Limitation Minimum	Limitation Maximum
Total aflatoxin (B1, B2, G1, G2) (ppb)	—	5
Estrogenic activity, ppb (DES eq)	—	1
Lindane (ppb)	—	20
Heptachlor (ppb)	—	20
Malathion (ppm)	—	2.5
Total DDT (ppb)	—	100
Dieldrin (ppb)	—	20
Cadmium (ppb)	—	160
Arsenic (ppm)	—	1.0
Lead (ppm)	—	1.5
Mercury (ppb)	—	100
Selenium (ppm)	0.1	0.6
PCB (ppb)	—	50
Nitrosamines (ppb)	—	10

From ref. 92.

Nutrition and diet can even affect drug metabolizing enzyme systems. For example, natural plant indoles and feed additives such as antioxidants can affect the mixed function oxidase system (340). It is beyond the scope of this chapter to discuss the effects of dietary constituents on the mixed function oxidase system. For a more in-depth discussion, the reader is referred to reviews listed in the reference section (50,164).

As noted in the above discussion, the influences of a wide variety of variables regarding diet can have significant impact on toxicology studies. Whether toxicologists should use dietary restriction depends on the goals and design of a given study. Obviously, the study director is "torn" between comparing lesions in a study with results from previous studies wherein rats were given feed *ad libitum* (historical controls) and whether to run a study with restricted diets whereby background nonneoplastic lesions and neoplasia will be at a lower incidence in control animals. Accordingly, the study director must decide whether to analyze diet for selected contaminants and levels of essential nutrients. Once again, the final decision is based on the goals and design of the study being planned.

DISEASE CONTROL

The presence of disease or parasitism can complicate interpretation of data in a given experiment. For example, in subchronic and chronic inhalation studies in rodents, infectious agents such as Sendai virus in mice or *Corynebacterium kutscheri* in rats might create difficulty in interpreting lung changes at terminal sacrifice. The use of sentinel animals in animal rooms (testing of serum for viral and bacteriological antibodies) will help the investigator determine to what extent background infections may have contributed to lesions and changes in body and organ weights, as well as clinical signs (141). Sentinel animals in a room during a chronic study can be sacrificed for serum, urine, and tissue sampling at intervals to help laboratory animal personnel keep a constant vigilance on the health of animals in a study. Other preventive measures will be discussed later.

It is beyond the scope of this chapter to present a lengthy discussion of infectious disease and parasitism in laboratory disease and the control of spread of these disorders. In other sections of this chapter, the importance of the quality of laboratory animals purchased is discussed. Obviously, these animals need to be as free of disease and parasites as possible. In the event of the arrival of diseased or parasitized animals at a facility, the use of proper quarantine and husbandry practices is mandatory for control of disease or spread of parasitism (11,162,191,205). The facility or institutional veterinarian is a resource to be utilized by the toxicologist and is an irreplaceable resource for providing prevention, diagnosis, and treatment of disease and parasitism. The reader is referred to the cited references for information on prevention and control of infectious disease (22,51,71,110,116). Also, there are excellent references cited for diagnosis, treatment, and prognosis of disease in laboratory animals (22,31,52,73,110,128,140,262,329).

However, for the purposes of this chapter, there are several specific areas with which the toxicologist should be familiar.

Some general discussions will be presented on the prevalence of possible background infections and infestations in laboratory animals, effects and changes disease can cause in a given study, and principles and practices suggested to prevent and/or minimize the complications that parasitism and disease can present to a given study. The main concept that toxicologists and other scientists should consider is that most disease outbreaks can be avoided and that any disease or parasite infestation could in and of itself cause complications attributed to stress or debilitation. In other words, the health status of animals could affect the outcome of a study by decreasing longevity or producing lesions or effects that would be difficult to discern from experimentally induced lesions or that could even interact with test material exposure to decrease or increase the effect (283). In a given experiment or study, the stress of disease may be "additive" with the overall stress of a high dose of a xenobiotic. The results of both biological burdens could be misinterpreted as the result of a specific toxicity or chemical interaction of the compound.

Mycoplasma sp. and eight different murine viruses cause the majority of problems in laboratory rodents (69). Commercial laboratories are available to run diagnostic tests for serum and other body fluids. Also bacteriological assays for such pathogens as *Corynebacterium kutscheri* in rats and *Pasteurella multocida* in rabbits are available. Several viral diseases can present problems in dogs and primates in toxicology laboratories. In the canine, distemper virus, canine hepatitus virus, parvovirus, and coronavirus are some of the viruses that could cause a disease outbreak in a kennel (116,128,163). However, these should not be a problem in reputable commercial laboratories that provide beagles and other breeds for toxicology laboratories. Primates can present problems with such viruses as the herpes complex and measles viruses. Tuberculosis bacterium can also be a problem in primates. These are but a few of the pathogenic microorganisms that can present problems to the toxicologists. In addition to complicating the results of a toxicology study, some disease pathogens can be transmitted to workers. An example of this is rat bite fever in laboratory personnel caused by being bitten by rats infected with *Streptobacillus moniliformis* (11).

Any scientist working with laboratory animals must be aware how prevalent pathogens can be in different colonies or laboratories. Even high quality laboratories may harbor several types of viruses in rats and mice (35,39,54,55,69,86,240,241), as well as in hamsters, guinea pigs, and rabbits (73,261).

In spite of a healthy appearance of laboratory animals, viruses or bacteria may be harbored silently or as latent infections. The stress of exposure to xenobiotics or commercial mixture of compounds could lead to outbreaks of disease. For mice, pathogenic viruses may include pneumonia virus of mice, minute virus of mice, Theiler's encephalomyelitis, reovirus type 3, K-virus, polyoma virus, mouse hepatitis virus, Sendai virus, adenovirus, lymphocytic choriomeningitis virus, and ectromelia (Table 6) (54,55,86,241). In rats, pathogenic viruses may include Sendai virus, Kilham virus, rat coronavirus, sialodacryoademitis, mouse hepatitis virus, pneumonia virus of mice, and reovirus type 3 (54,240,241). In the hamster, typical viruses may include pneumonia virus of mice, Sendai virus, Theiler's mouse encephalomyelitis,

TABLE 6. *Natural host range of rodent viruses*

Virus	Mouse	Rat	Hamster	Guinea pig
Sendai	+	+	+	+
PVM	+	+	+	+
Reo-3	+	+	+	+
LCM	+		+	+
MHV	+			
MVM	+			
Polyoma	+			
Mouse adeno	+	?		
Mousepox	+			
MEV	+			
EDIM	+			
Thymic agent	+			
LDH-E	+			
K	+			
Rat parvos[a]		+		
Rat coronas[b]	?	+		
Guinea pig herpes				+
SV-5			+	+
CMV[c]	+	+		+

From ref. 159, with permission.
[a] Includes RV, H-1 virus.
[b] Includes SDAV, Parker's rat coronavirus.
[c] Species-specific.

and SV-5 (240,241,261). Viruses that may be a problem in guinea pigs include Sendai virus, pneumonia virus of mice, reo virus type 3, and H1 virus (Toolan virus) (54). Viruses that can cause lesions in the lungs in laboratory rodents include Sendai and pneumonia virus of mice (45,138,335,352). Lesions include influx of inflammatory cells and, in the cases of Sendai virus and/or *Mycoplasma pulmonis,* chronic inflammation and squamous metaplasia of bronchial epithelium may also be seen (17,187,189,263,265). Sialodacryoadenitis virus can cause conjunctivitis in rats, which renders those animals unsuitable for ophthalmic studies (26,159,180,346).

Bacteria infections may also cause problems in laboratory animals either as opportunists in compromised animals as well as direct pathogens (73,104,113,117). Infectious disease may cause stress as indicated by increased adrenal weights in laboratory animals inoculated with *Salmonella typhimurium* and *Pneumoccocus sp.* The microorganism *Mycoplasma pulmonis* is particularly bothersome in the laboratory setting. As a pathogen, it can cause chronic respiratory disease, which can complicate the assessment of effects of a toxicant on rodent lungs because of the lesions caused by the organism (114,126,181,189,272). This organism may also affect such parameters as sperm motility as well as cause chronic disease of genital epithelium (56). Even bacteria that would be considered normal host microflora can complicate carcinogenesis studies. The pathogenicity of *M. pulmonis* is significantly increased by low levels of ammonia (44). In considering studies conducted to elucidate interactions between bacteria and toxicants, the toxicologist should be aware that some strains of animals may be more resistant to infection than other strains. For example, one investigator reported significant differences in the susceptibility of Sprague–Dawley, Long–Evans, and Wistar strains of rat to *Diplo-*

coccus pneumoniae, Escherichia coli, and *Staphlococcus aureus* (307).

Some of the bacteria in rodents and lagomorphs that may present problems include *Pasteurella multocida, Bacillus piliformis, Streptococcus pneumoniae, Corynebacterium kutscheri, Klebsiella pneumoniae, Salmonella sp.,* and *Mycoplasma pulmonis* (31,79,116,163). It is interesting to note that species of rodents may differ in resistance to infection (see Table 7).

Even metazoan parasites such as pinworms (*Syphacia muris*) can be readily spread from animal to animal or from species to species. Some investigators reported transmission of pinworms among rats, mice, hamsters, and gerbils (276). Infestation with pinworms can result in unhealthy animals that are unsuitable for research (312). Rickettsiae infestations alone or in conjunction with viruses can cause complications in research especially in immunology studies. These rickettsiae include *Haemobartonella* and *Eperythrozoon spp.* (see Table 8).

Even the circadian rhythm can have an effect on the resistance of rodents to infection. One example is mice intraperitoneally inoculated with pneumococci organisms in the light period were more apt to die in a shorter period of time than those mice inoculated during the dark cycle (358). Circadian rhythms will be discussed later in this chapter.

When one considers the impact of microorganisms and diseases, the subject of germfree and specific pathogenfree animals is invariably presented. The microbiological status of the animals to be used will be determined by the purpose of the studies and type of facility in which animals will be housed. However, scientists should be aware that germfree rodents such as rats may have depressed leucocyte count (48). Some investigators (204) have found lower incidence of hepatic tumors in germfree mice (39%) compared to con-

TABLE 7. *Selected pathogenic bacteria and mycoplasma*

Organism	Mouse	Rat	Guinea pig	Hamster
Bacillus piliformis	+	+	+	+
Bordetella bronchiseptica	+	+	+	+
Citrobacter freundii	+			
Corynebacterium kutscheri	+	+	+	+
Klebsiella pneumoniae	+	+	+	+
Mycoplasma spp.	+	+		
Pasteurella pneumotropica	+	+	+	+
Pseudomonas aeruginosa	+	+		
Salmonella spp.	+	+	+	+
Staphylococcus aureus (coagulase +)	+	+	+	+
Streptococcus, various groups	+	+	+	+
Streptococcus pneumoniae		+	+	+
Streptobacillus moniliformis	+	+		

From ref. 114, with permission.

TABLE 8. *Selected pathogenic endoparasites*

Organism	Mouse	Rat	Guinea pig	Hamster
Aspiculuris tetraptera	+	+		+
Capillaria hepatica	+	+		
Cysticercus fasciolaris	+	+		+
Eimeria spp.	+	+	+	
Encephalitozoon	+	+	+	+
Eperythrozoon coccoides	+			
Giardia muris	+	+		+
Haemobartonella muris	+	+		
Heterakis spumosa	+	+		
Hexamita muris	+	+		+
Hymenolepis diminuta	+	+		+
Hymenolepis nana	+	+		+
Syphacia muris	+	+		
Syphacia obvelata	+	+		+
Trichosomoides crassicauda		+		
Trypanosoma lewisi		+		

From ref. 114, with permission.

ventional mice (82%). Status of host microflora and infections can have significant effects on results of immunology and carcinogenicity studies (142,216).

Infection or clinical disease itself can affect the outcome of studies. One study (292) obtained a large increase frequency of lung tumors in male rats with chronic respiratory disease exposed to *N*-nitrosoheptamethyleneimine as to SPF and germfree animals exposed to the same carcinogen. This increase may be due to impaired mucociliary clearance or other defense mechanisms (216).

NOISE

The effects of noise in an animal facility can compromise data in unusual or extreme situations. The day-to-day activities of a typical vivarium are unavoidably noisy at times. These may include voices of animal technicians, noise from animals (e.g., dogs barking), metal cage parts, metal feed and water containers banging together, cleaning equipment dropped or clanging together, various alarm systems, cages and racks being moved during the cleaning process, and construction or maintenance noises. Personnel should be aware of the effects of noise on animals and react accordingly. There are good reviews in the scientific literature of the effects of noise on laboratory animals (102,120,243,256). Obviously, noise can produce stress. Although stress is discussed later in this chapter, some of the effects of noise will be discussed here.

Noise can affect organic weights, histopathology, clinical chemistry, hematology, and clinical signs, as well as reproductive performance. Levels above 68 db for 6 min caused a decrease in circulating eosinophils in rats in the first hour after exposure. In this same experiment, prolonged exposure to 73 db or greater (6 min/hr all day for 24 hr to 21 days) resulted in increased adrenal weights and serum cholesterol

(125). Rats exposed to typical noise caused by animal attendants had increased plasma corticosterone levels (24). This was true for singly housed and group-housed rats. The plasma corticosterone levels increased 33% in 20 min for singly housed animals and 64% for group-housed rats. Sudden intense sounds can induce epileptiform seizures in some strains of mice such as the DBA2 (158). Audiogenic stress can produce cardiac hypertrophy in the rat and rabbit (124). Guinea pigs exposed to the sound of firing caps or to 125 to 130 db of noise for 4 hr suffered destruction of the sensory hair cells of the organ of Corti (247). Auditory stress reduced fertility in both male and female mice and rats (102). Noise at levels from 83 to 95 db for 6 min/hr increased preimplantation failure and fertilization in Swiss mice (362). Sounds from a fire alarm system altered the cell cycle phases observed in vaginal smears of rats (119). Levels above 85 db reduced fertility in rodents (364) and increased blood pressure in nonhuman primates (242). High-pitched sound may cause urinary changes in rats (235).

To reduce noise in an animal facility, several measures can be taken, for example, the training of personnel to minimize noise, keeping loud species such as dogs and pigs away from other species, and locating noisy operations such as the cage wash area away from animal rooms. The use of cushioned casters and bumpers on carts, trucks, and racks is also helpful (71).

Noise in the animal room can vary according to the species on study (102). Consequently, it is recommended that noisy operations such as construction and cleaning should be broken up into small intervals (102). Although there is no set standards as to decibel level limitations for comfort for animals, all efforts should be taken to minimize sound. As a rule, the toxicologist should assume that animals are at least as sensitive to noise as humans (i.e., anatomical damage at 160 db, pain at 140 db, inner ear damage after prolonged exposures around 100 db) (16). On the basis of the studies quoted above, scientists should try to keep average levels of sound less than 70 db and try to avoid intermittent noises of more than 100 db. In the case of dog rooms, one might consider the practice of debarking dogs. However, locating dog rooms away from other species and issuing safety ear apparel (plugs or ear sets) to animal care technicians would probably be better alternatives.

STRESS

The most important factor the toxicologist and animal care staff must achieve is the minimization of stress in the animals. This encompasses a variety of factors discussed in other parts of this chapter (e.g., noise, diet, temperature, humidity). However, special consideration is given to stress because of its potential overriding influence on the results of an experiment. Special emphasis will be given to stress of isolation and overcrowding.

Methods of killing can result in stress based on the concentration of serum steroids. Chloroform inhalation to produce anesthesia before killing resulted in higher corticosterone levels than in animals decapitated (53). Capturing mice in their cages and transferring them to the bleeding area increased plasma corticosterone levels in less than 5 min (264). Movement of animals to another area before bleeding affects the serum value of luteinizing hormone and prolactin (95). Repeated blood sampling in rats by cardiac puncture caused an increase in prolactin and plasma glucose (30).

Immobilization of rats in the peak of their activities increases their susceptibility to gastric erosions (2). Increased susceptibility to gastric ulcers and tumors was reduced in rats by handling early in life (209). Pregnant mice (jax strain) shipped on days 12 and 13 of gestation had a 65% greater incidence of facial clefts in offspring than those shipped on days 14, 15, and 16 (202). "Boxing" of mice for shipment caused a 5% weight loss, which can be reduced by placing potatoes in the container (338). One study demonstrated that it takes weanling rats 48 hr to return to "equilibrate" after shipment stress (88). Monkeys kept in restraint chairs had consistently higher plasma levels of serum lactic dehydrogenase (294). Mice and rats subjected to immobilization stress have increased adrenal weights and decreased body weight (199).

Immunity and effects of disease can be influenced by stress. Stress induced by deprivation of feed, water, and bedding for 2 days resulted in higher numbers of salmonella organisms in the intestines of mice innoculated with *Salmonella typhimurium* (320). Chickens exposed to stress had a higher incidence of Marek's disease and a higher concentration of plasma corticosterone than less stressed chickens (135). Mice under stress are less able to reject transplanted tumors and more apt to succumb to virally induced tumors (264). The increased susceptibility of stressed laboratory rodents to neoplasia may be due to lymphopenia (especially lymphocytes), thymic involution, and loss of tissue mass in the spleen and peripheral lymph nodes. This effect on circulating lymphocytes and lymphoid organs appears to be the direct or indirect effect of increased circulating corticosterone (168,264,295). Grouping of mice can cause a decrease in circulating antibodies when compared to inbred mice (333). Other signs of stress to overcrowding in mice may include gastritis, decreased food consumption, and decreased body weights (62).

When considering ways to control unwanted stress in laboratory animals, one has to consider the effects of single animal housing (isolation stress), as well as overcrowding. The decision to house singly or group house depends on the species of animal, design of the experiment, and the biological systems expected to be studied in an experiment. The toxicologists will have to consider what physiological and psychological effects that single or group housing is apt to have on an experiment (51). In order to evaluate whether to house laboratory animals singly or in groups, a review of the literature should help the scientist reach a conclusion.

Mice housed singly had larger adrenal glands than those housed in groups of 10 (84). Rats housed singly had larger adrenal and thyroid glands but smaller spleens and thymus glands when compared with community-caged controls (147). Rats housed individually for 3 weeks showed decreased sleep time with barbiturates compared with group-housed rats. However, this effect disappeared after 6 weeks (82). Other effects of isolation may include increased serum gonadal hormones (41) and increased sensitivity to isoproterenol (23,206) in rats and increased movement and aggressiveness, as well as a decreased white blood cell count, in mice (348). For a more in-depth general review on isolation stress in

rodents, the reader should refer to the reference section (19,25,179).

Adverse effects caused by overcrowding in mice included increased adrenal gland weight, decreased testes weight, decreased fertility, increased intrauterine mortality, and decreased lactation with subsequent slowed growth of nursing young (60,61).

Crowding increased mortality in mice caused by malaria (246). Group-housing stress significantly increased the intensity of adjuvant-induced arthritis in Fischer rats (9). The *in vitro* response of sensitized splenic lymphocytes to thyroglobulin was increased by crowding and decreased by isolation in female rats and decreased in both isolated and overcrowded rats (160). Overcrowding in rats reduced the primary and secondary antibody response to bacterial antigen in male Fischer rats (303).

Singly housed mice responded to injected ascitic neoplastic cells with greater volumes of ascitic fluid than those housed in groups of 10 (84). Increased incidence of skin and tail lesions was seen with clustering, as well as with isolation of single mice (185). In isolation studies, housing rodents singly eliminates cannibalism and the tendency for rodents to filter out inhaled test material by breathing through cage mates' fur (283).

Amount of space and standardization of groups by age and sex have been practiced in the laboratory for many years. Through the breeding of commonly used strains of laboratory animals over many years, it is probable that these animals have become more adapted to the laboratory environment (211). The adverse psychological effects of isolation (single housing) can be offset by arranging cages so that animals can see each other and by increasing the level of careful human attention and handling (51).

If the toxicologist and laboratory animal care supervisor decide to group house animals, the minimum space requirements for laboratory animals should be consulted (71) (see Table 2). Special consideration should be given to how aggressive the species or strain of laboratory animal may be. Male mice, cats, or dogs may be overly aggressive, and special attention and precautions may have to be taken when group housing these animals.

SANITATION

Aspects of sanitation practices are discussed in other parts of this chapter. However, some general guidelines will be discussed in this section of the chapter. The toxicologist should refer to other cited literature for more details (51,71,80). Improper sanitation can lead to added stress of laboratory animals, the spread of disease, and more subtle effects such as decreased activity of hepatic enzyme systems (332).

There are basic practices that are universally accepted as far as sanitation is concerned. However, even if these practices are followed, the toxicologists and manager of the vivarium need to make a diligent effort to inspect facilities on a regular basis to evaluate the relative cleanliness of the facilities.

Sanitation of cages is one of the most important aspects of control of disease and stress. Bedding should be changed one to three times a week or as often as necessary to keep animals dry and clean. Soiled bedding and litter should be removed from cages and pans in areas other than the animal room to prevent dust and aerosolization of potentially infectious fomites. Cages should be washed and dried before the placement of animals in them. Solid bottom cages should be cleaned at least once a week, whereas wire bottom cages can be washed at least once every 2 weeks. Cage racks can be cleaned once every 2 weeks to once a month. Cleaning of cages can be accomplished by detergent and chemical cleansers followed by thorough rinsing to remove residues or by heat sterilization attained by water at least 180°F (82.2°C). Water at this temperature should be applied for at least 10 min or a sufficient time to kill pathogenic microorganisms. Washing and rinsing can be done by automatic tunnel washers and/or cage/rack washers or by hand in special sinks and specialized rooms with drains. If heat is used for sterilization, it has to be a minimum of 180°F (82.2°C). Feeders, containers, and bottles should be washed, cleaned, and changed at least once a week. Automatic waterers should be periodically flushed and cleaned, if necessary, to remove bacteria and other pathogens from water lines.

Rooms should be thoroughly cleaned between studies (ceiling, walls, and floors). During a given study, floors should be thoroughly cleaned at least once a week or as often as needed. The floors can be wet mopped or sanitized daily. Ideally, buckets, mops, sponges, and brooms should be available for each room and not taken to other animal rooms. If waste cans are in each room, they should be lined with plastic bags and have airtight lids.

VERMIN CONTROL

The presence of insects and wild rodents can compromise sanitation and the prevention of the spread of disease in the animal facility. Unfortunately, the toxicologist should not use any chemicals for vermin control without consideration of alternative measures and a thorough knowledge of the biological effects of any pesticide used. Many chemicals are inducers of hepatic microsomal enzymes and could alter results of animal experimentations (47,111,153,175,249). The immune system of laboratory animals can also be affected by insecticides (166,339). Any chemical used for vermin control should be evaluated for potential to alter the metabolic or immunologic status of the animals and for the potential to cause overt toxicity. In the case of cockroaches, relatively nontoxic materials such as boric acid or drying substances such as amorphous silica gel can be used (71). Keeping crevices and cracks sealed, as well as making walls and ceilings as smooth as possible, helps remove hiding places for insects.

WASTE DISPOSAL

Although more detailed discussions are available in other references (71,75,151), a brief overview is presented here to remind the toxicologists of some general principles. Waste should be removed as frequently as is reasonably possible.

Waste should be stored in sealed containers that are metal, plastic, or lined with plastic. Containers should be leakproof and have tight lids. These containers should be stored in a separate area until picked up for disposal.

Most local municipalities have statutes or ordinances controlling disposal of wastes. Hazardous and radioactive wastes must be disposed of according to government regulations. Animal carcasses and other biological wastes should be refrigerated until disposal. Bedding and litter is frequently put into sealed plastic bags and incinerated or carried to landfills. Noncontaminated bedding and litter can be flushed into a local sewer system. Where laboratories are conducting research on hazardous agents (radioactive substances, carcinogens, infectious agents, etc.), government regulations should be consulted. A local safety committee should be formed with knowledgeable members that oversee the disposal process and ensure that all personnel handling wastes are properly trained.

Chemical waste can usually be incinerated at high temperatures that will break down or destroy test chemicals or can be sent to government-approved disposal areas for burial in sealed containers. Methods of disposal of radioactive wastes vary as to half-life and nature of isotopes. Institutions can get licensed by the Nuclear Regulatory Commission to incinerate wastes with certain isotopes (C^{14} and H^3). The toxicologist should consult local, state, and federal regulations to determine the correct way to dispose of hazardous wastes.

GENERAL PRINCIPLES OF ANIMAL PROCUREMENT

Laboratory animals should be legally purchased from quality suppliers. The source of animals should be a proven supplier of quality, disease-free animals. Facilities of suppliers should adequately meet requirements for prevention of disease spread and provide environment necessary for healthy nonstressed animals (40). Ideally, such suppliers should provide records on the health status of the breeding colony, as well as records on husbandry practices. These records should include breeding records, and where pertinent, records on viral and bacterial antibody and culture information should be available (51,71,75). When selecting a supplier, method of transportation and efforts undertaken to minimize shipment stress should be considered. When possible, having a single quality source of a species helps minimize introduction and spread of disease. Choice of breed or strain of animals can be based on experience of investigators and the institution. The toxicology literature could be a helpful resource in selecting a strain and/or species of laboratory animal. As much as possible, species should be kept separate during shipment and quarantine (71). Animals can be classified as to their microbiological status (74). Most toxicologists use conventional or barrier-maintained animals. The choice between inbred versus outbred strains of rodents has been debated by different investigators (98,304). However, use of well-known strains or hybrids (e.g., Sprague-Dawley rats, Fischer rats, CD-1 mice, B_6C3F mice) provide the investigator with the advantage of historical data and scientific literature in interpreting data.

QUARANTINE

To provide additional assurance regarding control of spread of disease and utilization of healthy animals on study, a period of quarantine is required. Quarantine facilities should be separate from animal rooms. An alternative is that the test animal room serve as a quarantine room for the same animals that go on test. However, if animals break with disease during quarantine, the room has to be cleaned and disinfected before use as a test room. Quarantine also ensures stabilization of the animals' condition, as well as providing animals an opportunity to become acclimated to new facilities. If a complete history of animals is available from the supplier, a shorter quarantine can be implemented. Animals should be quarantined for at least a week (304). In the event a history on received animals is incomplete, the quarantine period should be long enough to allow expression of disease in the incubation stages (71). For rodents, a quarantine of 2 to 4 weeks for animals to be used in chronic studies should be sufficient. However, primates may require a quarantine of at least 3 months because of long incubation time to clinical disease caused by certain viruses, parasites, and tuberculosis (112,113,116,131).

INHERENT PRINCIPLES OF VARIABILITY

Selection of Species

In chronic studies (referred to as chronic bioassays), it is recommended that at least two species be used. Species should be selected on the basis of hardiness, longevity, genetic stability, background lesion incidence, and sensitivity to tumor induction (304). Other factors to consider in the selection of models are similar absorption, distribution, metabolism, and excretion of test chemicals (215), as well as similar toxicity to humans if that information is available (283). Unfortunately, this information is not always available, and choice of species will have to be made on other factors such as space availability, longevity, and the laboratory resources (costs, personnel, etc.).

The experienced toxicologist should be aware of specie differences in susceptibility to toxicity of compounds. Some differences in the susceptibility of rats and mice were reported in a review of 2-year bioassay carcinogenicity studies (145), although the correlation between these species is strong (146). Male rats exhibit a susceptibility of renal injury caused by volatile hydrocarbons (5). This is not generally seen in other species and probably explains the unique susceptibility of rats to kidney tumorigenicity with unleaded gasoline. The LD_{50} as well as carcinogenicity of aflatoxin B_1 vary from species to species. For example, aflatoxin B_1 is carcinogenic in rainbow trout and rats, whereas it is virtually noncarcinogenic in mice (272). It has been reported that some compounds (e.g., 1,2-dichloroethane) cause lung tumors in mice and not rats, whereas other compounds cause tumors in rats but not mice (e.g., 2,4,5-trimethyl aniline) (139). Another example is the carcinogenic response of beta napthalanine in primates, hamsters, and dogs in the urinary bladder; in mice, tests are negative or hepatic tumors are produced, and it is noncarcinogenic in most studies conducted in rats

(155,351). Dibutylnitrosamine causes liver tumors in rats and guinea pigs, but it causes bladder and esophageal neoplasia in mice. Teratogenicity of adrenal cortical hormones, thalidomide, trypan, and vitamin A vary as to species of animal studied (272).

Specie differences have been noted in upper respiratory tract deposition for acetone and ethanol in rats and guinea pigs (208). Differences in regenerative hyperplasia of urinary bladder epithelium following transurethral cauterization have been noted in rats, mice, hamsters, and guinea pigs (3). Species differences in susceptibility was noted in the sister chromatid exchange and micronucleus induction induced by cyclophosphamide in rats, mice, and Chinese hamsters. Carcinogenicity of azo dyes may be more similar in humans and the mouse, as compared to the rat (351). As a consequence of the specie differences mentioned above, as well as other factors reported in the literature, the toxicologist should consider potential strain differences when planning toxicity studies.

Strain of Animals

The toxicologist should be aware of strain, as well as specie, differences that exist in susceptibility of animals to toxicity of chemicals. An example of strain susceptibility of rats to N-2-fluorenylacetamide. In female Fischer rats, N-2-fluorenylacetamide produces liver tumors, whereas it produces mammary tumors in female Sprague-Dawley rats (272). Genetic differences as to strain of mice or rats and their metabolism of xenobiotics have been summarized (215). Distinct differences between different strains of mice and the metabolism of chemicals were noted. Hartley guinea pigs are more sensitive to acute anaphylaxis following subcutaneous injection of antigen than were 2 inbred strains of guinea pigs (186). Strain differences in mice in skin painting carcinogenicity studies have been noted and summarized. The strain sensitivity to complete skin carcinogenesis is Sencar>CD-1>C57BL/6>ICR/Ha Swiss≥C_3H≥BALB/C (299). These are just a few examples of how strain differences in a species can create problems.

Age and Sex

Other variables impacting susceptibility of animals to toxicity of xenobiotics include sex and age. Perhaps the best known sex-related toxicity is the sensitivity of male mice to renal necrosis with chloroform compared to female mice (93,94,129). Investigators have reported that very young and very old animals have increased susceptibility to noxious agents (363). Vinyl chloride in general causes more tumors (e.g., hemangiosarcomas) if rodents were exposed early in life (first 6–12 months) than those exposed later in life (87). Considering these examples, as well as others, toxicologists should not be surprised to see different incidences and severity of lesions in male and female animals or in different age animals.

CIRCADIAN RHYTHM

In scheduling injections of laboratory animals with xenobiotics, the toxicologist should be aware of circadian rhythms and what they may mean in biological systems. Daily rhythmic cycles could affect the interpretation of data on different effects of chemicals. Interaction of light cycle with circadian rhythm has been observed in hepatic drug metabolizing enzymes in the rat (214). A circadian rhythm of rat body temperature ranges from approximately 37.5°C to 38.5°C and is abolished in rats kept in total light or total darkness (100). Circadian rhythm can affect the LD_{50} for various drugs (148,207). The reader should refer to several review articles for more in-depth discussions of circadian rhythm (1,2,207,358). However, for certain kinds of experiments (e.g., LD_{50}'s and pharmacokinetics), the toxicologist should be aware of the influence that circadian rhythm may have on data.

PERSONNEL—TRAINING AND SAFETY

If a scientist had to choose between top quality facilities and well-trained and motivated personnel taking care of a vivarium, he/she would be wise to choose the personnel. A marginal facility can successfully provide an adequate environment if it is staffed by dedicated laboratory animal personnel and research staff. However, the best facilities will fail in providing a stress-free environment if staffed by unmotivated and inadequately trained individuals. To ensure success, qualified and experienced animal care technicians and technologists should be hired. Alternatively, a mixture of trained and experienced individuals along with an enthusiastic but less experienced staff who are willing to be trained will suffice.

New personnel hired to work in a vivarium should be properly oriented as to laboratory regulations; sanitation practices and requirements; instructions concerning maintenance of forms used for receipt of animals, quarantine of animals, care of animals and cages, and scheduling of feeding, water, and cage cleaning; instructions on handling of animals and minimizing stress; introduction to other scientists, toxicologists, technicians, and management; and for the more experienced technicians, instructions for obtaining fecal, urine, and blood samples, euthanasia and anesthesia techniques, and necropsy procedures (if those activities are conducted by animal care staff rather than toxicology staff). Having new personnel well oriented and "off to the right start" is invaluable in creating motivation and a high degree of morale.

Ongoing training of personnel, both laboratory animal care staff and scientific staff, is not only valuable but in compliance with recent federal regulations, policies, and guidelines (13,51,71,85,90–92,106,233). Two organizations provide training materials for laboratory animal care and experimental methods. These are the Institute of Laboratory Animal Resources (part of the National Research Council in Washington, DC) and the American Association of Laboratory Animal Science (AALAS) (7). AALAS also offers certification programs for three levels of certification: the assistant laboratory animal technician, the laboratory animal technician, and the laboratory animal technologist (12,18). AALAS is to be distinguished from AAALAC, which offers a program of accreditation for institutions whereby peer review teams evaluate facilities and programs to determine whether vivariums and research institutes and the husbandry practices of those institutes meet the criteria for accreditation. These inspection procedures evaluate the quality of animal care, humane treatment of animals, protection of personnel from hazards, and control of variables that could adversely affect animal research. This organization also provides suggestions for alleviating discrepancies. AAALAC uses the *Guide for the Care and Use of Laboratory Animals* (71) as a basic guide for specific standards of accreditation.

One of the most critical skills that personnel working with animals should have is the ability to evaluate laboratory animals for clinical signs of illness. Part of the laboratory staff's training should be recognition of these clinical signs. Some excellent resources are available for discussion of clinical signs as well as the hematology, clinical chemistry, gross pathology, and histopathology of various laboratory animal disease (51,71,113,116).

One very important aspect of personnel training as well as their working environment is the provision of a safe work environment. Instructions involving the hazards of biological, chemical, and physical agents with which the staff may come into contact should be provided (see Table 9). Instructions should be provided regarding use of protective clothing, sanitation practices including proper use of disinfectants and detergents, importance of personal hygiene, safety procedures for working with toxic chemicals and radioactive materials, and the techniques of zoonoses surveillance. Familiarization with institutional, local, state, and federal guidelines on the use of hazardous chemicals and biological waste should be part of any training program (51,52,71,304).

Occupational health procedures protecting the health of laboratory personnel should include periodic physical examination; records kept on animal bites, scratches, and allergies; immunization of personnel against tetanus; and appropriate immunization of personnel who work with animals at substantial risk to rabies and hepatitis B virus. Personnel working with primates should undergo regular tests for tuberculosis. Protective clothing (gloves, masks, and outer garments) for individuals working with primates and animals at risk for rabies should be required (71).

To provide instructions on health and safety, laboratory animal supervisors should obtain the aid of safety officers

---

TABLE 9. *Safety practices for storage and handling of hazardous chemicals[a]*

1. Identify and label all hazardous chemicals by affixing a "Biohazard Warning" label to them.
2. Store explosive chemicals in explosive-proof containers.
3. Provide safety equipment (protective clothing, respirators, showers, eye baths, etc.) for personnel handling hazardous substances.
4. Provide adequate training of personnel on hazards and safety protocol.
5. Store volatile chemicals so vapors cannot collect and create a hazard.
6. Maintain a current inventory of chemicals and store them under conditions that ensure stability.
7. Establish standard procedures for handling spills.
8. Limit access to the storage area.

[a] From ref. 157.

and/or radiation safety officers of the research institute. Additionally, supervisors should consult Occupational Safety and Health Administration (OSHA) guidelines and articles on zoonoses (114,116).

In summary, there is simply no substitution for well-trained, highly motivated staff and a safe, pleasant working environment to help ensure high quality research and data for scientists working in toxicology laboratories.

USE OF ANIMALS IN TOXICOLOGY AND EXPERIMENTATION

Every scientist has to recognize that a significant number of people oppose the use of animals in research. Some of these opponents (e.g., antivivisectionists) believe that animals should not be used in painful or even painless types of experiments, regardless of the benefit to humans or other animals. It is difficult to envision a toxicology research program based solely on alternate methods of research, and virtually all biological scientists consider animal research methods to be indispensable. Accordingly, no government has adopted the extreme position of banning all use of research animals, although there is a growing advocacy for the use of alternatives. Although it is beyond the scope of this chapter to discuss in depth the philosophical controversies surrounding the issue of the use of animals in research, additional reading in the area is recommended (15,118,155,156,184,190,305,306,349). It is advantageous for the investigator to be aware of the controversies that exist between biomedical scientists and antivivisectionists on laboratory animal use issues for several reasons. Such knowledge facilitates a greater understanding of the public concern for the humane care and use of animals in research facilities. It provides a perspective for (a) understanding the existence and stringency of federal regulations governing the use of laboratory animals, and (b) understanding the need for sound biomedical justification for the use of animals in research. There is nearly unanimous support for the view that animals in research should be provided high quality care, treated humanely, and exposed to as little pain and/or distress as possible, and therefore, the responsibility of each investigator to conduct animal research as humanely as possible cannot be overemphasized.

Several interdisciplinary societies have been founded for the primary purpose of promoting the humane and responsible use of laboratory animals. These organizations are excellent resources for investigators who plan to use research animals. AALAS, the Scientists Center for Animal Welfare (SCAW), and the Foundation for Biomedical Research are examples of such societies.

Toxicologists, veterinarians, and medical researchers are finding themselves under increasing pressure from animal rights groups and antivivisectionists. More now than ever, researchers must justify the use of animals in their experiments to themselves, as well as to those outside their laboratories expressing concern about the use of animals. The justification of animals in medical and toxicological research is similar to that rationale for the use of animals for food and clothing. All too often scientists are too unaware of the dependence of medicine, toxicology, biology, biochemistry, and governmental regulatory affairs on research conducted with laboratory animals. Scientists are very aware of developments in their own field but all too often woefully ignorant of the reliance of other branches of science and medicine on laboratory animals. The reader is referred to articles dealing with developments in the field relevant on use of animals (10,15,68,118,155,156,190,203,255,310,349).

In fact, considering all the breakthroughs and progress that has been made because of laboratory animal research, some may argue that it is unethical *not* to use laboratory animals for safety testing, as well as for drug and surgical research, until *in vitro* methods, mathematical modeling, structure activity relationships, and computer simulation reach a point of reliability whereby intact organisms may be substituted.

If animals are as irreplaceable in the laboratory as most scientists believe, what are our ethical responsibilities? Simply, they are as follows:

- Use *in vitro* systems in lieu of animals as much as possible.
- When possible, use isolated organs and tissue samples. (It should be remembered that these tissues are removed from animals that have been euthanized.)
- Use as few animals as possible in a given experiment. (However, enough animals should be used to have a valid study.)
- Use analgesics and anesthetics to relieve pain and suffering. Analgesics and anesthetics should be the most appropriate ones for that species.
- Provide euthanasia of animals that are in obvious pain or suffering wherein the use of analgesics or surgery would prohibit that animal's usefulness as data or results in that study.
- Use therapeutic drugs or methods to treat animals that are ill.
- Be aware that neither economics nor convenience is sufficient rationale for use of animals.
- Use animals only when it is expected that the study will contribute directly or indirectly to the well-being or protection and improvement of health for either humans or animals.
- Avoid experimental methods that require excessive restraint, excessive periods of withholding of food and water, or require absence of analgesics and other drugs in the event of pain or suffering.
- Adhere strictly to humane practices throughout all aspects of a given study.
- Do not use poisons or painful experiments to demonstrate symptomology or behavior solely for instructional purposes. Use lecture and films as a substitute for the use of live animals.
- Strive through literature review and dialogue with other scientists to select the most relevant animal model for a given experiment. The use of principles of pharmacokinetics and metabolism, structure activity relationships, and background tumor and lesion incidence for a given strain and species, as well as known toxic properties of compounds in the same chemical class, should help the toxicologist select the appropriate species for a given study.

The reader should refer to the reference section for more in-depth discussions of the principles listed above, as well as others concerning the appropriate judicious and humane use of laboratory animals (13,38,234,238,289,305,306,321). In addition to these articles, the reader is referred to other literature citations and presentations that discuss relevant legislation and guidelines, as well as the controversy that involves this legislation (116,156,281,311).

Number of Animals

Toxicologists should attempt to obtain the maximum amount of pertinent information from a given study in order to prevent repeating different studies of similar duration in a given species to determine different endpoints. For example, obtaining maximum volume blood and tissue samples from animals at terminal sacrifice in addition to specimens needed for routine clinical chemistry and hematology might prevent the necessity of doing additional studies. An example of this may be extra serum for complete lipid profiles in addition to routine serum chemistry in a caloric or nutrition study. This might require 2 to 5 ml of blood instead of 1 ml for more routine analysis. In addition, to maximize the use of animals at terminal sacrifice for analysis of biological changes, toxicologists should confer with statisticians to determine the minimum number of animals per sex per group to obtain necessary data. However, the toxicologist should not use so few animals such that insufficient survivors are left in groups to statistically evaluate the results. Additionally, toxicologists should also seek ways to avoid less meaningful designed studies. One example of this type of effort could be the use of approximate lethal dose studies that use small numbers of animals for determination of acute toxicity in lieu of LD_{50}'s using larger numbers of animals (169). The reader should be aware that the use of LD_{50}'s and other acute toxicity tests is becoming heavily scrutinized by the scientific community. In that way, the toxicologist could get a reasonable estimate of acute toxicity and at the same time derive information that would help determine doses for subacute and subchronic studies. Scientists should also consider ways to avoid unnecessary studies. In the case of strong acids or bases, the toxicologist might want to assume those agents are corrosive and report these agents as assumed to be corrosive instead of doing Draize tests or occluded skin irritancy tests. When feasible, the use of in vitro systems in lieu of Draize tests is recommended when such systems provide sufficient information to provide safety assessment (352–354).

Another area of considerable controversy is euthanasia and anesthesia. The scientist must select anesthetic and euthanasia agents that provide humane treatment and/or a state of analgesia to animals while not jeopardizing the quality and consistency of his/her data in a given study. Those scientists simply cannot render proper decisions without proper knowledge of pharmacological properties of the various drugs and agents available for these purposes. At the very least, those scientists should consult veterinarians or scientists knowledgeable in the pharmacology and utility of these agents, as well as their suitability for the species of laboratory animal being utilized. The reader is referred to the reference section for an in-depth discussion of anesthetic and euthanasia agents (49,52,101,167,193,301).

In closing, the only successful way to use laboratory animals in toxicology research is to use high quality laboratory animals; provide a clean, safe environment for those animals; provide an uncontaminated nutritious diet as well as uncontaminated drinking water; use well-trained conscientious staff; and through that staff and adequate facilities, provide an environment that is as stress-free as is reasonably possible. For this to occur, the veterinarian, scientist, toxicology technicians, laboratory animal care technicians, and IACUC must all understand their responsibilities. There are excellent articles in the literature that describe the responsibilities of all these personnel (51,71,116,165,233,237).

REFERENCES

1. Ader, R. (1967): Behavioral and physiological rhythms and the development of gastric erosions in the rat. Psychosom. Med., 29: 345–353.
2. Ader, R., and Friedman, S. B. (1968): Plasma corticosterone response to environmental stimulation: effects of duration of stimulation and the 24-hour adrenocortical rhythm. Neuroendocrinology, 3:378–386.
3. Akaza, H., Koseki, K., and Niijima, T. (1986): Species differences in regenerative hyperplasia of bladder urothelium after transurethral cauterization. Urol. Res., 14:223–225.
4. Albanes, D. (1987): Total calories, body weight, and tumor incidence in mice. Cancer Res., 47:1987–1992.
5. Alden, C. L. (1985): Species, sex, and tissue specificity in toxicologic and proliferative responses. Toxicol. Pathol., 13(2):135–140.
6. Allander, C., and Abel, E. (1973): Some aspects of the differences of air conditions inside a cage for small laboratory animals and its surroundings. Z. Versuchstierkd. Bd., 15:20–34.
7. American Association for Laboratory Animal Science (1975): Manual for Laboratory Animal Technicians, 216 pp., AALAS Publication 67-3, Joliet, IL.
8. American Institute of Nutrition (1977): Report of the American Institute of Nutrition Ad Hoc Committee on Standards for Nutritional Studies. J. Nutr., 107.
9. Amkraut, A. A., Solomon, G. F., and Kraemer, H. C. (1971): Stress, early experiences and adjuvant-induced arthritis in the rat. Psychosom. Med., (33)3:203–214.
10. Anchel, M. (1976): Beyond "adequate veterinary care." J. Am. Vet. Med. Assoc., 168(6):513–517.
11. Anderson, L. C., Leary, S. L., and Manning, P. J. (1983): Rat-bite fever in animal research laboratory personnel. Lab. Anim. Sci., 33(3):292–294.
12. Animal Technician Certification Board, American Association for Laboratory Animal Science (1975): The Animal Technician Certification Program, 5 pp. AALAS Publication 70-3, Joliet, IL.
13. The Animal Welfare Act of 1966, PL 89-544; as amended by Animal Welfare Act of 1970, PL 91-579; by the 1976 Amendments to the Animal Welfare Act, PL 94-297; and by the 1985 Food Security Act, PL 99-198.
14. Animal Welfare Institute (1979): Comfortable Quarters for Laboratory Animals. Washington, DC.
15. Anonymous (1972): Is Drug Toxicity in Animals a Valid Guide to Human Response? Lab. Anim., November/December.
16. Anthony, A. (1962): Criteria for acoustics in animal housing. Lab. Anim. Care, (13):340–347.
17. Appell, L. H., Kovatch, R. M., Reddecliff, J. M., and Gerone, P. J. (1971): Pathogenesis of Sendai virus infection in mice. Am. J. Vet. Res., 32:1835–1841.
18. Arnold, D. L., Fox, J. G., Thibert, P., and Grice, H. C. (1978): Toxicology studies. I. Support personnel. Food Cosmetics Toxicol., 16:479–484.
19. Baer, H. (1971): Long-term isolation stress and its effects on drug response in rodents. Lab. Anim. Sci., 21(3):341–349.
20. Baetjer, A. M. (1968): Role of environmental temperature and humidity in susceptibility to disease. Arch. Environ. Health, 16:565–570.
21. Baker, H. J., Lindsey, J. R., and Weisbroth, S. H. (1979): Housing to control research variables. In: The Laboratory Rat, Volume 1:

Biology and Diseases, edited by H. J. Baker, J. R. Lindsey, and S. H. Weisbroth, pp. 169–192. Academic Press, Orlando, FL.

22. Baker, H. J., Lindsey, J. R., and Weisbroth, S. H. (1979): *The Laboratory Rat,* Vol. 1: *Biology and Diseases.* Academic Press, Orlando, FL.

23. Balazs, T., and Dairman, W. (1967): Comparison of microsomal drug-metabolizing enzyme systems in grouped and individually caged rats. *Toxicol. Appl. Pharmacol.,* 10:409–411.

24. Barrett, A. M., and Stockham, M. A. (1963): The effect of housing conditions and simple experimental procedures upon the corticosterone level in the plasma of rats. *J. Endocrinol.,* (26):97–105.

25. Barrett, A. M., and Stockham, M. A. (1966): One or many animals in a cage? *Nutr. Rev.,* 24:116–119.

26. Barthold, S. W. (1986): Research complications and state of knowledge of rodent coronaviruses. In: *Complications of Viral and Mycoplasmal Infections in Rodents to Toxicology Research and Testing,* edited by T. E. Hamm, Jr., pp. 53–90. Hemisphere Publishing, Washington, DC.

27. Beall, J. R., Torning, F. E., and Runkle, R. S. (1971): A laminar flow system for animal maintenance. *Lab. Anim. Sci.,* 21(2):206–212.

28. Beck, R. W. (1963): The control of *Pseudomonas aeruginosa* in a mouse breeding colony by the use of chlorine in the drinking water. *Lab. Anim. Care,* 13(1) Part II:41–45.

29. Belin, R. P., and Banta, R. G. (1971): Successful control of snuffles in a rabbit colony. *J. Am. Vet. Med. Assoc.,* 159(5):622–623.

30. Bellinger, L. L., and Mendel, V. E. (1975): Hormone and glucose responses to serial cardiac puncture in rats. *Proc. Soc. Exp. Biol. Med.,* 148:5–8.

31. Benirschke, K., Garner, F. M., and Jones, T. C. (1978): *Pathology of Laboratory Animals,* Vols. I and II. Springer-Verlag, New York.

32. Berg, B. N., and Simms, H. S. (1960): Nutrition and longevity in the rat. II. Longevity and onset of disease with different levels of food intake. *J. Nutr.,* 71:255–263.

33. Berg, B. N., and Simms, H. S. (1961): Nutrition and longevity in the rat. III. Food restriction beyond 800 days. *J. Nutr.,* 74:23–32.

34. Besch, E. L. (1975): Animal cage-room dry-bulk and dew-point temperature differentials. *ASHRAE Trans.,* 88(II):549–557.

35. Bhatt, P. (1980): Virus infections of laboratory rodents. *Lab. Anim.,* May/June:43–47.

36. Binns, R., Clark, G. C., and Healey, P. (1971): Physiological and histopathological measurements on lungs of laboratory rats maintained under barrier and under conventional conditions. *Lab. Anim.,* 5:57–66.

37. Birt, D. F., and Conrad, R. D. (1981): Weight gain, reproduction, and survival of Syrian hamsters fed five natural ingredient diets. *Lab. Anim. Sci.,* 31(2):149–155.

38. Blackmore, W. M. (1982): Animal research ethics at the University of Southern California. *Lab. Anim.,* May/June, 41–47.

39. Boorman, G. A., Hickman, R. L., Davis, G. W., Rhodes, L. S., White, N. W., Griffin, T. A., Mayo, J., and Hamm, T. E., Jr. (1986): Serological titers to murine viruses in 90-day and 2-year studies. In: *Complications of Viral and Mycoplasmal Infections in Rodents to Toxicology Research and Testing,* edited by T. E. Hamm, Jr., pp. 11–24. Hemisphere Publishing, Washington, DC.

40. Box, P. G. (1976): Criteria for producing high quality animals for research. *Lab. Anim. Sci.,* 26(2):334–338.

41. Brain, P., and Benton, D. (1979): The interpretation of physiological correlates of differential housing in laboratory rats. *Life Sci.,* 24:99–116.

42. Brewer, N. R. (1964): Estimating heat produced by laboratory animals. New data on animal heat and vapor transmission account for activity and other factors to provide a more reliable basis for air conditioning design calculations. *Heating Piping Air Conditioning,* 36(10):139–141.

43. Brick, J. O., Newell, R. F., and Doherty, D. G. (1969): A barrier system for a breeding and experimental rodent colony: description and operation. *Lab. Anim. Care,* 19(1):92–97.

44. Broderson, J. R., Lindsey, J. R., and Crawford, J. E. (1976): The role of environmental ammonia in respiratory mycoplasmosis of rats. *Am. J. Pathol.,* 85(1):115–130.

45. Burek, J. D., Zurcher, C., Van Nunen, M. C. J., and Hollander, C. F. (1977): A naturally occurring epizootic caused by Sendai virus in breeding and aging rodent colonies. II. Infection in the rat. *Lab. Anim. Sci.,* 27(6):963–971.

46. Burkhart, C. A., and Robinson, J. L. (1978): High rat pup mortality attributed to the use of cedar-wood shavings as bedding. *Lab. Anim.,* 12:221–222.

47. Burns, J. J. (1968): Variation of drug metabolism in animals and the prediction of drug action in man. *Ann. N.Y. Acad. Sci.,* 151:959–967.

48. Burns, K. F., Timmons, E. H., and Poiley, S. M. (1971): Serum chemistry and hematological values for axenic (germfree) and environmentally associated inbred rats. *Lab. Anim. Sci.,* 21(3):415–419.

49. Bustad, L. K. (1982): An educator's approach to euthanasia. *Lab. Anim.,* May/June:37–39.

50. Campbell, T. C., and Hayes, J. R. (1974): Role of nutrition in the drug-metabolizing enzyme system. *Pharmacol. Rev.,* 26(3):171–197.

51. Canadian Council on Animal Care (1980): *Guide to the Care and Use of Experimental Animals,* Vol. 1. Ottawa, Canada.

52. Canadian Council on Animal Care (1984): *Guide to the Care and Use of Experimental Animals,* Vol. 2. Ottawa, Canada.

53. Carney, J. A., and Walker, B. L. (1973): Mode of killing and plasma corticosterone concentrations in the rat. *Lab. Anim. Sci.,* 23(5):675–676.

54. Carthew, P., Sparrow, S., and Verstraete, A. P. (1978): Incidence of natural virus infections of laboratory animals 1976–1977. *Lab. Anim.,* 12:245–246.

55. Carthew, P., and Verstraete, A. (1978): A serological survey of accredited breeding colonies in the United Kingdom for common rodent viruses. *Lab. Anim.,* 12:29–32.

56. Cassell, G. H., Wilborn, W. H., Silvers, S. H., and Minion, F. C. (1981): Adherence and colonization of *Mycoplasma pulmonis* to genital epithelium and spermatozoa in rats. *Isr. J. Med. Sci.,* 17:593–598.

57. Cayen, M. N., Givner, M. L., and Kraml, M. (1972): Effect of diurnal rhythm and food withdrawal on serum lipid levels in the rat. *Experientia,* 28:502–503.

58. Cheney, K. E., Liu, R. K., Smith, G. S., Leung, R. E., Mickey, M. R., and Walford, R. L. (1980): Survival and disease patterns in C57BL/6J mice subjected to undernutrition. *Exp. Gerontol.,* 15:237–258.

59. Cheney, K. E., Liu, R. K., Smith, G. S., Meredith, P. J., Mickey, M. R., and Walford, R. L. (1983): The effect of dietary restriction of varying duration on survival, tumor patterns, immune function, and body temperature in B10C3F₁ female mice. *J. Gerontol.,* 38(4):420–430.

60. Christian, J. J. (1955): Effect of population size on the adrenal glands and reproductive organs of male mice in populations of fixed size. *Am. J. Physiol.,* 182:292–300.

61. Christian, J. J., and Lemunyan, C. D. (1958): Adverse effects of crowding on lactation and reproduction of mice and two generations of their progeny. *Endocrinology,* 63:517–529.

62. Chvedoff, M., Clarke, M. R., Irisarri, E., Faccini, J. M., and Monro, A. M. (1980): Effects of housing conditions on food intake, body weight and spontaneous lesions in mice. A review of the literature and results of an 18-month study. *Food Cosmetics Toxicol.,* 18:517–522.

63. Cinti, D. L., Lemelin, M. E., and Christian, J. (1976): Induction of liver microsomal mixed-function oxidases by volatile hydrocarbons. *Biochem. Pharmacol.,* 25:100–103.

64. Clapp, M. J. L. (1980): The effect of diet on some parameters measured in toxicological studies in the rat. *Lab. Anim.,* 14:253–261.

65. Clarke, H. E., Coates, M. E., Eva, J. K., Ford, D. J., Milner, C. K., O'Donoghue, P. N., Scott, P. P., and Ward, R. J. (1977): Dietary standards for laboratory animals: report of the Laboratory Animals Centre Diets Advisory Committee. *Lab. Anim.,* 11:1–28.

66. Clough, G. (1982): Environmental effects on animals used in biomedical research. *Biol. Rev.,* 57:487–523.

67. Clough, G., and Gamble, M. R. (1976): *Laboratory Animal Houses. A Guide to the Design and Planning of Animal Facilities.* LAC Manual Series No. 4., Medical Research Council Laboratory Animals Centre, Abbey Press, Abingdon, Oxon.

68. Cohen, C. (1986): The case for the use of animals in biomedical research. *N. Engl. J. Med.,* 315(14):865–870.

69. Collins, M. J., Jr. (1986): Prevalence of pathogenic murine viruses and mycoplasma that are currently a problem to research. In: *Complications of Viral and Mycoplasmal Infections in Rodents to*

Toxicology Research and Testing, edited by T. E. Hamm, Jr., pp. 1–10. Hemisphere Publishing, Washington, DC.

70. Committee on Care and Use of Laboratory Animals, Institute of Laboratory Animal Resources, National Research Council (1978): *Guide for the Care and Use of Laboratory Animals.* U. S. Department of Health, Education and Welfare, Public Health Service, National Institutes of Health, DHEW Publication No. (NIH) 78-23rev.

71. Committee on Care and Use of Laboratory Animals, Institute of Laboratory Animal Resources, National Research Council (1985): *Guide for the Care and Use of Laboratory Animals.* U. S. Department of Health, Education and Welfare, Public Health Service, National Institutes of Health, DHEW Publication No. (NIH) 85-23.

72. Committee on Laboratory Animal Diets, Institute of Laboratory Animal Resources, Assembly of Life Sciences, National Research Council, National Academy of Sciences (1978): Control of diets in laboratory animal experimentation. *ILAR News,* 21(2):A1–A12.

73. Committee on Laboratory Animal Diseases, Institute of Laboratory Animal Resources, National Research Council (1974): A guide to infectious diseases of guinea pigs, gerbils, hamsters and rabbits. *ILAR News,* 17(4).

74. Committee on Long-Term Holding of Laboratory Rodents, Institute of Laboratory Animal Resources, National Academy of Sciences, National Research Council (1976): Long-term holding of laboratory rodents. *ILAR News,* 19(4):L1–L25.

75. Committee on Rodents, Institute of Laboratory Animal Resources, Assembly of Life Sciences, National Research Council (1977): Laboratory animal management: rodents. *ILAR News,* 20(3):L1–L15.

76. Conybeare, G. (1979): Effect of quality and quantity of diet on survival and tumour incidence in outbred Swiss mice. *Food Cosmetics Toxicol.,* 18:65–75.

77. Copeland, D. H., and Salmon, W. D. (1946): The occurrence of neoplasms in the liver, lungs, and other tissues of rats as a result of prolonged choline deficiency. *Am. J. Pathol.,* 22:1059–1067.

78. Coriell, L. L., and McGarrity, G. J. (1973): Biomedical applications of laminar airflow. In: *Germ-free Research Biological Effect of Gnotobiotic Environments,* edited by J. B. Henegham, p. 43. Academic Press, New York.

79. Cotchin, E., and Roe, F. J. C. (1967): *Pathology of Laboratory Rats and Mice.* Blackwell Scientific Publications, Oxford, England.

80. Cranmer, M. F. (1976): Advances in animal care technology at the National Centre for Toxicological Research. *Lab. Anim. Sci.,* 26:355.

81. Cunliffe-Beamer, T. L., Freeman, L. C., and Myers, D. D. (1981): Barbiturate sleeptime in mice exposed to autoclaved or unautoclaved wood beddings. *Lab. Anim. Sci.,* 31:672–675.

82. Dairman, W., and Balazs, T. (1970): Comparison of liver microsome enzyme systems and barbiturate sleep times in rats caged individually or communally. *Biochem. Pharmacol.,* 19:951–955.

83. Dashiell, O. L., and Kennedy, G. L., Jr. (1984): The effects of fasting on the acute oral toxicity of nine chemicals in the rat. *J. Appl. Toxicol.,* 4(6):320–325.

84. Dechambre, R. P., and Gosse, C. (1973): Individual versus group caging of mice with grafted tumors. *Cancer Res.,* 33:140.

85. Department of Agriculture (1987): Animal and plant health inspection service. 9 CFR Parts 1 and 2: Animal Welfare; Proposed Rules. *Fed. Reg.,* 52(61):10292–10322.

86. Descoteaux, J. P., Grignon-Archambault, D., and Lussier, G. (1977): Serologic study on the prevalence of murine viruses in five Canadian mouse colonies. *Lab. Anim. Sci.,* 27(5):621–626.

87. Drew, R. T., Boorman, G. A., Haseman, J. K., McConnell, E. E., Busey, W. M., and Moore, J. A. (1983): The effect of age and exposure duration on cancer induction by a known carcinogen in rats, mice and hamsters. *Toxicol. Appl. Pharmacol.,* 68(1):120–130.

88. Dymsza, H. A., Miller, S. A., Maloney, J. F., and Foster, H. L. (1963): Equilibration of the laboratory rat following exposure to shipping stresses. *Lab. Anim. Care,* 13:60–65.

89. Edwards, G. S., Fox, J. G., Policastro, P., Goff, U., Wolf, M. H., and Fine, D. H. (1979): Volatile nitrosamine contamination of laboratory animal diets. *Cancer Res.,* 39:1857–1858.

90. Environmental Protection Agency (1978): Proposed guidelines for registering pesticides in the U. S.: hazard evaluation: humans and domestic animals. *Fed. Reg.,* 43:37336–37403.

91. Environmental Protection Agency (1979): Proposed health effects test standards for toxic substances control act test rules. *Fed. Reg.,* 44:27334–27374.

92. Environmental Protection Agency (1979): Good laboratory practice standards for health effects. *Fed. Reg.,* July.

93. Eschenbrenner, A. B., and Miller, E. (1945): Induction of hepatomas in mice by repeated oral administration of chloroform with observations on sex differences. *J. Natl. Cancer Inst.,* 5:251–255.

94. Eschenbrenner, A. B., and Miller, E. (1945): Sex differences in kidney morphology and chloroform necrosis. *Science,* 102:302–303.

95. Euker, J. S., Meites, J., and Riegle, G. D. (1975): Effects of acute stress on serum LH and prolactin in intact, castrate and dexamethasone-treated male rats. *Endocrinology,* 96:85–92.

96. Everett, R. (1984): Factors affecting spontaneous tumor incidence rates in mice: a literature review. *CRC Crit. Rev. Toxicol.,* 13(3):235–251.

97. Ferguson, H. C. (1966): Effect of red cedar chip bedding on hexobarbital and pentobarbital sleep time. *J. Pharm. Sci.,* 55:1142–1143.

98. Festing, M. F. W. (1982): Commentary: genetic contamination of laboratory animal colonies: an increasingly serious problem. *ILAR News,* 25(4):6–10.

99. Fidler, I. J. (1977): Depression of macrophages in mice drinking hyperchlorinated water. *Nature,* 270:735–736.

100. Fioretti, M. C., Riccardi, C., Menconi, E., and Martini, L. (1974): Control of the circadian rhythm of the body temperature in the rat. *Life Sci.,* 14:2111–2119.

101. Flecknell, P. A. (1984): The relief of pain in laboratory animals. *Lab. Anim.,* 18:147–160.

102. Fletcher, J. L. (1976): Influence of noise on animals. In: *Control of the Animal House Environment—Laboratory Animal Handbooks,* Vol. 7, edited by T. McSheehy, pp. 51–62. Trevor Laboratory Animals Ltd., London.

103. Flynn, R. J. (1959): Studies of the etiology of ringtail of rats. *Proc. Anim. Care Panel,* 9:155–160.

104. Flynn, R. J. (1963): *Pseudomonas aeruginosa* infection and radiobiological research at Argonne National Laboratory: effects, diagnosis, epizootiology, control. *Lab. Anim. Care,* 13:25–35.

105. Flynn, R. J. (1973): *Parasites of Laboratory Animals.* The Iowa State University Press, Ames, Iowa.

106. Food and Drug Administration (1978): Nonclinical laboratory studies, good laboratory practice recommendations. *Fed. Reg.,* 43:59986–60025.

107. Ford, D. J. (1977): Effect of autoclaving and physical structure of diets on their utilization by mice. *Lab. Anim.,* 11:235–239.

108. Ford, D. J. (1977): Influence of diet pellet hardness and particle size on food utilization by mice, rats and hamsters. *Lab. Anim.,* 11:241–246.

109. Fortmeyer, H. P. (1982): The influence of exogenous factors such as maintenance and nutrition on the course and results of animal experiments. In: *Animals in Toxicological Research,* edited by I. Bartosek et al., pp. 13–32, Raven Press, New York.

110. Foster, H. L., Small, J. D., and Fox, J. G. (1982): *The Mouse in Biomedical Research,* Vol. II: *Diseases.* Academic Press, New York.

111. Fouts, J. R. (1970): Some effects of insecticides on hepatic microsomal enzymes in various animal species. *Rev. Can. Biol.,* 29(4):377–389.

112. Fox, J. (1979): Selected aspects of animal husbandry and good laboratory practices. *Clin. Toxicol.,* 15(5):539–553.

113. Fox, J. G. (1977): Clinical assessment of laboratory rodents on long term bioassay studies. *J. Environ. Pathol. Toxicol.,* 1:199–226.

114. Fox, J. G. (1986): Interrelationships of disease and environmental variables in laboratory animals. In: *Safety Evaluation of Drugs and Chemicals,* edited by W. E. Lloyd, pp. 91–114. Hemisphere Publishing, New York.

115. Fox, J. G., Aldrich, F. D., and Boylen, G. W., Jr. (1976): Lead in animal foods. *J. Toxicol. Environ. Health,* 1:461–467.

116. Fox, J. G., Cohen, B. J., and Loew, F. M. (1984): *Laboratory Animal Medicine.* Academic Press, Orlando, FL.

117. Fox, J. G., Niemi, S. M., Murphy, J. C., and Quimby, F. W. (1977): Ulcerative dermatitis in the rat. *Lab. Anim. Sci.,* 27(5):671–678.

118. Fox, M. A. (1986): *The Case for Animal Experimentation. An Evolutionary and Ethical Perspective.* University of California Press, Berkeley and Los Angeles, CA.

119. Gamble, M. R. (1976): Fire alarms and oestrus in rats. *Lab. Anim.,* 10:161–163.

120. Gamble, M. R. (1979): Effects of noise on laboratory animals. Ph.D. Thesis, University of London, England.

121. Gamble, M. R., and Clough, G. (1976): Ammonia build-up in animal boxes and its effect on rat tracheal epithelium. *Lab. Anim.,* 10:93–104.

122. Ganaway, J. R., and Allen, A. M. (1971): Obesity predisposes to pregnancy toxemia (ketosis) of guinea pigs. *Lab. Anim. Sci.,* 21(1): 40–44.

123. Gerber, W. F. (1970): Cardiovascular and teratogenic effects of chronic intermittent noise stress. In: *Physiological Effects of Noise,* edited by B. L. Welch and A. S. Welch, pp. 85–90. Plenum Press, New York.

124. Gerber, W. F., and Anderson, T. A. (1967): Cardiac hypertrophy due to chance audiogenic stress in the rat and rabbit. *Comp. Biochem. Physiol.,* 21:237.

125. Geber, W. F., Anderson, T. A., and Van Dyne, B. (1966): Physiologic responses of the albino rat to chronic noise stress. *Arch. Environ. Health,* 12:751–754.

126. Giddens, W. E., Jr., Whitehair, C. K., and Carter, G. R. (1971): Morphologic and microbiologic features of trachea and lungs in germfree, defined-flora, conventional, and chronic respiratory disease-affected rats. *Am. J. Vet. Res.,* 32:115–129.

127. Gillette, J. R. (1976): Environmental factors in drug metabolism. *Fed. Proc.,* 35(5):1142–1147.

128. Glickman, L. T. (1980): Preventive medicine in kennel management. *Curr. Vet. Ther.,* 7:67–76.

129. Goble, F. C. (1975): Sex as a factor in metabolism, toxicity, and efficacy of pharmacodynamic and chemotherapeutic agents. *Adv. Pharmacol. Chemother.,* 13:173–252.

130. Goodman, D. G., Ward, J. M., Squire, R. A., Chu, K. C., and Linhart, M. S. (1979): Neoplastic and nonneoplastic lesions in aging F344 rats. *Toxicol. Appl. Pharmacol.,* 48:237–248.

131. Grant, L., Hopkinson, P., Jennings, G., and Jenner, F. A. (1971): Period of adjustment of rats used for experimental studies. *Nature,* 232:135.

132. Greenman, D. L., Bryant, P., Kodell, R. L., and Sheldon, W. (1982): Influence of cage shelf level on retinal atrophy in mice. *Lab. Anim. Sci.,* 32(4):353–356.

133. Greenman, D. L., Kodell, R. L., and Sheldon, W. G. (1981): Association between cage shelf level and spontaneous and induced neoplasms in mice. *J. Natl. Cancer Inst.,* 73(1):107–113.

134. Greenman, D. L., Oller, W. L., Littlefield, N. A., and Nelson, C. J. (1980): Commercial laboratory animal diets: toxicant and nutrient variability. *J. Toxicol. Environ. Health,* 6:235–246.

135. Gross, W. B. (1972): Effect of social stress on occurrence of Marek's disease in chickens. *Am. J. Vet. Res.,* 33:2275–2279.

136. Halberg, F., Halberg, E., Barnum, C. P., and Bittner, J. J. (1959): Physiologic 24-hour periodicity in human beings and mice, the lighting regimen and daily routine. In: *Photoperiodism and Related Phenomena in Plants and Animals:* proceedings of a conference on photoperiodism, edited by R. B. Withrow, pp. 803–879. Publ. No. 55, American Association for the Advancement of Science, Washington, DC.

137. Hall, J. E., White, W. J., and Lang, C. M. (1980): Acidification of drinking water: its effects on selected biologic phenomena in male mice. *Lab. Anim. Sci.,* 30:643–651.

138. Hall, W. C., Lubet, R. A., Henry, C. J., and Collins, M. J., Jr. (1986): Sendai virus—disease processes and research complications. In: *Complications of Viral and Mycoplasmal Infections in Rodents to Toxicology Research and Testing,* edited by T. E. Hamm, Jr, pp. 25–52. Hemisphere Publishing, Washington, DC.

139. Hamm, T. E., Jr. (1983): The occurrence of neoplasm in long-term *in vivo* studies. In: *Applications of Biological Markers to Carcinogen Testing,* edited by H. Milman and S. Sell, pp. 9–23. Plenum Publishing, New York.

140. Hamm, T. E., Jr. (1984): *Complications of Viral and Mycoplasmal Infections in Rodents to Toxicology Research and Testing,* edited by T. E. Hamm, Jr. Hemisphere Publishing, Washington, DC.

141. Hamm, T. E., Jr., Raynor, T. H., and Sherrill, J. M. (1984): Procurement and management of rodents to minimize disease problems: The CIIT Animal Management Program. In: *Complications of Viral and Mycoplasmal Infections in Rodents to Toxicology Research and Testing,* edited by T. E. Hamm, Jr., pp. 175–184. Hemisphere Publishing, Washington, DC.

142. Hanna, M. G., Jr., Nettesheim, P., Richter, C. B., and Tennant, R. W. (1973): The variable influence of host microflora and intercurrent infections on immunological competence and carcinogenesis. *Isr. J. Med. Sci.,* 9:229–238.

143. Hardy, J. D. (1961): Physiology of temperature regulation. *Physiol. Rev.,* 41:521–606.

144. Harkness, J. E., Wagner, J. E., Kusewitt, D. F., and Frisk, C. S. (1977): Weight loss and impaired reproduction in the hamster attributable to an unsuitable feeding apparatus. *Lab. Anim. Sci.,* 27(1): 117–118.

145. Haseman, J. K., Crawford, D. D., Huff, J. E., Boorman, G. A., and McConnell, E. E. (1984): Results from 86 two-year carcinogenicity studies conducted by the National Toxicology Program. *J. Toxicol. Environ. Health,* 14:621–639.

146. Haseman, J. K., and Huff, J. E. (1987): Species correlation in long-term carcinogenicity studies. *Cancer Lett.,* 37:125–132.

147. Hatch, A. M., Wiberg, G. S., Zawidzka, Z., Cann, M., Airth, J. M., and Grice, H. C. (1965): Isolation syndrome in the rat. *Toxicol. Appl. Pharmacol.,* 7:737–745.

148. Haus, E., and Halberg, F. (1959): 24-Hour rhythm in susceptibility of C mice to a toxic dose of ethanol. *J. Appl. Physiol.,* 14:878–880.

149. Hemphill, F. E., Kaeberle, M. L., and Buck, W. B. (1971): Lead suppression of mouse resistance to *Salmonella typhimurium. Science,* 172:1031–1032.

150. Hermann, L. M., White, W. J., and Lang, C. M. (1982): Prolonged exposure to acid, chlorine, or tetracycline in the drinking water: effects on delayed-type hypersensitivity, hemagglutination titers and reticuloendothelial clearance rates in mice. *Lab. Anim. Sci.,* 32: 603–608.

151. Hessler, J. R., and Moreland, A. F. (1984): Design and management of animal facilities. In: *Laboratory Animal Medicine,* edited by J. G. Fox, B. J. Cohen, and F. M. Loew, pp. 505–526. Academic Press, Orlando, FL.

152. Hite, M., Hanson, H. M., Bohidar, N. R., Conti, P. A., and Mattis, P. A. (1977): Effect of cage size on patterns of activity and health of beagle dogs. *Lab. Anim. Sci.,* 27(1):60–64.

153. Hodgson, E. (1980): Chemical and environmental factors affecting metabolism of xenobiotics. In: *Introduction to Biochemical Toxicology,* edited by E. Hodgson and F. E. Guthrie, pp. 143–161. Elsevier, New York.

154. Holt, P. G., and Keast, D. (1977): Environmentally induced changes in immunological function: acute and chronic effects of inhalation of tobacco smoke and other atmospheric contaminants in man and experimental animals. *Bacteriol. Rev.,* 41(1):205–216.

155. Homburger, F. (1987): The necessity of animal studies in routine toxicology. *Comments Toxicol.,* 1(5):245–255.

156. Iglehart, J. K. (1985): Health policy report. The use of animals in research. *N. Engl. J. Med.,* 313(6):395–400.

157. Institute of Laboratory Animal Resources (1978): *Laboratory Animal Housing,* proceedings of a symposium held at Hunt Valley, MD, September 22–23, 1976. National Academy of Sciences, Washington, DC.

158. Iturrian, W. B. (1971): Effect of noise in the animal house on experimental seizures and growth of weanling mice. In: *Defining the Laboratory Animal,* proceedings of the IVth International Symposium on Laboratory Animals, pp. 332–352. National Academy of Sciences, Washington, DC.

159. Jacoby, R. O., and Barthold, S. W. (1981): Quality assurance for rodents used in toxicological research and testing. In: *Scientific Considerations in Monitoring and Evaluating Toxicological Research,* edited by E. J. Gralla, pp. 27–55. Hemisphere Publishing, Washington, DC.

160. Joasoo, A., and McKenzie, J. M. (1976): Stress and the immune response in rats. *Int. Arch. Allergy Appl. Immunol.,* 50:659–663.

161. Jonas, A. M. (1965): Laboratory animal facilities. *J. Am. Vet. Med. Assoc.,* 146:600–606.

162. Jonas, A. M. (1976): The research animal and the significance of a health monitoring program. *Lab. Anim. Sci.,* 26(2):339–344.

163. Jones, T. C., and Hunt, R. D. (1983): *Veterinary Pathology.* Lea & Febiger, Philadelphia.

164. Jose, D. G., and Good, R. A. (1973): Quantitative effects of nu-

tritional protein and calorie deficiency on immune responses to tumors in mice. *Cancer Res.,* 33:807–812.

165. Judge, F. J. (1967): The veterinarian's responsibilities under the Animal Welfare Act. *J. Amer. Vet. Med. Assoc.,* 151(12):1876–1882.

166. Keast, D., and Coales, M. F. (1967): Lymphocytopenia induced in a strain of laboratory mice by agents commonly used in treatment of ectoparasites. *Aust. J. Exp. Biol. Med. Sci.,* 45:645–650.

167. Keller, G. L. (1982): Physical euthanasia methods. *Lab. Anim.,* May/June:20–26.

168. Keller, S. E., Weiss, J. M., Schleifer, S. J., Miller, N. E., and Stein, M. (1981): Suppression of immunity by stress: effect of a graded series of stressors on lymphocyte stimulation in the rat. *Science,* 213:1397.

169. Kennedy, G. L., Jr., Ferenz, R. L., and Burgess, B. A. (1986): Estimation of acute oral toxicity in rats by determination of the approximate lethal dose rather than the LD^{50}. *J. Appl. Toxicol.,* 6(3):145–148.

170. Keplinger, M. L., Lanier, G. E., and Deichmann, W. B. (1959): Effects of environmental temperature on the acute toxicity of a number of compounds in rats. *Toxicol. Appl. Pharmacol.,* 1:156–161.

171. Knapka, J. J. (1983): Nutrition. In: *The Mouse in Biomedical Research,* Vol. III, edited by H. L. Foster, J. D. Small, and J. G. Fox, pp. 51–67. Academic Press, New York.

172. Knapka, J. J., Smith, K. P., and Judge, F. J. (1974): Effect of open and closed formula rations on the performance of three strains of laboratory mice. *Lab. Anim. Sci.,* 24(3):480–487.

173. Koller, L. D. (1973): Immunosuppression produced by lead, cadmium, and mercury. *Am. J. Vet. Res.,* 34:1457–1458.

174. Koller, L. D., and Kovacic, S. (1974): Decreased antibody formation in mice exposed to lead. *Nature,* 250:148–149.

175. Kolmodin, B., Axarnoff, D. L., and Sjoqvist, S. (1969): Effect of environmental factors on drug metabolism: decreased plasma half-life of antipyrine in workers exposed to chlorinated hydrocarbon insecticides. *Clin. Pharmacol. Ther.,* 10:638.

176. Kraft, L. M. (1958): Observations on the control and natural history of epidemic diarrhea of infant mice (EDIM). *Yale J. Biol. Med.,* 31:121–137.

177. Kraft, L. M., Pardy, R. F., Pardy, D. A., and Zeickel, H. (1964): Practical control of diarrheal disease in a commercial mouse colony. *Lab. Anim. Care.* 14:16–19.

178. Krichevsky, D., Weber, M. M., and Klurfeld, D. M. (1984): Dietary fat versus caloric content in initiation and promotion of 7,12-dimethylbenz(*a*)anthracene induced mammary tumorigenesis in rats. *Cancer Res.,* 44:3174–3177.

179. LaBarba, R. C. (1970): Experiential and environmental factors in cancer. A review of research with animals. *Psychosom. Med.,* 32(3):259–276.

180. Lai, Y.-L., Jacoby, R. O., Bhatt, P. N., and Jonas, A. M. (1976): Keratoconjunctivitis associated with sialodacryoadenitis in rats. *Invest. Ophthalmol.,* 15:538–541.

181. Lamb, D. (1975): Rat lung pathology and quality of laboratory animals: the user's view. *Lab. Anim.,* 9:1–8.

182. Lang, C. M. (1983): Design and management of research facilities for mice. In: *The Mouse in Biomedical Research,* Vol. III, edited by H. L. Foster, J. D. Small, and J. G. Fox, pp. 37–50. Academic Press, New York.

183. Lang, C. M., and Vesell, E. S. (1976): Environmental and genetic factors affecting laboratory animals: impact on biomedical research. Introduction. *Fed. Proc., Fed. Am. Soc. Exp. Biol.,* 35:1123–1124.

184. Langer, P. H. (1986): Animal welfare and ethical considerations in the use of animals in surgical research. Presented at the 2nd Annual Scientific Session of the Academy of Surgical Research, Clemson, SC.

185. Les, E. P. (1972): A disease related to cage population density: tail lesions of C3H/HeJ mice. *Lab. Anim. Sci.,* 22(1):56–60.

186. Levine, B. B. (1968): Genetic factors in hypersensitivity reaction to drugs. *Ann. N.Y. Acad. Sci.,* 151:988–996.

187. Lindsey, J. R., Baker, H. J., Overcash, R. G., Cassell, G. H., and Hunt, C. E. (1971): Murine chronic respiratory disease. *Am. J. Pathol.,* 64:675–716.

188. Lindsey, J. R., and Conner, M. W. (1978): Influences of cage sanitization frequency on intracage ammonia (NH_3) concentration

189. Lindsey, J. R., Davidson, M. K., Schoeb, T. R., and Cassell, G. H. (1986): Murine mycoplasmal infections. In: *Complications of Viral and Mycoplasmal Infections in Rodents to Toxicology Research and Testing,* edited by T. E. Hamm, Jr. pp. 91–122. Hemisphere Publishing, Washington, DC.

190. Loew, F. M. (1987): Using animals in research. What's going on here? *Invest. Radiol.,* 22:69–70.

191. Loew, F. M., and Fox, J. G. (1983): Animal health surveillance and health delivery systems. In: *The Mouse in Biomedical Research,* Vol. III, edited by H. L. Foster, J. D. Small, and J. G. Fox, pp. 69–82. Academic Press, New York.

192. Lu, F. C. (1985): Acute, short-term, and long-term toxicity studies. In: *Basic Toxicology. Fundamentals, Target Organs, and Risk Assessment,* pp. 99–112. Hemisphere Publishing, Washington, DC.

193. Lumb, W. V., and Moreland, A. F. (1982): Chemical methods for euthanasia. *Lab. Anim.,* May/June:29–35.

194. Madhavan, T. V., and Gopalan, C. (1968): The effect of dietary protein on carcinogenesis of aflatoxin. *Arch. Pathol.,* 85:133–137.

195. Madle, E., Korte, A., and Beek, B. (1986): Species differences in mutagenicity testing. II. Sister-chromatid exchange and micronucleus induction in rats, mice and Chinese hamsters treated with cyclophosphamide. *Mutagenesis,* 1(6):419–422.

196. Maeda, H., Gleiser, C. A., Masoro, E. J., Murata, I., McMahan, C. A., and Yu, B. P. (1985): Nutritional influences on aging of Fischer 344 rats: II. Pathology. *J. Gerontol.,* 40(6):671–688.

197. McDougall, P. T., Wolf, N. S., Stenback, W. A., and Trentin, J. J. (1967): Control of *Pseudomonas aeruginosa* in an experimental mouse colony. *Lab. Anim. Care,* 17(2):204–214.

198. McGarrity, G. J., and Coriell, L. L. (1976): Maintenance of axenic mice in open cages in mass air flow. *Lab. Anim. Sci.,* 26(5):746–750.

199. McGrady, A. V., and Chakraborty, J. (1983): Effects of stress on the reproductive system of male rats and mice. *Arch. Androl.,* 10:95–101.

200. McPherson, C. W. (1963): Reaction of *Pseudomonas aeruginosa* and coliform bacteria in mouse drinking water following treatment with hydrochloric acid or chlorine. *Lab. Anim. Care,* 13:737–744.

201. Megna, V. A. (1984): Engineering needs and trends of a toxicology laboratory. *Concepts Toxicol.,* 1:118–127.

202. Meskin, L. H., and Shapiro, B. L. (1971): Teratogenic effect of air shipment on A/Jax Mice. *J. Dent. Res.,* 50(1):169.

203. Miller, E. C. (1978): Some current perspectives on chemical carcinogenesis in humans and experimental animals: presidential address. *Cancer Res.,* 38:1479–1496.

204. Mizutani, T., and Mitsuoka, T. (1979): Effects of intestinal bacteria on incidence of liver tumors in gnotobiotic C3H/He male mice. *J. Natl. Cancer Inst.,* 63:1365.

205. Mohr, J. W. (1974): Health screening of incoming animals. *Lab Anim,* 3:22–30, 57.

206. Moore, K. E. (1968): Studies with chronically isolated rats: tissue levels and urinary excretion of catecholamines and plasma levels of corticosterone. *Can. J. Physiol. Pharmacol.,* 46(5):553–558.

207. Moore Ede, M. C. (1974): Circadian rhythms of drug effectiveness and toxicity. *Clin. Pharmacol. Ther.,* 14:925–935.

208. Morris, J. B., Clay, R. J., and Cavanagh, D. G. (1986): Species differences in upper respiratory tract deposition of acetone and ethanol vapors. *Fundam. Appl. Toxicol.,* 7:671–680.

209. Morton, J. R. (1968): Effects of early experience "handling and gentling" in laboratory animals. In: *Abnormal Behavior in Animals,* edited by M. W. Fox, pp. 261–292. Saunders, Philadelphia.

210. Mulder, J. B. (1971): Animal behavior and electromagnetic energy waves. *Lab. Anim. Sci.,* 21(3):389–393.

211. Mulder, J. B. (1977): Laboratory animal behaviour. *Synapse,* 10:26.

212. Mundy, L. A., and Porter, G. (1969): Some effects of physical environment on rats. *J. Inst. Anim. Tech.,* 20(2):78–81.

213. Murakami, H. (1971): Differences between internal and external environments of the mouse cage. *Lab. Anim. Sci..* 21(5):680–684.

214. Nair, V., and Casper, R. (1969): The influence of light on daily rhythm in hepatic drug metabolizing enzymes in rat. *Life Sci.,* 8(Part I):1291–1298.

215. Nebert, D. W., and Felton, J. S. (1976): Importance of genetic

factors influencing the metabolism of foreign compounds. *Fed. Proc., Fed. Am. Soc. Exp. Biol.*, 35:1133–1141.

216. Nettesheim, P., Schreiber, H., Creasia, D. A., and Richter, C. B. (1974): Respiratory infections and the pathogenesis of lung cancer. *Recent Results Cancer Res.*, 44:138–157.

217. Nevins, R. G. (1971): Design criteria for ventilation systems. In: *Proceedings of the Symposium on Environmental Requirements for Laboratory Animals*, edited by E. L. Besch, p. 28. Institute for Environmental Research Pub. IER-71-02. Kansas State University, Manhattan, KS.

218. Newberne, P. M. (1975): Influence on pharmacological experiments of chemicals and other factors in diets of laboratory animals. *Fed. Proc.*, 34:209–218.

219. Newberne, P. M. (1975): Diet: the neglected experimental variable. *Lab. Anim.*, 4:20–24.

220. Newberne, P. M., and Fox, J. G. (1978): Chemicals and toxins in the animal facility. In: *Laboratory Animal Housing*, proceeding of a symposium held at Hunt Valley, MD, September 22–23, 1976. National Academy of Sciences, Washington, DC.

221. Newberne, P. M., and Fox, J. G. (1980): Nutritional adequacy and quality control of rodent diets. *Lab. Anim. Sci.*, 30(2):352–365.

222. Newberne, P. M., and McConnell, R. G. (1979): Nutrition of the Syrian golden hamster. *Prog. Exp. Tumor Res.*, 24:127–138.

223. Newberne, P. M., and McConnell, R. G. (1980): Dietary nutrients and contaminants in laboratory animal experimentation. *J. Environ. Pathol. Toxicol.*, 4:105–122.

224. Newberne, P. M., and Rogers, A. E. (1973): Rat colon carcinomas associated with aflatoxin and marginal vitamin A. *J. Natl. Cancer Inst.*, 50:439–448.

225. Newberne, P. M., Rogers, A. E., and Wogan, G. N. (1968): Hepatorenal lesions in rats fed a low lipotrope diet and exposed to aflatoxin. *J. Nutr.*, 94:331–343.

226. Newell, G. W. (1980): The quality, treatment and monitoring of water for laboratory rodents. *Lab. Anim. Sci.*, 30:377–384.

227. Newton, W. M. (1978): Environmental impact on laboratory animals. *Adv. Vet. Sci. Comp. Med.*, 22:1–28.

228. Njaa, L. R., Utne, F., and Braekkan, O. R. (1957): Effect of relative humidity on rat breeding and ringtail. *Nature*, 180:290–291.

229. Noell, W. K., and Albrecht, R. (1971): Irreversible effects of visible light on the retina: role of vitamin A. *Science* (NY), 172:76.

230. Nolen, G. A., and Alexander, J. C. (1966): Effects of diet and type of nesting material on the reproduction and lactation of the rat. *Lab. Anim. Care*, 16(4):327–336.

231. Norris, M. L., and Adams, C. E. (1976): Incidence of pup mortality in the rat with particular reference to nesting material, maternal age and parity. *Lab. Anim.*, 10:165–169.

232. O'Dell, B. L., Vandepopuliere, J. M., Morris, E. R., and Hogan, A. G. (1956): Effect of a high phosphorus diet on acid-base balance in guinea pigs. *Proc. Soc. Exp. Biol. Med.*, 91:220–223.

233. Office for Protection from Research Risks (OPRR) (1986): *Public Health Service Policy on Humane Care and Use of Laboratory Animals*. National Institutes of Health, Bethesda, MD.

234. Office of Technology Assessment (1986): *Summary: Alternatives to Animal Use in Research, Testing, and Education*. Congress of the United States, Washington, DC.

235. Ogle, C. W., and Lockett, M. F. (1968): The urinary changes induced in rats by high pitched sound (20 kcyc./sec.). *J. Endocrinol.*, 42:253–260.

236. Oller, W. L., Greenman, D. L., and Suber, R. (1985): Quality changes in animal feed resulting from extended storage. *Lab. Anim. Sci.*, 35(6):646–650.

237. Orlans, F. B., Simmonds, R. C., and Dodds, W. J. (editors) (1987): *Effective Animal Care and Use Committees*. Published in collaboration with Scientists Center for Animal Welfare.

238. Oser, B. L. (1981): The rat as a model for human toxicological evaluation. *J. Toxicol. Environ. Health*, 8:521–542.

239. Otis, A. P., and Foster, H. L. (1983): Management and design of breeding facilities. In: *The Mouse in Biomedical Research*, Vol. III, edited by H. L. Foster, J. D. Small, and J. G. Fox, pp. 18–35. Academic Press, New York.

240. Parker, J. C., Hercules, J. I., and Von Kaenel, E. (1967): The prevalence of some indigenous viruses of rat and hamster breeder colonies. *Bacteriol. Proc. Abstract*, p. 163.

241. Parker, J. C., Tennant, R. W., and Ward, T. G. (1966): Prevalence of viruses in mouse colonies. *Natl. Cancer Inst. Monogr.*, 20:25–36.

242. Peterson, E. A., Augenstein, J. S., Tanis, D. C., and Augenstein, D. G. (1981): Noise raises blood pressure without impairing auditory sensitivity. *Science*, 211:1450–1452.

243. Pfaff, J. (1974): Noise as an environmental problem in the animal house. *Lab. Anim.*, 8:347–354.

244. Pick, J. R., and Little, J. M. (1965): Effect of type of bedding material on thresholds of pentylenetetrazol convulsions in mice. *Lab. Anim. Care*, 15(1):29–33.

245. Plank, S. J., and Irwin, R. (1966): Infertility of guinea pigs on sawdust bedding. *Lab. Anim. Care*, 16(1):9–11.

246. Plaut, S. M., Ader, R., Friedman, S. B., and Ritterson, A. L. (1969): Social factors and resistance to malaria in the mouse: effects of group vs. individual housing on resistance to *Plasmodium berghei* infection. *Psychosom. Med.*, 31:536–552.

247. Poche, L. B., Jr., Stockwell, C. W., and Ades, H. W. (1969): Cochlear hair cell damage in guinea-pigs after exposure to impulse noise. *J. Acoust. Soc. Am.*, 46:947–951.

248. Poiley, S. M. (1974): Housing requirements—general considerations. In: *Handbook of Laboratory Animal Science*, Vol. 1, edited by E. C. Melby, Jr., and H. H. Altman. CRC Press, Cleveland.

249. Poland, A. D., Smith, D., Knutzman, R., Jacobson, M., and Conney, A. H. (1970): Effect of intensive occupational exposure to DDT on phenylbutazone and cortisol metabolism in human subjects. *Clin. Pharmacol. Ther.*, 11:724.

250. Port, C. D., and Kaltenbach, J. P. (1969): The effect of corncob bedding on reproductivity and leucine incorporation in mice. *Lab. Anim. Care*, 19(1):46–49.

251. Porter, G., and Lane-Petter, W. (1965): The provision of sterile bedding and nesting materials with their effects on breeding mice. *J. Anim. Tech. Assoc.*, 16:5–8.

252. Profeta, M. L., Lief, F. S., and Plotkin, S. A. (1969): Enzootic Sendai infection in laboratory hamsters. *Am. J. Epidemiol.*, 89(3):316–324.

253. Prychodko, H. (1958): Effect of aggregation of laboratory mice (*Mus musculus*) on food intake at different temperatures. *Ecology*, 39:500.

254. Pucak, G. J., Lee, C. S., and Zaino, A. S. (1977): Effects of prolonged high temperature on testicular development and fertility in the male rat. *Lab. Anim. Sci.*, 27(1):76–77.

255. Rall, D. P. (1979): Relevance of animal experiments to humans. *Environ. Health Perspect.*, 32:297–300.

256. Ralls, K. (1967): Auditory sensitivity in mice: Peromyscus and Mus musculus. *Anim. Behav.*, 15:123–128.

257. Rao, G. N., and Knapka, J. J. (1987): Contaminant and nutrient concentrations of natural ingredient rat and mouse diet used in chemical toxicology studies. *Fundam. Appl. Toxicol.*, 9:329–338.

258. Rao, G. N., Piegorsch, W. W., and Haseman, J. K. (1987): Influence of body weight on the incidence of spontaneous tumors in rats and mice of long-term studies. *Am. J. Clin. Nutr.*, 45:252–260.

259. Raynor, T. H., White, E. L., Cheplen, J. M., Sherrill, J. M., and Hamm, T. E., Jr. (1984): An evaluation of a water purification system for use in animal facilities. *Lab. Anim.*, 18:45–51.

260. Reiter, R. J. (1973): Comparative effects of continual lighting and pinealectomy on the eyes, the Harderian glands and reproduction in pigmented and albino rats. *Comp. Biochem. Physiol.*, 44:503–509.

261. Renshaw, H. W., Van Hoosier, G. L., Jr., and Amend, N. K. (1975): A survey of naturally occurring diseases of the Syrian hamster. *Lab. Anim.*, 9:179–191.

262. Ribelin, W. E., and McCoy, J. R. (1965): *The Pathology of Laboratory Animals*. Charles C Thomas, Springfield, IL.

263. Richter, C. B. (1970): Application of infectious agents to the study of lung cancer: studies on the etiology and morphogenesis of metaplastic lung lesions in mice. In: *Morphology of Experimental Respiratory Carcinogenesis*, proceedings of Biol. Div., Oak Ridge Natl. Laboratory Conference, edited by P. Nettesheim, pp. 365–382. USAEC Symposium Series 21.

264. Riley, V. (1981): Psychoneuroendocrine influences on immunocompetence and neoplasia. *Science*, 212:1100–1109.

265. Robinson, T. W. E., Cureton, R. J. R., and Heath, R. B. (1968): The pathogenesis of Sendai virus infection in the mouse lung. *J. Med. Microbiol.*, 1:89–95.

266. Robison, W. G., Jr., and Kuwabara, T. (1976): Light-induced alterations of retinal pigment epithelium in black, albino, and beige mice. *Exp. Eye Res.*, 22(5):549–557.

267. Roe, F. J. C. (1981): Are nutritionists worried about the epidemic of tumours in laboratory animals? *Proc. Nutr. Soc.,* 40:57–65.

268. Roe, F. J. C. (1987): Some aspects of food toxicology: a personal view. In: *Toxicological Aspects of Food,* edited by K. Miller, pp. 59–72. Elsevier Applied Science Publishers, London.

269. Rogers, A. E. (1975): Variable effects of a lipotrope-deficient, high-fat diet on chemical carcinogenesis in rats. *Cancer Res.,* 35:2469–2474.

270. Rogers, A. E. (1977): Reduction of N-nitrosodiethylamine carcinogenesis in rats by lipotrope or amino acid supplementation of a marginally deficient diet. *Cancer Res.,* 37:194–199.

271. Rogers, A. E. (1979): Nutrition. In: *The Laboratory Rat,* Vol. 1: *Biology and Diseases,* edited by H. J. Baker, J. R. Lindsey, and S. H. Weisbroth, pp. 123–151. Academic Press, Orlando, FL.

272. Rogers, A. E. (1985): Factors influencing the results of animal experiments in toxicology. In: *Basic Toxicology: Fundamentals, Target Organs, and Risk Assessment,* edited by F. C. Lu, pp. 254–267. Hemisphere Publishing, Washington, DC.

273. Rogers, A. E., Herndon, B. J., and Newberne, P. M. (1973): Induction by dimethylhydrazine of intestinal carcinoma in normal rats and rats fed high or low levels of vitamin A. *Cancer Res.,* 33:1003–1009.

274. Rogers, A. E., and Newberne, P. M. (1971): Diet and aflatoxin B₁ toxicity in rats. *Toxicol. Appl. Pharmacol.,* 20:113–121.

275. Rogers, A. E., Sanchez, O., Feinsod, F. M., and Newberne, P. M. (1974): Dietary enhancement of nitrosamine carcinogenesis. *Cancer Res.,* 34:94–99.

276. Ross, C. R., Wagner, J. E., Wightman, S. R., and Dill, S. E. (1980): Experimental transmission of *Syphacia murin* among rats, mice, hamsters and gerbils. *Lab. Anim. Sci.,* 30(1):35–37.

277. Ross, M. H., and Bras, G. (1971): Lasting influences of early caloric restriction on prevalence of neoplasms in the rat. *J. Natl. Cancer Inst.,* 47:1095–1113.

278. Ross, M. H., and Bras, G. (1973): Influence of protein under- and overnutrition on spontaneous tumor prevalence in the rat. *J. Nutr.,* 103:944–963.

279. Ross, M. H., Bras, G., and Ragbeer, M. S. (1970): Influence of protein and caloric intake upon spontaneous tumor incidence of the anterior pituitary gland of the rat. *J. Nutr.,* 100:177–189.

280. Ross, M. H., Lustbader, E. D., and Bras, G. (1983): Body weight, dietary practices, and tumor susceptibility in the rat. *J. Natl. Cancer Inst.,* 71:1041–1046.

281. Rowsell, H. C., and McWilliam, A. A. (1983): Laboratory animal science: a global view. Presented at ICLAS/CALAS International Symposium on Laboratory Animal Science, Vancouver, British Columbia, Canada.

282. Sabine, J. R., Horton, B. J., and Wicks, M. B. (1973): Spontaneous tumors in C3H-Aʳʸ and C3H-AʳʸfB mice: high incidence in the United States and low incidence in Australia. *J. Natl. Cancer Inst.,* 50:1237–1242.

283. Salem, H. (1987): Factors influencing toxicity. In: *Inhalation Toxicology: Research Methods, Applications and Evaluation,* edited by H. Salem, pp. 35–57. Marcel Dekker, New York.

284. Sansone, E. B., and Fox, J. G. (1977): Potential chemical contamination in animal feeding studies: evaluation of wire and solid bottom caging systems and gelled feed. *Lab. Anim. Sci.,* 27(4):457–465.

285. Sansone, E. B., and Losikoff, A. M. (1978): Contamination from feeding volatile test chemicals. *Toxicol. Appl. Pharmacol.,* 46:703–708.

286. Sansone, E. B., and Losikoff, A. M. (1979): Potential contamination from feeding test chemicals in carcinogen bioassay research: evaluation of single- and double-corridor animal housing facilities. *Toxicol. Appl. Pharmacol.,* 50:115–121.

287. Sansone, E. B., and Losikoff, A. M. (1982): Environmental contamination associated with administration of test chemicals in drinking water. *Lab. Anim. Sci.,* 32(3):269–272.

288. Sansone, E. B., Losikoff, A. M., and Pendleton, R. A. (1977): Potential hazards from feeding test chemicals in carcinogen bioassay research. *Toxicol. Appl. Pharmacol.,* 39:435–450.

289. Schach von Wittenau, M. (1987): Strengths and weaknesses of long-term bioassays. *Regul. Toxicol. Pharmacol.,* 7:113–119.

290. Schoental, R. (1973): Carcinogenicity of wood shavings. *Lab. Anim.,* 7:47–49.

291. Schoental, R. (1974): Role of podophyllotoxin in the bedding and

292. Schreiber, H., Nettesheim, P., Lijinsky, W., Richter, C. B., and Walburg, H. E., Jr. (1972): Induction of lung cancer in germfree, specific-pathogen-free, and infected rats by N-nitrosoheptamethyleneimine: enhancement by respiratory infection. *J. Natl. Cancer Inst.,* 49:1107–1114.

293. Schroeder, H. A., Balassa, J. J., and Vinton, W. H., Jr. (1965): Chromium, cadmium and lead in rats: effects on life span, tumors and tissue levels. *J. Nutr.,* 86:51–66.

294. Scott, S. K., Kosch, P. C., and Hilmas, D. E. (1976): Serum lactate dehydrogenase of normal, stressed, and yellow fever virus-infected rhesus monkeys. *Lab. Anim. Sci.,* 26(3):436–442.

295. Seifter, E., Rettura, G., Zisblatt, M., Levenson, S. M., Levine, N., Davidson, A., and Seifter, J. (1973): Enhancement of tumor development in physically-stressed mice inoculated with an oncogenic virus. *Experientia,* 29:1379–1382.

296. Serrano, L. J. (1971): Carbon dioxide and ammonia in mouse cages: effect of cage covers, population, and activity. *Lab. Anim. Sci.,* 21(1):75–85.

297. Silverman, J., and Adams, J. D. (1983): N-Nitrosamines in laboratory animal feed and bedding. *Lab. Anim. Sci.,* 33(2):161–164.

298. Simmons, M. L., Robie, D. M., Jones, J. B., and Serrano, L. J. (1968): Effect of a filter cover on temperature and humidity in a mouse cage. *Lab. Anim.,* 2:113–120.

299. Slaga, T. J., and Fischer, S. M. (1983): Strain differences and solvent effects in mouse skin carcinogenesis experiments using carcinogens, tumor initiators and promoters. *Prog. Exp. Tumor Res.,* 26:85–109.

300. Small, J. D. (1983): Environmental and equipment monitoring. In: *The Mouse in Biomedical Research,* Vol. III, edited by H. L. Foster, J. D. Small, and J. G. Fox, pp. 83–100. Academic Press, New York.

301. Smith, A. W., Houpt, K. A., Kitchell, R. L., Kohn, D. F., McDonald, L. E., Passaglia, M., Jr., Thurmon, J. C., and Ames, E. R. (1986): Report of the AVMA panel on euthanasia. *J. Am. Vet. Med. Assoc.,* 188(3):252–268.

302. Smith, D. M., Rogers, A. E., and Newberne, P. M. (1975): Vitamin A and benzo(a)pyrene carcinogenesis in the respiratory tract of hamsters fed a semisynthetic diet. *Cancer Res.,* 35:1485–1488.

303. Solomon, G. F. (1969): Stress and antibody response in rats. *Int. Arch. Allergy,* 35:97–104.

304. Sontag, J. M., Page, N. P., and Saffiotti, U. (1976): *Guidelines for Carcinogen Bioassay in Small Rodents.* National Cancer Institute Technical Report Series No. 1, NCI-CG-TR-1, U.S. Department of Health, Education and Welfare, National Institutes of Health, DHEW Publication No. (NIH) 76-801.

305. Stevens, C. (1976): Humane considerations for animal models. In: *Animal Models of Thrombosis and Hemorrhagic Diseases,* pp. 151–158. U.S. Department of Health, Education, and Welfare, Public Health Service, National Institutes of Health, Washington, DC. DHEW Publication No. (NIH) 76-982.

306. Stevens, C. G. (1977): Humane perspectives. In: *The Future of Animals, Cells, Models, and Systems in Research, Development, Education, and Testing,* pp. 16–24. National Academy of Sciences, Washington, DC.

307. Stratman, S. L., and Conejeros, M. (1969): Resistance to experimental bacterial infection among different stocks of rats. *Lab. Anim. Care,* 19(5):742–745.

308. Subcommittee on Laboratory Animal Nutrition, Committee on Animal Nutrition, Agricultural Board, National Research Council (1972): *Nutrient Requirements of Laboratory Animals.* National Academy of Sciences, Washington, DC.

309. Subcommittee on Laboratory Animal Nutrition, Committee on Animal Nutrition, Board on Agriculture and Renewable Resources, National Research Council (1978): *Nutrient Requirements of Laboratory Animals.* National Academy of Sciences, Washington, DC.

310. Sun, M. (1983): Lots of talk about LD₅₀. *Science,* 222:1106.

311. Swindle, M. M. (1986): Controversies involving the use of animals in research. Presented at the Second Annual Scientific Session of the Academy of Surgical Research, Clemson, SC.

312. Taffs, L. F. (1976): Pinworm infections in laboratory rodents: a review. *Lab. Anim.,* 10:1–13.

313. Tannenbaum, A. (1942): The genesis and growth of tumors: II. Effect of caloric restriction per se. *Cancer Res.,* 2:460–467.

314. Tannenbaum, A. (1942): The genesis and growth of tumors: III. Effects of a high-fat diet. *Cancer Res.,* 2:468–475.

315. Tannenbaum, A. (1945): The dependence of tumor formation on the degree of caloric restriction. *Cancer Res.,* 5:609–615.

316. Tannenbaum, A. (1945): The dependence of tumor formation on the composition of the calorie-restricted diet as well as on the degree of restriction. *Cancer Res.,* 5:616–625.

317. Tannenbaum, A. (1959): Nutrition and Cancer. In: *The Physiopathology of Cancer,* 2d ed., edited by F. Homburger, pp. 517–562. Hoeber-Harper, New York.

318. Tannenbaum, A., and Silverstone, H. (1949): Effect of sodium fluoride, dinitrophenol, and low environmental temperature on the formation of spontaneous mammary carcinoma in mice. *Cancer Res.,* 6:499.

319. Tannenbaum, A., and Silverstone, H. (1949): Effect of low environmental temperature, dinitrophenol, or sodium fluoride on the formation of tumors in mice. *Cancer Res.,* 9:403–410.

320. Tannock, G. W., and Savage, D. C. (1974): Influences of dietary and environmental stress on microbial populations in the murine gastrointestinal tract. *Infect. Immun.,* 9(3):591–598.

321. Taylor, H. W., and Nettesheim, P. (1975): Influence of administration route and dosage schedule on tumor response to nitrosoheptamethyleneimine in rats. *Int. J. Cancer,* 15:301–307.

322. Teelman, K., and Weihe, W. H. (1974): Microorganism counts and distribution patterns in air-conditioned animal laboratories. *Lab. Anim.,* 8:109.

323. Thilsted, J. P., Newton, W. M., Crandell, R. A., and Bevill, R. F. (1981): Fatal diarrhea in rabbits resulting from the feeding of antibiotic-contaminated feed. *J. Am. Vet. Med. Assoc.,* 179(4):360–362.

324. Thompson, R. (1971): The water consumption and drinking habits of a few species and strains of laboratory animals. *J. Inst. Anim. Tech.,* 22(1):29–36.

325. Totton, M. (1958): Ringtail in new-born Norway rats. A study of the effect of environmental temperature and humidity on incidence. *J. Hyg.,* 56:190–196.

326. Tucker, M. J. (1979): The effect of long-term food restriction on tumours in rodents. *Int. J. Cancer,* 23:803–807.

327. Tucker, M. J. (1985): Effect of diet on spontaneous diseases in the inbred mouse strain C57B1/10J. *Toxicol. Lett.,* 25:131–135.

328. Turnbull, G. J., Lee, P. N., and Roe, F. J. C. (1985): Relationship of body-weight gain to longevity and to risk of development of nephropathy and neoplasia in Sprague-Dawley rats. *Food Chem. Toxicol.,* 23(3):355–361.

329. Van Hoosier, G. L., Jr., and McPherson, C. W. (1987): *Laboratory Hamsters.* Academic Press, Orlando, FL.

330. Vesell, E. S. (1967): Induction of drug-metabolizing enzymes in liver microsomes of mice and rats by softwood bedding. *Science,* 157:1057–1058.

331. Vesell, E. S., Lang, C. M., White, W. J., Passananti, G. T., Hill, R. N., Clemens, T. L., Liu, D. K., and Johnson, W. D. (1976): Environmental and genetic factors affecting the response of laboratory animals to drugs. *Fed. Proc.,* 35:1125–1132.

332. Vesell, E. S., Lang, C. M., White, W. J., Passananti, G. T., and Tripp, S. L. (1973): Hepatic drug metabolism in rats: impairment in a dirty environment. *Science,* 179:896–897.

333. Vessey, S. H. (1964): Effects of grouping on levels of circulating antibodies in mice. *Proc. Soc. Exp. Biol. Med.,* 115:225–255.

334. Vlahakis, G. (1977): Possible carcinogenic effects of cedar shavings in bedding of C3H-A^{vy}B mice. *J. Natl. Cancer Inst.,* 58:149–150.

335. Vogtsberger, L. M., Stromberg, P. C., and Rice, J. M. (1982): Histological and serological response of B$_6$C$_3$F$_1$ mice and F344 rats to experimental pneumonia virus of mice infection. *Lab. Anim. Sci.,* 32:419.

336. Wade, A. E., Holl, J. E., Hilliard, C. C., Molton, E., and Greene, F. E. (1968): Alteration of drug metabolism in rats and mice by an environment of cedarwood. *Pharmacology,* 1:317–328.

337. Walker, P. H. (1976): Monitoring control and alarm systems. In: *Control of the Animal House Environment—Laboratory Animal Handbooks,* Vol. 7, edited by T. McSheehy, pp. 277–290. Trevor Laboratory Animals Ltd., London.

338. Wallace, M. E. (1976): Effects of stress due to deprivation and transport in different genotypes of house mouse. *Lab. Anim.,* 10:335–347.

339. Wassermann, M., Wassermann, D., Gershon, Z., and Zellermayer, L. (1969): Effects of organochlorine insecticides on body defense systems. *Ann. N.Y. Acad. Sci.,* 160:393–401.

340. Wattenberg, L. W. (1975): Effects of dietary constituents on the metabolism of chemical carcinogens. *Cancer Res.,* 35:3326–3331.

341. Weichbrod, R. H., Hall, J. E., Simmonds, R. C., and Cisar, C. F. (1986): Selecting bedding material. *Lab. Anim.,* September:25–29.

342. Weihe, W. H. (1965): Temperature and humidity climatograms for rats and mice. *Lab. Anim. Care,* 15(1):18–28.

343. Weihe, W. H. (1973): The effect of temperature on the action of drugs. *Annu. Rev. Pharmacol.,* 13:409–425.

344. Weihe, W. H. (1976): The effect of light on animals. In: *Control of the Animal House Environment—Laboratory Animal Handbooks,* Vol. 7, edited by T. McSheehy, pp. 63–76. Trevor Laboratory Animals Ltd., London.

345. Weihe, W. H., Schidlow, J., and Strittmatter, J. (1969): The effect of light intensity on the breeding and development of rats and golden hamsters. *Int. J. Biometerol.,* 13(1):69–79.

346. Weisbroth, S. H., and Peress, N. (1977): Ophthalmic lesions and dacryoadenitis: a naturally occurring aspect of sialodacryoadenitis virus infection of the laboratory rat. *Lab. Anim. Sci.,* 27(4):466–473.

347. Weiss, I., Stotzer, H., and Seitz, R. (1974): Age- and light-dependent changes in the rat eye. *Virchows Arch. (A),* 362:145–156.

348. Weltman, A. S., Sackler, A. M., Schwartz, R., and Owens, H. (1968): Effects of isolation stress on female albino mice. *Lab. Anim. Care,* 18(4):426–435.

349. White, R. J. (1988): The facts about animal research. *Reader's Digest,* March.

350. Williams, G. M. (1984): The significance of environmental chemicals as modifying factors in toxicity studies. In: *Concepts in Toxicology,* Vol. 1. *Toxicology Laboratory Design and Management for the 80's and Beyond,* edited by A. S. Tegeris, pp. 14–19. S. Karger AG, Basel, Switzerland.

351. Williams, G. M., and Weisburger, J. H. (1986): Chemical Carcinogens. In: *Casarett and Doull's Toxicology. The Basic Science of Poisons,* edited by C. D. Klaassen, M. O. Amdur, and J. Doull, pp. 99–173. Macmillan Publishing Co., New York.

352. Williams, S. J. (1984): Prediction of ocular irritancy potential from dermal irritation test results. *Food Chem. Toxicol.,* 22(2):157–161.

353. Williams, S. J. (1985): Changing concepts of ocular irritation evaluation: pitfalls and progress. *Food Chem. Toxicol.,* 23(2):189–193.

354. Williams, S. J., Graepel, G. J., and Kennedy, G. L. (1982): Evaluation of ocular irritancy potential: intralaboratory variability and effect of dosage volume. *Toxicol. Lett.,* 12:235–241.

355. Wise, A. (1982): Interaction of diet and toxicity—the future role of purified diet in toxicological research. *Arch. Toxicol.,* 50:287–299.

356. Wise, A., and Gilburt, D. J. (1980): The variability of dietary fibre in laboratory animal diets and its relevance to the control of experimental conditions. *Cosmet. Toxicol.,* 18:643–648.

357. Wise, A., and Gilburt, D. J. (1981): Variation of minerals and trace elements in laboratory animal diets. *Lab. Anim.,* 15:299–303.

358. Wongwiwat, M., Sukapanit, S., Triyanond, C., and Sawyer, W. D. (1972): Circadian rhythm of the resistance of mice to acute pneumococcal infection. *Infect. Immun.,* 5(4):442–448.

359. Woods, J. E. (1975): Influence of room air distribution on animal cage environments. *ASHRAE Trans.,* 81:559–571.

360. Woods, J. E., Nevins, R. G., and Besch, E. L. (1975): Experimental evaluation of heat and moisture transfer in metal dog cage environments. *Lab. Anim. Sci.,* 25(4):425–433.

361. Yagil, R., Etzion, Z., and Berlyne, G. M. (1976): Changes in rat milk quantity and quality due to variations in litter size and high ambient temperature. *Lab. Anim. Sci.,* 26(1):33–37.

362. Zakem, H. B., and Alliston, C. W. (1974): The effects of noise level and elevated ambient temperatures upon selected reproductive traits in female Swiss-Webster mice. *Lab. Anim. Sci.,* 24:469–547.

363. Zbinden, G. (1973): Acute toxicity. In: *Progress in Toxicity, Special Topics,* Vol. 1, p. 23. Springer, Berlin, Heidelberg, New York.

364. Zondek, B., and Tamari, I. (1964): Effect of audiogenic stimulation on genital function and reproduction. III. Infertility induced by auditory stimuli prior to mating. *Acta Endocrinol.,* 45(Suppl. 90):227–234.

Principles and Methods of Toxicology, Second Edition, edited by A. Wallace Hayes, Raven Press, Ltd., New York © 1989.

CHAPTER 18

Methods for Behavioral Toxicology

Stata Norton

Department of Pharmacology, Toxicology, and Therapeutics, University of Kansas, College of Health Sciences and Hospital, Kansas City, Kansas 66103

Behavioral toxicology has become increasingly important in the evaluation of toxic compounds and in fact has been responsible for the development of some new tests for neurotoxicology. In addition, many psychopharmacological methods have been adapted to the special demands of the evaluation of central nervous system (CNS) function after exposure to toxic substances.

There are differences between behavioral pharmacology and its toxicological counterpart. When a drug or compound related to a known drug is administered, a specific type of action is often expected, and tests that measure the effects of known therapeutic agents can be selected for evaluating new drugs or exploring mechanisms. This approach has been the main thrust of psychopharmacology. In addition, drug effects are usually reversible, and most tests in psychopharmacology are designed to detect an effect that occurs rapidly after drug administration, followed by recovery of normal function within a few hours. Behavioral toxicology tests commonly are employed in a different context. No specific effect can be predicted in many studies. Because the effect of the toxic substance on brain tissue may be irreversible, associated with damage to or loss of some structural elements, rapid recovery may not occur.

The difference in the context in which testing is done in behavioral pharmacology and behavioral toxicology has a significant impact on the selection of test methods and interpretation of results. Four principles on which measurement of function of an organ depends have been stated (131):

1. Chemical and physical changes in cells govern all functional changes. In terms of behavior, this principle states that behavioral changes are caused by changes in brain tissue, regardless of whether such changes can be detected by given methods.
2. Organ damage can result in functional damage. This principle is essential, albeit obvious, if behavioral tests are to be used to evaluate toxicity.
3. Homeostatic (compensatory) mechanisms in an organ can obscure functional damage. This principle is also obvious. The CNS is an organ well endowed with compensatory mechanisms.
4. Homeostatic mechanisms include structural redundancy and tolerance. Structural redundancy is a significant mechanism for maintaining function in the brain when toxic substances cause death of a proportion of a neuronal population. Various hypotheses of mechanisms of tolerance to drug actions have been proposed. In a broad sense, tolerance is a form of learning, and the organism can learn not to respond to a stimulus, e.g., a toxic substance, as well as to respond to a stimulus by altering behavior.

These principles set limits on the ability of behavioral tests to detect alteration of the CNS by toxic substances and therefore have a cautionary role in the following discussion of methods for behavioral toxicology.

Under some conditions the information of importance to an investigator may be whether behavior has been altered, regardless of the presence of damage to the CNS. If compensatory mechanisms are adequate to restore function to normal in the presence of tissue damage, functional damage has not occurred. Consideration of this situation has led to an interest in tests that challenge these compensatory mechanisms and that, by placing an additional burden on a damaged system, may expose the loss of reserve capacity (180).

SELECTION OF BEHAVIORAL TESTS

Although various committees have been formed over the past 10 years for the purpose of selecting methods that, in the collective expertise of the committee, are appropriate for detection of behavioral toxicity from chemicals, inadequate information on the utility of different methods for different chemicals limits the value of recommended methods. In the selection of tests, various factors that affect results must be considered. Six major factors are described here briefly.

1. *Species.* The importance of selecting the appropriate species of animal for a particular test of a research goal cannot be overrated. There is a great deal to be gained by becoming familiar with the performance of a standard, commercially available strain of rat or mouse, but it is also important to be aware of the advantages that sometimes accrue from selecting a more novel organism with which to study a behavior.

2. *Sex.* The sex of animals used for testing is a critical variable. There are some marked variations related to the sex of an animal and performance in different tests. For example, it is well known that female rats can show estrus-associated hyperactivity when allowed to live in squirrel cages (running wheels). It is not so well known that estrus-associated hyperactivity is limited to squirrel cage environments and does not occur in other types of habitat. In many tests measuring locomotion, male rats are less active than female rats. However, male rats spend more time grooming than females (120) so that lack of locomotion does not necessarily mean inactivity.

It has been proposed that stimulant drugs are best detected using operant test schedules that result in low levels of responding, and that tests with high levels of responding are more sensitive to depressant drugs (51). The same consideration may well apply to other behaviors, even if only in the sense that if a decrease in a behavior is to be obtained, enough of the behavior must be present for the decrease to be meaningful.

Sex-related differences in metabolism are known to affect the choice of species for a behavioral test. The more rapid metabolism of amphetamine by male rats has been well documented (75), although differences in the male and female CNS appear also to be involved in the greater behavioral response of the female to amphetamine (156).

3. *Age.* The maturation of certain behaviors during the preweaning period is well known. However, age is a variable that is often overlooked in testing. Sexual maturity is an inaccurate guide to maturation of many behaviors. In the common laboratory strains of the Norway rat, onset of sexual function occurs at about 45 days in the female and 60 days in the male. At these ages the brain is far from mature. Surveys of the biochemistry of the developing rat brain, e.g., the volume by Friede (68), indicate that the CNS generally matures between 4 and 5 months after birth. Various aspects of behavior, of which grooming is an example, may alter progressively with age.

4. *Reliability.* When it is desired to test for the presence of a specific alteration in behavior, it may be important to use the most sensitive test or at least a test for which the reliability is known. That is, the test is selective and sensitive enough to be used to detect a specific type of behavioral change. This area is of crucial importance when selecting a test method. It is not possible to have a single behavioral test that answers the global question, "Has anything happened to the behavior of an animal by exposure to substance X?" It is possible, however, to ask more selective questions, such as, "Has the normal walking pattern been affected by exposure to substance X?" There are tests that are appropriate for addressing the latter question. A real lack in behavioral toxicology at present is in the number of reliable tests available, i.e., tests for which the ability to detect low level effects (sensitivity) and to detect certain kinds of damage (selectivity) is known.

5. *Reproducibility.* All good tests are reproducible, although the converse may not always be true. Sensitivity can be markedly influenced by reproducibility, as sensitivity involves the ability of a test to detect a range of doses, particularly the effects of relatively low doses. Detection of low level effects requires sorting a signal (behavioral alteration in this case) from random signals, and variability of results is inversely related to the detection of low signals. Variability in a test comes from within animals (if repeated measures are made on a single animal), from between animals (if more than one animal is tested), and between replicates of a test (because many factors can intervene when tests are repeated). It is important to consider the reproducibility of any test being performed. Generally, reproducibility can be improved by adequate attention to standardizing details that affect the outcome of a test. The number of animals used for each dose or condition is important in determining reproducibility. The number varies, depending on the degree of difference between treated and control populations and the variability in the populations.

6. *Validity.* Two aspects of validity are considered. The first is the meaning of the results of a test for the animal species being tested. If a behavioral test were specific for detecting damage to the mammillary bodies in the rat brain, for example, the interpretation of the results would be straightforward and valid for the rat. Unfortunately, such specific interpretation of results is rarely possible. The other aspects of validity concern extrapolation of results from one species to another. Here the situation is even more difficult, and the significance for one species of effects obtained in another species can only be estimated, at best. Some understanding of validity is critical for the rational selection of behavioral tests and interpretation of results.

An important consideration when evaluating a chemical for which the toxic effect is not known is the probability of a false-negative or false-positive result. In order to avoid or reduce the probability of a false negative, in which the method does not detect a change in behavior when behavior has been altered, a range of doses and adequate numbers of animals are required. The use of a chemical known to be detected by the test as a positive control is helpful for preventing false negatives resulting from unrecognized causes of variation. The best way to proceed to sort false-positive from true-positive results is to have a sequential strategy where a positive result in one test is followed by other tests that detect similar or more selective effects on the behavior under study.

Statistical Evaluation

Behavioral test results are usually subjected to statistical analysis, and there seems to be little need to emphasize the importance of probability statements when quantitative comparisons of experimental groups are made. For some tests, adequate statistical evaluations have been published and can serve as guides for investigators.

Two common failings in statistical analysis of behavioral tests are too small a sample size, including failure to use several groups to establish the dose response, and carrying out exploratory analysis, which increases the possibility of false-positive results. Exploratory statistical analysis or *post hoc* examination of data to look for significant effects in pilot studies is followed by confirmatory studies with prior selection of protocols.

There are numerous statistical books that emphasize analysis of behavioral data (e.g., 192) as well as articles specifically directed toward statistical analysis in toxicology (124; Gad and Weil, *this volume*).

METHODS

Testing methods for behavioral toxicology are available in great profusion. Some method of categorizing the tests is essential. One method, for which logical argument can be made, is to use the anatomical locus of the behavior under study as the source of the categories. Although current knowledge of the relation between structure and function in the CNS does not adequately serve as a basis for organizing the various types of behavioral test, the following outline is based on the way in which behavior is presumably a function of nervous system activity. The assumption is, of course, that a logical relation between structure and function can be defined. The nervous system is conventionally divided structurally into central, peripheral, and autonomic portions, each with distinct roles in the functioning of the intact organism. Neurotoxicology has, again conventionally, been limited to the central and peripheral nervous systems, and this limitation is followed here in reference to behavioral toxicology.

One of the first problems when attempting an anatomical-functional classification is that many human complaints from exposure to toxic agents are subjective. The most commonly reported effects of neurotoxic agents are headache, gastrointestinal disorders, dizziness, irritability, and fatigue (62). None of these symptoms is readily detected in animal behavior. However, they can be related to possible causes. Feldman (62) has proposed a fourfold classification of the behavioral effects of metals in humans: disorders of the cerebral hemispheres (headache, gastrointestinal complaints, and dizziness), disorders of the extrapyramidal system (altered posture and muscle tone), and disorders of the peripheral nervous system (weakness and sensory abnormalities). This classification could serve as a basis for animal tests to some extent,

but the emphasis on symptoms rather than signs leads to difficulties. A less subjective classification is used here, based on methods that involve various components of the nervous system. The categories are sensory, motor, sensorimotor integration, cognition, emotion, and reproductive behavior.

Strategies

The large number of behavioral tests that have been used to study an even greater number of toxic substances makes some strategy important for selecting the best test for the purpose (47,189). When the action of a toxic substance is predicted or known, the choice of test is simpler than when there is no predicted effect. In the first instance, either a specific action of the chemical is known or is of interest; all other possible effects are not considered. In the second instance, when no specific action is predicted, the strategy for selecting tests and evaluating them involves broader examination of the nervous system.

Strategy 1 (predicted effect). A test is selected that is specific for the type of effect predicted. Positive controls are used concurrently. A range of doses is usually important, as a quantitative evaluation may be desired. The risk of a false positive needs to be low, and conditions are chosen to ensure this.

Strategy 2 (no specific effect predicted). The primary consideration, when the behavioral effect of a toxic substance cannot be predicted, is to select a test that detects damage to various portions of the nervous system. Several tests may be employed, covering a range of actions.

Three major approaches to the analysis of behavior are generally identified: two types of "conditioned" behavior, in which behaviors are rigidly controlled, and "spontaneous" behavior in which the environments are controlled but behaviors are spontaneous. In fact, the distinction is probably more in the mind of the experimenter than in the functioning of the animals' nervous systems. Nevertheless, the tests are designed for special purposes, and the methodologies are different. The two types of conditioning, operant and Pavlovian, are described briefly.

Operant Behavior

Operant behavior tests, in which the experimental animals are trained to press (or peck) a lever to obtain a reward or to avoid unpleasant consequences, have had major use in psychopharmacology. In toxicology operant conditioning has been used to detect damage to components of sensory systems, to look in a general way for brain damage, and to evaluate learning and memory after exposure to toxic chemicals.

There is considerable interest in an operant test that can be used as a "general screen" for identification of deleterious effects of chemicals on the CNS. If the premise is accepted that behavioral changes are the most sensitive measure of CNS damage [for an evaluation of this premise, see Norton (131)], there is considerable value in deciding which behavioral tests can be used to detect damage anywhere in the CNS. Data are not available that can be used to decide with accuracy if there is a single operant test that is affected by various loci of damage and what the loci are. Those scientists who are attempting to delineate the unique relations of brain structures to functions may intuitively reject the idea that any one test is likely to serve the purpose of a global screen for brain damage. However, the need for a relatively simple way to evaluate damage to the CNS from substances with unknown toxic potential has resulted in the selection of some tests for this purpose, even though there is little convincing evidence that these tests are not subject to error of failure to detect various types of brain damage.

In the simplest operant procedure, rodents are trained to respond on a *fixed-interval (FI) schedule* in which one or more food or drink rewards are available at the end of a uniform period, e.g., 3 min, if the animal carries out a simple operant act such as pressing a lever. This schedule results in a "scallop-shaped" type of responding in which a period with no lever presses is followed by a burst of lever presses in a trained animal at a time when the animal has learned to expect the reward. A *fixed-ratio (FR) schedule* in which a reward is available after a fixed number of responses, e.g., 30 lever presses, results in a more uniform rate of lever pressing. With repeated experience, responding stabilizes to both schedules of reward. Different schedules may be combined so that it is possible to look at the effects of a single dose of a chemical on intermittent or low rates of responding (FI schedule) and high or steady responding (FR schedule). It is generally recognized that low levels of responding are more sensitive to effects of CNS stimulant drugs, and high rates are more sensitive to CNS depressants (52). This generalization has not been adequately tested for applicability to toxic exposures resulting in hyper- or hypoactivity and hyper- or hyporeflexia.

Mixed FI and FR schedules have been suggested as appropriate for general screening procedures (107) and have been used to evaluate the behavioral effects of diverse types of toxic substances, e.g., lead salts (18), mercury vapor (9), and methyl amyl ketone (6).

There is an extensive literature in psychopharmacology that contains data on the consequences of various FI and FR schedules of reward and punishment. Some introductory information is available in such books as the one by Thompson and Schuster (179). Applications to toxicology are available in reviews (25) and symposia (71).

Classical (Pavlovian) Conditioning

The primary feature of Pavlovian conditioning is the development of a conditioned response (CR) to a conditioning stimulus (CS) through repeated pairing of the CS with a stimulus (UCS) to which an animal makes an unconditioned response (UCR). Although there is no response initially to the CS, eventually the pairing of the CS with the UCS results in the transfer of the behavioral response to the previously ineffective stimulus. This principle underlies active and passive avoidance behaviors, which are studied in simple chambers such as shuttle boxes. The size and construction of these chambers varies among laboratories, but the basic learning

paradigm is the same. With active avoidance, the animal learns to move physically from one place to another (e.g., from the light side to the dark side of a two-compartmental box) in response to a CS (e.g., a buzzer) that precedes the onset of a UCS (e.g., shock delivered to the animal's feet through a grid floor) if the animal remains in the unsafe (e.g., light) side. If active avoidance is in one direction only (e.g., light to dark side), it is called one-way avoidance. With two-way avoidance, the two halves of the shuttle box are generally identical in appearance and the animal learns to move to the opposite side in the response to the CS. With passive avoidance, the animal performs a behavior (usually spontaneously) for a stated length of time after which it is punished (e.g., shocked) for performing that behavior. At intervals (2 min to 30 days) thereafter, the animal is retested for "learning" or withholding behavior based on the punishing experience. Active and passive avoidance have been used repeatedly for evaluating learning ability in rats. Duration of retention of a learned avoidance is often considered a measure of "memory." So long as learning and memory are operationally defined, the terms are useful. It is important to recognize that extrapolation to learning and memory under different conditions may be imprecise.

Spontaneous (Unconditioned) Behavior

Spontaneous, or unconditioned, behaviors differ from conditioned behavior in that the experimenter does not define the type of behavior the animal is expected to evince but measures the motor response an animal spontaneously performs in response to the stimulus. The stimulus for eliciting behavior may be a novel environment, a change in the environment such as circadian changes, or the initiation of a behavior by the animal in a stable environment. Thus no training by the experimenter is required to get the animal to perform the task, although there may be habituation or adaptation in the performance on repeated or prolonged exposure to the testing environment.

The following tests use all three types of behavior and involve various areas of the nervous system. One of the aims of the categories given in Table 1 and in the subsequent discussion is to suggest the areas of the nervous system for which the tests may monitor damage.

TABLE 1. *Methods for behavioral toxicology*

Adult behavioral tests
  Sensory
  Motor
  Sensorimotor integration
  Cognition, learning, and memory
  Social and emotional
  Reproductive
Postweaning behavioral tests
  Sensory
  Motor
  Cognition, learning, and memory
Prenatal behavioral tests
Invertebrate behavioral tests

Adult Behavioral Tests

Sensory system tests

Sensory system tests and examples of authors who have used them are as follows:

Startle response — Wecker and Ison (188)
Auditory discrimination — Stebbins and Rudy (171)
Visual discrimination — Evans (58)
Odor discrimination — Wood (193)
Vibration sensitivity — Maurissen et al. (112)

Damage to the sensory systems, in the absence of damage to motor systems, is well known following human exposures to some toxic substances. In tests for sensory damage in animals it is not easy to exclude damage to motor systems, as all animal behavioral tests depend on motor movement as the endpoint. In some cases electrophysiological tests, recording evoked potentials, may be more definitive than behavioral studies involving sensory discrimination by the animal. Nevertheless, valuable information can be obtained about sensory systems with some behavioral tests.

The auditory startle reflex appears in the postnatal development of rats at about day 12. In response to an intense auditory stimulus, a rapid sequence of anterior to posterior contractions of flexor muscles pulls the rat into a crouching position called the acoustic startle reflex. This reflex can be inhibited by selected stimuli. Modification of the acoustic startle reflex by other stimuli does not depend on learning, which enhances the usefulness of the procedure for examining the sensory systems involved (61). A typical apparatus for studying the reflex in rats consists of a small cage mounted in a way to record movement, a method for delivering controlled background noise, and devices for delivering sound pulses and other stimuli (64,85,91). In the rat the auditory startle response can be inhibited by light (158), and in the pigeon the visual startle response can be inhibited by sound (174). Interaction of acoustic and tactile sensations has also been monitored (195). The startle response is of interest as a method for testing development of sensory systems in animals exposed to toxic substances *in utero* (34), for detecting actions of toxic compounds on discrete brain areas receiving sensory impulses (60), and as a potentially useful method for examining damage to human sensory pathways (111).

Sensory discrimination procedures can be used to test the integrity of sensory systems after exposure to toxic substances, which is an important use of operant conditioning tests. It is possible not only to determine if an animal has impaired vision or hearing but if a chemical is present at an unpleasant level in the air and if the sensations caused by one chemical resemble another. Most of these tests require painstaking attention to details of training, and they are not tests that would be likely to be attempted unless the time and effort involved could be justified.

Auditory discrimination in monkeys and guinea pigs has been used by Stebbins and co-workers to detect partial hearing loss from some amino glycoside antibiotics (170,171). The method requires that the animal press a lever to avoid shock during the presentation of a sound. Both the frequency range over which hearing occurs and the threshold for sound can be evaluated. Recovery on withdrawal of the ototoxic substance can be examined in these tests. Salicylate ototoxicity has been studied in this way (125).

The intactness of the visual pathway also can be determined using comparable methods (79). Discrimination of both intensity of illumination and wave length can be tested using operant paradigms. However, some species, e.g., the dog and cat, are behaviorally insensitive to color and only the level of luminance can be used in these species. Other animals, notably birds and monkeys, do respond to color, and their discrimination of wave length can be studied. Crawford's studies with monkeys are an excellent example (48).

Olfaction in some species is a major component of sensory information. For example, rats learn olfactory discriminations and preferentially attend to odors when they are presented in conjunction with light or sound (128).

Sensory systems have been used in a different way from detection of sensory damage. It is possible to train animals to turn off a flow of irritant gas, and the percent of deliveries of the gas that are terminated by the trained animal are recorded. Details of such a system with controls for the possibility of nonspecific effect of the gas on response rate have been reported by Wood (193). Using an exposure chamber with one active and one inactive sensor (nose cones with photocells), mice are trained to poke their noses into one sensor to turn off a flow of ammonia and to turn on a flow of clean air. The inactive sensor serves as a control for nonspecific changes in nose-poking behavior. Such a system can be used to detect the lowest concentration of a gas that is irritating to normal mice.

Drugs and other chemicals when administered in doses that can be "detected" by the animal serve as sensory stimuli mediated through effects on the CNS (and probably not through effects on the peripheral nervous system). Thus some chemicals can serve as unconditional stimuli, either aversive or reinforcing (i.e., unpleasant or pleasant). They can be used as a discriminative stimulus in which the sensory effect of the chemical becomes a signal to the animal associated with reward or punishment in a conditioning test. An example of use of this phenomenon from pharmacology is the ability of rats to discriminate pentobarbital from chlordiazepoxide or saline (141). A review of the use of drugs as discriminative stimuli is available (16). Theoretically, the technique of using chemicals as discriminative stimuli has value for detecting toxic effects when there is interest in the degree of generalization of CNS effects of several chemicals. A serious limitation is that many toxic substances may not have the appropriate characteristics to act as discriminative stimuli.

Motor system tests

Motor system tests and examples of authors who have used them are as follows:

Balancing rods — Altman and Sudarshan (5)
Rotarod — Kaplan and Murphy (95)
Hindfoot splay — Edwards and Parker (54)
Gait — Mullenix et al. (122)
Grip strength — Cabe et al. (38)

Central nervous system control of motor performance has been extensively investigated in various species, particularly the rat, cat, and monkey. Three major brain areas are involved, each of which may be selectively damaged by toxic substances: Neurons of the corticospinal tract, the basal ganglia, and the cerebellum form an integrated system for complex motor activity. One species difference of interest in toxicology is the cortical representation of motor function. In the monkey (and in man) the cortical motor area is discrete from cortical sensory areas, whereas in the rat the topographic representation of motor functions is incorporated with the sensory areas in the posterior frontal and anterior parietal cortex (102). Damage to this area in the rat results in reduced ability in placing and hopping, with difficulty precisely positioning the feet (31,108,198). However, such rats do not develop marked ataxia. Damage to the basal ganglia and associated pathways results in muscle rigidity and poor control of fine movement (36), resembling parkinsonism in humans. Damage to the cerebellum results in marked ataxia, associated with loss of cerebellar Purkinje and granule cells (109).

When severe locomotor problems result from exposure to toxic agents, the cerebellar (83) or peripheral (95) motor systems may be involved. More subtle functional changes in gait result if damage is restricted to cortical motor areas or extrapyramidal areas (31,84,92). However, functional tests showing minor alterations in motor performance cannot be precisely interpreted as involving specific areas of the motor systems, as any or all systems can be involved. An analysis of swimming behavior in mice has shown that marked effects on this motor behavior can be associated with inner ear damage consisting of missing or malformed otoliths. Thus very specific and localized damage may result in gross alterations in motor function (74).

When rats walk on wide, flat surfaces, alterations in gait may not be obvious, but they may become apparent if the rat is trained to walk on a balancing rod or narrow pathway to a home cage or for food reward (84,110). The size of rods or narrow pathways must be appropriate to the size of the animal (e.g., a 12-mm flat pathway or 25-mm diameter rod for an adult rat). Locomotion on the narrow path may be recorded by observation, or it may be video-recorded for identification of loss of footing.

The rotating rod, or rotarod, has been used to detect motor system damage at various levels. The animal, usually a rat, is evaluated for the time its balance is maintained on a rod turning at a fixed rate. Training starts on a slowly revolving horizontal cylinder, and the speed is gradually increased during a short training period. Clearly, some learning is involved, as performance improves with training. The procedure has been used to detect various types of neurologic deficits, e.g., ataxia from CNS depressants (100), cerebellar deficits (33), and peripheral neuropathies (95). A modification of the rotarod is the accelerating rod, or accelerod, where the rate is rapidly increased (rate of increase is 1–3 rpm/sec) until the rat loses balance and falls off the rod. Various agents affecting motor function can be detected, e.g., ethanol and acrylamide (27) and soman (80). In the case of neuropathy from acrylamide, it has been proposed that simple measurement of the hindfoot spread of rats dropped from a height of 32 cm is as sensitive in detecting hindlimb disability as the rotarod procedure (54).

Gait, as noted above, may not appear grossly altered even with ablations of the motor cortex. However, quantitative

analysis of gait may reveal damage not noted by simple observation. Detailed analysis of locomotion has been carried out by various investigators. Descriptions of locomotion of various laboratory species are available (e.g., 73,84,87,172). A simple technique for obtaining the walking patterns of rats, described by Mullenix and co-workers (122), is a modification of an earlier report (151). This technique has been applied to studies of peripheral neuropathies (92). Rats are allowed to walk through a narrow corridor 80 cm long, lined on the bottom with ink-absorbent paper. The hindfeet of the rat are dipped in ink just before placing them at the beginning of the corridor, and gait is measured from the footprints left on the paper.

Peripheral neuropathies can be evaluated by the same tests as central neuropathies. A special case is the delayed neuropathy caused by some organophosphate compounds. The unique sensitivity of the hen, which resembles the human in sensitivity to organophosphates, makes the chicken the species of choice and mandates tests appropriate to this species. The simplest test is to observe locomotion of the hen on a smooth surface and to score the degree of weakness on a scale from 0 to 4 (1). However, more quantitative data on the gait of chickens can be obtained using a modification of the method described here for rats (164).

Operant conditioning techniques can be used to measure various aspects of motor control. Drugs have been shown to have predictable effects on motor control in lever pressing (59). This technique has been used to show the effects of ethanol on motor control in normal and dependent rats (152). Effects of drugs on the force of lever pressing (65,66) and grip strength (38) also have been examined. Although most of the studies to date have involved drugs, the extension of studies on motor discrimination to effects of substances toxic to the neuromuscular system is obvious. However, all these tests of motor control involve sensorimotor reflexes, and precise localization of damage must be confirmed by use of several tests or by demonstration of areas of morphological damage to the nervous system.

Sensorimotor integration tests

Sensorimotor integration tests and examples of authors who have used them are as follows:

Locomotor activity	Reiter and MacPhail (148)
Circadian activity	Reiter (146)
Conditioned active avoidance	Rodier et al. (150)
Conditioned passive avoidance	Sandstead et al. (153)

When evaluating human performance, tests of visuomotor coordination have been proposed as sensitive measures of brain damage and the acute effects of drugs, e.g., alcohol. Three components are involved in sensorimotor performance: the afferent (sensory) component, the efferent (motor) component, and a poorly defined integrative component that processes the sensory input and selects the appropriate motor response. When tests are used that involve various nervous system functions and the central and peripheral nervous systems, interpretation of the site of action of an agent may be limited unless the site can be inferred from other data. For example, if an animal shows progressive loss of high frequency sounds during continued exposure to a chemical, the inference may be drawn that the loss is occurring in the hair cells of the cochlea. However, the precise target cannot be identified by the behavioral findings, as damage might be occurring at various sites in the auditory pathway. Although it is difficult to distinguish with precision the damage to peripheral and central portions of sensory and motor systems using behavioral techniques, it is possible to distinguish effects on the afferent pathway from general effects on the motor function using other tests of motor function in conjunction with sensory evaluation.

The advantage of behavioral techniques that involve sensory, motor, and integration systems is that they are among the most generalized of the tests. That is, these techniques are more likely to detect effects when the target is not known, as the tests involve appropriate functioning of several systems. The major distinction between tests listed here as requiring integration differ from the tests of motor function primarily in the aspect of time. When sensorimotor integration involves complex behaviors, the animal is required to make a "decision" regarding activity. The inclusion of time as the essence of the test, or activity over time, presumably increases the CNS pathways involved over the previous two categories.

Locomotor activity seems to be a simple form of behavior, but it is likely that control of the amount of activity involves complex interpretations of the environment. Locomotor activity over a period of time in various environments has been measured utilizing several types of monitor. A review of the methods (148) offers a good introduction to the various techniques that have been tried. The principle involved is that an animal habituates to a novel environment in a regular way. Complex environments increase the amount of activity over simple spaces. Initial activity in a novel environment has been called "exploratory behavior" and is discussed below.

It has been pointed out in rats (19,187) and man (142) that the amount of activity is related to the method of measurement. Another important consideration is the duration of the exposure of the animals to the environment. Activity in an open field increases with repeated exposures (19), whereas in a maze-type environment activity decreases with habituation (49). When animals are allowed to live for days in an environment in which their activity can be recorded, circadian cycles of activity are marked for most species. Laboratory rats and mice are predominantly nocturnal animals, and most food and water consumption occurs at night. Some types of brain damage result in nocturnal hyperactivity but not diurnal hyperactivity in rats (129). Circadian activity is generally recorded in residential mazes (14,49) or conventional cages equipped with recording devices (41,119, 167,190).

Conditioning is readily demonstrated in complex environments requiring sensorimotor integration. Active avoidance conditioning requires that the animal perform a motor movement (escape) in response to a conditioning stimulus (sound or light) in order to avoid a shock. Positive rewards (food or water) may be used instead of the shock. In the positive reward test, the more general term used is "spatial discrimination" instead of "active avoidance" because the animal makes a choice of movements usually in a Y-maze or similar space to obtain a reward. Examples of both types of conditioning tests are readily available (40,183). Because UCS–CS pairing is involved, these tests utilize a kind of Pavlovian conditioning. With active avoidance the animals may be trained to move from one area to another through an opening (shuttle box), and the two compartments may be differently illuminated. An alternate method is to use a grid floor through which a shock is applied and an escape pole onto which the animal can climb or jump to avoid the shock. Latency to move and percent avoidance may be measured, and changes in the two parameters are correlated (101).

With Y-maze conditioning an animal is placed in a starting position (e.g., at the end of the long arm) and is trained to move into another arm, making the correct choice by negative reinforcement (e.g., foot shock) or reward (e.g., food). The USC is a buzzer or light preceding the onset of the CS. An example of the use of the Y-maze was described by Vorhees (184). An argument for using the Y-maze as a measure of learning was presented by Caul and Barrett (40).

Conditioned passive avoidance tests resemble active avoidance methods except that the animal is required to withhold movement rather than to initiate it. For example, a darker area acts as an incentive to rats to move from a lighter area to the darker space. However, if rats receive a shock upon entering the dark area, the animals may not enter the dark area a second time for a finite period, often proposed as a period of "memory." The test has been used extensively in psychology (42). In toxicology, conditioned avoidance tests have been used more as general tests of nervous system involvement by a toxic agent than as specific tests of learning deficits.

Cognitive tests: learning and memory

Cognitive tests of learning and memory and examples of authors who have used them are as follows:

Radial maze	Olton et al. (138)
Operant FI	Cory-Slechta et al. (45)
Operant FI/FR	Wenger et al. (190)
Spatial discrimination learning	Reiter (146)

Interpretation of tests of cognition in terms of damage to integrative pathways in the CNS involves poorly defined systems in the brain that are behaviorally categorized as learning and memory. The role of the hippocampal formation of the brain in memory has been under investigation for some time. In particular, the hippocampus has been proposed in association with learning in Pavlovian conditioning (97). The major difference between tests in the previous category and this one is the degree of complexity of the test for the rat.

Spatial learning and memory in conditioned animals in a radial maze has been related to hippocampal function (138). The radial arm maze consists of eight arms radiating from a central area. Access into an area is monitored, and animals obtain a food reward on the first entry of each arm. Subsequent entries into the same arm are errors and are not reinforced. Accuracy of selecting arms and activity (in number of times each arm is entered) is obtained. Altered performance is not limited to damage to the hippocampus, and damage to several brain areas causes the learning and performance deficits in this test (117).

One of the most commonly measured phenomena is the rate of learning, particularly in young animals that have been exposed to toxic chemicals during the perinatal period (30,32,89,169,197). Not all conditioning tests are useful for determining rates of learning. For some operant tests involving complex schedules, rates of acquisition of a response may be too variable between animals to allow any "average rate of learning" to be established for the experiment. Therefore simple schedules that most animals can master may be preferred, and the rate of acquisition of a behavior to a pre-established level, set as a criterion for learning, is determined.

Performance decrements and rates of learning are important measures of cognition in operant tests. It has been known for some time that different schedules of reinforcement generate different schedules of responding, and the effect of drugs is schedule-dependent (51). Schedules, rate of responding, and the effect of drugs have been carefully reviewed (154). Examples of schedules used in toxicology can be found in studies by Barthalmus and co-workers (18) using FR 30–FI 5 (a schedule where the pigeon received a reward once every 30 responses in blue light followed by a reward every 5 min in red light), the study by Anger and co-workers (6) using an FR 50–FI 3 schedule (a reward every 50 responses in red light and at the end of 3 min in yellow light), and an even more difficult schedule by Armstrong and co-workers (9), FR 60–FI 15 (a reward every 60 responses and a reward after 15 min). It might be thought that the more difficult the task, the more easily performance of it would be disrupted. However, an excessive variability can mask effects on performance. The value of various mixed schedules in detecting altered performance after exposure to toxic agents, particularly under chronic conditions, needs further study.

An example of variability among individual animals in operant performance was reported in a study of rats responding on a fixed interval when exposed to lead. Correlation between blood lead levels and response rates was also variable (45). However, some toxic exposures have resulted in good correlations between behavioral changes on an FR–FI schedule and CNS damage. Wenger and co-workers (190) reported that trimethyltin caused behavioral effects in circadian activity and an FR 30–FI 600 schedule that correlated with loss of granule cells in the hippocampal fascia dentata.

A high level of characterization of behavior deficits can be obtained with a series of conditioning tests which evaluate different aspects of intellectual function. Long-lived species such as the monkey are particularly appropriate to use in longitudinal studies. For example, deficits in performance of a discrimination paradigm were found in young monkeys exposed to low levels of lead from birth. The same animals, as adults, showed impairment in a complex spatial discrimination task in the presence, but not in the absence, of irrelevant stimuli (72).

The spatial distribution of activity in complex environments has been studied as spontaneous exploration as well as conditioned activity. With either type of study, the animal makes nonrandom choices of movement. Spontaneous activity, when no conditioning stimulus is used to structure behavior, is not always distributed randomly but may be altered by the varying spatial conditions (146). Exposure to toxic agents may distort the spatial distribution of activity

(129,146). There are interesting theoretical aspects to spatial distribution of insects in two- and three-dimensional environments that have not been studied experimentally in toxicology, although mathematical models and ecological information are available (3,10,70,81).

Tests of social and emotional behavior

Tests of social and emotional behavior and examples of authors who have used them are as follows:

Exploratory behavior	Walsh and Cummins (186)
Aggressive behavior	Perdue et al. (143)
Social investigation	Landauer et al. (104)
Complex behavior patterns	Mullenix et al. (123)

One of the most complicated issues in behavioral toxicology is the interpretation of tests that may involve subjective feelings on the part of experimental animals. Nevertheless, emotional alterations in humans are an important component of many toxic exposures, with symptoms ranging from sleepiness or fatigue to severe depression or confusion. The issue has been repeatedly addressed in behavioral experiments, as even the titles of some papers attest (26,63). The evidence for anatomical localization of subjective interpretations is imprecise in humans as well as experimental animals, although the concept of initiation of emotional behavior by the limbic system has been advanced. Various structures may be involved, including the olfactory cortex, amygdala, and hippocampus.

Certain behaviors in rodents have been inferred to be evidence of emotion on the part of the animal, e.g., defecation and urination. Arguments regarding this interpretation have been advanced (8). An alternative approach is to consider certain behaviors as generated in response to a stimulus, and the same behaviors may be generated by other stimuli. The concept of displacement reactions, where an animal behaves in apparently inappropriate ways, is well known in ethology. The tests included here may measure CNS functions that are not addressed in the tests described in the previous section on cognition. It does not follow from the lack of immediate cause and effect in the stimulus response, where behavioral acts are not specifically predictable from knowledge of the stimulus, that the reproducibility or reliability of these tests is lower than for conditioned behavior. We do not know how most behaviors are generated in mammals, but the available data suggest that in a stable environment there is a good deal of structure and constancy in spontaneous behavior. This point is illustrated by some of the tests included in this section.

One of the most commonly used behavioral tests is included in this section. The open field test has a long history of use for various reasons. This test has an appealing technical simplicity, but the data must be interpreted with caution. It is particularly important not to draw a generalization from a brief measure of locomotor acts in a special environment that an animal is "hyperactive" or "hypoactive." In order to measure locomotor activity in the open field test, the animal (usually a rat) is placed, usually, in the center of the field. The field is marked into squares, the size of which is appropriate to the size of the animal. Activity is measured by counting the number of squares entered or lines crossed in a brief period, often 15 min. The floor is cleaned before the next rat is tested. Latency to initiate movement may be scored. Latency to move and total activity are altered by repeated exposure to the open field. The response of a naive rat to the open field is sometimes called "exploratory behavior."

Exploratory behavior is defined as the sequence of locomotor acts when an animal is introduced to a novel environment. The amount of activity and the rapidity of habituation are dependent on the age of the animal as well as the spatial arrangement of the environment (19). Sex and strain differences and time of day may affect results in this test (46,82,175,182) as in many other tests. The significant characteristic of all methods of measuring exploratory behavior is that motor acts are recorded for short periods of time. In addition to the open field, closed environments such as mazes (46,90) or plastic cages resembling conventional laboratory cages may be used. Activity may be recorded by observation, as described by Streng (175), photocells (82), stabilimeter devices (119), electronic high frequency recorders (166), video recorders (147), and photographic records (130). An automated version of the open field has been described (88).

The behavior of a rat placed in an open field for the first time has often been described as fearful. Both latency to move ("freezing") and number of fecal pellets deposited over a short span of time have been used as measures of "emotionality." Tests for emotionality in rats and mice have been reviewed (8). The concept that the open field can be used to measure general autonomic reactivity, or "emotionality," is not substantiated by the evidence. For example, different measures of autonomic reactivity such as cardiac rate and defecation do not show parallel changes with habituation (39), nor is activity in the open field correlated with corticosterone levels (173). The open field as a test of "emotionality" has been reviewed by Walsh and Cummins (186).

Whether one wishes to ascribe emotion to the behavior of animals in novel or threatening situations is to some extent a matter of taste, but the risk of the use of general terms for classifying behaviors is that terms such as "fear" imply a relation between behaviors and species that is not justified by available data. Barnett and Cowan (13) have made this point clearly in a review of the reaction of rats to novel environments. Regardless of whether the latency to move or the rate of movement in a novel environment is influenced by fear or by any emotion in rats, the test is performed frequently. In addition to the open field, exploratory behavior has been recorded in maze-type environments such as the "plus maze" (15) and the "elevated maze" (139).

Although "emotionality" in the open field is perhaps the best known test of "emotion" in animals, tests of aggression, with the implication of parallels to emotion in humans, have received considerable attention. Aggression has been defined as "behavior which inflicts or threatens to inflict harm or damage to some goal entity" (162). However, even this simple operational definition depends on the intent of the act, and therefore two observers may interpret the same behavioral acts as aggressive or nonaggressive. For example, Michaelson and Sauerhoff (114) reported that 4-week-old rats treated with lead salts during the neonatal period showed increased aggressiveness toward other young rats. If aggressiveness is defined in terms of chasing, boxing, etc., the identification of an act as aggressive becomes uncertain, as these acts can also be termed components of "play" behavior in young rats.

The interpretation of the data thus depends in large measure on the decision by the observer of the intent of the rat.

Nevertheless, behavior designated "aggressive" has been extensively investigated in the past and will continue to be studied. Two types of aggression have been used, one of which relies on spontaneous attack behavior toward an animal of another species. This behavior is usually considered predatory. The other type of aggression is sometimes classed as "irritable aggression" and is usually induced by electric shocks to the feet of a rat. Predation may occur without overt autonomic signs, but irritable aggression is accompanied by marked autonomic activity. Aggressive behavior may be enhanced by isolation for several weeks prior to the test and by food restriction (86). Ambient noise level can affect aggression (163).

The spontaneous killing of white mice by the Norway rat was first described by Karli in 1956 (96). This interspecific behavior has been used somewhat less as a test of aggression than unavoidable foot shock, which is usually associated with nonspecific aggression. Examples of the use of this technique are numerous, e.g., studies by Halas and co-workers (77) and Thoa and co-workers (178).

Dominance behavior, which may result in a form of intraspecific aggression, also has been used as a test of aggression. With one test rats are trained to move to food through a Plexiglas tube of a size that only one rat can traverse at a time. When two trained rats are placed, one at each end of the tube, the "dominant" rat forces the "submissive" rat to back out of the tube. This test has been described and used by Miczek and co-workers (115,116).

Analysis of the behavior of animals in a social situation seems to have much to recommend it as a way of detecting subtle toxic effects on the CNS. It is possible that some of the most sensitive responses to brain damage would be altered social behaviors. However, this hope has not been realized yet in tests carried out on aspects of social behavior. A good deal is known about the social behavior of the wild Norway rat (e.g., 12), but only limited portions of the social repertoire of the albino or hooded variants have been studied in any detail. The simplest uses of social behavior have been in the study of activity of small groups. The activity of one, two, three, or four rats in a photocell residential maze has been recorded, and the biggest increment in activity was caused by adding the second rat (145). The open field also has been used as a measure of social behavior. Latané et al. (106) used a circular open field to measure "gregariousness," or distance between two rats, recorded every 10 sec for a 10-min test period. The Latané technique was subsequently used by Jonason and Enloe (93) to examine the effect of limbic system lesions on social attraction in hooded rats.

More complex social situations have been set up, notably those in which a "colony" of rats are allowed to live in a large arena, and various social behaviors are recorded. Two of these colonies are described by Gambill and Kornetsky (69) and Ellison (56). Both of these social situations have been used to examine the effects of chronic amphetamine treatment on social behaviors (57,69). In particular, Ellison (56) noted that behaviors of brain-damaged rats may be different after caging than after exposure to a more natural social setting.

Complex sequences of behavior are emitted by animals in stable environments where no unique stimuli are presented to alter the sequence. Behavioral patterns produced by rats in simple environments, e.g., Plexiglas boxes, have been scored from time-lapse film or video tapes (123,135,194). Control sequences are altered by low doses of various toxic agents and by brain lesions. Although the method is sensitive to many agents, additional automation is required to improve ease of data collection and analysis (148).

Tests of reproductive behavior

Tests of reproductive behavior and examples of authors who have used them are as follows:

Female estrus behavior   Birke and Archer (26)
Male mating behavior   Zenick et al. (196)

The focus of many studies of reproductive behavior has been endocrinological. The sequence of mating acts in female and male rats has been carefully described (2,21,22,105). Whereas mating tests are useful for studies relating hormone levels to reproductive function, these tests are not likely to be useful in broad strategies for detecting effects of toxic substances on the CNS. However, the potential usefulness of tests of reproductive behaviors in specific situations dealing with exposure to toxic substances is being explored.

Estrus behavior of rodents has been used in various ways. Persistent vaginal estrus and altered mating behavior suggest that the hypothalamic-pituitary-gonadal axis has been altered. Exposure of adult female rats (181) and prenatal exposure (76) to toxic agents may cause persistent estrus.

Estrus-associated activity changes in rats can be detected with the activity-measuring device known as the running wheel, or squirrel cage. The design, essentially in its present form, was reported in 1925 by Slonaker (167). It consists of the small cage with a large wheel in which the animal (usually a rat) can run. A sliding panel is used to control access from the cage to the wheel. The wheel is rotated by the animal as it runs, and each revolution is counted. Kennedy and Mitra (98) reported in 1963 that female rats became hyperactive about every fourth day, and that this increase in activity was associated with estrus as determined by vaginal washings. Estrus-associated hyperactivity was most reliable in rats maintained in these activity cages from weaning to adulthood. Estrus hyperactivity is apparently uniquely elicited by this environment. Female rats kept in conventional laboratory cages (28) or in more complex residential mazes (156) do not show hyperactivity during the estrus period. A detailed analysis of behavior patterns of the rat during estrus emphasizes that in nonstressful environments the estrus rat shows no significant increase in general activity (121).

The uniqueness of the running wheel recording cyclic activity of the female rat is often not appreciated. However, the running wheel can be used for measuring activity under other conditions. The most striking activity change, apart from the estrus cycle, is during the diurnal cycle. The activity of the rat in this cage, as well as in all other types of home cage, shows rhythmic alterations, decreasing with the onset of the light cycle and increasing with the onset of the dark cycle. The running wheel is not useful as a measure of general activity in rats for either long or short periods.

Male mating behavior consists in a series of acts that have

been quantified (21,105). Although many compounds are now known to affect reproductive outcome by their action on the male reproductive system (23), mating behavior of male animals has not been evaluated extensively in toxicology. In a standardized test of male rat mating behavior, an ovariectomized, hormonally primed female is placed with a male that has been acclimated to the cage or is in a home cage. Dim light or red light, to which the rat's eye is relatively insensitive, is preferred. Latency to mount, latency to ejaculation, number of mounts, and number of intromissions can be recorded. Effects on copulatory behavior may occur in the absence of changes in cauda epididymal sperm counts, testicular histology, or serum levels of testosterone, luteinizing hormone (LH), or follicle-stimulating hormone (FSH) (196).

Preweaning Behavioral Tests

Exposure of the fetus to toxic agents has long been known to damage various organs, including the nervous system. More recently, concern has developed for the possibility of damage below the levels that produce gross organ abnormalities. Specific concern for the integrity of the function of the nervous system has developed, and the term "behavioral teratology" has been used in this regard.

The prolonged development of the nervous system, throughout intrauterine development in the mammal and into the postnatal period in many mammals, makes the nervous system a potential target during both acute and chronic exposure of the pregnant mammal to toxic agents. An extensive literature is available for the evaluation of normal postnatal development of the mammal. Many studies have looked for developmental delays or alterations after pre- or postnatal exposure to toxic substances (149,150), and there are excellent sources of information on the developmental landmarks, acquisition of complex motor skills, and age at which spontaneous and conditioned performances achieve adult levels (5,29,67,133,136,144,168). A selection of some of the more significant developmental times for the rat is given in Table 2.

Most toxic agents that are expected to affect preweaning behaviors are administered to the pregnant animal during all or a specific portion of gestation. The perinatal period is sometimes the desired developmental target, and agents may be administered to the mother through parturition and lactation. The specific protocol for exposure is determined by the hypothesis being tested.

Sensory behavioral tests

Sensory behavioral tests and examples of authors who have used them are as follows:

Auditory startle   Comer and Norton (43)
Visual cliff   Sechzer et al. (159)
Olfactory discrimination Altman et al. (4)
Tactile placing   Hicks and D'Amato (84)

Various tests of early postnatal behavior rely on the development of sensory systems and integration with adequate motor coordination to perform the act. Motor reflexes de-

TABLE 2. *Developmental landmarks in laboratory rats*

Behavior tested	Postnatal age for successful performance (days)	Ref.
Earflap opening	3–5	11
Surface righting	7.7 ± 0.5	34
Cliff avoidance	7–9	11
Negative geotaxis	9–12	43
Jumping to home cage (12.5 cm)	10	11
Pivoting (nonambulatory homing)	10	5
Eruption lower incisors	11–14	11
Auditory startle	12.3 ± 0.3	49
Wire grasping without hindlimb support	10–15	43
Rearing	13–15	5
Eyelid opening	14.2 ± 0.1	49
Mid-air righting	17.1 ± 0.5	34
Narrow path traverse	17–19	5
Jumping to home cage (40 cm)	21	11
Vagina opening	34–40	11

velop early, and in some tests the limitation in time of normal development of the behavior is clearly the sensory system and its integration with the response.

Auditory startle, using methods similar to the test in adult animals, requires a sound with a sharp rise time to levels at which the animal makes an involuntary "jump." This reflex develops at about postnatal day 12.

Awareness of a visual cliff, in which the cliff appears to be a steep drop in the surface on which the animal stands, develops after the eyes open and requires interpretation of visual cues. The "cliff" is usually an illusion on a surface covered with clear plastic. Alterations in visual perception can be demonstrated following anoxia at birth in animals with highly developed visual abilities, e.g., monkeys (159).

Rats respond to olfactory cues at an early age and attempt to turn and move in the direction of the home litterbox (4).

Tactile placing in the forelimbs of rats develops at 4 to 7 days after birth and at 9 to 13 days in the hindlimbs (53). These reflexes develop with growth of corticospinal axons into the dorsal horn in the thoracic region of the spinal cord (day 4) to the coccygeal region (day 9). Data on responses of neurons in the somatosensory cortex of the postnatal rat suggest that the thalamic input develops in a similar time frame. The formation of synapses between corticospinal axons and spinal cord neurons may determine the time of development of corticospinal tract influence on placing reflexes (53).

Although sensory and motor tests during the preweaning period have been shown to be affected by various agents, association with specific damage to the CNS needs to be established.

Motor behavioral tests

Motor behavioral tests and examples of authors who have used them are as follows:

Negative geotaxis	Vorhees et al. (185)
Reflex suspension	Comer and Norton (43)

The ability to perform many complex motor acts develops during the second postnatal week for the rat. As noted above, it is not possible to distinguish clearly the roles of the developing sensory and motor systems in the performance of most early behaviors. Some tests require development of adequate motor coordination and strength. Two of these tests are listed here as motor tests, although functioning sensory pathways are also involved.

The *negative geotaxis* test is performed by placing the animal's head on an inclined screen. The screen (or other rough surface the animal can grasp securely) is at an angle of 25 to 30° from horizontal. The time required to turn 180° on the screen, so the animal is facing head upward, is recorded. Latency to initiate and time to complete the turn decrease with age. The number of animals achieving a stated criterion may be scored. The test is carried out in the rat prior to eye opening. Delays in performance have been caused by a variety of agents in rats (37), and similar delays have been reported in irradiated squirrel monkeys (140).

Reflex suspension ability is measured by allowing the young animal to grasp a rigid bar of appropriate diameter. Performance requires that the animal be able to support its body weight. The length of time grasp is maintained is the usual endpoint. Number of animals achieving a preset time may also be used. The test in the rat pup usually uses a 3 mm diameter rod. There is some evidence that performance in this test in control rats correlates with the negative geotaxis test (132). High correlations suggest that similar abilities may be involved in the measurements.

Tests of cognition, learning, and memory

Tests of cognition, learning, and memory and examples of authors who have used them are as follows:

Active avoidance	Sandstead et al. (153)
Passive avoidance	Rodier (149)

The ontogeny of active and passive avoidance behaviors in rats has been studied by several laboratories. Knowledge of the development of active and passive avoidance during the early postnatal period is of importance: These tests are often applied to young animals, and it may be important to know if a deficit in acquisition of a conditional behavior is a permanent alteration in behavior or a maturational delay.

It is generally conceded that the more difficult the task, the slower its acquisition; young rats (30 days or less old) take longer to learn tasks than older rats (up to old age). Optimum learning of one-way active avoidance is reached by 4 to 6 weeks postnatally (126). Two-way active avoidance peaks at about the same age in rats (20). Short-term and long-term retention (memory) in passive avoidance testing is not as good in 1-month-old rats as it is in 6- or 12-month-old rats (113), with a peak later than with active avoidance (55). However, rats as young as 15 days postnatal age can learn a passive avoidance response (157). Active (149,153) and passive (149) avoidance performances are affected by prenatal exposure to substances that damage proliferating cells. It has been proposed that relatively simple active-avoidance tasks, e.g., latency of escape, are easier and are learned earlier than more difficult tasks, e.g., one-way avoidance (20). This conclusion is supported by a study of rats exposed chronically to mercury vapor (101) in which response in a conditional avoidance task was affected before escape.

Prenatal behavior tests

Prenatal behavior tests have been conducted in the following species:

Rat   Narayan et al. (127)
Chick   Schmidt and Norton (155)

Complex motor behavior of mammals begins *in utero*, and it is not surprising that analyses of behavior can begin with the fetus. Spontaneous and evoked motility in the rat fetus has been studied extensively (e.g., 7,127,191). Angulo y Gonzalez (7) devised a numerical rating for various movements of the fetus. The technique most investigators have used is an examination of the fetus *in situ* after opening the uterus of a decerebrated pregnant rat immersed, except for the head, in warm Ringer-Locke's solution. Tactile stimulation with the tip of a fine wire evokes either movement of the regions stimulated or mass reactions in the fetus. The earliest movement, flexion of the head and neck in response to tactile stimulation, appears on the fifteenth day after insemination. Forelimb and mass movements of the trunk develop a day later. Head extension and hindlimb movement are present on the seventeenth day. Spontaneous activity also develops at this time (7,127).

The motility of the chick embryo has been recorded by various devices, both internally placed and located on the shell to sense motion externally (78). A valuable use of chick embryo activity has resulted in the demonstration that tolerance and withdrawal to opioids can be produced in the chick prior to hatching (103,155).

Invertebrate behavioral tests

Invertebrate behavioral tests have been conducted in the following species:

Drosophila (fly)	Tempel et al. (177)
Aplysia (mollusc)	Kandel et al. (94)
Formica (ant)	Ayre (10)
Boethcherisca (fly)	Mimura (118)
Tribolium (beetle)	Ogden (137)

Invertebrate behavior as a means of evaluating toxic substances has not been explored extensively. Nevertheless, the information obtained on some invertebrates to date suggests that this field of research may be of value.

Learning in honey bees has been known for some time and was investigated and made famous by Von Frisch (183). More recently learning has been demonstrated in *Drosophila* (81). Several mutant strains show marked differences in learning (176). In addition to studies in insects, learning has been demonstrated in *Aplysia*, a mollusc (94).

Motor behaviors of some ants, spiders, and beetles have

been investigated. As details of the nervous systems of invertebrates become better known, the analysis of behavior and study of effects of toxic agents may be rewarding. For some invertebrates, detailed analyses of the nervous systems are available (17,24,35).

EXAMPLES OF STRATEGIES AND PROTOCOLS

As noted earlier in the chapter, two basic strategies can be defined for evaluating the potential of a compound for adversely affecting behavior. The strategies differ, depending on the intent of the study and if there is evidence for a specific target in the nervous system. The more complicated situation exists when no type of effect is proposed and the aim of the experiment is a "fishing expedition" to see if the compound causes any kind of toxic behavioral effect.

When there is a hypothesized target or predicted behavioral effect, tests are selected that are expected to detect such an effect with low risk of false-positive results. However, when no specific effect is proposed, the strategy is more generalized and applicable to many situations. One approach used by some investigators is to do as many different tests as time and other constraints allow. For example, as many as 12 preweaning behavioral tests have been performed in a single study of a novel compound (50). When high correlations exist between tests on the same animals, there may not be much gain of information by carrying out all possible tests. Decisions regarding best strategies require good information on behavioral tests, and such information may be lacking.

Strategy I: Specific Type of Behavioral Toxicity Is Predicted

1. **Observation:** Related compounds have caused some ataxia and paralysis of unknown mechanism.

2. **Problem:** Does this compound cause neurotoxicity? If so, is the action on the central or the peripheral nervous system? Is it reversible?

3. **First test:** The *gait analysis test* was chosen as a general test of motor function: It can be repeated daily with little baseline change in control measurements. Three dose levels plus a control group were used. The *statistical test* was ANOVA for repeated measures, as the two measures of gait (width and length) were not correlated.

   a. *Experimental animal:* Male albino rats 2 months old were used in these experiments. Ten control and ten treated rats were examined per dose.

   b. *Apparatus:* Gait was measured by allowing each rat to walk through a corridor 10 cm^2 and 80 cm long with opaque sides and a clear top. The floor was covered with a sheet of ink-absorbent paper. The apparatus was at a 3° angle up from the starting end to the opposite end, which rested on the plastic home cage of the rats. A barrier was dropped at three places along the corridor as the rat walked up the corridor.

   c. *Procedure:* Each rat was given five trials, placing the rat at the low end of the corridor. During the first three trials the rat was removed and placed at the end by the home cage if it attempted to turn around or to loiter in the corridor. On the fourth and fifth trials, the hindfeet of the rat were dipped in India ink just before the trial.

d. *Results:* Length and width of stride were calculated from the ink record of the footprints. Six consecutive footprints from the center of the record were measured and averaged from the records of the fourth and fifth trials (Table 3).

e. *Analysis of data:* The treated rats had a wider and shorter stride. The difference in width was significant, based on comparison of control and treated rats.

f. *Discussion:* Direct comparisons of function using different tests rarely have been attempted, although the value of such comparisons is obvious. The test used here is more complicated than the hindfoot spread test and less time-consuming than the rotarod test, which requires some training of the rat (see previous sections for discussion of these two tests). With appropriate modifications of the apparatus, walking patterns also can be measured on chickens, which are uniquely sensitive to motor nerve damage from some compounds.

4. **Second test:** Grip strength test was considered, but *acoustic startle test* was chosen to evaluate motor function along with sensory processing time. The same doses were given to a new group of rats for this test. *Statistical test* was the same.

a. *Experimental animals:* Adult male albino rats, approximately 2 months old at the time of testing, were used.

b. *Apparatus:* Testing was carried out in a plastic cage 8 × 8 × 20 cm. Movement of the cage was recorded by a force transducer. White noise background at 70 dB was supplied by a white noise generator and speaker. The startle stimulus was supplied by an amplified oscillator at 117 dB. A light flash from a photostimulator could be delivered 100 msec before the tone. The apparatus was in a sound-attenuated box.

c. *Procedure:* Each animal received the startle stimulus ten times at 20-sec intervals, followed by ten presentations of the startle stimulus preceded by the light flash, followed by ten presentations of the startle stimulus alone. Amplitude of the startle response was measured from the dynograph record.

d. *Results:* The data in Table 4 were obtained by averaging the startle response for the first and last ten presentations of the startle stimulus alone and separately averaging the middle ten acoustic stimuli that were preceded by a light flash.

e. *Analysis of data:* Response to acoustic stimuli without light flash was significantly reduced in treated rats. The reduction in startle response by light was of a similar magnitude (about 45%) in treated and control rats.

f. *Discussion:* The background white noise level of 70 dB was chosen from the reports that startle magnitude increases with background noise of 50 to 90 dB (85). The prestimulus time of 100 msec for light was chosen from observations on the effect of light stimulus on the startle response (91,158).

TABLE 3. *Gait analysis*

Group	Width ± SE (mm)	Length ± SE (mm)
Control	37 ± 2	148 ± 4
Treated	43 ± 3	142 ± 5

TABLE 4. *Effect of light on the startle response*

Group	Response to acoustic stimuli alone (mm)	Response to acoustic stimuli preceded by light (mm)
Control rats	15.3 ± 2.4	8.1 ± 1.1
Treated rats	9.9 ± 3.0	5.2 ± 1.9

The doses of the agent appeared to have modified the magnitude of the startle response but not the effect of light on the startle response, suggesting an effect on the auditory or motor pathways involved in the response. A converse finding that there was a lesser response of treated rats to visual inhibition would have implied a deleterious effect of treatment on the visual pathway.

5. **Third test:** *Forelimb placing reactions to tactile stimuli* were evaluated in the second group of rats after acoustic startle test was completed. Again, changes from controls were noted in the rats and were scored as 0 (no placing reaction), 1 (slow or imprecise reaction), or 2 (normal). All rats were retested 4 weeks after exposure to the compound. Functional recovery to control values was rapid and complete.

6. **Supplementary tests:** Tissues were taken from the central and peripheral nervous systems for histological examination. Appropriate physiological and biochemical tests were considered.

7. **Conclusions:** Based on the behavioral data, it was considered probable that the chemical had caused reversible interference with various motor functions at the spinal level or on peripheral motor nerves. Histological examination of the nervous system and electrophysiological tests of neuromuscular function were required for confirmation.

Strategy II: No Specific Behavioral Toxicity Is Predicted

1. **Observation:** A chemical was to be used where workers could be exposed for prolonged periods. As part of a general toxicological evaluation, behavioral tests in experimental animals were needed, but no specific effect could be predicted.

2. **Problem:** The tests selected must minimize false negatives as a biological screen, and the risk of missing a positive result must be as low as feasible. Selection thus entails finding tests that demonstrate effects from a broad spectrum of chemicals, the use of an adequate number of animals, and the realization that any significant positive results are based on exploratory application of statistics and must be replicated in order to establish probability values correctly.

3. **First test:** A *measure of circadian activity* was chosen as a test with a low probability of false-negative results. The residential maze has been examined in detail for this purpose (146).

a. *Experimental animals:* Two-month-old female rats were kept on a 12-hr light/12-hr dark cycle. Females were chosen because a reproductive study was to be carried out with female rats at a later date using the same doses.

b. *Apparatus:* A figure-of-eight maze was used in which eight photocells were placed across corridors opening on a central raised area.

c. *Procedure:* Photocell counts were recorded hourly for 4 days while the rat remained continuously in the maze. Food and water were available *ad libitum.* Ten treated female rats were tested at each of two doses of the chemical; ten control rats were tested. Dosing was carried out for 2 weeks prior to placing the rats in the maze. Dosing was continued during the test.

d. *Results:* The data for the fourth day in the maze, after the rats had habituated to the maze, were examined. Counts were averaged per hour for each group of ten rats. There was typical circadian rhythm, with three peaks of activity during the 12-hr dark period, similar to the rhythm reported in the literature (130,147). The average activity in photocell counts for 12 hr of light and dark is shown in Table 5.

e. *Analysis of data:* Although the rats did not show a significant increase in activity during the light cycle, they were significantly hyperactive during the dark cycle. An analysis of variance was used to evaluate the effect of dose, which was not significant.

f. *Discussion:* Hyperactivity limited to the nocturnal period is not a novel finding in rats. Nocturnal hyperactivity after brain damage to several CNS areas has been reported (129), as has alteration in the peaks of nocturnal activity (147). The use of female rats in this test is not complicated by the estrous cycle. Estrus-associated changes in activity do not occur in the residential maze. The test was repeated, as proposed above, with similar results, confirming the original findings.

4. **Second test:** Coincident with the first test, histological data were obtained on organs from a separate toxicity study. Loss of cells in the hippocampal pyramidal cell layer was found. Based on the histological data and the fact that hyperactivity has been reported following hippocampal lesions, the second test was *passive avoidance* as a test of learning and memory.

a. *Experimental animals:* Sixteen male albino rats, aged 4 weeks at the start of the experiment, were used. Eight were exposed to the toxic substance and eight served as controls. Conditioning was started 24 hr after the last exposure, using the same doses and duration as in the first test.

b. *Apparatus:* A shuttle box composed of clear plastic with two chambers, one painted white and one painted black, was used. Illumination over the white side of the box was from a 22-watt circular fluorescent bulb at a distance of 6 inches above the top of the chamber. Each chamber was 20 × 20 × 25 cm high. The dark chamber had a grid floor of stainless steel rods, 0.5 inch apart. The sliding door between the chambers was 8 cm wide and was raised or lowered from above.

c. *Conditioning procedure:* Control and treated rats were alternated throughout. Each animal was placed in the white chamber and allowed to explore for 1 min. The door to the black chamber was then opened and the rat allowed to explore the chamber for 5 min. This regimen was repeated three more times on the first day. On the second day, three baseline trials were repeated as on the first day. On the fourth trial, when the rat entered the dark chamber the door was closed and the rat received a 4-mA shock lasting 2 sec. The rat then was removed to a holding cage for 2 min. The initial trial, postshock, was at 2 min. Three more tests were run without shock at 10-min intervals. Twenty-four hours later, four trials were run without shock, and four more trials without shock were done 30 days after the initial shock. A more critical experiment would use separate groups for 2-min, 24-hr, and 30-day passive avoidance measurements, with control groups receiving no shock or no training.

d. *Results:* The data in Table 6 give the results of the high dose in the experiment.

e. *Analysis of data:* The *analysis of variance* is used to evaluate the effect of exposure on time spent in the safe side using the summed or average data for four trials per rat as the unit of data or the analysis of variance for the repeated samples. In this experiment the differences between the exposed rats and the controls are not significant, although a significant decrease occurs with time. The use of the analysis of variance for biological data has been discussed at length by Winer (192). Analysis of the number of trials failed must take into account that four trials × eight rats does not equal 32 independent observations. Nonparametric tests (e.g., chi square or Fischer's exact test) could be used to analyze the data where the unit of data is the rat ($n = 8$) and not the trials ($n = 4 \times 8$). Discussions of nonparametric statistics for biological data are readily available (44,165).

f. *Discussion:* The characteristic of passive avoidance is that the animal withholds a preferred response (i.e., entrance into the dark compartment) as a consequence of a single foot shock. At 4 to 5 months of age, a significant effect of single shock may be retained for as long as 30 days. In young animals the response to a single shock disappears more rapidly. Various parameters may be measured in passive avoidance in addition to the ones given here, and details of the method vary in different studies (e.g., 113,149,157).

5. **Supplementary tests:** Additional histological evaluation of the CNS would be useful evidence regarding a causal relation between the observed damage to the hippocampus and the effect on passive avoidance. In particular, data about other areas would be interesting in order to see if the loss of cells in the hippocampus was unique. Unfortunately, it is difficult to detect loss of cells in the nonlayered brain areas, and cell loss in many other areas might go undetected unless marked gliosis was present.

TABLE 5. *Photocell counts*

| Group | Counts ± SE/hr | |
	Light	Dark
Control	20 ± 9	115 ± 21
Treated		
Dose A	21 ± 13	223 ± 38
Dose B	27 ± 10	289 ± 43

TABLE 6. *Passive avoidance data*

| Time tested after shock | Time spent in safe side (4 trials) per rat ± SE (min) | | No. of trials failed (entered dark chamber) for 8 rats | |
	Control	Exposed	Control	Exposed
2 min	4.2 ± 0.5	3.8 ± 0.7	2/32	7/32
24 hr	3.0 ± 0.7	2.5 ± 0.8	18/32	21/32
30 days	1.2 ± 0.6	1.3 ± 0.6	32/32	31/32

TABLE 7. *Examples of behavioral test results*

Test category	Toxic agents				
	TOCP[a]	MeHg	Hg (inorganic)	ETOH	Fetal irradiation
Sensory					
Central	0	++	+	+	0
Peripheral	++	++	+	+	0
Motor	++	+	+	+	±
Sensorimotor	+	+	+	++	±
Cognitive	0	+	+	++	±
Emotional	0	±	++	±	±
Reproductive	0	0	0	+	++

Scoring system: 0, no effect on most tests in this category; ±, occasional positive results with tests in this category; +, generally positive results with tests in this category; ++, readily detected by most tests in this category.

[a] TOCP = triorthocresylphosphate.

GUIDE TO BEHAVIORAL TESTING

The concept of strategies and the two examples given above lead to the suggestion that a guide to behavioral testing could be established based on compounds with known behavioral toxicity. An example of the way in which the guide could be set up is given in Table 7, using the categories of adult behavior tests in Table 1. When considering the data that would be appropriate for selection of toxic agents, a distinction must be made between chronic and acute effects. More data are needed on most of the tests described here in order to define the limits of the kinds of damage that can be detected. In the expansion of behavioral pharmacology since the discovery of "tranquilizers" in 1954, many new techniques and data have been developed in studying effects of drugs on the CNS. A similar expansion and modification of existing methodology is taking place now in behavioral toxicology in an attempt to cope with the need for more knowledge of the consequences of exposure to toxic substances.

Behavioral toxicology uses methods that serve various purposes. The aim of an experiment may be to collect scientific data regarding a hypothesis or generalization; it may be to collect information about a type of toxic substance or a group of related chemicals; or it may be to predict hazard for human exposure. The scientist using the method may be in academia, industry, or government. Although the reasons for selecting a test may vary, the need for reliable tests is the same for all.

The goal of any science is to achieve generalizations. The study of behavior has tended to be almost unique in that the function of an organ, the CNS, has been examined without direct attention to the organ itself. Development of powerful generalizations about the CNS and its functions requires synthesis of behavioral data with information from other areas of research: neuroanatomy, neurochemistry, and neurophysiology. Efforts to integrate these approaches to the CNS are being made, and the need for correlation of information from all these sources is generally recognized.

One final area of research activity in behavioral toxicology deserves comment. Automation of many behavior tests has become routine, and behaviors once labeled as too subjective for analysis can be quantified. Even complex behaviors, e.g.,

spontaneous movements of monkeys, can be digitized from video records and evaluated by computer (99). At the other end of the phylogenetic tree, the mollusc *Aplysia* has been shown to develop a form of Pavlovian conditioning, and the current interest in invertebrate behavior is expressed in two new compilations of research (17,160). New approaches to behavioral toxicology help establish the value of the discipline for two goals: to understand the mechanisms of action of toxic agents and to predict the consequences.

REFERENCES

1. Abou-Donia, M. B., Graham, D. G., Ashry, M. A., and Timmons, P. R. (1980): Delayed neurotoxicity of leptophos and related compounds: differential effects of subchronic oral administration of pure, technical grade and degradation products on the hen. *Toxicol. Appl. Pharmacol.* 53:150–163.
2. Adler, N. T., and Bell, D. (1969): Constant estrus in rats: vaginal, reflexive and behavioral changes. *Physiol. Behav.*, 4:151–153.
3. Ahmed, M. S. (1963): A stochastic model for the tunnelling and retunnelling of the flour beetle. *Biometrics*, 19:341–351.
4. Altman, J., Brunner, R. L., Bulut, F. G., and Sudarshan, K. (1974): The development of behavior in normal and brain-damaged infant rats, studied with homing (nest-seeking) as motivation. In: *Drugs and the Developing Brain*, edited by A. Vernadakis and N. Wiener, pp. 321–348. Plenum Press, New York.
5. Altman, J., and Sudarshan, K. (1975): Postnatal development of locomotion in the laboratory rat. *Anim. Behav.*, 23:896–920.
6. Anger, W. K., Jordan, M. K., and Lynch, D. W. (1979): Effects of inhalation exposures and intraperitoneal injections of methyl n-amyl ketone on multiple fixed-ratio, fixed-interval response rates in rats. *Toxicol. Appl. Pharmacol.*, 49:407–416.
7. Angulo y Gonzalez, A. W. (1932): The prenatal development of behavior in the albino rat. *J. Comp. Neurol.*, 55:395–442.
8. Archer, J. (1973): Tests for emotionality in rats and mice: a review. *Anim. Behav.*, 21:205–235.
9. Armstrong, R. D., Leach, L. J., Belluscio, P. R., Maynard, E. A., Hodge, H. C., and Scott, J. K. (1963): Behavioral changes in the pigeon following the inhalation of mercury vapor. *Am. Ind. Hyg. Assoc. J.*, 24:366–375.
10. Ayre, G. L. (1968): Comparative studies on the behaviour of three species of ants (Hymenoptera: Formicidae). *Can. Entomol.*, 100:165–172.
11. Barlow, S. M., Knight, A. F., and Sullivan, F. M. (1978): Delay in postnatal growth and development of offspring produced by maternal restraint stress during pregnancy in the rat. *Teratology*, 18:211–218.

12. Barnett, S. A. (1958): An analysis of social behaviour in wild rats. *Proc. Zool. Soc. Lond.*, 130:107–152.

13. Barnett, S. A., and Cowan, P. E. (1976): Activity, exploration, curiosity and fear: an ethological study. *Interdisc. Sci. Rev.*, 1:43–62.

14. Barnett, S. A., and McEwan, I. (1973): Movements of virgin, pregnant and lactating mice in a residential maze. *Physiol. Behav.*, 10:741–746.

15. Barnett, S. A., Smart, J. L., and Widdowson, E. M. (1971): Early nutrition and the activity and feeding of rats in an artificial environment. *Dev. Psychobiol.*, 4:1–15.

16. Barry, H., III, and Krimmer, E. G. (1978): Pharmacology of discriminative drug stimuli. In: *Drug Discrimination and State Dependent Learning*, edited by B. T. Ho, D. W. Richards III, and D. L. Chute, pp. 3–32. Academic Press, New York.

17. Barth, F. G., editor (1985): *Neurobiology of Arachnids.* Springer-Verlag, New York.

18. Barthalmus, G. T., Leander, J. D., McMillan, D. E., Mushak, P., and Krigman, M. R. (1977): Chronic effects of lead on schedule-controlled pigeon behavior. *Toxicol. Appl. Pharmacol.*, 42:271–284.

19. Bättig, K. (1969): Drug effects on exploration of a combined maze and open-field system by rats. *Ann. N.Y. Acad. Sci.*, 159:880–897.

20. Bauer, R. H. (1978): Ontogeny of two-way avoidance in male and female rats. *Dev. Psychobiol.*, 11:103–116.

21. Beach, F. A. (1947): A review of physiological and psychological studies of sexual behavior in mammals. *Physiol. Rev.*, 27:240–307.

22. Beach, F. A., and Jordan, L. (1956): Sexual exhaustion and recovery in the male rat. *Q. J. Exp. Psychol.*, 8:121–133.

23. Bernstein, M. E. (1984): Agents affecting the male reproductive system: effects of structure on activity. *Drug Metab. Rev.*, 15:941–996.

24. Berstein, S., and Bernstein, R. A. (1969): Relationships between foraging efficiency and the size of the head and component brain and sensory structures in the red wood ant. *Brain Res.*, 16:85–104.

25. Bignami, G. (1976): Behavioral pharmacology and toxicology. *Annu. Rev. Pharmacol. Toxicol.*, 16:329–366.

26. Birke, L. I. A., and Archer, J. (1975): Open-field behaviour of oestrous and dioestrous rats: evidence against an "emotionality" interpretation. *Anim. Behav.*, 23:509–512.

27. Bogo, V., Hill, T. A., and Young, R. W. (1981): Comparison of accelerod and rotarod sensitivity in detecting ethanol- and acrylamide-induced performance decrement in rats: review of experimental considerations of rotating rod systems. *Neurotoxicology*, 2:765–787.

28. Bolles, R. C. (1963): A failure to find evidence of the estrus cycle in the rat's activity level. *Psychol. Rep.*, 12:530.

29. Bolles, R. C., and Woods, P. J. (1964): The ontogeny of behaviour in the albino rat. *Anim. Behav.*, 12:427–441.

30. Brady, K., Herrera, Y., and Zenick, H. (1975): Influence of parental lead exposure on subsequent learning ability of offspring. *Pharmacol. Biochem. Behav.*, 3:561–565.

31. Brooks, C. M. (1933): Studies on the cerebral cortex. II. Localized representation of hopping and placing reactions in the rat. *Am. J. Physiol.*, 105:162–171.

32. Brown, D. R. (1975): Neonatal lead exposure in the rat: decreased learning as a function of age and blood lead concentrations. *Toxicol. Appl. Pharmacol.*, 32:628–637.

33. Brunner, R. L., and Altman, J. (1973): Locomotor deficits in adult rats with moderate to massive retardation of cerebellar development during infancy. *Behav. Biol.*, 9:169–188.

34. Brunner, R. L., McLean, M., Vorhees, C. V., and Butcher, R. E. (1978): A comparison of behavioral and anatomical measures of hydroxyurea induced abnormalities. *Teratology*, 18:379–384.

35. Bullock, T. H., and Horridge, G. A. (1965): *Structure and Function in the Nervous System of Invertebrates*, Vol. II. W. H. Freeman, San Francisco.

36. Butcher, L. L., and Hodge, G. K. (1979): Selective bilateral lesions of pars compacta of the substantia nigra: effects on motor processes and ingestive behaviors. *Adv. Neurol.*, 24:71–82.

37. Butcher, R. E., and Vorhees, C. V. (1979): A preliminary test battery for the investigation of the behavioral teratology of selected psychotropic drugs. *Neurobehav. Toxicol.*, 1(Suppl. 1):207–212.

38. Cabe, P. A., Tilson, H. A., Mitchell, C. L., and Dennis, R. (1978): A simple recording grip strength device. *Pharmacol. Biochem. Behav.*, 8:101–102.

39. Candland, D. K., and Nagy, Z. M. (1969): The open field: some comparative data. *Ann. N.Y. Acad. Sci.*, 159:831–851.

40. Caul, W. F., and Barrett, R. J. (1973): Shuttle-box versus Y-maze avoidance: value of multiple response measures in interpreting active-avoidance performance of rats. *J. Comp. Physiol. Psychol.*, 84:572–578.

41. Chahoud, I. (1977): Measurement of circadian rhythm in the motility of weaned rodents. In: *Methods in Prenatal Toxicology*, edited by D. Neubert, H. J. Merker, and T. E. Kwasigroch. Georg Thieme, Stuttgart.

42. Chorover, S. L., and Schiller, P. H. (1966): Reexamination of prolonged retrograde amnesia in one-trial learning. *J. Comp. Physiol. Psychol.*, 61:34–41.

43. Comer, C. P., and Norton, S. (1982): Effects of perinatal methimazole exposure on a developmental test battery for neurobehavioral toxicity in rats. *Toxicol. Appl. Pharmacol.*, 63:133–141.

44. Conover, W. J. (1971): *Practical Nonparametric Statistics.* Wiley, New York.

45. Cory-Slechta, D. A., Weiss, B., and Cox, C. (1983): Delayed behavioral toxicity of lead with increasing exposure concentration. *Toxicol. Appl. Pharmacol.*, 71:342–352.

46. Cowan, P. E. (1977): Neophobia and neophilia: new-object and new-place reaction of three Rattus species. *J. Comp. Physiol. Psychol.*, 91:63–71.

47. Cramer, G. M., Ford, R. A., and Hall, R. L. (1978): Estimation of toxic hazard—a decision tree approach. *Food Cosmet. Toxicol.*, 16:255–276.

48. Crawford, M. L. (1976): Behavioral control of visual fixation of the rhesus monkey. *J. Exp. Anal. Behav.*, 25:113–121.

49. Culver, B., and Norton, S. (1976): Juvenile hyperactivity in rats after acute exposure to carbon monoxide. *Exp. Neurol.*, 50:80–98.

50. Del Vecchio, F. R., and Rahwan, R. G. (1984): Teratological evaluation of a novel antiabortifacient, dibenzyloxyindanpropionic acid. II. Postnatal morphological and behavioral development. *Drug Chem. Toxicol.*, 7:357–381.

51. Dews, P. B. (1958): Analysis of the effect of pharmacological agents in behavioral terms. *Fed. Proc.*, 17:1024–1030.

52. Dews, P. B., and Wenger, G. R. (1977): Rate-dependency of the behavioral effects of amphetamine. In: *Advances in Behavioral Pharmacology*, Vol. 1, edited by T. Thompson and P. B. Dews. Academic Press, New York.

53. Donatelle, J. M. (1977): Growth of the corticospinal tract and the development of placing reactions in the postnatal rat. *J. Comp. Neurol.*, 175:207–232.

54. Edwards, P. M., and Parker, V. H. (1977): A simple, sensitive, and objective method for early assessment of acrylamide neuropathy in rats. *Toxicol. Appl. Pharmacol.*, 40:589–591.

55. Egger, G. J., and Livesey, P. J. (1972): Age effects in the acquisition and retention of active and passive avoidance learning by rats. *Dev. Psychobiol.*, 5:343–351.

56. Ellison, G. (1976): Monoamine neurotoxins: selective and delayed effects on behavior in colonies of laboratory rats. *Brain Res.*, 103:81–92.

57. Ellison, G., Eison, M. S., and Huberman, H. S. (1978): Stages of constant amphetamine intoxication: delayed appearance of abnormal social behaviors in rat colonies. *Psychopharmacology*, 56:293–299.

58. Evans, H. L. (1978): Behavioral assessment of visual toxicity. *Environ. Health Perspect.*, 26:53–57.

59. Falk, J. L. (1969): Drug effects on discriminative motor control. *Physiol. Behav.*, 4:421–427.

60. Fechter, L. D. (1974): The effects of L-DOPA, clonidine and apomorphine on the acoustic startle reaction in rats. *Psychopharmacologia*, 39:331–344.

61. Fechter, L. D., and Young, J. S. (1983): Discrimination of auditory from nonauditory toxicity by reflex modulation audiometry: effects of triethyltin. *Toxicol. Appl. Pharmacol.*, 70:216–227.

62. Feldman, R. G. (1982): Central and peripheral nervous system effects of metals: a survey. *Acta Neurol. Scand. [Suppl. 92]*, 66:143–166.

63. File, S. E., and Hyde, J. R. G. (1978): Can social interaction be used to measure anxiety? *Br. J. Pharmacol.*, 62:19–24.

64. Fleshler, M. (1965): Adequate acoustic stimulus for startle reactions in the rat. *J. Comp. Physiol. Psychol.*, 60:200–207.

65. Fowler, S. C., Filewich, R. J., and Leberer, M. R. (1977): Drug

effects upon force and duration of response during fixed-ratio performance in rats. *Pharmacol. Biochem. Behav.,* 6:421–426.

66. Fowler, S. C., Morgenstern, C., and Notterman, J. M. (1972): Spectral analysis of variations in force during a bar-pressing time discrimination. *Science,* 176:1126–1127.

67. Fox, M. W. (1965): Reflex-ontogeny and behavioural development of the mouse. *Anim. Behav.,* 13:234–241.

68. Friede, R. L. (1966): *Topographic Brain Chemistry.* Academic Press, New York.

69. Gambill, J. D., and Kornetsky, C. (1975): Effects of chronic d-amphetamine on social behavior of the rat: implications for an animal model of paranoid schizophrenia. *Psychopharmacologia,* 50:215–223.

70. Gardner, M. (1969): Mathematical games: random walks, by semi-drunk bugs and others, on the square and on the cube. *Sci. Am.,* 220:122–126.

71. Geller, I., Stebbins, W. C., and Wayner, M. J., editors (1979): Test methods for definition of effects of toxic substances on behavior and neuromotor function. *Neurobehav. Toxicol.,* 1(suppl. 1):1–215.

72. Gilbert, S. G., and Rice, D. C. (1987): Low-level lifetime lead exposure produces behavioral toxicity (spatial discrimination reversal) in adult monkeys. *Toxicol. Appl. Pharmacol.,* 91:484–490.

73. Gray, J. (1968): *Animal Locomotion.* Weidenfeld & Nicholson, London.

74. Gray, L. E., Jr., Rogers, J. M., Ostby, J. S., Kavlock, R. J., and Ferrell, J. M. (1988): Prenatal dinocap exposure alters swimming behavior in mice due to complete otolith agenesis in the inner ear. *Toxicol. Appl. Pharmacol.,* 92:266–273.

75. Groppetti, A., and Costa, E. (1969): Factors affecting the rate of disappearance of amphetamine in rats. *Int. J. Neuropharmacol.,* 8:209–215.

76. Gupta, C., Sonawave, B. R., and Yaffee, S. J. (1980): Phenobarbital exposure in utero: alterations in female reproductive function in rats. *Science,* 208:508–510.

77. Halas, E. S., Hanlon, M. J., and Sandstead, H. H. (1975): Intrauterine nutrition and aggression. *Nature,* 257:221–222.

78. Hamburger, V., and Oppenheim, R. (1967): Prehatching motility and hatching behavior in the chick. *J. Exp. Zool.,* 166:171–203.

79. Hanson, H. M. (1975): Psychophysical evaluation of toxic effects on sensory systems. *Fed. Proc.,* 34:1852–1857.

80. Harris, L. W., McDonough, J. H., Jr., Stitcher, D. L., and Lennox, W. J. (1984): Protection against both lethal and behavioral effects of soman. *Drug. Chem. Toxicol.,* 7:605–624.

81. Hay, D. A. (1975): Strain differences in maze-learning ability of *Drosophila melanogaster. Nature,* 257:44–46.

82. Henderson, N. D. (1963): Methodological problems in measuring ambulation in the open field. *Psychol. Rep.,* 13:907–912.

83. Hicks, S. P., D'Amato, C. J., Klein, S. J., Austin, L. L., and French, B. C. (1969): Effects of regional irradiation or ablation of the infant rat cerebellum on motor development. In: *Radiation Biology of the Fetal and Juvenile Mammal,* edited by M. R. Sikov and D. D. Mahlum, pp. 739–753. U.S. Atomic Energy Commission, Washington, D. C.

84. Hicks, S. P., and D'Amato, C. J. (1975): Motor-sensory cortex-corticospinal system and developing locomotion and placing in rats. *Am. J. Anat.,* 143:1–42.

85. Hoffman, H. S., and Searle, J. L. (1965): Acoustic variables in the modification of startle reaction in the rat. *J. Comp. Physiol. Psychol.,* 60:53–58.

86. Horovitz, Z. P., Raggozzino, P. W., and Leaf, R. C. (1965): Selective block of rat mouse-killing by antidepressants. *Life Sci.,* 4:1909–1912.

87. Hruska, R. E., Kennedy, S., and Silbergeld, E. (1979): Quantitative aspects of normal locomotion in rats. *Life Sci.,* 25:171–180.

88. Hughes, C. W. (1978): Observer influence on automated open field activity. *Physiol. Behav.,* 20:481–485.

89. Hutchings, D. E., and Gaston, J. (1974): The effects of vitamin A excess administered during the midfetal period on learning and development in rat offspring. *Dev. Psychobiol.,* 7:225–233.

90. Inglis, I. R. (1975): Enriched sensory experience in adulthood increases subsequent exploratory behaviour in the rat. *Anim. Behav.,* 23:932–940.

91. Ison, J. R. (1978): Reflex inhibition and reflex elicitation by acoustic stimuli differing in abruptness on onset and peak intensity. *Anim. Learn. Behav.,* 6:106–110.

92. Jolicoeur, F. B., Rondeau, D. B., and Barbeau, A. (1979): Com-

parison of neurobehavioral effects induced by various experimental models of ataxia in the rat. *Neurobehav. Toxicol.,* 1(suppl. 1):175–178.

93. Jonason, K. R., and Enloe, L. J. (1971): Alterations in social behavior following septal and amygdaloid lesions in the rat. *J. Comp. Physiol. Psychol.,* 75:286–301.

94. Kandel, E. R., Abrams, T., Bernier, L., Carew, F. J., Hawkins, R. D., and Schwartz, J. H. (1983): Classical conditioning and sensitization share aspects of the same molecular cascade in Aplysia. *Cold Spring Harbor Symp. Quant. Biol.,* 48:831–840.

95. Kaplan, M., and Murphy, S. D. (1972): Effect of acrylamide on rotarod performance and sciatic nerve β-glucuronidase of rats. *Toxicol. Appl. Pharmacol.,* 22:259–268.

96. Karli, P. (1956): The Norway rat's killing response to the white mouse, an experimental analysis. *Behaviour,* 10:81–103.

97. Kelso, S. R., and Brown, T. H. (1986): Differential conditioning of associative synaptic enhancement in hippocampal brain slices. *Science,* 232:85–87.

98. Kennedy, G. C., and Mitra, J. (1963): Hypothalamic control of energy balance and the reproductive cycle in the rat. *J. Physiol. (Lond.),* 166:395–407.

99. Kernan, W. J., Jr., Higby, W. J., Hopper, D. L., Cunningham, W., Lloyd, W. E., and Reiter, L. (1980): Pattern recognition of behavioral events in the nonhuman primate. *Behav. Res. Methods Instr.,* 12:524–534.

100. Kinnard, W. J., Jr., and Carr, C. J. (1957): A preliminary procedure for the evaluation of central nervous system depressants. *J. Pharmacol. Exp. Ther.,* 121:354–361.

101. Kishi, R., Hashimoto, K., Shimizu, S., and Kobayashi, M. (1978): Behavioral changes and mercury concentrations in tissues of rats exposed to mercury vapor. *Toxicol. Appl. Pharmacol.,* 46:555–566.

102. Kuhlenbeck, H. (1973): *The Central Nervous System of Vertebrates,* Vol. 3, Part II, pp. 652–661. Karger, Basel.

103. Kuwahara, M. D., and Sparber, S. B. (1981): Prenatal withdrawal from opiates interferes with hatching of otherwise viable chick fetuses. *Science,* 212:945–946.

104. Landauer, M. R., Tomlinson, W. T., Balster, R. L., and MacPhail, R. C. (1984): Some effects of the formamidine pesticide chlordimeform on the behavior of mice. *Neurotoxicology,* 5:91–100.

105. Lanier, D. L., Estep, D. Q., and Dewsbury, D. A. (1979): Role of prolonged copulatory behavior in facilitating reproductive success in a competitive mating situation in laboratory rats. *J. Comp. Physiol. Psychol.,* 93:781–792.

106. Latané, B., Eckman, J., Nesbitt, P., and Rodin, J. (1972): Long- and short-term social deprivation and sociability in rats. *J. Comp. Physiol. Psychol.,* 81:69–75.

107. Laties, V. G., Dews, P. M., McMillan, D. E., and Norton, S. E. (1977): Behavioral toxicity tests: In: *Principles and Procedures for Evaluating the Toxicity of Household Substances.* National Academy of Science, Washington, D. C.

108. Loucks, R. B. (1931): Efficacy of the rat's motor cortex in delayed alternation. *J. Comp. Neurol.,* 53:511–567.

109. MacDonald, J. S., and Harbison, R. D. (1977): Methylmercury-induced encephalopathy in mice. *Toxicol. Appl. Pharmacol.,* 39:195–205.

110. Maier, N. R. F. (1935): The cortical area concerned with coordinated walking in the rat. *J. Comp. Neurol.,* 61:395–405.

111. Marsh, R. R., Hoffman, H. S., and Stitt, C. L. (1978): Reflex inhibition audiometry: a new objective technique. *Acta Otolaryngol. (Stockh.),* 85:336–341.

112. Maurissen, J. P. J., Weiss, B., and Davis, H. T. (1983): Somatosensory thresholds in monkeys exposed to acrylamide. *Toxicol. Appl. Pharmacol.,* 71:266–279.

113. McNamara, M. C., Benignus, G., Benignus, V. A., and Miller, A. T., Jr. (1977): Active and passive avoidance in rats as a function of age. *Exp. Aging Res.,* 3:3–16.

114. Michaelson, A., and Sauerhoff, M. W. (1974): An improved model of lead-induced brain dysfunction in the suckling rat. *Toxicol. Appl. Pharmacol.,* 28:88–96.

115. Miczek, K. A. (1974): Intraspecies aggression in rats: effects of d-amphetamine and chlordiazepoxide. *Psychopharmacologia,* 39:275–301.

116. Miczek, K., Brykocozynski, T., and Grossman, S. P. (1974): Differential effects of lesions in the amygdala, periamygdaloid cortex, and stria terminalis on aggressive behaviors in rats. *J. Comp. Physiol. Psychol.,* 87:760–771.

117. Miller, D. B. (1984): Pre- and postweaning indices of neurotoxicity in rats: effects of triethyltin (TET). *Toxicol. Appl. Pharmacol.,* 72:557–565.

118. Mimura, K. (1986): Development of visual pattern discrimination in the fly depends on light experience. *Science,* 232:83–85.

119. Moorcroft, W. H., Lytle, L. D., and Campbell, B. A. (1971): Ontogeny of starvation-induced behavioral arousal in the rat. *J. Comp. Physiol. Psychol.,* 75:59–67.

120. Mullenix, P. (1977): Altered behavioral patterning in rats postnatally exposed to lead: the use of time-lapse photographic analysis. In: *Behavioral Toxicology: An Emerging Discipline,* edited by H. Zenick and L. Reiter. U.S. Environmental Protection Agency, Research Triangle Park, North Carolina.

121. Mullenix, P. (1981): Structure analysis of spontaneous behavior during the estrous cycle of the rat. *Physiol. Behav.,* 27:723–726.

122. Mullenix, P., Norton, S., and Culver, B. (1975): Locomotor damage in rats after x-irradiation in utero. *Exp. Neurol.,* 48:310–324.

123. Mullenix, P., Tassinari, M. S., and Keith, D. A. (1983): Behavioral outcome after prenatal exposure to phenytoin in rats. *Teratology,* 27:149–157.

124. Muller, K. E., Barton, C. N., and Benignus, V. A. (1984): Recommendations for appropriate statistical practice in toxicologic experiments. *Neurotoxicology,* 5:113–126.

125. Myers, E. N., and Bernstein, J. M. (1965): Salicylate ototoxicity: a clinical and experimental study. *Arch. Otolarygnol.,* 82:483–493.

126. Mysliveček, J., and Hassmanová, J. (1979): Ontogeny of active avoidance in the rat: learning and memory. *Dev. Psychobiol.,* 12:169–186.

127. Narayanan, C. H., Fox, M. W., and Hamburger, V. (1971): Prenatal development of spontaneous and evoked activity in the rat (Rattus norvegicus albinus). *Behaviour,* 40:100–134.

128. Nigrosh, B. J., Slotnick, B. M., and Nevin, J. A. (1975): Olfactory discrimination, reversal learning and stimulus control in rats. *J. Comp. Physiol. Psychol.,* 89:285–294.

129. Norton, S. (1976): Hyperactive behavior of rats after lesions of the globus pallidus. *Brain Res. Bull.,* 1:193–202.

130. Norton, S. (1977): The study of sequences of motor behavior. In: *Handbook of Psychopharmacology,* Vol. 7, edited by L. L. Iverson, S. D. Iverson, and S. H. Snyder. Plenum Press, New York.

131. Norton, S. (1978): Is behavior or morphology a more sensitive indicator of central nervous system toxicity? *Environ. Health Perspect,* 26:21–27.

132. Norton, S. (1986): Correlation of early postnatal behaviors in rats exposed to morphine in utero. *Toxicologist,* 6:218.

133. Norton, S., Culver, B., and Mullenix, P. (1975): Development of nocturnal behavior in albino rats. *Behav. Biol.,* 15:317–331.

134. Norton, S., and Kimler, B. F. (1987): Correlation of behavior with brain damage after *in utero* exposure to toxic agents. *Neurotox. Teratol.,* 9:145–150.

135. Norton, S., Mullenix, P., and Culver, B. (1976): Comparison of the structure of hyperactive behavior in rats after brain damage from x-irradiation, carbon monoxide and pallidal lesions. *Brain Res.,* 116:49–67.

136. Oakley, D. A., and Plotkin, H. C. (1975): Ontogeny of spontaneous locomotor activity in rabbit, rat and guinea pig. *J. Comp. Physiol. Psychol.,* 89:267–273.

137. Ogden, J. C. (1970): Artificial selection for dispersal in flour beetles (Tenebrionidae:Tribolium). *Ecology,* 51:130–133.

138. Olton, D. S., Becker, J. T., and Handelmann, G. E. (1979): Hippocampus, space and memory. *Behav. Brain Sci.,* 2:313–365.

139. Olton, D. S., Walker, J. A., and Gage, F. H. (1978): Hippocampal connections and spatial discrimination. *Brain Res.,* 139:295–308.

140. Ordy, J. M., Brizzee, K. R., Dunlap, W. P., and Knight, C. (1982): Effects of prenatal ^{60}Co irradiation on postnatal neural, learning and hormonal development of the squirrel monkey. *Radiat. Res.,* 89:309–324.

141. Overton, D. A. (1966): State-dependent learning produced by depressant and atropine-like drugs. *Psychopharmacologia,* 10:6–31.

142. Partington, M. W., Lang, E., and Campbell, D. (1971): Motor activity in early life. I. Fries' congenital activity types. *Biol. Neonate,* 18:94–107.

143. Perdue, V. P., Eastman, W. W., Burright, R. G., and Donovick, P. J. (1984): Behavioral analysis of kanamycin administration to mice. *Neurotoxicology,* 5:101–112.

144. Randall, P. K., and Campbell, B. A. (1976): Ontogeny of behavioral arousal in rats: effect of maternal and sibling presence. *J. Comp. Physiol. Psychol.,* 90:453–459.

145. Reiter, L. (1978): Use of activity measurements in behavioral toxicology. *Environ. Health Perspect.,* 26:9–20.

146. Reiter, L. W. (1983): Chemical exposures and animal activity: utility of the figure-eight maze. In: *Developments in the Science and Practice of Toxicology,* edited by A. W. Hayes, R. C. Schnell, and T. S. Miya, pp. 73–84. Elsevier, Amsterdam.

147. Reiter, L. W., Anderson, G. E., Ash, M. E., and Gray, L. E., Jr. (1977): Locomotor activity measurements in behavioral toxicology: effects of lead administration on residential maze behavior. In: *Behavioral Toxicology: An Emerging Discipline,* edited by H. Zenick and L. Reiter. U.S. Environmental Protection Agency, Research Triangle Park, North Carolina.

148. Reiter, L. W., and MacPhail, R. C. (1979): Motor activity: a survey of methods with potential use in toxicity testing. *Neurobehav. Toxicol.,* 1(suppl. 1):53–66.

149. Rodier, P. M. (1977): Correlations between prenatally-induced alterations in CNS cell populations and postnatal function. *Teratology,* 16:235–246.

150. Rodier, P. M., Reynolds, S. S., and Roberts, W. N. (1979): Behavioral consequences of interference with CNS development in the early fetal period. *Teratology,* 19:327–336.

151. Rushton, R., Steinberg, H., and Tinson, C. (1963): Effects of a single experience on subsequent reactions to drugs. *Br. J. Pharmacol.,* 20:99–105.

152. Samson, H. H., and Falk, J. L. (1974): Ethanol and discriminative motor control: effects on normal and dependent animals. *Pharmacol. Biochem. Behav.,* 2:791–801.

153. Sandstead, H. H., Fosmire, G. J., Halas, E. S., Jacob, R. A., Strobel, D. A., and Marks, E. O. (1977): Zinc deficiency: effects on brain and behavior of rats and rhesus monkey. *Teratology,* 16:229–234.

154. Sanger, D. J., and Blackman, D. E. (1976): Rate-dependent effects of drugs: a review of the literature. *Pharmacol. Biochem. Behav.,* 4:73–83.

155. Schmidt, M. B., and Norton, S. (1983): Relationship of dose to morphine tolerance in the chick embryo. *J. Pharmacol. Exp. Ther.,* 227:376–382.

156. Schneider, B. F., and Norton, S. (1979): Circadian and sex differences in hyperactivity produced by amphetamine in rats. *Physiol. Behav.,* 22:47–51.

157. Schulenberg, C. J., Riccio, D. C., and Stikes, E. R. (1971): Acquisition and retention of a passive-avoidance response as a function of age in rats. *J. Comp. Physiol. Psychol.,* 74:75–83.

158. Schwartz, G. M., Hoffman, H. S., Stitt, C. L., and Marsh, R. R. (1976): Modification of the rat's acoustic startle response by antecedent visual stimulation. *J. Exp. Psychol.* [*Anim. Behav.*], 2:28–37.

159. Sechzer, J. A., Faro, M. D., Barker, J. N., Barsky, D., Guiterrez, S., and Windle, W. F. (1971): Developmental behavior: delayed appearance in monkeys asphyxiated at birth. *Science,* 171:1173–1175.

160. Selverston, A. I., editor (1985): *Model Neural Networks and Behavior.* Plenum, New York.

161. Shapiro, R. E. (1987): Alternative testing methodologies—scientific updates. *Toxicol. Indus. Hlth.,* 3:307–309.

162. Sheard, M. H. (1977): Animal models of aggressive behavior. In: *Animal Models in Psychiatry and Neurology,* edited by I. Hanin and E. Usdin, pp. 247–258. Pergamon Press, New York.

163. Sheard, M. H., Astrachan, D., and Davis, M. (1975): Effect of noise on shock-elicited aggression in rats. *Nature,* 257:43–44.

164. Sheets, L., Hassanein, R. S., and Norton, S. (1987): Gait analysis of chicks following treatment with tri-ortho-cresyl phosphate *in ovo. J. Toxicol. Envir. Hlth.,* 21:445–453.

165. Siegel, S. (1956): *Nonparametric Statistics for the Behavioral Sciences.* McGraw-Hill, New York.

166. Silbergeld, E. K., and Goldberg, A. M. (1973): A lead-induced behavioral disorder. *Life Sci.,* 13:1275–1283.

167. Slonaker, J. R. (1925): Analysis of daily activity of the albino rat. *Am. J. Physiol.,* 73:485–503.

168. Smart, J. L., and Dobbing, J. (1971): Vulnerability of developing brain. II. Effects of early nutritional deprivation on reflex ontogeny and development of behavior in the rat. *Brain Res.,* 28:85–95.

169. Snowden, C. T. (1973): Learning deficits in lead-injected rats. *Pharmacol. Biochem. Behav.,* 1:599–603.
170. Stebbins, W. C., Green, S., and Miller, F. L. (1966): Auditory sensitivity in the monkey. *Science,* 153:1646–1647.
171. Stebbins, W. C., and Rudy, M. C. (1978): Behavioral ototoxicology. *Environ. Health Perspect.,* 26:43–52.
172. Stein, R. B., Pearson, K. G., Smith, R. S., and Redford, J. B., editors (1973): *Control of Posture and Locomotion.* Plenum Press, New York.
173. Stern, J. M., Erskine, M. S., and Levine, S. (1973): Dissociation of open-field behavior and pituitary-adrenal function. *Horm. Behav.,* 4:149–162.
174. Stitt, C. L., Hoffman, H. S., Marsh, R. R., and Schwartz, G. M. (1976): Modification of the pigeon's visual startle reaction by the sensory environment. *J. Comp. Physiol. Psychol.,* 90:601–619.
175. Streng, J. (1971): Open-field behavior in four inbred mouse strains. *Can. J. Psychol.,* 25:62–68.
176. Tempel, B. L., Bonini, N., Dawson, D. R., and Quinn, W. G. (1983): Reward learning in normal and mutant Drosophila. *Proc. Natl. Acad. Sci. USA,* 80:1482–1486.
177. Tempel, B. L., Livingstone, M. S., and Quinn, W. G. (1984): Mutations in the DOPA decarboxylase gene affect learning in Drosophila. *Proc. Nat. Acad. Sci. USA,* 81:3577–3581.
178. Thoa, N., Eichelman, B., Richardson, J., and Jacobowitz, D. (1972): 6-Hydroxydopa depletion of brain norepinephrine and the facilitation of aggressive behavior. *Science,* 178:75–77.
179. Thompson, T., and Schuster, C. R. (1968): *Behavioral Pharmacology.* Prentice-Hall, Englewood Cliffs, New Jersey.
180. Tilson, H. A., and Mitchell, C. L. (1983): Neurotoxicants and adaptive responses of the nervous system. *Fed. Proc.,* 42:3189–3190.
181. Uphouse, L., Mason, G., and Hunter, V. (1984): Persistent vaginal estrus and serum hormones after chlordecone treatment of adult female rats. *Toxicol. Appl. Pharmacol.,* 72:177–186.
182. Van Abeelen, J. H. F., and Strijbosch, H. (1969): Genotype-dependent effects of scopolamine and eserine on exploratory behaviour in mice. *Psychopharmacologia,* 16:81–88.
183. Von Frisch, K. (1967): *The Dance Language and Orientation of Bees,* translated by L. Chadwick. Howard University Press (Belknap), Cambridge, Massachusetts.
184. Vorhees, C. V. (1974): Some behavioral effects of maternal hypervitaminosis A in rats. *Teratology,* 10:269–275.
185. Vorhees, C. V., Butcher, R. E., Brunner, R. L., and Sobotka, T. J. (1979): A developmental test battery for neurobehavioral toxicity in rats: a preliminary analysis using monosodium glutamate, calcium carrageenan, and hydroxyurea. *Toxicol. Appl. Pharmacol.,* 50:267–282.
186. Walsh, R. N., and Cummins, R. H. (1976): The open-field test: a critical review. *Psychol. Bull.,* 83:482–504.
187. Weasner, M. H., Finger, F. W., and Reid, L. S. (1960): Activity changes under food deprivation as a function of recording device. *J. Comp. Physiol. Psychol.,* 53:470–474.
188. Wecker, J. R., and Ison, J. R. (1984): Acute exposure to methyl or ethyl alcohol alters auditory function in the rat. *Toxicol. Appl. Pharmacol.,* 74:258–266.
189. Weiss, B., Brozek, J., Hanson, H., Leaf, R. C., Mello, N. K., and Spyker, J. M. (1975): Effects on behavior. In: *Principles for Evaluating Chemicals in the Environment.* National Academy of Science, Washington, D. C.
190. Wenger, G. R., McMillan, D. E., and Cheng, L. C. (1984): Behavioral effects of trimethyltin in two strains of mice. I. Spontaneous motor activity. II. Multiple fixed ratio-fixed interval. *Toxicol. Appl. Pharmacol.,* 73:78–96.
191. Windle, W. F., and Baxter, R. E. (1935): Development of reflex mechanisms in the spinal cord of albino rat embryos: correlation between structure and function, and comparisons with the cat and the chick. *J. Comp. Neurol.,* 63:189–209.
192. Winer, B. J. (1971): *Statistical Principles in Experimental Design,* 2nd ed. McGraw-Hill, New York.
193. Wood, R. W. (1979): Behavioral evaluation of sensory irritation evoked by ammonia. *Toxicol. Appl. Pharmacol.,* 50:157–162.
194. Wootten, V., Brown, D. R., Poquette, M., and Schatz, R. A. (1986): Changes in behavioral pattern development in the neonate after maternal ingestion of ethanol. *Toxicologist,* 6:218.
195. Wu, M. F., Ison, J. R., Wecker, J. R., and Lapham, L. W. (1985): Cutaneous and auditory function in rats following methylmercury poisoning. *Toxicol. Appl. Pharmacol.,* 79:373–388.
196. Zenick, H., Blackburn, K., Hope, E., and Baldwin, D. (1984): An evaluation of the copulatory, endocrinologic, and spermatotoxic effects of carbon disulfide in the rat. *Toxicol. Appl. Pharmacol.,* 73:275–283.
197. Zenick, H., Padich, R., Thatcher, T., Santistevan, B., and Aragon, P. (1978): Influence of prenatal and postnatal lead exposure on discrimination learning in rats. *Pharmacol. Biochem. Behav.,* 8:347–350.
198. Zimmerman, E. A., Chambers, W. W., and Liu, C. N. (1964): An experimental study of the anatomical organization of the corticobulbar system in the albino rat. *J. Comp. Neurol.,* 123:301–324.

Principles and Methods of Toxicology, Second Edition, edited by A. Wallace Hayes, Raven Press, Ltd., New York © 1989.

CHAPTER 19

Biochemical Methods for Neurotoxicological Analyses of Neuroregulators and Cyclic Nucleotides

I. K. Ho and Beth Hoskins

Department of Pharmacology and Toxicology, University of Mississippi Medical Center, Jackson, Mississippi 39216

Neurotransmitters
  Biogenic Amines (Dopamine, Norepinephrine, Serotonin) and Metabolites • Related Enzymes • Neurotransmitter Receptors
Acetylcholine
  Gas Chromatographic Method • HPLC-EC Determination of ACh and Choline • Turnover • Related Enzymes • Receptors
γ-Aminobutyric Acid
  Enzymatic Fluorometry • Radioreceptor Assay • Mass

Fragmentographic Method • Turnover • Related Enzymes • GABA Receptors
Cyclic Nucleotides
  Cyclic Nucleotide Cyclases • Cyclic AMP and Cyclic GMP • Cyclic Nucleotide Assays
Conclusions
Acknowledgments
References

Most toxicants owe their toxicity to effects on the nervous system. Certain neurological and mental disorders induced by poisons can be related to specific defects in synaptic mechanisms. For example, the organophosphate and carbamate insecticides (inhibitors of cholinesterases) are believed to act at cholinergic synapses by reducing the rate of breakdown of acetylcholine (164). The neurotoxicity (e.g., hyperexcitability, tremor, and convulsions) induced by chlorinated hydrocarbons has been demonstrated to be related to the alteration of functional states of neurotransmitters (60).

Barchas et al. (7) have described the events of neurochemical function in terms of the neurotransmitters, which actually "convey information between adjacent nerve cells," and the neuromodulators, which act to "amplify or dampen neuronal activity." All of these substances have been termed neuroregulators in that they "play a key role in communication among nerve cells." As in the case of mediating hormone activities, the cyclic nucleotides, cyclic AMP and cyclic GMP, serve as second messengers in the central nervous system in that they "help to translate neurotransmitter or neuromodu-

lator signals into metabolic events." Evidence abounds for expanding the second messenger concept to include mediation of neuroregulator effects (30).

Because of the development of highly sensitive and specific procedures for estimation of tissue concentrations of neuroregulators and cyclic nucleotides and the activities of their synthetic and catabolic enzymes, assays of neurotransmitters, neuromodulators, and cyclic nucleotides have played key roles in neurochemical investigations of brain functions.

This chapter describes some of the techniques available for measuring the endogenous concentrations of the biogenic amines, acetylcholine, and γ-aminobutyric acid; the turnover rates of these neuroregulators; the activities of enzymes involved in their biosynthetic and degradative pathways; and receptor binding. Methods for determining endogenous levels of cyclic AMP and cyclic GMP and activities of the enzymes primarily responsible for the synthesis and breakdown of these cyclic nucleotides are also described.

We have not attempted to be inclusive but, rather, to select representative methods. The inescapable fact is that many excellent procedures have been omitted, as all methods currently available could not be listed, much less be selected for detailed description.

NEUROTRANSMITTERS

Biogenic Amines (Dopamine, Norepinephrine, Serotonin) and Metabolites

The biogenic amines dopamine (DA), norepinephrine (NE), and serotonin (5-HT) have played an important role as neurotransmitters in neurochemical investigations of brain functions. There are numerous combined methods available for two or more of the biogenic amines. Examples of such methods are those used to determine DA and NE (20); 5-HT and 5-hydroxy-3-indoleacetic acid (5-HIAA) (1,29); NE and 5-HT (87); NE, DA, and 5-HT (2,25,130,159); homovanillic acid and 5-HIAA (69); and NE, normetanephrine, DA, 3-methoxytyramine, and 5-HT (68). Developments in liquid chromatography-electrochemistry techniques have made possible the simultaneous detection of several biogenic amines and their metabolites in brain tissues with high sensitivity (36,89,90). We have chosen to describe three of these methods in some detail.

Determination of 5-HT and 5-HIAA

The method to determine 5-HT and 5-HIAA was reported a number of years ago (23).

Reagents

n-Butanol is acidified by adding 0.85 ml concentrated HCl to 1 liter of *n*-butanol (20). *o*-Phthaldialdehyde (OPT) 0.004% w/v in 10 N HCl, 0.1% w/v cysteine in 0.1 N HCl, 1% w/v cysteine in deionized water, and 0.1% w/v OPT in methanol are prepared immediately before use.

Procedures

Whole brain or cortex is homogenized in 10 volumes of cold acidified *n*-butanol. All other areas (weighing less than 300 mg) are homogenized in 3 ml of acidified *n*-butanol. After centrifugation for 5 min at 3,000 rpm (IEC model K), 2.5 ml of the supernatant fluid is pipetted into a 25-ml glass-stoppered tube and shaken mechanically for 5 min with 5 ml *n*-heptane and 0.4 ml 0.1 N HCl containing 0.1% L-cysteine. The phases are separated by centrifugation as before, and 5 ml of the organic phase is retained for the 5-HIAA determination.

To determine 5-HT, 0.1-ml samples of the aqueous phase are pipetted into 12 × 125 mm test tubes, and 0.6 ml of 0.004% OPT in 10 N HCl is added to each tube. After mixing and heating in a boiling waterbath for 15 min, the tubes are cooled in another waterbath. Contents of the tubes are transferred to microcuvettes, and fluorescence is measured using a spectrophotofluorometer. Activation and emission fluo-

rescence wavelengths are 360 and 470 nm, respectively. Standards are prepared as 60 *μ*g/ml solutions in deionized water (stored at −25°C), diluted 1:100 for use with 0.1 N HCl containing 0.1% cysteine; 0.1 ml is reacted with 0.6 ml of the 0.004% OPT in HCl solution. Blanks are prepared by reacting 0.6 ml of the OPT solution with 0.1 ml HCl–cysteine solution only. This reagent blank gives the same reading as tissue blanks prepared by reacting 0.1 ml of the aqueous phase with 0.6 ml 10 N HCl.

To determine 5-HIAA, the 5 ml of the organic phase remaining after the extraction of 5-HT is pipetted into a 25-ml glass-stoppered tube containing 0.6 ml of 0.5 M phosphate buffer (pH 7.0) and shaken mechanically for 10 min. After centrifuging for 3 min at 3,000 rpm, two 0.2-ml portions of the aqueous phase are pipetted into two test tubes, A and B. To A is added 0.02 ml of 1% cysteine solution and to B 0.02 ml of 0.02% sodium periodate solution. Then 0.4 ml of concentrated HCl is added to both A and B. After this, 0.02 ml of OPT solution (0.1% in methanol) and 0.02 ml of periodate solution are added to tube A. After 30 min, 0.02 ml of the cysteine and OPT solutions are added to tube B. Both tubes are then placed in a boiling waterbath for 10 min, cooled in water, and read at activation and emission fluorescence wavelengths of 360 and 470 nm, respectively. The reading obtained for tube B (blank) is subtracted from that of tube A (test). Standards are prepared as 15 *μ*g/ml solutions (stored at −25°C) and are diluted 1:100 in the pH 7.0 phosphate buffer for use, 0.2 ml being added to tubes A and B.

Simultaneous Determination of NE, Normetanephrine, DA, 3-Methoxytyramine, and 5-HT

Norepinephrine, normetanephrine (NM), DA, 3-methoxytyramine (3-MT), and 5-HT may be determined simultaneously (68).

Reagents

Norepinephrine, DA HCl, DL-normetanephrine HCl, 3-methoxytyramine HCl, and 5-HT creatinine sulfate are used for standards. Standard stock solutions of these amines are prepared in 0.001 N HCl, except for 5-HT creatinine sulfate, which is dissolved in water. The concentrations of the amines are expressed in terms of bases. Water is distilled and further purified by being run through an ion-exchange deionizer.

Preparation of columns

Woelm aluminum oxide, active W-200 neutral (M. Woelm, Eschwege, Germany), is used without prior acid washing or heat activation. Amberlite CG-50, type 2, 200 to 400 mesh (Rohm and Haas Co., Philadelphia, Pennsylvania), is washed by cycling through the acid, and sodium forms with 2 N HCl and 2 N NaOH, and finally with water. The resin is equilibrated with 0.1 M NaH₂PO₄-K₂PO₄ buffer (pH 6.1) and stored as a suspension in the same buffer. The concentration of the suspension is adjusted so that 1.0 ml of the resin slurry corresponds to about 90 mg dry resin.

Columns are constructed from Pyrex glass tubing of 0.6 cm diameter and 9 cm length. One end of the tube is narrowed to form a tip of conical shape, and the other end is connected by fusion to tubing 1.7 cm in diameter and 5 cm in length, which serves as a reservoir.

The apparatus for the double-column procedure is composed of two column racks made of transparent plastic. The two racks are of the same size, superimposable on the other. The heights of the racks are adjusted so the tips of the upper columns come just to the reservoirs of the lower columns. Using this apparatus, effluents from the upper columns (aluminum oxide column) can flow directly into the lower ones (Amberlite CG-50 column).

Preparation of tissue extracts

Tissue samples (up to 0.3 g) are homogenized in 3 ml of cold 0.4 N perchloric acid (PCA) using a Polytron homogenizer. The homogenates are centrifuged at $15,000 \times g$ at 2.5°C for 15 min in a refrigerated centrifuge. From the resultant supernatant fluids, 2.5-ml aliquots are taken and adjusted to pH 7.5 to 8.5 with 0.4 M K_2CO_3 while cooling in an icebath. The precipitated $KClO_4$ is removed by centrifugation at 0°C, and the clear supernatant fluid is placed on the double columns of aluminum oxide and Amberlite GC-50 for isolating the amines, as described below.

Double column procedure

The tips of the columns are plugged with small pledgets of cotton wool. Tightness of each plug is controlled so as to permit a solution to flow through the aluminum oxide column at the rate of 0.3 to 0.5 ml/min and through the Amberlite CG-50 column at the rate of 0.1 to 0.3 ml/min. The columns for aluminum oxide are filled with water to expel the air trapped around the cotton plugs and packed with about 150 mg aluminum oxide. Into the column for Amberlite CG-50 is poured 1 ml of the resin slurry prepared above, which forms a resin bed of about 0.35 ml. The columns are placed in a cold room (0°–5°C) and washed twice by filling the reservoirs with water. After the columns have been drained, the aluminum oxide columns are superimposed on the Amberlite CG-50 columns, each on each, by use of the column racks described above. The pH-adjusted supernatants of PCA extracts prepared above are put on the upper aluminum oxide columns. When the level of the sample solution has dropped just to the surface of the resin in the lower columns, 7 ml of cold water is poured into the reservoirs of the upper columns for wash. After the columns have been drained, the two column racks are separated, and another 7 ml of cold water is passed through both sets of columns. After complete draining of wash water, NE and DA are eluted from the aluminum oxide columns with 3 ml of cold 0.2 N HCl; and NM, 3-MT, and 5-HT are eluted from the Amberlite CG-50 columns with 3 ml of cold 0.5 N HCl.

Fluorometric assays

NE. A 1-ml aliquot of the acid eluate from an aluminum oxide column is mixed with 1 ml of 0.2 M phosphate buffer (pH 6.3). The mixture is adjusted to pH 6.3 with 0.5 N NaOH and diluted to a volume of 2.5 ml with water. The volume of 0.5 N NaOH necessary for the pH adjustment does not vary with different column eluates. The mixture is immersed in an icebath, and 0.1 ml of 0.1 N I_2-NaI is added. This mixture is left for 20 min at 0° to 4°C to oxidize NE to the intermediates of trihydroxyindole. The oxidation reaction is stopped by adding 0.5 ml of chilled alkaline sulfite solution (500 mg Na_2SO_3 and 200 mg EDTA-Na_2 in 20 ml of 2.5 N NaOH), which is prepared just prior to use. The mixture is left for 10 min at room temperature for tautomerization, followed by addition of 1 ml of 2.5 N acetic acid containing 0.01% cysteine HCl. The reaction mixture is allowed to stand for 60 min at room temperature before measurements at activation (380 nm) and emission (480 nm) wavelengths are made. An unoxidized tissue blank is prepared by reversing the order of addition of the iodine and alkaline sulfite reagents.

DA. To a 1-ml aliquot of the acid column eluate, 0.1 ml of 2% EDTA-Na_2 and 0.1 ml of 0.8% potassium ferricyanide are added. To this mixture, 0.5 ml of freshly prepared 1.6% Na_2SO_3 in 1 N NaOH is added, followed 6 min later by addition of 1 ml of 2.5 N acetic acid. All of the above reactions are conducted at room temperature. The reaction mixture is then heated at 75°C for 20 min and cooled in an icebath. The fluorescence is measured at 0°C using 330 nm activation and 370 nm emission wavelengths. Unoxidized tissue blanks are prepared as follows: 0.1 ml EDTA-Na_2 and 0.1 ml potassium ferricyanide reagents are mixed in a test tube, followed by 0.5 ml of the alkaline sulfite reagent. Six minutes later, 1 ml of 2.5 N acetic acid is added for acidification. Finally, 1 ml of the sample column eluate is added, and the tube is treated thereafter in parallel with the test samples.

NM and 3-MT. A 1-ml aliquot of the eluate from the Amberlite CG-50 column is mixed with 1 ml of 0.1 M pyrophosphate buffer (pH 8.4) with 0.6 N NaOH, and diluted to a volume of 2.5 ml with water. After the mixture is chilled in an icebath, 0.1 ml of 2×10^{-4} M pyrophosphate buffer (pH 8.4) is added. The mixture is adjusted to pH 8.4 with 0.6 N NaOH and diluted to a volume of 2.5 ml with water. After chilling in an icebath, 0.1 ml of 2×10^{-4} M alcoholic iodine is added to the mixture for oxidation to occur. After 8 min, 0.5 ml of alkaline sulfite reagent is added, and the mixture is allowed to stand for 10 min at room temperature for tautomerization, as described for the NE assay. After being acidified with 1 ml of 2.5 N acetic acid, the reaction mixture is left at room temperature for 60 min. The NM fluorescence is measured at activation/emission wavelengths of 380/480 nm, respectively. After the fluorescence measurements, the mixture is returned to the original test tube and heated at 75°C for 20 min. The tube is then cooled in an icebath, and the 3-MT fluorescence is read at 0°C using wavelengths of 330 and 370 nm. An unoxidized tissue blank is prepared as described above for the NE assay.

5-HT. A 1-ml aliquot of the column eluate is placed in a Pyrex glass test tube with a stopper, to which 0.3 ml of 1% cysteine HCl and 1.5 ml of OPT reagent (10 mg/dl in concentrated HCl) are added with mixing. The tube is stoppered and heated for 10 min at 75°C. After the contents of the tube return to ambient temperature, the fluorescence is measured at 355 and 480 nm. The tissue blank is prepared as follows: 1 ml of the sample eluate is oxidized with 0.02 ml of 0.1 N ethanolic iodine for 15 min at room temperature to destroy 5-HT. This step is followed by the addition of 0.3 ml of 1% cysteine HCl to reduce the residual iodine. OPT reagent is added. This blank is then treated in parallel with the test samples.

HPLC-EC Determination of Biogenic Amines and Metabolites

The high performance liquid chromatography-electrochemical (HPLC-EC) assay was described by Mayer and Shoup (90).

Reagents

The mobile phase is made by adding 0.15 M monochloroacetate buffer (pH 3.0) to 70 ml of acetonitrile to make 2 L. This mixture is filtered through a 0.2-μm membrane filter and degassed under vacuum. After filtering and degassing, 36 ml of tetrahydrofuran is added and gently mixed. Perchloric acid (0.05 M) for homogenization of tissue parts and for preparation of standards, is made by dilution of 70% perchloric acid. Norepinephrine bitartrate (NE), epinephrine bitartrate (E), DA, homovanillic acid (HVA), 5-HT, 5-HIAA, 3,4-dihydroxyphenylacetic acid (DOPAC), and 5-hydroxytryptophan (5-HTP) obtained from commercial sources are used as received. Stock standard solutions containing 50 μg of each solute per milliliter (as a mixture) are prepared in 0.05 M perchloric acid and kept refrigerated.

Equipment

A Bioanalytical Systems LC-304B liquid chromatograph is used as an example. The detector consists of two LC-4B electronic controllers operating in tandem and a modified LC-17 glassy carbon transducer. A 250 × 4.6 mm Biophase ODS-5 μm column (Bioanalytical Systems) is used. The flow rate is 1.6 ml/min.

Procedures

Brain regions, e.g., brainstem, hypothalamus, and striatum, are dissected according to the method of Glowinski and Iversen. Tissue parts are placed in 2 ml of ice-cold 0.05 M HClO$_4$ and sonicated for 3 min at 0°C, then centrifuged at 15,000 × g for 20 min at 4°C. The supernatant is removed and diluted, and 100 μl is injected onto the column. Quantitation is made by comparison of peak heights of sample components to those of known standards. The detection limit is about 0.2 pmol.

Turnover Rates

Nonisotopic methods are considered to be most popular for measuring turnover rates because of their low cost and simplicity. 5-HT turnover is generally considered to equal its rate of synthesis (4). The following assumptions are made for the estimation of 5-HT turnover (49): (a) 5-HT is formed by synthesis and lost by metabolism; (b) the rates of 5-HT synthesis and degradation are equal; (c) the turnover rates of tryptophan and 5-HT are constant; and (d) no discrimination is made between newly synthesized and preexisting molecules of 5-HT during degradation. The methods are based on the findings that (a) brain levels of 5-HT increase and those of 5-HIAA decrease linearly after the injection of monoamine oxidase (MAO) inhibitors, pargyline, or tranylcypromine (149); and (b) 5-HIAA is removed from brain by an acid transport process (101).

The nonisotopic method of Tozer et al. (149) is described here. This method is based on the assumption that 5-HT is converted solely to 5-HIAA and that 5-HT is the only precursor of the acid. Accordingly, the following reactions may be written:

$$\text{Synthesis} \rightarrow \text{5-HT} \xrightarrow{k_1} \text{5-HIAA}$$
$$\text{5-HIAA} \xrightarrow{k_2} \text{elimination}$$

If the rate of conversion of 5-HT to 5-HIAA is proportional to the level of 5-HT, the rates of 5-HT synthesis and catabolism are the same and are equal to k_1(5-HT)$_0$, where (5-HT)$_0$ is the normal molar concentration of the amine, and k_1 is the rate constant of 5-HT efflux. Therefore the rate of 5-HT synthesis also equals the rate of 5-HIAA loss, k_2(5-HIAA)$_0$, where (5-HIAA)$_0$ is the normal molar concentration of the acid, and k_2 is the rate constant of 5-HIAA loss. Hence:

$$k_1(\text{5-HT})_0 = k_2(\text{5-HIAA})_0 \qquad [1]$$

After the inactivation of monoamine oxidase, 5-HIAA is no longer produced and its level decreases. If the rate of decrease is proportional to the concentration, i.e., $[-d(\text{5-HIAA})/dt] = k_2(\text{5-HIAA})$, the decrease of the level with time is exponential, as seen from integration of the equation (5-HIAA)$_t$ = (5-HIAA)$_0$ e^{-k_2t} = (5-HIAA)$_0^{10-k_2t/2.3}$, where (5-HIAA)$_0$ is the initial level, and (5-HIAA)$_t$ is the level at time t. A plot of $\log_{10}$(5-HIAA)$_t$ versus time yields a straight line, the slope of which is 1/2.3 times the rate constant k_2 of 5-HIAA efflux. From Eq. 1, the product of k_2 and (5-HIAA)$_0$ yields the rate of 5-HT efflux, which in turn is equal to the rate of 5-HT synthesis.

For doing experiments, animals are killed at various intervals after intraperitoneal injection of pargyline 75 mg/kg. As the animals are killed, the brains are removed as rapidly as possible and stored in a freezer. Brain 5-HT and 5-HIAA levels are determined as described above. The values for the brain 5-HIAA levels are logarithmically transformed so that calculations of linearity of regression, standard error of the regression coefficients, and significance of differences between regression coefficients (137) may be performed. The values of 5-HT are statistically analyzed in the same manner as those of 5-HIAA but without the logarithmic transformation.

Catecholamine turnovers are assayed according to Brodie et al. (15), a method based on the assumption that brain levels of catecholamines disappear at an exponential rate after blockade of NE synthesis using α-methyltyrosine, an inhibitor of tyrosine hydroxylase (139).

The rate of NE synthesis (K) can be expressed as

$$K = k[NE]_0 \qquad [2]$$

where k is the rate constant of NE efflux, and $[NE]_0$ is the normal amine concentration. After blockade of synthesis, the concentration of NE decreases at a rate that is proportional to the concentration, i.e.,

$$-d[NE]/dt = k[NE]$$

Integrating this expression yields

$$[NE] = [NE]_0 e^{-kt}$$

and converting to $\log_{10}$ gives

$$\log[NE] = \log[NE]_0 - 0.434kt$$

where $[NE]_0$ is the initial level and $[NE]$ the level at time t. A plot of $\log[NE]$ versus time yields a straight line, the slope of which is $0.434 \times k$, the rate constant of NE efflux. Substituting in Eq. 2, the product of k and $[NE]_0$ gives the rate of NE efflux, which is equal to the rate of NE synthesis.

L-α-Methyltyrosine is dissolved in a small amount of 4 N NaOH, and the solution is adjusted with 4 N HCl to pH 9 and diluted with water to form a 2% solution. The amino acid (200 mg/kg) is injected intravenously via the tail vein. The animals are sacrificed at various times, and DA and NE are assayed as described above. The values for the tissue levels of NE and DA are logarithmically transformed for calculations of linearity of regression, standard error of the regression coefficients, and significance of differences between regression coefficients (134).

Isotopic methods used to determine the turnover rate of 5-HT are based on measurements of radiolabeled 5-HT synthesized from radiolabeled tryptophan. Examples of such methods include constant intravenous infusion of high specific activity of L-tryptophan and correlation of the change of specific activity in plasma tryptophan and brain 5-HT with time (81); injection of labeled tryptophan intraventricularly (6); and administration of an MAO inhibitor (pargyline) followed by L-^{3}H-tryptophan and measurement of the amount of ^{3}H-5-HT synthesis (131). Neff et al. (100) developed a procedure to measure the rates of synthesis of DA, NE, and 5-HT *in vivo* in the same group of animals after a pulse injection of tracer doses of radioactive tyrosine and tryptophan.

Related Enzymes

Enzymes involved in the biosynthesis of the biogenic amines (tyrosine hydroxylase, dopamine-β-hydroxylase, and tryptophan hydroxylase), as well as one involved in their destruction (monoamine oxidase), are often assayed in order to obtain additional (sometimes essential) information.

Tyrosine Hydroxylase

Three main methods are being used for the determination of tyrosine hydroxylase (TH) activity. The first method was introduced by Nagatsu et al. (98) and is based on the conversion of labeled tyrosine to DOPA; the DOPA formed is then absorbed onto alumina and eluted with acid. The radioactivity is determined using liquid scintillation spectrophotometry. The second method, introduced by Nagatsu et al. (97) and Pomerantz (112), is based on the release of tritiated water from 3,5-^{3}H-tyrosine. The third method is based on the coupled decarboxylation of the DOPA formed from L-1-^{14}C-tyrosine (156). The following two procedures are often used to determine TH activity in small tissue samples of different regions of the central nervous system.

Modified DOPA method

The DOPA method (98), as modified by Coyle (26), is as follows.

Preparation of tissue. Using a smooth glass homogenizer with a tightly fitting Teflon pestle (Kontes Glass, No. 88600), brain tissue is homogenized in 10 volumes (w/v) of ice-cold 0.05 M Tris-HCl buffer (pH 6.0) containing 0.2% Triton X-100 (v/v). The homogenates are centrifuged at 10,000 $\times$ g for 10 min, and the supernatant fluid is decanted for assay.

Purification of L-^{3}H-tyrosine. Side chain (2,3)-labeled L-^{3}H-tyrosine (specific activity, 13.5 Ci/mmol) is purified as follows: 1 mCi is diluted to 5 ml with 0.2 N sodium acetate buffer (pH 8.6) and stirred with 400 mg alumina. The alumina suspension is poured over a column of 400 mg of activated alumina and washed with 5 ml of water. The total effluent is titrated to pH 3 with 1 N HCl and applied to a Dowex-50 H$^+$ column (0.5 $\times$ 3.0 cm). The column is washed with 100 ml of water followed by 2 ml of 2 N HCl. The tyrosine is then eluted with 20 ml of 2 N HCl. The eluate is evaporated to dryness in a flash evaporator (Laboratory Glass Supply Co.), and the purified L-^{3}H-tyrosine is redissolved in 10 ml of absolute ethanol and stored until use at $-20°$C.

Immediately prior to an experiment, a portion of the ethanol solution of L-^{3}H-tyrosine (prepared as described above) is dried under a stream of nitrogen and redissolved in 0.2 N sodium acetate buffer (pH 8.6). After addition of approximately 1 mg of alumina, the suspension is mixed on a Vortex mixer. It is then centrifuged at 6,000 $\times$ g for 10 min, and a portion of the supernatant is mixed with an equal volume of a solution of 4 mM L-tyrosine in 0.2 N sodium acetate buffer (pH 8.6). ^{14}C-DOPA (specific activity 52 mCi/mmol), to be used as internal standard, is purified by chromatography over alumina and stored until use in 0.2 N HCl at $-20°$C.

Assay procedure. Fifty microliters of the supernatant of the brain homogenate are added to 15-ml glass-stoppered centrifuge tubes containing the following reaction mixture: 10 μl of 1 M KPO$_4$ buffer (pH 5.5), 10 μl of sheep liver dihydropteridine reductase, 11,000 units of catalase (Boehringer Chemical Co.) in 10 μl of glass-distilled water, 5 μl of 0.01 M TPNH (Boehringer), and 5 μl of 6.4 mM 2-amino-4-hydroxy-6,7-dimethyltetrahydropteridine (DMPH$_4$; Aldrich Chemical Co.) freshly prepared in ice-cold 0.005 M HCl. Blanks consisting of supernatant fluid heated to 95°C for 5 min are run in all experiments, as are internal standards consisting of 15,000 cpm of ^{14}C-DOPA in place of L-^{3}H-tyrosine. The reaction is initiated by the addition of 10 μl of

2.0 m*M* L-³H-tyrosine and is incubated for 10 to 60 min at 37°C in room air. The reaction is terminated by the addition of 6 ml of 0.4 *N* perchloric acid containing 6 μg of carrier L-DOPA.

The perchlorate-inactivated incubation mixture is centrifuged at 1,000 × g for 10 min. The resulting supernatant is added to a 20-ml beaker containing 30 mg of sodium bisulfate, 5 ml of 2% EDTA (w/v), 1.5 ml of 0.35 *M* KH₂PO₄, and 200 mg alumina. The mixture is stirred and titrated to pH 8.6 with 1 *N* NaOH. The suspension is then poured over columns containing 200 mg of activated alumina and washed with 20 ml of glass-distilled water. The ³H-DOPA is eluted with 2.5 ml of 0.2 *N* acetic acid, and the total eluate is collected in counting vials containing 15 ml of Triton phosphor. Radioactivity is determined in a liquid scintillation counter.

Modified tritiated water method

The tritiated water method (97), as modified by Cicero et al. (22), requires only milligram amounts of tissue, which makes it especially useful for studies in specific brain areas. The procedure is as follows: The incubation solution contains 0.1 m*M* L-tyrosine containing approximately 200,000 cpm of L-tyrosine [3,5-³H], 0.5 m*M* ferrous ammonium sulfate, 0.67 m*M* DMPH₄, 0.12 *M* 2-mercaptoethanol, and 0.2 *M* sodium acetate buffer (pH 6.0).

Incubation is initiated by the addition of 10 μl of tissue homogenates (equivalent to approximately 2 mg wet weight of tissue) to 110 μl of incubation solution. After incubation for 30 min at 37°C, the reaction is terminated by adding 400 μl of ice-cold trichloroacetic acid (TCA; 5% w/v). The mixture is then centrifuged at 2,000 rpm for 10 min, and the supernatants are transferred to chromatography columns (e.g., Bio-Rad). The incubation tubes are washed with 1,000 and 500 μl of water and the washings transferred to the columns. The combined eluates are collected in scintillation vials; after addition of scintillation cocktail, radioactivity is measured in a liquid scintillation counter. Enzyme activity is linear over a range of tissue weights from 0.5 to 3.0 mg.

Coupled decarboxylation of DOPA

Coupled decarboxylation of DOPA formed from 1-¹⁴C-L-tyrosine (156) may be performed. This assay is based on the differential affinity of aromatic L-amino acid decarboxylase for L-tyrosine and L-DOPA. By starting with carboxyl-labeled tyrosine as substrate, carboxyl-labeled DOPA is formed as product. An excess amount of decarboxylase is added to the tyrosine hydroxylase reaction medium, and the radioactive CO₂ preferentially liberated from the DOPA formed during the tyrosine hydroxylase catalyzed reaction is collected and measured. Crude brain enzyme is prepared as a 1:10 homogenate in glass-distilled water. The assay medium contains (in a total volume of 0.5 ml) 100 μmol of sodium acetate buffer (pH 6.1); 0.5 μmol of ferrous sulfate; 1 μmol of DMPH₄; 20 μmol of 2-mercaptoethanol; 1 μmol of sodium phosphate; 7.5 units of hog kidney aromatic L-amino acid decarboxylase; 5 nmol pyridoxal phosphate; brain homogenate; and 0.05 μmol 1-¹⁴C-L-tyrosine (10 μCi/μmol, 1.1 ×

10⁶ dpm). The reaction is carried out with shaking for various time intervals at 37°C in a 10-ml Erlenmeyer flask, which is covered by a rubber injection vial cap. A plastic vial (Kontes Glass Co., K-882320) is suspended from the rubber injection stopper and contains a folded paper wick and 0.2 ml NCS solubilizer to trap ¹⁴CO₂ formed in the decarboxylation step of the assay. The reaction is stopped by injection of 0.5 ml 10% TCA. Following the injection of TCA to terminate the reaction, acidified medium is shaken at 37°C for an additional 2 hr to recover all ¹⁴CO₂. The plastic vials are removed, wiped with absorbent tissue, placed in 15 ml of scintillation fluid (0.5 g of dimethyl POPOP and 4.0 g PPO/L of toluene), and counted by liquid scintillation spectrometry.

Dopamine-β-Hydroxylase

Dopamine-β-hydroxylase (DβH) is the enzyme that catalyzes the β-hydroxylation of DA in the biosynthesis of NE (70). The early assay procedures have measured the β-hydroxylated products formed from either DA or tyramine (28). When DA is used as the substrate, the NE formed may be measured either fluorometrically or chromatographically (79). If tyramine is the substrate, the resulting β-hydroxylated product, octopamine, can proceed to periodate cleavage, forming *p*-hydroxybenzaldehyde, which can be measured either spectrophotometrically (111) or radiometrically (42).

A relatively sensitive and rapid procedure for the determination of DβH activity was later developed by Molinoff et al. (95). The assay involves coupled enzymatic reactions in which the β-hydroxylated product of the DβH reaction is made radioactive by the transfer of a ¹⁴C-methyl group from *S*-adenosylmethionine methyl-¹⁴C (¹⁴C-SAM). The latter reaction is catalyzed by phenylethanolamine-*N*-methyltransferase (PNMT), an enzyme with high specificity for β-hydroxylated amines (3). The final reaction product is separated from the radioactive *S*-adenosylmethionine by solvent extraction, and its radioactivity is determined. The reaction sequence utilized in this assay when phenylethylamine is the substrate is shown as follows:

$$\text{Phenylethylamine} \xrightarrow{\text{D}\beta\text{H}} \text{phenylethanolamine}$$
$$\xrightarrow[\text{}^{14}\text{C-SAM}]{\text{PNMT}} {}^{14}\text{C-}N\text{-methylphenylethanolamine}$$

When tyramine is used as the substrate, the tyramine is converted to octopamine, which yields *N*-methyloctopamine (synephrine) in the presence of PNMT (3).

DβH assay

Tissues to be used for the DβH assay are weighed and then homogenized in 25 volumes of 0.005 *M* Tris buffer (pH 7.5) containing 0.1% Triton X-100. Homogenates are centrifuged at 10,000 × g for 10 min, and the liquid layer is removed by aspiration. Supernatant fluid, 200 μl, is added to a 15-ml glass-stoppered centrifuge tube containing the following reaction mixture: 25 μl of 0.048 *M* ascorbic acid (pH 6); 25 μl of 0.5 *M* sodium fumarate (pH 6); 20 μl of 0.006 *M* MAO inhibitor pargyline; 1,500 units of catalase in 10 μl of 0.03 *M* phenylethylamine; 10 μl of 1.0 *M* Tris buffer (pH 6); and

10 μl of 9.7×10^{-5} M $CuSO_4$. The reaction mixture (total volume 310 μl) is incubated at 37°C for 20 min. The DβH portion of the assay is then stopped and the PNMT reaction initiated by adding to each tube 100 μl of a mixture of 10 μl of purified PNMT, 10 μl of ^{14}C-SAM (1 μmol), and 80 μl of 1.0 M Tris buffer (pH 8.6). The PNMT reaction is allowed to proceed for 30 min at 37°C and then is terminated by the addition of 0.5 ml of borate buffer (pH 10). The ^{14}C-N-methylphenylethanolamine is extracted into 6 ml of toluene containing 3% isoamyl alcohol by vigorous shaking on a Vortex mixer for 15 sec. After centrifugation at low speed, 4 ml of the organic phase are transferred to a counting vial containing 10 ml of phosphor for determination of radioactivity in a liquid scintillation counter. Blanks consisting of tissue homogenates heated to 95°C for 5 min are run in all experiments, as are internal standards consisting of the reaction mixture and 100 ng of phenylethanolamine. The internal standard is used in the calculation of absolute amounts of DβH activity and corrects for any inhibition of PNMT.

When tyramine is used as the substrate, the assay is carried out in a similar way, except that 10 μl of 0.03 M tyramine is used as substrate and 40 ng of octopamine HCl is used as the internal standard. After the reaction is stopped with borate buffer, the ^{14}C-N-methyloctopamine formed is extracted into a mixture of toluene and isoamyl alcohol (3:2, v/v). After centrifugation, a 4-ml sample of the organic phase is transferred to a counting vial containing an additional 2 ml of toluene/isoamyl alcohol (3:2). The sample is then dried in a chromatography oven at 80°C. This drying step is necessary to remove volatile radioactive contaminants, which are extracted into the toluene/isoamyl alcohol (94). After drying, the residue is dissolved in 1 ml of ethanol; after the addition of 10 ml of phosphor, radioactivity is determined in a liquid scintillation counter.

Tryptophan Hydroxylase

Tryptophan hydroxylase occurs in extremely small amounts in most tissues; therefore its assay requires sensitive radiometric procedures. The following reasons also make the assay of tryptophan hydroxylase difficult: nonenzymatic hydroxylation of tryptophan occurs unless precautions are taken (48); when radioactive tryptophan is used as a substrate, it is difficult to separate and assay the product 5-HTP; and when the reaction proceeds to 5-HT, the risk of tryptophan decarboxylation to tryptamine and the contamination of 5-HT may be present.

There are at least three major procedures that are currently being used. Two are described briefly, and one is outlined in considerable detail.

1. Assay using DL-5-^{3}H-tryptophan as a substrate. This assay is based on the intramolecular migration of tritium during enzymatic tryptophan hydroxylation (118), when 5-^{3}H-tryptophan is converted to 5-(4-^{3}H)-hydroxytryptophan. The tritium atom in the 4-position of the 5-hydroxyindole exchanges readily with H_2O under acidic conditions. Renson (117), Lovenberg et al. (82), and Gal and Millard (43) have used this assay successfully.

2. Direct measurement of 5-HTP by the method of Freedman et al. (41). With this method, L-tryptophan is incubated with tissue preparations in the presence of an aromatic amino acid decarboxylase inhibitor. The product 5-HTP is then directly assayed by a fluorometric method. The method appears to work well with partially purified and rather active enzyme preparations. However, it may be difficult to use with crude brain preparations.

3. Incubation of tissue with carboxyl-labeled ^{14}C-tryptophan. This method was first described by Ichiyama et al. (62,63). After tryptophan hydroxylation has occurred, aromatic amino acid decarboxylase is added, and then labeled ^{14}CO_2 produced from the decarboxylation of 5-HTP is trapped and counted. This method has been successfully employed by Ichiyama et al. (63), Deguchi and Barchas (31), and Knapp and Mandell (74). The procedure is described in some detail below.

Preparation of enzyme

Brain tissue (usually brainstem) is homogenized with an appropriate volume of medium in a Potter-Elvehjem-type homogenizer with a Teflon pestle. All subsequent operations are carried out at 4°C. The crude mitochondrial fraction is prepared from the 10% homogenate in 0.32 M sucrose. The particulate fraction is pelleted by centrifugation for 20 min at $12,000 \times g$ and suspended in 0.32 M sucrose to make 3 ml of suspension from 1 g of the starting tissue using the homogenizer. Approximately 1 g of the starting tissue yields about 30 mg of protein in the crude mitochondrial fraction. The supernatant fraction is obtained from the 33% homogenate of the brainstem in 0.02 M Tris-acetate (pH 8.1) containing 10^{-3} M dithiothreitol by centrifugation for 30 min at $105,000 \times g$. Usually 1 g of the starting tissue yields 1.8 ml of the supernatant fluid containing approximately 15 mg of protein per milliliter.

Assay procedure

Tryptophan hydroxylase is assayed by measuring the rate of ^{14}CO_2 formation from the substrate L-tryptophan (side chain 1-^{14}C). Two standard assay systems are used. The first assay system is used for the homogenate or crude mitochondrial fraction. The reaction mixture (0.5 ml) contains 50 μmol of Tris-acetate (pH 8.1), 125 μmol of sucrose, 30 to 60 nmol of L-tryptophan-^{14}C (approximately 100,000 cpm), and 0.15 ml of the enzyme preparation. The second assay system is used for the soluble tryptophan hydroxylase. The reaction mixture (0.5 ml) contains 50 μmol of Tris-acetate buffer (pH 8.1), 0.3 μmol of DMPH$_4$, 1.2 μmol of dithiothreitol, 100 nmol of pyridoxal phosphate, 10 nmol of ferrous ammonium sulfate, L-tryptophan-^{14}C as in the first assay system, 30 μg of catalase, 5 to 10 units of aromatic L-amino acid decarboxylase, and 0.1 ml of the enzyme. The reaction is carried out for 60 min at 37°C in a test tube (diameter 1.6 cm, length 10 cm) that is connected via thick rubber tubing to a counting vial. The vial contains a filter paper strip (Whatman No. 3MM: width 1.7 cm, length 8 cm) that is immersed in 0.3 ml of a 20% solution of 2-phenylethylamine in methanol.

At the end of the incubation period, 0.8 ml of 4% perchloric acid containing 2×10^{-3} M triton is injected through the rubber tube. The acidified reaction mixture is incubated for an additional 3 hr at 37°C with gentle shaking or allowed to stand for 12 hr at 4°C. To each vial, 10 ml of scintillation solution consisting of 2.5 g PPO and 150 mg POPOP in 1 L of toluene is added. Radioactivity is determined in a liquid scintillation spectrometer. A blank incubation is carried out for all experiments; the blank contains all the ingredients listed above except that the enzyme preparation has been boiled for 5 min. The nonenzymic evolution of $^{14}CO_2$ is subtracted from the value for the experimental incubations. The amount of CO_2 formed is calculated from the specific activity of the 1-carbon atom, which is expected to be the same as that of the L-tryptophan (side chain 1-^{14}C) used as substrate.

Monoamine Oxidase

The enzymatic oxidation of amines is associated with the uptake of oxygen and the production of ammonia, hydrogen peroxide, and the corresponding oxidation products of the amine. All of these parameters and the disappearance of substrate have been used as a basis for assaying these enzymes (167). Greater sensitivity in assaying amine oxidases has been obtained, based either on the reaction of o-dianisidine with evolved hydrogen peroxide (46) or on the extraction of oxidation products of specific substrates and their determination by fluorometric (83) or radiometric (104,109,165) procedures. For further differentiation between two forms of monoamine oxidase—MAO-A and MAO-B (67)—the method of Garrick and Murphy is available (44). The sensitivity of the fluorescence assay procedure developed by Snyder and Hendley (137) is similar to that of the radiometric assays and permits the use of multiple substrates and continuous monitoring. The procedure of Snyder and Hendley (137) is described here.

The tissues are homogenized in 5 to 20 volumes of ice-cold 0.1 M Na-K phosphate buffer in a motor-driven glass homogenizer. Aliquots of whole homogenate are taken for monoamine oxidase assay. The assay mixture contains, in a final volume of 3 ml: 0.1 M Na-K phosphate buffer (pH 7.8); 0.04 mg of horseradish peroxidase (Calbiochem); 1 to 2 units of tissue enzyme preparation; 0.25 mg of homovanillic acid; and appropriate amine substrate. Before the addition of homovanillic acid and substrate, the reaction vessels (tubes) are preincubated for 10 min to remove endogenous substrates of H_2O_2-producing enzymes. Preincubation is performed in a Dubnoff metabolic shaker at 37°C. This procedure lowers tissue blanks 15 to 45%. After preincubation, homovanillic acid and substrate are added, and the tubes are incubated for 60 min at 37°C with shaking. The reaction is terminated by chilling the tubes to 4°C. Fluorescence intensity is measured in a spectrophotofluorometer (Aminco-Bowman) at an activation wavelength of 315 nm and an emission wavelength of 425 nm. The tubes are then centrifuged in the cold for 20 min at 12,000 $\times$ g before the fluorescence of the supernatant fraction is measured. Under these conditions, sampling aliquots at 10-min intervals showed that enzyme activity is linear for 90 min.

Blanks containing tissue enzyme but no added substrate are subtracted for calculation of enzyme activity. A calibration curve is determined in each experiment by adding increasing amounts of freshly prepared standard hydrogen peroxide solution, 1 mM, to a cuvette containing (in 3 ml): 0.1 M Na-K phosphate buffer (pH 7.8); horseradish peroxidase 0.04 mg; and homovanillic acid 0.25 mg. The exact molarity of the stock H_2O_2 solution is determined by titration with $KMnO_4$. The resultant fluorescence readings are used to calculate equivalent millimicromoles of substrate oxidized per hour. Fluorescence readings equivalent to twice the blank reading are obtained with 1 mmol of hydrogen peroxide.

Neurotransmitter Receptors

The biochemical characterization of receptors for neurotransmitters is a rapidly developing field. Different biogenic amines have multiple receptors (136) that may mediate different functions in the central nervous system (24). For example, D_1 and D_2 for dopamine, β, α_1, and α_2 for norepinephrine, and 5-HT$_1$ (62) and 5-HT$_2$ (61) for serotonin are being identified. The details of the characterization of various receptors are available (153). The following sections provide methods for biogenic amine receptor binding studies.

NE

α_1-Receptor

The method to measure α_1-receptors using [^{3}H]prazosin as ligand was described by Menkes et al. (93). It is a modification of a method described by Greengrass and Bremner (50). Brain regions are homogenized in 200 volumes of ice-cold 50 mM Tris HCl (pH 7.4) using a Brinkman Polytron (15 sec, setting 8). Following centrifugation at 39,000 $\times$ g, pellets are rehomogenized and centrifuged three times in the same buffer. For binding assays, membranes are resuspended in 50 mM Tris HCl (pH 8.0). Amount of protein needed for the assay depends on the regions studied. For instance, in thalamic membranes binding of [^{3}H]prazosin is linear with tissue concentration in the range of 0.25 to 1.80 mg protein/ml. For cerebral cortex, [^{3}H]prazosin binding to these membranes is linear with tissue concentration of 0.219 to 1.29 mg protein/ml.

Incubation mixtures (final volume 1 ml) contain [^{3}H]prazosin and 0.05% ascorbic acid, with or without 150 mM NaCl. The binding reaction is initiated by adding the membrane suspension (0.8 ml), and it is allowed to continue for 30 min at 25°C. The incubation is terminated by rapid filtration through Whatman GF/B filters, with three 6-ml rinses with ice-cold 50 mM Tris HCl (pH 7.4). Specific binding is defined as that displaceable by the α_1-antagonist (WB-4101 10^{-6} M; Ward-Blenkinsop). At ligand concentrations in the range of 1 nM, specific binding constitutes 75 to 80% of total binding. To estimate the density and affinity of [^{3}H]prazosin sites, concentrations ranging from 0.03 to 1.5 nM [^{3}H]prazosin are usually used. Samples are counted by liquid scintillation counter.

α_2-Receptor

The methods described by Cheung et al. (21) and Meller et al. (92) are outlined here. Tissues are homogenized in 20 volumes of ice-cold 5 mM Tris-HCl, 5 mM EDTA buffer, with an ultra-turrax homogenizer (two 10-sec bursts). The suspension is then centrifuged at 27,000 $\times$ g for 10 min at 4°C. The resulting pellet is washed once more with the same buffer by resuspension followed by centrifugation at 27,000 $\times$ g for 10 min at 4°C. One final washing is carried out by resuspending the pellet in ice-cold "assay buffer" [50 mM Tris-HCl, 0.5 mM EDTA, 0.1% ascorbate (pH 7.5)] and then centrifuging at 27,000 $\times$ g for 10 min at 4°C. The final pellet is resuspended in an appropriate volume (equivalent to 6 or 10 mg wet weight) for assay buffer.

Binding assays with [^{3}H]yohimbine are performed in a final volume of 250 ml assay buffer. This buffer is 50 mM Tris-HCl (pH 7.7), containing 0.5 mM Na$_2$EDTA. Following incubation at 25°C for 30 min, membranes are collected on Whatman GF/B filters under vacuum and rapidly washed three times with 5-ml ice-cold buffer. Nonspecific binding is estimated in the presence of 5 μM phentolamine HCl.

β-Receptor

The method of Schweitzer et al. (126) using [^{3}H]-dihydroalprenolol (^{3}H-DHA) as a ligand is described here.

The cerebral cortices are removed, homogenized using a Brinkmann Polytron (model PT-10 ST, setting 6, 20 sec) in 10 to 30 volumes of ice-cold 0.05 M Tris (pH 8.0 at 25°C), and centrifuged at 49,000 $\times$ g for 15 min. The pellet is re-homogenized in the same buffer and centrifuged again. The pellet is then resuspended in 97 ml of the buffer per gram of original wet weight of tissue. If catecholamines are to be used as ligands, 0.1% ascorbic acid and 1 μM pargyline are added to prevent destruction of the catecholamines. Inhibition of [^{3}H]DHA binding by (−)-alprenolol or 10^{-6} M (−)1-propranolol is the same with or without these additions.

[^{3}H]DHA binding is determined at 23°C by adding 10 μl of the appropriate concentration of the drug to 0.97 ml of the above particulate suspension (representing 10 mg of tissue, or about 0.4 mg of protein) followed by about 66,000 dpm of [^{3}H]DHA in 20 μl of water (final [^{3}H]DHA concentration, 1 nM). After 15 to 20 min the reaction mixtures are filtered under reduced pressure through Whatman glass fibers (GF/B). The filters are rinsed four times with 4 ml of ice-cold Tris buffer and placed in plastic vials along with 12 ml of Hydromix (Yorktown Research). The vials are mechanically shaken for 2 hr and then stored at 4°C for 6 to 24 hr, until the radioactivity is measured. The extent of nonspecifically bound [^{3}H]DHA is estimated from parallel assay tubes that contain a large excess (1 μM) of (−)-alprenolol. Specific binding, defined as the difference between total and nonspecific binding, is 70 to 80% of the total binding.

DA

D_1-DA receptor

The method of Porceddu et al. (113) using ^{3}H-SCH 23390 (13) as a ligand is described. Tissue is homogenized in 100 volumes of ice-cold 50 mM Tris-HCl buffer (pH 7.4). The homogenate is centrifuged (48,000 $\times$ g, 10 min), and the pellet is resuspended in the initial volume of the same buffer and recentrifuged. The final pellet is then resuspended in 50 mM Tris-HCl buffer (pH 7.4) containing 120 mM NaCl, 5 mM KCl, 2 mM CaCl$_2$, and 1 mM MgCl$_2$. For the binding assays 400-μl aliquots of the membrane preparations (approximately 250 μg protein) are incubated with different concentrations (0.098–6.000 nM) of ^{3}H-SCH 23390 (specific activity 80 Ci/mmol) in a final volume of 0.5 ml. Nonspecific binding is determined by adding 10^{-6} M unlabeled SCH 23390. After a 20-min incubation at 37°C the reaction is stopped by adding 4 ml of ice-cold 50 mM Tris-HCl buffer (pH 7.4), and the membranes are filtered under vacuum through Whatman GF/B filters. After three additional washings with 4 ml of the same buffer, the filters are placed in plastic vials containing 3 ml scintillation fluid. Specifically bound ^{3}H-SCH 23390 is defined as the difference between total binding and binding in the presence of 10^{-6} M unlabeled SCH 23390. The maximum number of binding sites (Bmax) and the apparent dissociation constant (KD) are calculated by linear regression analysis of Scatchard plots corresponding to saturation curves of specific ^{3}H-SCH 23390 binding.

D_2-DA receptor

Specific binding of D_2-DA receptor ligand [^{3}H]spiroperidol is determined following the methods used by Sivam et al. (133). Brain membranes are prepared according to the method of Zukin et al. (168) with slight modification as described (133). The samples are homogenized in 15 volumes of ice-cold 0.32 M sucrose using a Brinkman Polytron PT-10 at low speed (setting 3). The homogenate is centrifuged at 1,000 $\times$ g for 10 min; the pellet is discarded, and the supernatant fluid is centrifuged at 20,000 $\times$ g for 20 min to obtain a crude mitochondrial pellet. The crude mitochondrial pellet is then resuspended in double-distilled deionized water and dispersed with a Brinkman Polytron PT-10 (setting 6) for 30 sec. The suspension is centrifuged at 8,000 $\times$ g for 20 min. The supernatant including the buffer layer is collected and centrifuged at 48,000 $\times$ g for 20 min to obtain a pellet. The pellet is resuspended in water and centrifuged at 48,000 $\times$ g for 20 min. The final membrane preparation is suspended in 50 mM sodium phosphate buffer (pH 7.4).

Before the assays, the frozen membrane preparation is thawed and centrifuged at 25,000 $\times$ g for 15 min to obtain a pellet. The pellet is suspended in 50 mM Tris-HCl (pH 7.4) containing 5 mM EDTA (Tris-EDTA buffer). The suspension is incubated for 20 min at 37°C and centrifuged at 25,000 $\times$ g for 15 min. The supernatant is discarded, and the pellet is resuspended for final assay in a suitable volume of Tris-EDTA buffer.

Aliquots (0.2 ml) of the membrane preparation (2.0–2.5 mg/ml) are incubated with various concentrations (0.05–2.0 nM) of [^{3}H]spiroperidol in the presence of 10^{-7} M (+)- or (−)-butaclamol (127) in a final volume of 1 ml. Incubations are carried out for 20 min at 25°C. At the end of the incubation the samples are filtered under reduced pressure through glass fiber filters (GF/B, Whatman). The filters are then washed with 5 ml of Tris-EDTA buffer and after drying are placed in scintillation vials with 10 ml of Aquasol. After at least 45 min of shaking to equilibrate, the radioactivity is quantified by liquid scintillation spectrophotometry. Specific binding of spiroperidol is defined as the amount bound in the presence of $10^{-7} M$ (−)-butaclamol minus that bound in the presence of $10^{-7} M$ (+)-butaclamol.

5-HT

S_1-5-HT receptor

The methods of Bennet and Snyder (8), Nelson et al. (102), and Pedigo et al. (110) using [³H]5-HT as a ligand are described. The tissue is homogenized in 40 volumes of Tris-HCl buffer (0.05 M, pH 7.4) using a Brinkman Polytron. This homogenate is centrifuged at $48,000 \times g$ for 10 min. The pellet is resuspended and the process repeated three times. The membrane suspension is incubated at 37°C for 10 min between the second and third washes to facilitate removal of endogenous 5-HT. The final pellet is resuspended in Tris buffer (50–100 ml/g of original tissue weight) for use in the assay.

For the binding of [³H]5-HT, various concentrations (0.4–7.4 nM) of [³H]5-HT are added to glass tubes containing the tissue homogenate (0.5 ml) and Tris-HCl buffer (2 ml final volume). In addition to the [³H]5-HT and tissue homogenate, the tubes contain 5.7 mM ascorbate, 10 μM pargyline, 4 mM calcium chloride, and 50 mM Tris (pH 7.4) at 37°C. Incubations are carried out at 37°C for 7 min and are then terminated by vacuum filtration (Whatman GF/B filters). The filters are washed with three 5-ml volumes of the buffer. Radioactivity on the filters is measured by liquid scintillation spectrometry. Specific [³H]5-HT binding is defined as the difference between total binding and that occurring in the presence of either 0.3 μl unlabeled 5-HT or 1 μM metergoline (103). It represents 60 to 80% of the total radioactivity bound.

S_2-5-HT receptor

The method of Leysen et al. (80) using [³H]ketanserine as a ligand is described. The brain tissue is immediately placed in ice-cold 0.25 M sucrose (1:10, w/v) and homogenized with the use of a Potter Elvejhem conical glass tube and motor-driven Teflon pestle (four strokes at 120 rpm). Nuclei and cell debris are removed by centrifugation at $1,000 \times g$ for 10 min. The pellet is rehomogenized in 0.25 M sucrose (1:5, w/v) as above and centrifuged. Combined supernatants are diluted in Tris buffer (see below) to 1:40 (w/v). The suspension is centrifuged at $35,000 \times g$ for 10 min. The pellet is washed once by resuspension in the same volume of Tris buffer and centrifuged at $35,000 \times g$ for 10 min. The final pellet contains washed membranes of a total mitochondrial plus microsomal subcellular fraction. It is then suspended in Tris buffer using a motor-driven Teflon pestle and conical glass tube as above. The final concentration of the membrane suspension used for binding assays corresponds to 2.5 mg (original wet weight) of tissue per milliliter. The composition of Tris buffer is 50 mM Tris-HCl (pH 7.7).

With the standard procedure for [³H]ketanserin binding assays, the incubation mixture is composed of 4 ml of a freshly prepared membrane suspension in buffer and 0.2 ml of [³H]ketanserin (5.0–10.2 nM) in 10% ethanol. The mixture is incubated for 15 min at 37°C and rapidly filtered under reduced pressure through GF/B glass-fiber filter discs (2.5 cm diameter). Filters are rapidly rinsed three times with 5 ml of ice-cold Tris buffer. Filters are transferred to plastic counting vials, and 6 ml of Instagel (Packard) is added, followed by vigorous shaking for 10 min. The vials are stored for 12 hr at 4°C in the dark. Thereafter radioactivity is counted in a liquid scintillation spectrometer. Specific [³H]ketanserin binding is obtained by subtracting nonspecific binding, determined in assays containing (5 μM) unlabeled methysergide.

ACETYLCHOLINE

Bioassay procedures were once the only methods sensitive enough to be useful for determination of acetylcholine. Experimental details are given by MacIntosh and Perry (86) and Whittaker and Barker (162,163). The sensitive (2.0–20.0 pmol/ml) bioassay methods are those using guinea pig ileum and the dorsal muscle of the leech (144). Another method using the guinea pig ileum assay (61) has sensitivity in the 0.01 to 0.10 pmol range.

Fluorometric, polarographic, enzymatic radiochemical, gas chromatographic, and liquid chromatographic methods for the estimation of acetylcholine have been described. Fluorometric determination of the NADPH produced by coupled reactions has been described by Cooper (23), O'Neil and Sakamoto (108), and Browning (16). The sensitivity of these methods is in the range of 200 to 2,000 pmol. Fellman (37) has measured fluorescence of the salicylhydrazone formed from acetylcholine. The sensitivity of this method is also in the range of 200 to 2,000 pmol.

Two reaction sequences have been utilized in the enzymatic radiochemical assays. One is the quantitative acetylation of choline derived from enzymatic hydrolysis of acetylcholine by means of (acetyl-¹⁴C)-acetyl-CoA and choline acetyltransferase (35,129). The sensitivity of this assay is in the range of 50 to 2,000 pmol. The other procedure involves hydrolysis of acetylcholine followed by quantitative phosphorylation of the liberated choline using γ-³²P-ATP and choline kinase (45,116). This method, as described by Goldberg and McCaman (45), is about ten times more sensitive than the assay procedure using choline acetyltransferase. Because choline is a ubiquitous constituent of nervous tissues, it must be removed prior to the assay of acetylcholine by either of the above methods.

Gas chromatographic determination of acetylcholine involves conversion of the ester to a volatile compound. N-Demethylation with sodium benzene thiolate (66) or via pyrolysis (146) has been used to produce dimethylaminoethyl acetate from acetylcholine. The sensitivity of the procedure is dependent on the means of detection. With flame ionization detectors, the sensitivity of the demethylation technique is 50 to 10,000 pmol (64); that of the pyrolysis technique is 200 to 10,000 pmol (145). By using a mass spectrometer as a selective detector for the gas chromatogram, it is possible to identify fragments specifically originating from less than 1 pmol of acetylcholine (53). The mass spectrometer in conjunction with the gas chromatograph has been used to provide a definitive identification of acetylcholine in rat brain (52), as this method increases the already considerable specificity of the demethylation method.

A high performance liquid chromatographic (HPLC) method for the determination of acetylcholine (ACh) and choline levels has been described by Potter et al. (115). The method is based on the separation of ACh and choline by reverse-phase HPLC. The effluent is mixed with acetylcholinesterase and choline oxidase as it emerges from the column. In this way, endogenous choline and choline produced by the hydrolysis of ACh are converted to betaine and hydrogen peroxide. Production of hydrogen peroxide is continuously monitored electrochemically. The sensitivity of the procedure is 1 pmol for choline and 2 pmol for ACh. We have chosen to describe, in detail, a gas chromatographic assay and an HPLC-electrochemical (EC) method.

Gas Chromatographic Method

The principle of the gas chromatographic method of Jenden et al. (66) for the determination of ACh and other choline esters is based on prior N-demethylation with Na benzenethiolate.

Purification of Solvents

Glass-distilled water is used and is boiled before use. Butanone (J. T. Baker, AR) is purified and dried by slow distillation from a Linde type 4A molecular sieve using a 60-cm glass helix fractionating column. Chloroform (J. T. Baker, Spectroquality) is shaken with an equal volume of 2 N NH$_4$OH until both phases are clear (2–4 hr) and then washed twice with 2 N H$_2$SO$_4$ and three times with glass-distilled water. It is stored with 1% absolute ethanol in a dark bottle. Pentane (M. C. B., Spectroquality) is treated like chloroform, above, and is stored in pure form. All organic solvents are stored in tinted, ground-glass-stoppered vessels and kept in a cool, dark place.

Preparation of Sodium Benzenethiolate

Thiophenol (Aldrich, T3280-8; 83 g, 0.75 mol) and 20 g (0.50 mol) of sodium hydroxide are warmed in 100 ml of anhydrous ethanol until solution occurs. Toluene (700 ml) is added, and the mixture is distilled slowly at atmospheric pressure; the product is crystallized out as the ethanol and water are distilled. An additional 600 ml of toluene is added in aliquots of 100 ml to maintain the volume of the boiling mixture at 500 to 600 ml. The product is then filtered (Whatman No. 42) under dry nitrogen and washed with boiling toluene.

The steps that follow are necessary to obtain a quantitative yield of dimethylaminoethyl acetate from ACh at high dilutions. The product from the above reaction is added to 200 ml of absolute ethanol and 5 ml of ethyl acetate, shaken

in an atmosphere of nitrogen until dissolved, and allowed to stand at room temperature for 60 hr. It is then filtered, and the solvents are removed by distillation as before. The benzenethiolate salt is recovered by filtration under dry nitrogen and washed with boiling toluene. It is immediately placed in a vented desiccator (Aquasorb, Mallinckrodt) over P$_2$O$_5$ (Granusic, Baker) together with 100 to 200 g of Dry Ice and left for 65 hr. The product is then rapidly transferred to individually sealed vials for storage. For the demethylation reaction, a solution containing 6 mg/ml (50 mM) sodium benzenethiolate in butanone is freshly prepared each day and stored under nitrogen until used.

Preparation of Hexyldimethylamine

Bromohexane (K and K Labs; 0.2 mol) is added slowly to a 25% methanolic solution of dimethylamine (0.4 mol) at 0°C; the mixture is allowed to warm spontaneously to 35°C and is left at room temperature for 60 hr. After boiling for 30 min, 250 ml of water and 8 g of NaOH are added. The solution is extracted twice with 50 ml of diethyl ether and is then dried with anhydrous MgSO$_4$. The product is precipitated as the hydrochloride by adding an excess of dry ethereal hydrogen chloride followed by recrystallization from ethanol/ethyl acetate. The melting point of the product, hexyldimethylamine (HDA), is 169° to 171°C.

Procedure for Demethylation Reaction

The sample to be tested, containing 0.5 to 25.0 nmol of ACh and a precisely known amount (e.g., 10 nmol) of HDA hydrochloride, is placed in a conical centrifuge tube (Corning No. 8122) fitted with a Teflon-lined screw cap and is evaporated to dryness. The sodium benzenethiolate reagent (0.5 ml) is added, and air is displaced from the remainder of the tube with a gentle stream of dry nitrogen. The tube is then tightly capped and placed in a waterbath at 80°C for 30 min, with shaking at 5-min intervals.

Extraction of Dimethylaminoethyl Acetate

The following procedure removes excess benzenethiolate and undesired reaction products, and concentrates dimethylaminoethyl acetate into a minimum volume while retaining a high consistent yield.

Following completion of the demethylation reaction, the tube is cooled and opened. After adding 0.1 ml of aqueous citric acid (0.5 M) and 2 ml of pentane, the contents are shaken vigorously and centrifuged (International Clinical Centrifuge, model CL) to achieve complete separation of phases. The upper organic layer is discarded, and the aqueous phase is washed twice with 1 ml of pentane; the remaining traces of pentane are removed by evaporation with a gentle stream of dry nitrogen. To the aqueous residue, 50 μl of chloroform and 0.1 ml of ammonium citrate (2 M) in ammonium hydroxide (7.5 M) are added, shaken vigorously, and centrifuged. An aliquot (approximately 5 μl) of the lower (organic) phase is injected into the gas chromatograph.

Gas Chromatography

An F and M 5750A dual-column gas chromatograph equipped with flame ionization detectors is employed, using a silanized glass column (6 ft × 0.25 inch) containing 80/120 mesh Polypak 1 (F and M), coated with 1% (w/w) phenyldiethanolamine succinate (PDEAS; Analabs). Injections are made with a Hamilton No. 701-N 10-μl syringe. Chromatographic runs are performed isothermally, and the column temperature is maintained at 180°C. Injection port and flame detector temperatures are 204° and 200°C, respectively. Nitrogen is used as carrier gas, at a rate of 45 ml/min (80 psi). Airflow is maintained at 280 ml/min (30 psi) and hydrogen at 30 ml/min (26 psi). Each gas is passed through special drying tubes containing Molecular Sieve (Linde, type 5A) before coming in contact with each other and with the chromatographic apparatus. Peaks are recorded on a Varian Associates Recorder, model G-2000.

HPLC-EC Determination of ACh and Choline

The HPLC-EC assay for ACh and choline was described by Potter et al. (115).

Reagents

The mobile phase consists of 0.01 M sodium acetate buffered to pH 5 with 0.02 M citric acid and containing sodium octyl sulfate 4.5 mg/L and 1.2 mM TMA. The mobile phase is delivered at a rate of 0.8 ml/min. The enzyme solution consists of 0.2 M sodium phosphate buffer (pH 8.5) to which is added choline oxidase 1 U/ml and acetylcholinesterase 2 U/ml. The enzyme solution is delivered at a rate of 0.5 ml/min. Acetylcholine and choline standards are prepared using 0.02 M citrate-phosphate buffer (pH 3.5). Ethylhomocholine [EHC: N,N-dimethyl(N-ethyl)-3-amino-1-propanol] is used as the internal standard and is prepared in the laboratory by placing 0.25 ml of dimethyl-3-amino-1-propanol (8.45 M) in a glass tube and slowly adding an equal volume of iodoethane (12.5 M). After 30 min at room temperature, 12 ml of diethyl ether are added to form a white precipitate. The ether is poured off, and the crystals are dried under vacuum.

Equipment

The system consists of an Altex 110A pump (Beckman, Palo Alto, California), a Rheodyne 7125 injector with a 20-μl sample loop (Hamilton Co., Berkeley, California), a Bio-Rad ODS-5 guard column, and a 15-cm Bio-Rad Bio-Sil ODS-5S reverse-phase column (Bio-Rad Laboratories, Richmond, California). The enzyme reagent solution is pumped by a Rainin E-120 (Rainin Instrument, Wolburn, Massachusetts) intermediate-pressure pump. Electrochemical detection is by a Bio Analytical Systems LC-4A amperometric detector equipped with a platinum electrode (Bio Analytical Systems, West Lafayette, Indiana). Electrode potential is set at +0.5 V versus an Ag/AgCl reference electrode.

Procedures

Animals are killed by head-focused microwave irradiation. Brains are removed and dissected. Tissue parts are homogenized in 3 ml of 0.4 M HClO$_4$ containing 2 nmol of EHC and centrifuged for 20 min at 35,000 × g. The pH of the supernatant is adjusted to 4.2 with approximately 200 μl of 7.5 M potassium acetate. The samples are centrifuged at 35,000 × g for 20 min, after which 100 μl of 5 mM tetraethylammonium is added to the supernatant. Then 3 ml ice-cold reineckate solution (2%, w/v) is added to precipitate quaternary ammonium compounds. After 1 hr the samples are centrifuged at 1,000 × g for 10 min at 0°C. The supernatant is aspirated and the precipitate dried under vacuum overnight. The next day, 5 mM silver tosylate in HPLC-grade acetonitrile is added, and the samples are centrifuged at 1,000 × g for 2 min. The supernatant is dried under nitrogen, after which 200 μl of 0.02 M citrate phosphate buffer (pH 3.5) is added. Each sample is then injected onto the column.

Turnover

The simultaneous measurement of endogenous ACh and precursor is required for the estimation of steady-state turnover of ACh in $vivo$. Schuberth et al. (125) and Haubrich et al. (56) injected radiolabeled choline intravenously and estimated brain ACh turnover from the ratio of labeled choline to radiolabeled ACh in the brain at various times following injection. Hanin et al. (54) have estimated ACh turnover in rat salivary glands by a radio-gas chromatographic method. Jenden et al. (65) have coupled gas chromatography and mass spectrometry to estimate the turnover of ACh in brain in $vivo$ following a pulse intravenous injection of choline, using discrete deuterium-labeled variants of choline and ACh as tracer and internal standards. The method described by Schuberth et al. (125) is detailed here.

Tritium-labeled (Me-^{3}H) choline (100 μCi, 0.5 μmol) is injected intravenously via the mouse tail vein. Special efforts are made to standardize the injection procedure. The mice are killed at different times after injection by immersion in liquid nitrogen. The brains are chiseled out and ground to a fine powder in a mortar containing liquid nitrogen. The brain powder is then transferred to tared centrifuge tubes containing 2 ml ice-cold 7% TCA and 4 μmol each of unlabeled choline and ACh chloride. After thorough mixing, the tubes are weighed and left in the refrigerator for 30 min, after which they are centrifuged at 12,000 × g for 5 min. Each pellet is then suspended in 1 ml ice-cold 7% TCA, without added carrier, and centrifuged again. Supernatants resulting from the two centrifugations are combined; after portions have been taken for assay of total radioactivity, they are extracted six times with 3-ml portions of ether (pH then being adjusted to 4). After the removal of TCA, 2 ml of a freshly prepared saturated aqueous solution of ammonium reineckate is added. The precipitate formed is isolated by centrifugation, dissolved in 0.5 ml acetone/water (1:1, v/v), and applied to an anion-exchange column (Dowex 2-X8 in chloride form, 70 × 8 mm).

The column is eluted with acetone/water (1:1) and the first 6 ml of the eluate collected. The eluate is evaporated to dryness *in vacuo* and dissolved in 0.1 ml of water. The radioactive components in 10 μl of the solutions are then separated by high voltage electrophoresis in 0.2 M acetate buffer at pH 4.6. The choline and ACh spots are visualized by iodine vapor and cut out. The paper strips are combusted in oxygen flasks, which are then cooled to $-10°C$, and 14 ml of scintillation solution (dioxane/naphthalene/PPO/POPOP) is subsequently added. The radioactivity is measured in a liquid scintillation counter. The radioactivity can also be separated by paper chromatography in *n*-butanol/ethanol/water (5:1:4).

In contrast to paper electrophoresis, ACh in this system moves in front of choline. Good agreement between the two systems is found regarding the amount of labeled choline and ACh in the brain extracts.

Related Enzymes

Choline Acetyltransferase

The radiochemical procedures are the most useful assays for choline acetyltransferase (ChAc). In general, the enzyme in homogenates is released by treatment with detergent (38) or ether (17,57) and incubated with 0.1 mM (acetyl-^{14}C)acetyl coenzyme A (CoA), 10 mM choline, 300 mM NaCl, EDTA, phosphate buffer (pH 7.4), and 0.1 mM eserine to prevent hydrolysis of the ester by cholinesterases. The thiol groups of the enzyme are best protected by NaCN or thioglycolate; cysteine is inhibitory because it is acetylated by acetyl CoA (96). Separation of the radioactive ACh formed can be achieved by precipitation of the reineckate salt (91), passage over ion-exchange resins (124), or liquid-phase cation exchange using tetraphenylboron in an organic solvent (39).

The last method is convenient and is the most sensitive, being capable of the determination of the ChAc in 50 μg of brain (39). The method is described below.

Chemicals

Sodium (1-^{14}C) acetate (specific activity 52 mCi/mmol) is used. The radioactive acetate is dissolved in water and stored frozen. Acetone-dried pigeon liver (Sigma Chemical Co., St. Louis, Missouri) is extracted with 20 mM KHCO$_3$, and the clear supernatant is gel-filtered on a column (10 ml) of Sephadex G-25 (coarse grade) equilibrated with 20 mM sodium phosphate buffer (pH 7.4). Sodium tetraphenylboron (Kalignost) is obtained from E. Merek A. G., Darmstadt, Germany.

Enzyme preparations

Homogenates (5%, w/v) of brain are prepared in 1 mM EDTA buffer (pH 7.0) in a Potter-Elvehjem homogenizer. The clearance between pestle and wall is 0.2 mm, and the pestle is rotated at 1,440 rpm. To release full enzyme activity, samples are treated with 0.5% Triton X-100. The homogenates are diluted with 1 mM EDTA to a final concentration of 5 μg wet weight of tissue/μl.

Standard assay procedure for ChAc

The incubation volume is 1 ml in the macro procedure and 2 μl in the micro procedure. When the incubation volume is 2 μl, 10 μl of cyclohexane is added as a cover to prevent evaporation. The presence of cyclohexane does not affect the enzyme activity of the extraction procedures. The incubation temperature is 37°C for both procedures, which are described below.

Macro procedure. The macro procedure is generally used when reaction volumes are larger than 50 μl. The incubation mixture contains 5 mM sodium (1-^{14}C) acetate (10^6 cpm), 12.5 mM choline, 300 mM NaCl, 50 mM NaF, 10 mM ATP, 0.1 mM eserine salicylate, 0.5 mM KBH$_4$, 2.5 mM MgCl$_2$, and extract from 12 mg of acetone-dried pigeon liver. The incubation is carried out in 10-ml centrifuge tubes with ground-glass stoppers. The mixture is incubated for 10 min to form acetyl CoA, and the reaction is started by adding enzyme. The reaction is terminated by adding 7 ml of an ACh chloride solution (0.5 mg/7 ml), followed immediately by 1 ml of butyl ethyl ketone containing 25 mg of sodium tetraphenylboron. After being shaken gently for 4 min, the tubes are centrifuged at 3,000 $\times$ g for 4 min in a swinging bucket rotor to separate the aqueous and organic phases. After gently stirring the ketone layer, proteins soon separate out as a flat layer at the interface between the two phases. When more than 10 mg of brain homogenate is used, it is advisable to extract with 2 ml of ketone. The ketone layer, containing acetylcholine, is transferred by a Pasteur pipette to another tube and is washed once with 4 ml of 10 mM sodium phosphate buffer (pH 7.4) containing 2 mg of sodium tetraphenylboron. After recentrifugation, a sample of the ketone layer (usually 0.5 ml) is transferred to a scintillation vial containing 2 ml of acetonitrile and 10 ml of toluene scintillation mixture. The radioactivity is determined in a liquid scintillation spectrometer.

Micro procedure, based on (1-^{14}C) acetate. The micro procedure is used for reaction volumes of less than 50 μl. The incubation mixture contains 2 mM sodium (1-^{14}C) acetate, extracted from 2.5 μg of acetone-dried pigeon liver/μl of incubation mixture, and other components as described above for the macro procedure. The incubation mixture (100 μl) is preincubated for 10 min, and 1 μl is transferred via a pipette to a small conical tube (2 mm diameter) containing the enzyme preparation. After incubation the tube is transferred to a 10-ml centrifuge tube containing 7 ml of 10 mM sodium phosphate buffer (pH 7.5) and 0.25 mg of ACh chloride. The phosphate buffer solution is flushed into the conical micro tube three times using a Pasteur pipette. This step washes the contents of the micro tube into the large tube. The ACh is extracted with 1 ml of butyl ethyl ketone containing 15 mg of tetraphenylboron. The ketone layer is isolated by centrifugation, transferred to a new tube, and washed with 4 ml of 10 mM sodium phosphate buffer containing 2 mg of sodium tetraphenylboron. After recentrifugation, the radioactivity of the ketone layer is determined as described above.

Acetylcholinesterase

A wide variety of methods are available for the determination of acetylcholinesterase (AChE). The hydrolysis of the ester is accompanied by the release of one equivalent of acid. It can be measured by Warburg manometry as CO_2 liberated from a bicarbonate buffer by the acid (151) or determined titrimetrically with an automated pH-stat (73). Radiochemical assays in which the ^{14}C-acetic acid produced by hydrolysis of acetyl-1-^{14}C-ACh is measured also have been used (40,114). The most commonly used method is that of Ellman et al. (32). The method involves formation of the colored 5-thio-2-nitrobenzoate anion by the reaction of thiocholine with 5,5'-dithiobis-2-nitrobenzoic acid. This method is described below.

Solutions

The solutions used are the following:

Phosphate buffer, 0.1 M (pH 8.0)
Acetylthiocholine iodide, 0.075 M (21.67 mg/ml); this substrate solution is used successfully for 10 to 15 days if kept refrigerated
5,5'-Dithiobis-2-nitrobenzoic acid (DTNB), 0.01 M; 39.6 mg is dissolved in 10 ml of 0.1 M phosphate buffer (pH 7.0), and 15 mg of sodium bicarbonate is added (this reagent is made up in pH 7 buffer, in which it is more stable than in pH 8 buffer)

Tissue preparations

The tissue is homogenized (approximately 20 mg of tissue/ml phosphate buffer; pH 8.0, 0.1 M) in a Potter-Elvehjem homogenizer.

Assay procedure

A 0.4-ml aliquot of the homogenate is added to a cuvette containing 2.6 ml of phosphate buffer (pH 8.0, 0.1 M). DTNB reagent (100 μl) is added to the photocell. The absorbance is measured at 412 nm; when it has stopped increasing, the photometer slit is opened so that the absorbance is set to zero. Substrate (20 μl) is added, and changes in absorbance per minute are calculated. The rates are calculated as follows:

$$R = \frac{{\sim}A}{1.36 \times 10^4} \times \frac{1}{(400/3,120)C_0} = 5.74 \times 10^{-4}{\sim}A/C_0$$

where R is the rate (in moles of substrate hydrolyzed per minute per gram of tissue), ${\sim}A$ is the change in absorbance per minute, and C_0 is the original concentration of tissue (milligrams per milliliter).

Receptors

Muscarinic Receptors

Tritiated quinuclidinyl benzilate (QNB) is most often used as a ligand for studying muscarinic receptor binding (166).

For routine assay, brain membranes are prepared as previously described for D_2-DA receptor binding. The binding of [^{3}H]QNB is carried out according to the method of Yamamura and Snyder (166). The binding assay is performed in 50 mM sodium phosphate buffer (pH 7.4) with different concentrations (0.01–2.0 nM) of [^{3}H]QNB to generate saturation curves in a final volume of 1 ml. Specific binding is calculated as the total binding minus that occurring in the presence of 1 μM atropine. The binding is initiated by addition of 0.2 ml of membrane preparation (0.2–0.4 mg/ml), and incubations are carried out for 1 hr at 25°C in a shaking waterbath. The reaction is terminated by rapid filtering through Whatman GF/B glass fiber filters. Each filter is washed twice with 5 ml buffer, and the dried filter is transferred to scintillation vials containing 10 ml of Aquasol (New England Nuclear, Boston, Massachusetts). The radioactivity retained in the filters is determined by liquid scintillation spectrophotometry.

Nicotinic Receptors

Brain membrane preparations and binding assays are performed according to the method of Romano and Goldstein (121) with slight modification (88). The pooled samples are homogenized at 4°C in 10 volumes of buffer (w/v) using a Brinkman Polytron PT-10 at low speed. The buffer composition is as follows: 118 mM NaCl, 4.8 mM KCl, 2.5 mM $CaCl_2$, 1.2 mM $MgSO_4$, and 20 mM Hepes (pH 7.5). The homogenate is centrifuged at 48,000 $\times$ g for 30 min. The pellet is suspended in distilled water (5% w/v) and allowed to lyse for 60 min. The suspension is then centrifuged as previously described. The membrane pellets are suspended in buffer (15% w/v) for the assays.

Between 400 and 600 μg of protein in a final incubation volume of 250 μl is used in the binding assays. Binding is initiated by the addition of [^{3}H]nicotine (10–200 nM) to samples equilibrated at the final incubation temperature. Incubation is carried out for 2 hr in a shaking waterbath at 4°C (in a cold room). Specific binding is calculated as the total binding minus that which occurs in the presence of 1 $\times$ 10^{-5} M L-nicotine. At the end of incubation each sample is diluted with 4 ml of ice-cold wash buffer (composition identical with the incubation buffer, except that the Hepes concentration is reduced to 5 mM) and filtered under vacuum onto GF/C glass fiber filters that have been soaked in buffer containing 0.1% L-polylysine. The filters are subsequently washed three times with 4 ml of wash buffer. All dried filters are transferred to scintillation vials containing 10 ml of Aquasol. The radioactivity retained in the filters is determined by liquid scintillation spectrophotometry.

γ-AMINOBUTYRIC ACID

Tissue levels of γ-aminobutyric acid (GABA) and glutamate have been measured by various techniques: ion-exchange chromatography (128,138), paper chromatography-fluorometry (78), ligand-exchange chromatography (154), and most commonly an enzymatic-fluorometric technique (47,75) or a dansylation technique (135). More sensitive methods, e.g., radioreceptor assay (34) and mass fragmentography (11), have also been available. The most common method of enzymatic fluorometry, the radioreceptor assay and mass fragmentography, is described here.

Enzymatic Fluorometry

Enzymatic fluorometry was described by Graham and Aprison (47).

Preparation of Brain Extract

The animals are decapitated and the brains removed immediately and frozen in crushed Dry Ice. About 0.5 g of brain is weighed and homogenized in 3 ml of precooled 75% ethanol in a Nalgene centrifuge tube using a polytron. The homogenizer shaft is rinsed with 1 ml of 75% ethanol; and the polytron is turned on for an additional 5 sec to spin out the rinsings to the centrifuge tube. Homogenates are left at room temperature for several hours or are placed in a refrigerator overnight. After the homogenate is centrifuged at 20,000 × g for 30 min, the supernatant is dried under an air stream and then resuspended in exactly 10 ml of water and shaken at room temperature for 30 min. The slightly cloudy suspension is recentrifuged in an ultracentrifuge at 100,000 × g for 30 min. The clear supernatant is carefully transferred to a storage tube using a Pasteur pipette. This supernatant is used for GABA and glutamate assays. The GABA assay is described below.

Reagents

Sodium pyrophosphate buffer (pH 8.1, 0.2 M) is prepared by dissolving 8.92 g of $Na_2P_2O_7 \cdot 10\ H_2O$ in 90 ml of water. The pH is adjusted to 8.1 with 3 N HCl, and water is added to bring the volume to 100 ml. The solution is treated with 10 g Norit A (charcoal) and then filtered to remove fluorescent background. The α-ketoglutaric acid (α-KG) solution contains 4.6 mg α-KG in 2 ml of Na pyrophosphate buffer. The 2-mercaptoethanol solution is prepared by diluting 50 μl of 2-mercaptoethanol to a final volume of 7 ml with water. The NADP solution consists of 6 mg NADP in 6 ml of Na pyrophosphate buffer. The GABA stock standard is made by dissolving 10.3 mg of GABA in 100 ml of water (1 mM). GABAse is a partially purified cell-free preparation from *Pseudomonas fluorescens* containing GABA-α-ketoglutarate transaminase and succinic semialdehyde hydrogenase. It can be purchased from Sigma Chemical Co. The reaction mixture consists of the following: 5 ml of the NADP solution, 0.6 ml of the α-KG solution, 0.3 ml of the 2-mercaptoethanol solution, and 0.2 ml of GABAse. For sample blanks, 0.2 ml of water is used to replace the 0.2 ml of GABAse.

Assay Procedure

Using a pipette, 50 μl of brain extract is transferred to each of two 13 × 100 mm test tubes (one is used as a sample blank to measure background fluorescence due to the tissue extract itself). Na pyrophosphate buffer (50 μl) is added to each tube, and the tubes are placed in ice water. The appro-

priate reaction mixture, i.e., with or without GABAse, is added to each tube. Contents of tubes are mixed using a Vortex mixer, and each tube is covered with Parafilm. Incubation is carried out at 37°C for 50 min with constant shaking. The tubes are then placed in ice water, followed by incubation at 60°C for 30 min to stop the reaction. The tubes are allowed to stand for 20 min at room temperature; then 1 ml of water is added, and the contents are mixed well. Fluorescence is measured with an Aminco-Bowman spectrofluorometer at the excitation and emission wavelengths of 350 and 460 nm, respectively.

Standard Curve

In addition to experimental samples, a standard curve is prepared for each assay. Dilutions from the 1 mM GABA stock solution serve as standard curve solutions (e.g., 0.02, 0.04, 0.06, and 0.10 mM).

Radioreceptor Assay

The radioreceptor assay of Enna and Snyder (34) is based on the principle that the amount of ^{3}H-GABA bound to synaptosomal membrane fragments, in the presence of added GABA, is proportional to the logarithm of the added GABA.

Preparation of Synaptic Membranes

Crude synaptic membranes are isolated from rat brains. Male Sprague-Dawley rats (150–200 g) are decapitated and the brains removed rapidly and homogenized in 15 volumes of ice-cold 0.32 M sucrose in a Potter Elvehjem glass homogenizer fitted with a Teflon pestle. The homogenate is centrifuged at 1,000 × g for 10 min. The pellet is discarded, and the supernatant fluid is centrifuged at 20,000 × g for 20 min. The crude mitochondrial pellet is resuspended in distilled water and dispersed using a Brinkman Polytron PT-10 homogenizer (setting 6) for 30 sec. The suspension is centrifuged at 8,000 × g for 20 min. The supernatant is collected, and the pellet, a bilayer with a soft, buffy uppercoat, is rinsed carefully with the supernatant fluid to collect the upper layer. The combined supernatant fractions are then centrifuged at 48,000 × g for 20 min. The final crude synaptic membrane pellets are resuspended in water, centrifuged at 48,000 × g for 20 min, and then stored at −30°C for at least 18 hr. Prior to use, the frozen pellets are resuspended in water, maintained at 25°C for 20 min, centrifuged at 48,000 × g for 10 min, and suspended in the buffer for GABA binding assay. The ^{3}H-GABA binding capacity of frozen pellets remains intact for at least 90 days under these conditions. Storing frozen tissues enhances GABA postsynaptic receptor binding and markedly lowers sodium-dependent GABA binding, which is unrelated to receptor sites (33).

GABA Assay Procedure

Animals are decapitated and the brains rapidly removed (less than 30 sec) and placed into a beaker of methanol precooled to approximately −80°C on Dry Ice–acetone. The brain tissue is dispersed with a Polytron in 20 volumes of ice-cold distilled water, and the homogenate is centrifuged at 48,000 × g at 4°C for 10 min. For routine assays, a fraction of the supernatant is removed and diluted to the equivalent of 120 volumes with ice-cold distilled water. This solution, in 20-μl aliquots, is placed, in triplicate, in 16-ml Sorvall centrifuge tubes containing 1 ml of cold distilled water. To each tube is added 1 ml (0.7–1.2 mg protein) of the crude synaptic membrane suspended in 0.1 M Tris citrate buffer (pH 7.1 at 4°C) and 2 μl of a ^{3}H-GABA solution that in the 2-ml incubation mixture yields 25 nM ^{3}H-GABA (500,000 cpm). After mixing, the samples are incubated at 4°C for 5 min; the reaction is terminated by centrifugation at 48,000 × g for 10 min at 4°C. After centrifugation, the supernatant fluid is decanted, and the pellet is rinsed rapidly and superficially with 5 ml, then 10 ml, of ice-cold distilled water. Bound radioactivity is extracted into counting vials containing 1 ml of Protosol (New England Nuclear Corp.). Toluene phosphor (10 ml) is added and the radioactivity assayed by liquid scintillation spectrometry. Total specific ^{3}H-GABA binding is obtained by subtracting from the total bound radioactivity the amount displaced by 2 μmol GABA/2 ml.

Standard curves are determined routinely by placing 20-μl aliquots of various appropriate concentrations of unlabeled GABA into the incubation mixture and calculating the percent displacement of ^{3}H-GABA by each concentration relative to the blank value. For internal standards, 0.2 or 0.4 nmol of unlabeled GABA is added to the incubation mixture along with the tissue extract.

To determine percent recovery, brains from four rats are removed and frozen in the usual fashion. Each frozen brain is placed in a centrifuge tube and, prior to the addition of 20 volumes of ice-cold water, 20 μl of an aqueous solution containing 0.01 nmol ^{3}H-GABA (0.1 μCi) is placed in each tube. After the addition of cold water, the brain is homogenized with a Polytron for 1 min and the homogenate centrifuged for 10 min at 48,000 × g at 4°C. After centrifugation, recovery is determined by analyzing 20-μl aliquots of the aqueous supernatant for ^{3}H-GABA by liquid scintillation spectrometry.

Mass Fragmentographic Method

The mass fragmentographic method was described by Bertilsson and Costa (11).

Reagents and Reference Compounds

The following compounds are commercially available: pentafluoropropionic anhydride (PFPA, distilled before use) and 1,1,1,3,3,3-hexafluoroisopropanol (HFIP) from Pierce, Rockford, Illinois; L-glutamic acid and 5-amino-n-valeric acid (AVA) hydrochloride from K and K Labs, Plainview, New York; GABA from Calbiochem, LaJolla, California; L-2,3,3,4,4-^{2}H$_5$ glutamic acid (glutamic acid-d$_5$) from Merck, Sharp and Dohme, Montreal, Canada; deuterium chloride (20% in deuterium oxide; 100.0 atom %D) and deuterium oxide (99.7 atom %D) from Aldrich, Milwaukee, Wisconsin.

4,4-^{2}H$_2$-Glutamic acid (glutamic acid-d$_2$) and γ-amino-2,2-^{2}H$_2$-butyric acid (GABA-d$_2$) are synthesized by heating glutamic acid and GABA (200 mg of each), respectively, at 130°C in sealed tubes with 1 ml of 8% deuterium chloride in deuterium oxide. The solutions are reacted for three 12-day periods. After each period the solvent is evaporated by a stream of nitrogen gas and replaced by fresh deuterium chloride solution. After the last heating period, the crystals obtained are dissolved in protium water to replace active deuterium atoms with protium via exchange. When the water is evaporated, white crystals of glutamic acid-d$_2$ and GABA-d$_2$ are obtained.

Tissue Preparation

Rats (about 150 g) are killed by exposing their heads for 2.2 to 2.5 sec to a focused high-intensity microwave beam as described by Guidotti et al. (51). The brains are dissected out and immediately frozen in dry ice. The tissue can also be prepared as previously mentioned when a high-intensity microwave apparatus is not available. The tissue is homogenized in glass homogenizer tubes (Kontes, Vineland, New Jersey) in 80% aqueous ethanol containing the internal standards for the quantitations. Whole cerebella are homogenized in 500 μl of solution containing 380 and 750 nmol of glutamic acid-d$_5$ and AVA per milliliter, respectively.

After homogenization the tubes are centrifuged at 12,000 × g for 5 min at −2°C. The supernatant (only 50 μl from the whole cerebellum) is transferred to glass vials and evaporated to dryness under a stream of nitrogen. HFIP (50 μl) and PFPA (100 μl) are then added, and the vials are sealed, heated for 1 hr at 60°C, and stored at 4°C. Just before the mass fragmentographic analysis, the reaction mixture is evaporated to dryness. The residue is dissolved in 10 to 100 μl of ethyl acetate, and 1 to 3 μl of this solution is injected into the gas chromatograph–mass spectrometer.

Gas Chromatography–Mass Spectrometry

An LKB 9,000 gas chromatograph–mass spectrometer (GC-MS) with a multiple ion detector (LKB-Produkter, Bromma, Sweden) is used. The separations are made on a 2.5 m × 3.0 mm (inside diameter) silanized glass column packed with 3% OV-17 on Gas-Chrom Q, 100 to 120 mesh (Applied Science Labs, State College, Pennsylvania) maintained at a temperature of 115°C. The temperature of the flash heater is 200°C, and the ion source is kept at 270°C. The flow rate of the helium carrier is 25 ml/min. The ionizing potential and trap current are 80 eV and 60 μA, respectively. When mass spectra of reference compounds are recorded, the column temperature is 95°C.

Turnover

It is generally accepted that both GABA and glutamate play an important role in intermediary metabolism in addition to their postulated roles as neurotransmitters. Furthermore, neither glutamic acid nor GABA crosses the blood–

brain barrier. Therefore radioactive precursors of the tricarboxylic acid cycle have been used to label glutamic acid in brain (9,10,18,19,27,106,107,119,152). The labeling of the glutamic acid that functions as a GABA precursor is, however, complicated by the presence of different pools of glutamic acid in glial cells. In contrast, glucose preferentially labels a large pool of glutamate, which is associated with neuronal structures (5).

In 1977 Bertilsson et al. (12) selected ^{13}C-glucose as a precursor for glutamic acid and measured the incorporation of this stable isotope into glutamic acid and GABA. They further estimated the turnover rate of GABA after constant-rate intravenous infusion of ^{13}C-glucose.

Animal Treatments

Rats weighing 100 to 110 g are infused intravenously at a constant rate (0.10 ml/min) with ^{13}C-D-glucose (uniformly labeled with an isotopic enrichment of 75 to 85% (Merck, Sharp and Dohme, Montreal, Canada). The labeled glucose is dissolved in saline (155 mM NaCl) and infused into the tail vein at a rate of 50 μmol/kg body weight/min for 10 min. Labeling by constant rate infusion is necessary to obtain sufficient enrichment in the variant atomic species incorporated into glutamic acid and GABA at steady state. After the end of infusion, the rats are killed at 0, 2, 3.5, 5, 7, 10, 15, 25, 40, 70, and 100 min by exposing their heads for 2.2 sec to a focused high intensity microwave beam as described by Guidotti et al. (51). Rats infused intravenously with saline are used as controls. The brains are dissected from the skull and frozen on dry ice. On the average, the sample analyzed contains 40 to 80 μg protein, depending on the tissue. The ^{13}C enrichments of endogenous glutamic acid and GABA are measured in tissue by mass fragmentography.

Analytical Procedure

Tissues are homogenized in 1-ml glass homogenizers (Kontes Glass, Co., Vineland, New Jersey), with a solution of 100 μl of 80% aqueous ethanol containing the internal standards. This internal standard solution contains glutamic acid-d$_5$ and AVA hydrochloride in concentrations of 42 and 84 nmol/ml, respectively. After homogenization, the tubes are centrifuged at 12,000 $\times$ g for 5 min at $-2°C$. The supernatants are transferred to glass vials and evaporated to dryness under a stream of nitrogen. HFIP (50 μl) and PFPA (100 μl) are added. The vials are sealed, heated for 1 hr at 60°C, and then stored at 4°C. During this reaction the pentafluoropropionyl amide hexafluoropropyl esters of GABA, glutamic acid, and their internal standards are formed. Before measurement, the reagents are evaporated, and the residue is dissolved in 20 μl of ethyl acetate. A small aliquot (1–3 μl) of this solution is injected into a GC-MS (LKB model 9,000 with a multiple ion detector). Separations are made on a column (3% OV-17 on Gas-Chrom Q) maintained at 95°C.

By using the multiple ion detector, the following fragments are analyzed: m/e 398 from endogenous glutamic acid, m/e 403 from glutamic acid-d$_5$, m/e 399 from endogenous GABA, m/e 401 from ^{13}C-GABA, and m/e 413 from AVA.

Standard curves for the quantitation of endogenous glutamic acid and GABA are prepared by analyzing a series of standard solutions containing various amounts of natural forms of GABA and glutamic acid and constant amounts of the respective internal standards. The ratios of the ion currents generated by the characteristic ions monitored for glutamic acid/glutamic acid-d$_5$ and GABA/AVA are plotted against the various amounts of the natural compounds added to each tube. Pilot experiments carried out by these investigators have shown that after infusion with uniformly labeled ^{13}C-glucose, the maximal enrichment of ^{13}C occurs in two of the carbon atoms of glutamic acid and GABA. Therefore the peak height ratios of the m/e values, 400/398 and 401/399, measure the incorporation of ^{13}C into glutamic acid and GABA, respectively.

Calculation of GABA Turnover Rates

The finite differences (Eq. 3) of Neff et al. (100) have been used to calculate the turnover rates of GABA in substantia nigra, globus pallidus, nucleus caudatus, and nucleus accumbens. This equation refers to a kinetic situation where a precursor A (glutamic acid) is metabolized to the product B (GABA) in an open compartment system. The data obtained in these experiments indicate that recycling of ^{13}C may occur, which may present a problem when applying the principle of steady-state kinetics of GABA turnover rate measurements. Assuming that this perturbation is not important during the first 7 min of glucose infusion, Eq. 3 has been used to obtain an approximation of GABA turnover:

$$k_B = \frac{2[S_B(t_2) - S_B(t_1)]}{(t_2 - t_1)[S_A(t_1) + S_A(t_2) - S_B(t_1) - S_B(t_2)]} \quad [3]$$

The fractional rate constant (k_B) for GABA efflux is calculated for $(t_2 - t_1) = 1$ min. The experimental values, S_A and S_B, are the percent enrichment of ^{13}C in glutamic acid and GABA, respectively. The values of the rate constants (k_B) obtained between 1 and 7 min after the cessation of ^{13}C-glucose infusion are averaged and used in the steady-state equation (Eq. 4) to calculate turnover rate:

$$TR_B = k_B(B) \quad [4]$$

where TR_B is the turnover rate of GABA, and (B) is the steady-state concentration of GABA.

Related Enzymes

Glutamic Acid Decarboxylase

The method to assay glutamic acid decarboxylase (GAD) was developed by Roberts and Simonsen (120) and is generally used by investigators. This method is routinely used in our laboratory with minor modification (150).

The activity of GAD is determined by measuring the $^{14}CO_2$ formation from uniformly labeled ^{14}C-L-glutamic acid. Brain (0.5 g) is homogenized with a glass homogenizer immediately in 5 ml of ice-cold 0.1 M potassium buffer (pH 6.5) containing 0.03% reduced glutathione (GSH) at 4°C. Each assay mixture (total volume 1.0 ml) in an 18×150 mm test tube contains 100 μmol of potassium phosphate buffer (pH 6.5), 100 μmol L-glutamate (0.9 μCi), 4 μmol GSH, and 1 μmol pyridoxal-5-phosphate. Into a plastic vial (k-882320, Kontes, Vineland, New Jersey) hanging from a test tube is placed 0.2 ml of 1 M hyamine hydroxide solution in methanol. The reaction is started by injecting 2.5 mg of brain homogenate protein into the test tube. After 30 min of incubation at 37°C, 0.2 ml of $4\,N\,H_2SO_4$ is injected to stop the reaction and to release CO_2. After shaking another 90 min, the contents of the plastic vials are transferred to liquid scintillation counting vials that contain 10 ml Aquasol. The enzyme activity in micromoles glutamate decarboxylated/30 min/100 mg of protein of brain homogenate is calculated from the $^{14}CO_2$ liberated from ^{14}C-L-glutamate. The protein content of brain homogenate is determined by the method of Lowry et al. (84) with crystalline bovine serum albumin as a standard.

γ-Aminobutyric-α-ketoglutarate Transaminase

Isotopic assay

The isotopic assay of Waksman and Roberts (155) is useful for measuring low activities of γ-aminobutyric-α-ketoglutarate transaminase (GABA-T) because of the sensitivity of the method. The activity of GABA-T is measured by the formation of labeled glutamate from 5-^{14}C-α-ketoglutarate and nonradioactive GABA.

Animals are killed by decapitation, and whole brains or discrete brain areas are removed rapidly and placed in glass homogenizers containing precooled 0.01 M phosphate buffer (pH 7.2) with 1.5 μg/ml each of pyridoxal-5-phosphate and reduced GSH. Each assay mixture (total volume 1.0 ml) in a round-bottom, capped centrifuge tube contains 15 μmol of 5-^{14}C-α-ketoglutarate (0.1 μCi), 15 μg each of pyridoxal-5-phosphate and GSH, and 40 μmol of borate buffer (pH 8.2). The assay is started by adding homogenate containing 2 mg of protein. Incubations are performed in a Dubnoff metabolic shaker at 37°C for 30 min. Blanks are run in which GABA is omitted. After the reaction is stopped by adding one drop of concentrated HCl and heating at 100°C for 3 min, the pH of the reaction mixture is adjusted to between 3 and 4. The mixture is then transferred onto a 1×8 cm column of AG 50W-AX in the H^+ form. The unreacted α-ketoglutarate is washed out with 30 ml of water, and the labeled glutamic acid formed is eluted with 25 ml of 2 N NH_4OH. After the eluate is evaporated to dryness under an airstream, 1.5 ml of 1 M hyamine hydroxide in methanol is added. One milliliter of this final solution is pipetted into liquid scintillation counting vials containing 10 ml of Aquasol.

Spectrophotometric method

The spectrophotometric method of Schousboe et al. (123) is useful for routine and rapid assay of GABA-T. The GABA-T reaction is performed in a 100 mM Tris-HCl buffer (pH 8.0) containing 20 μM pyridoxal-5-phosphate, 100 μM 2-aminoethylisothiouronium bromide hydrobromide (AET),

50 mM GABA, and 10 mM α-ketoglutaric acid. This buffer plus enzyme is incubated in a waterbath with shaking for 30 min at 37°C. Under the above conditions, the reaction is linear with time for 1 hr. The reaction is terminated by adding aminooxyacetic acid to a final concentration of 100 μM, and the tubes are immediately transferred to an icebath. Blanks run either without enzyme or in the presence of 100 μM aminooxyacetic acid give comparable low values in the subsequent determination of glutamate.

The glutamate formed in the transaminase reaction is determined in aliquots of the reaction mixture using glutamate dehydrogenase and acetylpyridine-NAD^+ to catalyze the oxidation of glutamate to α-ketoglutarate. The increase in optical density at 363 nm attributable to acetylpyridine-NADH is measured. The buffer for this reaction contains 10 mM Tris-HCl (pH 8.0), 25 mM hydrazine, 1 mM aminooxyacetic acid, 750 μM acetylpyridine-NAD^+, and glutamate dehydrogenase (1.3 units/ml). The reaction is carried out at room temperature for 90 min. Acetylpyridine-NAD^+ is used instead of NAD^+, as it increases the equilibrium constant of the reaction by a factor of 100, and the reduced form has a 50% higher extinction coefficient than does NADH. Aminooxyacetic acid and hydrazine, which are carbonyl-trapping agents, are included to trap the α-ketoglutarate formed, thus ensuring completion of the reaction. Under these conditions, the conversion of glutamate to α-ketoglutarate is in excess of 95%.

The enzyme activity is expressed as units per milliliter of enzyme solution, and specific activities are units per milligram of protein. One unit is defined as that activity catalyzing the formation of 1 μmol of glutamate per minute at 37°C.

GABA Receptors

Two types of GABA receptor have been suggested, GABA-A and GABA-B. The GABA-A receptor binding is calcium-insensitive and is inhibited by the antagonist bicuculline, whereas GABA-B binding is calcium-dependent, baclofen is a specific ligand, and it is insensitive to bicuculline (14,58). When GABA binds to the GABA-A site, it causes a Cl^- ion channel in the membrane to open. The depressant drugs barbiturates and benzodiazepines also bind to the GABA-A site–Cl^- channel complex (105). The GABA-A receptor binding assay using ^{3}H-muscimol as a ligand and GABA-B receptor binding using ^{3}H-baclofen as a ligand are described below.

GABA-A Receptor

The specific binding of the GABA receptor ligand [^{3}H]muscimol is described below (132). The brain membranes are prepared as previously described for muscarinic receptor binding assay. The frozen membrane preparation is thawed and diluted with 10 volumes of 50 mM Tris-citrate buffer (pH 7.1) and centrifuged at $25,000 \times g$ for 20 min to obtain a pellet; the pellet is rehomogenized with a suitable volume of the Tris-citrate buffer and incubated at 37°C for 30 min to dissociate endogenous inhibitors (72). After incubation the suspension is recentrifuged at $25,000 \times g$ for

20 min to obtain a pellet that is resuspended in fresh buffer for assay. Binding of [³H]muscimol is initiated by the addition of 0.2 ml of the membrane preparation (1.0–1.5 mg/ml) to a mixture containing the required final concentration of [³H]muscimol (2–100 nM) in a total volume of 1.0 ml. Incubations are carried out at 4°C for 10 min. The reaction is stopped by rapidly filtering through Whatman GF/B filters; the filters are washed twice with 5 ml of ice-cold 50 mM Tris-citrate buffer (pH 7.1) and transferred to scintillation counting vials containing 10 ml of PCS (Phase Combining System, Amersham Co., Arlington Heights, Illinois). The vials are shaken for 60 min, and the radioactivity is then measured by liquid scintillation spectrophotometry. Nonspecific binding is determined by incubation in the presence of 1 mM unlabeled GABA.

GABA-B Receptor

For GABA-B binding, membranes are thawed, washed four times with 10 volumes of 50 mM Tris-HCl (pH 7.4) containing 2.5 mM CaCl$_2$. [³H]GABA or [³H]baclofen binding (16 concentrations, 10 nM to 6 µM) are determined at room temperature (20°–22°C) in the same buffer containing 40 µM isoguvacine, as described by Bowery et al. (14). Specific GABA-B binding is defined as that displaceable by 10^{-4} M (−)baclofen.

CYCLIC NUCLEOTIDES

Cyclic Nucleotide Cyclases

Adenylate Cyclase

Adenylate cyclase is the enzyme that catalyzes the formation of cyclic 3',5'-adenosine monophosphate (cyclic AMP) from its precursor nucleotide adenosine triphosphate (ATP). It is assayed *in vitro* by methods based on measuring the rate of formation of radioactively (¹⁴C, ³H, or ³²P) labeled cyclic AMP from the corresponding radioactively labeled substrate, i.e., ¹⁴C-, ³H-, or ³²P-ATP.

The major problem inherent in the assay is that of obtaining efficient separation of the radiolabeled cyclic AMP from the radioactive substrate and other radioactive contaminants. Because usually less than 0.05% of the substrate is converted to cyclic AMP, the sensitivity of the assay is directly proportional to and dependent on the efficiency of such separation.

General procedure

The tissue to be used (e.g., brain) is homogenized. Aliquots of the whole homogenate may be used in the assay, or subcellular fractions obtained through centrifugations may be used.

The reaction mixture contains radiolabeled ATP, magnesium, the required cofactor for adenylate cyclase activity, and nonradioactive cyclic AMP as "carrier" or theophylline. The "carrier" cyclic AMP prevents the destruction of newly formed labeled cyclic AMP by "trapping" it without interfering with its production. The use of theophylline is an alternate way to prevent the destruction of newly formed radioactive cyclic AMP, as it inhibits cyclic nucleotide phosphodiesterases. An aliquot of homogenate containing approximately 100 µg of protein is added to the above reaction mixture, the total reaction volume being small, and incubation is carried out at 30°C for 10 to 15 min. The reaction is stopped by immersing the reaction vessel in boiling water.

The procedures for isolating radioactive cyclic AMP that have been used with success are the following:

1. Adsorption onto and elution from Dowex ion-exchange columns, followed by addition of zinc sulfate and barium hydroxide solutions to the eluate to precipitate the remaining ATP and any residual trace contaminants. After centrifugation, aliquots of the supernatant are prepared for liquid scintillation counting of the radioactive cyclic AMP (158).
2. Adsorption onto and subsequent elution from columns containing neutral aluminum oxide followed by liquid scintillation counting of aliquots of the eluate (161).
3. Sequential chromatography on columns of Dowex cation-exchange resin and aluminum oxide, followed by liquid scintillation counting of aliquots of the final eluate (122).

The recovery of cyclic AMP can be determined either from measuring the optical density (260 mµ) of the final purified eluate (157) or by using a "marker" of cyclic AMP, i.e., cyclic AMP labeled with a radionuclide different from the label of the substrate. For example, if ³²P-ATP is used as the substrate, the "marker" would be ³H-cyclic AMP (122). Typical assays for brain adenylate cyclase are described in some detail below.

According to the method of Krishna et al. (76), brain tissue is homogenized gently in 10 volumes of 0.32 M sucrose. The crude homogenate is centrifuged at 3,000 × g for 10 min and the supernatant then recentrifuged at 10,000 × g for 20 min to obtain a crude mitochondrial fraction.

The incubation (reaction) medium contains Tris-HCl buffer (0.04 M, pH 7.3), magnesium sulfate (3.3 mM), sodium fluoride (10 mM), theophylline (10 mM), ATP (1–2 mM of ³H-, ¹⁴C-, or ³²P-labeled ATP; specific activity 5–50 mCi/mmol), and the mitochondrial enzyme preparation obtained above (1–10 mg of tissue) in a final total volume of 0.6 ml. Incubation is carried out at 30°C for specified time intervals. After the addition of 0.1 ml (0.5 mg) of a carrier cyclic AMP solution, the reaction is terminated by immersion in a boiling waterbath for 2 min.

The reaction vessel contents are centrifuged, and the supernatant is poured onto a previously prepared Dowex 50-H⁺ column. The column is eluted with water, and 2-ml fractions are collected. The ultraviolet (UV) absorption at 260 mµ is determined in each fraction. To the fraction(s) containing cyclic AMP, 0.2 ml of 0.25 M zinc sulfate and 0.2 ml of 0.25 M barium hydroxide are added, mixed, and the contents centrifuged. The supernatants are decanted into new tubes, and the barium–zinc precipitation step is repeated on these supernatants. After a final centrifugation, 0.5-ml aliquots are added to counting vials containing liquid scintillation fluor solution, and radioactivity is determined using liquid scintillation techniques.

Blanks are prepared by running the incubation without the enzyme preparation or with heat-denatured enzyme. UV absorption at 260 mμ of aliquots of the final supernatants is determined in order to calculate the recovery of cyclic AMP. Adenylate cyclase activity is expressed in terms of the amount of cyclic AMP formed per unit of time, e.g., micromoles of cyclic AMP per minute per gram of tissue wet weight, or per unit weight of tissue protein.

The procedure described by Salomon et al. (122) for the assay of adenylate cyclase activity in hepatic plasma membranes has been used successfully in our studies of whole brain and synaptic membranes. The details of this procedure are as follows: The incubation mixture contains 25 mM Tris-HCl (pH 7.5), 5 mM MgCl$_2$, 20 mM creatine phosphate, creatine phosphokinase 100 U/ml, 1 mM cyclic AMP, and 1 mM [α-^{32}P]-, [^{3}H]-, or [^{14}C]ATP (40–50 cpm/pmol). Increased activity is achieved by adding 20 mM sodium fluoride to the incubation medium. The reaction is initiated by the addition of brain tissue to give 10 to 250 μg of protein/ml in a final reaction volume of 100 μl. After incubation for 10 min at 30°C, the reaction is terminated by the addition of 5% trichloroacetic acid or of a "stopping solution" containing 2% sodium dodecylsulfate, 40 mM ATP, and 1.4 mM cyclic AMP at pH 7.5. Cyclic AMP containing a radionuclide different from that used as substrate (approximately 20,000 cpm) can then be added to monitor cyclic AMP recovery.

After addition of 0.8 ml water to each reaction tube, the tubes are mixed and decanted into columns (in our case, Bio-Rad Econo columns) containing 1 ml Dowex 50AG WX4 resin. The eluate from this and two successive 1-ml water washes are discarded. Water (3 ml) is then added to each column, and the eluate is collected in 13 × 100 mm test tubes. To each 3-ml fraction, 0.2 ml of 1.5 imidazole HCl (pH 7.2) is added. The tubes are mixed and decanted into columns containing 0.6 g neutral alumina [which has been previously washed with 8 ml of 0.1 M imidazole HCl (pH 7.5)]. The eluates from the columns are collected directly into scintillation vials containing a liquid scintillation cocktail. After the columns have completely drained, an additional 1 ml of the 0.1 M imidazole HCl (pH 7.5) buffer is added and collected in the scintillation vials.

At the completion of each experiment the columns can be regenerated by adding 2 ml of 1 N HCl to each Dowex column. Prior to their reuse the columns are washed with 10 ml of water. To regenerate the alumina columns, they are washed with 8 ml of 0.1 M imidazole HCl (pH 7.5).

Guanylate Cyclase

Guanylate cyclase is the enzyme that catalyzes the synthesis of cyclic 3′,5′-guanosine monophosphate (cyclic GMP) from its nucleotide precursor guanosine triphosphate (GTP). It is assayed by methods based on: (a) determination of cyclic GMP by enzymatic cycling methods; (b) determination of radioactive cyclic GMP separated by thin-layer chromatography; or (c) determination of radioactive cyclic GMP isolated with neutral aluminum oxide and Dowex-1 formate column. All three methods involve measurements of the rate of formation of cyclic GMP. After brief descriptive summaries of the first two methods, the third is described in some detail.

The principle of the *enzymatic cycling method* (55) is the conversion of cyclic GMP to GTP and then measurement of the orthophosphate that accumulates during incubation of GTP in a cycling system containing myosin, pyruvate kinase, and phosphoenolpyruvate as follows:

Stage 1: Samples (i.e., brain homogenates) containing cyclic GMP are incubated in the presence of purified cyclic nucleotide phosphodiesterase, which catalyzes the hydrolysis of cyclic GMP to form GMP, and in the presence of ATP: GMP phosphotransferase, which phosphorylates GMP to GTP at the expense of ATP.

Stage 2: A mixture of adenylate kinase and myosin is added to the above mixture, and the resulting mixture is incubated. This step reduces to negligible levels any remaining ADP or ATP left from stage 1 above.

Stage 3: A mixture of phosphoenolpyruvate, pyruvate kinase, and myosin is added to the above, and incubation is continued. The reaction is stopped by adding perchloric acid, and the orthophosphate resulting from the enzyme cycling system is measured in an aliquot of supernatant after centrifugation.

Thin layer chromatography, also used in the separation of cyclic GMP from GTP, has been described by White and Aurbach (160) and depends on detection of cyclic-^{32}P-GMP formed from α-^{32}P-GTP. The labeled product is separated from the labeled substrate by applying the reaction mixture to a Dowex-50 column and using ascending chromatography on silicic acid medium, i.e., ChromAR Sheet. The area corresponding to cyclic GMP is visualized with ultraviolet light, marked with a pencil, cut from the sheet, and prepared for liquid scintillation counting.

A third, sensitive method uses two *sequential chromatography* columns as described by Nakazawa and Sano (99). This method is outlined below.

The brain is quickly removed, chilled in an icebath, and homogenized with 10 volumes of a 0.25 M sucrose solution containing 0.02 M Tris-HCl buffer (pH 7.4), 1 mM EDTA, and 10 mM 2-mercaptoethanol. The homogenate is centrifuged at 10,000 × g for 10 min at 2°C. The supernatant is decanted and centrifuged at 105,000 × g for 60 min at 2°C. The resulting supernatant is used as the crude enzyme preparation.

The reaction (assay) mixture contains the following: 60 nM of ^{3}H-GTP (0.02 μCi/nmol), 0.3 μM of cyclic GMP, 0.3 μM of MnCl$_2$, 30 μM of Tris-HCl buffer (pH 7.7), and 30 to 80 mg of the enzyme protein in a total volume of 0.15 ml. Following addition of the enzyme preparation, incubation proceeds for 15 min at 30°C and is terminated by immersing the reaction vessel for 2 min in a boiling waterbath followed by chilling in ice.

To isolate the radioactive cyclic GMP, the reaction mixture is applied to a neutral aluminum oxide column. The column is then washed with 5 ml of 0.05 M Tris-HCl buffer (pH 7.4). The cyclic GMP passes through this column, whereas other guanine nucleotides remain adsorbed to the column. The eluate containing cyclic GMP is directly drained onto a Dowex 1-X2 column. After all of the eluate is drained from the alumina column, it is removed, and the Dowex column is washed with 10 ml of 0.05 N formic acid. The cyclic GMP is eluted from this column with 6 ml of 0.2 M ammonium formate in 4.0 N formic acid.

Using this method and ^{14}C-cyclic GMP as the marker, recovery of cyclic GMP is reported to be more than 85%. Units of enzyme activity are expressed in terms of the amount of cyclic GMP formed per unit time per weight of tissue or of tissue protein.

Finally, our laboratory has used the simple and sensitive assay described by Krishnan and Krishna (77), which is described in detail below.

Brain tissue is homogenized in 10 volumes of 40 mM Tris-HCl buffer (pH 7.4) using a Teflon pestle. After the homogenate is centrifuged at 12,000 × g for 10 min, the supernatant fraction is recentrifuged at 100,000 × g for 1 hr and the soluble fraction is used as the enzyme source. All operations are carried out at 4°C. The incubation mixture contains 40 mM Tris-HCl buffer (pH 7.4), 3.3 mM MnSO$_4$, 10 mM theophylline, 1 mM cyclic GMP, 1 nM GTP containing 0.5 to 5.0 μCi [^{32}P]- or [^{3}H]- or [^{14}C]GTP, and 10 to 100 μg of tissue protein. Following incubation at 37°C for 10 min, the reaction is terminated by adding 20 μl of a solution containing EDTA to attain a final concentration of 5 mM. After the reaction is stopped, cyclic GMP containing a radionuclide different from that used as substrate (approximately 25,000 cpm) is added to monitor recovery of cyclic GMP. The reaction mixtures are then diluted to 0.5 ml with water, mixed, and centrifuged at low speed and the supernatant fluids are transferred to Dowex 1-formate (or Bio-Rad AG 1-X8) columns (0.5 × 4.0 cm) freshly prepared by washing three times with five volumes of distilled water. The columns are first eluted with 10 ml of water and then with 10 ml of 2 N formic acid. After rinsing the column tips with water, cyclic GMP is eluted with 10 ml of 4 N formic acid, and the eluates are collected in clean 25 × 250 mm culture tubes and lyophilized. The lyophilized material is dissolved in 1 ml of 0.1 M Tris-HCl buffer (pH 7.4) and rechromatographed on dry neutral alumina columns (0.5 × 3.5 cm). The cyclic GMP is eluted from the alumina columns by an additional 2 ml of the Tris-HCl buffer, and the eluates are collected in scintillation vials.

Cyclic AMP and Cyclic GMP

The major problem encountered during assays of endogenous brain levels of cyclic AMP and cyclic GMP is that following decapitation the levels of these cyclic nucleotides increase. The postdecapitation changes in cyclic AMP are of a much greater magnitude than are the changes in cyclic GMP and thus present a major complication in the determination of brain cyclic AMP levels (71,141,143).

To obviate this difficulty by providing more rapid fixation of brain tissue, four methods have been tested in small animals for their usefulness in assays of endogenous cyclic AMP levels (85). The methods, used in order of decreasing effectiveness, were (a) microwave irradiation, (b) freeze-blowing (expulsion of brain tissue into liquid nitrogen), (c) immersion of the whole animal in liquid nitrogen, and (d) decapitation into liquid nitrogen. Guidotti et al. (51) have shown that microwave irradiation inactivates most enzymes in rat brain within 2 sec and has the same effect in mouse brain in 0.5 sec.

Cyclic Nucleotide Assays

The procedures for isolating cyclic nucleotides from brain are generally the same as described above for isolating the products of the cyclase reactions. Identification and quantitation of the endogenous cyclic nucleotides have been feasible only through the use of the radioimmunoassay developed by Steiner et al. (140–142).

The basic principle of radioimmunoassay is competition between radioactive antigen and nonradioactive antigen for a fixed number of binding sites on the antibody. In terms of the radioimmunoassay of cyclic nucleotides, the endogenous cyclic nucleotide to be measured is the nonradioactive antigen, which competes with a fixed amount of radioactive cyclic nucleotide for a fixed amount of specific antibody. This reaction is represented schematically below (CN = cyclic nucleotide).

Labeled antigen + specific antibody ⇌
(CN)   (Ab)

labeled antigen-antibody complex + unlabeled antigen ⇌
 (CN-Ab)   (tissue CN)

    unlabeled antigen–antibody complex
     (tissue CN-Ab)

The antigen–antibody complex is isolated and the radioactivity determined. The amount of radioactivity in the antigen–antibody complex is inversely proportional to the amount of cyclic nucleotide present in the tissue.

The radioimmunoassay of endogenous cyclic AMP and cyclic GMP has become so popular that commercial kits based on the method of Steiner et al. (140–142) are now available (e.g., New England Nuclear, Chicago, Illinois; Amersham; Becton-Dickinson Immuno-diagnostics, Orangeburg, New York; Calbiochem, La Jolla, California), containing all of the necessary components of the assays. The kits are highly specific, are sensitive, and provide excellent recoveries in addition to their involving easy and rapid procedures.

Cyclic Nucleotide Phosphodiesterase

The place of pride in assays of cyclic nucleotide phosphodiesterase (PDE) undoubtedly belongs to the two-stage enzymatic procedure developed by Thompson and Appleman (147). This procedure is outlined below.

Tissue preparation

Brain tissue is homogenized at 4°C in eight volumes of 10.9% sucrose for 1 min using a high speed tissue homogenizer (e.g., Sorval Omni-Mixer) at maximum speed. The homogenate is subjected to sonication in an icebath for 15 min per 30 ml of homogenate. The sonicated homogenate is maintained in the icebath while its pH is adjusted to pH 6.0 with 1 M acetic acid. After centrifugation at 20,000 × g for 20 min, the supernatant is used as the enzyme preparation.

PDE assay procedure

Stage 1 consists in hydrolysis of the cyclic nucleotide to the corresponding 5'-nucleotide by PDE. The reaction mixture contains, in a total volume of 0.4 ml, the following: ^{3}H-cyclic AMP or ^{3}H-cyclic GMP (approximately 200,000 cpm); unlabeled cyclic AMP (1.25×10^{-7} to 1×10^{-4} M) or unlabeled cyclic GMP (2.5×10^{-7} to 4.5×10^{-5} M); MgCl$_2$ (5 mM); Tris-HCl buffer (pH 8.0, 40 mM); 2-mercaptoethanol (3.75 mM); and the enzyme preparation. Incubation is carried out for 10 min at 30°C and is terminated by immersion in a boiling waterbath for 2.5 min.

Stage 2 consists in hydrolysis of the 5'-nucleotide to adenosine or guanosine using the nucleotidase in snake venom. To the contents of the reaction mixture in stage 1 is added 0.1 ml of snake venom (*Ophiophagus hannah*) solution (1 mg/ml in Tris-HCl buffer). Incubation is resumed for 10 min at 30°C and is then stopped by the addition of 1.0 ml of a 1:3 slurry of Bio-Rad resin, AG1-X2, 200 to 400 mesh, which binds all charged nucleotides, leaving only adenosine or guanosine. The contents of the reaction vessel are centrifuged in a low speed (clinical) centrifuge, and a 0.5-ml aliquot of the supernatant is used for measuring the radioactivity due to ^{3}H-adenosine or ^{3}H-guanosine by liquid scintillation counting techniques.

Thompson et al. (148) later modified this assay to obviate problems of nonspecific binding of adenosine, guanosine, and inosine to the anion-exchange resin. Details of the modified procedure are given below.

Tritiated cyclic AMP and tritiated cyclic GMP should have specific activities of 4 Ci/mmol or more, and the radionuclides are purified every 3 to 5 weeks on thin-layer plates (e.g., Baker-flex cellulose) developed with 2-propanol/ammonium hydroxide/water (7:1:2, v/v/v) and stored at −20°C in 50% ethanol. Lyophilized snake venom may be reconstituted to 1 mg/ml in water and stored at 4°C for several weeks. The anion-exchange resin, either Dowex 1-X8 or X2 (200–400 mesh) or AG1-X8 or X2 (200–400 mesh) is washed successively with 0.5 N HCl, water, 0.5 N NaOH, water, 0.5 N HCl, and repeated washings with water until pH 5 is reached.

The incubation medium is prepared as follows: 100 μl of 40 mM Tris-HCl buffer (pH 8) containing 4 mM 2-mercaptoethanol (the assay buffer) is added to 100 μl of tritiated cyclic nucleotide substrate in assay buffer containing 20 mM MgCl$_2$. Unlabeled cyclic nucleotide in assay buffer (100 μl) is added. After a brief equilibration of the medium at 30°C, 200 μl of the enzyme preparation (approximately 100 μg protein in assay buffer) is added to initiate the reaction. (Incubation is carried out at 30°C for 10 min and is terminated by immersion of the reaction tubes in a boiling waterbath for 45 sec (this step was shortened to reduce blank values). The tubes are then cooled in an icebath. Either of two methods may be used to separate the nucleosides from unreacted nucleotides: (a) "Batch method": 1.0 ml of a slurry consisting of 1 part resin plus 4 parts 100% methanol is added to each tube. The contents of the tubes are mixed thoroughly and equilibrated for 15 min at 4°C with occasional remixing. After centrifugation using a clinical centrifuge to sediment the resin, 0.5-ml aliquots of the supernatant are transferred to counting vials for determination of tritiated nucleoside liberated. (b) "Column method": 1.0 ml of 100% methanol

is added to the cooled tubes, and the entire contents are transferred to columns prepared by pipetting 1.0 ml of a 1:4 resin/methanol slurry into Pasteur pipettes or into Bio-Rad Econo columns. The reaction mixture is eluted from the columns with 1 ml of methanol, and the radioactivity of the eluate is determined after addition of the scintillation cocktail.

The units of PDE activity are in terms of the picomoles of cyclic AMP or cyclic GMP hydrolyzed per minute per milliliter of assay volume. Alternatively, one may express PDE activity as milliunits per gram of tissue wet weight, 1 mU corresponding to the hydrolysis of 1 nmol of cyclic nucleotide per minute (59).

CONCLUSIONS

A number of procedures for measuring levels, formation, and degradation of neurotransmitters, neuromodulators, and cyclic nucleotides in the central nervous system have been described—some in general, and others more specifically. It is hoped that the information presented will serve not only as a general guide for those embarking on studies involving the central nervous system but will also provide, in one place, specific procedural techniques described in sufficient detail to enable the researcher to perform neurotoxicological analyses with confidence.

Furthermore, it is hoped that this chapter will find utility as a reference tool; and to this end, we urge the reader to go directly to the original work referenced herein for more specific details on methodology. Finally, it is hoped that the chapter will nourish an ever-increasing awareness of the contributions that continue to advance the field of neurochemistry.

ACKNOWLEDGMENTS

This work was supported by grant DA-04480 from the National Institute of Drug Abuse. The authors are grateful to Mrs. Ann B. Porter for invaluable editorial assistance.

REFERENCES

1. Ahtee, L., Sharman, D. F., and Vogt, M. (1970): Acid metabolites of monoamines in avian brain; effects of probenecid and reserpine. *Br. J. Pharmacol.*, 38:72–85.
2. Ansell, G. B., and Beeson, M. F. (1968): A rapid and sensitive procedure for the combined assay of noradrenaline, dopamine, and serotonin in single brain sample. *Anal. Biochem.*, 23:196–206.
3. Axelrod, J. (1962): Purification and properties of phenylethanolamine-N-methyl transferase. *J. Biol. Chem.*, 237:1657–1660.
4. Axelrod, J., and Inscoe, J. K. (1963): The uptake and binding of circulating serotonin and the effect of drugs. *J. Pharmacol. Exp. Ther.*, 141:161–165.
5. Balazs, R., Patel, A. J., and Richter, D. (1973): Metabolic compartments in the brain: their properties and relation to morphological structure. In: *Metabolic Compartmentation in the Brain*, edited by R. Balazs and J. E. Cremer, pp. 167–184. Macmillan, London.
6. Bapna, J., Neff, N. H., and Costa, E. (1971): A method for studying norepinephrine and serotonin metabolism in small regions of rat brain; effect of ovariectomy on amine metabolism in anterior and posterior hypothalamus. *Endocrinology*, 89:1345–1349.

7. Barchas, J. D., Akil, H., Elliot, G. R., Holman, R. B., and Watson, S. J. (1978): Behavioral neurochemistry: neuroregulators and behavioral states. *Science,* 200:964–973.

8. Bennet, J. P., Jr., and Snyder, S. M. (1976): Serotonin and lysergic acid diethylamide binding in rat brain membranes: relationship to postsynaptic serotonin receptors. *Mol. Pharmacol.,* 12:373–389.

9. Berl, S., and Frigyes, T. L. (1968): Metabolism of ^{14}C leucine and ^{14}C acetate in sensorimotor cortex, thalamus, caudate nucleus and cerebellum of the cat. *J. Neurochem.,* 15:965–997.

10. Berl, S., and Frigyes, T. L. (1969): The turnover of glutamate, glutamine, aspartate and GABA labeled with [1-^{14}C] acetate in caudate nucleus, thalamus and motor cortex (cat). *Brain Res.,* 12:444–455.

11. Bertilsson, L., and Costa, E. (1976): Mass fragmentographic quantitation of glutamic acid and γ-aminobutyric acid in cerebellar nuclei and sympathetic ganglia of rats. *J. Chromatogr.,* 118:395–402.

12. Bertilsson, L., Mao, C-C., and Costa, E. (1977): Application of principles of steady-state kinetics to the estimation of γ-aminobutyric acid turnover rate in nuclei of rat brain. *J. Pharmacol. Exp. Ther.,* 200:277–284.

13. Billard, W., Ruperto, V., Crosby, G., Iorio, L. C., and Barnett, A. (1985): Characterization of the binding ^{3}H-SCH 23390, a selective D-1 receptor antagonist ligand, in rat striatum. *Life Sci.,* 35:1885–1893.

14. Bowery, N. G., Hill, D. R., and Hudson, A. L. (1983): Characteristics of GABA$_B$ receptor binding sites on rat whole brain synaptic membranes. *Br. J. Pharmacol.,* 78:191–206.

15. Brodie, B. B., Costa, E., Dlabac, A., Neff, N. H., and Smookler, H. H. (1966): Application of steady-state kinetics to the estimation of synthesis rate and turnover time of tissue catecholamines. *J. Pharmacol. Exp. Ther.,* 154:493–498.

16. Browning, E. T. (1972): Fluorometric enzyme assay for choline and acetylcholine. *Anal. Biochem.,* 46:624–638.

17. Bull, G., and Oderfeld-Nowak, N. (1971): Standardization of a radiochemical assay of choline acetyltransferase and a study of the activation of the enzyme in rabbit brain. *J. Neurochem.,* 18:935–941.

18. Busch, H. (1953): Studies in the metabolism of acetate-1-^{14}C in tissues of tumor bearing rats. *Cancer Res.,* 13:789–794.

19. Busch, H. (1955): Studies on the metabolism of pyruvate-2-^{14}C in tumor bearing rats. *Cancer Res.,* 15:365–374.

20. Chang, C. C. (1964): A sensitive method for spectrophotometric assay of catecholamines. *Int. J. Neuropharmacol.,* 3:643–649.

21. Cheung, Y. D., Barnett, D. B., and Nahorski, S. R. (1982): ^{3}H-Rauwolscine and ^{3}H-yohimbine binding to rat cerebral and human platelet membranes: possible heterogeneity of α_2-adrenoceptors. *Eur. J. Pharmacol.,* 84:79–85.

22. Cicero, T. J., Sharpe, L. G., Robins, E., and Grote, S. S. (1972): Regional distribution of tyrosine hydroxylase in rat brain. *J. Neurochem.,* 19:2241–2243.

23. Cooper, J. R. (1964): The fluorometric determination of acetylcholine. *Biochem. Pharmacol.,* 13:795–797.

24. Cooper, J. R., Bloom, F. E., and Roth, R. H. (1986): *The Biochemical Basis of Neuropharmacology,* 5th ed. Oxford University Press, New York.

25. Cox, R. H., and Perhach, J. L. (1973): A sensitive rapid and simple method for the simultaneous spectrophotofluorometric determination of norepinephrine, dopamine, 5-hydroxytryptamine and 5-hydroxy-indoleacetic acid in discrete areas of brain. *J. Neurochem.,* 20:1777–1780.

26. Coyle, J. T. (1972): Tyrosine hydroxylase in rat brain-cofactor requirements, regional and subcellular distribution. *Biochem. Pharmacol.,* 21:1935–1944.

27. Cremer, J. E. (1964): Amino acid metabolism in rat brain studied with ^{14}C labeled glucose. *J. Neurochem.,* 11:165–185.

28. Creveling, C. R., Daly, J. W., Witkop, B., and Udenfriend, S. (1962): Substrates and inhibitors of dopamine-β-oxidase. *Biochim. Biophys. Acta,* 64:125–134.

29. Curzon, G., and Green, A. R. (1970): Rapid method for the determination of 5-hydroxytryptamine and 5-hydroxyindoleacetic acid in small regions of rat brain. *Br. J. Pharmacol.,* 39:653–655.

30. Daly, J. (1977): *Cyclic Nucleotides in the Nervous System.* Plenum Press, New York.

31. Deguchi, T., and Barchas, J. D. (1973): Comparative studies on

32. Ellman, G. L., Courtney, K. D., Andres, V., Jr., and Featherstone, R. M. (1961): A new and rapid colorimetric determination of acetylcholinesterase activity. *Biochem. Pharmacol.,* 7:88–95.

33. Enna, S. J., and Snyder, S. H. (1975): Properties of γ-aminobutyric acid (GABA) receptor binding in rat brain synaptic membrane fractions. *Brain Res.,* 100:81–97.

34. Enna, S. J., and Snyder, S. H. (1976): A simple sensitive and specific radioreceptor assay for endogenous GABA in brain tissue. *J. Neurochem.,* 26:221–224.

35. Feigenson, M. E., and Saelens, J. K. (1969): An enzyme assay for acetylcholine. *Biochem. Pharmacol.,* 18:1479–1486.

36. Felice, L. J., Felice, J. D., and Kissinger, P. T. (1978): Determination of catecholamines in rat brain parts by reverse-phase ion-pair liquid chromatography. *J. Neurochem.,* 31:1461–1464.

37. Fellman, J. H. (1969): A chemical method for the determination of acetylcholine: its application in a study of pre-synaptic release and a choline acetyl-transferase assay. *J. Neurochem.,* 16:135–143.

38. Fonnum, F. (1966): A radiochemical method for the estimation of choline acetyltransferase. *Biochem. J.,* 100:479–484.

39. Fonnum, F. (1969): Isolation of choline esters from aqueous solutions by extraction with sodium tetraphenyl boron in organic solvents. *Biochem. J.,* 113:291–298.

40. Fonnum, F. (1969): Radiochemical micro assays for the determination of choline acetyltransferase and acetylcholinesterase activities. *Biochem. J.,* 115:465–472.

41. Freedman, P. A., Kappleman, A. H., and Kaufman, S. (1972): Partial purification and characterization of tryptophan hydroxylase from rabbit hindbrain. *J. Biol. Chem.,* 247:4165–4173.

42. Friedman, S., and Kaufman, S. (1965): 3,4-Dihydroxyphenylethylamine β-hydroxylase. *J. Biol. Chem.,* 240:4763–4773.

43. Gal, E. M., and Millard, S. A. (1972): Tryptophan 5-hydroxylase. *Methods Neurochem.,* 2:131–146.

44. Garrick, N. A., and Murphy, D. L. (1981): Monoamine oxidase type A: differences in selectivity towards l-norepinephrine compared to serotonin. *Biochem. Pharmacol.,* 31:4061–4066.

45. Goldberg, A. M., and McCaman, R. E. (1973): The determination of picomole amounts of acetylcholine in mammalian brain. *J. Neurochem.,* 20:1–9.

46. Gordon, A. R., and Peters, J. H. (1967): Plasma histaminase in various mammalian species: a rapid method of assay. *Proc. Soc. Exp. Biol. Med.,* 24:399–404.

47. Graham, L. T., and Aprison, M. H. (1966): Fluorometric determination of aspartate, glutamate, and β-aminobutyrate in nerve tissue using enzymatic methods. *Anal. Biochem.,* 15:487–497.

48. Grahame-Smith, D. G. (1964): Tryptophan hydroxylation in brain. *Biochem. Biophys. Res. Commun.,* 16:586–592.

49. Green, A. R., and Grahame-Smith, D. G. (1975): 5-Hydroxytryptamine and other indoles in the central nervous system. In: *Handbook of Psychopharmacology,* edited by L. L. Iversen, S. D. Iversen, and S. H. Snyder, Vol. 3, pp. 169–245. Plenum Press, New York.

50. Greengrass, P., and Bremner, R. (1979): Binding characteristic of ^{3}H-prazosin to rat brain α-adrenergic receptors. *Eur. J. Pharmacol.,* 55:323–326.

51. Guidotti, A., Cheney, D. L., Trabucchi, M., Doteuchi, M., Wang, C., and Hawkins, R. A. (1974): Focused microwave radiation: a technique to minimize postmortem changes of cyclic nucleotides, DOPA and choline and to preserve brain morphology. *Neuropharmacology,* 13:1115–1122.

52. Hammar, C-G., Hanin, I., Holmstedt, B., Kitz, R. J., Jenden, D. J., and Karlen, B. (1968): Identification of acetylcholine in fresh rat brain by combined gas chromatography–mass spectrometry. *Nature,* 220:915–917.

53. Hanin, I. (1969): A specific gas chromatography method for assaying tissue acetylcholine: present status. In: *Advances In Biochemical Psychopharmacology,* edited by L. E. Costa and P. Greengard, pp. 111–130. Raven Press, New York.

54. Hanin, I., Massarelli, R., and Costa, E. (1972): An approach to the in vivo study of acetylcholine turnover in rat salivary glands by radio gas chromatography. *J. Pharmacol. Exp. Ther.,* 181:10–18.

55. Hardman, J. G., Davis, J. W., and Sutherland, E. W. (1969): Effects of some hormonal and other factors on the excretion of guanosine

3',5'-monophosphate and adenosine 3',5'-monophosphate in rat urine. *J. Biol. Chem.*, 244:6354–6362.

56. Haubrich, D. R., Reid, W. D., and Gillette, J. R. (1972): Acetylcholine formation in mouse brain and effect of cholinergic drugs. *Nature [New Biol.]*, 238:88–89.

57. Hebb, C. O., and Smallman, B. N. (1956): Intracellular distribution of choline acetylase. *J. Physiol. (Lond.)*, 134:385–392.

58. Hill, D. R., and Bowery, N. G. (1982): [³H]Baclofen and [³H]GABA bind to bicuculline-insensitive GABA_B sites in rat brain. *Nature*, 290:149–152.

59. Hoskins, B., and Jackson, C. M. (1978): The mechanism of chlorothiazide-induced carbohydrate intolerance. *J. Pharmacol. Exp. Ther.*, 206:423–430.

60. Hrdina, P. D., Singhal, R. L., and Ling, G. M. (1975): DDT and related chlorinated hydrocarbon insecticides: pharmacological basis of their toxicity in mammals. *Adv. Pharmacol. Chemother.*, 12:31–88.

61. Hsu, S. Y., and Gerald, M. C. (1973): Determination of femtomole levels of acetylcholine by an improved bioassay procedure. *Eur. J. Pharmacol.*, 24:269–273.

62. Ichiyama, A., Nakamura, S., Nishizuka, Y., and Hayaishi, O. (1968): Tryptophan-5-hydroxylase in mammalian brain. *Adv. Pharmacol.*, 6A:5–17.

63. Ichiyama, A., Nakamura, S., Nishizuka, Y., and Hayaishi, O. (1970): Enzymic studies on the biosynthesis of serotonin in mammalian brain. *J. Biol. Chem.*, 245:1699–1709.

64. Jenden, D. J., Campbell, B., and Roch, H. (1970): Gas chromatographic estimation of choline esters in tissues: a modified procedure of submicrogram quantities. *Anal. Biochem.*, 35:209–211.

65. Jenden, D. J., Choi, L., and Silverman, R. W. (1974): Acetylcholine turnover estimation in brain by gas chromatography/mass spectrometry. *Life Sci.*, 14:55–63.

66. Jenden, D. J., Hanin, I., and Lamb, S. I. (1968): Gas chromatographic microestimation of acetylcholine and related compounds. *Anal. Chem.*, 40:125–128.

67. Johnston, J. P. (1968): Some observations upon a new inhibitor for monoamine oxidase in brain tissue. *Biochem. Pharmacol.*, 17:1285–1297.

68. Karasawa, T., Furukawa, K., Yoshida, K., and Shimizu, M. (1975): A double column procedure for the simultaneous estimation of norepinephrine, normetanephrine, dopamine, 3-methoxytyramine and 5-hydroxytryptamine in brain tissue. *Jpn. J. Pharmacol.*, 25:727–736.

69. Karasawa, T., Nakamura, I., and Shimizu, M. (1974): Simultaneous microdetermination of homovanillic acid and 5-hydroxyindoleacetic acid in brain tissue using Sephadex G-10 and GAE-Sephadex A-25. *Life Sci.*, 15:1465–1474.

70. Kaufman, S., and Friedman, S. (1965): Dopamine-β-hydroxylase. *Pharmacol. Rev.*, 17:71–99.

71. Kimura, H., Thomas, F., and Murad, F. (1974): Effects of decapitation, ether, and pentobarbital on guanosine 3',5'-phosphate and adenosine 3',5'-phosphate levels in rat tissues. *Biochim. Biophys. Acta*, 343:519–528.

72. Kingsbury, A. E., Wilkin, G. P., Patel, A. J., and Balázs, R. (1980): Distribution of GABA receptors in the rat cerebellum. *J. Neurochem.*, 35:739–742.

73. Kitz, R. J., and Ginsburg, S. (1968): The reaction of acetylcholinesterase (AChE) with some quaternary hydroxyaminophenols. *Biochem. Pharmacol.*, 17:525–532.

74. Knapp, S., and Mandell, A. J. (1973): Some drug effects on the functions of two measurable forms of tryptophan hydroxylase: influence of hydroxylation and uptake of substrate. In: *The Biochemical Basis of Neuropharmacology*, edited by J. R. Cooper, F. E. Bloom, and R. H. Roth, pp. 61–72. Oxford University Press, New York.

75. Kravitz, E. A., and Potter, D. D. (1965): A further study of the distribution of γ-aminobutyric acid between excitatory and inhibitory axons of the lobster. *J. Neurochem.*, 12:323–328.

76. Krishna, G., Weiss, B., and Brodie, B. B. (1968): A simple, sensitive method for the assay of adenyl cyclase. *J. Pharmacol. Exp. Ther.*, 163:379–385.

77. Krishnan, N., and Krishna, G. (1976): A simple and sensitive assay for guanylate cyclase. *Anal. Biochem.*, 70:18–31.

78. Levin, E., Lovell, R. A., and Elliot, K. A. (1961): The relation of γ-aminobutyric acid to factor I in brain extracts. *J. Neurochem.*, 7:147–154.

79. Levin, E. Y., Levenberg, B., and Kaufman, S. (1960): The enzymatic conversion of 3,4-dihydroxyphenyl-ethylamine to norepinephrine. *J. Biol. Chem.*, 235:2080–2086.

80. Leysen, J. E., Niemegeers, C. J. E., Van Nueten, J. M., and Laduron, P. M. (1982): [³H]-Ketanserin (R41468), a selective ³H-ligand for serotonin₂ receptor binding sites, binding properties, brain distribution, and functional role. *Mol. Pharmacol.*, 21:301–314.

81. Lin, R. C., Costa, E., Neff, N. H., Wang, C. T., and Ngai, S. H. (1969): In vivo measurement of 5-hydroxytryptamine turnover rate in the rat brain from the conversion of ¹⁴C-tryptophan to ¹⁴C-5-hydroxytryptamine. *J. Pharmacol. Exp. Ther.*, 170:232–238.

82. Lovenberg, W., Bensinger, R. E., Jackson, R. L., and Daly, J. W. (1971): Rapid analysis of tryptophan hydroxylase in rat tissue using 5-³H-tryptophan. *Anal. Biochem.*, 43:269–274.

83. Lovenberg, W., Levine, R. J., and Sjoerdsma, A. (1962): A sensitive assay of monoamine oxidase activity in vitro: application to heart and sympathetic ganglia. *J. Pharmacol. Exp. Ther.*, 135:7–10.

84. Lowry, O. H., Rosebrough, N. J., Farr, A. L., and Randall, R. J. (1951): Protein measurement with the Folin phenol reagent. *J. Biol. Chem.*, 193:265–275.

85. Lust, W. D., and Passonneau, J. V. (1973): Cyclic adenosine monophosphate, metabolites, and phosphorylase in neural tissue: a comparison of methods of fixation. *Science*, 181:280–282.

86. MacIntosh, F. C., and Perry, W. L. M. (1950): Biological estimation of acetylcholine. *Methods Med. Res.*, 3:78–92.

87. Maickel, R. P., Cox, R. H., Saillant, J., and Miller, F. P. (1968): A method for the determination of serotonin and norepinephrine in discrete areas of rat brain. *Int. J. Neuropharmacol.*, 7:275–281.

88. Marks, M. J., and Collins, A. C. (1982): Characterization of nicotine binding in mouse brain and comparison with the binding of α-bungarotoxin and quinuclidinyl benzilate. *Mol. Pharmacol.*, 22:554–564.

89. Maruyama, Y., Oshima, T., and Nakajima, E. (1980): Simultaneous determination of catecholamines in rat brain by reversed-phase liquid chromatography with electrochemical detection. *Life Sci.*, 26:1115–1120.

90. Mayer, G. S., and Shoup, R. E. (1983): Simultaneous multiple electrode liquid chromatographic-electrochemical assay for catecholamines, indoleamines and metabolites in brain tissue. *J. Chromatogr.*, 255:533–544.

91. McCaman, R. E., and Hunt, J. M. (1965): Microdetermination of choline acetylase in nervous tissue. *J. Neurochem.*, 12:253–259.

92. Meller, E., Bohmaker, K., Goldstein, M., and Friedhoff, A. J. (1985): Inactivation of D₁ and D₂ dopamine receptors by N-ethoxycarbonyl-2-ethoxy-1,2-dihydroquinoline in vivo: selective protection by neuroleptics. *J. Pharmacol. Exp. Ther.*, 233:656–662.

93. Menkes, D. B., Aghajanian, G. K., and Gallager, D. W. (1983): Chronic antidepressant treatment enhances agonist affinity of brain α₁-adrenoceptor. *Eur. J. Pharmacol.*, 87:35–41.

94. Molinoff, P. B., Landsberg, L., and Axelrod, J. (1969): An enzymatic assay for octopamine and other β-hydroxylated phenylethylamines. *J. Pharmacol. Exp. Ther.*, 170:253–261.

95. Molinoff, P. B., Weinshilboum, R., and Axelrod, J. (1971): A sensitive enzymatic assay for dopamine-β-hydroxylase. *J. Pharmacol. Exp. Ther.*, 178:425–431.

96. Morris, D. (1967): The effect of sulphydryl and other disulphide reducing agents on acetyltransferase activity estimated with synthetic acetyl-CoA. *J. Neurochem.*, 14:19–27.

97. Nagatsu, T., Levitt, M., and Udenfriend, S. (1964): A rapid and simple radioassay for tyrosine hydroxylase activity. *Anal. Biochem.*, 9:122–126.

98. Nagatsu, T., Levitt, M., and Udenfriend, S. (1964): Tyrosine hydroxylase—initial step in norepinephrine biosynthesis. *J. Biol. Chem.*, 239:2910–2917.

99. Nakazawa, K., and Sano, M. (1974): A new assay method for guanylate cyclase and properties of the cyclase from rat brain. *J. Biol. Chem.*, 249:4207–4211.

100. Neff, N. H., Spano, P. F., Groppetti, A., Wang, C. T., and Costa, E. (1971): A simple procedure for calculating the synthesis rate of noradrenaline, dopamine, and 5-hydroxytryptamine in rat brain. *J. Pharmacol. Exp. Ther.*, 176:701–710.

101. Neff, N. H., Tozer, T. N., and Brodie, B. B. (1967): Application

of steady-state kinetics of studies of the transfer of 5-hydroxy-in-doleacetic acid from brain to plasma. *J. Pharmacol. Exp. Ther.,* 158:214–218.

102. Nelson, D. L., Herbert, A., Bourgoin, S., Glowinski, J., and Hamon, M. (1978): Characteristics of central 5-HT receptors and their adaptive changes following intracerebral 5,7-dihydroxy-tryptamine administration in the rat. *Mol. Pharmacol.,* 14:983–995.

103. Nelson, D. L., Schnellmann, R., and Smit, R. (1983): [³H]-Serotonin binding sites: pharmacological and species differences. In: *Molecular Pharmacology of Neurotransmitter Receptors,* edited by T. Segawa, H. I., Yamamura, and K. Kuriyama, pp. 103–113. Raven Press, New York.

104. Okuyama, T., and Kobayashi, Y. (1961): Determination of diamine oxidase activity by liquid scintillation counting. *Arch. Biochem. Biophys.,* 95:242–250.

105. Olsen, R. W. (1982): Drug interactions at the GABA receptor ion-ophore complex. *Annu. Rev. Pharmacol. Toxicol.,* 22:245–277.

106. O'Neal, R. M., and Koeppe, R. W. (1966): Precursors in vivo of glutamate, aspartate, and their derivatives of rat brain. *J. Neurochem.,* 13:835–847.

107. O'Neal, R. M., Koeppe, R. E., and Williams, E. I. (1966): Utilization in vivo of glucose and volatile fatty acids by sheep brain for the synthesis of acidic amino acids. *Biochem. J.,* 101:591–597.

108. O'Neil, J. J., and Sakamoto, T. (1970): Enzymatic fluorometric determination of acetylcholine in biological extracts. *J. Neurochem.,* 17:1451–1461.

109. Otsuka, S., and Kobayashi, Y. (1964): A radioisotopic assay for monoamine oxidase determinations in human plasma. *Biochem. Pharmacol.,* 13:995–1006.

110. Pedigo, N. W., Yamamura, H. I., and Nelson, D. L. (1981): Discrimination of multiple [³H] 5-hydroxytryptamine binding sites by the neuroleptic spiperone in rat brain. *J. Neurochem.,* 36:220–226.

111. Pisano, J. J., Creveling, C. R., and Udenfriend, S. (1960): Enzyme conversion of p-tyramine to p-hydroxyphenylethanolamine (nor-synephrine). *Biochim. Biophys. Acta,* 43:566–568.

112. Pomerantz, S. H. (1964): Tyrosine hydroxylation catalyzed by mammalian tyrosine: an improved method of assay. *Biochem. Biophys. Res. Commun.,* 16:188–194.

113. Porceddu, M. L., Giorgi, O., Ongini, E., Mele, S., and Biggio, G. (1985): ³H-SCH 23390 binding sites in the rat substantia nigra: evidence for a presynaptic localization and innervation by dopamine. *Life Sci.,* 39:321–328.

114. Potter, L. T. (1967): A radiometric microassay of acetylcholines-terase. *J. Pharmacol. Exp. Ther.,* 156:500–506.

115. Potter, P. E., Meek, J. L., and Neff, N. H. (1983): Acetylcholine and choline in neuronal tissue measured by HPLC with electro-chemical detection. *J. Neurochem.,* 41:188–194.

116. Reid, W. R., Haubrich, D. R., and Krishna, G. (1971): Enzymic radioassay for acetylcholine and choline in brain. *Anal. Biochem.,* 42:390–397.

117. Renson, J. (1971): Development of monoaminergic transmissions in the rat brain. *Adv. Exp. Med. Biol.,* 13:175–184.

118. Renson, J., Daly, J., Weissbach, H., Witkop, B., and Udenfriend, S. (1966): Enzymatic conversion of 5-tritio-tryptophan to 4-tritio-5-hydroxytryptophan. *Biochem. Biophys. Res. Commun.,* 25:504–513.

119. Roberts, E., and Morelos, B. S. (1965): Regulation of cerebral metabolism of amino acid. IV. Influence of amino acid level on leucine uptake, utilization and incorporation into protein in vivo. *J. Neurochem.,* 12:373–387.

120. Roberts, E., and Simonsen, D. G. (1963): Some properties of L-glutamic decarboxylase in mouse brain. *Biochem. Pharmacol.,* 12:113–134.

121. Romano, C., and Goldstein, A. (1980): Stereospecific nicotine receptors on rat brain membranes. *Science,* 210:647–649.

122. Salomon, Y., Londos, C., and Rodbell, M. (1974): A highly sensitive adenylate cyclase assay. *Anal. Biochem.,* 58:541–548.

123. Schousboe, A., Wu, J-Y., and Roberts, E. (1973): Purification and characterization of the 4-aminobutyrate-2-ketoglutarate transaminase from mouse brain. *Biochemistry,* 12:2868–2873.

124. Schrier, B. K., and Shuster, L. (1967): A simplified radiochemical assay for choline acetyltransferase. *J. Neurochem.,* 141:977–985.

125. Schuberth, J., Sparf, B., and Sundwall, A. (1969): A technique for the study of acetylcholine turnover in mouse brain in vivo. *J. Neurochem.,* 16:695–700.

126. Schweitzer, J. W., Schwartz, R., and Friedhoff, A. J. (1979): Intact presynaptic terminals required for beta-adrenergic receptor regulation by desipramine. *J. Neurochem.,* 33:377–379.

127. Seeman, P., Lee, T., Chan-wong, J., Tedesco, J., and Wong, K. (1976): Dopamine receptors in human and calf brains using ³H-apomorphine and an antipsychotic drug. *Proc. Natl. Acad. Sci. USA,* 73:4354–4358.

128. Shaw, R. K., and Heine, J. D. (1965): Ninhydrin positive substances present in different areas of normal rat brain. *J. Neurochem.,* 12:151–155.

129. Shea, P. A., and Aprison, M. H. (1973): An enzymatic method for measuring picomole quantities of acetylcholine and choline in CNS tissue. *Anal. Biochem.,* 56:165–177.

130. Shellenberger, M. K., and Gordon, J. H. (1971): A rapid, simplified procedure for simultaneous assay of norepinephrine, dopamine, and 5-hydroxytryptamine from discrete brain areas. *Anal. Biochem.,* 39:356–372.

131. Shields, P. J., and Eccleston, D. (1972): Effects of electrical stimulation of rat midbrain on 5-hydroxytryptamine synthesis as determined by a sensitive radioisotope method. *J. Neurochem.,* 19:255–272.

132. Sivam, S. P., Nabeshima, T., and Ho, I. K. (1981): Alterations of regional GABA receptors in morphine tolerant mice. *Biochem. Pharmacol.,* 30:2187–2190.

133. Sivam, S. P., Norris, J. C., Lim, D. K., Hoskins, B., and Ho, I. K. (1983): Effects of acute and chronic cholinesterase inhibition with diisopropylfluorophosphate on muscarinic, dopamine and GABA receptors of rat striatum. *J. Neurochem.,* 40:1414–1422.

134. Snedecor, G. W. (1956): *Statistical Methods.* Iowa State College Press, Ames.

135. Snodgrass, S. R., and Iversen, L. L. (1973): A sensitive double isotope derivative assay to measure release of amino acids from brain in vitro. *Nature [New Biol.],* 241:154–156.

136. Snyder, S. H., and Goodman, R. R. (1980): Multiple neurotransmitter receptors. *J. Neurochem.,* 35:5–15.

137. Snyder, S. H., and Hendley, E. D. (1968): A simple and sensitive fluorescence assay for monoamine oxidase and diamine oxidase. *J. Pharmacol. Exp. Ther.,* 163:386–392.

138. Spackman, D. H., Stein, W. H., and Moore, S. (1958): Automatic recording apparatus for use in the chromatography of amino acids. *Anal. Chem.,* 30:1190–1206.

139. Spector, S., Sjoerdsma, A., and Udenfriend, S. (1965): Blockade of endogenous norepinephrine synthesis by α-methyl-tyrosine, an inhibitor of tyrosine hydroxylase. *J. Pharmacol. Exp. Ther.,* 147:86–95.

140. Steiner, A. L., Pagliara, A. S., Chase, L. R., and Kipnis, D. M. (1972): Radioimmunoassay for cyclic nucleotides. II. Adenosine 3′,5′-monophosphate and guanosine 3′,5′-monophosphate in mammalian tissues and body fluids. *J. Biol. Chem.,* 247:1114–1120.

141. Steiner, A. L., Parker, C. W., and Kipnis, D. M. (1970): The measurement of cyclic nucleotides by radioimmunoassay. *Adv. Biochem. Psychopharmacol.,* 3:89–112.

142. Steiner, A. L., Parker, C. W., and Kipnis, D. M. (1972): Radioimmunoassay for cyclic nucleotides. I. Preparation of antibodies and iodinated cyclic nucleotides. *J. Biol. Chem.,* 247:1106–1113.

143. Steiner, A. L., Rerrendelli, J. A., and Kipnis, D. M. (1972): Radioimmunoassay for cyclic nucleotides. III. Effect of ischemia, changes during development and regional distribution of adenosine 3′,5′-monophosphate and guanosine 3′,5′-monophosphate in mouse brain. *J. Biol. Chem.,* 247:1121–1124.

144. Szerb, J. C. (1962): The estimation of acetylcholine using leech muscle in a microbath. *J. Physiol. (Lond.),* 158:8P.

145. Szilagyi, P. I. A., Green, J. P., Monroe, B. O., and Margolis, S. (1972): The measurement of nanogram amounts of acetylcholine in tissue by pyrolysis gas chromatography. *J. Neurochem.,* 19:2555–2566.

146. Szilagyi, P. I. A., Schmidt, D. E., and Green, J. P. (1968): Microanalytical determination of acetylcholine, other choline esters, and choline by pyrolysis gas chromatography. *Anal. Chem.,* 40:2009–2013.

147. Thompson, W. J., and Appleman, M. M. (1971): Multiple cyclic

nucleotide phosphodiesterase activities from rat brain. *Biochemistry*, 10:311–316.

148. Thompson, W. J., Teraski, W. L., Epstein, P. M., and Strada, S. J. (1979): Assay of cyclic nucleotide phosphodiesterase and resolution of multiple molecular forms of the enzyme. *Adv. Cyclic Nucleotide Res.*, 10:69–92.

149. Tozer, T. N., Neff, N. H., and Brodie, B. B. (1966): Application of steady-state kinetics to the synthesis rate and turnover time of serotonin in the brain of normal and reserpine-treated rats. *J. Pharmacol. Exp. Ther.*, 153:177–182.

150. Tzeng, S. P., and Ho, I. K. (1977): Effects of acute and continuous pentobarbital administration of the γ-aminobutyric acid system. *Biochem. Pharmacol.*, 26:699–704.

151. Umbreit, W. W., Burris, R. H., and Stauffer, J. P. (1964): *Manometric Techniques*, 4th ed. Burgess, Minneapolis.

152. Van Den Berg, C. J., Mela, P., and Waelsch, H. (1966): On the contributions of the tricarboxylic acid cycle to the synthesis of glutamate, glutamine and aspartate in brain. *Biochem. Biophys. Res. Commun.*, 23:479–484.

153. Venter, J. C., and Harrison, L. C. (1984): *Membranes, Detergents, and Receptor Solubilization*, Vols. 1–4. Alan R. Liss, New York.

154. Wagner, F. W., and Liliedahl, R. L. (1972): A rapid method for the quantitative analysis of γ-aminobutyric acid in hypothalamus homogenates by ligand-exchange chromatography. *J. Chromatogr.*, 71:567–569.

155. Waksman, A., and Roberts, E. (1965): Purification and some properties of mouse brain γ-aminobutyric-α-ketoglutaric acid transaminase. *Biochemistry*, 4:2132–2138.

156. Waymire, J. C., Bjur, R., and Weiner, N. (1971): Assay of tyrosine hydroxylase by coupled decarboxylation of DOPA formed from 1-^{14}C-L-tyrosine. *Anal. Biochem.*, 43:588–600.

157. Weiss, B., and Costa, E. (1967): Adenyl cyclase activity in rat pineal gland: effects of chronic denervation and norepinephrine. *Science*, 156:1750–1752.

158. Weiss, B., and Costa, E. (1968): Regional and subcellular distri-

bution of adenyl cyclase and 3′,5′-cyclic nucleotide phosphodiesterase in brain and pineal gland. *Biochem. Pharmacol.*, 17:2107–2116.

159. Welch, A. S., and Welch, B. L. (1969): Solvent extraction method for simultaneous determination of norepinephrine, dopamine, serotonin, and 5-hydroxyindoleacetic acid in a single mouse brain. *Anal. Biochem.*, 30:161–179.

160. White, A. A., and Aurbach, G. D. (1969): Detection of guanyl cyclase in mammalian tissues. *Biochim. Biophys. Acta*, 191:686–697.

161. White, A. A., and Zenser, T. V. (1971): Separation of cyclic 3′,5′-nucleoside monophosphates from other nucleotides on aluminum oxide columns. *Anal. Biochem.*, 41:372–396.

162. Whittaker, V. P. (1963): Identification of acetylcholine and related esters of biological origin. In: *Handbuch der Experimentellen Pharmakologie Ergänzungswerk*, edited by G. B. Koelle, Vol. 15, pp. 1–39. Springer, Berlin.

163. Whittaker, V. P., and Barker, L. A. (1972): The subcellular fractionation of brain tissue with special reference to preparation of synaptosomes and their component organelles. In: *Methods of Neurochemistry*, edited by R. Fried, Vol. 2, pp. 1–52. Marcel Dekker, New York.

164. Wooley, D. E. (1976): Some aspects of the neurophysiological basis of insecticide action. *Fed. Proc.*, 35:2610–2617.

165. Wurtman, R. J., and Axelrod, J. (1963): A sensitive and specific assay for the estimation of monoamine oxidase. *Biochem. Pharmacol.*, 12:1439–1440.

166. Yamamura, H. I., and Snyder, S. H. (1974): Muscarinic cholinergic binding in rat brain. *Proc. Natl. Acad. Sci. USA*, 71:1725–1729.

167. Zeller, E. A. (1963): Diamine oxidases. In: *The Enzymes*, edited by P. D. Boyer, H. Lardy, and K. Myrbäck, Vol. 8, pp. 313–335. Academic Press, New York.

168. Zukin, S. R., Young, A. E., and Snyder, S. H. (1974): Gamma-aminobutyric acid binding to receptor sites in rat central nervous system. *Proc. Natl. Acad. Sci. USA*, 71:4802–4807.

Principles and Methods of Toxicology, Second
Edition, edited by A. Wallace Hayes,
Raven Press, Ltd., New York © 1989.

CHAPTER **20**

Detection and Evaluation of Chemically Induced Liver Injury

Gabriel L. Plaa and *William R. Hewitt

*Département de pharmacologie, Faculté de médecine, Université de Montréal, Montréal, Québec, Canada H3C 3J7; and *Department of Investigative Toxicology, Smith Kline & French Laboratories, Philadelphia, Pennsylvania 19101*

Liver injury induced by chemicals has been recognized as a toxicological problem for more than 100 years (256). During the late 1800s scientists were concerned about the mechanisms involved in the hepatic deposition of lipids following exposure to yellow phosphorus. Hepatic lesions produced by arsphenamine, carbon tetrachloride, and chloroform were also studied in laboratory animals during the first 40 years of the twentieth century. During the same period the correlation between hepatic cirrhosis and excessive ethanol consumption was recognized.

"Liver injury" is not a single entity; the lesion observed depends not only on the chemical agent involved but also on the period of exposure. After acute exposure, one usually finds lipid accumulation in the hepatocytes, cellular necrosis, or hepatobiliary dysfunction, whereas cirrhotic or neoplastic changes are usually considered to be the result of chronic exposures. Different biochemical alterations may lead to the same endpoint; no single mechanism governs the appearance of hepatocellular degenerative changes or alterations in function. Some forms of liver injury are reversible, whereas others result in a permanently deranged organ. The mortality associated with various forms of liver injury is variable. The incidence of injury can differ among species, and the presence of a dose-dependent relation may not always be apparent.

The marked vulnerability of the liver to chemically induced damage is a function of (a) its anatomical proximity to the blood supply from the digestive tract, (b) its ability to concentrate and biotransform foreign chemicals, and (c) its role in the excretion of xenobiotics or their metabolites into the bile. The diverse nature of the functional activity of the liver and its varied response to injury makes the selection of appropriate testing procedures a difficult task. The primary purpose of this chapter is to discuss the major tests that are useful in the detection and evaluation of liver injury in laboratory animals.

CLASSIFICATION OF CHEMICALLY INDUCED LIVER INJURY

The morphologic changes observed following hepatic injury produced by chemical and biological agents can be classified according to two parameters: location and type of lesion produced.

Location Within the Hepatic Parenchyma

An early system of describing pathologic lesions of the liver originated from the concept of the hexagonal lobule introduced by Kiernan in 1833 (111) (Fig. 1). This configuration, the classical manner of presenting the relations between the hepatic cell, its vascular supply, and the biliary system, was considered to represent the functional unit of the liver. The terminal hepatic venule (central vein) is found in the center of the lobule; and the portal space, containing

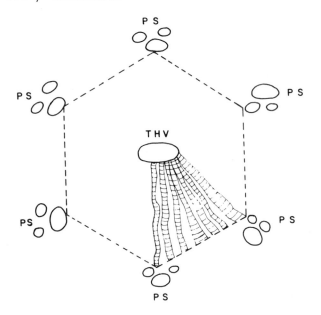

FIG. 1. Schematic representation of the traditional hexagonal lobule. (*PS*) portal space, consisting of a branch of the portal vein, hepatic arteriole, and a bile duct; (*THV*) terminal hepatic venule (central vein). [From Plaa (180), with permission.]

a branch of the portal vein, a hepatic arteriole, and a bile duct, is located at the periphery of the lobule. Based on this configuration, lesions of the hepatic parenchyma have been classified as centrilobular, midzonal, or periportal.

It is now clear that the hexagonal lobule configuration does not correspond to the functional unit of the liver. The hexagonal lobule is not conspicuous under microscopic examination. Injection of colored gelatin mixtures in the portal vein or hepatic artery shows that terminal afferent vessels supply blood only to sectors of adjacent hepatic lobules. These

sectors are situated around terminal portal branches and extend from the central vein of one hexagon to the central vein of an adjacent hexagon. Rappaport defined the parenchymal mass in terms of functional units called the liver acini (190,191). The simple liver acinus consists of a small parenchymal mass that is irregular in size and shape and is arranged around an axis consisting of a terminal portal venule, a hepatic arteriole, a bile ductule, lymph vessels, and nerves (Fig. 2). This acinus lies between two or more terminal hepatic venules (central veins) with which its vascular and biliary axis interdigitates. There is no physical separation between two liver acini. The hepatic cells of the simple acini are in cellular and sinusoidal contact with the cells of adjacent or overlapping acini. Even with this extensive communication, the hepatic cells of one particular acinus are preferentially supplied by their parent vessels. Three relatively discrete circulatory zones appear within each acinus (Fig. 2). Hepatocytes in close juxtaposition to the terminal afferent vessel constitute zone 1. These cells are the first to be supplied with fresh blood, rich in oxygen and nutrients. The higher order of zones 2 and 3 is indicative of the greater distance between the cells comprising these zones and the supply of fresh blood.

One of the interesting correlates of the concept of zonal acinar circulation is the growing realization that not all hepatic parenchymal cells within the liver lobule have the same kind of functional specificity. The intracellular characteristics of various organelles vary among zones (83). Areas of differing metabolic activity appear to exist within the liver and may correspond to the three acinar circulatory zones (83,191). Respiratory enzyme activity is particularly high in the zone closest to the terminal afferent vessel (zone 1) (Fig. 2), whereas the most distant zone (zone 3) is particularly rich in cytochrome P-450-dependent enzyme systems. The centrilobular cells, as seen in the classical hexagonal lobular configuration, are relatively rich in some NADPH-dependent enzymes, and peripheral cells are relatively poor (131,247). Sweeney and

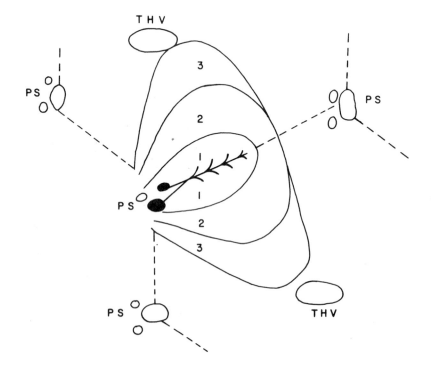

FIG. 2. Schematic representation of a simple hepatic acinus, according to A. M. Rappaport. (*PS*) portal space, consisting of a branch of the portal vein, a hepatic arteriole, and a bile duct; (*THV*) terminal hepatic venule (central vein); (*1, 2, 3*) zones draining off the terminal afferent vessel (in black). [From Plaa (180), with permission.]

co-workers (232,233), using sedimentation velocity analysis, found significant heterogeneity among populations of hepatocytes and suggested that the larger cells were richer in mixed function oxidase activity. Furthermore, enhancement of mixed function oxidase by two inducers (phenobarbital and 3-methylcholanthrene) resulted in different sedimentation-velocity patterns. The concept of "metabolic zonation" is based on differences observed between enzyme activities in periportal and centrilobular regions (108,241). Thurman and Kauffmann (241) reported on the lobular distribution of maximal enzyme activities measured by immunohistochemical or microchemical techniques; these parameters do not always correlate with metabolic flux rates as measured by microfluorometry and miniature O_2 electrodes (241). Oxygen uptake, gluconeogenesis, and glycolysis predictions based on enzyme distribution appear to agree reasonably well with measured flux rates, whereas ketogenesis does not. Monooxygenation and glucuronidation activity appear to follow the distribution of cytochrome P-450s and glucuronosyltransferases in livers from phenobarbital-treated rats but not from 3-methylcholanthrene-treated animals. The implications of such findings are not well understood. However, zonal and cellular enzymatic specificity and metabolic heterogeneity may permit the rationalization of differing mechanisms of action in the development of hepatic lesions associated with hepatotoxic agents.

The classical hexagonal descriptions of focal, midzonal, periportal, and centrilobular lesions, although functionally incorrect, are not incompatible with Rappaport's zonal acinar configuration. Centrilobular necrosis, for example, occurs in cells located in the distal acinar zone of Rappaport (zone 3) (Fig. 2). When several such zones are affected, a concentric lesion can be visualized. Regeneration is said to occur from cells located in the midzonal region of the hexagonal representation, which corresponds to the acinar zone closest to the terminal afferent vessel (zone 1), a zone shown to be particularly high in cytogenic activity. Therefore it appears that the acinal circulatory concept of the hepatic lobule does not come into serious conflict with the earlier descriptions of pathologic lesions.

Morphologic Classification

Morphologically, liver injury can manifest in different ways (180). The acute effects can consist of an accumulation of lipids (steatosis) and the appearance of degenerative processes, leading to cell death (necrosis). The necrotic process can affect small groups of isolated parenchymal cells (focal necrosis), groups of cells located in zones (centrilobular, midzonal, or periportal necrosis), or virtually all of the cells within a hepatic lobule (massive necrosis). The accumulation of lipids can also be zonal or more diffuse in nature. Although acute injury may consist in both necrosis and fat accumulation, it is not necessary that both features be present. The cholestatic type of lesion, resulting in diminution or cessation of bile flow with retention of bile salts and bilirubin, is also an important form of liver injury (172,177,184); this lesion leads to the appearance of jaundice. A type of massive necrosis that resembles a virus infection (256) is produced by certain chemicals. A number of drugs are also associated with a mixed

type of lesion, i.e., one that possesses both cholestatic and virus-like hepatic components (256). Chemically induced liver injury resulting from chronic exposure can produce marked alteration of the entire liver structure with degenerative and proliferative changes observed in the various forms of cirrhosis. Neoplastic changes may be another endpoint of chemical liver injury.

Through the years a number of classification systems have evolved to describe the chemicals involved (180,256). These schemes are beyond the scope of this chapter. In brief, however, some are based on morphologic changes (180), and others deal with the postulated mechanisms of action or the circumstances of exposure (256).

In the morphologic classifications, one finds those chemicals [e.g., carbon tetrachloride (CCl_4), chloroform ($CHCl_3$), phosphorus, tannic acid, ethionine, ethanol] that produce zonal hepatocellular alterations (necrosis, steatosis). Intrahepatic cholestasis is a lesion produced by a number of drugs (e.g., phenothiazine derivatives, antimicrobial agents, anabolic steroids, oral hypoglycemics) and is characterized by biliary dysfunction. In addition, a type of massive hepatocellular necrosis, which resembles that produced by virus infection, is also produced by other drugs (e.g., iproniazid, monoamine oxidase inhibitors, halothane).

In the classification schemes based on mechanism of action, one finds differences of opinion regarding which categories to include and how the various chemicals fit in these categories. It is clear, however, that in a number of instances the hepatic injury is an expression of individual susceptibility rather than the intrinsic toxicity of an offending agent; hypersensitivity (allergic reactions) and reactions involving an aberration in the metabolic handling of the chemical are important components in the elucidation of such lesions.

From these classifications, one can see that there are a variety of pathologic processes involved in what is called, in general terms, "liver injury." Furthermore, many kinds of substance can cause injury. Although these classification schemes assist in conceptualizing what is occurring, it should be understood that, with additional knowledge of the events actually involved in the elaboration of the biochemical lesion, changes in the classifications certainly occur. Regardless of this fact, the pathologic types of injury produced by hepatotoxicants largely determine the biochemical and functional manifestiation of injury and thus the battery of toxicological tests needed to detect and evaluate "liver injury."

EVALUATION OF HEPATIC INJURY

The major tests that have proved useful for evaluation of experimental hepatic injury in laboratory animals can be placed in four primary categories: (a) serum enzyme tests, (b) hepatic excretory tests, (c) alterations in the chemical constituents of the liver, and (d) histologic analysis of liver injury.

Serum Enzyme Techniques

Determination of the activity of hepatic enzymes released into the blood by the damaged liver is one of the most useful tools in the study of hepatotoxicity. The application of serum enzyme methodology to the detection of liver injury was introduced during the 1930s and 1940s with the demonstration of abnormal serum activities of alkaline phosphatase (213) and cholinesterase (23). However, the discovery during the 1950s that the activity of several serum aminotransferases was increased by tissue destruction represents the true advent of the serum enzyme methods. Subsequently, a number of other enzymes were identified in blood, several of which demonstrate abnormal activity in the presence of liver injury.

Zimmerman (256) identified four major categories of serum enzymes based on their specificity for and sensitivity to different types of liver injury. The first group contains enzymes such as alkaline phosphatase (AP), 5'-nucleotidase (5'-NT), and γ-glutamyltranspeptidase (γ-GT). Elevated serum activities of these enzymes appear to reflect cholestatic injury more effectively than parenchymal injury. In contrast, the second group of enzymes includes those that are more sensitive to cytotoxic hepatic injury. This group has been further subdivided into: (a) enzymes that are somewhat nonspecific and can reflect injury to extrahepatic tissue, e.g., aspartate aminotransferase (AST) and lactic dehydrogenase (LDH); (b) enzymes found mainly in the liver, e.g., alanine aminotransferase (ALT); and (c) enzymes that are almost exclusively located in the liver, e.g., ornithine carbamyl transferase (OCT) and sorbitol dehydrogenase (SDH). Assay of the latter, more hepatospecific subgroup of enzymes may be particularly useful when studying agents with unknown hepatotoxic potential. Although elevated serum activity of the aminotransferases may reflect injury to extrahepatic organs such as the heart, skeletal muscle, or kidney, elevated activities of OCT and SDH are reliable reflections of hepatic injury.

Zimmerman's third and fourth groups contain, respectively, enzymes that are relatively insensitive to hepatic injury but are elevated with extrahepatic diseases, e.g., creatine phosphokinase (CPK), and enzymes that demonstrate a depressed serum activity in liver disease, e.g., cholinesterase (ChE).

The selection of a battery of enzymes for evaluating the hepatotoxic potential of an unknown chemical in laboratory animals is complicated by the varying sensitivity of the enzymes to different types of lesion. In an early series of experiments, Molander et al. (160) found that the measurement of serum AST provided a more sensitive index of hepatocellular injury in rats treated with CCl₄ than did the measurement of either ChE or AP. A number of experimentally induced necrotic states are also detectable by an elevation in ALT activity. Balazs et al. (10) assessed serum ALT as a liver test in rats after treatment with ethionine, CCl₄, thioacetamide, dimethylnitrosamine, or allyl alcohol. Serum ALT elevation occurred following the acute administration of all of these agents, but with ethionine the elevation was not pronounced. This finding is understandable in that ethionine does not produce extensive centrilobular necrosis but usually results in fatty infiltration. Other investigators also found that ALT is an insensitive measure of hepatic steatosis (5,76). On the other hand, those agents that are associated with severe necrotic lesions produce pronounced elevation of serum ALT. Balazs et al. (9,10) found that when the gross pathological changes or the severity of the histopathology were compared to the elevation in ALT, there was a good correlation between the elevation in serum ALT and the severity of the lesion. Others showed (140,182) that there was an excellent correlation between the severity of quantified histologic damage produced by CHCl₃ or acetaminophen and the elevation in serum ALT activity in rats. Acetaminophen-induced elevation in plasma ALT activity and acetaminophen covalent binding to hepatocellular protein in mice have been shown to correlate well (248). Therefore it seems with ALT that not only is it possible to detect the presence of liver injury, but under some circumstances the severity of the lesion can be estimated by the elevation in serum enzyme activity.

Ornithine carbamyl transferase is found predominantly in the mitochondrial fraction of liver cells (48,201,202) and normally occurs only in minute amounts in serum. The mucosa of the small intestine contains a small amount, 1 to 2% that of the liver, and tissue such as brain and kidney contains only trace amounts (202–204). OCT serum activity is markedly elevated in both acute and chronic liver disease in humans (169,204). Furthermore, Reichard (204) suggested that OCT was a more sensitive test of liver injury in the human than either AST or ALT. With experimentally induced hepatotoxicity, Reichard (201) found that serum activity of OCT increased considerably more than those of the aminotransferases but followed a temporal phase similar to that of the aminotransferases. OCT was also as sensitive an index of liver injury as GDH and AST in cattle and sheep poisoned with CCl₄, dimidium bromide, or sporidesmin (70). Tegeris et al. (236) found that OCT activity was markedly elevated in dogs and swine poisoned with CCl₄, whereas the serum activity remained within normal limits in animals treated with uranyl nitrate, a nephrotoxicant. In addition, the peak serum activities of OCT (expressed as multiples of normal) in CCl₄-challenged animals were markedly greater that those of ALT, AST, LDH, or isocitric dehydrogenase (ICDH); the temporal pattern of OCT response was similar to that of the aminotransaminases. Serum OCT activity is a useful monitor of liver injury in rats treated with various hepatotoxicants (48,55,56,129). Indeed, Drotman (55) described a dose-dependent relation between the amount of CCl₄ administered to rats and serum OCT activity. In addition, a sixfold increase in OCT activity was found at a CCl₄ dose that did not produce distinctive liver damage upon light microscopic examination of the tissue, suggesting that OCT may be as sensitive an index of liver injury as histopathological examination (56). The correlation between elevation in serum OCT activity and quantified histological changes following CHCl₃ administration is good (182).

Sorbitol dehydrogenase, a cytoplasmic enzyme, is also relatively specific for liver (6,48), and an increase in the serum activity of this enzyme is a relatively sensitive index of hepatocellular damage. In an elegant series of experiments, Korsrud et al. (128) determined the serum activity of nine hepatic enzymes in CCl₄-poisoned rats in an attempt to identify those enzymes that would respond quantitatively to varying CCl₄ doses and would indicate minimal liver damage. They placed the enzymes in three groups based on the lowest dose of CCl₄ required to elevate serum activity and concluded that SDH was the most sensitive enzymic index of liver injury. A group of four enzymes [ICDH, fructose-1,6-aldolase (F-1,6-ALD), ALT, and AST] were less sensitive to CCl₄ than SDH but were more responsive to liver injury than were alcohol dehydrogenase (ADH), 6-phosphodigluconase (6-PDG), LDH, and malic dehydrogenase (MDH). However, histological alterations were observed at CCl$_4$ doses that did not elevate serum enzyme activity. Subsequently, Korsrud et al. (129) studied thioacetamide, dimethylnitrosamine, and diethanolamine. As before, serum SDH was the most sensitive enzymic index of liver necrosis. The dose of these hepatotoxicants required to elevate the serum activity of ICDH, F-1,6-ALD, ALT, and AST was less than that needed to elevate serum OCT, MDH, and LDH activity.

Sorbitol dehydrogenase was not a preferentially sensitive index of liver injury in diethanolamine-treated rats. Six enzymes (SDH, ICDH, F-1,6-ALD, ALT, AST, and MDH) were equally responsive to diethanolamine hepatotoxicity, whereas a higher dose of this compound was required to elevate the serum activity of OCT, GDH, and LDH. Based on these observations Korsrud et al. (129) suggested that SDH was the best enzymic index of liver injury when minimal damage or minimal changes are being assessed. However, as found in the previous study, histological changes characteristic of each hepatotoxicant were noted at doses that did not result in an elevation of serum activity. Thus the serum enzyme assays were less sensitive than histopathological examination for detecting liver damage.

The latter conclusions appear to conflict with those of Drotman and Lawhorn (55,56). These investigators found alteration in serum OCT activity at a dose of CCl$_4$ that did not produce distinctive liver damage in rats on light microscopic examination of the tissue. Interestingly, in one of these studies (56) the relative sensitivities of OCT and SDH were compared in rats poisoned with various doses of CCl$_4$ or diethylamine. At a low dose of CCl$_4$, elevations in serum OCT appeared prior to elevations in SDH activity; and relative to baseline serum activity, the maximum increase in OCT activity was greater than that for SDH. As the dose of CCl$_4$ was increased, the temporal appearances of OCT and SDH were similar; however, the maximum increase in serum enzyme activity was greatest for OCT regardless of the dose of CCl$_4$ administered. Essentially similar results were obtained in rats when diethylamine was used as the hepatotoxicant (56). OCT and SDH were generally more sensitive indices of liver injury than were ALT, AST, or ICDH. Although the discrepancies between the studies of Korsrud et al. (129) and Drotman and Lawhorn (56) cannot be resolved, it appears reasonable to suggest that one of these two enzymes (SDH or OCT) be used in conjunction with the aminotransferases when examining the hepatotoxic potential of an unknown chemical.

Analytical Determination of Aminotransferase Activity

There are essentially two major techniques employed for the measurement of serum aminotransferase activity (90). For AST, one measures the conversion of aspartic acid and α-ketoglutaric acid to glutamic acid and oxaloacetic acid; for ALT, one measures the conversion of alanine and α-ketoglutaric acid to glutamic acid and pyruvic acid. With the ultraviolet method of analysis, the enzyme processes are coupled with ones in which nicotinamide adenine dinucleotide (NAD) is converted from its reduced form (NADH) to the oxidized form (NAD). The course of the reaction is fol-lowed by the decrease in absorbance at 340 nm produced by the oxidation of NADH.

The colorimetric procedure involves the reaction of the product (oxaloacetic or pyruvic acid) with dinitrophenylhydrazine to form a colored hydrazone. This product can be determined by its absorbance in the visible range. The principal advantages of the colorimetric method are that an ultraviolet spectrophotometer is not required and temperature control of the enzymic reaction is more easily attained.

There has been a certain amount of controversy in the literature over the relative accuracies of both these procedures. However, most of the argument concerns the use of AST for the detection of coronary occlusion (3). For the detection of experimentally induced hepatic injury these objections do not seem to be as pertinent as they might be for the diagnosis of coronary occlusion. If one is primarily interested in following the kinetics of the enzyme reaction, the ultraviolet method is probably preferred. With this procedure, the product of the enzyme reaction does not accumulate because it is converted to another product through the use of either MDH or LDH. It is also true that when AST is measured by the colorimetric procedure one of the substrates (α-ketoglutaric acid) does interfere with the final colorimetric analysis. However, the primary use of serum aminotransferase activity in laboratory animals is for the detection of hepatic injury. In this situation one is not primarily interested in the absolute value of activity but, rather, in its general increase. Therefore the colorimetric procedure of Reitman and Frankel (206) is of sufficient accuracy. The relative ease of this procedure over the spectrophotometric method seems to make it more advantageous for use with laboratory animals, where large numbers of samples are to be analyzed. Wells and To (248) developed a microanalytical technique that allows repetitive plasma ALT measurements on tail vein blood from individual mice using the Reitman and Frankel procedure.

Note that the aminotransferase activity in different tissues varies and that distinct species differences occur (255). In most instances AST activity is greater than ALT activity. High AST activity occurs in skeletal muscle, diaphragm, heart muscle, and liver tissue. ALT is not as widely distributed; in humans the greatest activity is found in the liver. Cornelius (43) studied the hepatic distribution of ALT in various animals and found that a relation exists between body size and the amount of hepatic ALT activity. The smaller the animal is within the weight range studied, the greater the hepatic ALT activity. More than 90% of the ALT activity was found to be located within the liver of all mammals of small body size; this group includes the common laboratory animals used in toxicity studies. Cornelius et al. (44) showed that, whereas AST activity was present in almost all tissues of pigs, cattle, dogs, and horses, low activities of ALT were found in horses, cattle, and pigs. When these species were subjected to CCl$_4$ intoxication, significant elevation of serum ALT activity occurred only in the dog. On the other hand, when serum AST activity was used for measuring hepatotoxicity, all species exhibited an increase in serum enzyme activity after CCl$_4$. In the rat, both serum AST and ALT activities are markedly elevated after experimental injury; either enzyme could probably be used for detecting injury in this species. Hemolysis, however, has a marked effect on serum AST activity in the rat, whereas its effect is practically negligible in the case of serum ALT (178). This fact should be kept in mind when one is using rats for assessing liver function. Because serum ALT activity resides primarily in the liver, a better procedure might be to use this particular aminotransferase for determining the status of the liver rather than serum AST.

Alanine aminotransferase method. [ALT; EC 2.6.1.2, L-alanine: 2-oxoglutarate aminotransferase; glutamic pyruvic transaminase (GPT)]

The colorimetric procedure of Reitman and Frankel (206) is described. For use in mice and rats, the blood is drawn by cardiac puncture under light ether anesthesia, and plasma or serum is prepared as desired.

Reagents.

1. Phosphate buffer (0.1 M, pH 7.4): Mix 420 ml of 0.1 M disodium phosphate (26.81 g of $Na_2HPO_4 \cdot 7 H_2O/L$) and 80 ml of 0.1 M potassium dihydrogen phosphate (13.61 g of KH_2PO_4/L). The pH should be 7.4.
2. α-Ketoglutarate–alanine substrate: Dissolve 29.2 mg of α-ketoglutaric acid and 1.78 g of alanine in a small amount (1–2 ml) of 1 M NaOH. Adjust pH to 7.4 and bring to a final volume of 100 ml in a volumetric flask using the 0.1 M phosphate buffer.
3. Color reagent: Dissolve 19.8 mg of 2,4-dinitrophenylhydrazine in 100 ml of 1 N hydrochloric acid.
4. Sodium hydroxide (0.4 N): Dissolve 16 g of NaOH in distilled water to make 1 L.
5. Pyruvate standard (2 mM): Dissolve 22 mg of sodium pyruvate in 100 ml of phosphate buffer.

Procedure.

1. Pipette 0.5 ml of the substrate in a test tube. Incubate at 37°C for 5 min in a Temp-Blok module heater (Lab-Line Instruments). Prepare an extra tube for a blank.
2. Pipette an aliquot (0.1 ml) of plasma into the tube, mix by swirling, and incubate for exactly 30 min at 37°C.
3. At the end of the incubation, remove the tube from the heater, add 0.5 ml of the color reagent, and mix.
4. After 30 min, add 5.0 ml of 0.4 N NaOH and mix.
5. The absorbance of this solution is determined at 505 nm 30 min after the addition of NaOH. The units of enzyme are read from a standard curve after subtraction of the blank. If activities are too high to read on the standard curve, repeat the entire assay with an appropriate dilution of plasma.

Standard curve.

1. Set up a series of four tubes containing the amounts of the pyruvate standard, substrate, and water as indicated below:

Tube No.	Pyruvate standard (ml)	Substrate (ml)	H$_2$O (ml)	Calculated ALT units/ml
1	0.0	1.0	0.2	0
2	0.1	0.9	0.2	28
3	0.2	0.8	0.2	57
4	0.3	0.7	0.2	97

2. Add 1.0 ml of the color reagent to each tube, mix, and allow to stand at room temperature for 30 min.
3. At 30 min after the NaOH is added, add 10 ml of 0.4 N NaOH, mix, and determine the absorbance of the solution at 505 nm.
4. Plot the curve on linear graph paper using the calculated ALT units given above and their respective absorbance values.

Note that comparative studies have been made using commercially prepared reagents (Dade Reagents), and the results have been found to be comparable to those obtained with the individually prepared reagents.

Analytical Determination of Ornithine Carbamyl Transferase Activity

Mammalian OCT (EC 2.1.3.3) catalyzes the transfer of the carbamyl group from carbamyl phosphate to ornithine and results in the formation of citrulline. OCT activity may be measured directly by following the appearance of citrulline or indirectly by arsenolysis, in which the enzyme catalyzes the reverse reaction of citrulline to ammonia, carbon dioxide, and ornithine. In the forward reaction, citrulline is determined colorimetrically with diacetyl monoxime after destruction of serum urea with urease (33,34,244). In the reverse reaction, OCT activity is determined by production of $^{14}CO_2$ from [^{14}C-ureido]-L-citrulline (55,129,205) or by production of ammonia. The formation of ammonia can be analyzed by conversion to indophenol (127) or by a microdiffusion procedure in a Conway cell (200).

The isotopic method of Reichard (205) as modified by Korsrud et al. (129) and the colorimetric (indophenol) method of Konttinen (127,128) are described here. As in the assay of ALT activity, blood is drawn from ether anesthetized mice or rats by cardiac puncture, and plasma or serum is prepared as desired.

Ornithine carbamyl transferase activity: isotopic method

Reagents.

1. [^{14}C]Citrulline–arsenate reagent: Dissolve 1.75 g of L-citrulline and 15.6 g of dibasic sodium arsenate ($Na_2AsSO_4 \cdot 7 H_2O$) in distilled water. Add 45.45 μCi of [^{14}C-ureido]-L-citrulline. Adjust pH to 7.1 and dilute to a final volume of 100 ml with distilled water. This solution contains 50 μmol of [^{14}C]citrulline (0.004545 μCi/μmol, 10,000 dpm/μmol) in 0.5 ml of 0.5 M arsenate buffer (pH 7.1).
2. Sulfuric acid (9 N): Add 50 ml of concentrated H_2SO_4 to 40 ml of distilled water in a 100-ml volumetric flask. Let cool to room temperature and dilute to mark with distilled water.
3. Hyamine hydroxide (1 M): Obtain commercially.
4. Scintillation fluid: Dissolve 4 g of Omnifluor (New England Nuclear), containing 98% 2,5-diphenyloxazole and 2% p-bis-(O-methylstyryl)-benzene in 1,000 ml of toluene.

Procedure.
1. Add 0.5 ml of the [^{14}C]citrulline–arsenate reagent and plasma (up to 0.5 ml) to a 25-ml Erlenmyer flask (Kontes Glass Co., No. 882300).
2. Immediately cap the flask with a one-hole rubber septum stopper (Kontes, No. 882310) containing a polypropylene center well (Kontes, No. 882320).
3. Remove 20 ml of air from the flask (using a syringe and needle).
4. Incubate the flask, with gentle agitation, for 18 hr at 37°C.
5. At the end of the incubation period, stop the reaction by adding 0.5 ml of 9 *N* sulfuric acid [1.0-ml syringe fitted with a 20-gauge (1.5-inch) needle].
6. Add 0.25 ml of hyamine hydroxide to the center well (syringe and needle).
7. Incubate the flask for an additional 60 min to trap the evolved $^{14}CO_2$.
8. At the end of the trapping period, remove the center well and stopper from the flask, wipe the well free of condensation, and place it in a counting vial containing 15 ml of scintillation fluid.
9. Determine the activity of $^{14}CO_2$ by liquid scintillation spectrophotometry, correct for quench, and subtract the activity of the blank (flask containing all components minus plasma).
10. Express the results as nanomoles citrulline converted per minute per milliliter of plasma (129) or disintegrations per minute per milliliter of plasma (55).

The formation of $^{14}CO_2$ from [^{14}C-ureido]-L-citrulline is linear over a period of 24 hr. Drotman (55) used a modification of this method with success.

Ornithine carbamyl transferase activity: colorimetric method

With the colorimetric method, citrulline is decomposed by arsenolysis catalyzed by OCT. The liberated ammonia is determined as indophenol after reaction with phenolnitroprusside and alkaline hypochlorite (127).

Reagents.
1. Citrulline–arsenate reagent: Dissolve 3.5 g of DL-citrulline and 15.6 g dibasic sodium arsenate ($Na_2AsSO_4 \cdot 7\ H_2O$) in distilled water. Adjust the pH to 7.1 and dilute to 100 ml. This reagent can be obtained commercially from Sigma Chemical Co. (Cat. No. 108-1).
2. Phenol–nitroprusside reagents: Dissolve 10 g of phenol and 50 mg of sodium nitroprusside in distilled water and bring to a final volume of 400 ml. Store solution in an amber bottle at 4°C.
3. Alkaline hypochlorite: Dissolve 5 g of sodium hydroxide pellets in approximately 200 ml of distilled water. When cool, add 6 ml of sodium hypochlorite (10–14% Cl). Bring to a final volume of 400 ml with distilled water. Store in an amber bottle at 4°C.
4. Standard ammonia solution: Dissolve 464 mg of ammonium sulfate [$(NH_4)_2SO_4$] in approximately 600 ml of distilled water. Add 2 ml of concentrated sulfuric acid and dilute to a final volume of 1,000 ml with distilled

water. Dilute 10 ml of this stock solution to a final volume of 50 ml with distilled water. This solution contains 1.4 μmol ammonia/ml.

Procedure.
1. Prepare two tubes for each plasma sample. The first tube (S) is used to measure OCT activity, and the second tube (A) is used to determine endogenous plasma ammonia concentrations.
2. Add plasma (0.2–0.5 ml) to tubes S and A.
3. Add an equivalent volume of the citrulline–arsenate reagent to tube S, mix, and cap both tubes S and A.
4. Incubate the tubes for 24 hr at 37°C.
5. At the end of the incubation period, add the requisite volume of the citrulline–arsenate reagent to tube A and mix.
6. Transfer 0.05 ml of the reaction mixtures from tubes S and A to separate tubes; add 2.0 ml of the phenol–nitroprusside solution and mix.
7. Add 2.0 ml of the alkaline hypochlorite solution to each tube, mix, and incubate at 37°C for 15 min.
8. Prepare a blank and a standard by adding 0.05 ml of distilled water and the standard ammonia solution, respectively, to separate tubes. The color reaction is performed as in steps 6 and 7.
9. The absorbance of the colored solutions is determined at 630 nm.
10. The results are expressed as international units (IU) per liter of plasma according to the equation:

$$(Abs_S - Abs_A)/(Abs_{std} - Abs_B) \times 1.94 = IU/L\ of\ plasma$$

where Abs_S is the absorbance of tube S (NH_3 production from OCT activity), Abs_A is the absorbance of tube A (endogenous NH_3 in plasma), Abs_{std} is the absorbance of the standard, and Abs_B is the absorbance of the blank. One international unit (IU) is the activity of OCT that catalyzes the transformation of 1 μmol of citrulline to ornithine per minute.

This colorimetric determination of OCT activity has the advantage of not requiring a liquid scintillation spectrophotometer, and it eliminates the use of costly radiolabeled chemicals and scintillation cocktails.

Other Enzymes

Isoenzymes

In addition to serum enzyme activities, serum isoenzyme patterns have been utilized for the detection of organ damage in humans and laboratory animals (45,46,82,252). Isoenzymes are enzymatically active proteins that catalyze the same reactions and occur in the same species but differ in their physicochemical properties. The isoenzymes of LDH are used as diagnostic agents in clinical medicine (46) and in some instances have been evaluated for use in experimentally induced organ damage in laboratory animals. Cornish et al. (46) utilized LDH isoenzymes to detect specific organ damage in rats; they found that the serum isoenzyme patterns resulting from liver or kidney damage differed markedly and concluded that these differences could be utilized to distinguish the damaged organ. Liver damage resulted primarily in an increase in serum LDH-5 isoenzyme activity, whereas the activity of the LDH-1 and LDH-2 isoenzymes was elevated in rats with kidney injury. Grice et al. (82) treated rats with CCl_4, mercuric chloride, thioacetamide, or diethanolamine at doses that would produce either minimal or pronounced tissue damage. Although AST activity was a more sensitive indicator of organ damage than LDH, it did not provide isoenzyme patterns that could identify the specific target organ. In contrast, LDH isoenzyme patterns were capable of identifying the specific target organ; the LDH-5 bands indicative of liver injury were increased in rats poisoned with CCl_4, diethanolamine, and thioacetamide, whereas mercuric chloride, a potent nephrotoxicant, increased the activity of LDH-1 and LDH-2. Morphologic damage generally occurred at dosage levels considerably below those producing detectable serum enzyme alterations. Thus these authors concluded that serum enzyme activities and isoenzyme patterns are an important supplement to, but not a substitute for, histopathological examination of tissues.

A number of other enzymes of clinical interest occur in multiple forms, among which are AST and alkaline and acid phosphatase. Although these enzymes may have well-established roles in experimental toxicology, the use of their isoenzyme patterns does not yet have a definitive role.

Enzymes useful for detecting obstructive disorders

Most of the preceding discussion concerns the use of serum enzymes to detect necrotic or degenerative processes following the administration of toxicants. In general, these enzymes are not as useful for detecting those types of hepatic alteration that are associated with diminution or cessation of bile flow. The degree of change in serum enzyme activities that one can obtain by the induction of experimental hepatotoxicity in mice is demonstrated in Table 1. Three hepatotoxic procedures were employed in this study (178). One group of animals received α-naphthylisothiocyanate (ANIT), another received CCl_4, and the third group had their bile ducts ligated. Serum enzyme activities (ALT and AP) were determined 24 hr later. For comparative purposes, sulfobromophthalein (BSP) retention and serum bilirubin concentrations were also measured in these animals. It is evident (Table 1) that a necrotizing agent such as CCl_4 produces sufficient parenchymal injury to cause a large increase in serum ALT activity,

whereas those experimental procedures that markedly impair biliary excretion (ANIT treatment, bile duct ligation) causes only a mild increase in ALT activity. The reciprocal relation is obtained when serum AP activity is assessed; obstruction of biliary flow (bile duct ligation) markedly increases serum AP activity, whereas the necrotizing challenge (CCl_4) produces only a mild elevation.

Alkaline phosphatase is the prototype of those enzymes (Zimmerman's group 1) that reflect pathological reductions in biliary flow. In the rat this enzyme is found in the liver and the intestine. After bile duct ligation, the activity in the liver increases due to *de novo* synthesis of the membranous form of the enzyme (110,225). The use of this enzyme in chemically induced liver dysfunction has been fairly extensively investigated. In the dog the enzyme is useful for detecting biliary dysfunction. In the cat, however, ligation of the common bile duct results in only a slight increase in serum AP activity. The normal level of serum AP in the rat is exceptionally high, independent of growth, and unusually susceptible to variations in diet (84). Thus serum AP activity may not be useful for detecting cholestatic changes in the rat.

In addition to AP, other enzymes, e.g., 5'N, γ-GT, and leucine aminopeptidase (LAP), may be of use in assessing obstructive liver injury. The serum activity of these enzymes, which are localized in the membranes of hepatocytes and bile duct cells, is increased during extrahepatic cholestasis in humans (12,251). Kryszewski et al. (132) found a significant elevation in serum activity of AP, 5'N, and γ-GT 12 hr after bile duct ligation in the rat; AP and 5'N peaked at 24 hr and then gradually decreased, and γ-GT peaked at 48 hr and remained elevated even 192 hr after bile duct ligation. Thus changes in the serum activities of these enzymes are useful for detecting toxicant-induced cholestatic changes in laboratory animals.

Of interest is the observation of Moritz and Snodgrass (166) that acute obstruction of the bile duct in the rat produced a rapid rise in the serum activity of SDH and OCT. From 1 to 24 hr following bile duct ligation, the activities of these two enzymes increased in serum to levels approximating those found after a single dose of CCl_4, even though the histological degree of hepatic necrosis was substantially less with obstruction than with CCl_4 poisoning. This finding confirmed and extended the observation of Hallberg et al. (86) that bile duct obstruction in dogs resulted in increased serum OCT activity. These observations, if confirmed in other models of experimentally induced obstructive disorders,

TABLE 1. *Effect of various hepatotoxic procedures on four liver function tests in mice[a]*

Hepatotoxic procedure[b]	BSP retention (mg/dl)	Alkaline phosphatase (units)	Bilirubin concentration (mg/dl)	ALT activity (units/ml)
Control (no treatment)	0.3 ± 0.3	3.0 ± 0.5	0.2 ± 0.1	25 ± 5
ANIT (150 mg/kg p.o.)	45.0 ± 23	5.6 ± 2.6	1.1 ± 0.4	282 ± 126
CCl_4 (1 ml/kg p.o.)	13.0 ± 7	5.3 ± 1.3	0.4 ± 0.2	8,510 ± 1,930
Bile duct ligation	26.0 ± 3	19.0 ± 10	3.8 ± 0.8	655 ± 132

[a] Values are expressed as mean ± SE; each group contained ten mice.
[b] Hepatotoxic procedure was performed 24 hr before assessing function.
Data were obtained from Plaa (178).

suggest that OCT and SDH could serve to identify hepatic alterations associated with a diminution or cessation of bile flow.

Hepatic Excretory Function

Chemicals entering the systemic circulation are excreted by the liver unchanged or after modification within the hepatocyte. Compounds that undergo biliary excretion have been divided into three classes (A–C) based on the bile/plasma concentration ratios obtained during their excretion (22,119,126). Examples of class A substances include sodium, potassium, and chloride ions as well as glucose; these compounds have a bile/plasma ratio of about 1.0. Class B substances, e.g., bile salts, bilirubin, BSP, and many xenobiotics, achieve a bile/plasma ratio of more than 1.0, usually between 10 and 1,000. Among class C substances, which have a bile/plasma ratio of less than 1.0, are macromolecules such as inulin, phospholipids, mucoproteins, and albumin.

In terms of detecting and quantifying hepatic damage, the compounds of class B are of particular interest. Their biliary excretion is mediated by several multicomponent transport systems. For example, most organic acids, e.g., bilirubin and BSP, are believed to be excreted by a common transport system in the liver; however, a distinct system may exist for bile acids. In addition to the organic acid system, two other carrier systems—one for organic bases, e.g., procaineamide ethobromide (PAEB), and one for neutral organic molecules, e.g., ouabain—exist in the liver. Finally, a transport system(s) may exist for the biliary excretion of metals such as lead (119,126).

The most common class B chemical used in the detection of liver injury is BSP. This anionic phthalein dye was introduced into clinical medicine by Rosenthal and White in 1925 after preliminary tests with other phthalein dyes proved less satisfactory (215,216). Since its introduction, this substance has been used extensively for the assessment of liver function in humans and laboratory animals; the BSP clearance test has proved to be one of the most useful and sensitive indices for detection of hepatic dysfunction.

The use of BSP is based on the observation that dye removal from blood is delayed by hepatic dysfunction. Commonly, BSP concentration in plasma is determined at a specific time after a standard dose of dye (per unit of body weight) is administered intravenously. Selection of the optimal dose of BSP is essential for correct interpretation of functional impairment.

The removal of BSP from the plasma is dependent on the simultaneous operation of a number of hepatic processes, e.g., active transport across the plasma membrane into a storage compartment, metabolic transformation, and active transport across the canalicular membrane (119). The most critical step in this process is thought to be the transfer of BSP from liver to bile. Most important in terms of selecting an optimal BSP dose is that its biliary excretion can be saturated and a transport maximum (Tm) exists; the clearance of BSP by laboratory animals is dose-dependent (121). Usually one observes that small doses are rapidly removed from the circulation; this rate of removal continues as one increases the dose, until a dosage level of BSP is reached where the rate of disappearance becomes longer. For example, with the isolated perfused rat liver (183), 5, 10, and 20 mg of BSP are cleared at the same exponential rate; the capacity of the liver to extract BSP from the perfusate becomes saturated when 30 or 40 mg is injected. With the latter dose, the rate of disappearance becomes zero order, which indicates that the maximal capacity of the transport system is reached. This same type of phenomenon occurs in mice *in vivo* (58).

A marked species difference exists in the ability of the rat, rabbit, and dog to remove BSP from the plasma; this difference can be readily discerned by administering varying BSP doses to these laboratory animals (Fig. 3). Both the rat and the rabbit have a remarkable ability to clear BSP from the plasma, whereas the dog has a relatively poor capacity (121). Extrahepatic factors such as renal excretion or distribution apparently do not account for this species difference in plasma clearance (178). Rather, if the overall BSP Tm for biliary

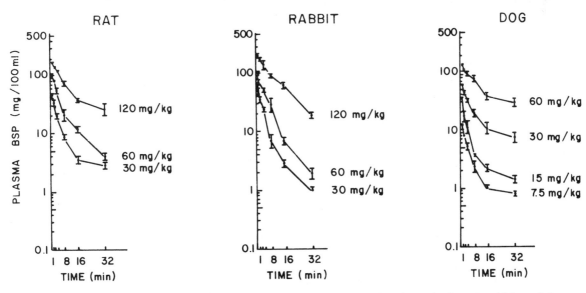

FIG. 3. Plasma disappearance curves for BSP administered in varying doses in the rat, rabbit, and dog. [From Klaassen and Plaa (121), with permission.]

excretion is measured, large differences are observed (121). The rat and rabbit excrete BSP at a rate of about 1 mg/min/kg, whereas the dog excretes it at a rate of about 0.2 mg/min/kg.

The significance of these findings is that the optimal dose of BSP for measuring liver function depends on the species employed. The dose should be one that is relatively close to the one that indicates BSP clearance capacity is being exceeded. For the rabbit, dog, and rat, these dosages are about 75, 15, and 50 mg/kg, respectively (121). In mice the optimal dosage depends on the strain employed but is somewhere between 75 and 100 mg/kg (178). The dose selected should result in about 2 to 3% retention at 30 min in normal animals.

Determination of the BSP Tm has been used as an index of hepatic function in humans. Wheeler et al. (250) devised a procedure that can be employed in unanesthetized dogs. With this technique, one infuses BSP at three different rates and measures the serum concentration at varying times. From the data, one can calculate the Tm and the relative storage capacity (S) for BSP. In addition, methods have been devised for making similar measurements in the rabbit and rat (120). Use of these techniques has not been widespread in laboratory animals. However, they are useful for assessing excretory capacity and are employed in mechanistic studies to determine specific functional lesions involved in the reduction of BSP clearance. For example, defects in (a) transfer of BSP from plasma to liver, (b) storage of BSP within the hepatocyte, (c) conjugation of BSP with glutathione, or (d) transfer of BSP from the liver cell into the bile could participate in the CCl_4-induced depression of BSP clearance. When these possibilities were evaluated, it appeared that the major effect of CCl_4 was to decrease the transfer of BSP from the hepatocyte to the bile (122,188). Klaassen and Plaa (122) found that 24 hr after a single intraperitoneal dose of CCl_4 both the BSP Tm and hepatic BSP conjugating activity were depressed; no change in hepatic BSP storage was detected. Because CCl_4 reduced plasma disappearance and the Tm of phenol-3,6-dibromophthalein disulfonate (DBSP), a nonmetabolized analog of BSP, and depressed excretion of both BSP and DBSP under submaximal conditions, it was concluded that the excretory parameter was probably the prime event altered by CCl_4. Subsequently, Priestly and Plaa (188) demonstrated that impaired BSP excretion, bile flow rate, relative hepatic storage, and BSP retention were observed as early as 3 hr after CCl_4 administration. Impaired BSP conjugation, however, was not unequivocally demonstrated until 12 hr after CCl_4. Thus although impairment of both conjugation and excretion contributes to BSP retention, the effect on excretion appears to be more important.

Although BSP was introduced in 1924, it was not until 1950 that it was realized that this dye is excreted in a conjugated form into the bile (24). Up to that time it was assumed that this material did not undergo biotransformation prior to its excretion. BSP is conjugated with glutathione in humans, rats, and dogs. A number of other conjugates, including BSP-cysteinylglycine and BSP-cysteine, are also formed, presumably by cleavage of glutamic acid and glycine from the glutathione moiety. BSP conjugation, catalyzed by a GSH-S-transferase, is a cytoplasmic process. Under certain conditions, impairment of BSP conjugation with hepatic glutathione can lead to depression of BSP excretion in the bile

without impairment of general excretory function (21,41, 187,189).

Although BSP is a useful and sensitive test of liver function, a variety of events can cause BSP retention. Diffuse and severe hepatocellular damage are associated with an increase in dye retention (87). Liver injury of the cholestatic type, however, usually decreases biliary excretion to a greater extent than does parenchymal cell injury (119). For example, using ANIT, Becker and Plaa (13) showed that the amount of BSP retained following such treatment is much greater than that observed after the necrotic effects of CCl_4. In this instance, ANIT affects BSP retention by decreasing the biliary excretion of BSP (181). In rabbits, treatment with anabolic steroids can result in BSP retention owing to a decrease in excretory capacity (139). In contrast, bunamiodyl [sodium 3-(3-butyramide-2,4,6-triiodophenyl)-2-ethylacrylate] seems to diminish uptake of BSP by the hepatocyte (18). Finally, decreased hepatic blood flow can also cause BSP retention (58).

Phenobarbital markedly enhances the excretion of BSP (123,179). This effect is apparently not related to an increase in BSP conjugation, as phenobarbital pretreatment also enhances the biliary excretion of DBSP (179). Klaassen showed (113–117) that when seven microsomal enzyme inducers were examined only phenobarbital produced a significant increase in bile flow and a significant increase in anion excretion; benzo(a)pyrene and 3-methylcholanthrene did not increase bile flow. Chlordane, nikethamide, phenylbutazone, and chlorcyclizine treatments tended to increase bile flow, but the increases were not statistically significant. These substances also failed to enhance BSP or DBSP biliary excretion (117). Subsequently, two other microsomal enzyme inducers, spironolactone and pregnenolone-16α-carbonitrile, increased bile flow and the biliary excretion of BSP and DBSP in rats (257). Thus the ability of various microsomal enzyme inducers to increase BSP and DBSP clearance appears to be related to their ability to increase bile flow (119).

BSP Clearance Procedure

Reagents

1. BSP injection solution: prepare a solution (50 mg/ml) of BSP in 0.9% NaCl.
2. Acidified NaCl: 100 ml of 0.9% NaCl plus 5 ml of 10% HCl.
3. Alkalinized NaCl: 100 ml of 0.9% NaCl plus 5 ml of 10% NaOH.

Procedure

1. Inject mice with BSP (75 mg/kg) via the tail vein.
2. Lightly anesthetize each mouse with ether and obtain a blood sample (0.6 ml) 30 min after BSP injection. A syringe rinsed with 1.6% sodium oxalate is used.
3. Add blood to a small test tube containing 1 mg of sodium oxalate, and centrifuge to separate plasma.
4. After centrifugation, place aliquots (0.1 ml) of the plasma into two tubes. Add 1.0 ml of acidified NaCl to one tube and 1.0 ml of alkalinized NaCl to the second tube. Mix each tube.

5. Determine the absorbance of the two solutions at 580 nm.
6. The concentration of BSP in plasma is determined by the difference between the absorbance of the alkalinized tube and that of the acidified tube followed by comparison with a BSP standard curve.

The test dose of BSP employed should be one that normal animals can readily clear in a 30-min period. Thus the amount of BSP retained by the mouse at 30 min is about 1% of the dose administered. As noted above, this procedure can be successfully used in several other species simply by altering the dose of BSP administered.

Biliary BSP Transport Maximum Procedure

Procedure

1. Anesthetize rats with sodium pentobarbital (50 mg/kg i.p.).
2. Restrain the rat in the supine position on a surgical board and cannulate the bile duct (PE-10 tubing) and a femoral vein (PE-50 tubing). The rectal temperature of the anesthetized rat is maintained at 37°C with a heat lamp to prevent hypothermic alterations in Tm (212).
3. A BSP solution in 0.9% NaCl is prepared to give an infusion of 2.5 mg BSP/kg/min at an infusion rate of 0.03 ml/min.
4. The infusion is continued for a period of 60 min, and bile is collected at 15-min intervals.
5. Measure the bile volume and determine the total biliary BSP concentration by alkalinizing an aliquot (50 μl) of bile with 0.01 M NaOH. The absorbance is determined at 580 mn.
6. The amount of BSP excreted ($min^{-1} kg^{-1}$) is calculated; the maximum value attained is the Tm. In the Sprague-Dawley rat the BSP Tm is about 1.0 mg/kg/min.

Several other compounds have been introduced into clinical medicine for the purpose of measuring liver function by the dye-clearance principle. The rose bengal test appeared in 1931 (50), and a third useful dye, indocyanine green (ICG), was introduced in 1959 (138).

Indocyanine green was originally introduced for the purpose of measuring cardiac output by the indicator-dilution technique. However, it was subsequently found (249) in the dog that 97% of the administered dose was eventually recovered from the bile in an unaltered form. No dye was found in the urine. ICG has about the same spectrum of sensitivity and specificity as BSP, but it has a number of properties that make it more desirable to employ under certain circumstances. Cherrick et al. (38) made a fairly comprehensive study of the material and found the following: (a) ICG is rapidly and completely bound to plasma protein, of which albumin is the principal carrier; (b) the dye is excreted in bile in an unconjugated form; (c) there seems to be no extrahepatic mechanism for removing the material; (d) ICG is nonirritating when inadvertently introduced subcutaneously, and it produces no untoward reactions upon single or repeated intravenous injections; and (e) the plasma disappearance of ICG is similar to that of BSP.

In laboratory animals, ICG is usually employed to supplement BSP tests. In the dog, Hunton et al. (97) found that: (a) the plasma disappearance rate of ICG is exponential for at least 15 min and usually for 30 to 60 min; (b) the amount removed per minute seems to be inversely related to the dose administered; (c) the maximal rate of excretion of ICG into the bile is about 0.4 mg/min/kg; and (d) substances such as bilirubin, rose bengal, and BSP interfere with ICG excretion. Klaassen and Plaa (125) found that over a 32-min period the rate of disappearance of ICG was exponential in the rat, rabbit, and dog (Table 2). The rabbit exhibited a greater capacity to remove ICG from plasma than did the rat, and the dog had the lowest capacity. It appears that the optimal dosage for ICG clearance in the dog is about 1.5 to 2.0 mg/kg; the optimal dosage in the rat is approximately 16 mg/kg; and it is 25 to 30 mg/kg in the rabbit.

Biliary excretory maximum and hepatic storage values for ICG could not be determined (125), as infusion rates sufficient to produce a biliary excretory Tm produced a marked decrease in bile flow. Decreased bile flow was observed in all three species but was most pronounced in the rat and least in the dog. Rapid administration of ICG, as used in plasma clearance experiments, does not produce marked alterations in bile flow. Other investigators (89) reported maximal biliary excretion rates for rats given ICG that were comparable to the peak excretion rates obtained by Klaassen and Plaa (125).

The major advantage of ICG in the detection and evaluation of hepatic function is that the material is not biotransformed prior to excretion. In addition, ICG is directly determined in plasma, without chemical treatment. In practice, it simply involves diluting an aliquot of plasma (0.1–1.0 ml) with water and determining the absorbance at 805 nm, the wavelength for peak ICG absorption. ICG, however, is unstable in aqueous solutions; this instability can be prevented by mixing ICG directly with serum or with an albumin solution. The dye is unstable when mixed with heparin solutions containing bisulfite (40), indicating that preservatives of the same type may also have an effect on ICG.

Although rose bengal was introduced before ICG, it has not been extensively employed in laboratory animals; in hu-

TABLE 2. *ICG plasma disappearance rates in rats, rabbits, and dogs*

ICG dose (mg/kg)	$T_{1/2}$ (min)	K (% removed/min)
Rat		
4	2.5	28
8	4.0	17
16	6.5	11
32	8.5	8
64	18.0	4
Rabbit		
8	1.5	46
16	3.5	20
32	7.0	10
Dog		
1	7.0	10
2	17.0	4
4	30.0	2

mans the dye is used to diagnose hepatic disorder, especially in children. Rose bengal, like ICG, has the advantage that it is apparently not biotransformed before excretion into the bile (118,133). It is available commercially in a radioactive form, so its concentration can be quantified in small blood samples. Klaassen (118) examined the pharmacokinetics of rose bengal in four species (rat, rabbit, dog, guinea pig) and found that, with the exception of biotransformation, the dye appears to be handled by the liver in a manner similar to BSP; it is a class B anion that is actively excreted into the bile. A marked species variation in the rate of biliary excretion of rose bengal exists (118). The rat and rabbit excrete rose bengal into the bile at comparable rates, whereas the guinea pig is much more efficient and the dog much less efficient.

Like BSP, the removal of rose bengal from the blood is altered by changes in hepatic excretory function (118,154,234), and Klaassen indicated that the dye could be used as a measure of hepatic excretory function in laboratory animals. Because it is not biotransformed, alterations in its clearance would reflect changes in its uptake into the liver or its excretion into the bile. However, if used as a hepatic function test by measuring the concentration of rose bengal in the blood at only one time after its administration, the selection of this time interval is critical; a blood sample at 15 to 20 min after administration appears optimal (118). Additional studies are needed to determine if rose bengal is as sensitive an index of hepatic dysfunction in laboratory animals as is BSP.

Other agents exist for monitoring hepatic excretory function. Mehendale and co-workers (151–153) used phenolphthalein glucuronide (PG), imipramine (IMP), and the polar metabolites of imipramine (PMIMP) as model compounds to characterize the hepatobiliary dysfunction produced by mirex. This pesticide did not suppress hepatic uptake and metabolism of IMP but inhibited the movement of PMIMP from the hepatocyte to bile; it also inhibited the biliary excretion of PG, a model anionic substrate that does not undergo biotransformation. These model substrates allowed the investigators to localize the site of mirex-induced dysfunction. In another report (47) they suggested that PG may be a more sensitive model compound than BSP for detection of hepatobiliary dysfunction. CCl_4 at 100 μl/kg depressed biliary excretion of PG in rats; hepatobiliary dysfunction was undetectable with BSP at this dosage of CCl_4 (25,122).

At least one endogenous substance, bilirubin, has been used to evaluate chemically induced hepatic injury. Normally, bilirubin is excreted into the bile. Elevation of serum bilirubin concentration accompanies sufficiently severe parenchymal injury, but it is a relatively insensitive measure of chemically induced hepatic injury. The degree of change in serum bilirubin that one obtains with experimental hepatotoxicity in mice is summarized in Table 1. CCl_4, although producing sufficient parenchymal injury to cause a large increase in serum ALT activity, does not affect bilirubin concentrations greatly. On the other hand, bile duct occlusion does elevate serum bilirubin considerably. ANIT also elevates serum bilirubin but not to the extent that bile duct occlusion does. The BSP retention values indicate that those experimental procedures that markedly impair biliary excretion also affect BSP retention, whereas CCl_4 causes a lesser degree of retention. However, if one assumes that BSP retention

and bilirubin concentrations measure relatively the same type of liver function, it is evident that the changes occurring with BSP are considerably greater that those occurring with bilirubin. A likely explanation is that the measurement of endogenous concentrations of bilirubin may not assess the total capacity of the liver to clear bilirubin, as does a load of BSP selected to be a near-capacity dose for the particular species of animal employed. Indeed, if one does administer exogenous amounts of bilirubin and follows its plasma disappearance, as with BSP, the sensitivity of the bilirubin clearance procedure can be increased. Nevertheless, BSP clearance is simpler and more sensitive than bilirubin and is therefore preferred for measurement of hepatocellular injury.

Techniques designed to assess bile secretory function are also available; however, these methods lend themselves more to specific research problems than to overall toxicological assessment. The methods applicable *in vivo* were reviewed by Fujimoto (73). The so-called bile acid-dependent and bile acid-independent fractions of total bile flow (60,126,172) have been studied extensively in several species; secretin-sensitive bile flow is thought to be small in the rat but more important in the rabbit and dog.

Fujimoto (73) developed a number of new techniques, where marker substances are injected retrogradely into the biliary tree to assess the permeability characteristics of the biliary system. ANIT, which produces intrahepatic cholestasis in rats, and bile duct ligation increase the distended capacity of the biliary tree, whereas another cholestatic agent, taurolithocholate, decreases the distended capacity; CCl_4 seems to exert no effect (72,175,176).

The retrograde technique has been modified to become the "segmented retrograde intrabiliary injection" (SRII) procedure (174). With the use of radioactive marker substances of varying molecular weights (D-glucose, mannitol, sucrose, inulin, or dextran), one can assess the "membrane" characteristics of the biliary tree (canalicular and tight-junction complexes). This procedure was used to study the hepatobiliary dysfunction produced by *Amanita phalloides* (72), taurolithocholate (73), colchicine (8), *S,S,S*-tributylphosphorotrithioate (8), manganese and manganese–bilirubin combinations (7), and sequential treatments with ketones and chloroform (91). These studies have been useful for discerning the site and possible mechanisms of action involved in their hepatobiliary effects.

SRII Method

Reagents

1. [^{3}H(G)]Inulin (133.0 mCi/g), diluted with 0.9% NaCl to give a 15 nmol/ml, 10 μCi/ml solution.
2. D-[1-^{3}H]Mannitol (27.4 Ci/mmol), diluted with 0.9% NaCl to give a 0.4 nmol/ml, 10 μCi/ml solution.

Procedure

1. Anesthetize rats with sodium pentobarbital (60 mg/kg i.p.).
2. Restrain the rat in the supine position on a surgical board and cannulate the bile duct with a 10-cm length of PE-

20 tubing just distal to the bifurcation of the biliary tree. Attach this tubing (via a stainless steel 26-gauge needle) to a longer piece of PE-20 tubing capable of containing exactly 40 μl of solution. The rectal temperature of the anesthetized rat should be maintained at 37°C with a heat lamp to prevent hypothermic alterations in bile flow (212).

3. Inject a "segment" (40 μl) of solution containing the radioactive marker compound (~0.4 μCi/animal; 0.60 nmol [³H]inulin or 0.02 nmol [³H]mannitol) into the bile duct, followed by 70 μl of 0.9% NaCl. A 200-μl Hamilton syringe attached to a Harvard infusion pump is used for the injection; the infusion rate is 2.3 μl/sec. The total volume injected is 110 μl.

4. Immediately after completion of the SRII, reestablish bile flow by disconnecting the 10-cm bile duct cannula from the infusion pump.

5. Collect 20 separate drops of bile serially (7.6 μl/drop, 152 μl of bile total) in vials containing 5 ml of Aquasol scintillation medium.

6. Calculate the bile flow rate by determining the time required to form each drop, assuming a volume of 7.6 μl/drop.

7. Determine radioactive content of each drop by liquid scintillation spectrometry.

8. Express the radioactive content of each drop as a percentage of the total radioactivity administered by SRII. Plot the percentage of marker recovered in each drop versus the cumulative volume of bile collected. Calculate the percentage of total marker recovered in the 152 μl of bile collected.

9. The volume of the distended biliary tree can also be evaluated by the SRII method (73,176).

Alterations in Chemical Constituents of the Liver

In addition to producing elevations in serum enzyme activities and altering hepatocyte transport processes, chemical hepatotoxicants can produce changes in structural and functional hepatic constituents that have been found useful for detecting and quantifying the degree of liver injury produced, as well as elucidating the mechanism(s) involved in producing the lesions.

Hepatic Lipid Content

A number of agents that produce liver injury also cause the accumulation of abnormal amounts of fat, predominantly triglycerides, in the parenchymal cells. In general, triglyceride accumulation can be thought of as resulting from an imbalance between the rate of synthesis and the rate of release of triglyceride by the parenchymal cells into the system circulation.

Nonesterified fatty acids (NEFAs) removed from the circulation or synthesized endogenously are processed through two major pathways in the liver: (a) mitochondrial β-oxidation for production of metabolic energy; and (b) incorporation into complex lipids, especially triglycerides, phospholipids, cholesteryl esters, and glycolipids (52). Once

synthesized, the complex lipids may be used for production of cellular membranes (structural lipids) or be continuously secreted from the liver into the blood. The latter pathway appears to be of greatest interest in the triglyceride accumulation observed in fatty liver.

Blockage of the secretion of hepatic triglyceride into the plasma is the basic mechanism underlying the fatty liver induced in the rat by CCl₄, ethionine, phosphorus, puromycin, or tetracycline, by feeding a choline-deficient diet, or by feeding orotic acid (52,95,144). When hepatic triglyceride is released into the plasma, it is not released as such but as a lipoprotein. The very low density fraction of the lipoproteins (VLDL) is the major transport vehicle for endogenously synthesized triglyceride; there is some evidence indicating that CCl₄ and ethionine cause a fall in the level of circulating lipoprotein, principally VLDL.

The composition of VLDL by weight is 8 to 10% protein and 90 to 92% lipid. Of the lipids, triglyceride is the most abundant component (56%); the average content of phospholipid is 19 to 21% and cholesterol 17% (101). Theoretically, decreased lipoprotein secretion may be the consequence of (a) a block in the synthesis of the protein moiety; (b) a defect in the assembly of the lipoprotein constituents due to either a change in their chemical structure and function or to an alteration in endoplasmic reticulum structure where the assembly seems to take place; and (c) a defect in the mechanism of release from liver cells of well formed lipoprotein micelles (52). CCl₄, ethionine, phosphorus, and puromycin can interfere with the synthesis of the protein moiety (63,214,230). Although there is evidence that all of these substances can affect synthesis of lipoproteins, it is by no means clear that it is the only mechanism involved. With ethionine and phosphorus, it appears to be the most likely defect; however, Recknagel (193) pointed out that the assembly phase of triglyceride secretion is probably affected by CCl₄. Dianzani (52) suggested that the assembly defect could be due to structural changes produced by CCl₄-induced peroxidation in either preexisting apoprotein molecules (i.e., denaturation of the protein molecule) or the lipid moiety of lipoproteins (e.g., incorporation of the trichlormethyl free radical into fatty acid side chains of phospholipids), thereby rendering the components nonfunctional. Peroxidative damage to the endoplasmic reticulum membrane, where the components are assembled, and defects in the lipoprotein secretion system should also be considered (52).

Orotic acid can produce fatty livers when fed to rats and also results in a large decrease in the release of lipoproteins into the blood (254). Total protein synthesis in the liver is slightly increased, but the incorporation of labeled amino acids into apoproteins from VLDL is strongly decreased by orotic acid administration. These results may be interpreted to indicate that in the presence of excess orotic acid proteins other than apolipoprotein are preferentially synthesized by the liver (52). In contrast, the impaired release of VLDL and associated fatty liver observed in animals fed a choline-deficient diet appears to result from impaired synthesis of phospholipid (145,173). With choline deficiency, phosphatidylcholine is replaced in the lipoprotein molecule by phosphatidylethanolamine and phosphatidylserine, which results in a molecule that is less efficient in binding and transporting triglycerides (52). With tetracycline, impaired release of VLDL occurs, but it is not known whether synthesis, assembly, or secretion is the phase affected (95).

Although the exact mechanism(s) by which lipoproteins are secreted from the cell has not been completely detailed, work suggests that microtubules may play a role in this process. A tubulin assembly–disassembly cycle exists in the liver, and interruption of the cycle by colchicine administration results in a blockage of VLDL secretion (103,231). The microtubule system could be a target site for hepatotoxicants that produce fatty liver by inhibition of lipoprotein secretion. Although this hypothesis has not been extensively tested, Gabriel et al. (74) provided some indirect evidence suggesting that aldehydes, known to be produced in the liver during CCl_4-induced lipid peroxidation, may functionally damage microtubules.

Elevated triglyceride could result because of an increase in the rate of synthesis of this substance. There is evidence that the rate of synthesis is directly proportional to the concentration of the substrates present (NEFAs and glycerophosphate), and so it is theoretically possible that increased hepatic triglyceride synthesis could occur because of increased NEFAs or increased glycerophosphate. Increased NEFAs could result from decreased oxidation, increased synthesis, or increased mobilization from peripheral stores. In the case of ethanol-induced fatty liver, impaired mitochondrial oxidation of NEFAs appears to be the primary abnormality seen in humans (95) due to a shift in redox potential (increased NADH/NAD ratio). It may be accompanied, however, by other abnormalities (100). There is little evidence to support the idea that fatty acid synthesis is involved in the development of fatty liver.

One can raise the question whether fat accumulation itself always represents an injurious response for the hepatocyte. A fatty liver does not necessarily lead to death of the hepatocytes: Ethionine, puromycin, and cycloheximide all cause fat accumulation without producing necrosis. Promethazine protects rats against the necrogenic effects of CCl_4 but does not abolish the fatty liver (199). Bucher and Malt (27) reviewed the biochemical and morphologic events associated with liver regeneration. Following partial hepatectomy in rats, there is a hormone-mediated mobilization of fat from adipose tissue. Neutral fat accumulates in the remainder of the liver within 18 to 24 hr, reaching a value ten times that of normal liver and bringing about distortion of the normal lobular pattern. The capacity to secrete triglycerides increases, but

liposomes begin to appear along with intracellular fat globules, indicating a relative delay in triglyceride secretion when compared with triglyceride accumulation. The hepatic cells, in the presence of this fat, still function as well as normal, if not more efficiently, while preparing for cell division at the same time. As Ingelfinger (99) pointed out, in the face of this finding, can one say that excessive fat accumulation in itself is damaging?

Determination of hepatic fat content remains a reliable technique for demonstrating alterations by agents that produce steatosis with little or no necrosis (ethionine, phosphorus, tetracycline) and that are poorly reflected by serum enzyme measurement (256). Alterations in hepatic triglyceride content have also been used as one of a battery of tests to determine the relative hepatotoxic potential of various halogenated hydrocarbons in rats (124) and to determine the ability of various alcohols or experimentally induced diabetes to potentiate the hepatotoxic actions of CCl_4 (88,242) (Table 3).

Determination of hepatic triglyceride content

The hepatic triglyceride assay described by Butler et al. (31) is an adaptation of the method of Van Handel and Zilversmit (243), originally developed for the direct determination of serum triglycerides. The procedure consists in five steps: (a) homogenization of tissue; (b) adsorption of phospholipids onto zeolite, followed by extraction of triglycerides into chloroform; (c) hydrolysis of triglycerides to fatty acids and glycerol; (d) oxidation of glycerol with $NaIO_4$ to formic acid and formaldehyde; and (e) formation of a colored complex of formaldehyde and chromotropic acid (31). The procedure is relatively simple and can be used to analyze a large number of tissue samples in a single day.

Reagents.

1. Phosphate buffer (67 mM, pH 7.0): Mix 67 mM dibasic sodium phosphate (Na_2HPO_4, 9.513 g/L water) and 67 mM monobasic potassium phosphate (KH_2PO_4, 9.118 g/L water) in the proportion 61.1:38.9.
2. Zeolite: Activate by heating at 125°C for 4 hr. Store desiccated.
3. Alcoholic potassium hydroxide (0.4%): Dissolve 2 g of reagent grade KOH in 95% ethanol and dilute to 100 ml.

TABLE 3. *Effect of alcohol pretreatment on CCl_4-induced hepatotoxicity in rats[a]*

Treatment	ALT activity (units/ml)	Triglycerides (mg/g liver)	G-6-Pase activity (mg Pi/g liver/20 min)
Ethanol (5.0 ml/kg)	50	8	6.7
Isopropanol (2.5 ml/kg)	50	6	6.2
CCl_4 (0.1 ml/kg)	100	9	6.0
CCl_4 (1.0 ml/kg)	500	17	3.8
Isopropanol + CCl_4 (0.1 ml/kg)	2,250[b]	22[b]	2.8[b]
Ethanol + CCl_4 (0.1 ml/kg)	500[b]	13[b]	4.8[b]

[a] The alcohol was given orally 18 hr before intraperitoneal CCl_4 administration. Liver function was assessed 24 hr after CCl_4 in ten rats.
[b] Significantly different from the group given alcohol alone; $p < 0.05$.
Data were obtained from Traiger and Plaa (242).

Dilute 10 ml of this stock solution to 50 ml with 95% ethanol on the day of use.

4. Sulfuric acid (0.2 N): Add 3 ml of concentrated H_2SO_4 to about 400 ml of distilled water. Let cool and dilute to 500 ml.

5. Sodium metaperiodate (0.05 M): Dissolve 1.07 g of $NaIO_4$ in distilled water and dilute to 100 ml.

6. Sodium arsenite (2.0 M): Dissolve 25.98 g of $NaAsO_2$ in distilled water and dilute to 100 ml.

7. Chromotropic acid (0.2%): Dissolve 2 g of 4,5-dihydroxy-2,7-naphthalenedisulfonic acid (chromotropic acid) in distilled water and dilute to 200 ml. Separately, add 600 ml of concentrated H_2SO_4 to 300 ml of distilled water chilled in an icebath. When cool, add the diluted H_2SO_4 to the chromotropic acid solution. Store in an amber bottle and prepare fresh every 2 to 3 weeks.

8. Triglyceride standard solution (0.05 mg/ml): Dissolve 0.5 g of commercial corn oil in chloroform and dilute to 100 ml with chloroform. Dilute this stock solution 1:100 with chloroform to prepare the working standard.

Procedure

1. Remove the liver from an ether-anesthetized rat, rinse in cold phosphate buffer, blot, and weigh.

2. Prepare a 10% (w/v) homogenate of liver in phosphate buffer using a minimum of 200 mg of liver.

3. Immediately after homogenization, add 1 ml of the homogenate to a 25-ml glass-stoppered tube containing 4 g activated zeolite moistened with 2 ml of chloroform.

4. Add 18 ml of chloroform and shake intermittently for at least 10 min.

5. Filter through Whatman No. 2 paper.

6. Transfer 0.5-ml (0.125–1.000 ml may be used) aliquots of the filtrate to each of three glass-stoppered tubes. Similarly, add aliquots (10 ml) of the corn oil standard to each of three glass-stoppered tubes.

7. Evaporate the chloroform from all tubes by heating at 80°C for about 30 min in a dry block heater.

8. Add 0.5 ml of alcoholic KOH to two of each three standards and unknowns (saponified sample). The third standard and unknown tube receives 0.5 ml of 95% ethanol (unsaponified sample). For each set of three standards, two samples will be saponified and one will be unsaponified. For each set of three unknowns, two samples will be saponified and one will be unsaponified.

9. Incubate all tubes at 65°C for 20 min.

10. Add 0.5 ml of 0.2 N H_2SO_4, mix, and heat tubes at 95°C for approximately 15 min to remove the ethanol.

11. After cooling, add 0.1 ml of the sodium metaperiodate to each tube and mix. Wait 10 min.

12. Add 0.1 ml of the sodium arsenite solution, mix, and wait 10 min.

13. Add 5.0 ml of the chromotropic acid reagent to each tube, mix, and incubate in the dark for 30 min at 95°C.

14. Determine the absorbance at 570 nm after the tubes have cooled.

Calculations are carried out as follows:

Triglyceride content (mg/g tissue)

$$= (A_{su} - A_{nsu})/(A_{ss} - A_{nss}) \times 0.05 \times (200/F)$$

where A_{su} is the average absorbance of saponified unknowns, A_{nsu} is the average absorbance of unsaponified unknowns, A_{ss} is the average absorbance of saponified standards, A_{nss} is the average absorbance of unsaponified standards, and F is the volume (ml) of chloroform extract used.

Measurement of Lipid Peroxidation

It is generally accepted that the toxicity of CCl_4 depends on the cleavage of a carbon–chlorine bond to generate a trichlormethyl free radical ($\cdot CCl_3$); this free radical reacts rapidly with oxygen to form a trichlormethyl peroxy radical ($\cdot CCl_3O_2$), which may contribute to the toxicity (37). The work of a number of investigators (37,159,195,196) demonstrates that: (a) the cleavage occurs in the endoplasmic reticulum and is mediated by the cytochrome P-450 mixed function oxidase system; (b) the product of the cleavage can bind irreversibly to hepatic proteins and lipids; and (c) the CCl_4-derived free radical(s) can initiate a process of autocatalytic lipid peroxidation by attacking the methylene bridges of unsaturated fatty acid side chains of microsomal lipids. The peroxidative process initiated by the $\cdot CCl_3$ radical, for example, is thought to result in early morphologic alteration of the endoplasmic reticulum, loss of activity of the cytochrome P-450 xenobiotic metabolizing system, loss of glucose-6-phosphatase activity, loss of protein synthesis, loss of the capacity of the liver to form and excrete VLDL, and eventually, through as yet unidentified pathways, to cell death (37,42,195,196). Alterations in these parameters have been used to monitor the course and extent of CCl_4-induced hepatic damage, and furthermore, have been applied to the evaluation of other hepatotoxicants.

Formation of lipid hydroperoxides, hydroxylated fatty acids, and aldehydes such as alkanals, alk-2-enals, and 4-hydroxyalkenals occurs during membrane peroxidation; some of these products have been used to estimate the extent of peroxidative membrane damage (159). Of potentially greater interest, however, is the possibility that one or more of these products may diffuse from their site of formation (e.g., the endoplasmic reticulum) and damage more distant cellular targets such as mitochondria and the plasma membrane. Comporti (42) reviewed the development of this concept and its supporting data. The hypothesis that soluble, stable cytotoxic products are formed during lipid peroxidation arose from studies where a target system (erythrocytes) were separated from a peroxidizing membrane (liver microsomes) by dialysis tubing. Despite the barrier provided by the tubing, relatively stable products (not free-radical intermediates) occurring during peroxidation of the microsomal preparation diffused to the erythrocytes and produced hemolysis. Subsequent studies demonstrated that the cytotoxic products could be isolated from the dialysate and fractionated chromatographically. The fraction containing a large concentration of carbonyl functions inhibited microsomal glucose-6-phosphatase activity, possessed hemolytic activity, and could lyse isolated hepatocytes (42); further characterization indicated that 4-hydroxy-trans-2,3-nonenal (4-HN) was the major compound produced. Synthetic 4-HN was shown to inhibit liver microsomal glucose-6-phosphatase activity, inhibit cytochrome P-450, hemolyze erthrocytes, and kill isolated hepatocytes. An increase in carbonyl functions, presumably derived from binding of 4-HN or related reactive aldehydes to protein sulfhydryl groups, was found in liver microsomal proteins and phospholipids from rats challenged *in vivo* with CCl_4 and $CBrCl_3$. These observations suggested that chemically induced lipid peroxidation may exert deleterious effects on hepatocellular function by a direct degradation of membranes at the site of peroxidation and by causing the generation of cytotoxic products that can produce dysfunction at cellular sites distant from the initial locus of peroxidative activity (42).

Initiation of lipid peroxidation is not unique to CCl_4 or the liver. Lipid peroxidation *in vivo* may be of importance in aging, damage to cells by air pollution, some phases of atherosclerosis, some forms of liver injury, and oxygen toxicity (42,159,185,196,198,235).

Several procedures for the detection and quantification of lipid peroxidation in tissue samples or whole animals have been developed (185,198). The reaction of malonaldehyde, a degradation product of peroxidized lipids, with thiobarbituric acid (TBA) to produce a TBA-malonaldehyde chromophore has been taken as an index of lipid peroxidation and is the most widely used method for detecting lipid peroxidation *in vitro*. Because malonaldehyde is rapidly metabolized in whole animals (185) and in whole liver homogenates (194), the failure to detect TBA-reacting material is not an indication of the absence of lipid peroxidation.

The determination of conjugated dienes in lipid extracts of hepatic subcellular fractions is a second approach for detecting lipid peroxidation (198). The ultraviolet difference spectra of peroxidized lipids show an absorption maximum at 233 nm with a secondary absorption maximum between 260 and 280 nm due to the presence of ketone dienes. The appearance of conjugated dienes after treatment *in vivo* with toxicants is an unmistakable indication that lipid peroxidation has taken place.

Several other methods for the measurement of lipid peroxidation have been described. For example, the iodometric procedure of Bunyan et al. (29) has been employed. A comparatively new approach is to measure the presence of fluorescent products. A variety of molecules that occur commonly in tissue may react with malonaldehyde and yield characteristic fluorescent chromophores (39). Malonaldehyde undergoes decomposition, and the decomposition products may also lead to fluorescent products when they react with proteins (226). Measurement of these fluorescent products seems to offer a workable way for detecting lipid peroxidation in biological systems and tissues (198). A second interesting approach is the measurement of hydrocarbon gases. These gases appear early in the course of autoxidation of edible fats (71,94). Two gases, ethane and pentane, are useful for measuring the peroxidative process *in vitro* and *in vivo*. Ethane is the predominant gas produced during autoxidation of linolenic acid (141), and pentane is the major gaseous hydrocarbon arising during thermal decomposition (61,62) and iron-catalyzed decomposition of linoleic and arachidonic acid hydroperoxides (57). Riely et al. (211) initiated the use of ethane analysis in biological systems. They observed that ethane production was a characteristic of spontaneously peroxidizing mouse tissue (liver and brain) and was found in mice injected with CCl_4. In addition, they found that CCl_4-induced ethane evolution *in vivo* was potentiated by prior administration of phenobarbital and diminished by α-tocopherol, an antioxidant. Several other groups of investigators used ethane production to monitor the course of lipid peroxidation *in vivo* (30,85,130,142). Dillard et al. (53) suggested that pentane expiration was a more sensitive index of lipid peroxidation than ethane in rats fed a vitamin E-deficient diet containing a high content of linoleic acid. Pentane production has also achieved considerable use as an index of the lipoperoxidative process (143,220,221). A method has been devised for monitoring lipid peroxidation in humans by quantifying the excretion of ethane and pentane in exhaled breath during a 2-hr period (246). Although the measurement of hydrocarbon gas production is an alternate procedure for the determination of lipid peroxidation, this technique cannot identify the tissue or subcellular organelle from which these substances arise. In addition, precautions must be taken to prevent or estimate the evolution of hydrocarbon gases by microorganisms in the gastrointestinal tract when *in vivo* studies are undertaken.

Because the procedures for measuring lipid peroxidation have been reviewed (28,198), no attempt is made to describe the individual procedures here.

Formation and Binding of Reactive Metabolites

Although the concept of lipid peroxidation is one of the truly important concepts of current experimental pathology and toxicology, it does not appear to serve as a universal mechanism of liver injury. A number of drugs and chemicals, e.g., acetaminophen (77,158), furosemide (77,158), 1,1-dichloroethylene (102,148,149), trichloroethylene (2), bromobenzene (77,209), and dimethylnitrosamine (77), produce hepatic damage but do not appear to promote lipid peroxidation. Rather, these agents are thought to be converted to highly reactive, electrophilic metabolites by the hepatic mixed function oxidase (MFO) system. Following formation, the metabolites, which are considered to be the ultimate toxicants, can interact with hepatic constituents (e.g., protein, lipid, RNA, DNA) to form alkylated or arylated derivatives. Various investigators postulate that the binding of reactive metabolites to hepatic macromolecules can initiate cellular damage through processes as yet unidentified.

A detailed discussion of the formation and detoxification of reactive metabolites and their interaction with hepatic constituents is beyond the scope of this chapter, and the reader is referred to several excellent reviews (37,77,78,147,155,156,158,159,227). However, the experimental work carried out to unravel the mechanisms by which several toxicants produce liver injury has led to some important observations that need to be discussed. One is that hepatotoxicity need not be correlated with the pharmacokinetics of the parent substance or even its major metabolites, but may be correlated with the formation of quantitatively minor, highly reactive intermediates. Assuming that a relation exists between the severity of the lesion and the amount of covalently bound metabolite, the covalent binding of the metabolite can be used as an index of its formation. Indeed, this parameter might well be the most reliable estimate of the availability of the metabolite for production of damage at the target site, as most of the metabolite may undergo decomposition or further metabolism before it can be isolated in body fluids or urine (155). Thus one widely used maneuver to assess the contribution of formation and binding of metabolites in chemically induced hepatotoxicity is to determine if radiolabeled chemicals administered to animals over a wide dosage range are covalently bound to macromolecular constituents in tissues that subsequently become necrotic (155).

A second concept is that a threshold tissue concentration of the metabolite must be attained before liver injury is elicited; if it is not attained, injury does not occur. Endogenous substances such as glutathione play an essential role in protecting hepatocytes from injury by chemically reactive metabolites. When low doses of acetaminophen (158) or bromobenzene (105) are administered, the toxic metabolite preferentially combines with glutathione, thereby preventing arylation of macromolecules and necrosis. As the dose is increased, the availability of glutathione is decreased; at a certain threshold dose, a sharp increase in covalent binding occurs and tissue necrosis results. Thus in the case of acetaminophen and bromobenzene, glutathione provides the cell with a means of preventing the reactive metabolite from attaining a critical, effective concentration. The mechanism that establishes a dose threshold, however, may vary from compound to compound. With furosemide, a dose threshold may exist for both necrosis and covalent binding, but the threshold in mice is not due to depletion of hepatic glutathione. Apparently, the threshold is caused by a change in the proportion of the unmetabolized compound that is eliminated. At subthreshold doses most of the furosemide is highly bound to plasma proteins and is eventually eliminated unchanged, whereas with high doses plasma binding becomes saturated and more furosemide becomes available for hepatic biotransformation (158). Finally, other enzymic pathways, e.g., glutathione-S-transferase and epoxide hydrolase, also play a role in protecting the hepatocyte by catalyzing the further degradation of the toxic reactive intermediates.

The studies mentioned above have provided relatively straightforward biochemical strategies for uncovering the possible existence of potentially toxic chemically reactive metabolites in new compounds (155). In general, a dose-response study employing the radiolabeled compound over a wide dosage range is perhaps the single most important facet of the overall study in that it can provide information relating to a dose threshold for toxicity, possible mechanisms for the threshold response (e.g., glutathione depletion), and the degree of covalent binding of metabolites to target organs or constituents with the target organ. This latter information, in conjunction with dose-response studies documenting the dosages required to produce necrosis (or other endpoint), provides strong presumptive evidence favoring toxicity mediated by a reactive metabolite. Subsequent efforts should include the use of inducers (e.g., phenobarbital, 3-methylcholanthrene) and inhibitors (e.g., SKF-525A, CoCl$_2$, piperonyl butoxide) of the MFO system. Enhancement of *in vivo* or *in vitro* covalent binding of the radiolabeled compound, as well as toxicity by an inducing agent, can provide support for the contention that a reactive metabolite mediates toxicity. A similar conclusion can be drawn if an inhibitor of the MFO system depresses covalent binding and toxicity. However, the observation that inhibitors increase the response or that inducers decrease the response does not preclude the possibility that the toxicant exerts its effect through the formation of chemically reactive metabolite (155). For example, an inducing agent may stimulate the activity of a detoxifying pathway to a greater extent that a toxifying pathway. In addition, manipulation of the concentration of hepatoprotective substances such as glutathione (e.g., depression of hepatic GSH concentration by diethylmaleate administration) can alter covalent binding or toxicity of a compound and support the likelihood that the toxic effects are mediated by a metabolite. Correlation of the data from several of these studies with a pharmacokinetic analysis can delineate the participation of a chemically reactive metabolite in the production of toxicity. For a more detailed discussion of these concepts, the reader is referred to the reviews cited above.

Hepatic Glucose-6-Phosphatase Activity

Regardless of the mechanism by which a chemical exerts its hepatotoxic effect, the biochemical sequelae may be useful in detecting and quantifying the damage produced. Glucose-6-phosphatase (G-6-Pase) is associated with the endoplasmic reticulum, and depression of its activity appears to specifically reflect injury to this organelle (195). The functional integrity of the enzyme is dependent on the presence of phospholipid; and peroxidative decomposition of microsomal lipids, as occurs with CCl$_4$, results in a significant loss of G-6-Pase activity (195–197).

Feuer et al. (68) administered a series of 19 compounds, including ten known hepatotoxicants, to rats and monitored their effects on eight hepatic enzymes. The enzymes selected represented the mitochondrial, microsomal (G-6-Pase), lysosomal, and cytoplasmic fractions. These investigators found that each of the ten known hepatotoxicants decreased hepatic G-6-Pase activity. Most of the other compounds, not known to affect the liver, did not alter G-6-Pase. Two compounds not considered to be hepatotoxicants, however, also reduced the activity of this enzyme. Based on these and other data, Grice (81) suggested that alterations in G-6-Pase activity might serve as an indicator of incipient liver damage and might occur in advance of histologically detectable organ damage. However, other data suggest that reduction of G-6-Pase is not the most sensitive test for detecting minimal hepatic damage: Klaassen and Plaa (124) found a significant depression of G-6-Pase in rat liver only at CCl$_4$ dosages of 0.3 mg/kg or greater, whereas hepatic triglyceride accumulation occurred at dosages of CCl$_4$ below 0.3 ml/kg; BSP retention occurs in rats after a CCl$_4$ dosage of 0.1 ml/kg (122); with light microscopy, morphologic changes are observed in rats treated with 0.13 ml CCl$_4$/kg (136).

Regardless of the relative sensitivity of this enzyme, it can be used as a diagnostic tool to quantify the effects of experimental maneuvers designed to increase or reduce the toxicity of known hepatotoxicants. An example is found in Table 3. This study (242) was designed to determine the ability of ethanol and isopropanol to potentiate CCl$_4$-induced hepatotoxicity. It is evident that the two alcohols themselves had no significant effect on ALT activity, triglyceride accumulation, or G-6-Pase activity. However, when pretreatment with either of these alcohols occurred 18 hr before the administration of the challenge dosage of CCl₄ (0.1 ml/kg), the response was greatly increased; it was evident using all three parameters of hepatotoxicity. The challenge dose of CCl₄ merely caused a slight hepatotoxic response when it was given alone. Increasing the challenge dose of CCl₄ tenfold (1.0 ml/kg) resulted in a response that was less than that produced with isopropanol plus CCl₄ (0.1 ml/kg). Ethanol plus CCl₄ resulted in a response that was about equal to the response exerted by the tenfold dose of CCl₄ given alone.

G-6-Pase has also been used to study mechanisms of CCl₄ and CHCl₃ liver injury. CHCl₃, which causes pathologic changes similar to those produced by CCl₄, does not alter hepatic G-6-Pase activity or the formation of conjugated dienes in hepatic microsomal lipids (124). These observations, along with others (185), suggest that CHCl₃ does not exert its hepatotoxic action by initiation of lipid peroxidation. Subsequently, CHCl₃ was found to produce conjugated dienes (26) and depress G-6-Pase activity (137) in phenobarbital-pretreated rats. Because CHCl₃-induced liver injury is more severe in phenobarbital-pretreated rats, the possibility exists that peroxidation is not the primary pathway by which CHCl₃ produces injury; rather, the putative initial lesion induced by CHCl₃ in these animals is only aggravated by the appearance of lipid peroxidation. Similarly, Jaeger et al. (102), using differences in the temporal sequences of serum (ALT) and hepatic (G-6-Pase) enzyme changes, found that CCl₄ and 1,1-dichloroethylene (1,1-DCE) have different modes of action. In conjunction with an analysis of the ability of 1,1-DCE to initiate lipid peroxidation, the enzyme data suggest that: (a) the initial site of injury differs for CCl₄ and 1,1-DCE; and (b) 1,1-DCE does not act through a lipoperoxidative mechanism. Thus as part of an integrative approach, G-6-Pase activity aided in distinguishing separate mechanisms of action for these hepatotoxicants.

Depression of G-6-Pase activity has been used to document microsomal damage produced by addition of agents to *in vitro* incubation systems. Glende et al. (80) and Benedetti et al. (17) used this enzyme (among other parameters) to demonstrate that the key event in CCl₄-induced alteration of microsomal enzyme activity is lipid peroxidation and not covalent binding of CCl₄-derived free radicals to microsomal lipids. Similarly, reduction of activity of this enzyme *in vitro* was used to document the destructive properties of degradation products of the lipoperoxidative process (19,96).

Analytical Determination of G-6-Pase Activity

The method to determine G-6-Pase (EC 3.1.3.9) activity to be described is based on the hydrolysis of glucose-6-phosphate to inorganic phosphate by an aliquot of whole rat liver homogenate. The procedure is patterned after that of Traiger and Plaa (242).

Reagents

1. Tris-maleate buffer (pH 6.2): Mix solutions of 0.1 *M* Tris [tris-(hydroxymethyl) aminomethane] (12.114 g/L water) and 0.1 *M* maleic acid (11.61 g/L water) together until the desired pH of 6.2 is obtained.
2. Glucose-6-phosphate: Dissolve 189 mg of glucose-6-

phosphate, monosodium salt (Sigma, No. G7879) in 25 ml Tris-maleate buffer (pH 6.2).
3. Trichloroacetic acid (TCA; 10%): Dissolve 100 g of TCA in about 700 ml of distilled water. Dilute to 1 L with distilled water.

Procedure

1. Livers are removed from ether-anesthetized rats, rinsed in cold Tris-maleate buffer, blotted, and weighed. A 20% (w/v) homogenate of liver is prepared in ice-cold Tris-maleate buffer (pH 6.2) using a glass homogenizer fitted with a Teflon pestle. An aliquot of the homogenate is subsequently diluted with cold buffer to yield a preparation containing 20 mg liver/ml buffer.
2. Pipette into 10-ml rounded centrifuge tubes 0.4 ml of buffer and 0.5 ml of the glucose-6-phosphate solution. Three tubes are prepared for each liver.
3. Equilibrate the tubes at 37°C in a Dubnoff metabolic shaking incubator.
4. Start the reaction by adding 0.2 ml of the 20 mg/ml liver homogenate and incubate for 20 min. Stop the reaction by adding 5.0 ml of 10% TCA. One tube per homogenate is used as a tissue blank either by adding 0.2 ml of boiled homogenate or adding TCA immediately after addition of the homogenate.
5. Remove precipitated protein by centrifugation and assay an aliquot (2.0 ml) of the supernatant for inorganic phosphorus by the method of Fiske and SubbaRow (69). Reagent kits prepared by Sigma (No. 670-C) can be used for this purpose.
6. Results are expressed as milligrams of inorganic phosphate (Pi) liberated per gram of liver every 20 min.

Alteration of Hepatic Drug Metabolizing Activity

Glucose-6-phosphatase is not the sole microsomal enzyme adversely affected by hepatotoxicants. A host of chemicals that produce liver injury can alter the activity of the hepatic MFO system, thereby changing the rate at which xenobiotics are metabolized. Alterations in the components of this system, xenobiotic metabolism per se, and alterations in the pharmacological effects of drugs can be used to provide qualitative, and in some instances quantitative, evidence of liver dysfunction.

The terminal oxidase of the MFO system, cytochrome P-450 (P-450), is particularly liable to damage by toxic chemicals, and depression of the content of this hemoprotein is becoming an increasingly popular index of damage to the endoplasmic reticulum. DeMatteis (51) described four properties of P-450 that may render it a preferential target for toxicants. First, P-450 plays a central role in drug oxidation and thus may serve as the binding site for several chemicals that are oxidized in the liver to reactive metabolites. Because these metabolites are produced at or near the P-450 site, the hemoprotein may be an early target for their action. Second, one of the coordination valences of the iron of the heme moiety is saturated by a thiol ligand from the apoprotein. This sulfur ligand is apparently responsible for the spectral characteristics as well as the stability and function of the hemoprotein. Oxidation of this thiol group or its blockage by sulfhydryl reagents results in the formation of cytochrome P-420, an unstable derivative of P-450, devoid of functional activity. Hence this thiol group may provide a locus for the effect of heavy metals and other sulfhydryl reagents on P-450. Third, maintenance of the structural integrity of the endoplasmic reticulum membrane is necessary for the normal structure and function of P-450. Agents that disrupt the organization of the hemoprotein within the hydrophobic environment of the endoplasmic reticulum membrane (e.g., detergents, solvents, lipolytic enzymes) convert P-450 to P-420. Therefore chemicals that initiate the autocatalytic peroxidative destruction of microsomal membrane lipids (e.g., CCl_4) would be expected to depress P-450 content. Fourth, the heme moiety of P-450 may serve as a substrate for heme oxygenase. Thus chemicals that markedly stimulate the activity of heme oxygenase (e.g., Co, other metals) depress P-450 content. In addition to these mechanisms, inhibition of the biosynthesis of P-450 by chemicals (e.g., 3-aminotriazole) can also reduce the hepatic content of this hemoprotein (237).

As might be expected, several rather diverse chemicals can reduce hepatic P-450 content. In addition to the examples given, a partial listing of agents that produce this effect includes allyl-containing compounds such as 2-allyl-2-isopropylacetamide (51), carbon disulfide and other sulfur-containing chemicals (51), acetaminophen, furosemide, thioactamide, N-hydroxy-2-acetylaminofluorene (158), vinyl chloride (210), and trichloroethylene (167). Furthermore, agents such as chloroform (26) and halothane (150,217), which apparently do not reduce P-450 content in naive animals, do so in induced animals under the appropriate conditions. Thus it appears that measurement of P-450 to detect

endoplasmic reticulum damage is applicable to a number of agents. Use of P-450, however, to quantify the degree of injury seems to be of limited usefulness (256).

Regardless of the mechanisms involved, destruction of cytochrome P-450 can be expected to lead to a concomitant decrease in the rate of metabolism of xenobiotics handled by this system. For example, Dingell and Heimburg (54) found that CCl_4 rapidly depressed (90% decrease within 8 hr) hepatic microsomal metabolism of aminopyrine, hexobarbital, and p-nitrobenzoic acid; microsomal enzyme activity required about 8 days to return to normal. These investigators established a dose-response relation between CCl_4 and MFO enzyme depression. Thus it appears that the activity of the MFO system can reflect incremental damage of the endoplasmic reticulum. Similar results have been obtained with other hepatotoxicants and MFO substrates (11,158,209,222). Loss of microsomal xenobiotic metabolizing activity on in vitro addition of agents that promote lipid peroxidation is also useful in the study of the peroxidative process. For example, loss of activity of aminopyrine N-demethylase (79,80,109,112,146,245,253), ethylmorphine N-demethylase (109,112,245), and aniline hydroxylase (112,245,253), among others, has been observed as a consequence of lipid peroxidation. Thus the activity of the MFO system can be used for mechanistic as well as diagnostic purposes.

Alterations in the pharmacological effects of drugs can be used to detect and in some instances quantify liver dysfunction. Plaa et al. (186) demonstrated that prolongation of pentobarbital sleeping time could be used to quantify the relative hepatotoxicity of seven haloalkanes (Fig. 4). In these exper-

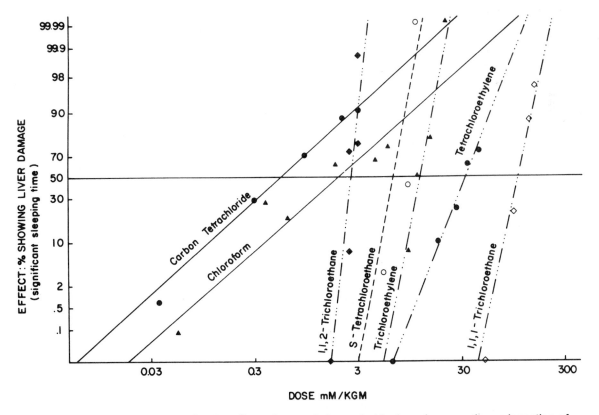

FIG. 4. Dose-response curves for the effect of seven halogenated hydrocarbons on the prolongation of pentobarbital sleeping time in mice. [From Plaa et al. (186), with permission.]

iments the upper limit of normalcy (mean sleeping time + 2 SD) for pentobarbital sleeping time was established in a large number of control mice. Subsequently, mice were administered various doses of one of the seven haloalkanes, and the pentobarbital sleeping time was determined 24 hr later. The frequency of abnormal sleeping times was then plotted against the haloalkane dose as one normally plots lethality data. These data permit comparison of dose-response curves, tests for parallelism, and statistical analyses of potency differences. Thus the relative hepatotoxic potential of these agents could be assessed. Kutob and Plaa (134) also used pentobarbital sleeping time in conjunction with BSP retention and liver succinic dehydrogenase activity to study the ability of ethanol to potentiate CHCl$_3$-induced liver damage in mice. Dingell and Heimburg (54), Lal et al. (135), Jaeger et al. (102), and Andersen et al. (4) have made use of barbiturate sleeping time to assess chemically induced hepatotoxicity.

Alteration of Hepatic Calcium Content

The role of calcium as a mediator of toxicant-induced hepatocyte death has been a matter of conjecture for more than 30 years (75). Reynolds and colleagues (207,208,238) found that CCl$_4$ produces striking alterations in calcium homeostasis in the liver. Calcium accumulation in the liver followed a biphasic pattern. During the initial phase, hepatic calcium doubled within 30 min following CCl$_4$ administration, reached a peak fourfold greater than normal by 1 hr, and returned to a near-normal value 4 hr after CCl$_4$ administration. The increased calcium appeared to be sequestered within the mitochondria. The second phase of calcium accumulation began approximately 8 hr after CCl$_4$ administration; hepatic calcium content was as large as 20-fold normal 48 hr after CCl$_4$ administration. Necrosis was observed 8 to 12 hr following CCl$_4$ administration and the extent of it increased in parallel with the rise in hepatic calcium content. The association between the increased hepatic calcium content and the appearance of necrosis suggests that an influx of Ca^{2+} into the hepatocyte initiates a series of cytotoxic events that results in cell death. The ability of CCl$_4$ to produce cell death in cultured rat hepatocytes supports this hypothesis. Casini and Farber (32) demonstrated that the extent of cell death induced by CCl$_4$ was dependent on the Ca^{2+} concentration of the incubation medium (0.3–3.6 mM).

Accumulation of calcium in the liver accompanies the cell death produced by a variety of other hepatotoxicants. For example, galactosamine increases hepatic calcium content (59), and the extent of galactosamine-induced cell death *in vitro* is dependent on the Ca^{2+} concentration of the medium (224). Chlorpromazine, which inhibits the flux of Ca^{2+} across membranes, reduced the galactosamine-induced death of cultured hepatocytes; the protective effect of chlorpromazine was overcome by increasing the Ca^{2+} concentration in the medium (224). Similarly, chlorpromazine protected against the hepatic calcium accumulation and cell necrosis produced by administration of galactosamine to rats *in vivo*. Incubation of cultured rat hepatocytes with ten membrane-active toxicants, e.g., A23187 (a Ca^{2+} ionophore), melittin, phalloidin, ethylmethanesulfonate (EMS), and silica, resulted in appre-

ciable cytotoxicity when hepatocytes were incubated with Ca^{2+}; cell death was dependent on extracellular Ca^{2+} (223); in the absence of added Ca^{2+}, none of these toxicants produced cytotoxicity.

These and other observations are consistent with the hypothesis that toxicant-induced injury to the hepatocyte plasma membrane results in the influx of Ca^{2+} into the cell, initiating a series of cytotoxic events that are common to a variety of hepatotoxicants and resulting in cell death (64,65). Although this hypothesis is attractive, a role for extracellular Ca^{2+} in hepatocyte death is not universally accepted. Smith et al. (229) demonstrated that CCl$_4$, bromobenzene, and EMS were appreciably more toxic to freshly isolated rat hepatocytes when incubated in the absence of extracellular Ca^{2+} than in its presence. Acosta and Sorenson (1) found that the presence of extracellular Ca^{2+} reduced cadmium-induced cytotoxicity in cultured rat hepatocytes. Perfusion of isolated rat livers with *t*-butylhydroperoxide (TBHP) or CCl$_4$ resulted in a similar degree of injury in the presence or absence of extracellular Ca^{2+} (228); cellular injury was independent of a rise or fall of total hepatic calcium content. Interestingly, Smith and Sandy (228) found that TBHP was more toxic to isolated hepatocytes incubated in the absence of extracellular Ca^{2+}. Fariss and Reed (66) demonstrated that bromobenzene, EMS, and the combination of Adriamycin plus 1,3-bis(2-chloroethyl)-1-nitrosourea (ADR-BCNU) produced an accelerated loss of viability in isolated hepatocytes incubated without extracellular Ca^{2+} compared to cells incubated with Ca^{2+}. Fariss et al. (67) proposed that the discrepancy between studies demonstrating that toxicant-induced hepatocyte death was dependent on extracellular Ca^{2+} and those demonstrating that extracellular Ca^{2+} had no role in cell death is due to the presence or absence of vitamin E in the incubation medium. The studies showing that toxicant-induced cell death occurred in the presence, but not the absence, of extracellular Ca^{2+} were performed with an incubation medium containing vitamin E. In contrast, vitamin E was not a component of the medium in the experiments that dismissed the role of extracellular Ca^{2+} in chemically induced cell death. When treated with EMS, A23187, or ADR-BCNU, protected cells incubated in Ca^{2+}-free medium with vitamin E contained substantially more vitamin E than unprotected cells incubated with extracellular Ca^{2+} and vitamin E. Thus the large increase in cellular vitamin E content, rather than the presence or absence of extracellular Ca^{2+}, appeared to be responsible for protecting hepatocytes against toxicant-induced injury (67). In total, these observations suggested that toxicant-induced hepatocyte death is not mediated by an influx of extracellular Ca^{2+}.

The intracellular distribution of calcium exerts a profound influence on cell metabolism, motility, and division (107,192). Thus intracellular calcium homeostasis is of importance to cell viability. The distribution of Ca^{2+} within hepatocytes is complex and involves binding to cell macromolecules (e.g., glycoproteins, proteins, and phospholipids) and compartmentation within subcellular organelles. The critically important cellular calcium pool for regulation of intracellular events is the free Ca^{2+} in the cytosol; the concentration of this pool is approximately 0.1 μM. The cytosolic free Ca^{2+} concentration is regulated by energy-requiring transport systems located in the plasma membrane, endoplasmic reticulum, and mitochondrion. An ATP-dependent Ca^{2+} pump in the plasma membrane extrudes Ca^{2+} from the cytoplasm. In addition, the membrane of the endoplasmic reticulum and the inner mitochondrial membrane have pump-leak systems that permit active extrusion of Ca^{2+} from the cytosol and a passive leak of Ca^{2+} back into the cytosol. About 65 to 80% of the total cell calcium may be contained within the mitochondria; this pool of calcium appears to serve as the primary buffer for the cytoplasmic free Ca^{2+} pool (107). As cytosolic free Ca^{2+} concentration increases, mitochondria accumulate calcium to maintain a normal concentration of free Ca^{2+} in the cytosol. Although the endoplasmic reticulum transporter has a relatively low capacity to accumulate calcium, especially when compared to mitochondria, sequestration of calcium by the endoplasmic reticulum does play a role in controlling cytosolic free Ca^{2+} concentration. Of importance in terms of the role of cell calcium in the pathogenesis of cell injury is the fact that substantial calcium is contained in the mitochondrial and endoplasmic reticular pools; the redistribution of calcium from these pools into the cytosol can elevate the cytosolic free Ca^{2+} concentration to the point where initiation of cell injury may occur.

t-Butylhydroperoxide, menadione, and acetaminophen are cytotoxic to isolated hepatocytes and appear to produce early alteration in intracellular calcium distribution (14,16,104,165,218,219,229,240). Exposure of isolated hepatocytes to TBHP results in marked blebbing of the plasma membrane (cell blebbing is associated with alterations in calcium homeostasis), leakage of lactate dehydrogenase, and uptake of trypan blue. TBHP biotransformation results in depletion of cellular glutathione content and ultimately oxidation of NADPH. Oxidation of NADPH appears to trigger release of Ca^{2+} from mitochondria, thereby increasing the cytosolic free Ca^{2+} concentration. Acetaminophen also appears to disrupt intracellular Ca^{2+} homeostasis (165). Incubation of hepatocytes with acetaminophen resulted in a dose-dependent increase in cell blebbing and trypan blue uptake. Depletion of mitochondrial and extramitochondrial calcium pools with an elevation of cytosolic free Ca^{2+} concentration was observed and preceded the loss of cell viability; the mitochondrial loss was quantitatively more important. Incubation of hepatocytes with *N*-acetyl-*p*-benzoquinone imine (NAPQI), the putative toxic metabolite of acetaminophen, produced a qualitatively similar pattern of alterations. Low concentrations of NAPQI caused complete release of calcium from isolated liver mitochondria, which was accompanied by pyridine nucleotide oxidation and preceded membrane damage; NAPQI also inhibited microsomal calcium uptake. NAPQI was associated with a rapid, dose-dependent depletion of both cytosolic and mitochondrial reduced glutathione and a loss of protein thiols. Moore et al. (165) suggested that acetaminophen and NAPQI exert their cytotoxic effects via disruption of intracellular calcium homeostasis secondary to the depletion of soluble and protein-bound thiols.

Alteration of the ability of the endoplasmic reticulum to sequester calcium has been implicated in cell death induced by other toxicants. The activity of the rat liver microsomal calcium pump is reduced by several hepatotoxicants including CCl_4, $CHCl_3$, 1,1-dichloroethylene, and carbon disulfide (161–164). Inhibition of Ca^{2+} pump activity is observed within minutes after administration of CCl_4, suggesting that

the reduction in pump activity is one of the earliest aberrations produced by this toxicant. In addition, pretreatments that modify the bioactivation of CCl_4 also modify its effect on the endoplasmic reticulum calcium pump. Isopropanol, for example, potentiates CCl_4-induced hepatotoxicity and alters CCl_4 biotransformation (180). Moore and Ray (163) demonstrated that isopropanol pretreatment significantly enhanced the ability of CCl_4 to inhibit microsomal calcium pump activity after *in vivo* or *in vitro* exposure.

The toxic effects of oxidative stress in isolated rat hepatocytes is associated with depletion of intracellular calcium pools, including the endoplasmic reticular pool (14,104). Interestingly, depletion of the endoplasmic reticular pool is preceded by the oxidation of cellular glutathione, suggesting that an alteration of the thiol redox status could be responsible for this process. In support of this hypothesis is the observation that inhibition of microsomal calcium sequestration by TBHP is prevented by thiol reducing agents such as glutathione and dithiothreitol (106). Thor et al. (240) demonstrated that calcium sequestration by the endoplasmic reticulum was inhibited by reagents that cause alkylation (*p*-chlormercuribenzoate) or oxidation (diamide) of protein sulfhydryl groups. Pretreatment of microsomes with cystamine, which results in formation of mixed disulfides with protein thiols, also resulted in the inhibition of calcium sequestration. These observations suggested that toxicants can inhibit calcium sequestration by the endoplasmic reticulum by affecting protein sulfhydryl groups. In the intact hepatocyte, such inhibition could reduce the ability of the endoplasmic reticulum to buffer the cytosolic free Ca^{2+} concentration, thereby resulting in an uncontrolled increase in cytosolic free Ca^{2+} and a rapid progression of toxic events (240).

The extrusion of calcium across the plasma membrane may also be a target for toxicants. TBHP is reported to cause inhibition of the plasma membrane Ca^{2+} translocase of the hepatocyte (15). In addition, Nicotera et al. (171) demonstrated that incubation of isolated rat hepatocytes with toxic concentrations of menadione inhibits plasma membrane Ca^{2+}-ATPase activity. Inhibition of calcium extrusion across the plasma membrane may be a critical event in that the hepatocyte would be unable to buffer the increased cytosolic free Ca^{2+} concentration resulting from release of Ca^{2+} from mitochondrial or endoplasmic reticular stores. This inability could result in a sustained elevation in cytosolic free Ca^{2+} concentration and cytotoxicity.

To summarize, toxicant-induced increases in the cytosolic concentration of free Ca^{2+} appear to initiate cytotoxic events that eventually result in death of the hepatocyte. Most of the data indicate that although the extracellular/intracellular concentration gradient of Ca^{2+} is large ($\approx 10,000:1$), death of the hepatocyte is not mediated primarily by influx of Ca^{2+} from the extracellular fluid. Rather, redistribution of calcium from pools maintained within subcellular organelles results in a rapid increase in the cytosolic free Ca^{2+}. Although extrusion of calcium across the plasma membrane could buffer the increased cytosolic free Ca^{2+} concentration, various toxicants are also capable of inhibiting the plasma membrane Ca^{2+} translocase system, thereby producing a sustained elevation in cytosolic free Ca^{2+}. Thus it appears that toxicant-induced alterations in one or more of the triumvirate of sys-

TABLE 4. *Histologic evaluation of the effects of pretreatment with various agents on CHCl₃-induced hepatotoxicity in male rats*[a]

Treatment	Normal hepatocytes (%)	Degenerated hepatocytes (%)	Necrotic hepatocytes (%)	ALT activity (units/ml)	Total bilirubin (mg/dl)
CHCl₃	99.7 ± 0.1	0.3 ± 0.1	0	37 ± 3	0.18 ± 0.01
n-Hexane + CHCl₃	97.9 ± 2.3	5.8 ± 0.9	6.3 ± 2.2	347 ± 100	0.24 ± 0.01
Acetone + CHCl₃	76.2 ± 4.7	9.2 ± 2.1	14.6 ± 3.0	1,177 ± 534	0.26 ± 0.02
2,5-Hexanedione + CHCl₃	51.9 ± 5.0	13.5 ± 2.6	34.7 ± 3.1	2,228 ± 477	0.82 ± 0.32
Methyl n-butyl ketone + CHCl₃	45.2 ± 2.0	17.5 ± 2.0	27.2 ± 1.8	4,910 ± 631	1.35 ± 0.17

[a] CHCl₃ (0.5 ml/kg i.p.) was administered 18 hr after a single oral dose (15 mmol/kg) of vehicle, n-hexane, acetone, 2,5-hexanedione, or methyl n-butyl ketone. The animals were killed 24 hr later. Values represent the mean ± SE determined in 4 to 15 rats.

Data were obtained from Hewitt et al. (93).

tems responsible for regulating cytosolic free Ca²⁺ concentration contribute to an elevation in this critical calcium pool.

Elucidation of the role of calcium in liver injury is complicated by the technical difficulties involved in the determination of calcium distribution within the hepatocyte. It seems clear that simple measurement of total cellular calcium content is an inadequate approach. Compartmentalization of cellular calcium can be estimated in hepatocytes with the metallochrome indicator arsenazo III (14,168) or fluorescent Ca²⁺ indicators such as Quin 2 (239). However, these techniques are complicated and may be invalid for use with some toxicants. An alternative method for estimating increases in cytosolic free Ca²⁺ concentration involves the determination of phosphorylase a activity (168). Phosphorylase a activity has been used to demonstrate changes in intracellular free Ca²⁺ concentration in hepatocytes induced by TBHP and acetaminophen (16,165,219). The utility of these various

techniques for assessing hepatic dysfunction is as yet undetermined.

Histological Analysis of Liver Injury

Analysis of the hepatotoxic potential of a chemical agent is incomplete without a histological description of the lesion produced. The characteristic hepatic lesions defined by light microscopy are mentioned above. The reader is referred to Zimmerman (256) and Newberne (170) for a more detailed discussion of the various expressions of hepatotoxicity as observed by light microscopy.

Quantification of the degree of injury observed by light microscopy can be achieved using the method of Chalkley (35) essentially as described by Mitchell et al. (157). One ocular of a microscope is fitted with a micrometer eyepiece

TABLE 5. *Linear regression analysis of the relation between histologic evaluation of severity of liver injury and alterations in various parameters of hepatic damage*

Correlation coefficient (r)	x-Axis (% hepatocytes)	y-Axis (parameter)	Regression line [y = m(x) + (b)]	Points/line
0.959	Abnormal	Log (ALT activity)	y = 0.0397(x) + (1.5538)	49
0.950	Necrotic	Log (ALT activity)	y = 0.0566(x) + (1.5881)	49
0.926	Degenerated	Log (ALT activity)	y = 0.1186(x) + (1.5386)	49
0.922	Necrotic	ALT activity	y = 99(x) + (−74)	49
0.903	Abnormal	ALT activity	y = 67(x) + (−106)	49
0.885	Abnormal	Log (OCT activity + 1)	y = 0.0550(x) + (0.5728)	47
0.879	Degenerated	Log (OCT activity + 1)	y = 0.1691(x) + (0.5281)	47
0.865	Necrotic	Log (OCT activity + 1)	y = 0.0773(x) + (0.6331)	47
0.830	Necrotic	Bilirubin concentration	y = 0.0025(x) + (0.15)	49
0.820	Abnormal	Bilirubin concentration	y = 0.017(x) + (0.14)	49
0.816	Degenerated	OCT activity	y = 116(x) + (−64)	47
0.813	Degenerated	ALT activity	y = 188(x) + (−69)	49
0.799	Abnormal	OCT activity	y = 37(x) + (19)	47
0.770	Necrotic	OCT activity	y = 51(x) + (27)	47
0.755	Degenerated	Bilirubin concentration	y = 0.049(x) + (0.14)	49
0.650	Abnormal	Relative liver weight[a]	y = 0.016(x) + (4.22)	49
0.645	Necrotic	Relative liver weight	y = 0.023(x) + (4.23)	49
0.628	Degenerated	Relative liver weight	y = 0.049(x) + (4.21)	49

[a] Relative liver weight = liver wt./body wt. × 100.

Data obtained from Plaa and Hewitt (182).

containing a grid on which 16 points of reference are chosen. A section of suitably stained liver tissue is selected from each animal and examined at ×400 magnification. In a study of acetaminophen hepatotoxicity in mice, Mitchell et al. (157) found that a single section of liver could be considered to be representative of the entire organ. Each section is evaluated by scanning a series of 25 microscopic fields chosen at random. In each field, the tissue element immediately underneath each of the 16 points of reference is termed a "hit"; thus 16 hits are examined per field. A total of 400 hits are examined in each section. The hits are categorized as: (a) normal parenchymal hepatocyte; (b) degenerated parenchymal hepatocyte; (c) necrotic parenchymal hepatocyte; and (d) other cellular structures (93). Hits on each of the first three categories are recorded and expressed as a percentage of the total number of hepatocytes examined in that section. Accumulation of the data from three to five animals in each treatment group provides a data base of sufficient size for statistical analysis.

This type of quantitative histological analysis was useful for determining the relative ability of various solvents to potentiate $CHCl_3$-induced hepatotoxicity (Table 4). In this study (93) rats were pretreated with an equimolar dose of n-hexane (H), acetone (A), 2,5-hexanedione (2,5-HD), or methyl n-butyl ketone (MBK); 18 hr later the rats received a small challenging dose of $CHCl_3$, calculated to produce minimal signs of liver injury. Hepatic damage was assessed 24 hr after $CHCl_3$ administration.

Although each of the solvents was capable of potentiating the hepatotoxic effects of $CHCl_3$, it is clear (Table 4) that a marked difference exists in the severity of the potentiation produced. Normal hepatocytes accounted for approximately 88, 75, 52, and 45% of the total of $CHCl_3$-challenged rats pretreated with H, A, 2,5-HD, or MBK, respectively. Degenerated hepatocytes accounted for approximately 6% of the total in rats receiving the combination of H + $CHCl_3$ and rose to approximately 18% in rats treated with MBK + $CHCl_3$. The percentage of necrotic hepatocytes was greatest in rats treated with MBK + $CHCl_3$ (37%) and decreased in the following order: 2,5-HD + $CHCl_3$ (35%), A + $CHCl_3$ (15%), and H + $CHCl_3$ (6%).

These results indicate that this method for quantifying histological alterations provides an index of toxicity sensitive enough to discern the varying potentiating capacities of the four solvents tested. It is also noteworthy that the use of histological criteria to rank these solvents in order of increasing potentiating ability (H < A < 2,5-HD ≈ MBK) provided results similar to those obtained via determination of serum ALT (Table 4) and serum OCT (93) activity. Furthermore, the quantitive histological analysis provided a greater degree of discrimination between the solvents tested than did determination of total plasma bilirubin content (Table 4). In general, this procedure for quantifying histological abnormalities correlates well with other indices of liver injury (182). An example of correlations between histopathologic alterations and changes in functional indices of liver injury is given

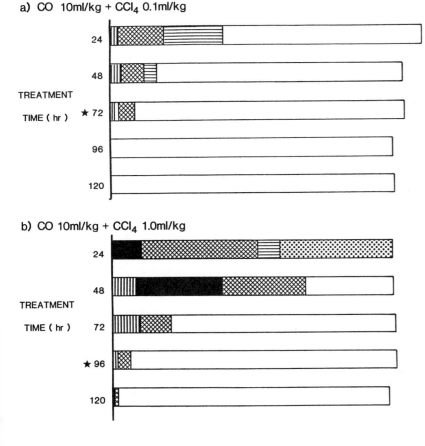

FIG. 5. Lobular morphologic patterns of CCl_4-induced liver injury for a 120-hr posttreatment period, according to the technique of Iijima et al. (98). The left side (0 μm) of the figure corresponds to the centrilobular region, whereas the right side (400 μm) corresponds to the periportal space of the hepatic lobule. ■, necrosis; ▥, inflammatory cell infiltration; ▨, swollen hepatocytes; ▤, ballooning of hepatocytes with pyknotic nuclei; ▦, accumulation of lipid droplets; and □, normal hepatocytes. [From Charbonneau et al. (36), with permission.]

in Table 5. The severity of the hepatic lesion, expressed as the percentage of degenerated hepatocytes, the percentage of necrotic hepatocytes, or the percentage of abnormal hepatocytes (necrotic plus degenerated) is compared to alterations in ALT and OCT or to the plasma content of bilirubin. Regardless of the parameters assessed, a linear correlation was observed between the extent of the lesion as quantified by light microscopy and the severity of the biochemical alteration. Marked differences, however, were observed in the strength of correlation between the different combinations of parameters examined. In general, elevations in the serum activity of ALT were most strongly correlated with the histopathologic alterations. The correlations between the severity of the lesion and alterations in relative liver weight, however, were not strong.

Minor modifications of this method have been used. Mitchell et al. (157) used an eyepiece containing eight points of reference and examined 50 random microscopic fields to collect 400 hits. It appears that the arrangement and number of reference points examined per field are of little consequence so long as a sufficient number of hits are collected for analysis. In one study (92), 30 points of reference per field and 50 fields were examined for a total of 1,500 hits/section. However, H. Miyajima (unpublished observations) found no statistical difference between the results obtained by examining 1,500 versus 400 hits per section. Thus for routine usage, it appears that collection of 400 hits per section is satisfactory.

The quantitative method described above does not allow one to visualize the lobular distribution relative to the zonal configuration of the hepatic lobule. Iijima et al. (98) devised a semiquantitative morphologic method that permits such visualization. To evaluate the morphologic patterns, ten hexagonal lobules are chosen randomly for each liver section. The distance of the injured area from the hepatocytes adjacent the terminal hepatic venule (THV; central vein) to the

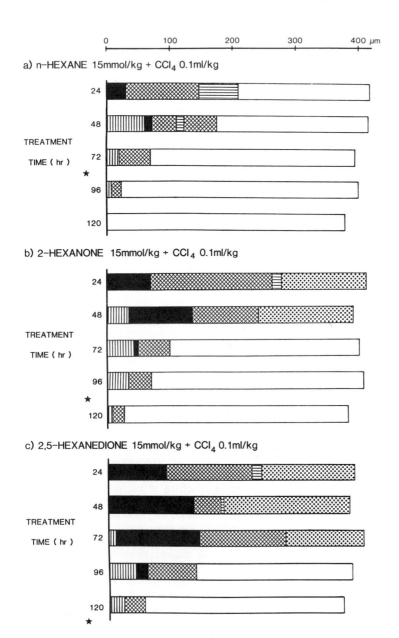

FIG. 6. Effect of potentiating agents (n-hexane, 2-hexanone, and 2,5-hexanedione) on the lobular morphologic pattern of CCl$_4$-induced liver injury for a 120-hr post-CCl$_4$ treatment observation period, according to the technique of Iijima et al. (98). See Fig. 5 for other details. [From Charbonneau et al. (36), with permission.]

portal area is measured in one fixed direction per lobule using a micrometer ocular disc containing 100 gradations of 5 mm each. This distance is measured at a magnification of ×100. The sections are then examined at a magnification of ×400 to classify the cellular changes observed. The damage is classified using six categories: (a) necrosis; (b) ballooning of hepatocytes; (c) swelling of hepatocytes; (d) inflammatory cell infiltration; (e) presence of lipid droplets; and (f) normal hepatocytes. The results are expressed in absolute mean distances (micrometers) from the THV. The mean distance for each category observed in a treatment group is calculated for four to six animals (total of 40–60 hexagonal lobules). The graphic representation of such an analysis is depicted in Fig. 5, where the lesions produced by two dosages of CCl_4 (0.1 and 1.0 ml/kg i.p.) were monitored over a 120-hr period (36). It is evident that the severity of the lesion and recovery were dose-dependent. Figure 6 demonstrates how pretreatment with a potentiating agent 18 hr before the CCl_4 challenge greatly enhanced the hepatic response to the smaller dosage (0.1 ml/kg) of CCl_4 (36). The major advantage of this semiquantitive morphologic procedure is that it permits the investigator to prepare a graphic representation of what is visualized after examination of many microscopic sections. It can be particularly useful for the preparation of toxicological reports.

Electron microscopy is also of value in toxicological studies, as it permits a correlation between the ultrastructural and functional changes induced by foreign chemicals. Grice (81) delineated several of the advantages and disadvantages encountered in the application of electron microscopic techniques to the study of chemically induced liver injury. In general, electron microscopy provides a much earlier demonstration of hepatocyte injury and is of value for detecting minimal and often reversible pathologic changes that may be evident before they are detectable by light microscopy. The ability to detect subtle ultrastructural defects early in the course of poisoning often permits identification of the initial site of the lesion and thus can provide clues to possible biochemical mechanisms involved in the pathogenesis of liver injury. In addition, the power of these techniques can be enhanced through a quantitative, morphometric analysis of chemical effects (20,49). However, serious restrictions involving proper fixation techniques, sampling procedures, and the complexity of sample preparation argue against the routine use of electron microscopy in the initial evaluation of the hepatotoxic potential of a new chemical. Rather, this technique is probably of greatest use for confirming a suspected alteration or defining a pathologic event (81).

CONCLUDING REMARKS

It can be seen that although techniques for determination of chemically induced liver injury in laboratory animals are readily available, no single technique is satisfactory for the detection and quantification of all forms of injury. Rather, a battery of procedures consisting of one or more of the biochemical/functional techniques coupled with a histological analysis of the liver is essential for the correct evaluation of the hepatotoxic potential of a chemical agent.

REFERENCES

1. Acosta, D., and Sorenson, E. M. B. (1983): Role of calcium in cytotoxic injury of cultured hepatocytes. *Ann. N.Y. Acad. Sci.,* 407: 78–92.
2. Allemand, H., Pessayre, D., Descatoire, V., Degott, C., Feldman, G., and Benhamou, J-P. (1978): Metabolic activation of trichloroethylene into a chemically reactive metabolite toxic to the liver. *J. Pharmacol. Exp. Ther.,* 204:714–723.
3. Amador, E., Frany, R. J., and Massod, M. F. (1966): Serum glutamic-oxaloacetic transaminase activity: diagnostic accuracy of the revised spectrophotometric and the dinitrophenylhydrazine methods. *Clin. Chem.,* 12:475–481.
4. Andersen, M. E., French, J. E., Gargas, M. L., Jones, R. A., and Jenkins, L. J., Jr. (1979): Saturable metabolism and the acute toxicity of 1,1-dichloroethylene. *Toxicol. Appl. Pharmacol.,* 47:385–393.
5. Asada, M. (1958): Transaminase activity in liver damage. I. Study on experimental liver damage. *Med. J. Osaka Univ.,* 9:45–51.
6. Asada, M., and Galambos, R. J. (1963): Sorbitol dehydrogenase and hepatocellular injury: an experimental and clinical study. *Gastroenterology,* 44:578–587.
7. Ayotte, P., and Plaa, G. L. (1986): Modification of biliary tree permeability in rats treated with a manganese-bilirubin combination. *Toxicol. Appl. Pharmacol.,* 84:205–303.
8. Bajwa, R. S., and Fujimoto, J. M. (1983): Effect of colchicine and S,S,S-tributyl phosphorotrithioate (DEF) on the biliary excretion of sucrose, mannitol and horseradish peroxidase in the rat. *Biochem. Pharmacol.,* 32:85–90.
9. Balazs, R., Airth, J. M., and Grice, H. C. (1962): The use of serum glutamic pyruvic transaminase test for the evaluation of hepatic necrotropic compounds in rats. *Can. J. Biochem. Physiol.,* 40:1–6.
10. Balazs, R., Murray, R. K., McLaughlan, J. M., and Grice, H. C. (1961): Hepatic tests in toxicity studies on rats. *Toxicol. Appl. Pharmacol.,* 3:71–79.
11. Barker, E. A., and Smuckler, E. A. (1972): Altered microsome function during acute thioacetamide poisoning. *Mol. Pharmacol.,* 8:318–326.
12. Batsakis, J. G., Kremers, B. J., Thiessen, M. M., and Shilling, J. M. (1968): Biliary tract enzymology—a clinical comparison of serum alkaline phosphatase, leucine aminopeptidase, and 5'-nucleotidase. *Am. J. Clin. Pathol.,* 50:485–490.
13. Becker, B. A., and Plaa, G. L. (1965): Quantitative and temporal delineation of various parameters of liver dysfunction due to α-naphthylisothiocyanate. *Toxicol. Appl. Pharmacol.,* 7:708–718.
14. Bellomo, G., Jewell, S. A., Thor, H., and Orrenius, S. (1982): Regulation of intracellular calcium compartmentation: studies with isolated hepatocytes and t-butylhydroperoxide. *Proc. Natl. Acad. Sci. USA,* 79:6842–6846.
15. Bellomo, G., Mirabelli, F., Richelmi, P., and Orrenius, S. (1983): Critical role of sulfydryl groups in ATP-dependent Ca^{2+} sequestration by the plasma membrane fraction from rat liver. *FEBS Lett.,* 163:136–139.
16. Bellomo, G., Thor, H., and Orrenius, S. (1984): Increase in cytosolic Ca^{2+} concentration during t-butylhydroperoxide metabolism by isolated hepatocytes involves NADPH oxidation and mobilization of intracellular Ca^{2+} stores. *FEBS Lett.,* 168:38–42.
17. Beneditti, A., Casini, A. F., Feralli, M., and Comporti, M. (1977): Studies on the relationships between carbon tetrachloride-induced alterations of liver microsomal lipids and impairment of glucose-6-phosphatase activity. *Exp. Mol. Pathol.,* 27:309–323.
18. Berthelot, P., and Billing, B. H. (1966): Effect of bunamiodyl on hepatic uptake of sulfobromophthalein in the rat. *Am. J. Physiol.,* 211:395–399.
19. Bertone, G., and Dianzani, M. U. (1977): Inhibition by aldehydes as a possible further mechanism for glucose-6-phosphatase inactivation during CCl_4-poisoning. *Chem. Biol. Interact.,* 19:91–100.
20. Bolender, R. P. (1978): Morphometric analysis in the assessment of the response of the liver to drugs. *Pharmacol. Rev.,* 30:429–443.
21. Boyland, E., and Grover, P. L. (1967): The relationship between hepatic glutathione conjugation and BSP excretion and the effect of therapeutic agents. *Clin. Chim. Acta,* 16:205–213.

22. Brauer, R. W. (1959): Mechanisms of bile secretion. *JAMA*, 169: 1462–1466.
23. Brauer, R. W., and Root, M. A. (1946): The effect of carbon tetrachloride induced liver injury upon the acetylcholine hydrolyzing activity of blood plasma of the rat. *J. Pharmacol. Exp. Ther.*, 88: 109–118.
24. Brauer, R. W., Krebs, J. S., and Pessotti, R. D. (1950): Bromsulfonphthalein as a tool for study of liver physiology. *Fed. Proc.*, 9: 259.
25. Brauer, R. W., Pessotti, R. L., and Krebs, J. S. (1955): The distribution and excretion of S^{35} labeled sulfobromophthalein sodium administered to dogs by continuous infusion. *J. Clin. Invest.*, 34: 35–43.
26. Brown, B. R., Jr., Sipes, I. G., and Sagalyn, A. M. (1974): Mechanisms of acute hepatic toxicity: chloroform, halothane and glutathione. *Anesthesiology*, 41:554–561.
27. Bucher, N. L. R., and Malt, R. A. (1971): *Regeneration of Liver and Kidney*. Little, Brown, Boston.
28. Buege, J. A., and Aust, S. D. (1978): Microsomal lipid peroxidation. *Methods Enzymol.*, 53:302–310.
29. Bunyan, J., Murrell, E. A., Green, J., and Diplock, A. T. (1969): On the existence and significance of lipid peroxides in vitamin E-deficient animals. *Br. J. Nutr.*, 21:475–495.
30. Burk, R. F., and Lane, J. M. (1979): Ethane production and liver necrosis in rats after administration of drugs and other chemicals. *Toxicol. Appl. Pharmacol.*, 50:467–478.
31. Butler, W. M., Jr., Maling, H. M., Horning, M. G., and Brodie, B. B. (1961): The direct determination of liver triglycerides. *J. Lipid Res.*, 2:95–96.
32. Casini, A. F., and Farber, J. L. (1981): Dependence of the carbon tetrachloride-induced death of cultured hepatocytes on the extracellular calcium concentration. *Am. J. Pathol.*, 105:138–148.
33. Ceriotti, G., and Gazzaniga, A. (1966): A sensitive method for serum ornithine carbamyltransferase determination. *Clin. Chim. Acta*, 14:57–62.
34. Ceriotti, G., and Gazzaniga, A. (1967): Accelerated micro and ultramicro procedure for ornithine carbamyltransferase (OCT) determination. *Clin. Chim. Acta*, 16:436–439.
35. Chalkley, H. W. (1943): Method for the quantitative morphologic analysis of tissues. *J. Natl. Cancer Inst.*, 4:47–53.
36. Charbonneau, M., Iijima, M., Côté, M. G., and Plaa, G. L. (1985): Temporal analysis of rat liver injury following potentiation of carbon tetrachloride hepatotoxicity with ketonic or ketogenic compounds. *Toxicology*, 35:95–112.
37. Cheeseman, K. H., Albano, E. F., Tomasi, A., and Slater, T. F. (1985): Biochemical studies on the metabolic activation of halogenated alkanes. *Environ. Health Perspect*, 64:85–101.
38. Cherrick, G. R., Stein, S. W., Leevy, C. M., and Davidson, C. S. (1960): Indocyanine green: observations on its physical properties, plasma decay and hepatic extraction. *J. Clin. Invest.*, 39:592–600.
39. Chio, K. S., and Tappel, A. L. (1969): Synthesis and characterization of the fluorescent products derived from malonaldehyde and amino acids. *Biochemistry*, 8:2821–2827.
40. Cobb, L. A. (1965): Effects of reducing agents on indocyanine green dye. *Am. Heart J.*, 70:145–146.
41. Combes, B. (1965): The importance of conjugation with glutathione for sulfobromophthalein sodium (BSP) transfer from blood to bile. *J. Clin. Invest.*, 44:1214–1224.
42. Comporti, M. (1985): Lipid peroxidation and cellular damage in toxic liver injury. *Lab. Invest.*, 53:599–623.
43. Cornelius, C. E. (1963): Relation of body weight to hepatic glutamic pyruvic transaminase activity. *Nature*, 200:580–581.
44. Cornelius, C. E., Bishop, J., Switzer, J., and Rhode, E. A. (1959): Serum and tissue transaminase activities in domestic animals. *Cornell Vet.*, 49:116–126.
45. Cornish, H. H. (1971): Problems posed by observations of serum enzyme changes in toxicology. *CRC Crit. Rev. Toxicol.*, 1:1–32.
46. Cornish, H. H., Barth, M. L., and Dodson, V. N. (1970): Isozyme profiles and protein patterns in specific organ damage. *Toxicol. Appl. Pharmacol.*, 16:411–423.
47. Curtis, L. R., Williams, W. L., and Mehendale, H. M. (1979): Potentiation of the hepatotoxicity of carbon tetrachloride following preexposure to chlordecone (Kepone) in the male rat. *Toxicol. Appl. Pharmacol.*, 51:283–293.
48. Curtis, S. J., Moritz, M., and Snodgrass, P. J. (1972): Serum enzymes derived from liver cell fractions. I. The response to carbon tetrachloride intoxication in rats. *Gastroenterology*, 62:84–92.
49. De la Iglesia, F. A., Sturgess, J. M., and Feuer, G. (1982): New approaches for the assessment of hepatotoxicity by means of quantitative functional-morphological interrelationships. In: *Toxicology of the Liver*, edited by G. L. Plaa and W. R. Hewitt, pp. 47–102. Raven Press, New York.
50. Delprat, G. D., and Stowe, W. P. (1931): The rose bengal test for liver function. *J. Lab. Clin. Med.*, 16:923–925.
51. DeMatteis, F. (1978): Loss of liver cytochrome P-450 caused by chemicals. In: *Heme and Hemoproteins*, edited by F. DeMatteis and W. N. Aldridge, pp. 95–128. Springer-Verlag, New York.
52. Dianzani, M. U. (1978): Biochemical aspects of fatty liver. In: *Biochemical Mechanisms of Liver Injury*, edited by T. F. Slater, pp. 45–96. Academic Press, New York.
53. Dillard, C. J., Dumelin, E. E., and Tappel, A. L. (1977): Effect of dietary vitamin E on expiration of pentane and ethane by the rat. *Lipids*, 12:109–114.
54. Dingell, J. F., and Heimburg, M. (1968): The effects of aliphatic halogenated hydrocarbons on hepatic drug metabolism. *Biochem. Pharmacol.*, 17:1269–1278.
55. Drotman, R. B. (1975): A study of kinetic parameters for the use of serum ornithine carbamoyltransferase as an index of liver damage. *Food Cosmet. Toxicol.*, 13:649–651.
56. Drotman, R. B., and Lawhorn, G. T. (1978): Serum enzymes as indicators of chemically induced liver damage. *Drug Chem. Toxicol.*, 1:163–171.
57. Dumelin, E. E., and Tappel, A. L. (1977): Hydrocarbon gases produced during in vitro peroxidation of polyunsaturated fatty acids and decomposition of preformed hydroperoxides. *Lipids*, 12:894–900.
58. Eckhardt, E. T., and Plaa, G. L. (1963): Role of biotransformation, biliary excretion and circulatory changes in chlorpromazine-induced sulfobromophthalein retention. *J. Pharmacol. Exp. Ther.*, 139:383–389.
59. El-Mofty, S. K., Scrutton, M. C., Serroni, A., Nicolini, C., and Farber, J. L. (1975): Early reversible plasma membrane injury in galactosamine-induced liver cell death. *Am. J. Pathol.*, 79:579–596.
60. Erlinger, S. (1982): Bile flow. In: *The Liver: Biology and Pathobiology*, edited by I. Arias, H. Popper, D. Schacter, and D. A. Shafritz, pp. 407–427. Raven Press, New York.
61. Evans, C. D., List, G. R., Doles, A., McConnell, D. G., and Hoffman, R. L. (1967): Pentane from thermal decomposition of lipoxidase-derived products. *Lipids*, 2:432–434.
62. Evans, C. D., List, G. R., Hoffman, R. L., and Moser, H. H. (1969): Edible oil quality as measured by thermal release of pentane. *J. Am. Oil Chem. Soc.*, 46:501–504.
63. Farber, E., Shull, K. H., Villa-Trevino, S., Lombardi, B., and Thomas, M. (1964): Biochemical pathology of acute hepatic adenosinetriphosphate deficiency. *Nature*, 203:34–40.
64. Farber, J. L. (1982): Calcium and the mechanisms of liver necrosis. *Prog. Liver Dis.*, 7:347–360.
65. Farber, J. L. (1982): Membrane injury and calcium homeostasis in the pathogenesis of coagulative necrosis. *Lab. Invest.*, 47:114–123.
66. Fariss, M. W., and Reed, D. J. (1985): Mechanisms of chemical-induced toxicity. II. Role of extracellular calcium. *Toxicol. Appl. Pharmacol.*, 79:296–306.
67. Fariss, M. W., Pascoe, G. A., and Reed, D. J. (1985): Vitamin E reversal of the effect of extracellular calcium on chemically induced toxicity in hepatocytes. *Science*, 227:751–754.
68. Feuer, G., Golberg, L., and LePelley, J. R. (1965): Liver response tests. I. Exploratory studies on glucose-6-phosphatase and other liver enzymes. *Food Cosmet. Toxicol.*, 3:235–249.
69. Fiske, C. H., and SubbaRow, Y. (1925): The colorimetric determination of phosphorous. *J. Biol. Chem.*, 66:375–400.
70. Ford, E. J. H. (1965): Changes in the activity of ornithine carbamyl transferase (OCT) in the serum of cattle and sheep with hepatic lesions. *J. Comp. Pathol.*, 75:299–308.
71. Frankel, E. N., Nowakowska, J., and Evans, C. D. (1961): Formation of methyl azelaaldehydate on autoxidation of lipids. *J. Am. Oil Chem. Soc.*, 38:161–162.
72. Fuhrman-Lane, C. L., Erwin, C. P., Fujimoto, J. M., and Dibben, M. J. (1981): Altered hepatobiliary permeability induced by

Amanita phalloides in the rat and the protective role of bile duct ligation. *Toxicol. Appl. Pharmacol.*, 58:370–378.

73. Fujimoto, J. M. (1982): Some in vivo methods for studying sites of toxicant action in relation to bile formation. In: *Toxicology of the Liver*, edited by G. L. Plaa and W. R. Hewitt, pp. 121–145. Raven Press, New York.

74. Gabriel, L., Bonelli, G., and Dianzani, M. U. (1977): Inhibition of colchicine binding to rat liver tubulin by aldehydes and by linoleic acid hydroperoxide. *Chem. Biol. Interact.*, 19:101–109.

75. Gallagher, C. H., Gupta, D. N., Judah, J. D., and Rees, K. R. (1956): Biochemical changes in liver in acute thioacetamide intoxication. *J. Pathol. Bacteriol.*, 72:193–201.

76. Ghoshal, A. K., Porta, E. A., and Hartroft, W. S. (1969): The role of lipoperoxidation in the pathogenesis of fatty livers induced by phosphorous poisoning in rats. *Am. J. Pathol.*, 54:275–291.

77. Gillette, J. R. (1975): Mechanisms of hepatic necrosis induced by halogenated aromatic hydrocarbons. In: *The Pathogenesis and Mechanisms of Liver Cell Necrosis*, edited by D. Keppler, pp. 239–254. MTP Press, Lancaster, United Kingdom.

78. Gillette, J. R. (1977): Kinetics of reactive metabolites and covalent binding in vivo and in vitro. In: *Biological Reactive Intermediates*, edited by D. J. Jollow, J. J. Kocsis, R. Snyder, and H. Vanio, pp. 25–41. Plenum Press, New York.

79. Glende, E. A., Jr. (1972): On the mechanism of carbon tetrachloride toxicity—coincidence of loss of drug-metabolizing activity with peroxidation of microsomal lipid. *Biochem. Pharmacol.*, 21:2131–2138.

80. Glende, E. A., Jr., Hruszkewycz, A. M., and Recknagel, R. O. (1976): Critical role of lipid peroxidation in carbon tetrachloride-induced loss of aminopyrine demethylase, cytochrome P-450 and glucose-6-phosphatase. *Biochem. Pharmacol.*, 25:2163–2170.

81. Grice, H. C. (1972): The changing role of pathology in modern safety evaluation. *CRC Crit. Rev. Toxicol.*, 1:119–152.

82. Grice, H. C., Barth, M. L., Cornish, H. H., Foster, G. V., and Gray, R. H. (1971): Correlation between serum enzymes, isozyme patterns and histologically detectable organ damage. *Food Cosmet. Toxicol.*, 9:847–855.

83. Gumucio, J. J., and Miller, D. L. (1982): Liver cell heterogeneity. In: *The Liver: Biology and Pathobiology*, edited by I. Arias, H. Popper, D. Schachter, and D. A. Shafritz, pp. 647–661. Raven Press, New York.

84. Gutman, A. D. (1959): Serum alkaline phosphatase activity in diseases of the skeletal and hepatobiliary systems: a consideration of the current status. *Am. J. Med.*, 27:875–901.

85. Hafeman, D. G., and Koekstra, W. G. (1977): Protection against carbon tetrachloride-induced lipid peroxidation in the rat by dietary vitamin E, selenium and methionine as measured by ethane evolution. *J. Nutr.*, 107:656–665.

86. Hallberg, D., Jonson, G., and Reichard, H. (1960): Serum alkaline phosphatases, transaminases and ornithine carbamyl transferase in biliary obstruction. *Acta Chir. Scand.*, 120:251–257.

87. Hallesy, D., and Benitz, K. F. (1963): Sulfobromophthalein sodium retention and morphological liver damage in dogs. *Toxicol. Appl. Pharmacol.*, 5:650–660.

88. Hanasono, G. K., Côté, M. G., and Plaa, G. L. (1975): Potentiation of carbon tetrachloride-induced hepatotoxicity in alloxan- or streptozotocin-diabetic rats. *J. Pharmacol. Exp. Ther.*, 192:592–604.

89. Hargreaves, T. (1966): Bilirubin, bromsulfophthalein and indocyanine green excretion in bile. *Q. J. Exp. Physiol.*, 51:184–195.

90. Henry, R. J. (1965): *Clinical Chemistry*. Hoeber, New York.

91. Hewitt, L. A., Ayotte, P., and Plaa, G. L. (1986): Modifications in rat hepatobiliary function following treatment with acetone, 2-butanone, 2-hexanone, mirex, or chlordecone and subsequently exposed to chloroform. *Toxicol. Appl. Pharmacol.*, 83:465–473.

92. Hewitt, W. R., Miyajima, H., Côté, M. G., and Plaa, G. L. (1979): Acute alteration of chloroform-induced hepato- and nephrotoxicity by mirex and Kepone. *Toxicol. Appl. Pharmacol.*, 48:509–527.

93. Hewitt, W. R., Miyajima, H., Côté, M. G., and Plaa, G. L. (1980): Acute alteration of chloroform-induced hepato- and nephrotoxicity by acetone, n-hexane, methyl n-butyl ketone and 2,5-hexanedione. *Toxicol. Appl. Pharmacol.*, 53:230–248.

94. Horvat, R. J., Lane, W. G., Ng, H., and Shepherd, A. D. (1964): Saturated hydrocarbons from autooxidizing methyl linoleate. *Nature*, 203:523–524.

95. Hoyumpa, A. M., Greene, H. L., Dunn, G. D., and Schenker, S. (1975): Fatty liver: biochemical and clinical considerations. *Dig. Dis.*, 20:1142–1170.

96. Hruszkewycz, A. M., Glende, E. A., Jr., and Recknagel, R. O. (1978): Destruction of microsomal cytochrome P-450 and glucose-6-phosphatase by lipids extracted from peroxidized microsomes. *Toxicol. Appl. Pharmacol.*, 46:695–702.

97. Hunton, D. B., Bollman, J. L., and Hoffman, H. N., II (1961): The plasma removal of indocyanine green and sulfobromophthalein: effect of dosage and blocking agents. *J. Clin. Invest.*, 40:1648–1655.

98. Iijima, M., Côté, M. G., and Plaa, G. L. (1983): A semiquantitative morphologic assessment of chlordecone-potentiated chloroform hepatotoxicity. *Toxicol. Lett.*, 17:307–314.

99. Inglefinger, F. J. (1971): Foreword. In: *Regeneration of Liver and Kidney*, by N. L. R. Bucher and R. A. Malt. Little, Brown, Boston.

100. Isselbacher, K. J. (1977): Metabolic and hepatic effects of alcohol. *N. Engl. J. Med.*, 296:612–616.

101. Jackson, R. L., Morrisett, J. D., and Gotto, A. M., Jr. (1976): Lipoprotein structure and metabolism. *Physiol. Rev.*, 56:259–316.

102. Jaeger, R. J., Trabulus, M. J., and Murphy, S. D. (1973): Biochemical effects of 1,1-dichloroethylene in rats: dissociation of its hepatotoxicity from a lipoperoxidative mechanism. *Toxicol. Appl. Pharmacol.*, 24:457–467.

103. Jeanrenaud, B., LeMarchand, Y., and Patzelt, C. (1977): Role of microtubules in hepatic secretory processes. In: *Membrane Alterations as Basis of Liver Injury*, edited by H. Popper, L. Bianchi, and W. Reutter, pp. 247–255. MTP Press, Lancaster, United Kingdom.

104. Jewell, S. A., Bellomo, G., Thor, H., Orrenius, S., and Smith, M. T. (1982): Bleb formation in hepatocytes during drug metabolism is caused by disturbances in thiol and calcium ion homeostasis. *Science*, 217:1257–1259.

105. Jollow, D. J., Mitchell, J. R., Zampaglione, N., and Gillette, J. R. (1974): Bromobenzene-induced liver necrosis: protective role of glutathione and evidence for 3,4-bromobenzene oxide as the hepatotoxic metabolite. *Pharmacology*, 11:151–169.

106. Jones, D. P., Thor, H., Smith, M. T., Jewell, S. A., and Orrenius, S. (1983): Inhibition of ATP-dependent microsomal Ca^{2+} sequestration during oxidative stress and its prevention by glutathione. *J. Biol. Chem.*, 258:6390–6393.

107. Joseph, S. K., Coll, K. E., Cooper, R. H., Marks, J. S., and Williamson, J. R. (1983): Mechanisms underlying calcium homeostasis in isolated hepatocytes. *J. Biol. Chem.*, 258:731–741.

108. Jungermann, K., and Katz, N. (1982): Functional hepatocellular heterogeneity. *Hepatology*, 2:385–395.

109. Kamataki, T., and Kitagawa, H. (1973): Effects of lipidperoxidation on activities of drug-metabolizing enzymes in liver microsomes of rats. *Biochem. Pharmacol.*, 22:3199–3207.

110. Kaplan, M. M. (1986): Serum alkaline phosphatase—another piece is added to the puzzle. *Hepatology*, 6:526–528.

111. Kiernan, F. (1833): The anatomy and physiology of the liver. *Philos. Trans. R. Soc. Lond.*, 123:711.

112. Kitada, M., Kamataki, T., and Kitagawa, H. (1974): Effects of lipid peroxidation on the microsomal electron transport system and the rate of drug metabolism in rat liver. *Chem. Pharm. Bull.*, 11:752–756.

113. Klaassen, C. D. (1969): Biliary flow after microsomal enzyme induction. *J. Pharmacol. Exp. Ther.*, 168:218–223.

114. Klaassen, C. D. (1970): Effects of phenobarbital on the plasma disappearance and biliary excretion of drugs in rats. *J. Pharmacol. Exp. Ther.*, 175:289–300.

115. Klaassen, C. D. (1970): Plasma disappearance and biliary excretion of sulfobromophthalein and phenol-3,6-dibromophthalein disulfonate after microsomal enzyme induction. *Biochem. Pharmacol.*, 19:1241–1249.

116. Klaassen, C. D. (1971): Does bile acid secretion determine canalicular bile production in rats? *Am. J. Physiol.*, 220:667–673.

117. Klaassen, C. D. (1971): Studies on the increased biliary flow produced by phenobarbital in rats. *J. Pharmacol. Exp. Ther.*, 176:743–751.

118. Klaassen, C. D. (1976): Pharmacokinetics of rose bengal in the rat, rabbit, dog, and guinea pig. *Toxicol. Appl. Pharmacol.*, 38:85–100.

119. Klaassen, C. D. (1977): Biliary excretion. In: *Handbook of Physiology, Sect. 9: Reactions to Environmental Agents*, edited by

D. H. K. Lee, H. L. Falk, S. D. Murphy, and S. R. Geiger, pp. 537–553. Williams & Wilkins, Baltimore.

120. Klaassen, C. D., and Plaa, G. L. (1967): Determination of sulfobromophthalein storage and excretory rate in small animals. *J. Appl. Physiol.*, 22:1151–1155.

121. Klaassen, C. D., and Plaa, G. L. (1967): Species variation in metabolism, storage, and excretion of sulfobromophthalein. *Am. J. Physiol.*, 213:1322–1326.

122. Klaassen, C. D., and Plaa, G. L. (1968): Effect of carbon tetrachloride on the metabolism, storage and excretion of sulfobromophthalein. *Toxicol. Appl. Pharmacol.*, 12:132–139.

123. Klaassen, C. D., and Plaa, G. L. (1968): Studies on the mechanism of phenobarbital-enhanced sulfobromophthalein disappearance. *J. Pharmacol. Exp. Ther.*, 161:361–366.

124. Klaassen, C. D., and Plaa, G. L. (1969): Comparison of the biochemical alterations elicited in livers from rats treated with carbon tetrachloride, chloroform, 1,1,2-trichloroethane and 1,1,1-trichloroethane. *Biochem. Pharmacol.*, 18:2019–2027.

125. Klaassen, C. D., and Plaa, G. L. (1969): Plasma disappearance and biliary excretion of indocyanine green in rats, rabbits and dogs. *Toxicol. Appl. Pharmacol.*, 15:374–384.

126. Klaassen, C. D., and Watkins, J. B. (1984): Mechanisms of bile formation, hepatic uptake, and biliary excretion. *Pharmacol. Rev.*, 36:1–67.

127. Konttinen, A. (1968): A further simplified method of ornithine carbamoyltransferase measurement. *Clin. Chim. Acta*, 21:29–32.

128. Korsrud, G. O., Grice, H. C., and McLaughlan, J. M. (1972): Sensitivity of several serum enzymes in detecting carbon tetrachloride-induced liver damage in rats. *Toxicol. Appl. Pharmacol.*, 22:474–483.

129. Korsrud, G. O., Grice, H. G., Goodman, R. K., Knipfel, J. E., and McLaughlan, J. M. (1973): Sensitivity of several serum enzymes for the detection of thioacetamide-, dimethylnitrosamine- and diethanolamine-induced liver damage in rats. *Toxicol. Appl. Pharmacol.*, 26:299–313.

130. Köster, U., Albrecht, D., and Kappus, H. (1977): Evidence for carbon tetrachloride- and ethanol-induced lipid peroxidation demonstrated by ethane production in mice and rats. *Toxicol. Appl. Pharmacol.*, 42:639–648.

131. Koudstall, J., and Hardouk, M. J. (1969): Histochemical demonstration of enzymes related to NADPH-dependent hydroxylating systems in rat liver after phenobarbital treatment. *Histochemie*, 20:68–77.

132. Kryszewski, A. J., Neale, G., Whitfield, J. F., and Moss, D. W. (1973): Enzyme changes in experimental biliary obstruction. *Clin. Chim. Acta*, 47:175–182.

133. Kubin, R. H., Grodsky, G. M., and Carbone, J. V. (1960): Investigation of rose bengal conjugation. *Proc. Soc. Exp. Biol. Med.*, 104:650–653.

134. Kutob, S. D., and Plaa, G. L. (1962): The effect of acute ethanol intoxication on chloroform-induced liver damage. *J. Pharmacol. Exp. Ther.*, 135:245–251.

135. Lal, H., Puri, S. K., and Fuller, G. C. (1970): Impairment of hepatic drug metabolism by carbon tetrachloride inhalation. *Toxicol. Appl. Pharmacol.*, 16:35–39.

136. Larson, R. E., Plaa, G. L., and Crew, L. M. (1964): The effect of spinal cord transection on carbon tetrachloride hepatotoxicity. *Toxicol. Appl. Pharmacol.*, 6:154–162.

137. Lavigne, J. G., and Marchand, C. (1974): The role of metabolism in chloroform hepatotoxicity. *Toxicol. Appl. Pharmacol.*, 29:312–326.

138. Leevy, C. M., Stein, S. W., Cherrick, G. R., and Davidson, C. S. (1959): Indocyanine green clearance: a test of liver excretory function. *Clin. Res.*, 7:290.

139. Lennon, H. D. (1966): Relative effects of 17α-alkylated anabolic steroids on sulfobromophthalein (BSP) retention in rabbits. *J. Pharmacol. Exp. Ther.*, 151:143–150.

140. Leonard, T. B., Hewitt, W. R., Dent, J. G., and Morgan, D. G. (1986): Serum alanine aminotransferase (ALT) as a quantitative indicator of hepatocyte necrosis. *Toxicologist*, 6:184.

141. Lieberman, M., and Mapson, L. W. (1964): Genesis and biogenesis of ethylene. *Nature*, 204:343–345.

142. Lindstrom, R. D., and Anders, M. W. (1978): Effect of agents known to alter carbon tetrachloride hepatotoxicity and cytochrome P-450 levels on carbon tetrachloride-stimulated lipid peroxidation and

ethane production in the intact rat. *Biochem. Pharmacol.*, 27:563–567.

143. Litov, R. E., Irving, D. H., Downey, J. E., and Tappel, A. L. (1978): Lipid peroxidation: a mechanism involved in acute ethanol toxicity as demonstrated by in vivo pentane production in the rat. *Lipids*, 13:305–307.

144. Lombardi, B. (1966): Considerations on the pathogenesis of fatty liver. *Lab. Invest.*, 15:1–20.

145. Lombardi, B., and Oler, A. (1967): Choline deficiency fatty liver: protein synthesis and release. *Lab. Invest.*, 17:308–321.

146. Masuda, Y., and Murano, T. (1977): Carbon tetrachloride-induced lipid peroxidation of rat liver microsomes in vitro. *Biochem. Pharmacol.*, 26:2275–2282.

147. Mazel, P., and Pessayre, D. (1976): Significance of metabolite-mediated toxicities in the safety evaluation of drugs and chemicals. In: *Advances in Modern Toxicology, Vol. 1, Part 1: New Concepts in Safety Evaluation*, edited by M. A. Mehlman, R. E. Shapiro, and H. Blumenthal, pp. 307–343. Hemisphere, New York.

148. McKenna, M. J., Zempel, J. A., Madrid, E. O., and Gehring, P. J. (1978): The pharmacokinetics of [14C]vinylidene chloride in rats following inhalation exposure. *Toxicol. Appl. Pharmacol.*, 45:599–610.

149. McKenna, M. J., Zempel, J. A., Madrid, E. O., Braun, W. H., and Gehring, P. J. (1978): Metabolism and pharmacokinetic profile of vinylidene chloride in rats following oral administration. *Toxicol. Appl. Pharmacol.*, 45:821–835.

150. McLain, G. E., Sipes, I. G., and Brown, B. R., Jr. (1979): An animal model of halothane hepatotoxicity: roles of enzyme induction and hypoxia. *Anesthesiology*, 51:321–326.

151. Mehendale, H. M. (1977): Mirex-induced impairment of hepatobiliary function: suppressed biliary excretion of imipramine and sulfobromophthalein. *Drug Metab. Disp.*, 5:56–62.

152. Mehendale, H. M. (1979): Modification of hepatobiliary function by toxic chemicals. *Fed. Proc.*, 38:2240–2245.

153. Mehendale, H. M., Ho, I. K., and Desaiah, D. (1979): Possible molecular mechanisms of mirex-induced hepatobiliary dysfunction. *Drug Metab. Disp.*, 7:28–33.

154. Meurman, L. (1960): On the distribution and kinetics of injected 131I-rose bengal. *Acta Med. Scand. [Suppl. 354]*, 167:7–85.

155. Mitchell, J. R., and Boyd, M. R. (1978): Dose thresholds, host susceptibility, and pharmacokinetic considerations in the evaluation of toxicity from chemically reactive metabolites. In: *Proceedings of the First International Congress on Toxicology*, edited by G. L. Plaa and W. A. M. Duncan, pp. 169–175. Academic Press, New York.

156. Mitchell, J. R., and Jollow, D. J. (1975): Metabolic activation of drugs to toxic substances. *Gastroenterology*, 68:392–410.

157. Mitchell, J. R., Jollow, D. J., Potter, W. Z., Davis, D. C., Gillette, J. R., and Brodie, B. B. (1973): Acetaminophen-induced hepatic necrosis. I. Role of drug metabolism. *J. Pharmacol. Exp. Ther.*, 187:185–194.

158. Mitchell, J. R., Nelson, S. D., Thorgeirsson, S. S., McMurty, R. J., and Dybing, E. (1976): Metabolic activation: biochemical basis for many drug-induced liver injuries. *Prog. Liver Dis.*, 5:259–279.

159. Mitchell, J. R., Smith, C. V., Lauterburg, B. H., Hughes, H., Corcoran, G. B., and Horning, E. C. (1984): Reactive metabolites and the pathophysiology of acute lethal cell injury. In: *Drug Metabolism and Drug Toxicity*, edited by J. R. Mitchell and M. G. Horning, pp. 301–319. Raven Press, New York.

160. Molander, D. W., Wroblewski, F., and LaDue, J. S. (1955): Serum glutamic oxalacetic transaminase as an index of hepatocellular injury. *J. Lab. Clin. Med.*, 46:831–839.

161. Moore, L. (1980): Inhibition of liver-microsome calcium pump by in vivo administration of CCl4, CHCl3, and 1,1-dichloroethylene (vinylidene chloride). *Biochem. Pharmacol.*, 29:2505–2511.

162. Moore, L. (1982): Carbon disulfide hepatotoxicity and inhibition of liver microsome calcium pump. *Biochem. Pharmacol.*, 31:1466–1467.

163. Moore, L., and Ray, P. (1983): Enhanced inhibition of hepatic microsomal calcium pump activity by CCl4 treatment of isopropanol-pretreated rats. *Toxicol. Appl. Pharmacol.*, 71:54–58.

164. Moore, L., Davenport, G. R., and Landon, E. J. (1976): Calcium uptake of a rat liver microsomal subcellular fraction in response to in vivo administration of carbon tetrachloride. *J. Biol. Chem.*, 251:1197–1201.

165. Moore, M., Thor, H., Moore, G., Nelson, S., Moldeus, P., and

Orrenius, S. (1985): The toxicity of acetaminophen and N-acetyl-p-benzoquinone imine in isolated hepatocytes is associated with thiol depletion and increased cytosolic Ca^{2+}. *J. Biol. Chem.*, 260: 13035–13040.

166. Moritz, M., and Snodgrass, P. J. (1972): Serum enzymes derived from liver cell fractions. II. Responses to bile duct ligation in rats. *Gastroenterology*, 62:93–100.

167. Moslen, M. R., Reynolds, E. S., Boor, P. J., Bailey, K., and Szabo, S. (1977): Trichloroethylene-induced deactivation of cytochrome P-450 and loss of liver glutathione in vivo. *Res. Commun. Chem. Pathol. Pharmacol.*, 16:109–120.

168. Murphy, E., Coll, K., Rich, T. L., and Williamson, J. R. (1980): Hormonal effects on calcium homeostasis in isolated hepatocytes. *J. Biol. Chem.*, 255:6600–6607.

169. Musser, A. W., Ortigoza, C., Vazquez, M., and Riddick, J. (1966): Correlation of serum enzymes and morphologic alterrations of the liver; with special reference to serum guanase and ornithine carbamyl transferase. *Am. J. Clin. Pathol.*, 46:82–88.

170. Newberne, P. (1982): Assessment of the hepatocarcinogenic potential of chemicals: response of the liver. In: *Toxicology of the Liver*, edited by G. L. Plaa and W. R. Hewitt, pp. 243–290. Raven Press, New York.

171. Nicotera, P., Moore, M., Mirabelli, F., Bellomo, G., and Orrenius, S. (1985): Inhibition of hepatocyte plasma membrane Ca^{2+}-ATPase activity by menadione metabolism and its restoration by thiols. *FEBS Lett.*, 181:149–153.

172. Oelberg, D. G., and Lester, R. (1986): Cellular mechanisms of cholestasis. *Annu. Rev. Med.*, 37:297–317.

173. Oler, A., and Lombardi, B. (1970): Further studies on a defect in the intracellular transport and secretion of proteins by the liver of choline-deficient rats. *J. Biol. Chem.*, 245:1282–1288.

174. Olson, J. R., and Fujimoto, J. M. (1980): Evaluation of hepatobiliary function in the rat by the segmented retrograde intrabiliary injection technique. *Biochem. Pharmacol.*, 29:205–211.

175. Olson, J. R., Fujimoto, J. M., and Peterson, R. E. (1977): Three methods for measuring the increase in the capacity of the distended biliary tree in the rat produced by α-naphthylisothiocyanate treatment. *Toxicol. Appl. Pharmacol.*, 42:33–43.

176. Peterson, R. E., Olson, J. R., and Fujimoto, J. M. (1976): Measurement and alteration of the capacity of the distended biliary tree in the rat. *Toxicol. Appl. Pharmacol.*, 36:353–368.

177. Phillips, M. J., Poucell, S., and Oda, M. (1986): Mechanisms of cholestasis. *Lab. Invest.*, 54:593–608.

178. Plaa, G. L. (1968): Evaluation of liver function methodology. In: *Selected Pharmacological Testing Methods, Medical Research Series*, Vol. III, edited by A. Burger, pp. 255–288. Marcel Dekker, New York.

179. Plaa, G. L. (1977): Factors influencing biliary excretion and apparent T_m for bilirubin and related anions. In: *Chemistry and Physiology of Bile Pigments*, edited by P. D. Berk and N. I. Berlin, pp. 396–403. National Institutes of Health, Bethesda.

180. Plaa, G. L. (1986): Toxic responses of the liver. In: *Casarett and Doull's Toxicology: The Basic Science of Poisons*, edited by C. D. Klaassen, M. O. Amdur, and J. Doull, pp. 286–309. Macmillan, New York.

181. Plaa, G. L., and Becker, B. A. (1965): Demonstration of bile stasis in the mouse by a direct and an indirect method. *J. Appl. Physiol.*, 20:534–537.

182. Plaa, G. L., and Hewitt, W. R. (1982): Quantitative evaluation of indices of hepatotoxicity. In: *Toxicology of the Liver*, edited by G. L. Plaa and W. R. Hewitt, pp. 103–120. Raven Press, New York.

183. Plaa, G. L., and Hine, C. H. (1960): The effect of carbon tetrachloride on isolated perfused rat liver function. *Arch. Industr. Health*, 21:114–123.

184. Plaa, G. L., and Priestly, B. G. (1976): Intrahepatic cholestasis induced by drugs and chemicals. *Pharmacol. Rev.*, 28:207–273.

185. Plaa, G. L., and Witschi, H. (1976): Chemicals, drugs and lipid peroxidation. *Annu. Rev. Pharmacol. Toxicol.*, 16:125–141.

186. Plaa, G. L., Evans, E. A., and Hine, C. H. (1958): Relative hepatotoxicity of seven halogenated hydrocarbons. *J. Pharmacol. Exp. Ther.*, 123:224–229.

187. Priestly, B. G., and Plaa, G. L. (1969): Effects of benziodarone on the metabolism and biliary excretion of sulfobromophthalein and related dyes. *Proc. Soc. Exp. Biol. Med.*, 132:881–885.

188. Priestly, B. G., and Plaa, G. L. (1970): Temporal aspects of carbon tetrachloride-induced alteration of sulfobromophthalein excretion and metabolism. *Toxicol. Appl. Pharmacol.*, 17:786–794.

189. Priestly, B. G., and Plaa, G. L. (1970): Sulfobromophthalein metabolism and excretion in rats with iodomethane-induced depletion of hepatic glutathione. *J. Pharmacol. Exp. Ther.*, 174:221–231.

190. Rappaport, A. M. (1969): Anatomic considerations. In: *Diseases of the Liver*, 3rd ed., edited by L. Schiff, pp. 1–49. Lippincott, Philadelphia.

191. Rappaport, A. M. (1979): Physioanatomical basis of toxic liver injury. In: *Toxic Injury of the Liver*, edited by E. Farber and M. M. Fisher, pp. 1–57. Marcel Dekker, New York.

192. Rasmussen, H., and Barrett, P. G. (1984): Calcium messenger system: an integrated view. *Physiol. Rev.*, 64:938–984.

193. Recknagel, R. O. (1967): Carbon tetrachloride hepatotoxicity. *Pharmacol. Rev.*, 19:145–208.

194. Recknagel, R. O., and Ghoshal, A. K. (1966): New data on the question of lipoperoxidation in carbon tetrachloride poisoning. *Exp. Mol. Pathol.*, 5:108–117.

195. Recknagel, R. O., and Glende, E. A., Jr. (1973): Carbon tetrachloride hepatotoxicity: an example of lethal cleavage. *CRC Crit. Rev. Toxicol.*, 2:263–297.

196. Recknagel, R. O., and Glende, E. A., Jr. (1977): Lipid peroxidation: a specific form of cellular injury. In: *Handbook of Physiology, Sect. 9: Reactions to Environmental Agents*, edited by D. H. K. Lee, H. L. Falk, S. D. Murphy, and S. R. Geiger, pp. 591–601. Williams & Wilkins, Baltimore.

197. Recknagel, R. O., and Lombardi, B. (1961): Studies of biochemical changes in subcellular particles of rat liver and their relationship to a new hypothesis regarding the pathogenesis of carbon tetrachloride fat accumulation. *J. Biol. Chem.*, 236:564–569.

198. Recknagel, R. O., Glende, E. A., Jr., Waller, R. L., and Lowrey, K. (1982): Lipid peroxidation: biochemistry, measurement, and significance in liver cell injury. In: *Toxicology of the Liver*, edited by G. L. Plaa and W. R. Hewitt, pp. 213–241. Raven Press, New York.

199. Rees, K. R., Sinha, P., and Spector, W. G. (1961): The pathogenesis of liver injury in carbon tetrachloride and thioacetamide poisoning. *J. Pathol. Bacteriol.*, 81:107–118.

200. Reichard, H. (1957): Determination of ornithine carbamyl transferase with microdiffusion technique. *Scand. J. Clin. Lab. Invest.*, 9:311–312.

201. Reichard, H. (1959): Ornithine carbamyl transferase in dog serum on intravenous injection of enzyme, choledochus ligation and carbon tetrachloride poisoning. *J. Lab. Clin. Med.*, 53:417–425.

202. Reichard, H. (1960): Ornithine carbamoyl-transferase activity in human tissue homogenates. *J. Lab. Clin. Med.*, 56:218–221.

203. Reichard, H. (1961): Ornithine carbamyl transferase activity in human serum in diseases of the liver and biliary system. *J. Lab. Clin. Med.*, 57:78–87.

204. Reichard, H. (1962): Studies on ornithine carbamoyl transferase activity in blood and serum. *Acta Med. Scand. [Suppl. 390]*, 172: 1–8.

205. Reichard, H. (1964): Determination of ornithine carbamoyl transferase in serum: a rapid method. *J. Lab. Clin. Med.*, 63:1061–1064.

206. Reitman, S., and Frankel, S. (1957): A colorimetric method for the determination of serum oxaloacetic and glutamic pyruvic transaminases. *Am. J. Clin. Pathol.*, 28:56–63.

207. Reynolds, E. S. (1963): Liver parenchymal cell injury. I. Initial alterations of the cell following poisoning with carbon tetrachloride. *J. Cell Biol.*, 19:139–157.

208. Reynolds, E. S. (1964): Liver parenchymal cell injury. II. Cytochemical events concerned with mitochondrial dysfunction following poisoning with carbon tetrachloride. *Lab. Invest.*, 13:1457–1470.

209. Reynolds, E. S. (1972): Comparison of early injury to liver endoplasmic reticulum by halomethanes, hexachloroethane, benzene, toluene, bromobenzene, ethionine, thioacetamide and dimethylnitrosamine. *Biochem. Pharmacol.*, 21:2555–2561.

210. Reynolds, E. S., Moslen, M. T., Szabo, S., Jaeger, R. J., and Murphy, S. D. (1975): Vinyl chloride-induced deactivation of cytochrome P-450 and other components of the liver mixed function oxidase system: an in vivo study. *Res. Commun. Chem. Pathol. Pharmacol.*, 12:685–694.

211. Riely, C. A., Cohen, G., and Lieberman, M. (1974): Ethane evolution: a new index of lipid peroxidation. *Science*, 183:208–210.

212. Roberts, R. J., Klaassen, C. D., and Plaa, G. L. (1967): Maximum biliary excretion of bilirubin and sulfobromophthalein during anesthesia-induced alteration of rectal temperature. *Proc. Soc. Exp. Biol. Med.,* 125:313–316.

213. Roberts, W. M. (1933): Blood phosphatase and the Van Den Bergh reaction in the differentiation of the several types of jaundice. *Br. Med. J.,* 1:734–738.

214. Robinson, D. S., and Seakins, A. (1962): The development in the rat of fatty livers associated with reduced plasma-lipoprotein synthesis. *Biochim. Biophys. Acta,* 62:163–165.

215. Rosenthal, S. M. (1922): An improved method for using phenotetrachlorphthalein as a liver function test. *J. Pharmacol. Exp. Ther.,* 19:385–391.

216. Rosenthal, S. M., and White, E. C. (1925): Clinical application of the Bromsulphalein test for hepatic function. *JAMA,* 84:1112–1114.

217. Ross, W. T., Jr., Daggy, B. P., and Cardell, R. R., Jr. (1979): Hepatic necrosis caused by halothane and hypoxia in phenobarbital-treated rats. *Anesthesiology,* 51:327–333.

218. Rush, G. F., Gorski, J. R., Ripple, M. G., Sowinski, J., Bugelski, P., and Hewitt, W. R. (1985): Organic hydroperoxide-induced lipid peroxidation and cell death in isolated hepatocytes. *Toxicol. Appl. Pharmacol.,* 78:473–483.

219. Rush, G. F., Yodis, L. A., and Alberts, D. (1986): Protection of hepatocytes from tert-butylhydroperoxide-induced injury by catechol. *Toxicol. Appl. Pharmacol.,* 84:607–616.

220. Sagai, M., and Tappel, A. L. (1978): Effect of vitamin E on carbon tetrachloride-induced lipid peroxidation as demonstrated by in vivo pentane production. *Toxicol. Lett.,* 2:149–155.

221. Sagai, M., and Tappel, A. L. (1979): Lipid peroxidation induced by some halomethanes as measured by in vivo pentane production in the rat. *Toxicol. Appl. Pharmacol.,* 49:283–291.

222. Sasame, H. A., Castro, J. A., and Gillette, J. R. (1968): Studies on the destruction of liver microsomal cytochrome P-450 by carbon tetrachloride administration. *Biochem. Pharmacol.,* 17:1759–1768.

223. Schanne, F. A. X., Kane, A. B., Young, E. E., and Farber, J. L. (1979): Calcium dependence of toxic cell death: a common final pathway. *Science,* 206:700–702.

224. Schanne, F. A. X., Pfau, R. G., and Farber, J. L. (1980): Galactosamine-induced cell death in primary cultures of rat hepatocytes. *Am. J. Pathol.,* 100:25–38.

225. Seetharam, S., Sussman, N. L., Komoda, T., and Alpers, D. H. (1986): The mechanism of elevated alkaline phosphatase activity after bile duct ligation in the rat. *Hepatology,* 6:374–380.

226. Shin, B. C., Huggins, J. W., and Caraway, K. L. (1972): Effects of pH, concentration and aging on the malonaldehyde reaction with proteins. *Lipids,* 7:229–233.

227. Sipes, I. G., and Gandolfi, A. J. (1982): Bioactivation of aliphatic organohalogens: formation, detection, and relevance. In: *Toxicology of the Liver,* edited by G. L. Plaa and W. R. Hewitt, pp. 181–212. Raven Press, New York.

228. Smith, M. R., and Sandy, M. S. (1985): Role of extracellular Ca^{2+} in toxic liver injury: comparative studies with the isolated perfused rat liver and isolated hepatocytes. *Toxicol. Appl. Pharmacol.,* 81:213–219.

229. Smith, M. T., Thor, H., and Orrenius, S. (1981): Toxic injury to isolated hepatocytes is not dependent on extracellular calcium. *Science,* 213:1257–1259.

230. Smuckler, E. A., Iseri, O. A., and Benditt, E. P. (1962): An intracellular defect in protein synthesis induced by carbon tetrachloride. *J. Exp. Med.,* 116:55–72.

231. Stein, O., and Stein, Y. (1973): Colchicine-induced inhibition of very low density lipoprotein release by rat liver in vivo. *Biochim. Biophys. Acta,* 306:142–147.

232. Sweeney, G. D., Garfield, R. E., Jones, K. G., and Latham, A. N. (1978): Studies using sedimentation velocity on heterogeneity of size and function of hepatocytes from mature male rats. *J. Lab. Clin. Med.,* 91:432–443.

233. Sweeney, G. D., Jones, K. D., and Krestynski, F. (1978): Effects of phenobarbital and 3-methylcholanthrene pretreatment on size, sedimentation velocity, and mixed function oxygenase activity of rat hepatocytes. *J. Lab. Clin. Med.,* 91:444–454.

234. Taplin, G. V., Meredith, O. M., and Kade, H. (1955): The radioactive (I^{131}-tagged) rose bengal uptake-excretion test for liver function using external gamma ray scintillation counting techniques. *J. Lab. Clin. Med.,* 45:655–678.

235. Tappel, A. L. (1973): Lipid peroxidation damage to cell components. *Fed. Proc.,* 32:1870–1874.

236. Tegeris, A. S., Smalley, H. E., Jr., Earl, F. L., and Curtis, J. L. (1969): Ornithine carbamyl transferase as a liver function test: comparative studies in dog, swine and man. *Toxicol. Appl. Pharmacol.,* 14:54–66.

237. Tephly, T. R. (1978): Inhibition of liver hemoprotein synthesis. In: *Heme and Hemoproteins,* edited by F. DeMatteis and W. N. Aldridge, pp. 81–94. Springer-Verlag, New York.

238. Thiers, R. E., Reynolds, E. S., and Vallee, B. L. (1960): The effect of carbon tetrachloride poisoning on subcellular metal distribution in rat liver. *J. Biol. Chem.,* 235:2130–2133.

239. Thomas, A. P., Alexander, J., and Williamson, J. R. (1984): Relationship between inositol polyphosphate production and the increase of cytosolic free Ca^{2+} induced by vasopressin in isolated hepatocytes. *J. Biol. Chem.,* 259:5574–5584.

240. Thor, H., Hartzell, P., Svensson, S-A., Orrenius, S., Mirabelli, F., Marinoni, V., and Bellomo, G. (1985): On the role of thiol groups in the inhibition of liver microsomal Ca^{2+} sequestration by toxic agents. *Biochem. Pharmacol.,* 34:3717–3723.

241. Thurman, R. G., and Kauffmann, F. C. (1985): Sublobular compartmentation of pharmacologic events (SCOPE): metabolic fluxes in periportal and pericentral regions of the liver lobule. *Hepatology,* 5:144–151.

242. Traiger, G. J., and Plaa, G. L. (1971): Differences in the potentiation of carbon tetrachloride in rats by ethanol and isopropanol pretreatment. *Toxicol. Appl. Pharmacol.,* 20:105–112.

243. Van Handel, E., and Zilversmit, D. B. (1957): Micromethod for the direct determination of serum triglycerides. *J. Lab. Clin. Med.,* 50:152–157.

244. Vassef, A. A. (1978): Direct micromethod for colorimetry of serum ornithine carbamoyltransferase activity, with use of a linear standard curve. *Clin. Chem.,* 24:101–107.

245. Vatsis, K. P., Kowalchyk, J. A., and Schulman, M. P. (1974): Ethanol and drug metabolism in mouse liver microsomes subsequent to lipid peroxidation-induced destruction of cytochrome P-450. *Biochem. Biophys. Res. Commun.,* 61:258–264.

246. Wade, C. R., and van Rij, A. M. (1985): In vivo lipid peroxidation in man as measured by the respiratory excretion of ethane, pentane, and other low-molecular-weight hydrocarbons. *Anal. Biochem.,* 150:1–7.

247. Wattenberg, L. W., and Leong, J. L. (1962): Histochemical demonstration of reduced pyridine nucleotide-dependent polycyclic hydrocarbon metabolizing systems. *J. Histochem. Cytochem.,* 10:412–420.

248. Wells, P. G., and To, E. C. A. (1986): Murine acetaminophen hepatotoxicity: temporal interanimal variability in plasma glutamic-pyruvic transaminase profiles and relation to in vivo chemical covalent binding. *Fundam. Appl. Toxicol.,* 7:17–25.

249. Wheeler, H. O., Cranston, W. I., and Meltzer, J. I. (1958): Hepatic uptake and biliary excretion of indocyanine green in the dog. *Proc. Soc. Exp. Biol. Med.,* 99:11–14.

250. Wheeler, H. O., Meltzer, J. I., and Bradley, S. E. (1960): Biliary transport and hepatic storage of sulfobromophthalein sodium in the unanesthetized dog, in normal man, and in patients with hepatic disease. *J. Clin. Invest.,* 39:1131–1144.

251. Whitfield, J. B., Pounder, R. E., Neale, G., and Moss, D. W. (1972): Serum γ-glutamyl transpeptidase activity in liver disease. *Gut,* 13:702–708.

252. Wilkinson, J. H. (1970): Clinical application of isoenzymes. *Clin. Chem.,* 16:733–739.

253. Wills, E. D. (1971): Effects of lipid peroxidation on membrane-bound enzymes of the endoplasmic reticulum. *Biochem. J.,* 123:983–991.

254. Windmueller, H. G., and von Euler, L. H. (1971): Prevention of orotic acid-induced fatty liver with allopurinol. *Proc. Soc. Exp. Biol. Med.,* 136:98–101.

255. Wroblewski, F. (1959): The clinical significance of transaminase activities of serum. *Am. J. Med.,* 27:911–923.

256. Zimmerman, H. J. (1978): *Hepatotoxicity.* Appleton-Century-Crofts, New York.

257. Zsigmond, G., and Solymoss, B. (1972): Effect of spironolactone, pregnenolone-16α-carbonitrile and cortisol on the metabolism and biliary excretion of sulfobromophthalein and phenol-3,6-dibromophthalein disulfonate in rats. *J. Pharmacol. Exp. Ther.,* 183:499–507.

Principles and Methods of Toxicology, Second Edition, edited by A. Wallace Hayes, Raven Press, Ltd., New York © 1989.

CHAPTER 21

Renal Methods for Toxicology

William O. Berndt and *Mary E. Davis

*Department of Pharmacology, College of Medicine, University of Nebraska Medical Center, Omaha, Nebraska 68105; and *Department of Pharmacology and Toxicology, West Virginia University Medical Center, Morgantown, West Virginia 26506*

This chapter presents methods of interest to the renal toxicologist. It exposes the reader to the state of the art with respect to renal function techniques as they apply to toxicology, including observations on data interpretation and pitfalls of the procedures. Specific detailed procedures are not given when they involve standard methods of renal physiology; these techniques can be found in well-known renal physiology texts (e.g., 21).

Background material on renal physiology and anatomy is given only briefly, as many excellent detailed text and reference books are available (3,11,19,22,27). A thorough background in renal physiology is essential for understanding the techniques and their application to renal toxicology.

Finally, it is not the intent of this chapter to be a "cookbook" of laboratory procedures. The focus is on evaluation of the techniques as they apply to toxicology and the interpretation of data generated from the various relevant procedures.

RENAL PHYSIOLOGY AND ANATOMY

The kidneys function to maintain water and electrolyte balance by removing large quantities of solutes and solvent from the plasma by filtration, and then selectively returning to the plasma the needed chemicals, including water (reabsorption), and further adding some chemicals to the tubular fluid (secretion). Despite processing a large volume of fluid, overall balance is maintained. The vascular tissue and tubular epithelia comprise the major tissue types of the kidneys. The

anatomical relationships between the blood vessels and the nephron are depicted in Figs. 1 and 2.

The blood supply to the kidney comes from the renal artery, which supplies the arcuate and interlobular arteries within the renal mass. The glomeruli arise from the interlobular arteries via the afferent arterioles. The glomeruli are unusual in that their capillaries are specialized for filtration and are the first of two capillary beds, in series within the kidney. Blood leaves the glomerulus via the efferent arterioles and then branches into capillary networks around the nephrons. The capillary networks are in the same general region as their parent glomeruli (the glomeruli from whence they arose). That is, efferent arterioles of glomeruli in the superficial cortex form the peritubular capillary network around the nephron tubules in the cortex while efferent arterioles from glomeruli in the midcortical area give rise to the peritubular capillaries in the midcortical area. Most of the glomeruli at the junction of the cortex and medulla (the juxtamedullary nephrons) have efferent arterioles that descend into the medulla, branching at various depths within the medulla to form capillary beds around the loop of Henle, the vasa rectae.

The glomerulus is a capillary bed specialized for filtering large amounts of water, electrolytes, and small molecules yet retaining proteins and formed elements within the vasculature (Fig. 3, A). The physical barrier separating plasma from urine is composed of three parts. The first is the fenestrae within the capillary endothelial cells. Fenestrae occupy approximately 20% of the endothelial wall; they are large (50–100 nm in diameter), and unlike other capillary fenestrae they do not have a diaphragm. The fenestrae have a negative charge; so although they are large in diameter, they can ob-

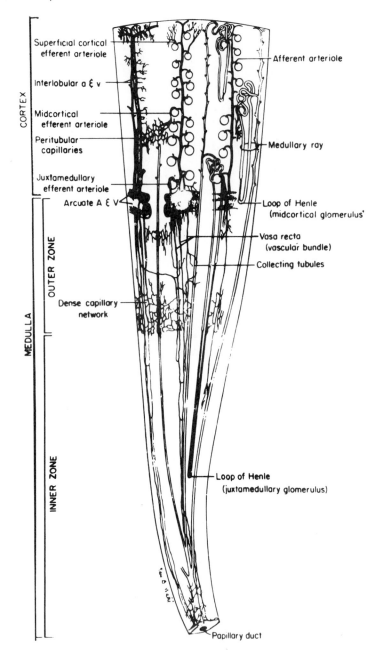

CORTEX

Superficial cortical
efferent arteriole

Interlobular a & v

Midcortical
efferent arteriole

Peritubular
capillaries

Juxtamedullary
efferent arteriole

Arcuate A & V

MEDULLA

OUTER ZONE

Dense capillary
network

INNER ZONE

Afferent arteriole

Medullary ray

Loop of Henle
(midcortical glomerulus)

Vasa recta
(vascular bundle)

Collecting tubules

Loop of Henle
(juxtamedullary glomerulus)

Papillary duct

FIG. 1. Intrarenal distribution of blood and its relation to the major nephron types. (From ref. 27.)

struct molecules, e.g., albumin, that have a negative charge. Dextran molecules of the same size as albumin cross the glomerulus, whereas anionic dextran sulfate molecules of the same size are trapped at the capillary fenestrae and do not reach the tubular urine (14,15,23,24). The second barrier to filtration is the basement membrane, a hydrated gel that excludes molecules based on size. The last barrier is the filtration slit formed by the interdigitation of finger-like processes of the epithelial cells that form the nephron capsule. The space between the two processes retards cationic molecules, and the slit constitutes the major hydraulic barrier.

Filtration occurs because the forces moving the fluid out of the capillary (hydrostatic pressure) exceed the forces preventing movement out of the capillary (oncotic pressure, due to the plasma proteins) and into the Bowman's space (hydraulic pressure within Bowman's capsule). The hydrostatic pressure derives from arterial blood pressure and decreases slightly over the length of the capillary, which permits the flow of blood through the glomerular capillary. As water is filtered out of the capillary, the proteins remaining behind are concentrated, and the plasma oncotic pressure increases. In most mammals the oncotic pressure exceeds the hydraulic pressure, and filtration stops before the blood reaches the end of the capillary; the remaining length of capillary can be thought of as a functional reserve.

The rate of filtration (glomerular filtration rate, GFR) is affected by changes of blood pressure, plasma protein concentration, and the ultrafiltration coefficient (K_f). GFR varies directly with blood pressure and inversely with protein concentration in the afferent arteriole. Increasing the rate of blood flow within the capillary increases the amount of water to be filtered, and the point of pressure equilibrium moves closer

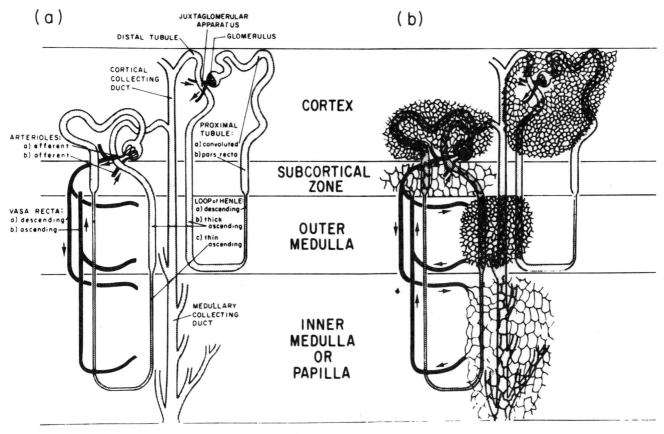

FIG. 2. a: Two major nephron types: superficial cortical and juxtamedullary nephrons. The early distal tubule segment near the glomerulus is the juxtaglomerular apparatus. **b:** The capillary networks surround all segments of the nephrons, including the collecting ducts. (From ref. 27.)

to the end of the capillary. In this way more filtration occurs. Conversely, decreasing the rate of glomerular blood flow allows more water to be filtered early along the length of the capillary, and less total fluid is filtered. Whereas GFR is highly blood flow-dependent, renal blood flow is normally independent of systemic blood pressure. Blood flow to the kidney is autoregulated, i.e., maintained approximately constant, so long as blood pressure is above about 80 mm Hg. Thus flow dependence occurs only when blood pressure falls, autoregulation fails, or intrinsic feedback mechanisms constrict the afferent arterioles (glomerular–tubular balance, see below).

The ultrafiltration coefficient (K_f) expresses the intrinsic permeability of the glomerulus and the surface area available for filtration. The coefficient is not constant but changes in response to agents such as angiotensin II, vasopressin, and norepinephrine. There are contractile elements within the connective tissue of the glomerulus (the glomerular mesangium), and contraction of these elements reduces the K_f (73). Decreases of K_f have been reported in acute renal failure caused by uranyl nitrate or gentamicin (32,90). The reduction of K_f is thought to be a major factor in the decrease of GFR but is not suggested as a mechanism of tubular toxicity (41). Alterations of K_f may be important in glomerular damage.

In addition to playing an important role in the regulation of GFR, plasma proteins also influence the rate of excretion of toxic chemicals and the effects of these chemicals on the kidneys. Only those substances of relatively small molecular

weight and in free solution pass the glomerular filter. If a chemical is partially bound to plasma proteins, only that portion not bound is filtered at the glomerulus. Therefore binding to plasma proteins can decrease excretion of the chemical and extend the duration of action (on the kidneys or other organs). The extent of binding is important when determining the concentration to which the tubular cells are actually exposed as well because materials bound to plasma proteins are neither filterable nor active while they are bound.

The distribution of glomeruli decreases from the outer

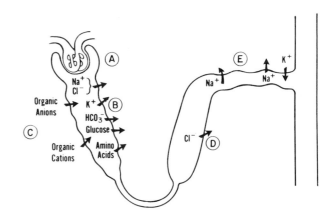

FIG. 3. Various transport functions of the nephron.

cortical to the inner cortical area. The rate of blood flow per glomerulus and the filtration rate per glomerulus are approximately equal throughout the cortex. Therefore the rate of blood flow parallels the distribution of glomeruli, being greater in the outer cortex and decreasing to the inner cortex. Still lesser amounts of blood are distributed to the medulla, renal papilla, perirenal fat, and connective tissue. Data from krypton or xenon washout studies suggest that as much as 85% of the total renal blood flow is associated with the cortical regions of the kidney. Total renal blood flow and distribution of blood within the kidney can be altered by chemical substances. The renal vasculature is a possible site of action for nephrotoxic chemicals or for chemicals that influence (either increase or decrease) nephrotoxicity.

The nephron tubule is a chain of segments that have different functions supported by different ultrastructure and enzymology (17). The proximal segments of the tubule can be differentiated by their gross appearance as either convoluted or straight. Ultrastructural studies have demonstrated three areas. The first segment (S1) is contained entirely within the proximal convoluted tubule and the last segment (S3) entirely within the straight segment. The second segment (S2) includes the end of the convoluted section and the beginning of the straight section. Both classification schemes are used because junctions between segments can be discerned only by ultrastructural techniques. The proximal convoluted tubule is a leaky epithelium that allows movement of solute between the cells, the paracellular path, as well as through cells, the transcellular route (Fig. 3, B). Approximately 60 to 70% of the filtrate is reabsorbed by the proximal convoluted tubule. Solutes are reabsorbed by transport processes, and water follows, passively, down the osmotic gradient; the tubular urine remains isosmotic to plasma (i.e., this process is an isosmotic reabsorptive one). The energy for this work is derived primarily from oxidation of fatty acids; both the convoluted and straight sections of the proximal tubule have relatively high concentrations of the enzymes of gluconeogenesis and low concentrations of those of glycolysis. Na^+,K^+-ATPase activity drives reabsorption and is found in all parts of the proximal tubules. The proximal tubule has glutathione and glutathione-S-transferase activity.

The cells of the S1 segment are tall and have a prominent brush border, extensive infoldings of the basal membrane, and interdigitations of lateral borders of adjacent cells. The interdigitating cell processes are filled with mitochondria, characteristic of Na^+-transporting epithelia. Sodium diffuses into the tubular cells and is actively extruded by Na^+,K^+-ATPase localized in the basolateral membrane. Within the S1 segment other osmolytes are co-transported with Na^+, including glucose, amino acids, and phosphate. Failure to reabsorb these osmolytes prevents reabsorption of an iso-osmotic amount of water, which is the cause of polyuria in patients with diabetes mellitus. In hyperglycemia the amount of glucose filtered overwhelms the capacity of the kidneys to reabsorb glucose, and glucose remains in the final urine. Each gram of glucose retains 21 ml of water in the urine. Glucosuria occurs in nephrotoxicity; in this situation the plasma glucose concentration is normal, but the damaged cells are not able to reabsorb the amount of glucose filtered. Amino acid reabsorption is handled by several transport systems that are selective for charge (acidic, basic, or neutral amino acids) or other structural features (imino acids, α-amino acids). Some amino acids are substrates for more than one system. Normally most (99%) of the filtered amino acids are reabsorbed; this percent is less in nephrotoxicity and certain congenital disorders, i.e., cystinurias (19).

The cells of the S2 segment are less complex than those of S1; the S2 cells have a shorter, less dense brush border and less basolateral interdigitation. Phosphate-dependent glutaminase (PDG), one of the enzymes catalyzing ammonia formation, is present in S2, and its activity is increased in the presence of acidosis (50). Glucose transport capability is about half that of S1; there are fewer glucose transporters available, but their affinity for glucose is greater, which is important because the concentration of glucose decreases along the length of the proximal tubule. The presence of high affinity transporters allows the remaining glucose to be reabsorbed more readily. A similar situation exists for glycine transport.

The rate of volume reabsorption is thought to decrease from S1 to S2, although in vitro studies using perfused tubules have demonstrated that S2 cells have approximately the same capacity as S1 cells. The rate decreases in vivo because the concentrations of the electrolytes driving volume reabsorption (Na^+, glucose, etc.) have been greatly decreased by reabsorption in the S1 segment. In contrast, transport of organic anions is much greater in S2.

The transport of organic anions and cations represents two types of secretory process (Fig. 3, C). Although both are found within the proximal tubule and both are active secretory processes, they are functionally distinct. That is, each transport system has its own substrates, competitors, and inhibitors. Transport of organic anions is not affected by organic cations; similarly organic cation transport is not decreased in the presence of either substrates or inhibitors of the organic anion transport system. The organic anion and cation transport systems are similar in that both are active processes and therefore both are subject to inhibition by metabolic inhibitors such as cyanide or iodoacetate. Tissue concentrations in excess of tenfold can be achieved by the organic ion transport system. Many of the organic ions also undergo reabsorption in the proximal segment; i.e., they undergo "bidirectional transport" in the proximal tubule. The degree of proximal tubular reabsorption is highly dependent on the compound in question and on the animal species (97). In addition, many organic ions undergo passive reabsorption, so-called nonionic diffusion, primarily in distal areas of the nephron (29). This process is highly dependent on the urine flow rate and the pH of the tubular urine.

The organic anion system has been studied more thoroughly and is better understood. The secretory process occurs in both the convoluted and straight sections of the proximal tubule; the specific segment having the highest activity depends on the species. Although several subsets of organic transport may exist (39), they all involve substances with anionic charges. The model substrate for the organic anion transport system is p-aminohippurate (PAH); model inhibitors are the organic anions probenecid and penicillin. In many species PAH is so effectively transported that its clearance is equal to, and used for measurement of, total renal blood flow. PAH excretion can be used to measure renal blood flow because filtration at the glomerulus and secretion by the tubule remove virtually all the PAH from the renal arterial blood. Actual measurements of PAH extraction (as the arteriovenous difference) in humans and dogs have shown PAH extraction to be 80 to 90% complete. Renal clearance of PAH is dependent on normal blood flow to the kidneys as well as a functioning transport system and intact tubule (maintaining normal imperviousness to passive reabsorption of PAH in the tubular urine). A nephrotoxic agent may affect PAH clearance by altering any of these three, i.e., decreasing renal blood flow, interfering with the organic anion transport system, or rendering the tubule leaky to PAH so that secreted PAH does not remain in the urine. Integrity of the transport system is readily assessed using in vitro techniques described later. With severe damage, the tubular epithelium is permeable to inulin (a polysaccharide with MW of 5,000 daltons), and leakiness can sometimes be assessed as the increased concentration of inulin in tissue.

Organic cations such as tetraethylammonium (TEA) or N-methylnicotinamide (NMN) also are secreted actively. This process occurs in the proximal tubule, as demonstrated with a variety of techniques (30,76,77). The details of the cellular mechanisms responsible for organic cation secretion are less well understood than those for organic anions. TEA or NMN transport can be blocked by organic cations such as quinine, cyanide No. 863 (a cationic dye), or phenoxybenzamine. It is likely that irreversible inhibition by haloalkylamines such as phenoxybenzamine occurs by formation of reactive ethylenimmonium intermediates that alkylate the transport carrier (89).

In general, metabolic inhibitors do not show selectivity for one transport system over the other; e.g., cyanide or iodoacetate blocks transport of both anions and cations. However, some selective effects of nephrotoxic substances have been reported (36,60).

There is little transition between the S2 and S3 segments, and the ultrastructure of S3 is different in rats and rabbits. In rabbits S3 cells are shorter and show less complexity than S2 cells; there are minimal lateral interdigitations and basal infoldings, and microvilli of the brush border are short and sparse. The S3 cells of rats have a well-developed brush border that is longer than the other proximal segments. Glucose reabsorptive capacity is about one-tenth that of S1. Organic anion and cation transport is high in S3. Xenobiotic biotransformation activity is localized to the S3 segment. Induction of renal cytochrome P-450 activity by TCDD is accompanied by proliferation of the smooth endoplasmic reticulum (SER) in the S3 segment (57). Fluorescence from NADPH-cytochrome P-450 reductase is more intense in S3 (52). Catabolism and synthesis of glutathione (GSH) occurs to a much greater extent in S3; γ-glutamyl transpeptidase is present in greater amounts in S3 than S1 or S2, and γ-glutamyl-cysteinyl-synthetase is localized to the S3 segment. γ-Glutamyl transpeptidase is attached to the brush border membrane, which juts into the lumen and catalyzes the first step in the breakdown of GSH or GSH conjugates that are present in the tubular urine. This action prevents excessive excretion of GSH precursors (GSH itself does not cross membranes). γ-Glutamyl transpeptidase is identical to phosphate-independent glutaminase (51); glutaminase activity predominates at low pH (6). Overall, the S3 segment has greater activity of enzymes associated with biotransformation of chemicals and high capacity to concentrate chemicals intracellularly. These factors may contribute to apparent sensitivity of this region to nephrotoxic chemicals.

Juxtamedullary nephrons have long, hairpin-like loops of Henle that extend into the medulla and papilla. In contrast, the loop of Henle segments of superficial nephrons do not descend into the medulla. The tubular epithelia of the descending and ascending portions have different permeabilities to water, urea, sodium, and chloride. These selective permeabilities allow the urine to become concentrated relative to plasma (3,11,19,27). In the kidneys of an animal producing concentrated urine, a gradient of tissue osmolality develops from the cortex (isosmotic with plasma) to the medulla (up to four times plasma osmolality). This gradient is initiated by reabsorption of chloride in the thick segment of the ascending limb (Fig. 3, D) and is magnified by counterflow exchange between the loop of Henle and the vasa recta, the vasa recta removing excess water during times of urine concentration. As the tubular fluid travels to the distal tubule, osmolytes are extruded and remain trapped in the interstitium. High tissue osmolality is achieved and maintained within the inner reaches of the medulla and papilla, and the urine is again concentrated as it passes through the collecting duct to the ureter. The chloride reabsorptive process results in movement of chloride ion against an electrochemical gradient and is therefore a thermodynamically active transport process, the details of which are not understood (88). In vitro studies have shown that the rate of chloride transport is increased in the presence of sodium or potassium. Possible mechanisms of transport include active transport of chloride and secondary active transport of two chlorides in conjunction with a sodium and potassium, the potassium leaking back into the lumen through the paracellular path (19). The thick ascending limb has the highest Na^+, K^+-ATPase activity and highest density of mitochondria of all the nephron segments. Energy for this work is derived from glycolysis (5). Chloride reabsorption is inhibited by the "high-ceiling" diuretics (45,46); and the result, excretion of large volumes of relatively dilute urine, is a common finding in chemical-induced acute failure. Inhibition of Cl transport by nephrotoxic agents has not been identified as a mechanism of nephrotoxicity; however, the osmotic gradient crucial to elaboration of concentrated urine may be "washed out" by high urine flow rates, possibly contributing to failure to concentrate urine. Furthermore, evidence suggests that most nephrotoxicants act on proximal tubule segments.

The distal tubule is a heterogeneous segment anatomically and functionally (Fig. 3, E). It appears to include as many as four distinct regions between the macula densa and the first confluence of the "distal" segment with another tubule segment (100). This complex distal segment has been referred to as the cortical diluting segment, partly because active sodium transport occurs essentially independently of fluid movement, leading to formation of a dilute tubular fluid.

Late in the distal tubule (or perhaps in the collecting duct) potassium ion enters the tubular fluid. Although net secretion of potassium can occur, the overwhelming body of evidence suggests that potassium entry into the nephron is largely a passive event. However, details of the mechanisms are not absolutely certain. Classically, potassium secretion was associated with a sodium reabsorptive process and referred to as a sodium–potassium exchange. Although the concept of a one-for-one exchange has been useful, there is little doubt that the active sodium reabsorptive component is not linked directly to the passive potassium secretory process. Apparently, the major role of the sodium reabsorption is to generate a favorable electrochemical gradient for potassium entry from the distal tubular cell, which has a high intracellular potassium concentration. Blockade of the sodium reabsorption with an appropriate diuretic or by the presence of a non-reabsorbable anion, reduces or eliminates potassium secretion (100).

It is also in the distal segment of the nephron that urinary acidification occurs. This consideration is important in that alterations in tubular fluid pH may greatly affect passive reabsorption (nonionic diffusion) of organic compounds in this nephron segment. Hence a nephrotoxic substance with an appropriate pKa might be recycled in the distal segment of the nephron through passive reabsorption of the un-ionized chemical moiety, which might then allow enhanced exposure of the distal tubular cells to an undesirable chemical, as well as permit a prolonged stay of the substance in the blood. Despite the potential exposure of distal tubular cells to nephrotoxic compounds, it is noteworthy that the proximal tubular segments are those most often affected.

Regulation of Renal Function

In addition to the extrinsic mechanisms that determine the rate of glomerular filtration, the kidneys have intrinsic feedback mechanisms that control GFR. This condition is referred to as glomerular tubular balance (GTB), and it apparently occurs for each nephron. The distal tubule of each nephron loops back and makes contact with the afferent and efferent arterioles of its own glomerulus. This area is called the juxtaglomerular apparatus (JGA) and is composed of specialized cells of the distal tubular epithelia called the macula densa cells, Goormaghtigh cells (which contain contractile fibrils), and granular cells, near the arterioles. The Goormaghtigh cells are between the macula densa and granula cells and are in contact with both. The macula densa cells sense a change in the composition of the distal tubular fluid associated with a change in the rate of fluid flow. The exact nature of the signal is the subject of some controversy; however, it is likely that it is chloride transport (possibly sodium-requiring) into the macula densa cells that initiates the feedback response. The Goormaghtigh cells convert the macula densa response into a signal that is sensed by the granular cells, stimulating synthesis and release of angiotensin II (AII). The increased release of AII causes contraction of the afferent arteriole, decreasing blood flow and therefore the rate of filtration in that nephron. The overall result is that the rate of filtration is decreased when the quantity of tubular fluid is increased; GTB can be thought of as a means for preventing massive fluid loss when the tubule cannot reabsorb the quantity of fluid delivered to it by filtration. Normally, approximately 99.6% of the glomerular filtrate is reabsorbed by the tubule. If filtration were to continue at normal rates when reabsorptive capacity is impaired, fluid losses and derangements of selectivity and balance would occur. Nephrotoxic

chemicals generally impair tubular function without affecting the glomeruli; yet decreased GFR is often observed (either directly or indirectly). When it occurs, GFR is decreased by feedback mechanisms. With severe damage, feedback regulation either is not complete or is impaired, and the urine output is increased even though the GFR is decreased. In this situation the reabsorption of water may fall to 80% of the filtered load (as happens with the tubular toxicant hexachloro-1,3-butadiene). If the GTB is perfect, the amount of filtrate formed, relative to the amount of plasma delivered [the filtration fraction, GFR/RPF (renal plasma flow)], is constant. Inhibition of the GTB allows excessive fluid losses and occurs with nephrotoxic agents (potassium dichromate) and diuretics. (It is probably important for the large diuresis seen with furosemide and other "high-ceiling" diuretics.) Because of GTB it is possible to see either an increase or a decrease of urine volume after damage to the tubule.

The control of renal function is an integral part of kidney activity, and these control mechanisms are possible targets for the action of toxic agents. The ability of the kidney to modulate renal hemodynamics complicates assessment of the actions of nephrotoxicants. Because the kidneys compensate for their own deficiencies, one must use relatively sophisticated, and usually invasive, techniques to monitor the early phases of renal failure. Only detection of relatively massive impairment is possible with routine screening procedures. Furthermore, a detailed understanding of nephrotoxicant action on renal control mechanisms has been relatively infrequently evaluated.

ROLE OF MORPHOLOGICAL STUDIES

It is accepted that all functional studies in toxicology should be coupled with appropriate histological studies. Although this approach is commonplace, it is important to know if information can be gained from morphological studies that is not available from the physiological or biochemical experiments.

Appropriate morphological studies are useful, especially for anatomical localization of the action of a nephrotoxin. Studies by Oliver and others (72) have demonstrated localization of the chromium ion in the proximal convoluted tubule of the kidney, whereas mercury produces its greatest morphological damage in the pars recta. These morphological observations were not helpful for understanding the mechanisms underlying the acute renal failure syndrome produced by these metals. In general, routine morphological studies with light microscopy are most useful for corroborating the data from appropriately planned physiological or biochemical studies. For example, if the action of a nephrotoxicant was thought to depend on renal metabolism of the chemical to a reactive form, evidence of damage to S3 cells would support that supposition and would be seen as damage to the corticomedullary junction (23).

Electron microscopic studies may prove more useful than routine light microscopy studies. With adequate sophistication, for example, it might be possible to identify a toxin effect on the plasma membrane before changes in other subcellular organelles were observed. Although not directly indicative of a mechanism of action, such studies might help localize toxin effects on specific cell types. In addition, subcellular sites of action might be observed with electron microscopy.

METHODS FOR MEASURING RENAL TOXICITY

To assess renal dysfunction as related to the toxic effects produced by xenobiotics properly, it is necessary to utilize a battery of techniques. The complexity and diversity of function at various sites along the nephron (sometimes referred to as intranephron heterogeneity) precludes the use of a single technique for examination of renal function, whether the assessment is for normal physiological function or renal toxicology. Hence it should be appreciated that under most circumstances more than one of the procedures discussed below is necessary to determine adequately the presence of renal toxicity.

Whole Animal Experiments

In general, studies involving whole animals utilize one or another form of "clearance experiment." The exact procedures vary from traditional clearance measurements to the use of micropuncture techniques. Some of the routine procedures discussed here also are useful with other experimental approaches and are not repeated subsequently.

Either anesthetized or conscious animals may be used for these experiments. With unanesthetized animals the rat is used commonly, although unanesthetized dogs have been used in pharmacological and physiological studies. An evaluation of overall renal function is facilitated greatly if small animals are used, as they can be housed individually in metabolism cages (1). This design permits not only the assessment of renal function by clearance procedures but also measurements of food and water intake.

The choice of anesthetic agent is important. Routine clearance procedures usually are performed with relatively short-acting anesthetics such as pentobarbital. Such agents are readily soluble, are administered easily, and are relatively inexpensive. Once injected (usually 30–60 mg/kg i.p., depending on species), the level of anesthesia remains relatively constant without frequent supplementation. If "minute-to-minute" control over the anesthesia is desired, volatile or gaseous agents can be administered with anesthesia machines. Such devices are available for small animals (48). However, less information concerning effects on renal function is available for the volatile agents. Although it is generally suggested that anesthetics do not alter blood flow to vital organs (7), caution should be taken with respect to the kidney. Walker et al. (96) studied the effects of anesthesia in trained, conscious, chronically catheterized rats. Pentobarbital and Inactin each produced an approximately 25% reduction in renal blood flow and GFR. Furthermore, in experiments where ether anesthesia was used, these same parameters failed to recover for several days after recovery from the anesthesia. These observations should be considered when anesthetized rats are used for renal function studies.

Because anesthetic agents may significantly affect renal function, such an experimental design may complicate a study of the effect of xenobiotics on renal function. That is, interaction of anesthetics with compounds that adversely affect renal function is possible. Little or no information is available concerning such interactions, but they may be important in renal toxicology studies.

The use of anesthetized animals permits greater precision in the conduct of clearance experiments, better control with respect to problems of fluid balance, achievement and maintenance of desired blood levels of a given test substance, assessment of early, direct toxic events, and so forth. Although precision with respect to the above parameters is greatly enhanced by the use of anesthetized animals, to some extent flexibility in experimental design is lost.

Clearance Experiments

A procedure fundamental to whole animal studies is the clearance technique. Details of clearance calculations as applied to renal physiology are discussed in any number of references (e.g., 13,27). These procedures involve the accurate assessment of the blood (P_x) and urine (U_x) concentrations of the substance under study as well as urine flow rates (V). Either glomerular or tubular function can be quantitated with the clearance techniques depending on which test substance is used. The renal clearance calculation is the same regardless of whether glomerular or tubular function is being determined. The classical clearance equation is:

$$C_x = \frac{U_x V}{P_x}$$

and defines the clearance (C) of compound x. The clearance represents the quantity of blood or plasma cleared of the substance per unit time and has units of volume (usually milliliters) $\times t^{-1}$.

The renal physiologist routinely uses the clearance procedure to calculate GFR by monitoring the renal handling of inulin or creatinine (Fig. 4). The effective renal plasma flow also can be measured if a marker is used that is excreted

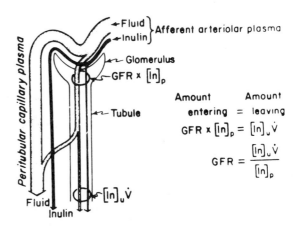

FIG. 4. Glomerular filtration process and calculation of the glomerular filtration rate in the physiology of the kidney. (From ref. 22.)

not only by filtration but by active tubular secretion as well. PAH is a good example of a substance whose clearance can be equated to the effective renal plasma flow if the organic anion transport system is intact.

Finally, note that the same clearance procedures can be applied to an analysis of the renal handling of any substance. If the clearance of substance x is greater than that calculated for a glomerular marker such as inulin, i.e., greater than the GFR, it may be concluded that substance x is added to the tubular fluid by mechanisms other than just filtration. Clearance values as large as those for PAH are suggestive of active tubular secretion, as well as glomerular filtration, with little or no reabsorption. Clearance values that are less than those for glomerular filtration suggest that tubular reabsorption may have occurred. The reabsorptive process may be either active or passive. Passive reabsorptive processes (nonionic diffusion) (27) are highly pH- and flow-dependent. For example, salicylate excretion can be greatly reduced by acidification of the urine or greatly increased by alkalinization. Excretion of a substance such as PAH is not affected by changes in urine pH. The basic methodology of clearance experiments requires that the test substance be administered so that a relatively constant concentration of the substance is maintained in the plasma. Urine samples are collected over a set period of time, and blood samples are taken contemporaneously (either at the midpoint of the urine collection or before and after the urine collection period). If anesthetized animals are used, a vein and artery are cannulated for infusion of test substance and collection of blood, respectively. Urine is obtained from either a large-diameter catheter placed in the bladder or by cannulating the ureters. (For a detailed discussion of clearance methods for the rat, see ref. 92.) For conscious animals, inulin can be administered as a subcutaneous bolus in gelatin (32%, w/v) (53). The solution is viscous and serves as a depot for inulin. The clearance period is begun 60 min after the injection; the rats are stimulated to urinate prior to placing them in metabolism cages to collect urine. Usually a 60-min collection period is sufficient to obtain an adequate sample. At the end of the period, a blood sample is taken from either the tail vein or the abdominal aorta (if the rat is to be killed).

Before the significance of clearance data can be determined, it is important to know about the plasma protein binding of the test substance. As indicated earlier, small-molecular-weight substances bound to plasma proteins are not filtered at the glomerulus. The magnitude of the protein binding is important for interpretation of clearance data, and several routine procedures are available for such measurements.

Toribara et al. (94) developed the procedure for ultrafiltration studies of calcium binding to plasma proteins. It involves placing a plasma sample in a dialysis bag, which in turn is placed in a glass centrifuge tube and supported on a frittered glass disk. The tube is gassed to maintain the pH and then centrifuged for a few hours. This method yields a few milliliters of plasma ultrafiltrate. Analysis of the ultrafiltrate and the original plasma for the compound under study gives information about binding. Procedures utilizing filter cones (Amicon Corporation, Lexington, Massachusetts) yield similar results. These cones do not prevent the passage of all plasma proteins. However, the leakage is small and does not complicate the overall analysis. Furthermore, these cones

have a loose matrix and relatively larger surface area, which permit rapid filtration. Because 1 ml or more of plasma ultrafiltrate can be obtained in a matter of minutes at low speed centrifugation ($<1,000 \times g$), gassing of samples to maintain pH is unnecessary. The speed and simplicity of this technique makes it useful for routine analyses. Equilibrium dialysis also is used for analysis of plasma protein binding. The method of McMenamy (78) is more rapid than older procedures and gives results comparable to those for ultrafiltration or older equilibrium dialysis procedures. Unquestionably, ultrafiltration is technically simpler and more rapid; and although somewhat expensive to initiate, it is preferred for routine use.

Computation of the GFR based on the clearance of a substance such as inulin is an important technique for assessing glomerular integrity. Substances such as inulin—which are not reabsorbed by the renal tubules, are not bound to plasma proteins, are small enough to pass the glomerular filter, and have no pharmacological effects—are ideal for the measurement of GFR. If inulin clearance values are below the expected normal, glomerular function may be compromised. Several chemical analyses for inulin are available and are discussed below and described in detail elsewhere (20). Inulin clearance also can be assessed with radiochemical procedures. Both ^{3}H-inulin and ^{14}C-inulin are available for use in experimental animals. Radioactivity in urine and plasma samples can be determined easily by standard liquid scintillation techniques.

Other ways to assess glomerular function involve the measurement of some normally occurring constituents of the blood. Blood urea nitrogen (BUN) may be the most commonly used procedure for assessing glomerular function. As filtration slows or ceases, BUN rises. The relation between BUN and glomerular function has been studied by many, and an example of this relation is seen in Fig. 5 (14). The plasma creatinine level parallels that of BUN and frequently is used as a marker for glomerular filtration. The relation depicted in Fig. 5 allows accurate assessment of remaining renal function for a given value of BUN or plasma creatinine. Figure 5 also shows that substantial loss of renal function can occur before BUN or plasma creatinine concentrations rise above normal. That is, BUN or plasma creatinine determinations do not detect a modest impairment of renal function. Control values for BUN are well established for every commonly used laboratory animal, and often a single value considerably in excess of known controls is predictive of renal dysfunction. These analyses are effective for both the chronic renal failure patient and the subject or animal that has ingested a nephrotoxic xenobiotic and is experiencing acute renal failure.

In general, elevations of BUN or plasma creatinine can be used as an index of decreased glomerular filtration. Ordinarily, the BUN/creatinine ratio is about 10:1. Hence a BUN measurement of 50 mg/dl or a creatinine measurement of about 5 mg/dl suggests that the GFR was approximately 25% of normal, as indicated in Fig. 5. Under some circumstances the BUN/creatinine ratio can be altered. For example, any situation that would increase the amount of protein that is metabolized to urea (e.g., high protein intake, increased catabolism) may cause a selective rise in BUN. Dehydration may also do it but not because of an effect on urea synthesis.

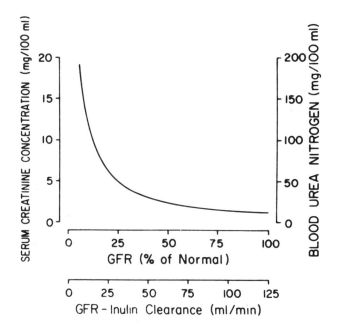

FIG. 5. Relation between plasma creatinine, BUN, and glomerular filtration rate. (From ref. 14.)

colorimetric analysis. Several methods are available (see ref. 20 for details) and are of approximately equal utility. Specific techniques for measurement of BUN are somewhat more complicated (33) but are used routinely. Indeed, some of these analyses have been developed into commercial kits [e.g., Urea Nitrogen (BUN) Rapid Stat Kit R, Pierce Co., Rockford, Illinois] intended for routine use. Note that although these kits are "cookbook"-like, there has been no loss of precision or sensitivity.

Although not strictly speaking a clearance procedure, measurement of the urinary excretion of proteins is important for the assessment of glomerular integrity (21). The selective permeability of the glomerular membranes is an important aspect of normal renal function (44). In general, the selectivity of the barrier is decreased by renal disease and by the actions of various nephrotoxic xenobiotics. Hence a common occurrence in renal failure is the excretion of excessive amounts of plasma proteins into the urine.

However, not all proteinurias should be interpreted as evidence of glomerular dysfunction. The so-called tubular proteinurias (21,47,74) probably are indicative of normal filtration of relatively small-molecular-weight proteins coupled with the failure of the tubular uptake mechanisms for these proteins. Protein also enters urine as a consequence of proximal tubule necrosis and loss of the brush border. The microvilli are sloughed into the lumen (and may coalesce, forming casts); this debris contains cellular protein and is excreted in the urine. Frequently, to resolve this problem it is necessary to use electrophoretic analyses of the urinary proteins, so that the specific proteins can be identified. However, any time an experimental animal excretes large amounts of protein in the urine after the administration of a suspected nephrotoxicant, one should be concerned about the possibility of glomerular dysfunction and attempt to confirm it with BUN or GFR measurements.

The renal clearance of PAH or similar organic ions is a quantitative expression of renal tubular secretory activity (Fig. 6) and is a measure of the effective renal plasma flow (if transport capacity has not been impaired by a tubular toxicant). However, renal extraction of PAH can be calculated from measurements of arterial and renal venous PAH concentrations and is used to correct the effective renal plasma flow. Correction of the plasma flow for hematocrit yields renal blood flow. Details of these procedures are given by Smith (20).

Dehydration results in a decreased tubular fluid flow rate, and under these conditions the percentage of the filtered urea reabsorbed is increased (28), a situation that does not occur with creatinine. Care should be taken in toxicological studies to ensure that these extraneous events are not disrupting the BUN or the BUN/creatinine ratio, either of which might be misleading with respect to glomerular function.

Plasma creatinine concentrations can be determined routinely and simply by a variety of methods, as can PAH and inulin. The details of these chemical analyses are presented elsewhere (20). PAH is determined by the method of Bratton and Marshall (43), as modified by Smith (20), which involves the diazotization of PAH with N-(2-naphthyl)-ethylenediamine dihydrochloride after nitrite reduction in acid. The color formed is stable for relatively long periods of time, and the color intensity, which can be determined spectrophotometrically, is directly related to PAH concentration.

The inulin analyses, in general, involve hydrolysis of the polysaccharide followed by determination of the fructose by

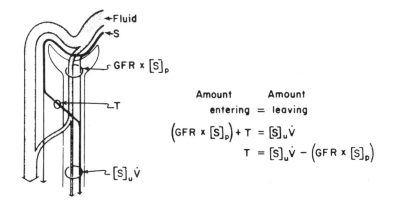

$$\text{Amount entering} = \text{Amount leaving}$$

$$\left(GFR \times [S]_p\right) + T = [S]_u \dot{V}$$

$$T = [S]_u \dot{V} - \left(GFR \times [S]_p\right)$$

FIG. 6. Renal tubular secretion and calculation of the amount of solute transported (T). (From ref. 22.)

$$\text{Renal plasma flow} = \frac{C_{PAH}}{E_{PAH}}$$

$$\text{Renal blood flow} = \frac{\text{renal plasma flow}}{1 - \text{hematocrit}}$$

where C_{PAH} is PAH clearance and E_{PAH} is PAH extraction by the kidney.

The intrarenal distribution of blood also may be altered by nephrotoxins. Whether such an action represents the primary disruption of renal function that leads to acute renal failure is unclear. Nonetheless, such effects might be important and suggest a vascular action of nephrotoxic compounds. Yarger et al. (101) examined procedures for measurement of both nutrient and glomerular blood flow, and their article should be reviewed for specific details. Rubidium-86 (^{86}Rb) distribution in the renal cortex and medulla gives an approximation of total renal blood distribution within the kidney. If a nephrotoxicant shunted blood flow from cortex to medulla, it might be expected that intrarenal ^{86}Rb distribution would become greater in medullary regions and lesser in cortical regions. The techniques involved are demanding. Injection of ^{86}Rb intravenously is followed immediately by the continuous collection of arterial blood samples to determine the arterial blood concentration curve. After 15 to 30 sec from the time of injection, the kidneys are removed and dissected into cortical and medullary regions. Blood and tissue samples are counted for radioactivity, and regional blood distribution is calculated as described by Yarger et al. (101).

The use of radioactive microspheres allows assessment of glomerular blood flow. The microspheres are tagged with a variety of short- and long-half-life gamma-emitting isotopes and are of such a size as to lodge in the glomerular capillaries. Hence by dissecting the renal cortex it is possible to learn whether glomerular flow has shifted, e.g., to the inner cortical regions in response to a nephrotoxicant. Both renal blood flow (from microsphere clearance) and regional (cortical) blood flow can be calculated as indicated by Yarger et al. (101).

Although nutrient and glomerular blood flow measurements may be helpful in toxicological studies, these techniques have been used relatively little. Rather than being connected with toxicology, these procedures usually are associated with studies in renal physiology. Although studies of renal blood or plasma flow have been useful for examining toxin effects on renal vascular effects (e.g., a suspected primary mechanism of action), emphasis should be placed on more standard clearance procedures.

Finally, alterations in the ability of the kidney to concentrate the urine are important. Frequently, it is noted that potential nephrotoxins reduce the ability of an animal to concentrate the urine (36,39). Even in those situations where urinary volume is reduced significantly by the nephrotoxin, the ability to concentrate urine still fails. Changes in urine osmolality occur early after administration of a nephrotoxin and frequently warn of more serious consequences to ensue. Measurements of urine osmolality are technically simple. Most commercially available osmometers measure osmolality by freezing point depression and provide "direct reading" (milliosmoles per liter) capability. Measurement of specific gravity yields similar information but not with as much accuracy or precision.

An important point with respect to effects on urine osmolality is that these actions are not nephrotoxicant-specific. Regardless of the xenobiotic (e.g., metals, solvents, drugs), decreased urinary osmolality occurs, usually as a prelude to other events. Hence nephrotoxicant-induced alteration of urine-concentrating ability has not proved useful for analyses of mechanisms of action.

Tubular Function

The variety of functions subserved by the tubular segments of the nephron are readily accessible to examination by the investigator. These tests can evaluate tubular secretory as well as tubular reabsorptive activities and, at least in part, may give insights into mechanisms of action.

One problem encountered in assessing the capacity of the tubule to reabsorb is that the tubule is limited by the quantity delivered by filtration, and thus decreases of GFR must be considered when evaluating reabsorptive capacity. Results can be expressed as the proportion of solute available to the nephron; it is calculated as the fractional excretion (FE): the amount of solute excreted, $[(U_x)(V)]$, divided by the amount of solute filtered $[(P_x)(GFR)]$. Fractional reabsorption is calculated as 1-FE. Values can be computed for solutes or volume. The reabsorptive capacity of a nephron for glucose is well established (see above) (Fig. 7). Frequently a nephrotoxicant causes increased excretion in the urine of moderate

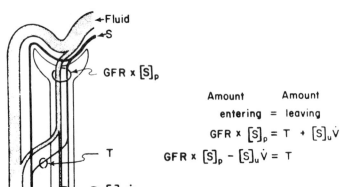

FIG. 7. Renal tubular reabsorption and calculation of reabsorptive events. (*T*) amount of solute transported in the reabsorptive direction. (From ref. 22.)

to large amounts of glucose in the absence of an elevated blood glucose. Fractional excretion of glucose is normally zero and can be increased to 100% of the filtered load after a nephrotoxic agent. Of course, it is important to establish that the blood glucose has remained normal and that the glucosuria observed is not the result of the production of a diabetes mellitus-like syndrome. Glucose determinations are accomplished most readily by the specific glucose oxidase procedure. This technique has been adapted to commercially available kits (e.g., Glucose Auto/State Kit R, Pierce Co., Rockford, Illinois) for routine use. The specificity of the technique is such that other reducing sugars do not interfere.

Secretory activity of the nephron can be monitored by examining the excretion of PAH as noted above. The clearance of this compound can be used to measure total renal blood flow because it is actively secreted by the proximal tubular cells into the tubular lumen. Hence the reduced excretion of PAH after the administration of a nephrotoxicant may be the result of interference with the active tubular secretory process or the direct disruption of blood flow to prevent the delivery of blood to the proximal tubular cells. Experimental protocols other than clearance experiments are needed to distinguish between these possible actions. For example, measurement of PAH transport by renal cortical slices, determination of the renal extraction of PAH with *in vivo* experiments, or measurement of total renal blood flow with an electromagnetic flow probe (e.g., Carolina Electronics) helps distinguish between these events. Animals (man, dog, rat) with normal renal function extract 80 to 90% of the PAH present in the arterial blood in a single passage through the kidney. Although PAH is filtered at the glomerulus, the major component in this extraction process is active tubular secretion (27). Measurement of renal extraction of PAH is facilitated by the use of large animals. Experiments can be done in rats, but care is required with the renal vein catheterization.

Another organic anion, phenolsulfophthalein (PSP), has been used by Plaa and Larsen (83) to assess tubular activity in mice. This anion is excreted in a manner similar to that for PAH; and although not used to assess renal blood flow as such, it has been useful in defining the functional integrity of the kidney. PSP is injected into control animals, and the rapidity of its urinary excretion by conscious, intact animals is compared to that by animals treated with the suspected nephrotoxicant. Although significant animal to animal variation occurs, this technique has proved useful for studies on certain nephrotoxic compounds. Although the procedure was first developed for studies in the mouse, it can be adapted to the rat as well. Its major utility is to allow the assessment of renal function in conscious, small animals. Details of the analytical procedures, described by Plaa and Larsen, essentially involve only urine collection on filter paper, extraction of the filter paper, and colorimetric determination of the PSP.

The effects of nephrotoxic compounds, particularly heavy metals, on renal tubular absorption of sodium and potassium also are of value in assessment of renal function. Frequently, metals interfere with sodium reabsorption and may produce dramatic effects on potassium excretion as well (10). However, there are no advantages to the assessment of tubular dysfunction by analysis of urinary sodium and/or potassium than by testing for PAH excretion or glucose reabsorption.

The sodium and potassium analyses (primarily by flame emission photometry), although not complex, offer no simplifications over routine colorimetric studies for glucose or PAH. Furthermore, no enhanced sensitivity with respect to the detection of renal dysfunction has been reported with measurements of urine concentration. Fractional excretion of sodium is an important index of renal reabsorptive capacity and can be used to demonstrate impaired reabsorptive capacity even in the presence of decreased urine output.

Renal Enzymes

Some investigators (35,82) have suggested that analysis of some "renal enzymes" might be useful in the early detection of nephrotoxicity induced by exogenous compounds. Specifically, maltase and alkaline phosphatase have been suggested as candidates for this role. These enzymes are located on the renal brush border, and maltase in the intestinal tract. Therefore the possibility of a nephrotoxicant causing a nonspecific, nonrenal release of, for example, maltase, is unlikely. Also, apparently release of maltase may be accomplished with only modest cellular damage. That is, the accessibility of the brush borders to potential nephrotoxicants appears to result in an early, relatively specific release of the enzyme. Many enzymes (e.g., lactic dehydrogenase, acid phosphatase) are known to be localized within certain renal tubular cells. Hence release of lysosomal or intracellular enzymes might indicate cell lysis or death, rather than a sensitive, early indicator of selective renal damage.

Although investigations of urinary enzymes as markers for nephrotoxicity have not been pursued vigorously, several workers (82,93) have demonstrated the possible utility of such an approach. Stroo and Hook (93) found that mercury caused increased urinary enzyme activities at doses lower than those that elevated BUN. Although neither chromium nor uranium showed selectivity for the brush border enzymes, the early onset of an effect caused by chromium can be interpreted as evidence of the sensitivity of the technique. Nonmetallic substances known to produce nephrotoxicity (e.g., carbon tetrachloride) did not release brush border enzymes at doses lower than those that elevated BUN. Nomiyama et al. (82) reported that changes in urinary enzymes (alkaline phosphatase, glutamic oxaloacetic transaminase) occur early after administration of uranyl nitrate. Unfortunately, measurements earlier than 24 hr after injection were not undertaken, so it is difficult to evaluate which urinary parameter (enzymes, inulin clearance, etc.) was first to respond.

In addition to the apparent lack of selectivity and perhaps sensitivity of this technique, there also are technical problems. In general, enzyme analyses are undertaken with well established procedures. Both maltase and alkaline phosphatase methods have been reported by Berger and Sacktor (35) with modifications by Stroo and Hook (93). Maltase activity is assessed by its ability to hydrolyze maltose, and alkaline phosphatase by hydrolysis of p-nitrophenylphosphate. With each enzyme, hydrolysis is monitored by spectrophotometric analysis for the hydrolysis product.

Care must be taken to ensure that the enzymes being measured are not inactivated in the urine during urine collection, which may extend over several hours. To avoid this problem, technical arrangements may be needed, for example, that permit collection of the urine in an icebath. Obviously, the collection of urine from rats in metabolism cages may be complicated if the collections are for more than a few hours. The presence of enzyme inhibitors in the urine may also prove troublesome. Frequently, however, this problem can be avoided by dialyzing the urine sample for 12 or 24 hr before making the enzyme measurement. Because the urinary concentration of some of the enzymes is relatively low, it may be necessary to concentrate the urine before the assays can be undertaken. Although all of the above technical difficulties are surmountable, they have contributed to a generalized lack of interest in this procedure for the routine assessment of urinary dysfunction.

In general, all of the analytical procedures required for the renal function tests discussed above (except enzyme analyses) are relatively straightforward. The chemical analyses for glomerular filtration or tubular function markers (e.g., inulin, PAH) have been described in great detail by many authors (20,27,28), and these specific chemical analyses have not been repeated here. Suffice it to say that all of the procedures involve standard colorimetric or spectrophotometric analyses of relatively stable, colored products. In some instances, efforts have been made to utilize radiochemical analyses rather than colorimetric tests. Once again, these tests are routine.

Finally, note that many of the above clearance-type procedures have considerable utility as screening methods for nephrotoxicity. Under these circumstances, individual animals are housed in metabolism cages, and urine samples are collected for 12 to 24 hr. For screening purposes it may be sufficient to measure urinary excretion of protein, glucose, etc. by standard "dip-stick" procedures that give a qualitative assessment of these substances in the urine. These procedures, coupled with assessment of urinary volume and urinary osmolality, reveal quickly the possibility of xenobiotic-induced nephrotoxicity. Although the "dip-stick" methods yield primarily qualitative results, there is no loss of specificity. The colorimetric procedures used are in every case just as specific as the quantitative analytical analyses; indeed, in many cases (e.g., glucose), the same procedures have been adapted to the "dip-stick" approach. These methods have been used for studies with metals (36) and various organic substances (37,38).

Stop-Flow Techniques

Although it is possible with clearance and excretion experiments to assess the tubular site of action of a nephrotoxic compound, these procedures are not ideal. Some years ago Malvin et al. (75) devised the stop-flow methodology to assess renal tubular sites of secretion and reabsorption. This procedure, as described and reviewed critically by Orloff and Berliner (11), is little used in modern renal physiology or pharmacology studies because of technical problems and difficulties in data interpretation. Details of this technique and the problems associated with it are available in the literature (11,75).

Stop-flow analysis has not been used in studies designed to examine nephrotoxicity phenomena. It is likely that such studies would be even more complex and the data more dif-

ficult to interpret than when used to study renal physiology. Administration of a nephrotoxic dose of mercuric chloride, for example, produces severe necrosis of the proximal tubule. How a severely necrotic tubule segment would respond to this trauma produced by the stop-flow occlusion is unclear; however, one might anticipate enhanced damage. These events and others would make data interpretation complex. Nonetheless, because few if any studies have been done, a brief investigation of the utility of this technique is appropriate.

Micropuncture Techniques

Micropuncture methodology is used to determine tubular sites of action and to quantitate transport processes in the single nephron. These techniques allow direct assessment of tubular fluid concentration, tubular fluid flow rates, and other renal functions in an intact, anesthetized animal. Because of the sophistication of this technology, micropuncture is especially susceptible to the introduction of technical errors and misinterpretation of results. These techniques are not to be adopted by the casual investigator or to be planned for routine screening procedures. Renal micropuncture methodology is not used routinely by toxicologists to assess renal function; rather, some micropuncture experts have adapted their techniques to the study of toxic substances (e.g., 31,40,72,87).

No attempt is made here to detail procedures or methods. Those interested in developing micropuncture techniques in their own laboratories would be required to train with a known micropuncturist. Only through such "on the job" training could one acquire the necessary skills and knowledge to develop the techniques in a new laboratory. A few general comments, however, are in order.

Although most barbiturates permit a satisfactory degree of anesthesia for renal experiments, many micropuncturists prefer a particular thiobarbiturate, Inactin, because of an apparently greater cardiovascular stability than with most barbiturates (8,16). Although there are disagreements concerning this point, it could be important because the sophisticated technology (see below) requires an unusual degree of physiological and mechanical stability.

Fundamental to many micropuncture procedures is the ability of the micropuncturist to collect measured samples of tubular fluid. The major problem with such collection procedures is adjusting the rate of collection so that the tubular fluid flow rate is neither accelerated nor impeded when relatively large volumes of fluid (and hence relatively long periods of time) are needed for analysis. Usually it is accomplished by injecting into the tubule a small volume of oil that is positioned slightly distal to the micropuncture pipette. It is assumed that if the collection rate is adjusted so that the oil droplet does not move from its position, the flow rate for the collection is exactly equivalent to the flow rate in the tubule. This technique requires that the oil droplet not be restricted in its movement so it will be a good marker for changes in fluid flow rate; on the other hand, the oil droplet must fit securely enough in the tubular lumen to prevent fluid from passing it from more distal areas. This problem is even more complex if one is trying to make distal tubular fluid collections, as tubular flow rates in the distal nephron are less than those in the proximal tubule.

Most workers try to obviate this problem by limiting their collections to very small volumes or collecting only a small fraction of the tubular fluid flow past a given point in the nephron. If these two restrictions are maintained, collections can be undertaken without the presence of an oil droplet. However, when these techniques are applied to the calculation of the single nephron filtration rate, a difficulty may be that the volume of fluid collected is so small that accurate fluid concentrations of the glomerular marker cannot be determined.

The stationary microperfusion or split oil droplet technique has been popular. This procedure allows assessment of tubular function in a restricted area of the nephron; and theoretically it might be advantageous to the toxicologist looking at the effects of toxins on tubular function. Gertz et al. (58) perfected this technique as follows. A droplet of castor oil is split by injection of the perfusion solution into the oil, and the change in the volume of the aqueous droplet is assessed photomicrographically as the two oil droplets approach each other. Because the osmolality of the proximal tubular fluid and proximal tubular reabsorbate are essentially isosmotic, observations on the rate of disappearance of the droplet from between the oil plugs allow estimation of proximal tubular sodium chloride transport.

Precise quantitation of reabsorptive characteristics may be difficult with this technique, however, because the miniscus of the oil droplet may disguise the actual surface area over which absorption occurred. Furthermore, the possibility exists that the oil droplets do not form a complete seal within the nephron and tubular fluid may leak beyond the oil droplets. It is important to note that this technique has not been applied to direct assessment of renal function in toxicological investigations. This technique, as with other micropuncture procedures, is a complicated, sophisticated one that has been directed mainly at a better understanding of mechanisms of proximal tubule fluid and electrolyte movement.

The tubular microinjection technique is one that has great utility for the assessment of tubular permeability characteristics and should be of considerable value to those with an interest in toxicology (8,16). With this procedure, a small volume of fluid containing radioactive inulin or other isotopes is injected into some part of the nephron during a free-flow situation. Serial urine samples are collected from the injected and contralateral kidneys and assayed for the compound injected. This technique is a relatively simple one for micropuncture studies and avoids such problems as the effects of oil on tubular function. The effects of nephrotoxins on tubular permeability could be assessed readily with such a technique. For example, if inulin recovery was greatly reduced after injection of a suspected nephrotoxin, it would probably mean that the inulin was leaking out of the injected nephron somewhere along its course. Although it would not prove that the nephrotoxicant was acting directly on the nephron as opposed to the vasculature, it would clearly indicate that the tubular permeability to inulin had been changed.

Finally, note that the value of all micropuncture technology depends to a large extent on the stability of the animal preparation. It is necessary to use an anesthetic that has minimal effects on renal blood flow, systemic blood flow, etc. In addition, one should take all necessary precautions to ensure that the surgical procedures involved, which are extensive, are as atraumatic as possible so as to preserve the stability of the animal. Once again, these techniques are best learned at the hands of the masters in the field and are essential for successful experiments. Detailed reviews on this methodology, its pitfalls, and its utilities are available (8,16).

Studies with Isolated Tissues: *In Vitro* Versus *In Vivo*

In general, studies with isolated tissues or subcellular fractions are directed at the mechanisms of action of nephrotoxic compounds rather than simply a description of a nephrotoxic event. Isolated tissue techniques offer several advantages over studies on intact animals. Specific transport studies can be undertaken without unwanted influences or alterations in GFR or renal blood flow, either of which may affect the availability of metabolites, substrates, etc., to the functional cells of the nephron. Although some nephrotoxins act at the level of the renal vasculature to produce their effects, frequently gross alterations in systemic circulation produce changes in renal blood flow that have only indirect effects on renal function. Noxious agents also may be tested *in vitro* without unwanted effects on other physiological systems. In addition, for the most part, precise control over the temperature, the gas atmosphere, and other factors can be maintained. Finally, and not insignificantly, a large number of experimental variables may be tested with the renal tissue from a single animal.

Specific transport studies can be accomplished for a variety of compounds using *in vitro* techniques. Organic substances (e.g., organic anions, organic cations, amino acids, sugars) can be examined with any number of the techniques discussed below. Furthermore, the transport of inorganic electrolytes can be monitored in certain experiments and their importance in supporting the transport of other substances tested. Finally, with most of the *in vitro* procedures to be described, the effects of toxins added directly to fresh tissue preparations can be studied. Animals also can be pretreated with toxic substances and the effects of these pretreatment regimens on discrete transport processes examined subsequently.

These isolated tissue techniques, as with all such procedures, present the problem of correlating *in vitro* studies with observations obtained *in vivo*. The difficulty is not unique to renal pharmacology and toxicology but frequently has been addressed more directly than in other disciplines. The direct correlation between *in vitro* renal transport and *in vivo* renal function has been studied most thoroughly with the renal cortical slice procedure (Table 1). In general, it appears that the accumulation of foreign organic anions and cations by renal slices is the *in vitro* counterpart of *in vivo* renal tubular secretion (2,49,79,80). From the literature, it is clear that substances added *in vitro* that enhance organic anion accumulation by slices, in general, increase the maximal transport rate for that anion *in vivo*. The early studies by Cross, Taggart, and Mudge (49,79,80) showed unequivocally that acetate enhanced renal slice uptake of PAH and the renal tubular transport maximum for that substance *in vivo*. Furthermore,

TABLE 1. *PAH transport by renal tissue*

Chemical substance	Response to exogenous chemical	
	In vivo (tubular transport)	*In vitro* (slice uptake)
Metabolic substrates		
Acetate 10^{-2} M	↑	↑
Lactate 10^{-2} M	↑	↑
Succinate 10^{-2} M	↓	↓
Fumarate 10^{-2} M	↓	↓
Metabolic inhibitors		
2,4-Dinitrophenol	↓	↓
2,4-Dinitro-6-phenylphenol	↓	↓
Organic anion competitors		
Probenecid	↓	↓
Carinamide	↓	↓
Iodopyracet	↓	↓
Penicillin	↓	↓

substances that decreased one parameter also decreased the other (e.g., probenecid or 2,4-dinitrophenol). Comparative studies also support the *in vivo–in vitro* comparison for the transport of organic substances. Diatrizoate, an iodinated organic anion, is accumulated actively by rabbit renal cortex slices and is actively secreted by the intact rabbit kidney, as demonstrated by both stop-flow and clearance techniques. On the other hand, dog renal cortex slices do not show net accumulation of diatrizoate, and whole animal stop-flow studies failed to demonstrate net tubular secretion. Inhibitor studies also support this dichotomy. For example, probenecid inhibited both *in vivo* secretion and *in vitro* accumulation of diatrizoate in the rabbit or rabbit cortical slices but had no effect in the dog (2).

Finally, the association between *in vivo* and *in vitro* function for organic anion transport is well substantiated by studies on the development of renal function in the newborn (55,56,61–63,66,67,85,86). Organic anion transport, whether assessed *in vivo* or *in vitro,* is absent or minimal in the newborn animal. Furthermore, organic anion transport, again whether assessed *in vivo* or *in vitro,* was inducible in the newborn by pretreatment of the pregnant dam with compounds such as penicillin. Both *in vivo* and *in vitro* transport developed over the same time scale as renal function developed in the newborn.

Hence with these studies there seems to be little doubt concerning the correlation between *in vivo* and *in vitro* studies. Other *in vitro* procedures need the same correlative approach but, in general, can be accepted as valid expressions of the *in vivo* function. Certainly, the isolated perfused tubule, which in practice is a segment of the intact functional unit of the nephron, can be utilized to obtain fundamental *in vivo* information. Isolated membrane vesicles are somewhat more removed than even the renal slices, but they are designed to examine parameters other than strictly renal function parameters. This technique was developed to learn fundamental aspects of membrane function, and the evidence suggests that the behavior of the vesicles reflects what intact membranes do in the intact animal.

Renal Cortex Slices, Tissue Fragments, Tubules

Renal cortical slices or tissue fragments may be prepared free-hand with the aid of a Stadie-Rigg microtome or a McIlwain tissue slicer. The slices or fragments prepared by these procedures (0.2–0.5 mm in thickness) are incubated in a balanced salt solution at a known temperature and with appropriate oxygenation. Frequently, the Cross-Taggart medium (49) is used, although other solutions [e.g., modified Cross-Taggart medium (9); bicarbonate-buffered medium (26)] are just as appropriate. Specific formulations are given by Umbriet et al. (26). Sodium chloride is the major constituent of these solutions, with calcium, magnesium, potassium, and so on present in concentrations that approximate those in rabbit or rat plasma. As a rule, albumin or other proteins are not used. Approximately 100 mg of tissue per incubation flask (25-ml Erlenmeyer) or beaker (30 ml) each containing 3 or 4 ml of buffer is usually sufficient for most studies. Incubations usually are undertaken in a Dubnoff shaking incubator or similar temperature-controlled, shaking waterbath. Unless the flasks are stoppered, a continual flow of the gas needed to establish the gas atmosphere is essential. For bicarbonate buffers 95% O_2 + 5% CO_2 is used, whereas 100% O_2 is satisfactory for phosphate buffers. An adult 250-g rat supplies enough renal tissue for 10 to 12 such flasks or beakers. The tissue from a single rabbit is sufficient for as many as 25 to 30 such flasks or beakers.

After an appropriate period of incubation under prescribed conditions, the tissue slices are removed from the beaker with forceps, blotted on moist filter paper, and weighed. The tissue slices are then processed, along with an aliquot of bathing solution, to determine the extent of uptake of whatever test substance is under study. For example, if radioactive substances are used, and it can be established that these compounds are not metabolized by the renal tissue, uptake of radioactivity by the slice can be monitored as a measure of accumulation. The tissue is homogenized in distilled water and an aliquot of the whole homogenate counted with standard liquid scintillation procedures. Similarly, an aliquot of the bathing solution is counted. The data obtained from such an experiment can be expressed in terms of the slice/medium ratio (S/M ratio), i.e., the amount of radioactivity per gram of tissue divided by the amount of radioactivity per milliliter of bathing solution. In general, it is agreed that S/M ratios of more than 1:1 are indicative of an active transport process. For example, with a substance such as PAH, the addition of a metabolic inhibitor can reduce the S/M ratio to less than 1:1.

This technique has particular utility for organic substances that are transported by the classical organic anion and organic cation systems. They also have proved useful for studies of amino acid transport (18). In general, the technique is a sensitive one for both the addition of toxic substances *in vitro* and the assessment of effects on transport after pretreatment. Specificity of the transport process can be assessed using various competitive transport inhibitors. For example, probenecid blocks selectively the renal slice accumulation of substances transported by the renal organic anion system. Probenecid does not block organic base or amino acid transport. In general, any organic anion transported by the anion system may serve as an inhibitor of the transport of other anions. A similar relation exists with the organic base transport system. Tetraethylammonium (TEA) and N′-methylnicotinamide (NMN) are examples of organic base transport substrates, and the basic dye cyanine No. 863 is a specific inhibitor of this system (12).

Although high S/M ratios usually reflect active accumulation, care must be taken with renal slices to ensure that the high ratios do not reflect nonspecific binding by renal tissue. With some substances (e.g., 2,4-dinitrophenol), nonspecific binding and specific tubular transport have been demonstrated (38). Even in the absence of renal tubular transport, 2,4-dinitrophenol accumulated to S/M ratios as high as 5:1, which apparently reflected nonspecific binding to cellular proteins and other macromolecules. Direct measurements of binding by cortical homogenates supported this contention, as did the failure of metabolic inhibitors to reduce the dinitrophenol S/M ratios to 1:1 or below.

Renal cortical slices have also been used to monitor sodium and potassium concentrations of renal tissue, total tissue water, and intracellular-extracellular water distribution. It is clear, however, that disruptions in cellular sodium and potassium content do not reflect changes in renal sodium or potassium reabsorption, or secretion by the nephron. Rather, alterations in the renal slice sodium or potassium content reflect changes in the general homeostatic function of the renal tubular epithelial cells. However, this analysis has utility in that it allows assessment of the general state of function of the renal tubular cells and may give insights into the mechanisms of action of toxins.

The techniques involved are relatively simple. The slices are incubated with inulin until a steady-state distribution is achieved (60–90 min). The tissues are then weighed wet, dried to a constant weight, and reweighed. The differences in weight reflect total tissue water. After the tissue has been dried, it is extracted with dilute nitric acid for several days. The nitric acid extract is used for inulin analyses (liquid scintillation counting or colorimetric analysis) and flame emission photometric analysis for sodium and potassium. The inulin is used for measurement of extracellular space and intra- and extracellular water, and intracellular electrolyte concentrations can be calculated by standard procedures (9).

Finally, renal cortical slice viability can be studied by monitoring oxygen consumption. Once again, this procedure does not give specific data on renal transport or renal function. The use of an oxygen electrode (e.g., Clark electrode) offers the greatest flexibility for such studies. The tissue is added to a small volume of balanced salt solution in the electrode chamber. The oxygen electrode is placed in the chamber (excluding the gas phase completely) to monitor the decrease in oxygen in the bathing solution. The reduction in oxygen tension in the bathing solution can be used to calculate oxygen consumption by the tissue. A complete measurement can be accomplished in 5 to 10 min utilizing as little as 15 to 30 mg of tissue.

It is important to have such assessments of tissue viability (electrolytes, oxygen consumption) so the investigator can distinguish between effects of toxins on specific renal transport processes and effects on the general metabolism within the tissue. Obviously, cessation of tissue metabolism would be expected to interfere with transport, but such an effect is not specific for one or another transport system. On the other hand, an action of a toxin on metabolism might represent an important mechanism of action.

Isolated Perfused Tubule

The isolated perfused tubule technique represents an attempt to develop an in vitro procedure that retains renal tubular function comparable to that in the intact animal. Furthermore, this technique can be used to analyze mechanisms of transport. Presumably, it would offer all the advantages of any in vitro procedure but with relatively little question of the comparability of this procedure to in vivo renal physiology, pharmacology, or toxicology. Unlike the renal slice procedure, this approach allows assessment of transepithelial transport.

Note, however, that despite all of the advantages of this technique for the assessment of renal function and the effects of xenobiotics on renal function, it has almost never been applied in the field of toxicology, no doubt in part because of difficulties encountered with dissection of the nephron segments from animals pretreated with nephrotoxicants. As with the micropuncture procedure, this technique is sophisticated and requires some significant dedication to the technique itself. It is not one that can be learned casually, but it is powerful enough to provide an understanding of renal function. Details of the procedure are not given here because they have been defined thoroughly by Burg and Orloff (4) and various other workers (see ref. 25 for a review). Some comments about advantages and disadvantages are appropriate, however.

A preparation of the tubule segment for perfusion is perhaps the most complicated and difficult part of the whole procedure. At present, such tubule segments are prepared for perfusion by manual dissection with the aid of a microscope. Earlier procedures utilizing enzymes, e.g., collagenase, have proved inappropriate because of damage to the basement membrane of the tubule segments. The rabbit kidney has proved the most useful for dissection of tubule segments, although kidneys from the dog, rat, mouse, hamster, frog, and human also have been studied. Indeed, although the rabbit remains the most popular species, improved techniques have permitted increased use of the rat. In any event, it is clear that certain species are more suitable for these dissection procedures than others, and some nephron segments are more easily isolated than others.

Minipipettes used for the perfusion procedure have become increasingly more sophisticated. The segment of nephron is suspended in a fluid bath of several milliliters between two such pipettes, one of which is the perfusion pipette and the other the collection pipette. Fluid transport out of the tubule segment is monitored by changes in the concentration of a nonpermeable marker in the perfusion solution. For example, ^{131}I-albumin or ^{14}C-inulin may be included in the perfusion solution. The collection pipette is used to obtain small volumes of perfusate, and both samples can be taken directly.

Each of the tubule segments studied has been shown to retain nearly its normal physiological function. For example, the proximal tubule shows no measurable osmotic gradient across it, the cortical collecting tubule responds to vasopressin, and electrolyte transport across the proximal tubule is similar to that seen with other techniques. Organic anion transport in the proximal tubule proceeds much as it does in renal slices and in micropuncture investigations. Indeed, it was with this technique that many of the details of organic anion transport across the tubule cell in the rabbit were established (95). These studies demonstrated that the primary active tubular transport mechanism in mammalian tissue was on the peritubular or plasma side of the cell, and that movement of material from cell to tubular lumen was primarily a passive process. Subsequent studies suggested that this passive process may be facilitated or mediated. Similar studies with glucose have shown the active transport step to be on the luminal side of the cell.

The major advantages of this technique over other *in vitro* procedures is that the relation between the *in vitro* and *in vivo* procedures is clear. The technique has demonstrated significant utility for studying the effects of pharmacological agents and should be as useful for toxicological studies. Of course, a dissected tubule is not in a normal environment and may differ from the *in vivo* situation because of that. Nonetheless, studies to date suggest that this model is a good one to study *in vivo* renal function. Unfortunately, little use has been made of this technique for studies of toxicological agents. In many ways it would be ideal to determine the action of toxicological agents on tubular cells versus glomerular events and localization of critical tubule segments. It would permit isolation of a nephron segment and study of that segment separate from the vasculature, glomerular problems, or the influences of other nephron segments. Presumably both pretreatment studies and direct *in vitro* addition studies would be possible.

A word of caution is indicated. As noted above, to date all studies have been done with rabbit nephron segments. Micropuncture and other studies [summarized by Weiner (97)] indicate that large species differences exist with respect to organic anion transport (both secretory and reabsorptive) on a segment-by-segment analysis of nephron function. Hence broad generalizations based on the isolated perfused nephron segments of rabbit kidney should be avoided.

Renal Cells in Culture

The use of cultured renal cells for the study of nephrotoxicity has obvious advantages. Under ideal circumstances large populations of specific cell types could be studied in circumstances where control of the environment would be maximized. Potentially, short- and long-term studies could be undertaken. A major complication in nephrotoxicity studies relates to the cellular heterogeneity of the kidney. Ideally this obstacle can be overcome with tissue culture studies. There is an excellent review of these techniques (6), and cell injury has been covered by Wilson (99).

A major approach to the use of cultured cells has involved established cell lines. These established lines (e.g., MDCK, LLC-PK$_1$) are available from tissue culture banks and are easily maintained in culture. The cells are not ideal, however, for studies of specific renal cell types. Often those cells were derived from cells of unknown origin, and all have been through many passages in culture. No doubt the cells have been modified from their original state as they adapted to

tissue culture. Even those cell lines that have been studied extensively and are well characterized do not perform ideally. The MDCK line (dog kidney) is thought of as a model for collecting duct or distal tubule epithelium and yet has some properties not normally associated with these cells. Furthermore, these cells may be tumorigenic in the nude mouse. The pig kidney cell line LLC-PK$_1$ does not behave under all circumstances as a proximal tubule cell line, which it is thought to represent, although it does retain some characteristics. For example, sodium-dependent glucose transport occurs, but certain amino acid transport functions appear to be absent (84). In addition, the LLC-PK$_1$ cell line shows a considerable biochemical response to vasopressin, a substance normally thought to exert its physiological effect on distal or collecting duct cells (91).

Primary cultures also have been used, and they often overcome some of the difficulties associated with the long-term cell lines. Often the exact cells of origin are not known in these studies as well, but at least the region of the nephron involved can be established easily, i.e., proximal tubule. In some studies, precise dissection of specific nephron segments has been undertaken and the cells explanted for further studies. Obviously these experiments are technically more complex than simple tissue culture studies.

Several studies have been undertaken to study chemical effects on renal tissue culture cells and have been summarized by Wilson (99). Various drugs, metabolic inhibitors, and metals have been examined in an attempt to better understand specific mechanisms of cell injury. A wide variety of metabolic and membrane perturbations have been reported, although how the effects related directly to the production of nephrotoxicity is unclear. It is equally unclear if the effects observed on tissue culture cells explain target organ selectivity of some nephrotoxic compounds. For example, mercuric chloride is known to damage a variety of cells, and the selectivity of this metal for the kidney *in vivo* is not seen in tissue culture studies.

Several studies have been undertaken to examine the role of calcium in cell injury; they also are summarized by Wilson (99). After anoxic damage, return of oxygen and substrates led to extensive cell damage that was prevented partially by removing calcium from the culture medium. Calcium channel blockers had a qualitatively similar effect. Enhanced toxicity was not observed, however, by agents that enhanced calcium entry into the cells. These and similar studies may give insights into mechanisms of cell injury.

The use of renal cells in culture holds promise for the future. Because of the technical problems associated with tissue culture, specialized laboratories are essential. Furthermore, the dominant issue of target organ selectivity must be addressed if the events of nephrotoxicity are to be understood. Finally, procedures must be developed to permit specific cell types to retain the well-recognized functions characteristic of a renal cell. Mechanistic studies with cells in culture cannot be achieved if the cells do not behave as renal tubule cells.

Isolated Membrane Vesicles

There has been an increase in the use of isolated membrane preparations for transport studies. Various techniques have been used to isolate these membranes, and in general the transport assays depend on the ability of the isolated membrane to separate two aqueous solutions. Obviously, these techniques are directed at understanding specific membrane functions rather than overall cellular transport processes. Presumably these membrane translocations involve the interactions of a particular solute with the membrane matrix that results in the movement of that substrate from one side of the membrane to the other. The movement may resemble simple diffusion, facilitated diffusion, coupled transport, or possibly some other process. The issue of the energetics of these systems is different from that in most transport studies. For the most part, the movement of a substrate depends on chemical energy supplied to the system or osmotic energy developed to fuel the transport process. Hence the usual concern for "active transport" becomes less clear-cut in this situation, as there are no cell energy-forming mechanisms associated with the membrane preparation. A detailed evaluation of this procedure with projections for the future was reported by Hopfer (65) in 1978. An examination of that assessment compared to the state of the art today is revealing.

A variety of techniques have been developed to facilitate preparation of renal membranes. Although initially the greatest effort was expended in the isolation of brush border or luminal membranes in pure form, this step is no longer a concern. These techniques have permitted the study of membrane function on both sides of the proximal tubular cell, for example, and it has been possible to note unquestionable distinctions between the transport characteristics of these two membrane types isolated from the same cell.

First attempts involved density gradient centrifugation techniques (54,68,69,81,98,102). Although useful, these techniques were far from ideal and did not allow a "clean" separation of brush border and basolateral membranes. Techniques by Sacktor and his group (34) perfected the isolation of brush border membranes but did not focus on basolateral membranes. Free flow electrophoresis (59) was demonstrated to have great utility in the separation of the two membrane types. This separation was based on the observation that the two membranes had a greater charge discrepancy than density discrepancy, but the utility of this technique is greatly limited by the cost of the apparatus and relatively small yield of membranes. Finally, Kinsella et al. (70) modified previously known cation precipitation techniques for a more efficient separation of basolateral and luminal membranes. This procedure, coupled with density gradient separation, has successfully isolated both types of membrane. However, this procedure has the limitation of requiring many hours to complete the separation. Boumendil-Podevin and Podevin (42) reported a technique of density gradient separation of both membrane types on a Percoll gradient. This procedure can be accomplished in a matter of 4 to 5 hr.

The vesicle system has a number of advantages over intact cells and renal slices. The absence of metabolism is important for the study of many compounds. For example, glucose transport is difficult to study in renal slices because of metabolism of the transport substrate itself. However, with the membrane preparation where metabolism has been eliminated, specific membrane transport functions are studied easily. Control over the composition of the aqueous bathing solution is maximized with the membrane preparation. It also is possible to establish artificial ion gradients in the membrane preparations for studying the movement of organic substances as well as the inorganic ions themselves. The heterogeneity of the membrane preparations is a distinct disadvantage. Even with the best separation techniques, contamination of basolateral with luminal, and luminal with basolateral, membranes, is unavoidable. Because there is heterogeneity of membranes in these preparations, absolutely precise quantitative data relating to flux measurements may be incorrect. However, general qualitative assessments are unquestionably valid. For example, sodium-driven glucose movement occurs in luminal membranes, not with basolateral membranes; and the major transport for PAH occurs in the basolateral membranes. Concern must be expressed as well about the orientation of the membranes. In every preparation some vesicles are "right side out" and some "inside out." Care must be taken to establish the extent of "right-sidedness" of the vesicles with each procedure.

To date, most of the efforts with isolated membrane preparations have dealt with the electrolyte-driven transport of organic substances, e.g., amino acids and glucose. Some studies with PAH, NMN, and other substances have been undertaken (64,71). Most striking is the absence of many studies, to date, on the effects of toxicologically important compounds on renal membrane transport. Clearly, preparations of this sort have great utility for determining whether a toxicologically important substance has actions directly on membrane function as opposed to cellular metabolism, for example. Metabolism as a factor is eliminated with these preparations, and any effects that might be noted must be related to the specific membrane transport process. It is likely that this technique will have greater utility for the fundamental understanding of basic physiological renal parameters than those related to toxicology. Nonetheless, it is important that specific membrane events related to toxicology be examined, and this technique offers that possibility.

SUMMARY

The kidney is a complicated organ. The functional unit of the kidney, the nephron, is in reality a series of functional units. This complexity of renal anatomy is amplified by physiological and biochemical studies. The importance of these observations to renal toxicological evaluations is that there is no single technique or procedure that allows an investigator to assess renal toxicity. A battery of renal tests is necessary to provide evidence of the existence of nephrotoxicity, although a standard screening procedure can be established to develop preliminary evidence. Such whole animal screening procedures are best undertaken with small animals and with a balance-study format.

Detailed clearance procedures on whole animals (conscious or anesthetized) can yield specific data about the time course of nephrotoxicity, glomerular versus tubular involvement, reversibility of the insult, and other processes. Experiments with anesthetized animals offer greater control and precision than those on conscious animals. On the other hand, studies conducted with metabolism cages offer greater flexibility. In either situation, however, the possibility of glomerular

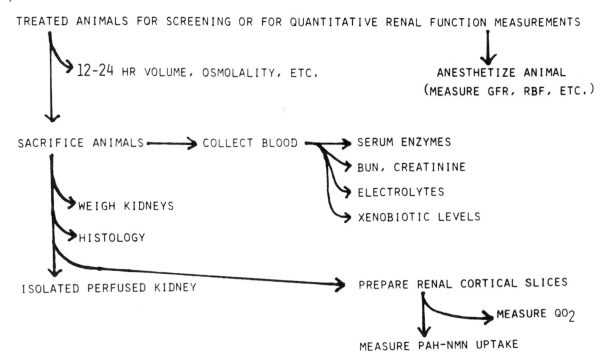

FIG. 8. Flow chart for *in vivo* and *in vitro* protocols for assessing effects of potential nephrotoxins on renal function.

and/or tubular involvement can be assessed. All of the techniques utilized in these studies are standard and readily learned by the novice.

Micropuncture procedures are powerful (potentially) tests for the analysis of nephrotoxicity. However, the cost and sophistication of these procedures precludes routine use as a screening technique. Micropuncture cannot be used by the novice.

Studies with isolated tissues are most useful for evaluating mechanisms and sites of action. Such studies eliminate problems with renal blood flow, systemic effects of toxins, etc. Although some investigators argue that *in vitro* procedures bear no relation to what occurs *in vivo,* this view is not shared by all. Renal slice studies are simple and easily learned. Isolated perfused tubule techniques are complicated and much more difficult to master but clearly resemble the *in vivo* situation more closely. Renal cells in culture hold promise for the future. The techniques are complex, and many technical problems exist; but this approach may become ideal for an understanding of mechanisms of action. Isolated cell membranes are useful for studies on membrane mechanisms free of cellular influences, e.g., energy production.

Overall, it is best first to apply a whole animal screening procedure (Fig. 8). This method allows a description of the time course of nephrotoxicity and its general characteristics. Subsequent studies with anesthetized animals allow more precise description of quantitative effects on renal function. Finally, studies with slices, tubules, isolated perfused kidney, or isolated membranes possibly permit an assessment of mechanisms and specific sites of action. This generalized approach, depicted in Fig. 8, offers an opportunity to acquire both *in vivo* and *in vitro* data from the same experimental protocol. If experiments are planned sequentially, whole an-

imal responses to nephrotoxins can be assessed first, followed by renal slice, isolated membrane experiments, etc. to investigate specific transport functions. In addition, any of the several *in vitro* or *in vivo* procedures can be used for various biochemical assessments. For example, involvement of nonprotein sulfhydryl groups (primarily glutathione), effects of toxins on specific enzymes, and so on involves procedures that are not unique to renal toxicology. Any of these analyses can be applied to studies of mechanisms of toxin action in the kidney.

REFERENCES

Monographs, Reviews, and Texts

1. Berndt, W. O. (1976): Renal function tests: what do they mean? A review of renal anatomy, biochemistry, and physiology. *Environ. Health Perspect.,* 15:55–71.
2. Berndt, W. O. (1976): Use of the tissue slice technique for evaluation of renal transport processes. *Environ. Health Perspect.,* 15:73–88.
3. Brenner, B., and Rector, F. (1986): *The Kidney,* 3rd edition. Saunders, Philadelphia.
3a. Brenner, B. M., and Lazarus, J. M. (1983): *Acute Renal Failure.* Saunders, Philadelphia.
4. Burg, M. B., and Orloff, J. (1973): Perfusion of isolated renal tubules. In: *Handbook of Physiology, Sect. 8: Renal Physiology,* Chap. 7, edited by J. Orloff and R. W. Berliner. American Physiological Society, Washington, D. C.
5. Cohen, J. J., and Kamm, D. E. (1976): Renal metabolism: relative to renal function. In: *The Kidney,* Vol. 1, Chap. 4, edited by B. M. Brenner and C. F. Rector. Saunders, Philadelphia.
6. Fine, L. G. (1986): Renal cells in culture. *Miner. Electrolyte Metab.,* 12:1–84.
7. Goodman, L. S., and Gilman, A., editors (1975): *The Pharmacological Basis of Therapeutics,* 5th ed., pp. 98–99, 109–110. Macmillan, New York.

8. Gottschalk, C. W., and Lassiter, W. E. (1973): Micropuncture methodology. In: *Handbook of Physiology, Sect. 8: Renal Physiology,* Chap. 6, edited by J. Orloff and R. W. Berliner. American Physiological Society, Washington, D. C.

9. Kleinzeller, A., Kostyuk, P. G., Kotyk, A., and Lev, A. A. (1969): Determination of intracellular ionic concentrations and activities. In: *Laboratory Techniques in Membrane Biophysics,* edited by H. Passow and R. Stampfli, pp. 69–84. Springer-Verlag, New York.

10. Magos, L., and Clarkson, T. W. (1977): Renal injury and urinary excretion. In: *Handbook of Physiology, Sect. 9: Reactions to Environmental Chemicals,* Chap. 17, edited by D. H. K. Lee. American Physiological Society, Bethesda.

11. Orloff, J., and Berliner, R. W. (1973): *Handbook of Physiology, Sect. 8: Renal Physiology.* Williams & Wilkins, Baltimore.

12. Peters, L. (1960): Renal tubular excretion of organic bases. *Pharmacol. Rev.,* 12:1–35.

13. Pitts, R. R. (1974): *Physiology of the Kidney and Body Fluids,* Chap. 13. Year Book, Chicago.

14. Relman, A. S., and Levinsky, N. G. (1971): Clinical examination of renal function. In: *Diseases of the Kidney,* 2nd ed., edited by M. B. Strauss and L. G. Welt, pp. 87–138. Little Brown, Boston.

15. Renkin, E. M., and Gilmore, J. P. (1973): Glomerular filtration. In: *Handbook of Physiology, Sect. 8: Renal Physiology,* edited by J. Orloff and R. W. Berliner, pp. 185–248. Williams & Wilkins, Baltimore.

16. Roch-Ramel, F., and Peters, G. (1979): Micropuncture techniques as a tool in renal pharmacology. *Annu. Rev. Pharmacol. Toxicol.,* 19:323–345.

17. Ross, B. D., and Guder, W. G. (1982): Heterogeneity and compartmentation in the kidney. In: *Metabolic Compartmentation,* edited by H. Sies, pp. 363–409. Academic Press, New York.

18. Segal, S., and Thier, S. O. (1973): Renal handling of amino acids. In: *Handbook of Physiology, Sect. 8: Renal Physiology,* Chap. 20. American Physiological Society, Washington, D. C.

19. Seldin, D. W., and Giebisch, G. (1985): *The Kidney, Physiology and Pathophysiology.* Raven Press, New York.

20. Smith, H. (1956): *Principles of Renal Physiology.* Oxford University Press, New York.

21. Strober, W., and Waldman, T. A. (1976): The role of the kidney in the metabolism of plasma proteins. In: *Proceedings of the 6th International Congress of Nephrology,* edited by S. Giovannetti, V. Bonomini, and G. D'Amico, pp. 392–405. Karger, Basel.

22. Sullivan, L. P. (1974): *Physiology of the Kidney.* Lea & Febiger, Philadelphia.

23. Tisher, C. C. (1976): Anatomy of the kidney. In: *The Kidney,* Vol. 1, edited by B. M. Brenner and F. C. Rector, Chap. 1. Saunders, Philadelphia.

24. Tisher, C. C., Giebisch, G. H., and Purcell, E. F. (1977): Glomerular morphology and its relationship to glomerular filtration. In: *Renal Function,* Section 1, edited by G. H. Giebisch and E. F. Purcell. Josiah Macy Jr. Foundation, New York.

25. Ullrich, K. J., and Greger, R. (1985): Approaches to the study of tubule transport functions. In: *The Kidney, Physiology and Pathophysiology,* Vol. 1, edited by D. G. Seldin and G. Geibisch, Chap. 20. Raven Press, New York.

26. Umbriet, W. W., Burris, R. H., and Stauffer, J. F. (1972): *Mamometric and Biochemical Techniques,* 5th ed., pp. 146–147. Burgess, Minneapolis.

27. Valtin, H. (1973): *Renal Function: Mechanisms Preserving Fluid and Solute Balance in Health.* Little Brown, Boston.

28. Valtin, H. (1979): *Renal Dysfunction: Mechanisms Involved in Fluid and Solute Imbalance.* Little Brown, Boston.

29. Weiner, I. M. (1973): Transport of weak acids and bases. In: *Handbook of Physiology, Sect. 8: Renal Physiology,* edited by J. Orloff and R. W. Berliner, pp. 415–502. Williams & Wilkins, Baltimore.

Research Articles

30. Acara, M., Roch-Ramel, F., and Rennick, B. (1979): Bidirectional renal tubular transport of free choline: a micropuncture study. *Am. J. Physiol.,* 236:F112–F118.

31. Bank, N., Mutz, E. F., and Aynedjian, H. S. (1967): The role of

32. Baylis, R., Rennke, H. R., and Brenner, B. M. (1977): Mechanisms of the defect in glomerular ultrafiltration associated with gentamicin administration. *Kidney Int.,* 12:344–353.

33. Beale, R. N., and Croft, D. N. (1961): A sensitive method for the colorimetric determination of urea. *J. Clin. Pathol.,* 14:418–424.

34. Beck, J. C., and Sacktor, B. (1978): The sodium electrochemical potential-mediated uphill transport of D-glucose in renal brush border membrane vesicles. *J. Biol. Chem.,* 253:5531–5535.

35. Berger, S. J., and Sacktor, B. (1970): Isolation and biochemical characterization of brush borders from rabbit kidneys. *J. Cell Biol.,* 47:637–645.

36. Berndt, W. O. (1975): The effect of potassium dichromate on renal tubular transport processes. *Toxicol. Appl. Pharmacol.,* 32:40–52.

37. Berndt, W. O. (1977): A further characterization of cytembena-induced nephrotoxicity. *Toxicol. Appl. Pharmacol.,* 39:207–217.

38. Berndt, W. O., and Grote, D. (1968): The accumulation of C^{14}-dinitrophenol by slices of rabbit kidney cortex. *J. Pharmacol. Exp. Ther.,* 164:223–231.

39. Berndt, W. O., and Hayes, A. W. (1977): Effects of citrinin on renal tubular transport functions in the rat. *J. Environ. Pathol. Toxicol.,* 1:93–103.

40. Biber, T. U. L., Mylle, M., Baines, A. D., and Gottschalk, C. W. (1968): A study by micropuncture and microdissection of acute renal failure in rats. *Am. J. Med.,* 44:664–705.

41. Blantz, R. C., and Pelayo, J. C. (1983): In vivo actions of angiotensin II on glomerular function. *Fed. Proc.,* 42:3071–3074.

42. Boumendil-Podevin, E. F., and Podevin, R. A. (1983): Isolation of basolateral and brush-border membranes from the rabbit kidney cortex. *Biochim. Biophys. Acta,* 735:86–94.

43. Bratton, A. C., and Marshall, E. K. (1939): A new coupling component for sulfanilamide determination. *J. Biol. Chem.,* 128:537–550.

44. Brenner, B. M., Hostetler, T. H., and Humes, H. D. (1978): Glomerular permselectivity; barrier function based on discrimination of molecular size and change. *Am. J. Physiol.,* 234:F455–F460.

45. Burg, M., and Green, N. (1973): Function of the thick ascending limb of Henle's loop. *Am. J. Physiol.,* 224:659–668.

46. Burg, M., Stoner, L., Cardinal, J., and Green, N. (1973): Furosemide effect on isolated perfused tubules. *Am. J. Physiol.,* 225:119–145.

47. Carone, F. A., Peterson, D. R., Oparil, S., and Pullman, T. N. (1979): Renal tubular transport and catabolism of proteins and peptides. *Kidney Int.,* 16:279–289.

48. Cooke, W. J. (1976): Small inexpensive anesthetic apparatus for rats. *J. Appl. Physiol.,* 41:429–430.

49. Cross, R. J., and Taggart, J. V. (1950): Renal tubular transport: Accumulation of p-aminohippurate by rabbit kidney slices. *Am. J. Physiol.,* 161:181–190.

50. Curthoys, N. P., and Lowry, O. H. (1973): The distribution of glutaminase isoenzymes in the various structures of the nephron in normal, acidotic and alkalotic rat kidney. *J. Biol. Chem.,* 248:162–168.

51. Curthoys, N. P., and Kuhlenschmidt, T. (1975): Phosphate-independent glutaminase from rat kidney: partial purification and identity with γ-glutamyl-transpeptidase. *J. Biol. Chem.,* 250:2099–2105.

52. Dees, J. H., Coe, L. D., Yasukochi, Y., and Masters, B. S. (1980): Immunofluorescence of NADPH-cytochrome C (-P450) reductase in rat and minipig tissues injected with phenobarbital. *Science,* 208:1473–1475.

53. Dicker, S. E., and Heller, H. (1945): The mechanisms of water diuresis in normal rats and rabbits analyzed by inulin and diodone clearances. *J. Physiol. (Lond.),* 103:449–460.

54. Ebel, H., Aulbert, E., and Merker, H. J. (1976): Isolation of the basal and lateral plasma membranes of rat kidney tubule cells. *Biochim. Biophys. Acta,* 443:531–546.

55. Ecker, J. L., and Hook, J. B. (1973): Accumulation of organic acids by isolated renal tubules from newborn rabbits. *Pharmacologist,* 15:187.

56. Ecker, J. L., and Hook, J. B. (1974): Analysis of factors influencing the in vitro developmental pattern of p-aminohippurate transport by rabbit kidney. *Biochim. Biophys. Acta,* 339:210–217.

57. Fowler, B. A., Hook, G. E. R., and Lucier, G. W. (1977): Tetra-

chlorodibenzo-p-dioxin induction of renal microsomal enzyme systems: ultrastructural effects on pars recta (S3) proximal tubule cells of the rat kidney. *J. Pharmacol. Exp. Ther.,* 203:712–721.

58. Gertz, K. H., Braun-Schubert, G., and Brandis, M. (1969): Methode der Messung der Filtrationsrate einzelner nohe der Nierenoberflache gelegener Glomeruli. *Arch. Ges. Physiol.,* 310:109–115.

59. Heidrick, H. G., Kinne, R., Kinne-Saffran, E., and Hanning, K. (1972): The polarity of the proximal tubule cell in rat kidney: different surface charges for the brush border microvilli and plasma membrane from the basal infoldings. *J. Cell Biol.,* 154:232–245.

60. Hirsch, G. H. (1973): Differential effects of nephrotoxic agents on renal organic ion transport and metabolism. *J. Pharmacol. Exp. Ther.,* 186:593–599.

61. Hirsch, G. H., and Hook, J. B. (1969): Maturation of renal organic acid transport: substrate stimulation by penicillin. *Science,* 165:909–910.

62. Hirsch, G. H., and Hook, J. B. (1970): Maturation of renal organic acid transport: substrate stimulation by penicillin and p-aminohippurate (PAH). *J. Pharmacol. Exp. Ther.,* 171:103–108.

63. Hirsch, G. H., and Hook, J. B. (1970): Stimulation of renal organic acid transport and protein synthesis by penicillin. *J. Pharmacol. Exp. Ther.,* 174:152–158.

64. Holohan, P. D., Pessah, N. I., Pessah, I. N., and Ross, C. R. (1979): Reconstitution of N'-methylnicotinamide and p-aminohippuric acid transport in phospholipid vesicles with a protein fraction isolated from dog kidney membranes. *Mol. Pharmacol.,* 16:343–356.

65. Hopfer, U. (1978): Transport in isolated membranes. *Am. J. Physiol.,* 234:F89–F96.

66. Horster, M., and Valtin, H. (1971): Postnatal development of renal function: micropuncture and clearance studies in the dog. *J. Clin. Invest.,* 50:779–795.

67. Horster, M., Kemler, B. J., and Valtin, H. (1971): Intracortical distribution of number and volume of glomeruli during postnatal maturation in the dog. *J. Clin. Invest.,* 50:796–800.

68. Kinne, R., Murer, H., Kinne-Saffran, E., Thees, M., and Sacks, G. (1975): Sugar transport by renal plasma membrane vesicles: characterization of the system in the brush border microvilli and basal-lateral plasma membranes. *J. Membr. Biol.,* 21:375–395.

69. Kinne, R., Schmitz, J.-E., and Kinne-Saffran, E. (1971): The localization of the Na$^+$-K$^+$-ATPase in the cells of rat kidney cortex: a study on isolated plasma membranes. *Pflugers Arch.,* 329:191–206.

70. Kinsella, J. L., Holohan, P. D., Pessah, N. I., and Ross, C. R. (1969): Isolation of luminal and antiluminal membranes from dog kidney cortex. *Biochim. Biophys. Acta,* 552:468–477.

71. Kinsella, J. L., Holohan, P. D., Pessah, N. I., and Ross, C. R. (1979): Transport of organic ions in renal cortical luminal and antiluminal membrane vesicles. *J. Pharmacol. Exp. Ther.,* 209:443–450.

72. Kramp, R. A., MacDowell, M., Gottschalk, C. W., and Oliver, J. R. (1974): A study in microdissection and micropuncture of the structure and the function of kidneys and the nephrons of rats with chronic renal disease. *Kidney Int.,* 5:147–176.

73. Kreisberg, J. I. (1983): Contractile properties of the glomerular mesangium. *Fed. Proc.,* 42:3053–3057.

74. Maack, T., Johnson, V., Kau, S. T., Figueinedo, J., and Sigulem, D. (1979): Renal filtration, transport, and metabolism of low-molecular-weight proteins: a review. *Kidney Int.,* 16:271–278.

75. Malvin, R. L., Wilde, W. S., and Sullivan, L. P. (1958): Localization of nephron transport by stopflow analysis. *Am. J. Physiol.,* 194:135–142.

76. McKinney, T. D., and Speeg, K. V., Jr. (1982): Cimetidine and procainamide secretion by proximal tubules in vitro. *Am. J. Physiol.,* 242:F672–F680.

77. McKinney, T. D., Myers, P., and Speeg, K. V., Jr. (1981): Cimetidine secretion by rabbit renal tubules in vitro. *Am. J. Physiol.,* 241:F69–F76.

78. McMenamy, R. H. (1968): Binding studies by dialysis equilibrium: a description of an accurate and rapid technique. *Anal. Biochem.,* 23:122–128.

79. Mudge, G. H., and Taggart, J. V. (1950): Effect of acetate on renal excretion of p-aminohippurate in the dog. *Am. J. Physiol.,* 161:191–197.

80. Mudge, G. H., and Taggart, J. V. (1950): Effect of 2,4-dinitrophenol on renal transport mechanisms in the dog. *Am. J. Physiol.,* 161:173–180.

81. Murer, H., Ammann, E., Biber, J., and Hopfer, U. (1976): The surface membrane of the small intestinal epithelial cell. I. Localization of adenyl cyclase. *Biochim. Biophys. Acta,* 433:509–519.

82. Nomiyama, K., Yamamoto, A., and Sato, C. (1974): Assay of urinary enzymes in toxic nephropathy. *Toxicol. Appl. Pharmacol.,* 27:484–490.

83. Plaa, G., and Larsen, R. E. (1965): Relative nephrotoxic properties of chlorinated methane, ethane, and ethylene derivatives in mice. *Toxicol. Appl. Pharmacol.,* 7:37–44.

84. Rabito, C. A. (1986): Sodium cotransport processes in renal epithelial cell lines. *Miner. Electrolyte Metab.,* 12:32–42.

85. Rennick, B. R. (1969): Development of renal accumulation of organic ions by chick embryo. *Am. J. Physiol.,* 217:247–250.

86. Rennick, B. R., Hamilton, B., and Evans, R. (1961): Development of renal tubular transports of TEA and PAH in the puppy and piglet. *Am. J. Physiol.,* 201:743–746.

87. Richards, A. N. (1929): Direct observations of change in function of the renal tubule caused by certain poisons. *Trans. Assoc. Am. Physicians,* 44:64–73.

88. Rocha, A. S., and Kokko, J. P. (1973): Sodium and water transport in the medullary thick ascending limb of Henle: evidence for active chloride transport. *J. Clin. Invest.,* 52:612–623.

89. Ross, C. R., Pessah, N. I., and Farah, A. (1968): Inhibitory effects of β-haloalkylamines on the renal transport of NMN. *J. Pharmacol. Exp. Ther.,* 160:375–384.

90. Schor, N., Ichikawa, I., Rennke, H. R., Troy, J. L., and Brenner, B. M. (1981): Pathophysiology of altered glomerular function in aminoglycoside-treated rats. *Kidney Int.,* 19:288–296.

91. Skorecki, K. L., Verkman, A. S., and Ausiello, D. A. (1986): Vasopressin receptor-adenylate cyclase interactions: studies in intact cultured renal epithelial cell line (LLC-PK$_1$). *Miner. Electrolyte Metab.,* 12:64–71.

92. Stitzer, S. A., and Martinez-Meldonado, M. (1978): Clearance methods in the rat. In: *Methods in Pharmacology,* Vol. 4B, edited by M. Martinez-Maldonado, pp. 23–40. Plenum Press, New York.

93. Stroo, W. E., and Hook, J. B. (1977): Enzymes of renal origin in urine as indicators of nephrotoxicity. *Toxicol. Appl. Pharmacol.,* 39:423–434.

94. Toribara, T. X., Terepka, A. R., and Dewey, A. A. (1957): The ultrafilterable calcium of human serum. I. Ultrafiltration methods of normal values. *J. Clin. Invest.,* 36:738–748.

95. Tune, B. M., Burg, M. B., and Patlak, C. S. (1969): Characteristics of p-aminohippurate transport in proximal renal tubules. *Am. J. Physiol.,* 217:1057–1063.

96. Walker, L. A., Buscemi-Bergin, M., and Gellai, M. (1983): Renal hemodynamics in conscious rats: effects of anesthesia, surgery and recovery. *Am. J. Physiol.,* 245:F67–F74.

97. Weiner, I. M. (1979): Urate transport in the nephron. *Am. J. Physiol.,* 237:F85–F92.

98. Wilfong, R. F., and Neville, D. M. (1970): The isolation of the brush border membrane fraction from rat kidney. *J. Biol. Chem.,* 245:6106–6112.

99. Wilson, P. D. (1986): Use of cultured renal tubular cells in the study of cell injury. *Miner. Electrolyte Metab.,* 12:71–84.

100. Wright, F. S., and Giebisch, G. (1976): Renal potassium transport: contributions of individual nephron segments and populations. *Am. J. Physiol.,* 235:F515–F527.

101. Yarger, W. E., Boyd, M. E., and Schrader, N. W. (1978): Evaluation of methods of measuring glomerular and nutrient blood flow in rat kidneys. *Am. J. Physiol.,* 235:H592–H600.

102. Zull, J. E., Malbon, C., and Chuang, J. (1977): Binding of tritiated bovine parathyroid hormone to plasma membrane from bovine kidney cortex. *J. Biol. Chem.,* 252:1071–1078.

Principles and Methods of Toxicology, Second Edition, edited by A. Wallace Hayes, Raven Press, Ltd., New York © 1989.

CHAPTER 22

Endomyocardial Biopsy Approach to Drug-Related Heart Disease

John J. Fenoglio Jr. and *Bernard M. Wagner

*Department of Pathology, Columbia University College of Physicians and Surgeons, New York, New York 10032, and *Office of the Director, Nathan Kline Research Institute, Orangeburg, New York 10962*

The dream of being able to biopsy the heart with the same ease that other organs are biopsied has fascinated cardiologists and to some extent pathologists, and numerous approaches have been attempted. Open cardiac biopsy has been feasible, but this technique is not applicable as a routine diagnostic procedure. Techniques for closed cardiac biopsy were developed in a canine model during the late 1950s and were subsequently applied in man (38,42). Initially a transthoracic approach was used, and a variety of biopsy needles were developed. There were several major drawbacks of these techniques, the most serious of which were the high mortality and morbidity rates reported from several large centers (40,45). Refinements in the biopsy needle and the technique minimized the risk of cardiac perforation; however, the initial reports of the high rate of complications doomed transthoracic cardiac biopsy, at least in the United States. In other countries, especially Brazil, transthorax cardiac biopsy was developed and used as a diagnostic tool, most successfully in the diagnosis of Chagas' disease.

By 1970 cardiac biopsy had been abandoned in the United States as a diagnostic procedure. Meanwhile, in Japan a new technique for endomyocardial biopsy was being widely used (39). The technique employed a biopsy forceps with which biopsy samples could be obtained from the endocardial surface of the right or left ventricle. The biopsy was done during cardiac catheterization under fluoroscopy and was relatively easy to perform. The Konno-Sakakibara bioptome was developed in 1962, and by 1971 the Japanese workers had biopsied more than 460 patients without serious complications (29). Despite the proved safety and success of this technique in Japan, it did not gain widespread acceptance.

In 1972 a modified Konno bioptome was developed at the Stanford University Medical Center as a diagnostic tool to monitor cardiac rejection in the cardiac transplantation program at that institution (11,12). The Caves-Schultz-Stanford bioptome provided a simple, safe technique for repeated performance of biopsies of the right ventricular septum. This bioptome was more flexible than the original Konno bioptome and could be introduced into the right internal jugular vein percutaneously under local anesthesia. Since its introduction the Caves-Schultz bioptome has proved a safe, reliable instrument (Fig. 1).

Today there is widespread and ever-increasing use of this technique (3,36,46). Numerous reports have clearly demonstrated the utility of biopsy in the diagnosis of restrictive cardiac disease, secondary cardiomyopathies, and myocarditis, and the technique has become an established diagnostic tool in the diagnosis of cardiac rejection and cardiotoxicity secondary to the anthracycline-derived chemotherapeutic agents. Although the biopsy technique has not been widely applied to the diagnosis of other forms of drug-related heart disease, the possible importance of the biopsy in the diagnosis of hypersensitivity myocarditis and toxic myocarditis has not escaped the notice of cardiologists and pathologists.

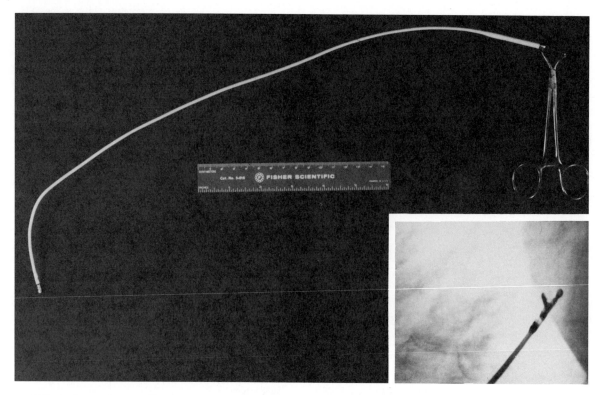

FIG. 1. Caves-Schultz-Stanford bioptome. **Inset:** The bioptome, under fluoroscopy, is positioned against the right side of the ventricular septum. The jaws of the bioptome are opened, and the bioptome is advanced to the septum. The jaws are then closed, evulsing a fragment of myocardium.

TECHNICAL CONSIDERATIONS

Proper handling and fixation of the biopsy specimen is crucial in order to obtain meaningful and reliable information. Excess handling of the specimen should be avoided and the tissue fragments fixed as rapidly as possible. It is convenient to fix all biopsy specimens in the cardiac catheterization laboratory at the time of biopsy. The biopsy specimen is removed from the bioptome with a sterile applicator, the end of a fine sterile forceps, or a sterile needle and immediately placed in fixative. Care must be used not to grasp the tissue fragment with forceps in order to avoid crush artifacts. Dividing the tissue fragments, even with a single stroke of a sharp blade, causes artifacts. Because the biopsy specimens are small, usually 2 to 3 mm², the specimens are best fixed in their entirety. Slightly larger tissue fragments, up to 4 mm², can be obtained from the right side of the ventricular septum with the Caves-Schultz-Stanford bioptome. Even with these larger tissue fragments, fixation is rapid and complete without dividing the tissue. Left ventricular biopsies are, as a rule, smaller than right ventricular biopsies and are also fixed in their entirety.

Because the biopsy specimens are small, it is recommended that a minimum of four samples be obtained at the time of the procedure. The utilization of the biopsy samples depends on the clinical indications for biopsy; i.e., in suspected cases of myocarditis or for monitoring transplant rejection, a minimum of three and preferably four samples should be examined histologically.

Fixation

Fixation with 2.5% phosphate-buffered (pH 7.35) glutaraldehyde is ideal for both light and electron microscopy. The biopsy specimen for light microscopy can also be fixed in 10% neutral buffered formaldehyde, which is the fixative of choice if immunoperoxidase stains are called for. Fixation is rapid with both fixatives because of the small size of the specimens. Fixation is done at room temperature rather than in chilled fixative, with either glutaraldehyde or formaldehyde, to minimize contraction artifacts. Other fixatives for both light and electron microscopy can be used with good results. We have used Bouin's fixative for light microscopy and 2.5% glutaraldehyde in 2% paraformaldehyde for electron microscopy.

The biopsy specimen for immunofluorescence or histochemistry is snap-frozen in isopentane and Dry Ice. It can be accomplished easily by placing the specimen in a large plastic Beem capsule filled with holding medium. Hank's solution can be used as the holding and embedding medium for frozen tissue specimens. The lid of the capsule is closed, and the whole capsule is immersed in the isopentane and Dry Ice mixture. The specimen can be stored indefinitely in the capsule at −70°C. Beem capsules of the type used for tissue embedding in electron microscopy are most convenient. This method is convenient and can be done easily in the catheterization laboratory immediately after the biopsy specimen is taken, or the tissue may be transported in Hank's solution to the pathology laboratory. The tissue can be readily retrieved by slicing the frozen capsule and mounting the frozen tissue in the medium directly on the cryostat chuck. Other methods of snap-freezing are equally acceptable, and liquid nitrogen can be used instead of isopentane and Dry Ice.

If needed, the frozen tissue can easily be retrieved for routine histology. The process of freezing and thawing, however, introduces additional artifacts of which the pathologist must be aware. Most importantly, there is extensive interstitial edema and separation of muscle fibers in specimens fixed for routine histology following snap-freezing. We have found 10% neutral buffered formaldehyde to be the best fixative in this situation. The frozen tissue is also useful for frozen sections for routine histology. This approach may be used in suspected cases of lipidosis or glycogen storage disease. In instances where rapid diagnosis is imperative, as in suspected cases of acute cardiac rejection following cardiac transplantation, sections can be prepared from the snap-frozen tissue without sacrificing the specimen for routine histology.

Histology

The biopsy specimen is processed in the routine manner following initial fixation. After paraffin embedding, sections are cut at 4-μm thickness. The entire block is ribboned and the ribbons of sections mounted so that each slide contains three to four sections. All sections are mounted. Three slides of sections from three depths in the block are routinely stained. An additional slide, preferably from the middle of the block, is routinely stained with Masson's trichrome. The remaining slides of sections are saved, unstained, for possible additional stains in selected cases or later use.

Three levels with multiple sections are routinely examined to minimize bias due to (a) the lack of orientation of the specimen prior to embedding and (b) the small specimen size. Because it is impossible to orient the biopsy, any single section may include only the endocardium or subendocardium and assessment of the degree of fibrosis or the myocardium is thus impossible. Because many disease processes are focal in nature, although the heart is diffusely involved, the entire biopsy specimen must be sampled. A connective tissue stain is essential for evaluating the degree of fibrosis in the biopsy specimen as well as for defining the vasculature. In our experience, Masson's trichrome or the Movat pentachrome stain are most helpful and most reliable.

Electron Microscopy

The biopsy specimen for electron microscopy is divided into three or four small blocks with a sharp blade after initial fixation. The small blocks are then returned to 2.5% glutaraldehyde and fixed for 4 hr or overnight. After fixation the tissue is rinsed in phosphate buffer and postfixed in 1.5% phosphate-buffered (pH 7.35) osmium tetroxide for 1 hr. The tissue is then dehydrated and embedded by any of a number of well-established procedures.

Tissue from every biopsy is collected for electron microscopy and processed to this point. In our laboratory electron microscopy is important for diagnostic purposes in approximately 20% of biopsies. Electron microscopy is done on all

cases in which a diagnosis cannot be established by light microscopy, in cases of suspected cardiotoxicity, and in cases of suspected small vessel disease. Specimens for these cases are processed immediately. In the remaining cases, the embedded blocks are stored for possible future use.

BIOPSY INTERPRETATION

The endomyocardial biopsy represents a small fragment of well-preserved myocardium, rather than the large section of autolyzed myocardium the pathologist is accustomed to evaluating. It requires that pathologists reorient their approach and view the endomyocardial biopsy in a manner similar to a liver or kidney biopsy. Diagnostic information can be derived from an appraisal of individual constituents of the endomyocardial biopsy. Individual cell morphology, interstitial tissue, and small vessels can be evaluated in biopsy specimens (Fig. 2). Even with careful handling of the biopsy specimen, however, there are several artifacts of which the pathologist must be aware when evaluating the endomyocardial biopsy. Contraction bands are frequent in endomyocardial biopsy specimens by both light and electron microscopy (Fig. 3). These contracted bands are an artifact of the procedure and cannot be used as evidence of myocardial ischemia. The most effective means of reducing contraction band formation is to fix the specimens at room temperature rather than in chilled fixative. This measure does not completely eliminate contraction band formation, however, so the pathologist must learn to "look past" the contraction bands when evaluating the biopsy.

When evaluating the biopsy in any patient who has had a previous endomyocardial biopsy, the pathologist must always

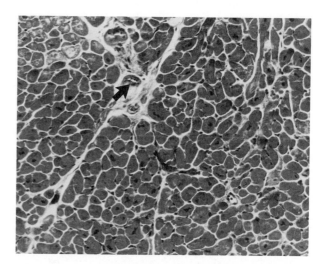

FIG. 2. Biopsy procedure yields a sample approximately 2 to 3 mm³. This sample is adequate to assess all myocardial components. In the normal right ventricle the myocardial cells are uniform in size with centrally placed ovoid nuclei. The interstitial connective tissue is delicate and barely perceptible at this magnification. The myocardium is divided into fascicles by fibrous tissue septa. Small arterioles (*arrow*), capillaries, and venules are readily apparent in these fibrous septa. Hematoxylin-phloxine-sulfarin. ×136.5.

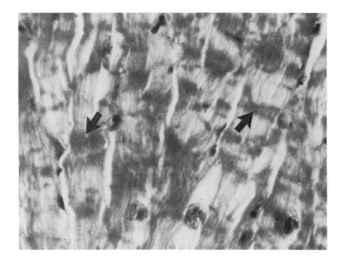

FIG. 3. Contraction bands (*arrows*) are an unavoidable artifact of the biopsy procedure. This artifact can be minimized but not eliminated by placing the biopsies in fixatives kept at room temperature rather than in cold fixative. Hematoxylin-phloxine-sulfarin. ×340.

be aware of the possibility of rebiopsying a previous biopsy site (Fig. 4). Although the possibility seems remote, in actuality it occurs frequently, probably because the bioptome is guided to the same site on the right ventricular septum by the configuration of the trabeculae. The rebiopsy specimen is then characterized by extensive granulation tissue. There is frequently an overlying mural thrombus if the biopsy was done within the previous week. A recent biopsy site is not difficult to recognize if the pathologist is aware of the possibility. Healed old biopsy sites, however, can easily be taken for extensive subendocardial fibrosis and pose a more difficult diagnostic problem. If in doubt, additional tissue (the snap-frozen specimen) is examined.

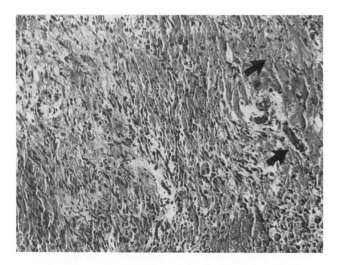

FIG. 4. Large areas of necrotic myocardial cells and granulation tissue are indicative of a previous biopsy site. Usually there is a distinct transition to normal, well-preserved myocardium (*arrows*) at the edge of the biopsy site. Hematoxylin-phloxine-sulfarin. ×96.

As with all biopsy specimens, it is helpful to examine the endomyocardial biopsy in a systematic fashion. The endocardium, myocardium, interstitial connective tissue, and vasculature are each assessed. Finally, it is important that the pathologist be fully apprised of the clinical information before establishing a final diagnosis.

DRUG-RELATED HEART DISEASE

Recognition of the structural changes associated with drug-induced disease has been hampered by the difficulty of differentiating drug-induced from naturally occurring cardiac disease (22). Our current knowledge of the morphological changes secondary to adverse drug reactions is derived primarily from individual case reports. Morphological changes are often assumed on the basis of previous reports but are rarely documented. Endomyocardial biopsy techniques will hopefully expand our knowledge of drug-induced heart disease and allow correlation between clinical findings and morphological changes.

Hypersensitivity Myocarditis

The exact incidence of hypersensitivity myocarditis is unknown, although it probably represents the most prevalent form of drug-induced heart disease. Our knowledge of this entity is based primarily on isolated case reports and clinical reviews. Clinically, the criteria for the diagnosis of drug hypersensitivity reactions are well established (33): (a) previous use of the drug without incident; (b) the hypersensitivity reaction bears no relation to the magnitude of the drug dose; (c) the reaction is neither the pharmacologic nor the toxic effect of the drug; (d) the reaction is characterized by classic allergic symptoms, symptoms of serum sickness, or syndromes suggesting infectious disease; (e) immunologic confirmation; and (f) persistence of symptoms until the drug is discontinued. The clinical diagnosis of drug-induced hypersensitivity myocarditis is made on the basis of these criteria plus signs and symptoms of cardiac disease that abate on withdrawal of the drug. It is presumed that the symptoms are secondary to drug-induced myocarditis, although the diagnosis is rarely confirmed morphologically. Without morphological confirmation it is impossible to classify these cases as drug-induced hypersensitivity myocarditis.

The morphological changes associated with hypersensitivity myocarditis were first described by French and Weller (18) in 1942 in their report of a specific myocarditis associated with sulfonamide administration (Figs. 5 and 6). Hypersensitivity myocarditis associated with drug therapy is characterized by an inflammatory infiltrate in the heart containing prominent eosinophils admixed with mononuclear cells, predominantly lymphocytes and plasma cells (16). The cellular infiltrate may be focal or diffuse and is most prominent interstitially. Focal myocytolysis is always present, although frequently sparse and obscured by the interstitial infiltrate. Foci of cellular necrosis are rarely seen. Evidence of interstitial fibrosis or replacement fibrosis is uniformly absent, and all of the lesions are similar in age and appearance. True granulomatous lesions are not a feature of hypersensitivity myo-

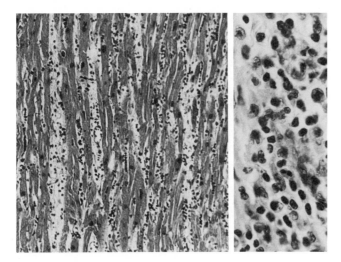

FIG. 5. Hypersensitivity myocarditis is characterized by a diffuse interstitial inflammatory infiltrate consisting of lymphocytes, macrophages, polymorphonuclear cells, and scattered eosinophils (*right panel*). The myocardial cells are separated by edema but appear intact even at this low magnification. Hematoxylin-phloxine-sulfarin. Left, ×112; right, ×380.

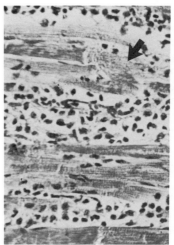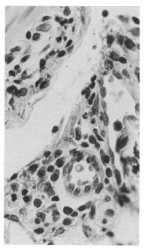

FIG. 6. **Left:** Although frank cellular necrosis is not usually a feature of hypersensitivity myocarditis, foci of myocytolysis are usually present. Myocytolysis is characterized by focal loss of myofilaments (*arrow*). **Right:** Vascular involvement is frequent in areas of extensive interstitial infiltrate. Hematoxylin-phloxine-sulfarin. Left, ×340; right, ×380.

carditis, although isolated giant cells, presumably of myocardial origin, are occasionally seen. Vascular involvement is frequent in areas of extensive interstitial infiltrates. The vascular involvement is identical to that seen in drug-related vasculitis and is characterized by a bland-appearing vasculitis involving small arteries, arterioles, and venules. Necrotizing vascular lesions are not associated with hypersensitivity myocarditis.

Drug-related hypersensitivity myocarditis is distinguished from other forms of myocarditis by the prominence of eosinophils, the absence of extensive myocardial necrosis, and the lack of replacement fibrosis. The lack of extensive necrosis or interstitial fibrosis suggests that this drug-induced disease is self-limiting. Once the offending agent is withdrawn, the myocarditis presumably resolves without residual cardiac damage. There are no reports of cardiac fibrosis or of a cardiomyopathy following drug-induced hypersensitivity myocarditis.

Numerous drugs have been implicated as the cause of hypersensitivity myocarditis (Table 1). A similar, presumably hypersensitivity myocarditis can also occur following injection of horse serum (14), tetanus toxoid (16), or smallpox vaccination (17). The pathogenesis of these myocardial lesions is still elusive. There is evidence that the allergic drug reactions to penicillin are immunologically mediated, and that a myocarditis, identical to that associated with drugs, can be produced in the rabbit by injection of rat anti-heart antiserum (25). This finding suggests that the myocarditis associated with drug therapy is a delayed hypersensitivity phenomenon.

Hypersensitivity drug reactions are not mediated through the drug but through chemically reactive metabolites (37). These metabolites, now acting as haptens, combine with endogenous macromolecules, especially protein, and it is the combination of the two molecules that is antigenic. The protein carrier is apparently able to interact with T lymphocytes,

initiating the immune response. Once T cells are activated, hapten-specific activation is produced in B lymphocytes, and anti-hapten antibodies are formed. The antigen must have multiple combining sites, permitting it to form a bridge between antibody molecules to elicit symptoms of hypersensitivity. This sequence of events permits soluble antibody molecules to react with complement and release cytoactive peptides. Bridging between cell-bound antibody molecules or antigen receptors on lymphocytes produces the change in cell membrane conformation required for mediator release or lymphocyte transformation. The requirement of multivalent haptens to initiate anti-hapten antibodies is one ex-

TABLE 1. *Drugs associated with various heart diseases*

Hypersensitivity Myocarditis

Methyldopa (34)	Streptomycin (13)
Penicillin (2)	Sulfonamides (18)
Phenindione (26)	Sulfonylureas (28)
Phenylbutazone (20)	Tetracyclines (28)

Toxic Myocarditis

Adriamycin (6)	Emetine hydrochloride (35)
Antimony compounds (21)	Fluorouracil (30)
Arsenicals (7)	Lithium carbonate (32)
Catecholamines (44)	Phenothiazines (19)
Cyclophosphamide (1)	Plasmocid (9)
Daunorubicin (1)	

Cardiomyopathy

Adriamycin (4)	Daunorubicin (10)
Amphetamine (41)	Ephedrine (47)
Arsenicals (15)	Lithium (43)
Catecholamines (endogenous) (27)	Rubidazone (3)

planation for the relative infrequency of allergic drug reactions. Most drugs and drug metabolites are univalent haptens that compete with multivalent antigens for antibody and thus inhibit the response. The organ-specific allergic reactions can also be explained by this theory. Conjugation of hapten with an organ-specific protein might produce an immunologic response with specificity for the protein as well as the haptenic group.

Toxic Myocarditis

In addition to eliciting an allergic response, drugs can cause myocardial damage by their toxic effects on the myocardial cell. The toxic effects result in cell death, which is expressed clinically as acute myocarditis or as a cardiomyopathy. The clinical expression depends on the extent of cell death and the speed with which it occurs. In this instance, drug toxicity is dose-related, and its effects are cumulative. The extent of cell damage then depends on the toxicity of the drug and the total dose administered. Cell damage also depends on drug absorption by the cell. It is the combination of these factors that determines the extent and speed of cell death. In acute myocarditis there is extensive, widespread cell death that occurs over a relatively short time—days to weeks. By contrast, in cardiomyopathy, cell death is slow, patchy, and ongoing over months.

Grossly, the heart in toxic myocarditis is not hypertrophied. The cardiac chambers are frequently dilated, and the myocardium is pale and soft. Microscopically, there is usually extensive but patchy cell death and an extensive inflammatory infiltrate. Areas of acute cell death alternate with foci of recent and healing myocardial cell damage. In areas of acute cell death, the myocardial cells are hypereosinophilic, and there is an infiltrate that is composed predominantly of

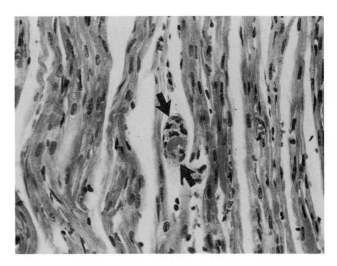

FIG. 8. Small fibrin–platelet thrombi (*arrows*) occluding an arteriole. Hematoxylin-phloxine-sulfarin. ×250.

polymorphonuclear cells. Foci of myofiber lysis, which represent areas of recent cell damage, are associated with a mixed inflammatory infiltrate consisting of lymphocytes, plasma cells, and polymorphonuclear cells. Healing areas of cell damage are characterized by proliferating fibroblasts and a sparse infiltrate of macrophages. Patchy areas of fibrosis, indicative of healed cell damage, are uncommon. Frequently, there is moderate interstitial edema and a sparse nonspecific interstitial infiltrate of lymphocytes, plasma cells, and macrophages. The endocardium and valves are usually not involved.

Toxic myocarditis is characterized by multifocal areas of cell death in various stages (Fig. 7). Although foci of recent and healing cell damage are seen, foci of acute cell death are usually predominant, and foci of fibrosis are usually not present. The inflammatory infiltrate in areas of acute cell death consists predominantly of polymorphonuclear leukocytes (Fig. 8). In areas of recent and healing myocardial damage, the inflammatory infiltrate is of mixed cell type. Eosinophils are notably absent. The lack of eosinophils and the varying stages of cell damage distinguish toxic from hypersensitivity myocarditis. The prominence of foci of acute cell death is diagnostic of toxic myocarditis. With toxic myocarditis cardiac symptoms appear suddenly, over days to weeks. Arrhythmias and electrocardiogram (ECG) abnormalities are frequent in toxic myocarditis usually in the absence of cardiomegaly.

The natural history of toxic myocarditis is not well understood. Our knowledge of this entity is derived from reports of fatal cases, which probably explains why areas of healed cell damage are not described in toxic myocarditis. It seems logical to assume, however, that ongoing cell damage would cease if the toxin or drug were withdrawn. The residuum would be focal myocardial scars, but such scarring might not be of sufficient magnitude to impair cardiac function. Focal myocardial scars are a frequent autopsy finding but are usually ascribed to subclinical ischemic heart disease.

Many drugs are suspected of being cardiotoxic. Toxic myocarditis, however, has been histologically documented for only a handful of drugs (Table 1). Digitalis and thyroid

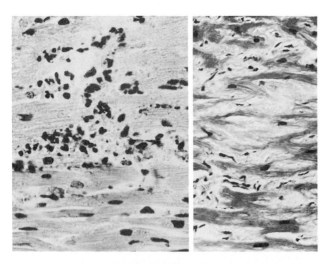

FIG. 7. Left: With toxic myocarditis the characteristic lesion is foci of acute cell death (left panel) associated with a polymorphonuclear leukocyte infiltrate. Areas of acute cell death alternate with foci of healing and healed cell damage. **Right:** Healed foci are marked by patchy areas of fibrosis that are often separate, individual myocytes. Hematoxylin-phloxine-sulfarin. Left, ×220; right, ×128.

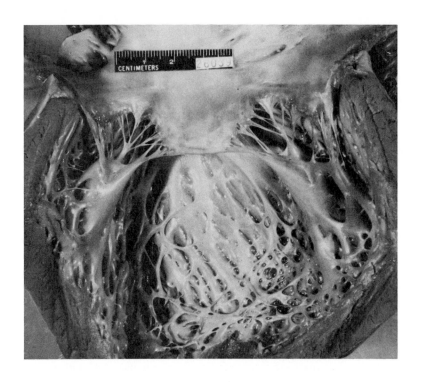

FIG. 9. With congestive cardiomyopathy, regardless of the etiology, the ventricular and atrial chambers are dilated. The heart is hypertrophied by weight, but the ventricular walls usually do not appear thickened. By definition, the cardiac valves are normal, and there is no evidence of coronary artery disease. Mural thrombi may be present in any of the cardiac chambers.

extract can produce a toxic myocarditis experimentally, but there is no evidence that these drugs produce a toxic myocarditis in man.

The mechanism of drug toxicity is varied and depends on the drug. Drugs may interfere with or inhibit cell metabolism, block or alter cell transport, or cause hemodynamic alterations that result in cell ischemia. The mechanism of drug toxicity is not clearly understood. However, the mechanisms of action and the resultant structural alterations caused by the cardiotoxic drugs emetine and cyclophosphamide are characterized in detail, and these drugs serve as models for other cardiotoxic drugs. Emetine is an inhibitor of oxidative phosphorylation (35). Structurally, its cardiotoxic effects are evidenced by mitochondrial swelling and widespread cell death. By contrast, the cardiotoxic effects of cyclophosphamide appear to be secondary to capillary endothelial damage and microthrombosis (8). Although microthrombosis is best appreciated by electron microscopy, small arterial thrombi are occasionally seen by light microscopy (Fig. 8). These microthrombi are thought to be secondary to drug-induced endothelial damage. The larger vessels are normal, and a true vasculitis is rarely present. The result is multifocal cardiac necrosis characterized structurally by extensive contraction bands, myofibrillar lysis, and electron-dense intramitochondrial inclusions—structural findings similar to those described for ischemia.

Drug-Related Cardiomyopathy

The sequela of chronic cardiac toxicity is cardiomyopathy. The underlying disease process is identical to that for toxic myocarditis; however, cell death is gradual and progressive rather than acute. The initial clinical findings are usually cardiomegaly and congestive heart failure rather than arrhythmias. The term cardiomyopathy should be reserved for cases that present with cardiomegaly and congestive heart failure rather than being applied generally to all cases of drug-related heart disease. Although a variety of drugs have been linked clinically and morphologically to the development of a cardiomyopathy (Table 1), this relation has been well established and documented only in anthracycline-induced cardiomyopathy (5,31).

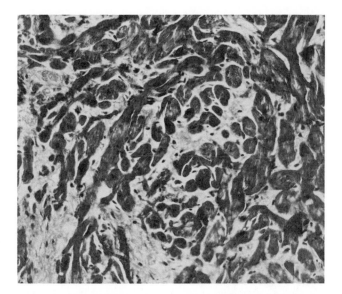

FIG. 10. Histologic findings in anthracycline-related cardiomyopathy are usually nonspecific. The most prominent finding is extensive interstitial fibrosis, which separates individual myocytes. The myocytes vary markedly in size, from large hypertrophied cells with irregular nuclei to small atrophic cells. Occasionally, vacuolated cells are present, but these changes are not reliable predictors of anthracycline damage at the light microscopy level. Hematoxylin-phloxine-sulfarin. ×225.

The anthracyclines daunorubicin and adriamycin are antitumor antibiotics. Both drugs are cardiotoxic and are associated with the development of cardiomyopathy. Symptoms usually appear weeks to months after treatment has been concluded. The clinical course is dominated by intractable congestive heart failure often preceded by the development of progressive cardiomegaly. Adriamycin cardiotoxicity is dose-related and occurs almost exclusively in patients receiving a total dose of more than 500 mg/M^2. As many as 30% of patients receiving more than this dose develop a cardiomyopathy, and mortality approaches 50% in this group. The data available do not suggest an increasing incidence with increasing dosage. Rather, the risk of developing a cardiomyopathy is roughly the same in patients receiving a total dosage of 600 mg/M^2 as in those receiving 1,000 mg/M^2, which suggests a considerable individual variation in the degree of anthracycline cardiotoxicity.

As with other forms of congestive cardiomyopathy, the heart is enlarged. All chambers are dilated, and mural thrombi are frequent in both ventricles (Fig. 9). Histologically, there are multifocal areas of patchy fibrosis and myocardial degeneration throughout the heart. Vacuolated myocardial cells are occasionally seen adjacent to areas of myocardial scarring. As with toxic myocarditis, foci of healing cell damage are associated with fibroblast proliferation and a histiocytic infiltrate. Areas of acute damage are infrequent, and foci of fibrosis predominate (Fig. 10).

Ultrastructurally, two types of cellular injury are seen: myofibrillar loss and vacuolar degeneration (4,24). Myofibrillar loss is characterized by either partial or total loss of myofibrils within the cell. Usually the nucleus is unaffected, and the mitochondria retain compact cristae. In vacuolar degeneration, the earliest change is distension of the sarcoplasmic reticulum and the T-tubular system. The distended vacuoles swell and eventually coalesce, forming large, membrane-bound spaces (Fig. 11). Frequently there is loss of the outer mitochondrial membranes and cristae. The nuclei demonstrate variable degrees of chromatin disorganization and partial replacement of the chromatin by pale-staining fibers and filaments. Myofibrillar loss and vacuolar degeneration can occur concomitantly in the same cell or in different cells. These changes are progressive, leading to cell death; and in severe cases of anthracycline cardiotoxicity, foci of frank cellular necrosis are apparent. As the myocytes die they are replaced by fibrous tissue that forms the patchy stellate scars characteristic of this cardiomyopathy.

These findings are not specific for anthracycline-induced or other drug-related cardiomyopathies. Nevertheless, these changes are characteristic of the drug-induced cardiomyopathy and can be produced experimentally. Rabbits treated

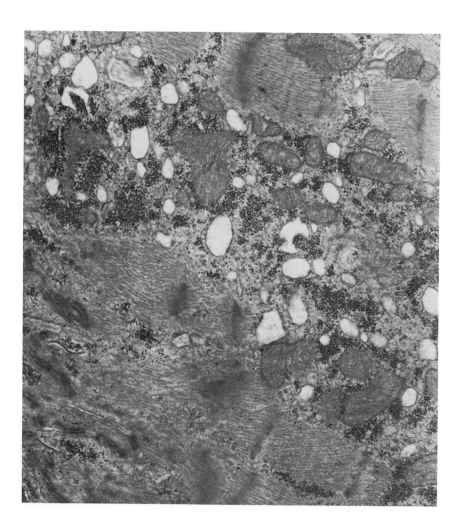

FIG. 11. The diagnosis of anthracycline-related cardiomyopathy is established by electron microscopy. The characteristic findings are dilation and coalescence of the tubules of the sarcoplasmic reticulum and focal myofibrillar loss. Both changes may be present in the same cell, as illustrated in this electron micrograph. The changes are graded as described in Table 2. The focal scant loss of myofibrils and dilated segments of sarcoplasmic reticulum illustrated are consistent with grade 1. ×17,000.

TABLE 2. *Histiopathologic grading system of anthracycline cardiotoxicity*

Grade	Criteria
0	Normal myocardial morphology.
1	Scanty, isolated myocytes affected with partial myofibrillar loss, a distended sarcotubular system, or both. (Anthracycline administration can continue.)
2a	Borderline of grade 1 and grade 2. (Anthracycline can be continued.)
2	Clusters of affected myocytes with definite change of marked or total myofibrillar loss, coalescing cytoplasmic vacuoles, or both. (Anthracycline administration can continue if hemodynamic data are satisfactory.)
2b	Borderline grade 3. (Only one more dose of anthracycline should be given.)
3	Diffuse myocyte damage with many severely affected cells including cell necrosis. (At this grade no further anthracycline should be administered, as heart failure invariably ensues.)

From ref. 4, with permission.

with both daunomycin and adriamycin develop a cardiomyopathy similar clinically and morphologically to the cardiomyopathy observed in man (23). The morphological changes are seen long before clinical signs and symptoms of cardiac disease are evident. The clear relation of the morphological changes to adriamycin administration and the lack of predictive clinical tests to identify patients at risk for the development of cardiomyopathy has led to the use of endomyocardial biopsy to monitor cardiotoxicity (3,4). The myofibrillar and vacuolar changes are graded from the biopsy (Table 2). By applying this scoring method it is possible to tailor treatment to the patient. Treatment can be stopped when morphological evidence of cardiotoxicity is observed before the patient develops irreversible congestive heart failure.

The experimental and morphological studies suggest several possible mechanisms of anthracycline-induced cardiotoxicity (5). The nuclear changes indicate a possible disturbance of nucleic acid metabolism induced by the known binding of these drugs to DNA. Alterations in nucleic acid metabolism, especially RNA transcription, could result in impaired protein synthesis with resultant myofiber lysis. The marked swelling of the sarcoplasmic reticulum suggests that cardiotoxicity is the result of generalized metabolic inhibition induced by the anthracyclines.

ACKNOWLEDGMENT

Supported in part by grant HL 26588 from the National Heart, Lung, and Blood Institute.

REFERENCES

1. Applebaum, F. R., Strauchen, J. A., and Graw, R. G., Jr. (1976): Acute lethal carditis caused by high-dose combination chemotherapy: a unique clinical and pathologic entity. *Lancet*, 1:58.
2. Banerjee, D. (1968): Myocarditis in penicillin sensitivity. *Indian Heart J.*, 20:72.
3. Billingham, M. E. (1979): Some recent advances in cardiac pathology. *Hum. Pathol.*, 10:367.
4. Billingham, M. E., Mason, J. W., Bristow, M. R., and Daniels, J. R. (1978): Anthracycline cardiomyopathy monitored by morphologic changes. *Cancer Treat. Rep.*, 62:865.
5. Bristow, M. R., Mason, J. W., Billingham, M. E., and Daniels, J. R. (1978): Doxorubicin cardiomyopathy: evaluation by phonocardiography, endomyocardial biopsy, and cardiac catheterization. *Ann. Intern. Med.*, 88:168.
6. Bristow, M. R., Thompson, P. D., Martin, P. R., et al. (1978): Early anthracycline cardiotoxicity. *Am. J. Med.*, 65:823.
7. Brown, C. E., and McNamara, D. H. (1940): Acute interstitial myocarditis following administration of arsphenamines. *Arch. Dermatol. Syph.*, 42:312.
8. Buja, L. M., Ferrans, V. J., and Graw, R. G., Jr. (1976): Cardiac pathologic findings in patients treated with bone marrow transplantation. *Hum. Pathol.*, 7:17.
9. Buja, L. M., Ferrans, V. J., and Roberts, W. C. (1974): Drug-induced cardiomyopathies. *Adv. Cardiol.*, 13:330.
10. Buja, L. M., Ferrans, V. J., Mayer, R. J., et al. (1973): Cardiac ultrastructural changes induced by daunorubicin therapy. *Cancer*, 32:771.
11. Caves, P. K., Schultz, W. P., Dong, E., Jr., Stinson, E. B., and Shumway, N. E. (1974): A new instrument for transvenous cardiac biopsy. *Am. J. Cardiol.*, 33:264.
12. Caves, P. K., Stinson, E. B., Graham, A. F., et al. (1973): Percutaneous transvenous endomyocardial biopsy. *JAMA*, 225:289.
13. Chatterjee, S. S., and Thakre, M. W. (1958): Fiedler's myocarditis: report of a fatal case following intramuscular injection of streptomycin. *Tubercle*, 39:240.
14. Clark, E. (1938): Serum carditis: the morphologic cardiac alterations in man associated with serum disease. *JAMA*, 110:1098.
15. Edge, J. R. (1946): Myocardial fibrosis following arsenical therapy. *Lancet*, 2:675.
16. Fenoglio, J. J., McAllister, H. A., and Mullick, F. G. (1981): Drug related myocarditis. I. Hypersensitivity myocarditis. *Hum. Pathol.*, 12:900.
17. Findlay-Jones, L. R. (1964): Fatal myocarditis after vaccination against smallpox: report of a case. *N. Engl. J. Med.*, 270:41.
18. French, A. J., and Weller, C. V. (1942): Interstitial myocarditis following the clinical and experimental use of sulfonamide drugs. *Am. J. Pathol.*, 18:109.
19. Giles, T. D., and Modlin, R. K. (1968): Death associated with ventricular arrhythmia and thioridazine hydrochloride. *JAMA*, 205:108.
20. Herman, J. E., Schwartz, Y., and Bassan, H. (1974): Primary cardiac involvement and painful salivary gland enlargement due to phenylbutazone. *Harefuah*, 86:246.
21. Honey, M. (1960): The effects of sodium antimony tartrate on the myocardium. *Br. Heart J.*, 22:601.
22. Irey, N. S. (1976): Tissue reactions to drugs. *Am. J. Pathol.*, 82:617.
23. Jaenke, R. S. (1974): An anthracycline antibiotic-induced cardiomyopathy in rabbits. *Lab. Invest.*, 30:292.
24. Jaenke, R. S., and Fajardo, L. F. (1977): Adriamycin-induced myocardial lesions: report of a workshop. *Am. J. Surg. Pathol.*, 1:55.
25. Kalikshtein, D. B., Okinokova, V. A., Paleev, N. R., and Gurevich, M. A. (1974): Hypersensitivity of delayed type manifested during the development of allergic lesions of the myocardium. *Bull. Exp. Biol. Med.*, 77:789.
26. Kerwin, A. J. (1964): Fatal myocarditis due to sensitivity to phenindione. *Can. Med. Assoc. J.*, 90:1418.
27. Kline, I. K. (1960): Myocardial alterations associated with pheochromocytomas. *Am. J. Pathol.*, 38:539.
28. Kline, I. K., Kline, T. S., and Saphir, O. (1963): Myocarditis in senescence. *Am. Heart J.*, 65:446.
29. Konno, S., Sekiguchi, M., and Sakakibara, S. (1971): Catheter biopsy of the heart. *Radiol. Clin. North Am.*, 9:491.
30. Lang-Stevenson, D., Mikhailidis, D. P., and Gillett, D. S., (1977): Cardiotoxicity of 5-flourouracil. *Lancet*, 2:406.
31. Lefrak, E. A., Pitha, J., Rosenheim, S., and Gottlieb, J. A. (1973): A clinicopathologic analysis of adriamycin cardiotoxicity. *Cancer*, 32:302.

32. Len Tseng, H. (1971): Interstitial myocarditis probably related to lithium carbonate intoxication. *Arch. Pathol.,* 92:444.

33. Lilienfeld, A., Hochstein, E., and Weiss, W. (1950): Acute myocarditis with bundle branch block due to sulfonamide sensitivity. *Circulation,* 1:1060.

34. Mullick, F. G., and McAllister, H. A. (1977): Myocarditis associated with methyldopa therapy. *JAMA,* 237:1699.

35. Murphy, M. L., Bullock, R. T., and Pearce, M. B. (1974): The correlation of metabolic and ultrastructural changes in emetine myocardial toxicity. *Am. Heart J.,* 87:105.

36. O'Connell, J. B., Subramanian, R., Robinson, J. A., and Scanlon, P. J. (1984): Endomyocardial biopsy: techniques and applications in heart disease of unknown cause. *Heart Transplant.,* 3:132.

37. Parker, C. W. (1975): Drug therapy: drug allergy. *N. Engl. J. Med.,* 292:511 and 292:732.

38. Price, K. C., Weiss, J. M., Hata, J. M., and Smith, J. R. (1955): Experimental needle biopsy of the myocardium of dogs with particular reference to histological study by electron microscopy. *J. Exp. Med.,* 101:687.

39. Sakakibara, S., and Konno, S. (1962): Endomyocardial biopsy. *Jpn. Heart J.,* 3:537.

40. Shirey, E. K., Hawk, W. A., Mukerji, D., and Effer, D. B. (1972): Percutaneous myocardial biopsy of the left ventricle: experience in 198 patients. *Circulation,* 46:112.

41. Smith, H. J., Roche, A. H. G., Jagusch, M. F., and Herdson, P. B. (1976): Cardiomyopathy associated with amphetamine administration. *Am. Heart J.,* 91:792.

42. Sutton, D. C., and Sutton, G. C. (1960): Needle biopsy of the human ventricular myocardium: review of 54 consecutive cases. *Am. Heart J.,* 60:364.

43. Swedberg, K., and Winblad, B. (1974): Heart failure as complication of lithium treatment. *Acta Med. Scand.,* 196:279.

44. Szakacs, J. E., and Cannon, A. (1958): l-Norephinephrine myocarditis. *Am. J. Clin. Pathol.,* 30:425.

45. Timmis, C. G., Gordon, S., Baron, R. H., and Brough, A. J. (1965): Percutaneous myocardial biopsy. *Am. Heart J.,* 70:499.

46. Ursell, P. C., and Fenoglio, J. J. (1984): Spectrum of cardiac disease diagnosed by endomyocardial biopsy. *Pathol. Annu.,* 19:197.

47. VanMieghem, W., Stevens, E., and Cosemans, J. (1978): Ephedrine-induced cardiomyopathy. *Br. Med. J.,* 1:816.

Principles and Methods of Toxicology, Second Edition, edited by A. Wallace Hayes, Raven Press, Ltd., New York © 1989.

CHAPTER 23

Methods in Gastrointestinal Toxicology

Carol T. Walsh

Department of Pharmacology and Experimental Therapeutics, Boston University School of Medicine, Boston, Massachusetts 02118

The gastrointestinal tract is an organ of considerable complexity, which is comprised of numerous tissue types and subserves multiple functions (61). There are consequently many possible loci for toxic effects by chemical substances (84,85,96). In addition, this organ, being the normal portal of entry of dietary substances, has considerable potential for exposure to toxic agents (84). This chapter will review selected methodology used in the assessment of the major structural and functional characteristics of this organ and their perturbation by toxic substances.

ASSESSMENT OF THE STRUCTURAL INTEGRITY OF THE GASTROINTESTINAL TRACT

Histology

Examination of gastrointestinal tissue by histologic techniques may be a useful approach for detection of toxic effects of some substances (132). In sectioning the stomach and small intestine, care must be exercised that cuts are made perpendicular to the longitudinal axis so that morphology of gastric pits and glands and intestinal villi can be inspected. Despite the importance of histologic assessment, altered function of the organ may be induced without changes in the microanatomy of the tissue. In addition, microscopic lesions may be highly localized so that they are missed by selective sampling techniques. For a review of the light microscopy of biopsies from stomach, duodenum, jejunum, ileum, and colon in humans, the reader should refer to Whitehead (145). The normal microanatomy of human small intestinal mucosal cells, including evaluation by electron microscopy, is described by Trier and Madara (134). Examples of depiction of the luminal surface of the gastrointestinal tract by scanning electron microscopy and cellular ultrastructure by transmission electron microscopy can be found in Pfeiffer et al. (87). This text covers the various regions of the gastrointestinal tract and includes tissue from several species of research animals including rat, mouse, and cat.

An important advance in clinical and experimental gastroenterology is the use of fiber optic instruments for visualizing the luminal surface of the gastrointestinal tract. In conjunction with endoscopy, biopsies of the gastrointestinal wall for histologic evaluation can be obtained with instrument attachments such as forceps or suction capsules. Animals should be fasted overnight and anesthetized before insertion of endoscopes or biopsy tools. The Olympus Bronchofibrescope Type BF-3C4 is suitable for use in rats (94).

Gross Evaluation: Extravasation of Nonerythrocytic Vascular Markers

Injury to the gastrointestinal wall may also be detected by sacrificing the animal and inspecting the mucosa for lesions or the serosa for perforations or adhesions (12,13,107). These methods are based on observations of hemorrhagic sites resulting from damage to mucosal cells and underlying vasculature. An example of semiquantitative methodology for assessing chemically induced ulcerogenesis is provided in the work of Szabo et al. (120). A *duodenal ulcer index* is generated as follows: The rat is killed and the duodenum is examined. The intensity of ulcerogenic effect, e.g., by cysteamine, is rated 0 to 3, where 0 = no ulcer, 1 = superficial mucosal erosion, 2 = deep ulcer or transmural necrosis, 3 = perforated or penetrated (into the pancreas or liver) ulcer. The mean of this value in a group of animals is added to the incidence (positive/total) of ulcer formation × 2. In evaluation of gastric lesions (122), the animal is killed and 4 ml of 10% aqueous buffered formaldehyde is instilled into the stomach via a rubber stomach tube. After 5 min, the stomach is removed, opened along the greater curvature, and pinned out with additional formaldehyde. The fixative was found to prevent loss of hemorrhagic fluid from the mucosal surface and thereby improve detection of sites of gastric lesions. The number of lesions are counted. The intensity of effect is assessed as 0 = normal mucosa; 1 = 1 to 4 small petechiae; 2 = 5 or more petechiae or hemorrhagic streaks up to 4 mm; 3 = erosions larger than 5 mm or confluent hemorrhages. Szabo et al. (122) also developed a more quantitative approach for measuring gastric lesions by using planimetry to determine the total area of lesions. The glandular portion of the stomach, which in the rat is separated from the more proximal nonglandular forestomach by the limiting ridge (10), is magnified with a stereomicroscope and projected onto the surface of the planimeter. The area of each lesion and total area involved are determined relative to the area of glandular tissue.

Visual inspection techniques can be made more sensitive by pretreating test animals with a nonerythrocytic vascular marker followed by its visualization on the mucosal surface or its quantitation in the gut lumen. One such marker found useful in the analysis of gastrointestinal effects of nonsteroidal anti-inflammatory agents is the dye pontamine sky blue 6 BX (Edward Gurr Ltd.) (13,124). This procedure, as applied by Brodie et al. (13), consists of injecting 1 ml of a 5% solution of the dye in 0.9% saline into the tail vein of 125- to 150-g rats. After 10 min the animal is sacrificed by intracardiac injection of pentobarbital. The gastrointestinal tract is then removed and opened and the mucosal surface inspected for foci of dark blue coloration. Under these conditions control animals are reported to have no sites of dye accumulation. In contrast, for example, animals treated orally with aspirin 4 hr previously exhibited dose-dependent incidences of these lesions. The sensitivity of animals to aspirin-induced lesions is markedly affected by 24-hr food deprivation. Fasting was found to increase the incidence of gastric lesions and to decrease the incidence of intestinal lesions.

A similar approach has been used with Evans blue dye administered intravenously in rats to characterize the pathologic effects on the stomach and duodenum of the ulcerogenic nonsteroidal anti-inflammatory agents, indomethacin, aspirin, and phenylbutazone (95). Just before killing the animals, 1 ml of a 1% Evans blue solution is injected via the tail vein. The stomach and small intestine are dissected and opened, along the greater curvature and antimesenteric side, respectively, and pinned out. The length or area of lesions was determined using a dissecting microscope with a 1-mm square-grid eyepiece (10×).

In an attempt to quantitate the extravasation of a vascular dye, another approach using pontamine sky blue entails injecting the 5% dye solution (0.2 ml/100 g) into the femoral vein of rats and, 2 to 3 hr after administration, measuring the gastric content of the dye (124). Quantitation is based on an extraction procedure using a solvent system of hyamine and chloroform followed by colorimetric assay. There is only a limited amount of published data on the factors influencing the gastric content of this dye after its intravenous administration. Among the questions that must be considered are the extent of emptying into the intestine during the experimental period and the effectiveness of the method used for collecting the stomach contents.

It should be noted that in testing for ulcerogenic effects of chemicals, the magnitude and site of lesions are dependent on a variety of factors including species, diet and feeding procedures, and dose, route, and time following chemical administration. Satoh et al. (95) presented evidence that the characteristics of lesions produced in humans by indomethacin are best mimicked in a rat model by fasting the animal for 48 hr, feeding rat chow pellets, administering indomethacin (30 mg/kg subcutaneous) 1 hr later, and sacrificing 6 hr later. Ulcerative lesions occur in the antrum and are inhibited by the prostaglandins PgE_2 and PgF_{2a} but not by procedures that reduce acid secretion. Results differed from the fasted or fed rat in which indomethacin, like stress (induced by cold, restraint, or water immersion), other nonsteroidal anti-inflammatory drugs, and acid secretagogues, primarily produced erosions in the corpus, not ulcers in the antrum.

Fecal Blood Loss

Another approach for monitoring the integrity of the mucosal lining of the gastrointestinal tract, which has the advantage of being noninvasive, is based on estimation of gastrointestinal bleeding by examination of the feces. This procedure entails the determination of occult blood in the feces by colorimetric or radioisotopic methods. The detection of fecal occult blood, an important clinical diagnostic tool (147), has application to the screening of substances for potential toxic effects on the gut and to the testing of agents with suspected or probable ulcerogenic properties, e.g., nonsteroidal anti-inflammatory agents.

There are a number of procedures available for assaying blood in the feces. Colorimetric techniques (3,57,91) are based on the use of phenolic compounds whose oxidation to color-emitting substances by hydrogen peroxide is catalyzed by hemoglobin. These reagents include *ortho*-tolidine, benzidine, guaiac, and 2,6-dichlorophenol-indophenol. Commercially available formulations for clinical application primarily use guaiac as the reagent (76), e.g., Hemoccult

(Smith, Kline Diagnostics) in which a slide is impregnated with guaiac.

There are numerous factors that affect a colorimetric assay (1,57). A primary variable is the peroxidase activity in the feces, which originates in the diet rather than from gastrointestinal bleeding. Boiling the fecal sample eliminates some of this activity but not that from hemoglobin. Consequently, hemoglobin from dietary sources such as red meat remains active in the assay. In contrast, certain dietary substances, e.g., ascorbic acid, decrease the reactivity of the colorimetric assay. In addition to interference from dietary factors, the results of this type of assay are dependent on the extent to which hemoglobin loses peroxidase activity by its metabolism in the gut lumen during transit from the site of bleeding (118). In addition, because bleeding may be intermittent, the results will depend on the fecal sampling technique. Results also depend on the extent of fecal hydration that affects the concentration of hemoglobin in the sample (1).

The reagents used in colorimetric assays differ in several respects. For one, their sensitivities differ, with guaiac being relatively less sensitive and o-tolidine being among the most sensitive. A second factor affecting their use is their carcinogenic potential, a property that has been demonstrated for benzidine and o-tolidine, necessitating caution in their handling. Usually this technique is only semiquantitatively applied, with results reported as negative, weakly positive, or strongly positive for occult blood. This approach is the most reasonable because of the various problems, described above, in relating the colorimetric response in a fecal sample to the amount of hemoglobin present because of gastrointestinal bleeding. In setting up such an assay for a given experimental animal population, the reagent concentration may be adjusted such that feces from control animals give negative color reactions within a standard time. For example, Nakamura et al. (81) used the following procedure in assessing fecal blood loss in mice. Three fecal pellets were homogenized in 1 ml of 30% acetic acid and extracted with 2 ml of ethyl ether. One volume of this extract was then added 1 min after combining 2 volumes of o-tolidine reagent and 1 volume of 3% H_2O_2. (The freshly prepared tolidine reagent was made by combining equal volumes of 4% o-tolidine in absolute ethanol, glacial acetic acid, and water.) This mixture was inspected 1 min later for color. Of 30 daily tests on each of seven control animals, all but two tests were reported as negative using this procedure.

An improved approach for measuring fecal blood is the new assay HemoQuant (1,101). The advantages of this technique are its increased sensitivity (compared to Hemoccult) and its capacity to detect degraded hemoglobin. The assay measures the fluorescence of porphyrin after removal of iron from the molecule. Direct measurement of stool samples detects porphyrins already released from hemoglobin by the action of intestinal and bacterial enzymes. Distinction can be made, therefore, between total and degraded hemoglobin, which may prove useful in determining the site of bleeding. A greater fraction of hemoglobin that is lost from proximal sites would be expected to be degraded than that lost distally. The general procedure is as follows: Remove heme iron to release free porphyrin by heating stool sample, e.g., 8 mg, for 90 min at 43°C in reducing acid (2.0 ml of 2.5 M oxalic acid and 0.09 M ferrous sulfate). Selectively extract iron-free

porphyrins of hemoglobin with series of solvent washes. Assay fluorescence with excitation setting at 402 nm and emission at 653 nm and compare to standard curve to determine milligrams of hemoglobin per milligrams of stool. The concentration of hemoglobin will depend on the degree of hydration of the stool sample.

A second approach for assessing gastrointestinal bleeding is based on quantitating radioactivity in the feces following radioisotopic labeling of erythrocytes with Fe^{59} or Cr^{51}. This procedure, which requires greater experimental intrusion than colorimetric methods, entails intravenous administration of Fe^{59}-sulfate for in vivo labeling of erythrocytes (66,88) or of erythrocytes prelabeled with Cr^{51} in vitro (22). These techniques, being based on the use of radioisotopes, require the experimenter to exercise considerably greater attention to the proper housing of animals, handling of excreta, disposal of carcasses, and other problems related to contamination and exposure. However, such approaches are more sensitive than older colorimetric methods and are not subject to invalid results caused by interference from dietary sources. In addition, metabolism of hemoglobin during its transit through the gut lumen has less of an effect on a radioisotopic assay than on the peroxidase-based colorimetric ones. Reabsorption of Fe^{59} liberated from erythrocytes metabolized in the gut lumen is believed, however, to explain the lower estimates of gastrointestinal bleeding obtained with this isotope as compared to those from Cr^{51} studies (66).

An example of the application of Fe^{59} in quantitating gastrointestinal bleeding in experimental animals has been detailed by Phillips (88). The procedure entails intravenous administration of 50 μCi of Fe^{59}-labeled ferrous sulfate in 1.0 ml isotonic saline to 10-kg dogs. Complete 24-hr fecal collections are made, diluted to a fixed volume (750 ml) in water, and homogenized. The entire sample is then assayed for radioactivity, using a gamma counter with a large-volume well. The radioactivity in 1 ml of whole blood is similarly determined. An estimate of the volume of 24-hr fecal blood loss is then computed by dividing the radioactivity in the stool by that found per milliliter of whole blood. An initial equilibration period is necessary for disposition of injected Fe^{59} not associated with erythrocytes; in the studies of Phillips, this delay was 7 days. Studies could then be carried out for as long as 68 days after Fe^{59} administration.

Cell Shedding

Another approach for quantitating structural damage to the gastrointestinal surface is to monitor the rate of cell loss into the gastrointestinal lumen. Exfoliation of mucosal cells from the gastric surface and intestinal villar apex is a normal component of the epithelial proliferative process in these organs (see below). Chemicals that induce mucosal injury may directly increase cell loss from these structures into the lumen.

One technique for quantitating the rate of cell loss is measurement of the DNA content of the luminal fluid. This approach met with limited success when colorimetric methods were used for assay of DNA; sensitivity was insufficient and was affected by other luminal contents, e.g., mucous glycoproteins. The use of a radioimmunoassay for DNA is reported to improve the feasibility of this procedure greatly (55). The assay is sufficiently sensitive that small samples of luminal fluid can be withdrawn at frequent intervals from an experimental animal or human subject. The procedure, as carried out by Hurst et al. (55), has been described for gastric and duodenal studies in anesthetized cats, dogs with exteriorized Pavlovian pouches, and patients intubated with multilumen gastroduodenal tubes. For example, with the anesthetized cat (previously fasted to reduce luminal DNA content from food sources), cannulas are inserted through the duodenal wall to form a 16-mm closed duodenal segment. Initially, luminal contents are rinsed out through the cannula. Test solutions in a 20-ml volume are perfused over 30 min, and 1-ml samples are removed for DNA measurement. Aliquots (50 μl) are assayed for DNA content. The assay procedure quantitates the extent to which the experimental samples displace ^{125}Iododeoxyuridine DNA from DNA antibodies. (The DNA antibody source in Hurst's experiments was plasma from patients with systemic lupus erythematosis.) In these studies each animal must serve as its own control. For purposes of summarizing the data, a crude estimate of surface area of the mucosal surface is obtained for each animal at the end of the experiments by planimetry of the dissected, opened organ. Hurst indicates quantitative and qualitative differences in responses of the stomach and duodenum from different species to acid and ulcerative agents. In the cat duodenal preparation, HCl and intravenous indomethacin (5 mg/kg) induced a significant increase in cell shedding. Further work with this preparation will be necessary to validate its efficacy in detecting chemicals with ulcerogenic potential.

ANALYSIS OF PROLIFERATION OF MUCOSAL CELLS

A potential effect of toxic substances on the gastrointestinal tract is alteration of the proliferative process, which occurs in the deeper regions of the gastric pits and in the intestinal crypts (32). This effect may be a primary event that occurs with antineoplastic agents that impair cell division. The effect may be, however, a secondary one that occurs in response to changes in one of the many factors regulating gastrointestinal renewal, e.g., hormones, microorganisms, food intake, and tissue injury (70). For a review of the proliferative characteristics of the many cell types in gastrointestinal tissue in normal and pathological states the reader is referred to Lipkin (70,71).

Alterations in intestinal crypt cell division and migration up the villar surface may in some cases be inferred from histologic evaluation of cell morphology and villar height. More definitive assessment is based on techniques of cell kinetic analysis (15). These procedures are based on pulse exposure of cells to tritiated thymidine, which is incorporated into DNA of crypt cells undergoing DNA replication. Tissue is collected at various times after thymidine exposure, and thin sections are processed using autoradiography. Specifically, in animal studies, ^{3}H-thymidine, 1 μCi/g body weight, is injected via the tail vein after an overnight fast (32). Bouin's solution is injected into the gastrointestinal lumen and the tissue of interest removed, cut open, flattened, and fixed in additional solution. After conventional alcohol dehydration and paraffin embedding, 5 μm sections are mounted on glass slides, dipped in Kodak NTB-2 or NTB-3 photographic emulsion (diluted 1:1 with distilled water), and enclosed in lightproof containers at 4°C for 2 to 4 weeks. Slides are then developed with Kodak D19, fixed, and stained (e.g., hematoxylin and eosin). From these samples it is possible to determine the time for complete migration of newly formed cells from the crypt to the site of extrusion on the villar tip. In addition, by evaluation of the fraction of mitoses in the crypt that are labeled with ^{3}H-thymidine as a function of time, one can estimate the characteristics of the cell cycle, including the duration of the various phases as well as the complete cell cycle time.

Methodology has recently been developed to analyze intestinal epithelial cell kinetics by flow cytometry. These procedures depend on separation and high recovery of crypt and villar cells from the intestinal wall (50). Cheng et al. (16,17) demonstrated the feasibility of incubation of intestinal tissue in calcium and magnesium free Hanks balanced salt solution containing 30 mM EDTA, followed by vibration, which removes the epithelial layer. Flow cytometry, which separates cells according to their DNA content, provides a much more rapid and precise approach to quantitation of cell kinetics than is possible with autoradiography.

As new columnar epithelial cells are formed in the intestinal crypts and subsequently migrate up the villus, they differentiate from proliferative, secretory cells into absorptive ones. There are numerous structural and functional indicators of this differentiation process (109). Several enzymes whose activities markedly differ in crypt cells and fully differentiated villar cells have been used as markers to assess the differentiation process. These tools also have application in verification procedures for methods of separating crypt and villar cells. Examples include thymidine kinase, whose activity is highest in proliferating crypt cells where DNA synthesis is occurring (56), and the oligosaccharidases, e.g., lactase and maltase (27), and fatty acid esterases (106), whose activity is highest in differentiated villar cells. The activity of these enzymes is dependent not only on their rate of formation but also on their rate of degradation. Recent studies have demonstrated, for example, that activity of sucrase, a disaccharidase on the brush border membrane of mucosal cells, can be altered by conditions that affect its degradation rate (43). This factor must be taken into account in interpretation of studies in which activity of a mucosal enzyme is altered.

DETERMINATION OF GASTRIC SECRETORY ACTIVITY

A primary function of the stomach is the secretion of hydrogen ions by the parietal cells that line the gastric glands. Gastric acidity is required for optimum activation of pepsinogen, elaborated and secreted by the chief cells of the stomach. This enzyme is responsible for initial digestion of proteins present in the diet. The acid secretory activity of the stomach provides one index of the functional status of this organ. Numerous physiologic factors affect basal and stimulated acid output, most notably neural and hormonal input to the parietal cell. The following are of importance to the toxicologist:

1. Agents with irritative effects on the gastric mucosa may, on chronic administration, produce gastritis characterized by inflammation, glandular atrophy, and reduction of secretory activity.
2. Agents that stimulate gastric acid secretion may cause acid-induced erosions and ulcers in the stomach and duodenum.

In Vivo Methodology

One approach to measurement of gastric acid secretion is invasive. Animals are fasted for 24 hr, and drinking water is withheld for 1 hr. The animal is then briefly anesthetized, e.g., with ether, the abdomen opened, and a tie placed around the pylorus to prevent gastric emptying. The gastric content is removed through a syringe and 22-gauge needle inserted through the gastric wall (121). The abdominal incision is sutured and the animals are unrestrained. After a fixed interval, e.g., 30 min, the animal is reanesthetized, the esophagus clamped, and the gastric contents aspirated again. After centrifugation to remove solid components, the fluid volume is determined. The sample is then assayed for the material under investigation. For determination of total titratable acidity, samples are titrated to pH 7.0 with 0.01 N NaOH, and results are usually expressed as millimoles per hour. [Use of pH 7.0 as an endpoint detects hydrogen ions associated with endogenous acidic compounds, e.g., mucoproteins. Titration to pH 3.5 may provide a better estimate of hydrochloric acid (129)]. An interval longer than 30 min is not advisable because pyloric ligation induces acid secretion, and after longer times a secretory effect of a chemical can be masked by the procedure itself (121).

A noninvasive approach developed by Segal et al. (103) entails quantitation of the liberation of azure A from an azure A-resin complex in the stomach, a reaction that is pH dependent. Azure A is absorbed from the intestine only after release from the resin and is substantially cleared into the urine. With this technique, animals are also fasted as described above. The dye (azuresin, Diagnex Blue, Squibb & Sons) is administered by gavage in a dose of 20 mg/100 g in 2 ml of 4% gelatin (Granular G-8, Fisher). Animals are individually housed in metabolism cages and urine is collected for 24 hr. (Food and water are withheld and the animals are subcutaneously injected with a total of 3 ml of 5% sucrose.) The 24-hr urine volume is measured and concentration of azure A is determined. The quantitation procedure is by spectrophotometry. In an experiment of this type, it is essential to verify that the experimental treatment does not affect the intestinal absorption or renal excretion of the unconjugated azure A. Azure A should therefore be administered to control and experimental animals to verify that once liberated from the resin its disposition is similar in the two groups.

A model that permits repeated study in an unanesthetized animal such as the dog is the use of the Heidenhain fundic pouch, which is surgically created with access to the body surface. The denervated preparation has the disadvantage of a low basal acid secretory rate. The preparation, however, permits controlled exposure of the gastric surface to toxic substances and repeated measurement of volume changes, electrolyte concentrations, hemorrhage, and mucosal blood flow. This technique has been used to demonstrate the damaging effect of aspirin in acid solution on the mucosa (142). Characteristically, the drug induces a decrease in hydrogen concentration in the luminal solution (increased inward flux) and an increase in Na^+ and K^+, blood, and plasma protein efflux into the lumen.

In Vitro Methods

Significant advances in elucidating physiological mechanisms of gastric secretion have resulted from use of *in vitro* preparations of this tissue (93,113). One approach is study of the epithelial tissue in a Ussing chamber. A segment of the stomach wall is removed from the animal, and the muscle layer is stripped off. The remaining tissue is mounted to separate two solutions. Acid secretion and electrolyte flux can be monitored. For improved definition of the physiology of individual cell types in the stomach, techniques have been developed to isolate the gastric gland as well as individual cell types. The gastric gland preparation is obtained by treatment of the intact mucosa with pronase or collagenase. This material is primarily composed of parietal and peptic cells in greater concentration than in the intact tissue. Advantages of this approach include the relatively good viability of the glands and the relatively normal intercellular connections, including tight junctions that remain between cells. Techniques have also been developed for isolation of the parietal cell from gastric glands (93,113). A calcium chelator, e.g., EDTA, increases dispersion of single cells from the gastric glands (113). A Percoll step gradient purification or centrifugal elutriation can be effectively used to separate parietal cells from other cell types in the tissue, based on the difference in their mass. With these single-cell preparations, unlike the intact tissue, no anatomical barrier exists between mucosal and serosal surfaces. Alternative approaches must therefore be used for measuring hydrogen ion secretion. Two techniques include quantitating oxygen consumption of the cells and measuring their accumulation of aminopyrine. Several types of studies have shown a close correlation between oxygen consumption and the energy-dependent process of acid secretion. Measurement of oxygen consumption with a Clark-type polarographic electrode or Gilson respirometer is one index of secretory activity. Another approach is based on monitoring the uptake of a weak base, aminopyrine, into the intracellular vesicular space of the parietal cell (112). Aminopyrine, which has a pKa of 5.0, readily traverses plasma membranes in its unionized form as it exists at neutral pH. In the parietal cell under conditions in which acid secretion is occurring, the compound becomes ionized in acid secretory vesicles and remains trapped in this acidic fluid. The cellular content of the compound relative to that in the media can be used as an index of acid formation by the parietal cell. The conventional approach is to use the ^{14}C isotope of aminopyrine and measure radioactivity in cells separated from media by filtration.

For a review of procedures to assess gastric secretion of other substances that play a role in chemically induced ulcerogenesis, e.g., mucins, prostaglandins, and bicarbonates, the reader is referred to texts by Harmon (45) and Allen et al. (2).

ASSESSMENT OF ABSORPTIVE FUNCTION OF THE GASTROINTESTINAL TRACT

The toxicologist is concerned with analysis of absorptive function of the gut for two primary reasons. One issue entails determination of the gastrointestinal absorption, metabolism and excretion of toxic substances, and factors that affect this process (47,58,84,86,90). The second problem is understanding the effect of toxic substances on the absorption of normal dietary constituents or orally administered therapeutic agents. Similar methodology may be applied to analysis of both problems.

There are numerous approaches for studying gastrointestinal absorption, both *in vivo* and *in vitro* (63,82). The technique chosen for a particular study will depend on the aspect of the absorption process that is of primary interest. Broadly speaking, the methodology can be categorized by the following:

1. the procedure by which the test substance is administered to the absorptive surface of the gut; and
2. the technique for quantitating the extent and/or rate of absorption.

The following discussion will detail several types of these procedures considered to be of greatest applicability.

In Vivo Determination of Overall Extent of Gastrointestinal Absorption

One approach, permitting the most overall assessment of gastrointestinal absorption, is based on oral administration of a test substance, followed by determination of its concentration in systemic fluids as a function of time. This technique is the least precise approach to quantitating gastrointestinal absorption kinetics in that numerous variables may influence the results. However, this methodology provides the best measure of the bioavailability of a xenobiotic and the impact of its absorption kinetics on systemic exposure. This approach is also useful as a screening procedure for determining whether a test substance induces malabsorption of nutrients.

Dosing

Several techniques for administering a test substance in an absorption study may be relevant. In certain cases, for example, in the determination of the gastrointestinal absorption of a toxic substance that may be a contaminant of the diet, the most meaningful analysis may entail appropriate incorporation of the substance into the diet of the experi-

mental animal. Not only will the rate of absorption differ from that following oral intubation but the extent of absorption may differ as well (136). Care must be exercised, using this approach, to ensure that the procedures required for dietary incorporation, especially into solid components of the diet, do not result in chemical modification of the test substance. Determination of the total ingested dose of the test substance must be made by careful measurement of the foodstuffs before and after presentation to the experimental animal. Such studies are greatly facilitated by use of commercially available metabolic cages, which restrict the area of the cage in which the animal has access to food. As a consequence, unconsumed food may be collected more easily and is not contaminated with urine, feces, or drinking water. Consideration must be made of the eating habits of the experimental animals. If consumption of the test substance over an extended period, e.g., hours, is undesirable, animals may be fasted and then presented with the diet for a short interval. A fasting procedure, however, may alter both the rate and extent of absorption.

A second technique for oral administration of a test substance is its intubation into the stomach of experimental animals. This procedure permits more precise control of the administered dose and allows the investigator to give the same dose (in absolute terms or on a per kilogram basis) to each experimental animal. With this technique the test substance is administered in a fluid vehicle, either in solution or as a suspension. Intubations are readily carried out in small animals, e.g., rats or mice, without use of sedative agents. The intubating needle must be passed into the stomach because delivery into the esophagus will often result in loss of the dose by regurgitation or aspiration into the lungs. Intubating needles for animals of a variety of sizes are commercially available. Care must be taken to ensure that the volume of the dose administered does not exceed the capacity of the stomach. The eating habits of the animal should be taken into consideration because the maximum dosing volume must be smaller when food is present in the stomach.

For many substances administered by the oral route, the rate of emptying from the stomach into the small intestine may be the determining factor in the overall rate and extent of systemic absorption (89). This phenomenon results from the generally lower rate of absorption of substances, whether acids, bases, or nonelectrolytes, from the stomach than from the small intestine because of the smaller surface area of the gastric region and the larger intraluminal distances. Consequently, in studies in which the question of interest is the relative rate and extent of absorption of an agent through the intestinal mucosal barrier, dosing in food or by intubation may be inappropriate. For such a study the test substance should be directly administered into the intestinal lumen. This procedure has been profitably used in the study of intestinal transport in humans through use of small-bore intubating tubes localized through radiographic techniques (35). In studies with small animals, dosing into the intestine is readily achieved by lightly anesthetizing the animal with ether, making a midline incision through the gut wall, and inserting a needle into the intestinal lumen through the gut wall opposite the attachment of the mesenteries. A tie should be made around the intestine to include the needle to prevent efflux of the injected substance at the site of insertion.

When administering a potentially toxic agent by the oral route to assess its absorption, the investigator must choose doses and their concentration with care. Preferably, a concentration range is achieved in the gastrointestinal lumen of the experimental animals, which includes levels likely to be reached during exposures in man. It is important to consider the possibility that an agent may produce direct effects on mucosal cells that alter its own absorption kinetics. Such a phenomenon would be expected to be highly dependent on the concentration of the agent achieved in the gastrointestinal lumen. A similar consideration applies in choosing doses of nutrients when testing the effects of chemicals on absorption of dietary substances. Many nutrients are absorbed by concentration-dependent mechanisms, e.g., facilitated diffusion and active transport. Effects of chemicals on absorption of a nutrient may therefore depend on the dose of both substances.

To quantitate the total amount of absorption from the oral route by sampling systemic fluids, the agent under study is also administered systemically (138). Ideally, the substance is given by the intravenous route, which provides a standard of complete systemic absorption for comparison to the situation after oral dosing. Where possible, the intravenous dose should be chosen to produce plasma concentrations in the range of those expected after oral administration. This adjustment is especially important in the case of a substance likely to produce acute toxic effects, especially effects that might alter the distribution, metabolism, or elimination of the agent itself.

Quantitation of Absorption

Sampling techniques and experimental design

In an investigation of the overall absorption of an agent following its acute oral administration, quantitation of the rate and extent of this process entails appropriate sampling and analysis of the concentration of the agent in a systemic fluid as a function of time. Relevant information may be derived from sampling not only systemic fluids such as plasma, but also saliva, urine, or breath (138). In addition, a more direct approach for analyzing absorption characteristics than the sampling of systemic or excreted body fluids entails the sampling of portal blood (83) or the collection of the mesenteric blood draining the sites of absorption of the test substance (5). These procedures require considerably more complicated surgical techniques than sampling of systemic blood. Furthermore, transfusions of blood into the animal may be required. An important advantage of this procedure is the capacity to determine the *in vivo* kinetics of metabolism of a test substance by intestinal tissues. An analogous approach for studying perturbations in mucosal uptake and metabolism of triglycerides and cholesterol (19) is to cannulate the mesenteric lymphatic vessel for sampling of lymph that carries these lipids from their absorption site. To assess the contribution of enterohepatic circulation of a substance to its systemic concentrations, studies can be carried out in animals with biliary cannulas that are exteriorized for complete biliary diversion or that fork to enter the gut lumen as well as provide an exterior sampling site (72).

Generally, collection of plasma samples is preferred as a relatively noninvasive procedure, which provides the most direct indication of systemic concentrations of the agent under study. A number of considerations dictate aspects of experimental design and procedure. First of all, samples must be collected over a sufficiently long time to determine the area under the plasma concentration versus time curve. Second, the volume of each sample must be large enough to permit detection of the agent by the method of quantitation. Third, the amount of blood withdrawn from the animal must not be so large as to affect blood volume and the subsequent kinetics of the agent under study. These factors will determine whether sequential samples can be taken from the same animal.

Data analysis

Under most circumstances, the extent of gastrointestinal absorption of a substance after acute administration is *proportional* to the area under the curve (AUC) of its concentration in plasma as a function of time. Consequently, assessment of extent of absorption, or bioavailability, can be determined by comparing the area achieved after oral administration to that after intravenous administration in which absorption is complete. Similarly, to determine whether a chemical induces malabsorption of a nutrient, the AUC of the latter is computed under control and test conditions. It is critical to recognize that the AUC is also a function of the distribution characteristics of the agent in the body and its elimination kinetics. Changes in these parameters may therefore be a source of error in the assessment of oral absorption by this method.

The area under the plasma concentration-time curve can be calculated by several techniques. A simple approach entails performing this integration by the trapezoidal rule (125,138). The plasma concentrations are connected by straight lines, thus forming a series of trapezoids. The area under each trapezoid is then computed from the expression $1/2(t_{n+1} - t_n)(C_n + C_{n+1})$, where t_n is the time of sampling and C_n is the plasma concentration at that time. These areas are then summed. Another more precise approach is the use of a Simpson's rule (125). These techniques have the advantage of not requiring a mathematical model to describe the kinetics observed. The ratio of the area observed after oral administration to that after the intravenous route is a measure of the systemic absorption of an agent (its bioavailability). The extent of absorption as determined by this procedure is dependent not only on the nature of the transport of a substance through the mucosal cell barrier but also on the first-pass effect, metabolism in the gastrointestinal lumen and mucosa and the liver that occurs after oral but not intravenous administration (38).

Malabsorption Tests for Dietary Substances

Carbohydrates

Monosaccharides: The D-xylose test. The functional integrity of the proximal small intestine can be assessed by quantitation of D-xylose absorption. D-xylose is a pentose monosaccharide that is absorbed by passive diffusion as well as by the Na^+-coupled carrier mechanism for dietary sugars, e.g., glucose and galactose. D-xylose has the advantage over glucose for testing purposes in that (a) its blood levels are insensitive to insulin, (b) its elimination pathway is primarily (although not exclusively) through renal excretion and not systemic metabolism, and (c) it is not normally present in blood or urine. Extensive injury to the luminal surface of the small intestine is reflected in reduction of the concentration of D-xylose in the blood and urine after its oral administration. Xylose is absorbed intact and is not dependent on mammalian luminal or brush border enzyme activity. The xylose test would generally not be abnormal in cases in which malabsorption, e.g., of fats or polysaccharides, results from defects in luminal or brush border enzyme activity. The test is carried out as follows: Animals are fasted, e.g., 12 hr, to minimize variability in results associated with stomach emptying and interactions with dietary contents. D-xylose is then administered by gavage (0.5 gm/kg body weight) in an aqueous solution. Blood samples are obtained every 30 min for 180 min. The concentration of D-xylose in plasma is determined by a spectrophotometric assay based on conversion of xylose to furfural under acidic conditions, which then reacts with p-bromoaniline to produce a pink color. Details of the assay are given by Tietz (129). A review of studies in dogs indicates that normal animals exhibit peak plasma levels of D-xylose greater than 45 mg/dl between 60 to 90 min (105). Malabsorption is characterized by reduced peak levels and AUC. Possible errors of interpretation occur if

1. gastric emptying is unusually slow, in which case the rate of absorption and therefore the peak plasma concentration will be low;
2. marked bacterial overgrowth exists in the proximal small intestine, in which case bacterial metabolism of D-xylose reduces its availability for absorption (41,130); and
3. renal clearance of D-xylose is depressed, which elevates the plasma levels and may mask an absorption defect. This source of error can be evaluated from urinary excretion data. The bladder must be empty at time of xylose administration and complete urine collections must subsequently be carried out.

Disaccharides. Disaccharides in the diet or released on starch digestion are absorbed only after cleavage into monosaccharides by the disaccharidases of the intestinal brush border. Malabsorption, including diarrhea and abdominal distension, may result from low activity of these enzymes, as occurs, for example, in lactase deficiency which is a genetically based phenomenon. In addition, the activity of disaccharidases may be selectively impaired by synthetic structural analogues of the endogenous substrates. Inhibition or deficiency of these enzymes can be assessed by oral administration of the disaccharide substrate and measurement of the subsequent rise in blood glucose. This rise is depressed under conditions of impaired disaccharidase activity. To prove the specificity of the abnormality, it is necessary to demonstrate that the absorption of glucose administered orally is normal. Numerous experimental variables can influence plasma glucose levels. In rats, for example, factors such as method and duration of restraint, method of blood

collection, animal handling, and fasting can alter baseline values (8), which average 98 to 152 mg/dl in plasma and serum (92). Experiments should be designed to minimize variability from these sources. Verification of altered brush border enzyme activity can be carried out by *in vitro* assays using intestinal homogenates or brush border membrane preparations (26).

Fats

Under normal conditions, fat in the diet is nearly completely digested and absorbed. Lipids that are excreted in the feces are primarily associated with intestinal bacterial cells and mucosal cells sloughed from the intestinal surface. Structurally, these lipids include mono-, di-, and triglycerides, fatty acids, phospholipids, glycolipids, sterols, and cholesterol esters. Numerous factors affect the process of digestion and absorption of dietary lipids. Fat malabsorption can therefore result from a variety of different toxic mechanisms. A primary goal in determining the cause of fat malabsorption is to distinguish between defects in the intraluminal digestion of fats to fatty acids from impairment in fatty acid absorption. Impaired digestion of lipids suggests a reduction in pancreatic lipase activity, which may result from a lack of the cholesytokinin signal for release, exocrine pancreatic insufficiency, or presence of a lipase inhibitor. Absorption defects may result from impaired micelle formation because of bile salt deficiency, reduced mucosal cell uptake because of cell damage or villous atrophy, impaired reesterification and chylomicron formation caused by reduced enzyme activities in the mucosa, and reduced chylomicron transport into the lymphatics because of cellular infiltration of the lamina propria or systemic lymphatic disease.

Crude screening for fat malabsorption can be effectively carried out by examination of the feces. Steatorrhea, an increase in fecal fat, can be qualitatively detected by use of the Sudan III preparation stain. A fresh sample of feces is smeared on a microscope slide. Two drops of glacial acetic acid and two drops of Sudan III are then added and a cover slip is placed on top. The slide is heated until the sample boils. The specimen is then examined for the presence of refractile orange droplets, which are fat globules. With high power magnification, the presence in a single field of many orange droplets the size of or larger than red blood cells is an indication of steatorrhea.

For a more quantitative assessment of steatorrhea, measurement of fecal lipid excretion should be carried out. For reliable results, total feces should be obtained over a 72-hr period and combined. Quantitative analysis can be accomplished gravimetrically or by titrimetric measurement of the total fatty acids. In the gravimetric method, a weighed sample is subjected to alkaline hydrolysis to convert lipids to fatty acids, salts, and sterols. The mixture is acidified, and the fatty acids and sterols are extracted into petroleum ether. After solvent evaporation, the sample is weighed to obtain a measure of the total lipids present. In the titrimetric procedure, the residue is dissolved in ethanol and titrated with a standard solution of sodium hydroxide to obtain a measure of total fatty acids present. For details of these procedures, refer to Ellefson and Caraway (33).

Once steatorrhea has been documented, additional tests are needed to determine the cause. The initial objective should be to distinguish maldigestion from malabsorption to isolate the mechanisms described above. One approach is oral dosing with a radiolabeled triglyceride, e.g., triolein, and on a separate occasion the constituent fatty acid (oleic acid). In clinical studies the validity of this approach has been demonstrated for use of the C^{13}- and C^{14}-labeled compounds with assay of the isotope in breath CO_2 at hourly intervals 3 to 6 hr after ingestion of the lipid (100). Reduction in the absorption of triglyceride but not of fatty acid is indicative of a defect in intraluminal metabolism. Impairment of fatty acid absorption, as well, suggests bile salt deficiency or mucosal cell injury.

In Vivo Intestinal Closed Segment Technique

Other approaches to quantitating absorption permit closer analysis of the transport process of a substance across the intestinal mucosa. Several procedures, e.g., the closed segment technique and perfusion methods, are based on monitoring the loss of an administered agent from the gastrointestinal tract as a measure of its absorption. The closed segment technique, which will be described in this section, is simple to carry out, requires a minimum of equipment, and provides a measurement of absorption rate under relatively physiologic conditions (139).

Dosing

With the in vivo closed segment technique, a solution of the agent under study is directly administered into the intestinal lumen. After etherization of the animal, the intestines are exposed. The region of the intestine of interest is identified, using landmarks such as the ligature of Trietz (just distal to the pylorus) and the ileocaecal junction. A segment is closed distally with a ligature. The needle for injection is then inserted at a more proximal site, and the gut lumen is closed around the needle with another tie. Care must be taken to ensure that the needle tip remains only with the lumen of the closed segment and does not puncture the gut wall. After the solution is injected, this tie is tightened and knotted as the needle is slowly withdrawn. To minimize variability in the results in a single experiment, segments should be located in the same part of the intestine in all animals, the length of the segment should be approximately the same, and the volume of fluid administered into the lumen should be identical. After dosing, the incision in the abdomen should be sutured, and the animal should be permitted to regain consciousness to minimize any possible influence of the anesthetic agent.

Quantitation of Absorption

At a predetermined time after the injection of the agent under study, the animal is rapidly anesthetized for removal of the entire closed intestinal segment. The amount of the injected substance remaining in this segment is then quantitated after the homogenization of the sample. The extent of absorption is determined as the difference between the total amount injected and the amount remaining in the segment at the end of the absorption period. This approach has the advantage of directly determining the entire systemic absorption from both the intestinal lumen and the mucosal cell. This method differs in this respect from perfusion techniques in which absorption of substances is quantitated from their loss out of the luminal fluid. Especially for substances that are highly bound in the intestinal mucosal cell, absorption out of the intestinal lumen cannot be equated with absorption into the systemic circulation.

The quantitation of absorption by determining the disappearance of a substance from a closed segment is only valid if loss does not occur, because of metabolism of the substance in the intestinal lumen or tissue. If metabolism of the substance does occur, assay of the intestinal closed segment for the parent compound and metabolites alone is inadequate for description of its absorption kinetics, unless metabolites are poorly absorbed and are all completely recovered in the gut samples. Consequently, analysis should be carried out to determine whether metabolite formation and absorption would be likely to occur before choosing this technique to assess the absorption rate of a compound.

Intestinal Perfusion Techniques

Another in vivo procedure for quantitating intestinal transport is based on infusing a solution at a constant rate into the intestinal lumen (69). The amount of the test substance in the effluent from a distal site is compared to the amount infused into the gut to determine its net absorption as a function of time. This technique, unlike the other in vivo procedures described above, is especially useful in studying the transport of water and its perturbations by toxicologic compounds. Quantitation of the net flux of water in the gut caused by absorptive and secretory processes can be carried out by monitoring the change in intraluminal concentration of a nonabsorbable marker. C^{14}-polyethylene glycol 4000 (PEG) is a frequently used marker substance that has been found suitable for these purposes (59,111). The validity of PEG 4000 as a volume marker in perfusion studies has been well documented (59). In contrast, methods based on recovery of fluid from closed segments of the gut by mechanical methods, e.g., draining the luminal content, have been found inadequate.

Before a perfusion study, animals should be fasted overnight to reduce luminal contents of the intestine. Animals are then anesthetized, and the proximal and distal ends of the region of the intestine of interest are cannulated. With rats, for example, PE-50 polyethylene tubing is inserted into the intestinal lumen of anesthetized animals. The marker is then infused into the proximal tubing using a peristaltic pump. The solution containing PEG, under most circumstances, should be made isotonic with the plasma of the species under study and should be heated to body temperature. An initial equilibration period of PEG infusion must be carried out; in studies using the rat and an infusion of 1.6 ml/min, 30 min has been found to be adequate to obtain constant output rates from the distal end of the small intestine (59).

After equilibration, fluid from the distal cannula is collected for fixed intervals, e.g., 10 min. Aliquots are removed for determination of the concentration of PEG in the effluent. The volume of the effluent can then be determined by computing the ratio of the amount of PEG infused during the collection period to its concentration in the collected fluid:

Effluent volume

$$= \frac{\text{Pump rate} \times \begin{array}{c}\text{collection}\\\text{period}\end{array} \times \begin{array}{c}\text{PEG concentration}\\\text{in infused fluid}\end{array}}{\text{PEG concentration in collected fluid}}$$

Comparison of the volume infused to that of the effluent then provides a measure of the net absorption or secretion of water by the intestinal segment.

In Vitro Methods

Numerous advances in the understanding of cellular mechanisms of electrolyte flux and nutrient absorption in the intestine have been made using in vitro, as opposed to in vivo, techniques. The review by Kimmich (63) illustrates the impact of development of in vitro techniques on elucidation of intestinal transport mechanisms of sugars. With in vitro procedures, physiological variables, e.g., intestinal motility and mesenteric blood flow, can be eliminated or controlled. In addition the experimenter has the option of control over factors such as the composition of the solutions bathing both the mucosal and the systemic side of the intestine and the electrochemical potential difference between the mucosal and serosal surfaces. Another advantage of certain in vitro techniques is the ability to control the stirring rate in the mucosal solution carefully. The stirring rate influences the thickness of the unstirred water layer, which can impose significant resistance to the mucosal uptake of substrates such as long-chain fatty acids, bile acids, cholesterol, and monosaccharides (127,148). Recent studies have also demonstrated that the layer of mucus that adheres to the mucosal cell surface can impede the diffusion of nutrients, e.g., disaccharides, small peptides (110), and cholesterol (75). The pronounced quantitative differences in the uptake rates of nutrients into various in vitro preparations of the small intestine (128) probably results, at least in part, from differences in the resistances conferred by the unstirred water layer and mucous coat. In vitro techniques include those analogous to in vivo methods already discussed. Investigators, for example, have studied the absorption of substances from isolated gut sections with perfusions of the lumen or with perfusions of the vasculature (49).

One in vitro method with no in vivo analogue is the everted sac technique (146). This method has been useful in the characterization of energy-dependent carrier-mediated transport processes. In this procedure small lengths of the intestine are everted, filled with fluid, and tied at both ends. Absorption is quantitated by monitoring the appearance of a test substance inside the sac in the fluid bathing the serosal surface of the intestine. Unlike the in vivo condition, therefore, absorption of a test substance in this model is considered equivalent to its passage not only through the mucosa but also through the submucosa, the external muscle layers, and

serosal tissue of the gut wall. Modifications have included cannulations permitting sequential sampling of the serosal fluid and control of the serosal fluid volume (25).

Problems with the everted segment technique include inadequate oxygen diffusion into the tissue and distension and hydration of the gut segment. Consequently, the preparation of the tissue and the experimental incubations must be short in duration. Everted sacs of the duodenum from rats exhibit structural abnormalities after 5-min incubation at 37°C (68). By 1 hour, marked distention of the villus as well as complete loss of the villar architecture occurs. These dramatic structural changes are associated, not surprisingly, with changes in transport kinetics. For example, with this preparation the absorption of large polar molecules, e.g., riboflavin, normally incompletely absorbed from the gut, begins to increase significantly within 30 min (39). One approach to improve tissue viability has been the use of intestinal segments from which the longitudinal and circular muscle layers and serosa have been stripped (149).

Other in vitro procedures include rings cut from the whole wall of the intestine (24). This approach is designed to improve oxygenation of the tissue but only permits measurement of the accumulation of test substances by all cell types of the intestinal wall. Several other methods have been developed for quantitating uptake of substances specifically by gut mucosal cells. Methods for recovering mucosal cells, e.g., scraping the inner surface of the gut with a glass slide (29) or vibrating a gut segment everted on a glass spiral (67), have been improved on to reduce contamination from cells of the lamina propria (131), as well as isolate crypt cells (46). In addition, of importance to analysis of carbohydrate digestion and absorption has been the isolation of mucosal brush border membranes recovered as vesicles after differential centrifugation (52,62,80,115). The preparation permits analysis of membrane transport kinetics uncontaminated by cytosolic metabolism of the permeant (51). In addition, production of membrane vesicles is reported to remove adherent mucous (110) so that this preparation, unlike in vivo and other in vitro models, is devoid of this diffusion barrier. Basal-lateral membranes of mucosal cells have also been isolated by use of differential and discontinuous sucrose-gradient centrifugation (30).

An additional in vitro preparation has been of major significance to the elucidation of mechanisms controlling electrolyte absorption and secretion (97). This procedure, the use of the Ussing chamber (135), entails in vitro short-term exposure of a segment of intestine to defined mucosal and serosal solutions (99). The electrical potential difference across the intestine is measured with a voltmeter and short-circuit current with an external microamp source. Flux of electrolytes is determined by addition of an isotope to the solution bathing one surface of the intestinal segment and monitoring its accumulation in the tissue or solution bathing the other surface. Similarly, the unidirectional flux chamber designed by Schultz et al. (98) exposes a defined area of luminal surface of the intestinal wall to solution containing the test permeant. Brief exposure times are used to permit measurement of influx through the mucosa. This methodology permits assessment of the integrity of brush border transport mechanisms. More recently, studies have been carried out using microelectrode impalement of individual cells of the intestinal wall to differentiate the active chloride secreting activity of crypt and villar cells (143). Possibly, this procedure could also be applied to distinguish cellular sites of action of toxic substances.

An *in vitro* preparation with the advantage of more prolonged viability is the organ culture of mucosal biopsies (53). This technique permits the *in vitro* maintenance of mucosal explants for 24 to 48 hr, depending on the species and region of the intestine biopsied (104,133). Modification of culture conditions may permit even greater longevity of samples. Autrup (4), for example, reported maintenance of human colonic mucosa for 28 days. A major advantage of this approach is that the normal anatomical arrangement of the villus and its mucosal cells is maintained and the processes of mucosal cell proliferation and differentiation can be studied. Although absorption studies are feasible, the greatest contributions with this preparation may well be in the study of colonic carcinogenesis and chemotherapy.

ROLE OF MICROFLORA IN GASTROINTESTINAL TOXICITY

The entire length of the gastrointestinal tract is populated by a diversity of microorganisms (14,20,108). The species composition and quantity of the gastrointestinal microflora differ markedly in the various regions of this organ. The stomach is relatively sparsely populated ($<10^3$ colony forming units/ml) with primarily gram positive, aerobic microorganisms, e.g., *Streptococci, Staphylococci,* and *Lactobacilli.* The large intestine, in contrast, is densely inhabited by gram negative anaerobes such that the luminal contents may contain 10^{12} colony forming units/ml. Among the more prominent species are *Bacteroides, Bifidobacterium,* and *Eubacterium.* Studies with animals that are delivered and reared under germfree conditions have clearly demonstrated that the indigenous microflora influences the structure and function of the gastrointestinal tract (21,37).

The gut microflora may mediate toxic effects on this organ by a variety of mechanisms. Pathogenic strains such as *Shigella* may elicit damage by their capacity to invade the mucosal epithelium and produce necrosis and hemorrhagic effects. Other types of microorganisms are capable of elaborating toxins that produce a secretory diarrhea by perturbing mucosal cell electrolyte and water flux. The toxin of *Vibrio cholerae,* for example, has become an important tool for elucidation of biochemical mechanisms regulating cyclic adenosine monophosphate (cAMP)-dependent chloride efflux. Overgrowth of the indigenous bacterial population in the small intestine may also produce malabsorption, most notably of fats and vitamin B_{12} (73). Another mechanism of toxicity mediated by intestinal microorganisms is an indirect one. The bacterial population is capable of catalyzing numerous chemical reactions that can alter the biologic activity of xenobiotics, which reach the more distal portions of the gut (40). Many examples exist of bacterial activation of chemicals to a form that exerts toxicity in the gut. A classic case is that of cycasin, a β-glucoside of methylazoxymethanol (MAM), which is contained in nuts of cycad plants (77). The β-glucosidase activity of indigenous bacteria cleaves the sugar

moiety and releases MAM, which is mutagenic and causes tumor formation in the colon, liver, and kidney (64).

Methods for Toxin Studies

A conventional technique for assessing the potential of a microorganism to perturb electrolyte and water flux in the gut is use of the rabbit ileal segment. Toxins of bacteria, e.g., *V. cholerae* and *E. coli,* that produce diarrhea in humans and experimental animals, cause fluid accumulation when injected into a closed segment of the small intestine. This technique provides a simple experimental approach for identifying the potential of a toxin for inducing intestinal secretory activity and estimating its potency (60). Young (12–24 week old) rabbits are fasted for 24 hr. The ileum, which is more sensitive and gives more consistent results than jejunum, is tied into three or four closed segments each 3 inches long. Segments are separated by 6 inches. Cultures or supernatants are injected into the segment with a 22-gauge needle. The animal is allowed to recover from anesthesia. Fluid distention is observable after 4 hr in cholera-toxin injected segments and does not occur in control segments (36). The experimenter can distinguish between toxicity induced by an exotoxin from that resulting from bacterial invasion of the mucosa. Cell-free preparations of bacterial suspensions, produced by selective filtration or by sonication and cell lysis, produce secretory responses in the ileal segment if an enterotoxin is produced but not if bacterial invasion of the mucosa is a prerequisite. For an elegant example of the experimental methodology useful in determining the etiology and basic mechanism of bacterially induced diarrhea, the reader should refer to Dupont et al. (31). Biochemical approaches that have permitted elucidation of the intestinal mucosal surface receptors for enterotoxins and their mechanism of activating chloride secretion by elevating mucosal adenylate cyclase are discussed by Fishman (34) and Moss and Vaughan (79).

Methods for Bacterial Metabolism Studies

An experimental approach for assessing the role of intestinal bacteria in mediating gastrointestinal or systemic toxicity is the use of germfree animals. Rats, for example, that have been aseptically delivered by cesarean section and reared under germfree conditions are available from animal suppliers. Procedures required for establishing and maintaining a germfree animal colony are described by Foster (37). To test whether bacteria are responsible for metabolic alteration of a compound, comparison can be made of its urinary and fecal elimination in germfree and conventional animals of the same strain. A difference in the composition of the metabolites of the compound in the urine or feces may suggest participation of bacterially mediated reactions in the biotransformation process. Absence of a particular metabolite of an administered compound in urine or feces from the germfree animal is presumptive evidence that the reaction is only catalyzed by bacterial and not mammalian enzymes.

Support for such a hypothesis can be obtained by examining the *in vitro* metabolic capability of defined bacterial cultures or of homogenates of the luminal gut contents. In experiments of this type, the culture conditions can markedly affect the experimental outcome. With studies of large intestinal contents or bacterial isolates from this source, it is especially important to carry out experiments using anaerobic conditions because the majority of organisms from this site are obligate anaerobes that are highly sensitive to even brief exposure to aerobic conditions. Demonstration of a particular enzymatic activity in a bacterial strain *in vitro* provides additional evidence of a possible bacterial role. However, it has frequently been difficult to predict *in vivo* routes of intestinal metabolism from *in vitro* studies. One possible reason for discrepancies of this type is offered by the work of Tasich and Piper (126). Their studies demonstrate a synergistic interaction between an extract from *Bacteroides fragilis,* which populates the distal intestine, and the microsomal enzyme activity of the colonic mucosa. Each component alone had minimal capacity to transform 2-aminoanthracene into a mutagen (with respect to a *Salmonella* tester strain). However, in combination, a substantial increase in mutagen formation occurred. The mechanism of this activating effect of a heat-labile component of the bacteria on the colonic microsomes is not known. This observation illustrates the complexity of interaction between bacteria, intestinal tissue, and xenobiotics and the potential limitations of *in vitro* studies.

ASSESSMENT OF THE PROPULSIVE FUNCTION OF THE GASTROINTESTINAL TRACT

A potential toxic effect of substances on the gastrointestinal tract is derangement of the propulsive function of this organ. Normal propulsion of the intraluminal contents of the gut is essential for the appropriate digestion of dietary constituents, delivery to their sites of absorption, and elimination of unabsorbed materials. There are numerous factors that influence the propulsive function of the gut and consequently many mechanisms by which substances can interfere with this aspect of gut physiology. For coverage of this subject, the reader should consult the reviews of Hunt (54), Weisbrodt (144), Mathias and Sninsky (74), and Christensen (18).

Methods used in the analysis of gastrointestinal propulsive function are of several types. One approach entails study of the transit of unabsorbable marker substances, the most direct approach for assessment of changes in propulsion (11,23). Other techniques involve analysis of the pressure in the gut lumen with a variety of devices used in the monitoring of pressure changes (23). More direct analysis of the properties of the smooth muscle of the gut is achieved by quantitation of its contractile activity (7) or its electrical activity (6,123), which may be determined *in vivo* or *in vitro*. The choice of the most suitable approach depends on the goal of the experimentation, a subject well-reviewed by Bass and Wiley (7) and Connell (23).

Measurement of the Transit of Luminal Contents

The propulsive activity of the gastrointestinal tract is readily assessed by monitoring the transit of a nonabsorbable intraluminal marker. Flow of the gut contents is influenced by a variety of factors, a critical one being the contractile activity of the gastrointestinal circular and longitudinal smooth muscle. Substances affecting the resting tone or frequency of contraction of the smooth muscle would therefore be expected to affect the transit characteristics. A second important factor that affects transit is the volume and viscosity of the intraluminal content. Flow can therefore also be altered by substances that act on mucosal cells of the gut and alter their absorptive and secretory activities. This technique can therefore serve as an effective screening device for substances that affect the gastrointestinal tract by numerous mechanisms.

The application of this method requires the choice of a valid marker. Among the initial characteristics of the ideal marker are lack of absorption from the gut, minimal adsorption onto the mucosal surface, lack of effect on gut function, and ease of precise quantitation. An additional consideration is the physical form of the marker. This factor is especially relevant to the study of gastric emptying, in which it has been shown that the contractile activity of the stomach has differing effects on solid as compared to liquid components of the stomach contents (65). Suitable markers for tracing the flow of substances in solution include sodium chromate, labeled with Cr^{51}, and polyvinyl pyrollidine, labeled with I^{125} or I^{131} (44). Markers used for solid components of the diet include ^{99m}technitium, incorporated into a chicken liver meal (65). The use of gamma-emitting radioisotopes has the advantage of allowing assay of the gastrointestinal segment and contents directly without any processing of the sample. The composition and volume of the solution or test meal containing a marker must be strictly controlled to minimize potential variability from this source. The composition of the solution used by Summers et al. (119), for example, consisted of 0.1 M Krebs phosphate buffer (pH 7.4) containing 100 mg glucose, 2.0 mg polyethylene glycol, 0.5 mg phenol red, and 100 μCi of Cr^{51} as Na_2CrO_4 per 100 ml of solution. For studies with 200- to 300-g rats, 1 ml of this solution is administered intragastrically or 0.5 ml intraduodenally.

A second critical factor in carrying out a transit study is the method of administering the marker. If the marker is administered by gastric intubation, the transit of the marker will be markedly affected by stomach emptying. If the experimenter is more interested in propulsion through the small intestine, the marker should be directly administered into the duodenum via an indwelling cannula. This technique avoids use of anesthesia or acute duodenal intubations, both of which would be expected to affect gastrointestinal contractility. The method (119) entails anesthetizing the animal and making a midline incision. A no. 15 spinal needle is then inserted through the back of the neck and fed subcutaneously to a ventral site where it is passed through the abdominal muscles and forestomach into the duodenum. PE 50 polyethylene tubing is then threaded through the needle and held in the duodenum as the needle is removed. The stomach is sutured to the abdominal wall at the site where the tubing has passed. A blunt 22-gauge needle is placed in the tubing opening at the back of the neck and sutured to the skin. Animals are used in transit studies 5 days later. The marker is injected at the neck and then flushed with air in a volume equivalent to the dead space of the tubing. A similar procedure has been described by Stewart et al. (117), using cannulation directly through the duodenal wall.

A third variable in this methodology is the procedure for quantitation of the location of the marker in the gastrointestinal tract. The animal should be rapidly anesthetized or killed for removal of the gut. A report by Scott and Summers (102) indicated that no major differences are observed in transit patterns after use of various procedures for rapid sacrifice of the animal. A technique should then be used to prevent movement of the marker in the gut before its assay. One approach, for example, is to put ligatures at 3- to 5-cm lengths of the small intestine. The number of tied segments created will, of course, depend on the length of the intestinal region to be individually assayed for marker content. The technique introduced by Derblom et al. (28) permits detection of radioactivity along the continuous length of the gastrointestinal tract. The gut is placed on a device that is moved at a constant rate under a scintillation detector, and radioactive counts are continuously recorded. Integration of the radioactive counts in a particular region, either instrumentally or by planimeter, then permits reporting of marker content as a percentage of the total amount detected. One commonly used approach is to describe the small intestinal radioactivity for 10 equal segments. Without equipment for continuous recording, the gut can be cut into segments that are individually counted in a conventional well-type gamma counter (117,141). Care must be taken, however, that the marker is not lost in the process of cutting the segments.

Several procedures have been used for summarizing data on marker distribution in order to facilitate comparisons among treatments. In studies of gastric emptying, the percent of the marker remaining in the stomach is calculated, and the mean for control animals is compared to those in the experimental group by appropriate statistical methods. In studies of intestinal transit, one approach is to identify the most distal site that 50% of the marker has reached. This site can then be expressed as a percent of the total distance of the small intestine, a value that is then used in statistical analyses. Another approach is to compute the geometric center of marker distribution (78). For each segment assayed, the marker content is determined, as a percent of the total recovered, and is multiplied by the segment number, 1 being the most proximal and n being the nth and most distal. These values are summed and divided by n to generate the geometric center.

Several additional points should be noted about the experimental design of a transit study. First of all, the time at which the animal is sacrificed should be chosen so that in control animals, half the marker has been emptied from the stomach or has traversed to the midpoint of the small intestine after gastric or intraduodenal administration, respectively. This approach improves the likelihood of demonstrating inhibition or acceleration of transit by test substances. Second, in an investigation of the effect of a substance on gastrointestinal transit, studies should be carried out at a series of times after various doses of the test substance. Because each animal provides only one measure of marker distribution, each experimental condition requires use of replicate animals.

Measurement of Contractility of Gastrointestinal Smooth Muscle *In Vitro*

Introduction

The contractile properties of gastrointestinal smooth muscle can be assessed with relative simplicity using *in vitro* preparations of this organ. Such *in vitro* techniques are of value in screening potentially toxic substances for effects on gastrointestinal smooth muscle and for elucidation of mechanisms of effects on propulsion observed with *in vivo* methodology. Use of *in vitro* techniques to study gastrointestinal motility has certain advantages over *in vivo* procedures. Generally, they are technically simpler to execute. They isolate the tissue from extrinsic neural and hormonal influences. The tissue can also be directly exposed to the test substance. These advantages are at the expense of loss of prediction of *in vivo* effects of a test substance (144).

The choice of a particular *in vitro* technique depends on the specific aim of the experimentation. Those techniques that are most commonly used differ in several ways. For one, the species from which the gut segment is taken markedly affect the basal contractile activity. The rabbit jejunum, for example, maintains rhythmic contractions *in vitro* (114) and is therefore especially useful for analysis of substances suspected of having inhibitory effects on gastrointestinal smooth muscle. The guinea pig ileum, in contrast, exhibits little spontaneous activity *in vitro*. This preparation is widely used, therefore, primarily in the bioassay of agents causing contraction of intestinal smooth muscle. To test for depressant effects, the investigator must induce contraction of this tissue with electrical stimulation, potassium depolarization, or pharmacologic agonists. Second, there are differences in the responses of gastrointestinal smooth muscle depending on the site of the gut under investigation. This limits the ability of the investigator to generalize from an experiment carried out with a muscle preparation from a single region of the gut and reinforces the importance of strictly controlling the tissue region studied in a series of experiments.

A recent advance in the *in vitro* study of gastrointestinal smooth muscle has been the isolation of myocytes and measurement of contractile events of single cells (9). This approach permits evaluation of the direct effects of chemicals on these cells in isolation from their intrinsic innervation via the myenteric and submucosal plexus that exist *in situ*. The isolated myocyte preparation has facilitated elucidation of membrane receptors, ionic channels, and excitation–contraction coupling mechanisms. This approach may prove useful, as well, in toxicologic studies for precisely defining mechanisms of altered gastrointestinal propulsion.

The Guinea Pig Ileum Preparation

Use of the guinea pig ileum preparation will be described in detail. This tissue has been extensively used in the study of the effects of chemicals on gut contractility (114). The guinea pig is killed by a blow on the head because use of drugs could alter responsivity of smooth muscles. The ileum is readily identified by locating the cecum to which the distal end is attached. Segments should be cut from the distal ileum, with care taken to avoid damaging the muscle layers with forceps. The location and length of these segments should be standardized in an experimental series; commonly, 1-cm segments are used, avoiding use of the most distal 10 cm of the ileum. The mesentery should be cut away from the gut segment, which is then placed in Tyrode's solution at 37°C. Once relaxed, the tissue should be gently flushed with solution at 37°C to remove the intraluminal contents. One approach is to insert a pipette filled with solution and raise the head by 1 to 2 cm. (The segment will maintain its viability for several hours if held in Tyrode's solution at just below 20°C.) Threads are then secured to the proximal and distal end of the segment without occluding the lumen. For studies in a single muscle type, the longitudinal muscle layer is readily dissected from the ileal segment (140). When obtained from the guinea pig, this tissue retains the myenteric plexus and is therefore useful for study of agents that affect neuronal conduction or neurotransmitter release, as well as smooth muscle contractility. The tissue is mounted with the proximal end up, in an organ bath containing Tyrode's solution, e.g., 25 ml, which is maintained at 37°C and gassed with 95% O_2 and 5% CO_2. The thread tied to the proximal end of the tissue is attached to a device for quantitating the contractile response of the tissue. Commonly, this apparatus consists of a Statham force-displacement transducer connected to an amplifier and chart recorder permitting continuous monitoring of response under isometric conditions.

Before attaching tissue, the instrumentation is calibrated by hanging weights on the transducer and generating a standard curve, relating weight to the height of pen deflection. Initially, tension, e.g., 1.0 g, should be applied to the tissue followed by an equilibration period, e.g., 30 min, before addition of test substances to the bath. The tension applied to the muscle should be chosen to stretch the tissue to a length that results in the greatest generated force on activation. This length, referred to as the optimum length, is determined by measuring the difference between passive and active tension for different lengths of the muscle with a maximally effective stimulus such as high potassium (110 mm)-induced depolarization (48). To reduce the contribution of spontaneous contractile activity and tone to "passive" tension, which may be confounding with intestinal muscle from some species, force-length relationships can be examined at low temperature (22°C), which minimizes this factor (42).

Modifications of this technique include electrical stimulation of the tissue and application of intraluminal pressure for eliciting peristaltic reflexes (137). The parameters chosen for electric stimulation of tissue determine the mechanism and characteristics of the contractile response. For electric field stimulation, muscle is hung between platinum electrodes connected to a stimulator, e.g., the Grass Model S-4. Stimuli of 1 Hz frequency for 1 msec at 100 V are likely to induce contractions mediated by neural stimulation. These contractions are sensitive to inhibition of neuronal conduction by sodium channel inactivators, e.g., tetrodotoxin (10^{-7} g/ml). Stimuli of higher frequency, e.g., 60 Hz, are likely to depolarize the muscle membrane directly, to be unaltered by tetrodotoxin, and to reflect the mechanical properties of the muscle itself.

Substances tested with this preparation should be added in a broad concentration range with washing of the tissue after each application. When a concentration of the test substance is found to cause contraction, additional concentrations should be tested to permit construction of a concentration-response curve that will facilitate analyses by use of such statistics as the EC50, the affinity, and the intrinsic activity (125). An additional consideration that may require evaluation is the development of tachyphylaxis to the test substance. This phenomenon may necessitate use of multiple tissue preparations, each exposed to only one concentration of the test substance in order to describe the dose-response relationship adequately.

REFERENCES

1. Ahlquist, D. A., McGill, D. B., Schwartz, S., Taylor, W. F., and Owen, R. A. (1985): Fecal blood levels in health and disease. A study using hemoQuant. *N. Engl. J. Med.*, 312:1422–1428.
2. Allen, A., Flemstrom, G., Garner, A., Silen, W., and Turnberg, L. A. (eds.) (1984): *Mechanisms of Mucosal Protection in the Upper Gastrointestinal Tract.* Raven Press, New York.
3. Andrews, J. S., and Oliver-Gonzalez, J. (1942): The quantitative determination of blood in human feces. *J. Lab. Clin. Med.*, 27: 1212–1217.
4. Autrup, H. (1980): Explant culture of human colon. In: *Methods in Cell Biology,* edited by C. C. Harris, B. F. Trump, and G. D. Stoner, pp. 385–401. Academic Press, London.
5. Barr, W. H., and Riegelman, S. (1970): Intestinal drug absorption and metabolism. I. Comparison of methods and models to study physiologic factors of *in vitro* and *in vivo* intestinal absorption. *J. Pharm. Sci.*, 59:154–163.
6. Bass, P. (1968): *In vivo* electrical activity of the small bowel. In: *Handbook of Physiology, Sect. 6; Alimentary Canal, Vol. IV., Motility,* edited by C. F. Code, pp. 2051–2076. Am. Physiol. Soc., Washington, DC.
7. Bass, P., and Wiley, J. N. (1972): Contractile force transducer for recording muscle activity in unanesthetized animals. *J. Appl. Physiol.*, 32:567–570.
8. Besch, E. L., and Chou, B. J. (1971): Physiological responses to blood collection methods in rats. *Proc. Soc. Exp. Biol. Med.*, 138: 1019–1021.
9. Bitar, K. N., and Makhlouf, G. M. (1982): Receptors on smooth muscle cells: characterization by contraction and specific antagonists. *Am. J. Physiol.*, 242(4):G400–G407.
10. Bivin, W. S., Crawford, M. P., and Brewer, N. R. (1979): Morphophysiology. In: *The Laboratory Rat, Vol. I: Biology and Diseases,* edited by H. J. Baker, J. R. Lindsey, and S. H. Weisbroth, pp. 77–83. Academic Press, New York.
11. Branch, W. J., and Cummings, J. H. (1978): Comparison of radioopaque pellets and chromium sesquioxide as inert markers in studies requiring accurate fecal collections. *Gut*, 19(5):371–376.
12. Brodie, D. A., Cook, P. G., Bauer, B. J., and Dagle, G. E. (1970): Indomethacin-induced intestinal lesions in the rat. *Toxicol. Appl. Pharmacol.*, 17:615–624.
13. Brodie, D. A., Tate, C. L., and Hooke, K. F. (1970): Aspirin: intestinal damage in rats. *Science,* 170:183–185.
14. Brown, J. P. (1977): Role of gut bacterial flora in nutrition and health: a review of recent advances in bacteriological techniques, metabolism, and factors affecting flora composition. *CRC Crit. Rev. Food Sci. Nutr.*, 8(3):229–336.
15. Cairnie, A. B., Lamerton, L. F., and Steel, G. G. (1965): Cell proliferation studies in the intestinal epithelium of the rat. I. Determination of the kinetic parameters. *Exp. Cell Res.*, 39:528–538.
16. Cheng, H., and Bjerknes, M. (1982): Whole population cell kinetics of mouse duodenal, jejunal, ileal and colonic epithelia as determined by radioautography and flow cytometry. *Anat. Rec.*, 203:251–264.
17. Cheng, H., Bjerknes, M., and Amar, J. (1984): Methods for the

determination of epithelial cell kinetic parameters of human colonic epithelium isolated from surgical and biopsy specimens. *Gastroenterology,* 86:78–85.

18. Christensen, J. (1987): Motility of the colon. In: *Physiology of the Gastrointestinal Tract,* vol. 1, edited by L. R. Johnson, pp. 665–694. Raven Press, New York.

19. Clark, S. B., and Tercyak, A. (1984): Reduced cholesterol transmucosal transport in rats with inhibited mucosal acyl CoA:cholesterol acyltransferase and normal pancreatic function. *J. Lipid Res.,* 25:148–159.

20. Clarke, R. T. J., and Bauchop, T. (1977): *Microbial Ecology of the Gut.* Academic Press, New York.

21. Coates, M. E. (ed.) (1968): *The Germfree Animal in Research.* Academic Press, New York.

22. Cohen, M. M., Cheung, G., and Lyster, D. M. (1980): Prevention of aspirin-induced faecal blood loss by prostaglandin E$_2$. *Gut,* 21:602–606.

23. Connell, A. M. (1971): Methodology of investigations of alimentary motility. In: *Gastrointestinal Motility,* edited by L. Demling and R. Ottenjann. Academic Press, New York.

24. Crane, R. K., and Mandelstam, P. (1960): The active transport of sugars by various preparations of hamster intestine. *Biochim. Biophys. Acta,* 45:460–476.

25. Crane, R. K., and Wilson, T. H. (1958): *In vitro* method for the study of the rate of intestinal absorption of sugars. *J. Appl. Physiol.,* 12:145–146.

26. Dahlqvist, A. (1968): Assay of intestinal disaccharidases. *Analytical Biochem.,* 22:99–107.

27. Dahlqvist, A., and Nordstrom, C. (1966): The distribution of disaccharidase activities in the villi and crypts of the small-intestinal mucosa. *Biochim. Biophys. Acta,* 113:624–626.

28. Derblom, H., Johansson, H., and Nylander, G. (1966): A simple method of recording quantitatively certain gastrointestinal motility functions in the rat. *Acta Clin. Scand.,* 132:154–165.

29. Dickens, F., and Weil-Malherbe, H. (1941): Metabolism of normal and tumor tissue. The metabolism of intestinal mucous membrane. *Biochem. J.,* 35:7–15.

30. Douglas, A. P., Kerley, R., and Isselbacher, K. J. (1972): Preparation and characterization of the lateral and basal plasma membranes of the rat intestinal epithelial cell. *Biochem. J.,* 128:1329–1338.

31. DuPont, H. L., Formal, S. B., Hornick, R. B., Snyder, M. J., Libonati, J. P., Sheahan, D. G., LaBrec, E. H., and Kaias, J. P. (1971): Pathogenesis of *Escherichia coli* diarrhea. *N. Engl. J. Med.,* 285:1–9.

32. Eastwood, G. L. (1981): Epithelial renewal in gastrointestinal mucosal injury. In: *Basic Mechanisms of Gastrointestinal Mucosal Cell Injury and Protection,* edited by J. W. Harmon, pp. 49–66. Williams and Wilkins, Baltimore.

33. Ellefson, R. D., and Caraway, W. T. (1976): Lipids and lipoproteins. In: *Fundamentals of Clinical Chemistry,* edited by N. Tietz, pp. 474–541. W. B. Saunders, Philadelphia.

34. Fishman, P. H. (1980): Mechanism of action of cholera toxin: events on the cell surface. In: *Secretory Diarrhea,* edited by M. Field, J. S. Fordtran, and S. G. Schultz, pp. 85–106. Am. Physiol. Soc., Bethesda, MD.

35. Fordtran, J. S., Rector, F. C. Jr., Ewton, M. F., Soter, N., and Kinney, J. (1965): Permeability characteristics of the human small intestine. *J. Clin. Invest.,* 44:1935–1944.

36. Formal, S. B., Kundel, D., and Schneider, H. (1961): Studies with *Vibrio cholerae* in the ligated loop of the rabbit intestine. *Br. J. Exp. Pathol.,* 42:504–510.

37. Foster, H. L. (1980): Gnotobiology. In: *The Laboratory Rat, Vol. II: Research Applications,* edited by H. J. Baker, J. R. Lindsey, and S. H. Weisbroth, pp. 43–57. Academic Press, New York.

38. Gibaldi, M., Boyes, R. N., and Feldman, S. (1971): Influence of first-pass effect on availability of drugs on oral administration. *J. Pharm. Sci.,* 60:1338–1340.

39. Gibaldi, M., and Grundhofer, B. (1972): Drug transport VI: functional integrity of the rat everted small intestine with respect to passive transfer. *J. Pharm. Sci.,* 61:116–119.

40. Goldman, P. (1978): Biochemical pharmacology of the intestinal flora. *Ann. Rev. Pharmacol. Toxicol.,* 18:523–539.

41. Goldstein, F., Karacadag, S., Wirts, C. W., and Kowlessar, O. D.

(1970): Intraluminal small-intestinal utilization of *d*-xylose by bacteria. A limitation of the *d*-xylose absorption test. *Gastroenterology,* 59:380–386.

42. Gordon, A. R., and Siegman, M. J. (1971): Mechanical properties of smooth muscle. I. Length-tension and force-velocity relations. *Am. J. Physiol.,* 221:1243–1249.

43. Gray, G. (1981): Carbohydrate absorption and malabsorption. In: *Physiology of the Gastrointestinal Tract,* edited by L. R. Johnson, pp. 1063–1072. Raven Press, New York.

44. Gustavsson, S., Jung, B., and Nelsson, F. (1977): Simultaneous measurement of the propulsion and mixing of small bowel contents in the rat. *Acta Clin. Scand.,* 143(6):359–364.

45. Harmon, J. W. (ed.) (1981): *Basic Mechanisms of Gastrointestinal Mucosal Cell Injury and Protection.* Williams and Wilkins, Baltimore.

46. Harrison, D. D., and Webster, H. L. (1969): The preparation of isolated intestinal crypt cells. *Exptl. Cell Res.,* 55:257–260.

47. Hartiala, K. (1977): Metabolism of foreign substances in the gastrointestinal tract. In: *Handbook of Physiology, Section 9: Reactions to Environmental Agents,* edited by D. H. K. Lee, H. L. Falk, S. D. Murphy, and S. R. Geiger, pp. 375–388. Am. Physiol. Soc., Bethesda, MD.

48. Herlihy, J. T., and Murphy, R. A. (1973): Length-tension relationship of smooth muscle of the hog carotid artery. *Circ. Res.,* 33:275–283.

49. Hohenleitner, F. J., and Senior, J. R. (1969): Metabolism of canine small intestine vascularly perfused *in vitro. J. Appl. Physiol.,* 26:119–128.

50. Holt, P. R., and Koss, L. G. (1984): Flow cytometry—biologic and clinical application of a powerful methodology (editorial). *Gastroenterology,* 86:196–198.

51. Hopfer, U. (1977): Isolated membrane vesicles as tools for analysis of epithelial transport. *Am. J. Physiol.,* 233(2):E445–E449.

52. Hopfer, U., Sigrist-Nelson, K., and Murer, H. (1975): Intestinal sugar transport: studies with isolated plasma membranes. *Ann. N.Y. Acad. Sci.,* 264:414–427.

53. Howdle, P. D. (1984): Organ culture of gastrointestinal mucosa. *Postgrad. Med. J.,* 60:645–652.

54. Hunt, J. N. (1983): Mechanisms and disorders of gastric emptying. *Ann. Rev. Med.,* 34:219–229.

55. Hurst, B. C., Rees, W. D. W., and Garner, A. (1984): Cell shedding by the stomach and duodenum. In: *Mechanisms of Mucosal Protection in the Upper Gastrointestinal Tract,* edited by A. Allen, G. Flemstrom, A. Garner, W. Silen, and L. A. Turnberg, pp. 21–26. Raven Press, New York.

56. Imondi, A. R., Balis, M. E., and Lipkin, M. (1969): Changes in enzyme levels accompanying differentiation of intestinal epithelial cells. *Exp. Cell Res.,* 58:323–330.

57. Irons, G. V. Jr., and Kirsner, J. B. (1965): Routine chemical tests of the stool for occult blood: an evaluation. *Am. J. Med. Sci.,* 249:247–260.

58. Israili, Z. H., and Dayton, P. G. (1984): Enhancement of xenobiotic elimination: role of intestinal excretion. *Drug Metab. Rev.,* 15:1123–1159.

59. Jacobson, E. D., Bondy, D. C., Broitman, S. A., and Fordtran, J. S. (1963): Validity of polyethylene glycol in estimating intestinal water volume. *Gastroenterology,* 44:761–767.

60. Jenkin, C. R., and Rowley, D. (1959): Possible factors in the pathogenesis of cholera. *Br. J. Exp. Pathol.,* 40:474–481.

61. Johnson, L. R. (ed.) (1987): *Physiology of the Gastrointestinal Tract,* vols. 1 and 2. Raven Press, New York.

62. Kessler, M., Acuto, O., Storelli, C., Murer, H., Muller, M., and Semenza, G. (1978): A modified procedure for the rapid preparation of efficiently transporting vesicles from small intestinal brush border membranes. *Biochim. Biophys. Acta,* 506:136–154.

63. Kimmich, G. A. (1981): Intestinal absorption of sugar. In: *Physiology of the Gastrointestinal Tract,* vol. 2, edited by L. R. Johnson, pp. 1035–1062. Raven Press, New York.

64. Laqueur, G. L., McDaniel, E. G., and Matsumoto, H. (1967): Tumor induction in germfree rats with methylazoxymethanol (MAM) and synthetic MAM acetate. *J. Natl. Cancer Inst.,* 39:355–371.

65. Lavigne, M. E., Wiley, Z. D., Meyer, J. H., Martin, P., and

MacGregor, I. L. (1978): Gastric emptying rates of solid food in relation to body size. *Gastroenterology, 74*:1258–1260.

66. Leonards, J. R. (1963): Aspirin and gastrointestinal blood loss. *Gastroenterology, 44*:617–619.

67. Levine, P. H., and Weintraub, L. R. (1970): Preparation of suspensions of small bowel mucosal epithelial cells. *J. Lab. Clin. Med., 75*:1026–1029.

68. Levine, R. R., McNary, W. F., Kornguth, P. J., and LeBlanc, R. (1970): Histological reevaluation of everted gut technique for studying intestinal absorption. *Eur. J. Pharmacol., 9*:211–219.

69. Lewis, L. D., and Fordtran, J. S. (1975): Effect of perfusion rate on absorption, surface area, unstirred water layer thickness, permeability, and intraluminal pressure in the rat ileum *in vivo. Gastroenterology, 68*:1509–1516.

70. Lipkin, M. (1987): Proliferation and differentiation of normal and diseased gastrointestinal cells. In: *Physiology of the Gastrointestinal Tract*, vol. 1, edited by L. R. Johnson, pp. 145–168. Raven Press, New York.

71. Lipkin, M. (1985): Growth and development of gastrointestinal cells. *Ann. Rev. Physiol., 47*:175–197.

72. Lipsky, M. H., and Berkley, S. (1977): Prolonged biliary fistulization in the rat without interruption of the enterohepatic cycle. *J. Surg. Res., 22*(1):65–68.

73. Mathias, J. R., and Clench, M. H. (1985): Review: pathophysiology of diarrhea caused by bacterial overgrowth of the small intestine. *Am. J. Med. Sci., 289*:243–248.

74. Mathias, J. R., and Sninsky, C. A. (1985): Motility of the small intestine: a look ahead. *Am. J. Physiol., 248*:G495–G500.

75. Mayer, R. M., Treadwell, C. R., Gallo, L. L., and Vahouny, G. V. (1985): Intestinal mucins and cholesterol uptake *in vitro. Biochim. Biophys. Acta, 833*:34–43.

76. *Med. Lett.* 28:5–6, (1986): Tests for occult blood.

77. Mickelsen, O. (1972): Introductory remarks, symposium on cycads. *Fed. Proc., 31*:1465–1546.

78. Miller, M. S., Galligan, J. J., and Burks, T. F. (1981): Accurate measurement of intestinal transit in the rat. *J. Pharmacol. Methods, 6*:211–217.

79. Moss, J., and Vaughan, M. (1980): Mechanism of activation of adenylate cyclase by choleragen and *E. coli* heat-labile enterotoxin. In: *Secretory Diarrhea*, edited by M. Field, J. S. Fordtran, and S. G. Schultz, pp. 107–126. Am. Physiol. Soc., Bethesda, MD.

80. Murer, H., Lucke, H., and Kinne, R. (1980): Isolated brush-border vesicles as a tool to study disturbances in intestinal solute transport. In: *Secretory Diarrhea*, edited by M. Field, J. S. Fordtran, and S. G. Schultz, pp. 31–43. Am. Physiol. Soc., Bethesda, MD.

81. Nakamura, W., Kankura, T., and Eto, H. (1971): Occult blood appearance in feces and tissue hemorrhages in mice after whole body x-irradiation. *Radiat. Res., 48*:169–178.

82. Parsons, D. S. (1968): Methods for investigation of intestinal absorption. In: *Handbook of Physiology, Section 6: Alimentary Canal*, vol. III, edited by C. F. Code, pp. 1177–1216. Am. Physiol. Soc., Washington, DC.

83. Pelzmann, K. S., and Havemeyer, R. N. (1971): Portal vein blood sampling in intestinal drug absorption studies. *J. Pharm. Sci., 60*:331.

84. Pfeiffer, C. J. (1977): Gastroenterologic response to environmental agents—absorption and interactions. In: *Handbook of Physiology, Section 9: Reactions to Environmental Agents*, edited by D. H. K. Lee, H. L. Falk, S. D. Murphy, and S. R. Geiger, pp. 349–374. Am. Physiol. Soc., Bethesda, MD.

85. Pfeiffer, C. J. (1985): Gastrointestinal tract. In: *Environmental Pathology*, edited by N. K. Mottet, pp. 230–247. Oxford University Press, New York.

86. Pfeiffer, C. J., and Hanninen, O. Alimentary excretion of environmental agents and unnatural compounds. In: *Handbook of Physiology, Section 9: Reactions to Environmental Agents*, edited by D. H. K. Lee, H. L. Falk, S. D. Murphy, and S. R. Geiger, pp. 513–535. Am. Physiol. Soc., Bethesda, MD.

87. Pfeiffer, C. J., Rowden, G., and Weibel, J. (1974): *Gastrointestinal Ultrastructure: An Atlas of Scanning and Transmission Electron Microscopy*. Academic Press, New York.

88. Phillips, B. M. (1973): Aspirin-induced gastrointestinal microbleeding in dogs. *Toxicol. Appl. Pharmacol., 24*:182–189.

89. Prescott, L. F., and Nimmo, W. S. (eds.) (1981): *Drug Absorption*. Adis Press, New York.

90. Reinhardt, M. C. (1984): Macromolecular absorption of food antigens in health and disease. *Ann. Allergy, 53*:597–601.

91. Rider, J. A., and Owens, F. J. (1954): Evaluation of an ortho-tolidine test (Fecatest) for determination of occult blood. *J.A.M.A., 156*:31–33.

92. Ringler, D. H., and Dabich, L. (1979): Hematology and clinical biochemistry. In: *The Laboratory Rat, Vol. 1: Biology and Disease*, edited by H. J. Baker, J. R. Lindsey, and S. H. Weisbroth, pp. 105–121. Academic Press, New York.

93. Sachs, G., and Berglindh, T. (1981): Physiology of the parietal cell. In: *Physiology of the Gastrointestinal Tract*, edited by L. R. Johnson, pp. 570–574. Raven Press, New York.

94. Salmon, G. K., and Leslie, G. B. (1985): The use of endoscopy in the induction and monitoring of gastric mucosal lesions in the rat. *The Toxicologist, 5*:9.

95. Satoh, H., Inada, I., Hirata, T., and Maki, Y. (1981): Indomethacin produces gastric antral ulcers in the refed rat. *Gastroenterology, 81*:719–725.

96. Schiller, C. M., Shoaf, C. R., and Chapman, D. E. (1984): Alteration of intestinal function by chemical exposure: animal models. In: *Intestinal Toxicology*, edited by C. M. Schiller, pp. 133–144. Raven Press, New York.

97. Schultz, S. G. (1981): Ion transport by mammalian large intestine. In: *Physiology of the Gastrointestinal Tract*, edited by L. R. Johnson, pp. 991–1002. Raven Press, New York.

98. Schultz, S. G., Curran, P. F., Chez, R. A., and Fuisz, R. E. (1967): Alanine and sodium fluxes across mucosal border of rabbit ileum. *J. Gen. Physiol., 50*:1241–1260.

99. Schultz, S. G., and Zalusky, R. (1964): Ion transport in isolated rabbit ileum. I. Short-circuit current and Na fluxes. *J. Gen. Physiol., 47*:567–584.

100. Schwabe, A. D., and Hepner, G. W. (1979): Breath tests for the detection of fat malabsorption. *Gastroenterology, 76*:216–218.

101. Schwartz, S., Dahl, J., Ellefson, M., and Ahlquist, D. A. (1983): The "HemoQuant" test: a specific and quantitative assay of heme (hemoglobin) in feces and other materials. *Clin. Chem., 29*:2061–2067.

102. Scott, L. D., and Summers, R. W. (1976): Correlation of contractions and transit in rat small intestine. *Am. J. Physiol., 230*:132–137.

103. Segal, H. L., Miller, L. L., and Plumb, E. J. (1955): Tubeless gastric analysis with an azure A ion-exchange compound. *Gastroenterology, 28*:402–408.

104. Shamsuddin, A. K. M., Barrett, L. A., Autrup, H., Harris, C. C., and Trump, B. F. (1978): Long term organ culture of adult rat colon. *Pathol. Res. Pract., 163*:362–372.

105. Sherding, R. G. (1983): Diseases of the small bowel. In: *Textbook of Veterinary Internal Medicine. Diseases of the Dog and Cat*, vol. II, edited by S. J. Ettinger, pp. 1278–1346. W. B. Saunders, Philadelphia.

106. Shiau, Y.-F., Boyle, J. T., Umstetter, C., and Koldovsky, O. (1980): Apical distribution of fatty acid esterification capacity along the villus-crypt unit of rat jejunum. *Gastroenterology, 79*:47–53.

107. Shriver, D. A., White, C. B., Sandor, A., and Rosenthale, M. E. (1975): A profile of the rat gastrointestinal toxicity of drugs used to treat inflammatory disease. *Toxicol. Appl. Pharmacol., 32*:73–83.

108. Simon, G. L., and Gorbach, S. L. (1984): Intestinal flora in health and disease. *Gastroenterology, 86*:174–193.

109. Smith, M. W. (1985): Expression of digestive and absorptive function in differentiating enterocytes. *Ann. Rev. Physiol., 47*:247–260.

110. Smithson, K. W., Millar, D. B., Jacobs, L. R., and Gray, G. M. (1981): Intestinal diffusion barrier: unstirred water layer or membrane surface mucous coat. *Science, 214*:1241–1244.

111. Soergel, K. H. (1968): Inert markers. *Gastroenterology, 54*:449–452.

112. Soll, A. H. (1980): Secretagogue stimulation of ^{14}C-aminopyrine accumulation by isolated canine parietal cells. *Am. J. Physiol., 238*:G366–G375.

113. Soll, A. H., and Berglindh, T. (1987): Physiology of isolated gastric gland and parietal cells: receptors and effectors regulating function.

In: *Physiology of the Gastrointestinal Tract,* edited by L. R. Johnson, pp. 883–909. Raven Press, New York.

114. Staff of the Department of Pharmacology, University of Edinburgh (1970): *Pharmacological Experiments on Isolated Preparations.* E. & S. Livingstone, Edinburgh.

115. Stevens, B. R., Kavnitz, J. D., and Wright, E. M. (1984): Intestinal transport of amino acids and sugars: advances using membrane vesicles. *Ann. Rev. Physiol.,* 46:417–433.

116. Stewart, J. J., Gaginella, T. S., and Bass, P. (1975): Actions of ricinoleic acid and structurally related fatty acids on the gastrointestinal tract. I. Effects on smooth muscle contractility *in vitro. J. Pharmacol. Exp. Ther.,* 195:347–354.

117. Stewart, J. J., Weisbrodt, N. W., and Burks, T. F. (1978): Central and peripheral actions of morphine on intestinal transit. *J. Pharmacol. Exp. Ther.,* 205:547–555.

118. Stroehlein, J. R., Fairbanks, V. F., McGill, D. B., and Go, V. L. W. (1976): Hemoccult detection of fecal occult blood quantitated by radioassay. *Am. J. Dig. Dis.,* 21(10):841–844.

119. Summers, R. W., Kent, T. H., and Osborne, J. W. (1970): Effects of drugs, ileal obstruction, and irradiation on rat gastrointestinal propulsion. *Gastroenterology,* 59:731–739.

120. Szabo, S. (1978): Animal model of human disease. Duodenal ulcer disease. Animal model: cysteamine-induced acute and chronic duodenal ulcer in the rat. *Am. J. Pathol.,* 93:273–276.

121. Szabo, S., Reynolds, E. S., Lichtenberger, L. M., Haith, L. R., and Dzau, V. J. (1977): Pathogenesis of duodenal ulcer. Gastric hyperacidity caused by propionitrile and cysteamine in rats. *Res. Commun. Chem. Pathol. Pharmacol.,* 16:311–323.

122. Szabo, S., Trier, J. S., Brown, A., Schnoor, J., Homan, H. D., and Bradford, J. C. (1985): A quantitative method for assessing the extent of experimental gastric erosions and ulcers. *J. Pharmacol. Methods.* 13:59–66.

123. Szurszewski, J. H. (1981): Electrophysiological basis of gastrointestinal motility. In: *Physiology of the Gastrointestinal Tract,* vol. 2, edited by L. R. Johnson, pp. 383–422. Raven Press, New York.

124. Takagi, K., and Kawashima, K. (1969): Effects of some anti-inflammatory drugs on capillary permeability of the gastric mucosa in the rat. *Jap. J. Pharmac.,* 19:431–439.

125. Tallarida, R. J., and Murray, R. B. (1981): *Manual of Pharmacologic Calculations with Computer Programs.* Springer-Verlag, New York.

126. Tasich, M., and Piper, D. W. (1983): Effect of human colonic microsomes and cell-free extracts of *Bacteroides fragilis* on the mutagenicity of 2-aminoanthracene. *Gastroenterology,* 85:30–34.

127. Thomson, A. B. R., and Dietschy, J. M. (1981): Intestinal lipid absorption: major extracellular and intracellular events. In: *Physiology of the Gastrointestinal Tract,* vol. 2, edited by L. R. Johnson, pp. 1147–1220. Raven Press, New York.

128. Thomson, A. B. R., and O'Brien, B. D. (1980): Uptake of homologous series of saturated fatty acids into rabbit intestine using three *in vitro* techniques. *Dig. Dis. Sci.,* 25:209–215.

129. Tietz, N. W. (1976): Gastric, pancreatic, and intestinal function. In: *Fundamentals of Clinical Chemistry,* edited by N. W. Tietz, pp. 1063–1099. W. B. Saunders, Philadelphia.

130. Toskes, P. P., King, C. E., Spivey, J. C., and Lorenz, E. (1978): Xylose catabolism in the experimental rat blind loop syndrome. Studies, including use of a newly developed *d*-[^{14}C]xylose breath test. *Gastroenterology,* 74:691–697.

131. Towler, C. M., Pugh-Humphreys, G. P., and Porteous, J. W. (1978):

132. Trier, J. S. (1971): Diagnostic value of peroral biopsy of the proximal small intestine. *N. Engl. J. Med.,* 285:1470–1473.

133. Trier, J. S. (1976): Organ-culture methods in the study of gastrointestinal-mucosal function and development. *N. Engl. J. Med.,* 295: 150–155.

134. Trier, J. S., and Madara, J. L. (1981): Functional morphology of the mucosa of the small intestine. In: *Physiology of the Gastrointestinal Tract,* vol. 2, edited by L. R. Johnson, pp. 925–962. Raven Press, New York.

135. Ussing, H. H., and Zerahn, K. (1951): Active transport of sodium as the source of electric current in the short-circuited isolated frog skin. *Acta Physiol. Scand.,* 23:110–127.

136. Van Harken, D. R., and Hottendorf, G. H. (1978): Comparative absorption following the administration of a drug to rats by oral gavage and incorporation in the diet. *Toxicol. Appl. Pharmacol.,* 43(2):407–410.

137. Van Nueten, J. M., Geivers, H., Fontaine, J., and Janssen, P. A. J. (1973): An improved method for studying peristalsis in the isolated guinea-pig ileum. *Arch. Int. Pharmacodyn.,* 203:411–414.

138. Wagner, J. G. (1975): *Fundamentals of Clinical Pharmacokinetics.* Drug Intelligence Publications, Inc., Hamilton, IL.

139. Walsh, C. T. (1982): The influence of age on the gastrointestinal absorption of mercuric chloride and methyl mercury chloride in the rat. *Environ. Res.,* 27:412–420.

140. Walsh, C. T., and Harnett, K. M. (1986): Inhibitory effect of lead acetate on contractility of longitudinal smooth muscle from rat ileum. *Toxicol. Appl. Pharmacol.,* 83:62–68.

141. Walsh, C. T., and Ryden, E. B. (1984): The effect of chronic ingestion of lead on gastrointestinal transit in rats. *Toxicol. Appl. Pharmacol.,* 75:485–495.

142. Warrick, M. W., and Lin, T.-M. (1977): Action of glucagon and aspirin on ionic flux, mucosal blood flow and bleeding in the fundic pouch of dogs. *Res. Commun. Chem. Pathol. Pharmacol.,* 16:325–335.

143. Welsh, M. J., Smith, P. L., Fromm, N., and Frizzell, R. A. (1982): Crypts are the site of intestinal fluid and electrolyte secretion. *Science,* 218:1219–1221.

144. Weisbrodt, N. W. (1987): Motility of the small intestine. In: *Physiology of the Gastrointestinal Tract,* vol. 1, edited by L. R. Johnson, pp. 631–664. Raven Press, New York.

145. Whitehead, R. (1979): *Mucosal Biopsy of the Gastrointestinal Tract,* 2d ed. W. B. Saunders, Philadelphia.

146. Wilson, T. H., and Wiseman, G. (1954): The use of sacs of everted small intestine for the study of the transference of substances from the mucosal to the serosal surface. *J. Physiol. (Lond.),* 123:116–125.

147. Winawer, S. J. (1976): Fecal occult blood testing. *Am. J. Dig. Dis.,* 21:885–888.

148. Winne, D. (1977): The influence of unstirred layers on intestinal absorption. In: *Intestinal Permeation,* Workshop Conferences, Hoechst, vol. 4., edited by M. Kramer and F. Lauterbach, pp. 58–64. International Congress Series, No. 391, Excerpta Medica, Amsterdam.

149. Wolfe, D. L., Forland, S. C., and Benet, L. Z. (1973): Drug transfer across intact rat intestinal mucosa following surgical removal of serosa and muscularis externa. *J. Pharm. Sci.,* 62:200–205.

Characterization of columnar absorptive epithelial cells isolated from rat jejunum. *J. Cell. Sci.,* 29:53–75.

Principles and Methods of Toxicology, Second Edition, edited by A. Wallace Hayes, Raven Press, Ltd., New York © 1989.

CHAPTER 24

Hormone Assays and Endocrine Function

John A. Thomas, *Michael J. Thomas, and *Dori J. Thomas

*Department of Pharmacology, University of Texas Health Science Center, San Antonio, Texas 78284; and *Department of Pharmacology and Toxicology, West Virginia University Medical Center, Morgantown, West Virginia 26506*

Pituitary Gland
Pituitary–Target Organ Relations • Adenohypophysis
Biochemical Assessments
Bioassay • Radioimmunoassay • Monoclonal Antibodies
Measurement of Anterior Pituitary Hormones
Adrenocorticotropin • Thyroid-Stimulating Hormone • Growth Hormone (Somatotropin) • Gonadotropins • Inhibin • Prolactin
Posterior Pituitary Hormones
Neurohypophyseal Peptides • Oxytocins • Vasopressin (Antidiuretic Hormone)
Thyroid Gland
Measurement of Thyroid Hormones

Parathyroid Gland
Adrenal Gland
Measurement of Corticoids • Plasma or Urinary Corticosteroids
Gonads
Male Hormones (Androgens) • Female Hormones (Estrogens)
Pancreas
Measurement of Insulin • Glucose Tolerance Tests • Cytological Evaluation of Pancreatic Islet Cells
Acknowledgments
References

Endocrine toxicology involves the study of chemicals and drugs that perturb the body's balance of hormonal secretions. Such chemicals and drugs can increase or decrease the secretory activity of various endocrine organs. Endocrine toxicology is not confined to the reproductive system, as nonsex hormones can also be altered by exogenous chemicals. In some instances a chemical interferes with a hormone's catabolism by a nonendocrine organ (e.g., liver, kidney) and results in secretory imbalances within the endocrine system itself. By some definitions, endocrine toxicology includes areas of teratology and neonatology. For example, some hormonal oral contraceptives not only suppress ovulation, they also produce virilizing side effects in the fetus. Reproductive toxicology (see Ch. 4) and teratology (see Ch. 5) are considered as separate topics, although they can be included under the larger umbrella of endocrine toxicology. Endocrine pharmacology, a discipline that involves the therapeutic and diagnostic use of hormones and other nonhormonally related agents, can also encompass a toxicologic component, as many of these medicinal products possess side effects that alter the biochemical activity or organs of internal secretion (98,128,136).

Although some endocrine organs appear to be more sensitive or vulnerable to toxicologic agents than others, hormone–target organ interrelations often lead to the substance causing multiple disruptions in the hormonal balance of the organism. It is not uncommon to witness chemically induced changes in gonadal function along with alterations in thyroid gland activity. In some species, chemically induced changes in sex steroids can affect pancreatic secretion of insulin. Chemically induced stress leading to increased secretion of glucocorticoids can also affect insulin secretion but more importantly can affect adrenocorticotropin (ACTH) levels and hence alter the pituitary-adrenal axis.

The thalidomide tragedy of the 1960s led to the formulation of toxicologic testing guidelines for the field of teratology. No such requirements have been invoked for the endocrine system. Pesticide-induced sterility (e.g., DBCP) has led to concern about the deleterious actions of such substances in both male and female reproductive systems (126,127). The inherent estrogenicity of *o,p*-DDT can affect the reproductive system, and concern has been expressed about the possible relation between diethylstilbestrol (DES) and the incidence of cervical cancer (79). Links have been suggested between 2,4,5-T and birth defects (22). Thus numerous examples of chemical-induced changes in the endocrine system have been reported. Many of these agents represent reproductive hazards in the workplace (127).

All chemically induced changes in the endocrine system cannot be considered undesirable. Indeed, synthetic steroids can be used to purposely inhibit pituitary gonadotropins, thereby providing a chemical method of birth control for millions of women. Chemical (or drug) suppression of target organ hormone secretion can also be therapeutically useful in such organs as the adrenal gland and the thyroid gland.

PITUITARY GLAND

Pituitary–Target Organ Relations

Endocrine toxicology necessitates an understanding of hormonal feedback systems when attempting to predict the effects of potentially toxic agents on a particular target organ. Although measurement of specific hormone levels might not be feasible or economical for the general toxicologic screening of a substance, some bioassays and microscopic techniques yield useful information. The reduction in animal growth rates, although in most instances caused by diminished nutritional intake, might be due to the suppression of pituitary growth hormone secretion. Similarly, a decrease in testicular weight following administration of certain chemicals can be due to interference with pituitary gonadotropins (32,96).

Generally, chemically induced changes that affect pituitary–target organ relations seldom manifest after a single administration of a toxic agent. Rather, compounds that have the potential to exert deleterious effects on the endocrine system ordinarily require longer durations of time before such changes are witnessed. Whereas chemically induced stress could provoke a rapid response in catecholamine secretion and an outpouring of glucocorticoids, other hormonal changes would not be as immediate. Those chemicals causing the induction of hepatic microsomal enzyme systems that affect hormone metabolism would most certainly require upward of a week before changes in the endocrine system are detected. Even those chemicals that are used as drugs and that are purposely designed to suppress a particular hormone target organ secretion may possess an onset of action consisting of several days (e.g., antithyroid drugs).

To appreciate chemically induced changes in the endocrine system, it is important to understand some of the classic hormonal relations between the adenohypophysis and the respective endocrine target organs (Fig. 1). Chemicals, including certain classes of therapeutically effective drugs, can interfere with the release of trophic hormones or can interfere with their synthesis. Still other toxic agents can exert inhibitory actions on the biosynthesis of target organ hormone secretions. Thus there are several sites of action of various chemicals on the adenohypophyseal–target organ feedback systems.

Depending on the particular chemical, the sites of action may differ in their sensitivity to toxic agents. Target organs such as the gonads are frequently sensitive to toxic substances, as rapidly dividing cells are often vulnerable to chemical destruction. Environmental stresses can affect the secretory activity of certain of the hypothalamic-releasing hormones and

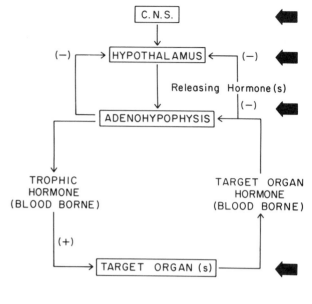

(−)   Inhibitory Action

(+)   Stimulatory Action

Possible Site of Hormonal Interference by Toxic Agents

FIG. 1. Relation between adenohypophyseal–hypothalmic axis and hormone target organs.

hence alter pituitary–target organ relations. Sometimes toxic agents bind to circulating blood proteins and alter the ratio of free/bound target organ hormones. Such changes in binding also can modify the pituitary–target organ relation.

Adenohypophysis

The adenohypophyseal trophic hormones and their hypothalamic-releasing hormones are depicted in Table 1. Because the trophic hormones are either protein or glycoprotein in chemical composition, they cannot be measured by standard spectrophotometric procedures. Such hormones must be either bioassayed or measured using radioimmunoassays (RIAs) or monoclonal antibody techniques. Although bioassays may be useful for certain of the adenohypophyseal hormones, such tests are often inaccurate or have been replaced by more sensitive methods. Bioassays, however, might be employed when there is only a secondary interest in determining if a particular toxicologic agent is affecting trophic hormone levels. Sometimes a target organ that is known to be directly influenced by a particular trophic hormone can be examined and hence provide some general insight into the nature of the chemically induced alterations in the endocrine system. Despite the more complex and involved RIA and monoclonal antibody methodologies, they are of immense value for measuring various hormones. RIA represents an analytical approach of great sensitivity, and such techniques have been applied to more than 200 biological substances, many of which cannot be assayed by other techniques (Table 2). Unlike bioassays that often require large amounts of tissue (or blood), the greater sensitivity of the RIAs or

TABLE 1. *Trophic hormones of the anterior pituitary gland and their respective hypothalamic releasing hormones*

Adenohypophyseal trophic hormone		Hypothalamic releasing hormone	
Abbreviation	Full name	Abbreviation	Full name
ACTH	Adrenocorticotropic hormone	CRH	Corticotropic-releasing hormone
TSH	Thyroid-stimulating hormone	TRH	Thyrotropic-releasing hormone
FSH	Follicle-stimulating hormone	FRH	Follicle-stimulating releasing hormone
LH	Luteinizing hormone	LRH	Luteinizing-hormone releasing hormone
GH	Growth hormone, somatotropin	SRH, GRH	Somatotropin-releasing hormone
		STH, GIH	Somatotropin-inhibitory hormone
Prl	Prolactin	PIH	Prolactin-inhibitory hormone
		PRH	Prolactin-releasing hormone
MSH	Melanocyte-stimulating hormone	MRH	Melanocyte-stimulating releasing hormone
		MIH	Melanocyte-inhibiting hormone

monoclonal antibody techniques can be achieved with small samples of biological fluids. Some of these RIA methodologies are more useful than others and to some extent depend on the degree of hormonal cross-reactions or, in the case of monoclonal antibody methods, their degree of sensitivity.

Some hormones can be measured by competitive assays utilizing either an immune system or a nonimmune system (29,58,63,95,137). In the immune system assay the antibody acts as the binding protein (e.g., insulin, ACTH), whereas in the nonimmune assay system the binding reagent is often a naturally occurring protein with a high affinity for the hormone being measured (e.g., cortisol, thyroxine).

BIOCHEMICAL ASSESSMENTS

Evaluation of endocrine function is an important aspect when determining mechanisms of drug toxicity on endocrine organs (41). Biochemical assessment of hormone levels in the blood can reveal much about sites of toxicity in the endocrine system. Potential sites of damage include the hormone-producing cell, the endocrine target cell, and circulatory pathways by which the hormones are transported to exert a positive or negative effect on the target cell or cell of hormone origin (i.e., feedback mechanism). Lastly, the status of hormonal receptors in the bloodstream (carrier proteins) and intracellular receptors can be studied.

Although such an appraisal of the endocrine system can reveal much about the pathophysiology of endocrine toxicity, biochemical assessment has limitations when studying toxicologic mechanisms. For instance, derangement of other factors that may have modulatory effects on endocrine target

TABLE 2. *Select hormones measured by competitive assays using immune or nonimmune systems*

Peptide hormones	Steroid hormones
ACTH	Aldosterone
FSH	Cortisol
STH (growth hormone)	Dihydrotestosterone
FSH	Estradiol
LH (and hCG)	Estrone
Oxytocin	Progesterone
Insulin	Testosterone
Prolactin	

cells cannot be identified by simple evaluation of hormone levels in the bloodstream. Thus biochemical assessment of the endocrine system offers a macroscopic survey of toxicologic mechanisms, but study of molecular mechanisms is difficult.

Currently, three techniques are employed to evaluate hormone levels in the bloodstream. Each has its own advantages and limitations, depending on the hormone(s) being evaluated. Principles and applications of each technique are considered for toxicologic assessment of endocrine status.

Bioassay

For many years bioassay was the only means for assessing endocrine status. Although the techniques of bioassay often involve laborious chemical assays, their approach still offers investigators a direct means of determining hormone levels. Under certain circumstances, use of bioassays can be more specific than RIA, as RIAs sometimes measure substances that have no biological (or hormonal) activity (e.g., cross-reactivity with precursors or metabolites of the hormone).

Chemical assays for hormonal levels are usually done on samples of blood, plasma, or urine. These assays offer direct measurement of the hormone or hormone metabolites. Chemical assays have proved most useful for nonpeptide hormones, mainly the steroid and thyroid hormones. For instance, cortisol can be evaluated using a fluorimetric assay based on the fact that steroid side groups (e.g., delta-4-3-ketone, 20-ketone, 11 β- and 21-hydroxyl groups) florescense. Another bioassay approach is to inject radiolabeled hormone into the bloodstream. Clearance rates of this substance can be measured in urine or blood samples, thereby evaluating metabolic degradation. By diluting the amount of radiolabeled hormone with unlabeled hormone, the production of the hormone can be determined by comparing the amount of labeled hormone to the total hormone in the sample.

Some of the problems associated with direct chemical bioassays include fluctuations in the amount of free hormone when compared to the total amount of hormone. Because many hormones are bound to plasma proteins, the degree of free hormone can vary according to the extent of hormone bound to carrier proteins. This situation is especially true for concentrations of thyroxine and cortisol. Furthermore, many hormones exhibit diurnal variation (or other cyclic patterns of release), so that the time of day becomes important when performing bioassays. Lastly, attention must be given to the metabolic status of the individual. For instance, blood glucose levels obviously affect hormonal levels of insulin, just as serum calcium levels should be considered for calcitonin and parathyroid hormone levels.

In selected instances, the bioassay approach for assessing endocrine status still offers viable alternatives to techniques involving RIAs or monoclonal antibody techniques.

Radioimmunoassay

Measurement of endocrine values was revolutionized in 1960 when Yalow and Berson developed the RIA to detect nanomolar concentrations of hormones in living subjects (141). Classic bioassays were surpassed in sensitivity, specificity, and facility by the RIA approach. In addition, RIA allowed measurement of materials not previously detectable by chromatographic or spectrophotometric techniques (40).

Radioimmunoassays can be used to measure hormones that cannot be radiolabeled to detectable levels *in vivo*. They are also used for hormones unable to fix complement when bound to antibodies, or they can be used to identify cross-reacting antigens that compete and bind with the antibody.

Competitive inhibition of radiolabeled hormone antibody binding by unlabeled hormone (either a standard or an unknown mixture) is the principle of most RIAs. A standard curve for measuring antigen (hormone) binding to antibody is constructed by placing known amounts of radiolabeled antigen and the antibody into a set of test tubes. Varying amounts of unlabeled antigen are added to the test tubes. Antigen–antibody complexes are separated from the antigen, and the amount of radioactivity from each sample is measured to detect how much unlabeled antigen is bound to the antibody. Smaller amounts of radiolabeled antigen–antibody are present in the fractions containing higher amounts of unlabeled antigen. Usually a standard curve is constructed that measures the percent of radiolabeled antigen bound with the concentration of unlabeled antigen present.

Although several methods exist for the separation of antigen–antibody complexes, two methods are most commonly employed in RIAs. The first, the double-antibody technique, precipitates antigen–antibody complexes out of solution by utilizing a second antibody, which binds to the first antibody. Although other means of antigen–antibody precipitation exist, they can sometimes chemically alter antigen–antibody binding properties. The drawback to the double-antibody technique is expense, which makes this technique uneconomical for RIA screening procedures.

The second most commonly used method is the dextran-coated activated charcoal technique. Addition of dextran-coated activated charcoal to the sample followed by quick centrifugation absorbs free antigen and leaves antigen–antibody complexes in the supernatant. Although most economical, some drawbacks to this technique are that it works best only when the molecular weight of the antigen is 30 kilodaltons or less. Also, sufficient carrier protein must be present to prevent adsorption of unbound antibody.

Once a standard curve has been constructed, the RIA can determine the concentration of hormone in a sample (usually plasma or urine). The values of hormone levels are usually accurate using the RIA. Certain parameters, e.g., pH or ionic concentrations, can affect antigen binding to the antibody. Thus similar conditions must be used for the standard and the sample.

Problems of RIAs include a lack of specificity. This problem is usually due to nonspecific cross-reactivity of antibody that binds antigen other than the hormone, or the antibody binds to a less biologically active form of antigen. In the first instance, nonspecific cross-reactivity of the antibody can result in binding of hormonal precursors or metabolites. The classic, well-studied example of this case is ACTH, a 39-amino-acid polypeptide that is proteolytically inactivated. Antibodies that recognize the inactive C-terminal portion react false positively with the inactive fragments, in addition to the 39-amino-acid hormone. Such cross-reactivity can be solved by utilizing an antibody that reacts only with the biologically active *N*-terminal of the hormone. Along similar lines, an antibody can recognize immunologically similar hormones that have different activity. For example, human placental lactogen in pregnant women cross-reacts with the antibody used in growth hormone RIAs. In the second instance, specificity can be compromised if the hormone exists in an altered, less biologically active state than the intact form of the hormone. Antiserum that cross-reacts with the less active hormone can give a falsely high value of "intact hormone" levels. Such is the case in subjects with chronic renal disease, where parathyroid hormone levels are high when determined by RIA. Thus the heterogenicity of peptide hormones is an important consideration when conducting an RIA. The problem can be circumvented by utilizing antiserum that recognizes certain determinants (see Monoclonal Antibodies, below).

A closely related technique employs proteins that can bind the hormone with high affinity and specificity. The radioreceptor assay can measure proteins that bind and transport the hormone in the bloodstream or exist at the endocrine target cell. Use of radioreceptor assays can provide another perspective on the pathogenesis of endocrine abnormalities.

Thus RIA offers the investigator a highly sensitive, specific means of determining hormone levels in a living subject. In the future, RIAs and radioreceptor assays should have their problems of specificity resolved by the use of monoclonal antibodies. As more is learned about the specificity of these techniques, the full capabilities of RIAs will be realized for studying the endocrine system.

Monoclonal Antibodies

Immunological techniques have long provided an approach to studying hormones (24,66,139). Because hormones possess a number of antigenic determinants, it is possible to produce antisera containing a variety of polyclonal antibodies that recognize and bind many parts of the hormone. Antibodies against hormones have been used in many types of RIAs and radioreceptor assays; but as discussed above, polyclonal antisera can create some nonspecificity problems such as cross-reactivity. Therefore it is sometimes desirable to produce a group of antibodies that selectively bind to a specific region of the hormone (i.e., antigenic determinant). In the past, investigators produced antisera to antigenic determinants of the hormone by cleaving the hormone and immunizing an animal with the fragment of the hormone containing the antigenic determinant of interest (e.g., ACTH immunization with the 24-amino-acid *N*-terminal end of the hormone). This approach solved some problems with cross-reactivity of antisera with other similar antigenic determinants, but problems were still associated with the heterogeneous collection of antibodies found in polyclonal antisera.

In 1975 Kohler and Milstein (64) devised an immunological method for producing monoclonal antibodies. The production of monoclonal antibodies offered investigators a homogeneous collection of antibodies that could selectively bind to a specific antigenic determinant with the same affinity. In addition to protein isolation and diagnostic techniques, monoclonal antibodies have contributed greatly to RIAs.

Because propagation of a single antibody-producing cell *in vitro* cannot occur, Kohler and Milstein took spleen cells from an immunized animal and fused them with myeloma cells (malignant lymphocytes) using a reagent that causes the cells to fuse (e.g., Sendai virus or polythylene glycol). The fused cells, hybridomas, share characteristics of their antibody-producing cells from the spleen and can be propagated *in vitro* using tissue culture techniques.

Unfused spleen cells die in tissue culture media. To separate unfused myeloma cells from hybridomas, the cells are placed in HAT medium (containing hypoxanthine, aminopterin, and thymidine). Myeloma cells used in the production of monoclonal antibodies lack the enzyme hypoxanthine-guanine-phosphoriboxyltransferase (HGPRT), whereas hybridomas contain the enzyme (contributed by fused spleen cells). Because the main pathway of DNA synthesis is blocked by aminopterin, only cells containing HGPRT can utilize hypoxanthine and synthesize DNA in order to propagate. Thus unfused myeloma cells die in HAT medium because they lack HGPRT. The hybridomas propagate.

In order to further isolate and separate variant myeloma cells that can overcome the aminopterin block (using thymidine kinase and exogenous thymidine), the cells are subjected to 5-bromodeoxyuridine, a pyrimidine analog that kills cells using this pathway:

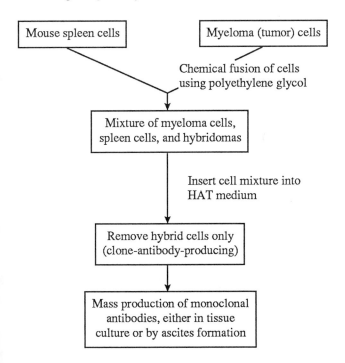

TABLE 3. *Advantages and disadvantages of monoclonal antibodies compared to polyclonal antisera*

Advantages	Disadvantages
Sensitivity	Overly specific
Quantifies available	Decreased affinity
Immunologically defined	Diminished complement fixation
Detection of neoantigens on cell membrane	Labor-intense; high cost

Modified from ref. 124a.

Once the hybridomas have been isolated from unfused cells, they are separated into individual colonies and the type of antibody they produce is characterized. Identification of a hybridoma clone that is producing a specific antibody to the antigen of interest allows the investigator to harvest large quantities of the monoclonal antibody.

Although monoclonal antibodies offer investigators a highly sensitive, specific method for detecting antigen, sometimes monoclonal antibody production are too specific, and affinity of the antibody for the antigen is compromised. In addition, there is usually decreased complement fixation, and costs are usually high for preparing and maintaining hybridomas that produce monoclonal antibodies (Table 3).

The monoclonal antibody technique offers the investigator a means of producing a specific antibody for binding antigen. This technique is useful for studying protein structure relations (or alterations) and has been used for devising specific RIAs. In the future, more efficient monoclonal antibodies will be produced, which will eliminate some of the present disadvantages.

MEASUREMENT OF ANTERIOR PITUITARY HORMONES

Adrenocorticotropin

The primary modulation of adrenal gland and secretory activity is done by adrenocorticotropin (ACTH). ACTH exerts a number of physiological actions including maintenance of the adrenal gland and stimulation of adrenal cortical steroid secretion. ACTH can cause depletion of adrenal gland ascorbic acid, an effect that was at one time employed as a measure of ACTH activity.

A number of pathologic states can alter ACTH secretion. Stress, caused by a variety of environmental or chemical stimuli, can cause a rapid elevation in ACTH blood levels.

Several methods are available for measuring ACTH, but most assays have indirectly assessed adrenal gland secretions. Gravimetric assay of adrenal glands represents one of the simplest methods for indirectly evaluating ACTH activity using hypophysectomized animals (e.g., rats); ACTH injections can maintain the weight of the adrenal glands. ACTH stimulates increases in plasma cortisol and corticosterone and elevates urinary 17-hydroxycorticosteroids and 17-ketosteroids, and these steroid levels can be used to assess this hormone. ACTH causes involution of the thymus gland and deposition of hepatic glycogen, and leads to a decrease in circulating eosinophils in hypophysectomized rodents. The latter ACTH-induced changes in such biological responses also have been used to assess ACTH activity.

In addition to those assays for ACTH that rely on adrenal gland responses (see section on adrenal glands), radioligand-receptor assays have been developed for ACTH (68). Often cortisol levels are used to assess ACTH. Cortisol can be determined using commercially available antibody-coated tube RIA kits. Several investigators have reported the use of a rapid ACTH test in normal subjects (30,80). Such ACTH tests have been reproducible (76).

Thyroid-Stimulating Hormone

Thyroid-stimulating hormone (TSH) is a glycoprotein capable of stimulating the growth and proliferation of cells of the thyroid gland. TSH can produce a number of biochemical and histological changes in the thyroid gland. TSH assays have, for example, employed the uptake of ^{32}P in the thyroid glands of baby chicks (108). Like ACTH, and for routine toxicologic assessment of TSH, many tests involve the measurement of target organ secretory responses. Hence the evaluation of TSH in routine toxicologic experiments often employs measurement of the thyroid hormones (viz., thyroxine and triiodothyronine; see section on the thyroid gland).

Several chemicals and drugs, environmental factors, and pathologic states can affect thyroid hormone secretion (20). Certain foodstuffs and plants contain chemicals that can act as antithyroidal agents. Most of these conditions or factors, however, seem to affect thyroid gland activity itself rather than impinge on TSH secretion.

Developments in immunochemistry have led to commercial kits for measuring TSH that have a much greater sensitivity for the hormone (47). Although cross-reactivity between TSH and luteinizing hormone (LH) or follicle-stimulating hormone (FSH) may not have been entirely eliminated (58), such interference has become less of a problem. A liquid-phase two-site immunoradiometric assay (IRMA) has been described for human TSH (hTSH). IRMA is based on the simultaneous addition of affinity purified sheep anti-hTSH IgG-^{125}I and rabbit anti-hTSH antiserum. This assay is specific for hTSH and exhibits no cross-reactivity with other pituitary glycoprotein (101). Thus the IRMA assays for TSH may be more specific than current RIAs for TSH. The one-step IRMA method involves the use of monospecific antibody against two immunogenic sites on the TSH molecule (109).

Growth Hormone (Somatotropin)

Growth hormone (GH) appears to exert a variety of complex metabolic actions leading to protein anabolism and stimulation of RNA synthesis. A deficiency in GH leads to a reduction in the incorporation of amino acids into protein. GH causes a marked stimulation of cartilaginous growth at the epiphyses of long bones.

Various agents can affect GH secretion (Table 4). Hypoglycemia or insulin can cause a sudden and dramatic increase in serum GH. Starvation can affect GH levels; and cold,

TABLE 4. *Effects of various agents on blood GH levels*

Increase GH levels	Decrease GH levels
Norepinephrine	Somatostatin
Epinephrine	
Serotonin	
TRH	
Vasopressin	
Substance P	
Endorphins	
Enkephalins	
Arginine[a]	
Prostaglandins	
Insulin (hypoglycemia)[a]	
α-Desoxyglucose	
Apomorphine	
L-DOPA[a]	
Clonidine[a]	

[a] Used a provocative test for the diagnosis of GH disorders.

stress, or surgical trauma can lead to an increase in serum GH. Drugs and chemicals that affect catecholamine neurotransmission and the autonomic nervous system can influence GH secretion.

Some GH assays simply use a 10-day body weight gain test in 100-g hypophysectomized female rats (100). The hormone also has been assayed by measuring the width of the tibial epiphysial growth plate.

Birge et al. (6) developed a sensitive RIA for rat GH. Human GH concentration can be measured with double-antibody RIA procedures (82,107).

Regardless of whether GH is assessed using bioassays or by the more accurate and sensitive RIA procedures, the experimental design of either acute or chronic toxicity tests must closely monitor the nutritional status of the animals. Many toxic agents can affect dietary intake and hence reduce body weight. Experimental designs using paired-feeding protocols is necessary for interpreting GH activity in any well-designed toxicology study.

Light microscopic immunocytologic assays for GH can also be performed on Epon-embedded, semi-thin sections using the avidin-biotin-peroxidase complex technique (53). Microdissection techniques (69) and other *in vitro* assays for the release of GH have been used (2).

Gonadotropins

The adenohypophysis secretes FSH and LH, whose principal actions are on the gonads. FSH stimulates follicular development in the ovary and spermatogenesis in the testes. LH, referred to as interstitial cell-stimulating hormone (ICSH) in the male subject, causes luteinization of the ovary and stimulates androgen production by testicular Leydig cells.

In the female human, blood levels of FSH and LH vary according to the phase of the menstrual cycle. In men, although there may be some diurnal fluctuation in FSH and LH, the blood levels are noncyclic. There is a paucity of information about the direct effects of chemicals and drugs on the ovary. Indeed, gonadotropin secretion in women is more complex to evaluate from a toxicologic standpoint. Conversely, the various secretory or cellular processes of the male gonad are more readily evaluated from the standpoint of toxicologic assessment. Figure 2 shows the major cellular sites of testicular toxins. In general, the Leydig cells (or interstitial cells) are somewhat resistant to chemical insult. However, the process of steroidogenesis can be used as an indicator of male sex steroid (e.g., testosterone, dihydrotestosterone) activity (see Gonads, below). Methods have been devised to examine isolated Leydig cell cultures as well as testicular perfusion systems in an effort to study androgen secretion by the male gonad. Spermatogenesis, on the other hand, is sensitive to chemical insult. Testicular sections (or biopsy) can be used to assess the degree of spermatogenic arrest as evidenced by the presence (or absence) of sterile or partial sterile seminiferous tubules. Electroejaculation methods and the use of an artificial vagina can be used for collecting semen for later examination that includes sperm counts, morphology, and motility. Such parameters are potential indicators of reproductive toxicity (7). Sertoli cells secrete a number of proteinaceous substances, and androgen-binding protein (ABP) has been used as an indicator of toxicologic insult following the administration of potentially damaging chemicals or drugs. Such Sertoli cell systems are *in vitro* tests (see Inhibin, below).

As for other adenohypophyseal hormones, FSH and LH levels can be assessed by direct measurement of the hormones or by indirect assays that reflect an influence of these hormones on their target tissues. RIAs are also available (81). Indirect measurement of gonadotropins in women might include the measurement of ovarian steroids or the study of vaginal cytology (see Gonads, below). In men, indirect assays might include the measurement of androgens or the histological assessment of spermatogenesis. Chromosome studies can also be of some value when assessing pituitary gonadal activity. Localization of FSH and LH and their receptors can be detected using immunoperoxidase techniques that employ antisera against the beta subunits of these gonadotropins (52).

Several methods are available for the bioassay of FSH and LH. FSH has been bioassayed by assessing its ability to enhance ovarian weight in immature rats treated with a placental gonadotropin: the "augmentation assay" (119) (Fig. 3). Early bioassays, assessing urinary gonadotropins that had

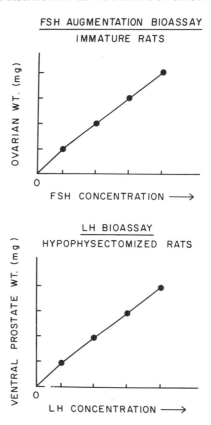

FIG. 3. Bioassay of gonadotropins.

been partially purified, often employed gravimetric responses of ovaries or uteri in immature rats or mice. The bioassay for FSH involving the reduction of tetrazolium by rodent vaginal tissue has not been satisfactory (5). Such bioassays failed to distinguish between FSH and LH, although the specificity of FSH could be enhanced by the presence of excess chorionic gonadotropin.

One of the more sensitive bioassays for LH involves the measurement of ovarian ascorbic acid (OAA) (99). This bioassay employs immature intact pseudopregnant rats that are injected with the test extract and the chemical measurement of LH-induced depletion of OAA. The greater the OAA depletion, the higher the concentration of LH in the tissue or serum extract. LH also can be bioassayed in hypophysectomized rats in which the ventral lobe of the prostate gland increases in weight in response to the gonadotropin (Fig. 3).

The bioassay of gonadotropins has largely been abandoned because of the lack of sensitivity and the great expense. The sensitivity of RIAs offers substantial advantages over bioassays even though the biological and immunological activities do not always correlate. Cross-reactivity between the gonadotropins and other hormones has, in some instances, reduced the accuracy of RIA. On the other hand, the cross-reactivity between LH and human chorionic gonadotropin (hCG) has been chemically exploited and has actually improved the accuracy of LH measurements. Stevens (124) made an exhaustive study comparing methods of LH measurement. Monroe et al. (84) developed a double-antibody RIA for rat LH. The RIA for LH has been quantified in various mam-

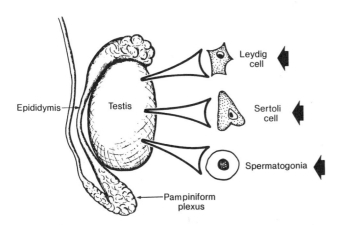

FIG. 2. Some possible sites of action of selected gonadotoxins.

malian species (61). Monoclonal antibodies to hCG have provided the basis for some assay systems (94).

Like RIAs for other glycoprotein hormones, the RIA for FSH stems from contaminated immunogens as well as immunologic similarities with other hormones. There are, in general, disparities between the values of FSH measured by RIA compared with the levels determined by bioassays. The RIA of FSH in urine is unreliable unless some attempt is made to partially purify the urine. The interpretation of pituitary gonadotropin assays is still a continuing challenge (108).

Inhibin

Inhibin is a proteinaceous substance found in the mammalian gonad that is involved in the negative feedback regulation of FSH secretion. In men, inhibin can be detected in the testes, seminal plasma, rete testes fluid, and spermatozoa. The Sertoli cells are the only testicular cells that secrete an inhibin-like substance referred to as Sertoli cell factor (SCF). Inhibin, as well as SCF, can suppress the pituitary secretion of FSH.

The biological activities of various inhibin preparations, including SCF, can be assessed *in vitro* using pituitary cell cultures (115,120). This *in vitro* assay consists in evaluating the degree of suppression of basal FSH release following a 3-day incubation with the test material relative to that of a control culture.

Prolactin

Prolactin causes initiation and maintenance of lactation in women. It has no known physiological function in men. In rodents, prolactin maintains the corpus luteum. In many species, milk ejection cannot be produced by suckling unless prolactin first stimulates the myoepithelial cells of the mammary glands.

Prolactin can be assessed by various bioassays, or it can be detected by the more sensitive RIA. With regard to bioassays, one of prolactin's more fascinating actions is its ability to stimulate the growth of the crop sac in pigeons and other birds (73,90). The bilaterally stimulated crop sacs are outpouchings of the esophagus. Prolactin can be assayed by injecting directly into one crop sac and comparing its size with the size of the contralateral uninjected control crop sac. Other bioassays for prolactin include the *in vitro* rabbit and mouse

TABLE 5. Conditions affecting the immunoassay of prolactin and GH in vitro

Duration of incubation
Incubation temperature
pH
Homogenate or tissue fraction
Concentration of test system constituents
Cysteamine
Reduce glutathione
EDTA
Urea
Sodium dodecyl sulfate
Iodoacetate

TABLE 6. Effect of various agents on blood prolactin levels[a]

Increase prolactin levels	Decrease prolactin levels
Reserpine	Acetylcholine
Methyl-DOPA	Apomorphine
α-Methyl-p-tyrosine	Dopamine
Chlorpromazine	L-DOPA
Atropine	Iproniazid
Perphenazine (and other	β-Hydroxy-GABA
phenothiazines)	Somatostatin
Haloperidol	Bromocriptine
Tricyclic antidepressants	
Sulpiride	
Diethyl ether	
Nicotine	
Vasopressin	
Estrogens	
Thyroxine (and T_3)	
Histamine	
Prostaglandin E	
β-Endorphin	
Met-enkephalin	
TRH	
Opiates	

[a] Response may vary quantitatively depending on the dose and the particular species.

mammary gland test (33). These bioassays might be adequate, but they are difficult to perform, time-consuming, and often costly.

An RIA has been developed for prolactin, although the availability of chemically pure human prolactin has curtailed the clinical usefulness of this assay relative to certain other pituitary hormones. RIAs have been developed for several species including humans (56), rats (89), and amphibians (21). Frantz and Turkington (34) developed an *in vitro* bioassay for ^{125}I-prolactin. Prolactin can also be identified in tissues using *in vitro* immunoassays, but there are a number of test system conditions *in vitro* that can affect the detectable levels of prolactin (Table 5) (72). It is important to determine the optimal conditions for assessing tissue prolactin. Thiol exposure increases the immunoassay ability of prolactin probably through the enhancement of thiol–disulfide interchange.

Several factors or chemicals can affect prolactin secretion, e.g., drugs (or chemicals) that affect dopaminergic mechanisms (Table 6). For example, α-methyldopa causes an elevation in blood prolactin. Certain tranquilizers, e.g., reserpine and phenothiazines, also produce hyperprolactinemia. Prolactin secretion can be increased by physical exercise, coitus, suckling, and surgical stress. Such factors must be taken into consideration when assessing prolactin levels in toxicologic protocols.

POSTERIOR PITUITARY HORMONES

Neurohypophyseal Peptides

The posterior pituitary gland, or neurohypophysis, contains a number of peptides of which only oxytocin and vasopressin (antidiuretic hormone, ADH) have been chemically identified. This gland also contains a group of peptides known as the neurophysins (116). The neurophysins appear to be synthesized in the same hypothalamic neurons as the octapeptides oxytocin and vasopressin. Whereas the physiological function of oxytocin and vasopressin are well established, less is known about the biological function of the neurophysins. The principal physiological function of vasopressin is conservation of fluids, which it exerts by affecting renal tubule reabsorption of water. Oxytocin's principal physiological functions are to stimulate uterine smooth musculature and to aid in the process of lactation.

Several drugs and other hormones affect the secretion of vasopressin or oxytocin (Table 7). Nonspecific stress also can stimulate the release of ADH and hence is an important variable to consider in any toxicologic protocol involved with monitoring water balance. Some chemicals and drugs affect the central release of the posterior pituitary hormones, whereas others block their peripheral action(s). Physiological factors also affect the secretory rate of oxytocin, and there are considerable differences among species. Suckling and mammary duct dilation lead to enhanced secretion of oxytocin. Estrogens and pregnancy enhance the sensitivity of the uterine smooth muscle to oxytocin.

Oxytocins

Oxytoxin may be measured by RIA or bioassay. Because oxytocin can stimulate the contraction of smooth muscles, several bioassays have been developed using isolated muscle strips. Oxytocin can be assayed by the method of Rydén and Sjöholm (111), which employs the mammotonic activity of the hormone on strips of lactating rat mammary gland. The increment of tension developed by the muscle strip is used as an index of oxytocic activity. A four-point assay can be carried out using USP posterior pituitary standard as a reference.

Chard (17) discussed the methodologies for RIA of both oxytocin and vasopressin. The RIA for oxytocin has been used primarily for studies on animal and human parturition. A sensitive and specific RIA for oxytocin reportedly measures

plasma levels in the order of 20 pg/ml (106). Chard et al. (18) and Kegan and Glick (60) reported being able to measure picogram amounts of the hormone. A solid-phase RIA for the direct measure of plasma oxytocin has been developed that is reported to be rapid, relatively sensitive, and reproducible, and does not require the prior extraction of plasma samples (12).

Vasopressin (Antidiuretic Hormone)

Vasopressin (ADH), like oxytocin, is an octapeptide. In some species ADH exerts a rather profound pressor action on vascular smooth muscle. In humans and most other mammals, however, the actions of ADH are primarily on the renal tubules, exerting a body fluid-sparing action.

The hormone can be measured by RIA or bioassay. With bioassay, ADH or extracts of posterior pituitary tissue can be measured for their antidiuretic activity in the rat under ethanol anesthesia and a constant water load (25); the diminution in urine flow is an index of antidiuretic activity. Unanesthetized trained dogs also have been employed in the bioassay, but any factor such as stress must be minimized because it can affect urinary output and hence the ADH assay.

The first RIA for an ADH was described by Roth et al. (110). Because vasopressin is present in biological fluids in low concentrations (picograms), tests must be sensitive. It ordinarily has been difficult to measure basal levels or small fluctuations resulting from particular experimental designs. Kamoi and Hama (59) reported a highly sensitive RIA for ADH. A solid-phase RIA for the determination of arginine vasopressin in urine has also been developed (65).

THYROID GLAND

To understand the thyroid as a target for toxicity, it is important to review the physiology of the gland. The primary secretions of the thyroid are thyroxine (T_4) and triiodothyronine (T_3). The initial step in the synthesis of these thyroid hormones is the uptake of iodide, derived from dietary iodine, into the follicular cells of the thyroid in response to the adenohypophyseal hormone thyrotropin (TSH). Once inside the cell, the iodide is oxidized, possibly through a free radical mechanism, and then combined with the tyrosine components of a protein, thyroglobulin, to form either monoiodotyrosyl or diiodotyrosyl residues. Two molecules of the latter can combine to form triiodothyronine. Under normal conditions, T_4 predominates over T_3 in the thyroid, although the ratio can be altered under certain physiological states.

The T_3 and T_4 remain incorporated in the thyroglobulin, which is stored in the follicular colloid material of the gland, until their release in response to TSH. The release, which involves lysosomes, results from the proteolytic cleavage of thyroglobulin into the thyroid hormones and component amino acids. Monoiodotyrosine and diiodotyrosine also are released at this stage; however, before reaching the circulation, they are enzymatically degraded, liberating iodide, which is reincorporated into protein by the gland. Normally, thyroglobulin does not reach the circulation but remains inside the thyroid cell (Fig. 4).

TABLE 7. *Effects of various drugs on the release or action of neurohypophyseal hormones*

Enhance release	Inhibit release	Block peripheral action
Vasopressin		
Acetylcholine	Ethanol	Lithium
Nicotine		β-Adrenergic agonists
α-Adrenergic agonists		Tetracyclines
β-Adrenergic agonists		
Vincristine		
Clofibrate		
Oxytocin		
Prostaglandin E_2	Ethanol	Propranolol
Prostaglandin $F_{1\alpha}$	Methallibure	Vasopressin analogues
		Oxytocin analogs

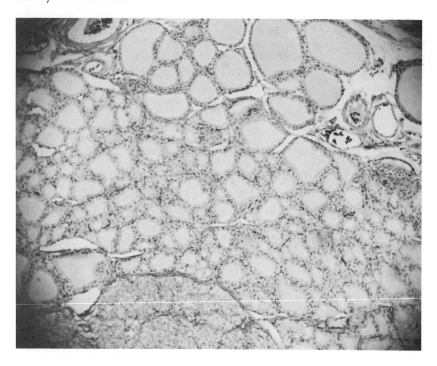

FIG. 4. Histology of rat thyroid/parathyroid gland. ×125.

Upon release into the circulation, T_3 and T_4 are transported in the plasma in association with proteins. Although there are species differences in the protein-binding patterns of the thyroid hormones (26), the primary binding protein in man is called thyroxine-binding globulin. It is an acidic glycoprotein (molecular weight 40,000) that binds T_4 with a relatively high binding affinity and T_3 with a lower binding affinity (123). A second transport protein, called thyroxine-binding prealbumin, although present in higher amounts than thyroxine-binding globulin, has a lower binding affinity for the thyroid hormones and is considered of secondary importance (92). In man and most other mammals, the thyroid hormones also can bind to albumin following occupation of the higher-affinity binding sites. As a consequence of this plasma protein binding, less than 0.1% of the total plasma thyroid hormones exist in a free, unbound form. Care must be exercised when monitoring thyroid function in a species such as the rat, which does not possess a thyroxine-binding globulin (i.e., high affinity binding protein) and which therefore has lower plasma levels of protein-bound thyroid hormone. Also, because it is the free hormone that is available for degradation, it is not unreasonable to expect that the plasma half-life for T_4 would

be longer in a species with a thyroxine-binding globulin than in a species without one. Such a correlation appears to exist. The T_4 plasma half-life in the human, which has a thyroxine-binding globulin, is 5 to 9 days (91,122); in the rat, which does not have a thyroxine-binding globulin, the T_4 plasma half-life is 12 to 24 hr (46,67).

It is thus evident that there are a number of steps where toxic chemicals might interfere with thyroid function (Table 8). In addition, experience with laboratory rats has revealed that a variety of physical and environmental factors (Table 9) also can alter circulating (i.e., plasma) levels of TSH, T_4, and T_3.

Measurement of Thyroid Hormones

Increased attention has been focused on the development of RIAs for the determination of serum T_3 and T_4 levels. However, both T_4 and T_3 can be measured using a competitive protein-binding assay that is based on the displacement of radiolabeled hormone from thyroxine-binding globulin (48,86). The amount of label displaced is proportional to the amount of hormone added to the assay in the sample serum.

TABLE 8. Chemicals producing abnormal thyroid function

Blocks iodide trapping	Blocks iodide oxidation	Mechanism not established
Chlorate	Amphenone	Acetazolamide
Hypochlorite	Carbimazole	Chlorpromazine
Iodate	Cobalt	Chlortrimeton
Nitrate	Methimazole	Thiopental
Perchlorate	p-Aminosalicylate	Tolbutamide
Thiocyanate	Phenylbutazone	
	Phenylindanedione	
	Propylthiouracil	
	Resorcinol	

TABLE 9. Factors influencing TSH, T_3, and T_4 levels in rat plasma

Sex of animal
Age of animal
Time of day
Stage of estrous cycle
Strain of animal
Environmental temperature
Blood collection technique
Animal handling
Locomotor activity of animal

In general, T$_4$ can be effectively measured using the competitive protein-binding assay; however, the hormone must first be extracted from the sample serum to eliminate any interference from endogenous binding proteins, which would tend to compete with the binding protein used in the assay.

There are a large number of laboratory tests that can be adapted to assess the function of the thyroid gland (Table 10). Assessment of laboratory tests can be divided into various categories including those that directly measure thyroid function (e.g., ^{131}I uptake), those that measure blood levels (free versus bound), those that measure metabolic actions (e.g., cholesterol lowering), and those that provide insight into the modulations of thyroid function by the adenohypophysis (e.g., thyroid suppression test).

Although T$_3$ also can be measured by the competitive protein-binding assay (88,121), the procedure is cumbersome. Because T$_4$ has a higher binding affinity than T$_3$ for thyroxine-binding globulin and the T$_4$/T$_3$ ratio is approximately 20:1, the determination of T$_3$ requires chromatographic separation of T$_4$ and T$_3$ as well as the extraction step discussed above. As these steps can be fairly involved, RIA procedures have been developed for the quantitation of T$_3$ (as well as T$_4$).

The RIA is based on the binding of endogenous hormone to a specific antibody, thereby displacing a proportional amount of radiolabeled hormone from that antibody. Obviously, the hormone-binding proteins in the sample (e.g., thyroxine-binding globulin, thyroxine-binding prealbumin and albumin) tend to compete with the antibody for the hormone. This interference can be prevented by extracting the serum prior to assay or adding chemical agents to block the binding of hormone to binding proteins (13,54). Another difficulty in measuring T$_3$ or T$_4$ by RIA is that the hormones are small and similar in structure, and hence it has been difficult to produce a specific antibody for T$_3$ that would not cross-react with T$_4$. Production of specific antisera with minimal cross-reactivity has been achieved (49,105) that now permits measurement of T$_3$ and T$_4$ without the need for prior chromatographic separation.

The "T$_3$ resin uptake" test measures the degree of saturation of the thyroxine-binding globulin in plasma. Radiolabeled T$_3$ and a resin are added to the test plasma, which normally contains thyroxine-binding globulin and an unknown amount of bound hormone. The greater the number of binding sites available on the globulin, the greater is the

amount of labeled T$_3$ bound. Because T$_4$ has a higher affinity for the thyroxine-binding globulin, T$_3$ should not displace endogenous T$_4$ from its binding sites. If the degree of saturation is calculated using this procedure, and if the total plasma levels of thyroid hormone are known, it is possible to calculate how much of the hormone exists in plasma in the free (unbound) state.

PARATHYROID GLAND

The balance of endogenous calcium is maintained by several intrinsic factors that modulate the remodeling of bone and the absorption and excretion of calcium. Parathyroid hormone (PTH), vitamin D, and calcitonin are the principal factors involved in calcium homeokinesis. PTH is a linear polypeptide with a molecular weight of about 10,000. There are species differences in its amino acid composition. About 98% of endogenous calcium resides in skeletal tissue, with the remainder sequestered in soft tissues and extracellular fluids. About 50% of serum calcium exists in an ionized form; ionized calcium is the biologically active form of the cation. Hypocalcemia provokes secretion of PTH.

Parathyroid hormone was originally bioassayed using a hormone-induced elevation in serum calcium in dogs. Several commonly used in vivo assays employ the measurement of serum calcium in parathyroidectomized rats or in calcium-injected chicks or quail. A commonly used in vitro assay is based on determining the activation of renal adenylate cyclase in response to PTH. This assay involves the conversion of ^{32}P-labeled ATP to radioactive cyclic AMP in vitro (93). PTH-stimulated cyclic AMP production in rat osteosarcoma cells cultured in vitro is still another highly sensitive bioassay.

Radioimmunoassays have been developed for PTH in numerous species, although the immunogenic determinants differ among the various peptide molecules (141). In addition, multiple types of immunoreactive fragments of PTH can be detected in the circulation. This immunoheterogeneity complicates the RIA for PTH. Thus RIAs for the carboxyl-terminal, midregion-terminal, and amino-terminal of PTH have been developed. The amino-terminal and the midregion assays show greater sensitivity. Efforts have been devoted to unifying PTH assay protocols and reagents (140). Hanley and Wellings (44) have described a carboxyl-terminal assay for PTH that purports to measure the intact molecule.

A monoclonal antibody assay for human vitamin D protein has also been reported (102). The anti-human vitamin-D-binding protein antibodies cross-react with monkey and pig vitamin-D-binding protein but not with vitamin-D-binding protein from the rat, mouse, or chicken.

ADRENAL GLAND

The adrenal gland is composed of an outer layer (adrenal cortex) and an inner layer (adrenal medulla). The inner and outer layers can be readily distinguished by histologic preparations (Fig. 5).

The adrenal medulla secretes epinephrine and norepinephrine in response to sympathetic stimulation, and the release of these hormones produces systemic effects that, in

TABLE 10. *Laboratory assessment of the thyroid*

Tests assessing metabolic effect of thyroid
 Serum cholesterol
 Basal metabolic rate
 Cardiac rate (i.e., systolic time intervals)
Tests assessing thyroid function
 TRH stimulation
 Thyroid suppression test
 Serum TSH
 ^{131}I uptake
Tests assessing blood levels (free and bound)
 Serum total T$_3$ and total T$_4$
 Serum free (unbound) T$_4$
 Resin T$_3$ uptake
 TBG (thyroxine-binding globulin)

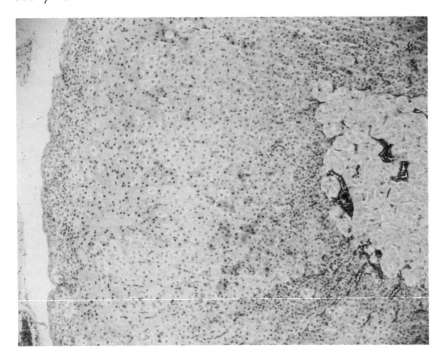

FIG. 5. Histology of rat adrenal cortex (outer area) and medulla (inner area). ×126.

turn, resemble generalized sympathetic stimulation. The adrenal cortex produces two major groups of hormones, the mineralocorticoids and the glucocorticoids, as well as smaller amounts of androgenic hormones.

In humans, the main mineralocorticoid is aldosterone, although deoxycorticosterone also exhibits mineralocorticoid activity; however, its potency is reported to be only one-thirtieth that of aldosterone. Cortisol, the major glucocorticoid produced in man, also exhibits a small amount of mineralocorticoid activity. The basic physiological effect of aldosterone is on electrolyte levels. It promotes the renal reabsorption of sodium in the ascending portion of the loop of Henle, the distal tubule, and the collecting tubule. Sodium reabsorption is accompanied by reabsorption of the chloride anion. In addition to stimulating sodium reabsorption, aldosterone enhances the urinary excretion of potassium and hydrogen ions. The increased elimination of hydrogen ions can lead to alkalosis and an increased extracellular content of bicarbonate ions, which when combined with an increased extracellular sodium and chloride content tends to promote tubular reabsorption of water.

The adrenal gland is essential for life, especially the salt-retaining properties of the mineralocorticoids. In the absence of mineralocorticoids, the extracellular fluid potassium concentration rises, and the sodium and chloride contents fall. Total lack of aldosterone secretion can cause the urinary elimination of 20% of the total body sodium in 1 day. The salt elimination can cause a dangerous reduction in the extracellular and blood volume, which if untreated leads to diminished cardiac output and death.

The principal glucocorticoid secreted in man is cortisol, or hydrocortisone, although both corticosterone and cortisone do possess some glucocorticoid activity. The three major systems regulated by the glucocorticoids are carbohydrate, protein, and fat metabolism. With carbohydrate metabolism, the glucocorticoids stimulate gluconeogenesis and decrease glucose utilization by the cells; both of these effects can lead to increased blood glucose levels. The glucocorticoids also produce a marked reduction in cellular protein content. An exception is the liver, where protein content increases as does the production of plasma protein by the liver. It is believed that the glucocorticoids interfere with the transport of amino acids into extrahepatic cells, and this action combined with continuing protein catabolism in these cells produces an increase in plasma amino acid content. Increased plasma amino acid levels and their subsequent transport into the liver probably promotes gluconeogenesis (i.e., the conversion of amino acids to glucose). The glucocorticoids also promote mobilization of fatty acids from adipose tissue, which raises plasma fatty acid levels. This effect plus increased oxidation of fatty acids in the cells is probably involved in the switch from glucose utilization to fatty acid utilization as a source of energy during periods of stress.

Corticosteroids are bound by two plasma protein fractions. A corticosteroid-binding globulin has a high affinity but a low binding capacity, whereas plasma albumin, the second protein fraction, has a low affinity and a relatively high binding capacity. Under normal conditions, most of the hormone is bound to the corticosteroid-binding globulin (CBG).

There is a paucity of data documenting the effects of chemicals on adrenocortical function, but many drugs are known to affect adrenocortical secretion (Table 11). Some drugs can specifically inhibit adrenocortical secretion (Fig. 6). If a test compound does not produce detectable morphologic damage to the adrenal following repeated administration, it is usually accepted that no adrenotoxicity has occurred. It is not to be assumed that severe malfunctions will pass undetected, however, particularly when one considers the influence the adrenocortical hormones have on plasma electrolytes, as well as on carbohydrate, protein, and fat metabolism. Such toxicity would probably be detected during routine clinical chemistry testing.

TABLE 11. *Drugs known to interfere with the measurement of corticosteroids and ketosteroids*

Antibiotics/antibacterial agents
   Nalidixic acid
   Sulfamerazine
   Triacetyloleandomycin
Sedatives/tranquilizers
   Chloral hydrate
   Chlordiazepoxide
   Chlorpromazine
   Ethinamate
   Hydroxyzine
   Meprobamate
   Paraldehyde
   Phenaglycodol
   Reserpine
Monoamine oxidase inhibitors
   Etryptamine
Oral hypoglycemic agents
   Acetohexamide
Miscellaneous drugs
   Colchicine
   Phenytoin (DPH)
   Quinidine
   Quinine
   Spironolactone

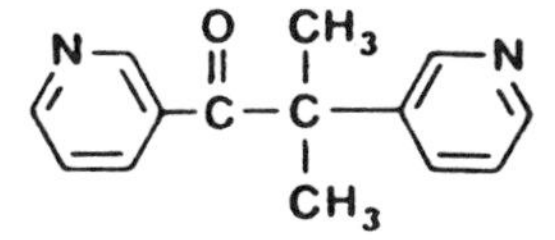

FIG. 6. Agents that inhibit adrenocortical steroid biosynthesis.

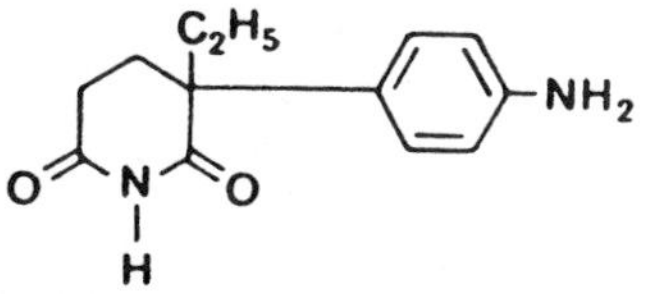

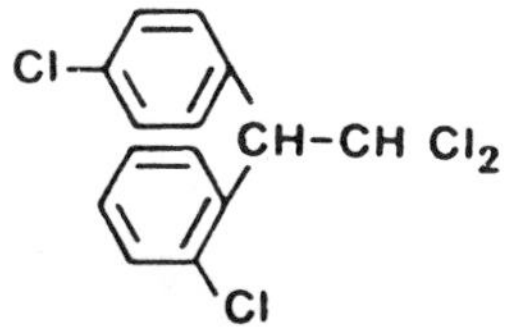

Measurement of Corticoids

Several methods have been used to quantitate plasma and urinary aldosterone levels. Among them are double-isotope dilution techniques (4,27,130), gas-liquid chromatographic techniques (1), and a number of RIAs (3,57,78,135). A difficulty associated with the RIA procedures is that aldosterone must be separated from other plasma steroids, which are normally present at far higher levels. This separation usually takes the form of paper or Sephadex R LH-20 chromatography prior to RIA. An interesting alternative was reported by Gomex-Sanchez et al. (38), who used an antibody to extract aldosterone from the plasma prior to the RIA.

Aldosterone levels can be altered without the need of a direct drug effect on the adrenal cortex. Three factors that could mediate an indirect drug effect on the adrenocortical secretion of aldosterone are (a) altered circulating levels of angiotension II, (b) altered ACTH levels, and (c) altered serum potassium levels (16).

Various analytical procedures have been used for the quantitation of glucocorticoids (42). One of the earliest procedures involved a colorimetric reaction between the glucocorticoid and a phenylhydrazine reagent (9,104). Other colorimetric methods also have been used (10,114). Both cortisol, which is the primary glucocorticoid in man, and corticosterone, which is the primary glucocorticoid in the rat, have been measured using a competitive protein-binding assay (15,85,87,133) that takes advantage of the binding affinity of the glucocorticoid-binding globulin found in the plasma. With the development of immunochemical techniques, it was found that plasma glucocorticoids could be effectively measured using the RIA (130,132). A complicating factor was the existence of competition between the endogenous glucocorticoid-binding globulin and the added antibody for the radioligand. To resolve this problem, investigators included an extraction step to remove both free and bound steroid from the serum prior to the assay; unfortunately, this additional step often led to loss of glucocorticoid. Gomez-Sanchez et al. (39) described the use of alcohol denaturation to destroy the glucocorticoid-binding globulin, a modification that permits the assay to be conducted without an extraction step.

Plasma or Urinary Corticosteroids

Stress can produce a rapid increase in ACTH production, which in turn promotes secretion of adrenocortical hormones (31). Thus the manner in which the animal is prepared for blood sampling can modify the corticoid levels. It has been demonstrated that under ether anesthesia blood corticoid levels are higher than those found after pentobarbital administration, which are higher than those found following decapitation. Likewise, the time elapsed following administration of pentobarbital influences blood hormone levels. Thus stress can be a major problem affecting the interpretation of results. An additional related problem is that fairly large volumes of blood must be drawn for adrenocortical hormone measurement. In chronic toxicity studies involving small animals, the sacrifice of these animals to routinely screen for adrenotoxicity would probably not be acceptable.

Adrenocortical function can be effectively monitored by measuring hormone levels in 24-hr urine samples (50,51). Major advantages to this approach are that (a) the animals can be housed stress-free in metabolic cages during toxicity testing, and (b) serial measurements can be conducted in the same animal by completely noninvasive techniques without sacrifice of the animal. A criticism of the approach can be illustrated using aldosterone secretion in the rat. The primary site of degradation for aldosterone is the liver, with only ap-

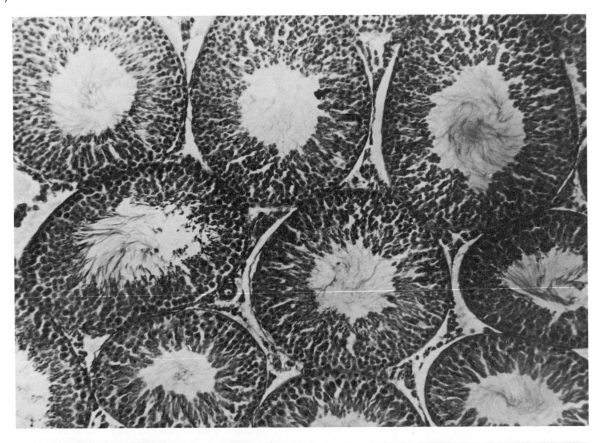

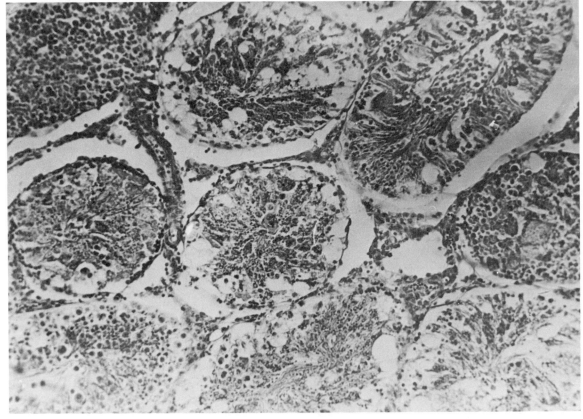

FIG. 7. Normal rat testes (**top**) and chemical-induced sterility in rat testes (**bottom**). Note the partially sterile seminiferous tubules.

proximately 1% of the secreted aldosterone being excreted unchanged by the kidneys. However, relative changes in the urinary corticosteroid patterns could certainly be of value as a screen for adrenotoxicity during chronic toxicity studies. RIA is the method of choice for the determination of urinary corticosteroids, keeping in mind the problems with cross-reactivity discussed earlier (42).

GONADS

Male Hormones (Androgens)

Aspects of male reproductive toxicology have been described elsewhere in this volume. Such discussions, however, have emphasized the process of spermatogenesis and to what extent various toxicologic agents can cause testicular damage (Fig. 7). Some cell types are more vulnerable than others with regard to toxic chemicals. Although chemical agents can readily produce testicular atrophy and spermatogenic arrest, some toxicologic testing protocols involve the assessment of testicular androgens. There are several sites of action of gonadal toxins in addition to the Leydig cells and the germinal epithelium (Fig. 2). Gonadotoxins may act directly on the testes or indirectly, e.g., via the central nervous system (CNS) (Table 12). Androgens, or male sex hormones, can be measured by several methods including spectrophotometric analyses, chromatographic procedures, and RIA. Androgens also can be detected in women, and not uncommonly represent pathological conditions depending on the levels detected in the tissues.

Androgens can be synthesized in a number of cellular sites, but the Leydig cells of the testes (also known as the interstitial cells) are the principal source of this hormone (Fig. 7). Relative to the germinal epithelium, the Leydig cells are not sensitive to the toxic effects of chemicals. Some physiochemical characteristics of gonadotoxins are delineated in Table 13.

Androgens are steroids (Fig. 8). Their molecular characteristics are such that they can be measured fluorometrically, by chromatography, and by RIA. They also can be bioassayed using various physiological responses such as the stimulation of accessory sex organ weights (e.g., prostate gland or seminal vesicles). Still other androgen assessments can be made by measuring male sex accessory gland constituents, e.g., seminal vesicle fructose levels (75) and zinc concentrations (43).

Androgens exert three main biological actions: (a) virilizing or masculinizing actions; (b) protein anabolic or myotropic and (c) antiestrogenic effects. All of these biological effects

TABLE 12. Sites of action of gonadotoxins

Indirect-acting (e.g., CNS)
  Hormonal
  Nonhormonal
Direct-acting (e.g., testes)
  Hormonal
  Nonhormonal
Mixed (i.e., indirect and direct)
  Hormonal
  Nonhormonal

TABLE 13. Some physicochemical characteristics of gonadotoxins

Usually lipophilic
Avidity for androgen receptor
Can permeate the testes–blood barrier
Diverse chemical structure
Molecular weight frequently less than 400
Propensity for rapidly dividing cells

can be bioassayed in experimental animals. Rodents are the most commonly used animal for the bioassay of androgens.

The androgenic actions of male sex hormones, i.e., their masculinizing actions, are usually bioassayed on the basis of the response of male sex accessory organs. Generally, either the rat seminal vesicle or its ventral lobes of the prostate gland are used to bioassay androgens (144). Figure 9 reveals the general anatomical relations of the rat sex accessory glands. For the bioassay, rats are castrated, and the sex accessory glands are allowed to regress in size for about 7 days. Using testosterone as a standard, castrate rats are injected for several days, the animals sacrificed, and either the seminal vesicles (empty) or the ventral prostate glands removed and weighed (Fig. 10). Sometimes immature rats are used for the bioassay instead of castrate animals.

Another bioassay that has been used to assess androgenic activity is the weight or the size of the comb of the castrated cock or immature cockerel. The direct application of testosterone (or other androgenic substances) to the comb causes it to increase in size and weight. After a 7-day treatment period with the androgen, the birds are sacrificed and autopsied on the eighth day. The combs are dissected out and weighed. At least ten chicks are used at each dose increment.

Stimulation of the rat levator ani muscle has been used to bioassay the protein anabolic actions of androgens. This "levator ani bioassay" was developed following observations on the myotropic and nitrogen-retaining activities of certain steroids. There is perhaps a lack of specificity of this test as a measure of protein anabolic activity. The levator ani test

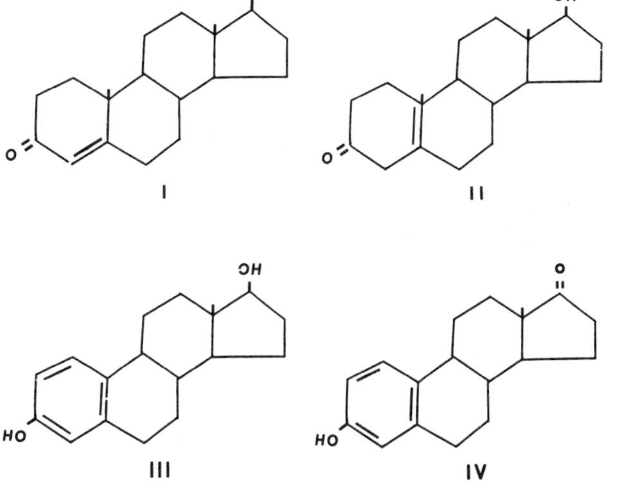

FIG. 8. I: Testosterone. **II:** Dihydrotestosterone. **III:** Estradiol-17β. **IV:** Estrone.

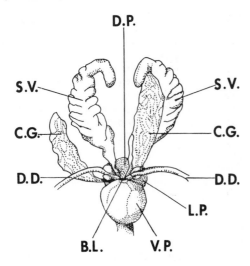

FIG. 9. Anatomical relation of components of rodent sex accessory glands. (*D.D.*) ductus deferens; (*B.L.*) bladder; (*V.P.*) ventral prostate; (*L.P.*) lateral prostate; (*C.G.*) coagulating gland (also called anterior prostate); (*S.V.*) seminal vesicle; (*D.P.*) dorsal prostate.

ordinarily uses immature castrate rats that have been treated for 1 week with the steroid (144). In addition to androgen bioassay methods using rodent sex accessory organs and muscles, as well as bird combs, the male sex hormones exert a renotropic action in mice. Androgens can stimulate the growth of the kidneys in castrate or immature mice.

Chemical indicator tests also have been used to assess androgen activity. Sex accessory organs contain several biochemical constituents that are androgen-dependent (75). For example, sex accessory fructose decreases following castration and can be restored by androgen administration. Sex accessory fructose has been used as a sensitive chemical indicator for testosterone and other androgens. Fructose can be measured spectrophotometrically by several techniques (129). Similarly, sex accessory organ citric acid can be used to assess androgenic activity (55). These chemical indicator tests for

androgens are more sensitive than the gravimetric responses used in bioassay procedures.

Testosterone levels have been determined using double-isotope derivative methods (36), gas liquid chromatography (23), and fluorometric procedures (28). Although these testosterone methods are specific and sensitive, elaborate purification is essential for accuracy, and routine application is often time-consuming. Competitive protein binding assays (77) and RIAs (35,62) are available. In the RIA, antiserum against testosterone can be produced in rabbits immunized with testosterone-3-oxime–beef serum albumin. Biological samples must undergo solvent extraction and be eluted on microcolumns. If the extraction and purification of the samples are appropriately carried out, the RIA of testosterone is highly sensitive and accurate; it is capable of detecting testosterone in nanogram to picogram amounts.

Circulating autoantibodies to androgen receptors (human and rat) are present in the blood of patients with prostatic disease. Hence monoclonal antibodies to androgen receptors are possible (70).

Female Hormones (Estrogens)

Female sex hormones, or estrogens, are biosynthesized by the theca interna cells of the ovarian follicles, the corpus luteum, the placenta, and in lesser amounts the adrenal cortex and the testes. Estradiol-17β is the major estrogen secreted, although some estrone is present in the circulation (Fig. 8). Estrone can be further metabolized to estriol by hepatic enzymes. Of these three main natural occurring estrogens, estradiol-17β is undoubtedly the most potent estrogen. All of these naturally occurring estrogens are steroids. Synthetic estrogens such as diethylstilbestrol are not steroids. Although steroidal and nonsteroidal estrogens can be bioassayed using similar tests, their different molecular structures do not allow them to be measured by similar chemical methodologies.

The two methods commonly used to bioassay estrogenic hormones involve either histological changes in the vaginal epithelium or an increase in the weight of the rodent uterus. Both bioassays require the use of ovariectomized animals.

In the mouse vaginal smear bioassay, ovariectomized animals (usually ten mice per group) are divided into about six groups consisting of various standard estradiol doses (0.005–0.050 μg), two doses of the unknown substance, and appropriate vehicle controls. Beginning at the second week postovariectomy, all mice are primed with 2 μg of estradiol to establish that the animals are responding, with a vaginal smear characterized by nucleated epithelial cells or cornified cells. Mice failing to exhibit a positive response to the priming dose of estradiol are discarded. The positive-responding mice then are subjected to daily injection of estradiol, and a dose-response curve is established (Fig. 11). Those with vaginal responses characterized by epithelial cornification are considered positive responders to the estradiol.

Estrogen bioassays also include using an increase in uterine weight in the ovariectomized rat or mouse. Uterine weight falls precipitously after ovariectomy (Fig. 12). At about 2 weeks postcastration, uterine weight loss begins to level off. The fall in uterine weight can be restored by daily injections of estradiol (Fig. 12). These ovariectomized mice (ten per

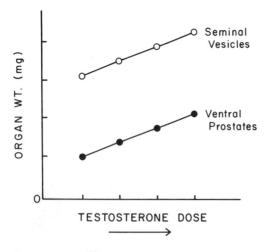

FIG. 10. Bioassay of androgens using rat seminal vesicles or ventral prostate glands from castrate rats.

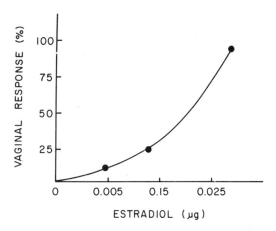

FIG. 11. Effect of estradiol on vaginal histology of the ovariectomized mouse.

group) are injected subcutaneously for a period of 7 days. On the eighth day, or 24 hr after the seventh daily injection, the mice are sacrificed and the uteri removed, trimmed of fat, and weighed. Like the vaginal smear bioassay, at least two dilutions of the unknown substance are run concurrently with the estradiol dose-response curve.

The immature chick can also be used to assess estrogenic potency. The immature chick bioassay is based on estrogens stimulating oviduct weights. A dose-response curve can be created by intramuscularly injecting immature chicks with varying doses of estradiol for a period of 7 days. Chicks are

sacrificed on the eighth day, and the oviducts are dissected and weighed.

Methods for measuring urinary metabolites of estrogens are available and have been used extensively to evaluate ovarian functions (11). The measurement of urinary estrogens is generally less reliable than measuring plasma levels of the hormone(s).

Radioligand binding and RIA for estrogens also are available (14). Vande Wiele and Dyrenfurth (131) compared various methods for the determination of estrogens. For the RIA of estradiol-17β, antiserum to estra-1,3,5(10)-triene-3,17β-diol 3-hemisuccinate–human serum albumin conjugate can be produced in ewes. Estradiol-17β standards may consist of 0, 1, 2, 5, 10, 25, 50, 100, and 200 pg in acetone. After the biological specimens containing estrogen(s) have been extracted with diethyl ether, the samples are separated on Sephadex columns (LH-20). Additional runs may be necessary to separate progesterone from estradiol.

Several methods for determining estrogen using monoclonal antibody assays have been reported (19,83).

PANCREAS

The pancreas secretes two important hormones: insulin and glucagon. These hormones are synthesized in the islets of Langerhans by alpha cells (glucagon) and beta cells (insulin). The morphologic arrangement of the pancreas is depicted on Fig. 13. A primary concern when testing for toxicity of an experimental drug is the potential for that compound to interfere with the normal functioning of the pancreatic beta cells. The signal that most often alerts the toxicologist to a possible pancreatic drug effect is hyperglycemia; and although this increased blood glucose content would normally be detected during routine clinical chemistry analyses, additional tests are required to pinpoint specific pancreatic toxicity.

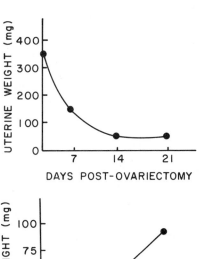

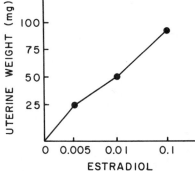

FIG. 12. A: Effect of ovariectomy on mouse uterine weights. **B:** Effect of daily injections of estradiol on uterine weight response in ovariectomized mice.

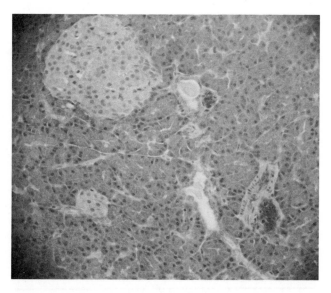

FIG. 13. Histology of rat pancreas. Note the acini ducts. ×256.

The relation between insulin and carbohydrate, fat, and protein metabolism represents some of the complexities seen in diabetes mellitus. Hyperglycemia may result from impaired utilization of glucose by cells due principally to insufficient production of insulin. The failure of glucose to penetrate adipose tissue mobilizes fat, producing a rise in the free fatty acid and triglyceride content of plasma and the triglyceride content of the liver (8). A diabetic fatty liver may result from the absence of lipoprotein synthesis brought on by accelerated gluconeogenesis. When glucose oxidation is impaired, fatty acids form the major source of energy; however, this situation generates an excess of intermediary metabolites, collectively described as ketone bodies (acetone, acetoacetic acid, and β-hydroxybutyric acid), which can lead to the development of metabolic acidosis.

Hyperglycemia also can lead to the appearance of glucose in the urine (glycosuria) when the blood glucose levels exceed the renal threshold of approximately 180 mg/dl. At lower levels, all the filtered glucose is normally reabsorbed by the renal tubules. It must be emphasized that blood glucose levels increased to the point of glycosuria also can be caused by emotional stress and the concomitant release of glucose from liver glycogen in response to epinephrine. Several drugs can affect blood glucose levels and can either increase or antagonize glycemic levels (Table 14). Glycosuria also can be the consequence of impaired renal tubular function caused by compounds such as the glycoside phlorizin. Renal glycosuria can produce an osmotic diuretic effect that leads to dehydration and polydipsia. Glycogenolysis and gluconeogenesis are increased in diabetes, generating glucose, which in turn increases blood glucose levels.

As was discussed earlier, the discovery of hyperglycemia during toxicity testing demands a more detailed investigation to determine the underlying mechanism(s). Such investigation focuses on the functional integrity of the pancreas and in particular of the beta cells. Experimental diabetes mellitus can be produced by destroying beta cell function with alloxan or streptozocin (Fig. 14).

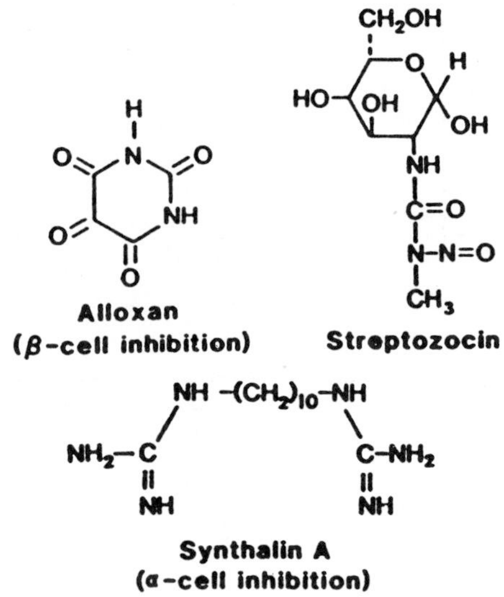

FIG. 14. Agents that inhibit pancreatic insulin and glucagon secretion.

Measurement of Insulin

Prior to RIAs, insulin was bioassayed using the rabbit hypoglycemia test. The biologic potencies of porcine, bovine, and human insulin using the rabbit bioassay requires that log-dose response curves be parallel (103).

Insulin was the first protein hormone to be measured by RIA (118,142,143). Although the RIA techniques that are available are similar with regard to the interaction between antigen and antibody, there are numerous variations in the methods for separating free insulin from antibody-bound insulin: gel filtration, salt precipitation, alcohol precipitation, precipitation with anti-γ-globulin serum, and adsorption on anion-exchange resin, cellulose, dextran-coated charcoal, antibody-coated tubes, and Sephadex-coupled antibodies. When measuring free plasma insulin, it is necessary to remove insulin antibodies by precipitation with polyethylene glycol (45).

An interesting method called the radioreceptor assay has been developed for quantitation of plasma insulin levels (71). This procedure uses insulin receptors isolated from a variety of sources, including placenta (97), rat liver plasma membranes (37), human lymphocytes (37), and guinea pig kidney (125). There are a number of advantages to this technique compared with the standard RIA. One is that the RIA exhibits varying degrees of cross-reactivity with proinsulin, which is not the case with the radioreceptor assay.

Plasma insulin levels may also be determined by enzyme-linked immunosorbent assay (ELISA) (138). Generally, this procedure has a number of drawbacks that preclude its routine use for the measurement of insulin, including a lower sensitivity than is seen with the RIA. Enzyme markers that have been utilized include alkaline phosphatase, glucoamylase, β-galactosidase, and peroxidase. Unfortunately, labeling and purification procedures are difficult, and assays tend to be more affected by nonspecific factors than are the RIA techniques.

TABLE 14. *Interaction of various drugs with oral hypoglycemic agents and insulin*

Enhanced effect (i.e., greater hypoglycemic action)	Antagonist effect
Ethanol	Acetazolamide
Anabolic steroids	D-Thyroxine
Chloramphenicol	Corticosteroids
Dihydroxycoumarin	Phenothiazines
Guanethidine	Epinephrine
Oxytetracycline	Phenytoin
MAO inhibitors	Marijuana
Phenylbutazone	Oral contraceptives
Phenyramidol	Diuretics
K$^+$ salts	(e.g. chlorthalidone,
Propranolol	ethracrynic acid,
Probenecid	furosemide, thiazides,
Salicylates	triamterene)
Sulfonamides	
Sulfinpyrazone	

Glucose Tolerance Tests

The glucose tolerance test, useful for evaluating endocrine pancreatic function, is based on the compensatory regulation of blood glucose levels by insulin following ingestion of a glucose load. The glucose load also can be administered orally or intravenously. Normally, in man the fasting blood glucose level is about 95 mg/dl. If 50 g of glucose is taken orally, the blood glucose level rises rapidly for approximately 30 to 60 min and then falls rapidly to obtain fasting levels by 2 to 3 hr. In situations where there is insufficient formation or release of insulin, there is an excessive rise in blood glucose levels following ingestion of the glucose load, and a slow, gradual fallback to preingestion levels.

Cytological Evaluation of Pancreatic Islet Cells

Alpha and beta islet cells can be differentiated using an aldehyde-fuchsin stain (Scott stain) following fixation of the tissue in Bouin's solution. The alpha cells stain light and the beta cells stain dark, permitting calculation of an alpha cell/beta cell ratio (113).

The use of pseudoisocyanic staining permits direct demonstration of insulin in the beta cells (112). The reaction involves the development of SO_2 groups formed by the oxidative splitting of the disulfide bridges of insulin with potassium permanganate.

Organ culture techniques for studying pancreatic islets have been investigated (74). The availability of suitably characterized dispersed islet cell preparation affords another *in vitro* test system to examine the effects of various drugs and chemicals on the pancreas (134). Monoclonal antibody methods are also available to assay for islet cell antibodies (117).

ACKNOWLEDGMENTS

The authors express their appreciation to Ms. Mary Rigoni for her assistance in typing and collating the manuscript as well as to Barbara Thomas for her grammatical and editing diligence.

REFERENCES

1. Aldercreutz, H. (1975): Determination of aldosterone in urine by gas-liquid chromatography. In: *Methods of Hormone Analysis*, edited by H. Breuer, D. Hamel, and H. L. Krüskemper, pp. 230–237. Wiley, New York.
2. Badger, T. M., Millard, W. J., McCormick, G. F., Bowers, C. Y., and Martin, J. B. (1984): The effects of growth hormone (GH)-releasing peptides on GH secretion in perifused pituitary cells of adult male rats. *Endocrinology*, 115:1432–1438.
3. Bayard, F., Bertlins, I. Z., Kowarski, A., and Migeon, C. J. (1970): Measurement of plasma aldosterone by radioimmunoassay. *J. Clin. Endocrinol.*, 31:1–6.
4. Bayard, F., Kowarski, A., Weldon, V. V., and Migeon, C. J. (1970): Appraisal of the double isotope dilution techniques for the measurement of plasma aldosterone. *J. Lab. Clin. Med.*, 75:347–354.
5. Bell, E. T., and Christie, D. W. (1970): Studies on the tetrazolium reduction assay for follicle stimulating hormone. *Acta Endocrinol. (Copenh.)*, 65:459–465.
6. Birge, C. A., Peake, G. T., Mariz, I. K., and Daughaday, H. (1967): Radioimmunoassayable growth hormone in the rat pituitary gland: effects of age, sex, and hormonal state. *Endocrinology*, 81:195–204.
7. Blazak, W. F., Ernst, T. L., and Stewart, B. E. (1985): Potential indicators of reproductive toxicity: testicular sperm production and epididymal sperm number, transit time, and motility in Fischer 344 rats. *Fundam. Appl. Toxicol.* 5:1097–1103.
8. Bondy, P. K. (1971): Disorders of carbohydrate metabolism: diabetes mellitus. In: *Cecil–Loeb Textbook of Medicine*, edited by P. B. Beeson and W. McDermott, pp. 1639–1658. Saunders, Philadelphia.
9. Bowman, R. (1975): Determination of cortisol in plasma as a Porter-Silber chromagen. In: *Methods of Hormone Analysis*, edited by H. Breuer, D. Hamel, and H. L. Krüskemper, pp. 211–218. Wiley, New York.
10. Braunsberg, H., and James, V. H. (1960): The fluorometric determination of adrenocortical steroids. *Anal. Biochem.*, 1:452–468.
11. Brown, J. B., and Mathews, J. D. (1962): The application of urinary estrogen measurements to problems in gynecology. *Recent Prog. Horm. Res.*, 18:337–385.
12. Burd, J. M., Weightman, D. R., and Baylis, P. H. (1985): Solid phase radioimmunoassay for direct measurement of human plasma oxytocin. *J. Immunoassay*, 6:227–243.
13. Burke, C. W., and Eastman, C. J. (1974): Thyroid hormones. *Br. Med. Bull.*, 30:93–99.
14. Butcher, R. L., Collins, W. E., and Fugo, N. W. (1974): Plasma concentration of LH, FSH prolactin, progesterone and estradiol-17β throughout the 4-day estrous cycle of the rat. *Endocrinology*, 94:1704–1708.
15. Cameron, E. H. D., and Scarisbrick, J. J. (1973): The determination of corticosterone concentration in rat plasma by competitive protein-binding analysis. *J. Steroid Biochem.*, 4:577–584.
16. Campbell, W. B., Pettinger, W. A., Keeton, K., and Brooks, S. N. (1975): Vasodilating antihypertensive drug-induced aldosterone release—a study of endogenous angiotensin-mediated aldosterone in the rat. *J. Pharmacol. Exp. Ther.*, 193:166–175.
17. Chard, T. (1974): Posterior pituitary peptides. *Br. Med. Bull.*, 30:74–79.
18. Chard, T., Kitau, M. J., and Landen, J. (1970): The development of radioimmunoassay for oxytocin: radioiodination, antibody production and separation techniques. *J. Endocrinol.*, 46:269–278.
19. Ciocca, D. R., and Dufau, M. L. (1984): Estrogen-dependent Leydig cell protein recognized by monoclonal antibody to MCF-7 cell line. *Science*, 226:445–446.
20. Clark, F., et al. (1985): The effect of drugs upon the assessment of thyroid function. *Adverse Drug React. Acute Poisoning Rev.*, 4(2):59–81.
21. Clemons, G. K., and Nicoll, C. S. (1977): Development and preliminary application of a homologous radioimmunoassay for bull frog prolactin. *Gen. Comp. Endocrinol.*, 32:531–535.
22. Collins, T. F. X., and Williams, C. H. (1971): Teratogenic studies with 2,4,5-T and 2,4-D in the hamster. *Bull. Environ. Contam. Toxicol.*, 6:559–567.
23. Collins, W. P., Sisterson, J. M., Koullapis, E. N., Mansfield, M. D., and Sommerville, I. F. (1968): The evaluation of a gas-liquid chromatographic method for the determination of plasma testosterone using nickel-63 electron capture detection. *J. Chromatogr.*, 37:33–45.
24. DePinho, R. A., Feldman, L. B., and Scharff, M. D. (1986): Tailor-made monoclonal antibodies. *Ann. Intern. Med.* 104:225–233.
25. Dicker, S. E. (1953): A method for the assay of very small amounts of antidiuretic titre of rats' blood. *J. Physiol. (Lond.)*, 122:149–157.
26. Döhler, K. D., Wong, C. C., and Mühlen, A. V. Z. (1979): The rat as model for the study of drug effects of thyroid function: consideration of methodological problems. *Pharmacol. Ther.*, 5:305–318.
27. Döllefeld, E., and Hamel, D. (1975): Determination of aldosterone in urine by double isotope derivative method. In: *Methods of Hormone Analysis*, edited by H. Breuer, D. Hamel, and H. L. Krüskemper, pp. 238–244. Wiley, New York.
28. Eechaute, W., Demeester, G., and Leusen, I. (1970): A sensitive

sulfuric acid ethanol induced fluorescence reaction for testosterone and androstenedione. *Steroids,* 16:277–287.

29. Ekins, R. P. (1974): Radioimmunoassay and saturation analysis—basic principles and theory. *Br. Med. Bull.,* 30:3–11.

30. El-Shaboury, A. H. (1965): Effect of a synthetic corticotrophin polypeptide on adrenal function in hypersensitive asthmatics. *Lancet,* 1:298–301.

31. Erbler, H. C. (1979): Measurement of corticosteroids as index for adrenal cortex function. *Pharmacol. Ther.,* 5:339–343.

32. Ewing, L. L., and Robaire, B. (1978): Endogenous antispermatogenic agents: prospects for male contraception. *Annu. Rev. Pharmacol. Toxicol.,* 18:167–187.

33. Forsyth, I. A., and Myers, R. P. (1971): Human prolactin: evidence obtained by the bioassay of human plasma. *J. Endocrinol.,* 51:157–168.

34. Frantz, W. L., and Turkington, R. W. (1972): Formation of biologically active ^{125}I-prolactin by enzymatic radioiodination. *Endocrinology,* 91:1545–1548.

35. Furuyama, S., Mayes, D. M., and Nugent, C. A. (1970): A radioimmunoassay for plasma testosterone. *Steroids,* 16:415–428.

36. Gandy, H. M., and Peterson, R. E. (1968): Measurement of testosterone and 17-ketosteroids in plasma by the double isotope dilution derivative technique. *J. Clin. Endocrinol. Metab.,* 28:949–977.

37. Gavin, J. R., Kahn, C. R., Gordon, P., Roth, J., and Neville, D. M. (1975): A radioreceptor assay of insulin: comparison of plasma and pancreatic insulins and proinsulins. *J. Clin. Endocrinol. Metab.,* 41:438–445.

38. Gomez-Sanchez, C. E., Kem, D. C., and Kaplan, N. M. (1973): A radioimmunoassay for plasma aldosterone by immunologic purification. *J. Clin. Endocrinol. Metab.,* 36:795–798.

39. Gomez-Sanchez, C. E., Murray, B. A., Kem, D. C., and Kaplan, N. M. (1975): A direct radioimmunoassay of corticosterone in rat serum. *Endocrinology,* 96:796–798.

40. Gorden, P., and Weintraub, B. D. (1985): Radioreceptor and other functional hormone assays. In: *Textbook of Endocrinology,* 7th ed., edited by J. F. Wilson and D. W. Foster. Saunders, Philadelphia.

41. Griffin, J. E. (1985): Dynamic tests of endocrine function. In: *Textbook of Endocrinology,* 7th ed., edited by J. D. Wilson and D. W. Foster. Saunders, Philadelphia.

42. Gross, H. A., Ruder, H. J., Brown, K. S., and Lipsett, M. B. (1972): A radioimmunoassay for plasma corticosterone. *Steroids,* 20:681–691.

43. Gunn, S. A., and Gould, T. C. (1956): The relative importance of androgen and estrogen in the selective uptake of Zn^{65} by the dorsolateral prostate of the rat. *Endocrinology,* 58:443–452.

44. Hanley, D. A., and Wellings, P. G. (1985): A "carboxyl terminal" clinical radioimmunoassay for parathyroid hormone with apparent recognition preference for the intact hormone. *J. Immunoassay,* 6:245–259.

45. Hanning, I., Home, P. D., and Alberti, K. G. M. M. (1985): Measurement of free insulin concentrations: the influence of the timing of extraction of insulin antibodies. *Diabetologia,* 28:831–835.

46. Harland, W. A., and Orr, J. S. (1969): A model of thyroxine metabolism based on the effects of environmental temperature. *J. Physiol. (Lond.),* 200:297–310.

47. Hermann, G. A., Sugiura, H. T., and Krumm, R. P. (1986): Comparison of thyrotropin assays by relative operating characteristic analysis. *Arch. Pathol. Lab. Med.,* 110:21–25.

48. Herrmann, J., and Krüskemper, H. L. (1975): Determination of total thyroxine in serum by competitive protein binding. In: *Methods of Hormone Analysis,* edited by H. Breuer, D. Hamel, and H. L. Krüskemper, pp. 118–125. Wiley, New York.

49. Hesch, R. K., Mühlen, A. V. Z., and Hufner, M. (1975): Radioimmunoassay of total triiodothyronine in plasma. In: *Methods of Hormone Analysis,* edited by H. Breuer, D. Hamel, and H. L. Krüskemper, pp. 150–155. Wiley, New York.

50. Hilfenhaus, M. (1977): Urinary aldosterone excretion rate and plasma aldosterone concentration in the rat: effect of ACTH, DOC, furosemide and of changes in sodium balance. *Acta Endocrinol. (Copenh.),* 85:134–142.

51. Hilfenhaus, M. (1977): Urinary excretion of corticosterone as a parameter of adrenal cortical function in rats. *Naunyn Schmiedebergs Arch. Pharmacol.,* 297(Suppl. 11):R41.

52. Hovatta, O., Huhtaniemi, I., and Wahlstrom, T. (1986): Testicular gonadotropins and their receptors in human cryptorchidism as revealed by immunohistochemistry and radioreceptor assay. *Acta Endocrinol. (Copenh.),* 111:128–132.

53. Hsu, S. M., Raine, L., and Fanger, H. (1981): A comparative study of the peroxidase-antiperoxidase method for studying polypeptide antibodies. *Am. J. Clin. Pathol.,* 75:734.

54. Hüfner, M., and Hesch, R. D. (1973): A comparison of different compounds of TBG-blocking used in radioimmunoassay for triiodothyronine. *Clin. Chim. Acta,* 44:101–107.

55. Humphrey, G. F., and Mann, J. (1949): Studies on the metabolism of semen. 5. Citric acid in semen. *Biochem. J.,* 44:97–105.

56. Hwang, P., Guyda, H., and Friesen, H. (1971): A radioimmunoassay for human prolactin. *Proc. Natl. Acad. Sci. USA,* 68:1902–1906.

57. Ito, T., Woo, J., Haning, R., and Horton, R. J. (1972): A radioimmunoassay for aldosterone in human peripheral plasma including a comparison of alternate techniques. *J. Clin. Endocrinol. Metab.,* 34:106–112.

58. Jacobs, H. S., and Lawton, N. F. (1974): Pituitary and placental glycopeptide hormones. *Br. Med. Bull.,* 30:55–61.

59. Kamoi, K., and Hama, H. (1977): Radioimmunoassay of the antidiuretic hormone. I. Methodology. *Acta Med. Biol.,* 25:101–108.

60. Kegan, A., and Glick, S. M. (1974): Oxytocin. In: *Methods of Hormone Radioimmunoassay,* edited by B. M. Jaffe and H. R. Behman, p. 173. Academic Press, New York.

61. Kennedy, J., and Chappel, S. (1985): Direct pituitary effects of testosterone and luteinizing hormone-releasing hormone upon follicle-stimulating hormone: analysis by radioimmuno- and radioreceptor assay. *Endocrinology,* 116:741–748.

62. Kimouchi, T., Pages, L., and Horton, R. A. (1973): A specific radioimmunoassay for testosterone in peripheral plasma. *J. Lab. Clin. Med.,* 82:309–316.

63. Kirkham, K. E., and Hunter, W. M., editors (1971): *Radioimmunoassay Methods.* Churchill Livingstone, Edinburgh.

64. Kohler, G., and Milstein, C. (1975): Continuous cultures of fused cells secreting antibody of predefined specificity. *Nature,* 256:495–497.

65. LaRose, P., Ong, H., and Du Souich, P. (1985): Simple and rapid radioimmunoassay for the routine determination of vasopressin in plasma. *Clin. Biochem.,* 18:357.

66. Larrick, J. W., and Buck, D. W. (1984): Practical aspects of human monoclonal antibody production. *Biotechniques,* Jan/Feb:6.

67. Larsen, P. R., and Frumess, R. D. (1977): Comparison of the biological effects of thyroxine and triiodothyronine in the rat. *Endocrinology,* 100:980–988.

68. Lefkowitz, R. J., Roth, J., and Pastan, Z. (1970): Radioreceptor assay of adrenocorticotropic hormone: new approach to assay of polypeptide hormones in plasma. *Science,* 170:633–635.

69. Leidy, J. W., and Robbins, R. J. (1986): Regional distribution of human growth hormone-releasing hormone in the human hypothalamus by radioimmunoassay. *J. Clin. Endocrinol. Metab.,* 62:372.

70. Liao, S., and Witte, D. (1985): Autoimmune anti-androgen-receptor antibodies in human serum. *Proc. Natl. Acad. Sci. USA,* 82:8345–8348.

71. Loffler, G., and Weiss, L. (1975): Radioimmunoassay of insulin in serum. In: *Methods of Hormone Analysis,* edited by H. Breuer, D. Hamel, and H. L. Krüskemper, pp. 85–100. Wiley, New York.

72. Lorsenson, M. Y. (1985): In vitro conditions modify immunoassayability of bovine pituitary prolactin and growth hormone: insights into their secretory granule storage forms. *Endocrinology,* 116:1399–1407.

73. Lyons, W. R., and Page, E. (1935): Detection of mammotropin in the urine of lactating women. *Proc. Soc. Exp. Biol. Med.,* 32:1049–1050.

74. Mandel, T. E., Hoffman, L., Collier, S., Carter, W. M., and Koulmanda, M. (1982): Organ culture of fetal mouse and fetal human pancreatic islets for allografting. *Diabetes,* 31(Suppl. 4):39–47.

75. Mann, T. (1964): *The Biochemistry of Semen and of the Male Reproductive Tract.* Wiley, New York.

76. May, M. E., and Carey, R. M. (1985): Rapid ACTH test in practice. *Am. J. Med.,* 79:679–684.

77. Mayes, D., and Nugent, C. A. (1968): Determination of plasma

testosterone by the use of competitive protein binding. *J. Clin. Endocrinol. Metab.*, 21:1169–1176.

78. Mayes, D., Furuyama, S., Kem, D. C., and Nugent, C. A. (1970): A radioimmunoassay for plasma aldosterone. *J. Clin. Endocrinol. Metab.*, 30:682–685.

79. McLachlan, J. A., and Dixon, R. L. (1977): Comparisons of experimental and clinical exposure to diethylstilbestrol during gestation. In: *Advances in Sex Hormone Research*, Vol. 3, edited by J. A. Thomas and R. J. Singhal, pp. 309–336. University Park Press, Baltimore.

80. Metcalf, M. C. (1963): A rapid method for measuring 17-hydroxy corticosteroids in urine. *J. Endocrinol.*, 26:415–423.

81. Millar, R. P., and Aehnelt, C. (1977): Application of ovine luteinizing hormone (LH) radioimmunoassay in the quantitation of LH in different mammalian species. *Endocrinology*, 101:760–768.

82. Millard, W. J., Sagar, S. M., Badger, T. M., and Martin, J. B. (1983): Cysteamine effects on growth hormone secretion in the male rat. *Endocrinology*, 112:509.

83. Moncharmont, B., and Parikh, I. (1983): Binding of monoclonal antibodies to the nuclear estrogen receptor in intact nuclei. *Biochem. Biophys. Res. Commun.*, 114:107.

84. Monroe, S. E., Parlow, A. F., and Midgley, A. R. (1968): Radioimmunoassay for rat luteinizing hormone. *Endocrinology*, 83:1004–1012.

85. Murphy, B. E. P. (1968): Clinical evaluation of urinary cortisol determinations by competitive protein-binding radioassay. *J. Clin. Endocrinol. Metab.*, 28:343–348.

86. Murphy, B. E. P., and Pattee, C. J. (1964): Determination of thyroxine utilizing the property of protein binding. *J. Clin. Endocrinol. Metab.*, 24:187–196.

87. Murphy, B. P., Engelberg, W., and Pattee, C. J. (1963): Simple method for the determination of plasma corticoids. *J. Clin. Endocrinol. Metab.*, 23:293–300.

88. Nauman, J. A., Nauman, A., and Werner, S. C. (1967): Total and free triiodothyronine in human serum. *J. Clin. Invest.*, 46:1346–1355.

89. Neill, J. D., and Reichert, L. E., Jr. (1971): Development of a radioimmunoassay for rat prolactin and evolution of the NIAMD rat prolactin radioimmunoassay. *Endocrinology*, 88:548–555.

90. Nicoll, C. S. (1967): Bioassay of prolactin: analysis of the pigeon crop-sac response to local prolactin injection by an objective and quantitative method. *Endocrinology*, 80:641–655.

91. Nicoloff, J. T., Low, J. C., Dussault, J. H., and Fisher, D. H. (1972): Simultaneous measurement of thyroxine and triiodothyronine peripheral turnover kinetics in man. *J. Clin. Invest.*, 51:473–483.

92. Nilsson, S. F., and Peterson, P. A. (1971): Evidence for multiple thyroxine-binding sites in human prealbumin. *J. Biol. Chem.*, 246:6098–6105.

93. Nissenson, R. A., Abbott, S. R., Teitelbaum, A. P., et al. (1981): Endogenous biologically active human parathyroid hormone: measurement by a guanyl nucleotide amplified renal adenylate cyclase assay. *J. Clin. Endocrinol. Metab.*, 52:840–846.

94. Norman, R. J., Poulton, T., Gard, T., and Chard, T. (1985): Monoclonal antibodies to human chorionic gonadotropin: implications for antigenic mapping, immunoradiometric assays, and clinical applications. *J. Clin. Endocrinol. Metab.*, 61:1031–1038.

95. Odell, W. D., and Daughaday, W. E., editors (1971): *Principles of Competitive Protein Binding Assays*. Lippincott, Philadelphia.

96. Odell, W. D., and Swerdloff, R. S. (1978): Abnormalities of gonadal function in men. *Clin. Endocrinol. (Oxf.)*, 8:149–180.

97. Ozaki, S., and Kalant, N. (1977): A radioreceptor assay for serum insulin. *J. Lab. Clin. Med.*, 90:686–699.

98. Palmer, A. K. (1981): Regulatory requirements for reproductive toxicology: theory and practice. In: *Developmental Toxicology*, edited by C. A. Kimmel and J. Buelke–Sam, p. 259. Raven Press, New York.

99. Parlow, A. F. (1961): Bioassay of pituitary luteinizing hormone by depletion of ovarian ascorbic acid. In: *Human Pituitary Gonadotropins*, edited by A. Albert, p. 300. Charles C Thomas, Springfield, Illinois.

100. Parlow, A. F., Wilhelmi, A. E., and Reichart, L. E., Jr. (1965): Further studies on the fractionation of human pituitary glands. *Endocrinology*, 77:1126–1134.

101. Piaditis, G. P., Hodgkinson, S. C., McLean, C., and Lowry, P. J.

(1985): Thyroid stimulating hormone. *J. Immunoassay*, 6:299–319.

102. Pierce, E. A., Dame, M. C., Bouillon, R., Van Baelen, H., and DeLuca, H. F. (1985): Monoclonal antibodies to human vitamin D-binding protein. *Proc. Natl. Acad. Sci. USA*, 82:8429–8433.

103. Pingel, M., Volund, A., Sorensen, E., Collins, J. E., and Dieter, C. T. (1985): Biological potency of porcine, bovine and human insulins in the rabbit bioassay system. *Diabetologia*, 28:862–869.

104. Porter, C. C., and Silber, R. H. (1950): A quantitative color reaction for cortisone and related 17,21-dihydroxy-20-keto steroids. *J. Biol. Chem.*, 185:201–207.

105. Prasad, J. A., and Hollander, C. S. (1979): Thyroxine and triiodothyronine. In: *Methods of Hormone Radioimmunoassay*, edited by B. M. Jaffe and H. R. Behrman, pp. 375–400. Academic Press, New York.

106. Raghavan, K. S., Singh, J., and Chhabra, J. K. (1977): Development of radioimmunoassay for oxytocin. *Indian J. Med. Res.*, 66:789–793.

107. Ratcliffe, J. E. (1974): Separation techniques in saturation analysis. *Br. Med. Bull.*, 30:32–37.

108. Hutchinson, J. S. M. (1988): The interpretation of pituitary gonadotropin assays—a continuing challenge. *J. Endocr.*, 118:169–171.

109. Rosenfeld, L., and Blum, M. (1986): Immunoradiometric (IRMA) assay for thyrotropin (TSH) should replace the RIA method in the clinical laboratory. *Clin. Chem.*, 32:No. 1.

110. Roth, J., Glick, S. M., Klein, L. A., and Peterson, M. J. (1966): Specific antibody to vasopressin in man. *J. Clin. Endocrinol. Metab.*, 26:671–675.

111. Rydén, G., and Sjöholm, I. (1962): Assay of oxytocin by rat mammary gland in vitro. *Br. J. Pharmacol.*, 19:136–141.

112. Schiebler, T. H., and Schiessler, S. (1959): Uber den Nachiweis von Insulin mit den metachromatisch Reagierenden Pseudoisocyaninen. *Histochemie*, 1:445–465.

113. Scott, H. R. (1952): Rapid staining of beta cell granules in pancreatic islets. *Stain Technol.*, 27:267–268.

114. Scriba, P. C., and Müller, O. A. (1975): Determination of cortisol in serum by fluorimetry. In: *Methods of Hormone Analysis*, edited by H. Breuer, D. Hamel, and H. L. Krüskemper, pp. 203–210. Wiley, New York.

115. Seethalakshmi, L., Steinberger, A., and Steinberger, E. (1984): Pituitary binding of ^{3}H-labeled Sertoli cell factor in vitro: a potential radioreceptor assay for inhibin. *Endocrinology*, 115:1289–1294.

116. Seif, S. M., and Robinson, A. G. (1978): Localization and release of neurophysins. *Annu. Rev. Physiol.*, 40:345–376.

117. Srikanta, S., Rabizadeh, A., Omar, M. A. K., and Eisenbarth, G. S. (1985): Assay for islet cell antibodies. *Diabetes*, 34:300.

118. Starr, J. I., Horwitz, D. L., Rubenstein, A. H., and Mako, M. E. (1979): Insulin, proinsulin and C-peptide. In: *Methods of Hormone Radioimmunoassay*, edited by B. M. Jaffe and H. R. Behrman, pp. 613–642. Academic Press, New York.

119. Steelman, S. L., and Pohley, F. M. (1953): Assay of follicle stimulating hormone based on the augmentation with human chorionic gonadotropin. *Endocrinology*, 53:604–616.

120. Hasegawa, Y., Miyamoto, K., Iwamura, S., and Igarashi, M. (1988): Changes in serum concentrations of inhibin in cyclic pigs. *J. Endocr.*, 118:211–219.

121. Sterling, K. (1975): Determination of total triiodothyronine in serum by competitive protein binding. In: *Methods of Hormone Analysis*, edited by H. Breuer, D. Hamel, and H. L. Krüskemper, pp. 134–149. Wiley, New York.

122. Sterling, K., and Lazarus, J. H. (1977): The thyroid and its control. *Annu. Rev. Physiol.*, 39:349–371.

123. Sterling, K., Hamada, S., Takemura, Y., Brenner, M. A., Newman, E. S., and Inada, M. (1971): Preparation and properties of thyroxine-binding alpha globulin (TBG). *J. Clin. Invest.*, 50:1758–1771.

124. Stevens, V. C. (1969): Comparison of FSH and LH patterns in plasma, urine and urinary extracts during the menstrual cycle. *J. Clin. Endocrinol. Metab.*, 29:904–910.

124a. Stites, D. P., Stobo, J. D., Fudenberg, H. H., and Wells, J. V. (1984): *Basic and Clinical Immunology*, 5th ed. Lange Medical Publications, Los Angeles, California.

125. Suzuki, K., Ohsawa, N., and Kosaka, K. (1976): Radioreceptor assay for insulin. *J. Clin. Endocrinol. Metab.*, 42:399–406.

126. Thomas, J. A. (1988): Occupational hazards and reproductive risks. In: *Hormones and Reproduction as Targets of Occupational Chemicals,* edited by S. Sezabo, and J. A. Thomas. Lewis Publishing Company.

127. Thomas, J. A. (1981): Reproductive hazards and environmental chemicals. *Rev. Toxic Substances J.,* 2:318.

128. Thomas, J. A., and Keenan, E. J. (1986): Drugs affecting the endocrine system. In: *Principles of Endocrine Pharmacology.* Plenum Press, New York.

129. Thomas, J. A., Mawhinney, M., and Mason, W. (1968): Sex accessory fructose: an evaluation of biochemical technique. *Proc. Soc. Exp. Biol. Med.,* 127:930–937.

130. Underwood, R. H., and Williams, G. H. (1972): The simultaneous measurement of aldosterone, cortisol, and corticosterone in human peripheral plasma by displacement analysis. *J. Lab. Clin. Med.,* 79:848–862.

131. Vande Wiele, R. L., and Dyrenfurth, I. (1973): Gonadotropins-steroid interrelationships. *Pharmacol. Rev.,* 25:189–217.

132. Vecsei, P. (1979): Glucocorticoids: cortisol, cortisone, corticosterone, compound S and their metabolites. In: *Methods of Hormone Radioimmunoassay,* edited by B. M. Jaffe and H. R. Behrman, pp. 767–796. Academic Press, New York.

133. Vermeulen, A. (1975): Determination of cortisol in plasma by competitive protein binding. In: *Methods of Hormone Analysis,* edited by H. Breuer, D. Hamel, and H. L. Kürskemper, pp. 195–202. Wiley, New York.

134. Weir, G. C., Halban, P. A., Meda, P., Wollheim, C. B., Orci, L., and Renold, A. E. (1984): Dispersed adult rat pancreatic islet cells in culture: A, B, and D cell function. *Metabolism,* 33:447–453.

135. Williams, G. H., and Underwood, R. H. (1979): Mineralocorticoids: aldosterone, deoxycorticosterone, 18-hydroxydeoxycorticosterone and 18-hydroxycorticosterone. In: *Methods of Hormone Radioimmunoassay,* edited by B. M. Jaffe and H. R. Behrman, pp. 743–766. Academic Press, New York.

136. Wilson, J. D., and Foster, D. W. (1985): *Textbook of Endocrinology,* 7th ed. Saunders, Philadelphia.

137. Wilson, M. A., and Miles, L. E. M. (1977): Radioimmunoassay of insulin. In: *Handbook of Radioimmunoassay,* edited by G. E. Abraham, pp. 275–297. Marcel Dekker, New York.

138. Wisdom, G. B. (1976): Enzyme immunoassay. *Clin. Chem.,* 22:1243–1255.

139. Wofsy, D. (1985): Strategies for treating autoimmune disease with monoclonal antibodies. *West J. Med.,* 143:804.

140. Worth, G. K., Nicholson, G. C., Retallack, R. W., Gutteridge, D. H., and Kent, J. C. (1985): Parathyroid hormone radioimmunoassay: the clinical evaluation of assays using commercially available reagents. *J. Immunoassay,* 6:277–298.

141. Yalow, R. S. (1985): Radioimmunoassay of hormones. In: *Textbook of Endocrinology,* 7th ed., edited by J. D. Wilson and D. W. Foster, pp. 123–321. Saunders, Philadelphia.

142. Yalow, R. S., and Berson, S. A. (1959): Assay of plasma insulin in human subjects by immunological methods. *Nature,* 21:1648–1649.

143. Yalow, R. S., and Berson, S. A. (1960): Immunoassay of endogenous plasma insulin in man. *J. Clin. Invest.,* 39:1157–1175.

144. Zarrow, M. X., Yochim, J. M., and McCarthy, J. L. (1964): *Experimental Endocrinology, A Source Book of Basic Techniques,* pp. 129–140. Academic Press, New York.

Principles and Methods of Toxicology, Second Edition, edited by A. Wallace Hayes, Raven Press, Ltd., New York © 1989.

CHAPTER **25**

Application of Isolated Organ Techniques in Toxicology

Harihara M. Mehendale

Department of Pharmacology and Toxicology, University of Mississippi Medical Center, Jackson, Mississippi 39216-4505

The concept of organ perfusion for physiological and biochemical studies is not new. Early accounts of organ perfusion techniques in biochemical and physiological studies may be found in the descriptions of Baglioni (14) and Muller (164). More detailed accounts of the historical development of organ perfusion techniques may be found in the works of Brodie (31) and Embden and Glaüssner (65). Systematic early developments in organ perfusion techniques have been reviewed by Skutul (234) and Kapfhammer (110). Increasing interest in the application of the techniques of perfusing isolated organs and tissues in biochemical and physiological investigations is apparent in the more recent works of Ross (215), Diczfalusy (57), and Ritchie and Hardcastle (213). An interest in the applications of the isolated perfused organ techniques in the studies on the toxicological mechanisms (151,153, 169,218,251) is apparent in the increasing number of reviews appearing in the literature. Some investigators have advanced the term "*ex vivo* perfusion" to refer to the technique of perfusing and maintaining functional isolated organs.

INTRODUCTION

The rationale for experimental studies using perfused organs and for trying to improve the technology of organ perfusion lies in the following physiological and biochemical considerations. We recognize homeostasis to be the outcome of many simultaneously occurring, interacting complex processes. It is recognized that when many simultaneously occurring processes interact, they may collectively take on functional properties that cannot be perceived in any of the individual component processes. In endocrine and metabolic systems, a basic experimental question arises at the organ level: How does the organ's uptake or output of some toxic substance depend on the composition of the arterial blood reaching the organ? The technique of organ perfusion can, if certain conditions are met, permit one to make controlled concentration changes in the perfusing blood while observing the time course of the organ's response in terms of its uptake or output of one or more substances. This kind of experimentation has several advantages. Mathematical models based on some convenient equations can be constructed relating the nature of a toxic compound(s) and its concentration in blood. The nature of the substances produced as a result of the biotransformation can be investigated and related to the specific organ, and the role of that organ in converting a substance into either a more harmful or a biochemically inert species can be effectively evaluated. Quantitative input on these pathways of biotransformation into the appropriate mathematical models can lead to the understanding and development of predictable values.

In the simplest terms, the essentials of isolated organ perfusion techniques are (a) the desirability of separating individual organs from the whole animal to permit the study of one in the absence of complex interaction by others; (b) the need for the tissue to be physiologically compatible to the *in vivo* situation; and (c) the desire to simulate the natural circulation through an organ. In the latter regard, the composition of the medium changes constantly, as in the whole body, at least with respect to the experimental toxic agent: Not all substances reenter the perfusion medium, nor are all substances entirely removed by the organ. Finally, an analytical study of the organ itself can be undertaken; artificial means of stimulating organ function may aid in magnifying the physiological role of, or effect on, the organ, thus enabling determination of such an interaction. Although use of autologous whole blood would be considered ideal for homeostatic mechanisms, substitution with artificial media is often necessary for technical reasons; an attempt is made to maintain the cell structure and function by following as many viability criteria as possible.

Choice of Donor Animal

A variety of factors may influence the choice of organ donor animals in perfused organ studies. Often the nature of the particular problem being investigated is the determining factor when choosing the experimental animal. Susceptibility or refractoriness to the toxic agent to be tested and the presence or absence of biotransformation pathways govern the selection of a particular species and often a particular strain. Other factors may influence the final selection of the experimental animal as well. Availability of pertinent background information in a particular animal model may compel the investigator in favor of that species in the interest of savings in time and resources. Availability, cost of animals, and maintenance or unique genetic characteristics may become important considerations. The rat has been most popular in this regard as a donor for perfusion experiments. Thus heart (9,143,163,167), liver (30,144,154,157), lung (37,135,180, 186,194), kidney (15,18,138,169), brain (3,69,124,249), and pancreas (89,113,187,188,243) perfused preparations obtained from the rat have been employed by many investigators for a variety of biochemical studies. Larger animals employed in perfusion experiments include the cat (4,44,80,115,189), dog (4,63,103,130,260,266), rabbit (4,43, 130,136,152,171,186,205,206,214), and monkey (4). Among the larger animals employed for perfusion experiments are calves (41), goats (142), pigs (63), and sheep (63,246).

All small animals have the disadvantage of small blood vessels, which pose difficulties in surgical procedures. In many instances the experimenter is interested in using autologous blood for perfusion, and small animals may not yield sufficient blood supply to prime the perfusion apparatus. The trend has been to utilize either diluted or reconstituted blood or completely artificial perfusion medium composed of natural or synthetic ingredients. Nevertheless, in a few instances the necessity of using autologous whole blood as a perfusate essentially eliminates the use of small experimental animals in perfusion experiments. Additional factors to be considered are the volume and number of the perfusate samples needed to carry out necessary analytical tests during the course of the experiment. These difficulties are clearly overcome by using large experimental animals. Large animals, however, have the distinct disadvantage of increased cost, on the one hand, and requisite chemicals, equipment, space, and other supplies on the other. Use of expensive isotopically labeled chemicals or limited availability of valuable samples of newly synthesized or isolated test drugs may make it necessary to restrict the perfusion experiments to organs from smaller animals.

Large or small, other considerations may also be important. Much fat, particularly in the abdominal areas of large animals or old small animals contributes to surgical difficulties. The presence or absence of some tissues, such as the gallbladder, which is absent in rat and present in the rabbit, might be an additional consideration. For the purpose of acquainting oneself with the techniques of organ perfusion, the size of the animal per se matters little. However, considerations of economy of space, equipment, small apparatus, and animal costs might make the choice of a small animal a prudent one. In view of these and other considerations discussed above, whenever possible, we consider the rat the animal of choice. However, it is important to bear in mind that most procedural and other technical considerations remain the same with minor modifications when a particular perfusion technique is intended to be applied to a large animal or to an animal of similar or smaller size.

In Situ and Isolated Organ Perfusion System

Isolated organ perfusion may be defined as the maintenance of an organ in vascular isolation from the rest of the tissues and organs of the body by mechanically assisted circulation of a suitable fluid through its vascular bed. In most cases, special apparatus is acquired, and each investigator has invariably adopted an individual approach to solving the technical problems associated with maintaining a particular organ in viable condition for a particular toxicological investigation. The resulting scattered literature and many technical variations introduced in the techniques of organ perfusion have to a large degree contributed to the difficulty of a newcomer to the field of isolated organ perfusion to readily adopt the application of these techniques toward investigating the special problems of toxicology. Often it is difficult to assess the merits of the available methods. Given the complexity of the problem, there is often reluctance on the part of some toxicologists to embark on isolated perfused organ studies, even in those areas of biochemical toxicology where these techniques offer unique and definitive advantages over other *in vitro* or *in vivo* techniques. Establishment of a set of standards for each organ perfusion system by an internationally composed committee might alleviate many of the problems arising out of infinitely varied perfusion techniques and methodology introduced by individual investigators in a scattered body of diverse literature.

One rather obvious prerequisite for isolated organ perfusion studies is that the organ to be perfused is capable of vascular isolation from the neighboring tissues, although physical isolation is not obligatory. A separate vascular bed is sufficient to ensure that only one tissue or organ is perfused in isolation. For instance, an organ may be perfused in isolation but may remain *in situ*, as in the case of lung (133), liver (96), intestine (112,191), or kidney (15). A principal advantage of perfusing the organ *in situ* is the time saved in surgical removal of the organ, thereby reducing the time of interrupted perfusion. An additional advantage is that it reduces physical damage to the organ, which may be inflicted during surgical removal of the organ.

Alternatively, the organ to be perfused may be physically isolated from the animal, as in the case of lung (173), liver (144,157), kidney (170), heart (163,167), intestine (61), and pancreas (89). The principal advantage of physically isolating an organ is the elimination of interactions between the organ being perfused and other tissues and organs present in the body. Although the vascular bed of the organ being perfused may be totally isolated, the endogenous substances being secreted may seep out of other tissues and organs and might come in physical contact with the organ being perfused, resulting in uncontrollable or even unanticipated interactions. Similarly, the compound being studied in the perfused organ may be secreted and absorbed by other surrounding tissues and organs by physical contact and hence may introduce experimental errors in the quantitative and qualitative aspects of the disposition of the toxic chemical being studied. Accuracy and reliability of mass-balance studies of toxic chemicals and hence the accountability of the chemical and possible metabolites are vastly better with isolated perfused organs.

Advantages of Isolated Perfused Organ Techniques

Isolated perfused organ preparations offer several advantages over experimentation with intact animals. Perfusion experiments lend themselves to a definitive evaluation of the role of a particular organ or tissue in the disposition of endogenous or exogenous chemicals. Although experimentation with whole animal preparations may provide clues implicating a possible role of a particular organ in regulating the levels of a test toxin or an endogenous substance in response to a toxin, decisive conclusions may not be feasible. A case in point is provided by the studies (71) that reported the presence of γ-aminobutyrate in the lungs of rats and mice after these animals were injected with radioactive putrescine. This finding cannot be taken as conclusive evidence for the formation of γ-aminobutyrate in the lungs, as it could have been transported from other sites of synthesis. Isolated, ventilated, and perfused lungs (207) and other tissue preparations were used to examine if rat and rabbit lungs were capable of metabolizing putrescine to γ-aminobutyrate (208), establishing that the lungs of these species are devoid of the diamine oxidase necessary for this metabolism. Isolated perfused organ studies provide opportunities to decisively ascertain or reject such possibilities.

Unlike the *in vitro* homogenate preparations, intact organ perfusion studies allow the experimenter to retain the structural and functional integrity of the organ in question during such experiments. Unlike in the intact animal, perfusion experiments allow the experimenter to retain control over several experimental parameters, e.g., perfusion pressure and blood flow; in the intact animals these measurements are likely to change during the course of an experiment, especially in response to administration of the experimental toxic chemical. The concentrations of endogenous or exogenous stimulatory substances and other factors can be under experimental control in isolated perfused organ studies. The isolated perfused organ would lend itself to a broader range

of concentrations of the experimental drug to be used in the study. That is, concentrations of drug at which the intact animal would not be expected to survive can be tested in isolated perfused organs. Determination of accurate and complete mass-balance of the toxic chemical in question is possible throughout the perfusion experiment, as the compound must either be in the perfusate or the tissue, or be excreted via excretory fluids such as bile and urine. Binding of the test drug to the glassware, tubing, and other components of the perfusion apparatus may occur, but this possibility can be explored in blank experiments from which appropriate correction factors are derived; moreover, removal of such interfering factors is often technically feasible. Another advantage of perfusion studies is the availability of large blood or perfusate samples; thus complete qualitative and quantitative analyses of minor and major biotransformation products of the test compound are feasible, as the volume of perfusate used in these experiments can be controlled. A further advantage of perfusion experiments in comparison with whole-animal experiments is the feasibility of tests with smaller quantities of toxic chemicals. This point is particularly noteworthy, as limitations of either the availability of small quantities of the toxins or the cost of isotopically labeled newly synthesized compounds can be formidable.

Another advantage of perfused organ studies is the maintenance of appropriate membrane barriers, not only between vascular and parenchymal sides but also between individual cells; hence the natural constraints of intact organs are retained throughout the experimental duration. Evidence has made it clear that one may not be able to predict the qualitative and quantitative aspects of biotransformation of a test drug by intact organ based only on the results of *in vitro* experiments with homogenate preparation (149). Factors governing the generation and availability of cofactors and transport of substrate to the site of biotransformation influence the final results in the intact perfused organ (101,149,250). These factors can remain operative in perfusion studies unlike with other *in vitro* techniques, thereby enabling realistic extrapolation of the results to *in vivo* situations. Finally, no matter how determined, experimental results have to be interpreted and extrapolated to the *in vivo* situation, where intact organs interact continuously; such interpretation and extrapolation are made easier by use of intact perfused organs in toxicological investigations.

Furthermore, the cell-to-cell interactions are preserved in an intact perfused organ, which might be either missing or at least compromised in isolated cells or other *in vitro* incubations. The collagenase trypsin or other proteases used in procedures to isolate cells might alter the plasma membrane, thereby altering the permeability and even receptor characteristics of isolated cells. For example, in freshly prepared hepatocytes, glutathione levels are only half of the normal values. Some essential and critical differences between the tissue slice experiments and perfusion studies are also of interest in this regard. Whereas the perfusion of intact organs allows entry of the chemical through the endothelium, which would be representative of what happens in the intact animal, tissue slice incubations permit entry of chemicals directly into the parenchymal cells through a direct contact. Studies using tissue slice incubations might not represent the *in vivo* situation, as some chemicals may not be taken up through the endothelial barrier altogether or be taken up to a small extent. Hepatocytes or slices incubated with the calcium channel blockers do not have any influence on cellular calcium, whereas the perfused liver is responsive to these same calcium blockers. The latter findings would be clearly more representative of the *in vivo* situation than the former.

Limitations

The present-day state of the art allows maintenance of isolated perfused organ preparations with adequate physiological and biochemical integrity for only short periods of time. Clinically, advances have allowed maintenance of the kidney for several days for later physical transplantation in patients. These procedures require subambient temperatures to preserve organ function. Such techniques are not generally useful in toxicological studies, as maintenance of the organ at optimal functional level is a prerequisite for most toxicological studies. Hence the principal limitation imposed by the isolated perfused organ preparations is the short duration of study. Critical and vital organ functions deteriorate in isolated perfused organs with time. For example, isolated perfused lung preparations can be maintained for a maximum of only 4 hr (173). Often it is not possible to determine the effect of therapeutic agents on the lung tissue in such a short period of time. Similarly, isolated perfused liver preparations cannot be maintained for longer periods without compromising liver function (114,142,218). A practical consideration of interest in this connection may also be the level of expertise required for setting up the perfusion experiments. Setting up and conducting successful perfusion experiments requires specially trained personnel in all aspects of the surgical procedures as well as the technical aspects of associated instrumentation. Unavailability of such personnel requires that the investigator allow valuable time for training.

Often a principal argument in favor of isolated perfused organ studies is the maintenance of natural membrane barriers, the integrity of the intact cells, and the complex and dynamic interrelations between individual and groups of cells. For certain studies this argument may represent a principal limitation. The complexity of a whole organ deprives the toxicologist of access to individual reactions that occur within the organ. Compartments and permeability barriers may prevent substrates and test drugs from exerting effects that are known to manifest when the particular toxic agent is allowed direct access to the enzyme or organelle of interest. *In vitro* experiments with homogenate preparations and tissue slice preparations would be the obvious choice of techniques when dissection of individual transport processes and biotransformation reactions is the principal objective. The size of a single experiment and time required to perform it may make organ perfusion a far less efficient use of time and resources than *in vitro* preparations that demonstrate the same effects. Another consideration is the availability of the experimental tissue or organs. Although access to valuable human tissues might be available, such access might be infrequent; and in any event, the available tissue would be limiting. Clearly, isolated cell techniques or other *in vitro*

techniques have the advantages of maximizing the use of such invaluable experimental material when designing and carrying out studies of utmost relevance. Schimmel and Knobil (227) pointed out the greater efficiency of establishing an experimental fact with tissue slices than with isolated perfused organ. Finally, despite all the refined techniques of maintaining the organ *in vitro* in as near a normal state as possible, the resulting preparation may differ in some highly significant manner from the organ *in vivo*, limiting the interpretation of results obtained in the organ perfusion system.

Scope of this Chapter

The principal purpose of this chapter is to acquaint the reader with generalized principles and methods for the isolation and perfusion of selected organs from experimental animals. Accordingly, the following discussion represents simplified and often idealized procedures, so a relative novice could undertake application of perfusion techniques to toxicological investigations. Sufficient references are included to serve as focal points for the benefit of those who are already engaged in perfusion of isolated organs and who seek advanced information. The principles governing the choice of isolated perfused organ studies, the experimental protocols (including the composition of perfusion media, duration of perfusion, considerations of recirculation, or single-pass circulation), and other related aspects are available in the examples of perfused organ studies employed in toxicology studies.

Thorough considerations of pumps and mechanical devices (22) used in perfusion of organs, application and testing of pharmacokinetic concepts to isolated perfused organs (219), and the mathematical considerations of single-pass studies in isolated organs (67,194) are available elsewhere. Similarly, use of radiolabeled microspheres to determine intraorgan and regional blood flows (220) may also be considered in isolated perfused organ studies. Excellent reviews on the application of perfusion techniques to biochemical studies (215), to the studies of reproductive endocrinology (57), and to other general consideration of perfusion techniques, especially in large experimental animals (213), are available elsewhere for those seeking additional and detailed considerations of organ perfusion techniques.

METHODOLOGY

Isolated Perfused Heart

Since Langendorff (130) described a procedure for isolation and perfusion of dog or rabbit heart, heart has been the model for studying the effects of toxic agents on metabolism in muscle. A succession of investigators (9,24,31,43,163,185) have demonstrated the stability and versatility of the preparation. The original method of Langendorff (130) has survived with only minor modifications and remains the standard preparation on which toxicological studies are performed (12,56,76,119).

Two procedures have been used for isolated perfused heart preparations. One uses the aortic perfusion described by Langendorff (130), and the other uses atrial perfusion, in which the left atrium is cannulated. The Langendorff preparation perfuses the muscle of both ventricles, although only the left ventricle produces any tension by contracting against the closed aortic valve. The atrial perfusion method gives a "working heart" preparation: It allows the left ventricle to fill, which results in normal systolic and diastolic cycles. The perfusion described by Morgan et al. (163) and later improvised by Neely et al. (167) provides for the working heart circulation (143,231). Several studies have compared the aortic perfusion of Langendorff and atrial perfusion of working heart preparations. One considerable advantage in the working heart preparation is the ease and accuracy with which myocardial performance can be quantified. In the Langendorff preparation, coronary flow and heart rate are the only available physical parameters of function. The "working heart," on the other hand, has aortic output as a quantifiable parameter of function, although it is dependent on the heart achieving an aortic pressure of at least 100 cm H_2O. Anoxia, lack of substrate, poison, and drugs may be qualitatively and quantitatively tested on this basis. Linearity of oxygen and substrate uptake is an additional means of assessing function in this preparation; and together with easily observed abnormalities of cardiac rhythm, which may also indicate failure of the preparation (66), the working heart preparation is easily and accurately assessed (143,231).

However, despite the completeness of description and advantages of the working heart, investigators in this field have experienced many difficulties establishing a viable working heart preparation for significant lengths of experimental time. Hence although quantitative differences do occur in many biochemical and functional measurements, the working and nonworking heart preparations are similar in many respects (122). Although with certain experimental protocols it is necessary to employ both preparations, it is doubtful if it will be necessary to carry out all toxicological tests on the heart in both Langendorff and working heart preparations. Because the former is so much simpler, its use will continue to be popular for some time to come.

Aortic Perfusion

Apparatus

The heart is suspended in a water-jacketed cylindrical chamber of 3 cm diameter and 20 cm length with a coarse sintered-glass filter disk sealed into the lower portion (Fig. 1). The aortic cannula is mounted in a Teflon stopper, through which pass the gas inlet tube and an outlet vent for the excess gases. The inflowing gas is delivered by means of a fine plastic tube extending into a small pool of perfusion medium, which collects on the surface of the sintered-glass filter. After passing through the filter, medium is recirculated by a peristaltic pump. This pumping arrangement results in a waveform applied to the heart, but it can be considerably dampened by passing the perfusate first through a bubble

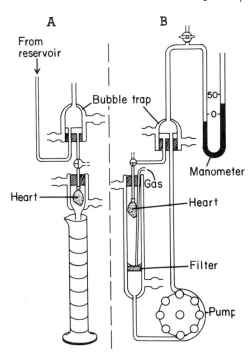

FIG. 1. "Langendorff" heart perfusion. A: Single-pass perfusion. B: Recirculating perfusion. (From ref. 163, with permission.)

trap containing 1 to 2 ml of air so that the characteristics of the pump waveform may be eliminated.

Operation procedure

Rats weighing approximately 250 to 300 g can be used for obtaining isolated heart preparations. The donor animal is killed by decapitation. It may be desirable to heparinize the animal by administering heparin intraperitoneally (5 mg) 1 hr before decapitation to prevent formation of large clots. Within 20 sec after decapitation, the thorax is widely opened by incisions to remove the anterior wall. The heart is removed immediately by means of a scissor cut across the great vessels about 5 mm from the heart. Earlier investigators (163) allowed a 1- to 2-min cooling period by immersing the heart in ice-cold Krebs-Ringer buffer solution. This step is not necessarily desirable, and in fact greater speed may help reduce the likelihood of anoxic damage to the heart. Ischemia and reperfusion are known to give rise to the formation of toxic free radical species that adversely affect the quality of the heart preparations (111,121,265). After blotting the heart with filter paper and weighing it, a small glass cannula (or polyethylene tubing, PE-200) can be inserted into the aorta, with the tip of the cannula positioned just above the semilunar valves. Instantaneously beating heart is then perfused through the aortic cannula. The heart preparation thus established may be allowed to equilibrate for a period of 15 to 20 min by means of a setup in which the perfusate is allowed to recirculate (Fig. 1). Oxygenation of the perfusate is accomplished using a mixture of oxygen and carbon dioxide (O_2/

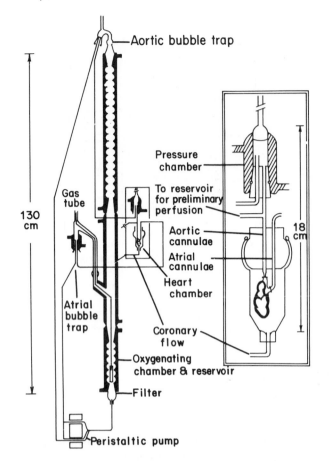

FIG. 2. Working rat heart preparation. Completely assembled apparatus is shown on the left. Heart chamber, cannula assembly, and pressure chamber are enlarged and illustrated on the right. The apparatus consists of the following components. *Heart chamber and cannula assembly.* The male portion of a size 35 ball joint is made up of Teflon and holds two stainless steel cannulas (0.134 in. o.d.) grooved to hold the ligatures. A tip of 0.109 in. o.d. tubing is soldered into the aortic cannula. The female portion of a 35/25 size ball joint is adopted for use as a heart chamber and held in place with a pinch clamp. *Aortic and atrial bubble traps and pressure chamber.* These parts are made from female portions of 14/35 standard taper joints. Male plugs are made of Teflon and fitted with neoprene "O" rings to facilitate sealing and removal of the stoppers. A side arm is sealed onto the arterial bubble trap, extended with Silastic tubing, and connected to the central portion of the apparatus by an 18/9 size ball joint. A side arm for the aortic bubble trap can be made from the male portion of a size 15 ball joint. This is connected to an adapter (size 28 ball, 29/42 standard taper), which in turn can be fitted into the iop condenser of the central portion of the apparatus. *Oxygenating chamber.* Three condensers with size 29/42 standard taper connections make up the central portion of the apparatus. Both the top condenser (60 cm long) and the bottom one (20 cm long) are ful-jak align condensers. An additional condenser can be used as the middle portion. It receives the overflow from the atrial bubble trap and coronary effluent from the heart chamber. A coarse-porosity, sintered glass filter is fitted into the bottom of the oxygenating chamber. A peristaltic pump is used to transport the blood to the top of the oxygenator via glass tubings. The shaded portion of the glass apparatus in-

CO_2, 95:5) that is humidified by passing through water at 37°C before entering the apparatus to prevent loss of perfusate volume by evaporation.

Atrial Perfusion of the Working Heart

Apparatus

Apparatus for the atrial perfusion of heart (167) is shown in Fig. 2. The glass components of the working heart perfusion apparatus are a double-jacketed oxygenator, a 100-cm bubble trap, a mixing column, connecting pieces, condensers, 100-cm reservoir, a heart chamber, and a second bottle trap. The filter used is a closed Millipore system adapted from that used in ultrafiltration. For example, a Millipore in-line filter holder may be used. Whenever possible, tubing components are composed of glass; connections between glass tubings are made with flexible tubing, with the exception of the compression tubing used in the roller pumps, for which siliconized medical grade tubing may be used. The apparatus is assembled as illustrated in Fig. 2.

Operating procedures

A rat weighing approximately 250 g is lightly anesthetized with ether. Without preparation of the skin, the first incision is made with large, pointed scissors around the lower margin of the ribs. The first cut is made across the upper abdomen, taking care not to injure the liver. This cut is extended laterally, and for this purpose the rat may be held in the left hand. The point of the scissors is then directed toward the head, and a single cut is made through the layers of the thorax, including the ribs up to the clavicle. Cuts are made on the left side and the right side, producing a free flap of the anterior chest, which is removed with a cut transversely at the level of the second rib. At this time the heart is fully exposed. The heart is grasped firmly between the thumb and forefinger of the left hand and lifted, drawing it to the animal's right. This step exposes the pulmonary veins and the site of entry into the left atrium. The point of the scissors is passed horizontally and behind the left atrium, pulmonary veins, and aortic arch. Before closing the blades to cut, the instrument is drawn well over the animal's left in order to leave the maximum length of pulmonary vein in continuity with the atrium. After cutting the pulmonary veins, the scissors are pointed downward and away from the operator, and the aorta is cut about 0.5 cm from the ventricle. This length is adequate for cannulation. If the cut is made too near the heart, a hole is made in the left atrium, rather than through the pulmonary veins, which makes cannulation difficult.

dicates double-jacket arrangement for circulating warm water to facilitate warming the perfusate. Fluid in bubble traps and the pressure chamber is indicated by stippling. (From ref. 167, with permission.)

The heart is thus removed and transferred rapidly to ice-cold Krebs-Ringer buffer, and aortic cannulation is carried out. The cannula is filled to the tip with oxygenated medium, making sure to avoid entrapping air bubbles. The aorta is grasped from opposite sides in two pairs of fine curved forceps and gently lifted over the straight cannula. The cannula may be retained by a single ligature around the aorta. It is important to watch that the tip of the cannula does not rest on the aortic valve because it is too far down the aorta. A flow of the medium at maximal rate is begun as soon as the ligature is tied, ending the unavoidable period of operative myocardial anoxia. The heart should begin to beat within 10 to 15 sec of starting the perfusion.

Arterial cannulation may be conducted at leisure, as the heart is fully perfused via the aorta and is no longer at risk of anoxia. The atrial wall is grasped by forceps as it lies on either side of the cannula, and by turning the wrist outward the wall is slightly averted. The atrium is then drawn over the cannula itself. The cannula is positioned and retained in this position by means of a ligature. The final step is to incise the right ventricle and its pulmonary trunk, which allows drainage of the medium that has accumulated in the right side of the heart from the minor coronary veins; otherwise such accumulation results in poor cardiac function. The incision is made with pointed scissors through the base of the ventricle and at the origin of the pulmonary trunk.

Perfusion Media

A variety of perfusion media with minor modifications have been used to perfuse isolated heart preparations. Use of whole blood (77,195), Krebs-Henseleit bicarbonate buffer medium (163,167), and Krebs-Ringer buffered solution (9,43) has been reported for maintaining successful perfused heart preparations. Many advantages have been pointed out for the use of whole blood to perfuse isolated heart preparations (77). However, whenever it has been done (77,161), circulation of whole blood through the isolated heart was maintained using support animals. In these preparations the circulation from the isolated heart enters the circulation of the support animal via the right jugular venous cannula and exits the support animal via the left carotid artery (77). Although satisfactory preparations are obtained, such isolated preparations may not adapt to all types of toxicological investigation. The principal limitation arises from introducing the support animal to the perfusion circuit. The support animal would clear the test chemical, making it difficult to correlate the effects of test toxins on cardiac function and to evaluate possible myocardial biotransformation. Hence artificial perfusates have been used most often in biochemical and toxicological investigations.

Various investigators have introduced minor variations in individual ion composition of the particular medium used in their own experimental setups. The medium of choice, however, seems to be the Krebs-Ringer bicarbonate-buffered solution of the following composition: NaCl 119 mM; KCl 4.75 mM; CaCl$_2$·2H$_2$O 2.54 mM; KH$_2$PO$_4$ 1.19 mM; MgSO$_4$·7H$_2$O 1.19 mM; NaHCO$_3$ 25.0 mM; glucose 5.5 mM. The solution may be sterilized by ultrafiltration to avoid microbial contamination. If autoclaving is used, addition of glucose is withheld until later. Equilibration with O$_2$/CO$_2$ (95:5) for at least 30 min before using the perfusate increases the viability of the perfused preparation as well as the buffering capacity of the perfusate during perfusion. The pH of the medium is adjusted to 7.4 by means of a dilute solution of NaOH.

Viability Criteria

A number of functional, biochemical, and histological determinations have been used to ensure the viability and validity of the perfused heart preparation. Physical measurements of cardiac function include electrocardiogram (ECG) recordings of the left ventricular pressure and left ventricular end-diastolic pressure, and the perfusion pressure of the isolated heart preparations (77). Other functional parameters that can be continuously recorded include the heart rate, isometric systolic tension, and coronary flow (9). Aronson and Serlick (9) examined the effect of perfusion time on a number of these parameters (Table 1). Changes in the heart rate were evident 15 min after the end of the initial equilibration period. However, after being perfused for as long as 4 hr, the heart rate was approximately 86% of the initial level, indicating the usefulness of the perfused heart preparation in toxicological studies. In contrast to the heart beat, coronary flow and isometric systolic tension (Table 1) appear to be more sensitive, as indicated by their decrease with perfusion time. A number of biochemical parameters can be examined in heart preparations as indices of viability (Table 2). Glycogen concentration was not significantly decreased until 3 hr but decreased to 33% of the zero time control values after 4 hr of perfusion. Likewise, adenosine-5′-triphosphate (ATP) concentrations remained stable for 3 hr but significantly decreased in hearts perfused for 4 hr. Creatine phosphate concentrations showed the greatest change during the first hour of perfusion; they diminished to 51% of the amount present at zero time in the control group. After perfusion for 4 hr, the creatine phosphate content of the tissue was 45% of the zero time control value. Histochemical evaluation of the heart preparations for viability can be useful initially in establishing the perfusion methodology (9). Tissues fixed by classical histological methods can be examined for any evidence of inflammatory infiltrate, edema, or hemorrhage.

Applications

Although isolated perfused heart preparations have been used in a variety of ways to study the mechanism and interaction of various drugs and hormones (8–10,56,85,90), as well as in biochemical investigations (111,215), these preparations are not generally used to screen drugs or toxic chemicals for potential cardiotoxicity. However, efforts (12,55, 68,76,115,119,121,143,204,205,231,265) have been directed toward using such preparations for toxicological investiga-

TABLE 1. *Effect of perfusion on heart rate, coronary flow, and isometric systolic tension in the isolated perfused rat heart*[a]

Perfusion time[b] (min)	No.[c]	Spontaneous heart rate ± SE (beats/min)	Coronary flow ± SE (ml/min)	Isometric systolic tension ± SE (g)
0	32	285 ± 5.9	7.9 ± 0.4	13.8 ± 0.7
15	26	280 ± 5.2	7.8 ± 0.4	15.0 ± 0.9[d]
30	26	270 ± 5.3[d]	7.7 ± 0.4	14.3 ± 0.9
45	26	267 ± 5.0[d]	7.8 ± 0.4	13.6 ± 0.9
60	26	270 ± 5.8[d]	7.9 ± 0.5	12.6 ± 1.0[d]
75	19	266 ± 6.0[d]	7.9 ± 0.6	12.3 ± 1.2[d]
90	19	263 ± 6.7[d]	7.5 ± 0.6	11.4 ± 1.2[d]
105	19	263 ± 6.7[d]	7.3 ± 0.6	10.6 ± 1.2[d]
120	19	262 ± 6.4[d]	7.0 ± 0.5[d]	9.6 ± 1.2[d]
135	12	272 ± 8.6	7.2 ± 0.6	8.2 ± 1.4[d]
150	12	272 ± 10.1	7.1 ± 0.5	7.7 ± 1.4[d]
165	12	275 ± 11.0	7.3 ± 0.7[d]	7.0 ± 1.4[d]
180	12	265 ± 9.7[d]	6.9 ± 0.5[d]	6.4 ± 1.3[d]
195	6	255 ± 10.2[d]	6.2 ± 0.2[d]	6.8 ± 2.0[d]
210	6	245 ± 9.2[d]	6.1 ± 0.6	6.0 ± 1.8[d]
225	6	245 ± 9.2[d]	5.7 ± 0.5[d]	5.3 ± 1.7[d]
240	6	245 ± 9.2[d]	5.2 ± 0.5[d]	4.8 ± 1.3[d]

[a] Hearts obtained from untreated normal male animals.
[b] Duration of perfusion after initial 15-min equilibration period.
[c] Total number of measurements.
[d] Significant ($p < 0.05$) compared to zero perfusion time by paired variate Student's *t*-test.
From ref. 9, with permission.

tions. For example, Autian (12) stressed the need for the development of reliable *in vitro* systems with which to screen large numbers of drugs and emphasized the advantages of using isolated perfused heart preparations. Gad et al. (76) used isolated perfused rat heart preparations to examine the inhibitory actions of the prooxidant butylated hydroxytoluene (BHT) on cardiac function. Cardiac contractility was depressed and leakage of creatine phosphate into the perfusate was found within 30 min of perfusion when BHT was included in the perfusion medium in concentrations ranging from 1 to 500 mg/L. Thus these investigations provided direct evidence that BHT depresses contractility and causes cellular damage of isolated heart as measured by the leakage of creatine phosphate from the myocardium.

Drug effects on myocardial contractile function are obviously of considerable practical importance for the toxicologist. The basic mechanism of such actions must reside at some point in the metabolism of cardiac muscle. Interference in the liberation of energy of the metabolic fuels utilized by the myocardial tissue may be implicated in many of the toxicological effects induced by drugs and other toxic chemicals. For instance, chlorpromazine (50 ng/ml) decreased isometric systolic tension and prolonged the QT interval in the ECG of the perfused rat heart (10). Fructose-1,6-diphosphate and pyruvate concentrations were elevated, suggesting aldolase inhibition and decreased pyruvate utilization. Anesthetic drugs that produce reversible depression of myocardial contractile function in a dose-dependent fashion have been shown to interfere with many of the mechanisms involving the generation and utilization of cellular energy in the heart

tissue (155). Use of isolated perfused heart preparations would be a valid and useful technique in the toxicological investigations related to drug-induced heart disease (10,13,53).

Dewildt and Speijers (55) studied the effects of dietary rapeseed oil and pure erucic acid on the mechanical behavior of the isolated rat hearts after 24 to 26 weeks. Neither compound caused any effects on the ECG changes in comparison to the control sunflower seed oil diet. After inotropic intervention, only the rapeseed oil group showed less contractile reserve capacity. The authors concluded that a fat-rich diet might result in reduced myocardial function during a state of energy demand, and that the erucic acid effects must be on the peripheral vascular system.

A number of studies (68,121,265) have examined the role of oxyradicals in myocardial damage due to ischemia and reperfusion using perfused heart preparations. Koster et al. (121) demonstrated the release of malonaldehyde (MDA) in the coronary effluent of hearts perfused with cumene peroxide (0.5 mM), indicating a susceptibility of the coronary vascular tissue preradical-induced lipid peroxidation. The possible role of oxygen preradicals in the development of reperfusion arrhythmias was investigated using a 10-min period of coronary ligation followed by reperfusion in the isolated rat heart (265). Glutathione (GSH) and a combination of superoxide dismutase, catalase, and mannitol reduced the incidence of reperfusion-induced ventricular fibrillation when given just prior to reperfusion. Because these oxyradical scavengers protected against the reperfusion-induced myocardial injury, such experiments have been employed to implicate the role of oxyradicals in reperfusion-induced arrhythmias (265).

TABLE 2. *Effect of perfusion time on metabolite concentrations in the isolated perfused rat heart*[a]

Metabolite	Concentration ($\mu m/g \pm SE$[b]) at various perfusion times[c]				
	0 hr	1 hr	2 hr	3 hr	4 hr
Glycogen	14.23 ± 1.25	11.83 ± 1.60	9.59 ± 1.60	5.44 ± 0.93[d]	4.75 ± 0.39[d]
D-Glucose-1-phosphate	0.0214 ± 0.0154	0.0142 ± 0.0141	0.0155 ± 0.0141	0.0018 ± 0	0.0062 ± 0
D-Glucose-6-phosphate	0.0336 ± 0.0141	0.0480 ± 0.0109	0.0343 ± 0	0.0410 ± 0.0063	0.0532 ± 0.0134
D-Fructose-6-phosphate	0.0252 ± 0.0134	0.0096 ± 0	0[d]	0.0018 ± 0[d]	0.0052 ± 0
Fructose-1,6-diphosphate	0.0380 ± 0.0161	0.0656 ± 0.0236	0.0248 ± 0.0091	0.0204 ± 0.0109	0.0258 ± 0.0118
D-Glyceraldehyde-3-phosphate	0.0750 ± 0.0218	0.0908 ± 0.0148	0.0626 ± 0.0276	0.0680 ± 0.0271	0.0732 ± 0.0373
Dihydroxyacetone phosphate	0.0438 ± 0.0271	0.0238 ± 0.0089	0.0320 ± 0.0091	0.0572 ± 0.0209	0.0134 ± 0.0077
Total triose phosphate	0.1188 ± 0.0223	0.1146 ± 0.0161	0.0946 ± 0.0294	0.1246 ± 0.0209	0.0866 ± 0.0313
L-(−)-Glycerol phosphate	0.1892 ± 0.0588	0.1764 ± 0.0331	0.2175 ± 0.0764	0.2326 ± 0.0399	0.4018 ± 0.1011
Pyruvate	0.0206 ± 0.0173	0.0146 ± 0.0099	0.0166 ± 0.0107	0	0.0300 ± 0.0299
L-(+)-Lactate	1.1458 ± 0.3296	0.6068 ± 0.1193	0.7733 ± 0.1505	0.6020 ± 0.0470	0.8980 ± 0.1961
Adenosine-5'-triphosphate	2.8882 ± 0.1258	2.4058 ± 0.2271	2.6448 ± 0.1670	2.3692 ± 0.1846	1.7400 ± 0.1290[d]
Adenosine-5'-diphosphate	0.1370 ± 0.0199	0.1688 ± 0.0503	0.1613 ± 0.0244	0.2118 ± 0.0354	0.2138 ± 0.0519
Adenosine-5'-monophosphate	0.0544 ± 0.0118	0.0776 ± 0.0138	0.0441 ± 0.0091	0.0364 ± 0.0126	0.0808 ± 0.0099
Total nucleotides	3.0796 ± 0.1174	2.6522 ± 0.1902	2.8503 ± 0.1650	2.6174 ± 0.1980	2.0346 ± 0.1140[d]
Creatine phosphate	3.7180 ± 0.1710[d]	1.8866 ± 0.3085[d]	2.3355 ± 0.2002[d]	1.4494 ± 0.0885[d]	1.6766 ± 0.1698[d]

[a] Hearts were obtained from untreated control animals. Results are from five or six hearts in each group.
[b] Expressed per gram of tissue (wet weight).
[c] Duration of perfusion after initial 15-min equilibration period.
[d] Significant at 5% level when compared to zero perfusion time by an independent Student's *t*-test.
From ref. 9, with permission.

Ferrari et al. (68) induced ischemia in isolated, perfused rabbit hearts by reducing the coronary flow from 25 to 1 ml/min for 90 min. The effects of postischemic reperfusion were also followed for 30 min. These studies provided evidence that severe ischemia induces a reduction of the protective mechanisms, e.g., GSH and protein SH groups and mitochondrial superoxide dismutase (SOD) activity. Reperfusion induces a massive release of reduced GSH, oxidized GSH (GSSG), and creatine phosphokinase (CPK), leading to a further decrease in tissue content of these important protective mechanisms, which in turn lead to loss of mechanical function. Interestingly, the CPK leakage associated with ischemia and reperfusion of the heart is augmented by arachidonic acid (111). In these studies the recovery of contractility was also suppressed by arachidonic acid (10 mg/ml). Arachidonic acid augmentation was protected by antioxidant vitamin E, indomethacin, a prostaglandin synthesis inhibitor, and nordihydroguarietic acid, a lipoxygenase inhibitor, observations that are consistent with the preradical mediation of ischemia-reperfusion injury of the myocardium. The studies demonstrated that isolated, perfused heart preparations have significantly advanced our understanding of the oxyradical involvement in myocardial injury.

Isolated, perfused heart preparations have also been employed to study mechanisms of specific toxic chemicals. McDonough et al. (143) employed the perfused working rat hearts to assess the intrinsic function after challenge with lethal or nonlethal doses of endotoxin to the rats. They concluded that the myocardial reserve was compromised by *in vivo* administration of endotoxin in a dose-dependent fashion.

Nahas and Trouve (165) employed Langendorff perfused rat heart preparations to assess the dose-response effects of natural cannabinoids on heart rate, coronary flow, and supraaortic differential pressure (ΔP). Δ^9-Tetrahydrocannabinol produced a biphasic increase in heart rate without any change in coronary flow, but ΔP was increased. Studies of the toxicity of doxorubicin (56), dantrolene (85), digitalis (115), chronic alcohol consumption (231), thioridazine-5-sulfoxide (90), acetone (204), and *n*-hexane (205) have also been studied toxicologically using perfused heart preparations.

For many toxicological studies it is necessary to determine the perfusate concentration of the experimental drugs with time. It is also necessary to determine the appearance and disappearance kinetics of possible metabolites of the test toxin. As is true in the case of most perfused organ studies, these experiments can be carried out employing either recirculating perfusate or a single-pass mode. In most experimental protocols, it is prudent to determine in advance which mode of circulation would be utilized. It will also be necessary to determine the size of the perfusate sample needed to carry out the analyses intended and the time course and total duration of the experiment. As indicated in Table 1, many enzymatic determinations can be carried out in the perfusate as well as in the heart tissue itself.

Isolated Perfused Liver

The isolated perfused liver preparation has enjoyed the longest-standing sustained attention in terms of functionally preserved isolated organs for biochemical, pharmacological,

and toxicological studies. The views of Miller et al. (157) concerning the perfused liver is that functional performance of the liver cells is best studied in the isolated liver perfused with continuously oxygenated whole, homologous blood under closely approximating physiological conditions. Earlier attempts to obtain viable, perfused liver preparations were marked by many problems, and in most cases the failure can be attributed to several factors (157): use of aqueous perfusion media such as Ringer's solution in place of whole blood; lack of adequate filtering devices to remove tiny fibrin clots that plug the hepatic circulatory system; relative unavailability of effective, nontoxic anticoagulants such as heparin, which result in ominous failure to carry out perfusion for more than 1 to 2 hr when whole blood is used as the perfusate. We have now witnessed the increased use of isolated liver preparations in a variety of pharmacological and toxicological investigations. Much credit for developing and standardizing isolated perfused liver techniques belongs to Miller et al. (157) and Schimassek (224).

There are two sources of blood supply to the liver: The portal vein supplies 80% and the hepatic artery 20% of the blood flow. Most workers have ignored the hepatic arterial supply when perfusing the rat liver. Although experiments confirm that the liver functions normally even in the absence of perfusion through the hepatic artery, techniques are now available that allow this small blood vessel to be perfused at normal arterial pressure, either under hydrostatic conditions (217) or by direct pumping (200). By and large, the rat has been the animal of choice for isolated perfused liver preparations (2,19,144,154,157,227,244,250,251), although livers from other experimental animals have been perfused for various investigations (4,41,63,153).

Apparatus

In the liver perfusion technique of Miller et al. (157), the liver is perfused at a constant hydrostatic pressure using diluted rat blood as the perfusion medium, which passes through a glass multibulb oxygenator. The perfusate enters the portal vein via a filter and drains from the liver through the inferior vena cava either via an indwelling cannula or through a free cut of the vena cava; it collects in a bottom reservoir. From the reservoir it is pumped to the top of the oxygenator, which it enters through a filter. The liver is removed from the animal after the cannulation procedure, and perfusion is conducted by connecting the portal cannula of the liver to the preprimed circulation of the apparatus housed in an enclosed liver chamber.

The apparatus designed by Miller has been almost universally adopted by workers using this technique, and it is also available commercially. The liver perfusion apparatus used in our laboratory (144) is based on Miller's (157) description and is illustrated in Fig. 3. The perfusion chamber is kept warm by means of a heater-fan assembly that is thermostatically controlled. The original description of Miller et al. (157) noted use of a heating coil that traversed the inner surface of the chamber. Cleaning the chamber becomes difficult with this arrangement. Hence the heating may be accomplished by installing a highly efficient heating coil inside a box, which would also house a fan (144). The glass mul-

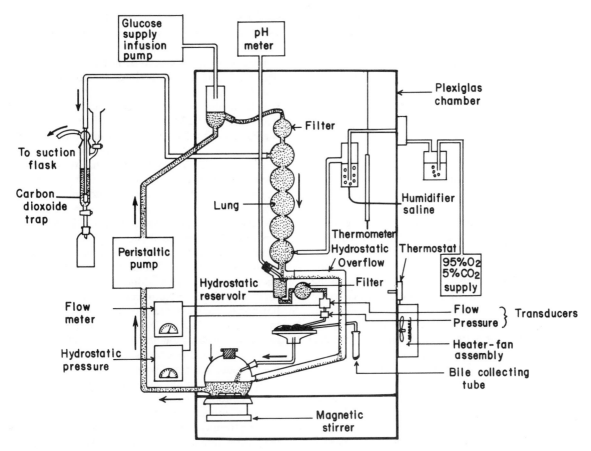

FIG. 3. Liver perfusion apparatus modified from that described by Miller et al. (157). Most of the circulation carrying the perfusate is housed inside a Plexiglas chamber fitted with a thermostatically controlled heater–fan assembly, which is connected to the top of the chamber to recirculate warm air from the chamber. In the center of the chamber a pair of vertical cylindrical rods (not shown) are fitted to facilitate securing various items inside the chamber by means of appropriate clamps. The bottom reservoir, liver platform, flow and pressure transducers, filter, multibulb glass lung hydrostatic reservoir, humidifier, and upper reservoir to dampen the peristaltic wave of the perfusate are held by means of suitable clamps on these vertical rods. The lever platform has a ground-glass joint that can fit the top of the bottom reservoir. A different arrangement is shown here that allows sampling the effusate directly from the liver by disconnecting the side-arm connection of the bottom reservoir. The inside of the chamber is accessible via two overlapping sliding doors (not shown) in the front of the chamber. (From ref. 144, with permission.)

tibulb oxygenator can be easily put together by connecting a series of 100-ml round-bottomed flasks (144). At the bottom of the multibulb glass oxygenator an inlet is provided for oxygen supply, and at the top of the oxygenator a side outlet is provided for the carbon dioxide to escape. The bottom reservoir is provided with a number of side arms and a principal opening at the top to connect the platform that supports the liver. A magnetic stirrer can be introduced into the bottom reservoir, and a magnetic stirring device can be placed below the reservoir under the chamber. The perfusate can be pumped by means of a peristaltic pump to avoid hemolysis of red blood cells when either whole blood or diluted blood is used as the perfusate. O_2/CO_2 (95:5) is passed through a water trap to humidify the gas mixture. The expired gas escaping from the top of the multibulb glass lung is passed through a carbon dioxide trapping device. This phase is especially useful in studies in which either labeled carbon dioxide or other volatile metabolic products are expected to be formed. Efficient filtration of the blood perfusion medium is considered to be crucial for successful perfusion. Two disks of Lucite are compressed together to hold a disk of white silk (100 × 150 mesh per inch), and two such filters are introduced into the perfusate circulation to clear broken cells, tiny fibrin clots, and any other debris in the perfusate.

Surgical Procedure

Surgical removal of the liver from the rat can be performed under ether anesthesia. With the animal lying on its back, the limbs are fixed in extension on a surgical board. The anterior abdomen is cleaned with 75% alcohol, and a ventrical longitudinal midline incision is made extending from pubis to upper chest. The common bile duct is cannulated with PE-10 tubing. The animal is heparinized with 1,000 units of sodium heparin by injecting the solution into the inferior vena cava anterior to the renal vein. Immediately after the injection the vena cava is ligated anterior to the site of injection. The portal vein is then cannulated with a PE-240 or a smaller cannula filled with the perfusate. An incision can be made in the thoracic vena cava using a PE-240 cannula. A loose ligature is placed around the inferior vena cava, and the outflow cannula is inserted through the right atrium. The inferior vena cava is cut between the heart and the cannula. The liver is then dissected out together with the diaphragm. Some investigators have suggested an incision through the anterior diaphragm, leaving only a collar of the diaphragm attached to the inferior vena cava.

The liver with or without the diaphragm is then lifted free of the abdomen together with its cannulas and transferred to a warm saline bath. Immersing the liver in the warm saline facilitates proper orientation of the lobes as well as cleaning the blood clots and debris that may be on the surface of the liver. Removing the liver and subsequent handling requires skill and should be accomplished with a minimum of handling of the organ itself. After ensuring that the lobes of the liver are properly oriented, the liver may be attached to the perfusion apparatus by connecting the portal cannula to the circulating perfusate. The liver is placed on the platform, making sure that the outflow cannula is let down through the central porthole of the platform extending into the neck of the bottom reservoir. Proper orientation of the common bile duct cannula ensures unhindered bile flow.

An equilibration period of 30 min is generally sufficient to establish proper perfusion flow and for the liver to recover from the brief period of anoxia it underwent during the surgical procedure. Glucose can be infused throughout the perfusion to replenish the glucose utilized by the liver. This procedure also allows replacing any fluid losses due to evaporation of the perfusate in the heated chamber (144).

Earlier investigators have used antibiotics (157,225) to prevent bacterial growth in the perfusate during the course of the perfusion. In many toxicological studies, it is important to keep the perfusion system free of drugs in view of the complexity of possible drug interactions. Most pieces of the perfusion apparatus can be autoclaved and sterilized. The perfusion chamber can be surface-sterilized using 75% ethanol. Other items that do not permit autoclaving can also be surface-sterilized with 75% ethanol. For instance, the perfusion flow transducer, pressure transducer, pH probe, and polyethylene cannulas and filters can be surface-sterilized using ethanol. Use of antibiotics has not been necessary under these conditions to obtain viable preparations up to 6 hr (144).

Perfusion Media

Miller used a medium of fresh, heparinized rat blood usually diluted with Ringer's solution to a hematocrit of 25 to 40%. By far the most variation introduced into a liver perfusion system is due to the differences in the composition of perfusate used. Whole rat blood would be the ideal physiological perfusate. Advantages of including whole blood are implicit in having hemoglobin and a natural oxygen carrier as well as natural protein and lipids to provide binding and carrier sites for experimental drugs. However, economic limitations make use of whole rat blood as a perfusate impractical. Moreover, certain experimental protocols such as single-

pass studies utilize large volumes of perfusate, and use of whole blood becomes exceedingly expensive and impractical. The following blood perfusate has the advantages of containing rat blood as well as being economical, as it is mixed with two parts of Krebs-Ringer bicarbonate-buffered solution (pH 7.4). Krebs-Ringer bicarbonate solution includes the following, in grams per liter: NaCl 6.896; KCl 0.354; $CaCl_2 \cdot 2H_2O$ 0.373; KH_2PO_4 0.162; $NaHCO_3$ 2.1; $MgSO_4 \cdot 7H_2O$ 0.293; bovine serum albumin (BSA) Cohn fraction V 45; and glucose 0.901. The solution is adjusted to pH 7.4 with 1 N NaOH solution. Freshly collected heparinized whole rat blood is mixed with this solution to obtain a 30% blood perfusate. The required volume of glucose solution (20% solution) is added to the perfusate to obtain a final glucose concentration of 3.2 g/L. The advantages of this type of medium are the physiological nature and high oxygen-supplying capacity. The disadvantages are the poorly defined nature of the blood with respect to the presence of hormones and substrates, and the difficulty of collecting blood from small animals. To circumvent the problem of uncertainty of hormones and substrates, some investigators have used human or bovine (225–227), or human (96) erythrocytes, which can be included in the perfusate after washing.

Triner et al. (254) demonstrated that isolated perfused liver preparations can be supported using artificial oxygen carriers such as fluorocarbon emulsions emulsified in electrolyte buffer solution. The use of fluorocarbon emulsion in the perfusion of isolated organs would have a number of advantages over erythrocyte suspension. Avoidance of possible antigenicity from nonautologous erythrocytes and simpler, more standardized, less expensive preparations of perfusion media are among the advantages. In experiments comparing the adequacy of fluorocarbon emulsions to replace erythrocytes in the perfusate, three kinds of fluorocarbon were evaluated (87,177,254). Urea nitrogen, glucose, sodium, potassium, and alanine aminotransferase in the medium, and incorporation of ^{14}C-lysine into the liver proteins, were found to be either normal or above normal compared to perfusate containing erythrocytes (177) when fluosol-43 was used as the fluorocarbon oxygen carrier. Using the fluorocarbon FC-47 emulsified in Krebs-Ringer bicarbonate-buffered solution, Goodman et al. (87) found that oxygen consumption, alanine aminotransferase gluconeogenesis, production of lactate and ketone bodies, and hepatic ATP concentrations were no different than when buffer or a medium containing suspended erythrocytes was used as perfusate. The cytosolic and mitochondrial redox states, as indicated by the hepatic lactate/pyruvate and β-hydroxybutyrate/acetic acid ratios, respectively, were also the same whether the medium contained erythrocytes or FC-47 (87).

Because of the varieties of perfusion media used for liver perfusion by various investigators (19,30,144,154,157,250,251) it is prudent to select the most appropriate perfusion medium for a particular experimental protocol. Many variables include the presence or absence of bovine or other serum albumin, erythrocytes, buffering agents, amino acids, glucose, vitamins, antibiotics, and heparin. These conditions in combination may or may not be appropriate for the particular experimental design. A study designed to examine the utilization of externally provided GSH may not be valid if BSA is included in the perfusion medium (107). Reduced GSH

(GSSG) is oxidized rapidly ($t_{1/2}$ 10 min) in Krebs-Ringer bicarbonate medium containing BSA (107). Replacing the albumin with high-molecular-weight dextran was found to preserve the GSSG. A perfusion system designed to study Ca^{2+} fluxes from the liver may not contain albumin or hemoglobin, as the ion-selective electrode used for measuring the change in perfusate Ca^{2+} might not be compatible with these constituents (154).

Viability Criteria

Certain viability criteria can be readily used to evaluate the perfused liver. For instance, bile flow can be used as a viability criterion. Here 1 to 1.5 $\mu l/min/g$ of liver can be expected from a normal rat liver, which can change depending on the experimental conditions. Bile flow can be expected to drop with the time of perfusion, as the endogenous bile acid pool would be depleted during bile collection. Some investigators have used an infusion of sodium taurocholate in the perfusate to maintain the bile flow throughout the perfusion time.

Another easily recognizable viability criterion is the perfusion flow rate. At a hydrostatic pressure of 15 to 20 cm H_2O, a flow rate of up to 60 ml/min can be obtained using diluted (30%) blood as perfusate. Even after allowing for a lower viscosity of the perfusate, this flow rate would be judged to be beyond the normal physiological range. Hence the perfusion flow rate should be controlled by means of a suitable clamp placed between the portal cannula and the hydrostatic reservoir. Once a stable flow is attained, the flow rate through the liver can be used as a readily available criterion for evaluating the viability of the organ.

Another easily detectable criterion is visual examination of the liver. Inadequately perfused liver gives a reddish appearance, indicating anoxia, as well as a blotchy appearance on the surface of the liver. Often, if the liver is not secured on the platform, the liver moves in such a way as to impede proper, continuous, uniform perfusion through the organ. The liver may move such that the flow of the liver through the outflow cannula may be impeded, resulting in swelling of the liver. Visually, this problem is easily recognized by the tensile and anoxic appearance of one or more lobes of the liver.

Oxygen consumption by the liver can be used as another criterion for viability. For instance, Schimassek (224) reported that oxygen consumption by the perfused liver was 2.2 nmol/min/g of tissue after the 30-min equilibration period, and it was maintained at this level thereafter. Oxygen consumption can be measured by following the oxygen tension of the perfusate before it enters the liver and sampling the oxygen content of the perfusate after it effuses from the liver (154).

A number of biochemical parameters can be used for ascertaining the viability of the perfused liver. Schimassek (225) has shown conclusively that the isolated perfused livers under standard conditions have glycolytic intermediate concentrations, a respiratory quotient, and adenine nucleotide levels close to those found in the liver fresh out of the animal (Table 3). Such determinations in the isolated perfused liver preparation have allowed several investigators to determine normal conditions of perfusion. A variety of other biochemical parameters have also been determined in isolated perfused liver preparations to establish the physiological validity of using such a preparation (126). Miller et al. (157) determined incorporation of ^{14}C-lysine into hepatic proteins as a biochemical index of optimum macromolecular synthetic activity during perfusion. Bock et al. (26) measured a number of biochemical parameters associated with the microsomal mixed function oxidase (MFO) and cytochrome P-450 system and found satisfactory preservation of the hepatic MFO sys-

TABLE 3. *Substrate content of isolated, perfused rat liver after various times of perfusion*

Metabolite	Content (μmol wet wt. of liver) under various conditions			
	In vivo	Before perfusion	After 30 min perfusion	After 120 min perfusion
Lactate (L)	1,450	12,000	3,570	3,400
Pyruvate (P)	145	50	277	345
α-Glycero-P	253	1560	304	450
DAP	38	21	45	67
Malate (M)	443	750	281	280
Oxaloacetate (O)	7	<1	4.2	4
FDP	22	17	20	41
F-6-P	75	—	—	41
G-6-P	370	986	141	206
Glucose	8,600	25,900	11,600	11,000
Glycogen	340,000	320,000	214,000	185,000
AMP	300	—	209	280
ADP	900	1853	684	620
ATP	2,900	710	2,270	2,060
L/P	10	239	13	10
G/D	6.7	72	6.7	6.5
M/O	64	—	70	70
ATP/ADP	3.3	0.4	3.3	3.3

Adapted from ref. 223.

tem after 4 hr of perfusion when erythrocyte-containing perfusate was used. Biliary excretion of sulfobromophthalein (BSP) and indocyanine green have also been useful as measures of the functional status of the isolated perfused liver. The disadvantage of using these markers for functional status is that the same perfused livers cannot be used for toxicological investigations after establishing that these livers are indeed viable. These tests are helpful for evaluating isolated perfused liver preparations, establishing the procedure, and subsequently evaluating the functional status of the liver preparations after treating with an experimental toxic agent. Phenolphthalein glucuronide (PG) has been used as a marker of biliary excretory function (154). The advantages of using PG are that it requires no further metabolism, it can be used at low concentrations, and it is sensitive for detecting hepatobiliary dysfunction and so can be used in livers being perfused for toxicological investigations (148,154).

Although histological examination of perfused livers is not done routinely, the technique is useful for setting up a perfused preparation. Several authors (30,221,225) have reported results of histological examinations of perfused livers, indicating the general usefulness of morphological examination in ascertaining the viability of perfused liver preparations. However, one should be aware that morphological examinations may be of limited usefulness, as cells that appear abnormal morphologically may exhibit normal cellular function; and conversely, normal-appearing cells may exhibit abnormal cellular functions (30,157). Oomen and Chamalarun (184) reported an excellent correlation between biochemical and histological parameters in their isolated perfused rat liver preparations.

Applications

Depending on the experimental protocol, the isolated perfused liver preparation can be used in either a single-pass or a recirculating mode (144,154,251). Many examples can be cited for the use of isolated perfused liver preparations in the evaluation of toxic responses to a variety of chemicals. It is instructive to consider a few examples of the use of isolated perfused liver preparations in toxicological investigations. Rice et al. (212) employed isolated perfused rat liver preparations to determine the effect of carbon tetrachloride (CCl$_4$) administered in vivo on the hemodynamics of the liver. Portal blood pressure and flow were recorded in perfused livers from either control or treated animals. The study concluded that although the primary lesion caused by CCl$_4$ was hepatocellular damage, subsequent effects included increased vascular resistance and enhanced response to norepinephrine. Iwamoto et al. (102) used perfused rat liver to establish the decreased intrinsic hepatic clearance of propranolol in CCl$_4$-injured liver. Another study used perfused liver to investigate the hepatic elimination of galactose in CCl$_4$-injured liver (259). Bullock et al. (34) utilized isolated perfused rat liver preparations to examine the effects of two fungal toxins, i.e., sporidesmin and icterogenin, on the mechanisms of bile secretion. Electron microscopic examination of livers perfused with these two toxins indicated that the cholestatic reaction was due to changes in canalicular membranes, which included extrusion of material into the canalicular lumen and aggregation of lysosomes in the cytoplasm. Abraham et al. (1)

examined the effect of hyperoxia on lysosomal enzymes using perfused liver preparations.

Radwan and Henschler (203) employed isolated liver preparations to study the uptake and metabolism of the hepatocarcinogen vinyl chloride. Using erythrocyte-suspension perfusion medium, they found that the solubility of vinyl chloride stayed constant at concentrations of 50 to 25,000 ppm. The amount metabolized, as determined by the difference between vinyl chloride concentration before and after passage through the liver was found to stay constant at 14.6% of the 50 to 25,000 ppm concentrations. Ethanol (12 mM) and pyrazole (200 mM) decreased the metabolism of vinyl chloride and was also modified by prior exposure of the animals to other inducing and inhibiting agents. It was concluded that vinyl chloride underwent a metabolic transformation via mixed function oxidation to reactive metabolites. The above study can be taken to represent how perfused liver preparations can be used to determine the metabolism of even volatile substances.

Lemaster et al. (134) used perfused liver to study hypoxic hepatocellular injury and concluded that shedding of cytoplasmic fragments resulting from the blebbing of centrilobular hepatocytes may represent a basis for the appearance of hepatic enzymes in the sera of patients with liver disease. Nastainczyk and Ullrich (166) used isolated perfused rat liver preparations to examine the effect of hypoxia on the metabolism of halothane. The study concluded that halothane is biotransformed via reductive in vivo metabolism to reactive intermediates when the oxygen concentration of the perfusate drops below a critical level (about 50 mM). These authors employed whole-organ spectrophotometry of isolated perfused livers to establish that a complex of macromolecules and halothane is formed under slightly hypoxic conditions, and that metyrapone, an inhibitor of MFO reactions, abolished the formation of this complex.

Use of isolated perfused liver preparations in the metabolism of toxic substances as well as the effect of the toxic substances on hepatic function are illustrated by a series of studies in which the hepatobiliary function was examined after the animals had been exposed to toxic chemicals (146–148). In these studies the effect of exposure to chlorocarbon pesticides, mirex and chlordecone (Kepone), was examined in isolated perfused liver preparations. Biliary excretion of anionic model compounds, BSP and imipramine were examined. These studies also illustrated the utility of isolated liver preparations in studying the biotransformation of chemicals. By assaying a series of perfusate samples as well as liver tissue at the end of a perfusion study, the metabolism of imipramine by control, as well as pretreated, livers was followed. Although both chlordecone and mirex were known to be inducers of hepatic mixed function oxidases, these experiments revealed that biliary excretion of endogenously formed metabolites of imipramine was suppressed by prior exposure to the above chlorocarbons. The pattern of imipramine metabolism indicated that the suppressed biliary excretory function was not related to alterations in metabolism of imipramine.

Other experiments (146,147), in which readily excretable polar metabolites of imipramine were introduced into the perfusate of control and treated liver preparations, indicated that biliary excretion of these metabolites was also hindered by prior exposure to mirex and chlordecone. Thus such experimental manipulations using isolated liver preparations were useful for evaluating the role of drug metabolism in hepatobiliary function. Isolated liver preparations can also be utilized to examine the role of hepatic uptake and metabolism in the disposition of toxic chemicals (145). In these studies the uptake, metabolism, and biliary excretion of polychlorinated biphenyls was examined using isolated perfused rat liver preparations. Similar preparations were useful in discovering the inhibitory effect of mirex on biliary excretion of polar metabolites of monochlorobiphenyl (147).

Thurman et al. (250) studied the kinetics of *p*-nitroanisole *O*-demethylation in hemoglobin-free perfused rat liver preparations. Using the isolated liver, these investigators were able to demonstrate that the rates of *p*-nitroanisole metabolism were linear for 30 min in normal livers and for 1 to 2 min in phenobarbital-induced livers. This reduced rate of metabolism could be reversed by infusing additional glucose, suggesting an intimate relation between drug and carbohydrate metabolism in the intact liver. Alteration in the rate of *p*-nitroanisole metabolism with various inducing agents of the MFO system produced parallel changes in rates of hepatic lactase production, reflecting the action of *p*-nitrophenol to uncouple oxidative phosphorylation. Thus these investigators were able to demonstrate that the reduction in the rate of *p*-nitroanisole metabolism in induced liver preparations was due to reduced availability of NADPH for MFO-catalyzed substrate oxidation. Using a similar noncirculating

liver perfusion system, Belinsky et al. (19) employed trypan blue to investigate the regiospecific hepatotoxic response of the liver. Periportal hepatocellular injury after allyl alcohol infusion to isolated perfused liver was readily evident from the stained nuclei only in the periportal zone. Takano et al. (244) described a technique similar to the one described by Thurman et al. (250), in which the dynamic effects of environmental agents on the hepatic drug-metabolizing system and on the energy metabolism could be monitored in the perfused liver. Such experiments with intact liver preparations have provided valuable insights into what might be occurring in terms of drug metabolism under *in vivo* conditions. These results demonstrated that despite the induced status of the liver, enhanced drug metabolism may not necessarily be the end result, as other factors, e.g., availability of cofactors, might become limiting and hence limit the quantitative aspects of drug metabolism.

There has been a significant interest in understanding the role of Ca^{2+} in chemical toxicity (222). Although it is generally agreed that a rising cytosolic Ca^{2+} level is detrimental to the cell, the source of the increased Ca^{2+} has been strongly debated (222,236). Because of the inherent disadvantages of working with isolated cells and organelles, intact perfused liver preparations offer the most suitable model. Such a perfusion setup, used by Mehendale et al. (154), is illustrated in Fig. 4. Infusion of menadione elicited an increased oxygen utilization by the liver, followed by a decrease in the perfusate Ca^{2+}. Hepatic accumulation of Ca^{2+} was accompanied by

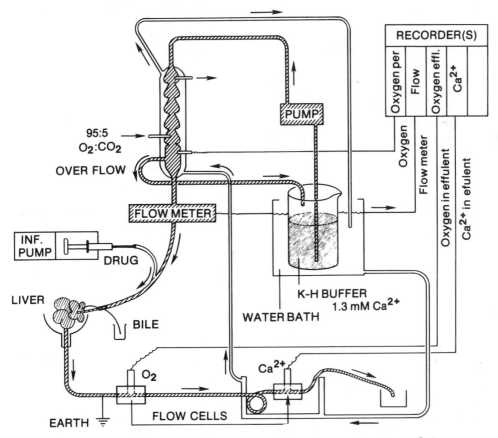

FIG. 4. Liver perfusion apparatus designed for on-line measurement of perfusate Ca^{2+} levels. (From ref. 154, with permission.)

stimulation of cytosolic phosphorylase a activity, indicating a rise in the cytosolic Ca^{2+} levels. A gradual recovery of perfusate Ca^{2+} to base levels was observed after cessation of menadione infusion. Leakage of lactate dehydrogenase (LDH) into the perfusate followed Ca^{2+} uptake, which was not accompanied by a decrease in reduced pyridine nucleotide or ATP level in the liver as evidenced by measurements either during maximal Ca^{2+} uptake or after recovery. However, Ca^{2+} uptake was correlated with decreased GSH and increased GSSG levels in the liver, both of which reversed during recovery from Ca^{2+} uptake. The amount of protein-bound mixed disulfides showed a striking relation to Ca^{2+} uptake, reaching a maximal value during Ca^{2+} uptake and reversing toward normal during recovery from Ca^{2+} accumulation. Depletion of hepatic GSH with prior diethylmaleate treatment resulted in increased Ca^{2+} accumulation during menadione infusion. These findings suggested that menadione-induced Ca^{2+} uptake is due to plasma membrane dysfunction as a result of loss of protein thiol groups, which are critical for maintaining the plasma membrane Ca^{2+} extrusion mechanism. This perfused liver model is particularly useful for studying the mechanisms underlying toxic disturbances in Ca^{2+} homeostasis in intact liver, as Ca^{2+} fluxes can be monitored under conditions in which cellular control mechanisms are not obliterated by excessive toxicity. The perfused liver preparations have also been useful for establishing the extracellular origin of Ca^{2+} seen to accumulate in livers of chlordecone-pretreated animals treated with CCl_4 (2). Livers obtained from rats at various points after the administration of CCl_4 were perfused for 30 min with ^{45}Ca-containing medium. More ^{45}Ca accumulation was demonstrated with the progression of toxicity during the time course, indicating the extracellular origin of the Ca^{2+} and the association between the Ca^{2+} accumulation and hepatocellular toxicity.

Use of the perfused liver for toxicity studies has increased. Examples of such studies include the study of hepatoprotective mechanism of silybin hemisuccinate on phenylhydrazine toxicity (258), hepatotoxicity of the hornet's venom sac extract (168) and galactosamine (209), metabolism of acetaminophen by liver after overdosage (199), lipid peroxidation associated with acetaminophen toxicity (248), isolation and characterization of the metabolites of T-2 toxin (78), and the hepatotoxicity of several cytotoxic agents (156). One report (160) described a technique of *in vivo* isolated perfusion of the rat liver to study the effect of hyperthermochemotherapy with 5-fluorouracil for possible clinical application in treating unresectable liver cancer in patients.

Isolated Perfused Lung

The heart–lung preparation of Knowlton and Starling (118) has been used extensively to study the respiratory functions of the lung in small and large animals. However, refinement of the isolated perfused lung preparation technique was expedited only after the nonrespiratory functions of the lungs were recognized. Popjak and Beeckmans (196) employed a rabbit perfused lung preparation to examine the utilization of oxygen and substrate incorporation into phospholipids of the lung tissue. A number of investigators have since refined the technique of perfusing lungs (16,37,133,135,173,179, 180,239).

A variety of methods have been used to perfuse lungs from experimental animals. Leary and Ledingham (133) described an *in situ* perfusion method with or without pulmonary ventilation. Similarly, Bakhle and co-workers (16) described an isolated perfused lung preparation without ventilation of the lung during perfusion. Isolated perfused lungs can be ventilated using either negative (173) or positive (183) pressure. Pulsatile perfusion was utilized by Hauge (92), and hydrostatic pressure was used for perfusion by Levey and Gast (135). Gillis and Iwasawa (83) and others have perfused right and left lungs as an intact organ (173,183).

An ideal perfused lung preparation is one that is totally isolated and in which respiratory and nonrespiratory functions can be tested. The isolated lung preparation has the advantage of being able to account for all the perfusion medium from the lung circulation at the end of perfusion experiments. Levey and Gast (135) pointed out that the *in situ* preparations result in some loss of perfusion medium through collateral vessels supplying the chest wall, and some fluid may be lost through exudation from the lung surface. Ventilation of the lung is essential for toxicological investigations in which maintaining a physiological route of gas exchange is important. Ventilation is an integral part of lung function, and hence nonventilating lung preparations represent less than desirable conditions, regardless of whether respiratory or nonrespiratory functions are being investigated. Retaining the ability of testing certain experimental drugs through the gaseous phase to simulate inhalational exposure would also be an additional advantage of maintaining a ventilating perfused lung preparation (150). Two types of isolated lung preparation are described here, one that utilizes negative-pressure ventilation and another that utilizes positive-pressure ventilation.

Apparatus

The perfusion system developed by Niemeier and Bingham (173), with small modifications, as is being presently used (5,37,51,86,152,180) is described (Fig. 5). The apparatus consists of a combination of pumps for ventilation, a peristaltic pump to drive the perfusate, an assembly of tubing for carrying the perfusate to and from the lung, and an artificial thorax kept warm by heated, circulating water. The thorax is made up of double-jacketed thick glass provided with an air-tight lid. Perfusate flow to the lung is maintained from the upper reservoir connected to the central porthole of the lid. The bottom of the reservoir has an opening through which the perfusate can be directed to the peristaltic pump. A small-animal respirator and a vacuum pump are connected to two of the portholes on the lid; these parts provide alternating negative pressure as a means of ventilating the perfused lung preparation. A magnehelic gauge or a simple manometer can be connected to another porthole on the lid in order to monitor the operating negative pressure in the thorax. At the center of the lid there are two portholes, one for a tracheal cannula and another for a pulmonary arterial cannula. The upper reservoir, which is also double-jacketed, connects to the central pulmonary arterial cannula by means of a stop-

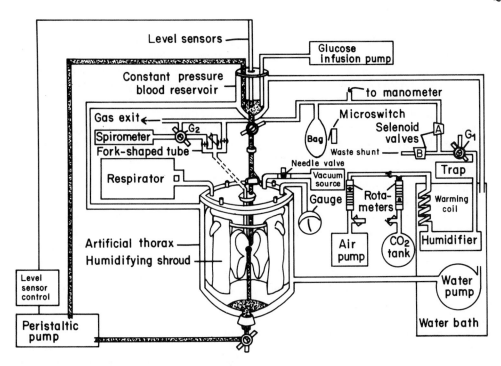

FIG. 5. Isolated perfused lung apparatus. This apparatus, originally developed by Niemeier and Bingham (173) for perfusion of rabbit lung, uses alternating negative pressure for ventilation. The apparatus can be scaled down to perfuse lungs from smaller animals (rats, guinea pigs) as well, using essentially the same procedure. (From ref. 173, with permission.)

cock arrangement and via pressure and flow transducers. The tracheal cannula is connected to a source of O_2/CO_2 (95:5), which is filtered and humidified by bubbling through warm saline. By means of appropriate one-way valves, provisions are made for inspiration as well as expiration of the ventilating lung. A spirometer is connected to measure the inspiration volume.

The perfusate from the upper reservoir passes through the assembly of transducers into the lung via the pulmonary arterial cannula. The perfusate empties into the bottom of the reservoir and is led to a peristaltic pump, which delivers it to the upper reservoir. A level-sensor controlling device can be introduced at the upper reservoir to maintain a constant level of the perfusate in the reservoir so as to provide constant hydrostatic pressure. This automatic sensing device regulates the peristaltic pump, maintaining a designated level of perfusate in the upper reservoir. An infusion pump can be used to infuse glucose, which replaces the glucose utilized by the perfusing lung. In the upper reservoir, a pH probe can be installed to monitor the pH of the circulating perfusate. The waterbath, equipped with a heater and a circulating water pump, provides a means for maintaining the thorax and the upper reservoir at physiological temperature (37°C).

Almost all components that come in direct contact with the perfusate are composed of glass, with the exception of small pieces of medical grade Silastic tubing used in the peristaltic pump, which requires flexible tubing. The glass components and flexible tubing of the apparatus are coated with Siliclad or a similar liquid silicone in order to avoid binding of experimental drugs to the tubing used for transporting the perfusate. The lid (thoracic roof) with a number of portholes

is composed of Plexiglas fitted with a rubber "O" ring and sealed with silicone high vacuum grease; the lid is held in place on the ground-glass rim of the thorax by appropriate clamps. The small-animal respirator is connected in reverse to the porthole on the lid for the purpose of generating alternating negative pressure in combination with the vacuum pump.

Prior to the surgical procedure to remove the lung, the apparatus is thoroughly cleaned, assembled, and rinsed with physiological saline. A measured volume of perfusate can be introduced into the upper reservoir, and the entire perfusate line can be primed with the perfusate. Precaution is taken to avoid entrapment of any air emboli in the perfusate anywhere in the apparatus. The remaining perfusate can be introduced into the upper reservoir.

Surgical Procedure and Preparation of Lung

Isolated perfused lung preparations can be obtained from almost any experimental animal. For the generalized description needed here, isolated perfused rabbit lung is used. The animal (New Zealand white rabbits weighing 2 to 3 kg) can be anesthetized using Nembutol (50 mg/kg), which is previously mixed with heparin (1,000 IU/kg), injected into the marginal ear vein. Upon reaching a proper level of anesthesia, the animal can be bled by means of a cardiac puncture with an 18-gauge needle connected to silicone tubing, which drains into a beaker held below the plane of the animal to facilitate flow by gravity. Bleeding the animal allows clean surgical procedures and decreases the amount of blood remaining in the vasculature of the lung. Therefore this procedure might be followed regardless of whether the blood is to be used as the perfusate. If the blood is intended for use in perfusion, it is collected in a heparinized container and immediately stirred. (Blood can also be used as a perfusate upon proper filtration.) When carrying out cardiac puncture, care is taken to enter between the sixth and seventh ribs next to the sternum so as to not damage the lungs.

A midline incision is made from the neck to the abdomen to expose the trachea and rib cage. The liver is retracted and the sternum grasped by means of a curved hemostat. The sternum is lifted upward to facilitate inflation of the lungs, at which time the trachea can be clamped by means of a hemostat to entrap the proper amount of oxygen in the lungs. An incision in the diaphragm at the midline area facilitates cutting the diaphragm on both sides along the rib cage. The rib cage can be cut laterally on both sides, making sure that the lung tissue is detached from the roof of the rib cage. The lungs and heart are thus exposed through a midline sternotomy, and the rib cage is retracted. The lungs and heart can be removed from the animal en bloc and transferred to a petri dish containing warm saline. All the subsequent operations can be carried out while the lungs rest in this petri dish.

The trachea is first cannulated using PE-300 tubing (PE-200 for the rat). At this time, the lungs can be ventilated artificially by means of a 100-cc syringe attached to the tracheal cannula by silicone tubing. Alternatively, the tracheal cannula can be attached to a small-animal ventilator so that the lungs can be ventilated during the subsequent cannulation procedure. The trachea, lungs, and heart are dissected free from their attachments, connective tissue, and other extraneous material, taking care not to puncture the lungs, and then rinsed with warm physiological saline. The pericardium is removed and the pulmonary artery cannulated with a PE-300 cannula (3 mm i.d., 5 cm in length) prefilled with perfusate. During this procedure, care must be taken not to introduce air emboli into the vasculature; if air is allowed in, immediate interruption of flow occurs upon perfusion. The entire right ventricle and the right atrium together with most of the left ventricle (up to 0.5 cm) below the atrioventricular septum is removed. The left atrium is cannulated by passing a PE-300 cannula (3 mm i.d., 6 cm in length, and curved) through the remaining left ventricle and bicuspid valves to the atrium. The cannula is secured with a ligature and the remaining tissue dissected free of the cannulated lung preparation. Throughout the procedure, a hemostat is retained on the pulmonary arterial cannula to avoid air bubbles entering the pulmonary artery. The cannulated lungs along with the hemostat, after blotting dry with filter paper, are weighed at this time.

The lung preparation is now suspended in the artificial thorax by connecting the tracheal and pulmonary arterial cannulas to the respective tubes, which extend to the inside of the Plexiglas lid. It is also important to avoid entrapment of any air bubbles, especially when the arterial cannula is connected to the perfusion apparatus. Flow is resumed through the arterial cannula after the lid is closed, and the perfusate line from the pump is connected to the top of the upper reservoir. Perfusion can be slowly established at this time, ensuring that no bubbles pass through into the pulmonary artery. The pumps can be activated to inflate the lung. The lungs are inflated by applying a negative pressure of 25 to 30 cm H_2O by activating the vacuum pump and increasing the vacuum. Once the collapsed lungs are inflated to a desired level, because the respirator is already turned on, the alternating negative–positive pressure automatically ventilates the lung. In the rabbit the frequency is kept at 50 respirations per minute. In the rat, respiration can be maintained at approximately 60 per minute. Once the ventilation cycle is initiated the apparatus is automatic, and perfusion and ventilation continue throughout the experiment. The perfusion flow rate increases quickly upon inflation of the lung and may steadily increase until steady-state ventilation is established. If the automatic level sensor is in operation, monitoring the perfusion flow rate is not necessary. However, if such an arrangement is not available, care must be exercised to maintain perfusate in the upper reservoir by manual control of the peristaltic pump. The lungs are usually allowed to equilibrate in the perfusion apparatus over a period of 15 to 20 min.

Positive-pressure ventilation procedure

The perfusion apparatus developed by O'Neil and Tierney (183) can be used to illustrate perfusion of lungs from smaller animals and by using a positive-pressure ventilation procedure. The apparatus and assembly are illustrated in Fig. 6.

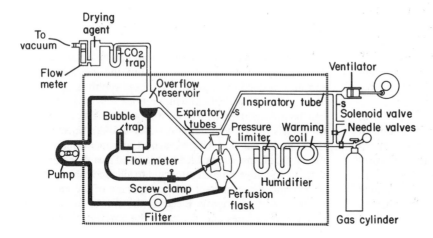

FIG. 6. Isolated perfused lung preparation of O'Neil and Tierney (183). This apparatus is used to perfuse lungs with positive-pressure ventilation. It can be scaled up to perfuse lungs from large animals as well. (S) solenid value; (O) needle valve. (From ref. 183, with permission.)

The lungs are ventilated directly by means of an animal respirator that is attached to the tracheal cannula. This procedure avoids the need for the additional vacuum pump that is required in the negative alternating-pressure ventilation method. Two selenoid valves (Fig. 6) are used to direct gas flow during the respiratory cycle. A tidal volume of approximately 3.5 ml is obtained for the rat and is adjusted to provide a maximum transpulmonary pressure of 12 cm H_2O. The end-expiratory pressure is set at 3.5 cm H_2O to keep the lung from collapsing during expiration. The rat lungs were perfused in this apparatus at a frequency of 13 respirations per minute. The procedure for isolating and cannulating the lung is essentially the same as described for the rabbit lung preparation, with the exception of smaller-diameter PE cannulas. The procedure for maintaining isolated perfused rat lung using positive-pressure ventilation has been described adequately by O'Neil and Tierney (183) and Young (267), who may be consulted for additional details. Lungs can also be perfused using a setup similar to the one described for the negative-pressure ventilation procedure with simple modifications. The vacuum pump is deleted, and the ventilator is connected directly to the trachea in a forward direction instead of the reverse direction used in the negative-pressure ventilation procedure. The procedure described by Camus and Mehendale (37) may be consulted for other details.

Perfusion Media

Nicolaysen (171) studied the effect of perfusate composition on edema development, and he found whole blood to be the most suitable perfusate. The perfusion procedure described by Niemeier and Bingham (173) included the use of autologous whole blood as a perfusate. This perfusate was practical in the case of a rabbit, as 100 ml or more of whole blood can be obtained by cardiac puncture from a rabbit weighing 3 kg or more. Blood is collected in a heparinized container and filtered to remove any debris, dead cells, or small blood clots. The blood is heparinized once again prior to circulation in the apparatus in order to avoid clotting. Using autologous whole blood is impractical, however, for perfusing rat lungs or lungs of other small animals. Blood may have to be collected from several animals in order to supply an adequate volume of perfusate for a single perfusion experiment. Furthermore, for certain experimental protocols such as single-pass experiments, several liters of perfusate may be required. For these reasons, use of artificially constituted medium as perfusate has been popular.

The widely used lung perfusate is the one described by Junod (109), which has the following composition in millimolar concentrations: NaCl 118; KCl 4.75; $CaCl_2$ 2.54; KH_2PO_4 1.19; $MgSO_4$ 1.19; and $NaHCO_3$ 25. BSA is added at a concentration of 4.5 g/L, and the final pH of the solution is adjusted to 7.4 with 1 N NaOH, so that the final Na^+ concentration of the standard medium is 161 mM. The medium is equilibrated with O_2/CO_2 (95:5) prior to priming the apparatus. This perfusate has been used by a number of investigators (5,37,51,84,152,153,180–183,186). The standard perfusion medium is Krebs-Ringer bicarbonate buffer solution, described by Umbreit et al. (256); it contains 5 mM of glucose and 4.5% BSA (Cohn fraction V). Several advantages

of using this artificial medium as a perfusate can be cited. First, in the one-pass perfusion experiments, large volumes of the perfusate are often used (196) and using whole blood as a perfusate becomes uneconomical. Second, manipulations of ionic changes in the perfusate can be introduced easily in an artificial medium. Introducing such changes in the perfusate is essential for studies aimed at mechanisms of pulmonary uptake of drugs (5–7,37,51,109,180–182). An additional advantage of artificial perfusate is the relative ease with which the test drug can be extracted and analyzed in the absence of erythrocytes and any interfering hemoglobin.

For some studies the presence or absence of BSA in the perfusate may become a critical factor. Albumin provides binding sites for drugs, which might be an important criterion for some studies of drug uptake and metabolism. Including albumin in the perfusate allows simulation of conditions of blood plasma *in vivo*. The absence of albumin results in a proportionately greater fraction of the drug being in a "free" state; consequently, drug uptake and metabolism might be expected to be greater. Studies have also indicated that albumin may interfere with GSH, cysteine, and similar thiol compounds (107,108). These thiol compounds are oxidized rapidly in the presence of albumin in Krebs-Ringer bicarbonate buffer (107,108). Replacing albumin with high-molecular-weight dextran ameliorated this particular difficulty. Other variations of the perfusion media include the use of 4.5% Ficoll 70 instead of BSA (62) and Hepes buffer with only 2% BSA (20).

A combination of either autologous or mixed whole blood and the Krebs-Ringer bicarbonate buffer artificial medium as a perfusate can also be used for perfusing lung preparations. Such a preparation has the advantage of including the natural constituents of blood so natural binding sites can be provided for the test drug. Differences in the uptake of drugs by the lung have been found between whole blood and artificial medium used as perfusate (5,186). Perfluorocarbons have not been used in the perfusate in isolated perfused lung preparations, although their successful usage in perfusing livers (87,178,254) suggests that fluorocarbon emulsions would also adequately support the isolated lung preparations. In the isolated lung preparations ventilated by positive pressure, Young (267) utilized Krebs-Ringer bicarbonate-buffered solution containing glucose and BSA, similar to the one described above. By and large, this erythrocyte-free medium has been widely used as a perfusate for maintaining viable preparations of isolated perfused lungs.

Viability Criteria

Niemeier and Bingham (173) measured a number of biochemical parameters in the circulating perfusate as well as in the lung to ascertain the viability of isolated perfused rabbit lung preparations. The concentrations of blood urea nitrogen (BUN), Ca^{2+}, albumin, total protein, and pyruvate in the perfusate changed little throughout the perfusion (Table 4). Inorganic phosphate, uric acid, lactic acid, and total bilirubin increased moderately during perfusion. LDH and serum glutamic oxaloacetic transaminase (SGOT) activities, as well as plasma hemoglobin, increased markedly during the 3-hr perfusion. Hematocrit levels decreased slightly, which may be

TABLE 4. *Biochemical changes and physiological values in the isolated perfused lung*

Parameter	Average concentration in plasma prior to perfusion	Average change in concentration per hour
Calcium (mg/dl)	13.8 ± 0.8	↓0.15 ± 0.29
Inorganic phosphate (mg/dl)	4.1 ± 0.4	↑0.78 ± 0.27
Glucose (mg/dl) adding 30 mg/hr	236 ± 35	↓34.5 ± 4.1
		± 2.3
BUN (mg/dl)	17.5 ± 3.2	↑0.14 ± 0.22
Uric acid (mg/dl)	0.62 ± 0.18	↑0.20 ± 0.12
Cholesterol (mg/dl) with vitamin E	37 ± 13	↑4.2 ± 0.7
		↑19.5 ± 7.1
Total protein (g/dl)	5.7 ± 0.4	↑0.10 ± 0.15
Albumin (g/dl)	0.53 ± 0.07	↓0.04 ± 0.03
Total bilirubin (mg/dl)	0.14 ± 0.06	↑0.12 ± 0.16
Alkaline phosphatase (mU/ml) with vitamin E	55 ± 36	↑4.8 ± 2.1
		↑0.6 ± 1.1
Lactate dehydrogenase (mU/ml)	135 ± 42	↑485 ± 201
SGOT (mU/ml)	58 ± 23	↑121 ± 58
Plasma hemoglobin (mg/dl)	0.19 ± 0.12	↑2.3 ± 0.6
Lactic acid (mg/dl)	173 ± 17	↑19.8 ± 5.2
Pyruvic acid (mg/dl)	1.19 ± 0.06	n.c.[a] 0.01
Hematocrit (%)	35.0 ± 5.0	↓1.63 ± 0.34
Weight gain (% hr)	↑2.81 ± 1.36	
Blood flow (ml/min)	160	
PO₂ (mm Hg), typical values	118 ± 6; 121 ± 10	
PCO₂ (mm Hg), typical values	39 ± 4; 34 ± 4	
pH range	7.35–7.45	
Tidal volume (ml)		
Typical values	11.7 ± 0.3; 11.0 ± 0.4	
Normal values	23.9 ± 5.5 (16)	

[a] No change.
From ref. 173, with permission.

a result of hemolysis, as autologous whole blood was used. In these experiments, sodium bicarbonate was added periodically to maintain the blood pH at 7.4, and heparin and epinephrine were added to maintain proper perfusion flow rates. These additions might have contributed to the decrease in hematocrit. Glucose levels decreased (34.5 ± 4.1 mg/hr) during perfusion, necessitating addition of glucose with an infusion pump at the rate of 30 mg/hr in 0.3 ml of water. Thus when glucose was replenished, the glucose concentration in the perfusate did not decrease significantly over the 3-hr period of perfusion. Cholesterol increased at a rate of approximately 11% per hour, but when α-tocopherol was added to the perfusate cholesterol increased markedly (53% per hour).

Lungs can be examined visually during perfusion for the appearance of translucent areas, which would indicate development of edema. Niemeier and Bingham (173) found that the lungs gained weight an average of 2.8% per hour over the 3-hr perfusion with autologous whole blood. Histopathological examination revealed no edema after 3 hr of perfusion, and the integrity of the pulmonary ultrastructure was well preserved (173,186).

Often after prolonged perfusion of lungs the lung preparations deteriorate, with the concomitant development of edematous areas characterized by a translucent appearance of the lung surface. After continued perfusion, the lung does not inflate and deflate with each respiratory cycle, and surfactant material might appear in the tracheal cannula. If the perfusion is continued after the lung appears to be edematous, large and copious flows of the surfactant material continue to appear through the tracheal cannula. Maintenance of perfusate pH can be a problem, and Niemeier and Bingham (173) maintained the pH by adding 1 mM sodium bicarbonate to the perfusate. However, they used room air mixed with 5% CO_2 to ventilate the rabbit lung preparations. If O_2/CO_2 (95:5) is used for ventilating the isolated lungs and the lungs are properly inflated, no problem is encountered in maintaining physiological pH of the perfusate (153).

An additional criterion of viability of the lung preparation is the evaluation of drug-metabolizing enzymes in the perfused lung (132). Various investigators have found that, after 2 to 3 hr of perfusion, microsomal drug-metabolizing activity of the lung remains unaltered, indicating satisfactory preservation of microsomal MFO activity of perfused lung preparation. ATP levels were measured in rat lungs perfused for 90 min by a positive-pressure ventilation procedure (267) and were found to be at or above the ATP levels in nonperfused lungs. By contrast, ATP content was decreased in lung slice incubations. Perfusion of rat (20) and rabbit (62,107) lungs results in only a slight decrease in the lung content of GSH, indicating that lungs can maintain GSH levels during perfusion.

Applications

Isolated perfused lung preparations have been used for a variety of studies, including drug uptake and metabolism and the disposition of various pharmacological and toxicological agents (153). Rhoades (211) described a technique of utilizing isolated perfused lungs ventilated by positive pressure for evaluating the effect of various gaseous environments on pulmonary biochemistry. Block and Cannon (25) investigated the effect of anoxia or hyperoxia on the ability of lungs to clear endogenous and exogenous chemicals. Use of isolated lung preparations has resulted in significant contributions to our understanding of the pulmonary role in uptake and metabolism of a variety of xenobiotics (23,37,42, 51,101,131,150,153,172,173,257). Examples of toxicological investigations using isolated perfused lung preparations include studies on the pulmonary uptake and disposition of aldrin and dieldrin (152,153), uptake of the herbicide paraquat (42), uptake and metabolism of trichloroethylene (50), and uptake and metabolism of benzo(a)pyrene (23,257). Although this list is by no means a survey of toxicological investigations utilizing isolated perfused lung preparations, these preparations have been useful for determining the pulmonary contribution to the disposition of toxic chemicals.

Perfused lung preparations have been useful for demonstrating epoxidase activity in the lung tissue (149,152,153). Aldrin is a cyclodiene pesticide that is readily epoxidized to dieldrin and in the liver can be further metabolized by epoxide hydrase to dihydrodiol metabolites. In the lung, aldrin could be readily epoxidized to dieldrin, which is a stable epoxide and can be quantitated as a measure of aldrin epoxidase activity. This finding represented the first direct demonstration of epoxidase capability of lung tissue. Aldrin is thus metabolized to dieldrin irrespective of whether it enters via airways or through the vascular system, and the metabolite appears in the perfusate rapidly (149). In these studies, it was demonstrated that intact perfused lung preparations were able to turn over aldrin to dieldrin at a lesser rate than the *in vitro* incubations of lung homogenate preparations. These studies serve to illustrate the utility of perfusing intact organs in order to realistically evaluate the biochemical metabolic contribution by the organ to the metabolism and disposition of a test chemical. Thus turnover of aldrin to dieldrin was four to seven times greater in *in vitro* preparations than in *ex vivo* preparations using perfused intact lungs (149). Although the reason for such a discrepancy between *in vitro* and intact organ perfusion systems is incompletely understood, Itakura et al. (101) demonstrated that the availability of necessary cofactors might be limiting in intact perfused lung preparations. They observed that demethylation of *p*-nitroanisole by the perfused rabbit lung preparations was limited by the availability of the cofactor NADPH, the generation of which could be stimulated by introducing glucose to the perfusion medium. Even in the presence of excessive glucose in the perfusate, aldrin epoxidation, a reaction requiring NADPH, was saturable (152), suggesting that the cofactor availability can be limiting in intact lungs, an observation that would not be apparent from the idealized *in vitro* incubations.

Perfused lung preparations of rat and rabbit (179–182) have also been helpful in identifying a flavin monooxygenase

capable of *N*-oxidizing chlorpromazine and imipramine. Most interestingly, these studies established that although the rat lung is capable of *N*-oxidation of both of these substrates, rabbit lung is devoid of this activity. Curiously, rabbit lung does contain a flavin monooxygenase capable of *N*-oxidizing *N,N*-dimethylaniline (151). These studies also established the absence of any significant cytochrome P-450-mediated metabolism of these substrates. Furthermore, the remarkable species differences between rats and rabbits in pulmonary flavin monooxygenase activities became apparent from these perfusion studies (151,179–182).

The study of Dalbey and Bingham (50) illustrates the utility of isolated perfused lung preparations for studying the uptake and disposition of gaseous toxic substances. They studied the uptake and metabolism of trichloroethylene in isolated perfused rat lung preparations by introducing trichloroethylene vapors through the trachea. Perfused rat lung preparations metabolized trichloroethylene to trichloroethanol, and guinea pig lungs were even more active in the metabolism of trichloroethylene to the alcohol. In future, it should be anticipated that more experimentation will be carried out utilizing isolated perfused lung preparations for such toxicological investigations (150).

The use of isolated perfused lung preparations to study the metabolism of carcinogenic chemicals such as benzo-(a)pyrene is another example of the development of perfused lung preparations, aiding the advancement in this area. Bingham and associates (23) studied the metabolism of benzo(a)pyrene and reported the formation of several metabolites of this chemical including the formation of carcinogenic reactive epoxide and dihydrodiol metabolites in the lung. In addition to containing the necessary enzyme systems for carrying out oxidative metabolism of these toxic chemicals, lungs contain enzyme systems that catalyze phase II reactions such as epoxide hydrase and glucuronyl transferase and GSH-S-transferase using 1-chloro-2,4-dinitrobenzene as substrate, which can be demonstrated using intact perfused lung preparations (52,257). The use of isolated lung preparations for determining other physiological effects of toxic chemicals mediated via the endogenous hormone system is illustrated by the studies of Seiler et al. (232). They examined the effect of certain anorexic agents, including chlorphentermine, on the clearance of 5-hydroxytryptamine (5-HT; serotonin) and observed that the anorexic agents enhanced the vasoconstrictor effects of 5-HT in the pulmonary circulation. Subsequent studies by Angevine and Mehendale in perfused rabbit (6) and rat (7) lungs revealed the mechanism. Chlorphentermine was found to inhibit the pulmonary deactivation of 5-HT (6,7,151), consequently allowing the action of the vasoactive 5-HT to prevail. Another example of the use of isolated perfused lung preparations to evaluate the effect of foreign toxic chemicals on pulmonary clearance of endogenous chemicals is the study of Gillis and Roth (84) in which they examined the turnover of endogenous hormones, e.g., 5-HT and norepinephrine.

Isolated perfused rabbit lungs were employed by Dunbar et al. (62) to examine the GSH status of the lung upon perfusion with 420 μM paraquat or nitrofurantoin. Significant increases in lung GSSG were observed, which provided evidence for the preoxidant nature of the lung injury caused by these agents. Possible utilization of externally provided

GSH by rat (20) and rabbit (107) lungs was studied by determining the GSH status of the isolated, ventilated, and perfused lungs with or without prior GSH depletion. The rat lungs appeared to be able to utilize external GSH (20), whereas the rabbit lungs failed to do so (107). The question of whether externally provided GSH can be utilized by the lung tissue is of significance for many toxicological considerations. The role of the GSH redox cycle as a defense system against H_2O_2-induced prostanoid formation and vasoconstriction was investigated in perfused rabbit lungs (230).

Oxyradicals generated by xanthine–xanthine oxidase also interfere with the endothelial removal of 5-HT in perfused rabbit lungs (46). The question of hydroxyl radical ('OH) involvement in granulocyte-mediated oxidant lung injury was examined in perfused rat lungs using dimethylthiourea (DMTU) as the radical scavenger (74). When isolated rat lungs were perfused with polymorphonuclear neutrophils (PMNs) activated by phorbal myristate acetate (PMA) to produce 'OH, lung weights were increased significantly. Because the increase in lung weights was preventable by 10 mM DMTU, the findings are supportive of the role for the 'OH radical in acute granulocyte-mediated lung injury. Evidence for a protective role of intact human erythrocytes against H_2O_2-mediated damage (253) and the finding that DMTU treatment might be helpful for treating acute edematous lung injury such as seen in adult respiratory distress syndrome have provided some insights into the origin and mechanism of such lung injury.

Additional examples of the use of perfused lungs are available (27,38,93,128,198,229). These studies include the effect of asbestos (38), staphylococcal α-toxin (229), and the haloalkanes (198) on the pulmonary metabolism of vasoactive substances. Pulmonary uptake and release of morphine (51,93) and metabolism and macromolecular binding of the carcinogenic nitropyrene (27) are additional examples of the applications of the perfused lung preparations. Lafranconi et al. (129) employed perfused rat lungs to investigate the toxic effects of equinatoxin, a peptide of 147 amino acid residues isolated from the venom of the sea anemone *Actinia equina*. In this study, equinatoxin was found to adversely affect fluid regulation in the lung tissue, suggesting that it might become an important tool for the investigation of fluid regulation in the lung.

Although the recirculation apparatus was illustrated above, simple modification allows one to perform experiments using a single-pass perfusion system. A number of investigators have utilized single-pass perfusion to investigate the mechanisms of drug uptake and release from the lung (83). For example, Junod (109) examined the mechanisms of pulmonary uptake of imipramine using a single-pass mode of perfusion. Likewise, single-pass kinetics were used to determine the uptake, metabolism, and release mechanism of aldrin and dieldrin in the rabbit perfused lung preparations (152). Single-pass experiments can be expensive in terms of both materials (albumin used for preparing the perfusate) and the technical assistance required to conduct these experiments. An ideal single-pass experiment requires the assistance of three individuals to work in swift coordination and usually involves analyzing a large number of samples. Hence the information to be gained from such experimental protocols must be weighed against the expense involved. Often equally

valuable information results from recirculating perfusion experiments at a fraction of the effort and resources expended. For additional interest, the reader may wish to refer to Roth (218) for a review of the methodology and applications of perfused lung preparations.

Isolated Perfused Kidney

Although a number of methods for obtaining perfused kidney preparations from various mammalian species have been devised, use of isolated kidney preparations in toxicological studies has been infrequent. Historically, most workers in this field have been concerned with the study of autoregulation, excretion, and reabsorption functions of the organ (15,18). Isolated perfused kidney preparations have been used in such studies from the rat (15,18,29,138,216), dog (11,223,260,266), rabbit (72,214), pig (33), monkey and sheep (246), and human (125). Considerable variation has existed among the various investigators concerning the specific techniques used for perfusing kidneys. The kidney may be perfused via the dorsal aorta or the renal artery. Pulsatile or nonpulsatile perfusate flow can be used, and perfusion pressure may be exerted either with the pump (95) or by means of a hydrostatic pressure head (21).

As with other perfused organ systems, the most important variable has been the perfusion medium, and a considerable range of varying compositions have now been tested. Argument persists in the literature relating to whether pulsatile flow is preferred as a simulation of the *in vivo* situation (216). A second major problem has been vasoconstriction and deterioration of the kidney preparations associated with the use of whole blood as a perfusion medium. By and large, to circumvent this problem, investigators have used either diluted blood, a reconstituted blood perfusate, or an erythrocyte-free medium containing various electrolytes, glucose, and albumin. Most investigators are content with the use of a Krebs-Ringer bicarbonate-buffered solution containing albumin and glucose. As in the case of other organs, kidneys can also be perfused either *in situ* or in total isolation in chambers that can be kept warm for normothermic conditions. A further variation can be in the mode of perfusion; kidneys can be perfused either using recirculating perfusate or in a single-pass mode.

Apparatus

The apparatus used for perfusing kidney preparations is similar to the one described for perfusing livers (Fig. 7). It includes the outer chamber used for perfusing the liver and is fitted with a heater–fan assembly for maintaining the desired temperature inside the chamber. A multibulb glass lung can be used to oxygenate the perfusate. Perfusate is led to a roller type or peristaltic pump and is transported to the top of the oxygenator via glass tubing. A filter placed between the lung and the glass tubing ensures trapping fat droplets and any other particulate material, including cell debris, from the perfusate before it enters the kidney. A major difference between the liver and kidney is the higher (120 cm) hydrostatic pressure used for perfusing the kidney. Oxygenated

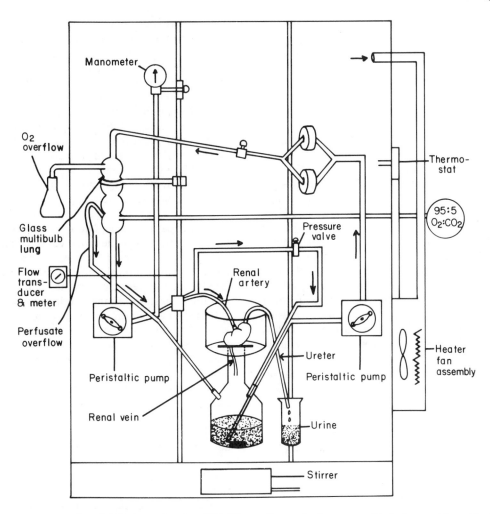

FIG. 7. Isolated perfused kidney apparatus (15). The entire perfusion assembly is housed in a Plexiglas chamber fitted with a heater–fan assembly (21,144). The circulation of the perfusate is accomplished by two peristaltic pumps: One directs the perfusate via a Millipore filter device into a multibulb glass lung for oxygenation, and the other directs the perfusate to the renal artery at a desired perfusion pressure. The perfusion pressure can be adjusted by imposing a clamp on the arterial diverticulum, which can be opened to reduce perfusion pressure or closed to increase it. The perfusion pressure is monitored by placing a manometer in the system. An outflow arrangement is provided at the bottom of the lung, and this tube drains the excess oxygenated fluid into the central reservoir, which also receives the venous flow from the kidney. Additions or sampling can be done in the central reservoir. The perfused kidney rests on a platform made up of a petri dish with a central porthole for the venous flow. A muslin cloth stretched across the mouth of the petri dish and held by a rubber band provides the platform for the perfused kidney.

blood by means of glass tubing then enters the renal arterial cannula. A set of perfusion pressure and flow transducers can be placed between the arterial cannula and the glass tubing in order to measure the perfusion pressure and flow rates. Similarly, electrodes can be placed before and after the kidney to monitor oxygen levels of the perfusate. A pH probe can be placed anywhere in the circulation to monitor pH continuously. The effusate from the kidney is guided back to the reservoir to complete the recirculation. An overflow arrangement from the hydrostatic reservoir to the central reservoir allows maintenance of a constant hydrostatic pressure. The kidney rests on a nylon mesh stretched over a ring approximately 7.5 cm in diameter. The stainless steel strip is mounted about 2.5 cm above the tray to support the arterial cannula. The temperature of the cabinet can be maintained

at approximately 38°C, thereby allowing the kidney and the perfusate temperature to equilibrate at 37°C.

Most of the tubing used in the assembly of the apparatus can be replaced by glass in order to minimize binding of test drugs to rubber or plastic tubing used in earlier perfusion setups. The arterial cannula is composed of glass tubing (2.8 mm i.d.; 3.5 mm o.d.) drawn to a taper of 1.3 mm o.d. and 1 mm i.d. It is bent to a right angle 1.5 cm from the tip, and the short limb of the cannula has little or no taper. The tip of the cannula is leveled slightly to facilitate its insertion into the renal artery. The venous cannula, consisting of a 3 cm long size PE-270 (2 mm i.d., 3 mm o.d.) cut off at an angle to form a short tip, is placed in the inferior vena cava. When the cannula is in position, its opening lies opposite the right renal vein. It might be advantageous to prepare several cannulas of varying sizes, as there is considerable variation in the renal artery from animal to animal. The renal arterial cannula is filled with heparinized perfusate in order to avoid any clots or air embolus during cannulation.

Surgical Procedure

The surgical procedure for isolating and perfusing the rat kidney is described here, as this animal appears to be the most popular experimental animal for toxicological investigation (46,169,216,217). Kidneys can be surgically removed from rats weighing 300 to 400 g, preferably starved overnight to decrease rates of gluconeogenesis and possibly reduce perinephric fat. After anesthetizing the rat with an injection of pentobarbital (50 mg/kg), an abdominal incision is made in the midline and extended laterally. The intestines can be swept to the animal's left to facilitate the next steps. Because of the anatomical advantage of the mesenteric artery arising from the aorta at the same level as the renal artery, the right kidney is used for perfusion. This technique facilitates passing the cannula through the aorta into the renal artery with loss of little blood and no interruption of blood flow to the kidney. Figure 8 illustrates the principal blood vessels encountered in the cannulation and surgical preparation of the right rat kidney.

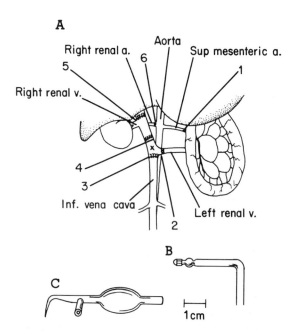

FIG. 8. A: Peripheral blood vessels in the upper abdomen of a rat with the position of ligatures in the preparation for cannulation of the kidney. Intestines are swept to the left of the animal, and the liver is retracted to expose the superior mesenteric artery. **B:** Venous cannula. **C:** Arterial cannula. Cannulation procedure is described in the text. Briefly, ligature 1 is tied, a clamp is placed on the superior mesenteric artery near its origin, and an incision is made into the artery proximal to the ligature. Ligatures 2 and 3 are tied, the venous cannula is introduced into inferior vena cava at X; ligature 4 is tied around the venous cannula. The right renal artery is cannulated via the superior mesenteric artery, and ligations 5 and 6 are completed. (From ref. 138, with permission.)

To expose the major abdominal vessels and the right kidney, fat and perivascular tissue are cleared away by teasing the tissues around the blood vessels. The adrenal branch of the right renal artery is ligated, and loose ligatures are placed around the vessels as follows: one on the inferior vena cava just distal to the liver, one on the aorta above the mesenteric artery, two on the mesenteric artery near the aorta separated by 0.5 cm, three on the inferior vena cava, one between the right and left renal vein, one distal to the left renal vein, and one further down on the inferior vena cava. Finally, a ligature is placed on the left renal vein. The ureter is cannulated by means of PE-10 tubing, and a ligature is placed around the ureter to hold the cannula in place.

The animal is heparinized by injecting approximately 200 units of heparin into the inferior vena cava, after which the opening in the wall of the vein is closed by means of a ligature passed over the point of the injecting needle. After tying the ligature on the left renal vein, the venous cannula is inserted into the inferior vena cava and tied in place by means of the two upper ligatures on the inferior vena cava. The cannula is turned such that the opening lies opposite the right renal vein. The other end of the cannula can be temporarily closed by a loose plug of tissue paper. The distal ligature on the mesenteric artery is tied, the artery is grasped at its origin with fine curved forceps, and an incision is made on the wall. The cannula filled with perfusion medium is inserted and passed to meet the forceps, which are then removed. The tip of the cannula is advanced into the aorta and then into the renal artery, which takes off on the opposite side of the aorta, allowing the perfusion medium to flow to the kidney. The cannula is tied in place by means of the anterior ligature on the renal artery and the ligature on the mesenteric artery as well.

With all the cannulas intact and in place, the kidney is surgically removed. The isolated kidney is transferred to the kidney platform in the perfusion chamber, and perfusion is resumed by connecting the arterial cannula to the perfusion flow of the preprimed apparatus. With practice, the total time required for the surgical procedure can be reduced to approximately 15 min, starting from the initial midline incision.

Perfusion Media

As indicated earlier, the perfusion medium of choice appears to be a cell-free perfusion fluid with adequate buffering capacity and containing salts, glucose, and albumin (15,29,138,169,217). The perfusion medium described earlier for liver and lung, containing Krebs-Ringer bicarbonate-buffered solution, appears to be satisfactory for perfusing kidney preparations. Earlier attempts to utilize blood as a natural perfusate have met with problems relating to vasoconstriction, whether the blood was defibrinated (260) or heparinized (174). Another cause of impaired renal flow was found to be embolization of fat droplets, especially at later stages of perfusion using whole blood (174) as a perfusate. An additional disadvantage of using whole blood as a perfusate is the unavailability of a requisite volume of blood, especially in small experimental animals such as the rat. A volume of 100 ml of perfusate is often necessary to conduct an isolated perfused kidney experiment, and several animals would be required to obtain the volume of blood needed for perfusing the rat kidney. In addition to the economic considerations, other problems may be encountered when mixing blood from several animals. One is the possibility of immunological interactions in blood pooled from several animals. Finally, in certain experiments it is essential to have one-pass circulation through the kidney. This method requires greater volumes of perfusate, and using blood would be impractical in such studies.

A major advance in the development of isolated perfused kidney preparations was made with the use of artificial, cell-free perfusion fluids such as buffered saline solutions supplemented with serum albumin (15,29,54,138,169,217) or macromolecular plasma substitutes (75,228,241,261). A principal disadvantage of using a perfusion fluid devoid of red blood cells is the relatively high perfusate flow rates observed under these conditions (15) and the relative anoxia due to the limitation of oxygen-carrying capacity of the cell-free medium (75). Second, an absence of natural components of blood in perfusion medium devoid of whole blood may alter the disposition of the test chemical. Although Krebs-Ringer bicarbonate-buffered solution containing glucose and albumin can be used for perfusing kidneys, investigators have found it necessary to dialyze the BSA (Cohn fraction V) to obtain satisfactory kidney preparations that are being perfused for longer durations (138). Third, Millipore filters must be used to filter out any cellular debris that may enter the circulation. Fourth, higher flow rates are necessary to ensure an adequate oxygen supply to the kidney when an artificial medium is used for perfusion.

In addition to the composition for artificial perfusate given above, Fonteles et al. (72) found that addition of GSH (500 mg/L) to the perfusate prevented depletion of endogenous cortical and medullary GSH. Furthermore, GSH supplementation of the perfusate decreased renal vascular resistance and increased perfusate flow. GSH extraction studies revealed a progressive decrease in renal extraction with time, ranging from complete extraction at 10 min to a value of 38% at 60 min (72). Including GSH in the perfusate might be especially relevant for toxicological investigations in view of the reports that many toxic agents deplete endogenous GSH levels in various tissues. Thus far, only kidney has been shown to be able to use external GSH to any significant extent. As was pointed out earlier, rat lung is reportedly able to utilize external GSH (20) but rabbit lung cannot (107).

Viability Criteria

To date most of the isolated perfused kidney studies have dealt with the mechanism of autoregulation and physiological functions of the kidney. Because of such a background on which perfused kidney preparations have been refined, techniques for evaluating adequacy and viability of the perfused kidney are abundant. Renal blood flow can be measured by placing a flow transducer prior to the kidney. Alternatively, a flow transducer can also be placed after the perfusate exits the kidney. Blood flow through the kidney can reach 6 to 7 ml/min/g of tissue, depending on perfusion pressures varying from 90 to 130 mm Hg (174). With the artificial perfusate,

flow through the kidney can reach as much as 30 to 60 ml/min/g of tissue. One problem associated with using perfusion flow rate as an index of viability is not knowing the intrarenal distribution of the flow. The regional distribution of the blood flow within the kidney can change markedly with artificial perfusion, with a striking increase in flow to the medulla and inner cortex (220). This fact is especially important for any toxicological investigations, as blood flow through an organ can be either shunted or altered in other ways as a result of toxic action of a test drug. Radiolabeled microspheres (10–15 μm) introduced into the circulation of a perfused organ may be used to assess the regional distribution of flow through the organ. Detailed accounts of such techniques are available (220).

Another criterion used for viability of perfused kidney preparations is the glomerular filtration rate (GFR). During the initial phase of perfusion, the GFR is at a lower limit (46–50 ml/min/100 g) of the normal range (174,260). Better values have been obtained with difibrinated blood at 69 ml/min/100 g tissue. GFR decreases progressively after 2 to 3 hr of perfusion. Often when blood is used as a perfusate, this impairment has been attributed to the embolization of fat droplets in the glomeruli (260). In unsuccessful experiments, when the weight of the kidney increases it is often due to retention of fluid in the tubules and interstitial edema (174,260).

Urine concentration and excretion of water are other criteria used for establishing the viability of perfused kidney preparations. During the first period of up to 1 hr, urine may reach an osmolality of 800 mosm, which is later reduced (60–150 mosm) owing to increased urine flow. The water diuresis in the kidney preparation can be suppressed by administration of vasopressin in the perfusate. After 3 to 4 hr the urine concentration approaches isotonicity (125,260,266). When observed, loss of urine concentrating power is probably due to medullary edema and disturbances of deep cortical and medulla blood flow (174). Sodium excretion can be used as an additional parameter of viability. In contrast to frequent statements in the literature, the fractional reabsorption of sodium can be normal (21) in perfused kidney preparations. In Berndt's experiments (*unpublished data, 1980*), sodium excretion exceeded 0.4% of the filtered load after 2 hr of perfusion using the Krebs-Ringer bicarbonate buffer type of artificial medium. After prolonged perfusion, however, sodium rejection may develop unless the perfusate is replaced, which may be due to accumulation of metabolic end products such as ammonia in the perfusate (125,260).

Acidification of urine is yet another functional viability criterion used for evaluating perfused kidney preparations. The loss of ability to excrete acidic urine represents a major functional abnormality of isolated kidney (125,260). An additional functional parameter that can be applied to perfused kidney preparations is the determination of insulin as well as paraaminohippurate (PAH) clearance values. A disadvantage of using these clearances as determinants of viability is that, depending on the experimental conditions, these tests may or may not be compatible with the original intended use of the perfused preparation. Hence many functional tests may have to be carried out infrequently rather than routinely as an internal check of the perfused preparation.

Finally, the kidney preparations can be sampled for electron microscopy as well as light microscopy, and morphological examination can be used as a determinant of functional abnormality. However, routine morphological examination at the light microscopic or ultrastructural level might not be practical for several reasons. Whether the preparation was viable cannot be determined until after the perfusion experiment. Facilities or expertise for routine morphological examination may not be available, and when available might be prohibitively expensive for routine use in experimental work. Often the validity of using morphological alterations as indicative of functional abnormality is questionable because other functional parameters might be optimal despite the morphological alterations at the cellular or subcellular level. Conversely, despite the normal morphological appearance, distinct functional aberrations may be observed. At least in part, such discrepancies can be explained on the basis of the relatively short time required for a functional abnormality to be detected, whereas longer periods may be required for the observed morphological alterations to develop and vice versa. At any rate, as pointed out earlier for the liver and lungs, morphological observation should be helpful initially for establishing a viable perfused preparation in any laboratory (72,260,268). Second, it is useful for examining the effects of toxic chemicals on perfused kidney preparations (46,60).

Applications

Historically, the isolated perfused kidney preparations have not been utilized in pharmacological and toxicological investigations despite the availability of refined techniques for some time (138,174). The bulk of the isolated perfused kidney work can be seen in the physiological literature. One reason might be increased attention devoted to establishment of the physiological parameters such as GFR, autoregulation of blood flow through the kidney, absorption–reabsorption mechanisms in the kidney tubules, and hormonal regulation of renal tubular functions. However, the utility of isolated perfused kidney preparations can be demonstrated by the nature of the information that can be obtained using this technique (174). For instance, the control of GFR by an endogenously released humoral factor was definitively demonstrated using isolated kidney preparations (174).

Using isolated erythrocyte-free, perfused rat kidney preparations, Schureck et al. (228) demonstrated that sodium reabsorption can be increased by including glucose as the sole energy source of the kidney. The nature of glucose handling by the kidney has also been investigated using perfused kidney (29). Because the tubular transport maximum (Tm) for glucose is proportional to GFR in the perfused kidney preparations, it was concluded that the Tm for glucose is not controlled by extrarenal factors.

Many physiological parameters of kidney function have been studied and are understood; and in many cases the renal control mechanism has been confirmed using isolated perfused kidney preparations (174). Use of the perfused kidney to investigate the toxicological mechanisms has increased (46,105,158,159,238,241), and these and other applications of the perfused kidney are briefly discussed.

Study of GSH extraction from the circulating perfusate by isolated perfused kidney preparations is an example of a biochemical study that can be useful in toxicological investigations (72). Including GSH in the circulating perfusate at a concentration of 500 mg/L resulted in the preservation of cortical and medullary GSH. Perfusion without the addition of GSH consistently resulted in depletion of tissue levels of this important tripeptide. In addition, including GSH in the perfusate resulted in decreased renal vascular resistance and increased perfusion flow. Whether the increased flow is due to intrarenal alterations in flow patterns is unclear. It appears that GSH storage in the kidney can level off, as indicated by the above study, in which complete extraction of added GSH was seen at 10 min; this uptake was reduced to 38% of administered GSH at 60 min. These studies of Fonteles et al. (72) indicated a high affinity of rabbit kidney for GSH and a relatively large net reabsorption of this important tripeptide. In view of the many toxicological molecular events being related to alterations in the endogenous pools of GSH, this observation might be important in toxicological studies using isolated perfused kidney preparations.

Another example of using the isolated perfused kidney in toxicological investigations lies in the studies of Dovrak et al. (60), in which they examined the effects of high doses of methylprednisolone on the isolated perfused dog kidney. They noted several histological changes in the kidneys perfused with methylprednisolone for 20 hr or longer. The primary changes consisted in necrosis of capillary loops, inclusion of eosinophilic material in Bowman's space, thickening of the basement membrane, and endothelial cell damage. Arterial changes consisted primarily of inclusion of afferent arterioles with dense eosinophilic material. Tubular changes consisted in inclusion of tubular lumens and damage to tubular epithelial cells. These studies demonstrated that administration of high doses of methylprednisolone can produce irreversible hemodynamic and histological changes in the kidney.

Summerfield et al. (240) utilized isolated perfused kidney preparations to examine conjugating reactions involved in the elimination of certain bile acids in urine. These investigators demonstrated that lithocholic and chenodeoxycholic acids can be metabolized by the perfused kidney to their monosulfate conjugates; the disulfate metabolites of these bile acids were not detected in the urine. These findings supported the hypothesis that renal synthesis of monosulfate conjugates may account for at least some of the bile acid sulfates present in urine in the cholestatic syndrome of man. The results further suggested that in chemically induced hepatic injury the kidney may be able to conjugate some of the bile acids, and they demonstrated the presence of sufficient biochemical machinery within the renal tissue for conjugating endogenous substrates. The experiments also demonstrated the possibility of conjugation of foreign chemicals in the renal tissue, facilitating their elimination in urine.

Jaffe et al. (105) employed perfused rabbit kidney to evaluate the genotoxic potential of the S-(trans-1,2-dichlorovinyl)-L-cysteine (DDVC). The proposed mechanism of renal toxicity of this and other vinyl cysteine conjugates is activation by β-lyase, an enzyme in the renal brush border membrane of the renal tubular epithelial cells. This enzyme converts the halogenated vinyl cysteine conjugate to reactive thiovinyl intermediates, which alkylate subcellular macromolecules such as DNA. In these rabbit kidney perfusion studies, a dose-dependent (0.01–1.00 mM DDVC) effect of DDVC on DNA single-strand breaks was demonstrated.

The study of Tark et al. (245) may be cited as an example of yet another use of isolated perfused kidney in toxicological investigations. These investigators examined substrate metabolism in the isolated perfused dog kidney and established that free fatty acids (FFAs) and glucose serve as significant substrates for providing energy for sodium transport in the kidney. Second, their studies suggested that glucose may substitute for FFAs as an energy source at times when FFAs in the circulation are decreased. The effect of toxic chemicals in the renal circulation on substrate metabolism in the kidney can be examined using the methods described by Tark et al. (245).

Johannesen et al. (106) employed perfused kidney preparations to study the renal energy metabolism inhibitor 2,4-dinitrophenol.

There has been an increase in the use of isolated perfused kidney preparations in toxicological investigations. Perfused rat kidney has been used to investigate the mechanism of gentamicin toxicity (46,158,159). Mitchell et al. (158) established that a specific effect of gentamicin on potassium secretion is responsible for clinically observed hypokalemia during gentamicin therapy. This study and those of Hook and associates (46) have established that reduced water and electrolyte reabsorption were the earliest effects of gentamicin on the kidney. Perfusion of the rat kidneys with gentamicin induced a dose-dependent decrease in reabsorption and metabolism of lysozyme (46). The basis of the sex differences in renal toxicity was the subject of additional inquiry (159). The sex differences could not be demonstrated in the perfused rat kidneys exposed to gentamicin, suggesting that the sex differences in the susceptibility to this antibiotic *in vivo* might be due to some extrarenal factors.

Koschier et al. (120) perfused rat kidneys to study the effects of bis-(p-chlorophenyl) acetic acid (DDA), the principal water-soluble metabolite of DDT. At a concentration of 1 mM DDA in the perfusate, the GFR, urine volume, and fractional excretion of sodium were decreased, suggesting a direct action of DDA on nephron function. Sumpio et al. (241) employed isolated perfused rat kidneys to characterize the renal toxicity of cis-diaminedichloroplatinum (CDDP) and to determine if treatment with ATP-MgCl$_2$ could prevent or reduce the nephrotoxic effect of CDDP. After 2 hr of perfusion, CDDP (100 μg/ml) treatment led to marked inhibition of protein reabsorption with only a minimal decrease in sodium and water reabsorption. Despite a marked diuresis, GFR was not significantly altered. Posttreatment with ATP-MgCl$_2$ (2 mM) led to partial alleviation of the nephrotoxic effect of CDDP. After 1 hr of perfusion, simultaneous treatment with ATP-MgCl$_2$ (0.3 mM), however, fully protected the protein reabsorptive capacity of CDDP-treated kidneys. Because the CDDP-induced toxicity simulates the acute renal failure seen clinically, these findings are suggestive of a new therapeutic modality for clinical management.

Isolated Perfused Brain

Brain does not lend itself to simple and totally isolated perfusion, and all the preparations to date include more or less extraneural tissue. Perfusion has found little place in many of the biochemical and toxicological studies with brain tissue, as the technique presents great difficulty even when effort is not made to exclude extraneural tissue. In addition, the brain is heterogeneous, and the contribution by both neuronal and nonneuronal tissue of the brain to drug uptake and turnover in perfusion causes difficulties in duplicating the results. The blood–brain barrier is one aspect of brain metabolism in particular that remains noticeably obscure, and it has been the subject of studies with perfused brain preparations (3,70,80,82,249). The heterogeneity of the preparation together with the many neural tissues represented in the brain make perfusion a somewhat less valuable technique for toxicological investigations than other individual organs. Nevertheless, several investigators have been able to maintain a viable perfused brain preparation that can be utilized for drug metabolism and investigations on the effects of toxic chemicals that may adversely affect the central nervous system. The difficulty of maintaining the isolated perfused brain preparation coupled with the readily available *in vitro* and *in vivo* techniques have resulted in underutilization of perfused brain preparations for pharmacological and toxicological investigations.

Comparatively simple techniques of perfusing the rat brain are described here. The "perfused rat head" preparation of Thompson et al. (249), in which the entire head is perfused with no attempt to limit the circulation to the brain, is not described in detail. However, such a technique may be useful in some toxicological investigations and may be considered before setting up more difficult preparations. Far more elaborate and therefore technically more difficult is the preparation described by Andjus et al. (3), which attempts to exclude the muscle of the head and neck from the perfusion circuit; this method is described because of the obvious superiority of the technique. The preparation is based on the more elaborate perfusion technique developed in the cat by Geiger and Magnes (80), which may be consulted if larger animal models are suitable to meet the particular need. Readers may refer to White (262) for a total isolated, vascularly perfused monkey brain preparation or to Gilboe et al. (82) for a dog brain perfusion preparation.

Apparatus

Figure 9 shows the schematics of the equipment used for oxygenating the venous drainage from the brain and perfusion of the isolated rat brain described by Andjus et al. (3). The bubble oxygenator and reservoir are made from two disposable plastic drug administration sets combined and fitted with connectors and plastic tubing. A small volume of recirculating fluid pumped by a peristaltic pump is used to perfuse the brain. The perfused brain preparation is held in a funnel from which the effluent perfusate drips to the oxygenator and passes through a filter to complete one circulation. If a single-pass circulation is desired, the peristaltic pump is disconnected, and a reservoir of perfusate is used at a height sufficient to provide satisfactory perfusion pressure and flow.

Surgical Procedures

After the animal is anesthetized using a proper anesthetic agent, both common carotid arteries are exposed, and the

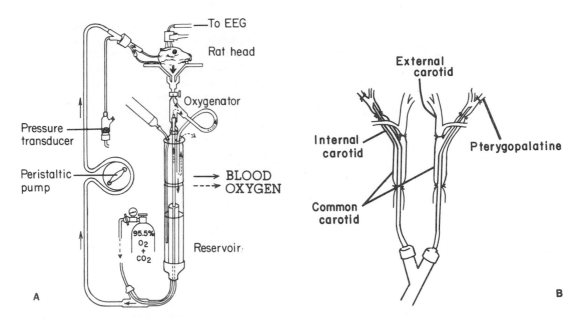

FIG. 9. A: Perfusion system for the isolated perfused rat brain preparation. Venous blood from the preparation flows by gravity into the collecting funnel and then is dispersed by the stream of gas (O_2/CO_2, 95:5) into short segments and carried through the side branch of the oxygenator into the reservoir. The stream of gas is prevented from escaping through the collecting funnel by adjusting the rate of flow of gas and the screw clamp just below the funnel. Fixed in the lower part of the reservoir is a metal-mesh filter. For perfusion without recirculation, the blood from the collecting funnel drains into a bottle, and fresh blood is added at the top of the oxygenator as needed. The peristaltic pump has a continuously variable speed with maximum delivery of 2 ml/min. The perfusion pressure is monitored by a pressure transducer. Substances can be added to or samples taken from the reservoir by means of the syringe and attached tubing shown to the left of the oxygenator. The solid arrows show the direction of flow of blood, the dashed arrows the direction of flow of gas. **B:** Relation of the perfusion cannulas to the cannulated and adjacent arteries. (From ref. 3, with permission.)

trachea is intubated via a tracheostomy. The animal is heparinized by injecting 500 IU of sodium heparin through the jugular vein, which is then ligated by means of a suture. The external carotid and pterygopalatine arteries are ligated. In the rat the pterygopalatine artery is a branch of the internal carotid artery, which supplies blood to various extracranial structures. A plastic cannula filled with perfusion fluid is then inserted into each common carotid, advanced into the internal carotid artery, and tied in position so its tip is near the origin of the previously ligated pterygopalatine artery. The arrangement of the vessels and the cannulas are illustrated in Fig. 9.

A slow perfusion is initiated, and then the skin and the muscles of the head, face, and neck are removed together with the mandible. A sturdy ligature is placed around the vertebral column, which is transected just below the ligature. The transected vertebral canal is packed with a cotton or tissue paper plug, and the canal is sealed with melted wax. The completed preparation consists of the skull and its contents with the upper cervical vertebrae and small remnants of muscle tissue attached. Toward the end of the surgical procedure, the perfusion flow is gradually increased. After severing the vertebral column, the perfusion flow rate is adjusted to a desired value (1.4 ml/min). The cannulated preparation is then mounted above the collecting funnel. The entire preparation and the apparatus can be housed in a heating chamber to facilitate maintenance of the proper temperature. The chamber used for liver preparations (144,157) may be used for this purpose.

Thompson et al. (249) described a technique of *in situ* perfusion of the rat head. They used the apparatus reminiscent of that of Miller et al. (157). The aortic arch of the rat is perfused, and the inferior vena cava is cannulated for the outflow. Recirculation of the perfusion medium, made up of diluted rat blood, maintains the preparation for up to 3 hr. The isolated perfused rat brain preparation described by Andjus et al. (3) can be maintained for 2 hr with satisfactory CNS function. Geiger and Magnes (80) described an isolated perfused brain from the cat that is similar to the preparation described above for the rat. The Geiger–Magnes preparation has been used for various studies by other investigators. For example, Barrett et al. (17) used it to evaluate the effect of a number of centrally acting drugs on cat brain. In addition, Otsuki et al. (189) used the cat brain preparation to evaluate the suitability of using various perfusion media.

Perfusion Media

Andjus et al. (3) used pooled rat blood obtained from several rats as the perfusion medium. However, they found that when blood was used it did not support the spontaneous electrical activity of the isolated brain. After several trials they concluded that an artificial perfusion fluid similar to that described by Geiger (79) should be used.

The fluid portion of the artificial perfusate is Krebs-Ringer bicarbonate buffer solution, described earlier for perfusion of the liver, lung, and kidney. BSA (Cohn fraction V) is dissolved in distilled water and deionized by passing it through a column of Amberlite MB-3 before mixing it with the Krebs-Ringer bicarbonate-buffered solution. Erythrocytes obtained from dog blood were washed and used in this perfusion fluid. The cells are washed four times with cold, buffered (0.01 M, pH 7.4) isotonic sodium chloride solution and finally with isotonic Krebs-Ringer bicarbonate-buffered solution prior to use. The final perfusate contains 7 to 8% BSA, a hematocrit of 20 to 25%, and pH adjusted to 7.3. The perfusate is always best freshly prepared just prior to use. The glucose concentration of the blood for perfusion is adjusted to 200 mg/dl by adding a requisite volume of 5% glucose in normal saline solution.

The perfusate and the isolated brain preparation described by Andjus et al. (3) remained at room temperature (23° to 27°C) throughout the experiment; most of the perfusion experiments were conducted at 25°C. However, maintaining the entire perfusion at body temperature should be considered. It can be easily done by employing a heated chamber such as the one used for perfusing the liver (144,157). The total volume of perfusate is 100 ml, and perfusion is carried out at a constant arterial pressure of 100 to 120 mm Hg. The perfusion rate is 3 to 5 ml/min and should be maintained at this rate throughout the experiment. The temperature of the brain can be maintained at 30°C using a heated chamber as indicated above.

Otsuki et al. (189) compared a number of perfusion media using Krebs-Ringer bicarbonate buffer as the solution and either low-molecular-weight (40,000) or high-molecular-weight (70,000) dextran as the substituent for BSA. They also compared the effect of including a number of amino acids in the perfusion medium. Their study concluded that dextran could replace BSA in the perfusion medium and that the low-molecular-weight dextran was superior to the high-molecular-weight dextran. Furthermore, including glutamic acid in the perfusate along with low-molecular-weight dextran improved functional performance of the isolated perfused cat brain.

Viability Criteria

Spontaneous electrical activity was recorded by Andjus et al. (3) as a functional parameter of brain activity. The isolated rat brain preparation had spontaneous electroencephalographic (EEG) activity that persisted as long as 5 hr with single-pass perfusion and about 2 hr when recirculating perfusion was conducted. Although the reason for the shorter period of viability in a recirculation is not well understood, it is possible that endogenous biochemical products of intermediary metabolism may accumulate in the recirculating perfusion, to the detriment of the perfused brain. Addition of pentylenetetrazol to the perfusing blood evoked characteristic EEG signs of convulsive activity either before or after spontaneous EEG activity had ceased. Otsuki et al. (189) carried out a similar study using EEG measurements to compare the suitability of altering the perfusion medium to perfuse cat brain. Response to loud sounds can also be observed by EEG recordings and can be used as a viability criterion. After perfusion for 5 hr, Andjus et al. (3) reported that the rat brain was nonresponsive to sound, indicating deterioration of the preparation. Thus although EEG recordings indicated viability of the rat brain preparations, response to loud noise was lost after 5 hr of perfusion (3), suggesting that not all the criteria are satisfied, especially during a perfusion that lasts several hours. Gilboe and associates (82) have used oxygen utilization and EEG pattern as satisfactory criteria for dog brain perfusion.

An additional criterion for viability is the rate of glucose utilization by the isolated brain preparation. It can be measured as the decrease in glucose concentration in the perfusing blood and should be linear during the first hour of the experiment; later it tends to decrease with the deterioration of the preparation. Lactate accumulates in the circulating perfusate, but the rate at which it accumulates does not appear to be directly related to glucose utilization (3). Otsuki et al. (189) also used rates of glucose utilization as a measure of viability for evaluating the various perfusion media to support isolated perfused cat brain preparations.

Applications

Although the use of isolated perfused brain preparations for toxicological investigations had been infrequent, examples can be cited where isolated perfused brain preparations have been used for such studies. The principal reason for the relatively infrequent use of isolated perfused brain preparations seems to be relatively slow development of the techniques (3,17,80,189). Hein et al. (94) investigated the effect of thiopental anesthesia on the energy metabolism of the isolated perfused rat brain. They perfused the rat brain in the presence and absence of 5 to 15 mM thiopental and investigated glucose turnover as well as a number of indicators of the glycolytic pathway. They noted that glucose uptake by the brain preparation was increased when thiopental was included in the perfusate. However, the glycolytic pathway remained inhibited, indicating the sensitivity of the glycolytic pathway to thiopental. They also noted that this effect was not mediated via hindered uptake of glucose. In another study, Dirks et al. (58) investigated the effect of piracetam and methohexital on rat brain energy metabolism and concluded that piracetam had no acute effect on energy metabolism, and methohexital protected the rat brain from ischemic effects. Thus these reports demonstrated the usefulness of the perfused brain preparation for studying intermediary metabolism (58,123) of the brain as affected by the presence of toxic drugs or chemicals in the circulating perfusion medium. Similar preparations should be useful for studying the effect of centrally acting toxic chemicals such as industrial solvents and gaseous substances as well as other neurotoxins. For example, Krieglstein and Stock (124) described the effect of chloral hydrate and trichloroethanol on cerebral intermediary metabolism. Fink et al. (69) used perfused rat brain to study the central activity of valtrate, following the EEG activity of brains perfused with or without valtrate. Fitzpatrick and Gilboe (70) used perfused dog brain to study the effects of nitrous oxide on the cerebrovascular tone, oxygen consumption, and EEG, and demonstrated that nitrous oxide reduces cerebral vascular tone but exhibits no effects on central oxygen metabolism.

The applicability of isolated rat brain preparations to study central neurological mechanisms can be illustrated by the study of Kilbinger and Krieglstein (114). They found that physostigmine caused a rise in the acetylcholine concentration of both the isolated perfused rat brain and the rat brain *in vivo*. Oxotremorine, on the other hand, produced an increase in acetylcholine content in the brain *in vivo* but was ineffective in the isolated rat brain at the same dosage. These investigations were carried out by recording the EEG as well as determining perfusate and brain levels of acetylcholine. These studies suggested the feasibility of using brain preparations to evaluate the effect of toxic chemicals on alterations of endogenous neurohormones and neurotransmitters.

In addition to the studies mentioned above, the technique of perfusion has also been used to aid histological fixation (190,252) of brains from experimental animals. For this purpose, the arch of the aorta is perfused with a balanced salt solution followed by a fixative. A distinct advantage of the perfusion technique to fix the brain preparation for histological examination is the delivery of oxygen through the oxygenated perfusion medium to the brain in order to achieve better preservation of the tissue.

Although the isolated perfused brain preparations described to date include extraneural tissue and many types of nerve centers within the brain itself, the perfusion technique should nevertheless be valuable for examining the specific effects of centrally active toxic chemicals. The state of the art in this area has developed to a degree to which the technique should prove useful in toxicological investigations.

Isolated Perfused Intestine

Over the years there have been several attempts to study the mammalian intestine as an isolated tissue sustained by a vascular perfusion. Mainly because of the nature of the tissue itself, there has been ambiguity in the use of the term "perfusion" in the field of intestinal research. Intraluminal circulation of fluid for the purpose of studying the transport of small molecules across the intestinal mucosa has often been referred to as intestinal perfusion (235,237). Intraluminal perfusion experiments can be performed *in vivo* for subacute toxicity studies (139) or for shorter periods of time (210), or *in vitro* with excised segments of intestine (141). A full range of experimental techniques are available for work with intestinal tissue, and the topic has been reviewed (192), including the technique of vascular perfusion (104). No single experimental technique provides information about all phases of the absorptive processes involved in the removal of a substance from the lumen of the small intestine, its transport across the intestinal wall, and its entry into either blood or the lymphatic circulation. Techniques such as intraluminal perfusion and everted sac described by Wilson and Wiseman (263) are discussed elsewhere in this book. This particular discussion deals with the vascular perfusion of small intestine.

Isolated vascular perfusion of intestine has not been prominent in gastrointestinal research because of the many problems encountered obtaining sustained viability (264). It is clear that vascular resistance, spasmodic bowel contractions, tissue edema, and progressive destruction of the mucosal epithelium were the principal problems encountered during earlier attempts to establish a vascularly perfused intestinal preparation. Second, because most investigators were concerned with the mechanisms of intestinal absorption and were dealing with the mucosal layer, these investigators found it convenient to use intraluminal perfusion with fluid containing the experimental drug to study the intestinal absorption. In addition to supplying the experimental drugs through the intraluminal fluid, such fluid could also carry the necessary oxygen for supporting the mucosal layer (28). However, arguments can be made for developing a viable, vascularly perfused intestinal preparation (112,264). The role played by other layers of intestinal wall such as the muscle can be studied in a vascularly perfused intestinal preparation. Also, the disadvantages of everted gut preparation, in which only transport across the wall is studied (rather than transport into the blood circulation), are overcome by utilizing an isolated vascularly perfused preparation. Thus anatomically and functionally distinct compartments, e.g., lumen, lymph, and bloodstream, are kept separated and can be studied individually. These arguments and the need to separate intestinal tissue to describe those absorptive, distributive, and metabolic functions of the tissue fully justify the development and use of the isolated, vascularly perfused intestinal preparation.

As has been observed for other isolated perfused organs, intestine can be perfused *in situ* (112,191,264) or in complete isolation (35,73,100). In addition, the perfused preparation can be used with an intraluminal flow maintained in the natural direction of peristalsis (61,112) or without the intraluminal flow (73,81,100). If the intestine is perfused without the intraluminal flow, two dynamic compartments (perfusion fluid and lymph) can be sampled for an experimental test chemical in addition to the intestinal tissue itself. If intraluminal flow is maintained, however, three dynamic compartments (perfusion fluid, lymph, intraluminal fluid) and the static compartment of intestine tissue can be sampled for an experimental test chemical. For most practical purposes, maintaining intraluminal flow would introduce another dynamic variability in the experimental condition so that analysis and interpretation of the experimental results from analyzing all four compartments would be difficult if not impossible. The following description of an isolated perfused intestinal preparation is based on the procedure of Kavin et al. (112), later improvised by Windmueller et al. (264).

Apparatus

An acrylic plastic box (75 cm high, 60 cm wide, 50 cm deep) houses the apparatus (Fig. 10). Temperature in the chamber is maintained at 37°C by means of a heater and fan assembly that is thermostatically controlled. The chamber is kept humidified by a small jet of steam blown inside the chamber. The acrylic plastic cyclical oxygenator-reservoir (7 cm diameter, 15 cm high) contains a thin acrylic disk with a gently sloping convex upper surface and separated edges supported by three equidistant flanges about 3.7 cm from the top. The tip of the Silastic tubing that carries venous and bypassed blood rests on the disk so that it flows on the disk

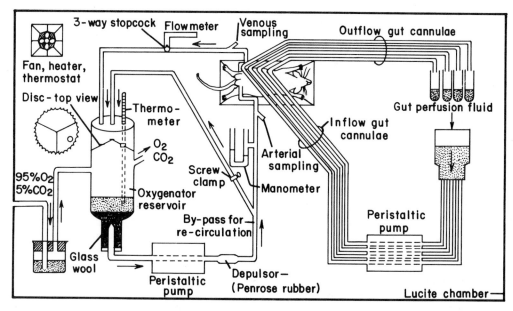

FIG. 10. Apparatus for vascular perfusion of small intestine. (From ref. 112, with permission.)

and spreads out to the serrated edges and finally down the inner wall of the cylinder as a thin film, thereby exposing a maximum surface area for oxygenation. O_2/CO_2 (95:5) is bubbled through distilled water and led into the gas inlet of the oxygenator-reservoir via the thin Silastic tubing. An appropriate blood filter can be placed at the bottom of the reservoir to filter out any broken cells or other debris before the blood circulation is pumped via a peristaltic pump to the animal. From the plastic filter, blood is led to a peristaltic pump via silicone tubing (4.60 mm o.d., 3.35 mm i.d.). A hydrostatic reservoir is maintained between the peristaltic pump and the animal to provide a constant perfusion pressure. A bypass flow from the hydrostatic reservoir to the central reservoir facilitates maintaining a constant hydrostatic head. Blood flow is determined by means of a transducer connected to the venous circuit by a three-way stopcock. Blood is sampled from the arterial and venous channel via polyethylene tubing, using Y connections near the arterial and venous cannulas. Thus blood is in contact with Silastic tubing, a hydrostatic reservoir, and polyethylene connections (Fig. 10). Most of the silicone tubing could be replaced by glass in the apparatus, and use of the silicone tubing should be restricted to glass tube connections and the peristaltic pump. If intraluminal flow is desired in the experimental protocol, an infusion pump can be used to introduce a fluid, with or without the test chemical, into the intestinal lumen. A peristaltic pump can be used for this purpose, giving a peristaltic wave motion for the intraluminal flow. Fluid effusing out of the intestine can be collected as desired or recirculated after sampling.

Perfusion Procedure

The rat is anesthetized with a mixture of ether and oxygen or an intraperitoneal injection of pentobarbital (50 mg/kg). Through an L-shaped abdominal incision, the small intestine, cecum, and proximal large intestine are gently exteriorized and supported on a plastic platform that is covered with gauze soaked in warm 0.9% NaCl. The intestine is covered with saline-soaked gauze in a plastic sheet and kept at 37°C by means of a heat lamp. Both ends of the intestine are ligated using an appropriate suture: proximally at the duodenum about 1.5 cm from the pylorus and distally near the midpoint of the descending colon. Included in the proximal ligature are the common bile duct and the mesentery between the duodenum and superior mesenteric vein. A PE-90 cannula is placed in the duodenal lumen and secured by the same ligature in those experiments in which intraluminal infusion is required.

Lymph is collected from a polyethylene cannula of 0.023 in. i.d. and 0.0238 in. o.d. and secured with a ligature in the main intestinal lymph duct. Loose ties are placed around the superior mesenteric artery, about 5 mm from the aorta, and around the superior mesenteric vein just below the junction with the pyloric and coronary veins. The mesenteric artery can be cannulated using a PE-50 cannula filled with perfusion fluid and connected to a syringe with perfusate at the other end. Insertion of the PE-50 cannula is facilitated by introducing the beveled end of the cannula via a V-shaped cut made in the mesenteric artery using fine scissors. After the cannula is secured by a ligature, flow of the perfusate can be started by disconnecting the syringe and connecting the cannula to the perfusate of the preprimed perfusion apparatus. Immediate resumption of perfusate flow is essential, as the isolated small intestinal loop has been ischemic throughout the surgical procedure. At this point, a flow of 8 to 9 ml/min would ensure adequate oxygen supply to the tissue.

The rat is then exsanguinated by severing the left jugular vein and carotid artery. The superior mesenteric vein is cannulated by means of another PE-50 cannula in a manner analogous to the above procedure and secured by means of a suitable suture. The venous effluent is recycled through the perfusion apparatus to the oxygenator-reservoir. Once recirculation of the perfusate is established, arterial flow is increased until an arterial pressure of approximately 95 mm Hg is reached. The venous pressure is adjusted to 150 mm H$_2$O by an adjustable clamp on the outflow cannula. With experience, total surgical time can be minimized to 30 min or less. All of these procedures are easier with large animals; the isolated, vascularly perfused canine intestine is described in the literature (35,100,176).

Perfusion Media

The semiartificial perfusion medium consists of 80 to 120 ml fresh heparinized rat blood drawn by abdominal aortic puncture from an ether-anesthetized animal (264). The blood is heparinized with 10,000 to 25,000 IU of sodium heparin. Windmueller et al. (264) used antibiotics in the blood (penicillin G, streptomycin), but often use of these compounds is undesirable as they may interfere with the test drug. If the perfusion chamber and all of the components of the apparatus are sterilized, antibiotics have not been necessary for the isolation and perfusion of organs such as the lung and liver (144,153,154). Use of antibiotics should be avoided unless it becomes critical in a particular experimental protocol. Norepinephrine is used continuously at a rate of 1.0 to 2.2 ml/min as a 0.153 mg/ml solution in order to alleviate increased vascular resistance noted by earlier investigators. A glucocorticoid (dexamethasone, 6×10^{-7} M) is added in a single dose as a solution (25 mg/dl) in the perfusate to the reservoir. A combination of the glucocorticoid and norepinephrine aids in maintaining the low vascular resistance and improved tissue preservation.

The perfusate described for other perfusate organs containing Krebs-Ringer bicarbonate-buffered solution with glucose and BSA can be used for perfusing intestinal preparations with satisfactory results. Kavin et al. (112) utilized a similar perfusate with low-molecular-weight dextran instead of albumin in their perfusion fluid. Addition of norepinephrine and a glucocorticoid to this perfusate would make it comparable to Windmueller et al.'s (264) preparation. The fluid for intraluminal flow is 0.9% saline containing glucose (220 mM) and sodium taurocholate (10 mM) infused at 2.6 ml/hr. Regardless of whether intraluminal flow is intended, use of the Krebs-Ringer bicarbonate-buffered solution with glucose and albumin or low-molecular-weight dextran should be considered for toxicological investigations. The perfusion flow rate of 16 to 20 ml/min is obtained under these conditions at an arterial pressure of 95 mm Hg. *In vivo* flow in rats was found to be 8 to 10 ml/min (264), approximately half of that observed with the heparinized blood as perfusate. This rate is an indication of low vascular resistance; and when the intestinal vasculature is isolated, this resistance may persist during the remainder of the perfusion period.

Viability Criteria

Histological examination of the intestine after 5 hr of perfusion (264) indicated that the integrity of the vascularly perfused tissue was well preserved. Cross-sections through the duodenum showed that the brush border of the intestinal wall and the base epithelium of the duodenum were well preserved after 5 hr of perfusion (112,264). Additional parameters used for determining the viability of vascularly perfused intestinal preparations include the perfusion flow rate, uptake of glucose by tissue, and production of lymph and continued satisfactory oxygen consumption. In general, the preparation can be maintained viable for at least 5 hr, as indicated by its gross and microscopic appearance and by the continued oxygen consumption, peristaltic motility, water transport, and vascular responsiveness to norepinephrine. The perfused intestine is capable of glucose transport, and in most experiments lymph flow continues without reduction for 5 hr (264). The rate of lymph flow is increased by infusing intraluminal fluid and by increasing venous pressure. An additional parameter used for evaluating the perfused intestinal preparation is fat transport and lipoprotein biosynthesis (264). Morphological examination of the intestinal tissue by light and electron microscopy (112,264) is useful for ascertaining viability.

Applications

The effects of bolus intraarterial doses of heroin and other stimulant drugs were studied (176) in vascularly perfused isolated segments of canine dog small intestine. Heroin caused dose-related increases in intraluminal pressure similar to those caused by morphine. Perfusion with Krebs bicarbonate solution containing naloxone selectively abolished intestinal responses to heroin. Perfusion with cinanserin, a 5-HT antagonist, decreased intestinal responses to 5-HT and heroin without affecting responses to dimethylphenylpiperazinium or bethanechol. Atropine antagonized the contractile responses. The authors concluded that heroin interacts with a conventional opiate receptor in the intestine and that the intestinal stimulatory effect of heroin is mediated by the release of endogenous 5-HT, which activates intramural cholinergic neurons. In other studies, perfused canine intestines were used to evaluate the proposed k receptor agonists such as ethylketoxyclazocine, nalorphine, and bremazocine (100) and concluded that k receptors did not appear to be involved in the contractile response of the canine small intestine to opioids.

Isolated vascularly perfused intestinal preparations have been used in toxicological investigations infrequently. It is not readily apparent as to why it is so, but difficulty developing the techniques for maintaining a viable perfused preparation and the requirement for a thoroughly elaborate set of equipment must have some deterrent influence on the use of this technique. The preparation should prove especially useful in studies relating to drug absorption and the interaction of drugs as it relates to intestinal absorption and transport mechanisms. It might also be useful for evaluating the role of intestinal metabolism and overall disposition of various drugs and toxic chemicals. The preparation should also prove useful for testing reported intestinal elimination of a number of chlorinated hydrocarbon compounds via the luminal surface. All of these aspects relate to toxicology of a particular test drug. Finally, the effect of toxic chemicals on absorption of nutrients, generation and preservation of mucosal cell lining, and various drug-metabolizing enzymes can also be evaluated using the perfused intestinal preparations.

The effect of toxic chemicals on endogenous biochemical parameters that are related to the intermediary metabolism of the intestine itself can also be investigated.

Isolated Perfused Pancreas

The pancreas is a highly vascular endocrine organ in which the anatomy of the blood supply lends itself to isolated vascular perfusion. Compared to the isolated islet incubation (127), pancreatic slices (137), and tissue fragments (48), the superfusion method of Burr et al. (36) for the isolated perfused pancreas is the most satisfactory and ideal approach to study the interrelations between pancreatic and other hormones as well as the effect of toxic chemicals on pancreatic function. The perfused pancreas is preferred over all the other tissue preparations for these studies in view of the following advantages offered by the isolated perfused pancreas preparation (140). Superficial and deep islets are equally provided with oxygen, which is constantly replenished; and the substrates and effectors arrive at the cell in a physiologically normal way. The islets remain in an anatomical relation with other cells and tissues of the organs, including blood vessels and nerves. Only extrinsic nerve control is lost, and many intrinsic factors that actively regulate the gland's function may be preserved in an isolated perfused pancreatic preparation. Maintenance of the tissue's cellular integrity can be confirmed at the end of the experiment by light and electron microscopic examination. There is a possibility of a control and experimental period of study in the same pancreas preparation. Such controls in other *in vitro* systems require multiple incubations.

Of greater significance might be the ability to maintain the exocrine secretions of the pancreas from getting back into contact with the islet cells, as cannulation of the segment of duodenum into which the exocrine secretions drain allows collection of these secretions separately. Thus the enzymes and other secretions produced are kept separate from the cells that produce them, and the well-known digestive effect of pancreatic enzymes on the pancreatic tissue is avoided. Despite the overwhelming superiority of vascularly perfused pancreatic preparations, there has been a lag in the development of perfusion techniques with this endocrine tissue. The lag can be attributed to the technical difficulties encountered with surgical preparations and the heterogeneity of the tissue in the isolated pancreatic preparation.

The location of the pancreatic duct entering the duodenum might be of some significance, especially in studies related to exocrine function such as protein synthesis. The pancreatic ducts are multiple, and their entry into the intestine is variable (45). Doerr and Becker (59) reported the main pancreatic duct as emptying into the bile duct rather than into the duodenum in the rat. In the guinea pig and rabbit (59), the main pancreatic duct enters the duodenal tract. The general rule is that in carnivores the ducts empty near or into the common bile duct, whereas in herbivores they empty more distally into the duodenum.

A limited literature is available on the technique of isolated perfused pancreatic preparation, although excellent descriptions of feline (39,64) and canine (97,103,117) pancreas preparations are available. The principal descriptions are those of Grodsky et al. (89), Sussman et al. (243), and Loubatieres et al. (140). The following is a description of a combination of the better features of all three perfusion preparations.

Apparatus

The apparatus used by Sussman et al. (243) is adequate for perfusion of the isolated pancreas and is described here. The chamber of the perfusion apparatus is based on the original description of that used by Miller et al. (157). The details of the apparatus are given in Fig. 11. Perfusate is pumped from the reservoir through Silastic tubing to a multibulb glass lung for oxygenation. The perfusate is then pumped by means of a peristaltic pump through a flow transducer, after which it courses through a filter to the enclosed perfusion chamber. The perfusate enters the pancreatic circulation through the arterial cannula, and the pressure is measured in millimeters of mercury using a aneroid manometer. The arterial blood may be sampled through another, similar arrangement (Fig. 11). O_2/CO_2 (95:5) is directed to the lung after bubbling it through a humidifier. The pancreas is kept moist with either the same solution used as perfusate or normal saline. The pancreas is perfused using Krebs-Ringer bicarbonate-buffered solution (pH 7.4) containing glucose and BSA, as described for the liver, which is circulated through the glass lung for oxygenation. A pediatric plastic cannula (1.5 mm o.d.) is used to cannulate the arterial side with an attachment for measuring intraluminal pressure. The venous cannula is PE tubing (2 mm o.d.). The duodenal cannula, an arrangement similar to the one described earlier for perfusion of the intestine would be adequate.

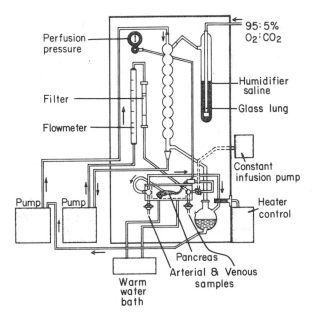

FIG. 11. Apparatus for perfusion of an isolated pancreas preparation, described by Sussman et al. (243). It is a modification of the apparatus described by Miller et al. (157) and adapted to the perfusion of the rat pancreas. (From ref. 243, with permission.)

Surgical Procedure

The animal may be starved overnight to facilitate the operation by depleting the omental fat. Although this method facilitates surgical procedures, the investigator may wish to avoid starving the animal as starvation is known to cause increased toxicity of some chemicals, which might also mean that pancreatic effects are altered. The animal is anesthetized by appropriate means (e.g., pentobarbital 50 mg/kg i.p.). A lateral incision and a midline incision through the skin and linea alba and through the skin over the inferior thorax are made as described for the surgical procedure to isolate the liver. The intestine is moved to the animal's left and covered with a wet saline gauze, and the aorta with the superior mesenteric branch is clearly made visible. The descending colon is easily identified as it remains attached to the lower posterior abdominal wall by a short mesentery. The fine layer of connective tissue is cut along the length of the colon in a plane in which no blood vessels are found, thereby mobilizing the lower gut, which is later removed. Using blunt-end dissection scissors, the pancreas is separated from the overlying colon. The jejunum is ligated and severed just behind its pancreatic attachment. This ligature will be useful for orientation later. The distal jejunum has a copious blood supply, and its vessels are tied for the last 0.5 in. of the distal segment to facilitate its later removal.

At this time the superior mesenteric vein, which runs into the portal vein, can be seen over the surface of the pancreas. The superior mesenteric vein is tied just below the pancreas with double ligatures and cut between them. Any other attachments of the pancreas to the descending colon are ligated and cut. At this stage the superior mesenteric artery and celiac axis can be identified and are preserved through the following dissection. The fine membrane covering the spleen and any other closely adherent tissue is carefully picked off with sharp forceps. The main splenic vessels, entering toward the upper pole, are tied twice and cut between the ligatures. A whole set of vessels curve through the mesentery to cross between the pancreatic tail and the spleen. If tied together, these pedicles can bunch the vessels in the tail of the pancreas. It is better to tie each of them individually with additional investments of time. A marker thread may be left to denote the tail of the pancreas for relative ease in orienting it upon its isolation

The stomach is pulled downward, and the major left gastric artery, which runs into the upper and medial aspect of stomach near the esophagus, is tied. One ligature encloses both the vessels and the esophagus, and second and third ligatures include the vessel and esophagus separately higher up. The vessels and esophagus are cut between ligatures. Lifting the stomach to the right exposes vascular connections to the posterior wall, which can be tied, using a single distal tie and then cut. Finally, the pylorus is tied twice and cut between the ligatures, releasing the stomach, which can now be checked. At this stage the animal can be heparinized by means of an injection via the inferior vena cava. The right renal pedicle (containing artery, vein, ureter) is cleared with blunt dissection and a ligature passed behind the artery and vein with curved forceps. Double ligatures allow the vessels to be cut and the kidney removed.

By careful dissection, the aorta is exposed at this level to clear it from the inferior vena cava between the left renal artery and superior mesenteric artery. A ligature passed behind the aorta at this level can now be tied. Three loose ligatures are passed around the portal vein as it leaves the pancreas for the liver. The uppermost ligatures should include all structures of the portal tract (vein, hepatic artery, bile duct), whereas the other two include only the vein. Cannulation is delayed until the aorta has been cleared along its length, preserving the celiac and mesenteric branches. This step entails passing ligatures around and tying particularly the lumbar arteries. The aorta is free from the inferior vena cava from the level of the diaphragm to the ligature below the left renal artery. Loose ligatures are positioned around the aorta just below the diaphragm, avoiding the origin of the celiac artery.

The portal vein can be cannulated in a retrograde manner by tying the uppermost ligatures first and making an incision in the anterior wall of the vein. The cannula (made from PE-140 to PE-100 tubing) is filled with heparinized perfusion medium before insertion. When flow through a portal cannula is ensured, aortic cannulation is performed. The rat is turned around with the head toward the operator, and a midline incision is made through the thorax, cutting the diaphragm through the edge. The anoxic phase begins from the moment of entering, and speed of surgical procedure is essential (it comes with practice). The thoracic walls are spread apart by means of appropriate retractors, and the thoracic aorta is separated from behind the esophagus. The cannula is inserted and advanced until its tip just passes the diaphragm. The abdominal aortic ligature is tightened, and with the cannula in place the flow should commence. The final step is to complete the isolation of the pancreatic circulation by tying the ligature, which has already been prepared, around the lower inferior vena cava.

The perfusing pancreas is now transported to the organ chamber. The inferior vena cava is cut distal to the last tied ligature, and removal of the cannulated pancreas should be possible by grasping the two cannulas and the loop of duodenum to lift the pancreas clear of the rat. The organ is oriented on the platform in the perfusion chamber by means of identifying ligatures that were placed during the preparation; successful uniform perfusion is obtained if this step is carefully undertaken. There should be a flow of 2 ml/min with a perfusion pressure of about 40 mm Hg. It may be wise to reject preparations if pressures above 80 mm Hg are obtained, as it usually results in further deterioration of the perfused pancreatic preparation. The entire surgical procedure takes roughly 60 to 75 min, assuming familiarity with surgical techniques (49).

With the method of Grodsky et al. (89), perfusion of the pancreas is performed together with perfusion of the stomach, spleen, and duodenum as a unit, which is removed from the rat through a vertical abdominal incision and transferred to the prewarmed chamber. The celiac axis is cannulated for the inflow and the portal vein for the outflow. A peristaltic pump supplies the perfusion medium to the celiac axis at a pressure of 40 to 100 mm Hg, and the flow is adjusted to 10 ml/min. The principal disadvantage of Grodsky's procedure is that it involves perfusion of additional tissues so that ascribing a particular biochemical function to the pancreas would be more difficult when perfusion is used. The principal advantage is that the surgical procedure is much simpler. Procedures for the cannulation and perfusion of feline and canine pancreas are available. Figure 12 shows the constant perfusion system of the blood-perfused canine pancreas (103).

Perfusion Media

Grodsky et al. (89) used whole rat blood mixed with an artificial medium as a perfusate, but they, as well as others who utilized whole blood, encountered hemolysis of the red blood cells, which resulted in complications of the perfusion. Hence the use of artificial media has become more popular for perfusion of the pancreas. The medium containing 4% dextran in Krebs-Henseleit medium prepared and gassed with O_2/CO_2 (95:5) is satisfactory. This medium is the standard one mentioned in the subsequent work of Grodsky as well as by many other investigators. Alternatively, 4% human serum albumin or BSA can be used instead of dextran with no apparent difference in insulin production, medium flow, and rate of circulation of perfusion (49). The pH is adjusted to 7.4, and the addition of sodium bicarbonate and adequate bubbling with the O_2/CO_2 ensures maintaining the appropriate pH. If the pH seems to fluctuate during the experiment, addition of sodium bicarbonate solution to the perfusate helps stabilize its pH.

Khayambashi and Lyman (113) used a medium containing fresh rat plasma diluted 1:1 with Ringer's saline or 0.9% saline with satisfactory results. Costiner et al. (49) used diluted heparinized rat blood as perfusate to support satisfactory pancreatic function. Advantages of perfusing pancreas with whole blood have been pointed out (91), and the advantage of the larger animal size has been noted by several investigators when using autologous blood (32,91,103,117).

Viability Criteria

Several parameters of physiological and biochemical function were reported by Grodsky et al. (89). Histological examinations at the end of the perfusion period indicated that well-preserved granules diminished in number roughly in proportion to the measured release of insulin into the medium (89). Oxygen consumption by the perfused pancreas can be used as a comparatively rough indicator of viability. However, in the preparation of Grodsky et al. (89), because other tissues are involved in the perfusion circulation, oxygen consumption may not be an exclusive indicator of viability of the perfused pancreas. In the preparation of Sussman and Vaughn (242), because less peripheral tissue is involved, oxygen consumption might represent a better viability criterion. In any case, production of insulin by the preparation, consumption of glucose, and the analysis of exocrine secretion collected through the duodenal cannula can be used as adequate criteria for the viability of the perfused pancreas. The pH of the circulating perfusate can be monitored and adjusted if necessary by regulating the O_2/CO_2 when oxygenating the perfusate. Second, appropriate amounts of sodium bicarbonate solution can be added to adjust the pH of the circulating perfusate.

Amylase formation has been shown to be linear for 40 min in the preparation used by Khayambashi and Lyman (113), and an amylase assay might be a reasonable parameter for viability. However, they observed that the rate of amylase production fell beyond 40 min despite the linearity of the perfusion flow rate. This decrease may be a reflection of the discharge of existing enzymes rather than the inability for the isolated perfused organ to synthesize enzymes. In the work of Khayambashi and Lyman (113), the composition of the perfusion medium was demonstrated to have a definite effect on the secretion of the amylase type of enzymes by the pancreas. Hence such a criterion may have to be established in conjunction with other parameters of perfused preparation.

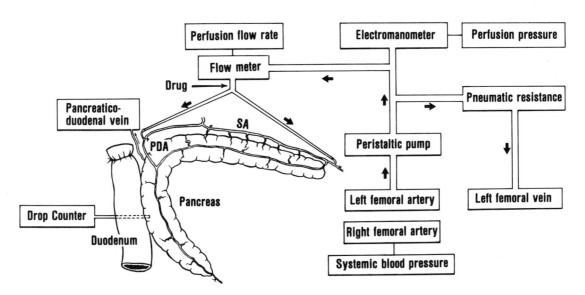

FIG. 12. Constant perfusion system of the blood-perfused canine pancreas preparation. Arterial cannulas are inserted into the pancreaticoduodenal (*PDA*) and splenic (*SA*) arteries. (From ref. 103, with permission.)

Sampling of the tissue to demonstrate effects that may be reflected in the medium or related to a particular treatment of perfusion is clearly important in the assessment of the perfused organ. In this connection, it may be pointed out that the dendritic form of the rat pancreas lends itself to sampling when a single arm of the pancreas is tied off and perfusion is continued in the remaining tissue. However, if a portion of the organ is sampled, the biochemical study done with the same perfused organ may be compromised, especially with respect to later time points, as all of the organ would not be present at later times, especially if such sampling is carried out repeatedly.

Applications

The perfused pancreas has not been used in toxicological investigations. The development of sensitive radioimmunoassays for insulin and glucagon in biological fluids has enabled quantitative measurement of their secretion and has led to the use of pancreas perfusion techniques in such studies (233). Clearly, the perfused pancreas can be used to evaluate the effect of drugs and drug interactions that affect pancreatic function. Drugs not having exclusive action on the pancreas may mutually interact within the body to produce an action on pancreatic function (193). Peterson and Fujimoto (193) have demonstrated increased pancreatic secretory activity after exposure to such agents as ethanol and CCl_4. The mechanism of such enhanced pancreatic secretory activity is not understood. Use of a perfused pancreatic preparation obtained from control and treated animals may be useful in the elucidation of the underlying mechanisms.

Examples of the use of isolated perfused pancreas for a number of pharmacological (88,103,191), physiological (64,188), and toxicological (32,117) studies are available. The studies of Kimura et al. (117) provide one example of the utility of the perfused pancreas in mechanistic toxicological investigations. Although steroid administration has long been suspected of causing acute pancreatitis, clinical and experimental data have failed to firmly establish the association or to uncover a pathogenic mechanism. The acute effects of large doses of methylprednisolone on the pancreas were evaluated utilizing an isolated, perfused, canine pancreas (117). Using a dose of 200 mg of methylprednisolone, there were no significant differences between the control and steroid-treated preparations over a 4-hr perfusion period. When the dose of methylprednisolone was increased to 400 mg, again there were no significant differences in gross appearance, weight gain, or serum amylase during a 3-hr perfusion period. However, pancreatic secretion was initially depressed in the steroid-treated preparations. Following a maximal secretory stimulus (secretin), secretion markedly increased during the fourth hour of perfusion but again was significantly less in the steroid-treated glands. Viscosity of pancreatic secretions was significantly increased in the steroid-treated glands. These studies suggest a mild inhibitory effect of steroids on pancreatic secretion, which might be mediated through an increase in viscosity. Another example is provided by the studies of Broe and Cameron (32).

Controlled clinical trials have documented the development of acute pancreatitis in 5% of patients receiving aza-thioprine for Crohn's disease, by far the highest incidence of drug-induced pancreatitis recorded to date. The isolated, perfused canine pancreas was used to evaluate the effects of azathioprine on the pancreas. No significant changes in gross appearance, weight, or serum amylase were observed in azathioprine-treated glands compared to controls. Azathioprine administration, however, resulted in a twofold increase in secretory volume and bicarbonate output as well as a profound depression of trypsin output compared to controls. These preliminary studies demonstrate that azathioprine has a marked effect on pancreatic function in this model (32).

ACKNOWLEDGMENTS

The author is the recipient of the 1988 Burroughs Wellcome Toxicology Scholar Award.

This effort was supported in part by U.S. Public Health Service grant (HL-20622) from the National Heart, Lung and Blood Institute and by U.S. Environmental Protection Agency grant R-811072. The excellent assistance of Margaret Nicholas, Pamela Banks, Gloria Griffis, and Shirley Gray in the preparation of this manuscript is greatly appreciated. The fine contributions of my colleagues included in the work referenced in this manuscript are also appreciated.

REFERENCES

1. Abraham, R., Dawson, W., Grasso, P., and Goldberg, L. (1968): Lysosomal changes associated with hyperoxia in the isolated perfused rat liver. *Exp. Mol. Pathol.*, 8:370–387.
2. Agarwal, A. K., and Mehendale, H. M. (1986): Effect of chlordecone on carbon tetrachloride induced increase in calcium uptake in isolated perfused rat liver. *Toxicol. Appl. Pharmacol.*, 83:342–348.
3. Andjus, R. K., Suhara, K., and Stoviter, H. A. (1967): An isolated, perfused rat brain preparation, its spontaneous and stimulated activity. *J. Appl. Physiol.*, 22:1033–1039.
4. Andrews, W. H. H., Hecker, R., and Maegraith, B. G. (1956): The action of adrenaline, noradrenaline, acetylcholine and histamine on the perfused liver of the monkey, cat and rabbit. *J. Physiol. (Lond.)*, 132:509–521.
5. Angevine, L. S., and Mehendale, H. M. (1980): Chlorphentermine uptake by isolated perfused rabbit lung. *Toxicol. Appl. Pharmacol.*, 52:336–346.
6. Angevine, L. S., and Mehendale, H. M. (1980): Effect of chlorphentermine on the pulmonary disposition of 5-hydroxytryptamine in the isolated perfused rat lung. *Am. Rev. Respir. Dis.*, 122:891–898.
7. Angevine, L. S., and Mehendale, H. M. (1982): Effect of chlorphentermine treatment on 5-hydroxytryptamine disposition in the isolated perfused rat lung. *Fundam. Appl. Toxicol.*, 2:306–312.
8. Aronson, C. E. (1976): Effects of thyroxine pretreatment and calcium on the isolated, perfused rat heart. *Arch. Int. Pharmacodyn.*, 222:351–360.
9. Aronson, C. E., and Serlick, E. R. (1976): Effects of prolonged perfusion time on the isolated perfused rat heart. *Toxicol. Appl. Pharmacol.*, 38:479–488.
10. Aronson, C. E., and Serlick, E. R. (1977): Effects of chlorpromazine on the isolated rat heart. *Toxicol. Appl. Pharmacol.*, 39:157–176.
11. Auda, S. P., Kesner, L., Butt, K., and Dountz, S. L. (1975): Continuous single pass perfusion of the isolated kidney. *Trans. Am. Soc. Artif. Intern. Organs*, 21:84–88.
12. Autian, J. (1975): In vitro toxicity testing gains strength. *Forum Advancement Toxicol.*, 8:1–2 (newsletter).
13. Aviado, D. M. (1975): Drug action, reaction, and interaction. II. Teratogenic cardiopathies. *J. Clin. Pharmacol.*, 15:641–655.

14. Baglioni, D. E. (1910): Stoffwecheseluntershugangen and Uberlebenden organen. *Hand. Biol. Arb. Meth.,* 3:364.
15. Bahlmann, J., Giebisch, G., Ochwady, B., and Schoeppe, W. (1967): Micropuncture study of isolated perfused rat kidney. *Am. J. Physiol.,* 221:77–82.
16. Bakhle, T. S., Reynard, A. M., and Vane, J. R. (1969): Metabolism of the angiotensins in isolated perfused tissues. *Nature,* 222:956–958.
17. Barrett, J. P., Ingenito, A. J., and Procita, L. (1969): A brain perfusion technique adapted for the study of drugs which may affect the peripheral circulation through a central action. *J. Pharmacol. Exp. Ther.,* 170:199–209.
18. Bauman, A. W., Clarkson, T. W., and Miles, E. M. (1963): Functional evaluation of isolated perfused rat kidney. *J. Appl. Physiol.,* 18:1239–1246.
19. Belinsky, S. A., Popp, J. A., Kauffman, F. C., and Thurman, R. G. (1984): Trypan blue uptake as a new method to investigate hepatotoxicity in periportal and pericentral regions of the liver lobule: studies with allyl alcohol in the perfused liver. *J. Pharmacol. Exp. Ther.,* 230:755–760.
20. Berggren, M., Dawson, J., and Moldéus, P. (1984): Glutathione biosynthesis in the isolated perfused rat lung: utilization of extracellular glutathione. *FEBS Lett.,* 176:189–192.
21. Deleted.
22. Bernstein, E. F. (1971): Evaluation of mechanical systems used in perfusion. In: *Perfusion Techniques,* edited by E. Diszfalusy, pp. 44–73. Karolinska Institute, Stockholm.
23. Bingham, E., Warshawsky, D., and Niemeier, R. W. (1978): Metabolism of benzo(*a*)pyrene in the isolated perfused rabbit lung following N-dodecane inhalation. In: *Carcinogenesis: Mechanisms of Tumor Production and Carcinogenesis,* edited by T. J. Slaga, A. Sivak, and R. K. Boutwell, Vol. 2, pp. 509–516. Raven Press, New York.
24. Bleehan, N. M., and Fisher, R. B. (1954): The action of insulin on the isolated rat heart. *J. Physiol. (Lond.),* 123:260–276.
25. Block, E. R., and Cannon, J. K. (1978): Effect of oxygen exposure on lung clearance of amines. *Lung,* 155:287–295.
26. Bock, K. W., Forhling, W., and Scholte, W. (1972): Activity and stability of microsomal mixed function oxidase and NAD glycohydrolase in isolated perfused rat liver. *Naunyn Schmiedebergs Arch. Pharmacol.,* 273:193–203.
27. Bond, J. A., and Mauderly, J. L. (1984): Metabolism and macromolecular covalent binding of [^{14}C]-1-nitropyrene in isolated perfused and ventilated rat lungs. *Cancer Res.,* 44:3924–3929.
28. Boyd, C. A. R., Parsons, D. S., and Thomas, A. V. (1968): The presence of K$^+$ dependent phosphatase in intestinal epithelial cell brush borders isolated by a new method. *Biochim. Biophys. Acta,* 150:723–726.
29. Bowman, R. H., and Maack, T. (1972): Glucose transport by the isolated rat kidney. *Am. J. Physiol.,* 222:1499–1504.
30. Brauer, R. W., Pessotti, R. L., and Pizzolato, P. (1951): Isolated rat liver preparation: bile production and other basic properties. *Proc. Soc. Exp. Biol. Med.,* 78:174–185.
31. Brodie, T. G. (1903): The perfusion of surviving organs. *J. Physiol. (Lond.),* 29:266–275.
32. Broe, P. J., and Cameron, J. L. (1983): Azathioprine and acute pancreatitis: studies with an isolated perfused canine pancreas. *J. Surg. Res.,* 34:159–163.
33. Brull, L., and Louis-Bar, D. (1957): Toxicity of artificially circulated heparinized blood on the kidney. *Arch. Int. Physiol. Biochem.,* 65:470–476.
34. Bullock, G., Eakins, M. N., Sawyer, B. C., and Slater, T. F. (1974): Studies on bile secretion with the aid of the isolated perfused rat liver. I. Inhibitory action of sporidesmin and icterogenin. *Proc. R. Soc. Lond.,* 186:333–356.
35. Burks, T. F. (1974): Vascularly perfused isolated perfused intestine. In: *Fourth International Symposium on Gastrointestinal Motility.* Mitchell Press, Vancouver.
36. Burr, I. M., Stauffacher, W., Balant, L., Renold, A. E., and Grodsky, G. (1969): Dynamic aspects of proinsulin release from perfused rat pancreas. *Lancet,* 2:882–883.
37. Camus, Ph., and Mehendale, H. M. (1986): Pulmonary sequestration of amiodarone and desethylamiodarone. *J. Pharmacol. Exp. Ther.,* 237:867–873.
38. Cardieux, A., Masse, S., and Sirois, P. (1983): Effect of asbestos in the metabolism of vasoactive substances in isolated perfused guinea pig lungs. *Environ. Health Perspect.,* 51:287–291.
39. Case, R. M., Harper, A. A., and Scratcherd, T. (1968): Water and electrolyte secretion by the perfused cat pancreas. *J. Physiol. (Lond.),* 196:133–149.
40. Cesarone, C. F., Fugassa, E., Gallo, G., Voci, A., and Orunesu, M. (1984): Collagenase perfusion rat liver induces DNA damage and DNA repair in hepatocytes. *Mutat. Res.,* 141:113–116.
41. Chapman, N. D., Saint George, S., and Ishida, T. (1960): Small volume perfusion system of the isolated rat liver. *J. Appl. Physiol.,* 15:128–136.
42. Charles, J. M., Abou-Donia, M. B., and Menzel, D. B. (1978): Absorption of paraquat and diquat from the airways of the perfused rat lung. *Toxicology,* 9:59–67.
43. Chiong, M. A., Berenzy, G. M., and Winton, T. L. (1978): Metabolism of the isolated perfused rabbit heart. I. Responses to anoxia and reoxygenation. II. Energy stores. *Can. J. Physiol. Pharmacol.,* 56:844–856.
44. Chuté, A. L., and Smyth, D. H. (1939): Metabolism of the isolated perfused cat's brain. *Q. J. Exp. Physiol.,* 29:379–394.
45. Cohrs, P., Jaffe, R., and Meesen, H. (1958): *Pathologie der Laboratoriumstiere,* Vol. 1. Springer-Verlag, Berlin.
46. Cojocel, C., Docius, N., Maita, K., Smith, J. H., and Hook, J. B. (1984): Renal ultrastructural and biochemical injuries induced by aminoglycosides. *Environ. Health Perspect.,* 57:293–299.
47. Cook, D. R., Howell, R. E., and Gillis, C. N. (1982): Xanthine oxidase-induced lung injury inhibits removal of 5-hydroxytryptamine from the pulmonary circulation. *Anesth. Analg.,* 61:666–670.
48. Coore, H. G., and Randle, P. J. (1964): Regulation of insulin secretion studied with pieces of rabbit pancreas incubated in vitro. *Biochem. J.,* 93:66–78.
49. Costiner, E., Ghiea, D., Simionescu, L., and Oprescu, M. (1975): Modified technique of perfusion of isolated rat pancreas tested by insulin release after glucose administration. *Endocrinol. Exp.,* 9:197–204.
50. Dalbey, W., and Bingham, E. (1978): Metabolism of trichloroethylene by the isolated perfused lung. *Toxicol. Appl. Pharmacol.,* 43:267–277.
51. Davis, M. E., and Mehendale, H. M. (1979): Absence of metabolism of morphine during accumulation by isolated perfused rabbit lung. *Drug Metab. Dispos.,* 7:425–428.
52. Dawson, J. R., Vapakangas, K., Jernstrom, B., and Moldeus, P. (1984): Glutathione conjugation by isolated lung cells and isolated perfused lung: effect of external glutathione. *Eur. J. Biochem.,* 138:439–443.
53. Deglin, S. M., Deglin, J. M., and Chung, E. K. (1977): Drug-induced cardiovascular diseases. *Drugs,* 14:29–40.
54. DeMello, G., and Maack, T. (1976): Nephron function of the isolated perfused rat kidney. *Am. J. Physiol.,* 231:1699–1707.
55. De Wildt, D. J., and Speizers, G. J. A. (1984): Influence of dietary rapeseed oil and erucic acid upon myocardial performance and hemodynamics in the rat. *Toxicol. Appl. Pharmacol.,* 74:99–108.
56. De Wildt, D. J., De Jong, Y., Hillen, F. C., Steerenberg, P. A., and Van Hoesel, Q. G. C. M. (1985): Cardiovascular effects of doxorubicin-induced toxicity in the intact Lou/M Wsl rat and isolated heart preparations. *J. Pharmacol Exp. Ther.,* 235:234–240.
57. Diczfalusy, E. (1971): *Perfusion Techniques.* Karolinska Institute, Stockholm.
58. Dirks, V. B., Seibert, A., Sperling, G., and Krieglstein, J. (1984): Comparison of the effects of piracetam and methohexital on brain energy metabolism. *Azneimittelforschung,* 34:258–266.
59. Doerr, W., and Becker, V. (1958): Bauchspeicheldruse (pancreas). In: *Pathologie der Laboratariumstierre,* Vol. 1, edited by P. Cohrs, R. Jaffe, and Hm Messen, p. 130. Springer-Verlag, Berlin.
60. Dovrak, K. J., Braun, W. E., Magnusson, M. O., Stowe, N. T., and Banowsky, L. H. W. (1976): Effect of high methylprednisolone on the isolated perfused canine kidney. *Transplantation,* 21:149–157.
61. Dubois, R. S., Vaughn, G. D., and Roy, C. C. (1968): Isolated rat small intestine with intact circulation. In: *Organ Perfusion and Perservation,* edited by J. C. Norman. pp. 863–868. Appleton Century Crofts, New York.
62. Dunbar, J. R., Delucia, A. J., and Bryant, L. R. (1984): Glutathione

status of isolated rabbit lungs: effects on nitrofurantoin and paraquat perfusion with normoxic and hyperoxic ventilation. *Biochem. Pharmacol.*, 33:1343–1348.

63. Eisman, B., Knipe, P., McColl, H., and Orloff, M. J. (1961): Isolated liver perfusion for reducing blood ammonia. *Arch. Surg.*, 83:356–363.

64. Elisha, E. E., Hutson, D., and Seratcherd, T. (1984): The direct inhibition of pancreatic electrolyte secretion by noradrenaline in the isolated perfused cat pancreas. *J. Physiol. (Lond.)*, 351:77–85.

65. Embden, G., and Glaüssner, K. (1902): Uber den ortder atherschwefelsaurebildung im tierkorpen. *Hoffmlisters Beituug 2 Chem. Phys. Band.*, 1:310–327.

66. Enser, M. B., Kunz, F., Borenstanjn, J., Opie, L. H., and Robinson, D. S. (1967): Metabolism of biglyceride fatty acids by perfused rat heart. *Biochem. J.*, 104:306–317.

67. Evans, G. H., Wilkinson, G. R., and Shand, D. G. (1973): The disposition of propranolol. IV. A dominant role of tissue uptake in the dose dependent extraction of propranolol by the perfused rat liver. *J. Pharmacol. Exp. Ther.*, 186:447–456.

68. Ferrari, R., Ceconi, C., Curello, S., Guarnieri, C., Caderara, C. M., Albertini, A., and Visioli, O. (1985): Oxygen-mediated myocardial damage during ischemia and reperfusion: role of the cellular defenses against oxygen toxicity. *J. Mol. Cell Cardiol.*, 17:937–945.

69. Fink, V. C., Hölzl, J., Riegger, H., and Kriegelstein, J. (1984): Effects of valtrate on the EEG of the isolated perfused rat brain. *Azneimittelforschung*, 34:170–174.

70. Fitzpatrick, J. H., Jr., and Gilboe, D. D. (1982): Effects of nitrous oxide on the cerebrovascular tone, oxygen metabolism, and electroencephalogram of the isolated perfused canine brain. *Anesthesiology*, 57:480–484.

71. Fogel, W. A., Bieganski, T., Schayer, R. W., and Maslinski, C. (1981): Involvement of diamine oxidase in catabolism of ^{14}C-putrescine in mice in vivo with special reference to the formation of γ-aminobutyric acid. *Agents Actions*, 11:679–684.

72. Fonteles, M. C., Pillion, D. J., Jeske, A. H., and Leibach, F. H. (1976): Extraction of glutathione by the isolated perfused rabbit kidney. *J. Surg. Res.*, 21:169–174.

73. Forth, W. (1968): Eisen und Kobalt-Resorption am perfundierten Dendarmasegment. In: *3 Konfder Gesellschaft fur Biologische Chemie*, edited by W. Staib and R. Scholz, pp. 242–254. Springer-Verlag, Berlin.

74. Fox, R. B. (1984): Prevention of granulocyte-mediated oxidant injury in rats by a hydroxyl radical scavenger, dimethylthiourea. *J. Clin. Invest.*, 74:1456–1464.

75. Franke, H., and Weiss, C. (1976): The O_2 supply of the isolated cell-free perfused rat kidney. *Adv. Exp. Med. Biol.*, 75:425–432.

76. Gad, S. C., Leslie, S. W., and Acosta, D. (1979): Inhibitory actions of butylated hydroxytoluene on isolated ileal, atrial and perfused heart preparations. *Toxicol. Appl. Pharmacol.*, 49:45–52.

77. Gamble, W. J., Conn, P. A., Edalji-Kumer, A., Pleuge, R., and Monroe, R. G. (1970): Myocardial oxygen consumption of blood-perfused, isolated supported rat heart. *Am. J. Physiol.*, 219:604–612.

78. Gareis, M., Hashem, A., Bauer, J., and Gedek, B. (1986): Identification of glucuronide metabolites of T-2 toxin and diacetoxyscirpinol in the bile of isolated perfused rat liver. *Toxicol. Appl. Pharmacol.*, 84:168–172.

79. Geiger, A. (1958): Correlation of brain metabolism and function by the use of a brain perfusion in situ. *Physiol. Rev.*, 38:1–20.

80. Geiger, A., and Magnes, J. (1947): The isolation of the cerebral circulation and the perfusion of the brain in the living cat. *Am. J. Physiol.*, 149:517–537.

81. Gerber, G. B., and Remy-Defraigne, J. (1966): DNA metabolism in perfused organs. II. Incorporation in DNA and catabolism of thymidine at different levels of substrate by normal and x-irradiated liver and intestine. *Arch. Int. Physiol. Biochem.*, 74:785–794.

82. Gilboe, D. D., Betz, A. L., and Langebartel, D. A. (1973): A guide for the isolation of the canine brain. *J. Appl. Physiol.*, 34:534–537.

83. Gillis, C. N., and Iwasawa, Y. (1972): Technique for measurement of norepinephrine and 5-hydroxytryptamine uptake by rabbit lung. *J. Appl. Physiol.*, 33:404–408.

84. Gillis, C. N., and Roth, J. A. (1976): Pulmonary disposition of circulating vasoactive hormones. *Biochem. Pharmacol.*, 25:2547–2553.

85. Gollan, F., and McDermott, J. (1979): Effect of skeletal muscle relaxant dantrolene sodium on the isolated, perfused heart. *Proc. Soc. Exp. Biol. Med.*, 160:42–45.

86. Gonmori, K., Prasada Rao, K. S., and Mehendale, H. M. (1986): Pulmonary synthesis of 5-hydroxytryptamine in isolated perfused rabbit and rat lung preparations. *Exp. Lung Res.*, 11:295–306.

87. Goodman, M. N., Parrilla, R., and Toews, C. J. (1973): Influence of fluorocarbon emulsions on hepatic metabolism in perfused rat liver. *Am. J. Physiol.*, 225:1384–1388.

88. Goto, Y., Seino, Y., Note, S., and Imura, H. (1980): The dual effect of alloxan modulated by 3-O-methylglucose or somatostatin on insulin secretion in the isolated perfused rat pancreas. *Horm. Metab. Res.*, 12:140–143.

89. Grodsky, G. M., Batts, A. A., Bennett, L. L., Veella, C., McWilliams, N. B., and Smith, D. F. (1963): Effects of carbohydrates on secretion of insulin from isolated rat pancreas. *Am. J. Physiol.*, 205:638–644.

90. Hale, P. W., Jr., and Poklis, A. (1984): Thioridazine-5-sulfoxide cardiotoxicity in the isolated, perfused rat heart. *Toxicol. Lett.*, 21:1–8.

91. Hashimoto, K., Satoh, S., and Takeuchi, O. (1971): Effect of dopamine on pancreatic secretion in the dog. *Br. J. Pharmacol.*, 43:739–746.

92. Hauge, A. (1968): Conditions governing the pressor response to ventilation hypoxia in isolated perfused rat lungs. *Acta Physiol. Scand.*, 72:33–44.

93. Heaton, J. D., McAnalley, B. H., Gardiner, T. H., and Johnson, A. R. (1982): Uptake and release of ^{14}C-morphine by pulmonary endothelium and cultured pulmonary endothelial cells. *Gen. Pharmacol.*, 13:105–110.

94. Hein, H., Krieglstein, J., and Stock, R. (1975): The effects of increased glucose supply and thiopental anesthesia on energy metabolism of the isolated perfused rat brain. *Naunyn Schmiedebergs Arch. Pharmacol.*, 289:399–407.

95. Hemingway, A. (1931): Some observations on the perfusion of the isolated kidney by a pump. *J. Physiol. (Lond.)*, 71:201–213.

96. Hems, R., Ross, B. D., Berry, M. N., and Krebs, H. A. (1966): Gluconeogenesis in the perfused rat liver. *Biochem. J.*, 101:284–292.

97. Herman-Taylor, J. (1973): The isolated perfused canine pancreas. In: *Isolated Organ Perfusion*, edited by H. D. Ritchie and J. D. Hardcastle, pp. 171–190. University Park Press, Baltimore.

98. Hilliker, K. S., Imlay, M., and Roth, R. A. (1984): Effects of monocrotaline treatment on norepinephrine removal by isolated, perfused rat lungs. *Biochem. Pharmacol.*, 33:2692–2695.

99. Hilliker, K. S., and Roth, R. A. (1985): Injury to the isolated, perfused lung by exposure in vitro to monocrotaline pyrrole. *Exp. Lung Res.*, 8:201–212.

100. Hirning, L. D., Porreca, F., and Burks, T. F. (1985): μ But not k, opioid agonists induce contractions of the canine small intestine ex vivo. *Eur. J. Pharmacol.*, 109:49–54.

101. Itakura, N., Fisher, A. B., and Thurman, R. G. (1977): Cytochrome P450-linked p-nitroanisole O-demethylation in the perfused lung. *J. Appl. Physiol.*, 43:238–245.

102. Iwamoto, K., Watanabe, J., Araki, K., Satoh, M., and Deguchi, N. (1985): Reduced hepatic clearance of propranolol induced by chronic carbon tetrachloride treatment in rats. *J. Pharmacol. Exp. Ther.*, 234:470–475.

103. Iwatsuki, K., Ikeda, K., and Chiba, S. (1982): Effects of nitroprusside on pancreatic juice secretion in the blood perfused canine pancreas. *Eur. J. Pharmacol.*, 79:53–60.

104. Jacobs, F. A. (1968): Continuous radioactivity monitoring of perfusion in the small intestine of the intact animal. *Adv. Tracer Methodol.*, 4:255–272.

105. Jaffe, D. R., Hassal, C. D., Gandolfi, A. J., and Brendel, K. (1985): Production of DNA single strand breaks in rabbit renal tissue after exposure to 1,2-dichlorovinylcysteine. *Toxicology*, 35:25–33.

106. Johannesen, J., Lie, M., and Kiil, F. (1977): Renal energy metabolism and sodium reabsorption after 2,4-nitrophenol administration. *Am. J. Physiol.*, 233:207–217.

107. Joshi, U. M., Dumas, M., and Mehendale, H. M. (1986): Glutathione turnover in perfused rabbit lung. *Biochem. Pharmacol.* (in press).

108. Joshi, U. M., Prasada Rao, K. S., and Mehendale, H. M. (1987):

Glutathione status in constituted physiological fluid containing albumin. *Intern. J. Biochem.*, 19:1129–1135.

109. Junod, A. F. (1972): Accumulation of ^{14}C-imipramine in isolated perfused rat lungs. *J. Pharmacol. Exp. Ther.*, 183:182–187.

110. Kapfhammer, J. (1927): Die leber im Stoffwechzel. In: *Handbuch der Biochemie*, edited by K. Oppenheimer, 2nd ed., Vol. 9, pp. 98–150. Jena. G. Fischer.

111. Karmazyn, M., and Moffat, M. P. (1985): Toxic properties of arachidonic acid in normal, ischemic and reperfused hearts: indirect evidence for free radical involvement. *Prostaglandins Leukotrienes Med.*, 17:251–264.

112. Kavin, H., Levin, N. W., and Stanley, M. M. (1967): Isolated perfused rat small bowel-technique: studies of viability, glucose absorption. *J. Appl. Physiol.*, 22:604–611.

113. Khayambashi, H., and Lyman, R. L. (1969): Secretion of rat pancreas perfused with plasma from rats fed soybean trypsin inhibitor. *Am. J. Physiol.*, 217:646–651.

114. Kilbinger, H., and Krieglstein, J. (1974): Applicability of the isolated perfused rat brain for studying central cholinergic mechanisms. *Naunyn Schmiedebergs. Arch. Pharmacol.*, 285:407–411.

115. Kim, D.-H., and Akera, T. (1984): Effects of myocardial hypoxia on digitalis-induced toxicity in the isolated heart of guinea pigs and cats. *Eur. J. Pharmacol.*, 104:303–312.

116. Kim, J. H., and Miller, K. L. (1969): The functional significance of changes in activity of the enzymes, tryptophan pyrrolase and tyrosine transaminase after induction in intact rats and isolated perfused rat liver. *J. Biol. Chem.*, 244:1410–1416.

117. Kimura, T., Zuidema, G. D., and Cameron, J. L. (1979): Steroid administration and acute pancreatitis studies with an isolated, perfused canine pancreas. *Surgery*, 85:520–524.

118. Knowlton, F. P., and Starling, E. H. (1912): The influence of variations in temperature and blood pressure on the performance of the isolated mammalian heart. *J. Physiol. (Lond.)*, 44:206–219.

119. Kopp, S. J., Daar, A. A., Prentice, R. C., Tow, J. P., and Feliksik, J. M. (1986): ^{31}P-NMR studies of the intact perfused rat heart: a novel analytical approach for determining functional-metabolic correlates, temporal relationships, and intracellular actions of cardiotoxic chemicals nondestructively in an intact organ model. *Toxicol. Appl. Pharmacol.*, 82:200–210.

120. Koschier, F. J., Gigliotti, P. J., and Hong, S. K. (1980): The effect of bis(p-chlorophenyl) acetic acid on the renal function on the rat. *J. Environ. Pathol. Toxicol.*, 4:209–217.

121. Koster, J. F., Slee, R. G., Essed, C. E., and Stam, H. (1985): Studies on canine hydroperoxide-induced lipid peroxidation in the isolated perfused rat heart. *J. Mol. Cell. Cardiol.*, 17:701–708.

122. Kraupp, O., Adler-Kastner, L., Niessner, H., and Plank, B. (1967): The effects of starvation and acute and chronic alloxan diabetes on myocardial substrate levels and on liver glycogen in the rat in vivo. *Eur. J. Biochem.*, 2:197–214.

123. Krieglstein, G., Krieglstein, J., and Stock, R. (1972): Suitability of the perfused rat brain for studying effects on cerebral metabolism. *Naunyn Schmiedebergs. Arch. Pharmacol.*, 275:124–134.

124. Krieglstein, J., and Stock, R. (1973): Comparative study of the effects of chloral hydrate and trichloroethanol on cerebral metabolism. *Naunyn Schmiedebergs. Arch. Pharmacol.*, 277:323–332.

125. Kulatilake, A. E. (1967): Isolated perfusion of canine and human kidneys. *Br. J. Surg.*, 54:877–882.

126. Kvetina, J., and Guaitani, A. (1969): A versatile method for the in vitro perfusion of isolated organs of rats and mice with particular reference to liver. *Pharmacology*, 2:65–81.

127. Lacy, P. E., and Kostianowsky, M. (1967): Method for isolation of intact islets of Langerhans from the rat pancreas. *Diabetes*, 16:35–39.

128. Lafranconi, W. M., Ferlan, I., Russell, F. E., and Huxtable, R. J. (1984): The action of equinatoxin, a peptide from the venom of the sea anemone, Actinia equinia, on the isolated lung. *Toxicology*, 22:347–352.

129. Lafranconi, W. M., and Huxtable, R. J. (1984): Hepatic metabolism and pulmonary toxicity of monocrotaline using isolated perfused liver and lung. *Biochem. Pharmacol.*, 33:2479–2484.

130. Langendorff, O. (1895): Untersuchungen am Uberleberden Saügertierzen. *Pflugers Arch. Ges. Physiol.*, 61:291–332.

131. Law, F. C. P. (1978): Metabolism and disposition of 4′-tetrahydro-

cannabinol by the isolated perfused rabbit lung. *Drug Metab. Dispos.*, 6:154–163.

132. Law, F. C. P., Eling, T. E., Bend, J. R., and Fouts, J. R. (1974): Metabolism of xenobiotics by the isolated perfused lung. *Drug Metab. Dispos.*, 2:433–442.

133. Leary, W. P. P., and Ledingham, J. G. (1969): Removal of angiotensin by isolated perfused organs of the rat (1969). *Nature*, 222:959–960.

134. Lemaster, J. J., Ji, S., Stemkowski, C. J., and Thurman, R. G. (1983): Hypoxic hepatocellular injury. *Pharmacol. Biochem. Behav.*, 18:455–459.

135. Levey, S., and Gast, R. (1966): Isolated perfused rat lung preparation. *J. Appl. Physiol.*, 21:313–316.

136. Levin, N. W., Ryan, W. G., Hayashi, J., and Kark, R. M. (1965): Studies on the isolated perfused rabbit kidney. *S. Afr. J. Med. Sci.*, 30:78–79.

137. Light, A., and Simpson, M. S. (1966): Studies on the biosynthesis of insulin. I. The paper chromatographic isolation of ^{14}C-labeled insulin from calf-pancreas slices. *Biochem. Biophys. Acta*, 20:251–261.

138. Little, J. R., and Cohen, J. J. (1974): Effect of albumin concentration on function of isolated perfused rat kidney. *Am. J. Physiol.*, 226:512–517.

139. Lorenz-Meyer, H., Roth, H., Elsässer, P., and Hahn, R. (1985): Cytotoxicity of lectins on rat intestinal mucosa enhanced by neuraminidase. *Eur. J. Clin. Invest.*, 15:227–234.

140. Loubatieres, A., Mariani, M. M., Chapal, J., and Portal, A. (1967): Action penatrice de faibles doses d'adrenaline et de noradrenaline sur l'insulino secretion etadiee sur le pancreas isole et perfuse du rat. *C. R. Soc. Biol. (Paris)*, 161:2578–2586.

141. Lyons, D. E., Beery, J. T., Lyons, S. A., and Taylor, S. L. (1983): Cadaverine and aminoguanidine potentiate the uptake of histamine in vitro in perfused intestinal segments of rats. *Toxicol. Appl. Pharmacol.*, 70:445–458.

142. McCarthy, R. D., Shaw, J. C., and Lakshmanan, S. (1958): Metabolism of volatile fatty acids by the perfused goat liver. *Proc. Soc. Exp. Biol. Med.*, 99:560–564.

143. McDonough, K. H., Brumfield, B. A., and Lang, C. H. (1986): In vitro myocardial performance after lethal and nonlethal doses of endotoxin. *Am. J. Physiol.*, 250:H240–H246.

144. Mehendale, H. M. (1976): Uptake and disposition of chlorinated biphenyls by isolated perfused rat liver. *Drug Metab. Dispos.*, 4:124–132.

145. Mehendale, H. M. (1976): Effect of preexposure to Kepone on the biliary excretion of polychlorinated biphenyl compounds. *Toxicol. Appl. Pharmacol.*, 36:369–381.

146. Mehendale, H. M. (1977): Mirex-induced impairment of hepatobiliary function: suppressed biliary excretion of imipramine and sulfobromophthalein. *Drug Metab. Dispos.*, 5:56–62.

147. Mehendale, H. M. (1977): Effect of preexposure to Kepone on the biliary excretion of imipramine and sulfobropthalein. *Toxicol. Appl. Pharmacol.*, 40:247–259.

148. Mehendale, H. M. (1978): Pesticide-induced modification of hepatobiliary function: hexachlorobenzene, DDT and toxaphene. *Food Cosmet. Toxicol.*, 16:19–25.

149. Mehendale, H. M. (1980): Aldrin epoxidase activity in the developing rabbit lung. *Pediatr. Res.*, 14:282–285.

150. Mehendale, H. M. (1982): Use of isolated perfused lung in determining pulmonary disposition and potential toxicological significance of inhaled environmental pollutants. *J. Environ. Toxicol. Chem.*, 1:231–244.

151. Mehendale, H. M. (1984): Pulmonary disposition of pneumophilic agents and possible relationship to pulmonary hypertension. *Fed. Proc.*, 43:2586–2591.

152. Mehendale, H. M., and El-Bassiouni, E. A. (1975): Uptake and disposition of aldrin and dieldrin by isolated perfused rabbit lung. *Drug Metab. Dispos.*, 3:543–556.

153. Mehendale, H. M., Angevine, L. S., and Ohmiya, Y. (1981): The isolated perfused lung—a critical evaluation. *Toxicology*, 21:1–36.

154. Mehendale, H. M., Svensson, S. Ä., Baldi, C., and Orrenius, S. (1985): Accumulation of Ca^{2+} induced by cytotoxic levels of menadione in the isolated perfused rat liver. *Eur. J. Biochem.*, 149:201–206.

155. Merin, R. G. (1978): Myocardial metabolism for the toxicologist. *Environ. Health Perspect.*, 26:169–174.

156. Merker, G., Helling, H. J., Krahl, M., and Aigner, K. (1983): Ultrastructural changes in the dog liver cell after isolated liver perfusion with various cytotoxins. *Recent Results Cancer Res.*, 86:103–109.

157. Miller, L. L., Bly, C. G., Berry, M. N., and Krebs, H. A. (1951): The dominant role of the liver in plasma protein synthesis: a direct study of the isolated perfused rat liver with the aid of lysine-[14]C. *J. Exp. Med.*, 94:431–453.

158. Mitchell, C. J., Bullock, S., and Ross, B. D. (1977): Renal handling of gentamicin and other antibiotics by the isolated perfused rat kidney: mechanism of nephrotoxicity. *J. Antimicrob. Chemother.*, 3:593–600.

159. Miura, K., Pasino, D. A., Goldstein, R. S., and Hook, J. B. (1985): Effects of gentamicin on renal function in isolated perfused kidneys from male and female rats. *Toxicol. Lett.*, 26:15–18.

160. Miyazaki, M., Makowka, L., Falk, R. E., Falk, W., Venturi, D., Ambus, U., and Falk, J. A. (1983): Hyperthermochemotherapeutic in vivo isolated perfusion of the rat liver. *Cancer*, 51:1254–1260.

161. Monroe, R. G., Larfarge, C. G., Gamble, W. J., Honda, S., and Kevy, S. W. (1968): Ventricular performance and coronary flow of isolated hearts when perfused through isolated lungs and membrane oxygenators. In: *Organ Perfusion and Preservations*, edited by J. C. Norman, pp. 779–979. Appleton-Century-Crofts, New York.

162. Moore, G. K., and Hook, J. B. (1978): Hemodynamic effects of furosemide in isolated perfused rat kidneys. *Proc. Soc. Exp. Biol. Med.*, 158:354–358.

163. Morgan, H. E., Henderson, M. J., Regen, D. M., and Park, C. R. (1961): Regulation of glucose uptake in muscle. I. The effect of insulin and anoxia on glucose transport and phosphorylation in isolated perfused heart of normal rats. *J. Biol. Chem.*, 235:253.

164. Muller, F. (1910): Dir kunslitche Durchbluntung resp. durchspulung von orgen. *Hand 6 Biol. Arb. Meth.*, 3:327.

165. Nahas, G., and Trouve, R. (1985): Effects of interactions of natural cannabinoids on the isolated heart. *Proc. Soc. Exp. Biol. Med.*, 180:312–316.

166. Nastainczyk, W., and Ullrich, V. (1978): Effect of oxygen concentration of the reaction of halothane with cytochrome P-450 in liver microsomes and isolated perfused rat liver. *Biochem. Pharmacol.*, 27:387–392.

167. Neely, J. R., Liebermiester, H., Battersby, E. J., and Morgan, H. E. (1967): Effect of pressure development on oxygen consumption by isolated rat heart. *Am. J. Physiol.*, 212:804–814.

168. Neuman, M. G., Eshchar, J., Cotariu, D., Ben-Sason, R., Ziv, E., Baron, H., and Ishay, J. S. (1985): Hepatotoxicity of hornet's venom sac extract in isolated perfused rat liver. *Acta Pharmacol. Toxicol. (Copenh.)*, 56:133–138.

169. Newton, J. E., and Hook, J. B. (1981): Isolated perfused kidney. *Methods Enzymol.*, 77:94–105.

170. Nichiitsutsuiji-Uwo, J. M., Ross, B. D., and Dribs, H. A. (1967): Metabolic activation of the isolated perfused rat kidney. *Biochem. J.*, 103:852–862.

171. Nicolaysen, G. (1971): Perfusate qualities and spontaneous edema formation in an isolated perfused lung preparation. *Acta Physiol. Scand.*, 83:563–570.

172. Niemeier, R. W. (1976): Isolated perfused rabbit lung: a critical appraisal. *Environ. Health Perspect.*, 16:67–71.

173. Niemeier, R. W., and Bingham, E. (1972): An isolated perfused lung preparation for metabolic studies. *Life Sci.*, 11:807–820.

174. Nizet, A. (1975): The isolated perfused kidney: possibilities, limitations and results. *Kidney Int.*, 7:1–11.

175. Norman, J. C., editor (1978): *Organ Perfusion and Perservation*. Appleton-Century-Crofts, New York.

176. Northway, M. O., and Burks, T. F. (1979): Indirect intestinal stimulatory effects of heroin: direct action on opiate receptors. *Eur. J. Pharmacol.*, 59:237–243.

177. Novakova, V., Birke, G., Plantin, L. O., and Wretland, A. (1976): A perfluorochemical oxygen carrier (Fluosol-43) in a synthetic medium used for perfusion of isolated rat liver. *Acta Physiol. Scand.*, 98:356–365.

178. O'Brien, R. F., Makarski, J. S., and Rounds, S. (1985): Studies on the mechanism of decreased angiotensin. I. Conversion in rat lungs injured with alpha-naphthylthiourea. *Exp. Lung Res.*, 8:243–259.

179. Ohmiya, Y., Angevine, L. S., and Mehendale, H. M. (1983): Effect of drug-induced phospholipidosis on pulmonary disposition of pneumophilic drugs. *Drug Metab. Dispos.*, 11:25–30.

180. Ohmiya, Y., and Mehendale, H. M. (1979): Uptake and accumulation of chlorpromazine in the isolated perfused rabbit lung. *Drug Metab. Dispos.*, 7:442–443.

181. Ohmiya, Y., and Mehendale, H. M. (1980): N-Oxidation of imipramine by isolated perfused rat and rabbit lung. *Life Sci.*, 26:1411–1421.

182. Ohmiya, Y., and Mehendale, H. M. (1980): Uptake and metabolism of chlorpromazine by rat and rabbit lungs. *Drug Metab. Dispos.*, 8:313–318.

183. O'Neil, J. J., and Tierney, F. (1974): Rat lung metabolism, glucose utilization by isolated perfused lungs and tissue slices. *Am. J. Physiol.*, 226:867–873.

184. Oomen, H. A. P. C., and Chamalarun, R. A. F. M. (1971): Correlation between histological and biochemical parameters of isolated perfused rat liver. *Virchows Arch.*, 8:243–251.

185. Opie, L. H. (1965): Coronary flow rate and perfusion pressure as determinants of mechanical function and oxidative metabolism of isolated perfused rat heart. *J. Physiol. (Lond.)*, 180:529–541.

186. Orton, T. C., Anderson, M. W., Pickett, R. D., Eling, T. E., and Fouts, J. R. (1973): Xenobiotic accumulation and metabolism by isolated perfused rabbit lungs. *J. Pharmacol. Exp. Ther.*, 186:482–497.

187. Otsuki, M., Nakamura, T., Okabayashi, Y., Oka, T., Fuji, M., and Baba, S. (1985): Comparative inhibitory effects of pirenzapine and atropine on cholinergic stimulation of exocrine and endocrine rat pancreas. *Gastroenterology*, 89:408–414.

188. Otsuki, M., Sakamoto, C., Ohki, A., Akabayashi, Y., Suehiro, I., and Baba, S. (1983): Effect of acarbose on exocrine and endocrin pancreatic function in the rat. *Diabetologia*, 24:445–448.

189. Otsuki, S., Watanabe, S., Morimistu, J., and Edamatsu, N. (1967): Regulatory effects of blood constituents on the function and metabolism of the cat brain perfusion experiments. *Acta Med. Okayama*, 21:279–296.

190. Palay, S. L., McGee-Russell, S. M., Gordon, S., and Grillo, M. A. (1962): Fixation of neural tissues for electron microscopy by perfusion with solutions of osmium tetroxide. *J. Cell Biol.*, 12:385–410.

191. Pang, K. S., Yuen, V., Fayz, S., Tekopple, J. M., and Mulder, G. J. (1986): Absorption and metabolism of acetaminophen by the in situ perfused rat small intestine preparation. *Drug Metab. Dispos.*, 14:102–111.

192. Parsons, D. D., and Prichards, J. S. (1968): A preparation of perfused small intestine for the study of absorption in amphibia. *J. Physiol. (Lond.)*, 198:405–434.

193. Peterson, R. E., and Fujimoto, J. M. (1976): Increased "bile duct-pancreatic fluid" flow in rats pretreated with carbon tetrachloride. *Toxicol. Appl. Pharmacol.*, 35:29–39.

194. Pickett, R. D., Anderson, M. W., Orton, T. C., and Eling, T. E. (1975): The pharmacodynamics of 5-hydroxytryptamine uptake and metabolism by the isolated perfused rabbit lung. *J. Pharmacol. Exp. Ther.*, 194:545–553.

195. Pitzele, S., Sze, S., and Dosell, A. R. C. (1971): Hypothermic plasma perfusion of the isolated heart. *Surgery*, 70:407–412.

196. Popjak, G., and Beeckmans, M. (1950): Extra-hepatic lipid synthesis. *Biochem. J.*, 47:233–238.

197. Post, C., Anderson, R. G. G., Ryfeldt, Å., and Nilsson, E. (1978): Transport and binding of lidocaine by lung slices and perfused lung of rats. *Acta Pharmacol. Toxicol. (Copenh.)*, 43:156–163.

198. Post, C., and Hede, A. R. (1982): Trichloroethylene and halothane inhibit uptake or 5-hydroxytryptamine in the isolated perfused rat lung. *Biochem. Pharmacol.*, 31:353–358.

199. Poulsen, H. E., Lerche, A., and Skovgaard, L. T. (1985): Acetaminophen metabolism by the perfused rat liver twelve hours after acetaminophen overdose. *Biochem. Pharmacol.*, 34:3729–3733.

200. Powis, G. (1970): Perfusion of rat liver with blood: transmitter overflows and gluconeogenesis. *Proc. R. Soc. Lond.*, B174:503–515.

201. Prasada Rao, K. S., and Mehendale, H. M. (1987): Precursor utilization for 5-hydroxytryptamine biosynthesis in isolated perfused rabbit and rat lungs. *Can. J. Physiol. Pharmacol.*, 65:2117–2123.

202. Prasada Rao, K. S., and Mehendale, H. M. (1988): Precursor utilization of [^{14}C]-L-tryptophan and [^{14}C]-5-hydroxytryptophan for pulmonary biosynthesis of [^{14}C]-5-hydroxythryptamine: a review. *Ind. J. Pharmacol. (in press).*

203. Radwan, Z., and Henschler, D. (1977): Uptake and rate of metabolism of vinyl chloride by the isolated perfused rat liver preparation. *Int. Arch. Occup. Environ. Health,* 40:101–110.

204. Raje, R. R. (1980): In vitro toxicity of acetone using coronary perfusion in isolated rabbit heart. *Drug Chem. Toxicol.,* 3:333–342.

205. Raje, R. R. (1983): In vitro toxicity of n-hexane and 2,5-hexanedione using isolated perfused rabbit heart. *J. Toxicol. Environ. Health,* 11:879–884.

206. Rao, M. M., and Elmslie, R. G. (1970): A modified technic of isolated pancreatic perfusion. *J. Surg. Res.,* 10:357–362.

207. Rao, S. B., and Mehendale, H. M. (1987): Uptake and disposition of putrescine, spermidine, and spermine by isolated perfused rabbit lungs. *Drug Metab. Dispos.,* 15:189–194.

208. Rao, S. B., Rao, K. S. P., and Mehendale, H. M. (1986): Absence of diamine oxidase activity from rabbit and rat lungs. *Biochem. J.,* 234:733–736.

209. Rasenack, J., Koch, H. K., Lesch, R., and Decker, K. (1980): Hepatotoxicity of D-galactosamine in isolated perfused rat liver. *Exp. Mol. Pathol.,* 32:264–275.

210. Reichelderfer, M., Pero, B., Lorenzsonn, V., and Olsen, W. A. (1984): Magnesium sulfate-induced water secretion in hamster small intestine. *Proc. Soc. Exp. Biol. Med.,* 176:8–13.

211. Rhoades, R. A. (1976): Perfused lung preparation for studying altered gaseous environments. *Environ. Health Perspect.,* 16:73–75.

212. Rice, A. J., Roberts, R. J., and Plaa, G. L. (1967): The effect of carbon tetrachloride administered in vivo on the hemodynamics of the isolated perfused rat liver. *Toxicol. Appl. Pharmacol.,* 11:422–431.

213. Ritchie, H. D., and Hardcastle, J. D. (1973): *Isolated Organ Perfusion.* University Park Press, Baltimore.

214. Rosenfeld, S., Sellers, A. L., and Katz, J. (1959): Development of an isolated perfused rabbit kidney. *Am. J. Physiol.,* 196:115–159.

215. Ross, B. D. (1972): *Perfusion Techniques in Biochemistry.* Clarendon Press, Oxford.

216. Ross, B. D., Epstein, F. H., and Leaf, A. (1973): Sodium reabsorption in the perfused rat kidney. *Am. J. Physiol.,* 225:1165–1171.

217. Ross, B. D., Hems, R., and Krebs, H. A. (1967): The rate of gluconeogenesis from various precursors in the perfused rat liver. *Biochem. J.,* 102:942–951.

218. Roth, J. A. (1979): Use of the isolated perfused lung in biochemical toxicology. *Rev. Biochem. Toxicol.,* 1:287–310.

219. Rowland, M. (1972): Application of clearance concepts to some literature data on drug metabolism in the isolated perfused liver preparation and in vivo. *Eur. J. Pharmacol.,* 17:352–356.

220. Rudolph, A. M., and Hyemann, M. A. (1971): Measurement of flow in perfused organs using microsphere techniques. In: *Perfusion Techniques,* edited by E. Diczfalusy, pp. 112–117. Karolinska Institute, Stockholm.

221. Ryoo, H., and Tarver, H. (1968): Studies on plasma protein synthesis with a new liver perfusion apparatus. *Proc. Soc. Exp. Biol. Med.,* 128:760–772.

222. Schanne, F. A. X., Kane, A. B., Young, E. E., and Farber, J. L. (1979): Calcium dependence of toxic cell death: a final common pathway. *Science,* 206:700–702.

223. Schermann, J., Stowe, N., Yarimizu, S., Magnusson, M., and Tingwald, G. (1977): Feedback control of glomerular filtration rate in isolated, blood perfused dog kidneys. *Am. J. Physiol.,* 223:217–224.

224. Schimassek, H. (1962): Perfusion of rat liver with a semisynthetic medium and control of liver function. *Life Sci.,* 1:629–637.

225. Schimassek, H. (1963): Metabolite des kohlendydrastoffwechels der isoliert perfundierten rattenleber. *Biochem. Z.,* 336:460–467.

226. Schimassek, H., and Gerok, W. (1965): Control of the levels of free amino acids in plasma by the liver. *Biochem. Z.,* 343:407–415.

227. Schimmel, R. J., and Knobil, E. (1969): Role of free fatty acid in stimulation of gluconeogenesis during fasting. *Am. J. Physiol.,* 217:1803–1808.

228. Schureck, J., Brecht, J. P., Lofert, H., and Hierholzer, K. (1975): The basic requirements for the function of the isolated cell free perfused rat kidney. *Pflugers Arch.,* 354:349–365.

229. Seeger, W., Bauer, M., and Bhakdi, S. (1984): Staphylococcal α-toxin elicits hypertension in isolated rabbit lungs: evidence for thromboxane formation and the role of extracellular calcium. *J. Clin. Invest.,* 74:849–858.

230. Seeger, W., Suttrop, N., Schmidt, F., and Neuhof, H. (1986): The glutathione redox cycle as a defense system against hydrogen-peroxide induced prostanoid formation and vasoconstriction in rabbit lungs. *Am. Rev. Respir. Dis.,* 133:1029–1036.

231. Segel, L. D., Rendig, S. V., and Mason, D. T. (1979): Left ventricular dysfunction of isolated working rat hearts after chronic alcohol consumption. *Cardiovasc. Res.,* 13:136–146.

232. Seiler, K. U., Tamm, G., and Wasserman, O. (1974): On the role of serotonin in the pathogenesis of pulmonary hypertension induced by anorectic drugs: an experimental study in the isolated perfused rat lung. *Clin. Exp. Pharmacol. Physiol.,* 1:463–471.

233. Seiver, B. R., and Whitney, J. E. (1967): Biosynthesis of insulin by the isolated perfused dog pancreas. *Diabetes,* 16:647–651.

234. Skutul, K. (1908): Uber durchstromunsapporate. *Pflugers. Arch.,* 123:249–273.

235. Sladen, G. E. (1968): Perfusion studies in relation to intestinal absorption. *Gut,* 9:624–628.

236. Smith, M. T., Thor, H., and Orrenius, S. (1981): Toxic injury to isolated hepatocytes is not dependent on extracellular calcium. *Science,* 213:1257–1259.

237. Soergel, K. H. (1971): Intestinal perfusion studies: values, pitfalls, and limitations. *Gasteroenterology,* 61:261–263.

238. Southard, J. H., Senzig, K. A., Hoffman, R. M., and Belzer, F. O. (1980): Toxicity of oxygen to mitochondrial respiratory activity in hypothermically perfused canine kidneys. *Transplantation,* 29:459–461.

239. Sperling, F., and Marcus, W. L. (1968): Turpentine-induced histological changes in isolated rat and guinea-pig lungs. *Arch. Int. Pharmacodyn. Ther.,* 175:330–338.

240. Summerfield, J. A., Gollan, J. L., and Billing, B. H. (1976): Synthesis of bile acid monophosphates by the isolated perfused rat kidney. *Biochem. J.,* 156:339–345.

241. Sumpio, B. E., Chandry, I. H., and Baue, A. E. (1985): Reduction of the drug-induced nephrotoxicity by ATP-MgCl$_2$. I. Effects of the cis-diaminedichloro platinum-treated isolated perfused kidneys. *J. Surg. Res.,* 38:429–437.

242. Sussman, K. E., and Vaughn, G. D. (1967): Insulin release after ACTH, glucagon and adenosine 3',5'-phosphate (cyclic AMP) in the perfused isolated rat pancreas. *Diabetes,* 16:449–454.

243. Sussman, K. E., Vaughn, G. D., and Timmer, R. F. (1966): An in vitro method for studying insulin secretion in perfused rat pancreas. *Metabolism,* 15:466–476.

244. Takano, T., Miyazaki, Y., and Motohashi, Y. (1983): A method to evaluate the dynamic effects of environmental chemical agents on intracellular functions: the real time observations of changes in the spectra of mitochondrial cytochromes, cytochrome P-450, and catalase and in the fluorescence or reduced pyridine nucleotides in perfused rat liver. *Jpn. J. Hyg.,* 38:649–656.

245. Tark, M., Randall, Jr., H. M., and Hoffer, T. L. (1976): Substrate metabolism in the isolated perfused kidney. *Invest. Urol.,* 14:132–136.

246. Telander, R. L. (1964): Prolonged monothermic perfusion of the isolated primate and sheep kidney. *Surg. Gynecol. Obstet.,* 118:347–353.

247. Terao, N., and Shen, D. D. (1985): Reduced extraction of I-propranolol by perfused rat liver in the presence of uremic blood. *J. Pharmacol. Exp. Ther.,* 233:277–284.

248. Thelen, M., and Wendel, A. (1983): Drug-induced lipid peroxidation in mice. V. Ethane production and glutathione release in the isolated liver upon perfusion with acetaminophen. *Biochem. Pharmacol.,* 32:1701–1706.

249. Thompson, A. M., Cavert, H. M., and Lifson, N. (1968): A rat head-perfusion technique developed for the study of brain uptake of materials. *J. Appl. Physiol.,* 24:407–411.

250. Thurman, R. G., Marazzo, D. P., Jones, L. S., and Kauffman, F. C. (1977): The continuous kinetic determination of p-nitroanisole o-demethylation in hemoglobin-free perfused rat liver. *J. Pharmacol. Exp. Ther.,* 201:498–506.

251. Thurman, R. G., Reinke, L. A., and Kauffman, F. C. (1979): The isolated perfused liver: a model to define biochemical mechanisms of chemical toxicity. *Rev. Biochem. Toxicol.*, 1:249–286.

252. Torack, R. M. (1969): Sodium demonstration in rat cerebellum following perfusion hydroxyadipaldehyde antimonate. *Acta Neuropathol. (Berl.)*, 12:173–182.

253. Toth, K. M., Clifford, D. P., Berger, E. M., White, C. W., and Repine, J. E. (1984): Intact human erythrocytes prevent hydrogen peroxide-mediated damage to isolated perfused rat lungs and cultured bovine pulmonary artery endothelial cells. *J. Clin. Invest.*, 74:292–295.

254. Triner, L., Verosky, M., Habif, D. V., and Nahas, G. G. (1970): Perfusion of isolated liver with fluorocarbon emulsions. *Fed. Proc.*, 29:1778–1781.

255. Tsuji, M., and Nakajima, T. (1978): Studies on the formation of γ-aminobutyric acid from putrescine in rat organic purification of its synthesis enzyme from rat intestine. *J. Biochem. (Tokyo)*, 83:1407–1420.

256. Umbreit, W. W., Burris, R. H., and Stauffer, J. F. (1972): *Manometric Biochemical Techniques*, 5th ed., p. 146. Burguess, Minneapolis.

257. Vähäkangas, K., Nevasaari, K., Pelkonen, O., and Karki, N. T. (1977): The metabolism of benzo(a)pyrene in isolated perfused lungs from variously treated rats. *Acta Pharmacol. Toxicol. (Copenh.)*, 41:129–140.

258. Valenzuela, A., and Guerra, R. (1985): Protective effect of the flavonoid silybin dihemisuccinate on the toxicity of phenyl hydrazine on rat liver. *FEBS Lett.*, 181:291–294.

259. Vilstrap, H. (1983): Effects of acute carbon tetrachloride intoxication on kinetics or galactose elimination by perfused rat livers. *Scand. J. Clin. Lab. Invest.*, 43:127–131.

260. Waugh, W. A., and Kubo, T. (1959): Development of an isolated perfused dog kidney with improved function. *Am. J. Physiol.*, 217:227–290.

261. Welbourne, T. C. (1974): Ammonia production and pathways of glutamine metabolism in the isolated perfused rat kidney. *Am. J. Physiol.*, 226:544–548.

262. White, R. J. (1971): Preparation and mechanical perfusion of the isolated monkey brain. In: *Perfusion Techniques*, edited by E. Diczfalusy, pp. 200–216. Karolinska Institute, Stockholm.

263. Wilson, T. H., and Wiseman, G. (1954): Use of sacs of everted small intestine for study of transference of subtrances from the mucosal to serosal surface. *J. Physiol. (Lond.)*, 123:116–125.

264. Windmueller, H. G., Spaeth, A. E., and Ganote, C. E. (1970): Vascular perfusion of isolated rat gut: norepinephrine and glucocorticoid requirement. *Am. J. Physiol.*, 218:197–204.

265. Woodward, B., and Zakaria, M. N. M. (1985): Effect of some free radical scavengers on reperfusion induced arrhythmias in the isolated rat heart. *J. Mol. Cell. Cardiol.*, 17:485–493.

266. Yamamoto, K., Hasegawa, T., and Ueda, J. (1968): Renin secretion in the perfused dog kidney. *Jpn. J. Pharmacol.*, 18:1–8.

267. Young, S. L. (1976): An isolated perfused rat lung preparation. *Environ. Health Perspect.*, 16:61–66.

268. Youngman, R. C., Klugo, R. C., Cruickshank, R. D., and Cerny, J. C. (1976): A technique for isolated in vivo renal perfusion. *Invest. Urol.*, 14:187–190.

Principles and Methods of Toxicology, Second Edition, edited by A. Wallace Hayes, Raven Press, Ltd., New York © 1989.

CHAPTER 26

Immune System: Evaluation of Injury

Jack H. Dean, Joel B. Cornacoff, *Gary J. Rosenthal, and *Michael I. Luster

*Department of Toxicology, Sterling-Winthrop Research Institute, Rensselaer, New York 12144; and *Immunotoxicology Group, National Institute of Environmental Health Sciences, National Institutes of Health, Research Triangle Park, North Carolina 27709*

The immune system is comprised of several cell types (e.g., granulocytes, macrophages, lymphocytes, natural killer cells, and mast cells) that can be found in the peripheral blood, lymphatic fluid, and organized lymphoid tissues, including bone marrow, spleen, thymus, lymph nodes, tonsils, and gut-associated lymphoid tissue. The system, in a constant state of self-renewal and maturation, exists to defend against invasion by infectious agents and spontaneously arising neoplasms. It is a highly regulated network of cells that must discriminate self from nonself and react to nonself with pleiotropic defensive responses (111).

IMMUNE MECHANISMS IN HOST DEFENSE

The functions of the immune system are provided by two major mechanisms: a *nonspecific (constitutive) mechanism,* which does not require prior sensitization with the inducing agent to elicit a response and lacks specificity, and a *specific (adaptive) mechanism* directed against a specific elicitating agent to which it has been previously sensitized. Penetrance of the epithelial defense barriers by an invading microorganism first results in nonspecific reactions involving phagocytic cells (e.g., granulocytes and macrophages) followed by specific

responses involving antibody production and the induction of effector lymphocytes, which respond through mediators to seek out and destroy the invading agent. Both antibody-producing lymphocytes (B cells) and thymus-dependent lymphocytes (T cells) are triggered by mechanisms in which the foreign antigen is recognized, digested, and presented to lymphocytes by macrophages. Following antigen-induced activation, B cells proliferate and differentiate into plasma cells (PCs), which produce large quantities of specific antibodies, e.g., immunoglobulins (Igs). The antibodies enter the circulation where they bind the foreign material and either neutralize, lyse, or facilitate phagocytosis of the agent. Antibody–antigen interactions are expanded by a series of complement (C') proteins and other mediators of inflammation (e.g., prostaglandins and leukotrienes). Fever, opsonization, and lytic factors released by activated lymphoid cells also contribute to the process.

Nonspecific and Specific Mechanisms of Immunity

Two categories of phagocytic leukocytes—the polymorphonuclear phagocyte (PMN), or granulocyte, and the mononuclear phagocyte, or macrophage—are involved with nonspecific mechanisms of host resistance. Both cell types originate from the same myeloid progenitor cells in the bone marrow, pass through several developmental stages, and enter the bloodstream (25). PMNs readily traverse blood vessels and provide the primary line of defense against infectious agents. Both PMNs and macrophages exhibit phagocytic activity toward foreign material, especially in the presence of specific opsonic antibodies and complement, and can destroy most microorganisms. Macrophages are recruited to the site in the event that PMNs either cannot contain or are destroyed by the infectious agent, as in the case with certain bacteria (e.g., *Listeria*). Macrophages can be activated to a state of enhanced bactericidal or tumoricidal activity by soluble lymphocyte products produced by T lymphocytes (e.g., lymphokines) sensitized to the microbial agent (21).

The immune response involved with adaptive host resistance represents a series of complex events that occur after the introduction of a foreign antigenic material into the host. There are two major types of immune response: (a) cell-mediated immunity (CMI), which is a response by specifically sensitized T cells and is generally associated with delayed-type hypersensitivity (DTH), rejection of tumors or foreign grafts, and resistance to persistent infectious agents; and (b) humoral immunity (HI), which involves the production of specific antibodies by B cells following sensitization to a specific antigen.

Organization and Function of Primary Lymphoid Tissue

The cellular elements of the immune system arise from pluripotent stem cells, a unique group of unspecialized cells that have self-renewal capacity. During fetal development, pluripotent stem cells are found in the blood islands of the embryonic yolk sac in the liver of the fetus and later in the bone marrow. The pluripotent stem cell differentiates along several pathways, giving rise to either erythrocytes, myeloid

series cells (i.e., macrophages and PMNs), megakaryocytes (platelets), or lymphocytes. Maturation generally occurs within the bone marrow, although lymphoid progenitor cells are disseminated by the vasculature to the primary lymphoid organs, where they often undergo further differentiation under the influence of the hormonal microenvironment of these organs (Fig. 1).

The primary lymphoid organs include the thymus in all vertebrates and the bursa of Fabricius in birds, or bursa-equivalent tissue, probably bone marrow and gut-associated lymphoid tissue in mammals (Table 1). Primary lymphoid organs are lymphoepithelial in origin, derived from ectoendodermal junctional tissue in association with gut epithelium. During the second half of embryogenesis (days 12 to 13 in the mouse), stem cells migrate into the epithelia of the thymus and bursa-equivalent areas, where they differentiate independent of antigenic stimulation into immunocompetent T cells and B cells, respectively (Fig. 1). The thymus, which is derived embryologically from the third and fourth pharyngeal pouches, is an organization of lymphoid tissue located in the chest, above the heart. Thymus development occurs during the sixth week of embryologic development in humans and day 9 of gestation in the mouse. The thymus reaches its maximum size at birth or shortly thereafter in most mammals and then begins a gradual involution that is complete between 5 to 15 years in humans. Histologically, the thymus consists of multiple lobules, each containing a cortex and medulla. Lymphocyte precursors from bone marrow proliferate in the cortex of the lobules and then migrate to the medulla, where they further differentiate, under the influence of thymic epithelium and hormonal factors, into mature T lymphocytes before emigrating to secondary lymphoid tissues. The neonatal/postnatal thymus has an endocrine function associated with the nonlymphoid thymic epithelium cells. These cells are believed to produce a family of thymic hormones essential for T-lymphocyte maturation and differentiation (111).

B cell differentiation occurs in the bursa of Fabricius in

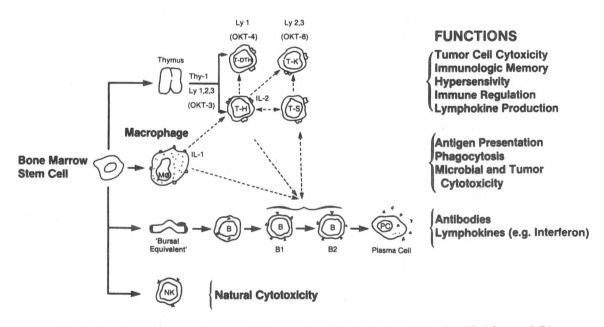

FIG. 1. Development, interactions, and effector cells of the immune system. (Modified from ref. 7.)

TABLE 1. *Origin and characteristics of primary and secondary lymphoid tissue*

Parameter	Primary lymphoid organs	Secondary lymphoid organs
Lymphoid organs	Thymus Bursa of Fabricius (birds) Fetal liver (mammals) Adult bone marrow	Spleen Lymph nodes Gut-associated lymphoid tissue Bronchial-associated lymphoid tissue
Embryonic origin and development	Ectoendodermal junction Thymus: days 9–10, mouse; week 6, man Bursa-equivalent: days 10–13, mouse; week 10, man	Mesoderm
Lymphoid cell proliferation	Independent of antigenic stimulation	Dependent on antigenic stimulation
Germinal center formation	Nonexistent	Occurs after antigenic stimulation
Cells repopulating after depletion	Stem cells only	Differentiated lymphocytes
Early surgical or chemical removal	Depressed numbers of T and B cells; depressed immune responses	No significant effect on immune function

birds, a lymphoepithelial organ that develops from a diverticulum of the posterior wall of the cloaca. It is divided into a medullary region, containing lymphoid follicles, and a cortical region. The mammalian bursa-equivalent is believed to be the fetal liver, neonatal spleen, gut-associated lymphoid tissue, and adult bone marrow. Mature B lymphocytes migrate from the bursa-equivalent tissue to populate the B-dependent areas of the secondary lymphoid tissues.

Neonatal removal or chemical destruction of primary lymphoid organs prior to the maturation of lymphocytes into T or B cells or prior to their population of secondary lymphoid tissue dramatically depresses the immunologic capacity of the host. However, removal of these same organs in adults has little influence on immunologic capacity. In addition, neonatal thymectomy in mammals dramatically impairs the development of CMI but does not generally influence the generation of immunoglobulin-producing cells involved in HI unless they require T-lymphocyte help for induction of antibody production. In contrast to the removal of primary lymphoid organs, removal of secondary lymphoid organs does not inhibit the development of immunocompetence, although it may suppress the magnitude or alter the tissue location of the responsive cells.

Organization and Function of Secondary Lymphoid Tissue

In the above section the origin of the primary lymphoid tissues was discussed in the context of lymphoid cell differentiation. Also of extreme importance for immunocompetence and in host defense is the organization and function of secondary lymphoid organs (Table 1). The organized areas of secondary lymphoid tissues are the spleen, lymph nodes, gut-associated lymphoid tissue (GALT), and bronchial-associated lymphoid tissue (BALT). The anatomic organization of these tissues provides a microenvironment for functional development of lymphoid cells and immune responses.

Because the spleen is the major filter of blood-borne antigens, it is also the major site of immunologic responses to these antigens. In addition, the spleen is a site of extramedullary hematopoiesis and removal of damaged blood cells. There are two major histologic regions within the spleen: the red pulp and the white pulp. These areas have been named for their color in a freshly cut spleen. The white pulp consists of numerous white blood cell aggregates and lymphoid follicles. The red pulp contains cords and venous sinuses analogous to the medullary region of lymph nodes. The spleen has no afferent lymphatic vessels; and thus all antigenic material or cells enter the spleen through the blood vasculature. The marginal sinus in the spleen is structurally and functionally similar to the subcapsular sinus of the lymph node.

Lymph nodes are discrete, organized secondary lymphoid organs that serve as filtering devices for lymphatic fluid, much like the spleen serves as the major filter for the blood. Lymph nodes are divided structurally into three areas: cortex, paracortex, and medulla (Fig. 2). Each lymph node is served by several afferent lymphatic vessels collecting lymphatic fluid from distal tissue sites. This fluid, or lymph, may contain foreign antigens. The efferent lymphatic vessel, which drains lymph from the node, contains antibodies, lymphokines, and lymphocytes produced in response to foreign antigenic stimulation. The cortex, located underneath the subcapsular sinus, receives the afferent lymph and serves as the major site of B-lymphocyte localization. The cortex consists of a narrow rim of small lymphocytes in the absence of antigenic stimulation. Also located in the cortex are aggregations of small lymphocytes, termed lymphoid follicles, which contain dendritic reticulum cells capable of retaining antigens on their plasma membranes. When the lymphocytes comprising the lymphoid follicles are stimulated by antigen, they proliferate, giving rise to dense aggregations of lymphocytes, termed *germinal centers,* which serve as sites for differentiation of B lymphocytes to plasma cells capable of antibody production. Following antigenic stimulation, germinal centers are easily detectable as spherical or ovoid structures containing many large and medium-sized lymphocytes, predominantly B lymphocytes. The paracortex, lying between the cortex and the medulla, is composed predominantly of T cells and is a major site of macrophage–T cell interactions. Neonatal thymectomy or lymphocyte depletion by cytolytic drugs reduces paracortical lymphocytes, leading to depressed immune capacity. In addition, the paracortex contains a specialized blood vasculature, termed postcapillary venules, which serve as points of entry for recirculating lymphocytes from the bloodstream. The medulla of the lymph node is composed primarily of networks of cords and sinuses; it serves as an effective filter for removing particulate material from lym-

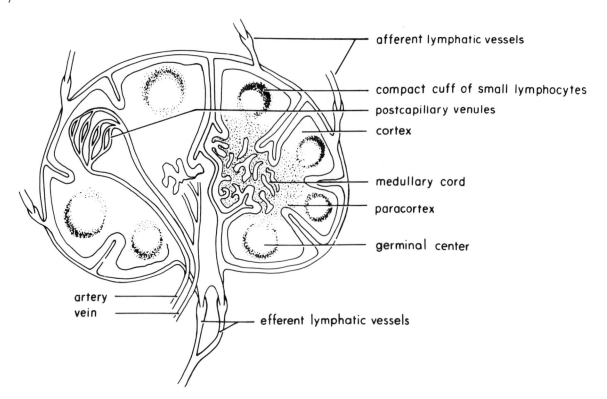

FIG. 2. Cross-section of a lymph node showing architectural organization. (Modified from ref. 25.)

phatic fluid. Following antigenic stimulation a major portion of the antibody is produced by plasma cells found within these medullary cords.

Cell-Mediated Immunity

Whether an antigen induces CMI, antibody production, or both depends on the physical and chemical nature of the antigen, the mode of presentation of the antigen to lymphocytes, the localization pattern of the antigen within lymphoid tissue, and the molecular configuration of the antigen. Those antigens that generally elicit CMI include tissue-associated antigens, chemical agents and drugs that covalently bind to autologous proteins, and antigenic determinants on persistent intracellular microorganisms. The route of exposure also plays a major role in the type of response generated. For example, sheep erythrocytes elicit antibody production but not CMI when injected intravenously, but elicit both when injected intracutaneously.

The induction of CMI proceeds when small lymphocytes differentiate into large pyroninophilic cells and ultimately divide, giving rise to cells responsible for immunologic memory and effector function. T cells can further differentiate into effector cells endowed with cytotoxic potential (i.e., cytotoxic T cells); helper cells (T_H), which facilitate antibody responses by B lymphocytes and aid in some T lymphocyte responses; or T-suppressor cells (T_S) capable of inhibiting both T and B cell responses. The steps involved in T cell activation and the humoral factors elaborated by T cells that regulate and amplify CMI are shown in Fig. 1 (7). These

factors, termed lymphokines, include, among others, γ-interferon, chemotactic factor, macrophage activation factor, interleukins (e.g., IL2 and IL4), and B-cell growth factors.

Humoral Immunity

The main function of B lymphocytes is production of antibody, which is produced in response to antigenic stimulation and reacts with specific antigenic determinants. Based on chemical structure and biologic function, there are five classes of antibody molecule: IgM, IgG, IgA, IgD, and IgE. Table 2 lists some of the physical and biologic characteristics of these classes.

Over a period of 3 to 5 days following the introduction of antigens into an immunocompetent host, B lymphocytes sequentially differentiate into lymphoblasts, immature plasma cells, and finally antibody-secreting plasma cells. HI can be characterized by an early rise in IgM antibody titer in the serum, followed several days later by the appearance of IgG antibodies. During this differentiation process, some of the lymphocytes develop into memory cells so that when the antigen is encountered a second time, an enhanced response is observed. The secondary response is characterized by a shorter latency for the appearance of IgG, increased production of Ig, and sustained production of IgG antibodies.

Antibody molecules have three basic functions in protecting the host from infectious agents: (a) virus neutralization (i.e., antibodies bind and prevent virus particles from infecting target cells); (b) opsonization (i.e., antibody molecules react with infectious agents and enhance phagocytosis of the

TABLE 2. *Biological properties of major immunoglobulin classes in the mouse*

Class	Serum concentration (mg/dl)	Mol. wt.	Placental transfer	Half-life (days)	Biological function	Abnormalities
IgG	670 ± 33	150,000	+	23	Primarily synthesized during secondary immune response. Readily diffuses into extravascular tissue. Fixes complement.	Increased in liver disease, chronic infection. Reduced in B cell depression.
IgM	61 ± 5	890,000	−	5	Produced early in immune response. Isoagglutinins. Fixes complement.	Increased in infection. Reduced in B cell depression.
IgA	40 ± 4	170,000	−	6	Major Ig in seromucous secretion.	Increased in liver disease. Increased or decreased in sinopulmonary infection.
IgD	—	150,000	−	2.8	Lymphocyte receptor.	Decreased following thymectomy.
IgE	0.02	196,000	−	1.5	Mediator of allergic reactions and atopic diseases.	Increased in parasitic and allergic diseases, homocytropic.

antibody-coated agent); and (c) antibody-dependent cellular cytotoxicity (i.e., antibody-coated target cells are killed by Fc receptor-bearing leukocytes).

Mononuclear Phagocyte System

In most instances antigen is initially processed by macrophages and then presented to lymphocytes through cell surface interactions via specific surface proteins (e.g., Ia molecules). Once macrophages are activated by antigen they secrete interleukin-1 (IL1), which signals the T-helper/inducer cells to produce interleukin-2 (IL2). IL2 interacts with specific receptors on T cells to help develop T-effector cells including suppressor and cytotoxic T cells. Some T cells secrete other lymphokines, including γ-interferon, which along with IL2 can modulate natural killer (NK) cells. NK cells are important cytotoxic effector cells in immune defense against malignancy, infectious agents, and the regulation of immunoglobulin production by B cells.

Mononuclear phagocytes must cope with many xenobiotics, as their location results in interactions with drugs, chemicals, and physical agents entering the organisms via the air, food, or blood. Once a xenobiotic has gained entry to the host, extensive tissue damage can result from macrophage-mediated responses to the agent (21). Many believe that silicosis and asbestosis may represent examples of diseases resulting from macrophage-induced injury.

CHEMICAL-INDUCED IMMUNE DYSFUNCTION

Immunosuppression

Immunosuppressive therapy has been used to treat certain autoimmune, collagen-vascular, and chronic inflammatory diseases, as well as to prevent rejection of transplanted organs. Unfortunately, therapeutic immunosuppression frequently causes complications from bacterial, viral, fungal, and par-

asitic infections. Another complication of immunosuppression in transplant patients has been a high frequency of secondary cancer. Partial or complete regression of the secondary cancers often occurs if the therapy is terminated. In a large sampling of renal transplant patients who survived 10 years, approximately 50% developed cancer (102). The types of tumors observed were heterogeneous and included skin and lip cancer (21-fold increase over the general population), non-Hodgkin's lymphomas (28- to 49-fold increase), Kaposi's sarcoma (400- to 500-fold increase), and carcinomas of the cervix (14-fold increase).

Additionally, a large body of information has developed demonstrating that xenobiotic exposure can produce immune dysfunction and altered host resistance in experimental animals following acute and chronic exposure (23,25,88,147), although only a limited number of reports indicate immune dysfunction following human exposure to xenobiotics (23,25). Taken together these findings suggest that an increased frequency of infectious disease and neoplasia might be an expected consequence of immune modulation following inadvertent exposure to xenobiotics. A detailed review of immune dysfunction induced by selected xenobiotics and their proposed mechanism are discussed in a later section.

Autoimmunity

The immune system can adequately defend against infectious agents and prevent adverse reactions to self because of the exquisitely regulated network of interacting, discriminatory components. Much of this regulation is carried out through the delicate balance achieved between helper and suppressor T cells and macrophages. Autoimmunity arises when there is a perturbation or imbalance such that helper–suppressor cell function is inappropriate.

Autoimmune diseases are disorders of immunologic regulation in which many predisposing factors (e.g., viral, genetic, hormonal, environmental, and emotional) may play an etiological role. The pathogenesis of autoimmune disease includes production of autoantibodies, destructive inflam-

TABLE 3. *Drugs and chemicals inducing an autoimmune syndrome*

Autoimmune syndrome	Compound
Systemic lupus erythematosus	Hydralazine
	Procainamide
	Chlorpromazine
	Anticonvulsants
	Isoniazid
	Penicillamine
Hemolytic anemia	Methyldopa
	Penicillin
	Mefenamic acid
	Sulfa
Thrombocytopenia	Acetazolamide
	Chlorothiazide
	Gold salts
	p-Aminosalicylic acid
	Rifampin
	Quinidine
Scleroderma-like disease	Vinyl chloride
Pemphigus	Penicillamine

TABLE 4. *Industrial materials known or presumed to cause allergic problems*

Material	Industry
Platinum salts	Metal-refining
Cotton dusts	Textile
Castor bean, green coffee bean, papain, pancreatic extracts, organic dusts, molds	Oil, food
Formaldehyde	Garment, laboratory
Grain and flour	Farmers, bakers, mill operators
Hog trypsin, ethylenediamine phthalic anhydride, trimellitic anhydride, diisocyanates (TDI, HDI, MDI)	Chemical, plastic, rubber, resin
Phenylglycine acid chloride sulfone chloramides, ampicillin, spiramycin, piperazine, amprolium hydrochloride, antibiotic dust	Pharmaceutical
Wood dusts	Wood mills, carpenters
Vegetable gums (acacia, karaya), natural resins	Printers
Organophosphate insecticides	Farmers
Pyrolysis products of polyvinyl chloride, label adhesives	Meat wrappers

Modified from ref. 87.

matory cell infiltrates in target tissues, and deposition of immune complexes in vascular sites. Several xenobiotics capable of inducing an autoimmune syndrome are shown in Table 3.

There is a general impression that the incidence of autoimmune diseases, e.g., systemic lupus erythematosus and rheumatoid arthritis, may be increasing for reasons not well understood. The well-documented examples of drug-induced autoimmune syndromes suggest that exposure to xenobiotics could contribute to the incidence of these diseases through interference with normal immunoregulation. Whether xenobiotics significantly contribute to altered immune regulation requires further investigation.

Hypersensitivity/Allergy

Acute hypersensitivity or allergy is a pathological state resulting from prior sensitization to a specific molecule or structurally related compound. A number of industrial chemicals and drugs or their metabolites have been shown to induce hypersensitivity reactions (Table 4) (23). These compounds are sometimes directly antigenic, but more often

they covalently bind to macromolecules present in the lung, gastrointestinal tract, bone marrow, or skin. Individuals with potential occupational exposure (e.g., chemical manufacturing workers and farmworkers) are at a higher risk than the general public for development of respiratory and cutaneous contact hypersensitivity to chemicals.

Hypersensitivity diseases are among the most common and costly health problems in the United States, afflicting at least 35 million Americans. The indirect costs, such as wages lost because of illness, are estimated in excess of $800 million annually for asthma alone, with more than 35 million sick days lost each year (168). Industry produces or uses materials capable of inducing occupational immunological lung disease or contact hypersensitivity in workers (Table 4). Studies in

TABLE 5. *Immunological classification of hypersensitivity diseases*

Type	Target organs	Clinical manifestations	Mechanisms responsible
Anaphylactic I	GI tract, skin, lungs, vasculature	GI allergy, urticaria, dermatitis, asthma, shock	IgE and other Igs
Cytotoxic II	Circulating blood elements	Hemolytic anemia, leukopenia, thrombocytopenia	IgG, IgM
Arthus or immune complex disease III	Blood vessels, skin, joints, kidneys, lungs	Serum sickness, systemic lupus, chronic glomerulonephritis	Ag–Ab complexes (IgG)
Cell-mediated or delayed-type hypersensitivity IV	Skin, lungs, CNS, thyroid, other organs	Contact dermatitis, tuberculosis, allergic encephalitis, thyroiditis, primary homograft	Sensitized T cells

the metal-refining industry, for example, suggest that many workers regularly exposed to the complex salts of platinum develop disorders of the upper or lower respiratory tract. A study of workers exposed to toluene diisocyanate (TDI), a substance used in manufacturing polyurethane, revealed that 5% of those surveyed developed occupational asthma to TDI. Studies of the detergent industry indicate that about 2% of exposed employees developed asthma symptoms from inhaling enzymes used in detergents (168). Contact or skin hypersensitivity can occur as a result of exposure to certain drugs and chemicals, cosmetics, consumer products, and various metals including nickel and chromium following repeated skin exposure. Coombs and Gell (19) have provided a working classification of hypersensitivity responses that is useful for assessing the immune responses to specific xenobiotics (Table 5). This classification is used for chemical agents shown to produce one of the four types of hypersensitivity reaction described.

IMMUNOTOXICITY ASSESSMENT IN RODENTS

Manifestations of immune system toxicity following xenobiotic exposure in experimental animals can appear as: (a) alterations in lymphoid organ weights or histology; (b) quantitative or qualitative changes in the cellularity of lymphoid tissue, peripheral blood leukocytes, or bone marrow; (c) impairment of cell function at the effector or regulatory level; or (d) increased susceptibility to infectious agents or tumors. The sensitivity and utility of the analysis of immune function for detecting subclinical toxic injury is well recognized. Any agent that alters the delicate regulatory balance of the immune system may affect the functions of several cell types or alter their proliferation or differentiation.

No single immune function assay can conclusively demonstrate the deleterious or enhancing effects of a chemical or drug on the immune system. Hence a testing configuration composed of in vivo and in vitro assays has been proposed for assessing immunosuppression in rats (147) and mice (23,126). Based up these configurations a panel has been refined, evaluated, and validated in four laboratories (92) under sponsorship by the National Toxicology Program (NTP). This flexible approach to immunotoxicity assessment, which is currently used at the Chemical Industry Institute of Toxicology and in the NTP, consists in a two-level panel (Table 6) that enables rapid identification of compounds that may produce immune alterations. The assays in level I would be applied to mice or rats in a subchronic dosing protocol for chemicals that demonstrate suspicious structure–activity relations, pharmacokinetic properties or indicator "flags" (Table 7) that suggest potential immunotoxicity. In its simplest form, immunotoxicity assessment includes both in vivo and ex vivo/in vitro measures of quantitative and functional changes in immune status: immunopathology, cell-mediated immune function, antibody production, and NK cell function.

Agents that are immunomodulatory in some aspect of the level I screening can be further evaluated with assays selected from the more comprehensive level II panel, which enables

TABLE 6. *Approach for detecting immunotoxic alterations*

Parameters	Procedures
LEVEL I (MOUSE OR RAT)	
Immunopathology	Routine hematology
	Lymphoid organ weights (spleen, thymus)
	Histology (spleen, thymus, lymph nodes)
	Cellularity (spleen, bone marrow)
Cell-mediated immunity Proliferation	Mixed leukocyte and mitogenic response
Tumoricidal	Natural killer cell activity
Humoral-mediated immunity	IgM antibody plaque-forming cells (PFCs)
	Specific antibody concentrations
LEVEL II (MOUSE ONLY)	
Immunopathology	Quantification of lymphocyte subpopulations using surface markers (monoclonal antibody reagents)
Host resistance challenge models	PYB6 sarcoma
	B16F10 melanoma
	Listeria monocytogenes
	Streptococcus
	Influenza virus
	Plasmodium yoelli
Cell-mediated immunity	Delayed hypersensitivity or cytotoxic lymphocyte (CTL)-mediated tumor cell cytolysis
Humoral-mediated immunity	IgG antibody PFCs
Macrophage function	Phagocytosis
	Ectoenzymes

confirmation of immune modulation, assessment of host susceptibility to disease, and determination of the cell populations affected.

Design of Immunotoxicity Assessment Protocols

When designing protocols for assessing immunotoxicity, special attention should be given to the choice of species and

TABLE 7. *Possible indicators of immunotoxic effect observed during toxicological evaluation of chemicals*

Increased mortality due to infectious agent
Type of neoplasia
Altered hematology parameter
Changes in lymphoid organ/body weight ratio (thymus, spleen)
Changes in lymphoid organ cellularity (bone marrow, spleen)
Changes in histology of lymphoid organs (thymus, nodes, spleen, bone marrow)

age of the animals; the duration, dosage, and route of exposure; and the pharmacokinetics and disposition of the compound. The rationale for selecting the inbred B6C3F1 mouse for immunotoxicity studies at the NTP (101) was based on the fact that the immune system of inbred mice is the best characterized of all rodents; there is less variation in organ weights and organ function measurements in inbred species; functional assays and tumor and infectious agent challenge models are better defined; and monoclonal antibody reagents are available to analyze and isolate lymphoid subpopulations. It should be noted that the rat is frequently used for toxicity assessment and can accommodate assays in level I, although the level II assays (Table 6) are more difficult in the rat. The high degree of homology between the proteins of man and nonhuman primate species and the potential for sequential monitoring of hematological and immunological parameters appear to make these species ideal for safety assessment of biotherapeutics produced by recombinant DNA methods.

The exposure interval required for a chemical to produce an immune alteration depends on the disposition, metabolism requirements, pharmacokinetics, the type of immunological injury, and the functional reserve of the immune parameter affected. In general, a repeat-dosing protocol of 14 to 30 days is recommended in young adult animals (6–8 weeks) for assessing chemical-induced alterations in immune competence, although longer exposure is sometimes necessary with certain chemicals to achieve a steady state (e.g., metals).

Dose selection involves consideration of known information about the effect of the chemical on general toxicological parameters (e.g., LD_{50}, LD_{10}) and the type of acute or subchronic toxicity observed. Careful dose selection is critical for assessing immunomodulatory compounds; high doses producing overt toxicity or severe weight loss should be avoided, as severe stress and malnutrition may modulate certain immune functions. The intended therapeutic range of the compound is also an important consideration when testing immunoenhancing agents, and multiples of the therapeutic dose are generally recommended. To establish dose-effect relations, three or more exposure levels are recommended. Ideally, the highest dose approaches the maximum tolerated dose (MTD) and has minimal associated mortality; dilutions of this dose (e.g., one-half MTD, one-tenth MTD) are suggested.

The route of exposure should, when possible, mimic the expected route of exposure in man. For many chemicals, oral exposure (i.e., feeding or gavage) is preferred. When an accurately delivered dose is desirable, parenteral, subcutaneous, or intraperitoneal exposure can also be used. In the case of airborne agents, inhalation exposure is recommended.

Our laboratories are beginning to investigate a third-level tier in which human peripheral blood lymphocytes (PBLs) are preincubated *in vitro* with the chemical under study prior to analysis in various humoral and cell-mediated immune function assays. Human PBLs may be isolated from anticoagulated peripheral blood of normal volunteers by centrifugation on a number of standard density gradient separation media. These assays can also be coupled with microsomal preparations where metabolism of the compound is required to demonstrate the immunomodulatory effect(s).

Methods Utilized for Level I Immunotoxicology Assessment

Immunopathology

Routine histopathology of bone marrow, thymus, spleen, and lymph node, a hemogram (complete blood count and differential), and the cellularity of the spleen are useful for assessing the immunomodulatory activity of a drug or nondrug chemical, particularly when these data are combined with effects observed in lymphoid organ weights (e.g., spleen, thymus, lymph node). Because of the structural division of the spleen and lymph nodes into thymus-dependent and thymus-independent compartments, careful microscopic examination may indicate preferential effects of the chemical for T or B cells. Likewise, microscopic examination of the thymus may reveal a compound that alters T cell maturation.

The following functional tests are performed in our laboratories for level I assays in the B6C3F1 mouse; they are applicable for other rodent species with some modification. The authors have avoided recommendations with regard to specific vendors for reagents.

Mixed Lymphocyte Response Assay

The proliferative response of T lymphocytes in the spleen to surface antigens on allogeneic cells (e.g., Ia and H-2 antigens) provides a sensitive indicator for cell-mediated immune competence and for detecting chemical-induced immunosuppression. From a clinical viewpoint, the mixed lymphocyte response (MLR) assay measures responses involved in graft rejection and graft-versus-host reactions. The assay has been shown to be predictive of host response to organ transplants; it represents the recognition phase for the generation of cytotoxic T lymphocytes and is believed to assess general immunocompetence (49). The MLR is generally performed in a unidirectional assay where the stimulator cells are inactivated by mitomycin C or irradiation prior to addition to culture.

Materials and reagents

RPMI-1640 medium with 25 mM Hepes supplemented with 5×10^{-5} M 2-mercaptoethanol (2-ME), 2 mM glutamine, gentamicin or penicillin/streptomycin, and 5 to 10% heat-inactivated serum [human AB serum, fetal calf serum (FCS), or a combination of AB and FCS may be used]. The investigator should evaluate a number of test lots of serum and perform checkerboard titrations to optimize the assay for their specific application; mitomycin C; ^{3}H-TdR (6.7 Ci/mM); trypan blue (0.08%); balanced salt solution (BSS); concanavalin A (Con A); aqueous counting scintillant; and round-bottomed 96-well tissue culture treated plates are also needed.

Procedure

1. Prepare single cell suspensions (SCSs) from spleens of control and chemically exposed mice in RPMI medium. These cells are referred to as the "responder" population.
2. Determine the cell concentration and correct for viability. Bring the SCSs to a final concentration of 1×10^6 cells/ml and add 0.1 ml of this suspension (1×10^5 cells total) to a minimum of four wells of a 96-well round-bottomed tissue culture plate.
3. Prepare SCSs from spleens of DBA/2 mice. For a typical assay splenocytes from four or five animals may be pooled. These cells are referred to as the "stimulator" population.
4. Bring cells to a volume of 1×10^7 to 2×10^7 cells/ml in serum-free RPMI. Add 50 μg of mitomycin C (MMC) (100 μl of 0.5 mg/ml stock) per milliliter of cell suspension. Cover tube with foil to prevent light inactivation of MMC and incubate in a waterbath shaker at 37°C for 45 min.
5. Wash cells three times in an excess of BSS or RPMI. Perform a cell count and correct for viability. Bring to a final concentration of 3×10^6 to 4×10^6 cells/ml.
6. Stimulator cells are added (0.1 ml) to quadruplicate wells of responder cells prepared above (3×10^5 to 4×10^5 total) to give an optimum stimulatory ratio of 3:1 or 4:1, which should be predetermined prior to assay. Include control rows for DBA/2 cells to which 0.1 ml of an optimum concentration of Con A is added to ensure nonproliferation of MMC-treated stimulator cells.
7. Incubate cultures for 120 hr at 37°C in an atmosphere of 5% CO_2 with 95% relative humidity. At 18 hr prior to termination, pulse each well with 1 μCi of ^{3}H-TdR in a volume of 10 to 50 μl. Each laboratory should determine the optimum time of cell harvest (e.g., 4–6 days of culture) and optimum stimulator/responder cell ratio (3:1 to 4:1).
8. Harvesting of each microculture is accomplished with an automatic cell harvester, and incorporation of ^{3}H-TdR is determined in a β-scintillation counter. Data are expressed as average counts per minute (cpm) of MLR wells minus the cpm of control wells, which contain responder but not stimulator cells. The MLR response is then compared between control and chemically exposed groups for statistical changes using Dunnett's multicomparison test.

Sources of error and variability

1. Different lots of FCS and human AB serum may vary in their ability to support the proliferation of responder cells in the assay. A variety of vendors, test lots, and serum concentrations should be evaluated.
2. Mitomycin C is cytotoxic, and it is critical that the stimulator cells are washed exhaustively prior to adding the responding population.
3. Mitomycin C may cause cell clumping, which may interfere with accurate quantitation and dispensing, or may decrease the yield of treated cells. Irradiation with cobalt (^{60}Co) or cesium (^{137}Cs) is often used as an alternative (2,000 rad).
4. The age and health status of the mice used as a source of stimulator cells is an important consideration. Animals

should be approximately 8 to 12 weeks of age and maintained under specific pathogen-free conditions.

Lymphocyte Blastogenesis to Mitogens

The lymphocyte blastogenesis assay is a relatively simple and reproducible procedure employed to measure the proliferative capacity of splenic or peripheral blood T and B lymphocytes to selected plant lectins (mitogens) or bacterial lipopolysaccharides. Decreased lymphocyte proliferation is thought to represent impaired host immune competence and to be indicative of an immunotoxic effect by the chemical being tested.

Materials and reagents

They are the same as for the MLR assay with the following exceptions or additions: No 2-ME; flat bottom 96-well tissue culture plates; Con A and lipopolysaccharide (LPS). The mitogens are diluted, filter-sterilized, and stored frozen at −70°C in small aliquots that are 100 to 1,000 times the working concentration.

Procedure

1. Prepare SCSs from spleens of control and treated mice in RPMI medium and determine cell number and viability. Dilute the SCSs to a final concentration of 2×10^6 cells/ml. The serum concentration should be doubled if the mitogen solutions are prepared in serum-free medium.
2. Aliquot 0.1 ml of cell suspension into quadruplicate flat-bottomed wells of a 96-well tissue culture plate (2×10^5 cells/well).
3. Dilute mitogen in RPMI medium. The optimal mitogen concentrations are determined by titration. Generally, three concentrations of Con A and two concentrations of LPS are used. Add 0.1 ml of mitogen solution at each concentration to quadruplicate samples as prepared above.
4. Incubate cultures for 72 hr at 37°C in an atmosphere of 5% CO_2 with 95% relative humidity. Eighteen hours prior to termination, pulse each well with 1 μCi of ^{3}H-TdR in a volume of 10 to 50 μl.
5. Harvest cultures with an automatic harvesting system and determine incorporation of ^{3}H-TdR in a β-scintillation counter. Data are expressed as the averaged cpm of each mitogen concentration for each exposure group compared to the corresponding cpm for control animals.

Sources of error and variability

1. The comments made with regard to serum for the MLR assay apply for mitogen proliferation as well.
2. Mitogens are variable among vendors and lots relative to the amount required for the optimum blastogenic dose. A dose-response curve consisting of five concentrations

should be developed for each new lot to select the optimum, suboptimum, and supraoptimum concentrations.

NK Cell Assay

Natural killer cells are lymphoid cells that are capable of lysing tumor cells without prior immunological memory or class I or II antigen restriction. These cells play a major role in inhibiting the growth of primary tumors and the development of metastases. In addition, NK cells may be involved in the control of microbial infections, and they play a role in immune regulation.

Materials and reagents

They are the same as for the MLR assay with the following exceptions and additions: sodium chromate-51 (sp. act. 200–500 mCi/mg); Triton X-100; and YAC-1 cell line (ATCC No. TIB-160).

Procedure

Radiolabeling of target cells for in vitro cytolysis.
1. Label 2×10^6 to 4×10^6 log phase YAC-1 cells in 0.2 ml of serum with 150 μCi sodium chromate-51 by incubation for 45 min at 37°C in a shaking waterbath.
2. Pellet the labeled cells, discard the supernatant in a radioactive waste container, and wash three times with BSS.
3. Resuspend cells in complete medium after the final wash. Determine cell viability and number by trypan blue dye exclusion in a hemacytometer designated for use with radiolabeled cells.
4. Prepare suspension of ^{51}Cr-YAC-1 at 1×10^5 viable cells/ml for addition to wells containing effector cells (final target cell density is 1×10^4 cells/well).

Preparation of effector cells and in vitro NK cytolysis assay.
1. Prepare single-cell suspensions in the medium and adjust the final density to 1×10^7 viable cells/ml.
2. Make a twofold dilution of the cell suspension (to yield 5×10^6/ml) so that the final effector/target cell ratios are 100:1 and 50:1.
3. Dispense 0.1 ml of each cell aliquot prepared in step 2 to quadruplicate wells to complete a row of 12 wells.
4. Dispense 0.1 ml medium per well to one row not containing murine effector cells for determining spontaneous releasable (SR) counts.
5. Dispense 0.1 ml 0.05% Triton-X to another row of empty wells for determining total releasable (TR) counts.
6. Add 0.1 ml ^{51}Cr-YAC-1 target cells prepared as above to all wells and centrifuge for 10 min at 1,200 rpm.
7. Incubate the plate 4 hr at 37°C in a humidified 5% CO_2 incubator.
8. Supernatants are harvested using a semiautomatic harvesting system.
9. Radiolabel released into the supernatants is quantitated

in a gamma counter, and the percent specific cytolysis is determined using the formula

% Specific cytolysis

$$= \frac{\text{exptl. release} - \text{spontaneous release}}{\text{total release} - \text{spontaneous release}} \times 100$$

Sources of error and variability

1. NK activity is greatest in relatively young mice, being maximal in mice up to 12 weeks of age. Basal NK activity may be undetectable in mice over 20 weeks old.
2. The YAC-1 cell line must be in the log phase of growth in order to achieve adequate labeling with ^{51}Cr. Sufficient cells are maintained in liquid nitrogen for reintroduction to culture if difficulty is noted in labeling cells that have been passed in culture for an extended period of time. In addition, the YAC-1 cell lines are assessed for *Mycoplasma* contamination at periodic intervals.

IgM Plaque-Forming Cell Response

Within a few days following *in vivo* injection of a foreign antigen, antibody molecules of the IgM class are produced and released from plasma cells into the systemic circulation. The antibody plaque-forming cell (PFC) assay quantitates the production of specific antibody through enumeration of antibody-producing cells in the spleen following a primary antigenic stimulus such as sheep red blood cells (SRBCs). Although the antibody PFC response to SRBCs is a measure of B cell function, it is an excellent functional parameter to examine, as it requires cell–cell interaction and regulation by macrophages and T cells.

Materials and reagents

Sheep red blood cells, a Cunningham slide chamber, and guinea pig complement are required.

Procedure

1. Mice are immunized intravenously with 0.2 ml of a 5% suspension of SRBCs (5×10^8 cells) 4 days prior to PFC analysis. Each laboratory should run a time course study to determine the optimum day of response between 3 and 5 days.
2. Prepare SCSs from the immunized spleens of control and chemically exposed mice in complete medium.
3. Wash SRBCs three times in BSS and adjust to 12% (v/v) in complete medium.
4. Reconstitute guinea pig complement, absorb each milliliter with 100 μl of packed SRBCs for 20 min at 4°C. Centrifuge for 5 min at 4°C and remove the complement from the RBC pellet and store in an ice bucket. Dilute the preparation from 1:2 to 1:4 for use. Each new test lot of complement should be titrated prior to use.

5. Mix 0.1 ml of complement, 0.3 ml of 12% SRBCs, and 1×10^6 viable splenocytes; adjust to 1.0 ml with complete medium.

6. Pipette 25 μl of each splenocyte mixture into two to four chambers and seal with Vasoline. Include control slides containing splenocytes obtained from mice that were not injected with SRBCs. Incubate for 1.0 to 1.5 hr at 37°C until PFCs are fully visible.

7. Count the number of plaques per chamber and determine the average of the replicate chambers. Determine the number of PFCs per 10^6 splenocytes by using a correction factor (i.e., 1000 μl added to chamber) of 40, as only 25 μl of a 1 ml preparation was analyzed per chamber. The number of PFCs per spleen may be calculated by correcting for the original volume of SCSs obtained.

Sources of error and variability

1. The PFC response varies greatly depending on the day of analysis following immunization. Each species and strain should be evaluated for the optimum PFC response.

2. The dose and route of antigen exposure alter the peak PFC response. Intravenous injections shift the optimum response to an earlier time, whereas an intraperitoneal injection delays the peak response.

3. Complement must be absorbed with packed SRBCs at 4°C and diluted properly to maintain consistency.

4. The day of antibody induction relative to the last dose of chemical exposure should be considered.

XENOBIOTICS PRODUCING IMMUNOTOXICITY: MECHANISMS OF ACTION

A substantial data base exists demonstrating that a broad spectrum of environmental pollutants and drugs can alter immune function in laboratory animals as well as in humans occupationally or accidentally exposed (Table 8). This identification of the immune system as a sensitive target organ for chemicals has prompted additional research into the subcellular and molecular events responsible for the immunotoxicologic manifestation of certain xenobiotics. The following represent some examples of compounds shown to modulate immune function and is representative of those xenobiotics that have been examined in depth.

Polycyclic Aromatic Hydrocarbons

Polycyclic aromatic hydrocarbons (PAHs) form a class of widely disseminated compounds consisting of fused benzene rings sharing an anthracene nucleus. These compounds are formed as products of incomplete combustion of fossil fuels and can be found as environmental contaminants in tobacco smoke, soot, coke, and automobile exhaust (169). A lesser quantity is also produced via bacteria and plants. Human exposures occur primarily through inhalation or ingestion. Human health risks associated with PAHs have centered pri-

TABLE 8. *Selected examples of chemical exposure in rodents and humans associated with immunological disturbance*

Chemical class	Example[a]	Immune disturbance	
		Rodent	Man
Polyhalogenated	TCDD	+	+
aromatic	PCB	+	+
hydrocarbons	PBB	+	+
	HCB	+	+
Heavy metals	Lead	+	+
	Cadmium	+	+
	Methyl mercury	+	+
Polycyclic aromatic	DMBA	+	N.K.[b]
hydrocarbons	BaP	+	N.K.
Organotins	DOTC	+	N.K.
	DBTC	+	N.K.
Aromatic amines	Benzidines	+	+
Oxidant gases (air	NO$_2$		
pollutants)	O$_3$	+	+
	SO$_3$		
Aromatic hydrocarbons	Organic solvents	+	+
Others	Asbestos	+	+
	DMN	+	+
	DES	+	+

[a] TCDD, 2,3,7,8-tetrachlorodibenzo-*p*-dioxin; PCB, polychlorinated biphenyls; PBB, polybrominated biphenyls; DOTC, di-*n*-octyltin dichloride; DBTC, di-*n*-butyltin dichloride; HCB, hexachlorobenzene; DMBA, 7,12-dimethylbenz(a)anthracene; BaP, benzo(a)pyrene; DMN, dimethylnitrosamine; DES, diethylstilbestrol.

[b] N.K. = not known.

marily around their carcinogenic potential. A correlation that has emerged following examination of their immunotoxicity indicates that PAHs that are carcinogenic possess potent immunosuppressive properties, whereas those that are not carcinogenic lack substantial immunosuppressive effects (156). This finding has led to the suggestion that a chemical's potential to cause immunosuppression may serve as a cofactor for carcinogenicity by altering immunocompetence and allowing tumor neoantigens to bypass normal host immune surveillance and, once established, prevent normal immune mechanisms from inhibiting tumor growth and metastasis.

In experimental studies, suppression of humoral immunity has been a frequent observation following exposure to a number of PAHs, including benzo(*a*)pyrene [B(*a*)P], 7,12-dimethylbenzanthracene (DMBA), and 3-methylcholanthrene (3-MC) (25,88,156). These three substances have been shown to suppress the antibody response to T-dependent (SRBCs) as well as T-independent (TNP-carrier) antigens (24,139,158,160). In the case of DMBA, the suppression in antibody-forming cell responses persisted more than 8 weeks after exposure (157). Although humoral immunosuppression following DMBA exposure may reside at the level of T cell regulation, reduced progenitor B cells (CFU-BL) in exposed animals suggest that B cells may be directly targeted early in their maturational process (158). B(*a*)P has been shown to also impair production of IL1, implicating chemical-induced defects in accessory cell function as a contributing factor in decreased antibody-forming cell production (93).

Cell-mediated immunity is also inhibited by PAHs. Cytotoxic T cell activity is suppressed by DMBA or 3-MC following *in vitro* as well as *in vivo* exposure in mice (27,28,84,166). Additional measures of CMI suppressed following DMBA, B(a)P, and 3-MC exposure include mixed lymphocyte responsiveness and NK cell activity (27,28, 84,144,158). Apparently, because of more pronounced CMI effects, DMBA, but not B(a)P, demonstrated a marked increase in host susceptibility to *Listeria monocytogenes* and PYB6 sarcoma challenges (158). Lack of immunomodulatory effects on cell-mediated immunocompetence were previously reported for B(a)P (22). Addition of IL2 or T-helper cells, but not IL1, to cultures of DMBA-exposed lymphocytes restored cytotoxic T lymphocyte (CTL) function, suggesting that T-helper cells may be a sensitive target following *in vitro* and *in vivo* exposure (54).

Halogenated Aromatic Hydrocarbons

Halogenated aromatic hydrocarbons (HAHs) form a family of compounds with widespread environmental distribution. Primary sources of HAHs are commercial ventures that produce industrial chemicals, pesticides, flame retardants, and heat conductors; HAHs are also by-products during the manufacture of halogenated biphenyls or phenols and at commercial incinerators. Laboratory studies have demonstrated that a number of HAHs possess immunomodulatory potential, including specific chlorinated dibenzo-*p*-dioxins, dibenzofurans, hexachlorobenzene, polychlorinated biphenyls (PCBs), and polybrominated biphenyls (127,141). Additionally, selected isomers of this class of compounds have been associated with teratogenic, carcinogenic, neurotoxic, and hepatotoxic effects (68).

The first indication that PCBs affected the immune system stemmed from observations of altered weight and histology of lymphoid organs in experimental animal studies (153). Functionally, PCB-mediated immunotoxicity in laboratory animals is characterized by suppressed humoral immunity. Administration of Aroclor or highly chlorinated biphenyls to guinea pigs (153), rabbits (73), rhesus monkeys (142), or mice (125,163) inhibits antibody production. The effects on CMI are less clear. PCBs have been reported to suppress DTH reactions in guinea pigs (151) but not mitogenic responses, MLRs, graft-versus-host reactions, or cytotoxic T lymphocyte activity of spleen cells in mice (126). PCBs also alter host resistance to a number of infectious agents including *Plasmodium berghei* (86), *Listeria monocytogenes* (130), *Salmonella typhimurium* (142), and herpes simplex (56). Increased tumor growth following inoculation with Walkers 256 carcinoma cells (67) and Ehrlich's ascites tumor (64), but not Moloney leukemia virus (69) or MKSA or L1210 tumor cell implants (85), occurs in PCB-exposed animals. Immunological changes consistent with those seen in animal studies have been reported in individuals accidentally exposed in Japan and Taiwan to PCBs and PCDFs through consumption of contaminated rice oil (82,167).

2,3,7,8-Tetrachlorodibenzo-*p*-dioxin (TCDD) has been the most widely studied HAH. Predominant features of TCDD toxicity include myelosuppression, immunodysregulation, and thymic atrophy; these reactions occur in most species examined thus far and at concentrations that preclude overt toxicity (22,88,141,153). TCDD administered to mice has been associated with thymic atrophy, myelotoxicity, inhibition of complement system components, suppression of lymphocyte function, and impaired host resistance to challenge with *Salmonella bern* and *Plasmodium yoelii,* but not *Listeria monocytogenes* (89,91). It appears that macrophage and NK functions are spared any measurable effect (80,96). As probably occurs with a number of immunosuppressive HAHs, the specific effects of TCDD on the immune system can vary depending on the age of the animal relative to chemical exposure. For example, the primary effect following perinatal TCDD exposure is persistent suppression of cellular immunity, a condition mimicking neonatal thymectomy (150). In contrast to perinatal exposure, TCDD exposure in adult mice, although still inducing deterioration of thymic tissue (predominantly cortical lymphoid depletion), causes a transient antiproliferative response in rapidly dividing cell populations including progenitor hematopoietic cells and B lymphocytes (35,143). The marked and persistent suppression of T cell function seen in neonates is not manifested following adult exposure, although suppression of the cytotoxic T lymphocyte response is reported to occur (15).

Regardless of the status of maturity at the time of exposure, immunosuppression by TCDD, as well as PCBs, is believed to be mediated via stereospecific and irreversible binding to an intracellular receptor protein found in the cellular targets for TCDD, including lymphoid tissue, bone marrow cells, and thymic epithelium (141). This receptor is termed the *Ah* receptor and is controlled by the *Ah* locus, which is also responsible for microsomal enzyme production. Evidence for the association of TCDD immunotoxicity with *Ah* genotype was derived from immune studies comparing inbred strains of *Ah*-responsive and *Ah*-nonresponsive mice in which the ability of TCDD to cause immunotoxicity coordinated with the presence of the *Ah* locus (143,145). Additionally, a good correlation exists between the binding affinities of various HAHs and their ability to induce immunotoxicity (128,143).

The role, if any, of microsomal enzyme induction in the cellular mechanism(s) responsible for inducing immunotoxicity following the binding of TCDD to its receptor are unknown. The observation that thymic epithelium contains relatively high concentrations of receptor suggests that TCDD may be inducing maturational defects in developing thymocytes (47). Studies performed using thymic epithelial cell cultures have shown that binding of TCDD to the *Ah* receptor results in the terminal differentiation of these cells and the loss of supportive microenvironment required for thymocyte maturation (47). Data suggest that cellular targets other than T cells (e.g., bone marrow cells and B cells) may be susceptible to similar patterns of altered cell proliferation and maturation following TCDD binding to the *Ah* receptor found in these cells (92). Studies examining the effects of TCDD on B cell maturation have shown that TCDD selectively inhibited late stages of the cell cycle and the development of B cells into plasma cells. TCDD was required at the time of initial lymphoid cell activation to be effective, suggesting that TCDD may interfere with early activation events of these cells (90).

Pesticides

A number of pesticides have been examined for immunotoxic potential in laboratory animals, including organochlorines and organophosphates (34a,149). The literature to date suggests that organochlorine compounds, including DDT, captan, and chlordane, can modulate immune function (4,5,44,63,137,140). Additionally, methylparathion has been shown to suppress immune function (140) and host resistance (37). Although the toxicity of most organophosphate pesticides is relatively low owing to their rapid detoxification by carboxyesterases, certain contaminants formed during their manufacture and storage have the capacity to inhibit carboxyesterase activity, and they have been shown to be immunotoxic (30,109,110). *O,O,S*-Trimethylphosphorothioate (*OOS*-TMP), a contaminant found in malathion, fenitrothion, and acephate, is immunotoxic at concentrations lower than those observed for other manifestations of its toxicity. Rodgers et al. (109,110) demonstrated that murine exposure to *OOS*-TMP, but not malathion, caused lymphocytopenia, thymic atrophy, suppression of antibody synthesis, and decreased CTL activity. Interestingly, neither IL2 production nor lymphoproliferative responses were affected. Macrophages treated with *OOS*-TMP have shown evidence of chemical-induced activation (e.g., inflammatory macrophages), suggesting that the immunosuppressive profile demonstrated with *OOS*-TMP *in vivo* may relate to alterations in tissue macrophages. Although the molecular mechanisms involved in *OOS*-TMP immunosuppression have not been elucidated, alterations in cholinesterase activity do not seem to play a role, as *O,O,S*-trimethylphosphorodithioate, a structural analog of *OOS*-TMP, modulates cholinesterase activity without affecting immunocompetence (30,110).

Metals

Inorganic Metals

Heavy metals, including lead, cadmium, and mercury, have been shown by a number of investigators to be capable of altering immune responsiveness in laboratory animals (71,81). This literature indicates that although immunosuppression is a frequent manifestation of exposure, immunopotentiation may also result. This apparent divergence may stem from differences in animal species used, the dose and route of administration, and the type of assay system employed. Alterations in B lymphocyte function have been the most frequent observation following exposure to lead and cadmium, although T cell and macrophage dysfunctions have also been described (8,36,66). Studies examining the effects of heavy metals on host resistance have shown a strong correlation between metal exposure and impaired ability to resist bacterial or viral challenges, an observation that does not always correlate with alterations in B cell or T cell activity. Along these lines, heavy metals have been shown to synergize with injected bacterial endotoxin in mice and dramatically increase the likelihood of endotoxin shock (17,18). Lead acetate exposure in mice altered endotoxin-induced reticuloendothelial cell activities (117), including lipid peroxidation, reactive oxygen intermediates, and glutathione-associated

enzymes, findings that may account for increased susceptibility following bacterial and viral challenge.

The divergent data reported on inorganic metal interactions with the immune system suggest that more than one mechanism may be operable in the immunotoxicity and impaired host resistance associated with this class of compounds. Although defects in B cell function have been suggested to reside at the level of plasma cell development (70), impaired accessory cell function or deficient complement system components have also been implicated (34,58). The subcellular mechanism involved in metal-induced immunotoxicity is complex. Lead as well as cadmium are sulfhydryl alkylating agents with high binding affinity for cellular sulfhydryl groups, and it has been suggested that these metals alter lymphocyte function by modulating membrane-bound thiols (8). This observation is strengthened by the fact that suppressive effects of lead, at least *in vitro*, can be reversed by the addition of exogenous thiol reagents (8).

The augmentation of B or T cell responsiveness discussed above could precipitate autoimmunity, and metals have been implicated in influencing autoimmune disorders, although the precise cellular mechanism is poorly understood (81). Glomerulonephritis, arthritis, and interstitial nephritis have been suggested to have an immunologic pathogenesis and have been associated with exposure to mercury, gold, and lead, respectively (81). Experimentally, administration of mercury has been shown to induce polyclonal activation of B cells, resulting in increased antibody synthesis to self-antigens (52). Thus metal-induced tissue damage resulting in altered self-antigens and loss of tolerance or stimulation of immune system components may be partially responsible for metal-induced autoimmune diseases.

Evidence suggesting that human exposure to metals may result in immune system defects has been reported. Workers in the lead industry with blood lead levels of 52 μg/100 g have demonstrated decreased levels of serum complement components as well as depressed levels of secretory IgA (34). Children with elevated blood lead levels and infected with the gram-negative bacterium *Shigella enteritis* had prolonged manifestations of the illness (116). Additionally, lead smelters have been reported to have a greater incidence of influenza infections (34). The cationic heavy metals mercury, gold, and lead have been associated with immune complex diseases in humans (81,95).

Organotins

Organotin compounds are utilized primarily as heat stabilizers, industrial and agricultural biocides, and industrial catalysts in the production of foams and rubbers. Immunotoxic properties have been attributed to a number of organic tin compounds (122,154). Rats fed dibutyltin exhibited a dose-related decrease in thymus, spleen, and lymph node weights histologically associated with depletion of lymphocytes (74) in the periarteriolar lymphocyte sheath (spleen and thymus) and paracortical areas (lymph nodes). Depletion of lymphocytes from the thymic cortex occurs without causing cytolysis, myelotoxicity, or nonlymphoid toxicity (98). Immune function of rats exposed to dialkyltins demonstrated suppression of CMI parameters including increased skin graft rejection time, suppressed DTH, and decreased T cell mitogenesis (121). These immunologic defects appear to be species-specific, as neither immune function nor lymphoid atrophy is impaired in mice or guinea pigs fed dialkyltins.

A cellular depletion mechanism may be partly responsible for observed decreases in CMI, as decreased T cell mitogen responsiveness correlated with decreased numbers of circulating lymphocytes with T cell surface markers. Additionally, suppression of T-helper cells resulting in altered regulation may account for the decreases observed in the T-dependent humoral immunity in these studies (121,123). Another class of organotin compounds, triorganotins (e.g., tri-n-butyltin; TBT) have been shown to induce thymic atrophy and suppress CMI (133,152). However, following oral administration in the rat, these compounds are rapidly dealkylated, and thymus atrophy is mediated by the dealkylated metabolite of tributyltin, dibutyltin (132).

Studies examining the mechanisms involved in organotin-induced thymic atrophy demonstrated a significant increase in the consumption of glucose and accumulated pyruvate and lactate in thymocytes incubated with a number of dialkyltins (103). This class of compounds has been indirectly shown to inhibit α-keto acid-oxidizing enzyme complexes in mitochondria: pyruvate dehydrogenase and α-ketoglutarate dehydrogenase (103,105). Thus organotins may interfere directly with lymphocyte function or thymocyte maturation by inhibiting glucose metabolism via disturbances in mitochondrial respiration. Apart from inhibiting cellular energetics, alterations found in DNA, RNA, and protein synthesis in isolated rat thymocytes may also account for the particular sensitivity of this primary lymphoid organ (99,104).

Inhaled Pollutants

The respiratory tract is a major route of exposure for many industrial and environmental xenobiotics. Consequently, the lungs and associated pulmonary defense mechanisms are often targets of airborne chemicals. Because of their strategic location within the lung, alveolar macrophages provide a first-line defense mechanism against inhaled pollutants. An extensive data base exists on xenobiotic-induced alterations in alveolar macrophage function (11). Additional immunologic defense mechanisms also operable in the respiratory tract include HI and CMI responses of lung bronchial associated lymphoid tissue (6) as well as NK activity in interstitial lung tissue (138). However, much less information is available on the mechanism by which inhaled pollutants modulate these immunologic processes. Of the multitude of pollutants that exist in the ambient or industrial atmosphere, only a few have been examined for their immunotoxic potential. The following discussion represents some of those xenobiotics that have been studied in depth.

Benzene

The toxicity of benzene has been the subject of considerable research for more than a century, with particular emphasis on its hematologic and leukemogenic potential (135). In humans, the predominant hemopathy associated with benzene

exposure is pancytopenia, with associated bone marrow hypoplasia (45). Although hematopoietic progenitor cells are particularly susceptible to benzene, the mature circulating lymphocyte also responds to benzene via an antiproliferative response (134). For example, suppression of B and T cell mitogenesis and mixed leukocyte responsiveness has been reported following benzene inhalation in rodents (114,115). Additionally, Wierda and Irons (162) demonstrated that administration of benzene or the hydroquinone and catechol metabolites to mice resulted in suppression of mitogenesis and antibody production. Host resistance studies have demonstrated impaired resistance to *Listeria monocytogenes* in mice exposed to benzene concentrations as low as 30 ppm (113). Studies employing PYB6 tumor cell challenge similarly demonstrated increased susceptibility at concentrations of benzene that also impaired CTL-mediated tumor cell cytolysis (114). Additional evidence of increased host susceptibility was supported from early studies demonstrating increased susceptibility to tuberculosis (161) and pneumonia (165) in benzene-exposed rabbits. These studies are consistent with reports of severe benzene toxicity in humans, which has been characterized by acute, overwhelming infections (57). Additional evidence for the immunotoxic potential of benzene in humans includes reports of depressed levels of serum complement and IgG and IgA circulating immunoglobulins in chronically exposed workers (77,131), although these populations were exposed to other vapors as well.

The mechanism of benzene's toxic effects on immune system components remains unknown, partly because the precise toxic metabolite(s) responsible for immunotoxicity remain unidentified. The polyphenol and quinone metabolites of benzene have been shown to alter macrophage function, possibly through disruption of signal transduction systems (83a). A cellular depletion mechanism may be at least partially responsible for observed immunotoxicity, although evidence for defective B cell and T cell function also exists. The antiproliferative effects of benzene may relate to its ability to alter cytoskeletal development through inhibition of microtubule assembly. Polyhydroxy metabolites of benzene (*p*-benzoquinone and hydroquinone) have been shown to bind to sulfhydryl groups on proteins necessary for the integrity and polymerization of microtubules (106), which may alter cell membrane fluidity and may explain the sublethal effect of benzene on lymphocyte function.

Pollutant Gases

Ozone (O_3) is a photochemical oxidant resulting from atmospheric reactions of hydrocarbons and nitrogen oxides catalyzed by sunlight. The immunotoxicologic data on O_3 indicate marked impairment of the pulmonary host defense mechanisms (46). Laboratory studies have shown that mice exposed to concentrations as low as 0.1 ppm show decreased host resistance to bacterial challenge (16). Additionally, O_3 has been shown to increase the incidence of pulmonary infections induced by a number of other pathogenic organisms, including *Streptococcus* sp., *Pasteurella haemolytica*, and *Mycobacterium tuberculosis* (46). The increased susceptibility may relate to O_3-induced impairment in alveolar macrophage function. Studies supporting this supposition have demonstrated that exposure to O_3 can significantly decrease the number of alveolar macrophages (39), impair the phagocytic ability of alveolar macrophages (39), and decrease the ability of macrophages to secrete reactive oxygen intermediates (2) and interferon (124). O_3-induced systemic immune dysfunction has also been demonstrated (3) and cannot be ruled out as an additional factor in impaired host defense. Alterations in rabbit alveolar macrophage production of arachidonic acid metabolites [increased prostaglandin E_2 (PGE_2)] following *in vitro* and *in vivo* O_3 exposure has also been reported (31,118). These authors suggested that increased PGE_2 production represents a potential mechanism for the impaired alveolar macrophage function consistently observed in O_3-exposed animals. Nonimmunologic mechanisms may contribute to decreased host resistance. O_3-induced impairment in mucociliary clearance and increased mucous secretions could result in an accumulation of pathogenic organisms in a controlled study (65,79).

Nitrogen dioxide (NO_2) exposure appears to result in patterns of altered host resistance similar to those seen with O_3 exposure. Animals exposed to NO_2 respond to experimentally induced pulmonary infections in a concentration-dependent manner (46). Many parameters of alveolar macrophage function are impaired by NO_2 exposure, including phagocytosis (136), interferon production (41), recognition of tumorigenic cells (136), and bactericidal capacity (32). Morphological alterations observed in alveolar macrophages following NO_2 exposure most likely underlie the functional deficits observed in these cells (14). Systemically, NO_2 has been shown to suppress splenic T and B cell mitogenic responses (94) as well as the primary antibody response to SRBCs (38). However, the role of systemic immunity in pulmonary infectivity models is not fully understood.

Asbestos

Asbestos exposure in humans has long been associated with respiratory diseases, including fibrosis, asbestosis, and mesothelioma. Often associated with these conditions are alterations in cellular and humoral immune responses (97). Asbestos-associated impairments in CMI in humans are characterized by decreases in DTH responses, numbers of circulating T cells, and T cell mitogen proliferation (42,50,61,83). In contrast to the T cell suppression that is often observed in asbestosis patients, hyperactive B cell functions are observed that are manifested by increased levels of serum immunoglobulins (IgA, IgM, and IgG) and increased secretory IgA production (55,62,178). Kagan et al. (60) described a number of cases demonstrating an association between asbestos exposure and B cell lymphoproliferative disorders including neoplasia. Additionally, NK cell reactivity has been reported to be altered in individuals exposed to asbestos (43,76). Experimental studies have confirmed the immunomodulatory potential of asbestos, particularly at the level of the alveolar macrophage (97). Asbestos fibers reaching the distal airways are readily phagocytized by alveolar macrophages, eventually resulting in cell lysis and release of inflammatory products and lysosomal enzymes (100). In this regard, fiber size (length) has been shown to be an important factor in inducing macrophage toxicity, with decreased tox-

icity associated with reduced fiber length (13,155). Additionally, direct T cell–fiber interactions have been reported to result in altered immunoregulation (9). Suppression of *in vitro* T-dependent antibody responses following addition of chrysotile asbestos to spleen cell cultures has also been shown (159), a finding that was associated with dysfunction of an adherent cell population.

The data concerning modulation of immune function in humans exposed to asbestos are consistent with the loss of immunoregulatory control of alveolar macrophages. Macrophages are generally thought to down-regulate immune function in the respiratory tract under normal physiological circumstances (53). In a situation analogous to that described for silica, asbestos may exert an adjuvant-like response resulting in augmentation of immune system reactivity (97). However, the reported increased release of prostaglandins by macrophage cell lines and primary alveolar macrophage cultures (12,129) would be more consistent with asbestos-induced immunosuppression. Experimental studies examining the interactions of murine alveolar macrophages have shown that asbestos-exposed alveolar macrophages lose the capacity to suppress or down-regulate both T cell (10) and B cell mitogenesis and production of antibody to sheep red blood cells (112). A more thorough understanding of the role of asbestos in immunotoxicity will result as the immunoregulatory function of alveolar macrophages becomes better defined.

Beryllium

Beryllium is an industrial pollutant used in the manufacture of copper, nonsparking tools, lightweight alloys, and nuclear reactor components. Environmental beryllium contamination arises from coal combustion and to a lesser extent from its use as a rocket propellant. In humans, beryllium is associated with a number of diseases that clearly have an immunologic pathogenesis, i.e., beryllium dermatitis, acute beryllium pneumonitis, and chronic pulmonary granulomatosis (berylliosis) (107). Whereas beryllium-induced neoplasia in humans is controversial (119,120), osteocarcinoma and adenocarcinoma have been reported in experimental studies following administration of beryllium oxide and beryllium sulfate, respectively (40,146).

Immune system abnormalities associated with beryllium are believed to result from the antigenicity of various chemical forms of beryllium. Current dogma states that beryllium, a poorly soluble particle, is essentially a hapten that associates with tissue protein(s) resulting in a complete antigen (107). Evidence to support this statement can be found in studies showing that in $BeSO_4$-sensitized guinea pigs beryllium complexed with serum albumin resulted in a more intense cutaneous reaction than that produced by $BeSO_4$ alone (75). Clinical evidence of beryllium exposure is most often associated with blast-like transformation of T lymphocytes obtained from bronchoalveolar lavage as well as peripheral blood (48,59). The correlation of T lymphocyte blast transformation and beryllium hypersensitivity is so strong that for practical purposes the test has been used as a surveillance tool for berylliosis (29,164). Lymphocytes from beryllium workers restimulated with beryllium demonstrated an increased production of macrophage migration inhibitory factors (51), and this test has also been used to diagnose beryllium hypersensitivity. Additionally, cutaneous hypersensitivity demonstrated by positive patch test results has been often reported in beryllium-exposed workers (20). In light of the recognition of beryllium as a tissue antigen, increased levels of circulating immunoglobulins have been detected in beryllium workers and berylliosis patients; however, these antibodies were not shown to be specific for beryllium (108).

The precise mechanisms involved in beryllium-induced hypersensitivity remain poorly understood. The granulomatous hypersensitivity associated with beryllium is associated with a specific immune response to tissue contact and is mediated and perpetuated by the accumulation and proliferation of reticuloendothelial cells. It has been hypothesized that the pulmonary granuloma may represent a state of hypersensitivity induced by macrophage migration inhibitory factor, impeding the mobility of these cells in the presence of antigen (107). Increased numbers of T cells in bronchoalveolar lavage fluid of patients suffering from beryllium disease strengthen this theory (33). In fact, evidence of free activated pulmonary T cells is so frequent that berylliosis is often confused with sarcoidosis. Although the human data demonstrating the immunotoxic capacity of this compound are overwhelming, more experimental work is needed to increase our understanding of the molecular mechanisms involved in beryllium diseases.

CONCLUSIONS AND FUTURE DIRECTION

The immune system is composed of several cell populations where maturation of each is subject to orderly control by *endogenous* hormones and *exogenous* bacterial product. These mediators possess activation, growth-promotion, or differentiation properties and are under the influence of potent but not well understood regulators. From observations in rodents and limited studies in humans inadvertently exposed, it is apparent that a number of xenobiotics adversely affect the immune system through disruption of cell maturation, regulation, or cytotoxic processes. These examples and our current knowledge about the pathogenesis of disease support the possibility that chemical-induced damage to the immune system may be associated with a wide spectrum of diverse pathological conditions, some of which may become detectable only after a long latency. Likewise, exposure to immunoalterative xenobiotics might represent additional risk to individuals with already fragile immune systems (e.g., malnutrition, infancy, old age). However, it is important that caution be exercised when attempting to extrapolate meaningful conclusions from experimental data or isolated epidemiological studies to risk assessment for low-level human exposure.

Because of the functional heterogeneity of the immune system, efforts to assess chemical-induced immunotoxicity in laboratory animals have historically been performed using a tiered approach with multiple assays (23,72,148). The testing configuration described in this chapter (i.e., level I screening assays) is derived from a more comprehensive panel taken from the NTP's guidelines for immunotoxicity evaluation in mice (92). A similar configuration has been included in the Environmental Protection Agency's FIFRA regulations for immunotoxicity testing of biochemical pesticides. Each of the assays in level I has undergone extensive scrutiny in order to determine intra- and interlaboratory reproducibility, accuracy, sensitivity, and predictability (92). The configuration (level I) represents a limited screening effort that includes immunopathology as well as functional assays for CMI, HMI, and NK cell function. Although the probability of detecting potent immunotoxicants in level I is high, the likelihood of detecting weaker immunotoxicants, such as those that may affect only a specific cell population or subpopulation, is presumably less. Nonetheless, based on the data from compounds that have undergone a more stringent testing battery, almost all compounds that can be considered immunotoxic alter at least one parameter in level I. Thus although level I provides little information on the specific cell type responsible for the immune defect or its relevance to the host, it can readily discern immune alterations resulting from chemical exposure.

The value of incorporating immunological rodent data for the toxicological assessment of drugs, chemicals, and biologicals for human risk assessment has been increasingly accepted. The preceding decade of research has provided a data base of immunotoxic and nonimmunotoxic compounds, studies correlating immune dysfunction and altered host resistance, and a better standardized panel of methods for detecting immunomodulatory chemicals. In the near future, research related to methodology is needed to: (a) further refine and validate immune function tests and host resistance assays, particularly in the rat; (b) develop, refine, and validate better testing methods to evaluate the effects of chemical inhalation on lung immunity; (c) determine the need and relevance of methods for assessing hematopoietic and polymorphonuclear leukocyte functions; (d) develop and evaluate *in vitro* methodology as screens for detecting chemical-induced immunotoxicity using rodent and human immune cells; (e) develop improved methods for evaluating chemical-induced hypersensitivity and autoimmunity; and (f) develop a testing battery to examine dysfunction in humans occupationally or environmentally exposed to chemicals shown to be immunotoxic in laboratory animals.

REFERENCES

1. Alfred, L. J., and Wojdani, A. (1983): Effects of methylcholanthrene and benzanthracene on blastogenesis and aryl hydrocarbon hydroxylase induction in splenic lymphocytes from three inbred strains of mice. *Int. J. Immunopharmacol.*, 5:123–129.
2. Amoruso, M. A., Witz, G., and Goldstein, B. D. (1981): Decreased superoxide anion radical production by rat alveolar macrophages following inhalation of ozone or nitrogen dioxide. *Life Sci.*, 28:2215–2221.
3. Aranyi, C., Vana, S. C., Thomas, P. T., Bradof, J. N., Fenters, J. D., Graham, J. A., and Miller, F. J. (1983): Effects of subchronic exposure to a mixture of O_3, SO_2, $(NH_4)_2SO_4$, on host defenses in mice. *Environ. Res.*, 12:55–71.
4. Barnett, J. B., Spyker-Cranmer, J. M., Avery, P. C., and Hoberman, A. M. (1980): Immunocompetence over the lifespan of mice exposed in vitro to carbofuran or diazinon. *J. Environ. Pathol. Toxicol.*, 4:53–63.
5. Beggs, M., Menna, J. H., and Barnett, J. B. (1985): Effects of chlordane on influenza type A virus and herpes simplex type 1 virus replication in vitro. *J. Toxicol. Environ. Health.*, 16:173–188.

6. Bice, D. E. (1985): Methods and approaches for assessing immunotoxicity of the lower respiratory tract. In: *Immunotoxicology and Immunopharmacology,* edited by J. H. Dean, M. I. Luster, A. E. Munson, and H. Amos, pp. 145–157. Raven Press, New York.

7. Bick, P. H. (1985): The immune system: organization and function. In: *Immunotoxicology and Immunopharmacology,* edited by J. H. Dean, M. I. Luster, A. E. Munson, and H. Amos, pp. 1–10. Raven Press, New York.

8. Blakely, B. R., and Archer, D. L. (1981): The effects of lead acetate on the immune response of mice. *Toxicol. Appl. Pharmacol.,* 61: 18–26.

9. Bozelka, B. E., Gaumer, H. R., Nordberg, J., and Salvaggio, J. E. (1983): Asbestos-induced alterations of human lymphoid cell mitogenic responses. *Environ. Res.,* 30:281–290.

10. Bozelka, B. E., Sestini, P., Hammad, Y., and Salvaggio, J. E. (1986): Effects of asbestos fibers on alveolar macrophage-mediated lymphocyte cytostasis. *Environ. Res.,* 40:172–180.

11. Brain, J. D. (1986): Toxicological aspects of alterations of pulmonary macrophage function. *Annu. Rev. Pharmacol. Toxicol.,* 26:547–565.

12. Brown, R. C., and Poole, A. (1980): Arachidonic acid release and prostaglandin synthesis in a macrophage-like cell line exposed to asbestos. *Agents Actions,* 15:336–340.

13. Brown, R. C., Chamberlain, M., Griffiths, M., and Timbrell, V. (1978): The effect of fiber size on the in vitro biological activity of three types of amphibole asbestos. *Int. J. Cancer,* 22:721–727.

14. Brummer, M. E. G., Schwartz, L. W., and McQuillen, N. K. (1977): A quantitative study of lung damage by scanning electron microscopy: inflammatory cell responses to high ambient levels of ozone. *Scan. Electron Microsc.,* 2:513–518.

15. Clark, D. A., Gauldie, J., Szewcyk, M. R., and Sweeney, G. (1981): Enhanced suppressor cell activity as a mechanism of immunosuppression by TCDD. *Proc. Soc. Exp. Biol. Med.,* 168:290–299.

16. Coffin, D. L., and Gardner, D. E. (1972): Interactions of biological agents and chemical air pollutants. *Ann. Occup. Hyg.,* 15:219–235.

17. Cook, J. A., and Karns, L. (1978): Effects of RES stimulation and suppression on lead sensitization to endotoxin shock. *J. Reticuloendothel. Soc.,* 24:1A.

18. Cook, J. A., Hoffman, E. D., and DiLuzio, N. R. (1975): Influence of lead and cadmium on the susceptibility of rats to bacterial challenge. *Proc. Soc. Exp. Biol. Med.,* 150:741–747.

19. Coombs, R. R. A., and Gell, P. G. H. (1975): Classification of allergic reactions responsible for clinical hypersensitivity and disease. In: *Clinical Aspects of Immunology,* edited by P. G. H. Gell, R. R. A. Coombs, and P. J. Lachman, p. 761. Lippincott, Philadelphia.

20. Curtis, G. H. (1959): The diagnosis of beryllium disease with special reference to the patch test. *Arch. Industr. Health,* 19:150–153.

21. Dean, J. H., and Adams, D. O. (1986): The effects of environmental agents on cells of the mononuclear phagocyte system. In: *The Reticulo-Endothelial System: A Comprehensive Treatise, Vol. V: Immunopharmacology of the Reticulo-endothelial System,* edited by J. Hadden and A. Szentivany, pp. 389–409. Plenum Press, New York.

22. Dean, J. H., and Lauer, L. D. (1983): Immunological effects following exposure to 2,3,7,8-tetrachlorodibenzo-p-dioxin: a review. In: *Public Health Risks of the Dioxins,* edited by W. W. Lowrance, pp. 275–294. Rockefeller University, New York.

23. Dean, J. H., Luster, M. I., and Boorman, G. A. (1982): Immunotoxicology. In: *Immunopharmacology,* edited by P. Sirois and M. Rola-Pleszczynski, pp. 349–397. Elsevier/North Holland, Amsterdam.

24. Dean, J. H., Luster, M. I., Boorman, G. A., Lauer, L. D., Luebke, R. W., and Lawson, L. (1983): Selective immunosuppression resulting from exposure to the carcinogenic congener of benzopyrene in B6C3F1 mice. *Clin. Exp. Immunol.,* 52:199–206.

25. Dean, J. H., Murray, M. J., and Ward, E. C. (1986): Toxic modification of the immune system. In: *Casarett and Doull's Toxicology: The Basic Science of Poisons,* 3rd ed., edited by J. Doull, C. D. Klaassen, and M. O. Amdur, pp. 245–285. Macmillan, New York.

26. Dean, J. H., Padarathsingh, M. L., and Jerrells, T. R. (1979): Assessment of immunobiological effects induced by chemicals, drugs and food additives. I. Tier testing and screening approach. *Drug Chem. Toxicol.,* 2:5–17.

27. Dean, J. H., Ward, E. C., Murray, M. J., Lauer, L. D., and House,

R. V. (1985): Mechanisms of dimethylbenzanthracene-induced immunotoxicity. *Clin. Physiol. Biochem.,* 3:98–110.

28. Dean, J. H., Ward, E. C., Murray, M. J., Lauer, L. D., and House, R. V. (1986): Immunosuppression following 7,12-dimethylbenz(a)anthracene exposure in B6C3F1 mice. II. Altered cell-mediated immunity and tumor resistance. *Int. J. Immunopharmacol.,* 8:189–198.

29. Deodhar, S. D., Barna, B., and VanOrdstrand, H. S. (1973): A study of the immunologic aspects of chronic berylliosis. *Chest,* 63: 309–313.

30. Devans, B. H., Grayson, M. H., Imamura, T., and Rodgers, K. E. (1985): O,O,S-trimethyl phosphorothioate effects on immunocompetence. *Pesticide Biochem. Physiol.,* 24:251–259.

31. Driscoll, K. (1986): Doctoral dissertation, New York University Medical Center, Department of Environmental Health. University Microfilms.

32. Environmental Criteria and Assessment Office (1982): *Air Quality for Nitrogen Oxides,* Chap. 15, pp. 22–39. EPA-600/8-82-026. U.S. Environmental Protection Agency, Research Triangle Park, North Carolina.

33. Epstein, P. E., Dauber, J. H., Rossman, M. D., and Daniele, R. P. (1982): Bronchoalveolar lavage in a patient with chronic berylliosis: evidence for hypersensitivity pneumonitis. *Ann. Intern. Med.,* 97: 213–216.

34. Ewers, U., Stiller-Winkler, R., and Idel, H. (1982): Serum immunoglobulin complement C3 and salivary IgA levels in lead workers. *Environ. Res.,* 29:351–357.

34a. Exon, J. H., Kirkvliet, N. I., and Talcott, P. A. (1987): Immunotoxicity of carcinogenic pesticides and related chemical. *Environ. Carcin. Rev. (J. Environ. Sci. Health),* C5:73–120.

35. Faith, R. E., and Luster, M. I. (1979): Investigations on the effects of 2,3,7,8-tetrachlorodibenzo-p-dioxin on parameters of various immune functions. *Ann. N.Y. Acad. Sci.,* 320:564–571.

36. Faith, R. E., Luster, M. I., and Kimmel, C. A. (1979): Effect of chronic developmental lead exposure on cell mediated immune functions. *Clin. Exp. Immunol.,* 35:413–420.

37. Fan, A., Street, J. C., and Nelson, R. M. (1978): Immune suppression in mice administered methyl parathion and carbofuran by diet. *Toxicol. Appl. Pharmacol.,* 45:235–242.

38. Fujimaki, H., Shimizu, F., and Kubota, K. (1981): Suppression of antibody response in mice by acute exposure to nitrogen dioxide: in vitro study. *Environ. Res.,* 26:490–496.

39. Gardner, D. E., and Graham, J. A. (1976): Increased pulmonary disease mediated through altered bacterial defenses. In: *Pulmonary Macrophage and Epithelial Cells,* edited by C. L. Sanders, R. P. Schneider, G. E. Doyle, and H. A. Ragan, pp. 1–21. Proceedings Sixteen Annual Hanford Biology Symposium, ERDA Symposium Series, Richland, Washington.

40. Gardner, L. U., and Heslnigton, H. F. (1946): Osteo-sarcoma from intravenous beryllium compounds in rabbits. *Fed. Proc.,* 5:221.

41. Gardner, D. E., Graham, J. A., Illing, J. W., Blommer, E. J., and Miller, F. J. (1979): Impact of exposure patterns on the toxicological response to NO₂ and modifications by added stressors. In: *Proceedings, U.S.-USSR 3rd Joint Symposium on Problems in Environmental Health,* pp. 17–40. NIEHS, Research Triangle Park, North Carolina.

42. Gaumer, H. R., Doll, N. Y., Kaimmal, Y., Schuyer, M., and Salvaggio, Y. E. (1981): Diminished suppressor cell function in patients with asbestosis. *Clin. Exp. Immunol.,* 44:108–116.

43. Ginns, L. C., Ryo, J. H., Rogol, P. R., Sprince, N. L., Oliver, L. C., and Larsson, C. L. (1985): Natural killer cell activity in cigarette smokers and asbestos workers. *Annu. Rev. Respir. Dis.,* 131: 831–834.

44. Glick, B. (1974): Antibody-mediated immunity in the presence of mirex and DDT. *Poultry Sci.,* 53:1476–1485.

45. Goldstein, B. D. (1977): Hematotoxicity in humans. *J. Toxicol. Environ. Health,* 2(Suppl.):69–106.

46. Graham, J. A., and Gardner, D. E. (1985): Immunotoxicity of air pollutants. In: *Immunotoxicology and Immunopharmacology,* edited by J. H. Dean, M. I. Luster, and A. E. Munson, pp. 367–380. Raven Press, New York.

47. Greenlee, W. F., Dold, K. M., Irons, R. D., and Osborne, R. (1985): Evidence for direct action of 2,3,7,8-tetrachlorodibenzo(p)dioxin on thymic epithelium. *Toxicol. Appl. Pharmacol.,* 19:112–120.

48. Hanifin, J. M., Epstein, W. L., and Cline, M. J. (1970): In vitro

studies of granulomatous hypersensitivity to beryllium. *J. Invest. Dermatol.,* 55:284–288.

49. Harmon, W. E., Parkman, R., Gavin, P. T., Grupe, W. E., Ingelfunger, J. R., Yunis, E. J., and Levey, R. H. (1982): Comparison of cell-mediated lympholysis and mixed lymphocyte culture in the immunologic evaluation for renal transplantation. *J. Immunol.,* 129:1573–1577.

50. Haslam, P. L., Lukoszek, A., Merchant, J. A., and Turner-Warwick, M. (1978): Lymphocyte responses to phytohemagglutinin in patients with asbestosis and pleural mesothelioma. *Clin. Exp. Immunol.,* 31:178–188.

51. Henderson, W. R., Fukuyama, K., Epstein, W. L., and Spitler, L. F. (1972): In vitro demonstration of delayed hypersensitivity in patients with berylliosis. *J. Invest. Dermatol.,* 58:5–8.

52. Hirsch, F., Couderc, J., Sapin, C., Fournie, G., and Druet, P. (1982): Polyclonal effect of HgCl$_2$ in the rat, its possible role in an experimental autoimmune disease. *Eur. J. Immunol.,* 12:620–625.

53. Holt, P. A. (1986): Down regulation of immune responses in the lower respiratory tract: the role of alveolar macrophages. *Clin. Exp. Immunol.,* 63:261–270.

54. House, R. V., Lauer, L. D., Murray, M. J., and Dean, J. H. (1987): Suppression of t-helper cell function in mice following exposure to the carcinogen 7,12-dimethylbenz(a)anthracene and its restoration by interleukin 2. *Int. J. Immunopharmacol.,* 9:85–87.

55. Huuskonen, M. S., Rasanen, Y. A., Hankonen, H., and Asp, S. (1978): Asbestos exposure as a cause of immunologic stimulation. *Scand. J. Respir. Dis.,* 59:326–332.

56. Imanishi, J., Nomura, H., Matsubara, M., Kita, M., Won, S. J., Mizutani, T., and Kishida, T. (1980): Effect of polychlorinated biphenyl on viral infections in mice. *Infect. Immun.,* 29:275–277.

57. International Agency for Research on Cancer (1982): Evaluation of the carcinogenic risk of chemical to humans: some industrial chemicals and dye stuffs. *IARC Monogr.,* 29:93–148.

58. Ito, Y., Kurita, H., Yoshida, T., Shima, S., Niiya, Y., Tariumi, H., Nakayasu, T., Kamori, Y., and Sarai, S. (1982): Studies on serum specific protein levels in lead exposed workers. *Jpn. J. Industr. Health,* 24:390–391.

59. Jones, J. M., and Amos, H. E. (1975): Contact sensitivity in vitro: the effect of beryllium preparations on the proliferative response of specifically allergized lymphocytes and normal lymphocytes stimulated with PHA. *Int. Arch. Allergy,* 48:22–29.

60. Kagan, E., Jacobson, R. J., Yeung, K. Y., Haildale, D. J., and Machnani, G. H. (1979): Asbestos-associated neoplasms of B-cell lineage. *Am. J. Med.,* 67:325–331.

61. Kagan, E., Solomon, A., Cochrane, J. C., Beissmer, E. K., Gluckman, J., Rocks, P. H., and Webster, I. (1977): Immunological studies of patients with asbestosis. I. Studies of cell mediated immunity. *Clin. Exp. Immunol.,* 28:261–267.

62. Kagan, E., Solomon, A., Cochrane, J. C., Kuba, P., Rocks, P. H., and Webster, I. (1977): Immunological studies of patients with asbestosis. II. Studies of circulating lymphoid numbers and humoral immunity. *Clin. Exp. Immunol.,* 28:268–275.

63. Kaminsky, N. E., Wells, D. S., Dauterman, W. C., Roberts, J. F., and Guthrie, F. (1986): Macrophage uptake of lipoprotein sequestered toxicant: a potential route of immunotoxicity. *Toxicol. Appl. Pharmacol.,* 82:474–480.

64. Keck, G. (1982): Effets de la contamination par les polychlorobiphenyles sur le developpement de la tumeur d'Ehrlich chez la souris Swiss. *Toxicol. Eur. Res.,* 3:229–236.

65. Kenoyer, J. L., Phalen, R. F., and Davis, J. R. (1981): Particle clearance from the respiratory tract as a test of toxicity: effect of ozone exposure on short and long term clearance. *Exp. Lung Res.,* 2:111–120.

66. Kerkvliet, N. I., and Baecher–Steppan, L. (1982): Immunotoxicology studies on lead: effect of exposure on tumor growth and cell-mediated immunity after syngeneic or allogeneic stimulator. *Immunopharmacology,* 4:213–224.

67. Kerkvliet, N. I., and Kimeldorf, D. J. (1977): Antitumor activity of a polychlorinated biphenyl mixture, Aroclor 1254, in rats inoculated with Walker 256 carcinocoma cells. *J. Natl. Cancer Inst.,* 59:951–955.

68. Kimbrough, R. D. (1980): *Halogenated Biphenyls, Terphenyls, Naphthalenes, Dibenzodioxins and Related Products.* Elsevier/North Holland, New York.

69. Koller, L. D. (1977): Enhanced polychlorinated biphenyl lesions in moloney leukemia virus infected mice. *Clin. Toxicol.,* 11:107–116.

70. Koller, L. D. (1979): Effects of environmental contaminants on the immune system. *Adv. Vet. Sci. Comp. Med.,* 23:267–295.

71. Koller, L. D. (1980): Immunotoxicity of heavy metals. *Int. J. Immunopharmacol.,* 2:269–279.

72. Koller, L. D., and Exon, J. H. (1985): The rat as a model for immunotoxicity assessment. In: *Immunotoxicity and Immunopharmacology,* edited by J. H. Dean, M. I. Luster, A. E. Munson, and H. Amos, pp. 99–112. Raven Press, New York.

73. Koller, L. D., and Thigpen, J. E. (1973): Reduction of antibody to pseudorabies virus in polychlorinated biphenyl-exposed rabbits. *Am. J. Vet. Res.,* 34:1605–1606.

74. Krajns, E. I., Wester, P. W., Loeber, J. G., van Leeuwen, F. X. R., Vos, J. G., Vaessen, H. A. M. G., and van der Heijden, G. A. (1984): Toxicity of bis(tri-n-buthyltin)oxide in the rat. I. Short-term effects on general parameters and on the endocrine and lymphoid systems. *Toxicol. Appl. Pharmacol.,* 75:363–386.

75. Krivanek, N. D., and Reeves, A. L. (1972): The effect of chemical forms of beryllium on the production of the immunologic response. *Am. Industr. Hyg. Assoc. J.,* 33:45–52.

76. Kubota, M., Kagamimori, S., Yokoyama, K., and Okada, A. (1985): Reduced natural killer activity of lymphocytes from patients with asbestosis. *Br. J. Industr. Med.,* 42:276–280.

77. Lange, A., Smolik, R., Zatonski, W., and Szymanska, J. (1973): Serum immunoglobulin levels in workers exposed to benzene, toluene, and xylene. *Int. Arch. Arbeitsmed.,* 32:37–44.

78. Lange, A., Smolik, R., Zatonski, W., and Szymanska, Y. (1974): Autoantibodies and serum immunoglobulin levels in asbestos workers. *Int. Arch. Arbeitsmed.,* 32:313–325.

79. Last, J. A., Jennings, M., Schwartz, L. W., and Cross, C. E. (1977): Glycoprotein secretion by tracheal explants cultured from rats exposed to ozone. *Am. Rev. Respir. Dis.,* 116:695–703.

80. Lauer, L. D., Tucker, A. N., House, R. V., Barbera, P. W., Fenters, J. D., Ehrlich, J. P., Burleson, G. R., and Dean, J. H. (1987): Altered B cell function is a predominant feature of TCDD exposure in adult mice. (*Submitted.*)

81. Lawrence, D. A. (1985): Immunotoxicity of heavy metals. In: *Immunotoxicology and Immunopharmacology,* edited by J. H. Dean, M. I. Luster, A. E. Munson, and H. Amos, pp. 341–353. Raven Press, New York.

82. Lee, T. P., and Chang, K. J. (1985): Health effects of polychlorinated biphenyls. In: *Immunotoxicology and Immunopharmacology,* edited by J. H. Dean, M. I. Luster, A. E. Munson, and H. Amos, pp. 415–422. Raven Press, New York.

83. Lew, F., Tsang, P., Holland, J. F., Warner, N., Selikoff, I. J., and Bekesi, J. G. (1986): High frequency of immune dysfunctions in asbestos workers and in patients with malignant mesothelioma. *J. Clin. Immunol.,* 6:225–233.

83a. Lewis, J. T., Odom, B., and Adams, D. O. (1988): Toxic effects of benzene metabolites on mononuclear phagocytes. *Toxicol. Appl. Pharmacol.,* 92:246–254.

84. Lill, P. H., and Gangemi, J. D. (1986): Suppressive effects of 3-methylcholanthrene on the in vitro antitumor activity of naturally cytotoxic cells. *J. Toxicol. Environ. Health,* 17:347–356.

85. Loose, L. D., Silkworth, J. B., Charbonneau, T., and Blumenstock, F. (1981): Environmental chemical-induced macrophage dysfunction. *Environ. Health Perspect.,* 39:79–91.

86. Loose, L. D., Silkworth, J. B., Pittman, K. A., Benitz, K. F., and Mueller, W. (1978): Impaired host resistance to endotoxin and malaria in polychlorinated biphenyl- and hexachlorobenzene-treated mice. *Infect. Immun.,* 20:30–35.

87. Luster, M. I., and Dean, J. H. (1982): Immunological hypersensitivity resulting from environmental or occupational exposure to chemicals: a state-of-the-art workshop summary. *Fundam. Appl. Toxicol.,* 2:327–330.

88. Luster, M. I., Blank, J. A., and Dean, J. H. (1987): Molecular and cellular basis of chemically induced immunotoxicity. *Annu. Rev. Pharmacol. Toxicol.,* 27:23–49.

89. Luster, M. I., Boorman, G. A., Dean, J. H., Harris, M. W., and Luebke, R. W. (1980): Examination of bone marrow immunologic parameters and host susceptibility following pre- and postnatal exposure to 2,3,7,8-tetrachlorodibenzo(p)dioxin. *Int. J. Immunopharmacol.,* 2:301–310.

90. Luster, M. I., Germolec, D. R., Clark, G., Wiegand, G., and Ro-

senthal, G. J. (1988): Selective effects of 2,3,7,8-tetrachlorodibenzo-p-dioxin and corticosteroid on in vitro activation, proliferation and differentiation of murine B-lymphocytes. *J. Immunol.*, 140:928–935.

91. Luster, M. I., Hong, L. H., Tucker, A. N., Clark, G., Greenlee, W. F., and Boorman, G. A. (1985): Acute myelotoxic responses in mice induced in vivo and in vitro by 2,3,7,8-tetrachlorodibenzo-p-dioxin. *Toxicol. Appl. Pharmacol.*, 81:156–165.

92. Luster, M. I., Munson, A. E., Thomas, P. T., Holsapple, M. P., Fenters, J. D., White, K. L., Lauer, L. D. D., Germolec, D. R., Rosenthal, G. J., and Dean, J. H. (1988): Development of a testing battery to assess chemical-induced immunotoxicity: National Toxicology Program's guidelines for immunotoxicity evaluation in mice. *Fundam. Appl. Toxicol.*, 10:2–19.

93. Lyte, M., and Bick, P. H. (1986): Modulation of interleukin 1 production by macrophages following benzo(a)pyrene exposure. *Int. J. Immunopharmacol.*, 8:377–381.

94. Maigetter, R. Z., Fenters, J. D., Findlay, J. C., Ehrlich, R., and Gardner, D. E. (1978): Effects of exposure to nitrogen dioxide on T and B cells in mouse spleen. *Toxicol. Lett.*, 2:157–161.

95. Makker, S. P., and Aikawa, M. (1979): Mesangial glomerulonephropathy with deposition of IgG, IgM and Cb induced by mercuric chloride. *Lab. Invest.*, 41:45–50.

96. Mantovani, A., Vecchi, A., Luini, W., Sironi, M., Candiani, G., Spreafico, F., and Garattini, S. (1980): Effect of 2,3,7,8-tetrachlorodibenzo-p-dioxin on macrophage and NK cell mediated cytotoxicity in mice. *Biomedicine*, 32:200–204.

97. Miller, K., and Brown, R. C. (1985): The immune system and asbestos associated disease. In: *Immunotoxicology and Immunopharmacology*, edited by J. H. Dean, M. I. Luster, A. E. Munson, and H. Amos, pp. 429–440. Raven Press, New York.

98. Miller, K., and Scott, M. P. (1985): Immunologic consequences of dioctyltin dichloride (DOTC)-induced thymic injury. *Toxicol. Appl. Pharmacol.*, 78:395–403.

99. Miller, R. P., Hartung, R., and Cornish, H. H. (1980): Effects of diethyltindichlorides on amino acids and nucleoside transport in suspended rat thymocytes. *Toxicol. Appl. Pharmacol.*, 55:564–571.

100. Miller, K., Weintraub, Z., and Kagan, E. (1979): Manifestations of cellular immunity in the rat after prolonged asbestos inhalation. I. Physical interactions between alveolar macrophages and splenic lymphocytes. *J. Immunol.*, 123:1029–1038.

101. Moore, J. A., Huff, J. E., and Dean, J. H. (1982): The National Toxicology Program and immunological toxicology. *Pharmacol. Rev.*, 34:13–16.

102. Penn, I. (1985): Neoplastic consequences of immunosuppression. In: *Immunotoxicology and Immunopharmacology*, edited by J. H. Dean, A. Munson, I. Luster, and H. Amos. Raven Press, New York.

103. Penninks, A. H., and Seinen, W. (1980): Toxicity of organotin compounds. IV. Impairment of energy metabolism of rat thymocytes by various dialkyltin compounds. *Toxicol. Appl. Pharmacol.*, 56:221–231.

104. Penninks, A. H., Kuper, F., Spit, B. J., and Seinen, W. (1985): On the mechanisms of dialkyltin induced thymus involution. *Immunopharmacology*, 10:1–10.

105. Penninks, A. H., Verschuren, P. M., and Seinen, W. (1983): Di-n-butyltindichloride uncouples oxidative phosphorylation in rat liver mitochondria. *Toxicol. Appl. Pharmacol.*, 70:115–120.

106. Pfeifer, R., and Irons, R. D. (1981): Inhibition of lectin-stimulated lymphocyte agglutination and mitogenesis by hydroquinone: reactivity with intracellular sulfhydryl groups. *Exp. Mol. Pathol.*, 35:189–198.

107. Reeves, A. L., and Preuss, O. P. (1985): The immunotoxicity of beryllium. In: *Immunotoxicology and Immunopharmacology*, edited by J. H. Dean, M. I. Luster, A. E. Munson and H. Amos, pp. 441–455. Raven Press, New York.

108. Resnik, H., Roche, M., and Morgan, W. K. C. (1970): Immunoglobulin concentrations in berylliosis. *Am. Rev. Respir. Dis.*, 101:504–510.

109. Rodgers, K. E., Imamura, T., and Devans, B. H. (1985): Effects of subchronic treatment with O,O,S-trimethyl phosphorothioate on cellular and humoral immune response systems. *Toxicol. Appl. Pharmacol.*, 81:310–318.

110. Rodgers, K. E., Imamura, T., and Devans, B. H. (1985): Investigations into the mechanism of immunosuppression caused by acute treatment with O,O,S-trimethyl phosphorothioate. I. Characterization of the immune cell population affected. *Immunopharmacology*, 10:171–180.

111. Roitt, I. M., Brostoff, J., and Male, D. K. (1985): *Immunology*, pp. 1.1–25.9. Gower, London.

112. Rosenthal, G. J., and Luster, M. I. (1987): Asbestos-induced reversal of the normal down regulatory function of alveolar macrophages. *Fed. Proc.*, 46:539.

113. Rosenthal, G. J., and Snyder, C. A. (1985): Modulation of the immune response to Listeria monocytogenes by benzene inhalation. *Toxicol. Appl. Pharmacol.*, 80:502–510.

114. Rosenthal, G. J., and Snyder, C. A. (1987): Inhaled benzene reduces aspects of cell-mediated tumor surveillance in mice. *Toxicol. Appl. Pharmacol.*, 88:35–43.

115. Rozen, M. G., Snyder, C. A., and Albert, R. E. (1984): Depressions in B- and T-lymphocyte mitogen-induced blastogenesis in mice exposed to low concentrations of benzene. *Toxicol. Lett.*, 20:343–349.

116. Sachs, H. K. (1978): Intercurrent infections in lead poisoning. *Am. J. Dis. Child.*, 32:315–316.

117. Sakaguchi, O., Abe, H., Sakaguchi, S., and Hsu, C. C. (1982): Effect of lead acetate on superoxide anion generation and its scavengers in mice given endotoxin. *Microbiol. Immunol.*, 26:767–778.

118. Schleshinger, R. B., and Driscoll, K. E. (1987): Respiratory tract defense mechanisms and their interaction with air pollutants. In: *Current Topics in Pharmacology and Toxicology, Volume 4*, edited by M. A. Hollinger, Elsevier, New York.

119. *Science* (1977): Occupational cancer: government challenged in beryllium proceedings. 198:898–901.

120. *Science* (1981): Beryllium report disputed by listed author. 211:556–557.

121. Seinen, W. (1981): Immunotoxicity of alkyltin compounds. In: *Immunologic Considerations in Toxicology*, edited by R. P. Sharma, Vol. 1, pp. 103–119. CRC Press, Boca Raton, Florida.

122. Seinen, W., and Penninks, A. (1979): Immune suppression as a consequence of a selective cytotoxic activity of certain organometallic compounds on thymus dependent lymphocytes. *Ann. N.Y. Acad. Sci.*, 320:499–517.

123. Seinen, W., Vos, J. G., Van Krieken, R., Penninks, A. H., Brands, R., and Hooykaas, H. (1977): Toxicity of organotin compounds. III. Suppression of thymus-dependent immunity in rats by di-n-butyltin dichloride. *Toxicol. Appl. Pharmacol.*, 42:213–224.

124. Shingu, H., Sugiyama, M., Watanabe, M., and Nakajima, T. (1980): Effects of ozone and photochemical oxidants on interferon production by rabbit alveolar macrophages. *Bull. Environ. Contam. Toxicol.*, 24:433–438.

125. Silkworth, J. B., and Grabstein, E. M. (1982): Polychlorinated biphenyl immunotoxicity: dependence on isomer planarity and the Ah gene complex. *Toxicol. Appl. Pharmacol.*, 65:109–115.

126. Silkworth, J. B., and Loose, L. D. (1981): Assessment of environmental contaminant-induced lymphocyte dysfunction. *Environ. Health Perspect.*, 39:105–128.

127. Silkworth, J., and Vecchi, A. (1985): The role of the Ah receptor in halogenated aromatic hydrocarbon immunotoxicity. In: *Immunotoxicology and Immunopharmacology*, edited by J. H. Dean, M. I. Luster, A. E. Munson, and H. Amos, pp. 263–275. Raven Press, New York.

128. Silkworth, J. B., Antrim, L., and Grabstein, E. M. (1984): Correlations between polychlorinated biphenyl immunotoxicity: the aromatic hydrocarbon locus, and liver microsomal enzyme induction in C57BL/6 and DBA/2 mice. *Toxicol. Appl. Pharmacol.*, 75:156–165.

129. Sirois, P., Rola-Pleszczynski, M., and Begin, R. (1980): Phospholipase A activity and prostaglandin synthesis from alveolar macrophages exposed to asbestos. *Prostaglandins Med.*, 5:31–37.

130. Smith, S. H., Sanders, V. M., Barrett, B. A., Borzelleca, J. F., and Munson, A. E. (1978): Immunotoxicological evaluation on mice exposed to polychlorinated biphenyls. *Toxicol. Appl. Pharmacol.*, 45:A336.

131. Smolik, R., Grzybek–Hryncewicz, K., Lange, A., and Zatonski, W. (1973): Serum complement level in workers exposed to benzene, toluene and xylene. *Int. Arch. Arbeitsmed.*, 31:243–247.

132. Snoeij, N. J., Penninks, A. H., and Seinen, W. (1987): Toxicity of triorganotin compounds: species-dependency, dose-effect relation-

ships and kinetics of the thymus atrophy induced by tri- and diorganotin compounds. (*Submitted.*)

133. Snoeij, N. J., Van Iersel, A. A. J., Penninks, A. H., and Seinen, W. (1986): Triorganotin-induced cytotoxicity to rat thymus, bone marrow, and red blood cells as determined by several in vitro assays. *Toxicology,* 39:71–83.

134. Snyder, C. A., Goldstein, B. D., Sellakumar, A. R., Bromberg, I., Laskin, S., and Albert, R. E. (1980): The inhalation toxicology of benzene: incidence of hematopoietic neoplasms and hematotoxicity in AKR/J and C57BL/6 mice. *Toxicol. Appl. Pharmacol.,* 54:323–331.

135. Snyder, R., and Kocsis, J. J. (1975): Current concepts of chronic benzene toxicity. *CRC Crit. Rev. Toxicol.,* 3:265–288.

136. Sone, S., Brennan, L. M., and Creasia, W. A. (1983): In vivo and in vitro NO_2 exposure enhances phagocytic and tumoricidal activities of rat alveolar macrophages. *J. Toxicol. Environ. Health,* 11:151–163.

137. Spyker-Cranmer, J. M., Barnett, J., Avery, D. L., and Cranmer, M. F. (1982): Immunoteratology of chlordane: cell mediated and humoral immune responses in adult mice exposed in utero. *Toxicol. Appl. Pharmacol.,* 62:402–408.

138. Stein-Streilein, J., Bennett, M., Mann, D., and Kumar, V. (1983): Natural killer cells in mouse lung: surface phenotype target preference, and response to local influenza virus protection. *J. Immunol.,* 131:2699–2704.

139. Stjernsward, J. (1966): Effect of noncarcinogenic and carcinogenic hydrocarbons on antibody forming cells measured at the cellular level. *J. Natl. Cancer Inst.,* 36:1189–1195.

140. Street, J. C., and Sharma, R. P. (1975): Alteration of induced cellular and humoral immune responses by pesticides and chemicals of environmental concern: qualitative studies of immunosuppression by DDT, Arochlor 1254, carbaryl, carbofuran, and methylparathion. *Toxicol. Appl. Pharmacol.,* 32:587–602.

141. Thomas, P., and Faith, R. (1985): Adult and perinatal immunotoxicity by halogenated aromatic hydrocarbons. In: *Immunotoxicology and Immunopharmacology,* edited by J. H. Dean, M. I. Luster, A. E. Munson, and H. Amos, pp. 305–313. Raven Press, New York.

142. Thomas, P. T., and Hinsdill, R. D. (1978): Effect of polychlorinated biphenyls on the immune responses of rhesus monkeys and mice. *Toxicol. Appl. Pharmacol.,* 44:41–51.

143. Tucker, A. N., Vore, S. J., and Luster, M. I. (1986): Suppression of B cell differentiation by 2,3,7,8-tetrachlorodibenzo-p-dioxin. *Mol. Pharmacol.,* 29:372–377.

144. Urso, P., Gengozian, N., Rossi, R. M., and Johnson, R. A. (1986): Suppression of humoral and cell mediated immune responses in vitro by benzo(a)pyrene. *J. Immunopharmacol.,* 8:223–241.

145. Vecchi, A., Sironi, M., Canegrati, M. A., Recchia, M., and Garattini, S. (1983): Immunosuppressive effects of 2,3,7,8-tetrachlorodibenzo-p-dioxin in strains of mice with different susceptibility to induction of aryl hydrocarbon hydroxylase. *Toxicol. Appl. Pharmacol.,* 68:434–441.

146. Vorwald, A. J., Pratt, P. C., and Urban, E. J. (1955): The production of pulmonary cancer in albino rats exposed by inhalation to an aerosol to beryllium sulfate. *Acta Un. Int. Contra Cancrum,* 11:735.

147. Vos, J. G. (1977): Immune suppression as related to toxicology. *CRC Crit. Rev. Toxicol.,* 5:67–101.

148. Vos, J. G. (1980): Immunotoxicity assessment: screening and function studies. *Arch. Toxicol. [Suppl.],* 4:95–108.

149. Vos, J. G., and Krajnc, E. I. (1983): Immunotoxicology of pesticides. In: *Developments in the Science and Practice of Toxicology,* edited by A. W. Hayes, R. C. Schnell, and T. S. Miya, pp. 229–239. Elsevier, New York.

150. Vos, J. G., and Moore, J. A. (1974): Suppression of cellular immunity in rats and mice by natural treatment with 2,3,7,8-tetrachlorodibenzo-p-dioxin. *Int. Arch. Allergy Appl. Immunol.,* 47:777–789.

151. Vos, J. G., and van Driel Grootenhuis, L. (1972): PCB-induced suppression of the humoral and cell-mediated immunity in guinea pigs. *Sci. Total Environ.,* 1:289–302.

152. Vos, J. G., de Klerk, A., Krannc, E. I., Kruizinga, W., van Ommen, B., and Rozing, J. (1984): Toxicity of bis(tri-n-butyltin)oxide in the rat. II. Suppression of thymus dependent immune responses and of parameters of nonspecific resistance after short term exposure. *Toxicol. Appl. Pharmacol.,* 75:387–408.

153. Vos, J. G., Faith, R. E., and Luster, M. I. (1980): Immune alterations. In: *Halogenated Biphenyls, Terphenyls, Naphthalenes, Dibenzodioxins and Related Products,* edited by Kimbrough, pp. 241–266. Elsevier, Amsterdam.

154. Vos, J. G., Krajnc, E. I., and Wester, P. W. (1985): Immunotoxicity of bis(tri-n-butyltin)oxide. In: *Immunotoxicology and Immunopharmacology,* edited by J. H. Dean, M. I. Luster, A. E. Munson, and H. Amos, pp. 327–340. Raven Press, New York.

155. Wade, M. J., Lipkin, L. E., Stanton, M. F., and Frank, A. L. (1980): P388D1 in vitro cytotoxicity assay as applied to asbestos and other minerals: its possible relevance to carcinogenesis. In: *The In Vitro Effects of Mineral Dusts,* edited by R. C. Brown, I. P. Gormly, M. Chamberlain and R. Davis. Academic Press, New York.

156. Ward, E. C., Murray, M. J., and Dean, J. H. (1985): Immunotoxicity of nonhalogenated polycyclic aromatic hydrocarbons. In: *Immunotoxicology and Immunopharmacology,* edited by J. H. Dean, M. I. Luster, A. E. Munson, and H. Amos, pp. 291–304. Raven Press, New York.

157. Ward, E. C., Murray, M. J., Lauer, L. D., House, R. V., and Dean, J. H. (1986): Persistent suppression of humoral and cell mediated immunity in mice following exposure to the polycyclic aromatic hydrocarbon 7,12-dimethylbenzanthracene. *Int. J. Immunopharmacol.,* 8:13–22.

158. Ward, E. C., Murray, M. J., Lauer, L. D., House, R. V., Irons, R., and Dean, J. H. (1984): Immunosuppression following 7,12-dimethylbenzanthracene exposure in B6C3F1 mice. I. Effects on humoral immunity and host resistance. *Toxicol. Appl. Pharmacol.,* 75:299–308.

159. White, K. L., and Munson, A. E. (1986): Suppression of the in vitro humoral immune response by chrysotile asbestos. *Toxicol. Appl. Pharmacol.,* 82:493–504.

160. White, K. L., Lysy, H. H., and Holsapple, M. P. (1985): Immunosuppression by polycyclic aromatic hydrocarbons: a structure activity relationship in B6C3F1 and DBA/2 mice. *Immunopharmacology,* 9:155–164.

161. White, W. C., and Gammon, A. M. (1914): The influence of benzol inhalations on experimental pulmonary tuberculosis in rabbits. *Trans. Assoc. Am. Physicians,* 29:332–337.

162. Wierda, D., and Irons, R. D. (1982): Hydroquinone and catechol reduce the frequency of progenitor B lymphocytes in mouse spleen and bone marrow. *Immunopharmacology,* 4:41–54.

163. Wierda, D., Irons, R. D., and Greenlee, W. F. (1981): Immunotoxicity in C57Bl/6 mice exposed to benzene and Aroclor 1254. *Toxicol. Appl. Pharmacol.,* 60:410–417.

164. Williams, W. R., and Jones-Williams, W. (1982): Development of beryllium lymphocyte transformation tests in chronic beryllium disease. *Int. Arch. Allergy,* 67:175–180.

165. Winternitz, M. C., and Hirschfelder, A. D. (1913): Studies upon experimental pneumonia in rabbits. Parts I–III. *J. Exp. Med.,* 17:657–665.

166. Wojdani, A., and Alfred, L. J. (1984): Alterations in cell mediated immune functions induced in mouse splenic lymphocytes by polycyclic aromatic hydrocarbons. *Cancer Res.,* 44:942–945.

167. Wu, J. C., Lu, Y. C., Kao, H. Y., Pan, C. C., and Lin, R. Y. (1984): Cell-mediated immunity in patients with polychlorinated biphenyl poisoning. *J. Formosa Med. Assoc.,* 83:419–429.

168. Young, P. (1980): *Asthma and allergies: an optimistic future (Based on the "Report on the Task Force on Asthma and the Other Allergic Diseases").* NIH Publ. No. 80-388. U.S. Government Printing Office, Washington, D. C.

169. Zedeck, M. S. (1980): Polycyclic aromatic hydrocarbons: a review. *J. Environ. Pathol. Toxicol.,* 3:537–567.

Principles and Methods of Toxicology, Second Edition, edited by A. Wallace Hayes, Raven Press, Ltd., New York © 1989.

CHAPTER 27

Techniques in Membrane Toxicology

Timothy D. Phillips and *A. Wallace Hayes

*Department of Veterinary Public Health, Texas A & M University, College Station, Texas 77843; and *Center for Toxicology, RJR Nabisco, Winston-Salem, North Carolina 27102*

Membranes and membrane-associated transport systems are intimately associated with the integrity of vital cellular and subcellular processes. Their significance in such fundamental biochemical events as cell–cell communications, respiration, excretion, secretion, nerve transmission, muscle contraction, hormonal control, reproduction, vision, hearing, and smell continues to be elucidated (24). It is apparent from the extant scientific literature that membranes are important biological targets for a wide variety of toxic agents. However, the fundamental mechanisms of action/interaction of toxins on membrane architecture, transport-mediated events, and membrane function have not been clearly delineated. Much remains to be discovered in this dynamic area of research, i.e., membrane transport perturbation as a progenitor of toxicity.

Cell membranes inhabit a uniquely important and clearly vulnerable biological location, compartmentalizing the extrastructural and intrastructural cellular environments. The basic framework for all membranes consists of a double layer of lipid molecules (commonly referred to as a phospholipid bilayer) containing different kinds of proteins adsorbed to the surface or integrated in the lipid bilayer imparting a distinctive identity and specialized function to the membrane (10,91). Thus, the cell membrane, as an external barrier functioning to translocate biologically important molecules, is the first component of the cell that is exposed to toxic materials. In separating both the extracellular and intracel-

lular components of cells, membranes can be acted on or may act themselves to confirm sensitivity or resistance to a particular toxin (24,45).

STRUCTURAL ASPECTS OF MEMBRANES

The phospholipid matrix of membranes possesses intrinsic macromolecules (lipoproteins and glycoproteins) of different shape and assemblage that carry out specific functions (37,83). Proteins, embedded in the lipid bilayer, consist of two general types—Type I and Type II (Fig. 1). Type I proteins are (for the most part) contained outside of the cytoplasm and thus resemble secreted proteins in many aspects. They typically function as specific receptor sites or as distinctive cellular markings (10,37). Examples of Type I proteins are sialoglycoproteins of erythrocyte membranes, histocompatibility antigens, e.g., H2 in mice and human leukocyte antigen (HLA) in humans, surface immunoglobulin receptors on B lymphocytes, and components of enveloped viruses (10,37). Cell surface proteins may also extend across the bilayer as a hydrophobic chain of amino acids coiled in an alpha helix and linked to the cytoplasm via a hydrophilic segment (10). Type II proteins, on the other hand, contain most of their mass in the cytoplasm. Type II proteins may be divided into two major groups. The first group is represented by cytochrome b_5, the corresponding reductase, and stearyl-CoA

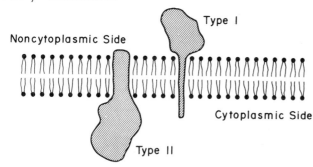

Type I

Noncytoplasmic Side

Cytoplasmic Side

Type II

FIG. 1. Diagrammatic illustration of the arrangement in the membrane of Type I and Type II intrinsic membrane proteins. (From ref. 37, with permission.)

desaturase. The second group is represented by macromolecules (transmembrane oligomers) that are involved in membrane transport processes and in maintaining the structural integrity of the membrane, e.g., Na^+-K^+ adenosine triphosphatase (ATPase)—the enzyme mediator of active cation transport, Ca^{2+} ATPase, anion exchange protein, acetylcholine receptor, and vertebrate rhodopsin (Table 1) (37).

Membrane architecture and chemistry result in regional polarization, i.e., inward hydrophobic and peripheral hydrophilic regions that act to constrain passive transmembrane diffusion of molecules and produce a flexible, semiliquid consistency allowing for lateral movement and assisting in transport (10). Biogenesis, assemblage, and degradation of integral membrane components play an important role in the conformation and maintenance of the cell membrane surface, resulting in steady states that are required for integrity, orderly function, and viability (24,30).

FUNCTIONAL COMPONENTS OF MEMBRANE TRANSPORT

The basic processes of transport have been generally represented by three levels of organization (19):

Primary order—the movement of a substance across a single biological membrane;

Secondary order—transcellular or transepithelial transport; and

Tertiary order—transport resulting from integrated organ function.

The first level is usually characterized by movement with or against an electrochemical potential gradient. Simple diffusion and active transport are representative examples. In simple diffusion, movement of the substance occurs with an electrochemical gradient without the expenditure of energy. In the membrane of the red blood cell, a globular transport protein, referred to as the *anion channel,* functions as a passageway for negatively charged ions such as chloride and bicarbonate between the blood to the cell cytoplasm (10). On the other hand, active transport consists of movement against an electrochemical gradient at the expense of cellular energy. This type of "uphill" transport is directly coupled to the hydrolysis of ATP and is represented by the sodium pump (Na^+-K^+ ATPase) mechanism. Facilitated diffusion or "downhill" active transport is also a primary process. It is not energy dependent. Solute movement is facilitated by a carrier, possibly through permeability modification, thus enhancing membrane translocation. Glucose uptake by erythrocytes is thought to occur by this process (19,78). Most of the molecules needed for growth of the cell are produced through intrinsic biosynthesis or absorption from the blood via transport; however, some essential nutrients are not available by either mechanism. For example, cholesterol (a vital component for the synthesis of membrane) and ferric ion (which is needed to build cyctochromes) are present in the blood as large complexes, low density lipoprotein (LDL) and transferrin, respectively. These cannot pass through a channel and are not transported into the cell by common mechanisms. Instead, they are internalized by a membrane process of receptor-mediated endocytosis. In growing cells, LDL and transferrin have been shown to bind at specific receptors (pits in the membrane coated on the cytoplasmic side with a lattice of a large fibrous protein called clathrin). The pit containing LDL and transferrin deepens, invaginates, and breaks off to form a coated vesicle in the cell. Next, the vesicle sheds its coat and fuses with an endosome. A change in pH results in the release of LDL from the receptor and ferric ions from transferrin, which are further transported to

TABLE 1. *Properties of membrane transport proteins[a]*

	Na^+-K^+ ATPase	Ca^{2+} ATPase	Anion exchange protein	Acetylcholine receptor	Rhodopsin
Molecular weights of component polypeptides	α-90,000 β-40,000	α-100,000	α-90,000	α-40,000 β-48,000 γ-58,000 δ-64,000 ϵ-105,000	α-38,000
Glycoproteins	β		α	$\alpha(\beta$-$\epsilon)$?	α
Probable structure and molecular weight of the protein part of the enzyme	$\alpha_2\beta_2$ 260,000	$(\alpha_2$?) (200,000?)	α_2 180,000	ϵ_2 or $\alpha_2\beta_2$ 240,000	$(\alpha_2$ to α_4?) (76,000–152,000?)
Transmembrane arrangement	α		α		α
Detergent binding (mg/mg of protein)	0.28	0.20	0.77	0.7	1.10
Relative hydrophobic surface area of subunit	0.20–0.24	0.2–0.25	0.5–0.65	0.5–0.6	0.54

[a] Adapted from ref. 37.

lysosomes, which degrade LDL producing cholesterol (10,35,65).

Secondary order processes represent more than one process operating in sequence in many cases. They may represent excretion or absorption, according to cell polarity and associated organ systems. Basically, this type of transport involves movement "uphill" indirectly coupled to metabolic energy, i.e., potential energy of an ionic gradient. Intestinal absorption of nutrients or reabsorption in the kidneys of nutrients mainly occurs by this type of mechanism (19). This process usually involves movement of molecules across an epithelial sheet of cells, e.g., those lining the gut, the dividing cells of the skin, and the cells of internal organs and the urinary bladder. Epithelial sheets are composed of cells joined by "tight junctions" that prevent leaks and separate the cell membrane into two distinctive regions: the apical surface and the basolateral surface. This separation results in a functional asymmetry necessary to transport molecules in *only one direction,* e.g., transport of useful molecules from the intestine to the blood (10).

Tertiary transport involves a multiplicity of primary and secondary transport processes, the net result being excretion of a substance by an organ system representing the complex summation of many sequential processes of transport. An excellent example of this level of transport is the countercurrent multiplier system of the mammalian and avian kidney.

All of the transport processes mentioned above, in addition to Na^+ transport, are important and clearly deserving of further attention. Yet reviewing the entire scope of transport is not the objective of this chapter. For the interested reader, a number of excellent reviews on membrane theory and active transport are available (3,7,12,13,26,30–34,38,48,57,60,92–96). The remaining discussion will examine model systems representative of primary and secondary transport and review the methodology and techniques that may be employed in studying these systems as potential indicators of toxicity.

TOXICOLOGICAL IMPORTANCE

The membrane (as the outermost barrier of the cell) is uniquely vulnerable to insult by toxic agents. Its exposed location makes it an ideal target for reactive chemicals such as toxins, drugs, and hormones (45). Toxic substances may react either with the protein or lipid components (or both) and, as a consequence, significantly alter transport function and cellular integrity. Membrane toxicity may be expressed through perturbation of a variety of critical functions. For example, the transport-related enzyme complexes referred to as Na^+-K^+ ATPase, Ca^{2+} ATPase, and mitochondrial ATPase are important components of most membranes. Their biological involvement ranges from ATP synthesis and oxidative phosphorylation to the translocation of cations.

The stability of these enzyme systems is essential in maintaining a variety of physiological and biochemical functions, including primary active transport, salt homeostasis and osmoregulation, cellular and organelle integrity, bioelectric potential, regulation of mitochondrial metabolism, and muscle contraction. Membrane interaction with chemically diverse substances, e.g., cardiotonic glycosides, mycotoxins,

heavy metals, organochlorine pesticides, phenoxyacetic acid herbicides, antibiotics, fatty acids, biotoxins, phenothiazine tranquilizers, and neurotransmitters, may be linked to a variety of pharmacologic and toxicologic effects. For example, inhibition of cardiac Na^+-K^+ ATPase may indirectly affect calcium transient, leading to ionotrophy and cardiotoxicity (11). Inhibition of renal ATPase may produce tubular transport defects, resulting in diuresis and natruiresis (62), possibly leading to Fanconi syndrome (49). Vanadium, an environmentally important metallic element of the first transition series, can produce marked alterations in renal function as the inorganic oxyanion vanadate and is a potent inhibitor of Na^+-K^+ ATPase from a variety of sources (Table 2) (72). It is conceivable that vanadate's effects on membrane transport may result in the expression of certain toxic phenomena in the kidneys.

In the liver, inhibition of ATPase may produce abnormal degenerative changes in hepatocytes, thus affecting metabolism/detoxification and biliary excretion. Such hepatic changes may result in a buildup of free fatty acids and ammonia. Elevated ammonia has been shown to alter brain Na^+-K^+ ATPase and may be related to hepatic coma (1). Because there is an interaction between mitochondrial Mg^{2+}-oligomycin-sensitive ATPase and oxidative phosphorylation (77), inhibition of this component may result in effects on energy metabolism and respiration (21,67). Because the plasma membrane is intimately involved in the movement of cells during normal growth and development, it has been postulated that chemical alterations in membrane function may play a role in the induction of cancerous growth in which cell multiplication and migration are uncontrolled

TABLE 2. *Concentrations of vanadate required to produce 50% inhibition of Na^+-K^+ ATPase*

Source	Tissue	Preparation	I_{50} vanadate, $\times 10^{-8}$ M
Human	Whole kidney	Microsomes	9
	Whole kidney	Homogenate	20
Dog	Kidney cortex	Microsomes	20
	Kidney outer medulla	Microsomes	10
	Brain	Microsomes	50
	Heart	Microsomes	20
	Liver	Microsomes	30
	Kidney cortex	Homogenate	100
	Kidney outer medulla	Homogenate	50
Cat	Whole kidney	Microsomes	6
	Brain	Microsomes	30
	Heart	Microsomes	20
Rabbit	Whole kidney	Microsomes	10
	Brain	Microsomes	30
	Heart	Microsomes	7
Rat	Whole kidney	Microsomes	10
	Brain	Microsomes	50
	Heart	Microsomes	10
Chicken	Whole kidney	Homogenate	180
	Brain	Homogenate	600
	Heart	Homogenate	800
	Liver	Homogenate	1000

Adapted from ref. 72.

(59,82). These examples adequately demonstrate the importance of membranes as potential receptors for toxic chemicals. The widely diverse manifestations of toxin–membrane interactions provide a basis for elucidating the fundamental mechanisms of membrane toxicity as they relate to transport phenomena. Furthermore, a thorough understanding of such mechanisms will greatly enhance our basic knowledge of cellular processes.

METHODOLOGICAL ASPECTS OF TRANSPORT AND TRANSPORT-ASSOCIATED ENZYME SYSTEMS

ATPases are transport enzymes found in all animal cells, in plants, and in bacteria. Although each ATPase may differ in its ultimate cellular role, they all have several common characteristics. All are structure-bound enzymes that hydrolyze the terminal phosphate in ATP, releasing adenosine diphosphate (ADP) and orthophosphate; this ATP splitting function is allostearically regulated. All are mechanochemical enzymes, i.e., they translocate other molecules or allostearic effectors across themselves. Gain of potassium intracellularly and loss of sodium are achieved by this mechanism with Na^+-K^+ ATPase (60).

The ATPase systems of plasma membranes will be reviewed in detail because so much interest has been focused in this area. The chapter is not intended to be comprehensive but rather representative of experimental methodology that can be used to evaluate the toxic effects of chemicals on transport.

Sodium-Potassium-Activated ATPase

It is now generally recognized that the Mg^{2+}-dependent, Na^+-K^+-stimulated ATPase, or ATP phosphohydrolase (EC 3.6.1.3), found structurally bound in plasma membranes, is the system responsible for active cation transport across cell membranes and the biochemical manifestation of the sodium pump (84,85). Although the molecular mechanisms responsible for transport are still not fully understood, data suggest the possibility of a series of reversible conformational shifts in a system of allostearically linked proteins in a cyclic expression of the total reaction. A schematic diagram illustrating the cyclic nature of this overall reaction is presented below:

$$\text{Step 1: } E_1 + ATP \underset{\phantom{Na^+,Mg^{2+}}}{\overset{Na^+,Mg^{2+}}{\rightleftarrows}} E_1 \cdot P + ADP$$

$$\text{Step 2: } E_1 \cdot P \overset{Mg^{2+}}{\rightleftarrows} E_2 \cdot P$$

$$\text{Step 3: } E_2 \cdot P \overset{K^+}{\rightarrow} E_1 + P_1$$

In the presence of free enzyme (E_1), Na^+, ATP, and Mg^{2+}, the $E_1 \cdot$ phosphoenzyme ($E_1 \cdot P$) complex is formed (step 1). This complex undergoes a change in conformation to form an $E_2 \cdot$ phosphoenzyme ($E_2 \cdot P$) complex (step 2), which is sensitive to hydrolysis by K^+ (step 3) (25). These reactions can be separately analyzed via proper adjustment of substrate concentrations to the point where interaction is minimized. The effects of a particular chemical can then be assessed at different states of substrate and cationic activation of the enzyme to determine a specific site of action.

From the literature on Na^+-K^+ ATPase, it is apparent that significant variations in the extent of purification, optimal activation parameters, and specific activities can be expected. Much of this variability may be readily attributed to differences in the source and type of Na^+-K^+ ATPase preparations as well as the analytical methods of measuring the enzymatic reaction.

Isolation and Purification

This section will briefly illustrate a few of the basic techniques used to isolate and purify Na^+-K^+ ATPase from selected tissues. Many of the techniques for one type of tissue are also applicable to other tissue sources. Na^+-K^+ ATPase has been purified to varying degrees from mammalian kidney (41,50,51), eel electroplax organ (23), rectal gland of the spiny dogfish (39), and various rabbit tissues (61). Important structural differences may exist among Na^+-K^+ ATPases because they are not equal in sensitivity to specific inhibitors such as ouabain (81).

One of the most difficult Na^+-K^+ ATPases to purify is from cardiac muscle. However, analysis of this enzyme is important for evaluation of agents such as the cardiac glycosides that display cardiotoxicity and specificity. Initial attempts to isolate Na^+-K^+ ATPase from cardiac muscle yielded enzymes with very low specific activities. Pitts and Schwartz (73) developed an improved method that yielded approximately 60 mg of ATPase from 800 g of cardiac tissue with specific activities in the range of 340 to 400 μmol inorganic phosphate/mg protein/hr (units/mg). This procedure is outlined as follows:

1. Fresh beef hearts are trimmed, chopped into small pieces, and blended for 30 sec with 300 ml 0.25 M sucrose/1 mM Tris–EDTA (pH 7.0).
2. Sucrose–EDTA is added (300 ml), and the suspension is blended for an additional 45 sec. Further dilution with 600 ml of the sucrose solution is followed by filtration through cheesecloth.
3. The filtrate is then centrifuged at 12,000 g for 10 min, and the pellet is resuspended in 400 ml sucrose–EDTA and blended for 60 sec.
4. Sodium deoxycholate (40 ml of a 5% solution in sucrose–EDTA) is slowly added to the homogenate, stirred for 20 min, and centrifuged at 96,000 g for 60 sec.
5. The supernatant fluid is recovered and diluted to 850 ml with 1 mM EDTA (pH 7.0) and centrifuged at 96,000 g for 90 min.
6. The pellet is resuspended in 80 ml of 1 mM EDTA and stored at −20°C. Storage for more than 4 days results in a loss of activity.
7. Fragmented membrane suspensions are pooled and washed with an equal volume of 1 mM EDTA and centrifuged at 40,000 g for 30 min.
8. The pellet is resuspended in a volume of 120 ml EDTA solution.

9. A solution of 6 M NaI (containing 15 mM EDTA and 150 mM Tris base, pH 8.4) is added dropwise over 1 min (30 ml), then diluted with 240 ml EDTA and centrifuged at 96,000 g for 25 min.

10. The pellet is resuspended in 390 ml of 25 mM imidazole-HCl/1 mM EDTA (pH 7.0) and centrifuged at 96,000 g for 20 min. The pellet is resuspended in 40 ml of the buffer and adjusted to 10 mg protein/ml.

11. The NaI-treated enzyme is further purified by treatment with deoxycholate-citrate. See Pitts and Schwartz (73) for details.

12. The final enzyme (third pellet) is dialyzed overnight against imidazole-EDTA and stored at 0 to 4°C because considerable loss of activity occurs on freezing.

A highly purified renal Na^+-K^+ ATPase preparation from rabbit kidney outer medulla has been described by Jorgensen (41) and Depont et al. (20). The microsomal fraction obtained after differential centrifugation of tissue homogenate is treated with deoxycholate and yields a Na^+-K^+ ATPase activity of 200 to 250 units/mg protein. Further purification is achieved by isopycnic zonal centrifugation followed by removal of endogenous ATP, extensive washing, and recentrifugation. The final preparation is free of basal Mg^{2+} ATPase activity and is 95% pure by sodium dodecyl sulfate gel electrophoresis. Average specific activities of this preparation are 1300 units/mg protein. The proteins of this preparation are organized in particles of maximum diameter of 50 Å, each containing one alpha subunit (MW 104,000) and one beta subunit (MW ~40,000). Both subunits possess extracellular portions, whereas only the alpha subunit protrudes on the intracellular side of the membrane. Approximately 20–40% of the transport protein has been estimated to be embedded in the lipid bilayer using either infrared spectroscopy or detergent binding methods (42). Data from studies on the purified protein indicate that significant structural changes (but not rotation or translation of major protein portions) occur at the alpha subunit and are coupled to the basic reactions of the sodium pump. These changes include (a) position changes of residues forming lysyl or arginyl peptide bonds at three different positions on the alpha subunit, (b) position changes of tryptophanyls and an amino group near the ATP binding site, (c) change in alpha unit structure by phosphorylation and transition between the phosphoforms (involving sulfhydryl groups of unknown number and location), and (d) change in structure of the alpha subunit by ouabain (42).

Highly purified enzyme preparations possess certain advantages over crude preparations in kinetic studies designed to determine the specificity and binding affinities of a particular ligand or the molecular mechanism of action of a transport inhibitor. However, ATPase purification can be time consuming and may require a fair amount of laboratory sophistication. Also, the final product is usually not as stable as ATPase from partially purified membrane preparations. The latter preparations are by far the most popular.

An excellent example is the NaI-treated pig brain microsomal preparation of Nakao et al. (61). This enzyme can be prepared from tissues other than brain (e.g., kidney, intestine, and heart) resulting in highly specific and relatively stable Na^+-K^+ ATPase preparations. In this procedure, microsomes are obtained from the white matter of cerebral hemispheres or from the kidney cortex according to the method outlined by Schwartz et al. (80). The microsomes are then treated using the following procedure:

1. Microsomal pellets are washed three times with 0.32 M sucrose containing 5 mM EDTA, then suspended in cold water at a concentration of 3–5 mg protein/ml.

2. An NaI solution (10 ml) containing 6 ml of 6.6 M NaI (pH 8.0 with Tris-HCl), 50 mM cysteine, 5 mM $MgCl_2$, 3 mM ATP, and 5 mM EDTA is slowly added at 0°C to 10 ml of the microsomal suspension.

3. The solution is diluted (after 30 min) with water to 0.8 M NaI and centrifuged for 30 min at 20,000 g.

4. The pellet is washed three times with an aqueous solution containing 5 mM EDTA and 5 mM NaCl (pH 7.4).

5. The final pellet is suspended in water to a concentration of approximately 2 mg/ml and stored at −20°C.

Specific activities for Na^+-K^+ ATPase activity from rabbit tissues have varied from as high as 208 units/mg protein in brain microsomal enzyme preparations to 14 units/mg protein from stomach homogenate enzyme preparations. Basal Mg^{2+}-activated ATPase is greatly reduced in all tissues following NaI treatment. Thus, this procedure (or modifications) may be applicable for the selective study of Na^+-K^+ ATPase from many different sources.

A rapid isolation procedure for canine, cat, rabbit, chicken, and human kidney ATPase has been described by Nechay and co-workers (63,64). The procedure has been used effectively to study the role of Na^+-K^+ ATPase in natriuresis and the mechanism of action of various cardiac glycosides, ethacrynic acid, and heavy metals. Canine whole kidney homogenates and fractions are isolated in the following manner:

1. Kidneys are removed and placed in beakers on ice. Perfusion is not necessary.

2. Capsules are stripped and kidneys are dispersed in a Waring blender for 1 min. Initial homogenates are prepared in 0.5 M sucrose solution containing 5 mM EDTA and 0.1% sodium deoxycholate adjusted to pH 6.8 with Tris and 10% (wt/vol) dilutions. The homogenate is further homogenized in all-glass tissue grinders and then filtered through a double layer of cheesecloth.

3. Homogenates are diluted 1:10 with 0.25 M sucrose in 1 mM Tris at pH 7.4 and centrifuged at 1,000 g for 20 min.

4. The supernatant fluid is fractionated by spinning at 10,000 g for 20 min and then at 80,000 g for 45 min.

5. Pellets are resuspended in 2 ml of sucrose-Tris solution, stored at −20°C, and assayed within 24 hr.

Whole canine kidney homogenates contain a total ATPase activity of approximately 69 units/mg protein with a ouabain sensitivity >50%. Resuspended cell fractions vary according to the percentage of the total homogenate activity and protein, with the 10,000 g fraction containing the greatest activity (46.4%) of the whole kidney homogenate.

Another fractionation technique has been used to isolate crude mixtures of mitochondria, endoplasmic reticulum, and nerve endings, as well as microsomes from brain, liver, and kidney for in vitro and in vivo analysis of ATPase activity (67). It is a rapid isolation technique that avoids the use of detergents and extensive washing procedures, thus minimizing the potential for dissociation of bound ligand and facilitating ATPase analysis *in vivo*. This procedure can be used to screen and differentiate the effects of toxic chemicals on major enzymatic components of mitochondrial-associated Mg^{2+} ATPase (oligomycin sensitive and insensitive) and membrane Na^+-K^+ ATPase.

Briefly, animals are euthanized by decapitation, and the brain, kidneys, and liver are quickly removed and stored in ice-cold 0.32 M sucrose solution, pH 7.5, containing 1 mM EDTA and 10 mM imidazole. Tissues are separately homogenized in 10 ml of the sucrose solution with a ground-glass homogenizer. Homogenates are fractionated by first spinning at 900 *g* for 10 min to eliminate nuclei and heavy cellular fragments. The supernatant fluid is then centrifuged at 13,000 *g* for 20 min. The resulting pellet obtained after this centrifugation is resuspended in cold 0.32 M sucrose solution. This fraction (B) contains a mixture of nerve endings, endoplasmic reticulum, and mitochondria. The Mg^{2+}-stimulated component can be delineated into oligomycin sensitive (mitochondrial) and insensitive ATPase by adding 5×10^{-6} M oligomycin to reaction mixtures. Microsomal fractions are prepared from the supernatant fluid (B fraction) by centrifugation at 100,000 *g* for 1 hr. The resulting pellet (fraction C) is resuspended in the same manner as B. The preparations are appropriately diluted (0.5–1.0 mg/ml) and divided into small aliquots, which are immediately quick frozen in liquid nitrogen. Samples can be stored at −80°C, and they remain stable for at least 6 months.

Specific activities for ATPase from mouse and rat tissues obtained by this method are dependent on the tissue type and source. They typically range from nondetectable to very low (for Na^+-K^+ ATPase in liver B and C fractions) and 30 to 50 units/mg protein (for Na^+-K^+ ATPase in brain B and C fractions). Magnesium ATPase activities associated with B fractions range from 5 to 30 units/mg protein (oligomycin sensitive) and 15 to 20 units/mg protein (oligomycin insensitive). The inhibitory effects of a variety of mycotoxins have been investigated using B and C fractions from mouse and rat brain and a highly specific Na^+-K^+ ATPase from swine brain cerebral cortex microsomes (66,68,70,71,88). Numerous methods for the isolation and preparation of a variety of ATPases, including reconstituted sodium pumps from sources such as kidney, brain, and rectal gland, have also been reviewed (3,30,31,60,77,81,86).

Calcium and Magnesium-Activated ATPase and Sodium/Calcium Exchange

Calcium continuously penetrates cells and must be pumped out to prevent an intracellular overload. Two such pumping mechanisms have been identified: a specific ATPase and a sodium/calcium exchange mechanism. Although the exchange mechanism has been considered as the major mode of removal of calcium from excitable tissues, both systems coexist in excitable and nonexcitable tissues (12).

Calcium transport occurs in the plasma membrane as well as subcellular organelles such as the mitochondria and sarcoplasmic reticulum (SR) of the muscle fiber. The enzyme that plays a major role in this transport event is Ca^{2+}-Mg^{2+}-

activated ATPase (Ca^{2+}-Mg^{2+} ATPase). Its occurrence has been reported in red blood cells, blood platelets, brain microsomes, nerve, salivary gland, placenta, gill, renal tubular cells, and sarcolemma and has been reviewed in detail by Stekhoven and Bonting (86) and Bronner and Peterlik (12). There are indications that calcium maintenance may play a role in the control of gene expression during the development of fertilized eggs, the transformation of lymphocytes, the replication of hemopoietic stem cells, in embryonic induction, and in fusion and differentiation of muscle cells; however, much of this evidence has been indirectly derived and is not clearly understood at this time. Ca^{2+}-Mg^{2+} ATPase also has been reported to play a major role in avian egg-shell thickness. Reproductive failure has been attributed to the thinning of the egg shell in a number of bird species after exposure to dichlorodiphenyltrichloroethane (DDT). The mechanism of action has been determined to be an inhibition of Ca^{2+}-Mg^{2+} ATPase by dichlorodiphenyldichloroethene (DDE) (common metabolite of DDT), which significantly alters Ca^{2+} transport from the blood to the shell (18,58).

Research on the sodium/calcium exchange mechanism from isolated vesicles of heart sarcolemma (SL) indicates that the carrier is electrogenic with a probable stoichiometry of three sodiums exchanged per one calcium, based on direct flux measurements during exchange activity. Thus the exchanger couples transmembrane movements of calcium to sodium in the opposite direction. This conclusion has originated from several lines of evidence. The time course of sodium-stimulated calcium efflux from SL vesicles has also been studied using stopped-flow spectrophotometry and the calcium-sensitive dye, Arsenazo III (14). In the absence of sodium, calcium efflux occurred very slowly (i.e., <0.01 nmol/mg protein/sec); however, as the concentration of sodium was increased, there was a significant rise in the velocity of calcium release (>2 nmol/mg protein/sec at 80 mM NaCl) (14). Interestingly, the exchanger appeared to be calmodulin insensitive and was not inhibited by vanadate at concentrations that completely disrupt Ca^{2+} ATPase activities (12).

Sarcoplasmic Reticulum and Ca^{2+}-Mg^{2+} ATPase

Calcium and magnesium-activated ATPase plays an important role in the maintenance of normal muscle contraction. It has been proposed that changes in free cytoplasmic calcium concentrations during development of muscle may influence the rate of synthesis of SR Ca^{2+} ATPase and other calcium binding proteins by calcium-dependent regulation of relevant classes of translatable messenger ribonucleic acids (mRNAs). Cytoplasmic calcium concentration may be modulated through nuclear calcium binding proteins serving as selective inducers or repressors of gene transcription (56). Vesicular fragments of sarcoplasmic reticulum (subcellular organelles of the muscle fiber) display an active and specific Ca^{2+} pump action. This active transport process is thought to be mediated by a Mg^{2+}-dependent Ca^{2+} ATPase (60,86). A phosphorylated intermediate in the ATPase reaction, much like that of the Na^+-K^+ ATPase, has been postulated. Structural studies of isolated SR vesicles have suggested the presence of three major proteins (Ca^{2+}-Mg^{2+} ATPase, calsequestrin, and M_{55}) and various phospholipids. The ATPase enzyme constitutes approximately 80% of the total SR protein and represents the pump mechanism, whereas the calsequestrin and M_{55} proteins probably serve to bind calcium in the SR (44). Bastide and co-workers (5) proposed that similarities of the primary sequence of the active sites of Na^+-K^+ ATPase from plasma membranes and Ca^{2+}-Mg^{2+} ATPase from SR of muscle suggest evolution of these two enzymes from a common ancestor. Many methods for isolation and purification of SR ATPase have been published with estimated molecular weights ranging from 80,000 to 190,000 daltons (30,40).

Inesi et al. (40) employed an extraction procedure for rabbit muscle that appears to remove minor protein components completely from the SR membrane. The main component remains with the membrane particles, which retain all of the ATPase activity. The residual particles are then solubilized with Triton X-100 to give a solution of pure, active ATPase with almost 100% yield.

A variety of methods for determining calcium and phosphate transport across mitochondrial membranes, renal and intestinal epithelial cell membranes, and hormonal regulation of transport have been reported (12).

Basal Mg^{2+} ATPase Activity of Plasma Membrane

When Na^+, K^+, and Ca^{2+} are not present in reaction mixtures, membrane preparations still have a residual ability to hydrolyze ATP. This component, which significantly varies in activity according to tissue source and isolation technique, has been designated as Mg^{2+}-stimulated ATPase. Its physiological role and/or interrelationship to the other ATPases is not currently understood. It may represent a distinct enzyme system or merely a different functional state of the Na^+-K^+- and/or Ca^{2+}-stimulated complex. Mg^{2+} is required for both Na^+-K^+ ATPase and Ca^{2+} ATPase activity, but Mg^{2+} is not transported under conditions that are optimal for these enzymes. Mg^{2+} ATPase is not affected by a variety of chemicals that are potent inhibitors of Na^+-K^+ ATPase. Its activity can be altered by nonspecific agents such as ethacrynic acid and p-chloromercuribenzoate, but inhibition constants are usually higher than for other ATPase components. More research is warranted to determine the nature of this indigenous component of enzyme transport.

Gastric Mucosal ATPase

A thiocyanate (SCN^-)-inhibited bicarbonate-stimulated ATPase has been observed in the gastric mucosa of the frog, and its involvement in the process of hydrochloric acid secretion has been postulated (43). The location of this ATPase has been confirmed in the smooth vesicular membrane of oxyntic cells of the hog stomach. The proposed model for its mechanism of action resembles the theory of chemiosmotic coupling of oxidative phosphorylation with CO_3^{2-} substituting for O^{2-}. A type of ATPase has been described that is K^+ stimulated, ouabain insensitive, and Mg^{2+} dependent (29). The ability of these mammalian preparations to perform vectorial ATP-driven proton (H^+) transport suggests

their participation in the process of acid secretion in the stomach (75).

Proverbio and Michelangeli (75) have suggested that Ca^{2+} acts as a second messenger in stimulus-secretion coupling in the parietal cell. Their protocol for the preparation of hog gastric microsomes (with activities of Ca^{2+}-activated H^+/K^+ ATPase on the order of 467 nmolP_i/mg protein/hr) is outlined as follows:

1. Empty hog stomachs are obtained fresh from a slaughterhouse.
2. The antral and cardiac regions are cut away, and the mucosa is removed from the outer muscle by scalpel dissection.
3. Mucosal cells are scraped off from the underlying connective tissue and each gram of tissue is immediately homogenized (5 strokes at 2,000 rpm) at 0°C in 5 ml of a 0.25-M sucrose solution buffered with 10 mM Tris-HCl (pH 7.4) in a Teflon ground-glass homogenizer.
4. The homogenate is spun at 500 g for 10 min.
5. The resulting supernatant fluid is centrifuged at 20,000 g for 20 min. The final supernatant fluid is spun at 100,000 g for 120 min.
6. Microsomal pellets are resuspended in sucrose solution to a final suspension of 5 to 8 mg protein/ml. Twenty milliliters are used for assay of the ATPase activity.

These preparations contain a basal Mg^{2+}-dependent ATPase activity that is stimulated by K^+ and low levels of Ca^{2+} (10 μM). High concentrations of Ca^{2+} (>100 μM) inhibit the K^+-stimulated component of ATPase activity. For further information on gastric proton-transport ATPase, the reader is referred to an excellent review of the topic by Sachs and co-workers (20).

METHODS OF ATPase ANALYSIS

ATPase activity has been routinely determined using two methods of analysis, both involving hydrolysis of ATP to ADP and inorganic phosphate. The two methods are (a) discontinuous or chemical endpoint phosphate analysis and (b) continuous or enzyme-linked analysis. The chemical endpoint method utilizes the formation of a reduced phosphomolybdate complex and colorimetric analysis to determine ATPase activity, although the linked or coupled enzymatic method utilizes the formation of ADP to drive a sequence of reactions resulting in oxidation of reduced nicotinamide adenine dinucleotide (NADH) with a concomitant decrease in absorbance at 340 nm (which is spectrophotometrically followed).

There are advantages and disadvantages to both methods. In the discontinuous method, many agents may react with the molybdate reagent or chemicals other than inorganic phosphate, yielding erroneous results. These possibilities must be spectrophotometrically eliminated. In the continuous assay, many compounds that inhibit ATPase may inhibit reaction-dependent enzymes such as pyruvate kinase and lactic acid dehydrogenase, thus altering results. The main advantage of the continuous method, as the name implies, is that the reaction can be continuously monitored with time, and a constant steady state level of ADP is maintained, thus avoiding negative feedback, which occurs at levels approaching 0.5 to 0.7 μmol in the chemical method. Both methods, however, warrant attention in this chapter, and for means of comparison and confirmation, both can be employed in the same study. It has been shown that no significant differences occur between the two assay methods when employed under exacting conditions (22).

Discontinuous Method

Many methods for determining inorganic phosphate in the ATPase assay have been based on color formation from the reduction of a phosphomolybdate complex. Probably the most widely used method is that of Fiske and Subbarow (27). However, many modifications of this method have been employed to enhance stability and to increase sensitivity. An ascorbic acid method has been reported by Lowry and associates (53) and modified by Chen and co-workers (16). Sensitive automated techniques utilizing the discontinuous method have also been reported (9,76). Grindley and Nichol (36) have combined essential methodology with solvent extraction of inorganic phosphate complexes.

The method of Lowry and Lopez (52) as modified (67) will be described in more detail. It does not require numerous and complex reagents; however, good technique is critical. Determination of Na^+-K^+ and Mg^{2+} ATPase activity is accomplished in a 1.0-ml reaction mixture containing, in final concentration, 5.0 mM ATP, 5.0 mM Mg^{2+}, 100 mM Na^+, 20 mM K^+, 135 mM imidazole/HCl buffer (pH 7.5), and 10 to 50 μg enzyme protein. The total cationic ligand-stimulated ATPase activity of enzyme aliquots is measured with Na^+, K^+, and Mg^{2+} present in the reaction mixture. The basal Mg^{2+} component is measured by omitting both Na^+ and K^+. Thus, delineation of the Na^+-K^+-activated component of ATPase is obtained from the difference between total ATPase (Na^+ + K^+ + Mg^{2+}) and basal Mg^{2+} ATPase (Mg^{2+} only) activity. The Na^+-K^+ ATPase activity is consistently ouabain

sensitive. Treated and control preparations, reagent, and enzyme blanks (to correct for inherent phosphate present in samples) are simultaneously incubated at 37°C for 10 min before initiation of the reaction with ATP. Incubation is stopped after 10 to 20 min with the addition of trichloroacetic acid (TCA) at a final concentration of 5% wt/vol in the reaction mixture. Samples are assayed for inorganic phosphate by the modified Lowry and Lopez method. Protein is determined by the method of Lowry et al. (54) with bovine serum albumin as the standard. A specific outline of this procedure is given in Table 3.

Assay

Reagent, solvent vehicle, and enzyme blanks should always be determined (and subtracted if necessary). Volumes must be maintained at 0.9 ml through step 6 (see below), and "assays" should be run in triplicate and independently reproduced, according to the following steps:

1. Pipette buffer with salts (Na^+, K^+, Mg^{2+}, and Mg^{2+} only) and H_2O or buffer for dilution (as needed) into 13 × 100-cm disposable tubes.
2. Add the enzyme preparation (usually 10–50 μg protein/0.050 ml) and mix thoroughly.
3. Add any chemicals to be tested in as small a volume as possible for addition of the enzyme preparation, using a Hamilton microsyringe, and mix. This can be accomplished by carefully inserting the tip of the syringe under the center swirl. (Do not forget the solvent blank and solvent control.)
4. Preincubate if desired at 37°C in a water bath.
5. Start the incubation reaction by adding substrate (ATP) into each tube at 10- to 15-sec timed intervals (e.g., sample no. 1, 0 sec; no. 2, 10 sec; no. 3, 20 sec).
6. Immediately mix each tube and incubate in a water bath at 37°C for 10 to 20 min, depending on protein and/or

TABLE 3. *Discontinuous ATPase procedure*

Stock reagents	Final concentration reaction mixture
A. Refrigerator (0–4°C)	
1. Buffer: imidazole	135 mM
2. Salts:	
NaCl	100 mM
KCl	20 mM
MgCl	5 mM
Prepare all salts in 1.0 L of buffer (pH 7.5) (=total reaction mixture).	
Prepare Mg^{2+} only in 1.0 L of buffer (pH 7.5) (=basal Mg^{2+} reaction mixture).	
Ascorbic acid (Sigma), 1% solution	
TCA (Sigma), 50% solution	
B. Freezer (−20°C)	
ATP (vanadium free, Sigma). Solutions are not stable.	
C. Shelf	
1. Ammonium molybdate, 2% solution (wt/vol)	
Stir well and filter if necessary (avoid contaminated glassware with this and all solutions).	
2. H_2SO_4 (1.0 N)	
Mix C1 and C2 just before use at 1:1 ratio to give 0.5 N H_2SO_4 and 1% molybdate solution.	
This solution should not be used after 15 min postmixing.	
3. Sodium acetate (0.1 N)	

cation-substrate concentration and specific activity of the preparation.

7. Stop the reaction with 0.1 ml of the 50% TCA solution (ice cold) by adding it to the reaction mixture and mixing. Addition of TCA should be in the same order and interval used to start the reaction.
8. If a precipitate is formed, centrifuge the tubes at 3,000 rpm for 5 min and remove aliquots of the supernatant fluid for the assay. No more interval timing is required at this point.
9. Add 3.0 ml of 0.1 N sodium acetate solution per 1.0 ml reaction mixture to each tube as soon as possible after stopping the reaction.
10. Add 0.4 ml of the molybdate/H_2SO_4 solution to each tube.
11. Add 0.4 ml ascorbic acid solution to each tube.
12. Mix all tubes and start the timer.
13. Read absorbance at 800 nm after 25 min.
14. The Na^+-K^+-activated component of the ATPase activity is equal to the difference between total ATPase (Na^+ + K^+ + Mg^{2+}) and basal Mg^{2+} ATPase (Mg^{2+} only).

Check the following:

1. Final pH should be between 4.0 and 4.6; if not, adjust acetate solution.
2. Spectrophotometer zero with sample blanks and killed enzyme blanks, etc., should be established.
3. The phosphomolybdate complex develops as a function of time and plateaus in approximately 15 min; however, this time varies with concentration of protein and enzyme source, etc. Check on the spectrophotometer if in doubt about stability time for the phosphomolybdate complex.

Specific Activity

Construct a standard curve. Final concentrations of phosphate from 0.0625 to 1.0 mM in 1.0 ml buffer solution are prepared from a stock solution of 0.0025 M phosphate. The color is developed as above (from the TCA step), and the optical density (OD) is read after 25 min. Phosphate in the samples is calculated and expressed as specific activity in μmoles inorganic phosphate formed per milligram protein per hour (μmol P_i/mg/hr).

Continuous Method

As previously described, the continuous or linked enzymatic method of analysis of ATPase utilizes the formation of ADP, which drives a coupled reaction forward with subsequent oxidation of NADH and a resultant decrease in absorbance at 340 nm. The reactions are summarized in the following scheme:

Step 1. ATP $\xrightarrow{\text{ATPase}}$ ADP + inorganic phosphate

Step 2. ADP + phosphoenol pyruvate $\xrightarrow{\text{pyruvate kinase (PK)}}$ pyruvate + ATP

Step 3. Pyruvate + NADH $\xrightarrow{\text{lactate dehydrogenase (LDH)}}$ lactate + NAD^+

A modified version of the enzymatic method (28) for analysis of ATPase has been described by Koch (46) and Desaiah and coworkers (22). In this procedure, a 3-ml reaction mixture contains 4.5 mM ATP, 5 mM Mg^{2+}, 100 mM Na^+, 20 mM K^+, 135 mM imidazole-HCl buffer (pH 7.5), 0.2 mM NADH, 0.5 mM phosphoenol pyruvate (PEP), 0.02% bovine serum albumin (BSA), 9 units of PK, 12 units of LDH, and 20–50 μg enzyme protein. Absorbance changes in the reaction mixture are measured at 340 nm in a recording ultraviolet (UV)-visible spectrophotometer with the temperature controlled at 37°C. The change in absorbance at 340 nm over a period of 10 min is used to calculate the specific activity. Enzyme activities are expressed as μmoles P_i per milligram protein/per hour. Protein is determined by the method of Lowry et al. (54) with BSA as the standard. Total ATPase activity is measured with Mg^{2+}, Na^+, and K^+ in the reaction mixture. Mg^{2+} activity is measured in the presence of 1 mM ouabain, which is a specific inhibitor of Na^+-K^+ ATPase. Na^+-K^+-activated ATPase activity (ouabain-sensitive) is obtained by the difference between total ATPase activity and Mg^{2+} ATPase activity. The Mg^{2+} ATPase also can be differentiated into mitochondrial oligomycin sensitive and insensitive components by adding 5×10^{-6} M oligomycin (based on a combined molecular weight of 401.2 from 15% oligomycin A and 85% oligomycin B in ethanol) to Mg^{2+} reaction mixtures. Oligomycin is a potent inhibitor of the mitochondrial Mg^{2+} ATPase activity involved in oxidative phosphorylation (77). A detailed protocol for this assay is given in Table 4.

Many other methods of ATPase analysis have been reported. Albers and Koval (2) described a pH stat method for measuring ATPase activity. Another procedure directly monitors enzymatic activity as the amount of radiolabeled ^{32}P liberated from (^{32}P) ATP during the hydrolysis reaction (17,55). Excellent methods for measurement of phosphorylation and transphosphorylation have been reported (4,55,74). Kinetic analysis has been successfully used to characterize the mechanisms of action by numerous chemicals. Techniques for the determination of effects of mycotoxins on Na^+-K^+ ATPase (66,68,71) have been previously described.

SHORT-CIRCUIT CURRENT TECHNIQUE

Much of our present state of knowledge concerning the transport of specific ions (e.g., sodium) has been derived from studies conducted with the epithelial membranes of frog skin and toad bladder. The intrinsic ability of these types of tissues to generate a biopotential difference (PD) between external and internal surfaces has been recognized for a significant period of time. For a detailed review, see Kotyk and Janacek (48).

Ussing and Zerahn (90) developed a novel method whereby frog skin preparations could be mounted between chambers separating each surface of the skin with aqueous phases. The PD was measured across the intact skin and reduced to zero (short-circuited) by the application of a current from a small battery in an external circuit. In the presence of identical solutions on both sides of the skin (which were used to eliminate chemical gradients) and zero potential difference, net movement of Na^+ ions occurred indicating active, electro-

TABLE 4. *Continuous ATPase procedure*

Stock reagents		Final concentration in reaction mixture
Refrigerator (0–4°C)		
Buffer: 200 mM imidazole (MW 68.1)		135 mM
13.62 g/L H$_2$O; adjusted to pH 7.5 with HCl		
Salts		
1.7 M NaCl (FW 58.45)	24.85 g	100 mM
0.34 M KCl (FW 74.56)	6.35 g } dissolved in 250 ml buffer	20 mM
0.085 M MgCl (6 H$_2$O) (FW 203.3)	4.32 g	5 mM
PK + LDH		
PK = 400 U/ml		
LDH = 900 U/ml; 0.2 ml PK + 0.1 ml LDH + 0.7 ml H$_2$O		
Ouabain (8 H$_2$O) (FW 728.6); 1.1664 g/100 ml H$_2$O		1 mM
Oligomycin; 6 mg/ml EtOH		
Sucrose solution: adjust pH to 7.5 with HCl		
Sucrose 109.536 g		
Imidazole 0.681 g } dissolved in 1 L redistilled H$_2$O		
EDTA 0.3362 g		
Freezer (−20°C; in individual vials)		
BSA; 6 mg/ml H$_2$O (2 ml/vial)		0.02%
PEP (see below for preparation) (2 ml/vial)		0.5 mM
ATP (see below for preparation)		4.5 mM
ATP: 3 H$_2$O		0.5144 g/10 ml redistilled water
ATP: 3.5 H$_2$O		0.5221 g/10 ml redistilled water
ATP: 4 H$_2$O		0.5348 g/10 ml redistilled water
ATP: 5 H$_2$O		0.5450 g/10 ml redistilled water
PEP: 4 H$_2$O		0.04590 g/10 ml redistilled water
PEP: 4.5 H$_2$O		0.04725 g/10 ml redistilled water
PEP: 5 H$_2$O		0.04896 g/10 ml redistilled water
PEP: 5.5 H$_2$O		0.04956 g/10 ml redistilled water
PEP: 6 H$_2$O		0.05052 g/10 ml redistilled water
PEP: 7 H$_2$O		0.05402 g/10 ml redistilled water
Shelf		
NADH: required amount to be added to the buffer before making the reaction mixture		

Reaction mixture	For batch of:	
	10	20
Buffer	24 ml	42 ml
Salts	1.76 ml	3.52 ml
BSA	1 ml ($\frac{1}{2}$ vial)	2 ml (1 vial)
PEP	1 ml ($\frac{1}{2}$ vial)	2 ml (1 vial)
NADH	3.5 mg	6.5 mg

Assay	Vial I	Vial II	Vial III
Reaction mixture	2.50 ml	2.50 ml	2.50 ml
PK-LDH	0.01 ml	0.01 ml	0.01 ml
H$_2$O	0.20 ml		
Ouabain		0.20 ml	0.20 ml
Oligomycin			0.001 ml
ATP	0.15 ml	0.15 ml	0.15 ml
Let mixtures warm in water bath for 15 min			
Enzyme fraction	0.10 ml	0.10 ml	0.10 ml
Reaction volume	2.96 ml	2.96 ml	2.96 ml

Start timer; mix; pour into cuvettes; let stand 5 min and record the Δ absorbance for 10 to 15 min at 340 nm and 37°C.

genic sodium transport. The current (SCC) required to short circuit the PD was shown to be equivalent to the amount of Na$^+$ transported, thus establishing a simple method for analyzing the sodium pump. Koefoed-Johnsen and Ussing (47) (Fig. 2) defined the PD across the epithelial layer of frog skin as a passive Na$^+$ entry step followed by an active extrusion of sodium through a pump located in the epithelial serosa (the last step being associated with Na$^+$-K$^+$ ATPase). Further evidence indicates that the pump and Na$^+$-K$^+$ ATPase are intimately related (5,8).

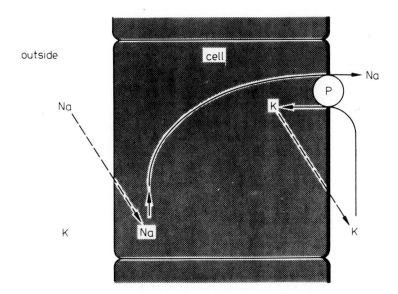

FIG. 2. Schematic illustration of the two-membrane hypothesis of Koefoed-Johnson and Ussing (47) to explain the origin of electric potential of frog skin. In this model, the inner membrane is specifically permeable to K$^+$ and possesses the sodium-potassium exchange pump, whereas the outer membrane is much more permeable to Na$^+$ than K$^+$. A potential difference (inside positive) is generated because of the asymmetry of the inner and outer membranes (32).

Figure 3 illustrates the classical SCC device of Ussing and Zerahn. It has been reported that the entry process of sodium exhibits saturation kinetics at approximately 60 mM Na$^+$ in the mucosal medium. Therefore, the active extrusion process is proportional to the amount of Na$^+$ in the transport pool and is limited by a saturable (possibly carrier-mediated) entry of Na$^+$ into the cells. Biber and Mullen (6) suggested that entry occurs via a transcellular pathway that interacts with the active transport pathway in frog skin. Recent research has indicated that cell-cell coupling between adjacent cell layers in frog skin may vary (according to the functional state of the tissue) and that the whole epithelium may function as

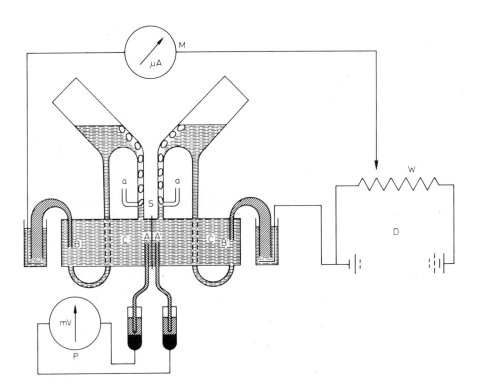

FIG. 3. Diagram of basic short-circuit apparatus of Ussing and Zerahn (90) for determining ionic fluxes across a single skin or bladder, S; a, air inlets; A and A', salt bridges connecting inside and outside bathing solutions via calomel electrodes; B and B', salt bridges for applying external EMF; D, battery; W, potential divider; M, microammeter; P, high-impedance millivoltmeter.

a syncytium (where all cells could participate in the pumping of sodium), and/or the outermost cell layer pumps most of the sodium (89).

Similar methods have been used to measure SCC and PD across epithelial sheets of other tissues, including turtle urinary bladder, gastric mucosa, and artificial secretory membranes. Because of their structural simplicity (only two cell layers thick), the intact urinary bladders of the turtle and toad represent an excellent *in vitro* model with which to study the effects of toxic agents on epithelial function, i.e., ion transport, ATPase activity, permeability, and hormonal control (49).

Methods

The two chambers required for SCC technique can be constructed from Plexiglas or glass and held together by a variety of clamping devices, screws with wing nuts, or elastic bands. Well-designed chambers and minimal pressure applied to the skin or bladder are desirable to prevent edge damage (97,98). This problem can be eliminated through the use of soft, inert gasket materials around the opening of each cell chamber and appropriate clamps. The chambers can be aerated and mixed by "bubble lifts" connected in line with each half cell (87). Efficiency of mixing and time required for total mixing should be checked with dyes. The chambers can be continuously perfused with fresh aerated solutions, if preferred, over the bubble lift. The biopotential difference across the tissue source can be monitored by calomel electrodes or silver-silver chloride electrodes connecting each half cell chamber via salt bridges. The bridges are placed as near to the surface of the membrane as possible and are made from small diameter polyethylene tubing filled with agarose (1–3%)-3 M KCl solution or Ringer's solution (which is used to bathe the tissue). The agarose-salt solution can be liquified in a hot water bath and quickly drawn into the polyethylene tubing by suction. On cooling, the tubing can be sliced into salt bridges of appropriate length using a razor blade or scalpel, making sure to expose the surface of the gel at an angle for maximal contact with solutions. A millivoltmeter, appropriate recording device, or electrometer with sufficiently high input impedance can be used to measure PD at predetermined intervals (48).

Electrical PD is localized on the membrane because the efficiency of the salt bridges in suppressing liquid junction potentials is the same in both halves of the circuit. By using the electromotive force of a small battery (6 V), an electrical current of measured strength is passed through the membrane until the PD is equal to zero. This SCC value is equivalent to Na$^+$ transport. This relationship can be verified via bidirectional flux measurements with radioactive sodium. Net flux (mucosal to serosal) is comparable to SCC. The SCC to Na$^+$ transport rate equivalency can then be readily calculated for any SCC apparatus (given the area of membrane surface exposed to the chamber solutions). A commonly used expression of rate is μEq or μmoles Na$^+$ per hour per square centimeter membrane. The rate equivalency of SCC can be derived as follows:

1. One faraday or 96,500 coulombs is equal to the charge carried on 1.0 mole Na$^+$ ions.

2. Current is equal to the rate of transfer of charge, and 1 μA is equal to 1.0363×10^{-11} moles/sec.

3. This value must be related to a unit area. Assuming the exposed area through which current flowed is 2.01 cm^2,

$$1 \ \mu A = \frac{1.0363 \times 10^{-11} \ \text{moles/sec}}{2.01 \ \text{cm}^2}$$

$$= 0.516 \times 10^{-11} \ \text{moles/sec/cm}^2$$

4. Conversion of SCC to hours and moles to μmoles gives

$$1 \ \mu A \ \text{SCC} = 0.0186 \ \mu\text{mol Na}^+/\text{cm}^2/\text{hr}$$

Therefore, an observed SCC of 40 μA would be equivalent to 0.75 μmol Na$^+$ transported per square centimeter membrane per hour in an apparatus with an exposed area of 2.01 cm^2.

Short-circuit current can be applied to the intact membrane using silver-silver chloride electrodes either connected via salt bridges to the half chambers or directly included in the medium bathing the membrane. The connections in either case should be as far away from the surfaces of the tissue source as possible. Silver wire can be easily anodized with silver chloride to form silver-silver chloride electrodes. Care must be taken that the silver is rigorously cleaned and that anodization is carried out slowly under controlled conditions. Major technical improvements and evolving strategies have been described for SCC analysis, e.g., multiple chambers for simultaneously monitoring paired hemibladders or paired sections of the same membrane, as well as an apparatus that automatically maintains the PD at zero while constantly recording SCC. We have designed and tested a microchamber for the measurement of SCC in anuran urinary bladder preparations and have demonstrated that the mycotoxin patulin impairs Na$^+$ transport and Na$^+$-K$^+$ ATPase activity (69). Inhibition of SCC was time dependent (Fig. 4) and of a second-order nature (Fig. 5). The linear response between Na$^+$ transport and Na$^+$-K$^+$ ATPase activity at different concentrations of patulin (Fig. 6) suggested that inhibition of Na$^+$ ion transport and the enzyme Na$^+$-K$^+$ ATPase were interrelated.

The rate of Na$^+$ transport can be quite variable. The investigator should be aware that many confounding factors can influence the rate of Na$^+$ transport, including temperature and pH fluctuations, edge damage, pressure and concentration variations in the chambers, and ground loop in the circuitry (48,97,98). Studies employing SCC technique should be rigorously controlled and initiated only after stable, reproducible baseline parameters are achieved. This may vary from preparation to preparation and season to season, but usually 1 to 4 hr is sufficient equilibration time. As previously mentioned, SCC is yet another useful method whereby toxic chemical-induced effects on the sodium pump can be investigated.

OTHER METHODS

Most functional aspects of membranes are mediated by specific receptors with a propensity for certain molecules or related classes of molecules. Thus, the ability to identify membrane receptor sites for toxic chemicals may greatly facilitate an understanding of molecular mechanisms of mem-

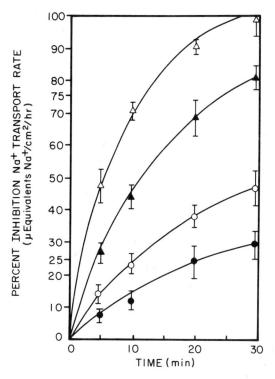

FIG. 4. Time course of inhibition of Na$^+$ transport by patulin. Data represent the percent inhibition ($\bar{X} \pm$ SE) of control rates (μEq Na$^+$/cm^2/hr) from three separate experiments (●, 1 × 10^{-4} M patulin; ○, 5 × 10^{-4} M patulin; ▲, 1 × 10^{-3} M patulin; △, 3 × 10^{-3} M patulin). (From ref. 69, with permission.)

brane toxicity. An impressive array of "cutting edge" techniques, applicable to membrane receptor research, have emerged from the forefronts of a variety of disciplines. Several excellent methodological reviews (detailing many of these approaches) have been published (92–94) and are recommended reading for the membrane toxicologist. Techniques discussed include methods of membrane receptor solubilization, e.g., organic solvent extraction, analysis of membrane phospholipids, photoaffinity labeling of receptors, erythrocyte sedimentation rate (ESR) spectroscopy of membranes; methods of purification of receptors, e.g., affinity chromatography, affinity phase partitioning, high performance liquid chromatography of membrane proteins, isoelectric focusing, autoantibodies as receptor probes; and methods of molecular and chemical characterization of receptors, e.g., monoclonal antibodies, immunoprecipitation, peptide mapping, reconstitution of membrane receptors, and recombinant DNA techniques.

SUMMARY

This chapter has detailed only a few of the numerous techniques available to the toxicologist interested in investigating the effects of toxins on membrane transport function. In addition to the cited literature, the reader is referred to the five excellent volumes of *Membrane Transport in Biology* edited by Giebisch et al. (30–34). These volumes consider in detail such aspects as transport across erythrocyte membranes, axon membranes, skeletal muscle fibers, mitochondrial mem-

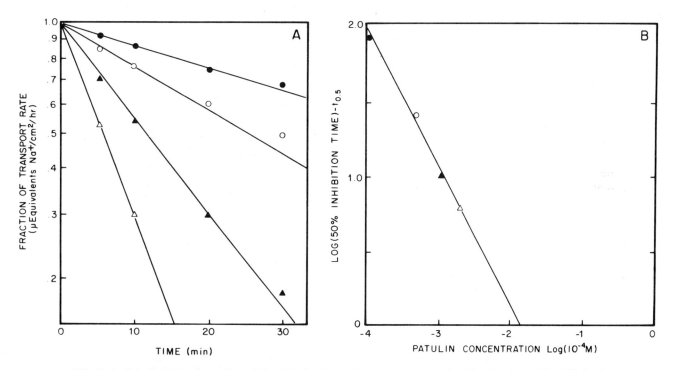

FIG. 5. A: Semilog transformation of the data in Fig. 4. Data are expressed as the fraction of the initial rate of transport (μEq Na$^+$/cm^2/hr). **B:** Log-log plot of the time for 50% inhibition ($t_{0.5}$) vs patulin concentration. (From ref. 69, with permission.)

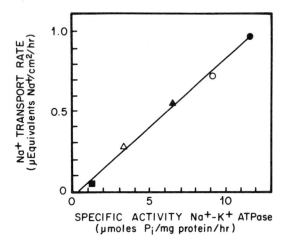

FIG. 6. Effect of patulin on toad bladder Na^+-K^+ adenosine triphosphatase (ATPase) activity (μmol P_i/mg protein/hr) and on the rate of Na^+ transport. Each value represents the $\bar{X}$ of three experiments. Linear regression analysis of the data gave $r = 0.996$ (●, control; ○, 1×10^{-4} M patulin; ▲, 5×10^{-4} M patulin; △, 1×10^{-3} M patulin; ■, 3×10^{-3} M patulin). (From ref. 69, with permission.)

branes, lysosomal membrane, plant and algal cells, insect excretory and gut epithelium, eye epithelia, choroid plexus, capillary endothelium, renal tubules, salivary and salt glands, gastric mucosa, small and large intestine, exocrine pancreas, gallbladder, hepatocytes, amphibian skin, and urinary bladder. The reader is also referred to the text *Impedance Measurements in Biological Cells,* edited by Ceretti (15), the text *Membranes, Molecules, Toxins and Cells* (7), Volumes 1 and 2 of *Receptor Biochemistry and Methodology* (which review cutting edge procedures for isolation, purification, and detection of membrane receptors), and the chapter by Kinter and Pritchard (45) in the *Handbook of Physiology, Reactions to Environmental Agents,* which further describe techniques in membrane toxicology.

In conclusion, membranes and associated transport systems are clearly vulnerable to insult by many different toxins. Evidence indicates that heavy metals and organochlorines (45), as well as numerous drugs and reactive toxins (21,22,67,69), may have as their primary mode of toxicity effects on membrane structure and/or transport. Still, a "membrane theory of toxicity" (45) is vaguely perceived. Large gaps exist in our knowledge of (a) the molecular interactions of toxins and cell membranes, (b) diagnostic indicators of membrane perturbation, and (c) the mechanisms of membrane toxicity. Much remains to be discerned in this dynamic area of research. The pursuit of such studies by the toxicologist will not only enhance our understanding of the basic chemical mechanisms of membrane toxicity but will increase our knowledge of molecular events governing membranes and membrane-associated transport phenomena that are critical to life processes.

REFERENCES

1. Ahmed, K., and Thomas, B. S. (1971): The effects of long chain fatty acids on sodium plus potassium ion-stimulated adenosine triphosphatase of rat brain. *J. Biol. Chem.,* 246:103–109.

2. Albers, K. W., and Koval, G. J. (1972): Sodium-potassium-activated adenosine triphosphatase VII. Concurrent inhibition of Na^+-K^+-adenosine triphosphatase and activation of K^+-nitrophenylphosphatase activities. *J. Biol. Chem.,* 247:3088–3092.

3. Askari, A. (editor) (1974): *Properties and Functions of ($Na^+ + K^+$)-Activated Adenosinetriphosphatase.* New York Academy of Sciences, New York.

4. Banerjee, S. P., Khanna, V. K., and Sen, A. K. (1970): Inhibition of sodium and potassium-dependent adenosine triphosphatase by ethacrynic acid: two modes of action. *Mol. Pharmacol.,* 6:680–690.

5. Bastide, F., Meissner, G., Fleischer, S., and Post, R. L. (1973): Similarity of the active site of phosphorylation of the adenosine triphosphatase for transport of sodium and potassium ions in kidney to that for transport of calcium ions in the sarcoplasmic reticulum of muscle. *J. Biol. Chem.,* 248:8385–8391.

6. Biber, T. U. L., and Mullen, T. J. (1976): Saturation kinetics of sodium efflux across isolated frog skin. *Am. J. Physiol.,* 231:995–1001.

7. Bloch, K., Bolis, L., and Tosteson, D. C. (1981): *Membranes, Molecules, Toxins and Cells.* PSG, Boston.

8. Bonting, S. L., and Canady, M. R. (1964): Na-K activated triphosphatase and sodium transport in toad bladder. *Am. J. Physiol.,* 207:1005–1009.

9. Bornancin, M., and De Renzis, G. (1976): A sensitive automated method for adenosine triphosphatase kinetics. *Anal. Biochem.,* 755:374–381.

10. Bretscher, M. S. (1985): The molecules of the cell membrane. *Sci. Am.,* 253:100–108.

11. Brody, T. M., and Akera, T. (1977): Relations among Na^+, K^+-ATPase activity, sodium pump activity, transmembrane sodium movement, and cardiac contractility. *Fed. Proc.,* 36:2219–2224.

12. Bronner, F., and Peterlik, M. (1981): *Calcium and Phosphate Transport Across Biomembranes.* Academic Press, New York.

13. Callingham, B. A. (editor) (1974): *Drugs and Transport Processes.* University Park Press, Baltimore.

14. Carfoli, E. (1981): Ca^{2+} pumping systems in the plasma membrane. In: *Calcium and Phosphate Transport Across Biomembranes,* edited by F. Bonner and M. Peterkik, pp. 9–13. Academic Press, New York.

15. Ceretti, S. R. P. (editor) (1978): *Impedance Measurements in Biological Cells.* John Wiley & Sons, New York.

16. Chen, P. S., Toribara, T. Y., and Warner, H. (1956): Microdetermination of phosphorus. *Anal. Chem.,* 28:1756–1758.

17. Chignell, C. F., and Titus, E. (1966): Effect of adrenal steroids on a Na^+- and K^+-requiring adenosine triphosphatase from rat kidney. *J. Biol. Chem.,* 241:5083–5089.

18. Cooke, A. S. (1973): Shell thinning in avian eggs by environmental pollutants. *Environ.,* 4:84–152.

19. Davis, R. P. (1969): Biochemical and metabolic aspects of transport. In: *Biological Membranes,* edited by R. M. Dowben, p. 109. Little, Brown, Boston.

20. Depont, J. J. H. H. M., Eeden, A. V. P. V., and Bonting, S. L. (1978): Role of negatively charged phospholipids in highly purified ($Na^+ + K^+$)-ATPase from rabbit kidney outer medulla. Studies on ($Na^+ + K^+$)-ATPase. *Biochim. Biophys. Acta,* 508:464–477.

21. Desaiah, D., Hayes, A. W., and Ho, I. K. (1977): Effects of rubratoxin B on adenosine triphosphatase activities in the mouse. *Toxicol. Appl. Pharmacol.,* 39:71–79.

22. Desaiah, D., Phillips, T. D., Hayes, A. W., and Ho, I. K. (1979): Effects of the aflatoxins on ATPase activities in mouse and rat liver. *J. Environ. Sci. Health,* B14:265–278.

23. Dixon, J. F., and Hokin, L. E. (1974): Studies on the characterization of the sodium-potassium transport adenosine triphosphatase. Purification and properties of the enzyme from the electric organ of *Electrophorus electricus. Arch. Biochem. Biophys.,* 163:749–758.

24. Dowben, R. M. (editor) (1969): *Biological Membranes.* Little, Brown, Boston.

25. Fahn, S., Koval, G. J., and Albers, R. W. (1966): Sodium-potassium-activated adenosine triphosphatase of *Electrophorus* electric organ. *J. Biol. Chem.,* 241:1882–1889.

26. Featherstone, R. M. (editor) (1973): *A Guide to Molecular Pharmacology-Toxicology* (1). Marcel Dekker, New York.

27. Fiske, C. H., and Subbarow, Y. (1925): The colorimetric determination of phosphorus. *J. Biol. Chem.,* 66:375–400.

28. Fritz, P. J., and Hamrick, M. E. (1966): Enzymatic analysis of adenosine triphosphatase. *Enzymologia,* 30:57.

29. Ganser, A. L., and Forte, J. G. (1973): K⁺-stimulated ATPase in purified microsomes of bullfrog oxyntic cells. *Biochim. Biolphys. Acta,* 307:169–180.

30. Giebisch, G., Tosteson, D. C., and Ussing, H. H. (editors) (1978): *Membrane Transport in Biology. I. Concepts and Models.* Springer-Verlag, New York.

31. Giebisch, G. Tosteson, D. C., and Ussing, H. H. (editors) (1979): *Membrane Transport in Biology. II. Transport Across Single Biological Membranes.* Springer-Verlag, New York.

32. Giebisch, G., Tosteson, D. C., and Ussing, H. H. (editors) (1978): *Membrane Transport in Biology. III. Transport Across Multi-Membrane Systems.* Springer-Verlag, New York.

33. Giebisch, G., Tosteson, D. C., and Ussing, H. H. (editors) (1979): *Membrane Transport in Biology IVA. Transport Organs.* Springer-Verlag. New York.

34. Giebisch, G., Tosteson, D. C., and Ussing, H. H. (editors) (1979): *Membrane Transport in Biology. IVB. Transport Organs.* Springer-Verlag, New York.

35. Golstein, J. L., Anderson, R. G. W. and Brown, M. S. (1979): Coated pits, coated vesicles and receptor-mediated endocytosis. *Nature,* 279: 679–685.

36. Grindley, G. B., and Nichol, C. A. (1970): Microprocedure for determination of pyrophosphate and orthophosphate. *Anal. Biochem.,* 33:114–119.

37. Guidotti, G. (1977): The structure of intrinsic membrane proteins. *J. Struct.,* 7:489–497.

38. Hatefi, Y., and Djavadi-Ohaniance, L. (editors) (1976): *The Structural Basis of Membrane Function.* Academic Press, New York.

39. Hokin, L. E., Dahl, J. L., Deupree, J. D., Dixon, J. F., Hackney, J. F., and Perdue, J. F. (1973): Studies on the characterization of the sodium-potassium transport of adenosine triphosphatase X. Purification of the enzyme from the rectal gland of *Squalus acanthias.* *J. Biol. Chem.,* 248:2593–2605.

40. Inesi, G., Blanchet, S., and Williams, D. (1973): ATPase and ATP binding sites in the sarcoplasmic reticulum membrane. In: *Organization of Energy-Transducing Membranes,* edited by M. Nakao and L. Packer, pp. 93–105. University Park Press, Baltimore.

41. Jorgensen, P. L. (1974): Purification and characterization of (Na⁺ + K⁺) ATPase. III. Purification from outer medulla of mammalian kidney after selective removal of membrane components by sodium dodecyl sulphate. *Biochim. Biophys. Acta,* 356:36–52.

42. Jorgensen, P. L. (1982): Topology in the membrane and principal conformations of the alpha subunit of Na⁺/K⁺ ATPase. In: *Membranes and Transport* (Vol. 1), edited by A. N. Martonosi, pp. 537–546. Plenum Press, New York.

43. Kasbekar, D. K., and Durbin, R. P. (1965): An adenosine triphosphatase from frog gastric mucosa. *Biochim. Biophys. Acta,* 105:472–482.

44. Katz, A. M., and Takenaka, H. (1981): Calcium transport across the sarcoplasmic reticulum. In: *Calcium and Phosphate Transport Across Biomembranes,* edited by F. Bronner and M. Peterlik, pp. 59–66. Academic Press, New York.

45. Kinter, W. B., and Pritchard, J. B. (1977): Altered permeability of cell membranes. In: *Handbook of Physiology* (Sec. 9), *Reactions to Environmental Agents,* edited by D. H. K. Lee, H. L. Falk, S. D. Murphy, and S. R. Geiger, pp. 563–576. Williams & Wilkins, Baltimore.

46. Koch, R. B. (1971): Biochemical studies of olfactory tissue: responses of ATPase activities to octanol and ascorbic acid. *Chem. Biol. Interact.,* 4:195–208.

47. Koefoed-Johnson, V., and Ussing, H. H. (1958): The nature of the frog skin potential. *Acta Physiol. Scand.,* 42:298–308.

48. Kotyk, A., and Janacek, K. (editors) (1970): *Cell Membrane Transport, Principles and Techniques.* Plenum Press, New York.

49. Kramer, H. J., and Gonick, H. C. (1970): Experimental Fanconi Syndrome 1. Effect of maleic acid on renal cortical Na-K-ATPase activity and ATP levels. *J. Lab. Clin. Med.,* 76:799–808.

50. Kyle, J. (1971): Purification of the sodium- and potassium-dependent adenosine triphosphatase from canine renal medulla. *J. Biol. Chem.,* 246:4157–4165.

51. Lane, L. K., Copenhaver, J. H., Lindenmayer, G. E., and Schwartz, A. (1973): Purification and characterization of and (H³) ouabain

binding to the transport adenosine triphosphatase from outer medulla of canine kidney. *J. Biol. Chem.,* 248:7197–7200.

52. Lowry, O. H., and Lopez, J. A. (1946): The determination of inorganic phosphate in the presence of labile phosphate esters. *J. Biol. Chem.,* 162:421–428.

53. Lowry, O. H., Roberts, N. R., Leiner, K. Y., Wu, M. L., and Farr, A. L. (1954): Quantitative histochemistry of brain. Chemical methods. *J. Biol. Chem.,* 207:1.

54. Lowry, O. H., Rosebrough, N. J., Farr, A. L., and Randall, R. J. (1951): Protein measurement with the Folin phenol reagent. *J. Biol. Chem.,* 193:265–275.

55. Mardh, S., and Post, R. L. (1977): Phosphorylation from adenosine trisphosphate of sodium and potassium-activated adenosine triphosphatase. *J. Biol. Chem.,* 252:633–638.

56. Martonosi, A. N. (1981): A possible role for cytoplasmic Ca²⁺ in the regulation of the synthesis of sarcoplasmic reticulum proteins. In: *Membranes and Transport* (Vol. 1), pp. 593–600. Plenum Press, New York.

57. Martonosi, A. N. (editor) (1982): *Membranes and Transport* (Vol. 1). Plenum Press, New York.

58. Miller, D. S., Kinter, W. B., and Peakall, D. B. (1976): Enzymatic basis for DDE-induced eggshell thinning in a sensitive bird. *Nature,* 259:122–124.

59. Miller, E. C. (1978): Some current perspectives on chemical carcinogenesis in humans and experimental animals. *Cancer Res.,* 38: 1479–1496.

60. Nakao, M., and Packer, L. (editors) (1973): *Organization of Energy-Transducing Membranes.* University Park Press, Baltimore.

61. Nakao, T., Tashima, Y., Nagano K., and Nakao, M. (1965): Highly specific sodium-potassium-activated adenosine triphosphatase from various tissues of rabbit. *Biochem. Biophys. Res. Commun.,* 19:755–758.

62. Nechay, B. R. (1977): Biochemical basis of diuretic action. *J. Clin. Pharmacol.,* 17:626–641.

63. Nechay, B. R., and Nelson, J. A. (1970): Renal ouabain-sensitive ATPase activity and Na⁺ reabsorption. *J. Pharmacol. Exp. Ther.,* 175:717–726.

64. Nechay, B. R., Nelson, J. A., Contreras, R. R., Sarles, H. E., Remmers, A. R., Beathard, G. A., Fish, J. C., Lindley, J. D., Brady, J. M., and Lerman, M. J. (1975): Ouabain-sensitive adenosine triphosphatase from human kidneys. *J. Pharmacol. Exp. Ther.,* 192: 303–309.

65. Pearse, B. M. F., and Bretscher, M. S. (1981): Membrane recycling by coated vesicles. *Annu. Rev. Biochem.,* 50:85–101.

66. Phillips, T. D., Chan, P. K., and Hayes, A. W. (1980): Inhibitory characteristics of the mycotoxin penicillic acid on (Na⁺-K⁺)-activated adenosine triphosphatase. *Biochem. Pharmacol.,* 29:19–26.

67. Phillips, T. D., and Hayes, A. W. (1977): Effects of patulin on adenosine triphosphatase activities in the mouse. *Toxicol. Appl. Pharmacol.,* 42:175–187.

68. Phillips, T. D., and Hayes, A. W. (1978): Effects of patulin on the kinetics of substrate and cationic ligand activation of adenosine triphosphatase in mouse brain. *J. Pharmacol. Exp. Ther.,* 205:606–616.

69. Phillips, T. D., and Hayes, A. W. (1979): Inhibition of electrogenic sodium transport across toad urinary bladder by the mycotoxin patulin. *Toxicology,* 13:17–24.

70. Phillips, T. D., and Hayes, A. W. (1979): Structural modification of polyfunctional rubratoxin B: effects on mammalian adenosine triphosphatase. *J. Environ. Pathol. Toxicol.,* 2:853–860.

71. Phillips, T. D., Hayes, A. W., Ho., I. K., and Desaiah, D. (1978): Effects of rubratoxin B on the kinetics of cationic and substrate activation of (Na⁺-K⁺)-ATPase and *p*-nitrophenyl phosphatase. *J. Biol. Chem.,* 253:3487–3493.

72. Phillips, T. D., Nechay, B. R. and Heidelbaugh, N. D. (1983): Vanadium: chemistry and the kidney. *Fed. Proc.,* 42:2969–2973.

73. Pitts, B. J. R., and Schwartz, A. (1975): Improved purification and partial characterization of (Na⁺, K⁺)-ATPase from cardiac muscle. *Biochim. Biophys. Acta,* 401:184–195.

74. Post, R. L., Toda, G., and Rogers, F. N. (1975): Phosphorylation by inorganic phosphate of sodium plus potassium ion transport adenosine triphosphatase. *J. Biol. Chem.,* 250:691–701.

75. Proverbio, F., and Michelangeli, F. (1978): Effect of calcium on the H⁺/K⁺ ATPase of hog gastric microsomes. *J. Membr. Biol.,* 42:301–315.

76. Putnins, R. F., and Yamada, E. W. (1975): Colorimetric determination of inorganic pyrophosphate by a manual or automated method. *Anal. Biochem.,* 68:185–195.

77. Racker, E. (1975): Reconstitution, mechanism of action and control of ion pumps. *Biochem. Soc. Trans.,* 3:785–802.

78. Rothstein, A., Takesita, M., and Knauf, P. A. (1972): Chemical modification of proteins involved in the permeability of the erythrocyte membrane to ions. *Biomembranes,* 3:393–413.

79. Sachs, G., Koelz, H. R., Berglindh, T., Rabon, E., and Saccomani, G. (1981): Aspects of gastric proton-transport ATPase. In: *Membranes and Transport* (Vol. 1), pp. 633–643. Plenum Press, New York.

80. Schwartz, A., Bachelard, H. S., and McIlwain, H. (1962): The sodium-stimulated adenosine-triphosphatase activity and other properties of cerebral microsomal fractions and subfractions. *Biochem. J.,* 84:626–637.

81. Schwartz, A., Lindenmayer, G. E., and Alka, J. C. (1972): *Current Topics in Membrane Transport,* edited by F. Bronner and A. Kleinzweller, pp. 1–83. Academic Press, New York.

82. Schen, S. S., Hamamoto, S. T., Bern, H. A., and Steinhardt, R. A. (1978): Alteration of sodium transport in mouse mammary epithelium associated with neoplastic transformation. *Cancer Res.,* 38:1356–1361.

83. Singer, S. J., and Nicholson, G. L. (1972): The fluid mosaic model of the structure of cell membranes. *Science,* 175:720–731.

84. Skou, J. C. (1961): Symposium on membrane transport and metabolism, Prague. In: *Membrane Transport and Metabolism,* edited by A. Kleinzeller and A. Kotyk, p. 228. Academic Press, New York.

85. Skou, J. C. (1964): Enzymatic aspects of active linked transport of Na^+ and K^+ through the cell membrane. *Prog. Biophys.,* 14:131–166.

86. Stekhoven, F. S., and Bonting, S. L. (1981): Transport adenosine triphosphatases. *Physiol. Rev.,* 61:1–76.

87. Toom, P. M., and Phillips, T. D. (1975): Effects of purified components of jellyfish toxin (*Stomolophus meleagris*) on active sodium transport. *Toxicon,* 13:261–271.

88. Unger, P. D., Phillips, T. D., and Hayes, A. W. (1978): Conversion of rubratoxin B to its carboxylic acid derivative and its effect on adenosine triphosphatase activity and toxicity to mice. *Fd. Cosmet. Toxicol.,* 16:463–467.

89. Ussing, H. H., and Nielsen, R. (1981): Coupling between epithelial cells in frog skin. In: *Membranes, Molecules, Toxins and Cells,* edited by K. Bloch, L. Bolis, and D. C. Tosteson, pp. 243–254. PSG, Boston.

90. Ussing, H. H., and Zerahn, K. (1951): Active transport of sodium as the source of electric current in the short-circuited isolated frog skin. *Acta Physiol. Scand.,* 23:110–127.

91. Van Le, A., and Doyle, D. (1984): General theory of membrane structure and function. In: *Membranes, Detergents and Receptor Solubilization* (Vol. 1), edited by J. C. Venter and L. C. Harrison, pp. 1–25. Alan R. Liss, New York.

92. Venter, J. C., and Harrison, L. C. (1984): *Receptor Biochemistry and Methodology: Membranes, Detergents and Receptor Solubilization* (Vol. 1). Alan R. Liss, New York.

93. Venter, J. C., and Harrison, L. C. (1984): *Receptor Biochemistry and Methodology: Receptor Purification Procedures* (Vol. 2). Alan R. Liss, New York.

94. Venter, J. C., and Harrison, L. C. (1984): *Receptor Biochemistry and Methodology: Molecular and Chemical Characterization of Membrane Receptors* (Vol. 3). Alan R. Liss, New York.

95. Venter, J. C., and Harrison, L. C. (1984): *Receptor Biochemistry and Methodology: Monoclonal and Anti-Idiotypic Antibodies as Probes for Receptor Structure* (Vol. 4). Alan R. Liss, New York.

96. Wallach, D. F. H., and Winzler, R. J. (editors) (1974): *Evolving Strategies and Tactics in Membrane Research.* Springer-Verlag, New York.

97. Walser, M. (1969): Reversible stimulation of sodium transport in the toad bladder by stretch. *J. Clin. Invest.,* 48:1714–1723.

98. Walser, M. (1970): Role of edge damage in sodium permeability of toad bladder and a means of avoiding it. *Am. J. Physiol.,* 219:252–255.

Principles and Methods of Toxicology, Second Edition, edited by A. Wallace Hayes, Raven Press, Ltd., New York © 1989.

CHAPTER **28**

Analysis and Characterization of Enzymes

F. Peter Guengerich

Department of Biochemistry and Center in Molecular Toxicology, Vanderbilt University School of Medicine, Nashville, Tennessee 37232

Analytical Procedures
Preparation of Microsomal and Cytosolic Fractions • Protein Determination • Assay of Cytochrome P-450 • Assay of NADPH-Cytochrome P-450 Reductase • Cytochrome P-450-Linked Activities • Other Cytochrome P-450-Linked Activities • Microsomal Flavoprotein Oxidase • Heme Oxygenase • Epoxide Hydrolase • Other Conjugating Enzymes

Isolation of Enzymes
Cytochrome P-450 • NADPH-Cytochrome P-450 Reductase • Epoxide Hydrolase • Other Enzymes • Methods for Determination of Enzyme Purity • Reconstitution of Enzyme Activity • Immunochemical Techniques • Immunoinhibition of Catalytic Activity • Quantitation of Proteins by Immunoblotting
References

Our knowledge in the field of toxicology has been advanced by investigations at a number of levels of organism complexity, including whole animal, organ perfusion, single cell, subcellular organelle, and isolated enzyme studies. The purpose of this chapter is to review *in vitro* assay procedures as well as techniques associated with preparation and utilization of purified enzymes important in toxicology. Such highly purified systems have been used to address a number of questions that could not have been definitively answered otherwise. For instance, although a number of studies strongly suggested the existence of multiple forms of cytochrome P-450 and other drug-metabolizing enzymes, isolation and characterization studies have provided the strongest evidence for this hypothesis and demonstrated exactly how the individual enzymes differ. Moreover, isolated enzyme systems have been used to define the roles of individual enzymes in various metabolic processes.

Almost a half-century has elapsed since the concept of bioactivation of chemicals to ultimate toxic forms originated (195). Such activation of many chemicals is now widely accepted as the first step leading to toxic and carcinogenic effects. By far the most common mechanism for such activation is mixed-function oxidation by cytochrome P-450. This enzyme system was discovered during the late 1950s and has attracted a great deal of interest ever since. A number of enzyme forms appear to exist within each species; some are tissue-specific as well as species-specific. The different forms preferentially oxidize different substrates, and this specificity contributes to the preferential bioactivation and detoxication of chemicals by different enzyme forms. Many of the basic principles discussed here also apply to other drug-metabolizing enzymes found in multi-gene families.

With a general catalytic mechanism involving abstraction of electrons or hydrogen atoms followed by oxygen rebound (88), one can explain the apparently diverse oxidative reactions catalyzed by cytochrome P-450, which can be classified as (a) carbon hydroxylation, (b) heteroatom oxygenation, (c) heteroatom release, (d) epoxidation, (e) oxidative group migration, and (f) suicidal inactivation by olefins (Figs. 1 and 2). These basic mechanisms can also explain the suicidal inactivation observed with other substrates such as cyclopropyl heteroatoms and aminobenzotriazole; variation of structural features has allowed the selective inactivation of individual isozymes by mechanism-based (suicide) inhibitors (212). Cytochrome P-450 also appears to reduce some compounds such as azo dyes and carbon tetrachloride.

The total number of cytochrome P-450 substrates easily runs into the thousands (292). The broad specificity is due in part to the existence of multiple forms, but even a single purified form (rat P-450$_{PB-B}$) has been shown to oxidize more than 70 substrates (82). The active site must be large enough to accommodate all of these substrates. However, a number of larger substrates, e.g., warfarin, testosterone, and debrisoquine, and other drugs are stereo- and regioselectively ox-

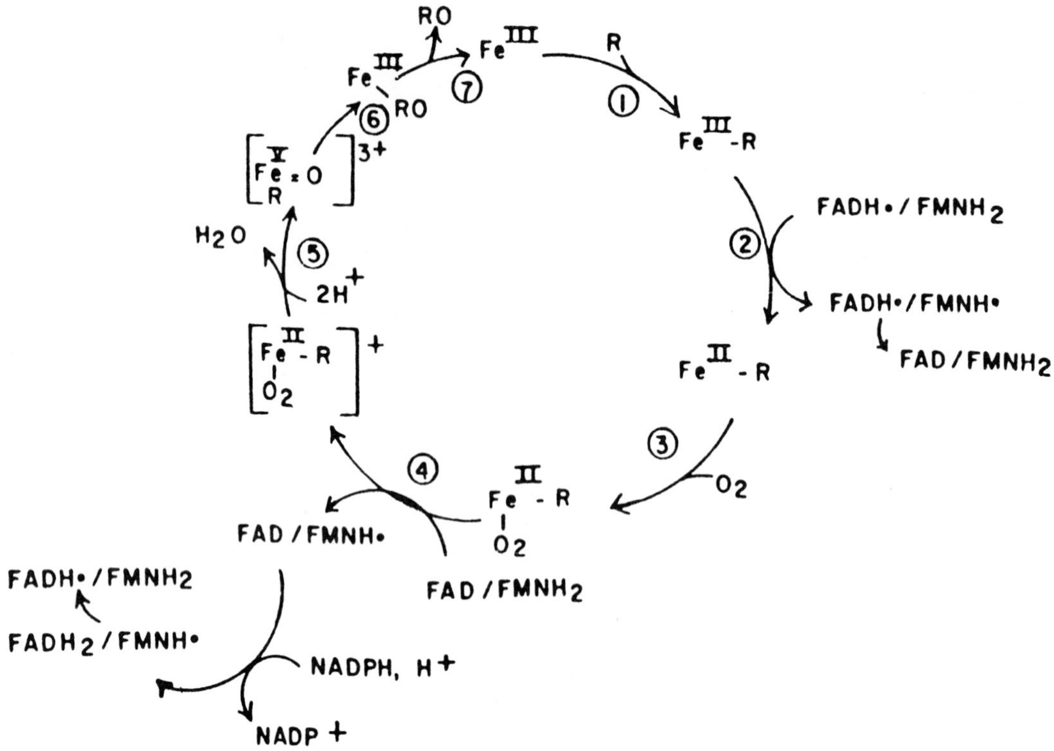

FIG. 1. Working scheme for the catalytic mechanism of cytochrome P-450. See ref. 88.

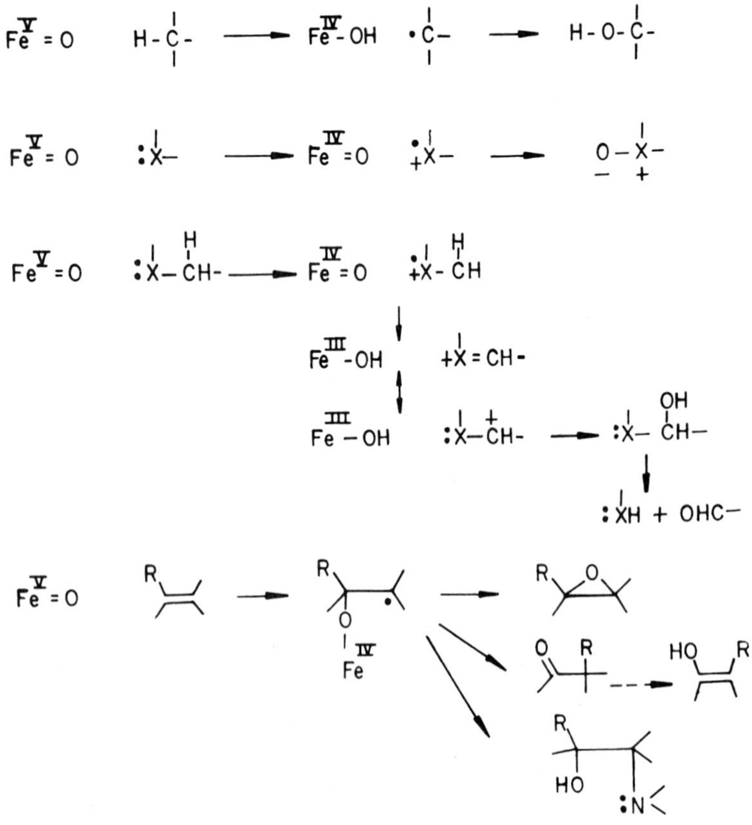

FIG. 2. Mechanisms of cytochrome P-450 reactions rationalized by electron abstraction (88). See text for discussion.

idized by cytochrome P-450 enzymes, indicating that the binding sites do have some distinct features. The smaller substrates apparently fit into these sites, and the sites of oxidation on them are probably governed more by chemical than spatial (physical) properties (Figs. 3–5). The view is widespread that cytochrome P-450 enzymes exist for the metabolism of specific endogenous substrates such as fatty acids, steroids, and eicosanoids; however, others believe that the purpose of these enzymes is the clearance of ingested foreign chemicals (e.g., terpenes, pyrolysis products).

One of the major reasons for the widespread study of cytochrome P-450 is that these enzymes are involved in the activation and detoxication of xenobiotics. However, much of the direct evidence is circumstantial. The literature is filled with examples in which one can directly demonstrate covalent binding of a chemical to protein or DNA with a cytochrome P-450 or produce mutagenesis in bacterial strains. Known cytochrome P-450-generated metabolites can be found bound to macromolecules *in vivo,* and in some cases administration of known products of cytochrome P-450 oxidation can produce the toxicity observed with the parent substrate (e.g., fluoroxene and trifluoroacetic acid) (87). Often the administration of chemicals known to induce (or inhibit) forms of cytochrome P-450 can increase or decrease the toxicity of a certain chemical in experimental animals. Unfortunately, the usefulness of this approach is limited because of the ability of these chemicals to alter the levels of several cytochromes P-450 concomitantly, alter the content of other

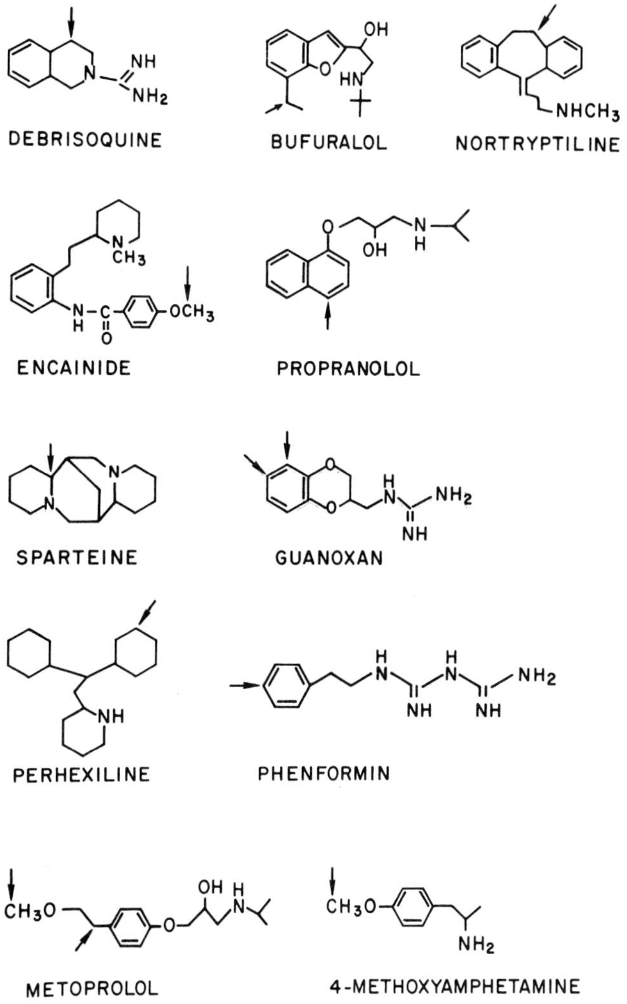

FIG. 4. Structures of drugs associated previously with debrisoquine 4-hydroxylation. The major hydroxylation sites thought to be involved are indicated with *arrows* (99).

enzymes as well, and affect the physiological parameters (e.g., blood flow) that contribute to endpoints under consideration. The problem of knowing exactly *how* metabolites exert toxic effects also obfuscates the problem. Although cytochromes P-450 do appear to play a role in the generation of ultimate toxicants and carcinogens, efforts to show the importance of changes in the composition of individual forms on the effects are not clear.

Today no doubt exists concerning the existence of distinct forms of cytochrome P-450 in experimental animals or man. Approximately 20 have been purified from rat liver and another set of 10 from rabbit liver. The purified proteins differ in electrophoretic properties, immunochemical aspects, primary sequence, and other criteria, including catalytic specificity (Fig. 6). The assignment of the proteins as separate gene products has been done using recombinant DNA technology as well as protein sequencing in some cases. Several of the rat cDNAs have been cloned, and this approach has

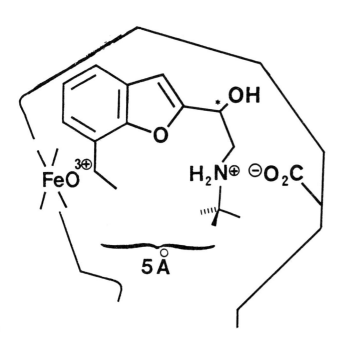

FIG. 3. Active site of the cytochrome P-450 involved in the metabolism of debrisoquine, bufuralol, sparteine, and other compounds. Bufuralol is shown in the active center. The asterisk denotes the chiral center of bufuralol. The distance between the nonbonding electrons of the basic nitrogen and the site of hydroxylation is about 5 Å. The phenyl ring is postulated to fit in a hydrophobic region of the enzyme (99).

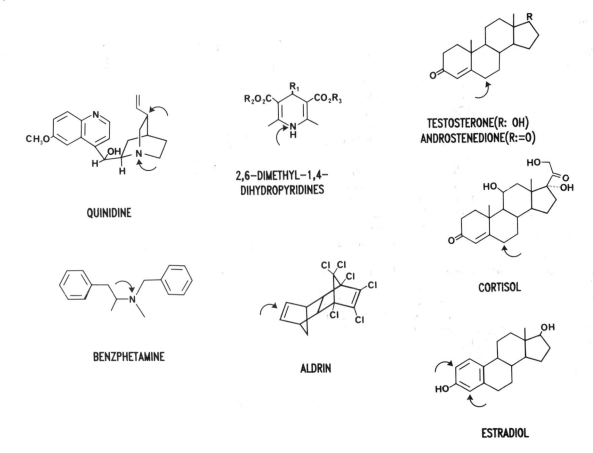

FIG. 5. Structures of substrates for human liver P-450_NF (99,101). Arrows indicate primary sites of oxidation. In the N-dealkylation reactions, the initial site of oxidation is presumed to be the nitrogen (nonbonded electrons) (88). See text for further discussion.

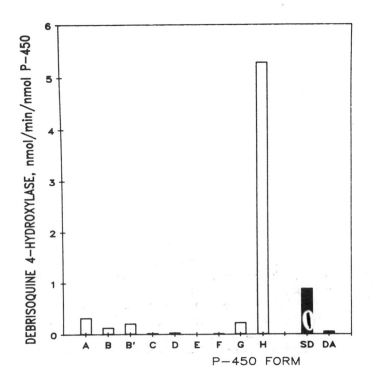

FIG. 6. 4-Hydroxylation of debrisoquine by rat liver cytochromes P-450. Open bars indicate rates of hydroxylation by individual forms of cytochrome P-450 in reconstituted systems: A, P-450_UT-A; B, P-450_PB-B; B', P-450_βNF-B; C, P-450_PB-C; D, P-450_PB-D; E, P-450_PCN-E; F, P-450_UT-F; G, P-450_ISF-G; H, P-450_UT-H. The filled bars show the activities with liver microsomes isolated from male Sprague-Dawley (SD) and female dark Agouti (DA) rats.

been used, in the main part, to establish the amino acid sequences of many of the rat cytochromes P-450. In addition, some genomic DNA sequences encoding rat cytochromes P-450 have been established. Similar efforts have been applied to some of the rabbit and mouse cytochromes P-450 as well.

The number of cytochrome P-450 forms has been a matter of speculation. About 20 forms have been purified from a single tissue (liver), and some of them appear, in turn, to be members of multigene families. Cytochrome P-450 forms known to catalyze certain key reactions (e.g., several steps in cholesterol formation) have not yet been isolated. Thus the total number of cytochrome P-450 genes could easily be in the range of 25 to 50 (2). There is no evidence to support the view that gene translocations have made cytochrome P-450 a very large supergene family like the immunoglobulins.

In some cases considerable conservation of cytochrome P-450 structure is found between species. Small differences among the cytochromes P-450 that have been sequenced, however, can generate large differences in catalytic activity and substrate specificity, as shown in several notable examples in rat and mouse liver: a 3% difference can lower catalytic activity by an order of magnitude (P-450$_{PB-B}$ versus P-450$_{PB-D}$) or specifically abolish a certain activity (warfarin 8-hydroxylase in mice) (82).

Several human cytochromes P-450 have now been purified (99), and they have been shown to have specificity in catalyzing the oxidation of drugs and other chemicals (Fig. 5). In every case some structural similarity with certain cytochrome P-450 forms isolated from experimental animals has been shown; however, this homology can be misleading in ascertaining catalytic specificity in some cases. As in the case of experimental animal models, immunochemical methods have been of use to establish the roles and catalytic specificities of the human cytochromes P-450. Probes for cytochromes P-450 from experimental animals have been used to identify several cDNAs for human cytochromes P-450 and derive their sequences, although in many cases the sequence of cytochromes P-450 deduced from these cDNA clones have not been correlated to cytochrome P-450 proteins that occur *in vivo*.

There are several levels at which overall catalytic activity can be influenced (80). Cofactor supply can be important: NADPH levels can be altered by starvation, and oxygen gradients exist in the liver. The different cytochrome P-450 forms also are localized preferentially in different regions of the liver (and in different cell types in liver and extrahepatic tissues). Heme is necessary as a prosthetic group for cytochrome P-450, and heme deficiency can lower activity. Furthermore, it is not known if there is any effect of heme on the regulation of cytochrome P-450 genes. NADPH-cytochrome P-450 reductase is present at an order of magnitude lower than that of cytochrome P-450 and is needed for activity. Although reconstituted cytochrome P-450 systems are stimulated by phospholipid, *in vivo* changes in lipid composition probably do not have any significant effect.

In experimental animals, the major way in which activities, or at least rather specific catalytic activities, are modulated is via changes in the amounts of individual cytochrome P-450 forms present (98). Such changes have been clearly demonstrated to involve *de novo* synthesis and seem to generally involve specific increases in rates of nuclear DNA transcrip-

tion. The list of cytochrome P-450 inducers is nearly as long as the list of substrates. Only in a few cases does one see induction of only one cytochrome P-450; more commonly several are induced. In some cases the level of one protein is depressed while others are induced (39,98). Several of the rodent liver cytochromes P-450 are also regulated by steroid hormones. There are two aspects of such modulation (apparently by androgens in both sexes), neonatal imprinting, and a later maintenance effect (41,281). The cytochrome P-450 proteins have similar half-lives (about 24 hr); however, some evidence exists for a stabilizing effect of certain classic "inducers" on mRNA and protein stability. Only in the case of one cytochrome P-450 does evidence exist for an intracellular receptor. The receptor has only recently been purified, but the structural gene for that polycyclic hydrocarbon-inducible cytochrome P-450 has been sequenced, and some information is available about the 5'-flanking regions that control expression (142).

Another aspect of regulation is polymorphism, which is observed with certain catalytic activities in both experimental animals and man. Although most of the catalytic activities associated with cytochromes P-450 are affected at least somewhat by environmental factors, genetic polymorphisms are distinct and not so readily influenced by other factors. They can be produced by variations in structural genes or in other proteins that regulate expression. Several polymorphisms have been mapped to chromosomes in humans, rats, and mice, but structural details underlying the polymorphisms have not been elucidated. In humans, genetic polymorphisms in the metabolism of certain drugs have been identified. Correlations have been made between individuals expressing one of the phenotypes and susceptibility to chemical carcinogenesis. The author's own laboratory has purified several human liver microsomal cytochromes P-450 that are involved in genetic polymorphisms of oxidative metabolism, and we are trying to establish the basis of the polymorphisms and their relevance to chemical toxicity and carcinogenesis (51,84,99,101,242). Others have characterized the DNA coding for human adrenal microsomal 21-hydroxylase, which is altered in a genetic disease of glucocorticoid metabolism, and found that the gene is located in the midst of the genes coding for a complement factor (289).

Although the cytochromes P-450 have received considerable attention, one should realize that the existence of isozymes is not unusual nor is a multigene family. These situations probably occur with many enzymes, including some that are involved in other aspects of metabolism of xenobiotic chemicals. For instance, at least ten forms of glutathione (GSH) *S*-transferase exist and have been shown to be distinct gene products. Again, the catalytic specificities of these enzyme forms differ, and many are under differential regulatory control. Considerable evidence supports the view that several forms of UDP-glucuronyl transferase and epoxide hydrolase are distinct gene products. Studies indicate that distinct forms of microsomal flavin-containing monooxygenase are found in various tissues, specifically the liver and lung (290). However, in other instances only one gene appears to be involved, e.g., NADPH-cytochrome P-450 reductase (222).

As mentioned above, cytochrome P-450-catalyzed oxidation can result in bioactivation or detoxication of a potential toxicant. (In general, reduction reactions catalyzed by either cytochrome P-450 or NADPH-cytochrome P-450 usually lead to more reactive products.) Oxidations by other enzymes (i.e., microsomal flavin-containing monooxygenase, alcohol and aldehyde dehydrogenases) can also result in bioactivation or detoxication. For instance, oxidation of allylic alcohols by alcohol dehydrogenase yields acrolein derivatives, which react rapidly with soft nucleophiles. In classical drug metabolism, oxidation–reduction reactions are usually considered "phase I," and conjugation reactions, which usually follow oxidation or reduction, are termed "phase II." Most of these "phase II" conjugation processes detoxicate chemicals, and therefore increases in the concentrations of the protein that catalyzes these reactions or increases in the concentrations of cofactors (cosubstrate) tend to render an organism at decreased risk to protoxicants. However, many exceptions to this generalization can be found. For example, epoxide hydrolase action on benzo-(a)pyrene-7,8-oxide leads to formation of a substrate that is efficiently converted to 9,10-oxo-7,8-dihydroxy-7,8-dihydrobenzo(a)pyrene, which reacts rapidly with DNA and is a potent mutagen and carcinogen. GSH-S-transferase, as indicated later, can activate vic-dihaloalkanes to yield DNA damage. Glucuronides formed by action of UDP-glucuronyl transferase on hydroxylamines can break down in the acidic environment of the bladder to release nitrenium ions, which can alkylate DNA. Thus we see that metabolic transformations must be viewed in a global manner to put the importance of individual steps into context.

What can studies on metabolic transformations tell us about the toxicity of chemicals? Comparison of the actions of a series of small industrial compounds provides some examples.

$$CH_2{=}CH{-}CN$$
$$CH_2{=}CH{-}Cl$$
$$Br{-}CH_2{-}CH_2{-}Br$$

Acrylonitrile is acutely toxic and causes several types of general toxicity problems as well when administered at high doses in chronic studies (i.e., nausea, weight loss, gastric disturbances). The compound is not particularly carcinogenic, causing only tumors of the forestomach, brain, and possibly Zymbal's gland at high doses. These actions can be understood when the various pathways for acrylonitrile are measured using in vitro assays. Acrylonitrile reacts rapidly and nonenzymatically with sulfhydryls, in both proteins and GSH (Fig. 7). Conjugation with GSH is the major fate of acrylonitrile and renders it innocuous. Reaction with proteins is considerable and probably accounts for the toxic effects of acrylonitrile. About 10% of acrylonitrile is oxidized by cytochrome P-450 to its epoxide, which can (a) release cyanide (which does not appear to play a role in toxicity), (b) be conjugated with GSH, (c) alkylate protein, or (d) alkylate nucleic acids. The latter reaction occurs and, although the tumorigenic potential of acrylonitrile is low, it is probably involved in the phenomenon (63,100,120).

Vinyl chloride may look similar to acrylonitrile but behaves differently. Only high doses are acutely toxic, and this toxicity is probably unrelated to metabolism. However, vinyl chloride is carcinogenic, causing a peculiar hemangiosarcoma that is almost unique to vinyl chloride production workers and can be reproduced in laboratory animals. Unlike acrylonitrile, vinyl chloride does not react directly with thiols, and its metabolism proceeds strictly through oxidation. The epoxide 2-chloroethylene oxide can react with nucleic acids, including $1,N^6$-ethenoadenine, $1,N^3$-ethenocytidine, and N^7-(2-oxoethyl)guanine, to form several lesions. Which of these reactions is most intimately related to tumorigenesis is yet unclear, although some evidence favors the latter adduct. The epoxide also spontaneously rearranges to form 2-chloroacetaldehyde, and 2-chloroacetaldehyde could also be formed by direct oxidation (167,196). 2-Chloroacetaldehyde is more like acrylonitrile, reacting rapidly and nonenzymatically with GSH and protein thiols. It reacts only slowly with nucleic acids and is probably not relevant to tumor initiation. The major site of vinyl chloride oxidation is the parenchymal cells of the liver. However, hepatic tumors originate in the reticuloendothelial cells, which have little if any oxidation capacity. A possible explanation is that the epoxide is formed

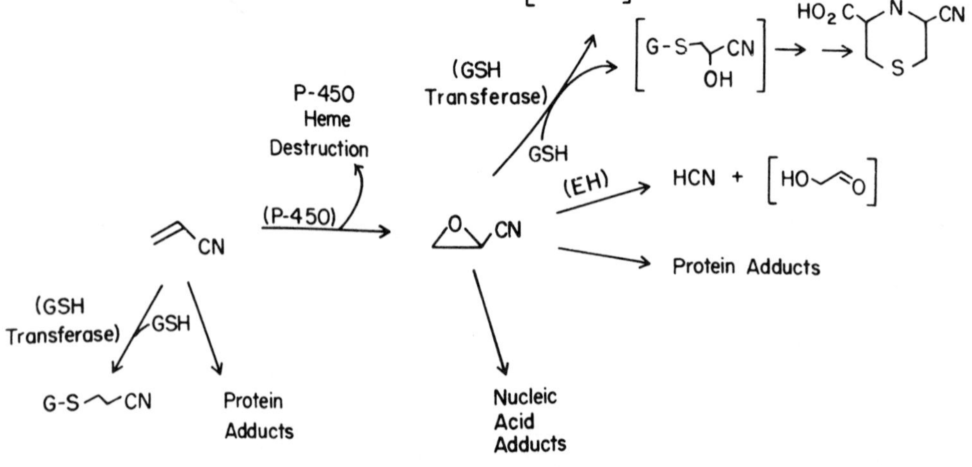

FIG. 7. Proposed scheme for hepatic metabolism of acrylonitrile (63).

in the parenchymal cells and is stable enough to migrate to other cells [some experimental evidence supports this view (102)]; the differential susceptivity to the alkylating agent may be explained by variations in rates of DNA adduct repair among the cell types.

The next compound to consider in this series is ethylene dibromide (1,2-dibromoethane). This compound causes kidney toxicity and is carcinogenic at a number of sites. Oxidation by cytochromes P-450 yields 2-bromoacetaldehyde, which behaves in the same way as 2-chloroacetaldehyde (*vide supra*) and depletes sulfhydryls. GSH S-transferase-catalyzed conjugation of ethylene dibromide with GSH also occurs; the ratio of ethylene dibromide metabolized through the oxidative and conjugative pathways is about 4:1 (270). In this case the GSH conjugate is unstable, however, because of the leaving group still present (Br) (Fig. 8). Spontaneous dehydrohalogenation produces an episulfonium (or thiiranium) ion, which also has several fates. If hydrolyzed, S-(2-hydroxyethyl)GSH is formed, and this innocuous product is degraded and excreted. The putative episulfonium ion can also react with another GSH to form the ethylene-bis GSH adduct, which is also innocuous. Another possibility is elimination to yield GSH plus ethylene, another mode of detoxication. However, another reaction (of the episulfonium ion) occurs with DNA to yield S-[N^7-(2-guanyl)-ethyl]GSH as the major product (213). This GSH pathway appears to be related to carcinogenesis because *in vitro* DNA binding and mutagenesis are much more dependent on cytosolic than microsomal enzymes; *in vivo* studies support this view (130,156).

Thus GSH conjugation can become a major bioactivation pathway.

The above three compounds share some apparently similar features, yet further analysis indicates that they differ widely in terms of their chemical properties, the manner in which they are handled by the body, and the biological effects that are exerted. Much of our understanding of these chemicals has come from *in vitro* studies using assays of the type described here. What can we learn from studies that focus on identification and quantitation of individual enzymes?

One example involves suppression of a particular cytochrome P-450 in rat liver. Polycyclic hydrocarbons such as 3-methylcholanthrene, β-naphthoflavone, and isosafrole induce increased synthesis of at least two forms of cytochrome P-450 in rat liver: P-450$_{\beta NF-B}$ and P-450$_{ISF-G}$. Increases in microsomal catalytic activities following administration of such compounds has generally been held to support the involvement of these inducible forms in a particular transformation, and in many *in vivo* studies alterations in acute toxicity of compounds by these inducers has been interpreted in the same terms. We purified a particular form of cytochrome P-450 in our laboratory, P-450$_{UT-A}$, and found that levels of this particular protein (measured with a specific antibody) were decreased when these compounds were given to rats that induced P-450$_{\beta NF-B}$ and P-450$_{ISF-G}$ (which were also measured immunochemically) (98). The decrease was as much as tenfold when certain polybrominated biphenyl congeners were administered to rats (39). Subsequent investigations established that P-450$_{UT-A}$ is male-specific (41,281)

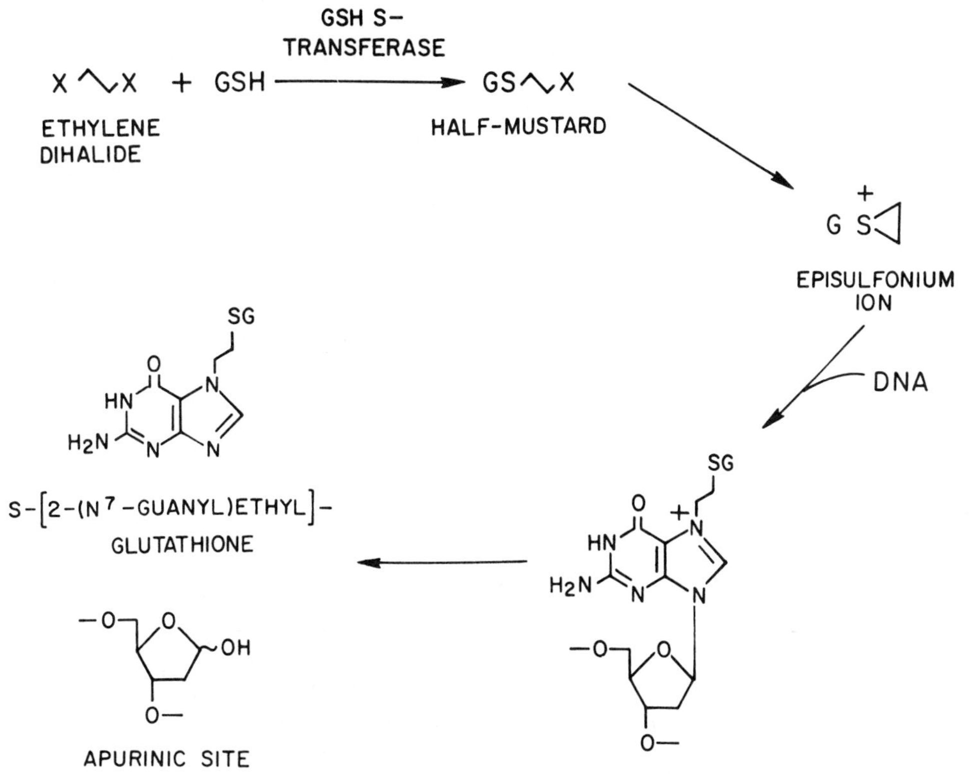

FIG. 8. Scheme showing formation of the major DNA adduct from ethylene dibromide and ethylene dichloride and the breakdown of the adduct (130).

and is responsible for the bulk of certain catalytic activities, including testosterone 2α-hydroxylation (281) and generation of the potentially toxic quinoneimine derivative of acetaminophen (112). If formation of a reactive metabolite is mediated by P-450$_{UT-A}$ and neither P-450$_{\beta NF-B}$ nor P-450$_{ISF-G}$ acts on the parent compound, one might (without knowledge of the complexity of the situation) conclude that if administration of polycyclic hydrocarbons such as 3-methylcholanthrene to rats decreases toxicity and total cytochrome P-450 levels, cytochrome P-450 must have a detoxicating role in metabolism. As we see here, that view could be totally erroneous and lead to unsound predictions for other situations. The basic information underlying the phenomenon presented here, e.g., the suppression of individual forms of cytochrome P-450, could only have been obtained with the use of purification, enzyme reconstitution, and immunochemical techniques.

Does the identification and assay of individual enzyme forms have any relevance in clinical settings? The answer is yes, and several examples are given from the realm of drug toxicity and therapeutic effectiveness. The antituberculosis drug rifampicin is a potent enzyme inducer and appears to increase the cytochrome P-450 form(s) that catalyzes the A ring hydroxylation of ethynylestradiol, an oral contraceptive. Such oxidation renders the drug ineffective, and cases have been reported where rifampicin administration to women has led to unexpected pregnancy (16). In other clinical cases, genetic deficiency in debrisoquine 4-hydroxylase activity has led to the accumulation of certain drugs and the production of undesirable side effects, such as the neuropathy associated with perhexiline and captopril-induced agranulocytosis (204). The suggestion has been made that dangers associated with chemicals in the environment may be affected by some of the same factors that influence drug clearance; for instance, phenotypic slow debrisoquine metabolizers appear to be less prone to tumors related to aflatoxin B$_1$ and cigarette smoking (6,124). The molecular basis of the debrisoquine hydroxylase polymorphism is not known, but several pieces of information suggest that mutation in structural genes may be involved (30). If such is the case, we may ultimately be able to understand interindividual variations in response to potentially toxic chemicals at the level of specific sequence changes. Toward this end, methods in enzymology are necessary and need to be applied in the field of toxicology.

For many of these enzymes, a number of purification techniques have been developed independently, and the reader is referred to the original literature for details. Different procedures for the purification of each enzyme have often been developed; the choice of the purification scheme often depends on the investigator's research situation. When describing the general assay procedures for use with microsomal and purified fractions, an effort has been made to deal with those most commonly used in the author's and other laboratories.

ANALYTICAL PROCEDURES

Preparation of Microsomal and Cytosolic Fractions

Microsomal fractions have been prepared from a variety of tissues using procedures developed for use with rat liver.

The following procedure (74,272) has been found to be useful in this laboratory for the preparation of microsomes from a variety of animal and human tissues.

Reagents

1. KCl 1.15%
2. Buffer A: 0.1 M Tris-acetate buffer (pH 7.4) containing 0.1 M KCl, 1 mM EDTA, and 20 μM butylated hydroxytoluene (BHT)
3. Buffer B: 0.1 M potassium pyrophosphate buffer (pH 7.4) containing 1 mM EDTA and 20 μM BHT
4. Buffer C: 10 mM Tris-acetate buffer (pH 7.4) containing 1 mM ethylenediamine tetraacetic acid (EDTA) and 20% (w/v) glycerol

Procedure

Rats are killed by decapitation; livers are excised and placed in cold 1.15% KCl. All subsequent steps are carried out at 0° to 4°C. The livers are trimmed of debris and washed with 1.15% KCl; if desired, hemoglobin contamination can be lowered by perfusing livers with KCl via the portal vein. The livers are blotted and weighed, placed in four times that weight of buffer A, and minced with scissors. The method of homogenization depends on the scale of the preparation. If only a few livers are used, a mechanically driven Teflon-glass homogenizer (four or five vertical passes) is preferred. For larger preparations, two 40-sec bursts in a Waring blender are more efficient.

The homogenate is centrifuged at 10,000 × g for 20 min, and the supernatant is saved. If the yield of microsomes is a factor, the precipitate can be homogenized in buffer A again and recentrifuged to obtain additional supernatant. The supernatant is centrifuged for 60 min at 100,000 × g (35,000 rpm in a Beckman 45 Ti rotor) to yield a microsomal pellet. After discarding the supernatant, a volume of buffer B equal to that of the discarded supernatant is added, and microsomes are removed from the clear glycogen pellet by gentle swirling or, if necessary, using a rubber policeman. The suspended microsomes are homogenized with four passes of a mechanically driven Teflon-glass homogenizer and recentrifuged at 100,000 × g for 60 min; the resulting pellets are homogenized and recentrifuged (60 min at 100,000 × g). The pellet is homogenized (with four strokes of the Teflon-glass system) in a minimum volume of buffer C (to give 20–50 mg protein ml^{-1}) and stored at −20° or −70°C.

Several comments are in order. BHT and EDTA are added to retard lipid peroxidation, and the pyrophosphate buffer is useful for removing hemoglobin and nucleic acids (272). If proteases are a potential problem, as is often the case in extrahepatic tissues, phenylmethylsulfonyl fluoride (PMSF) or other protease inhibitors can be used. PMSF is unstable in water; therefore a stock 0.1 M solution should be prepared in absolute ethanol or n-propanol, stored at −20°C, and added to buffers to give a final concentration of 0.1 mM immediately prior to their use. The use of dithiothreitol has also been reported to be necessary for the preparation of functional rat colon microsomes (56).

Buffers containing 0.25 M sucrose can be substituted for

buffers A and B in the procedure. If an ultracentrifuge is not available, precipitation of microsomes can be done at lower speeds when 8 mM CaCl$_2$ is added to buffers (31). Alternatively, microsomes can be isolated using gel exclusion chromatography (137,253). More sophisticated techniques are available for the separation of rough and smooth endoplasmic reticulum and Golgi apparatus fractions. Some workers prefer to store microsomes as frozen pellets. For many enzyme activities, microsomes are functional for at least several months when stored either as pellets or frozen in buffer C.

Protein Determination

The most commonly used method for protein determination is probably that of Lowry et al. (170).

Reagents

1. Bovine serum albumin, ca. 1 mg ml^{-1} (determined accurately using $E_{278}^{1\%} = 6.67$)
2. Buffer A: Na$_2$CO$_3$(20 mg ml^{-1}) and NaOH (4 mg ml^{-1})
3. Buffer B$_1$: 2% sodium potassium tartrate (Fisher No. S-387)
4. Buffer B$_2$: 1% CuSO$_4 \cdot$7H$_2$O
5. Folin reagent (2 N phenol solution; Fisher No. S-O-P24)
6. Buffer C: 1 part each of buffers B$_1$ and B$_2$ added to 100 parts buffer A; prepared just before use

Procedure

A series of clean (preferably new) test tubes are prepared containing 0, 10, 20, 30, 40, and 50 μg albumin (in duplicate) plus buffer containing the same amount of each component (salt, glycerol, detergent, etc.) present in the sample. The total volume in each tube is brought to 0.1 ml, and 2.0 ml of buffer C is added while mixing the sample with a vortex device. After exactly 10 min at room temperature, 0.2 ml of Folin reagent is added to each tube while mixing. After 30 min, the A$_{750}$ of each tube is read, and a standard curve is constructed.

All standards and samples are done in duplicate, and samples are preferably done at more than one dilution. A standard curve is constructed for each set of samples.

In our laboratory we have replaced the above procedure with the *Pierce bicinchoninic acid (BCA) method,* using the manufacturer's instructions (Pierce, Rockford, Illinois). Specifically, we heat samples at 60°C for 30 min. This assay is more sensitive than the above procedure and, perhaps more importantly, is not so subject to interference by salts, detergents, and the like.

The *biuret procedure* (161) is less sensitive to interfering materials but requires much larger amounts of sample. The *Coomassie blue G-250 binding assay* (20) can also be used; this assay gives values similar to those of the Lowry assay for microsomes but gives varying values for purified preparations of cytochrome P-450 and other enzymes because of detergent interference. The *fluorescamine assay* (268) is sensitive but has not been as widely used with proteins.

Assay of Cytochrome P-450

The most generally used method to measure cytochrome P-450 is that of Omura and Sato (210), which utilizes the reduced-CO versus reduced difference spectrum.

Reagents

1. Potassium phosphate buffer 0.1 M (pH 7.4) containing 1 mM EDTA, 20% glycerol, 0.5% (w/v) sodium cholate, and 0.4% (w/v) Triton N-101, Renex 690, or Emulgen 913
2. Na$_2$S$_2$O$_4$ (sodium dithionite, sodium hydrosulfite), reagent grade (keep bottle tightly closed when not in use)
3. CO gas, reagent purity; *store and use in fume hood*

Procedure

Microsomes (or other preparations) are added to the buffer to give a final concentration of 0.05 to 5.00 μM cytochrome P-450; the material is mixed, divided into two portions, and placed in 1.0-ml glass cuvettes (10 mm path length). A baseline is recorded between 400 to 500 nm using a split-beam spectrophotometer. The sample cuvette is saturated with 30 to 40 bubbles of CO at a rate of about 1 bubble sec^{-1}. A few crystals of Na$_2$S$_2$O$_4$ (1–2 mg) are added to each cuvette; the cuvettes are covered with Parafilm, inverted several times to mix the Na$_2$S$_2$O$_4$, and placed in the spectrophotometer again after checking for drops on the sides of the cuvettes; spectra are recorded (400–500 nm) until the 450-nm peak reaches a maximum.

A$_{490}$ (isobestic point) serves as a reference point. Cytochrome P-450 content is determined as follows:

$$[(A_{450\text{-}490})_{observed} - (A_{450\text{-}490})_{baseline}]/0.091$$

$$= \text{nmol cytochrome P-450 ml}^{-1}$$

Cytochrome P-420 represents denatured forms of cytochrome P-450 and is determined using the following formulas:

$$(\text{Cytochrome P-450, nmol ml}^{-1}) \times (-0.041)$$

$$= (A_{420\text{-}490})_{theoretical}$$

$$(A_{420\text{-}490})_{observed} - (A_{420\text{-}490})_{theoretical} - (A_{420\text{-}490})_{baseline}/0.110$$

$$= \text{cytochrome P-420 mol ml}^{-1}$$

For an example see Fig. 9.

The extinction coefficient ($\Delta E_{450\text{-}490}$) of 91 m$M^{-1}$ cm^{-1} has been verified using highly purified rat and rabbit liver cytochrome P-450 preparations (113,230). The second set of formulas is based on the observation that cytochrome P-450 has an extinction coefficient of -41 mM^{-1} cm^{-1} ($\Delta E_{420\text{-}490}$) in the difference spectrum (i.e., the A$_{420}$ of the reduced-CO complex is less than the A$_{420}$ of reduced cytochrome P-450) (211).

Rat liver microsomes can be routinely prepared with minimal hemoglobin contamination, but many other preparations cannot. The procedure of Matsubara et al. (189) for assaying cytochrome P-450 in liver homogenates is then use-

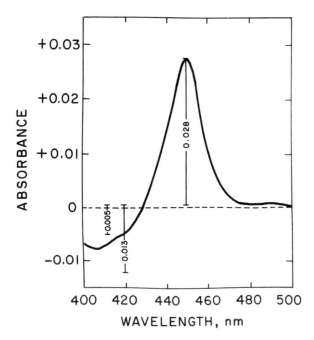

FIG. 9. Calculation of cytochrome P-450 and P-420 concentrations. A sample of rat liver P-450$_{\beta NF-B}$ was diluted tenfold with 0.1 M potassium phosphate buffer (pH 7.7) containing 1 mM EDTA, 40% glycerol, 0.2% Emulgen 913, and 0.5% sodium cholate. The sample was divided and placed in two cuvettes, which were balanced in a Cary 219 spectrophotometer using the automatic baseline correction mode. The corrected baseline was recorded (*broken line*). After addition of CO and Na$_2$S$_2$O$_4$, as indicated in the text, the final difference spectrum was obtained. The calculations are as follow: 0.028 ÷ 0.091 = 0.31 nmol P-450 ml^{-1}. 0.31 × (−0.041) = −0.013 (A$_{420}$). −0.013 − (−0.005) = −0.008. 0.008 ÷ 0.110 = 0.073 nmol P-420 ml^{-1}. 0.31 × 10 = 3.1 nmol P-450 ml^{-1}. 0.073 × 10 = 0.73 nmol P-420 ml^{-1}. See text for more discussion.

ful. With this method two cuvettes are prepared as before, but both are equilibrated with CO, and the baseline is recorded. Na$_2$S$_2$O$_4$ is added *only* to the sample cuvette to obtain a reduced-CO versus oxidized-CO difference spectrum; the extinction coefficient (ΔE$_{450-490}$) is 106 mM^{-1} cm^{-1}. Distinguishing between methemoglobin and cytochrome P-420 is difficult, although Johannesen and De Pierre (138) reported that methemoglobin can be specifically reduced by ascorbate and phenazine methosulfate.

Detergents are routinely used in the assay of cytochrome P-450 in this laboratory, as they solubilize the microsomal membranes to reduce light scattering and do not denature cytochrome P-450 in the presence of glycerol (272). The buffer also prevents settling of any insoluble particles. If one desires to carry out determinations in the absence of detergents, a spectrophotometer should be used that is capable of handling turbid solutions. The limit of detection of cytochrome P-450 in extrahepatic tissues is influenced more by the presence of hemoglobin than by instrumental considerations. In our own laboratory, we use Varian 635 M and Cary 219 spectrophotometers for such measurements; each handles turbid solutions well, and the latter has the advantage of having an automatic baseline correction system. Other instruments are suitable, however; the Aminco DW-2a instrument has been popular among investigators.

Assay of NADPH-Cytochrome P-450 Reductase

NADPH-cytochrome P-450 reductase is conveniently measured by its NADPH-cytochrome c reductase activity (219).

Reagents

1. Horse heart cytochrome c (0.5 mM) in 10 mM potassium phosphate (pH 7.7)
2. Potassium phosphate buffer (0.3 M, pH 7.7)
3. NADPH (10 mM); fairly stable for ≤7 days at 4°C in the dark; however, for the most accurate work, solutions should be prepared fresh daily

Procedure

Into a 1.0-ml glass cuvette (10 mm path length) are pipetted 0.08 ml cytochrome c, the enzyme sample, and sufficient 0.3 M phosphate buffer to bring the total volume to 0.99 ml. The components are mixed and preincubated at 30°C in a recording spectrophotometer; the recorder is adjusted to zero absorbance at 550 nm (full scale 1.0; slit width 1 nm). After recording the baseline for 3 min, 0.01 ml of NADPH is added, and A$_{550}$ is followed for about 3 min. Activity is calculated as follows:

$$\frac{\Delta A_{550} \text{min}^{-1}}{0.021} = \text{nmol cytochrome } c \text{ reduced min}^{-1}$$

An amount of enzyme should be used such that the initial ΔA$_{550}$ does not exceed 0.2 min^{-1}. The assay is an indirect measure of NADPH-cytochrome P-450 reductase activity; measurement of the actual NADPH-cytochrome P-450 reductase activity requires anaerobic conditions and rapid reaction techniques (218). A small peptide of the reductase is required for NADPH-cytochrome P-450 reductase activity but not cytochrome c reductase activity; if no proteolysis has occurred, the two activities are closely correlated (275).

NADPH-cytochrome c reductase activity is stimulated by the high salt concentration used in the assay (219). If activity is assayed in the presence of mitochondria, KCN (1 mM) may be added as a precautionary measure to block nonmicrosomal activity. The reduction of several other compounds, e.g., dichlorophenolindophenol, ferricyanide (275), or a tetrazolium dye (226), may also be used to assay activity. Spectrophotometers with automatic sample positioners may be used to carry out four or five assays simultaneously.

Cytochrome P-450-Linked Activities

The assay of benzphetamine N-demethylase activity is popular because of its ease and sensitivity, especially with microsomes prepared from animals treated with phenobarbital or polyhalogenated biphenyls. Three assays are commonly used. HCHO is released during the reaction and forms the basis for the first two assays.

Colorimetric Measurement of HCHO

For studies on colorimetric measurement of HCHO, see refs. 32, 177, and 200.

Reagents

1. Potassium phosphate buffer 1 M (pH 7.7)
2. $NADP^+$ 10 mM
3. Yeast glucose-6-phosphate dehydrogenase 10^3 IU ml^{-1}
4. Glucose-6-phosphate 0.1 M
5. d-Benzphetamine HCl 10 mM (d-benzphetamine HCl is a controlled substance and can be obtained through Dr. P. W. O'Connell of the Upjohn Co., Kalamazoo, Michigan)
6. $HClO_4$ 17%
7. Nash reagent [30 g ammonium acetate, 0.4 ml acetylacetone (2,4-pentanedione), and 0.6 ml glacial acetic acid per 100 ml]

Procedure

Incubations are carried out in 1.5 ml total volume, which includes 0.5 to 2.0 mg microsomal protein, 50 mM phosphate buffer, 0.5 mM $NADP^+$, glucose-6-phosphate dehydrogenase 1 IU ml^{-1}, and 1.0 mM benzphetamine HCl (which is added after the other components from a 10 mM aqueous stock). Tubes are preincubated for 3 min at 37°C, and then glucose-6-phosphate is added to 10 mM to start incubations. After shaking the tubes (150 rpm) for 10 min at 37°C, the incubations are stopped by adding 0.5 ml of 17% $HClO_4$; they are then chilled on ice for 5 to 10 min. (Because of the short incubation time, it is convenient to start and stop individual tubes every 10 sec.) Tubes are centrifuged at 1,000 × g for 5 min, and 1.0 ml of each supernatant is transferred to a new tube. To each of these tubes is added 0.4 ml of Nash reagent. The tubes are heated at 60° to 70°C for 20 min in a waterbath (covered to prevent evaporation). The tubes are cooled in tap water, and A_{412} values are read versus a water blank. Minus benzphetamine and minus NADPH-generating system blanks are prepared; the A_{412} values for these blanks, which should be similar, are subtracted from the experimental values. A standard curve can be prepared using HCHO; we find that such curves routinely yield factors of 460 to 480, which when multiplied by net A_{412} give the total nanomoles of HCHO produced. If microcuvettes are used for reading A_{412}, the entire procedure can be scaled down tenfold.

Extraction of H^{14}CHO

Extraction of H^{14}CHO necessitates the use of [N-methyl-^{14}C]-benzphetamine but offers increased sensitivity (94,230). This material can be synthesized commercially from d-ben-

zylamphetamine (available from Upjohn). The synthesis has been carried out in this laboratory as follows (86).

Benzylamphetamine (free base) (1 mmol) is stirred with 1.1 mmol of $^{14}CH_3I$ (2 mCi) and 1.1 mmol of K_2CO_3 in 30 ml of acetone overnight. The solvent is removed *in vacuo*, and the residue is suspended in water. The pH is adjusted to ≥10 with K_2CO_3 if necessary; the solution is extracted three times with $CHCl_3$. The $CHCl_3$ layers are combined, dried with anhydrous $MgSO_4$, and saturated with dry HCl gas. Solvent is removed *in vacuo*, and the residue is crystallized from ethyl acetate to give [N-methyl-^{14}C]-benzphetamine HCl in about 50% yield. Purity can be checked by nuclear magnetic resonance and mass spectrometry; the melting point appears to be sensitive to the crystallization procedure but should be sharp.*

Assays are set up as in the colorimetric procedure, but the volume is reduced to 0.75 ml, and the protein concentration may be reduced to fit the situation. Incubations are stopped by adding 0.25 ml 1 N NaOH and 5 ml $CHCl_3$. Tubes are mixed using a vortex device and centrifuged (1,000 × g for 5 min). The aqueous upper layer is transferred to a clean tube, 5 ml of $CHCl_3$ is added, and the mixing, centrifugation, and transfer are repeated. The above step is repeated once more, and a 0.5-ml aliquot of the aqueous phase is transferred to a miniscintillation vial. The contents are neutralized by adding 0.5 ml of 0.1 M sodium citrate buffer (pH 6.5) to which has been added 0.0625 N HCl; 5 ml of ACS cocktail (Amersham-Searle, Arlington Heights, Illinois) is added. Vials are capped, mixed, and counted (10 min usually produces satisfactory counting deviation). Blanks contain all components except NADPH or protein.

The efficiency of extraction is usually more than 90%. HCHO remains in the aqueous phase, and residual substrate is extracted in the $CHCl_3$ layers at the basic pH.

Enhancement of NADPH Oxidation or O$_2$ Uptake

Because of high rates of endogenous oxidase activity, procedures that enhance NADPH oxidation or O_2 uptake are more commonly used with reconstituted enzyme systems than with microsomes (181,203).

With the oxygen electrode procedure, experiments are set up as before and a background rate of O_2 uptake is observed. The differences in the rates obtained with substrates are measured; each nanomole of O_2 consumed corresponds to one nanomole of substrate metabolized (203).

The NADPH oxidation assay is carried out in a similar way. The NADPH-generating system is deleted. Incubations, containing all components except NADPH, are preincubated for 3 min at 37°C in 1.0-ml glass cuvettes in a recording spectrophotometer set at 340 nm (1.0 full scale absorbance). NADPH (0.015 ml of a 10 mM solution) is added, and the rate of decrease in A_{340} is observed. Blank incubations contain all components except benzphetamine. Rates are determined

---

* The melting point of a sample obtained from Upjohn was 152° to 154°C. The value listed in the *Merck Index* is 129° to 130°C (crystallization from ethyl acetate). For material synthesized in this laboratory it was 194° to 195°C (uncorrected).

by dividing net ΔA_{340} min^{-1} by 0.00622 to obtain nanomoles of NADPH oxidized min^{-1}. The benzphetamine demethylase rate determined by this procedure has been found to be identical to that obtained by the HCHO assay under some conditions (146) but not others (203) and should be checked before routine use.

7-Ethoxycoumarin O-Deethylase

The assay for 7-ethoxycoumarin O-deethylase is sensitive, convenient, and applicable to a wide variety of samples (71,76).

Reagents

1. 7-Ethoxycoumarin 30 mM (Aldrich Chemical Co., Milwaukee, Wisconsin), dissolved in methanol (avoid exposure to light)
2. Potassium phosphate buffer 1 M (pH 7.4)
3. NADP$^+$ 10 mM
4. Yeast glucose-6-phosphate dehydrogenase 10^3 IU ml^{-1}
5. Glucose-6-phosphate 0.1 M
6. Sodium borate 0.2 M (pH 9.6)
7. 7-Hydroxycoumarin 1 mM (Aldrich), dissolved in 0.1 N NaOH/0.1 M NaCl (prepare fresh solution each day; avoid exposure to light)

Procedure

An appropriate amount of enzyme is placed in a test tube along with 50 mM phosphate buffer, 0.5 mM NADP$^+$, glucose-6-phosphate dehydrogenase 1 IU ml^{-1}, and 0.3 mM 7-ethoxycoumarin, plus water to bring the volume to 0.9 ml. After a 3-min preincubation at 37°C, glucose-6-phosphate is added to 10 mM to start incubations. (As in the case of benzphetamine, reactions are conveniently started and stopped each 15 sec.) After 5 to 10 min, incubations are stopped by adding 0.1 ml of 2 N HCl and 2 ml CHCl$_3$. Tubes are mixed and centrifuged for 5 min at 1,000 × g. One milliliter of the lower CHCl$_3$ phase (containing both substrate and product) is transferred to a clean tube, and 2 ml of 0.2 M sodium borate buffer is added. The tubes are mixed and centrifuged 5 min at 1,000 × g. The upper phase, containing the phenolic product, is transferred to a new tube and fluorescence is read versus a standard curve in a fluorimeter with the excitation wavelength set at 338 nm and the emission wavelength at 458 nm.

Benzo(a)pyrene Hydroxylase

The assay for benzo(a)pyrene hydroxylase activity has been widely used because of the sensitivity of the assay, the widespread occurrence of the enzyme's activity, and an interest in the carcinogenic aspects of benzo(a)pyrene. This substrate is carcinogenic and light-sensitive, and gives rise to many metabolites. The following procedure measures primarily the 3- and 9-hydroxy derivatives (202).

Reagents

1. Potassium phosphate buffer 1 M (pH 7.4)
2. NADP$^+$ 10 mM
3. Yeast glucose-6-phosphate dehydrogenase 10^3 IU ml^{-1}
4. Benzo(a)pyrene 8 mM, dissolved in acetone
5. Quinine 2 mg ml^{-1} in 0.1 N H$_2$SO$_4$
6. 3-Hydroxybenzo(a)pyrene 1 mM (can be obtained from the National Cancer Institute Chemical Repository, Bethesda, Maryland)

Procedure

An appropriate amount of enzyme is placed in a test tube along with 50 mM phosphate buffer (pH 7.4), 0.5 mM NADP$^+$, glucose-6-phosphate dehydrogenase 1 IU ml^{-1}, 80 μM benzo(a)pyrene, and sufficient water to bring the total volume to 1.0 ml. (All procedures are carried out in dim light (or under yellow light), and appropriate precautions are taken to prevent exposure of skin to benzo(a)pyrene or its metabolites. When solid material is being handled, precautions are taken to avoid breathing dust.) After 3 min preincubation at 37°C, glucose-6-phosphate is added to 10 mM to initiate reactions (conveniently done every 15 sec). After 5 to 10 min, reactions are stopped by adding 1.0 ml of cold acetone and mixed. Hexane (3.25 ml) is added, and mixing is repeated. Two milliliters of the upper layer is transferred to a clean tube with a pipette, and 4 ml of 1 N NaOH is added. After vortex mixing and centrifugation for 3 to 5 min at 1,000 × g, the aqueous phase is carefully transferred to a clean tube.

Fluorescence is read with excitation at 396 nm and emission at 522 nm. A standard curve is prepared in 0.1 N NaOH using 3-hydroxybenzo(a)pyrene. Because solutions of the standard are unstable, a convenient method involves setting up the standard curve, changing the wavelength setting to 350 nm (excitation) and 450 nm (emission) without adjusting other settings and preparing a standard curve using serial dilutions of quinine sulfate. The quinine sulfate can then be used as a secondary standard for subsequent experiments, and 3-hydroxybenzo(a)pyrene levels can be calculated by reference to the original curves.

An alternative procedure, devised by Dehnen et al. (44), is comparable in terms of convenience and sensitivity. Incubations are set up as before (1.0 ml volume) and stopped by the addition of 2.3 ml of a fresh mixture of 1 mM EDTA, 10% (w/v) Triton X-100, and 1.2% (w/v) triethylamine. After mixing, tubes are capped until fluorescence measurements are made. The excitation wavelength is set at 435 nm, and fluorescence emission is scanned (and a chart recorded) between 450 and 650 nm. Residual substrate gives a large peak near the 450 nm region of the chart, and the product appears as a peak at 522 nm. A baseline is drawn between the trough [between benzo(a)pyrene and 3-hydroxybenzo(a)pyrene] and the point at which the 3-hydroxybenzo(a)pyrene peak tails into a baseline at about 575 nm. The distance between this slanted baseline and the top of the 522 nm peak can be calibrated against the quinine sulfate curve prepared as described above.

Other benzo(a)pyrene metabolism assays can be carried out with radioactive substrate to measure total polar metabolites (46), individual metabolites [after separation by high-pressure liquid chromatography (HPLC)] (240,257), or metabolites covalently bound to protein or added nucleic acids (47).

Mephenytoin 4-Hydroxylase

Many aromatic substrates are converted to phenols via hydroxylation by cytochrome P-450 enzymes; in addition, many aryl ethers are O-dealkylated to form phenols. In many cases advantage can be taken of the increased polarity of the (deprotonated) phenolic product to aid in measuring its formation in *in vitro* assays. The general principle involves incubation of radioactive substrate with enzyme and separation of product from substrate by thin-layer chromatography (TLC) using a solvent containing NH_4OH to deprotonate the phenol, thereby increasing its polarity and decreasing its mobility. Of course, more rigorous identification of the chemistry of the reaction products may be necessary, particularly in the case of substrates that can be hydroxylated at any of several positions. However, in many cases essentially only *para*-hydroxylation occurs, and the separation is relatively easy. We have utilized this general approach to measure S-mephenytoin 4-hydroxylation (Fig. 10) (243), acetanilide 4-hydroxylation (89), and phenacetin O-deethylation (51).

In practice the assays are set up in the same general manner as others involving cytochrome P-450 enzymes (*vide supra*).

Reagents

S-Nirvanol (20.4 mg, 0.1 mmol), synthesized as described elsewhere (119), is dissolved in a small amount of acetone (about 1 ml) containing 6.17 mg KOH (0.11 mmol). $^{14}CH_3I$ (15.6 mg, 0.11 mmol; specific activity of about 10 mCi mmol^{-1}; New England Nuclear, Boston, Massachusetts) is added at 0°C, and the reaction is stirred at 0°C. The reaction is allowed to warm to 23°C and is nearly complete after about 4 hr. The mixture is filtered through glass wool, and the filtrate is evaporated to dryness under nitrogen; the resulting [*methyl*-^{14}C]mephenytoin is redissolved in a small amount of acetone and crystallized by careful addition of H_2O. The product is collected by centrifugation, washed with acetone-water, and dried *in vacuo* over Drierite overnight. The typical yield of crystalline product (first crop) is 8 to 10 mg (37–46%). Radiopurity is more than 99% as judged by

TLC (Whatman LK6DF silica; CHCl$_3$/MeOH/concentrated NH$_4$OH, 90:10:1, v/v/v).

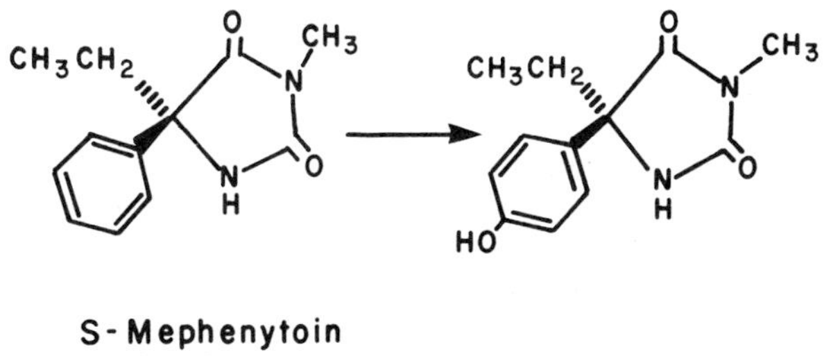

Procedure

The mephenytoin 4-hydroxylation activity of human liver microsomes is assayed as follows. The standard reaction mixture (final volume 100 μl) contains liver microsomes (about 100 pmol of cytochrome P-450) or a reconstituted monooxygenase system containing 100 pmol of partially purified cytochrome P-450, 100 pmol of NADPH-cytochrome P-450 reductase, and 6 nmol of sonicated dilauroyl glyceryl 3-phosphorylcholine; an NADPH-generating system consisting of 50 nmol of NADP$^+$, 1 μmol of glucose-6-phosphate, and 0.2 IU of yeast glucose-6-phosphate dehydrogenase; 10 μmol of potassium phosphate buffer (pH 7.4); and 40 nmol of S-[*methyl*-^{14}C]mephenytoin. The reaction is started by adding the glucose-6-phosphate, continued for 30 min at 37°C, and stopped with 50 μl of ice-cold tetrahydrofuran containing 0.2 mM unlabeled 4-hydroxymephenytoin. Fifty microliters of the mixture is applied to the loading zone of a Whatman LK6DF chromatography plate using a plastic-tipped pipetting device. After separation by TLC in the solvent system used for analyzing the substrate purity (*vide supra*) and detection with 254-nm light, zones containing 4-hydroxymephenytoin are scraped from the thin-layer plate. Alternatively, autoradiography under x-ray film can be used to locate the product zones. CH$_3$OH (1 ml) is added to elute the product. After 10 min, 4 ml of 4a20 cocktail (Research Products International, Elk Grove Village, Illinois) is added. Radioactivity is measured by liquid scintillation spectrometry. Enzyme activities are expressed as picomoles of product formed per minute per nanomole of cytochrome P-450.

Figure 11 shows the results of chromatographic analysis of [*methyl*-^{14}C]mephenytoin and its 4-hydroxy metabolite after incubation with human liver microsomes (containing 100 pmol of cytochrome P-450) for 0, 20, and 40 min at 37°C. The figure shows clearly the gradual formation of the 4-hydroxylation metabolite of mephenytoin (4.5 cm migration) with increasing incubation time. In the TLC analysis no radioactive metabolites of mephenytoin other than 4-hydroxymephenytoin were detected. Furthermore, the only products of such incubates detected using HPLC (159) were 4-hydroxymephenytoin and nirvanol.

Nifedipine Oxidase

A description of the assay for nifedipine oxidase is included to serve as an example of how modern HPLC methods may be utilized efficiently. Nifedipine is a widely used calcium channel blocker, and oxidation by cytochrome P-450 renders it inactive (101).

Nifedipine oxidation [from the dihydropyridine to the pyridine metabolite (Fig. 12)] is measured in the following manner. *All incubation, extraction, and other handling of samples is done in amber vials because of the light sensitivity of nifedipine solutions.* These vials are available from the Pierce Chemical Co., Rockford, Illinois. Typical incubations include liver microsomes containing 10 to 100 pmol of cy-

FIG. 10. 4-Hydroxylation of S-mephenytoin (241,242).

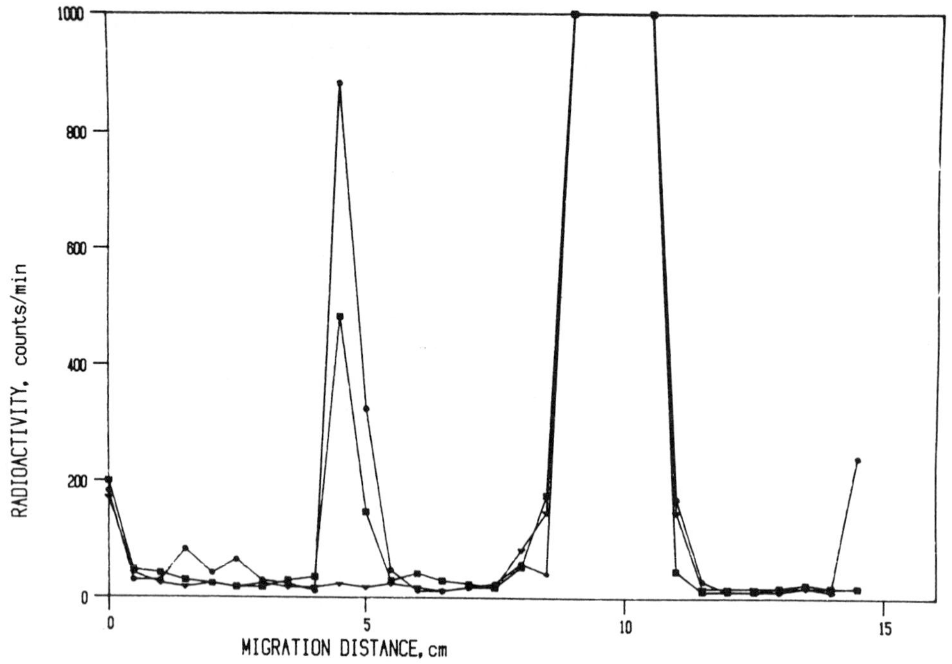

FIG. 11. TLC analysis of the formation of 4-hydroxymephenytoin from mephenytoin with human liver microsomes. S-[*Methyl*-^{14}C]mephenytoin was incubated with human liver microsomes containing 100 pmol cytochrome P-450 for 0 min (▼), 20 min (■), and 40 min (●) in the presence of the NADPH-generating system, and the hydroxylated metabolite was determined as described in the text (243).

tochrome P-450, 0.1 M potassium phosphate buffer (final pH 7.85), and 0.2 mM nifedipine (added from a stock solution of 20 mM in acetone) in a final volume of 0.50 ml. The components are equilibrated for 3 min at 37°C, and the reaction is initiated by adding an NADPH-generating system consisting of (final concentrations) 10 mM glucose-6-phosphate, 0.5 mM NADP$^+$, and yeast glucose-6-phosphate dehydrogenase 0.33 IU ml^{-1}. The reaction proceeds for 10 min at 37°C and is then quenched by adding 1.0 ml of CH$_2$Cl$_2$. Na$_2$CO$_3$ buffer, 100 μl (1 M, pH 10.5), containing 2 M NaCl is added to each vial. The content of each vial is mixed using a vortex device, and the two layers are separated by centrifugation at 3,000 × g for 10 min. From each lower organic layer, 0.7 ml is transferred to an amber "Reacti-vial" (Pierce Chemical Co., Rockford, Illinois); 1.0 ml of CH$_2$Cl$_2$ is added to the remaining contents. The vortex mixing and centrifugation steps are repeated, and an additional 0.9 ml of each organic layer is combined with the original 0.7 ml extract. The total 1.6 ml is reduced to dryness at 23°C under an N$_2$ stream. The contents are dissolved in 50 μl of CH$_3$OH, and

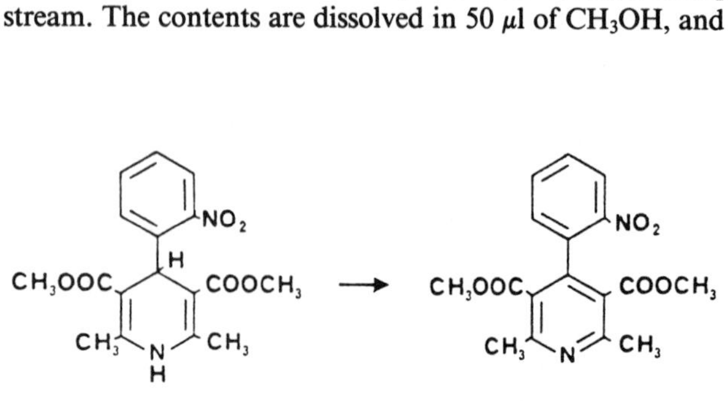

20 μl is injected onto an octyldecylsilyl (C18) reverse-phase HPLC column (DuPont Zorbax Golden Series, 3 μm particle size, 6.2 mm × 8.0 cm; DuPont Company, Wilmington, Delaware) placed in line following a 1 cm long octyldecylsilyl guard column. The column is eluted with an isocratic mixture of 64% CH$_3$OH/36% H$_2$O (v/v) at a flow rate of 3.0 ml min^{-1}. Detection is at 254 nm (found to be optimal by previous scanning). Quantitation is usually done with external standards and by the use of peak heights. Alternatively, nitrendipine can be used as an internal standard. Typically a 20 ng sample of the metabolite (59 pmol) yields a maximal A$_{254}$ of about 0.015 under these conditions. A typical chromatogram resulting from injection of a human liver microsomal incubation extract is shown in Fig. 13.

Assay conditions were optimized with a human liver microsomal sample. Product formation was linear up to a time of 20 min, the pH optimum was 7.85 (Tris-HCl yielded lower rates than did potassium phosphate buffer), the rate of product formation per unit enzyme was constant over a range of 5 to 1,000 pmol cytochrome P-450 ml^{-1}, and a substrate concentration of 200 μM was optimal (K_m = 10 μM; substrate inhibition observed at concentrations of more than 500 μM; no evidence for multiphasic behavior was observed using concentrations of 2 to 1,000 μM).

When purified cytochrome P-450 fractions are assayed for activity, the microsomes are replaced with 20 to 100 pmol of cytochrome P-450, 250 pmol of rabbit NADPH-cytochrome P-450 reductase, and 15 nmol of L-α-dilauroylglyceryl-3-phosphocholine. These components are mixed and then incubated for 30 min at 23°C prior to addition of other materials. Examination of experimental conditions indicated that the NADPH-cytochrome P-450 reductase, substrate, and

FIG. 12. Oxidation of nifedipine to its pyridine metabolite (101).

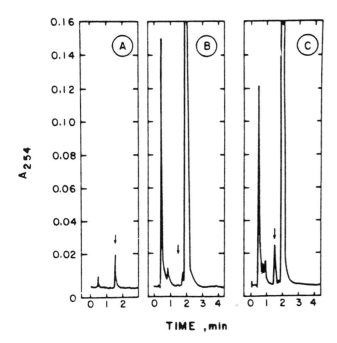

FIG. 13. HPLC separation of the oxidized (pyridine) product of nifipidine oxidation from human liver microsomes. A typical 10-min incubation with 100 pmol of human liver microsomal cytochrome P-450 was done, and 20 μl of the total extract was chromatographed as described. The retention time of the nifedipine metabolite is indicated with an arrow. **A:** Authentic standard of the metabolite (200 ng). **B:** Extract of an incubation devoid of NADPH. **C:** Complete incubation (101).

phospholipid concentrations used are optimal. However, product formation is not linear for more than 5 min.

The separation of the product from the substrate is efficient with the reverse-phase system used. The only solvent components needed are methanol and water, thereby eliminating problems with salts. The product elutes before the substrate, enhancing sensitivity of the assay. There is no need to have more than baseline separation, and interfering peaks are absent. Thus a short column and high flow rate can be used without a buildup of back pressure. As shown in Fig. 13, the total HPLC time for each assay is less than 3 min.

The efficiency of analysis could also be improved with the use of an automated injector system. Although the analysis time could be reduced if incubations were only deproteinized and not extracted prior to HPLC analysis, the sensitivity would also be reduced.

A final point is that the sensitivity of many HPLC assays can be enhanced by use of a fluorescence monitor if the compounds of interest are fluorescent. A number of good grating and filter systems are available. These instruments are convenient to use, are relatively inexpensive, and can increase the sensitivity of appropriate compounds by several orders of magnitude, as well as reduce the interference by other eluting materials.

Sparteine Δ^5-Oxidase

The measurement of sparteine Δ^5-oxidase activity is an example of a tritium release assay. In the process of oxidation,

a tritium atom is released from the substrate and appears with water. If the substrate is nonpolar, it can be extracted and the radioactivity in the water determined. In addition to the measurement of sparteine Δ^5-oxidase activity, we have also utilized this assay to measure the 2- and 4-hydroxylation of 17β-estradiol in collaborative experiments with Nelson (40,101) and the oxidation of an analog of nifedipine (Fig. 14).

$\Delta^{5,6}$-Dehydrosparteine can be prepared from sparteine by mercuric acetate oxidation; reduction with NaB^{3}H$_4$ gives only the correct stereoisomer of sparteine (81,163). The [5-^{3}H] material can be easily crystallized as the hydrosulfate or perchlorate salt. These salts are water-soluble, and assays are set up as in the general manner with 1.0 mM concentrations of the substrate. After 20 min at 37°C, the pH of the incubation (total volume 200 μl) is raised to more than 12, and the mixture is extracted three times with 1.0-ml aliquots of CH$_2$Cl$_2$, with brief intermediate centrifugation to separate the layers. The aqueous phase (100 μl) is counted in 5 ml of ACS scintillation cocktail, with care taken to allow any chemiluminescence to decay in the dark.

In the case of 17β-estradiol hydroxylation a similar procedure was used, except that acid was added prior to extraction to protonate the phenol (40).

With these approaches the results should be corrected for the kinetic tritium isotope effect if one exists (163). One cannot always be certain that this isotope effect is constant among the various enzyme samples.

Covalent Binding of Metabolites to Protein

The irreversible binding of reaction products to protein was observed 40 years ago (195). Although there is no clear consensus about the importance of individual targets or how such modification of proteins leads to death of cells, in vitro binding of chemicals to protein provides an index of bioactivation processes and can be useful in the characterization of reactive intermediates.

In general, the enzyme system under investigation is incubated with the radioactive substrate for a fixed amount of time, during which the rate of production of species binding covalently should remain constant. In practice it is usually less than 1 hr. Incubations are terminated, and binding to protein is measured. Several approaches are available for measuring binding.

1. One method involves precipitation of the protein with organic solvent (ethanol or methanol, more than two volumes) or trichloroacetic acid (5% final concentration) and collection of the pelleted material after centrifugation (10^4

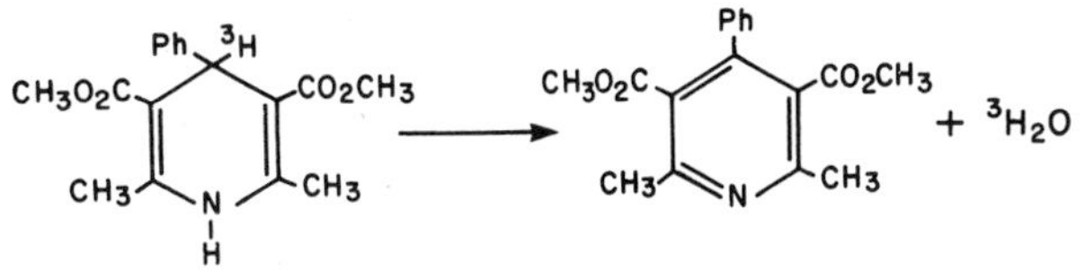

FIG. 14. Example of a tritium release assay: release of tritium from 2,6-dimethyl-4-phenyl-3,5-bis(carbomethoxy)-1,4-dihydropyridine during oxidation by cytochrome P-450.

$\times g$, 15 min). The sensitivity of the residual substrate to the solvent must be considered, as well as the solubility. The supernatant is decanted, and more acid or solvent is added; the protein pellet is washed by vigorous mixing or homogenization. We have found that carrying out the entire procedure in stainless steel centrifuge tubes is convenient because the vessels can be centrifuged in a Sorvall SS-34 or SA-600 rotor and homogenized with a Sorvall Omni-mixer (DuPont Instruments, Wilmington, Delaware) without the need to transfer contents. The process of homogenization, centrifugation, and decantation of supernatant is repeated several times until significant radioactivity no longer appears in the wash fractions. At that point the protein samples are dried by heating at 60°C for 2 hr. The protein is dissolved in 1 N NaOH (about 1–2 ml) for 1 hr at 60°C. Insoluble material is removed by centrifugation, and the protein in an aliquot of *each* sample is measured [by the Lowry et al. (170) or Pierce (*vide supra*) method], as the recovery is variable. A larger aliquot of each sample is added to 5 to 10 ml of a scintillation cocktail capable of holding water, and chemiluminescence is allowed to decay overnight at room temperature in the dark prior to counting. The results are expressed in terms of nanomoles of adduct (mg protein)$^{-1}$, with subtraction of the values obtained with an inactive enzyme (e.g., without NADPH in the case of mixed-function oxidases).

2. Another approach is extensive dialysis of protein samples against buffer containing sodium dodecyl sulfate (SDS). This procedure was developed by Sun and Dent (250). We have utilized the method with hydrophilic materials such as acrylonitrile (63,100,120) but have not obtained reliable results with hydrophobic, water-insoluble materials.

3. A third method involves the adsorption of protein to glass fiber filters, such as those used for *in vitro* protein translation experiments (277). These disks can be washed with organic solvents in a shaking device to remove unbound material. We have usually used five to eight changes of the wash solvent, with wash times of 30 min (usually with ethanol as the solvent). The capacity of these filters is limited, so that such an approach may not be satisfactory if considerable amounts of protein must be used. However, if satisfactory sensitivity can be achieved with the use of milligram amounts of protein, the method is considerably easier than the other approaches. In our experience with trichloroethylene, we have found that recovery of protein on the filters is nearly quantitative when no more than 1 mg of protein is used (checks on binding can be done with radiolabeled proteins) (196).

Covalent Binding of Metabolites to DNA

Like the binding of reaction products to protein, binding to DNA provides an index of bioactivation. One must remember that binding to naked DNA in such a system may be much higher than in the presence of chromosomal proteins, which are removed from the site of electrophile production by membrane layers. Binding to protein is not to be equated with nucleic acid binding: Notable examples demonstrate that different enzymes and pathways can be involved in the generation of the various types of adducts (cf. acrylonitrile, ethylene dibromide—*vide supra*) (97).

Calf thymus DNA has been used in many *in vitro* binding experiments. Herring sperm DNA is considerably less expensive and more soluble; its fragmented nature does not cause a problem in this type of work. In general, DNA, at a concentration of 1 to 2 mg ml^{-1}, is added to incubations containing a radioactive substrate, with other components as used in standard procedures (*vide supra*).

Several methods can be used to purify the DNA for measurement of bound adducts. The choice depends on the situation.

1. One approach involves initial extraction of the aqueous solution with water-saturated butanol to remove small compounds (144). Brief centrifugation may be required to separate the layers after each step. Extraction with phenol is useful for removing proteins (131). The DNA solution is shaken gently with an equal volume of phenol/isoamyl alcohol/CHCl$_3$, 24:1:25 (v/v/v), with 1.0 g of 8-hydroxyquinoline and 140 ml of *m*-cresol added per liter of phenol prior to mixing. Brief centrifugation after each step may be required to separate the layers: DNA remains in the upper phase. The step is repeated one or two times. NaCl is added to the DNA layer to a concentration of 0.1 M. The DNA is precipitated by adding 2 volumes of cold ($-20°C$) ethanol and is recovered by centrifugation; the material, dried under an N$_2$ stream, can be dissolved in any of a number of low-ionic-strength buffers, although shaking or other agitation may be necessary.

2. Another procedure that has been used as an alternative to the butanol and phenol extractions involves sedimentation of DNA by ultracentrifugation (129). This process is usually done following the metabolic incubation: SDS is added to a final concentration of 1% (w/v) (from a stock 10% solution). The incubation buffer should not contain potassium ions because potassium SDS is rather insoluble. The preparations are centrifuged at $10^5 \times g$ for 16 hr at 20°C to pellet the DNA. The recovery is generally good (more than 80%), and most proteins remain soluble and are decanted in the supernatant. Although the procedure is limited by availability of rotor spaces in the ultracentrifuge, the effort involved in manipulations is minimal. Note that ultracentrifugation will not precipitate highly fragmented DNA samples such as herring sperm DNA (see above).

3. Sometimes these procedures do not completely remove unbound materials; for instance, some GSH adducts tend to persist (156). A useful procedure for further purification is hydroxylapatite chromatography. The method used in this laboratory is outlined: For a sample containing 1 mg of DNA, 1 g of dry hydroxylapatite (Calbiochem DNA grade) is suspended in 5 mM sodium phosphate buffer (pH 6.8) and swirled to hydrate the particles. The suspension is evacuated (at 40°C) to remove gas bubbles using an aspirator and poured into a column (1.6 cm diameter), where 5 mM sodium phosphate buffer (pH 6.8) is pumped through the column at a flow rate of 2.0 ml min^{-1} using a peristaltic pump. The DNA is applied to the column (using the pump), and the column is sequentially eluted with 100, 200, and 300 mM sodium phosphate buffers (pH 6.8). EDTA should *not* be included. The eluate is monitored at 254 nm, and the elution buffer is not changed until A$_{254}$ has decreased nearly to the baseline. Eluted fractions are collected. Proteins are then eluted with 100 mM phosphate, RNA with 200 mM phos-

phate, and DNA with 300 mM phosphate. Aliquots of fractions can be assayed for radioactivity after mixing with a cocktail containing a detergent and designed for aqueous samples. When large volumes of water and high phosphate concentrations are used, the conditions needed for formation of a stable gel should be checked carefully beforehand.

If concentration of peak fractions is necessary, it is conveniently achieved by removing the salt from the pooled samples via extensive dialysis and subsequent lyophilization. In some cases further treatment of DNA with RNase (heating at 80°C for 10 min prior to use to destroy DNase) or pronase may be desired, with subsequent recovery of DNA by phenol extraction and ethanol precipitation. Analyses for RNA can be done using the orcinol procedure (48). Protein can be measured with any of several assays or, if necessary, by amino acid hydrolysis (120). (*Note:* purine decomposition leads to abnormally high levels of glycine). DNA itself can be estimated with the diphenylamine procedure (25), with Hoechst 33258 dye using a fluorimeter (26), or using the approximate relation $E_{260}^{1\%} = 200$ cm^{-1}.

If major DNA adducts have been identified for a particular substrate, the best approach is to hydrolyze the DNA and measure the adduct by a specific method, e.g., chromatography or immunoassay.

Other Cytochrome P-450-Linked Activities

The assays described above are among the most widely used. However, the activities that have been examined are much more extensive. Some of these activities are presented in Table 1, along with appropriate references. The table acquaints the reader with the wide variety of cytochrome P-450 substrates and the assays available for use. Many of these assays can be modified to permit determination of almost any activity.

Microsomal Flavoprotein Oxidase

Microsomal flavoprotein oxidase, a mixed-function oxidase, consists of a single flavoprotein (299,300). The best source of the enzyme appears to be porcine liver, and the activity appears to be less stable than cytochrome P-450-

TABLE 1. *Survey of microsomal mixed function oxidase activities and assays*

Substrate	Methods	Refs.	Substrate	Methods	Refs.
Acetanilide	Colorimetry Radiometry TLC HPLC	89,157,263	7-Ethoxycoumarin Ethanol	Fluorimetry Colorimetry	71,269
2-Acetylaminofluorene	Colorimetry Radiometry TLC HPLC	17	Ethoxyresorufin Furans	Radiometry GLC Fluorimetry Radiometry (covalent binding)	197 23 73,74
Aflatoxin B$_1$	HPLC Radiometry (covalent binding)	201	Lauric acid	Radiometry HPLC	55,177
Alkanes	Radiometry NADPH oxidation GLC	177,203	Methyl azodyes	Colorimetry Radiometry (covalent binding)	72,144,245
Aminopyrine	Radiometry	221		GLC	
Aniline	Colorimetry Radiometry	115,128,175	N-Methylchloroaniline	Fluorescence derivation	271
Benzo(a)pyrene	Fluorimetry Radiometry HPLC Mutagenic method	44,46,47, 202,240, 257,294	N-Nitrosopyrrolidine Parathion	HPLC Radiometry (TLC) Radiometry (covalent binding)	27 145,146
Benzphetamine	Colorimetry Radiometry NADPH oxidation Oxygen uptake	94,203,227	Pyrroles	Radiometry (covalent binding)	91
Biphenyl	Fluorimetry GLC TLC	23,24,225	Pyrrolizidine alkaloids	Colorimetry HPLC	73
			Terpenes	GLC	166
Carbon disulfide	Radiometry (covalent binding)	45	Testosterone	Radiometry TLC HPLC	35,259,281
Carbon tetrachloride	Radiometry (covalent binding)	244	Thioureas	TLC Oxygen uptake	223
Chlorcyclizine	Radioisotope derivative	158	Vinyl chloride	Radiometry Mutagenic method	93 186
Chloroform	GLC	244	Warfarin	HPLC	57,147–149
Dimethylnitrosamine	Colorimetry Radiometry Mutagenic method	29,37,169	Zoxazolamine	Radiometry	262

linked activities (224). The enzyme is often assayed by measuring the methimazole or *N*-methylaniline-stimulated rate of NADPH oxidation or oxygen uptake (223) (see section under benzphetamine); activity is stimulated by certain amines (299). The enzyme may oxidize the alkaloid slaframine in a rather novel manner (85), although roles for other oxidases need to be further investigated.

Heme Oxygenase

Microsomal heme oxygenase is an enzyme that binds free heme and, coupled with NADPH-cytochrome P-450 reductase, catalyzes the mixed-function oxidation of heme to biliverdin IXα (255,297,298). Spleen is a principal source of this enzyme; the enzyme is also found in liver, and its concentration is elevated by certain divalent metal ions. The enzyme can be assayed by coupling the activity to the cytosolic enzyme biliverdin reductase and measuring bilirubin production spectrophotometrically (255).

Reagents

1. Hemin chloride [dissolve in 1 part 0.1 N KOH; quickly add 9 parts of 50 mM potassium phosphate buffer (pH 7.0) and filter through glass wool to give a solution of ca. 1 mM]
2. Rat liver cytosol
3. NADP$^+$ 10 mM
4. Yeast glucose-6-phosphate dehydrogenase 10^3 IU ml^{-1}
5. Glucose-6-phosphate 0.1 M
6. Potassium phosphate buffer 1 M (pH 7.4)

Procedure

A 2 ml mixture of 24 μM hemin chloride, microsomal enzyme, rat liver cytosol (2 mg ml^{-1}), 0.5 mM NADP$^+$, 10 mM glucose-6-phosphate, and 50 mM phosphate buffer is prepared, divided, and placed in two 1.0-ml cuvettes. The cuvettes are equilibrated at 37°C in a split-beam spectrophotometer (capable of handling the turbidity), and a baseline is recorded between 350 and 600 nm. Glucose-6-phosphate dehydrogenase (1 IU ml^{-1}) is added to the sample cuvette, and spectra are recorded. The bilirubin formed has an extinction coefficient of 56 mM^{-1} cm^{-1} at 456 nm (255). Alternatively, the spectrophotometer can be set at 456 nm, and direct kinetic measurements can be made if the baseline remains stable, or biliverdin IXα production can be followed directly at 650 nm in the absence of cytosol (297,298).

Epoxide Hydrolase

Epoxide hydrolase is active toward a wide variety of alkyl and aryl epoxides (79,190,205). The most commonly used substrate is [7-^{3}H]styrene oxide, which can be obtained from New England Nuclear (Boston, Massachusetts) or Amersham-Searle (Des Plaines, Illinois).

Reagents

1. [7-^{3}H]Styrene oxide, 16 mM in tetrahydrofuran containing 0.1% triethylamine (*Note:* purity should be checked by TLC prior to use.)
2. Tris-HCl buffer 0.5 M (pH 8.7 at 37°C; pH 9.0 at 25°C)
3. 2,5-Diphenyloxazole (PPO) 0.4% and 1,4-*bis*-[2-(4-methyl-5-phenyloxazolyl)]benzene (POPOP) 0.001% in toluene or equivalent commercial scintillation cocktail

Procedure

Incubations containing enzyme, 0.17 M Tris-HCl, and water to give a total volume of 300 μl are initiated (every 15 sec) by adding 20 μl of styrene oxide; they are then shaken for 5 to 10 min at 37°C. The reactions are stopped by adding 5 ml petroleum ether [boiling point (bp) 30°–60°C], mixed with a vortex device, centrifuged for 5 min at 1,000 $\times$ g, and immersed in a Dry Ice–acetone bath. After the aqueous phase has frozen, the upper phase is decanted, the tubes are thawed in a lukewarm waterbath, and the extraction procedure is repeated twice. Ethyl acetate (2 ml) is added to each tube, and the tubes are mixed and centrifuged as before. A 0.3-ml portion of each ethyl acetate phase (containing the styrene glycol) is transferred to a miniscintillation vial, and 5 ml of scintillation cocktail is added. Vials are counted (2–10 min is usually sufficient), and rates of glycol production are determined; blanks contain all components except enzyme (or enzyme boiled for 10 min) (207).

An alternative procedure is more convenient, especially if a large number of samples are involved (136). Incubations are scaled down to a total volume of 80 μl. Reactions are stopped by adding 25 μl of tetrahydrofuran containing 0.4 M styrene glycol (Aldrich Chemical Co., Milwaukee, Wisconsin) and placed on ice. A 35-μl portion of each incubation is applied to the loading portion of a Whatman LK6DF TLC plate (Whatman, Clifton, New Jersey). Plates are dried briefly in air and developed in a 4:1 (v/v) mixture of CHCl$_3$/ethyl acetate. When the solvent reaches the top of the plate, styrene glycol regions ($R_f \sim 0.1$) are marked after visualization with short-wavelength (254 nm) ultraviolet (UV) light. The plates are allowed to stand under room light for 2 hr to lower the resulting chemiluminescence. The regions containing styrene glycol are scraped into miniscintillation vials and shaken briefly after adding 1.0 ml of CH$_3$OH. Scintillation cocktail (4 ml) is added, and the vials are counted. Chemiluminescence may still be a problem, and raising the floor of the channel window is useful; alternatively, overnight decay in the dark may be necessary.

The TLC procedure has been modified for a number of other radioactive substrates (136). Oesch's group described a generalized extraction procedure for a number of radioactive epoxides (9), and we have found that this assay procedure can be used with these unlabeled epoxides when the diols are quantitated using fluorescence measurements (106). Assays based on spectrophotometric measurement of residual substrate (safrole and chloroethylene oxide) have been used, but they suffer from a lack of sensitivity (93,106,111,280).

Spectrophotometric Assay with NAD⁺ Reduction

Spectrophotometric Assay with NAD⁺ Reduction

We have devised an alternative spectrophotometric assay for the assay of epoxide hydrolase utilizing the reduction of NAD⁺ by glycols in the presence of alcohol dehydrogenase (90).

Reagents

1. Octene-1,2-oxide 50 mM in tetrahydrofuran containing 0.1% (v/v) triethylamine (90)
2. NAD⁺ 0.1 M
3. Horse liver alcohol dehydrogenase, 5 mg ml⁻¹ [desalted by gel filtration and dialyzed versus 50 mM Tris-chloride (pH 8.0) containing 0.1 M KCl]
4. Potassium phosphate buffer 1 M (pH 7.7)

Procedure

Incubations containing enzyme, 0.1 M phosphate buffer, alcohol dehydrogenase 0.5 mg ml⁻¹, and 5 mM NAD⁺ are preincubated for 3 min at 37°C in a recording spectrophotometer set at 340 nm. The octene oxide solution (10 μl ml⁻¹) is added, and the sample is mixed. Hydrolase activity is monitored by the increase in A$_{340}$ (1 nmol glycol formed produces an absorbance change of 0.00622 in a 1-ml volume). A convenient concentration of rat liver microsomes to use is 0.25 mg ml⁻¹.

This assay is not as sensitive as the radiometric and fluorimetric assays but has a number of advantages, especially when the number of assays to be carried out is limited: The need for purchasing or synthesizing radiolabeled substrates is precluded, and results can be obtained quickly without the need for extraction, chromatography, or scintillation counting. The linearity of the assay can be directly observed using a single sample; this point can be important when working with purified preparations. The assay was developed using octene-1,2-oxide because the resulting diol is a good substrate for alcohol dehydrogenase, but many other diols are substrates, and the assay can probably be used to assay hydrolase activity toward many other epoxides as well (90).

Other Conjugating Enzymes

The methodologies for assaying each of the other conjugating enzymes are not elaborated here. The reader should bear in mind that many of these enzymes exist in different forms and that an assay for one may not be applicable to others.

A variety of assays for UDP-glucuronyl transferase have been utilized and are reviewed by Kasper and Henton (151). They include radiometric, colorimetric, fluorimetric, and chromatographic methods. This microsomal enzyme exhibits considerable latency; that is, its activity is increased considerably after solubilization of the membrane with detergent.

The most popular assays of GSH S-transferases are spectrophotometric, such as that involving conjugation of 1-chloro-2,4-dinitrobenzene (108). Other spectrophotometric, titrimetric, and chromatographic assays have been developed and are reviewed by Jakoby and Habig (132). Many of the reactions catalyzed by GSH S-transferase occur at finite rates in the absence of the enzyme, and control reactions are needed in which enzyme is absent. In addition to the conjugating activities, some forms of the enzyme also catalyze steroid double-bond epimerization and peroxide reduction (132).

γ-Glutamyl transpeptidase cleaves the glutamate moiety of GSH and GSH conjugates. The enzyme is most abundant in the kidney and intestinal plasma membranes. The activity can be measured as described by Meister et al. (193).

After the γ-glutamyl transpeptidase reaction occurs, hydrolysis of the glycine moiety gives a cysteine conjugate. These cysteine conjugates can undergo β-elimination by a pyridoxal phosphate-containing enzyme found in liver and kidney, cysteine conjugate β-lyase. The assay is not convenient: S-(2,4-dinitrophenyl)-L-[³⁵S]-cysteine is incubated with the enzyme, and one of the products, 2,4-dinitrobenzethiol, is methylated with CH₃I and analyzed by TLC (251).

A number of enzymes form sulfate monoesters by transferring the sulfate group from 3′-phosphoadenosine-5′-phosphosulfate (PAPS) to a hydroxyl group. Because the acceptor substrates vary, so do the assays that can be used. One of the more common assays involves chromatographic separation after incubation with ³⁵S-PAPS (1,134,237).

Methyltransferases are most conveniently assayed with radiolabeled methyl donors (5,18,286). Transfers can involve N, O, or S atoms. Other chromatographic, fluorometric, and spectrophotometric assays have also been used but are generally not as sensitive or rapid (18).

Another moiety that is often transferred in biological reactions of interest is the acetyl group. The physiological donor group is acetyl coenzyme A (CoA), and a variety of colorimetric (285), fluorimetric (192), spectrophotometric (135,282,283), and radiometric (69) assays have been described.

ISOLATION OF ENZYMES

Cytochrome P-450

Cytochrome P-450 is the enzyme that has probably received most of the attention of those concerned with microsomal metabolism to date. Early studies on the role of the enzyme system and its inducibility in carcinogenesis and toxicology have been reviewed elsewhere (33,34,64,68) as well as more recently (83,292). Other reviews of progress in purification and reconstitution techniques have also appeared (78,83,172).

Liver microsomal cytochrome P-450 was first solubilized and partially purified by Lu and Coon and their associates (171,177); since that time a number of advances have been made. Because a variety of forms of cytochrome P-450 are found in various tissues of different animals, a number of procedures have been developed for purification of individual forms (98,113,115,147–149,152,220,231). Major features of some of the purification schemes are presented, and the reader is referred to the original literature for details. The choice of a purification system depends on the animal species of choice, if simultaneous purification of other enzymes is desired, and other factors. Most of the procedures discussed here are carried out at 0° to 4°C in the presence of 20% glycerol for stabilization. A number of alkyl phenyl ether-based detergents have been used in the purification process, including Emulgen 911 and 913 (Kao-Atlas, Tokyo), Triton N-101 (Sigma, St. Louis, Missouri), Renex 690 (Imperial Chemical Industries, Wilmington, Delaware), and Non-Idet NP40 (Shell Chemical Co., New York). Our work (76) and that of others (36,139–141) suggests that these nonionic detergents are relatively interchangeable, although some differences exist.

The following procedure for purification of rat liver microsomal cytochrome P-450 was developed in our laboratory. It represents a modification of early methods (73,76); the major inducible liver microsomal cytochromes P-450 of phenobarbital- or β-naphthoflavone-treated rats can be highly purified in good yield using two basic chromatography steps (89).

Preparation of n-Octylamino-Sepharose 4B

Reagents

1. Pharmacia Sepharose 4B, 400 ml wet volume, washed with distilled H_2O and suspended in 1,000 ml H_2O
2. CNBr 100 g dissolved in 300 ml dioxane immediately before use
3. 1,8-Diaminooctane 114 g dissolved in 400 ml H_2O

Procedure

The entire procedure is carried out in a fume hood with adequate ventilation. The Sepharose is stirred in a 2-L beaker, and a pH electrode and a thermometer are inserted into the suspension. The CNBr solution is added in a dropwise manner with a separatory funnel over a period of 10 min, and NaOH is added to maintain a pH of 11. Ice is added to keep the temperature at 20° to 25°C. After a total of 20 min has elapsed, about 600 ml of crushed ice is added to quench the reaction, and the contents are poured into a large sintered glass funnel attached to a water aspirator. The gel is washed in vacuo with 4 L of cold water and added to the 1,8-diaminooctane solution. The solution is adjusted to pH 10 with 6 N HCl, and the mixture is stirred (as slowly as possible with a magnetic stirrer) overnight at 4°C. The gel is filtered in vacuo, washed with 10 L of distilled H_2O, then 2 L of 0.2 M potassium phosphate buffer (pH 7.25), and then another 10 L of H_2O. About 200 ml of the washed gel is suspended in 300 ml of H_2O, deaerated in vacuo for 15 min, and poured into a 2.5 cm diameter column designed for use with a peristaltic pump. The column is allowed to settle for 20 min and then filled to a height of 40 cm. The column is equilibrated with 300 ml of 0.1 M potassium phosphate buffer (pH 7.25) containing 1 mM EDTA, 20% glycerol, and 0.6% (w/v) sodium cholate (see below).

Purification of Cytochrome P-450

Reagents

1. Microsomes, prepared from phenobarbital- or β-naphthoflavone-treated rat livers
2. Lubrol PX 20% (Sigma Chemical Co., St. Louis, Missouri)
3. Sodium cholate 20%

Procedure

Cholic acid (Sigma Chemical Co.) is recrystallized twice (as the free acid) from 50% aqueous ethanol using charcoal in the first step. The free acid is dried to constant weight in vacuo in a desiccator, mixed with 0.1 part NaOH pellets (w/w), dissolved in water, slowly adjusted to pH 7.5 with acetic acid, made up to volume with water, and filtered through paper.

All steps are carried out at 0° to 4°C. Microsomes are suspended to 2 mg protein ml^{-1} in 0.1 M potassium phosphate (pH 7.25) solution containing 20% glycerol, 1 mM EDTA, and 20 μM butylated hydroxytoluene; sodium cholate is added dropwise (from a separatory funnel) over 20 min to a final concentration of 0.6% (w/v) while stirring. After stirring an additional 30 min, the clarified solution is centrifuged at 100,000 $\times$ g (35,000 rpm in a Beckman 45 Ti rotor). An amount of the supernatant equivalent to 3,000 nmol of cytochrome P-450 is applied to the equilibrated octylamino-Sepharose 4B column at a flow rate of 1 ml min^{-1}. A safe guide to follow is to have cytochrome P-450 bound only to the top one-third of the column. The column is washed with 800 ml of 0.1 M potassium phosphate buffer (pH 7.25) containing 1 mM EDTA, 20% glycerol, and 0.42% (w/v) sodium cholate. Cytochrome P-450 is eluted using about 1,500 ml of 0.1 M potassium phosphate buffer containing 1 mM EDTA, 20% glycerol, 0.33% (w/v) cholate, and 0.06% (w/v) Lubrol PX (89) (Fig. 15). NADPH-cytochrome P-450 reductase is eluted with 1,500 ml of 50 mM potassium phosphate buffer (pH 7.25) containing 0.1 mM EDTA, 20% glycerol, 0.15% (w/v) sodium deoxycholate, and 0.35% (w/v) sodium cholate (the cholic acid need not be recrystallized for this final buffer) (126). The fractions eluted with the last two buffers are monitored for cytochrome P-450 (A_{417}) and NADPH-cytochrome c reductase activity (Fig. 1). The A_{417} peak tubes are pooled, concentrated to 50 ml using an Amicon PM-30 ultrafiltration apparatus, and dialyzed versus 1 L of a 20% glycerol/0.1 mM EDTA solution and then versus 1 L of 10 mM potassium phosphate buffer (pH 7.7) containing 0.1 mM EDTA, 20% glycerol, 0.1% (w/v) Lubrol PX, and 0.2% (w/v) sodium cholate (not recrystallized). The yield of cytochrome P-450 at this step is 40 to 70%, and the specific content is usually about 6 to 9 nmol mg^{-1} protein.

The cytochrome P-450 is further purified by DEAE-cellulose chromatography. Several points should be noted: The procedure is carried out at room temperature for convenience, as suggested by other workers (231,287). Lubrol PX, in contrast to the phenyl ether detergents, does not have optical absorbance at 280 nm and permits protein to be mon-

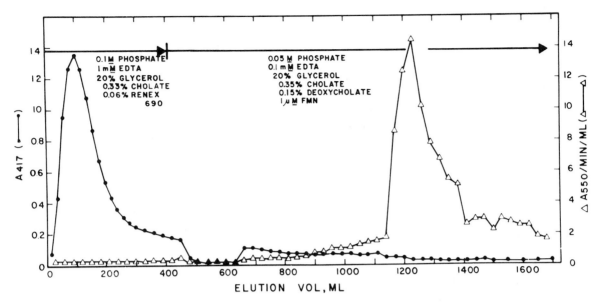

FIG. 15. Separation of rat liver microsomal cytochrome P-450 (A_{417}) and NADPH-cytochrome P-450 reductase on *n*-octylamino-Sepharose 4B (73,89,126). The procedure utilized solubilized microsomes derived from phenobarbital-treated rats as described in the text.

itored at this wavelength; sodium cholate is also added but is not recrystallized. Different brands of DEAE-cellulose behave somewhat differently.

The cytochrome P-450 is applied to a 2.5 × 50 cm column of Pharmacia DEAE-Sephacel previously equilibrated with 1 L of 10 mM potassium phosphate buffer (pH 7.7) containing 0.1 mM EDTA, 20% glycerol, 0.1% (w/v) Lubrol PX, and 0.2% (w/v) sodium cholate. The column is washed with 700 ml of the equilibration buffer and then eluted with a 2 L linear gradient of the equilibration buffer to the same containing 0.25 M NaCl (Fig. 16). With either β-naphthoflavone- or phenobarbital-treated rat liver microsomes, the last major A_{417} peak contains the bulk of the cytochrome P-450 (Fig. 2). The peak fractions are pooled, concentrated with an

Amicon PM-30 ultrafiltration device, stirred with Bio-Beads, SM-2 (Bio-Rad Laboratories, Richmond, California) or Amberlite XAD-2 polystyrene beads (Sigma Chemical Co., St. Louis, MO) to remove excess detergent (~0.5 g/mg protein for 2 hr) (272), filtered through glass wool, and dialyzed overnight versus 50 volumes of 10 mM Tris-acetate buffer (pH 7.4) containing 0.1 mM EDTA and 20% glycerol. Alternatively, detergent can be removed using calcium phosphate gel or hydroxylapatite (272). Preparations contain 13 to 18 nmol cytochrome P-450 (mg protein)$^{-1}$ and are electrophoretically homogeneous (160). Yields are 25 to 45% for the DEAE column; thus overall yields range from 10 to 30% depending on the source of microsomes, with the higher yields for phenobarbital-treated rats.

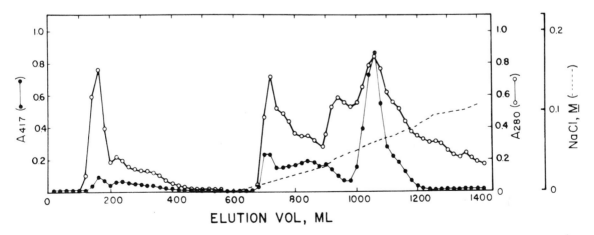

FIG. 16. Purification of rat liver microsomal cytochrome P-450 using DEAE-cellulose chromatography in the presence of sodium cholate and Lubrol PX. The cytochrome P-450 fraction obtained in Fig. 15 was chromatographed as described in the text; NaCl concentrations were estimated by conductivity measurements (89).

Comment

Many individual forms of cytochrome P-450 have now been purified and characterized from a number of species, including humans. A complete discussion of these preparations is beyond the scope of this chapter, and the reader is referred to other references (50,82,83,98,99).

One of the reasons for purifying individual forms of cytochrome P-450 is to determine which individual forms are involved in particular reactions. This task has been made somewhat easier in the light of current knowledge available concerning cytochromes P-450.

The first step is the development of an *in vitro* assay for the particular activity under consideration. It must be developed with liver microsomes, and the sensitivity should be optimized, along with conditions such as pH, time, and protein and substrate concentrations.

The next step involves comparison of rates of oxidation with microsomes isolated from (untreated) male and female rats and male rats treated with various inducing agents. A considerable body of knowledge now exists concerning the effects of gender and inducing agents on individual cytochrome P-450 forms, and this information can be used to advantage (41,82,83,98,281). For example, male (adult) rats have P-450$_{UT-A}$ and P-450$_{PCN-E}$ but not P-450$_{UT-I}$. Phenobarbital administration induces P-450$_{PB-B}$, P-450$_{PB-C}$, P-450$_{PB-D}$, and P-450$_{PCN-E}$. Pregnenolone 16α-carbonitrile and dexamethasone induce only P-450$_{PCN-E}$ (and any closely related forms). Levels of P-450$_{UT-A}$ are suppressed by administration of any of several of the typical inducers, particularly polycyclic aromatic hydrocarbons. From information obtained in such experiments one can begin to hypothesize which forms are involved.

The next step involves examination of the relative abilities of individual forms of cytochrome P-450 to catalyze the reaction. Reconstitution conditions are described elsewhere.

The last step involves using specific antibodies with microsomal preparations to determine which ones inhibit the reaction. This approach is discussed later in the chapter. The results should agree with and confirm those obtained in the above experiments.

When specific inhibitors are known for individual forms of cytochrome P-450 (e.g., 7,8-naphthoflavone for rat P-450$_{\beta NF-B}$) they can also be used to advantage.

NADPH-Cytochrome P-450 Reductase

Procedures have been described by Yasukochi and Masters (295) and Strobel and Dignam (154,249) for the purification of NADPH-cytochrome P-450 reductase from rat and hog liver using detergent extraction from microsomes, DEAE-cellulose chromatography, and 2',5'-ADP- or NADP$^+$-agarose affinity chromatography. 2',5'-ADP-agarose is commercially available from Pharmacia (Uppsala) and P-L Biochemicals (Milwaukee, Wisconsin). The ion-exchange chromatography or some initial purification procedure appears to be necessary for binding the reductase to the affinity column (295). Alternatively, the polyethylene glycol–ammonium sulfate fraction from Coon's procedure for rabbit cytochrome P-450

purification (272,273) or the *n*-octylamino–Sepharose 4B reductase fraction from rabbit, rat, or human liver cytochrome P-450 purification procedures (72,73,76,89,126,127,278) can be applied directly to the affinity column. The column is washed with 0.25 *M* potassium phosphate buffer (pH 7.7) containing 0.1 m*M* EDTA, 20% glycerol, and 0.2% Renex 690 (or other nonionic detergent) to remove other proteins. The detergent is then removed by washing the column with 30 m*M* potassium phosphate containing 0.1 m*M* EDTA, 20% glycerol, and 0.1% (w/v) sodium cholate. The reductase is eluted with the latter buffer containing 10 m*M* 2'-AMP or NADP$^+$ (and 0.1 m*M* phenylmethylsulfonyl fluoride) and dialyzed (48 hr) versus 100 volumes of 10 m*M* Tris-acetate buffer (pH 7.4) containing 0.1 m*M* EDTA and 20% glycerol to remove cholate and 2'-AMP (or NADP$^+$) (75,89,98).

This procedure has been used to obtain NADPH-cytochrome P-450 reductase in yields as high as 50%; specific activities for cytochrome *c* reduction range from 40 to 70 μmol min^{-1} (mg protein)$^{-1}$ (75,249,295). Spectra show the absence of nonflavin components: The A_{455}/A_{380} ratios are 1.10:1 to 1.15:1 (75,89). The apparent monomeric molecular weight is 74,000 [the protein sequence has now been deduced from a DNA clone, and the actual weight is somewhat different (222)]. Sometimes proteolysis is a problem and results in cleavage of a peptide necessary for activity toward cytochrome P-450 (but not cytochrome *c*). This problem can be avoided by adding phenylmethylsulfonyl fluoride (from a stock ethanolic solution) to 0.1 m*M* to buffers immediately prior to use in order to inhibit serine-active proteases. Some preparations appear to lose some flavin mononucleotide (FMN), as evidenced by stimulation by 10 μM FMN. This problem can be minimized by including 1 μM concentrations of FMN in buffers and minimizing exposure to light (126).

Epoxide Hydrolase

Highly purified rat, rabbit, and human liver enzymes have been prepared in a number of laboratories (8,106,155,173,179). In general, purification procedures are carried out at 0° to 4°C using nonionic detergents, and styrene-7,8-oxide hydrolase activity is usually monitored. The procedure presented below was developed in our laboratory and is based on the original work of Knowles and Burchell (155); this procedure routinely yields apparently homogeneous enzyme in reasonably good yield (89,106).

Procedure

Liver microsomes prepared from phenobarbital-treated rats (ca. 4 g protein) are suspended at 4 mg ml^{-1} in 0.2 *M* potassium phosphate buffer (pH 7.4) containing 0.1 m*M* EDTA. A 20% (w/v) aqueous solution of Lubrol PX (Sigma Chemical Co., St. Louis, Missouri) is added while stirring at 0° to 4°C to yield a final detergent concentration of 1% (w/v). After 30 min of additional stirring, the clarified solution is centrifuged for 60 min at 100,000 × *g* (35,000 rpm in a Beckman 45 Ti rotor). The pellets are discarded, and the combined supernatants are dialyzed twice (8 hr) against 15 volumes of 5 mM potassium phosphate buffer (pH 7.25) containing 0.05% (w/v) Lubrol PX. The dialysate is applied to a 5 × 50 cm column of DEAE-cellulose (Whatman DE-52) equilibrated with the dialysis buffer. The column is washed with the same buffer; no activity remains bound to the column. Because Lubrol PX does not absorb in the UV region, fractions are monitored at 280 nm, and those fractions showing significant absorbance (>0.05) are pooled and dialyzed versus 10 volumes of 5 mM potassium phosphate buffer (pH 6.5) containing 0.05% Lubrol PX. The dialysate is applied to a 4 × 30 cm CM-cellulose (Whatman CM-52) column equilibrated with dialysis buffer. The column is eluted with 500 ml more of the dialysis buffer and then with a 1 L linear phosphate gradient (5–300 mM) containing 0.05% Lubrol PX. The void volume fractions are monitored for absorbance at 280 nm and constitute one peak of epoxide hydrolase activity denoted fraction "A"; the other (located by styrene oxide activity assays) is eluted with the gradient at about 100 mM phosphate. The second fraction, denoted "B," is dialyzed versus 5 mM phosphate buffer (pH 7.25), and both fractions are applied to 3 × 15 cm hydroxylapatite columns. The individual columns are washed with 500 ml of 5 mM phosphate buffer (pH 7.25) containing 0.05% Lubrol PX. A 750-ml linear phosphate gradient (50–500 mM, pH 7.25, with 0.05% Lubrol PX present) is applied to each column, and individual fractions are assayed for styrene oxide hydrolase activity and A$_{280}$. Peak activity fractions are pooled and stirred with Bio-Beads SM-2 (ca. 0.5 g/mg protein) for 2 hr; beads are removed by filtration through glass wool or nylon mesh. Alternatively, detergent can be removed using a hydroxylapatite column, with washing using buffer devoid of detergent and elution with 0.5 M phosphate buffer. Final preparations are concentrated by ultrafiltration using Amicon PM-30 membranes and stored at −20°C.

The overall yields are 10 to 20% for the "A" fraction and 5 to 10% for the "B" fraction. Preparations are apparently homogeneous as judged by SDS-polyacrylamide gel electrophoresis and have varying activities toward a variety of epoxides. The procedure has also been used successfully with microsomes prepared from stilbene oxide- and 3-methylcholanthrene-treated and untreated rats. The enzymes of human liver behave differently, and this procedure is not directly applicable (106).

Multiple forms of epoxide hydrolase exist, although some aspects of the multiplicity remain unclear (79). The liver microsomal epoxide hydrolase activity toward substrates such as styrene-7,8-oxide, octene-1,2-oxide, and others can be chromatographed into different fractions (42,105,106,208). These fractions have somewhat different properties, including their electrophoretic migration (106), although the contribution of lipids and detergents to the difference has been reported (21). Immunochemical sensitivity of different catalytic activities to antibodies (206,261) and the homogeneity of an N-terminal sequence of a purified preparation (52) have been cited as evidence for the existence of a single form of the enzyme. Lyman et al. (183) presented evidence for different forms of microsomal epoxide hydrolase in inbred mouse strains, and this work suggested that more than one form might also be expressed in outbred animals of other species (although not necessarily in each individual). Cholesterol-5α,6α-oxide hydrolation has been reported to be catalyzed by a distinct form of liver microsomal epoxide hydrolase (164). A distinct cytosolic form of epoxide hydrolase has been purified from mouse (109,191) and human (279) liver. Rabbit liver microsomal epoxide hydrolase has been sequenced (117).

Other Enzymes

Microsomal flavin-containing monooxygenase has been isolated from porcine liver using detergent extraction, gel exclusion chromatography, and preparative electrophoresis (300). The enzyme is inherently less stable than the others discussed above. The enzyme has been purified from rat (153) and mouse (232) liver and from rabbit lung (290). The lung enzyme appears to be different from that in the liver.

Heme oxygenase has been obtained in highly purified form from porcine (297) and bovine (298) spleen and from CoCl$_2$-induced rat liver (184). The properties of the two isolated preparations suggest that they are similar enzymes. However, evidence for multiple forms of the rat liver enzyme has been reported (185).

A number of transferases are involved in the overall metabolism of xenobiotics. Most are cytosolic enzymes and exist in multiple forms. References for the purification and characterization of the following enzymes are given: GSH S-transferase (60,108,116,132,133,162,187,198,254,266,274), UDP-glucuronyl transferase (15,227,267), N-acetyltransferase (3,284), metallothionein (actually more of a "sink" for trapping electrophiles and metals than an enzyme) (291), methyltransferases (4,18,286), sulfotransferase (134,235,236), and cysteine conjugate acetyltransferase (53).

Other redox-active enzymes of interest (and appropriate references) include alcohol dehydrogenase (19,125,143,194), aldehyde dehydrogenase (118,168), cysteine conjugate β-lyase (247,251,252), monoamine oxidase (234,288), DT-diaphorase (54,121), cytochrome b_5 (246), and NADPH-cytochrome b_5 reductase (214).

Methods for Determination of Enzyme Purity

As in the case of other chemicals, no single technique can be used to establish purity; moreover, purity is defined as a lack of heterogeneity in a given analytical system, and one can argue that nothing is really "pure." However, some techniques are more useful than others for ruling out heterogeneity and are discussed here.

1. An obvious criterion of homogeneity is the absence of suspected contaminants. For instance, cytochrome P-450 preparations should be devoid of NADPH-cytochrome c reductase activity, epoxide hydrolase preparations should be devoid of heme, and so on. Of course, such impurities must always be defined in terms of detectable limits of contamination. A point to be considered here is that an experimental situation may call for the absence of lipid or detergent con-

tamination as well as protein contamination, and the limit of such impurity must be determined.*

2. Specific activity or specific content of the isolated enzyme is a guidepost to follow in purification. For instance, cytochrome P-450 preparations should contain x nanomoles of cytochrome P-450 (mg protein)$^{-1}$, where $x = 10^6 \div$ subunit molecular weight (i.e., $x = 16$–22); NADPH-cytochrome P-450 reductase preparations should catalyze the reduction of 40 to 70 μmol of cytochrome c min^{-1} (mg protein)$^{-1}$ under optimal conditions; and epoxide hydrolase preparations should catalyze the hydrolysis of 500 to 1,000 nmol of styrene oxide min^{-1} (mg protein)$^{-1}$ (8,155,179). However, such measurements are dependent on the accuracy of the protein estimation, which may be a problem. Specific activities are sometimes more variable than expected. In the case of cytochrome P-450, some forms exist *in vivo* without a full complement of heme (233). Nevertheless, these general guidelines are useful for the evaluation of purity.

3. SDS-polyacrylamide gel electrophoresis (160) has been used as one of the main criteria for homogeneity. This technique has been useful for the determination of homogeneity; moreover, the subunit molecular weight estimates appear to be reasonably valid for cytochrome P-450 (13,76,86) and NADPH-cytochrome P-450 reductase (154,222). The reader should remember, however, that even this powerful technique has its limitations. Evidence has been presented that different microsomal enzymes cannot always be distinguished by this technique (11,12,38,98). Furthermore, the results obtained with this technique are dependent on the exact procedure used, and the methods vary in resolving abilities (76,98). Finally, apparent molecular weights also vary depending on the procedure and the standards used, and the reader is cautioned to compare results from different laboratories carefully and allow for as much as 3,000- to 4,000-dalton differences in molecular weights.

Electrophoresis in the absence of detergents has been used far less, primarily because of the tendency of many of these proteins to aggregate and not migrate in gels. However, agarose gel electrophoresis has been used in the author's laboratory to distinguish between forms of cytochrome P-450 (78) and epoxide hydrolase (106) and to estimate their isoelectric points.

Isoelectric focusing offers a great potential for resolution of enzymes and has been used for studying cytochromes P-450. However, a number of artifacts are related to the use of this methodology, and at the present time one should view data obtained using isoelectric focusing of membrane proteins with caution (77,78,82,209,276). Nevertheless, the technique has been useful in certain cases.

Staining of electrophoretograms is usually done with protein stains. In the absence of SDS, NADPH-cytochrome P-450 reductase can be stained using tetrazolium dyes (104), and cytochrome P-450 can be stained using benzidine de-

rivatives and H_2O_2 (105,260). The latter method has also been used to tentatively identify cytochrome P-450 in SDS-polyacrylamide gel electrophoresis. However, much of the heme leaves the enzyme, even in the absence of reducing agents. Although others have claimed that heme does not bind to other proteins, Thomas et al. (260) found that heme was bound to albumin; thus one must be cautious when interpreting data involving such a technique. Immunochemical techniques have been developed for the identification of cytochrome P-450 separated from microsomal membranes by SDS-polyacrylamide gel electrophoresis; these methods have proved useful for answering a number of questions about cytochrome P-450 induction (*vide infra*).

4. *N*-Terminal analysis should produce single residues at each step of automated Edman degradation for homogeneous proteins. This technique has been used for some of the microsomal enzymes (13,114).

5. A variety of immunological criteria have been used to assess homogeneity (8,43,98,103–105,140,149,155,231). An antibody should produce a single precipitin line when diffused against the antigen if the antigen is homogeneous. Immunoelectrophoresis of a crude preparation should show only the antigen (*vide infra*). Cross-reactivity of related proteins does exist, and many of the isolated microsomal proteins do not induce production of monospecific antibodies.

6. Hydrodynamic criteria have been used to assess the homogeneity of the various isolated microsomal proteins; because all of these proteins tend to aggregate, velocity and equilibrium studies carried out to examine homogeneity must be done in the presence of detergents or other strong denaturants (8,86).

Reconstitution of Enzyme Activity

Epoxide hydrolase activity toward a wide variety of substrates is observed with the purified enzyme. Many of the activities have slightly basic pH optima (176,179). The presence of phospholipid enhances activity of the purified enzyme toward some substrates but not others; these results have been interpreted in terms of a model in which the phospholipid micelles bind substrate (176).

Reconstitution of mixed-function oxidase activity has been reviewed by Lu and West (174). The following general statements can be made. The optimum rate of enzyme activity, based on cytochrome P-450, is obtained when NADPH-cytochrome P-450 reductase is present at an equimolar concentration or in slight excess. Phospholipid enhances the rates of most activities; this phospholipid can be in the form of a microsomal extract or synthetic dilauroylglyceryl-3-phosphorylcholine. Some nonionic detergents partially replace phosphatidylcholine at low concentrations (172,178,180). The activity toward some substrates can be further enhanced by small amounts of cholate or deoxycholate (174). The role of phospholipid is not completely understood, but a dual role has been postulated (59): Dilauroylglyceryl-3-phosphorylcholine increases the affinity of rabbit liver cytochrome P-450 LM2 for *both* organic substrate and NADPH-cytochrome P-450 reductase; all four components are complexed during catalysis. In the rat liver systems that have been studied, lipid does not appear to enhance substrate binding. Several investigators have studied synthetic liposomal systems; how-

---

* Phospholipid can be determined by thoroughly dialyzing the enzyme versus Tris buffer and then water; lipids are extracted as described by Bligh and Dyer (14), and phosphate is determined according to Chen et al. (28). Ethylene oxide-based detergents (including Emulgens 911 and 913, Renex 690, Triton N-101, and Lubrol PX) can be extracted and assayed by the method described by Garewal (62) and subsequently modified by Goldstein and Blecher (70).

ever, no such system has been prepared to date that is more active in hydroxylation than a system reconstituted in the presence of subcritical micelle concentration levels of phospholipid. Neither cytochrome b_5 nor NADH is required for activity in many reactions, although some are definitely enhanced considerably by cytochrome b_5. The effect of the phospholipid appears to be kinetic and can be overcome with high protein concentrations and extended preincubation conditions (199).

A basic procedure for reconstituting mixed-function oxidase activity is outlined below. Equimolar concentrations of cytochrome P-450 and NADPH-cytochrome P-450 reductase [both of which have been stripped of excess detergent by treatment with beads, calcium phosphate gel, or both (272)] are first mixed in the presence of 40 μM sonicated dilauroylglyceryl-3-phosphorylcholine, and after 5 min an appropriate buffer (i.e., 50–100 mM potassium phosphate or other buffer, pH 7.0–7.7) is added plus a sufficient volume of water. The substrate is then added, in water if possible. [If not, the substrate should be dissolved in acetone, dimethylsulfoxide, or methanol such that the final concentration of organic solvent is ≤1% (v/v) for the enzymes. Some forms of cytochrome P-450 metabolize these compounds (e.g., rat P-450j, rabbit P-450 LM3a), and caution must be exercised.] The system is preequilibrated at 37°C for 3 to 5 min, and the reaction is initiated by the addition of NADPH (0.15–0.5 mM) or a NADPH-generating system. [The organic substrate should not be the last addition, as prior addition of NADPH results in the generation of H_2O_2, which can destroy cytochrome P-450 (75).] The length of the time for which the reaction is linear depends on the substrate; in general, rapidly metabolized substrates do not give long periods of linearity, and some substrates are converted to metabolites that destroy cytochrome P-450 rapidly. Table 2 presents some of the substrates that have been used in reconstituted cytochrome P-450 systems.

Flavin-containing monooxygenase activity requires only the single protein, of course, but the enzyme is dramatically less heat-stable than others (223,299). The enzyme is stabilized by pyridine nucleotides, so NADPH is added to the enzyme before incubation at 37°C, after which the organic substrate is added. Heme oxygenase activity has been reconstituted in the presence of NADPH-cytochrome P-450 reductase (185,297,298). NADPH-cytochrome P-450 reductase has other enzyme activities in the absence of cytochrome P-450, many of which require no special conditions but may be stimulated, as is the case for lipid peroxidation, by high salt concentrations.

Immunochemical Techniques

Antibodies have been raised to cytochrome P-450, NADPH-cytochrome P-450 reductase, epoxide hydrolase, and many of the other enzymes considered here. For instance, these antibodies have been used to show the involvement of cytochrome P-450 (43,49,139,145,147–149,258,259) and its reductase (104,188) in a number of reactions. Antibodies have also been used to examine the homogeneity of isolated enzyme fractions, the multiplicity of enzymes in microsomes, and the amounts of individual enzyme formed in microsomal

preparations (8,38,39,43,98,140,141,155,231,258). The topical location of the enzymes in microsomal membranes has also been studied with immunological techniques (43,259), as have several aspects of enzyme biosynthesis. Antibodies have also been used to study the localization of the enzymes in various sections of individual organs (7).

All three of the above enzymes are antigenic, and antibodies have been raised in rabbits using less than 100 μg of protein. Sheep, goats, and guinea pigs have also been used for antibody production. A number of immunization schedules can be used, depending on the animal and the dose. Antisera can be used in some procedures, but immunoglobulin G (IgG) fractions are more useful (43,149). To prepare these fractions, antisera are heated 20 min at 56°C and centrifuged at 10,000 × g for 10 min. The supernatants are mixed with equal volumes of 50% (w/v) ammonium sulfate and recentrifuged. The pellets are washed with 25% (w/v) ammonium sulfate to remove most of the color and then dissolved in 10 mM potassium phosphate buffer (pH 8.0) and dialyzed against the same buffer. The dialysates are passed through columns of DEAE-cellulose equilibrated with the same buffer. The void volume fractions (measured by absorbance at 280 nm) are pooled, retreated with ammonium sulfate as above to remove color if necessary, concentrated by ultrafiltration (up to 50 mg ml^{-1}), and stored at −20°C.

The list of immunochemical techniques that can be used with such antibodies is lengthy, and the reader is referred to texts on the general subject (67). The procedures include double-diffusion analysis, radial diffusion quantitation, inhibition of enzyme activity, complement fixation, radioimmune assay, crossed gel electrophoresis, immunoprecipitation, immunoaffinity column chromatography, and immunohistochemical localization. These techniques should continue to be useful in future studies of the roles of individual forms of these microsomal enzymes in various processes.

Immunoinhibition of Catalytic Activity

With immunoinhibition of catalytic activity one adds an antibody to an enzyme preparation and determines if that antibody preparation can block catalytic activity (Fig. 17). This approach is most useful with a crude enzyme system, such as a subcellular organelle preparation. Thus one can ask what fraction of total activity is the result of the enzyme specifically recognized by the antibody (if the antibody completely inhibits the activity of the antigen itself). Such an approach has been useful in a number of cases in our own laboratory (49,51,82,242) as well as in many others.

Antibodies to some proteins tend to be more inhibitory than others. In general, polyclonal antibodies raised against cytochromes P-450 are usually inhibitory. However, inhibitory antibodies have not been reported for microsomal flavin-containing monooxygenase, and only occasionally has inhibitory anti-epoxide hydrolase been prepared (206). Some of the difference may be due to the size of the substrate or accessory protein that interacts with the antigen in catalysis. Thus one would expect binding of an antibody to block binding of large substrates (viz., other proteins) more readily than small compounds. In support of this view, anti-NADPH-

TABLE 2. *Substrates for reconstituted liver microsomal cytochrome P-450 systems*

Substrate	Refs.	Substrate	Refs.
Acetanilide	98,141,238	Ethylmorphine	82,98,113
2-Acetylaminofluorene	82	Fluroxene (→ trifluoroethanol) (and other vinyl ethers)	82
Acrylonitrile	100		
Aflatoxin B$_1$	73	Glu-P-1(2-amino-6-methyldipyrido	82
Aldrin	101,293	(1,2-*a*:3',2'-*d*)imidazole)	
4-Aminobiphenyl	82	Hexane (and other alkanes)	82,180,203
Aminofluorene	58	Hexobarbital	82
2-Amino-3-methylimidazo[4,5-*f*]-quinoline	82	7α-Hydroxy-4-cholesten-3-one	10
		Iodobenzene	82,88
Aminopyrine	82,98	4-Ipomeanol	73
5α-Androstane-3α,17β-diol	107	Iproniazid	82
Androstenedione	82,281	Isopropylhydrazine	82
Aniline	98,115,127,175	Isosafrole	82
Anthracene	82	Lasiocarpine	73
Arachidonic acid	82	Lauric acid	66,171
Azoprocarbazine *N*-oxygenation	82	Lithocholic acid	11
Benz[*a*,*h*]anthracene	82	*N*-Methyl-4-aminoazobenzene	73
Benzo(*a*)pyrene	47,58,82,98,122, 123,139,228,294	8-Methylbenz[*a*]anthracene	82
		Naphthalene	82
Benzo(*a*)pyrene-4,5-oxide (reduction)	82	1-Naphthylamine	110
Benzphetamine	98,115,123,145,150, 177,203,231,278	2-Naphthylamine	110
		p-Nitroanisole	98,115
Biphenyl	115	*p*-Nitrophenetole	82
3-*t*-Butyl-4-hydroxyanisole	82	1-Nitropropane	82
Chlorobenzene	239	Octanoic acid	181
1-(2-Chloroethyl)-3-(cyclohexyl)-1-nitrosourea	82	Parathion	73,145,146
		Pentoxyresorufin	182
1-(2-Chloroethyl)-3-(*trans*-4-methyl cyclohexyl)-1-nitrosourea	82	*trans*-1-Phenyl-1-butene	82
		Progesterone	82
Cholesterol	12	7-Propoxycoumarin	82
Coumarin	123	Scoparone	199
Cyclohexane	82,203	Taurodeoxycholic acid	11
Cyclopropylamines and cyclopropyl ethers	82	Testosterone	82
		1,1,2,2-Tetrachloroethane	82
Dichlorinated biphenyls	82	Toluene	82
1,2-Dichloroethane	97	*p*-Tolylethyl sulfide	82
N,*N*-Dimethyl-4-aminoazobenzene	73	1,1,2-Trichloroethane	61
N,*N*-Dimethylaniline	22,82	Trichloroethylene	196
7,12-Dimethylbenz[*a*,*h*]anthracene	82	1,3,4-Trimethylpyrrole	91
Dimethylnitrosamine	73,98,169	Trp-2(3-amino-1-methyl-5*H*-pyrido-[4,3-*b*]indole)	82
17β-Estradiol 2-hydroxylation	82		
Ethanol	197,256	Vinyl chloride	92,93,96
7-Ethoxycoumarin	82,98,123,199,231	Vinylidene chloride	82
Ethoxyresorufin	23,98,139,199	Warfarin	57,82
2-(*N*-Ethylcarbamoylhydroxymethyl)-furan	73	Zoxazolamine	262

cytochrome P-450 reductase blocks reduction of cytochrome *c* but not ferricyanide or neotetrazolium blue (104). Another general trend is that only a limited fraction of monoclonal antibodies are inhibitory, even in cases where polyclonal antisera are strongly inhibitory (215,216).

Analyzing for antibody inhibition is a relatively straightforward process. In general, the enzyme preparation of interest is mixed with the antibody and incubated for 20 to 30 min at room temperature. Other components are then added, and catalytic activity is measured in the usual manner.

A good way to properly assess enzyme inhibition is to run several incubations, varying the amount of antibody and holding the amount of enzyme constant. Parallel assays are done in which a nonimmune antibody preparation prepared in the same way is added at the same levels to the enzyme preparation of interest (Fig. 17). (Alternatively, one can mix varying ratios of immune and nonimmune antibodies with each aliquot of enzyme, maintaining a constant *total* amount of antibody added.)

Most assays of this type are done with IgG antibody fractions. Serum and ascites fluid contain other materials that can cause nonspecific inhibition. However, if the antibody

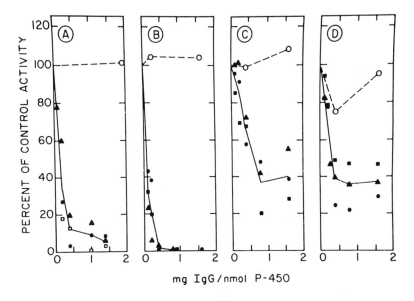

FIG. 17. Inhibition of mixed-function oxidation of debrisoquine, sparteine, encainide, and propranolol in human liver microsomes by anti-P-450$_{UT-H}$. Incubations were carried out with microsomes prepared from liver samples 17 (△), 25 (□), 31 (●), 32 (▲), 34 (■), 72 (◇), and 86 (◆), which contained 0.32, 0.55, 0.77, 0.50, 0.55, 0.61, and 0.30 nmol P-450 (mg protein)$^{-1}$, respectively. The microsomes were incubated with indicated amounts of anti-P-450$_{UT-H}$ (IgG fraction) for 30 min at 23°C in the appropriate buffer, and other incubation components were then added. Results are expressed as percent of the control activity (obtained in the absence of antibody) for debrisoquine 4-hydroxylation (**A**), formation of Δ^5-dehydrosparteine from sparteine (**B**), encainide O-demethylation (**C**), and propranolol 4-hydroxylation (**D**). The solid lines are drawn connecting the means of the values obtained with the various samples, and the broken lines connect the means of the values obtained with IgG prepared from preimmune antisera (individual values not shown). Control activities of debrisoquine 4-hydroxylation were 0.16, 0.060, and 0.19 pmol min^{-1} (nmol cytochrome P-450)$^{-1}$ for samples 25, 31, and 32, respectively. Control activities of Δ^5-dehydrosparteine formation were 26.6, 20.4, and 2.0 pmol min^{-1} (nmol cytochrome P-450)$^{-1}$ for samples 31, 32, and 34, respectively. Control activities of encainide O-demethylation were 0.044, 0.072, and 0.039 nmol min^{-1} (nmol cytochrome P-450)$^{-1}$ for samples 31, 32, and 34, respectively. Control activities of propranolol 4-hydroxylase were 0.17, 0.12, and 0.081 nmol min^{-1} (nmol cytochrome P-450)$^{-1}$ for samples 31, 32, and 34, respectively (49).

titer is high (with regard to inhibition) or if the catalytic assay is so sensitive that little antibody is needed for inhibition, such crude materials may be used.

In general, little can be said about inhibition that is less than about 15% of the total unless enough careful replicates are done and the difference between immune and nonimmune serum incubates is reproducible, concentration-dependent, and statistically significant. To the first approximation the percentage of inhibition is a reflection of the fraction of the total catalytic activity in the preparation due to the protein that reacts with the antibody. The antibody should completely inhibit the purified enzyme itself, however, for this analysis to be valid, as the possibility exists that non-inhibitory antibodies may hinder the binding of inhibitory antibodies, and total inhibition may never be achieved.

Quantitation of Proteins by Immunoblotting

In many cases the absolute concentration of a particular protein in a sample is derived, apart from its catalytic activity. The most direct way to obtain such measurements is with the use of specific antibodies. A variety of immunochemical techniques are available for use, including various types of radioimmune assays (RIAs) and enzyme-linked immune absorbent assays (ELISAs) (217). However, knowledge concerning the specificity of the antigen–antibody reaction must be available. Probably the single most reliable technique for evaluating specificity is coupled SDS–polyacrylamide gel electrophoresis/immunoperoxidase staining, or immuno-

blotting (which also goes by the trivial term "Western blotting"), where a crude mixture of protein is separated by electrophoresis and the resolved proteins are transferred to a thin sheet of nitrocellulose paper where they can be detected after binding antibodies and antibodies coupled to enzymes with chromogenic substrates (Fig. 18). In our early studies with this system, we found that the intensity of the staining of protein bands was proportional to the amount of antigen electrophoresed, and that such a procedure could be utilized for making quantitative measurements (Fig. 19). We still continue to use such a system to quantify many proteins for several reasons. Under appropriate conditions the method is accurate and relatively sensitive. It provides a check on the specificity of antigen–antibody interaction in each individual antigen sample and provides data even when cross-reactive materials are present (if they can be resolved in a single electrophoretic dimension). The method is relatively rapid and straightforward; and even when new systems are explored, little optimization is required.

Samples of roughly 5 μg of microsomal or cellular homogenate protein are solubilized by heating with SDS and β-mercaptoethanol. The samples are electrophoresed in a typical system based on the procedure of Laemmli (160): A slab gel is used with up to 25 samples. Five or six lanes are used to prepare a standard curve for each gel; the lanes contain, for example, 0.5, 1, 2, 3, 5, and 10 pmol of the purified antigen. Crude protein samples to be analyzed are loaded into the wells for the other lanes. Typically, 1 to 20 μg of microsomal protein might be loaded per well for analysis of cytochromes P-450. Protein samples are dissolved in a mix-

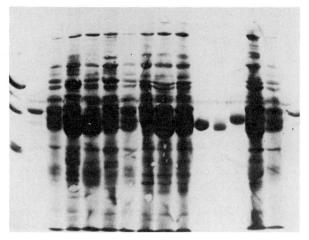

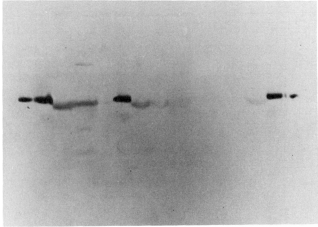

1 2 3 4 5 6 7 8 9 10 11 12 13 14 15 16

A

B

C

FIG. 18. Electrophoresis and immunoelectrophoresis of liver microsomes and purified microsomal proteins (38). In all parts of the figure (**A–C**), the individual wells contained the same samples. Electrophoresis was carried out according to the method of Laemmli (160), with the anode at the bottom of the gel. *Lanes 1,17:* M_r standards (M_r STDS): 1.0 μg each of bovine serum albumin (accepted M_r 68,000), *Escherichia coli* L-glutamate dehydrogenase (M_r 53,000), and rabbit muscle aldolase (M_r 40,000). *Lanes 2,16:* 0.5 μg of purified hog liver microsomal flavin-containing monooxygenase (ENZ). *Lanes 3,7,15:* 10 μg of porcine liver microsomal protein (μS). *Lane 4:* 20 μg of rabbit liver microsomal protein. *Lane 5:* 20 μg of dog liver microsomal protein. *Lane 6:* 20 μg of human liver microsomal protein (sample HL 22). *Lane 8:* 20 μg of microsomal protein prepared from untreated rats. *Lane 9:* 20 μg of liver microsomal protein prepared from phenobarbital (PB)-treated rats. *Lane 10:* 20 μg of liver microsomal protein prepared from β-naphthoflavone (BNF)-treated rats. *Lane 11:* 0.5 μg of purified rat liver microsomal epoxide hydrolase (EH). *Lane 12:* 0.5 μg of purified rat liver microsomal cytochrome P-450$_{(PB-B_2)}$. *Lane 13:* 0.5 μg of purified rat liver microsomal cytochrome P-450$_{(BNF-B_2)}$. *Lane 14:* 20 μg of mouse liver microsomal protein. Unless noted otherwise, all microsomes were prepared from untreated male animals (human microsomes were from a female patient). **A:** The gel was stained for protein using Coomassie brilliant blue R-250. **B:** Proteins were transferred from the gel to a sheet of nitrocellulose, and the sheet was stained for flavin-containing monooxygenase in the described manner (38). The rabbit anti-hog liver flavin-containing monooxygenase antiserum was diluted 1:100. **C:** Proteins were transferred from the gel to a sheet of nitrocellulose, and the sheet was treated with a mixture of rabbit antiserum prepared to hog liver flavin-containing monooxygenase (diluted 1:100), rat liver cytochrome P-450$_{PB-B}$ (diluted 1:100), rat liver cytochrome P-450$_{BNF-B}$ (diluted 1:100), and rat liver epoxide hydrolase (diluted 1:100) prior to treatment with goat anti-rabbit IgG, peroxidase–rabbit antiperoxidase complex, and 3,3'-diaminobenzidine/H_2O_2 in the usual manner (103). In **B** and **C** protein concentrations were similar to those used for Coomassie blue staining (**A**) except that 0.2 μg of purified porcine liver microsomal flavin-containing monooxygenase was used.

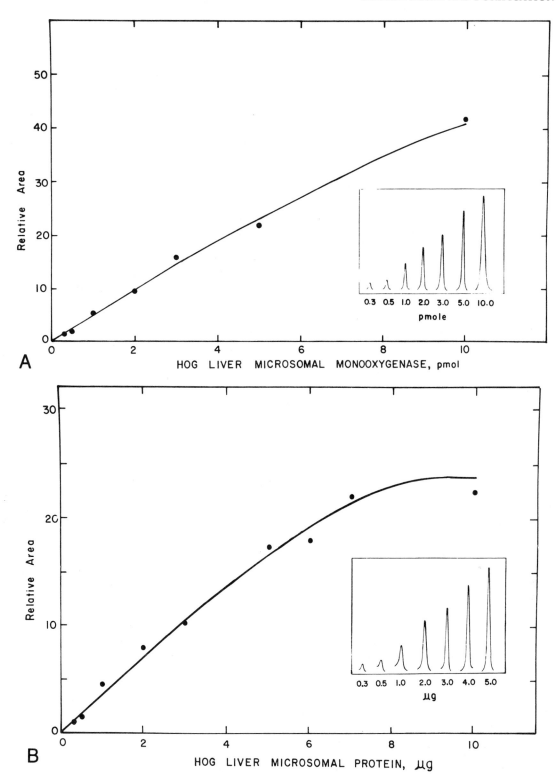

FIG. 19. Immunoelectrophoresis and densitometry of flavin-containing monooxygenase in purified samples and porcine liver microsomes (38). **A:** Area under the densitometric peak as a function of the amount of purified porcine liver flavin-containing monooxygenase electrophoresed. **Inset:** Actual densitometric traces. **B:** Area under the densitometric peak as a function of the amount of porcine liver microsomal protein electrophoresed. **Inset:** Actual densitometric traces.

ture of 63 mM Tris-HCl buffer (pH 6.8) containing 10% glycerol (v/v), 1.0% (w/v) SDS, 0.001% (w/v) pyronin Y, and 5% (v/v) 2-mercaptoethanol; they are then heated for 60 sec at 95°C. Aliquots are loaded into the wells of a 1.5 mm × 16 cm × 20 cm gel (Protean II, Hoefer, San Francisco, California). The separating gel is poured from a mixture of 0.375 M Tris-HCl buffer (pH 8.8) containing 7.5% (w/v) acrylamide, 0.03% (v/v) tetramethyl ethylenediamine (TEMED), 0.1% (w/v) SDS, and 0.0425% (w/v) ammonium persulfate; the stacking gel, in which the wells are formed, is poured from a mixture of 0.14 M Tris-HCl buffer (pH 6.8) containing 3.5% (w/v) acrylamide, 0.057% (v/v) TEMED, 0.65% (w/v) sucrose, 0.11% (w/v) SDS, and 0.045% (w/v) ammonium persulfate. The electrode buffer (pH 8.3) contains 190 mM glycine, 25 mM Tris, and 0.1% SDS. Power is applied to the system at a constant current setting of 24 mA per gel to move the samples through the separating gel. Cooling the system is usually not necessary. The electrophoresis takes about 4 hr. When the pink dye front has moved to within about 1 cm of the edge of the gel, the power is turned off, and the system is separated. One of the glass plates on the gel is removed, and water is sprinkled on the surface. A wetted piece of nitrocellulose paper (0.45 µm; Scheicher and Schull, Keene, New Hampshire) is laid over the wet gel. Care is taken (and enough water used) to avoid trapping air bubbles. Two sheets of Whatman No. 3 paper, prewetted with water, are laid over the nitrocellulose. The glass plate is removed from the other side of the gel and replaced by a wet sheet of Whatman No. 3 paper. The entire "sandwich" is placed between two wet sponges and then enclosed between the two electrode baffles of a Hoefer electrotransfer apparatus with the nitrocellulose closer to the anode than the cathode. The apparatus, with the gel and nitrocellulose between the baffles, is filled with 0.025 M Tris-HCl buffer (pH 8.2) containing 0.192 M glycine and 20% CH_3OH (v/v). Constant current (400 mA for 1 hr or 200 mA for 2 hr) is applied to the system. If a commercial electroblotting apparatus is not available, household sponges ("Brillo," Purex Corp., Lakewood, California) and a pair of stainless steel plates (attached to electrodes) can be substituted, with the device held by rubber bands and immersed in a beaker. Satisfactory results can be obtained (103,265), although the cathode plate tends to pit and corrode, especially if not washed thoroughly.

After the blotting operation, the polyacrylamide gel and the filter papers are discarded, and the nitrocellulose sheet is placed in 25 ml of a solution of phosphate-buffered saline [PBS: 10 mM potassium phosphate buffer (pH 7.4) containing 0.9% NaCl] containing 10% calf serum and 3% (w/v) bovine serum albumin (BSA). The sheet is conveniently placed in a plastic box of only slightly larger dimensions (13 × 18 × 3 cm) with a lid. The gel is shaken in a 37°C waterbath for 30 min to block reactive sites on the nitrocellulose sheet with serum proteins so that antibodies will not be bound in subsequent steps. After the blocking step, the nitrocellulose sheet is washed twice with 60 ml of PBS at room temperature. In practice, the box is rocked on a platform rocker (Bellco Glass, Inc., Vineland, New Jersey) for 5 min, the buffer is decanted, and 60 ml of fresh PBS is added each time.

In the next step, 25 ml of PBS containing 10% calf serum, 3% BSA, and an appropriate dilution of the antiserum of choice is poured into the box over the nitrocellulose sheet. The system is shaken (or rocked) at 37°C for 30 min and then overnight at 4°C; alternatively, 37°C for 2 hr is usually satisfactory. Typical antisera dilutions range from 1:25 to 1:500 (some monoclonal antibodies have been successfully used at 10^{-6} dilutions of ascites fluid). Then the nitrocellulose sheet is washed six times (5 min each at room temperature) with 60 ml of PBS. The next addition is 25 ml of PBS containing 10% calf serum, 3% BSA, and 0.2% (v/v) goat anti-rabbit IgG antiserum (if the primary antiserum was made in rabbits) (Research Biogenics, Inc., Bastrop, Texas). This solution is rocked or shaken with the nitrocellulose sheet at room temperature for 30 min, and the sheet is then washed again six times with PBS as before. The next addition to the sheet is 25 ml of a solution of PBS containing 10% (v/v) calf serum, 3% (w/v) BSA, and 0.2% (v/v) horseradish peroxidase–rabbit anti-horseradish peroxidase complex (Miles Laboratories, Elkhart, Indiana). The sheet is rocked in this solution at room temperature for 30 min and washed six times with PBS as before.

Development of the stain is done in the following manner. 4-Chloro-1-naphthol (32 mg) is dissolved in 12 ml of CH_3OH and diluted with 60 ml of PBS. A 30% H_2O_2 solution (120 µl) is added, and the solution is poured over the nitrocellulose sheet; bands usually appear within a few minutes. The solution is removed; the nitrocellulose sheet is washed three times with PBS and twice with H_2O. Sheets can be dried between two layers of Whatman No. 3 filter paper, with a uniform weight applied.

When the gel is dry (within 1–2 hr), the bands can be scanned using a densitometer. In our own laboratory we use a Kontes Fiber-optic instrument in the reflectance mode, and the signal output (1 volt) is entered into a recording integrator (Hewlett Packard 3320A). The integrals are used to construct standard curves and estimate the amount of antigen in each sample.

In practice, a standard curve is constructed on each nitrocellulose sheet. An additional way to reduce error is to include an internal standard in each protein sample. We have used equine alcohol liver dehydrogenase for this purpose, adding 0.2 µg to each sample prior to electrophoresis. The buffer containing the primary antiserum is fortified with a 1:500 dilution of rabbit antiserum raised against equine alcohol dehydrogenase. When the nitrocellulose sheets are visualized, the cytochrome P-450 band in the 50,000 to 60,000 region is accompanied by a second band migrating with an apparent molecular weight of 43,000. The integrals of both bands are obtained from the densitometer. The ratio of the areas of the two bands can be compared to the ratios found with the standard antigen samples.

Even if the antigen–antibody system is not specific enough to visualize only a single electrophoretic band, useful information can be obtained if the antigens are electrophoretically separable. For instance, rat P-450$_{\beta NF-B}$ and P-450$_{ISF-G}$ cross-react but can be separated and quantified (39,98). The same situation exists with human P-450$_{MP-1}$ and P-450$_{MP-2}$ (242).

Since the original immunoblotting work was done (265), a number of variations of the procedure have been reported, many of which are cited in reviews (65,264). For instance, different additives can be used in the buffers for blocking the sheets. Nylon membranes, e.g., Zeta-Probe (Bio-Rad, Richmond, California), have increased capacity and can be used to increase the sensitivity of the methods. *Staphylococcus aureus* protein A conjugates can be bound to the primary antibody. Other enzymes, e.g., alkaline phosphate, can replace peroxidase; alternatively, ^{125}I-labeled antibodies can be used with autoradiography, as described in the original Towbin et al. paper (265). If monoclonal antibodies are used, the methods must be adapted by including a step with rabbit anti-mouse IgG (215,216) or an equivalent procedure; many monoclonal antibodies give poor responses in this system because the individual epitopes do not have sufficient affinity constants.

In our laboratory we have now applied this approach to rat and human microsomal epoxide hydrolase, rat NADPH-cytochrome P-450 reductase, ten forms of rat cytochrome P-450, two forms of rabbit cytochrome P-450, five forms of human cytochrome P-450, and flavin-containing monooxygenase. The method can be utilized with cells (248) or tissue homogenates (38) as well as with subcellular organelles.

REFERENCES

1. Adams, J. B., and Poulos, A. (1967): Enzymatic synthesis of steroid sulfates. III. Isolation and properties of estrogen sulphotransferase from bovine adrenal gland. *Biochim. Biophys. Acta,* 146:493–508.
2. Adesnik, M., and Atchison, M. (1986): Genes for cytochrome P-450 and their regulation. *CRC Crit. Rev. Biochem.,* 19:247–306.
3. Allaben, W. T., and King, C. M. (1984): The purification of rat liver arylhydroxamic acid N,O-acyltransferase. *J. Biol. Chem.,* 259:12128–12134.
4. Ansler, S. S., and Jakoby, W. B. (1986): Amine N-methyltransferases from rabbit liver. *J. Biol. Chem.,* 261:3996–4001.
5. Axelrod, J. (1962): Catechol-O-methyltransferase from rat liver. *Methods Enzymol.,* 5:748–751.
6. Ayesh, R., Idle, J. R., Ritchie, J. C., Crothers, M. J., and Hetzel, M. R. (1984): Metabolic oxidation phenotypes as markers for susceptibility to lung cancer. *Nature,* 312:169–170.
7. Baron, J., Kawabata, T. T., Redick, J. A., Knapp, S. A., Wick, D. G., Wallace, R. B., Jakoby, W. B., and Guengerich, F. P. (1983): Localization of carcinogen-metabolizing enzymes in human and animal tissue. In: *Extrahepatic Drug Metabolism and Chemical Carcinogenesis,* edited by J. Rydström, J. Montelias, and M. Bengtsson, pp. 73–88. Elsevier, New York.
8. Bentley, P., and Oesch, F. (1975): Purification of rat liver epoxide hydratase to apparent homogeneity. *Fed. Eur. Biol. Soc. Lett.,* 59:291–295.
9. Bentley, P., Schmassmann, H., Sims, P., and Oesch, F. (1976): Epoxides derived from various polycyclic hydrocarbons as substrates of homogeneous and microsome-bound epoxide hydratase. *Eur. J. Biochem.,* 69:97–103.
10. Bernhardsson, C., Björkhem, I., Danielsson, H., and Wikvall, K. (1973): 12α-Hydroxylation of 7α-hydroxy-4-cholesten-3-one by a reconstituted system from rat liver microsomes. *Biochem. Biophys. Res. Commun.,* 54:1030–1038.
11. Björkhem, I., Danielsson, H., and Wikvall, K. (1974): Hydroxylations of bile acids by reconstituted systems from rat liver microsomes. *J. Biol. Chem.,* 249:6439–6445.
12. Björkhem, I., Danielsson, H., and Wikvall, K. (1974): 7α-Hydroxylation of cholesterol by reconstituted systems from rat liver microsomes. *Biochem. Biophys. Res. Commun.,* 61:934–941.
13. Black, S. D., and Coon, M. J. (1986): Comparative structures of P-450 cytochromes. In: *Cytochrome P-450: Structure, Mechanism, and Biochemistry,* edited by P. R. Ortiz de Montellano, pp. 161–216. Plenum Press, New York.
14. Bligh, E. G., and Dyer, W. J. (1959): A rapid method of total lipid extraction and purification. *Can. J. Biochem. Physiol.,* 37:911–917.
15. Bock, K. W., Burchell, B., Dutton, G. J., Hänninen, O., Mulder, G. J., Owens, I. S., Siest, G., and Tephley, T. R. (1983): UDP-glucuronyl transferase activities: guidelines for consistent interim terminology and assay conditions. *Biochem. Pharmacol.,* 32:953–955.
16. Bolt, H. M. (1979): Metabolism of estrogens—natural and synthetic. *Pharmacol. Ther.,* 4:155–181.
17. Booth, J., and Boyland, E. (1964): The biochemistry of aromatic amines. 10. Enzymic N-hydroxylation of arylamines and conversion of arylhydroxylamines into o-aminophenols. *Biochem. J.,* 91:362–369.
18. Borchardt, R. (1980): N- and O-methylation. In: *Enzymatic Basis of Detoxication,* Vol. 2, edited by W. B. Jakoby, pp. 43–62. Academic Press, New York.
19. Bosron, W. F., Magnes, L. J., and Li, T-K. (1983): Kinetic and electrophoretic properties of native and recombined isoenzymes of human liver alcohol dehydrogenase. *Biochemistry,* 22:1852–1857.
20. Bradford, M. M. (1976): A rapid and sensitive method for the quantitation of microgram quantities of protein utilizing the principle of protein-dye binding. *Anal. Biochem.,* 72:248–254.
21. Bulleid, N. J., Graham, A. B., and Craft, J. A. (1986): Microsomal epoxide hydrolase of rat liver: purification and characterization of enzyme fractions with different chromatographic characteristics. *Biochem. J.,* 233:607–611.
22. Burka, L. T., Guengerich, F. P., Willard, R. J., and MacDonald, T. L. (1985): Mechanism of cytochrome P-450 catalysis: mechanism of N-dealkylation and amine oxide deoxygenation. *J. Am. Chem. Soc.,* 107:2549–2551.
23. Burke, M. D., and Mayer, R. T. (1975): Inherent specificities of purified cytochromes P-450 and P-448 toward biphenyl hydroxylation and ethoxyresorufin deethylation. *Drug Metab. Dispos.,* 3:245–253.
24. Burke, M. D., and Prough, R. A. (1978): Fluorimetric and chromatographic methods for measuring microsomal biphenyl hydroxylation. *Methods Enzymol.,* 52:399–407.
25. Burton, K. (1956): A study of the conditions and mechanisms of the diphenylamine reaction for the colorimetric estimation of deoxyribonucleic acid. *Biochem. J.,* 62:315–323.
26. Cerasone, C. F., Bolognesi, C., and Santi, L. (1979): Improved microfluorometric DNA determinations in biological material using 33258 Hoechst. *Anal. Biochem.,* 100:188–197.
27. Chen, C. B., McCoy, G. D., Hecht, S. S., Hoffman, D., and Wynder, E. L. (1978): High pressure liquid chromatographic assay for alpha hydroxylation of n-nitrosopyrrolidine by isolated rat liver microsomes. *Cancer Res.,* 38:3812–3816.
28. Chen, P. S., Jr., Toribara, T. Y., and Warner, H. (1956): Microdetermination of phosphorus. *Anal. Chem.,* 28:1756–1758.
29. Chin, A. E., and Bosmann, H. B. (1976): Microsome-mediated methylation of DNA by N,N-dimethylnitrosamine in vitro. *Biochem. Pharmacol.,* 25:1921–1926.
30. Churchill, P. F., Churchill, S., Martin, M. V., and Guengerich, F. P. (1987): Characterization of a rat liver cytochrome P-450_{UT-H} cDNA clone and comparison of mRNA levels with catalytic activity. *Mol. Pharmacol.,* 31:152–158.
31. Cinti, D. L., Moldeus, P., and Schenkman, J. B. (1972): Kinetic parameters of drug-metabolizing enzymes in Ca^{+2}-sedimented microsomes from rat liver. *Biochem. Pharmacol.,* 21:3249–3256.
32. Cochin, J., and Axelrod, J. (1959): Biochemical and pharmacological changes in the rat following chronic administration of morphine, nalorphine, and normorphine. *J. Pharmacol. Exp. Ther.,* 125:105–110.
33. Conney, A. H. (1967): Pharmacological implications of microsomal enzyme induction. *Pharmacol. Rev.,* 19:317–366.
34. Conney, A. H. (1971): Environmental factors influencing drug metabolism. In: *Fundamentals of Drug Metabolism and Drug Disposition,* edited by B. N. La Du, H. G. Mandel, and E. L. Way, pp. 253–278. Williams & Wilkins, Baltimore.
35. Conney, A. H., Levin, W., Jacobsson, M., and Kuntzman, R. (1969): Specificity in the regulation of the 6β, 7α, and 16α-hydroxylation of testosterone by rat liver microsomes. In: *Microsomes and Drug Oxidations,* edited by J. R. Gillette, pp. 279–301. Academic Press, New York.
36. Coon, M. J., van der Hoeven, T. A., Dahl, S. B., and Haugen, D. A. (1978): Two forms of liver microsomal cytochrome P-450,

P-450$_{LM-2}$, and P-450$_{LM-4}$ (rabbit liver). *Methods Enzymol.,* 52:109–117.

37. Czygan, P., Greim, H., Garro, A. J., Hutterer, F., Schaffner, F., Popper, H., Rosenthal, O., and Cooper, D. Y. (1973): Microsomal metabolism of dimethylnitrosamine and the cytochrome P-450 dependency of its activation to a mutagen. *Cancer Res.,* 33:2983–2986.

38. Dannan, G. A., and Guengerich, F. P. (1982): Immunochemical comparison and quantitation of microsomal flavin-containing monooxygenases in various hog, mouse, rat, rabbit, dog, and human tissues. *Mol. Pharmacol.,* 22:787–794.

39. Dannan, G. A., Guengerich, F. P., Kaminsky, L. S., and Aust, S. D. (1983): Regulation of cytochrome P-450: immunochemical quantitation of eight isozymes in liver microsomes of rats treated with polybrominated biphenyl congeners. *J. Biol. Chem.,* 258:1282–1288.

40. Dannan, G. A., Porubek, D. J., Nelson, S. D., Waxman, D. J., and Guengerich, F. P. (1986): 17β-Estradiol 2- and 4-hydroxylation catalyzed by rat hepatic cytochrome P-450: roles of individual forms, inductive effects, developmental patterns, and alterations by gonadectomy and hormone replacement. *Endocrinology,* 118:1952–1960.

41. Dannan, G. A., Waxman, D. J., and Guengerich, F. P. (1986): Hormonal regulation of rat liver microsomal enzymes: role of gonadal steroids in programming, maintenance, and suppression of Δ^4-steroid 5α-reductase, flavin-containing monooxygenase and sex-specific cytochromes P-450. *J. Biol. Chem.,* 261:10728–10735.

42. Dansette, P. M., Yagi, H., Jerina, D. M., Daly, J. W., Levin, W., Lu, A. Y. H., Kuntzman, R., and Conney, A. H. (1974): Assay and partial purification of epoxide hydrase from rat liver microsomes. *Arch. Biochem. Biophys.,* 164:511–517.

43. Dean, W. L., and Coon, M. J. (1977): Immunochemical studies on two electrophoretically homogeneous forms of rabbit liver microsomal cytochrome P-450: P-450$_{LM-2}$ and P-450$_{LM-4}$. *J. Biol. Chem.,* 252:3255–3261.

44. Dehnen, W., Tomingas, R., and Roos, J. (1973): A modified method for the assay of benzo(a)pyrene hydroxylase. *Anal. Biochem.,* 53:373–383.

45. De Matteis, F. (1974): Covalent binding of sulfur to microsomes and loss of cytochrome P-450 during the oxidative desulfuration of several chemicals. *Mol. Pharmacol.,* 10:849–854.

46. DePierre, J. W., Johannesen, K. A. M., Moron, M. S., and Seidegard, J. (1978): Radioactive assay of aryl hydrocarbon monooxygenase and epoxide hydrase. *Methods Enzymol.,* 52:412–418.

47. Deutsch, J., Leutz, J. C., Yang, S. K., Gelboin, H. V., Chiang, Y. L., Vatsis, K. P., and Coon, M. J. (1978): Regio- and stereoselectivity of various forms of purified cytochrome P-450 in the metabolism of benzo(a)pyrene and (−)trans-7,8-dihydroxy-7,8-dihydrobenzo(a)pyrene as shown by product formation and binding to DNA. *Proc. Natl. Acad. Sci. USA,* 75:3123–3127.

48. Dische, Z. (1955): Color reactions of nucleic acid components. In: *The Nucleic Acids,* Vol. 1, edited by E. Chargoff and J. N. Davidson, pp. 285–305. Academic Press, New York.

49. Distlerath, L. M., and Guengerich, F. P. (1984): Characterization of a human liver cytochrome P-450 involved in the oxidation of debrisoquine and other drugs by using antibodies raised to the analogous rat enzyme. *Proc. Natl. Acad. Sci. USA,* 81:7348–7352.

50. Distlerath, L. M., and Guengerich, F. P. (1987): Enzymology of human liver cytochromes P-450. In: *Mammalian Cytochromes P-450,* edited by F. P. Guengerich, pp. 133–198. CRC Press, Boca Raton, Florida.

51. Distlerath, L. M., Reilly, P. E. B., Martin, M. V., Davis, G. G., Wilkinson, G. R., and Guengerich, F. P. (1985): Purification and characterization of the human liver cytochromes P-450 involved in debrisoquine 4-hydroxylation and phenacetin O-deethylation, two prototypes for genetic polymorphism in oxidative drug metabolism. *J. Biol. Chem.,* 260:9057–9067.

52. DuBois, G. C., Appella, E., Armstrong, R., Levin, W., Lu, A. Y. H., and Jerina, D. M. (1979): Hepatic microsomal epoxide hydrolase: chemical evidence for a single polypeptide chain. *J. Biol. Chem.,* 254:6240–6243.

53. Duffel, M. W., and Jakoby, W. B. (1982): Cysteine S-conjugate N-acetyl-transferase from rat kidney microsomes. *Mol. Pharmacol.,* 21:444–448.

54. Ernster, L., Davidson, L., and Ljunggren, M. (1962): DT diaphorase. I. Purification from the soluble fraction of rat-liver cytoplasm, and properties. *Biochim. Biophys. Acta,* 58:171–188.

55. Fan, L. L., Masters, B. S. S., and Prough, R. A. (1976): Microsomal lauric acid 11- and 12-hydroxylation: a new assay method utilizing high pressure liquid chromatography. *Anal. Biochem.,* 71:265–272.

56. Fang, W-F., and Strobel, H. W. (1978): The drug and carcinogen metabolism system of rat colon microsomes. *Arch. Biochem. Biophys.,* 186:128–138.

57. Fasco, M. J., Vatsis, K. P., Kaminsky, L. S., and Coon, M. J. (1978): Regioselective and stereoselective hydroxylation of R and S warfarin by different forms of purified cytochrome P-450 from rabbit liver. *J. Biol. Chem.,* 253:7813–7820.

58. Frederick, C. B., Mays, J. B., Ziegler, D. M., Guengerich, F. P., and Kadlubar, F. F. (1982): Cytochrome P-450 and flavin-containing monooxygenase-catalyzed formation of the carcinogen N-hydroxy-2-aminofluorene, and its covalent binding to nuclear DNA. *Cancer Res.,* 42:2671–2677.

59. French, J. S., Guengerich, F. P., and Coon, M. J. (1980): Interactions of cytochrome P-450, NADPH-cytochrome P-450 reductase, phospholipid, and substrate in the reconstituted liver microsomal enzyme system. *J. Biol. Chem.,* 255:4112–4119.

60. Friedberg, T., Milbert, U., Bentley, P., Guenther, T., and Oesch, F. (1983): Purification and characterization of a new cytosolic glutathione S-transferase (glutathione S-transferase X) from rat liver. *Biochem. J.,* 215:617–625.

61. Gandolfi, A. J., and Van Dyke, R. A. (1973): Dechlorination of chloroethane with a reconstituted liver microsomal system. *Biochem. Biophys. Res. Commun.,* 53:687–692.

62. Garewal, H. S. (1973): A procedure for the estimation of microgram quantities of Triton X-100. *Anal. Biochem.,* 54:319–324.

63. Geiger, L. E., Hogy, L. L., and Guengerich, F. P. (1983): Metabolism of acrylonitrile by isolated rat hepatocytes. *Cancer Res.,* 43:3080–3087.

64. Gelboin, H. V. (1967): Carcinogens, enzyme induction and gene action. *Adv. Cancer Res.,* 10:1–81.

65. Gershoni, J. M., and Palade, G. E. (1983): Protein blotting: principles and applications. *Anal. Biochem.,* 131:1–15.

66. Gibson, G. G., and Schenkman, J. B. (1978): Purification and properties of cytochrome P-450 obtained from liver microsomes of untreated rats by lauric acid affinity chromatography. *J. Biol. Chem.,* 253:5957–5963.

67. Gill, T. J., III (1972): The chemistry of antigens and its influence on immunogenicity. In: *Immunogenicity,* edited by F. Borek, pp. 5–44. American Elsevier, New York.

68. Gillette, J. R. (1966): Biochemistry of drug oxidation and reduction by enzymes in hepatic endoplasmic reticulum. *Adv. Pharmacol.,* 4:219–261.

69. Glowinski, I. B., Radtke, H. E., and Weber, W. W. (1978): Genetic variation in N-acetylation of carcinogenic arylamines by human and rat liver. *Mol. Pharmacol.,* 14:940–949.

70. Goldstein, S., and Blecher, M. (1975): The spectrophotometric assay for polyethoxy nonionic detergents in membrane extracts: a critique. *Anal. Biochem.,* 64:130–135.

71. Greenlee, W. F., and Poland, A. (1978): An improved assay of 7-ethoxycoumarin O-deethylase activity: induction of hepatic enzyme activity in C57BL/6J and DBA/2J mice by phenobarbital, 3-methylcholanthrene and 2,3,7,8-tetraclorodibenzo-p-dioxin. *J. Pharmacol. Exp. Ther.,* 205:596–605.

72. Guengerich, F. P. (1977): Preparation and properties of highly-purified cytochrome P-450 and NADPH-cytochrome P-450 reductase from pulmonary microsomes of untreated rabbits. *Mol. Pharmacol.,* 13:911–923.

73. Guengerich, F. P. (1977): Separation and purification of multiple forms of microsomal cytochrome P-450: activities of different forms of cytochrome P-450 towards several compounds of environmental interest. *J. Biol. Chem.,* 252:3970–3979.

74. Guengerich, F. P. (1977): Studies on the activation of a model furan compound: toxicity and covalent binding of 2-(N-ethylcarbamoylhydroxymethyl)-furan. *Biochem. Pharmacol.,* 26:1909–1915.

75. Guengerich, F. P. (1978): Destruction of heme and hemoproteins mediated by liver microsomal reduced nicotinamide adenine dinucleotide phosphate-cytochrome P-450 reductase. *Biochemistry,* 17:3633–3639.

76. Guengerich, F. P. (1978): Separation and purification of multiple forms of microsomal cytochrome P-450: partial characterization of three apparently homogeneous cytochromes P-450 isolated from liver microsomes of phenobarbital- and 3-methylcholanthrene-treated rats. *J. Biol. Chem.*, 253:7931–7939.

77. Guengerich, F. P. (1979): Artifacts in isoelectric focusing of the microsomal enzymes cytochrome P-450 and NADPH-cytochrome P-450 reductase. *Biochim. Biophys. Acta*, 577:132–141.

78. Guengerich, F. P. (1979): Isolation and purification of cytochrome P-450, and the existence of multiple forms. *Pharmacol. Ther.*, 6:99–121.

79. Guengerich, F. P. (1982): Epoxide hydrolase: properties and metabolic roles. *Rev. Biochem. Toxicol.*, 4:5–30.

80. Guengerich, F. P. (1984): Effects of nutritive factors on metabolic processes involving bioactivation and detoxication of chemicals. *Annu. Rev. Nutr.*, 4:207–231.

81. Guengerich, F. P. (1984): Oxidation of sparteines by cytochrome P-450: evidence against the formation of N-oxides. *J. Med. Chem.*, 27:1101–1103.

82. Guengerich, F. P. (1986): Enzymology of rat liver cytochromes P-450. In: *Mammalian Cytochromes P-450*, edited by F. P. Guengerich, pp. 1–54. CRC Press, Boca Raton, Florida.

83. Guengerich, F. P. (1986): Cytochrome P-450 enzymes and drug metabolism. In: *Progress in Drug Metabolism, Volume 10*, edited by J. Bridges, L. F. Chasseaud, and G. G. Gibson, pp. 1–54. Taylor & Francis, London.

84. Guengerich, F. P. (1986): Activation of organic compounds by cytochrome P-450 isozymes. In: *Mechanisms of Cell Injury: Implications for Human Health*, Dahlem Konferenzen, edited by B. Fowler, pp. 7–17. John Wiley & Sons, Chicester, U.K.

85. Guengerich, F. P., and Aust, S. D. (1977): Activation of the parasympathomimetic alkaloid slaframine by microsomal and photochemical oxidation. *Mol. Pharmacol.*, 13:185–195.

86. Guengerich, F. P., and Holladay, L. A. (1979): Hydrodynamic characterization of highly-purified and functionally-active liver microsomal cytochrome P-450. *Biochemistry*, 18:5442–5449.

87. Guengerich, F. P., and Liebler, D. C. (1985): Enzymatic activation of chemicals to toxic metabolites. *CRC Crit. Rev. Toxicol.*, 14:259–307.

88. Guengerich, F. P., and Macdonald, T. L. (1984): Chemical mechanisms of catalysis by cytochromes P-450: a unified view. *Acct. Chem. Res.*, 17:9–16.

89. Guengerich, F. P., and Martin, M. V. (1980): Purification of cytochrome P-450, NADPH-cytochrome P-450 reductase, and epoxide hydratase from a single preparation of rat liver microsomes. *Arch. Biochem. Biophys.*, 205:365–379.

90. Guengerich, F. P., and Mason, P. S. (1980): Alcohol dehydrogenase-coupled spectrophotometric assay of epoxide hydrolase. *Anal. Biochem.*, 104:445–451.

91. Guengerich, F. P., and Mitchell, M. B. (1980): Metabolic activation of model pyrroles by cytochrome P-450. *Drug. Metab. Dispos.*, 8:34–38.

92. Guengerich, F. P., and Strickland, T. W. (1977): Metabolism of vinyl chloride: destruction of the heme of highly purified liver microsomal cytochrome P-450 by a metabolite. *Mol. Pharmacol.*, 13:993–1004.

93. Guengerich, F. P., and Watanabe, P. G. (1979): Metabolism of [^{14}C]- and [^{36}Cl]-labeled vinyl chloride in vivo and in vitro. *Biochem. Pharmacol.*, 28:589–596.

94. Guengerich, F. P., Ballou, D. P., and Coon, M. J. (1975): Purified liver microsomal cytochrome P-450: electron-accepting properties and oxidation-reduction potential. *J. Biol. Chem.*, 250:7405–7414.

95. Deleted.

96. Guengerich, F. P., Crawford, W. M., Jr., and Watanabe, P. G. (1979): Activation of vinyl chloride to covalently-bound metabolites: roles of 2-chloroethylene oxide and 2-chloroacetaldehyde. *Biochemistry*, 18:5177–5182.

97. Guengerich, F. P., Crawford, W. M., Jr., Domoradzki, J. Y., Macdonald, T. L., and Watanabe, P. G. (1980): In vitro activation of 1,2-dichloroethane by microsomal and cytosolic enzymes. *Toxicol. Appl. Pharmacol.*, 55:303–317.

98. Guengerich, F. P., Dannan, G. A., Wright, S. T., Martin, M. V., and Kaminsky, L. S. (1982): Purification and characterization of rat liver microsomal cytochromes P-450: electrophoretic, spectral, catalytic, and immunochemical properties and inducibility of eight isozymes isolated from rats treated with phenobarbital or β-naphthoflavone. *Biochemistry*, 21:6019–6030.

99. Guengerich, F. P., Distlerath, L. M., Reilly, P. E. B., Wolff, T., Shimada, T., Umbenhauer, D. R., and Martin, M. V. (1985): Human liver cytochromes P-450 involved in polymorphism of drug oxidations. *Xenobiotica*, 16:367–378.

100. Guengerich, F. P., Geiger, L. E., Hogy, L. L., and Wright, P. L. (1981): In vitro metabolism of acrylonitrile to 2-cyanoethylene oxide, conjugation with reduced glutathione, and irreversible binding to proteins and nucleic acids. *Cancer Res.*, 41:4925–4933.

101. Guengerich, F. P., Martin, M. V., Beaune, P. H., Kremers, P., Wolff, T., and Waxman, D. J. (1986): Characterization of rat and human liver microsomal cytochrome P-450 forms involved in nifedipine oxidation, a prototype for genetic polymorphism in oxidative drug metabolism. *J. Biol. Chem.*, 261:5051–5060.

102. Guengerich, F. P., Mason, P. S., Stott, W. T., Fox, T. R., and Watanabe, P. G. (1981): Roles of 2-haloethylene oxides and 2-haloacetaldehydes derived from vinyl bromide and vinyl chloride in irreversible binding to protein and DNA. *Cancer Res.*, 41:4391–4398.

103. Guengerich, F. P., Wang, P., and Davidson, N. K. (1982): Estimation of isozymes of microsomal cytochrome P-450 in rats, rabbits, and humans using immunochemical staining coupled with sodium dodecyl sulfate-polyacrylamide gel electrophoresis. *Biochemistry*, 21:1698–1706.

104. Guengerich, F. P., Wang, P., and Mason, P. S. (1981): Immunological comparison of rat, rabbit, and human liver NADPH-cytochrome P-450 reductases. *Biochemistry*, 20:2379–2385.

105. Guengerich, F. P., Wang, P., Mason, P. S., and Mitchell, M. B. (1981): Immunological comparison of rat, rabbit, and human microsomal cytochromes P-450. *Biochemistry*, 20:2370–2378.

106. Guengerich, F. P., Wang, P., Mitchell, M. B., and Mason, P. S. (1979): Rat and human liver microsomal epoxide hydrolase: purification and evidence for the existence of multiple forms. *J. Biol. Chem.*, 254:12248–12254.

107. Gustafsson, J-A., and Ingleman-Sundberg, M. (1976): Multiple forms of cytochrome P-450 in rat liver microsomes: separation and some properties of different hydroxylases active on free and sulphoconjugated steroids. *Eur. J. Biochem.*, 64:35–43.

108. Habig, W. H., Pabst, M. J., and Jakoby, W. B. (1974): Glutathione S-transferases: the first enzymatic step in mercapturic acid formation. *J. Biol. Chem.* 249:7130–7139.

109. Hammock, B. D., Prestwich, G. D., Loury, D. N., Cheung, P. Y. K., Eng, W-S., Park, S-K., Moody, D. E., Silva, M. H., and Wixtrom, R. N. (1986): Comparison of crude and affinity purified cytosolic epoxide hydrolases from hepatic tissue of control and clofibrate-fed mice. *Arch. Biochem. Biophys.*, 244:292–309.

110. Hammons, G. J., Guengerich, F. P., Weis, C. C., Beland, F. A., and Kadlubar, F. F. (1985): Metabolic oxidation of carcinogenic arylamines by rat, dog, and human hepatic microsomes and by flavin-containing and cytochrome P-450 monooxygenases. *Cancer Res.*, 45:3578–3585.

111. Hanzlik, R. P., and Hilbert, J. M. (1978): Synthesis of epoxides with electronegative substituents: photometric substrates for epoxide hydrase. *J. Organic Chem.*, 453:610–614.

112. Harvison, P. J., Guengerich, F. P., Rashed, M. S., and Nelson, S. D. (1988): Cytochrome P-450 isozyme selectivity in the oxidation of acetaminophen. *Chem. Res. Toxicol.*, 1:47–52.

113. Haugen, D. A., and Coon, M. J. (1976): Properties of electrophoretically homogeneous phenobarbital-inducible and β-naphthoflavone-inducible forms of liver microsomal cytochrome P-450. *J. Biol. Chem.*, 251:7929–7939.

114. Haugen, D. A., Armes, L. G., Yasunobu, K. T., and Coon, M. J. (1977): Amino-terminal sequence of phenobarbital-inducible cytochrome P-450 from rabbit liver microsomes: similarity to hydrophobic amino-terminal segments of preproteins. *Biochem. Biophys. Res. Commun.*, 77:967–973.

115. Haugen, D. A., van der Hoeven, T. A., and Coon, M. J. (1975): Purified liver microsomal cytochrome P-450: separation and characterization of multiple forms. *J. Biol. Chem.*, 250:3567–3570.

116. Hayes, J. D., and Clarkson, G. H. D. (1982): Purification and characterization of three forms of glutathione S-transferase A: a comparative study of the major YaYa-, YbYb- and YcYc-containing glutathione S-transferases. *Biochem. J.*, 207:459–470.

117. Heinemann, F. S., and Ozols, J. (1984): The covalent structure of

hepatic microsomal epoxide hydrolase. II. The complete amino acid sequence. *J. Biol. Chem.*, 259:797–804.

118. Hempel, J., Bahr-Lindström, H., and Jörnvall, H. (1984): Aldehyde dehydrogenase from human liver: primary structure of the cytoplasmic isoenzyme. *Eur. J. Biochem.*, 141:21–35.

119. Henze, H. R., and Isbell, A. F. (1954): Researches on substituted 5-phenyl hydantoins. *J. Am. Chem. Soc.*, 76:4152–4156.

120. Hogy, L. L., and Guengerich, F. P. (1986): In vivo interaction of acrylonitrile and 2-cyanoethylene oxide with DNA. *Cancer Res.*, 46:3932–3938.

121. Höjeberg, B., Blomberg, K., Stenberg, S., and Lind, C. (1981): Biospecific adsorption of hepatic DT-diaphorase on immobilized dicoumarol. I. Purification of cytosolic DT-diaphorase from control and 3-methylcholanthrene treated rats. *Arch. Biochem. Biophys.*, 207:205–216.

122. Holder, G., Yagi, H., Dansette, P., Jerina, D. M., Levin, W., Lu, A. Y. H., and Conney, A. H. (1974): Effects of inducers and epoxide hydrolase on the metabolism of benzo(a)pyrene by liver microsomes and a reconstituted system: analysis by high pressure liquid chromatography. *Proc. Natl. Acad. Sci. USA*, 71:4356–4360.

123. Huang, M-T., West, S. B., and Lu, A. Y. H. (1976): Separation, purification, and properties of multiple forms of cytochrome P-450 from the liver microsomes of phenobarbital-treated mice. *J. Biol. Chem.*, 251:4659–4665.

124. Idle, J. R., Mahgoub, A., Sloan, T. P., Smith, R. L., Mbanefo, C. O., and Bababunmi, E. A. (1981): Some observations on the oxidation phenotype status of Nigerian patients presenting with cancer. *Cancer Lett.*, 11:331–338.

125. Ikuta, T., Fujiyoshi, T., Kurachi, K., and Yoshida, A. (1985): Molecular cloning of a full-length cDNA for human alcohol dehydrogenase. *Proc. Natl. Acad. Sci. USA*, 82:2703–2707.

126. Imai, Y. (1976): The use of 8-aminooctyl-Sepharose for the separation of some components of the hepatic microsomal electron transfer system. *J. Biochem. (Tokyo)*, 80:267–276.

127. Imai, Y., and Sato, R. (1974): A gel-electrophoretically homogeneous preparation of cytochrome P-450 from liver microsomes of phenobarbital-pretreated rabbits. *Biochem. Biophys. Res. Commun.*, 60:8–14.

128. Imai, Y., Ito, A., and Sato, T. (1966): Evidence for biochemically different types of vesicles in the hepatic microsomal fraction. *J. Biochem. (Tokyo)*, 60:417–428.

129. Inskeep, P. B., and Guengerich, F. P. (1984): Glutathione-mediated binding of dibromoalkanes to DNA: specificity of rat glutathione S-transferases and dibromoalkane structure. *Carcinogenesis*, 5:805–808.

130. Inskeep, P. B., Koga, N., Cmarik, J. L., and Guengerich, F. P. (1986): Covalent binding of 1,2-dihaloalkanes to DNA and stability of the major DNA adduct, S-[2-(N⁷-guanyl)ethyl]glutathione. *Cancer Res.*, 46:2839–2844.

131. Irving, C. C., and Veazy, R. A. (1968): Isolation of deoxyribonucleic acid and ribosomal ribonucleic acid from rat liver. *Biochim. Biophys. Acta*, 166:246–248.

132. Jakoby, W. B., and Habig, W. H. (1980): Glutathione transferases. In: *Enzymatic Basis of Detoxication*, Vol. 2, edited by W. B. Jakoby, pp. 63–94. Academic Press, New York.

133. Jakoby, W. B., Ketterer, B., and Mannervik, B. (1984): Glutathione transferases: nomenclature. *Biochem. Pharmacol.*, 33:2539–2540.

134. Jakoby, W. B., Sekura, R. D., Lyon, E. S., Marcus, C. J., and Wang, J-L. (1980): Sulfotransferases. In: *Enzymatic Basis of Detoxication*, Vol. 2, edited by W. B. Jakoby, pp. 199–228. Academic Press, New York.

135. Jenne, J. W., and Boyer, P. D. (1962): Kinetic characteristics of the acetylation of isoniazid and p-aminosalicylic acid by a liver enzyme preparation. *Biochim. Biophys. Acta*, 65:121–127.

136. Jerina, D. M., Dansette, P. M., Lu, A. Y. H., and Levin, W. (1977): Hepatic microsomal epoxide hydrase: a sensitive radiometric assay for hydration of arene oxides of carcinogenic aromatic hydrocarbons. *Mol. Pharmacol.*, 13:342–351.

137. Jernström, B., Capdevila, J., Jakobsson, S., and Orrenius, S. (1975): Solubilization and partial purification of cytochrome P-450 from rat lung microsomes. *Biochem. Biophys. Res. Commun.*, 64:814–822.

138. Johannesen, K. A. M., and De Pierre, J. W. (1978): Measurements of cytochrome P-450 in the presence of large amounts of contam-

inating hemoglobin and methemoglobin. *Anal. Biochem.*, 86:725–732.

139. Johnson, E. F., and Muller-Eberhard, U. (1977): Multiple forms of cytochrome P-450: resolution and purification of rabbit liver aryl hydrocarbon hydroxylase. *Biochem. Biophys. Res. Commun.*, 76:644–651.

140. Johnson, E. F., and Muller-Eberhard, U. (1977): Purification of the major cytochrome P-450 of liver microsomes from rabbits treated with 2,3,7,8-tetrachlorodibenzo-p-dixoin (TCDD). *Biochem. Biophys. Res. Commun.*, 76:652–659.

141. Johnson, E. F., and Muller-Eberhard, U. (1977): Resolution of two forms of cytochrome P-450 from liver microsomes of rabbits treated with 2,3,7,8-tetrachlorodibenzo-p-dioxin. *J. Biol. Chem.*, 252:2839–2845.

142. Jones, P. B. C., Galeazzi, D. R., Fisher, J. M., and Whitlock, J. P., Jr. (1985): Control of cytochrome P₁-450 gene expression by dioxin. *Science*, 227:1499–1502.

143. Jörnvall, H., Hempel, J., Vallee, B. L., Bosron, W. F., and Li, T-K. (1984): Human liver alcohol dehydrogenase: amino acid substitution in the β₂β₂ oriental isozyme explains functional properties, establishes an active site structure, and parallels mutational exchanges in the yeast enzyme. *Proc. Natl. Acad. Sci. USA*, 81:3024–3028.

144. Kadlubar, F. F., Miller, J. A., and Miller, E. C. (1976): Microsomal N-oxidation of the hepatocarcinogen N-methyl-4-aminoazobenzene and the reactivity of N-hydroxy-N-methyl-4-aminoazobenzene. *Cancer Res.*, 36:1196–1206.

145. Kamataki, T., Belcher, D. H., and Neal, R. A. (1976): Studies of the metabolism of diethyl p-nitrophenyl phosphorothionate (parathion) and benzphetamine using an apparently homogeneous preparation of rat liver cytochrome P-450: effect of a cytochrome P-450 antibody preparation. *Mol. Pharmacol.*, 12:921–932.

146. Kamataki, T., Lee-Lin, M. C. M., Belcher, D. H., and Neal, R. A. (1976): Studies of the metabolism of parathion with an apparently homogeneous preparation of rabbit liver cytochrome P-450. *Drug Metab. Dispos.*, 4:180–189.

147. Kaminsky, L. S., Fasco, M. J., and Guengerich, F. P. (1979): Comparison of different forms of liver, kidney, and lung microsomal cytochrome P-450 by immunological inhibition of regio- and stereoselective metabolism of warfarin. *J. Biol. Chem.*, 254:9657–9662

148. Kaminsky, L. S., Fasco, M. J., and Guengerich, F. P. (1980): Comparison of different forms of purified cytochrome P-450 from rat liver by immunological inhibition of regio- and stereoselective metabolism of warfarin. *J. Biol. Chem.*, 255:85–91.

149. Kaminsky, L. S., Fasco, M. J., and Guengerich, F. P. (1981): Production and application of antibodies to rat liver cytochrome P-450. *Methods Enzymol.*, 74:262–272.

150. Kaschnitz, R. M., and Coon, M. J. (1975): Drug and fatty acid hydroxylation by solubilized human liver microsomal cytochrome P-450:phospholipid requirement. *Biochem. Pharmacol.*, 24:295–297.

151. Kasper, C. B., and Henton, D. (1980): Glucuronidation. In: *Enzymatic Basis of Detoxication*, Vol. 2, edited by W. B. Jakoby, pp. 3–36. Academic Press, New York.

152. Kawalek, J. C., Levin, W., Ryan, D., Thomas, P. E., and Lu, A. Y. H. (1975): Purification of liver microsomal cytochrome P-448 from 3-methylcholanthrene-treated rabbits. *Mol. Pharmacol.*, 11:874–878.

153. Kimura, T., Kodama, M., and Nagata, C. (1983): Purification of mixed-function amine oxidase from rat liver microsomes. *Biochem. Biophys. Res. Commun.*, 110:640–645.

154. Knapp, J. A., Dignam, J. D., and Strobel, H. W. (1977): NADPH-cytochrome P-450 reductase: circular dichroism and physical studies. *J. Biol. Chem.*, 252:437–443.

155. Knowles, R. G., and Burchell, B. (1977): A simple method for purification of epoxide hydratase from rat liver. *Biochem. J.*, 163:381–383.

156. Koga, N., Inskeep, P. B., Harris, T. M., and Guengerich, F. P. (1986): S-[2-(N⁷-Guanyl)ethyl]glutathione, the major DNA adduct formed from 1,2-dibromoethane. *Biochemistry*, 25:2192–2198.

157. Krisch, K., and Staudinger, H. J. (1961): Untersuchungen zur enzymatischen Hydroxylierung: Hydroxylierung von Acetanilid und

deren Beziehungen zur mikrosomalen Pyridinnucleotidoxydation. *Biochem. Z.*, 334:312–327.

158. Kuntzman, R., Tasi, I., and Burns, J. J. (1967): Importance of tissue and plasma binding in determining the retention of norchlorcyclizine and norcyclizidine in man, dog and rat. *J. Pharmacol. Exp. Ther.*, 158:332–339.

159. Küpfer, A., James, R., Carr, K., and Branch, R. (1982): Analysis of hydroxylated and demethylated metabolites of mephenytoin in man and laboratory animals using gas-liquid chromatography and high performance liquid chromatography. *J. Chromatogr.*, 232: 93–100.

160. Laemmli, U. K. (1970): Cleavage of structural proteins during the assembly of the head of bacteriophage T$_4$. *Nature*, 227:680–685.

161. Layne, E. (1957): Spectrophotometric and turbidimetric methods for measuring proteins. *Methods Enzymol.*, 3:447–454.

162. Lee, C-Y., Johnson, L., Cox, R. H., McKinney, J. D., and Lee, S-M. (1981): Mouse liver glutathione S-transferases: biochemical and immunological characterization. *J. Biol. Chem.*, 256:8110–8116.

163. Leonard, N. J., Thomas, P. D., and Gash, V. W. (1955): Unsaturated amines. IV. Structures and reactions of the dehydrosparteines and their salts. *J. Am. Chem. Soc.*, 77:1552–1558.

164. Levin, W., Michaud, D. P., Thomas, P. E., and Jerina, D. M. (1983): Distinct rat hepatic microsomal epoxide hydrolases catalyze the hydration of cholesterol 5,6α-oxide and certain xenobiotic alkene and arene oxides. *Arch. Biochem. Biophys.*, 220:485–494.

165. Levin, W., Ryan, D., West, S., and Lu, A. Y. H. (1974): Preparation of partially purified, lipid-depleted cytochrome P-450 and reduced nicotinamide adenine dinucleotide phosphate-cytochrome c reductase from rat liver microsomes. *J. Biol. Chem.*, 249:1747–1754.

166. Licht, H. J., and Cosica, C. J. (1978): Cytochrome P-450 LM$_2$ mediated hydroxylation of monoterpene alcohols. *Biochemistry*, 17:5638–5646.

167. Liebler, D. C., and Guengerich, F. P. (1983): Olefin oxidation by cytochrome P-450: evidence for group migration in catalytic intermediates formed with vinylidene chloride and trans-1-phenyl-1-butene. *Biochemistry*, 22:5482–5489.

168. Lindahl, R., and Evces, S. (1984): Rat liver aldehyde dehydrogenase. II. Isolation and characterization of four inducible isozymes. *J. Biol. Chem.*, 259:11991–11996.

169. Lotlikar, P. D., Baldy, W. J., Nyce, J., and Dwyer, E. N. (1976): Phospholipid requirement for dimethylnitrosamine demethylation by hamster hepatic microsomal cytochrome P-450 enzyme system. *Biochem. J.*, 160:401–404.

170. Lowry, O. H., Rosebrough, N. J., Farr, A. L., and Randall, R. J. (1951): Protein measurement with the Folin phenol reagent. *J. Biol. Chem.*, 193:265–275.

171. Lu, A. Y. H., and Coon, M. J. (1968): Role of hemoprotein P-450 in fatty acid ω-hydroxylation in a soluble enzyme system from liver microsomes. *J. Biol. Chem.*, 243:1331–1332.

172. Lu, A. Y. H., and Levin, W. (1974): The resolution and reconstitution of the liver microsomal hydroxylation system. *Biochim. Biophys. Acta*, 344:205–240.

173. Lu, A. Y. H., and Levin, W. (1978): Purification and assay of liver microsomal epoxide hydrase. *Methods Enzymol.*, 52:193–200.

174. Lu, A. Y. H., and West, S. B. (1978): Reconstituted mammalian mixed-function oxidases: requirements, specificities, and other properties. *Pharmacol. Ther.*, 2:337–358.

175. Lu, A. Y. H., Jacobson, M., Levin, W., West, S. B., and Kuntzman, R. (1972): Reconstituted liver microsomal enzyme system that hydroxylates drugs, other foreign compounds and endogenous substrates. IV. Hydroxylation of aniline. *Arch. Biochem. Biophys.*, 153: 294–297.

176. Lu, A. Y. H., Jerina, D. M., and Levin, W. (1977): Liver microsomal epoxide hydrase: hydration of alkene and arene oxides by membrane-bound and purified enzymes. *J. Biol. Chem.*, 252:3715–3723.

177. Lu, A. Y. H., Junk, K. W., and Coon, M. J. (1969): Resolution of the cytochrome P-450-containing ω-hydroxylation system of liver microsomes into three components. *J. Biol. Chem.*, 244:3714–3721.

178. Lu, A. Y. H., Levin, W., and Kuntzman, R. (1974): Reconstituted liver microsomal enzyme system that hydroxylates drugs, other foreign compounds and endogenous substrates. *Biochem. Biophys. Res. Commun.*, 60:266–272.

179. Lu, A. Y. H., Ryan, D., Jerina, D. M., Daly, J. W., and Levin, W.

(1975): Liver microsomal epoxide hydrase: solubilization, purification, and characterization. *J. Biol. Chem.*, 250:8283–8288.

180. Lu, A. Y. H., Strobel, H. W., and Coon, M. J. (1969): Hydroxylation of benzphetamine and other drugs by a solubilized form of cytochrome P-450 from liver microsomes: lipid requirement for drug demethylation. *Biochem. Biophys. Res. Commun.*, 36:545–551.

181. Lu, A. Y. H., Strobel, H. W., and Coon, M. J. (1970): Properties of a solubilized form of the cytochrome P-450-containing mixed-function oxidase of liver microsomes. *Mol. Pharmacol.*, 6:213–220.

182. Lubet, R. A., Mayer, R. T., Cameron, J. W., Nims, R. W., Burke, M. D., Wolff, T., and Guengerich, F. P. (1985): Dealkylation of pentoxyresorufin: a rapid and sensitive assay for measuring induction of cytochrome(s) P-450 by phenobarbital and other xenobiotics in the rat. *Arch. Biochem. Biophys.*, 238:43–48.

183. Lyman, S. D., Poland, A., and Taylor, B. A. (1980): Genetic polymorphism of microsomal epoxide hydrolase activity in the mouse. *J. Biol. Chem.*, 255:8650–8654.

184. Maines, M. D., Ibrahim, N. G., and Kappas, A. (1977): Solubilization and partial purification of heme oxygenase from rat liver. *J. Biol. Chem.*, 252:5900–5903.

185. Maines, M. D., Trakshel, G. M., and Kutty, R. K. (1986): Characterization of two constitutive forms of rat liver microsomal heme oxygenase: only one molecular species of the enzyme is inducible. *J. Biol. Chem.*, 261:411–419.

186. Malaveille, C., Bartsch, H., Barbin, A., Camus, A. M., Montesano, R., Croisy, A., and Jacquignon, P. (1975): Mutagenicity of vinyl chloride, chloroethylene oxide, chloroacetaldehyde, and chloroethanol. *Biochem. Biophys. Res. Commun.*, 63:363–370.

187. Mannervik, V., Alin, P., Guthenberg, C., Jenson, H., Tahir, M. K., Warholm, M., and Jörnvall, H. (1985): Identification of three classes of cytosolic glutathione transferase common to several mammalian species: correlation between structural data and enzymatic properties. *Proc. Natl. Acad. Sci. USA*, 82:7202–7206.

188. Masters, B. S. S., Baron, J., Taylor, W. E., Isaacson, E. L., and LoSpalluto, J. (1971): Immunochemical studies on electron transport chains involving cytochrome P-450. I. Effects of antibodies to pig liver microsomal reduced triphosphopyridine nucleotide-cytochrome c reductase and nonheme iron protein from bovine adrenocortical mitochondria. *J. Biol. Chem.*, 246:4143–4150.

189. Matsubara, T., Koike, M., Touchi, A., Tochino, Y., and Sugeno, K. (1976): Quantitative determination of cytochrome P-450 in rat liver homogenate. *Anal. Biochem.*, 75:596–603.

190. Maynert, E. W., Foreman, R. L., and Watabe, T. (1970): Epoxides as obligatory intermediates in the metabolism of olefins to glycols. *J. Biol. Chem.*, 245:5234–5238.

191. Meijer, J., and DePierre, J. W. (1985): Properties of cytosolic epoxide hydrolase purified from the liver of untreated and clofibrate-treated mice. *Eur. J. Biochem.*, 148:421–430.

192. Meisler, M. H., and Reinke, C. (1979): A sensitive fluorescent assay for N-acetyltransferase activity in human lymphocytes from newborns and adults. *Clin. Chim. Acta*, 96:91–96.

193. Meister, A., Tate, S. S., and Griffith, O. W. (1981): γ-Glutamyl transpeptidase. *Methods Enzymol.*, 77:237–253.

194. Mezey, E., and Potter, J. J. (1983): Separation and partial characterization of multiple forms of rat liver alcohol dehydrogenase. *Arch. Biochem. Biophys.*, 225:787–794.

195. Miller, E. C., and Miller, J. A. (1947): The presence and significance of bound aminoazo dyes in the livers of rats fed p-dimethylaminoazobenzene. *Cancer Res.*, 7:468–480.

196. Miller, R. E., and Guengerich, F. P. (1983): Metabolism of trichloroethylene in isolated hepatocytes, microsomes, and reconstituted enzyme systems containing purified cytochromes P-450. *Cancer Res.*, 43:1145–1152.

197. Miwa, G. T., Levin, W., Thomas, P. E., and Lu, A. Y. H. (1978): The direct oxidation of ethanol by a catalase- and alcohol dehydrogenase-free reconstituted system containing cytochrome P-450. *Arch. Biochem. Biophys.*, 187:464–475.

198. Morgenstern, R., and DePierre, J. W. (1983): Microsomal glutathione transferase: purification in unactivated form and further characterization of the activation process, substrate specificity and amino acid composition. *Eur. J. Biochem.*, 134:591–597.

199. Müller-Enoch, D., Churchill, P., Fleischer, S., and Guengerich, F. P. (1984): Interaction of liver microsomal cytochrome P-450

and NADPH-cytochrome P-450 reductase in the presence and absence of lipid. *J. Biol. Chem.*, 259:8174–8182.

200. Nash, T. (1953): The colorimetric estimation of formaldehyde by means of the Hantzsch reaction. *Biochem. J.*, 55:416–421.

201. Neal, G. E., and Colley, P. J. (1978): Some high-performance liquid-chromatographic studies of the metabolism of aflatoxins by rat liver microsomal preparations. *Biochem. J.*, 174:839–851.

202. Nebert, D. W., and Gelboin, H. V. (1968): Substrate-inducible microsomal aryl hydroxylase in mammalian cell culture. I. Assay and properties of induced enzyme. *J. Biol. Chem.*, 243:6242–6249.

203. Nordblom, G. D., and Coon, M. J. (1977): Hydrogen peroxide formation and stoichiometry of hydroxylation reactions catalyzed by highly purified liver microsomal cytochrome P-450. *Arch. Biochem. Biophys.*, 180:343–347.

204. Oates, N. S., Shah, R. R., Drury, P. L., Idle, J. R., and Smith, R. L. (1982): Captopril-induced agranulocytosis associated with an impairment of debrisoquine hydroxylation. *Br. J. Pharmacol.*, 14:601P.

205. Oesch, F. (1973): Mammalian epoxide hydrases: inducible enzymes catalysing the inactivation of carcinogenic and cytotoxic metabolites derived from aromatic and olefinic compounds. *Xenobiotica*, 3:305–340.

206. Oesch, F., and Bentley, P. (1976): Antibodies against homogeneous epoxide hydratase provide evidence for a single enzyme hydrating styrene oxide and benz(a)pyrene-4,5-oxide. *Nature*, 259:53–55.

207. Oesch, F., Jerina, D. M., and Daly, J. (1971): A radiometric assay for hepatic epoxide hydrase activity with [7-^{3}H] styrene oxide. *Biochim. Biophys. Acta*, 227:685–691.

208. Oesch, F., Jerina, D. M., and Daly, J. W. (1971): Substrate specificity of hepatic epoxide hydrase in microsomes and in a purified preparation: evidence for homologous enzymes. *Arch. Biochem. Biophys.*, 144:253–261.

209. O'Farrell, P. Z., Goodman, H. M., and O'Farrell, P. H. (1977): High resolution two-dimensional electrophoresis of basic as well as acidic proteins. *Cell*, 12:1133–1142.

210. Omura, T., and Sato, R. (1964): The carbon monoxide-binding pigment of liver microsomes. I. Evidence for its hemoprotein nature. *J. Biol. Chem.*, 239:2370–2378.

211. Omura, T., and Sato, R. (1967): Isolation of cytochromes P-450 and P-420. *Methods Enzymol.*, 10:556–561.

212. Ortiz de Montellano, P. R., and Correia, M. A. (1983): Suicidal destruction of cytochrome P-450 during oxidative drug metabolism. *Annu. Rev. Pharmacol. Toxicol.*, 23:481–503.

213. Ozawa, N., and Guengerich, F. P. (1983): Evidence for formation of an S-[2-(N^7-guanyl)ethyl]glutathione adduct in glutathione-mediated binding of 1,2-dibromoethane to DNA. *Proc. Natl. Acad. Sci. USA*, 80:5266–5270.

214. Ozols, J., Korza, G., Heinemann, F. S., Hediger, M. A., and Strittmatter, P. (1985): Complete amino acid sequence of steer liver microsomal NADPH-cytochrome b₅ reductase. *J. Biol. Chem.*, 260:11953–11961.

215. Park, S. S., Fujino, T., Miller, H., Guengerich, F. P., and Gelboin, H. V. (1984): Monoclonal antibodies to phenobarbital-induced rat liver cytochrome P-450. *Biochem. Pharmacol.*, 33:2071–2081.

216. Park, S. S., Fujino, T., West, D., Guengerich, F. P., and Gelboin, H. V. (1982): Monoclonal antibodies to 3-methylcholanthrene-induced rat liver microsomal cytochrome P-450. *Cancer Res.*, 42:1798–1808.

217. Paye, M., Beaune, P., Kremers, P., Frankinet-Collignon, C., Guengerich, F. P., Goujon, F., and Gielen, J. (1984): Quantification of two cytochrome P-450 isoenzymes by enzymoimmunoassay using monoclonal antibodies. *Biochem. Biophys. Res. Commun.*, 122:137–142.

218. Peterson, J. A., Ebel, R. E., and O'Keefe, D. H. (1978): Dual-wavelength stopped-flow spectrophotometric measurement of NADPH-cytochrome P-450 reductase. *Methods Enzymol.*, 52:221–226.

219. Phillips, A. H., and Langdon, R. G. (1962): Hepatic triphosphopyridine nucleotide-cytochrome c reductase: isolation, characterization, and kinetic studies. *J. Biol. Chem.*, 237:2652–2660.

220. Philpot, R. M., and Arinc, E. (1976): Separation and purification of two forms of hepatic cytochrome P-450 from untreated rabbits. *Mol. Pharmacol.*, 12:483–493.

221. Poland, A. P., and Nebert, D. W. (1973): A sensitive radiometric

222. Porter, T. D., and Kasper, C. B. (1985): Coding nucleotide sequence of rat NADPH-cytochrome P-450 oxidoreductase cDNA and identification of flavin-binding domains. *Proc. Natl. Acad. Sci. USA*, 82:973–977.

223. Poulsen, L. L., Hyslop, R. M., and Ziegler, D. M. (1974): S-Oxidation of thioureylenes catalyzed by a microsomal flavoprotein mixed-function oxidase. *Biochem. Pharmacol.*, 23:3431–3440.

224. Poulsen, L. L., Sofer, S. S., and Ziegler, D. M. (1976): Properties and applications of an immobilized mixed-function hepatic drug oxidase. *Methods Enzymol.*, 44:849–856.

225. Raig, V. P., and Ammon, R. (1972): Nachweis einiger neuer phenolischer Stoffwechselprodukte des biphenyls. *Arzneimittelforschung*, 22:1399–1404.

226. Roerig, D. L., Mascaro, L., Jr., and Aust, S. D. (1972): Microsomal electron transport: tetrazolium reduction by rat liver microsomal NADPH-cytochrome c reductase. *Arch. Biochem. Biophys.*, 153:475–479.

227. Roy Choudhury, J., Roy Choudhury, N., Falany, C. N., Tephley, T. R., and Arias, I. M. (1986): Isolation and characterization of multiple forms of rat liver UDP-glucuronate glucuronyltransferase. *Biochem. J.*, 233:827–837.

228. Ryan, D., Lu, A. Y. H., and Levin, W. (1978): Purification of cytochrome P-450 and P-448 from rat liver microsomes. *Methods Enzymol.*, 52:117–123.

229. Ryan, D., Lu, A. Y. H., Kawalek, J., West, S. B., and Levin, W. (1975): Highly-purified cytochrome P-448 and P-450 from rat liver microsomes. *Biochem. Biophys. Res. Commun.*, 64:1134–1141.

230. Ryan, D., Lu, A. Y. H., West, S., and Levin, W. (1975): Multiple forms of cytochrome P-450 in phenobarbital- and 3-methylcholanthrene-treated rats: separation and spectral properties. *J. Biol. Chem.*, 250:2157–2163.

231. Ryan, D. E., Thomas, P. E., Korzeniowski, D., and Levin, W. (1979): Separation and characterization of multiple forms of highly purified forms of liver microsomal cytochrome P-450 from rats treated with polychlorinated biphenyls, phenobarbital, and 3-methylcholanthrene. *J. Biol. Chem.*, 254:1365–1374.

232. Sabourin, P. J., Smyser, B. P., and Hodgson, E. (1984): Purification of the flavin-containing monooxygenase from mouse and pig liver microsomes. *Int. J. Biochem.*, 16:713–720.

233. Sadano, H., and Omura, T. (1983): Reversible transfer of heme between different molecular species of microsome-bound cytochrome P-450 in rat liver. *Biochem. Biophys. Res. Commun.*, 116:1013–1019.

234. Salach, J. I. (1979): Monoamine oxidase from beef liver mitochondria: simplified isolation procedure, properties, and determination of its cysteinyl flavin content. *Arch. Biochem. Biophys.*, 192:128–137.

235. Sekura, R. D., and Jakoby, W. B. (1979): Phenol sulfotransferases. *J. Biol. Chem.*, 254:5658–5663.

236. Sekura, R. D., and Jakoby, W. B. (1981): Aryl sulfotransferase IV from rat liver. *Arch. Biochem. Biophys.*, 211:352–359.

237. Sekura, R. D., Marcus, C. J., Lyon, E. S., and Jakoby, W. B. (1979): Assay of sulfotransferases. *Anal. Biochem.*, 95:82–86.

238. Selander, H. G., Jerina, D. M., and Daly, J. W. (1974): Metabolism of acetanilide with hepatic microsomes and reconstituted cytochrome monoxygenase systems. *Arch. Biochem. Biophys.*, 164:241–246.

239. Selander, H. G., Jerina, D. M., and Daly, J. W. (1975): Metabolism of chlorobenzene with hepatic microsomes and solubilized cytochrome P-450 systems. *Arch. Biochem. Biophys.*, 168:309–321.

240. Selkirk, J. K., Croy, R. G., Roller, P. P., and Gelboin, H. V. (1974): High-pressure liquid chromatographic analysis of benzo(a)pyrene metabolism and covalent binding and the mechanism of action of 7,8-benzoflavone and 1,2-epoxy-3,3,3-trichloropropane. *Cancer Res.*, 34:3474–3480.

241. Shimada, T., and Guengerich, F. P. (1985): Participation of a rat liver cytochrome P-450 induced by pregnenolone 16α-carbonitrile and other compounds in the 4-hydroxylation of mephenytoin. *Mol. Pharmacol.*, 28:215–219.

242. Shimada, T., Misono, K. S., and Guengerich, F. P. (1986): Human liver microsomal cytochrome P-450 mephenytoin 4-hydroxylase, a prototype of genetic polymorphism in oxidative drug metabolism:

assay of aminopyrine N-demethylation. *J. Pharmacol. Exp. Ther.*, 184:269–277.

purification and characterization of two similar forms involved in the reaction. *J. Biol. Chem.,* 261:909–921.

243. Shimada, T., Shea, J. P., and Guengerich, F. P. (1985): A convenient assay for mephenytoin 4-hydroxylase activity of human liver microsomal cytochrome P-450. *Anal. Biochem.,* 147:174–179.

244. Sipes, I. G., Krishna, G., and Gillette, J. R. (1977): Bioactivation of carbon tetrachloride, chloroform, and bromotrichloromethane: role of cytochrome P-450. *Life Sci.,* 20:1541–1548.

245. Sladek, N. E., and Mannering, G. J. (1969): Induction of drug metabolism. II. Qualitative differences in the microsomal N-demethylating systems stimulated by polycyclic hydrocarbons and by phenobarbital. *Mol. Pharmacol.,* 5:186–199.

246. Spatz, L., and Strittmatter, P. (1971): A form of cytochrome b_5 that contains an additional hydrophobic sequence of 40 amino acid residues. *Proc. Natl. Acad. Sci. USA,* 68:1042–1046.

247. Stevens, J., and Jakoby, W. B. (1983): Cysteine conjugate β-lyase. *Mol. Pharmacol.,* 23:761–765.

248. Steward, A. R., Dannan, G. A., Guzelian, P. S., and Guengerich, F. P. (1985): Changes in the concentration of seven forms of cytochrome P-450 in primary cultures of adult rat hepatocytes. *Mol. Pharmacol.,* 27:125–132.

249. Strobel, H. W., and Dignam, J. D. (1978): Purification and properties of NADPH-cytochrome P-450 reductase. *Methods Enzymol.,* 52:89–96.

250. Sun, J. D., and Dent, J. G. (1980): A new method for measuring covalent binding of chemicals to cellular macromolecules. *Chem. Biol. Interact.,* 32:41–61.

251. Tateishi, M., and Shimizu, H. (1980): Cysteine conjugate β-lyase. In: *Enzymatic Basis of Detoxication,* Vol. 2, edited by W. B. Jakoby, pp. 121–130. Academic Press, New York.

252. Tateishi, M., Suzuki, S., and Shimizu, H. (1978): Cysteine conjugate β-lyase in rat liver: a novel enzyme catalyzing formation of thiol-containing metabolites of drugs. *J. Biol. Chem.,* 253:8854–8859.

253. Taugen, O., Jonasson, J., and Orrenius, S. (1973): Isolation of rat liver microsomes by gel filtration. *Anal. Biochem.,* 54:597–603.

254. Telakowski-Hopkins, C. A., Rodkey, J. A., Bennett, C. D., Lu, A. Y. H., and Pickett, C. B. (1985): Rat liver glutathione S-transferase: construction of a cDNA clone complementary to a Yc mRNA and prediction of the complete amino acid sequence of a Yc subunit. *J. Biol. Chem.,* 260:5820–5825.

255. Tenhunen, R., Marver, H. S., and Schmid, R. (1969): Microsomal heme oxygenase: characterization of the enzyme. *J. Biol. Chem.,* 244:6388–6394.

256. Teschke, R., Hasumura, Y., and Lieber, C. S. (1974): Hepatic microsomal ethanol-oxidizing system: solubilization, isolation and characterization. *Arch. Biochem. Biophys.,* 163:404–415.

257. Thakker, D. R., Yagi, H., and Jerina, D. M. (1978): Analysis of polycyclic aromatic hydrocarbons and their metabolites by high-pressure liquid chromatography. *Methods Enzymol.,* 52:279–296.

258. Thomas, P. E., Koreniowski, D., Ryan, D., and Levin, W. (1979): Preparation of monospecific antibodies against two forms of rat liver cytochrome P-450 and quantitation of these antigens in microsomes. *Arch. Biochem. Biophys.,* 192:524–532.

259. Thomas, P. E., Lu, A. Y. H., West, S. B., Ryan, D., Miwa, G. T., and Levin, W. (1977): Accessibility of cytochrome P-450 in microsomal membranes: inhibition of metabolism by antibodies to cytochrome P-450. *Mol. Pharmacol.,* 13:819–831.

260. Thomas, P. E., Ryan, D., and Levin, W. (1976): An improved staining procedure for the detection of the peroxidase activity of cytochrome P-450 on sodium dodecyl sulfate polyacrylamide gels. *Anal. Biochem.,* 75:168–176.

261. Thomas, P. E., Ryan, D. E., von Bahr, C., Glaumann, H., and Levin, W. (1982): Human liver microsomal epoxide hydrolase: correlation of immunochemical quantitation with catalytic activity. *Mol. Pharmacol.,* 22:190–195.

262. Thomaszewski, J. E., Jerina, D. M., Levin, W., and Conney, A. H. (1976): A highly sensitive radiometric assay for zoxazolamine hydroxylation by liver microsomal cytochrome P-450 and P-448: properties of the membrane-bound and purified reconstituted system. *Arch. Biochem. Biophys.,* 176:788–798.

263. Thorgeirsson, S. S., Jollow, D. J., Sasame, H. A., Green, I., and Mitchell, J. R. (1973): The role of cytochrome P-450 in N-hydroxylation of 2-acetylaminofluorene. *Mol. Pharmacol.,* 9:398–404.

264. Towbin, H., and Gordon, J. (1984): Immunoblotting and dot immunoblotting—current status and outlook. *J. Immunol. Methods,* 72:313–340.

265. Towbin, H., Staehelin, T., and Gordon, J. (1979): Electrophoretic transfer of proteins from polyacrylamide gels to nitrocellulose sheets: procedure and some applications. *Proc. Natl. Acad. Sci. USA,* 76: 4350–4354.

266. Tu, C-P. D., Lai, H-C. J., Li, N-Q., Weiss, M. J., and Reddy, C. C. (1984): The Yc and Ya subunits of rat liver glutathione S-transferases are the products of separate genes. *J. Biol. Chem.,* 259: 9434–9439.

267. Tukey, R. H., and Tephley, T. R. (1981): Purification and properties of rabbit liver estrone and p-nitrophenol UDP-glucuronyl transferases. *Arch. Biochem. Biophys.,* 209:565–578.

268. Udenfriend, S., Stein, S., Böhlen, P., Dairman, W., Leimgruber, W., and Weigele, M. (1972): Fluorescamine: a reagent for assay of amino acids, peptides, proteins, and primary amines in the picomole range. *Science,* 178:871–872.

269. Ullrich, V., and Weber, P. (1972): The O-dealkylation of 7-ethoxycoumarin by liver microsomes. *Z. Physiol. Chem.,* 353:1171–1177.

270. Van Bladeren, P. J., Breimer, D. D., van Huijgevoort, J. A. T. C. M., Vermuelen, N. P. E., and van der Gen, A. (1981): The metabolic formation of N-acetyl-S-2-hydroxyethyl-L-cysteine from tetradeutero-1,2-dibromoethane: relative importance of oxidation and glutathione conjugation in vivo. *Biochem. Pharmacol.,* 30:2499–2502.

271. Van der Hoeven, T. (1977): A sensitive, fluorometric method for the assay of microsomal hydroxylase: N-demethylation of p-chloro-N-methylaniline. *Anal. Biochem.,* 77:523–528.

272. Van der Hoeven, T. A., and Coon, M. J. (1974): Preparation and properties of partially purified cytochrome P-450 and reduced nicotinamide adenine dinucleotide phosphate-cytochrome P-450 reductase from rabbit liver microsomes. *J. Biol. Chem.,* 249:6302–6310.

273. Van der Hoeven, T. A., Haugen, D. A., and Coon, M. J. (1974): Cytochrome P-450 purified to apparent homogeneity from phenobarbital-induced rabbit liver microsomes: catalytic activity and other properties. *Biochem. Biophys. Res. Commun.,* 60:569–575.

274. Vander Jagt, D. L., Hunsaker, L. A., Garcia, K. B., and Roger, R. E. (1985): Isolation and characterization of the multiple glutathione S-transferases from human liver: evidence for unique heme-binding sites. *J. Biol. Chem.,* 260:11603–11610.

275. Vermilion, J. L., and Coon, M. J. (1978): Purified liver microsomal NADPH-cytochrome P-450 reductase: spectral characterization of oxidation-reduction states. *J. Biol. Chem.,* 253:2694–2704.

276. Vlasuk, G. P., and Walz, F. G., Jr. (1980): Liver endoplasmic reticulum polypeptides resolved by two-dimensional gel electrophoresis. *Anal. Biochem.,* 105:112–120.

277. Wallin, H., Schelin, C., Tunek, A., and Jergil, B. (1981): A rapid and sensitive method for determination of covalent binding of benzo(a)pyrene to proteins. *Chem. Biol. Interact.,* 38:109–118.

278. Wang, P., Mason, P. S., and Guengerich, F. P. (1980): Purification of human liver cytochrome P-450 and comparison to the enzyme isolated from rat liver. *Arch. Biochem. Biophys.,* 199:206–219.

279. Wang, P., Meijer, J., and Guengerich, F. P. (1982): Purification of human liver cytosolic epoxide hydrolase and comparison to the microsomal enzyme. *Biochemistry,* 21:5769–5776.

280. Watabe, T., and Akamatsu, K. (1974): Photometric assay of hepatic epoxide hydrolase activity with safrole oxide (SAFO) as substrate. *Biochem. Pharmacol.,* 23:2839–2844.

281. Waxman, D. J., Dannan, G. A., and Guengerich, F. P. (1985): Regulation of rat hepatic cytochrome P-450: age-dependent expression, hormonal imprinting, and xenobiotic inducibility of sex-specific isoenzymes. *Biochemistry,* 24:4409–4417.

282. Weber, W. W. (1971): N-Acetyltransferase (mammalian liver). *Methods Enzymol.,* 17B:805–811.

283. Weber, W. W., and Cohen, S. N. (1968): The mechanism of isoniazid acetylation by human liver N-acetyltransferase. *Biochim. Biophys. Acta,* 151:276–278.

284. Weber, W. W., and Hein, D. W. (1985): N-Acetylation pharmacogenetics. *Pharmacol. Rev.,* 37:25–29.

285. Weber, W. W., Miceli, J. N., Hearse, D. J., and Drummond, G. S. (1976): N-Acetylation of drugs: pharmacogenetic studies in rabbits selected for their acetylator characteristics. *Drug Metab. Dispos.,* 4:904–911.

286. Weisiger, R. A., and Jakoby, W. B. (1979): Thiol S-methyltransferase from rat liver. *Arch. Biochem. Biophys.,* 196:631–637.

287. West, S. B., Huang, M-T., Miwa, G. T., and Lu, A. Y. H. (1978): A simple and rapid procedure for the purification of phenobarbital-inducible cytochrome P-450 from rat liver microsomes. *Arch. Biochem. Biophys.,* 193:42–50.

288. Weyler, W., and Salach, J. I. (1985): Purification and properties of mitochondrial monoamine oxidase type A from human placenta. *J. Biol. Chem.,* 260:13199–13207.

289. White, P. C., Grossberger, D., Onufer, B. J., Chaplin, D. D., New, M. I., DuPont, B., and Strominger, J. L. (1985): Two genes encoding steroid 21-hydroxylase are located near the genes encoding the fourth component of complement in man. *Proc. Natl. Acad. Sci. USA,* 82:1089–1093.

290. Williams, D. E., Hale, S. E., Muerhoff, A. S., and Masters, B. S. S. (1985): Rabbit lung flavin-containing monooxygenase: purification, characterization, and induction during pregnancy. *Mol. Pharmacol.,* 28:381–390.

291. Winge, D. R., Nielson, K. B., Zeikus, R. D., and Gray, W. R. (1984): Structural characterization of the isoforms of neonatal and adult rat liver metallothionein. *J. Biol. Chem.,* 259:11419–11425.

292. Wislocki, P. G., Miwa, G. T., and Lu, A. Y. H. (1980): Reactions catalyzed by the cytochrome P-450 system. In: *Enzymatic Basis of Detoxication,* Vol. 1, edited by W. B. Jakoby, pp. 135–182. Academic Press, New York.

293. Wolf, T., Greim, H., Huang, M-T., Miwa, G. T., and Lu, A. Y. H. (1980): Aldrin epoxidation catalyzed by purified rat-liver cytochromes P-450 and P-448: high selectivity for cytochrome P-450. *Eur. J. Biochem.,* 111:545–551.

294. Wood, A. W., Levin, W., Lu, A. Y. H., Yagi, H., Hernandez, O., Jerina, D. M., and Conney, A. H. (1976): Metabolism of benzo(a)pyrene and benzo(a)pyrene derivatives to mutagenic products by highly purified hepatic microsomal enzymes. *J. Biol. Chem.,* 251:4882–4890.

295. Yasukochi, Y., and Masters, B. S. S. (1976): Some properties of a detergent-solubilized NADPH-cytochrome c(cytochrome P-450) reductase purified by biospecific affinity chromatography. *J. Biol. Chem.,* 251:5337–5344.

296. Yoshida, T., and Kikuchi, G. (1978): Features of the reaction of heme degradation catalyzed by the reconstituted microsomal heme oxygenase system. *J. Biol. Chem.,* 253:4230–4236.

297. Yoshida, T., and Kikuchi, G. (1978): Purification and properties of heme oxygenase from pig spleen microsomes. *J. Biol. Chem.,* 253:4224–4229.

298. Yoshinaga, T., Sassa, S., and Kappas, A. (1982): Purification and properties of bovine spleen heme oxygenase: amino acid composition and sites of action of inhibitors of heme oxidation. *J. Biol. Chem.,* 257:7778–7785.

299. Ziegler, D. M. (1980): Microsomal flavin-containing monooxygenase: oxygenation of nucleophilic nitrogen and sulfur compounds. In: *Enzymatic Basis of Detoxication,* Vol. 1, edited by W. B. Jakoby, pp. 201–227. Academic Press, New York.

300. Ziegler, D. M., and Mitchell, C. H. (1972): Microsomal oxidase. IV. Properties of a mixed-function amine oxidase isolated from pig liver microsomes. *Arch. Biochem. Biophys.,* 150:116–125.

Principles and Methods of Toxicology, Second Edition, edited by A. Wallace Hayes, Raven Press, Ltd., New York © 1989.

CHAPTER **29**

Organelles as Tools in Toxicology

Bruce A. Fowler, George W. Lucier, and *A. Wallace Hayes

*National Institute of Environmental Health Sciences, National Institutes of Health, Research Triangle Park, North Carolina 27709; and *Center for Toxicology, R.J.R. Nabisco, Winston-Salem, North Carolina 27102*

Cells are composed of a number of organelle compartments that play crucial roles in facilitating metabolic processes essential to cellular viability (Fig. 1). The effects of many toxic agents on cells are mediated via damage to one or more of these specialized subcellular compartments. Specific organelle systems may become damaged by toxic agents when they perform a primary role in the metabolism of a particular toxicant, when a toxicant is stored intracellularly, or as a result of an inherent sensitivity of some essential biochemical pathway in the organelle to perturbation. In terms of understanding the mechanisms of cellular toxicity, it is clear that evaluation of organelles as basic units of subcellular function may provide useful insights into the basis of toxicant action. It should also be obvious that the ability to detect damage within particular organelle systems depends on the sensitivity and nature of the parameters measured.

The following discussion examines some of the current ultrastructural and biochemical methods available for evaluation of specific organelles, and reviews some of the ways in which these techniques have aided understanding the mechanisms of toxicity. A critical examination of these techniques will also be presented to aid the reader in assessing the potential value of a given procedure for delineating information about a specific toxic process.

MITOCHONDRIA

Mitochondria are essential organelles which play an important role in cell metabolism by mediating a number of metabolic functions (Fig. 2). Enzymes involved in energy production, carbohydrate metabolism, heme biosynthesis, and the urea cycle are found in this organelle. These enzymes are not randomly distributed within the mitochondria but are localized within specific subcompartments such as the outer and inner membranes and matrix (Table 1).

In terms of the effects of toxicants on this organelle, it is important to understand the relationship between particular metabolic functions and the physical integrity of the mitochondrion as a structure, because frequently *in vivo* biochemical perturbations result directly from structural damage. The following examination of ultrastructural and biochemical methods for mitochondrial evaluations utilizes examples of some well-known toxicants to illustrate how each technique aided in understanding the mechanisms of toxicity.

Ultrastructural Techniques

Fixation and Embedding

Preservation of mitochondria within intact cells is routinely carried out by rapid chemical fixation using glutaraldehyde- or glutaraldehyde–formaldehyde-based fixatives. Tissues may be either placed in these fixatives or perfused via the blood vasculature for optimal preservation of cellular structure. Electron density is imparted to the mitochondrial membranes by post fixation in a 1% solution of osmium tetroxide (OsO_4) followed by dehydration in a graded series of alcohol from 70 to 100%. Dehydrated tissues are then placed in solutions

Hepatocyte Organelles

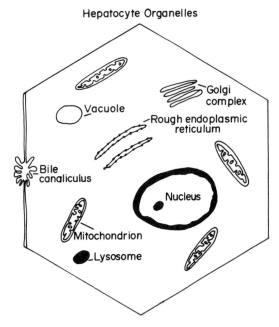

FIG. 1. Diagrammatic representation of a hepatocyte showing nucleus, mitochondria, lysosomes, endoplasmic reticulum, and Golgi apparatus.

TABLE 1. Activity and function of enzymes in mitochondria

Enzyme activities	Function
Outer membrane	
Fatty acid CoA synthetase	Fatty acid metabolism
Mononamine oxidase	Catecholamine metabolism
Inner membrane	
NADH oxidase	Transport
Succinic dehydrogenase	TCA substrate
β-hydroxybutyrate dehydrogenase	Oxidation
Mg^{+2} ATPase	Generation of ATP
Coproporphyrinogen oxidase	
Ferrochelatase	Heme biosynthesis
ALA synthetase	
Anion and cation transport systems	Mitochondrial conformation
Matrix	
Pyruvate DH complex	
Malate DH	
Isocitric DH	
Citrate synthetase	Intermediary metabolism
Fumarase	
Glutamic DH	
Glutamic transaminases	Ammonia metabolism
Ornithine carbamoyl transferase	
Carbamoyl PO_4 synthetase	Urea synthesis

Mitochondrial Functions

Cellular energy production (ATP)

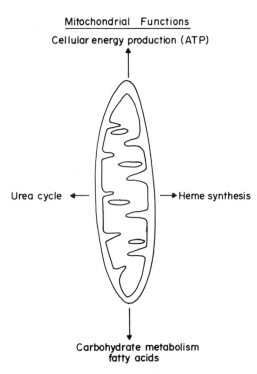

Urea cycle ← → Heme synthesis

Carbohydrate metabolism
fatty acids

FIG. 2. Diagrammatic representation of a mitochondrion showing outer membrane, inner membrane with infoldings (cristae) and matrix. This multifunctional organelle has enzyme systems that are concerned with the production of ATP, carbohydrate metabolism, heme biosynthesis, and the urea cycle, and which are specifically localized in the outer membrane, inner membrane, or matrix. (From ref. 31, with permission.)

of propylene oxide and embedded in plastic resins such as Epon. A stepwise routine procedure for fixation and embedding of tissues for electron microscopy is as follows:

1. Place tissue blocks (1 mm³) in fixative [2% glutaraldehyde, 2.6% formaldehyde in 0.07 M cacodylate buffer (pH 7.4) and 3% sucrose] for 2 hr in a refrigerator.
2. Decant fixative and place blocks in above cacodylate buffer overnight in a refrigerator.
3. Post-fix blocks in 1% OsO_4 (*Caution:* volatile toxicant) in 0.1 M phosphate buffer (pH 7.4) for 2 hr and then decant in a fume hood.
4. Dehydrate tissue blocks in 70, 90, 95 (two changes), and 100% alcohol at room temperature for 15 min at each step.
5. Decant final 100% alcohol solution and place blocks in two changes of propylene oxide.
6. Place blocks in 50:50 propylene oxide plastic resin mixture overnight to infiltrate tissue blocks.
7. Place tissue blocks in final plastic resin mixture and embed in Teflon capsules.
8. Place in curing oven (60°C) to harden plastic before sectioning.

Ultrastructural Morphometry

This technique, which is essentially an approach to quantitating the dimensions of organelle compartments within intact cells based on evaluation of their surface area in a large number of electron micrographs, has been extensively reviewed (5,7,104,105). The method may be readily employed to determine the overall volume of organelles such as mitochondria within cells (volume density), but determinations of mitochondrial membrane surface area (surface density) and numbers of mitochondria (numerical density) require the application of correction factors that have recently undergone revision (5,7,104). The specific steps in this technique, as well as the equations necessary for evaluation of generated data, are given in an article by Weibel et al. (107) and will not be repeated here.

The application of morphometry to evaluation of mitochondria following *in vivo* exposure to arsenate (29,32), cortisone (108), methyl mercury (28), and vitamin E deficiency (34) has been successfully employed to document increases or decreases in this organelle system and the relationship of these effects to observed biochemical changes.

The primary value of ultrastructural morphometry in delineating toxic mechanisms for organelles such as the mitochondrion rests with the ability to quantitatively assess changes in mitochondrial structure within the intact cell. Such data have proven invaluable not only in interpreting the results of biochemical studies on this organelle (30) but also in suggesting new and more integrative hypotheses which consider change in the biochemical functionality of the mitochondrion in relation to concomitant chemical-induced alterations in other organelle systems (e.g., the endoplasmic reticulum) within the same cells (26). In other words, this technique has provided a rigorous approach for simultaneously assessing whether changes are occurring in more than one organelle system and thereby minimizing the possibility of erroneously concluding that a chemical is acting at only one site within a target cell population, which is one of the great pitfalls in contemporary mechanistic toxicology. It should be noted (22,23) that the application of this technique to toxicology is extremely labor-intensive and requires a serious commitment of resources in order for successful utilization. This aspect requires serious consideration by those contemplating use of this powerful morphological technique.

Ultrastructural Evaluation of Mitochondrial Fractions

Evaluation of mitochondria from tissues following homogenization and isolation in sucrose (see below) by electron microscopy provides one method for evaluating the purity of the samples and the degree of structural integrity. This technique also has been employed to examine changes in mitochondrial conformational behavior during respiration following *in vitro* exposure to uncoupling agents such as dinitrophenol (43) or *in vivo* following exposure to lead (38) or arsenate (32).

The technique essentially involves utilizing the chemical fixation and embedding process described above to process pellets of mitochondria and other organelles. A more quantitative approach to evaluation of isolated organelles has been recently described by Deter (18).

Negative Staining of Isolated Mitochondria

The technique of negative staining (47) involves uranyl acetate, phosphotungstic acid, or ammonium molybdate, to stain the Formvar grid backing so that isolated organelles, such as mitochondria, stand out against the dark background. This method has proven extremely useful for high resolution microscopy studies of mitochondrial membrane preparations and has been used to evaluate changes in mitochondrial membranes following *in vitro* exposure to these organelles to uncoupling agents (78). A general flow sheet for this technique follows, and a more complete discussion is given elsewhere (47). As with the other morphological techniques discussed in this section, the main value of this procedure rests with providing correlative structural information about change in the internal structure of this organelle in relation to biochemical alterations within these intramitochondrial compartments (23).

Techniques

1. Isolate mitochondria (See Fig. 3).
2. Final dilution of mitochondria to 60 mg/ml.
3. Pipet sample on the Formvar-coated grids and allow to dry in covered dish.
4. Cover grids with a drop of negative stain (pH 7.4) at 1–2% concentration.
5. Blot excess stain from edge of grid with filter paper.
6. Examine sample with transmission electron microscope.

Scanning Electron Microscopy

Application of scanning electron microscopy to evaluation of mitochondrial conformational behavior or the conformational behavior of the intact inner membrane (mitoplast) has been employed by Andrews and Hackenbrock (2) to confirm findings obtained by transmission electron microscopy.

Technique

1. Place mitochondrial or mitoplast sample (1–2 mg/ml) on Formvar-coated grids and cover with one drop 2% glutaraldehyde in 0.1 M phosphate buffer (pH 7.4).
2. Place grids in perforated vials and dehydrate in acetone; follow with critical point drying.
3. Coat samples with a 150-Å layer of palladium–gold in a vacuum evaporator.
4. Examine in a scanning electron microscope.

Freeze-Etch Analysis

The technique of freeze-etching has been employed to study the three-dimensional structure of mitochondrial membranes during different energy states (42,58) and their relationship to localization of protein complexes within the membrane. This method essentially involves chemical fixation and rapid freezing of biological samples in Freon prior to fracturing in a freeze-etch device (57). The fracture plane is thought to primarily cleave across the hydrophobic regions of the membranes, thereby exposing both inner and outer

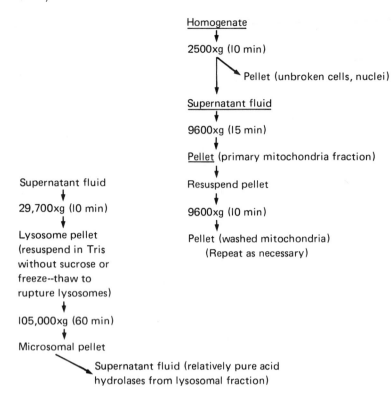

FIG. 3. Standard isolation procedure for mitochondria and other organelles such as lysosomes and microsomes by differential centrifugation in 0.25 M sucrose–0.05 M Tris buffer (pH 7.4).

surfaces. The surfaces are then sputter-coated with metals such as platinum and carbon to form replicas that are floated off the tissue and collected on standard electron microscopy grids for evaluation in a transmission electron microscope. A detailed examination of the techniques and known artifacts has been given elsewhere (57). To date, this technique has not been applied to evaluation of toxicant action on mitochondria.

Techniques

1. Fix tissue in the glutaraldehyde fixative described above.
2. Incubate tissue in 10–20% glycerol until tissue is impregnated.
3. Place specimen on specimen carrier and immerse in Freon 22 cooled to −165°C with liquid nitrogen.
4. Place specimen in freeze-etch device and fracture with steel blade.
5. Etch cleaned surface of specimen by allowing ice to sublime from sample.
6. Shadow specimen surface with carbon–platinum to form replica and cover replica with carbon backing layer.
7. Remove specimen and replica from evaporator and place in an aqueous solution similar to original glycerol freezing solution to release replica from specimen surface.
8. Clean replica in 5% sodium hypochlorite solution.
9. Rinse replicas in several changes of water and mount on 150-mesh grids.

Overall Assessment

The primary value of the various ultrastructural techniques described in this section rests with delineating the organelle system within a target cell population that is being affected by a given toxicant within an intact tissue. These techniques may be further extended to provide information about changes in organelle infrastructure that may point to a molecular site of action, which may be approached by biochemical techniques. In this regard, these techniques have also proven highly useful in interpreting results of biochemical studies on various organelle systems following either *in vivo* or *in vitro* chemical treatment. Thus, although these procedures do not by themselves delineate mechanisms, they are extremely valuable techniques for detecting molecular sites of action and correctly interpreting biochemical studies which examine chemical mechanisms at those loci.

Biochemical Procedures

There are a variety of biochemical parameters that can be used to assess the effects of toxicants on mitochondrial function. In part, the effectiveness of these techniques depends on the procedures used to isolate mitochondria prior to evaluation. A relatively standard procedure is given in Fig. 3 that essentially involves Tris (0.05 M)–sucrose (0.25 M) with subsequent pelleting of mitochondria by centrifugation. In addition to this basic procedure, resuspension and recentrifugation may be used to "wash" the mitochondria and to remove contamination by microsomes. In the process of reducing mitochondrial contamination, it should be noted that mitochondria from different tissues vary in their sensitivity to physical damage or chelating agents such as EDTA. This means that caution must be exercised in order to separate toxicant effects on these organelles from other effects derived from the isolation procedures. A more complete examination of problems encountered in the isolation of mitochondria and other organelles has been given by Deter (18).

In addition, mitochondria may be separated into the outer mitochondrial membrane and inner mitochondrial membrane plus matrix (mitoplast) by treatment with controlled digitonin digestion (93) or use of a pressure cell (39) with subsequent pelleting of membranes by centrifugation. This technique has been successfully used to identify the submitochondrial localization of a host of marker enzyme activities (Table 1).

General Mitochondrial Isolation Procedures

1. Homogenize tissues in 0.25 M sucrose or mannitol in 0.07 M Tris–HCl buffer (pH 7.4) at 1 g tissue 9 ml of Tris–sucrose. Agents such as EDTA may also be added to aid disruption of cells.
2. Place in centrifuge tubes and spin at $2500 \times g$ for 10 min to remove nuclei and unbroken cells.
3. Decant supernatant fluid into centrifuge tubes and spin at $10,000 \times g$ for 10 min to form primary mitochondrial pellet.
4. Decant supernatant fluid and gently resuspend pellet in 10-ml Tris–sucrose for washing. Recentrifuge pellet and decant supernatant fluid. This washing cycle may be repeated a number of times depending on the tissue involved and the degree of mitochondrial purity desired.
5. Resuspend final mitochondrial pellet (1 ml Tris–sucrose/ 1 g of original sample) (1).

Separation of Outer and Inner Mitochondrial Membranes

1. Place washed mitochondria (30–60 mg protein/ml) in a precooled French pressure cell and subject to 1500 psi. Extruded material is taken up in an equal volume of double strength medium and centrifuged at $12,100 \times g$ for 10 min.
2. Resuspend the resultant pellet in the previous volume and recentrifuge at $12,100 \times g$ for 10 min.
3. Combine supernatant material from the above pellets and centrifuge at $27,100 \times g$ for 10 min.
4. Supernatant fluid from this pellet is centrifuged at $144,000 \times g$ for 90 min to obtain the outer membrane (pellet) and intermembrane fraction (supernatant fluid).

Respiratory Function

One of the primary functions of mitochondria within intact cells is the oxidation of substrates with subsequent generation of adenosine triphosphate (ATP). There are two major classes of oxidizable substrates that are capable of causing electron flow through the mitochondrial electron transport chain. The first of these involves those substrates (pyruvate, malate, and β-hydroxybutyrate) that use nicotinamide-adenine dinucleotide (NAD) as an acceptor of protons and is capable of generating three moles of ATP per molecule oxidized. Succinate is the other substrate type and generates two moles of ATP per molecule oxidized. Methods employed for the evaluation of mitochondrial respiratory function include War-

burg respirometry and the oxygen electrode; each measures oxygen consumption by mitochondria in the presence of oxidizable substrates. The advantage of the first type of measurement rests with its ability to measure oxygen consumption within intact tissue slices, whereas the latter is capable of detecting changes in respiration during different states of respiration.

Techniques (oxygen electrode)

1. Isolated mitochondria in Tris–sucrose medium (10–20 mg/ml) are placed into a 1–3-ml oxygen electrode cell with stirrer containing a reaction mixture composed of 40 mM Tris HCl (pH 7.5), 5 mM K_2HPO_4, 5 mM $MgSO_4$, and 100 mM KCl with 1–2 mg mitochondrial protein per ml.
2. A stable recorder baseline is obtained and initial state 4 respiration is initiated by adding succinate or NAD-linked substrates to yield a final concentration in the cell of 5 mM.
3. After 1–2 min of state 4 respiration, state 3 respiration is initiated by adding 2–5 μmoles adenosine diphosphate (ADP).
4. Following complete utilization of the added ADP, a return of state 4 respiration will be observed.
5. Respiratory control ratios (RCR) are calculated by dividing the state 3 rate by the state 4 rate. ADP/O ratios are calculated by dividing the amount of ADP added by the calculated amount of oxygen consumed as described by Estabrook (19).

As an approach to the toxicity assessment of mitochondria, respiratory function is an essential index of mitochondrial function which is easily damaged by many toxic agents. Toxic trace metals such as arsenic (29,31–32), lead (38,39), mercury (21,28,97), and cadmium (53) inhibit mitochondrial respiration. For lead and arsenic, this inhibition is relatively specific for NAD-linked substrates such as pyruvate/malate (29,31–32,38). This process is thought to be due to inhibition of mitochondrial dehydrogenases for these substrates which are located in the mitochondrial matrix. In addition, alteration of mitochondrial conformation behavior has been reported in relation to these phenomena (32,38), indicating that the well-known energy-linked transformation (41–43) of these organelles is also altered. Organic toxicants such as pesticides (79) and others (11,52) also damage mitochondrial respiratory function leading to diminished production of ATP.

Obviously, as the primary energy source for most cells, mitochondrial respiration and ATP generation are essential to cell survival. While impairment of mitochondrial respiration implies the reduced availability of ATP for maintaining essential cellular processes, it should be noted that quantitation of cellular ATP levels is essential to confirming such a mechanism since ATP appears to be present in excess within cells. Chemical methods for quantitating ATP require an extraction process which in our experience usually *added* to the variability in these measurements by such procedures. Such methodological problems increase standard deviations, which reduces the ability to discriminate effects between treatment groups on a statistical basis. More recently, the advent of *in vivo* ^{31}P-nuclear magnetic resonance (NMR) spectroscopy has permitted more specific measurement of the three ATP resonances as well as inorganic phosphorus, NAD, and sugar phosphates and other phosphorylated chemical species (Fig. 4). A major advantage to this technique is the ability to monitor changes in ATP concentrations in major target organs such as the liver in real time without sacrificing an animal by placing an NMR surface coil over the organ of interest (61) while the anesthetized animal rests inside the large bore NMR magnet. We have recently employed this technique (12) to study the effects of acute arsenite (As^{3+}) treatment on hepatic ATP content following a single intravenous dose. The data demonstrate not only the expected decrease in hepatic ATP and rise in Pi but the attendant increased phosphorylation of several other chemical species. These latter events would never have been appreciated via simple extraction and measurement of ATP.

Carbohydrate Metabolism

Many of the enzymes involved in intermediary metabolism are localized in the mitochondrial matrix. Dehydrogenases for pyruvate, malate, and glutamate are localized in this portion of the organelle. A typical assay procedure for malate dehydrogenase has been extensively described elsewhere (80). Toxicant damage to this aspect of mitochondrial function has been demonstrated for agents such as arsenic (29,31–33) and methyl mercury (69).

Heme Biosynthesis

Three of the key enzymes in the heme biosynthesis pathway are localized in the mitochondrion and are associated with the inner mitochondrial membrane. Ferrochelatase coproporphyrinogen oxidase and δ-aminolevulinic acid synthetase are highly sensitive to the action of toxic trace metals (111–114,116) with resultant increases in the urinary excretion of

porphyrin precursors that have proven to be useful biological indicators of toxicity. Assay procedures for these mitochondrial enzymes have also been extensively described (112) and will not be described here.

The value of measuring mitochondrial heme biosynthetic pathway enzymes rests with determining enzymatic mechanisms for specific chemical-induced porphyrinuria patterns which have widespread use as biological indicators for both organic (101) and inorganic (30) chemicals. Measurement of these enzymes in target tissues such as the liver (101,112,114) and kidney (111,113) has provided valuable insight into the tissue source of the excreted porphyrins which are among the most useful biological indicators available of chemical exposure and toxicity. If other parameters of mitochondrial structure and function are measured (28–32) along with these enzyme activities, then a rather complete picture of the nature and mechanism of the mitochondrial toxicity emerges. In other words, both the biochemical mechanism and tissue/organelle localization of the chemical-induced injury are identified. Since these events usually precede the onset of overt clinical disease, they offer the prospect of detecting target tissue toxicity at an early stage.

Mitochondrial Protein Synthesis

Studies on the synthesis of mitochondrial proteins have been extensively reviewed (13) and may be generally regarded as divisible into two categories: structural and enzymatic. Beattie (3) showed that these two categories of protein could be separated biochemically on the basis of solubility in dilute acetic acid into proteins synthesized within the mitochondria for structural purposes, and those enzymes synthesized outside the mitochondria in the endoplasmic reticulum with subsequent incorporation into the mitochondria.

Mitochondrial protein synthesis studies are essential for determining whether changes in the specific activities of mitochondrial marker enzymes following *in vivo* chemical exposure are the result of a direct chemical–enzyme interaction, a change in the synthesis of that enzyme, or both. We have

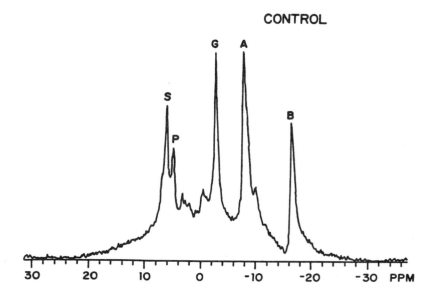

CONTROL

FIG. 4. *In vivo* ^{31}P-NMR spectra from a control rat liver showing three ATP peaks (G, A, B) and inorganic phosphorus (P) and sugar (S) compounds. (Courtesy of Dr. Benjamin Chen.)

also found these studies of value for interpreting structural changes in mitochondria delineated by ultrastructural morphometry. Protein synthesis studies in this organelle are thus extremely valuable for interpreting the results of morphological as well as other biochemical studies.

Techniques

Application of this technique to toxicology studies has shown that prolonged *in vivo* exposure of fetal rat liver mitochondria to methyl mercury produced preferential suppression of membrane but not enzymatic protein synthesis (28). In contrast, exposure of adult rats to arsenate (32) produced an increased synthesis of both protein compartments and morphometric increases in the surface density of the inner mitochondrial membrane. The changes in protein synthesis were associated with increases in the specific activities of the mitochondrial marker enzymes monoamine oxidase cytochrome oxidase and Mg^{+2} ATPase.

Technique—Mitochondrial protein biosynthesis

1. Give the rat an intraperitoneal injection of ^{14}C-leucine (20 μCi) and kill 10 min later.
2. Liver tissue is excised and mitochondria are isolated as described above.
3. Isolated mitochondria are placed in 1.4% acetic acid in capped ultracentrifuge tubes and shaken for 30 min in the cold (4°C).
4. Centrifuge tubes at 90,000 × g for 1 hr to pellet acid-insoluble proteins. Rinse pellet with ice-cold water and suspend in 0.4 N NaOH followed by shaking at 37°C in an incubator until material is dissolved.
5. Pipet supernatant fluid into new centrifuge tubes and neutralize solution while shaking with 2 N NaOH.
6. Centrifuge solutions at 105,000 × g for 1 hr to pellet acid-soluble proteins.
7. Wash pellet in ice-cold water and suspend in 0.4 N NaOH followed by shaking at 37°C in an incubator until material is dissolved.
8. Pipet 0.2 ml of each fraction into counting vials, add 20 ml of scintillation fluid, shake, and count in a liquid scintillation counter.

Conformation Behavior

The technique of following mitochondrial swelling and contraction by measurement of light scattering in a spectrophotometer was developed by Tedeschi and Harris (104). This method is based on the increased optical density of mitochondria in a contracted state and decreased density in a swollen or orthodox configuration due to cation influx. Agents such as arsenic (32) and phosphate (70) produce detectable alterations of swelling and contraction behavior that can be detected by measurement of light scattering at 520 nm. Data from these studies are useful functional tests of mitochondrial membrane integrity following *in vivo* or *in vitro* exposure to a chemical agent. It is also useful for discriminating between high and low amplitude mitochondrial swelling.

Technique

1. Place a solution of 0.12 M KCl in 0.02 M Tris–Cl (pH 7.4) in spectrophotometer cuvettes and add isolated mitochondria to a final concentration of 2 mg/ml.
2. Mitochondrial swelling is measured as a decrease in optical density at 520 nm with time.
3. Maximal swelling is usually achieved by 15 min with liver mitochondria.
4. Initiate contraction of the mitochondria after about 15 min by adding Mg^{+2} + ATP (5 mM), which produces a corresponding increase in the optical density of the sample to near its original reading.

Ion Translocation by Specific Ion Electrode

During mitochondrial respiration or changes in conformation, the transport of H^+, Na^+, K^+, or Ca^{+2} occurs (76,82,84). Movement of these cations between isolated mitochondria and the surrounding medium may be monitored by specific ion electrodes as described in a review by Pressman (84) that contains specific details for application of this technique. Application of this approach to measuring mitochondrial membrane functionality following exposure to mercurials (6,60) and lead (83) has provided useful information about the nature of mercury–mitochondrial membrane interactions. Other studies have shown energy-dependent mitochondrial uptake of arsenic. Data from such investigations are highly useful in more specifically delineating which ion transport systems are altered by agents which affect mitochondrial membrane integrity.

LYSOSOMES

Lysosomes are spherical structures that play a central role in the storage and catabolism of many substances. Biochemically, these organelles are characterized by the presence of several acid hydrolases. In terms of understanding the impact of toxicants on this organelle system, it is useful to discern the various categories of lysosomes by both ultrastructural and biochemical techniques.

Ultrastructural Techniques

Cytochemistry

Active lysosomes (secondary lysosomes) may be cytochemically distinguished from inactive (teleolysosomes) or autophagic vacuoles by the presence of acid phosphatase activity (Fig. 5). This technique gives a clear demonstration of this enzyme activity provided development time of the reaction is carefully monitored to minimize spurious or nonspecific deposition of lead–phosphate reaction product. Though the technique is largely qualitative, it does provide

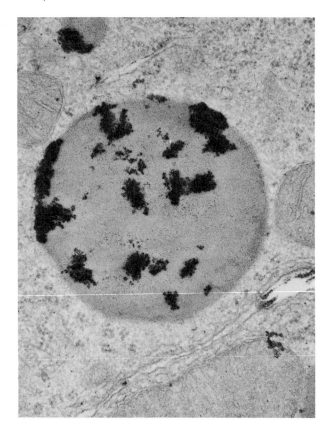

FIG. 5. Cytochemical demonstration of acid phosphatase activity at the electron microscope level showing positive (dense, lead phosphate precipitate) over a secondary lysosome in a renal proximal tubule cell of a rat exposed to methyl mercury in its drinking water. ×46,000.

essential information for delineating lysosomes from other subcellular structures.

Technique—Histochemical determination of acid phosphatase

1. Remove tissue under light ether anesthesia.
2. Cut into thick (2–3 mm) slices on plate of dental wax.
3. Fix at approximately 4°C for 2–3 hr in 2.5% glutaraldehyde in 0.1 M Na–cacodylate buffer containing 7.5% sucrose. Final pH 7.1 or standard glutaraldehyde–formaldehyde fixative described above.
4. Rinse slices in cold Na–cacodylate buffer, pH 7.4, containing 0.33 M sucrose.
5. Transfer pieces to stage of tissue chopper and cut 10–50-μ sections.
6. Collect in cold Na–cacodylate, pH 7.4, containing 0.33 M sucrose.
7. Rinse 20 min to 2 hr in two changes of sucrose buffer.
8. Warm Gomori medium to 60°C for 1 hr; cool to room temperature for 4 min, filter through one piece of Whatman #1.
9. Incubate sections 15 min to 2 hr at 37°C in medium (depending on reactivity of tissue).
10. Rinse twice for 1 min in cold 0.05 M acetate buffer, pH 5.0, containing 7.5% sucrose and 4% formaldehyde.
11. For light-microscopic monitoring of reaction development, expose sections to $(NH_4)_2S$ [two drops of 45% $(NH_4)_2S$ in 10 ml H_2O].
12. Transfer to glass slides and mount in water-soluble embedding medium.
13. For electron microscopy: post fix for 30–60 min in 1% O_sO_4 in acetate–veronal buffer, pH 7.4, containing 49 mg/ml sucrose.
14. Rapidly dehydrate starting with 70% ethanol.
15. Embed in plastic resin as described above.

Gomori medium

1. 0.12 g $Pb(NO_3)_2$.
2. 100 ml 0.05 M NaAc buffer, pH 5.0, containing 7.5% sucrose.
3. Add slowly with gentle mixing, 10 ml of 3% sodium-β-glycero phosphate or cytidine monophosphate (CMP).

Glutaraldehyde fixative

1. 0.1 M Cacodylate buffer, pH 7.4, 97.5 ml, containing 7.5% sucrose.
2. Ultrapure glutaraldehyde (70%), 2.5 ml.

Buffer rinse

1. 0.1 M Cacodylate buffer, pH 7.4, containing 0.33 M sucrose (11.2%).

Formaldehyde rinse

1. 0.05 M Acetate buffer, pH 5.0, 40 ml.
2. 37% Formaldehyde (formalin solution), 10 ml 7.5 g sucrose.

Acetate buffer

1. 15 ml N HCl.
2. 50 ml N NaAc.
3. Adjust to pH 5.0; dilute to 1300 ml.

Localization of Substances Within Lysosomes

There are several ultrastructural techniques available for demonstrating the presence of particular substances within lysosomes of intact cells. X-ray microanalysis (Fig. 6) has been used by several investigators (10,24,27,36,100) to demonstrate the presence of toxic trace metals within lysosomes following in vivo exposure. This method essentially utilizes the focused electron beam of the electron microscope to displace orbital electrons from the atoms present in the sample with resultant generation of characteristic X-rays from within

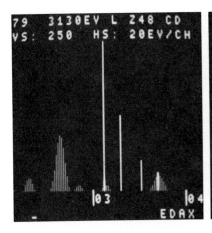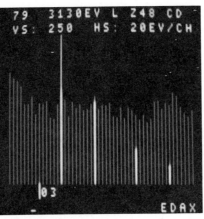

FIG. 6. Energy-dispersive X-ray spectrum from a renal proximal tubule lysosome of a rat injected with 0.6 mg/kg cadmium (Cd) as Cd-metallothionein before (*left*) and following (*right*) background subtraction. The presence of a Cd L$_\alpha$ X-ray peak (3.13 keV) is indicated by the first vertical marker bar.

the sample that are separated by wave-length or energy dispersive techniques. Major problems with the technique for analysis of biological samples are related to extraction or translocation of elements during tissue processing (45), volatilization of elements by specimen heating (10), and detection of elements within biological thin sections due to insufficient excitation or low concentrations of the elements within the tissue (45). The obvious chief advantage to this technique is that it provides a clear means of placing the toxic element of concern in structures such as lysosomes within target cell populations, thus providing evidence that could not be readily generated by subcellular fractionation studies.

Techniques—X-ray Microanalysis (thin section: ≤2500 Å)

1. Section blocks of tissue embedded for electron microscopy (as described above) at 2500 Å or less using an ultramicrotome. Place on carbon-coated grids made of carbon, beryllium, or some other element with X-ray emission lines different from those in the sample to be analyzed.
2. Place sample grid in specimen holder of transmission or scanning electron microscope fitted with energy dispersive or wave-length dispersive spectrometers.
3. Perform X-ray microanalysis of lysosomes (or other organelles of interest) by condensing the electron beam onto the site to be analyzed and monitoring the elemental X-rays generated.
4. Problems associated with extraction of elements from the tissue during fixation, dehydration, and embedding may be circumvented to some degree by use of cryosectioning of frozen samples and liquid nitrogen-cooled cold stages.
5. Vaporization of elements by specimen-heating from the condensed electron beam may be dealt with to some degree by altering the accelerating voltage of the electron microscope and reducing counting times.
6. A more complete description of this technique and the available instrumentation has been given elsewhere (45).

Ultrastructural Autoradiography

Autoradiography of compounds labeled with ^{125}I or ^{3}H is another sensitive tool that requires great care in application

due to translocation of label and insufficient grain development. This technique has been successfully applied to detection of proteins within lysosomes of intact cells to show uptake into this cellular compartment. At the light microscope level, lysosomal uptake of fluorescent dyes has been demonstrated by fluorescence microscopy (1). Histochemical staining methods (8) have also been used to demonstrate lysosomal uptake of metals in cells of metal-exposed animals. These techniques like X-ray microanalysis provide useful approaches for localizing chemicals of interest in lysosomes of target cell populations.

Ultrastructural Morphometry

In terms of quantitating *in vivo* changes in the lysosomal compartment, ultrastructural morphometry has been employed to evaluate changes in the lysosome system with prolonged methyl mercury (25) and age (15) and cadmium metallothionein (99). Application of this method to lysosomes is subject to some of the same constraints and limitations noted previously for mitochondria.

Biochemical Methods

Isolation procedures for lysosomes by centrifugation are given in Fig. 1 and have been extensively described elsewhere (94). Changes in lysosomal sedimentation characteristics have been reported (18) following loading with metals such as iron. This effect as well as alterations of lysosomal membrane stability (59) should be carefully considered when evaluating lysosomes in toxicity studies. In addition, consideration should also be given to distribution of lysosomes within different cell types within a given organ since not all cells will be equally affected.

Lysosomal Protein Degradation

Protein degradation by lysosomes has been monitored by following release of ^{125}I from labeled protein following either *in vitro* (72–75) or *in vivo* (68) incubations. *In vitro* exposure of lysosomes to agents such as toxic metals (68,72,74) or mycotoxins (75) has been found to alter the ability of lysosomes to perform this basic function.

Marker Enzyme Assays

Measurement of the various acid hydrolase activities found in lysosomes is another means for assessing lysosome functionality. As noted in Fig. 3, these assays are frequently performed on lysed lysosomes so that activities of the lysosomal enzymes may be more clearly separated from those present in the microsomal fraction. Marker enzymes frequently measured are the cathepsin A, B, C, and D (94), acid phosphatase, aryl sulfatase, glycosidases, and acid RNAase. Exposure of animals by intravenous injection of protein (66–67) activates a number of the above enzymes in kidney lysosomes. As with the protein degradation procedure, these assays provide essential information about changes in lysosome functionality following chemical exposure. The metabolic consequences of lysosomal enzyme inhibition are varied but may include proteinuria or a number of lysosomal storage diseases.

Techniques

Acid phosphatase assay

1. 0.1 ml 0.004 M Citrate buffer, pH 4.8.
2. 0.1 ml p-Nitrophenylphosphate 100 mg/25 ml (kept frozen).
3. 0.1 ml Enzyme extract.
4. Incubate at 37°C for various times.
5. Stop reaction by adding 5 ml and 0.2 M glycine, pH 10.4.
6. Centrifuge in tabletop centrifuge for 5 min.
7. Read optical density at 405 nm.
8. Report specific activity in terms of nmoles/min/mg.
9. Prepare standard curve of OD_{405} versus nmoles p-nitrophenol/5.4 ml of reaction mixture.

Cathepsin D assay

1. 1.0 ml 0.2 M Acetate, pH 4.5.
2. 0.5 ml 2% Hemoglobin.
3. Add 0.5 ml enzyme solution.
4. Incubate at 37°C for 1 hr.
5. Stop reaction by adding 8 ml 5% TCA.
6. Centrifuge at 1400 rpm for 5 min.
7. Read at 280 nm.
8. Report specific activity as ΔOD_{280}/mg protein.

RNAase assay

1. 0.2 ml 0.03 M Acetate–0.15 M NaCl, pH 5.8.
2. 0.1 ml Homogenate.
3. 0.1 ml H_2O.
4. 0.2 ml 1% RNA.

The reaction mixture is shaken at 37°C for 20 min. After incubation the tubes are placed in ice. To precipitate the protein and RNA, add 0.9 ml of a mixture of 10 volumes of 76% ethanol in 1 N HCl and 1 volume of 0.75% uranyl acetate in 2.5 N $HClO_4$. After allowing the mixture to stand for 10 min, centrifuge at $1000 \times g$ for 10 min. The absorbance of a 1:10 dilution of each supernatant is read at 260 nm. Specific activity is reported as ΔOD_{260}/min/mg. *Caution: The RNA is unstable and needs to be prepared just before use to prevent high reading in the blank.*

β-Glucuronidase assay using p-nitrophenyl-β-glucuronide as the substrate

1. 1.0 ml 0.2 M Acetate, pH 5.0.
2. 0.6 ml p-Nitrophenyl β-D-glucuronide (15 mM).
3. 0.2 ml Lysosomal protein.
4. Incubate at 37°C for 15–30 min.
5. Stop the reaction by adding 3 ml 0.2 M glycine, pH 10.4.
6. Centrifuge in tabletop centrifuge for 5 min.
7. Read at 405 nm.
8. Obtain nmoles of p-nitrophenol from standard curve.
9. Report activity in terms of nmoles/min/mg of protein.

ENDOPLASMIC RETICULUM

The endoplasmic reticulum is comprised of a complex pattern of membranes or cisternae that permeates the cytoplasmic matrix, and the centrifugal fraction containing fragmented endoplasmic reticulum is called the microsomal fraction. Two distinct forms of endoplasmic reticulum have been characterized by histological as well as biochemical and centrifugal techniques. The rough endoplasmic reticulum (RER) is a complex of granular basophilic membranes distinguished by extensive ribosomal units on the outer surface of the membrane. In mammals, the RER forms layered stacks of cisternae. The smooth endoplasmic reticulum (SER) is essentially agranular and forms a myriad of branching interconnecting tubules extending to all areas of the cytoplasmic matrix. In general, protein synthesis occurs in the RER, whereas the SER functions in protein transport and glycogen storage. Both the RER and SER function in drug metabolism as evidenced by the detection of bioactivation/detoxification enzyme systems in both microsomal subfractions.

The heterogeneous microsomal fraction is commonly employed to assess the capacity of the endoplasmic reticulum to bioactivate and/or detoxify a variety of foreign chemicals, as well as some endogenous compounds such as the steroid hormones. The role that microsomal enzymes play in chemical toxicity is extremely difficult to evaluate since a single enzyme system might activate or deactivate a chemical depending on the molecular structure of the chemical, animal age (state of development or differentiation), site of metabolism (as related to organ-specific toxicity), and interactions with other chemicals (potentiation or antagonism). To study microsomal metabolism of chemicals, standard techniques are employed to prepare heterogeneous microsomal fractions or to separate SER and RER. Much of the information presented in this section will deal with hepatic microsomal function because of the wealth of methodological information available for this tissue. However, the relative lack of time spent on extrahepatic tissues should not detract from the contribution of extrahepatic pathways to pharmacokinetics and toxic reactions.

Ultrastructural Methods

Ultrastructural Morphometry

The surface area or more precisely the surface density (S_v) of smooth and rough endoplasmic reticulum may be estimated by application of morphometric techniques to intact cell (99,104,105). This approach has been used to quantitate changes in the endoplasmic reticulum of hepatocytes following exposure of rats to phenobarbital (99). Studies of this type provide useful *in situ* correlations with the biochemical evaluations of microsomal enzyme preparations described below, as well as a means for estimating membrane recoveries from intact cells (4,6). The labor-intensive nature discussed in reference to the mitochondria above also applies to surface density (S_v) measurements of the endoplasmic reticulum but the data generated have proven extremely useful in interpreting changes in microsomal enzyme activities produced by metals such as indium (26) and thallium (26,115,117).

Ultrastructural Evaluation of Microsomal Fractions

Ultrastructural examination of microsomal fractions may be conducted to assess the purity of the preparation in a manner similar to that previously described for mitochondria. Fixation, dehydration, and embedding procedures for microsomal pellets are essentially similar to those used for other organelle fractions. The value of these procedures for assessing relative microsomal purity and determining the efficiency of RER and SER centrifugal separations cannot be understated.

Biochemical Methods

Preparation of Microsomes

Standard method

The most common method used to prepare microsomes from a variety of tissues involves tissue and cell disruption followed by differential centrifugation. A general procedure for rat liver is as follows:

1. Liver is removed, minced, and homogenized in 1.15% KCl buffered with 0.02 M *N*-2-hydroxyethylpiperazine-*N*-2-ethane-sulfonic acid (HEPES), pH 7.5, at 5°C to make a 20% (w/v) mixture. Homogenization is accomplished by using six strokes in a motor-driven Potter-Elvehjem homogenizer.
2. Nuclei and cell debris are removed by centrifugation at $670 \times g$ for 10 min.
3. Mitochondria are removed by centrifugation of the 670-g supernatant fluid at $10,000 \times g$ for 15 min.
4. Microsomes are pelleted by centrifugation of the postmitochondrial supernatant fluid at $105,000 \times g$ for 60 min, washed once with HEPES-KCl buffer, and finally resuspended in the buffer so that 1.0 ml of microsomal

suspension contains material from 0.5 g liver (wet wt). The 10,000-g pellet can be homogenized by hand and recentrifuged to avoid loss of microsomes in unbroken cells and sedimented microsomal vesicles.

There are some points that need to be considered when experimental protocols are being developed. For example, depending on the tissue, microsomal fragments may pellet with the nuclear or mitochondrial fraction. Although it appears that extramicrosomal drug metabolism does occur (20,50,54), many researchers have mistakenly reported the subcellular distribution of microsomal enzymes because of tissue differences in fragmentation of the endoplasmic reticulum. Preliminary experimentation must therefore include a thorough examination of the effect of various disruption techniques (homogenization, sonication, etc.) on the disruption of the endoplasmic reticulum.

Calcium aggregation method

Recently, a new method was developed to prepare microsomes from rat liver that does not require ultracentrifugation (56,91,92). This procedure results in aggregation of microsomes following the addition of Ca^{2+} ions to the postmitochondrial supernatant fluid. In addition to eliminating the need for an ultracentrifuge, this method greatly reduces the time needed to prepare microsomes. The procedure is outlined as follows:

1. Liver is removed, minced, and homogenized in 10 mM Tris HCl containing 250 mM sucrose, pH 7.4, to make a 20% (w/v) mixture. Homogenization is accomplished by using six strokes in a motor-driven Potter–Elvehjem homogenizer.
2. Nuclei and cell debris are removed by centrifugation at $670 \times g$ for 10 min.
3. Mitochondria are removed by centrifugation of the 670-g supernatant fluid at $10,000 \times g$ for 15 min.
4. Solid $CaCl_2$ is added to the postmitochondrial supernatant fluid to achieve a final concentration of 8 mM. The suspension is stirred and the microsomes pelleted by centrifugation at $25,000 \times g$ for 15 min.
5. The microsomal pellet is resuspended in 150 mM KCl–10 mM Tris HCl, pH 7.4, and centrifuged at $25,000 \times g$ for 15 min, which sediments the washed microsomal pellet.

Many studies have compared the activities of microsomal enzymes prepared by the two methods. In general, specific activities of rat liver microsomes were similar in preparations derived by either method (92). However, the calcium aggregation method cannot be applied to all tissues or species. Researchers have found markedly different enzyme activities in preparations derived by the two methods as a function of species and tissue. These findings emphasize the need to determine whether the calcium aggregation method is a viable method before applying it to preparation of microsomes from a source other than rat liver.

Although many xenobiotics induce the specific activity of microsomal enzymes, these chemicals do not generally cause great changes in total microsomal protein content. However, some changes do occur in the relative distribution of SER and RER, and significant changes also occur in SER:RER specific activity ratios of enzymes. For example, the potent inducing agent 2,3,7,8-tetrachlorodibenzo-p-dioxin (TCDD) reduces the SER:RER activity ratio for aminopyrine demethylation, benzo[a]pyrene hydroxylation, p-nitrophenol glucuronidation, and microsomal protein (62). These biochemical and pharmacological changes are associated with concomitant alterations in the cellular distribution of SER and RER in hepatocytes following *in vivo* exposure to TCDD as well as to a wide range of organohalogens, some of which are hepatotoxins.

The following discontinuous sucrose gradient method is commonly used to isolate SER from RER in liver (16):

1. Liver is homogenized in 0.25 M sucrose to make a 20% (w/v) mixture.
2. The postmitochondrial supernatant fluid is prepared as described earlier in this section.
3. 2.0 ml 1.3 M Sucrose (not containing CsCl) is added to a centrifuge tube.
4. 0.5 ml 0.6 M Sucrose (also not containing CsCl) is layered on the heavy sucrose.
5. The postmitochondrial supernatant fluid is made 15 mM with respect to CsCl and 4.0 ml of the suspension layered above the 0.6 M sucrose. The three-layered system is then centrifuged at $105,000 \times g$ for 90 min. The RER is pelleted at the bottom of the centrifuge tube and the SER forms a band at the top of the 1.3 M sucrose.
6. The SER fraction can be aspirated off and pelleted by dilution with buffer and centrifugation at $105,000 \times g$ for 60 min.

Several other methods are available to further subfractionate SER and RER including rate-differential centrifugation and isopycnic density gradient centrifugation (16).

In Vitro *Methods for Evaluating Microsomal Function*

Isolated organs

Although the use of isolated microsomes has many advantages in the characterization of individual enzyme systems and the quantitation of the response of these systems to inducers, inhibitors, or repressors, it is difficult to develop a good pharmacokinetic model using such preparations. Accordingly, many investigators have used isolated perfused organs to evaluate the complex interrelationships among heterogeneous cell types, different metabolic pathways, variations in substrate concentrations, and time–course relationships. This system represents an open metabolic system capable of generating important information in "steady state" pharmacokinetics. Several organ systems have been used extensively including the liver, lung, intestine, kidney, and testes. Detailed methods for conducting isolated organ studies have been reviewed by Sies (95) and Mehendale (*this Volume*).

Isolated cells

The use of isolated hepatocytes as an experimental model to study drug biotransformations and toxicity has increased over the past few years. Isolated cells are often selected as an experimental model to study microsomal function because they provide a reasonable intermediate between perfused organ systems and preparation of subcellular organelles and reconstituted systems. Now that many of the technical problems have been resolved for the isolation and maintenance of isolated hepatocytes, it is possible to use this system to investigate the activity and products of complex bioactivation/detoxication enzyme systems and also to investigate, in a more precise way, organelle interactions that might qualitatively and/or quantitatively alter the metabolic capacity of microsomal enzyme systems. References (40,77) are available that detail and summarize procedures for evaluating metabolism and toxicity in isolated cells.

Of particular importance is the requirement that (a) the cells remain viable for a sufficient period of time to evaluate a biochemical or pharmacological parameter and (b) the isolated cells retain the characteristics and functions present *in vivo*. Cell viability is commonly determined by the trypan blue exclusion test or by leakage of cytosolic enzymes (indication of membrane dysfunction or damage) such as lactate dehydrogenase into the cell-free medium (77). Following the maintenance of isolated hepatocytes for relatively long periods of time (more than 2 days), liver cells have been reported to revert to a more fetal form (97). The relative contribution of fetal type cells can be monitored by biochemical indicators such as α-fetoprotein, alkaline phosphatase, and λ-glutamyl transpeptidase. Although most studies are conducted on liver cells, other organ systems can be investigated by analogous techniques.

Isolated cells, in general, seem to provide an excellent experimental model to study microsomal activation/deactivation of chemicals and the subsequent reactivity of metabolites to cellular macromolecules such as DNA, RNA, and protein, and thereby allow the investigator to gain insight into the mechanisms to toxicity of some carcinogens, mutagens, teratogens, and organ-specific toxins.

MICROSOMAL ACTIVATION/DEACTIVATION SYSTEMS

Microsomal Cytochromes

The endoplasmic reticulum contains a series of flavoproteins and cytochromes that function in electron transport, ultimately resulting in the activation and reduction of molecular oxygen. An enormous number of studies have focused on the behavior and characterization of cytochrome P-450, a microsomal cytochrome, which functions in oxidative biotransformation reactions such as epoxide formation, hydroxylation of aromatics N-hydroxylation, C-hydroxylation, N-dealkylation, O-dealkylation of xenobiotics, and many endogenous compounds such as the steroid hormones and fatty acids. The enzymes catalyzing these reactions are cytochrome P-450-dependent and are collectively termed mixed-function oxidases (MFO). A schematic representation of P-450-dependent oxidations is presented in Figs. 7 and 8.

The function of the cytochrome P-450 system involves a series of sequential reactions: (a) the formation of a substrate–ferric heme complex; (b) flavoprotein NADPH–cytochrome P-450 reductase mediated reduction of this complex; (c) for-

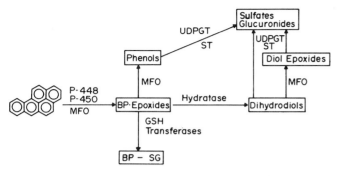

FIG. 7. Metabolic pathways for benzo[a]pyrene. BP, benzo[a]pyrene; MFO, mixed function oxidases; GSH, glutathionine; UDPGT, UDP glucuronyl transferase; ST, sulfotransferase; BP-SG, glutathione conjugate of benzo[a]pyrene. (From ref. 61a, with permission.)

mation of an oxycytochrome P-450 substrate complex following interaction of oxygen with reduced heme protein; (d) activation of oxygen for interaction with the organic substrate; and (e) dissociation of the less lipophilic product and regeneration of the ferric heme protein. (See ref. 35 for more detail on the nature and function of this system.) The net effect of this series of coupled reactions is the generation of a metabolite less lipophilic than the parent compound and therefore more excretable. However, electrophilic, reactive, and highly toxic metabolites can also be formed by this system.

Determination of P-450 by Difference Spectra

The most common method of measuring cytochrome P-450 content of a microsomal preparation is by the appearance of an absorbance band at 450 nm for the CO adduct of the reduced cytochrome. The procedure is as follows:

1. Dilute the microsomal suspension with the homogenizing buffer to achieve a protein concentration of approximately 1.5 mg/ml.
2. The baseline of equal light absorbance is determined by placing equal volumes of diluted microsomal suspension into two cuvettes.
3. Gently gas the sample cuvette with CO, and record the spectrum that quantifies oxyhemoglobin contamination.
4. Add sodium dithionite (about 1 mg solid) to the sample cuvette, and record the difference spectrum of the CO adduct of the reduced cytochrome P-450.
5. Add sodium dithionite to the reference cuvette, and record the difference spectrum of the CO complex of reduced cytochrome P-450 minus the spectral contribution of reduced cytochrome P-450.
6. Convert the change in absorbance at 450 nm relative to 490 nm to cytochrome P-450 concentration using a millimolar extinction coefficient of 91.

Administration of many compounds such as phenobarbital to intact animals results in induced levels of cytochrome P-450. Exposure to another class of chemicals, such as the polycyclic hydrocarbons, results in induced levels of a closely related cytochrome, P-448. This change in absorbance maximum can be detected by sophisticated double-beam spectrophotometers. Lists of those chemicals that selec-

tively induce P-450 (phenobarbital type) or P-448 (3-methylcholanthrene type) are provided elsewhere (14,37).

In addition to measurement of cytochrome P-450 content, difference spectra are also used to study substrate interactions with cytochrome P-450 and to investigate mechanisms of inhibition of mixed function oxidation reactions. Depending on the substrate, three types of spectral interactions can be detected *in vitro:* Type I spectral change, which is characterized by a peak at 385 nm and a trough at 420 nm; Reverse-Type I spectral change, which is the mirror image of Type I spectral change; and Type II spectral change, which is characterized by a broad trough between 390 and 410 nm and a peak between 425 and 435 nm (91).

Detection of Hemoproteins by SDS Gels

During recent years convincing evidence has accumulated to support the idea that microsomal cytochrome P-450 consists of multiple forms. Several hemoproteins have been detected using a variety of electrophoresis techniques (89,108). Analysis of hemoprotein profiles has provided considerable insight into the ability of chemicals to selectively induce or repress specific forms of microsomal hemoproteins.

Reconstituted and Purified Systems

The use of crude microsomal preparations allows only limited characterization of individual components in the complex sequences of reactions involved in cytochrome P-450-dependent oxidative reactions. To better understand the nature of this system, researchers have utilized a variety of techniques to purify individual components of the system and to reconstitute the electron transport chain (48,88). Prior to purification of the cytochrome P-448 system, animals are induced with 3-methycholanthrene or an appropriate P-448 inducer, whereas greater yields of P-450 can be obtained using phenobarbital-treated rats. Using purification/reconstitution techniques, basic differences have been observed in microsomal hemoproteins of different species and from different tissues of the same species.

Synthesis/Degradation of Hemoproteins

One common method used to study the turnover characteristics of hepatic hemoproteins involves pulse-labeling of the heme moiety with ^{3}H-δ-aminolevulinic acid, partially

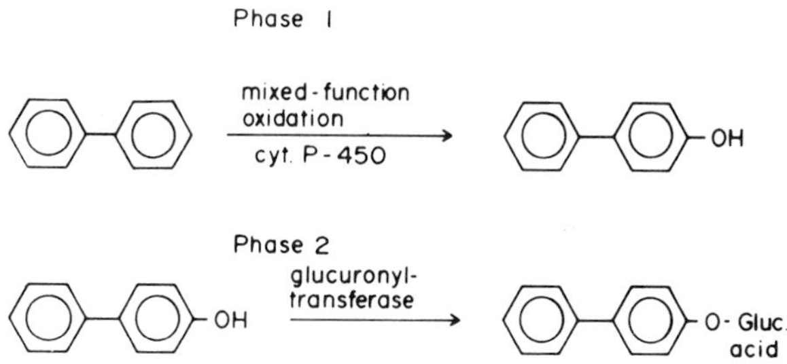

FIG. 8. Schematic representation of glucuronidation of hydroxylated biphenyl. (From ref. 61a, with permission.)

purifying (removal of the other microsomal cytochrome, b_5) the CO-binding particles (P-450) and measuring synthesis/degradation characteristics of the cytochrome. These kinds of studies have identified a fast-phase component and a slow-phase component of P-450, and each component exhibits selective responses to inducive or repressive agents (63) and is age- and sex-dependent.

Other Methods

In addition to the methods described above, basic information on P-450–substrate interactions has been generated using electron spin resonance spectroscopy (87) and immunochemical techniques (118).

Microsomal Enzymes

Cytochrome P-450-Dependent Enzymes

One of the most common assays is oxidative demethylation using aminopyrine, ethylmorphine, or benzphetamine as the substrate. This method measures the production of formaldehyde which is an intermediate in oxidative demethylation reactions (107). The assays for aminopyrine as the substrate is conducted as follows:

1. Add buffer (50 mM Tris–HCl, pH 7.5, 1.5 ml) to incubation tube.
2. Add saturating levels of NADPH (3.1 mM) in 0.5 ml Tris buffer.
3. The incubation medium is made 20 mM with respect to $MgCl_2$.
4. Add ammopyrine to achieve a substrate concentration of 2.5 mM.
5. After prewarming the incubation contents to 37°C, initiate the reaction by adding approximately 0.5–1.5 mg microsomal protein.
6. After a 10-min incubation, stop the reaction by adding 1.0 ml 10% trichloroacetic acid.
7. Sediment the protein by low-speed centrifugation, and add 2 ml of supernatant fluid to 1 ml of NASH reagent (2 M ammonium acetate, 0.05 M acetic acid, 0.02 M acetylacetone).
8. Heat the solution for 8 min at 60°C. Measure the formaldehyde concentration at 405 nm and read against a standard curve. Blank values are obtained by omitting microsomes from the incubation medium.

The reaction rate is linear with respect to time and microsomal protein under these incubation conditions, although each investigator should assess these parameters as part of preliminary investigations. Ethylmorphine and benzphetamine demethylation rates can be determined using the same method. A radiolabel assay has been devised for aminopyrine demethylation that can be used when increased sensitivity is required to detect low enzyme activity as a function of tissue, developmental stage, or toxic or disease state (85).

Cytochrome P-448-Dependent Enzymes

Aryl hydrocarbon hydroxylase (AHH) is an indicator of P-448 function. AHH is often used as an indicator of the capacity of biological systems to form reactive electrophilic metabolites, which are frequently in the form of arene oxide intermediates produced in hydroxylation reactions. However, AHH assays often are a measure of total hydroxylated or polar metabolites and are not necessarily indicative of metabolic activation. For example, polycyclic hydrocarbons such as benzo[a]pyrene produce large numbers of microsomal oxidative metabolites possessing widely different capacities for binding to cellular macromolecules in in vitro systems. Information on the rates of formation of specific active metabolites capable of eliciting biochemical lesions is needed to achieve a valid toxicokinetic evaluation. However, such a definitive evaluation is not feasible for each toxicant. Therefore, determinations of AHH activity by using benzypyrene, biphenyl, or another suitable substrate may provide approximate data on the capacity of some biological systems to activate some substrates (those activated by the microsomal monooxygenase system).

A general scheme illustrating benzo[a]pyrene metabolism is presented in Fig. 7. AHH can be measured by a fluorometric method as described below:

1. Add buffer (50 mM Tris–HCl, pH 7.5, 0.075 ml) to incubation vessel.
2. Add benzpyrene suspension (0.25 ml, 60 mM in 2.5% carboxymethyl-cellulose).
3. Add microsomes (0.25 ml) so that the final incubation medium contains approximately 1 mg protein/ml.
4. Equilibrate the reaction mixture at 37°C for 3 min and initiate the reaction by adding 0.25 ml NADPH solution to achieve a concentration of 3.1 mM in the incubation medium.
5. After 10 min, stop the reaction by adding 2 ml ice-cold acetone.
6. Add hexane (20 ml) to stoppered 45-ml shaking tubes.
7. Wash the incubation mixtures into the shaking tubes with water (three times with 0.5 ml).
8. Shake the tubes 10 min and store overnight at 4°C or freeze.
9. Centrifuge the tubes for 15 min at $600 \times g$.
10. Transfer the hexane layer (upper 15 ml) by pipette to a clean 45-ml shaking tube.
11. Add NaOH (5 ml, 0.1 M) and shake the tubes for 10 min followed by centrifugation for 10 min.
12. Read fluorescence of the aqueous layer (excitation 400 nm; emission 525 nm). Determine the concentration of phenolic metabolites by using 3-hydroxybenzpyrene as the standard.

In addition to the fluorometric assay for AHH, a radioactive assay is available (17) that uses ^{3}H-benzopyrene as the substrate. For those investigators who wish to avoid carcinogenic substrates, a direct fluorometric method with 7-ethoxyresorufin as the substrate is available (71). This assay method is an extremely good indicator of cytochrome P-448 levels. Another fluorometric method, that has the advantage of simultaneously measuring biphenyl-2-hydroxylase (P-448-dependent) and biphenyl-4-hydroxylase (P-450-dependent), is available (9). Epoxide hydrase is an important microsomal enzyme system that functions in the deactivation of reactive epoxides/arene oxides and can be measured by the method of Oesch (81).

The scientific value of measuring the above enzyme systems rests with gathering information about changes in the functional activity of metabolic systems which are capable of activating a host of endogenous and xenobiotic organic chemicals. Changes in the activity of these enzymes produced by one agent may also greatly influence the subsequent toxicity of another which is either activated or inactivated by these enzyme systems. The value of such measurements is hence greatly increased under conditions where mixtures of chemicals are present.

Toxicant–Receptor Interactions

The findings that (a) some xenobiotics selectively induce cytochrome P-448-dependent enzymes; (b) precise structure–activity relationships can be described for selective induction; and (c) some inducers are extremely potent suggested that polycyclic hydrocarbons such as 3-MC and TCDD may initiate their inductive actions by interaction with a cytosolic receptor protein in a manner analogous to steroid hormone action. Researchers have characterized such a receptor (86), which has a finite capacity, pronounced selectively, high dissociation constant, and the ligand–receptor complex appears to undergo nuclear translocation. The receptor was characterized using high specific activity ^{3}H-TCDD.

Microsomal Conjugative Enzymes

On simplification, and depending on the chemical substrate, the drug biotransformation process may be divided into two parts: first, an oxidative reaction, such as hydroxylation, that results in the formation of a free hydroxyl group; this is then rapidly conjugated with glucuronic acid, sulfate, or another conjugate as indicated in Fig. 8. This series of reactions renders the molecule more polar and generally more excretable and less toxic. However, conjugation reactions may also function in the formation of reactive electrophilic intermediates.

UDP Glucuronyltransferase

One of the more important routinely measured conjugative enzymes is UDP glucuronyltransferase. This enzyme system appears to consist of multiple forms, and it functions in the metabolism/excretion of many endogenous compounds (i.e., steroid hormones) as well as xenobiotics. Recent evidence has demonstrated functional (64) as well as biochemical heterogeneity (4) of UDP glucuronyltransferase. Depending on molecular structure, substrates appear to be conjugated either by Group I or Group II glucuronyltransferase. A general method of measuring p-nitrophenol glucuronidation (Group I) is shown below:

1. Incubation medium contains 1.5 mM UDPGA (cofactor), 0.5 mM MgCl$_2$, 0.8 mM p-nitrophenol (substrate) in 1.4 ml 40 mM Tris–HCl, pH 7.5.
2. Warm the incubation mixture at 37°C for 3 min.
3. Start the reaction by adding 0.25–1.0 mg Triton X-100-activated microsomes. Microsomal suspensions are activated prior to addition to the incubation medium by mixing 0.2 μl Triton X-100/mg microsomal protein.
4. The reaction is stopped by adding 5.0 ml 0.2 M glycine buffer containing 0.15 M NaCl, pH 10.4.
5. Measure p-nitrophenol concentration spectrophotometrically at 405 nm. Blank values are obtained by omitting UDPGA from the reaction medium.

Group II substrates can be measured by a rapid radiometric method (65). This procedure is especially useful for the study of steroid conjugation reactions.

The incubation system for glucuronidation measurements is added to liquid scintillation vials and consists of the following: 1.2 ml 75 mM Tris–HCl buffer (pH 7.4), 1.0 μmol UDPGA, 10.0 μmol unlabeled substrate in 50 μl methanol and 1×10^5 dpm-labeled substrate in 50 μl methanol. This volume of methanol is used to insure substrate solubilization and has no apparent effect on glucuronyltransferase activity. The incubation contents are warmed at 37°C for 3 min, and then 0.4–0.6 mg microsomal protein is added. The incubation period is approximately 10 min. The reaction is stopped by the addition of 10 ml nonaqueous scintillation fluid prepared by mixing 43 ml liquiflour (New England Nuclear) per liter of toluene. Samples are capped, shaken for 10 sec on a vortex mixer, and radioactivity is counted in the same vials in which the incubation reactions are performed. Addition of the toluene-based scintillation fluid results in a two-phase mixture (toluene on top and the aqueous fraction on the bottom). Unreacted substrate partitions into the toluene and this radioactivity is detected in a Packard Tri-Carb liquid scintillation counter equipped with an Automatic Quench Analyzer. Glucuronides remain in the aqueous fraction and, since ^{14}C and ^{3}H in a water medium do not scintillate, radioactivity associated with glucuronides is not detectable by liquid scintillation spectrometry. This phenomenon enables steroid glucuronidation rates to be measured by substrate disappearance. Blank values are obtained by omitting UDPGA from the reaction mediums. The incubation blanks represent 0% activity and correct for the amount of substrate remaining in the aqueous fraction (incubation medium). Glucuronides detected after addition of scintillation fluid to incubation mediums reflect the amount of radioactivity detected after 100% glucuronidation of substrate. Enzyme activity using 300 nmol substrate in the incubation medium is expressed by the equation:

$$1 - \frac{\text{radioactivity after incubation} - \left[\text{radioactivity after incubation} \times \text{fraction of respective } \beta\text{-D-glucuronide detected}\right]}{\text{radioactivity in blank}}$$

$$\times 300 \text{ nmol} = \text{nmol substrate conjugated}$$

This assay procedure is applicable to a wide range of substrates and enzyme reactions in which the polarity of the product is significantly different than the substrates.

Hydrolytic Enzymes

The endoplasmic reticulum also contains a variety of hydrolytic enzymes that exhibit a dual localization in that they are also active in lysosomes. These enzymes include β-glucuronidase (performs the reverse reaction of UDP glucuronidase by liberating the free aglycone from β-D-glucuronic acid conjugates), acid and alkaline phosphatase, and aryl sulfatase. The function of these microsomal enzymes is not clear, although they appear to play a role in the regulation of steroid metabolism and in some cases may represent structural proteins of the endoplasmic reticulum. Bacterial β-glucuronidase plays an important role in the absorption and toxicity of many chemicals including some carcinogens. One possible explanation for the dual localization of these enzyme systems is that they are synthesized in the RER, transported through the membranous cisternae of the SER and fragments of the SER are incorporated into lysomes. Reviews describing the potential role of these lysosomal/microsomal systems are available (44,105). Hydrolytic enzymes such as β-glucuronidase can be detected by histochemical or biochemical methods. One simple method for measuring mammalian β-glucuronidase activity is as follows:

1. The incubation medium contains 1.0 mM substrate (β-D-glucuronide of p-nitrophenol, 4-methylumbelliferone, or phenolphthalein) in 50 mM acetate buffer, pH 4.5.
2. Warm the incubation mixture for 3 min at 37°C.
3. Initiate the reaction by adding 1.0 mg microsomal protein.
4. After a 10-min incubation period, stop the reaction by adding 5 ml glycine buffer (see p-nitrophenol glucuronidation assay).
5. Remove protein by low-speed centrifugation, and measure the formation of the product spectrophotometrically (p-nitrophenol, 405 nm; phenolphthalein, 550 nm; and methylumbelliferone, 365 nm).

The value of measuring conjugation–deconjugation enzyme activities rests with assessing the potential capacity of a cell or organ to deactivate/activate potentially toxic reactive intermediates. While these measurements are an indirect approach to assessing tissue/cell susceptibility to these highly toxic chemical species, the data generated from past studies has proven highly useful toward predicting cellular potential for injury.

PROTEIN SYNTHESIS

Although much of the pharmacological/toxicological research on microsomes focuses on their role in metabolic activation/deactivation reactions, the main function of this organelle involves protein synthesis. Increasingly, researchers are attempting to identify sensitive biochemical indicators of toxicity (usually protein) that have predictive/diagnostic value and also provide insight into the mechanisms of toxic actions of these chemicals. Although a survey of the genetics and molecular biology of protein synthesis is not in the scope of this chapter, there are some general useful methods that can be applied to investigations on the effects of chemicals on overall and/or specific protein synthesis. These methods involve injection of radiolabeled amino acids into intact animals (usually tail vein); the incorporation of radiolabel into specific organelles or specific proteins is then determined. Obviously, protein purification or immunochemical procedures must be undertaken to assess synthesis/degradation of

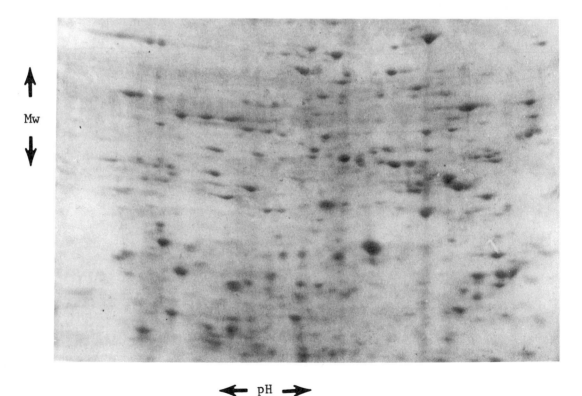

FIG. 9. Coomassie blue stained 2-D gel of rat kidney showing numerous gene product spots.

individual protein. When conducting such pulse-label experiments, it is essential that samples are taken over a wide range of sample periods so that meaningful and valid conclusions can be made concerning alterations either in synthetic or degradative phases for a particular protein. For example, if a toxic chemical selectively alters protein degradation and a pulse label is taken during the synthetic phase, the investigator could miss critical information. If possible, it is desirable to conduct pulse-label experiments with carbon rather than tritium in order to avoid nonspecific redistribution of label during homogenization and purification.

Another method, termed 2-dimensional gel electrophoresis, is being used to determine protein synthesis profiles (51). This procedure involves administration of high specific activity ^{35}S-methionine to intact animals or isolated cells, and the subsequent electrophoretic mapping of labeled proteins by SDS in one direction and isoelectric focusing in the second direction. This procedure is now commonly used in studies investigating the role of specific protein synthesis tissue differences in response to chemical exposure, "stress proteins," and in development and differentiation, and can resolve as many as 1000 proteins (Fig. 9).

PHOSPHOLIPIDS AND LIPOPROTEINS

Phospholipids and lipoproteins provide important permeability properties to membrane structures such as the endoplasmic reticulum. These membrane phospholipids and lipoproteins are synthesized on the endoplasmic reticulum and often play an integral role in enzyme activity by regulating the membrane environment of enzymes that are imbedded in the endoplasmic reticulum. The production of certain forms of lipoproteins seems to be associated with specific toxic and disease states. For example, the relative amount of very low density lipoproteins produced by the liver appears to play a critical role in the development and susceptibility of cardiovascular disease.

Phospholipid and lipoprotein synthesis can be studied by measuring ^{32}P or ^{14}C incorporation into these compounds as outlined earlier in this section (protein synthesis).

REFERENCES

1. Allison, A. C., and Young, M. R. (1964): Uptake of dyes and drugs by living cells in culture. *Life Sci.*, 3:1407–1414.
2. Andrews, P. M., and Hackenbrock, C. R. (1975): A scanning and stereographic ultrastructural analysis of the isolated inner mitochondrial membrane during change in metabolic activity. *Exp. Cell Res.*, 90:127–136.
3. Beattie, D. S. (1968): Studies on the biogenesis of mitochondrial protein components in rat liver slices. *J. Biol. Chem.*, 243:4027–4033.
4. Billings, R. F., Tephly, T. R., and Tukey, R. H. (1978): The separation and purification of estrone and *p*-nitrophenol UDP glucuronyltransferase activities. In: *Conjugation Reactions in Drug Biotransformation*, edited by A. Aitio, pp. 365–376. Elsevier, The Netherlands.
5. Blouin, A., Bolender, R. P., and Weibel, E. R. (1977): Distribution of organelles and membranes between hepatocytes and nonhepatocytes in the rat liver parenchyma: A stereological study. *J. Cell Biol.*, 72:441–455.
6. Bogucka, K., and Wojtczak, L. (1979): On the mechanism of mer-

curial induced permeability of mitochondrial membrane to K$^+$. *FEBS Lett.*, 100:301–304.
7. Bolender, R. P., Paumgartner, D., Losa, G., et al. (1978): Integrated stereological and biochemical studies on hepatocytic membranes. I. Membrane recoveries in subcellular fractions. *J. Cell Biol.*, 77:565–583.
8. Brun, A., and Brunk, U. (1970): Histochemical inducations for lysosomal localization of heavy metals in normal rat brain and liver. *J. Histochem. Cytochem.*, 18:820–827.
9. Burke, M. D., Bridges, J. W., and Parke, D. V. (1975): The effects of nonionic detergent Tween 80 on hepatic microsomal hydroxylation. *Xenobiotica*, 5:261–277.
10. Carmichael, N. G., and Fowler, B. A. (1979): Effects of separate and combined chronic mercuric chloride and sodium selenate administration in rats: Histological, ultrastructural and X-ray microanalytical studies of liver and kidney. *J. Env. Pathol. Toxicol.*, 3:399–412.
11. Cederbaum, A. I., Lieber, C. S., and Rubin, E. (1974): The effect of acetaldehyde on mitochondrial function. *Arch. Biochem. Biophys.*, 161:26–39.
12. Chen, B., Burt, C. T., Goering, P. L., Fowler, B. A., and London, R. E. (1986): *In vivo* ^{31}P nuclear magnetic resonance studies of arsenite-induced changes in hepatic phosphate levels. *Biochem. Biophys. Res. Commun.*, 139:228–234.
13. Christensen, E. I., and Madsen, K. M. (1978): Renal age changes: Observations on the rat kidney cortex with special reference to structure and function of the lysosomal system in the proximal tubule. *Lab. Invest.*, 39:289–297.
14. Chuha, N.-H., and Schmidt, G. W. (1979): Transport of proteins into mitochondria and chloroplasts. *J. Cell Biol.*, 8:461–483.
15. Conney, A. M. (1967): Pharmacological implications of microsomal enzyme induction. *Pharmacol. Rev.*, 19:317–366.
16. Dallner, G. (1978): Isolation of microsomal subfractions by use of density gradients. In: *Methods in Enzymology, Vol. 52, Biomembranes*, Part C, edited by S. Fleischer and L. Packer, pp. 71–83. Academic Press, New York.
17. DePierre, J. W., Moron, M. S., Johannesen, K. A. M., and Ernster, L. (1975): A reliable, sensitive, and convenient radioactive assay for benzpyrene monooxygenase. *Anal. Biochem.*, 63:470–484.
18. Deter, R. L. (1973): Electron microscopic evaluation of subcellular fractions obtained by ultracentrifugation. In: *Principles and Techniques of Electron Microscopy: Biological Applications, Vol. 3*, edited by M. A. Hayat, pp. 199–235. Van Nostrand Reinhold, New York.
19. Estabrook, R. W. (1967): Mitochondrial respiratory control and the polarographic measurement of ADP:O ratios. In: *Methods in Enzymology, Vol. 10*, edited by S. Colowick and N. O. Kaplan, pp. 41–47. Academic Press, New York.
20. Fouts, J. R. (1972): Comments on microsomal hepatic and extrahepatic toxication–detoxication systems. *Environ. Hlth. Perspect.*, 2:55–60.
21. Fowler, B. A., and Woods, J. S. (1977): Ultrastructural and biochemical changes in renal mitochondria during chronic oral methyl mercury exposure: The relationship to renal function. *Exp. Molec. Pathol.*, 27:403–412.
22. Fowler, B. A. (1983): The role of ultrastructural techniques in understanding mechanisms of metal-induced nephrotoxicity. *Fed. Proc.*, 42:2957–2964.
23. Fowler, B. A. (1980): Ultrastructural morphometric/biochemical assessment of cellular toxicity. In: *Proceedings of the Symposium on the "Scientific Basis of Toxicity Assessment,"* edited by H. P. Witschi, pp. 211–218. Elsevier, The Netherlands.
24. Fowler, B. A., Brown, H. W., Lucier, G. W., and Beard, M. E. (1974): Mercury uptake by renal lysosomes of rats ingesting methyl mercury hydroxide: Ultrastructural observations and energy dispersive X-ray analysis. *Arch. Pathol.*, 98:297–301.
25. Fowler, B. A., Brown, H. W., Lucier, G. W., and Krigman, M. R. (1975): The effects of chronic oral methyl mercury exposure on the lysosome system of rat kidney: Morphometric and biochemical studies. *Lab. Invest.*, 32:313–322.
26. Fowler, B. A., Kardish, R., and Woods, J. S. (1983): Alterations of hepatic microsomal structure and function by acute indium administration: Ultrastructural morphometric and biochemical studies. *Lab. Invest.* 48:471–478.
27. Fowler, B. A., and Nordberg, G. F. (1978): The renal toxicity of cadmium metallothionein: Morphometric and X-ray microanalytical studies. *Toxicol. Appl. Pharmacol.*, 46:609–623.

28. Fowler, B. A., and Woods, J. S. (1977): The transplacental toxicity of methyl mercury to fetal rat liver mitochondria: Morphometric and biochemical studies. *Lab. Invest.,* 36:122–130.

29. Fowler, B. A., and Woods, J. S. (1979): The effects of prolonged oral arsenate exposure on liver mitochondria of mice: Morphometric and biochemical studies: *Toxicol. Appl. Pharmacol.,* 50:177–187.

30. Fowler, B. A., and Woods, J. S. (1987): Metal and metalloid-induced porphyrinurias: Relationship to cell injury. *Ann. N.Y. Acad. Sci.,* 514:172–182.

31. Fowler, B. A., Woods, J. S., and Schiller, C. M. (1977): Ultrastructural and biochemical effects of prolonged oral arsenic exposure on liver mitochondria of rats. *Environ. Hlth. Perspect.,* 19:197–204.

32. Fowler, B. A., Woods, J. S., and Schiller, C. M. (1979): Studies of hepatic mitochondrial structure and function: Morphometric and biochemical evaluation of *in vivo* perturbation by arsenate. *Lab. Invest.,* 41:313–320.

33. Frenkel, R., and Cobo-Frenkel, A. (1973): Differential characteristics of the cytosol and mitochondrial isozymes of malic enzyme from bovine brain: Effects of dicarboxylic acids and sulfhydryl reagents. *Arch. Biochem. Biophys.,* 158:323–330.

34. Frigg, M., and Rohr, H. P. (1976): Ultrastructural and stereological study on the effects of vitamin E on liver mitochondrial membranes. *Exp. Molec. Pathol.,* 24:236–243.

35. Gillette, J. R., and Jollow, D. R. (1974): Drug metabolism in liver, In: *The Liver: Normal and Abnormal Functions,* edited by F. Becker, pp. 165–195. Dekker, New York.

36. Goldfischer, S. (1965): The localization of copper in the pericanalicular granules (lysosomes) of liver in Wilson's Disease (hepatolenticular degeneration (1)). *Am. J. Pathol.,* 46:977–983.

37. Goldstein, J. A., Hickman, P., Bergman, H., et al. (1977): Separation of pure polychlorinated biphenyl isomers into two types of inducers on the basis of induction of cytochrome P-450 or P-448. *Chem. Biol. Interact.,* 17:69–87.

38. Goyer, R. A., and Krall, R. (1969): Ultrastructural transformation in mitochondria isolated from kidneys of normal and lead-intoxicated rats. *J. Cell Biol.,* 41:393–400.

39. Greenwalt, J. W. (1979): Survey and update of outer and inner mitochondrial membrane separation. In: *Methods in Enzymology,* edited by S. Fleischer and L. Packer, pp. 88–98. Academic Press, New York.

40. Grisham, J. W., Charlton, R. K., and Kaufman, D. G. (1978): *In vitro* assay of cytoxicity with cultured liver: Accomplishments and possibilities. *Environ. Hlth. Perspect.,* 25:161–172.

41. Hackenbrock, C. R. (1972): States of activity and structure in mitochondrial membranes. *Ann. N.Y. Acad. Sci.,* 195:492–505.

42. Hackenbrock, C. R. (1972): Energy-linked ultrastructural transformations in isolated liver mitochondria and mitoplasts. Preservation of configurations by freeze-cleaning compared to chemical fixations. *J. Cell Biol.,* 53:450–465.

43. Hackenbrock, C. R., and Caplan, A. I. (1969): Ion-induced ultrastructural transformations in isolated mitochondria. The energized uptake of calcium. *J. Cell Biol.,* 42:221–234.

44. Hadd, M. E., and Blickenstaff, R. T. (1969): *Conjugates of Steroid Hormones.* Academic Press, New York.

45. Hall, T. A. (1971): The microprobe assay of chemical elements. In: *Physical Techniques in Biological Research, Vol. 1A,* edited by G. Oster, pp. 157–275. Academic Press, New York.

46. Harris, E. J., and Achenjang, F. M. (1977): Energy-dependent uptake of arsenite by rat liver mitochondria. *Biochem. J.,* 168:129–132.

47. Haschemeyer, R. H., and Myers, R. T. (1973): Negative staining. In: *Principles and Techniques of Electron Microscopy, Vol. 2,* edited by M. A. Hayat, pp. 99–147. Van Nostrand Reinhold, New York.

48. Haugen, D. A., Van der Hoever, T. A., and Conn, M. J. (1975): Purified liver microsomal cytochrome P-450 separation and characterization of multiple forms. *J. Biol. Chem.,* 250:3567–3570.

49. Holtzman, D., and Hsu, J. S. (1976): Early effects of inorganic lead on immature rat brain mitochondrial respiration. *Ped. Res.,* 10:70–75.

50. Hook, G. E. R., Haseman, J. K., and Lucier, G. W. (1975): Induction and suppression of hepatic and extrahepatic microsomal foreign compound metabolizing enzyme systems by 2,3,7,8-tetrachlorodibenzo-p-dioxin. *Chem. Biol. Inter.,* 10:199–214.

51. Illsley, N. P., Lamartiniere, C. A., and Lucier, G. W. (1979): Analysis of sex-specific changes in rat hepatic cytosol protein patterns using two-dimensional electrophoresis. *J. Appl. Biochem.,* 1:385–395.

52. Inouye, B., Ogino, Y., Ishida, T., Ogata, M., and Utsumi, K. (1978): Effects of phthalate esters on mitochondrial oxidative phosphorylation in the rat. *Toxicol. Appl. Pharmacol.,* 43:189–198.

53. Jacobs, E. E., Jacob, M., Sanadi, D. R., and Bradley, L. B. (1956): Uncoupling of oxidative phosphorylation by cadmium ion. *J. Biol. Chem.,* 223:147–156.

54. James, M. O., Foureman, G. L., Law, F. C., and Bend, J. R. (1977): The perinatal development of epoxide-metabolizing enzyme activities in liver and extrahepatic organs of guinea pig and rabbit. *Drug. Metab. Dispos.,* 5:19–28.

55. Kagawa, Y., and Kagawa, A. (1969): Accumulation of arsenate-76 by mitochondria. *J. Biochem.,* 65:105–112.

56. Kupfer, D., and Levin, R. (1972): Monooxygenase drug metabolizing activity in CaCl₂-aggregated hepatic microsomes from rat liver. *Biochem. Biophys. Res. Commun.,* 47:611–618.

57. Koehler, J. K. (1973): The freeze-etching technique. In: *Principles and Techniques of Electron Microscopy, Vol. 2.,* edited by M. A. Hayat, pp. 51–98. Van Nostrand Reinhold, New York.

58. Lang, R. D. A., and Bronk, J. R. (1978): A study of rapid mitochondrial structural changes *in vitro* by spray-freeze-etching. *J. Cell Biol.,* 77:134–147.

59. Lauwerys, R., and Buchet, J. P. (1972): Study on the mechanism of lysosome labilization by inorganic mercury *in vitro. Eur. J. Biochem.,* 26:535–542.

60. Lee, M. J., Harris, R. A., and Green, D. E. (1969): Action of fluorescein mercuric acetate upon mitochondrial-energized processes. *Biochem. Biophys. Res. Commun.,* 36:937–946.

61. London, R. E., Galvin, M. J., Thompson, M., Jeffreys, L., and Mester, T. (1985): An approach to NMR studies of the metabolism of internal organs using surface coils. *J. Biochem. Biophys. Meth.,* 11:21–29.

61a.Lucier, G. W. (1981): In: *Developmental Toxicology,* edited by C. A. Kimmel and J. Buelke-Sam, Raven Press, New York.

62. Lucier, G. W., McDaniel, O. S., Hook, G. E. R., et al. (1973): TCDD-induced changes in rat liver microsomal enzymes. *Environ. Hlth. Perspect.,* 5:199–211.

63. Lucier, G. W., Matthews, H. B., Brubaker, P. E., et al. (1973): Effects of methylmercury on microsomal mixed-function oxidase components of rodents. *Mol. Pharmacol.,* 9:237–246.

64. Lucier, G. W. (1974): Microsomal glucuronidation of steroids using a rapid radioassay. *J. Ster. Biochem.,* 5:681–687.

65. Lucier, G. W., and McDaniel, O. S. (1977): Steroid and non-steroid UDP glucuronidation of synthetic estrogens as steroids. *J. Ster. Biochem.,* 8:867–873.

66. Maack, T. (1967): Changes in the activity of acid hydrolases during reabsorption of lysozyme. *J. Cell Biol.,* 35:268–273.

67. Maack, T., Mackensie, D. D. S., and Kinter, W. D. (1971): Intracellular pathways of renal reabsorption of lysozyme. *Am. J. Physiol.,* 221:1609–1616.

68. Madsen, K. M., and Christensen, E. I. (1978): Effects of mercury on lysosomal protein digestion in the kidney proximal tubule. *Lab. Invest.,* 38:165–174.

69. Magnaval, R., Batti, R., and Thiessard, J. (1975): Methyl mercury effect on rat liver mitochondrial dehydrogenases. *Experientia,* 31:406–407.

70. Matlib, M. A., and Srere, P. A. (1976): Oxidative properties of swollen rat liver mitochondria. *Arch. Biochem. Biophys.,* 174:705–712.

71. Mayer, R. T., Jermyn, J. W., Burke, M. D., and Prough, R. A. (1977): Methoxyresorufin as a substrate for the fluorometric assay of insect microsomal O-dealkylases. *Pestis. Biochem. Physiol.,* 7:349–354.

72. Mego, J. L., and Barnes, J. (1973): Inhibition of heterolysosome formation and function in mouse kidneys by injection of mercuric chloride. *Biochem. Pharmacol.,* 22:373–381.

73. Mego, J. L., and Cain, J. A. (1973): The effect of carbon tetrachloride on lysosome function in kidneys and livers of mice. *Biochim. Biophys. Acta,* 297:343–345.

74. Mego, J. L., and Cain, J. A. (1975): An effect of cadmium on heterolysosome formation and function in mice. *Biochem. Pharmacol.,* 24:1227–1232.

75. Mego, J. L., and Hayes, A. W. (1973): Effects of fungal toxins on uptake and degradation of formaldehyde-treated ¹²⁵I-albumin in mouse liver phagolysosomes. *Biochem. Pharmacol.,* 22:3275–3286.

76. Mintz, H. A., Youen, D. H., Safer, B., et al. (1967): Morphological and biochemical studies of isolated mitochondria, from fetal neonatal and adult liver and from neoplastic tissues. *J. Cell Biol.,* 34: 513–525.

77. Moldeus, P., Hogberg, J., and Orrenius, S. (1978): Isolation and use of liver cells. In: *Methods in Enzymology, Vol. 52,* Biomembranes, *Part C,* edited by S. Fleischer and L. Packer, pp. 60–70. Academic Press, New York.

78. Muscatello, U., Guarriero-Bobyleva, V., Pasquali-Ronchetti, I., and Ballotti-Ricci, A. M. (1975): Configurational changes in isolated rat liver mitochondria as revealed by negative staining III. Modifications caused by uncoupling agents. *J. Ultrastruc. Res.,* 52:2–12.

79. Nelson, B. D. (1975): The action of cyclodiene pesticides on oxidative phosphorylation in rat liver mitochondria. *Biochem. Pharmacol.,* 24:1485–1490.

80. Ochoa, S. (1955): Malic dehydrogenase from pig heart. In: *Methods in Enzymology, Vol. 1,* edited by S. Colowick and N. O. Kaptan, pp. 735–739. Academic Press, New York.

81. Oesch, R. (1973): Mammalian epoxide hydrases: Inducible enzymes catalysing the inactivation of carcinogenic and cytotoxic metabolites derived from aromatic and olefinic compounds. *Xenobiotica,* 3: 305–340.

82. Papa, S., Guerrieri, F., Simone, S., et al. (1973): Mechanisms of respiration-driven proton translocation by the inner mitochondrial membrane. *Biochim. Biophys. Acta,* 292:20–28.

83. Parr, D. R., and Harris, E. J. (1976): The effect of lead on the calcium-handling capacity of rat heart mitochondria. *Biochem. J.,* 158:289–294.

84. Pressman, B. C. (1967): Biological applications of ion-specific glass electrodes. In: *Methods in Enzymology, Vol. 10,* edited by S. Colowick and N. O. Kaplan, pp. 714–726. Academic Press, New York.

85. Poland, A., and Nebert, D. W. (1973): A sensitive radiometric assay of aminopyrine *N*-demethylation. *J. Pharmacol. Exp. Ther.,* 184: 269–277.

86. Poland, A., and Glover, E. (1976): Stereospecific, high affinity binding of 2,3,7,8-tetrachlorodibenzo-*p*-dioxin by hepatic cytosol. *J. Biol. Chem.,* 251:4936–4946.

87. Randolph, M. L. (1972): Biological application of electron spin resonance. In: edited by H. M. Swartz, J. R. Bolton, and D. C. Borg, p. 119. Wiley (Interscience), New York.

88. Ryan, P., Lu, Y. H., and Levin, W. (1978): Purification of cytochrome P-450 and P-448 from rat liver microsomes. In: *Methods in Enzymology, Vol. 52,* Biomembranes, *Part C,* edited by S. Fleischer and L. Packer, pp. 117–123. Academic Press, New York.

89. Ryan, P., Lu, A. Y. H., Kawalek, J., et al. (1975): Highly purified P-448 and P-450 from rat liver microsomes. *Biochem. Biophys. Res. Commun.,* 64:1134–1141.

90. Schenkman, J. B., Remmer, H., and Estabrook, R. W. (1967): Spectral studies of drug interaction with hepatic microsomal cytochrome. *Mol. Pharmacol.,* 3:113–123.

91. Schenkman, J. B., and Cinti, D. L. (1972): Hepatic mixed function oxidase activity in rapidly prepared microsomes. *Life Sci.,* 11:247–257.

92. Schenkman, J. B., and Cinti, D. L. (1978): Preparation of microsomes with calcium. In: *Methods in Enzymology, Vol. 52,* Biomembranes, *Part C,* edited by S. Fleischer and L. Packer, pp. 83–89. Academic Press, New York.

93. Schnaitman, C., Erwin, V. G., and Greenawalt, J. W. (1967): The submitochondrial localization of monoamine oxidase, an enzymatic marker for the outer membrane of rat liver mitochondria. *J. Cell Biol.,* 32:719–735.

94. Shibko, S., and Tappel, A. L. (1965): Rat kidney lysosomes: Isolation and properties. *Biochem. J.,* 95:731–741.

95. Sies, H. (1978): The use of perfusion of liver and other organs for the study of microsomal electron-transport and cytochrome P-450 systems. In: *Methods in Enzymology, Vol. 52,* Biomembranes, *Part C,* edited by S. Fleischer and L. Packer, pp. 48–60. Academic Press, New York.

96. Silbergeld, E. K., and Fowler, B. A. (1987): Mechanisms of chemical-induced porphyrinopathies. *Ann. N.Y. Acad. Sci.,* 514:1–352.

97. Sirica, A. E., Richards, W., Tsukada, Y., et al. (1979): Fetal phenotypic expression by adult rat hepatocytes on collagen gel/nylon meshes. *Proc. Natl. Acad. Sci.,* 76:282–287.

98. Southard, J. H., and Nitisewojo, P. (1973): Loss of oxidative phosphorylation in mitochondria isolated from kidneys of mercury poisoned rats. *Biochem. Biophys. Res. Commun.,* 52:921–927.

99. Squibb, K. S., Pritchard, J. B., and Fowler, B. A. (1984): Cadmium metallothionein nephropathy: Ultrastructural/biochemical alterations and intra-cellular cadmium binding. *J. Pharmacol. Exp. Ther.,* 228:311–321.

100. Stabuli, W., Hess, R., and Weibel, E. R. (1969): Correlated morphometric and biochemical studies on the liver cell. II. Effect of phenobarbital on rat hepatocytes. *J. Cell Biol.,* 41:92–112.

101. Strik, J. J. T. W. A. (1987): Porphyrias associated with chlorinated organic exposure. *Ann. N.Y. Acad. Sci.,* 514:219–221.

102. Stuve, J., and Galle, P. (1970): Role of mitochondria in the handling of gold by the kidney: A study by electron microscopy and electron probe microanalysis. *J. Cell Biol.,* 44:667–676.

103. Suda, T., Horiuchi, N., Ogata, E., et al. (1974): Prevention by metallothionein of cadmium-induced inhibition of vitamin D activation reaction in kidney. *FEBS Lett.,* 42:23–26.

104. Tedeschi, H., and Harris, D. L. (1958): Some observations on the photometric estimation of mitochondrial volume. *Biochim. Biophys. Acta,* 28:392–402.

105. Wakabayashi, M. (1970): β-Glucuronidase in metabolic hydrolysis. In: *Metabolic Conjugation and Metabolic Hydrolysis,* edited by W. Fishman, pp. 520–592. Academic Press, New York.

106. Weibel, E. R., and Paumgartner, D. (1979): Integrated stereological and biochemical studies on hepatocyte membranes. II. Correction of section thickness effect and volume and surface density estimates. *J. Cell Biol.,* 77:584.

107. Weibel, E. R., Staubli, W., Gnagi, H. R., and Hess, F. A. (1969): Correlated morphometric and biochemical studies on the liver cell. I. Morphometric model, stereologic methods, and normal morphometric data for rat liver. *J. Cell Biol.,* 42:68–91.

108. Welton, A. F., and Aust, S. D. (1974): Multiplicity of cytochrome P-450 hemoproteins in rat liver microsomes. *Biochem. Biophys. Res. Commun.,* 56:898–906.

109. Werringloer, J. (1978): Assay of formaldehyde generated during microsomal oxidation reactions. In: *Methods in Enzymology, Vol. 52,* Biomembranes, *Part C,* edited by S. Fleischer and L. Packer, pp. 297–302. Academic Press, New York.

110. Wiener, J., Loud, A. V., Kimberg, D. V., and Sprio, D. (1968): A quantitative description of cortisone-induced alterations in the ultrastructure of rat liver parenchymal cells. *J. Cell Biol.,* 37:47–62.

111. Woods, J. S., Eaton, D. L., and Lukens, C. B. (1984): Studies of porphyrin metabolism in the kidney. Effects of trace metals and glutathione on renal uroporphyrinogen decarboxylase. *Mol. Pharmacol.,* 26:336–341.

112. Woods, J. S., and Fowler, B. A. (1977): Effects of chronic arsenic exposure on hematopoietic function in adult mammalian liver. *Environ. Hlth. Perspect.,* 19:209–213.

113. Woods, J. S., and Fowler, B. A. (1977): Renal porphyrinuria during chronic methyl mercury exposure. *J. Lab. Clin. Med.,* 90:266–272.

114. Woods, J. S., and Fowler, B. A. (1978): Altered regulation of mammalian hepatic heme biosynthesis and urinary porphyrin excretion during prolonged exposure to sodium arsenate. *Toxicol. Appl. Pharmacol.,* 43:361–371.

115. Woods, J. S., and Fowler, B. A. (1986): Alterations of hepatocellular structure and function by thallium chloride: Ultrastructural morphometric and biochemical studies. *Toxicol. Appl. Pharmacol.,* 83: 218–229.

116. Woods, J. S., and Fowler, B. A. (1987): Metal alterations of uroporphyrinogen decarboxylase and cophoporphyrinogen oxidase. *Ann. N.Y. Acad. Sci.,* 514:55–64.

117. Woods, J. S., Fowler, B. A., and Eaton, D. L. (1984): Studies on the mechanisms of thallium-mediated inhibition of hepatic mixed function oxidase activity: Correlation with inhibition of NADPH-cytochrome with (P-450) reductase. *Biochem. Pharmacol.,* 33:571–576.

118. Yasukochi, Y., and Masters, B. S. S. (1976): Some properties of a detergent-solubilized NADPH-cytochrome c (cytochrome P-450) reductase purified by biospecific affinity chromatography. *J. Biol. Chem.,* 251:5337–5344.

Principles and Methods of Toxicology, Second Edition, edited by A. Wallace Hayes, Raven Press, Ltd., New York © 1989.

CHAPTER **30**

Pharmacokinetics in Toxicology

Andrew Gordon Renwick

Department of Clinical Pharmacology, University of Southampton, Southampton, SO9 3TU, United Kingdom

The term pharmacokinetics is derived from the Greek words *pharmako* (medicine, drug, or poison) and *kinetikos* (motion or movement). Thus pharmacokinetics is the study of the movement of drugs within the body, i.e., the absorption, distribution via the blood, metabolism, and excretion. This term is in contrast to *pharmacodynamics,* which is concerned with the pharmacological actions of the drug within the body. The word drug is popularly associated with medicines or therapeutic agents, although for certain subjects, e.g., drug metabolism, this word has long been applied to any environmental anutrient, i.e., drugs, pesticides, environmental contaminants, plant products. Because the processes concerned with the absorption, distribution, and elimination of therapeutic drugs are nonspecific and shared with other types of anutrients, the principles of pharmacokinetics apply to any environmental anutrient. It is thus valid to apply the term pharmacokinetics to all foreign compounds, and it is preferable to the use of semantically correct but unrecognized terms such as "chemobiokinetics" (22) to describe the application of these principles to nontherapeutic substances.

Toxicokinetics is receiving increasing and even international (86) usage; it has useful connotations with respect to the nonspecific nature of the toxicant and the implicit requirement for kinetic data at toxic doses. However, most of the basic texts are concerned with "pharmacokinetics," and any subdivision into toxicokinetics is both unnecessary and open to "tunnel vision."

Pharmacokinetic studies are important in the development of useful compounds, and such information is regarded as necessary before proceeding with long-term and carcinogenicity tests. Frequently, if the pharmacokinetic evidence indicates tissue accumulation on prolonged dosing, saturation of elimination at subtoxic doses, or the formation of chemically reactive metabolites, chemical analogs without these problems would be selected for study, as the above criteria mitigate against a high therapeutic index or acceptable daily intake.

The severity of toxicity of a compound is related to two variables: the sensitivity of the target organ and the concentration at the site of action (19). Frequently the compound has to pass many lipid and metabolic barriers prior to reaching the target, as shown in Fig. 1. An understanding of the extent and nature of these processes may be derived from serial analysis of the concentrations of the chemical in the plasma and urine. A knowledge of the concentrations of the parent compound and any metabolites in plasma and tissue, allied to the rate of change on further dosing or cessation of administration, allows us the opportunity to rationalize both the species of animal most appropriate for testing a compound and the extrapolation of any toxicity observed in animals to the likely risk for man (2,19,86).

The aim of this chapter is to introduce the underlying principles in both biological and mathematical terms and subsequently to describe methods of obtaining suitable sam-

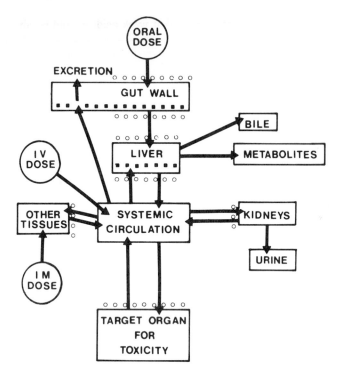

FIG. 1. Toxicity in relation to pharmacokinetics. The chemical may be given orally or by injection or inhalation. The concentration at the target organ is in equilibrium with that in the systemic circulation, which is itself in dynamic equilibrium with a large number of other physiological processes tending to increase or decrease that concentration. The transfer from one tissue to another usually involves transfer across a lipid membrane (*open circles*) and frequently entails entering a tissue with high metabolic capacity (*solid squares*) such as the liver.

ples from certain animal species, primarily the rat. The final section of the chapter covers the analysis of data, with examples to illustrate the type of information and insights that may be obtained using these techniques. In all cases, the examples and data processing described have been restricted to analysis of results that can be performed using a simple calculator, graph paper, and so on. References are provided for further reading, as the analysis of data using computer programs and more complex mathematical models are not covered in this chapter.

In the past, animal and human disposition studies during drug development utilized slightly different approaches, with animal data usually including tissue distribution, 24-hr radiolabeled balance studies, and *in vitro* and *in vivo* metabolism studies, and human data including excretion and *in vivo* metabolism studies and plasma concentration–time curves. The basis for the development of the last approach, i.e., plasma concentration–time curves, was the formulation of suitable mathematical models that allowed the derivation of rates of absorption, metabolism, and excretion in man. It was thus possible, using pharmacokinetic methods, to gain a degree of insight into the extent of processes in man that had been shown to occur in animals using serial sacrifice and tissue analysis, and that had been seen in metabolic studies

(measurement of 24-hr urinary metabolites or incubation of the drug with liver microsomes).

However, with the development of analytical techniques of high sensitivity and specificity (such as HPLC) and the expansion of laboratories undertaking plasma drug analyses, the full potential of pharmacokinetics to reveal information on *in vivo* drug absorption, distribution, and elimination has resulted in these techniques being applied increasingly to toxicology problems in laboratory animals. Problems of accumulation on repeated dosing and saturation of elimination are particularly pertinent to high dose animal toxicity studies, and information on these areas can be obtained only from suitably designed pharmacokinetic studies. It must be emphasized at the outset that the key to successful pharmacokinetic studies is the development of an assay of high specificity that measures the chemical without interference by its metabolites and that is of sufficient sensitivity to define the terminal slope accurately (see later).

BIOLOGICAL PRINCIPLES

Certain general principles governing the disposition of drugs may be applied to most foreign compounds that are not substrates for normal intermediary metabolism. These general properties of absorption, distribution, and elimination are valuable concepts, but it should be emphasized that they are not universally applicable, and investigators must be alert for exceptions. This situation is especially likely if the foreign compound is structurally similar to an endogenous body constituent, as it may then undergo specific carrier-mediated uptake processes, metabolism, and so on. Good examples of compounds showing this characteristic include the antiparkinsonian drug levodopa, the intense sweetener aspartame, and the purine and pyrimidine base analogs used in cancer chemotherapy, many of which not only undergo active uptake into cells but also may be metabolized to phosphorylated products, which accumulate within the cells of the body.

Absorption

Absorption describes the processes involved in the transfer of the drug from the site of administration to the systemic blood circulation. Because most toxicity studies are performed by the oral route, absorption from the gut is of greatest importance, although absorption from other sites is appropriate for certain toxicological studies.

Absorption from the Gut

The extent of drug absorption is largely determined by the pH of the gut lumen and the pKa and lipid solubility of the drug. Other biological variables, e.g., the presence of food, gastric emptying time, intestinal transit time, and the gut microflora, may also play important roles in limiting the amount of unchanged drug absorbed. The absorption of drugs requires passage across lipoid membranes, which can involve (a) passive diffusion through the membrane, (b) passage through membrane pores, and (c) specialized carrier-mediated processes.

The rate of diffusion of a drug across a membrane, given by Fick's law, is proportional to the concentration gradient, the membrane surface area, and the permeability coefficient of the compound. The permeability coefficient depends on the diffusivity of the molecule through the membrane, the membrane/aqueous medium partition coefficient, and the thickness of the membrane (14), and thus it is a characteristic for that particular compound and corresponds to a rate constant. Most environmental anutrients are absorbed in the small intestine because of the large surface area. For weak acids and bases the membrane/aqueous partition coefficient, however, varies with the pH of the medium. For such compounds, the diffusivity and partition coefficient of the ionized molecular species may be regarded as insignificant compared with the uncharged species, and thus the following system may be regarded as applying:

$$Acid^{\ominus} \underset{\text{High pH}}{\overset{\text{Low pH}}{\rightleftarrows}} Acid\text{-}H$$

$$Base\text{-}H^{\oplus} \underset{\text{Low pH}}{\overset{\text{High pH}}{\rightleftarrows}} Base$$

| Ionized | Nonionized |
| Water soluble | Lipid soluble |

Because it is the uncharged species that readily diffuses across membranes, absorption is faster under conditions in which ionization is suppressed, i.e., low pH for acids and high pH for bases. When the two compartments separated by the lipoid membrane are kept at different pH values, the total concentrations in each compartment at equilibrium are different. The extent of ionization of a weak acid may be related to the environmental pH and its pKa by the Henderson-Hasselbalch equation:

$$pH = pKa + \log \frac{[\text{conjugate base}]}{[\text{conjugate acid}]}$$

At equilibrium, the concentrations of the diffusible form (nonionized) on each side of the membrane are equal, and the concentration of the ionized form is given by the Henderson-Hasselbalch equation (Fig. 2).

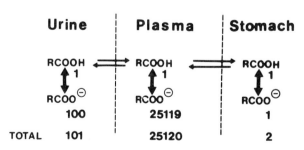

FIG. 2. pH partitioning. The numbers give the relative concentration of un-ionized and ionized species in each compartment, as determined by the Henderson-Hasselbalch equation, for a weak acid (pKa 3.0) at the pH of stomach (3.0), plasma (7.4), and urine (5.0). The total concentration is the concentration of compound in each compartment at equilibrium assuming that the ionized form undergoes negligible diffusion.

It is apparent from Fig. 2 that weak acids should be absorbed rapidly and extensively in the low pH of the stomach, whereas weak bases should undergo absorption in the intestine. Although it is undoubtedly true for bases, absorption from the stomach is limited, even for simple acids, possibly due to the relatively small surface area of the gastric mucosa. Strong organic acids and bases frequently show incomplete absorption from the gut, as they are extensively ionized at all pH values of the gut. The absorption of drugs by passage through membrane pores, which are about 4 Å diameter, is largely applicable to small (less than 200 daltons) water-soluble molecules (14). The bulk passage of water across the membrane may act as a driving force and carry small molecules with it (45). This fact should be borne in mind when studying the absorption kinetics of large doses of sparingly water-soluble compounds. Under such circumstances, the oral administration of high doses in large volumes of hypotonic solution could result in enhanced absorption. This situation is the opposite of the case for compounds undergoing carrier-mediated absorption because here the carrier may be saturated and the absorption rate reduced at high doses. Food may also affect carrier-mediated absorption by competition of the natural substrate for the carrier. Examples of foreign compounds undergoing active absorption are rare and usually apply when the drug resembles a nutrient (e.g., levodopa).

A number of factors may limit the amount of drug that reaches the systemic blood after oral administration (bioavailability):

1. Extremes of pH, which may affect the stability of the compound. Species differences may then arise between rats (gastric pH 3.8–5.0) and rabbits (gastric pH 1.9) (68).
2. Hydrolytic enzymes. The gut is rich in nonspecific proteases and lipases, which may affect drugs.
3. Gut microflora. The gut flora can perform a wide range of largely degradative metabolic reactions on foreign compounds (62), which may reduce the amount of drug available for absorption or result in the formation of potentially toxic metabolites (48). The flora show species differences in both types of organism present and their distribution along the gut (68).
4. Metabolism by the gut wall. The gut wall has the capacity to inactivate metabolically certain compounds prior to their reaching the hepatic portal vein (first-pass effect) (10).
5. Metabolism by the liver. Many compounds are effectively removed from the hepatic portal vein at a single passage (first-pass effect) (26).
6. Food present in the gut lumen, which may affect the absorption rate, gastric pH, or gut motility.

These barriers to the establishment of effective plasma levels of the compound may be associated with suppression of systemic pharmacological and toxic properties (25) and thus render dietary administration an inappropriate route for the toxicity testing of compounds for which exposure is parenteral, i.e., via the lungs, skin, and so on.

Absorption from the Nasal Cavity

The nasal cavity has received increasing interest, as it possesses various potentially useful properties. Although it has relatively small surface area, the mucous membrane is highly permeable, so that even quaternary ammonium compounds, e.g., clofilium tosylate, that are poorly absorbed from the gut show blood levels approaching those produced by intravenous administration (72). In addition, the nature of this site and its venous drainage directly into the systemic circulation allow increased absorption of compounds extensively metabolized in the gut lumen (e.g., proteins) or in the liver (e.g., the β-blocker propranolol). Local toxicity may be a problem with this route at high doses (72).

Absorption from the Lung

The lung represents a poor barrier to a chemical entering the blood, as it has a large surface area of thin membrane, a limited capacity to metabolize foreign compounds, and an excellent blood supply. The epithelium acts as a limited permeability barrier, allowing only slow absorption of highly water-soluble compounds (75) although the rate may be greater than that from the gastrointestinal tract. The lung is a major site of inactivation of circulating local hormones such as peptides and prostaglandins; however, for toxicity testing, similar substances would not be likely to be given by this route. Major problems exist with the quantitative analysis of the extent and rate of absorption from the lung due to poor measurement of the dose given by this route. Particulate matter is largely trapped by the cilia and passed back to be absorbed in the gut. Volatile compounds are absorbed only partially, and the unabsorbed fraction is eliminated in the expired air and not retained for subsequent absorption, as in the gut (27).

Percutaneous Absorption

The extent of percutaneous absorption of drugs is highly dependent on the lipophilicity of the compound, as the stratum corneum of the epidermis acts as an effective barrier (27,36). This route is important for both the therapeutic administration of potent lipophilic drugs that undergo extensive first-pass metabolism (e.g., organic nitrates in angina) and the environmental exposure of workers using aerosols. Studies in animals and man suggest that the rate-limiting step is the initial penetration of the stratum corneum (28), which may result in "flip-flop" kinetics (see later).

Distribution

Drugs are distributed largely via the blood, although the lymphatic system may be important in the initial distribution of some lipid-soluble drugs given orally. The rate of uptake of a drug by the tissues may be limited by diffusion or perfusion rates.

1. Diffusion rate: If the diffusion of the chemical across membranes is slow, the rate of entry of the drug into tissues is limited by this property of the molecule.
2. Perfusion rate: If the diffusion of the chemical across membranes is rapid, the rate of entry of the drug is limited by the rate of delivery to the tissue, i.e., the perfusion rate.

As a generalization, diffusion rate limitation applies to highly water-soluble compounds, whereas perfusion rate limitation applies to the entry of lipid-soluble compounds into slowly perfused systems such as adipose tissue. The perfusion rates of the major organ systems of man (Table 1) can be readily divided into well and poorly perfused tissues.

The extent to which drugs leave the blood and enter tissues depends on their relative affinities for each system. Thus compounds highly bound to plasma protein but not to tissue show a relatively high concentration in the plasma, whereas drugs with a high affinity for tissue components such as proteins or fat have a low plasma concentration. However, it should be remembered that it is the *relative* affinity that determines the extent of distribution to tissues. Thus Evans blue dye has a high affinity for plasma protein, and its distribution (Table 2) is restricted to the plasma volume (3 L in man); however, the β-blocker propranolol is also highly bound to plasma protein (95%), but it shows a higher affinity for the tissues, and little remains in the plasma after distribution.

The volumes of body fluids and drugs that distribute in them are given in Table 2. However, only rarely do compounds distribute to a single physiologically recognizable volume, and usually some degree of tissue selectivity is observed. Thus a compound may appear to have dissolved in total body water because the apparent volume of distribution (see below) corresponds to about 60% of body weight, but it may actually show a nonuniform tissue distribution.

Many foreign compounds bind reversibly to plasma proteins, with albumin being of the greatest importance, although acid glycoproteins may be important for certain organic bases

TABLE 1. *Relative organ perfusion rates in man[a]*

Organ	% Body weight[b]	Blood flow[c] (ml/min)	% Cardiac output[b,c]	Blood flow[b,c] (ml/min/ 100 g)
Well perfused				
Lung	1.2	5,000	100	1,000
Adrenals	0.02	25	1	550
Kidneys	0.4	1,260	23	450
Thyroid	0.04	50	2	400
Liver				
Total	2	1,350	25	75
Via portal				
vein		1,050	20	60
Heart	0.4	252	5	70
Intestines	2	1,050	20	60
Brain	2	750	15	55
Poorly perfused				
Skin	7	462	9	5
Skeletal				
muscle	40	840	16	3
Connective				
tissue	7			1
Fat	15	95	2	1

[a] The results are for an adult male under resting conditions and are approximate values only.
[b] Adapted from ref. 9.
[c] Adapted from ref. 4.

TABLE 2. *Volumes of body fluids with drugs showing restricted distribution*

Fluid	Volume (L)	% Body weight	Drug[a]
Total body water	41	58	D_2O, antipyrine, ethanol, urea
Extracellular water	12	17	Na^+, Br^-, tubocurarine, sucrose
Plasma	3	4	Evans blue, ^{131}I-albumin

[a] Drugs for which the distribution is restricted to a particular body fluid.
Adapted from refs. 9,27.

(46). Foreign compounds bind at specific sites in a reversible, saturable fashion, and the bound drug represents a pharmacologically inactive depot of the chemical. Extensive protein binding lowers the concentration of unbound drug in the blood, which may increase the concentration gradient and thus the rate of diffusion into blood from the gut or kidney tubules (38). The rate of dissociation of the drug–protein complex is measured in milliseconds and by comparison with tissue perfusion times may be regarded as instantaneous. Thus for tissues in which the free plasma concentration is lowered rapidly by an active uptake process within the tissue (i.e., liver or kidney), the drug can be effectively stripped off the plasma protein in a single passage. The plasma protein binding of foreign compounds has been reviewed and discussed by several authors (12,16,34,38,41).

Elimination

There are two main mechanisms by which the circulating levels of a foreign compound may be reduced: metabolism and excretion. *Metabolism* and its toxicological consequences are discussed in an earlier chapter. Certain mathematical implications are discussed below.

Excretion

The principal routes of drug excretion are via the urine and feces, and in the case of volatile compounds the expired air.

Excretion via urine

There are three major processes affecting drug elimination in the kidney.
Glomerular filtration. The glomerular membrane has pores of 70 to 80 Å; and under the positive hydrostatic conditions in the glomerulus, all molecules smaller than about 20,000 daltons are filtered. Thus proteins and protein-bound drugs remain in the plasma, and about 20% of the nonbound drug is carried with 20% of the plasma water into the glomerular filtrate.
Reabsorption. Because the glomerular filtrate contains many important body constituents (e.g., glucose), there are

specific active uptake processes for them. Although not substrates for these transport processes, many lipid-soluble drugs diffuse back from the tubule into the blood, especially as the urine becomes more concentrated because of water reabsorption. The pH of the urine is generally lower than that of the plasma, and therefore pH partitioning (see above) tends to increase the reabsorption of weak acids. The pH of the urine can be altered appreciably by treating the animal with ammonium chloride (decreases pH) or sodium carbonate (increases pH); the buffered plasma shows little change. It is thus relatively easy to affect the pH partitioning of foreign compounds between tubule contents and plasma and either increase or decrease the elimination rate. This possibility should be considered when preparing dose solutions, as the use of excess acid or alkali to dissolve the test compound may alter its renal elimination.
Tubular secretion. Foreign compounds may be secreted actively into the renal tubule against a concentration gradient by anion and cation carrier processes. These processes are saturable and of relatively low specificity; many basic or acidic drugs and their metabolites (especially the phase 2 or conjugation products) are removed by them (17). Because the dissociation rate for the drug–albumin complex is rapid, it is possible for highly protein-bound drugs to be almost completely cleared at a single passage through the kidney.

Excretion via the gut

The most important mechanism allowing circulating foreign compounds to enter the gut is in the bile. The biological aspects of this mechanism have been reviewed (69), and certain pertinent points have emerged. The bile may be regarded as a complementary pathway to the urine, with small molecules being eliminated by the kidney and large molecules in the bile. Thus the bile becomes the principal excretory route for many drug conjugates. Species differences exist in the molecular weight requirement for significant biliary excretion, which has been estimated as 325 ± 50 in the rat, 440 ± 50 in the guinea pig, and 475 ± 50 for the rabbit (31). In the rat, small molecules (less than 350 daltons) are not eliminated in the bile or large molecules (more than 450 daltons) in the urine, even if the principal excretory mechanism is blocked by ligation of the renal pedicles or bile duct, respectively. Compounds of intermediate molecular weight (350–450 daltons) are excreted by both routes, and ligation of one pathway results in increased use of the other (30).
Foreign compounds may also enter the gut by direct diffusion or secretion across the gut wall, elimination in the saliva, pH partitioning of bases into the low pH of the stomach, and elimination in the pancreatic juice. In most cases these routes are quantitatively of minor importance, although they may play an important role in toxicity by allowing a foreign compound to undergo metabolism by the gastrointestinal flora (20,50). The toxicological implications of the gut microflora have been reviewed by Scheline (62).

MATHEMATICAL PRINCIPLES

In order to describe adequately the changes in blood plasma levels of foreign compounds, it is necessary to assign a suitable mathematical model that accurately predicts the slope of the plasma concentration–time curve. However, certain aspects of drug handling are model-independent and are considered first, as these considerations are usually built into the various models. In addition, there has been a marked trend away from multicompartmental analysis, which offers little apart from mathematical predictability, toward physiologically more relevant model-independent concepts such as clearance (84).

Model-Independent Considerations

Biochemical and physiological processes are usually either zero-order or first-order reactions. In zero-order reactions the rate of change in concentration occurs at a fixed amount per time, i.e.,

$$\frac{dC}{dt} = k$$

where C is concentration, t is time, and k is a constant with units of amount per time, e.g., micrograms per minute. In first-order reactions the rate of change in concentration is proportional to the concentration of chemical available for the reaction, i.e.,

$$\frac{dC}{dt} = kC$$

where k is a constant that represents a proportional change with time and has units of time^{-1}, e.g., min^{-1}.

Most processes (e.g., diffusion, carrier-mediated uptake, metabolism, excretion) are first-order reactions at low concentrations. Most of the equations given below make this assumption. Zero-order reactions are particularly important at high concentrations when enzymes are working at maximum rate and an increase in C cannot result in an increase in rate. This situation produces nonlinear, or saturation kinetics, which can assume considerable importance in toxicity studies.

First-order reactions can be described by equations employing exponential functions. In many cases the entry of a foreign substance into the body or individual tissues follows an exponential increase, which may be described mathematically by

$$\text{Uptake} = 1 - e^{-kt} \qquad [1]$$

where the uptake is the concentration present at time t divided by the final concentration when all the compound has entered the body or tissue. This equation assumes that there is no elimination process occurring. The elimination of a compound (by a single mechanism) once it has entered the body or tissue may be described by

$$C = C_0 e^{-kt} \qquad [2]$$

where C is the concentration present at time t, and C_0 is the initial concentration. In both cases k is the rate constant for that process. Exponential equations of the type given in Eq. 2 may be solved as

$$\ln C = \ln C_0 - kt$$

or

$$\log C = \log C_0 - \frac{kt}{2.303}$$

which represents an equation of the generalized form

$$y = C + mx$$

where m and C are constants, and x and y are variables. In such cases, a plot of x against y gives a straight line graph with a slope of m and an intercept of C. Thus for pharmacokinetics, a graph of $\log C$ against time gives a slope of $-k/2.303$ and an intercept of $\log C_0$. If such a graph is drawn using log-linear graph paper, the slope must be calculated by taking the logs of the concentration terms and dividing by the time (see below).

Frequently, the equation necessary to describe the kinetics of a compound in the body requires the use of two exponential rate terms, i.e., absorption into a single compartment or elimination from a two-compartment system (see below). In such cases the early time points in the concentration–time curve are influenced by both rates. However, provided the rate constants are sufficiently dissimilar, eventually the influence of the component with the higher rate becomes negligible, whereas the smaller rate constant still affects the concentration. Thus the terminal phase of the concentration–time curve is determined by the process with the smaller rate constant and the earlier phase by the sum of both processes. This process allows both rate constants to be determined by the procedure known as the *method of residuals*, stripping, or feathering (see below).

Tissue Extraction

Removal of a drug from the blood by a tissue is schematized in Fig. 3. On constant infusion, the rate of entry into the tissue may be regarded as equivalent to a first-order absorption rate (52):

$$\text{Uptake} = 1 - e^{-kt} \qquad [1]$$

where uptake = the fractional uptake = Ct/Ct(equilibrium).

In *perfusion limited uptake,* the value k is related to the flow rate (Q) as follows (Fig. 3):

$$\text{Fractional uptake} = 1 - e^{-\left(\frac{Q}{PV_t}\right)t} \qquad [3]$$

(Note that Q/V_t is the volume-adjusted flow rate.) The uptake half-time may be derived as described below for Eq. 19:

$$t_{1/2} \text{ uptake} = \frac{0.693}{k} = \frac{0.693PV_t}{Q} = \frac{0.693P}{Q/V_t} \qquad [4]$$

For *diffusion limited uptake,* the value k is related to the diffusion rate constant and thus is not readily measurable.

Plasma Protein Binding

The extent of protein binding may be represented by an equilibrium reaction:

$$P^r + C_u \rightleftharpoons C_b$$

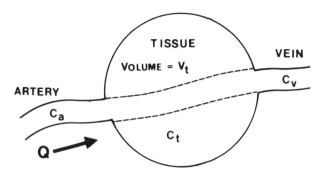

FIG. 3. Tissue uptake of foreign compounds. Q is the blood flow, C_a is the arterial concentration, C_v is the venous concentration, C_t is the concentration in tissue, and V_t is the volume of tissue. We define the following parameters: rate of delivery of drug = QC_a, rate of outflow of drug = QC_v, and rate of uptake = $QC_a - QC_v$. The units for these rates are wt time^{-1} (i.e., μg min^{-1}, etc.). Thus

$$\text{Extraction ratio } (E) = \frac{\text{rate of uptake}}{\text{rate of delivery}}$$

$$= \frac{QC_a - QC_v}{QC_a} = \frac{C_a - C_v}{C_a}$$

$$\text{Partition ratio } (P) = \frac{\text{concentration in tissue}}{\text{concentration in blood supply}}$$

$$= \frac{C_t}{C_a}$$

where P^r is the free protein, C_u is the unbound drug, and C_b is the drug–protein complex. The equilibrium constant K is given by

$$\frac{[C_b]}{[P^r][C_u]} = \frac{[\text{product}]}{[\text{reactants}]} \quad [5]$$

The fraction unbound is given by

$$\alpha = \frac{C_u}{C_u + C_b} = \frac{C_u}{C_p} \quad [6]$$

where C_p is total plasma concentration. Scatchard plots of r/C_u against r (where r is the moles of drug bound per mole of protein, and C_u is the free drug concentration in moles) can be used to derive the number of binding sites and their association or affinity constants (16). Normally, for the binding of organic compounds to albumin, two or more binding sites are revealed. This approach is valuable for detailed studies on binding to and displacement from albumin, but it could yield multiple binding sites if applied to a complex protein mixture such as plasma, containing different proteins at different concentrations.

Because it is the unbound drug in plasma that undergoes equilibration with the unbound drug in tissues (Fig. 4), adequate information may be obtained from a knowledge of α, or the percentage bound. Detailed knowledge is not required for pharmacokinetic analysis of the plasma data. However, because plasma protein binding is a saturable process (see later) *in vitro* binding studies should be performed over a range of concentrations.

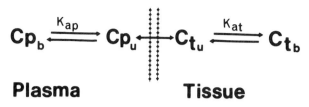

FIG. 4. Protein binding and tissue distribution. C_p is the plasma concentration, C_t is the tissue concentration, u = unbound, b = bound, K_{ap} is the association constant for plasma protein binding, and K_{at} is the association constant for tissue protein binding. At equilibrium, $C_{pu} = C_{tu}$; and the relative distribution between plasma and tissue is determined by the values of K_{ap} and K_{at}.

Clearance

Clearance (Cl) may be defined as the ratio

$$\frac{\text{Rate of drug elimination}}{\text{Plasma concentration}}$$

and may be regarded as the volume of plasma or blood that is cleared of drug in unit time by the route under consideration. The units are volume · time^{-1} e.g., usually ml min^{-1} because if rate is μg min^{-1} and plasma concentration is μg ml^{-1} the plasma clearance must be ml min^{-1}.

Renal clearance

The renal clearance (Cl_R) is given by

$$Cl_R = \frac{\text{rate of elimination in urine}}{\text{plasma concentration}} = \frac{C_U \times F_U}{C_p} \quad [7]$$

where C_U is the urine concentration, F_U is the urine flow (volume in unit time), and C_P is the plasma concentration at the midpoint of the urine collection period. The concentration in urine is dependent on a number of variables, which are now described.

Glomerular filtration. The rate of drug filtration is given by

$$\text{GFR} \times C_{pu} = \text{GFR} \times C_p \times \alpha \quad [8]$$

where GFR is the glomerular filtration rate, C_{pu} is the unbound drug concentration, C_p is the total plasma concentration, and α is the fraction unbound.

Thus compounds binding extensively to plasma protein show limited clearance by glomerular filtration. The protein binding equilibrium is not disturbed in the glomerulus, because after loss of 20% free drug and 20% water, C_{pu} is unaltered, whereas the concentrations of both free protein and drug protein complex increase by 20%, i.e.,

	Before filtration	After filtration
$K_{ap} =$	$\dfrac{[\text{complex}]}{[C_{pu}][P^r]}$	$= \dfrac{[1.2 \text{ complex}]}{[C_{pu}]1.2[P^r]}$

where K_{ap} is the protein binding association constant. Thus the drug–protein complex does not dissociate in the glomerulus. The complex dissociates to give more free drug when the plasma is diluted by water reabsorbed in the distal parts of the tubule. Under such circumstances, about 99% of the plasma water is reabsorbed, so that the concentrations of the protein and complex return to almost the initial levels, whereas the concentration of unbound drug represents about 80% of its former level, i.e., after reabsorption:

$$K_{ap} \neq \frac{[\text{complex}]}{0.8[C_{pu}][P^r]}$$

Therefore the complex dissociates to restore the equilibrium. The glomerular filtration rate is about 130 ml min^{-1} in men and 120 ml min^{-1} in women, or approximately 2 ml min^{-1} kg^{-1}, which is lower than that of the Wistar rat (3.4 ml min^{-1} kg^{-1}) (70).

Reabsorption. The reabsorption process is variable and dependent on the lipid solubility of the drug, the pH of the urine, and the extent of concentration of the urine (i.e., water reabsorption). Mathematical quantitation is impracticable, but an indication of the extent of reabsorption may be obtained (see below). In certain instances the administered foreign compound may be a substrate for carrier-mediated reabsorption, in which case the renal elimination is greater at high doses when this reuptake is saturated. Such a process is obviously ideal for maintaining a constant low body load of an essential compound, e.g., glucose or riboflavin, which might show adverse effects at high body concentrations.

Tubular secretion. These saturable carrier-mediated processes show a relatively low substrate specificity, and the extent of their involvement for a particular compound is dependent on the affinity between the compound and the carrier protein. The extent of clearance by these active processes may be regarded as analogous to hepatic clearance, which is another active saturable process. The specificity of the carriers, especially the anion mechanism, has been discussed, and structural requirements such as

$$\begin{array}{c} \text{R}-\text{C}-\text{N}-(\text{CHR}')_n-\text{COOH} \\ \| \quad | \\ \text{O} \quad \text{X} \end{array}$$

have been proposed (17). However, until further studies on intersubstrate competition are completed, it cannot be known whether one or more carriers is involved (82).

All three processes described above can simultaneously and independently alter the value of C_U for a given value of C_p, and the final renal clearance may be regarded as a composite expression:

Renal excretion = glomerular filtration

− reabsorption + tubular secretion

Rate of excretion = GFR $C_p\alpha$ − rate of reabsorption

+ rate of tubular secretion

The values of GFR, C_p, and α can be determined experimentally. Measurement of inulin clearance (or creatinine clearance in man) determines the GFR, as this compound does not undergo significant reabsorption, tubular secretion, or protein binding; thus for inulin:

Rate of renal excretion = GFR C_p

and because

$$Cl_R = \frac{\text{rate of excretion}}{C_p}$$

$$Cl_R = \text{GFR}$$

The extent of reabsorption and secretion of a compound may be inferred from a comparison of renal clearance with the value of GFR $\times \alpha$, i.e.,

If $Cl_R <$ GFR $\times \alpha$ Reabsorption must be occurring and is greater than secretion (which may or may not be present).

If $Cl_R =$ GFR $\times \alpha$ Reabsorption, which may or may not be present, is negated by an equal rate of secretion.

If $Cl_R >$ GFR $\times \alpha$ Tubular secretion must be occurring and is greater than reabsorption (which may or may not be present).

The mathematical implications of the renal elimination process have been the subject of a number of reviews (21,81).

Hepatic clearance. The clearance of a compound by the liver may be regarded as dependent on the rate of delivery to the organ (blood flow) and the efficiency of removal from the blood (extraction ratio; see Fig. 3). Thus

$$Cl_H = QE \qquad [9]$$

where Cl_H is the hepatic (metabolic) clearance, Q is the hepatic blood flow, and E is the extraction ratio.

This simple relationship has been verified experimentally for a number of drugs. However, it is complicated by the finding that the variables Q and E are not independent, because for certain compounds the extraction efficiency decreases with an increase in blood flow. This finding led Rowland et al. (59) to propose the following relation, known as the *perfusion limited model*:

$$Cl_H = Q\left[\frac{\alpha Cl_{int}}{Q + \alpha Cl_{int}}\right] \qquad [10]$$

where α is the fraction unbound in plasma, Cl_{int} is the intrinsic metabolic clearance by the hepatocytes from the cell water, and Q is the blood flow (as plasma). Further analysis of this equation (see ref. 83 for discussion) indicates that

$$Cl_{int} = \frac{V_{max}}{K_m + C_{pu}} \qquad [11]$$

where V_{max} and K_m are Michaelis-Menton constants for the enzyme metabolizing the foreign compound, and C_{pu} is the hepatic venous concentration of unbound compound.

If C_{pu} is much less than the K_m for the enzyme (i.e., well below saturation levels), this term may be ignored and

$$Cl_{int} = \frac{V_{max}}{K_m} = \text{constant}$$

Thus using Eq. 10, if the metabolic clearance (Cl_{int}) is high, the value in parentheses, equivalent to the term E in Eq. 9, approaches unity, and the hepatic clearance approximates to the hepatic blood flow and thus is dependent on the blood flow. However, if the metabolic clearance is low, $Q + Cl_{int}$ approximates to Q, and the hepatic clearance remains relatively constant, as the extraction ratio (E) decreases with an increase in blood flow. These equations adequately explain the effects of changes in perfusion rate on the extraction ratio and clearance of compounds that show a range of extraction ratios. In addition, comparison of the hepatic clearance (calculated by measurement of Q and E) with nonrenal clearance [calculated as plasma clearance (see below) − renal clearance] can indicate the role of extrahepatic tissues in the elimination of the compound.

When the value of C_{pu} approaches or exceeds K_m, the substrate concentration is sufficient to saturate the enzyme, and the kinetics are grossly altered and become nonlinear. This situation is a distinct possibility in high-dose toxicity testing and is discussed later in more detail.

Biliary clearance

The clearance via the bile Cl_B is given, by analogy with renal clearance, as

$$Cl_B = \frac{\text{rate of elimination in bile}}{C_p} = \frac{C_B F_B}{C_p} \qquad [12]$$

where C_B is the concentration in bile, and F_B is the volume of bile in unit time (bile flow).

Plasma clearance

Plasma clearance (Cl) may be defined as

$$Cl = \frac{\text{rate of elimination from plasma}}{C_p}$$

The plasma clearance is the sum of the various contributory clearance processes:

$$Cl = Cl_R + Cl_H + Cl_B + \text{etc.} \qquad [13]$$

Plasma clearance, which is one of the most valuable pharmacokinetic constants, is determined from the plasma concentration–time curve and is discussed in detail later. It may be used to derive other model-independent variables, e.g., mean residence time, which are given later under Statistical Moment Analysis.

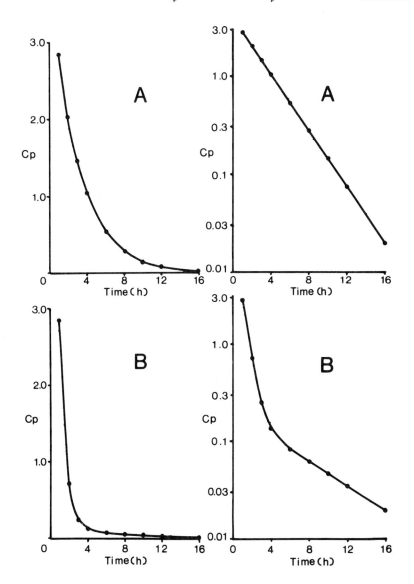

FIG. 5. Plasma concentration–time data for two compounds; results were plotted using linear and semilogarithmic paper. The data used to generate the curves are given in Table 3.

Compartmented Systems: Modeling

In order to describe plasma concentration–time curves mathematically, the data have to be fitted to an appropriate predictive model. The correlation between the actual data and the concentration–time curve generated using the model selected shows the suitability of the model in describing the experimental results.

Thus considering the data presented in Fig. 5 and Table 3, it is apparent that a single model is inadequate to describe the properties of both compounds, although in both cases the initial and final plasma measurements were the same. The differences in the plasma concentration–time profiles originate in the number of rates at which the compound may leave and enter the plasma. If the tissues show instantaneous equilibration with plasma, the compound leaves the plasma by a single process (Scheme 1,A), an elimination process. Alternatively, the compound may leave the plasma to enter "other tissues" at measurable rates, as well as undergoing elimination from the plasma. Under such circumstances, the "other tissues" may be adequately described mathematically by one compartment in addition to the plasma (or the central compartment). In some cases, two or more additional compartments are required. It is important to realize that these "other tissues" share only one criterion, i.e., their associated rate constants, and that biologically diverse tissues may be part of the same compartment. In addition, elimination may occur from compartments other than the central compartment (Scheme 1,C,D,E,G). In most cases the processes of elimination and distribution of foreign compounds are by first-order reactions; i.e., the rate of the reaction is proportional to the amount of substrate available for the reaction.

Wagner (78) reviewed the number of possible models and showed that 17 linear models existed to describe one-, two-, and three-compartment systems, i.e., models in which the plasma concentration–time curve could be resolved into a number of linear components (see below). However, if the input into the model was noninstantaneous, additional models would be generated. Wagner (78) concluded that there were 760 possible pharmacokinetic models comprising up to three distribution compartments and two input compartments, but that in many cases and for many calculations a knowledge of the best fit model was not necessary. Because the aim of this chapter is to provide an introduction to pharmacokinetics (i.e., samples needed, data handling, and the

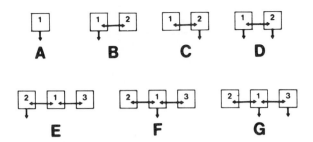

SCHEME 1. Compartmental models. Linear disposition models showing one (A), two (B, C, D), or three (E, F, G) compartments. Only 3 of the 13 possible three-compartment models are shown; others are derived by variable elimination from any or all compartments and by compartment 3 equilibrating via compartment 2, not compartment 1. In all cases, compartment 1 is taken as the blood and tissues undergoing essentially instantaneous equilibration.

type of information that can be obtained), only simple models are discussed in detail. Readers are referred to standard texts on pharmacokinetics if the plasma data or other factors do not fit either of the two models discussed here. However, the two models selected show widespread applicability, and an understanding of the principle of these simple models is essential if the numbers (e.g., rate constants) generated by computer analysis of more complex models are to have any meaning. In addition, more complex models contain greater numbers of variables, and blood sampling must be increased to define these constants accurately.

Texts recommended for further reading include those by Rescigno and Segre (52), a mathematical approach with few drug illustrations; Gibaldi and Perrier (26), a mathematical approach that is well explained and illustrated using actual experimental data; Rowland and Tozer (58), a well-written, readable text with many excellent illustrations and study problems at the end of each section; and Wagner (79), an approach similar to that of Gibaldi and Perrier but with a useful "biological" introductory chapter and expanded sections on dosage regimen calculations, pharmacological response, and automated pharmacokinetic analysis. All volumes provide references, either at the end of each chapter or for each illustration.

One-Compartment Open Model

Intravenous Bolus Dose

The drug is dissolved in and evenly distributed within a single compartment of volume V. Elimination of the drug, by both excretion and metabolism, is by first-order processes, and changes in plasma concentration are reflected in similar and simultaneous decreases in the tissue concentrations, as all tissues represent part of the single compartment (Schemes 1,A and 2). In Scheme 2, V is the volume of distribution, k_{ex} is the excretion rate constant, and k_m is the metabolism rate constant. The plasma concentration–time curve for a one-compartment system is given in Fig. 6; the data are presented in Table 4. In mathematical terms, such a system may be adequately described by a simple first-order equation, where

TABLE 3. Data used for Figure 5

Time after i.v. dosing (hr)	C_p (μg/ml)	
	Compound A	Compound B
1	2.850	2.850
2	2.040	0.705
3	1.470	0.250
4	1.050	0.136
6	0.540	0.082
8	0.280	0.062
10	0.145	0.047
12	0.075	0.035
16	0.020	0.020

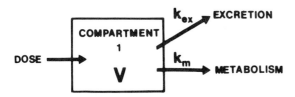

SCHEME 2. One-compartment model.

TABLE 4. Data used for Figure 6[a]

Time (hr)	C_p (μg ml^{-1})	ln C_p	
1	80.0	4.382	
2	41.5	3.726	$k = 0.656$ hr^{-1}
3	21.5	3.068	$t_{1/2} = 1.06$ hr
4	11.2	2.416	
5	5.8	1.758	$C_{p0} = 154.3$ μg ml^{-1}
6	3.0	1.099	$V = 324$ ml kg^{-1}

[a] The plasma concentrations were obtained after an intravenous bolus dose of 50 mg/kg.

the rate of removal of a drug from the body (in milligrams per hour) is proportional to the body load (in milligrams):

$$\frac{dAb}{dt} = kAb \qquad [14]$$

where Ab is the amount of drug in the body, and k is the elimination rate constant. A solution to this equation to give the amount of drug remaining in the body at time t after injection is given by

$$Ab_t = Ab_0 e^{-kt} \qquad [15]$$

where Ab_t is the amount of drug at time t, and Ab_0 is the amount of drug at time zero.

Assuming uniform distribution within a single compartment, the concentration in the plasma (Cp) may be related to Ab by the *apparent volume of distribution* (V). This volume may be regarded as the volume of plasma in which the drug would have to be dissolved to give the plasma concentration measured. Thus for a drug that is lipid-soluble or that readily binds to tissue components, the plasma concentration represents a small fraction of the dose, and thus the drug appears to have been dissolved in a large volume of plasma (see below):

$$C_p = \frac{Ab}{V} \qquad [16]$$

where C_p is the plasma concentration, and V is the apparent volume of distribution. Thus Eq. 15 may be rewritten in its more usual form,

$$C_p = C_{p0} e^{-kt} \qquad [17]$$

For such a system we can define certain parameters as follows.

Apparent volume of distribution

The apparent volume of distribution (V) is the apparent volume into which the dose would have been dissolved to give the initial plasma concentration, C_{p0}, i.e.,

$$V = \frac{Ab}{C_p} = \frac{\text{dose}}{C_{p0}} \qquad [18]$$

The units are in liters, milliliters, liters per kilogram, or milliliters per kilogram.

Elimination rate constant

The elimination rate constant (k) represents the *fractional* loss of drug from the body, i.e.,

$$k = \frac{\text{amount of drug eliminated in unit time}}{\text{amount of drug in the body}} = \frac{(dAb/dt)}{Ab}$$

Equation 17 may be rewritten

$$\log C_p = \log C_{p0} - \frac{kt}{2.303}$$

Thus a graph of log C_p against time has a slope of $-k/2.303$ and an intercept of log C_{p0} (Fig. 6). The units are hr^{-1} or min^{-1}. Thus if the elimination rate constant is determined as 0.4 hr^{-1}, it means that 40% of the body load is removed each hour. The value of k is the summation of component elimination rate constants (e.g., k_{ex}, k_m).

Elimination half-life

The elimination half-life is the time taken for the amount in the body (Ab) or the plasma concentration (Ab/V) to decrease to one-half. Thus after one half-life, C_p in Eq. 17 equals $C_{p0}/2$, i.e.,

$$\frac{C_{p0}}{2} = C_{p0} e^{-kt_{\frac{1}{2}}} \quad \text{or} \quad \frac{1}{2} = e^{-kt_{\frac{1}{2}}}$$

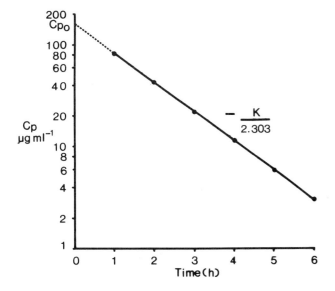

FIG. 6. Plasma concentration–time curve after a bolus intravenous dose for a one-compartment system. The data are given in Table 4.

Therefore, $\ln 2 = kt_{\frac{1}{2}}$ or $t_{\frac{1}{2}} = \ln 2/k$, and

$$t_{\frac{1}{2}} = \frac{0.693}{k} \qquad [19]$$

where the units are hours or minutes.

Plasma clearance

Plasma clearance (Cl) is the amount of drug eliminated in unit time related to the plasma concentration and may be regarded as the amount of blood that is cleared of drug in unit time. In many respects, this measurement is a better reflection of the inherent capacity of the tissues to eliminate the drug than is the half-life or elimination rate constant:

$$Cl = \frac{\text{rate of elimination}}{\text{plasma concentration}}$$

$$Cl = \left(\frac{dAb/dt}{C_p}\right) \qquad [20]$$

Substituting from Eq. 14,

$$Cl = \frac{kAb}{C_p}$$

The amount of drug in the body at any time (Ab) is given by Eq. 16; therefore

$$Cl = \frac{kC_pV}{C_p} = kV \qquad [21]$$

where the units are in liters hr^{-1}, liters min^{-1}, ml hr^{-1}, or ml min^{-1}. Rearranging,

$$k = \frac{Cl}{V}$$

This equation shows clearly that the elimination rate constant (k) is derived from two independent variables that can be related to physiological processes: the *clearance*, which reflects the capacity of the organs of elimination to remove drug from the plasma, and the *apparent volume of distribution*, which reflects the proportion of the total body burden that is circulated to the organs of elimination. Plasma clearance may approach plasma flow to the principal organs of elimination and can thereby provide useful insights.

Clearance may also be obtained without knowing the value of V. Rearranging Eq. 20,

$$\frac{dAb}{dt} = ClC_p$$

or in time dt, the amount lost $dAb = ClC_p dt$. Therefore integrating between 0 and infinity (∞) during which time the total dose will have been eliminated,

$$\text{Dose} = Cl \int_0^\infty C_p dt$$

$$= Cl \times \text{AUC}$$

$$Cl = \text{dose}/\text{AUC} \qquad [22]$$

where AUC is the area under the plasma concentration–time curve, or from Eq. 21,

$$V = \frac{\text{dose}}{\text{AUC} \times k} \qquad [23]$$

The value of Eqs. 22 and 23 is that both the clearance and the apparent volume of distribution can be derived from infusion or parenteral drug administration, where the determination of V using Eq. 18 is not possible because the total dose is not present in the central compartment at $t = 0$. These equations may also be applied to oral administration, providing that allowance is made for incomplete absorption of the dose. This method of calculating Cl is also applicable to multicompartment linear systems with elimination from the central compartment.

Information obtainable from urinary data

From Eq. 7, we obtain

$$\text{Rate of urinary excretion} = Cl_R C_p$$

where Cl_R is the renal clearance. Thus

$$Cl_R C_p = k_R V C_p = k_R Ab$$

from Eqs. 21 and 18, where k_R is the renal excretion rate constant. However, Ab at any time = dose e^{-kt}. Therefore

$$\text{Rate of urinary excretion} = k_R \text{ dose } e^{-kt} \qquad [24]$$

or

$$\log(\text{Rate of excretion}) = \log k_R \text{ dose} - \frac{kt}{2.303} \qquad [25]$$

A plot of rate of excretion (amount excreted per time interval) against time gives a straight line on log-linear graph paper, the slope of which is $-k/2.303$, and the intercept is $\log k_R$ dose. It is important to note that the slope gives the overall elimination rate constant, not the specific urinary elimination rate constant. In other words, the decrease in the amount appearing in the urine mirrors the overall decrease in the plasma concentration. It is not possible to obtain information regarding other kinetic parameters without sampling the central compartment. The value of k_R may be derived from the values of renal clearance

$$Cl_R = \frac{C_U \times F_U}{C_p} \qquad [7]$$

and the apparent volume of distribution, V, when $Cl_R = k_R V$.

The above approach is subject to considerable fluctuations in the excretion rate due to such factors as incomplete bladder emptying. To overcome this problem, the rate constant can be derived from the amount remaining to be excreted, using the *sigma-minus* method. This method is based on the equation below, which is derived from integration of Eq. 24:

$$A_{ex} = \frac{k_R \text{ dose}}{k}[1 - e^{-kt}] \qquad [26]$$

where A_{ex} is the total amount excreted up to time t. At infinite time, $[1 - e^{-kt}]$ equals unity. Therefore

$$A_{ex}^\infty = \frac{k_R \, \text{dose}}{k}$$

where A_{ex}^∞ is the cumulative total amount excreted in urine up to time infinity. Substituting back into Eq. 26 therefore

$$A_{ex} = A_{ex}^\infty [1 - e^{-kt}]$$

or

$$A_{ex}^\infty - A_{ex} = A_{ex}^\infty e^{-kt} \qquad [27]$$

The left-hand side of Eq. 27 is equivalent to the amount finally excreted minus the amount excreted up to that time (ΔA_{ex}). Taking logs

$$\log \Delta A_{ex} = \log A_{ex}^\infty - \frac{kt}{2.303} \qquad [28]$$

Thus the semilog plot of the ΔA_{ex} against time gives a straight line of slope $k/2.303$. An example of this method is described below under Data Handling.

By analogy with Eq. 22 Cl_R may be calculated from the total amount excreted and the plasma AUC

$$Cl_R = \frac{A_{ex}}{\text{AUC}}$$

where A_{ex} and AUC refer to the same time interval.

Constant Intravenous Infusion

During infusion the plasma concentration (C_p) rises to reach a plateau or steady-state concentration (C_{pss}) when the rate of infusion equals the rate of elimination. By analogy with Eq. 1,

$$\frac{C_p}{C_{pss}} = (1 - e^{-kt})$$

or

$$C_p = C_{pss}(1 - e^{-kt}) \qquad [29]$$

The various pharmacokinetic parameters may be derived from the plasma concentration–time curve for infusion (as given in Fig. 7).

Decrease at end of infusion

The slope equals $-k$ because on cessation of entry into the single compartment, $C_p = C_{p0} e^{-kt}$. The same slope would be obtained if the infusion was stopped at any stage during the infusion.

C_{pss}

At steady state, the rate of infusion (R) equals the rate of elimination:

$$R = Cl C_{pss}$$

or

$$Cl = \frac{R}{C_{pss}} = Vk$$

Increase to plateau

Rearranging Eq. 29,

$$(C_{pss} - C_p) = C_{pss} e^{-kt}$$

Therefore, a plot of $\ln (C_{pss} - C_p)$ against time gives a straight line with a slope equal to k. The time taken to peak is therefore similar to the time taken to eliminate the compound, or about 97% of the final level within five half-lives.

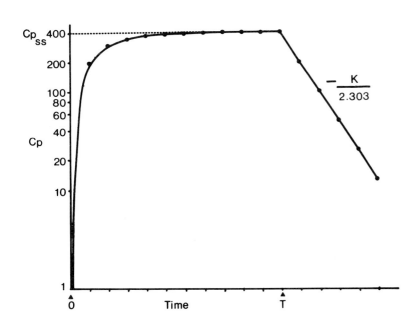

FIG. 7. Plasma concentration–time curve for constant intravenous infusion into a single-compartment system. The foreign compound was infused at a constant rate from time = 0 to time = T when the infusion was stopped.

Area under the curve

Both Cl and V may be derived using Eqs. 22 and 23.

Oral Administration

The absorption of drugs frequently obeys first-order kinetics (54) but may involve a lag time due to delayed gastric emptying. The plasma concentration–time profile may thus resemble Fig. 8 (see also Table 5), and the various pharmacokinetic parameters are related by the equation

$$C_p = \frac{F \times \text{dose} \times k_a(e^{-kt} - e^{-k_a t})}{V(k_a - k)} \qquad [30]$$

where F is the fraction of the dose absorbed and k_a is the absorption rate constant.

Decrease after peak

The decrease after the peak is determined by the slower of two processes (absorption or elimination), but it is usually elimination, and the slope is equal to $-k$. (Note that for a polar compound showing slow absorption and rapid elimination, this decrease is equivalent to k_a, a situation described by Gibaldi and Perrier (26) as "flip-flop" kinetics.)

Peak plasma concentration

The peak plasma concentration is determined by the relative rates k_a and k and may be of toxicological importance, as the extent of toxicity is frequently related to the peak plasma concentration rather than to the area under the curve. An increase in the absorption rate may be as important toxicologically therefore as a decrease in elimination rate.

Area under the curve

Both Cl and V may be derived using Eqs. 22 and 23, providing the dose used in the calculation is adjusted for the fraction absorbed (F), i.e.,

$$Cl = \frac{\text{dose} \times F}{\text{AUC}}$$

It is common to see Cl_{oral} calculated in the absence of any information on F. Such a term is meaningless; and if F is unknown, oral AUC data should be compared as such. Attempts to relate an altered AUC at high oral doses to altered clearance or F requires intravenous data.

The value of F may be determined by comparison of oral with intravenous dosing, as Cl remains constant:

$$Cl = \frac{\text{dose}_o}{\text{AUC}_o} \times F = \frac{\text{dose}_{iv}}{\text{AUC}_{iv}}$$

$$F = \frac{\text{dose}_{iv}\, \text{AUC}_o}{\text{AUC}_{iv}\, \text{dose}_o} \qquad [31]$$

where o relates to oral, and iv relates to intravenous dosing. These relationships are valid only if the AUC/dose ratio is constant; if not, the value of either F or Cl must alter with an increase in dose, suggesting saturation of absorption or elimination.

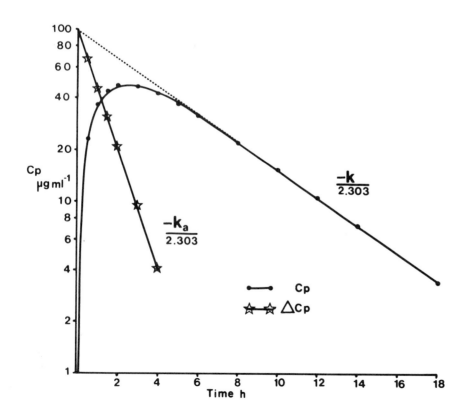

FIG. 8. Use of the method of residuals to calculate the absorption rate constant for a one-compartment system. The dose was given at time 0, and plasma levels (C_p) were measured at intervals. The linear terminal phase was extrapolated to yield the values corresponding to the measurement times. The difference values (C_p extrapolated − C_p measured) are plotted (ΔC_p) to yield a line of slope $-ka/2.303$ or $-k/2.303$; see text. The data are given in Table 5.

TABLE 5. *Data used for Figure 8*

Time (hr)	C_p	$\ln C_p$	$\ln C_{pex}$	C_{pex}	ΔC_p	$\ln \Delta C_p$	
0.5	23.0		4.501	90.1	67.1	4.206	⎫
1	36.5		4.406	82.0	45.5	3.818	⎪
1.5	43.9		4.312	74.6	30.7	3.424	⎪
2	47.2		4.218	67.9	20.7	3.030	⎬ $k_a = 0.797\ hr^{-1}$
3	46.8		4.029	56.2	9.4	2.241	⎪
4	42.4		3.840	46.5	4.1	1.411	⎭
5	36.7		3.652	38.5	1.8		
6	31.1		3.463	31.9	0.8		
8	21.8	3.082					⎫
10	15.0	2.708					⎪
12	10.3	2.332	$k = 0.1887\ hr^{-1}$				⎬
14	7.1	1.960					⎪
18	3.3	1.194					⎭

$\ln C_{pex}$: data generated by linear regression analysis of the terminal phase of $\ln C_p$ against time.
C_{pex}: antilogs.
ΔC_p: the values $(C_{pex} - C_p)$ used to draw the residuals line.
Note: The 5 and 6 hr points are not included in the residuals analysis, as an error of 3% in the original value of C_p would translate into an error of 61 and 117%, respectively, for the ΔC_p value.

Alternatively, the fraction F may be derived from the cumulative urinary excretion:

$$F = \frac{\text{dose}_{iv}\, A_{exo}^{\infty}}{\text{dose}_o\, A_{exiv}^{\infty}} \qquad [32]$$

Increase to peak

The increase to peak is determined by the more rapid of the two processes, i.e., usually absorption. Measurement of the rate constant must make allowance for the excretion occurring throughout the postdosing period; the method of residuals is used [see Gibaldi and Perrier (26) for the mathematical basis of this method]. The method is illustrated and explained in Fig. 8 and Table 5. In cases where the absorption is slow, the increase may be determined by the elimination rate constant. Thus the value of k_a can be assigned to the increase to peak only after demonstration that the value of k for the decrease is similar to that seen after intravenous dosing.

Metabolite Kinetics

As discussed in a previous chapter, the biotransformation of xenobiotics is often associated with the formation of a toxic metabolite, and thus measurement of the rate of metabolism *in vivo* can provide much useful information. In nearly all cases, the rate of metabolite formation is governed by *in vivo* enzyme kinetics, which are first order only over a limited substrate concentration range. Saturation of metabolism is discussed in more detail below, and the following analysis relates to metabolite formation under first-order reaction conditions.

The measurements that are available for analysis of metabolite kinetics include plasma levels of unchanged drug (C_p) and metabolite (C_p^m). Discussing further the system given earlier, we consider Scheme 3, where V, k_{ex}, and k_m are, respectively, the apparent volume of distribution, excretion rate, and metabolism rate constants for the parent compound, and V^m, k_{ex}^m, and k_m^m are the same parameters for the metabolite. The time course for the metabolite is given by

$$\frac{dM}{dt} = k_m Ab - k^m M$$

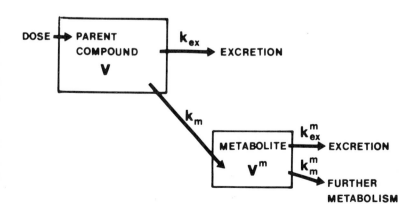

SCHEME 3. One-compartment model with metabolite formation.

where Ab and M are the amount of parent compound and metabolite in the body, respectively, and k^m is the overall elimination rate constant for the metabolite, i.e., $k^m = k_{ex}^m + k_m^m$. This equation may be solved to yield

$$C_p^m = \frac{k_m \text{ dose } (e^{-k^m t} - e^{-kt})}{V^m (k - k^m)} \quad [33]$$

In many cases the overall elimination rate of the metabolite (k^m) is greater than the overall elimination rate of the parent compound (k) (i.e., in the case of the formation of a more polar metabolite). In such cases the term $e^{-k^m t}$ approaches zero before e^{-kt}, and thus at late time points Eq. 33 may be rewritten and solved omitting e^{-k^m}, when it becomes

$$\log C_p^m = \log \frac{k_m \text{ dose}}{V^m (k^m - k)} - \frac{kt}{2.303} \quad [34]$$

Thus the log plasma concentration of the metabolite–time curve has a terminal slope similar to that of the parent compound (i.e., $-k/2.303$) (Fig. 9). In this case the rate of elimination of the metabolite is limited by the elimination of the parent drug, and the metabolite/drug ratio remains constant during the elimination phase (Fig. 9).

In those cases where the elimination rate of the metabolite (k^m) is less than that of the parent compound (k), the term e^{-kt} approaches zero before $e^{-k^m t}$, and thus Eq. 33 may be written

$$\log C_p^m = \log \frac{k_m \text{ dose}}{V^m (k - k^m)} - \frac{k^m t}{2.303} \quad [35]$$

and a plot of log plasma concentration of the metabolite–time curve has a slope of $-k^m/2.303$. In this case the ratio metabolite/drug increases during the elimination phase (Fig. 9). The latter case is of particular interest to toxicologists because on repeated exposure the concentrations of metabolite at steady state may exceed the parent compound.

The overall elimination rate constants may also be derived from urinary metabolite levels as described above for the parent compound, although again the derived rate may be either k or k^m, and the identity can be determined only by measuring k and k^m separately after administration of both the parent compound and the metabolite. However, if metabolite kinetics are based solely on urinary excretion data, the formation of more lipid-soluble metabolites may be missed. For example, the active thioether metabolite of sulfinpyrazone is a major circulating metabolite of which negligible amounts are excreted in the urine (71).

Two-Compartment Open Model

Mathematically and physiologically, it is often more appropriate to regard the body as representing a simple two-compartment open system in which the distribution to certain peripheral tissues is not an instantaneous process. In such a system the drug initially enters a central compartment (the plasma and tissues, in which drug distribution is instantaneous) and is subsequently distributed to a second, peripheral compartment. Elimination occurs from the central compartment, so that drug in the peripheral compartment must transfer back to the central compartment to be eliminated (Scheme 1,B or Scheme 4). In Scheme 4, k_{12} and k_{21} are the rate constants for transfer from compartment 1 to 2 and from 2 to 1, respectively, and k_{10} is the elimination rate from the central compartment.

Intravenous Bolus Dose

After a single intravenous bolus dose into a two-compartment system, the plasma concentration (C_p) at time t may be described by

$$C_p = Ae^{-\alpha t} + Be^{-\beta t} \quad [36]$$

where A and B may be regarded as analogous to C_{p0} for each compartment, and $A + B = C_{p0}$; α and β correspond to hybrid rate constants, each influenced by all the individual distribution, redistribution, and elimination rate constants, i.e., k_{12}, k_{21}, and k_{10} (26). The shape of a typical plasma concentration–time curve following a bolus intravenous dose is given in Fig. 10 (see also Table 6) with the plasma data and the method of derivation of the various constants. As with the determination of absorption rate constants discussed

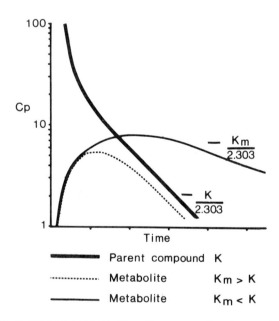

FIG. 9. Plasma concentration–time curves for drug and metabolite after intravenous dosing. The parent drug was given as an intravenous bolus dose at time 0.

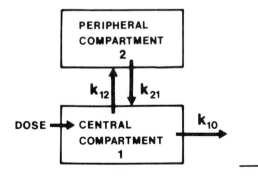

SCHEME 4. Two-compartment model.

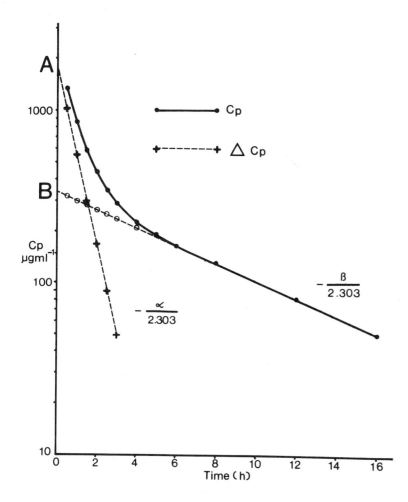

FIG. 10. Plasma concentration–time curve for two-compartment system. The data are given in Table 6.

above, the method of residuals or line stripping is used. In the terminal phase, $Ae^{-\alpha t}$ approaches zero, and the data are described by $C_p = Be^{-\beta t}$. For example, using the data in Table 6, when $t = 8$ hr, $Be^{-\beta t} = 346e^{-0.121 \times 8} = 131$ µg/ml, and $Ae^{\alpha t} = 1,875e^{-1.214 \times 8} = 0.1$ µg/ml; therefore the contribution of the latter term is negligible. The terminal phase is therefore extrapolated back to time 0 when the intercept is equal to B

and the slope of log C_p against time is $-\beta/2.303$. As described in Table 6, the values of B and β may also be derived by least-squares linear regression analysis of the terminal phase, after graphical analysis to determine the point at which linearity commences.

At early time points, the difference between the actual C_p values and the concentrations derived by back-extrapolation

TABLE 6. Data used for Figure 10

Time (hr)	C_p (µg/ml)	ln C_p	ln C_{pex}	C_{pex}	ΔC_p	ln ΔC_p	
0.5	1,345		5.788	326	1,019	6.927	By linear regression
1	864		5.727	307	557	6.323	$\alpha = 1.214$ hr⁻¹
1.5	593		5.666	289	304	5.717	ln $C_{p0} = 7.537$
2	438		5.606	272	166	5.112	$\therefore A = 1,875$ µg/ml
2.5	346		5.545	256	90	4.500	
3	290		5.485	241	49	3.892	
4	228		5.364	214	15	2.708	
5	193		5.243	189	4	1.386	
6	168	5.122	Terminal phase;				
8	131	4.879	by linear regression $\beta = 0.1210$ hr⁻¹				
12	81	4.395	ln $C_{p0} = 5.848$				
16	50	3.911	$\therefore B = 346$ µg/ml				

ln C_{pex}: data generated by linear regression analysis of the terminal phase data for ln C_p against time.

C_{pex}: antilogs of these extrapolated points; similar values may be obtained from the extrapolated line on the graph.

ΔC_p: the values of $(C_p - C_{pex})$; they may be used to derive the residuals line (slope $- \alpha/2.303$) or may be converted to natural logarithms and analyzed by linear regression.

of the $Be^{-\beta t}$ line are due to the component arising from $Ae^{-\alpha t}$. The values of A and α may be similarly derived by calculated linear regression or graphical analysis of the residuals (C_p actual $- C_p$ extrapolation). In the analysis of the residuals (Table 6), the ΔC_p values for 4 and 5 hr were not included, as these values represent only about 5% or less of the original value of C_p and thus are subject to large inaccuracies (up to $\pm 100\%$) owing to the errors inherent in all methods of analysis of foreign compounds in biological fluids.

Thus the plasma concentration–time curve in Fig. 10 may be represented by the equation

$$C_p = 1{,}875\,e^{-1.214t} + 346\,e^{-0.1210t}$$

The rate constants α and β are composite rate constants, from which it is possible to derive k_{12}, k_{21}, and k_{10} given in Scheme 4 using the following equations (see refs 26 and 79 for derivations):

$$C_{p0} = A + B$$

$$\alpha + \beta = k_{12} + k_{21} + k_{10}$$

$$V_1 = \frac{\text{dose}}{A + B} \qquad [37]$$

where V_1 is the volume of the central compartment, and

$$k_{21} = \frac{A\beta + B\alpha}{A + B} \qquad [38]$$

$$k_{10} = \frac{\alpha\beta}{k_{21}} \qquad [39]$$

$$k_{12} = \alpha + \beta - k_{21} - k_{10} \qquad [40]$$

For the example given in Fig. 10,

$$k_{21} = \frac{(1{,}875 \times 0.1210) + (346 \times 1.214)}{(1{,}875 + 346)} = 0.291$$

$$k_{10} = \frac{(1.214 \times 0.1210)}{0.291} = 0.505$$

$$k_{12} = 1.214 + 0.1210 - 0.291 - 0.505 = 0.539$$

It is important to note that k_{10} (0.505) and β (0.121) do not relate to the same process, as k_{10} refers to the elimination from the central compartment, whereas β refers to the overall elimination from the body. The relation between β and k_{10} is given by Eq. 40, which may be rewritten as

$$\beta = k_{10} + k_{21} + k_{12} - \alpha$$

which clearly shows that β is a hybrid rate constant. It is, however, a valuable constant and can be used to derive the half-life ($0.693/\beta$).

As with the one-compartment system, an intravenous bolus allows derivation of most pertinent pharmacokinetic parameters:

1. A, B, α, and β may be derived from plasma data (see above).
2. k_{10}, k_{12}, k_{21}, and V_1 may be derived by manipulation of α, β, etc. (see above).
3. α, β, k_{10}, k_{12}, and k_{21} may be derived from urine by plotting the excretion rate against time. In this case, the intercept values ($A' + B'$) do not equate to $A + B$, and thus

V_1 cannot be deduced. However, k_{10}, k_{12}, and k_{21} can be obtained from Eqs. 38 to 40 by substitution of A and B by A' and B'. The renal elimination rate constant (k_R) is given by

$$k_R = \frac{A' + B'}{\text{dose}}$$

4. α, β, k_{10}, k_{12}, and k_{21} may be derived from urine by the sigma-minus method, where $\log (A_{ex}^\infty - A_{ex}^t)$ is plotted against time. Again α and β may be derived by the method of residuals; k_{10}, k_{12}, and k_{21} from α and β; and the intercepts (A'' and B'') by substitution in Eqs. 38 to 40. The renal elimination rate constant (k_R) is given by

$$k_R = \frac{A_{ex}^\infty}{\text{dose}} \times k_{10}$$

5. The renal elimination constant, k_R, may be derived also from the renal clearance

$$Cl_R = \frac{C_U \times F_U}{C_p} \qquad [7]$$

and the value of V_1, as $Cl_R = k_R V_1$.

6. The amount of drug in the peripheral compartment may be calculated from the following equation (which is similar to Eq. 30 for absorption into a single compartment):

$$C_2 = \frac{\text{dose} \times k_{12}(e^{-\beta t} - e^{-\alpha t})}{V_2(\alpha - \beta)} \qquad [41]$$

where C_2 and V_2 are the concentrations in and volume of the peripheral or deep compartment.

During the terminal phase of the concentration–time curve, $e^{-\alpha t}$ approaches zero and therefore Eq. 41 may be simplified as

$$C_2 = \frac{\text{dose} \cdot k_{12} e^{-\beta t}}{V_2(\alpha - \beta)}$$

Therefore, a graph of $\log C_2$ against time has a slope of $-\beta/2.303$. Thus the terminal rate of decrease in the peripheral compartment of a two-compartment system is identical to the decrease in the central compartment. However, in absolute terms, calculation of C_2 is not particularly valuable, as the peripheral tissues comprising the deep compartment are not homogeneous and may not show a uniform concentration. Thus C_2 should not be regarded as the effective drug concentration even if the target organ lies within the deep compartment. Rather, the concentration in the target organ is measured, from which subsequent concentrations may be calculated using β defined from the central compartment.

A further useful parameter (V_β), which relates the total amount of drug in the body to the plasma concentration, is given by the equation

$$V_\beta\beta = V_1 k_{10} = \frac{\text{dose}}{\text{AUC}} = Cl$$

Just as β is a hybrid term reflecting overall drug elimination from the body, so V_β is a composite but valuable function.

$$V_\beta = \frac{\text{dose}}{\text{AUC} \times \beta}$$

Intravenous Infusion

The shape of the plasma concentration–time curve on intravenous infusion into a two-compartment open system is given in Fig. 11. The pharmacokinetic parameters may be derived from the graph similarly to the one-compartment model, as follows.

Increase to plateau

The increase to plateau follows a complex exponential function with 90 and 99% of the steady-state concentration being reached after four and seven half-lives, respectively.

Plateau level (C_{pss})

At steady state the rate of infusion (R) equals the rate of elimination. Therefore

$$\frac{R}{C_{pss}} = Cl = V_1 k_{10} = V_B \beta$$

Decrease after plateau

The decrease after plateau follows the equation

$$C_p = A^* e^{-\alpha t*} + B^* e^{-\beta t*}$$

where

$$A^* = \frac{AR}{\alpha \, dose}$$

$$B^* = \frac{BR}{\beta \, dose}$$

t^* = time since cessation of infusion

Thus it may be possible to derive values of α, β, A^*, and B^*; however, in many cases, two-compartment characteristics seen after a bolus dose are obscured in postinfusion data, as differences between the constants A and B are reduced.

Area under the curve

The AUC can be used to derive the plasma clearance using Eq. 22.

Oral Administration

Assuming first-order absorption into compartment 1, the plasma concentration at time t is given by

$$C_p = A^\ddagger e^{-\alpha t} + B^\ddagger e^{-\beta t} + C^\ddagger e^{-k_a t}$$

Graphical analysis by a semilogarithmic plot of log C_p against time may reveal three separate phases from which α, β, and k_a should be measurable using the method of residuals. However, in practice, the value of k_a is frequently similar to α, and compounds that require a two-compartment model after intravenous administration appear to fit first-order absorption into a one-compartment model following oral dosing (11). Thus analysis is not possible without reference to intravenous data to determine which rate constant refers to the absorption rate. An example of linear regression analysis to obtain the three rate constants was given by Wagner (79). An alternative method (deconvolution method) may be used that derives the absorption rate constant by a comparison of plasma concentrations for intravenous and oral administration; it does not require fitting the data to a particular one-, two-, or three-compartment model. This method (26,79) does, however, require analysis of the plasma concentrations at the same time points after both oral and intravenous dosing. Various

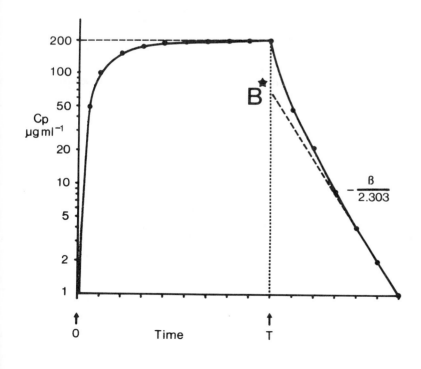

FIG. 11. Plasma concentration–time curve for intravenous infusion in a two-compartment open system. The foreign compound was infused at a constant rate between time 0 and time T, at which time the infusion was stopped.

methods of calculating the absorption rate are discussed in Gibaldi and Perrier (26).

The absorption rate is likely to be of greatest importance in acute toxicity studies, whereas the bioavailability (F) may be more significant in chronic studies; the latter may be measured using model-independent equations (Eq. 31 or 32). However, absorption from the gastrointestinal tract is complex, as it involves physiologically different membranes at differing luminal pH values. Thus the process may involve more than one first-order rate, a zero-order component, or both.

Metabolite Kinetics

Frequently metabolites of foreign compounds fit a two-compartment open model, in which case Scheme 5 applies. Under such circumstances, the elimination of the metabolite is given by an equation analogous to Eq. 36, in which

$$C_p^m = Ae^{-\alpha t} + Be^{-\beta t} + De^{-\gamma t} + Ee^{-\delta t}$$

However, in practice, the concentration–time curve often appears as a biexponential function determined by the slowest rates, i.e., β or δ. In the terminal phase, the slower of these rates is seen; and for a plot of the C_p^m against time, the slope is either $-\beta/2.303$ or $-\delta/2.303$. Application of the method of residuals does not yield further meaningful information, as the single faster rate is a composite of the other rate constants (α, γ, and β or δ). Values of γ and δ may be determined by intravenous administration of the metabolite.

Multiple Dosing: Chronic Administration

On multiple dosing or continuous intake, the plasma levels increase over a period of four to five half-lives to establish a plateau concentration similar to that seen with intravenous

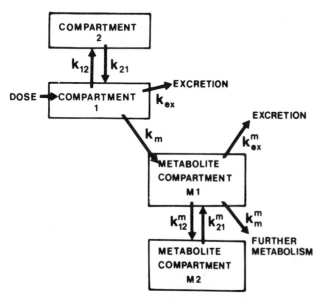

SCHEME 5. Two-compartment model with metabolite formation.

infusion (Figs. 7 and 11). The average plateau level is subject to variations around a mean as material is eliminated between "doses." In oral toxicity studies, these "doses" may represent either repeated single gavage doses or the feeding habits of the animals if the test compound is incorporated into the diet and fed *ad libitum*. On cessation of chronic intake, the rate of decrease in blood levels is usually but not always similar to that seen after a single dose (15).

One-Compartment Open Model

The time taken to reach plateau plasma levels is four to five times the half-time of the terminal phase of the plasma concentration–time curve. The average plateau level is given (by analogy with intravenous infusion) as

$$C_{p\ mean} = \frac{dose \times F}{VkT} \qquad [42]$$

where F is the fraction absorbed, T is the dose interval, and k is the elimination rate constant. However, it is important to realize that this apparently simple relationship holds a number of possible pitfalls. The value k is appropriate only if the terminal phase following oral administration is due to elimination of the drug. If the drug exhibits slow absorption and rapid elimination, the decrease in plasma levels is determined by the slower absorption rate. An alternative equation can be derived from the fact that at steady state the rate of input ($F \times dose/T$) is balanced by the rate of elimination ($C_{p\ mean} \times Cl$); therefore

$$C_{p\ mean} = \frac{dose \times F}{T \times Cl}$$

The fluctuations around the mean plateau level depend on the dosing interval in relation to the terminal elimination rate. Thus compounds with a short half-life show much larger fluctuations, as more of the drug is eliminated between each dose. In the case of drugs with a short half-life (2–3 hr), single daily dosing gives plasma levels approaching zero prior to each dose. These interdose fluctuations may be reduced and blunted by slow absorption. The equations relating to these processes were detailed by Gibaldi and Perrier (26) and Wagner (79). In summary, at steady state after repeated intravenous doses, the minima and maxima are given by

$$C_{p\ minimum} = \frac{dose}{V}\left(\frac{e^{-kT}}{1 - e^{-kT}}\right) \qquad [43]$$

$$C_{p\ maximum} = \frac{dose}{V}\left(\frac{1}{1 - e^{-kT}}\right) \qquad [44]$$

When absorption from the gut occurs as a first-order process with a rate constant that is not many times larger than the value of k, the fluctuations in the steady-state concentration–time curve can be described by the following equation:

$$C_p = \frac{F \times dose \times k_a}{V(k_a - k)} \times \left[\left(\frac{1}{1 - e^{-kT}}\right)e^{-kt} - \left(\frac{1}{1 - e^{-k_aT}}\right)e^{-kt}\right]$$

$$[45]$$

where C_p is the concentration at time t and T is the dose interval. The similarity between this equation and Eq. 30 for absorption of a single dose is readily apparent.

The value of the mean plasma concentration at steady state ($C_{p\,mean}$) may, however, be calculated without knowledge of F, V, k_a, or k by measuring the area under the plasma concentration–time curve for a single oral dose, as

$$\text{AUC}_{\text{oral}} = \frac{\text{dose} \times F}{Vk} = \frac{\text{dose} \times F}{Cl} \qquad [23]$$

where AUC_{oral} is the area under the plasma concentration–time curve between $t = 0$ and $t = $ infinity for a single oral dose (units in $\mu g\ ml^{-1}$ hr, etc.). Substituting into Eq. 42,

$$C_{p\,mean} = \frac{\text{AUC}_{\text{oral}}}{T} \qquad [46]$$

It is important to realize, however, that substitution of Eq. 23 into Eq. 42 assumes that the AUC is directly proportional to the dose, i.e., that dose-dependent kinetics are absent and that Cl does not alter during chronic administration of the compound. The latter possibility may be assessed by comparison of the $\text{AUC}_{0-\infty}$ for a single dose with the AUC_{0-T} for chronic administration. If AUC_{0-T} (chronic) is less than $\text{AUC}_{0-\infty}$ (single), either induction of metabolism or decreased bioavailability is indicated.

The extent of accumulation on repeated intake may be measured by the average amount in the body at steady state Ab_{mean} divided by the amount in the body after a single dose, i.e.,

$$\frac{Ab_{mean}}{Ab} = \frac{Ab_{mean}}{\text{dose} \times F}$$

The amount in the body at the plateau is given by Eq. 42:

$$Ab_{mean} = VC_{p\,mean} = \frac{F\,\text{dose}}{kT}$$

Therefore

$$\text{Extent of accumulation} = \frac{1}{kT} = \frac{1}{0.693/t_{\frac{1}{2}}T} = \frac{1.44t_{\frac{1}{2}}}{T} \qquad [47]$$

Two-Compartment Open Model

The equations giving the plasma concentration at time t at steady state into a two-compartment system with first-order absorption are considerably more complex than those for the one-compartment system. However, the simplified equation (Eq. 42) applies in the form

$$C_{p\,mean} = \frac{\text{dose} \times F}{V_1 k_{10} T} = \frac{\text{dose} \times F}{V_B \beta T}$$

and the value of $C_{p\,mean}$ may still be derived from Eq. 46:

$$C_{p\,mean} = \frac{\text{AUC}_{\text{oral}}}{T} = \frac{\text{dose} \times F}{ClT}$$

Statistical Moment Analysis

Pharmacokinetic studies have moved away from compartmental analyses because they involve multiple variables, which require numerous properly timed blood samples to characterize them adequately. Also, curve fitting is dependent on the terminal slope, which is frequently measured using plasma concentrations that approach the limit of detection of the assay method, i.e., the weakest data. In contrast, terms such as clearance are measured from dose and AUC, the latter being determined largely from the highest and most accurately measured concentrations. Such "time-averaged" parameters may be extended to "time-related" parameters by the use of statistical moment theory, which allows assessment of additional useful pharmacokinetic parameters such as *mean residence time* (MRT). The plasma concentration–time curve may be regarded as a statistical distribution curve for which the zero and first moments are the AUC and MRT, respectively:

$$\text{AUC} = \int_0^{\infty} C_p\,dt$$

$$\text{MRT} = \frac{\text{AUMC}}{\text{AUC}} \qquad [48]$$

Where AUMC is the area under the first moment of concentration time curve, i.e., $\int_0^{\infty} t \cdot C_p\,dt$. The AUMC may be calculated using the trapezoid rule, which is illustrated under Data Handling (see Table 17, below). Whereas the AUC from the last data point to infinity can be calculated as $C_{p\,last}/\beta$, the AUMC from the last data point to infinity has to be calculated as

$$\frac{t_{last} \cdot C_{p\,last}}{\beta} + \frac{C_{p\,last}}{\beta^2}$$

Clearly any inaccuracy in the value of β affects the value of AUMC more than the value of AUC. This situation is shown clearly in data given in Table 17 (see below), where the extrapolated area is 17% of the AUMC but only 3% of the AUC.

In the same way that AUC can be related to Cl, k and V, β and V_β, etc. so AUMC can be used to derive useful parameters.

Intravenous Administration

Following an intravenous bolus dose MRT can be calculated by Eq. 48 as illustrated in Table 17 (below). The *apparent volume of distribution at steady state* (V_{ss}) may be regarded as the volume of drug containing plasma that has to be "removed" from the body, i.e., the product of clearance (ml min^{-1}) and MRT (min):

$$V_{ss} = Cl \cdot \text{MRT} = \frac{\text{dose}}{\text{AUC}} \times \frac{\text{AUMC}}{\text{AUC}} = \frac{\text{dose} \cdot \text{AUMC}}{\text{AUC}^2} \qquad [49]$$

Attempts to separate the MRT, which refers to the whole body, into central and peripheral components (77) may prove to be of value but are dependent on the data fitting a two-compartment model.

If the compound is too toxic to be given as an instantaneous bolus, the MRT can be calculated from the AUMC determined following an intravenous infusion using the equation:

$$\text{MRT}_{\text{infusion}} = \text{MRT} + \frac{T}{2} \qquad [50]$$

where $\text{MRT}_{\text{infusion}}$ is calculated from the AUMC and AUC by Eq. 48 from the infusion data, and T is the infusion time.

The V_{ss} cannot be derived directly from these AUMC and AUC data, as the AUMC value contains a component due to the infusion time. The following equation therefore applies.

$$V_{ss} = \frac{\text{infused dose} \cdot \text{AUMC}}{\text{AUC}^2} - \frac{\text{infused dose} \cdot T}{2 \cdot \text{AUC}} \qquad [51]$$

In the same way that Cl may be related to V by the rate constant k (Eq. 21) so it may be related to V_{ss} by the first-order rate constant K_{ss} (6,26).

$$Cl = K_{ss}V_{ss} = \frac{V_{ss}}{\text{MRT}}$$

Therefore K_{ss} is equivalent to $1/\text{MRT}$, and for a two-compartment system it is intermediate between α and β. The half-life derived from K_{ss} ($0.693/K_{ss}$ or $0.693 \cdot \text{MRT}$) is therefore a composite half-life that may usefully be regarded as the "effective" half-life, which is shown clearly in the data analyzed later (see Table 17, below). The half-life derived from K_{ss} ($0.693 \times 25 = 17$ min) is intermediate between that calculated from α ($0.693/0.0705 = 10$ min) and β ($0.693/0.0240 = 34$ min).

Oral Administration

A strength of the statistical moment theory is its ability to derive meaningful data following oral administration, and it is both more reliable and easier to use than most other methods (11). The most useful parameter is the *mean absorption time* (MAT), which is the difference between the mean residence times following oral and intravenous dosing:

$$\text{MAT} = \text{MRT}_{\text{oral}} - \text{MRT}_{\text{iv}} \qquad [52]$$

The MAT may be used to derive apparent first-order rate constants and half-lives:

$$k_a = \frac{1}{\text{MAT}}$$

$$\text{Absorption } t_{\frac{1}{2}} = 0.693 \cdot \text{MAT}$$

Alternatively, if absorption appears to be zero order, by analogy with Eq. 50

$$\text{MAT} = \frac{T}{2}$$

where T is the duration of the absorption process.

The measurement of MAT is generally applied to absorption from a solution. If a sparingly soluble compound is given,

$$\text{MRT}_{\text{oral}} = \text{MRT}_{\text{iv}} + \text{MAT} + \text{MDT}$$

where MDT is the mean dissolution time.

The statistical moment theory is a valuable technique for comparisons on the influence of dosage formulations on absorption (11,53).

During Chronic Administration

As discussed previously the increase to steady state for multicompartment models is complex. AUC data may be applied in the absence of compartmental analysis to derive the proportion of steady state reached at any time after dosing. This proportion is simply equal to the proportion of the total AUC calculated to infinity ($\text{AUC}_{0-\infty}$) represented by the AUC to that time (AUC_{0-t}), i.e.,

$$\% \text{ Steady state} = 100 \times \frac{\text{AUC}_{0-t}}{\text{AUC}_{0-\infty}}$$

There is, however, a complication in the use of statistical moments for analysis of steady-state data because, unlike AUC data, $\text{AUMC}_{0-\infty}$ for a single dose does not equal AUMC_{0-T} during regular dosing (5). A simple way to overcome this difficulty is to apply a method of residuals to the steady-state plasma concentration prior to the regular dose (C_{min}). Assuming that this level decreases by a single first-order rate (β) determined from the terminal phase of the interdose period (or the terminal phase following a single dose), the contribution of this residue to each subsequent sample can be calculated as $C_{\text{min}}e^{-\beta t}$, where t is the time of that particular sample after C_{min}. The calculated residue is then subtracted from the measured value at each time to derive pseudo-single dose data that can be used to calculate AUMC.

Dose-Dependent or Nonlinear Kinetics

Whereas simple diffusion obeys first-order kinetics at all concentrations, many of the other processes fundamental to pharmacokinetics involve an interaction between the foreign chemical and a specific site on a protein (examples being active transport across the gut, plasma and tissue protein binding, metabolism, and renal tubular secretion). These processes have a finite capacity for interaction between the chemical and the protein; and thus at high concentrations of chemical, all the specific sites on the protein are occupied. Addition of further chemical cannot result in further interaction between chemical and protein, and the concentration of free compound increases rapidly. Depending on the nature of the protein–chemical interaction, there are a number of possible consequences, which are summarized in Table 7. This table represents a considerable simplification, as the effect of saturation at one site may affect another protein–chemical interaction. For example, saturation of renal tubular secretion gives increased AUC/dose and elevated plasma levels. However, the resultant high concentrations may saturate plasma protein binding, resulting in an increase in free drug and increased glomerular filtration or hepatic clearance. Thus the decreased elimination in the tubule may be overcome to some extent by increased elimination elsewhere.

Almost all the processes listed in Table 7 may be described

TABLE 7. *Consequences of saturation of drug–protein interactions*

Site	Interaction	Possible consequences of saturation at high dose
Absorption	Active uptake	Reduced plasma levels and AUC after oral but not i.v. doses.
	First-pass metabolism	Increased plasma levels and AUC after oral but not i.v. doses.
Distribution	Plasma protein	Increased volume of distribution; increased glomerular filtration; increased hepatic clearance if extraction ratio is low.
	Tissue protein	Decreased volume of distribution; a graph of C_t/C_p against C_p will be nonlinear.
Metabolism	Metabolizing enzyme (saturation by substrate, depletion of cofactors, product inhibition)	Decreased clearance; AUC/dose ratio increases for parent compound, whereas AUC of metabolite/dose ratio may decrease for both oral and i.v. doses; enzymes with high Km values may handle a larger proportion of the dose.
Excretion	Renal tubular secretion	Decreased renal clearance; AUC/dose ratio increases for oral and i.v. doses; nonrenal routes of elimination become of more importance; total excretion in urine per dose may decrease depending on the availability of other routes of elimination.
	Renal tubular reabsorption (rare)	Opposite of effects for saturation of renal tubular secretion.
	Biliary excretion	Decreased biliary clearance; decreased enterohepatic recirculation; renal route may become more important; AUC/dose ratio increases for oral and i.v. doses.

by a Michaelis-Menten equation of the type introduced into Eq. 11, i.e.,

$$-\frac{dC}{dt} = \frac{V_m C}{K_m + C} \quad [53]$$

where V_m is the theoretical maximum rate of the reaction, and K_m is the Michaelis constant (which reflects the concentration giving 50% saturation of the protein). At low concentrations, $C \ll K_m$, and Equation 53 may be approximated to

$$-\frac{dC}{dt} = \frac{V_m C}{K_m}$$

and V_m/K_m is equivalent to the first-order rate constant k. At higher concentrations, $C \gg K_m$, and Eq. 53 may be approximated to

$$-\frac{dC}{dt} = \frac{V_m C}{C} = V_m$$

and thus the elimination is a zero-order reaction. The shape of the plasma concentration–time curve for a hypothetical compound showing saturation kinetics is given in Fig. 12, which clearly shows that although low doses are indistinguishable from first-order elimination, the decrease at high plasma levels shows zero-order and then first-order reaction components.

It is important to note that the terminal slope and half-life are derived from low plasma concentrations and do not provide evidence of dose dependence. However, the plasma clearance, which is derived from AUC data and which reflects the capacity of the organs of elimination to remove the chemical from plasma, provides the best evidence of saturation. It is shown clearly for the example given in Fig. 12 by derivation of the appropriate rate constants, etc. (Table 8), which shows a fivefold change in Cl; it also illustrates the power of the statistical moment approach, which shows a

fourfold increase in MRT. The value of k (0.0485) approximates (V_{max}/K_m) (0.050).

An increased understanding of saturation kinetics can be obtained by the determination of K_m and V_{max} from *in vivo* data. The value of K_m, which reflects the plasma concentration necessary to give 50% saturation of the active process, is particularly useful. These constants can be determined following a single intravenous bolus dose using various equations, provided the elimination is by a single saturable process (see below). The simplest method applicable to a one-compartment model is by calculation directly from the plasma concentration–time curve using the equations

$$\ln C_p = \ln C_{p0e} - \frac{V_{max} \cdot t}{K_m}$$

and

$$K_m = \frac{C_{p0a}}{\ln (C_{p0e}/C_{p0a})}$$

where C_{p0e} is the value of C_p at $t = 0$ derived by back-extrapolation of the terminal linear phase, and C_{p0a} is the actual concentration measured at $t = 0$.

Thus a plot of $\ln C_p$ against time has a terminal "first-order" slope of V_{max}/K_m. Applying these equations to the data in Fig. 12 for the highest dose gives values of 0.0486 for the slope, 200 for C_{p0a}, and 2,701,271 for C_{p0e}. Thus

$$K_m = \frac{200}{\ln (2,701,271/200)} = 21 \ \mu g \ ml^{-1}$$

and

$$V_{max} = 0.0486 \times 21 = 1.0 \ \mu g \ min^{-1}$$

Alternative equations for the calculation of K_m and V_{max} require calculation of the rate of change of concentration from one sample to the next ($\Delta C_p/\Delta t$) as well as the plasma concentration at the midpoint (C_{pm}).

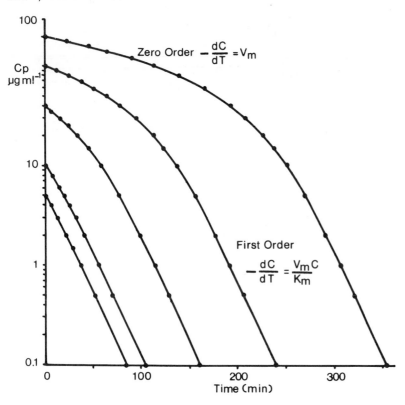

FIG. 12. Plasma concentration–time curve for a compound showing saturation kinetics. The data were generated using an apparent V_{max} of 1 μg/min and a K_m of 20 μg/ml for initial concentrations of 5, 10, 40, 100, and 200 μg/ml. Data points were obtained using a derivative of Eq. 53, i.e., $V_{max}(t - t_0) = C_{p0} - C_p + K_m \ln(C_{p0}/C_p)$.

Lineweaver-Burk plot

$$\frac{1}{\Delta C_p/\Delta t} = \frac{K_m}{V_{max} \cdot C_{pm}} + \frac{1}{V_{max}}$$

Therefore a plot of $1/(\Delta C_p/\Delta t)$ against $1/C_{pm}$ has a slope of K_m/V_{max} and an intercept of $1/V_{max}$.

Hanes-Woolf plot

$$\frac{C_{pm}}{\Delta C_p/\Delta t} = \frac{K_m}{V_{max}} + \frac{C_{pm}}{V_{max}}$$

Therefore a plot of $C_{pm}/(\Delta C_p/\Delta_t)$ against C_{pm} has a slope of $1/V_{max}$ and an intercept of K_m/V_{max}.

Woolf-Augustinsson-Hofstee plot

$$\frac{\Delta C_p}{\Delta t} = V_{max} - \frac{(\Delta C_p/\Delta t)K_m}{C_{pm}}$$

Therefore a plot of $\Delta C_p/\Delta t$ against $(\Delta C_p/\Delta t)/C_{pm}$ has a slope of $-K_m$ and an intercept of V_{max}.

TABLE 8. *Pharmacokinetic parameters derived from data showing saturation kinetics: Figure 12*

Parameter	Curve 1	Curve 2	Curve 3	Curve 4	Curve 5
Dose (mg/kg)	5	10	40	100	200
C_{p0} (μg/ml)	5	10	40	100	200
k (min^{-1})[a]	0.0486	0.0486	0.0486	0.0485	0.0486
Half-life (min)[a]	14.3	14.3	14.3	14.3	14.3
AUC (μg ml^{-1} min)[b]	115	254	1614	7020	24,027
AUMC (μg ml^{-1} min^2)[b]	2,437	5,702	50,682	355,788	2,002,493
Cl (ml min^{-1} kg^{-1})[c]	43.5	39.4	24.8	14.2	8.3
MRT (min)[d]	21.2	22.4	31.4	50.7	83.3

The parameters were calculated assuming a one-compartment model with a volume of distribution of 1 L/kg, which is not dose-dependent.

[a] Derived from data between 2.0 and 0.1 μg/ml for each dose.

[b] Calculated by the trapezoid rule with extrapolation to infinity. (See Table 17 for a worked example.)

[c] Cl, dose/AUC (Eq. 22).

[d] MRT, AUMC/AUC (Eq. 48).

When the data for the highest dose in Fig. 12 are analyzed by these techniques (Table 9) the following values were obtained (Fig. 13):

Lineweaver-Burk plot

$$x\text{-intercept} = \frac{-1}{K_m} = -0.0537; \quad K_m = 18.6 \ \mu g \ ml^{-1}$$

$$y\text{-intercept} = \frac{1}{V_{max}} = 1.04; \quad K_m = 0.96 \ \mu g \ min^{-1}$$

$$\text{Slope} = \frac{V_{max}}{K_m} = 0.0517; \quad \frac{0.96}{18.6} = 0.0516$$

Hanes-Woolf plot

$$\text{Slope} = \frac{1}{V_{max}} = 0.999; \quad V_{max} = 1.001$$

$$\text{Intercept} = \frac{K_m}{V_{max}} = 19.85; \quad K_m = 19.9$$

Woolf-Augustinsson-Hofstee plot

$$\text{Slope} = -K_m = -20.3; \quad K_m = 20.3$$

$$\text{Intercept} = V_{max} = 1.005$$

The values of V_m and K_m may be derived from plateau levels on intravenous infusion, providing elimination is essentially by a saturable process only, as rate of input = rate of elimination:

$$R = \frac{V_m C_{pss}}{K_m + C_{pss}}$$

where R is the rate of infusion, or

$$R = V_m - K_m \times \frac{R}{C_{pss}}$$

Thus a plot of R against R/C_{pss} gives a straight line with a slope of K_m and an intercept of V_m on the R axis.

Frequently, the rate of elimination can be described by a combination of saturable and nonsaturable processes when

$$-\frac{dC}{dt} = \frac{V_m C}{K_m + C} + k'C$$

where k' is the rate constant for the nonsaturable process. k' may be replaced by Cl'/V, where Cl' is the clearance by nonsaturable processes, e.g., glomerular filtration, in which case $GFR\alpha/V$ may be substituted for k'.

However, of greatest importance for toxicology is the clear demonstration of saturation at high doses, an estimation of the plasma concentration above which first-order kinetics cease to apply, and the plasma level present in animals showing overt toxicity. Wagner (79) proposed five tests for the establishment of saturation or nonlinear kinetics.

1. Graphs of C_p/dose against time should be superimposable for linear kinetics at different doses. Although considerable scatter is seen, an overall trend to increased or decreased levels at higher doses should be apparent for nonlinear systems.
2. Administer different intravenous doses and estimate C_{p0} by fitting only the first two or three early time points to the equation $\ln C_p = \ln C_{p0} - kt$. Graphs of C_p/C_{p0} against time should be superimposable if linear kinetics apply.
3. Fit each set of concentration–time data to a linear model and derive the appropriate kinetic parameters (Cl, V, k, k_{12}, k_{21}, V_1, etc). A dose-dependent change in a parameter indicates nonlinearity or saturation kinetics.
4. If Michaelis-Menten kinetics apply, the percentage me-

TABLE 9. *Calculation of K_m and V_{max} from plasma concentration time data*

Time[a]	C_p[a]	$\Delta C_p/\Delta t$[b]	C_{pm}[c]	$1/\Delta C_p/\Delta t$	$1/C_{pm}$	$C_{pm}/(\Delta C_p/\Delta t)$	$(\Delta C_p/\Delta t)/C_{pm}$
0	200	0.905	188	1.10	0.0053	207.7	0.0048
22.1	180	0.893	168	1.12	0.0060	188.1	0.0053
44.5	160	0.885	147	1.13	0.0068	166.1	0.0060
67.1	140	0.865	127	1.16	0.0079	146.8	0.0068
90.2	120	0.844	107	1.18	0.0093	126.8	0.0079
113.9	100	0.820	87	1.22	0.0115	106.1	0.0094
138.3	80	0.775	68	1.29	0.0147	87.7	0.0114
164.1	60	0.712	49	1.40	0.0204	68.8	0.0145
192.2	40	0.637	34.2	1.57	0.0292	53.7	0.0186
207.9	30	0.549	24.5	1.82	0.0408	44.6	0.0224
226.1	20	0.467	17.7	2.14	0.0565	37.9	0.0264
236.8	15	0.382	12.5	2.62	0.0800	32.7	0.0306
249.9	10	0.265	7.3	3.77	0.1370	27.5	0.0363
268.8	5	0.141	3.3	7.09	0.3030	23.4	0.0427
290.1	2	0.067	1.4	14.93	0.7140	20.9	0.0479
305.0	1	0.035	0.70	28.57	1.4286	20.0	0.0500
319.3	0.5	0.012	0.225	83.33	4.44	18.8	0.0530
351.9	0.1						

[a] Raw data.
[b] Calculated as 200 − 180/22.1 − 0 = 0.905, etc.
[c] Read off the concentration time curve at midpoint of interval.

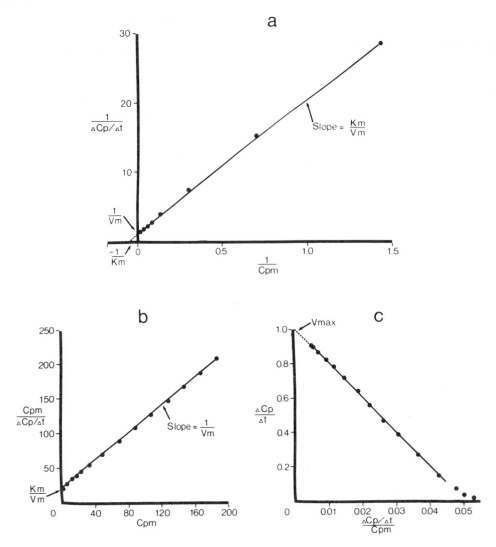

FIG. 13. Analysis of the maximum dose given in Fig. 12 to derive K_m and V_{max} using the data in Table 9 and the methods of **(a)** Lineweaver-Burk, **(b)** Hanes-Woolf, and **(c)** Woolf-Augustinsson-Hofstee.

tabolized by that pathway decreases with an increase in dose (provided other elimination routes are available), the value of AUC/dose is not constant, and plots of log C_p against time curve downward, as shown in Fig. 12.

5. Measure the tissue and unbound plasma concentrations over a range of doses. As suggested by Fig. 4, a plot of tissue concentration against unbound concentration should be a straight line for a linear tissue extraction. Saturation of tissue binding is shown by the tissue concentration having a smaller increase at higher concentrations. Alternatively, the value C_t/C_{pu} is a reflection of the tissue association constant and should be constant for a linear system. Nonlinearity of tissue binding is shown by this value becoming smaller at high doses.

A consequence of nonlinear kinetics is that the time to reach steady state is also dose-dependent. In simple terms, it is because the "effective half-life," calculated by 0.693 × MRT, increases with an increase in dose (e.g., Table 8) so that the time to steady state (four to five half-lives) must also

increase. This situation should be borne in mind when planning short-term studies. The importance of nonlinear kinetics in toxicology is discussed in greater detail after Data Handling, below.

PRACTICAL METHODS

General information on techniques may be obtained from the texts by Waynforth (80) and Cocchetto and Bjornsson (13). Waynforth described practical methods ranging from how to hold the animal for injection to such specialist techniques as renal transplantation. The other work, which contains 501 references, is an extensive and invaluable literature review of methods for the collection of body fluids. A number of modifications applicable to other species are given below.

The methods for dosing, blood sampling, urine collection, etc., described below are largely related to the rat, as it is the species most commonly used in toxicological studies.

Administration Techniques

Oral Dosing

Because a number of lipid and metabolic barriers separate the lumen of the gastrointestinal tract from the systemic circulation (Fig. 1), plasma levels of test compounds usually increase gradually after oral administration to reach a maximum. It is thus possible to give higher doses by this route than by intravenous injection, and this technique is aided by the capacity of the stomach to hold a large bulk of liquid. For pharmacokinetic studies, the oral route can provide valuable information on elimination and clearance values, provided the extent of absorption from the gut is known. The latter may be determined by measuring either the area under the curve or the total amount of the test substance excreted in the urine unchanged after oral and intravenous administration at low doses. The fraction absorbed is given by Eq. 31, and this figure can then be used to measure the clearance as described in the derivative of Eq. 22. The possibility of saturation of absorption may be determined by plotting the value C_p/dose against time for doses up to and including those producing overt toxicity.

Rats, guinea pigs, and mice may be dosed orally using a syringe fitted with a suitable intubation needle; in rabbits a polythene cannula is passed into the stomach while the jaws are held open by a gag. Certain precautions should be taken to prevent artifacts. For example, it is important that the test chemical is completely dissolved. If the chemical is given in suspension, the apparent absorption rate must include a component due to dissolution of the chemical. If this factor is rate-limiting, the measured absorption rate reflects the dissolution rate and is not related to the biological availability of the chemical. The vehicle for dissolution ideally is water or a small volume of a water-miscible solvent such as ethanol, propylene glycol (propane-1,2-diol), or dimethylsulfoxide. Excess acids or bases should not be used to dissolve the test compound, and the pH of the dose solution should be near pH 7 to avoid affecting pH partitioning in either the gut or the renal tubule, which could alter the measured absorption or elimination rate constants. If an organic solvent is used to dissolve the chemical, water should be added to reduce the dehydrating effect of the solvent within the gut lumen. The volume of water or solvent/water used to dissolve the chemical should be kept low, as excess quantities may distend the stomach and cause rapid gastric emptying. In addition, large volumes of water may carry the chemical through membrane pores and increase the absorption rate. Thus if dose-dependent absorption is suspected, it is important that the different doses are given in the same volume of solution.

The maximum volume of aqueous solution that can be administered without the possibility of gross interference with absorption is approximately 5 to 10 ml/kg. Larger volumes may be given, although nonlinear kinetics seen under such circumstances may be due to solvent-induced alteration of intestinal function. The use of water-immiscible solvents such as corn oil, which are sometimes used for gavage doses, should be avoided, as it is possible that mobilization from the vehicle is rate-limiting. However, such a solvent would obviously be appropriate if it was the method of administration used in toxicity studies, as it would give information on the rate of absorption and bioavailability under the conditions of the toxicity study.

Nasal Administration

Methods have been described for assessing absorption from the nasal cavity based on plasma pharmacokinetics following intranasal and intravenous dosing and by *in situ* perfusion experiments (32,72).

Rectal Administration

Because a number of therapeutic compounds are given in the form of suppositories, an indication of the bioavailability after rectal administration is sometimes required. Normally, toxicity studies and initial drug formulations of such compounds are performed by the oral route, and the rectal formulation comes late in development and marketing. In view of the differences between laboratory animals and man in the anatomy and microflora of the colon and rectum, animal bioavailability studies late in drug development are of limited value. However, in cases where an indication of rectal bioavailability is required, the compound may be introduced into the rectum of the rat using an oral dosing needle to prevent tissue damage. To avoid rapid excretion of the unabsorbed dose, anesthetized animals are used and the dose is retained with an inert plug or bung.

Inhalation

As indicated previously, the major problem associated with the kinetics of inhalation concerns the measurement of the extent to which the drug is absorbed across the lung rather than passed back into the mouth to be swallowed, exhaled in the expired air, or absorbed across the skin. Comparison of the area under the plasma concentration–time curve, or the total urinary excretion of unchanged drug, after a period of inhalation with this parameter after a known intravenous dose can be used to determine the total dose entering via the lungs and gut.

A method used successfully by McKenna et al. (40) to obtain kinetic data involved a 6-hr exposure to the vapor of [^{14}C]vinylidene chloride in rats, after which the animals were transferred to a metabolism cage. The body load at the time of removal was determined by the total recovery of radioactivity in the expired air, excreta, cage washings, and carcass. This method is appropriate, as the nonspecific measurement of ^{14}C includes parent compound and all metabolites. If the parent compound alone is measured, the inhalation data must be related to intravenous data to measure the exposure after inhalation. The approach of McKenna et al. (40) was capable of revealing differences between fasted and fed animals in their capacity to metabolize vinylidene chloride, which correlated well with the toxicity of this compound. The absorption of most compounds tested by this route is rapid, although certain compounds, e.g., the antiasthmatic drug sodium cromoglycate, may by their structures be expected to show a measurable first-order absorption across the lungs. However, after instillation of a micronized powder into the trachea, the observed rate may be that of the formulation, not of the chemical moiety itself.

An interesting method used by Andersen et al. (1) to study the rate constants of 1,1-dichloroethylene metabolism on inhalation was based on measurement of the rate of removal of the compound from circulating air in a closed chamber system containing the experimental animal. The air was recirculated and oxygen was added to maintain the concentration at 19 to 21%. The air was sampled at regular intervals and analyzed for unabsorbed 1,1-dichloroethylene by gas-liquid chromatography. The rate of removal showed two phases: a rapid phase proportional to the mass of the animal and the concentration of chemical, and a slow phase, which represented metabolism of the compound. The slow phase showed saturation (Michaelis-Menten) kinetics; and rate constants (K_m and V_{max}) were derived in terms of the concentration of chemical in the chamber. This approach is interesting as the data are obtained by a noninvasive method. Also, the kinetic constants are derived in terms of vapor or gas concentrations, which are most appropriate when considering the possible dangers of human exposure to volatile agents.

Percutaneous Absorption

The percutaneous route is likely to be of increasing importance in drug formulation in the future. Animals may be used as suitable models, and an added pharmacokinetic advantage to this route is that the fraction absorbed may be measured as described above for the oral route (i.e., AUC data) and by analysis of the amount remaining at the site of administration. The dermal absorption of vapors can be assessed in rats using a body-only chamber (39).

Intravenous Injection

The bolus intravenous dose is the most important single technique for deriving information concerning the kinetics of the distribution and elimination of chemicals. As with oral administration, aqueous or aqueous miscible solvents should be used, although the volume is considerably reduced, i.e., about 2 ml/kg for aqueous and 1 ml/kg for solvent–aqueous mixtures. Ideally, the solution is made isotonic by the addition of sodium chloride, although in practice dissolution of low doses in isotonic saline is adequate.

There are two important parameters to be considered in such studies. First, the data processing assumes that the material was administered instantaneously at time 0. In practice, a rapid injection may produce considerable toxicity, which a slower injection can prevent. Generally, a "bolus" dose, given over a finite period of up to a few minutes, is regarded as instantaneous provided the total injection time does not represent more than about 5% of the half-life of the most rapid phase of the plasma concentration–time curve. The other parameter to be considered is the true location of the dose, as in kinetic studies it is important that 100% of the dose is intravenous and none ends up in a perivascular site. The following techniques have proved successful.

Rat

The tail and hind paw veins are convenient for dosing but neither is particularly easy to use or gives 100% intravascular dosing repeatedly and routinely without the necessary expertise. The following technique, although more complex, is preferable because it overcomes the problems experienced with the above routes, and the cannula can be used subsequently for sample collection (providing that the chemical is not adsorbed onto the tubing). The animal is anesthetized with ether, and an incision is made through the skin of the neck to the right of the midline. Blunt dissection is used to separate the thin layer of muscle covering the external jugular vein, which is exposed and cleaned (Fig. 14). Thread is passed under the vein at both anterior and posterior ends of the exposed section but is not tied off posteriorly. A small incision is made in the vein, and a length of polythene cannula tubing, connected to the dosing syringe, is passed into the vein toward the heart for a distance of about 2 cm.

The dose solution is injected and the cannula rinsed with isotonic saline. The tubing may then be removed and the

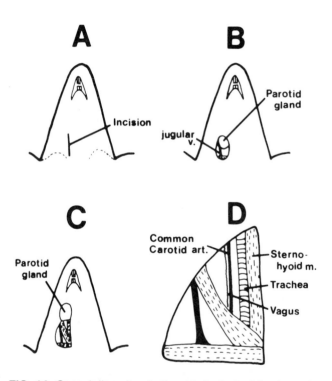

FIG. 14. Cannulation sites in the rat. **A:** An incision is made to the left of the midline, slightly anterior to the limbs. Subcutaneous tissue is removed by blunt dissection to reveal the vein. **B:** The *external jugular vein* is cleared and cannulated as described in the text. **C:** The incision is enlarged and the parotid gland displaced forward. The common carotid artery is found by blunt dissection between the sternohyoid muscle and the diagonal sternocleido-mastoid group of muscles. **D:** The *common carotid artery* is separated from the parallel nerve tract; one thread is tied loosely around the anterior end, and two threads are tied loosely around the posterior end. Blood flow is prevented by tension on the anterior and second posterior tie, and the cannula tubing is inserted as described in the text.

vein tied off or the cannula tubing tied *in situ* for subsequent sampling, providing that the compound does not adhere to the cannula (see below). In anesthetized rats that will not regain consciousness during the study, an alternative site of injection is the femoral vein, which may be exposed by an incision into the ventral surface of the top of the hind leg.

Guinea pig

A modification of the external jugular method described above may be used for the guinea pig. The external jugular vein of an anesthetized animal is exposed but not cleaned of connective tissue. The dose is injected directly using a fine needle (0.5 mm gauge) bent inward through about 45°, which allows the needle to be positioned without undue stretching or movement of the vein. The vein is clamped, above and below the injection site, as the needle is withdrawn. The vein is subsequently ligated and the incision sutured.

Rabbit

It is relatively easy to administer intravenous doses to rabbits, as the vein running around the periphery of the ear lobe can be readily exposed by shaving with a scalpel blade. This vein is of sufficient size and visibility to give reliable intravenous dosing.

Intravenous Infusion

For intravenous infusion studies the dose must be given via an indwelling cannula, and the external jugular vein is an excellent site. If the infusion period is prolonged, such that recovery from anesthesia is envisaged, the cannula can be run under the skin from the ventral surface of the neck and exteriorized on the dorsal surface behind the ears. If the cannula is then secured on the dorsal surface, the animal is prevented from damaging it during infusion while being permitted a degree of restricted movement. This method of exteriorization is also valuable as a method of long-term sampling (see below).

The delivery of compound during intravenous infusion must be at a constant but low rate such that the animal is not subjected to excessive hemodilution. To date, the standard method has been to use a high quality infusion pump (e.g., Harvard Compact Infusion Pump). The development of osmotically driven minipumps (Alzet), which can be implanted into the animal and deliver a constant rate as low as 0.5 μl/hr for up to 2 weeks, opened up exciting possibilities. Minipumps allow investigations of steady-state plasma and tissue levels associated with toxicity and the pharmacokinetics under similar steady-state conditions. Such devices have been used to study the renal clearance of ^{63}Ni under steady-state conditions; and, interestingly, these studies revealed diurnal fluctuations in the steady-state levels, probably due to metabolic changes that were not suspected from earlier studies (64).

Sampling Techniques

Blood (Plasma and Serum)

When considering the frequency, timing, and duration of blood sampling, it is important that an adequate number of samples are taken to define each section of the plasma concentration–time curve (Fig. 5). It has been suggested that plasma samples be collected during the first four to five half-lives, during which time 93 to 97% of the compound will have been eliminated (85). However, it is possible that such a restriction may mask a quantitatively minor component on single dosing capable of significant accumulation on continuous ingestion as part of a toxicity test. Such a component could be perfusion- or diffusion-limited distribution to a tissue in which the tissue affinity (Fig. 4) was high. If such a tissue was the site of overt toxicity on chronic administration, the pharmacokinetic investigation would have failed to throw any light on the process involved. Thus as a general guideline the plasma concentration should be measured until the limit of detection of the analytical method is reached. Obviously, if the limit of detection allows analysis over a large number of half-lives, less frequent sampling is required during the slow terminal phase, which can be adequately defined by about six linear samples. Thus a three-compartment system can be accurately analyzed by 15 to 18 samples provided that they are correctly timed. The corollary to this situation is that a relatively insensitive analytical method is incapable of yielding full pharmacokinetic data. Thus considering Fig. 5, if the limit of detection for compounds A and B were 0.1 μg/ml, both would appear to be represented adequately by a one-compartment model, with different values of k. Indeed, under these circumstances the plasma concentration of both A and B would fall from 2.85 to 0.10, a decrease of 97%, equivalent to about five half-lives.

Using the methods described below, it is possible to withdraw a significant fraction of the total blood volume (64 ml/kg in the rat), thereby modifying the perfusion of the organs of elimination and corrupting the derived pharmacokinetic data. This problem can be avoided by taking the smallest samples consistent with accurate analysis and the minimum number of samples necessary to adequately define the various phases (i.e., smaller samples at early time points). As a general rule, individual blood samples should be restricted to a maximum of about 0.5 ml/kg body weight, providing the total number of samples is small (i.e., less than ten). This general rule takes no account of the duration of the experiment, which may indicate either smaller or larger sample sizes.

Rat

Various methods have been successfully used to obtain small serial blood samples from anesthetized and conscious rats.

Tail vein. Whole blood samples (approximately 70 μl) are obtained on cutting the tail vein with a scalpel blade and collecting the blood into heparinized capillary tubes. This method is widely used and was employed by Sauerhoff et al. (61) in their study of the dose-dependent kinetics of 2,4,5-trichlorophenoxyacetic acid.

Toe vasculature. Blood samples (up to 500 μl) may be collected by clipping the toenail into the vascular bed and allowing the blood to run into heparinized capillary tubes (29).

Cardiac puncture. Multiple cardiac sampling is possible but involves more trauma than the above methods, as (ether) anesthesia is essential. However, provided that a fine (0.5 mm) needle is used, it is possible, with practice, to obtain a number of samples without evidence of extravascular blood loss.

Orbital sinus. The animal is anesthetized with ether and held down by gentle pressure with thumb and forefinger behind the head. A heparinized capillary tube is inserted into the orbit at the anterior apex and moved to rupture the sinus membrane in the anterior dorsal region at the back of the orbit. A considerable blood flow is obtained, which stops on removal of the tube and the pressure at the back of the neck.

External jugular vein. Methods have been described in which silicon medical grade cannula tubing (Silastic; 0.05 cm i.d., 0.09 cm o.d.) implanted in the external jugular vein (Fig. 14) has remained patent for blood sampling for periods up to 2 months (76). The use of silicon tubing is preferred to polyethylene for such long-term studies because it is more flexible for exteriorization on the dorsal surface and less apt to cause thrombosis.

The tubing is inserted into the vein by either of two methods. First, a suitable size syringe needle shaft is attached, which is passed into the vein and then pushed back out again about 5 mm lower down. The needle shaft is then removed, and the cannula tubing is gently pulled back until it reenters the vein. Alternatively, the end of the cannula is made into a point by a steep diagonal cut and inserted via a small incision in the vein. A shallow diagonal cut (i.e., almost parallel with the longitudinal axis of the tubing) aids insertion but is more prone to obstruction by the vein wall during sampling. Careful positioning of the end of the cannula tubing by gentle maneuvering may be necessary to achieve optimal sampling, which usually involves passing the cannula toward the heart for a distance of about 2 cm. A similar technique has been described (3) in which the cannula is then exteriorized and secured behind the head of the animal. However, under such circumstances a collar may be necessary to prevent the animal damaging the tubing (13).

Common carotid artery. In anesthetized animals in which the external jugular vein is used for infusion, the ipsilateral carotid artery can be used for sampling (Fig. 14). The artery lies deep below the sternohyoid muscle and may be reached using blunt dissection. The artery is a robust structure and can be brought to the surface by curved forceps. Cotton ties are placed anterior and posterior to the intended site of incision and tied loosely. The artery is then placed under tension by artery forceps attached to the anterior tie and to the posterior tie nearer the heart so as to prevent blood loss during incision. A small incision is made in the artery, and a length of cannula tubing, attached to a saline-filled syringe, is inserted and passed toward the heart, through the first posterior tie. It is tied firmly, and the tension on the second posterior tie is released. The cannula can now be slid through the second posterior tie, which is then tied securely. The anterior tie is now tightened and the artery forceps removed. Blood may be sampled by removing the syringe when the blood pressure is sufficient to expel the saline. The sampling is stopped by clamping the tubing, replacing the syringe, and passing saline back up the tubing. It is important to keep the artery under tension during insertion of the cannula, or significant blood loss may occur. An alternative method of applying tension is to insert a pair of forceps underneath the artery and allow them to open and stretch the artery.

Other species

For experiments performed under anesthesia, a major vein or artery (e.g., jugular, carotid, femoral) can be cannulated. For multiple sampling under temporary ether anesthesia, cardiac puncture has been used successfully for rats and guinea pigs; however, the orbital sinus is a more appropriate site for the mouse, and the marginal ear vein can be used for the rabbit without anesthesia.

Urine

A knowledge of the urinary excretion rate is necessary for calculating the overall renal clearance of a compound. The bladder causes variable slowing of the output; and for compounds with a short half-life, a method of overcoming sporadic urination is necessary. Calculating results by the sigma-minus method rather than using excretion rate data reduces the importance of incomplete bladder emptying and the resultant scatter in the data.

However, for compounds with a half-life of many hours, sufficiently frequent samples may be obtained merely by placing the animals in a metabolism cage, which gives adequate separation of urine and feces, and by encouraging reflex urination (13). Under anesthesia, the effect of the bladder may be overcome by (a) inserting and tying a cannula into the bladder via the urethra or directly across the bladder wall, and emptying and rinsing the bladder with isotonic saline using a syringe; (b) inserting a cannula via the urethra and allowing the urine to be expelled naturally or with the aid of gentle massage (8); or (c) cannulation of both ureters and collection of the urine without it passing through the bladder (51).

The third technique was used to analyze the extent of reabsorption of saccharin from the rat urinary bladder but was found to be technically difficult as both ureters had to be cannulated with polyethylene tubing stretched to give a suitable taper while slight twisting of the ureter effectively blocked the urine flow. This technique is not recommended for routine investigations. However, these studies did reveal that although the intact urinary bladder was relatively impermeable to saccharin (which is highly ionic) manipulation of the bladder with forceps produced a slight increase in permeability and bladder cannulation (as described above) produced a marked increase in permeability and reabsorption. Thus any damage or irritation caused by the cannula should be kept to a minimum; and if a cannula is inserted across the wall into the apex of the bladder, it is essential that the contents are removed and rinsed at frequent intervals, i.e., at least every 15 min. Similarly, any palpation used in method (b), above, should not be excessive, or increased reabsorption from the bladder may occur and cause a decreased apparent renal clearance. In addition, cannulas passed via the urethra, which is particularly suitable for female animals, should be positioned carefully such that they do not enter too far into the bladder lumen and damage the epithelium.

Renal clearance studies may be performed either after single doses or during infusion at steady state (when the clearance can be related to total clearance and plasma concentration). Insights into the extent of reabsorption and tubular secretion can be obtained by measuring the renal clearance of inulin given simultaneously (1–20 μCi of [^{14}C]inulin/kg or 50 to 100 μCi of [^{3}H]inulin/kg).

Bile

Bile may be collected from a cannula inserted into the common bile duct such that the tip is located at the point of bifurcation near the hilar region of the liver. The common bile duct is found by making an incision through the midline into the anterior part of the body cavity. Slight tension on the proximal part of the duodenum reveals the bile duct running through the pancreatic tissue. The bile duct is cleaned, a thread is placed loosely around it, and cannula tubing is inserted via a small incision and tied in place. The bile flow is usually 0.5 to 1.0 ml/hr in the rat. Bile may be collected by either placing the animal in a restraining cage and collecting from the exteriorized cannula or passing the tubing into a suitable container (sealed plastic sachet) placed subcutaneously. The test chemical is usually given soon after establishing the cannula, as changes in bile composition occur if the bile salts, etc., are not allowed to recirculate. A modified technique avoiding the use of animals still under the stress of surgery has been demonstrated by Light et al. (37). With this technique the bile cannula was exteriorized and joined to a second cannula, which passed back into the body cavity and entered the duodenum via the greater curvature of the stomach. The animals were then left for 4 days, after which constant food intake and body weight were observed. This method could be useful for studies after intravenous dosing or possibly for studies with chronic dietary intake of the chemical. However, more than 4 days would be necessary after surgery to reestablish steady-state intake, which may be different from that of normal animals.

In animal species that possess a gallbladder (i.e., guinea pig and rabbit), it is necessary to prevent this organ from acting as a variable capacitance vessel by ligation around its base so that bile has to pass directly down the cannula.

DATA HANDLING

The type of information that can be obtained from pharmacokinetic studies and its derivation from raw plasma and urine data is illustrated by results obtained by the author and T. W. Sweatman as part of an investigation into the pharmacokinetics of saccharin. This synthetic nonnutritive sweetener has been shown to cause an increased incidence of tumors of the urinary bladder in male rats when fed at high dietary concentrations (more than 3%) for two generations (60) or from birth (63). The possibility of nonlinear

kinetics at such high doses was investigated using the Charles River CD derived rat, because this strain showed detectable tumorigenicity. The study, which has been published elsewhere (74), investigated the concentrations of saccharin in the tissues of animals fed saccharin-containing diets and used the pharmacokinetic techniques outlined above to investigate details of the disposition of this compound. Previous studies using [^{14}C]saccharin had shown that it was incompletely absorbed from the gut and eliminated in the urine and feces without undergoing detectable metabolism (49).

On feeding rats saccharin-containing diets *ad libitum* for a period of 22 days, significant nonlinearity was apparent in the concentrations of saccharin in the plasma and tissues, with elevated concentrations at high dietary levels (Fig. 15). The following studies were performed in an attempt to investigate the cause of this phenomenon.

Intravenous Bolus Dose: Plasma Analysis

Saccharin is a strong organic acid (pKa about 2) that forms a highly water-soluble sodium salt. [5-^{3}H]Saccharin was used in these studies, and the concentrations in plasma and urine samples were determined by measuring the total radioactivity present (*because saccharin does not undergo metabolism*). A range of doses of saccharin were given (1–1,000 mg/kg as a

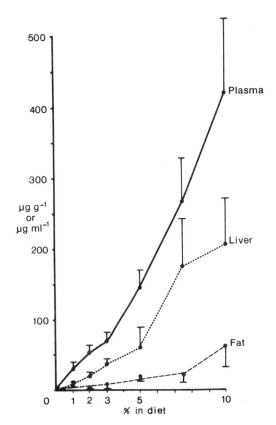

FIG. 15. Concentrations of saccharin in the plasma and tissues of rats given saccharin-containing diets. Adult male rats were given saccharin-containing diets *ad libitum* for 22 days prior to sacrifice at 6 a.m. The results are the means with standard deviations represented by vertical bars. (From ref. 74, with permission.)

TABLE 10. *Concentrations of saccharin in the plasma and urine of a rat given a single intravenous bolus dose[a]*

Plasma		Urine	
Time of sample (min)	Concentration ($\mu g\ ml^{-1}$)	Collection period (min)	Amount excreted (μg)
5	184.3	0–5	7,518
15	102.0	5–15	6,275
30	50.5	15–30	4,989
45	24.9	30–45	2,580
60	14.1	45–60	1,485
75	8.0	60–75	861
90	5.7	75–90	561
105	4.0	90–105	363
120	2.9	105–120	300

[a] The animal (body weight 570 g) was given a single intravenous bolus dose of saccharin (50 mg/kg) at time 0.

single intravenous bolus over a period of 30 sec) to anesthetized male rats via a cannula inserted into the jugular vein. The dead volume in the cannula was displaced with saline. Plasma samples were subsequently withdrawn from the same cannula, as saccharin showed no tendency to adhere to the polyethylene tubing used. The bladder was cannulated, emptied, and rinsed at each plasma collection period. The results for an individual animal given 50 mg/kg are presented in Table 10.

A graph of plasma concentration against time (Fig. 16) clearly shows a biphasic decrease, which may be analyzed graphically using the method of residuals as shown in Table 11. Alternatively, the β phase can be analyzed by linear regression analysis to yield the extrapolated values, which can then be analyzed by linear regression to give the values of A, B, α, and β as shown in Table 11. The data selected for this discussion were for an individual animal that showed

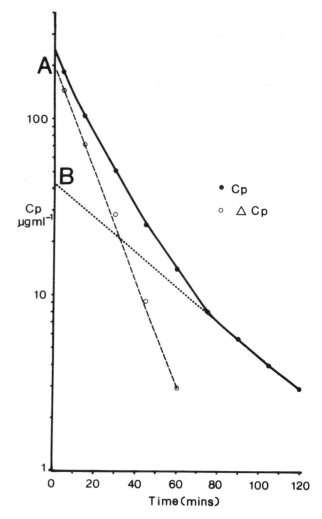

FIG. 16. Plasma concentration–time curve after a bolus of saccharin (50 mg/kg i.v.) into a male rat. The data used are given in Tables 10 and 11.

TABLE 11. *Data from Figure 16*

Analysis	Graphical		Linear regression
75–120 min			
β	$= \dfrac{(\log 11.1 - \log 2.9)}{120 - 60} \times 2.303 = 0.0224\ min^{-1}$		$0.0226\ min^{-1}$
B	$= 42\ \mu g\ ml^{-1}$		$43.7\ \mu g\ ml^{-1}$
Residuals			
	Time (min)	*Conc. ($\mu g\ ml^{-1}$)*	*Conc. ($\mu g\ ml^{-1}$)*
	5	184.3 − 37.5 = 146.8	184.3 − 39.0 = 145.3
	15	102.0 − 30.0 = 72.0	102.0 − 31.1 = 70.9
	30	50.5 − 21.6 = 28.9	50.5 − 22.1 = 28.4
	45	24.9 − 15.5 = 9.4	24.9 − 15.8 = 9.1
	60	14.1 − 11.1 = 3.0	14.1 − 11.2 = 2.9
5–45 min			
α	$= \dfrac{(\log 198 - \log 10) \times 2.303}{45 - 0} = 0.0664\ min^{-1}$		$0.0683\ min^{-1}$
A	$= 198\ \mu g\ ml^{-1}$		$204.5\ \mu g\ ml^{-1}$

TABLE 12. *Urinary excretion of saccharin after a single bolus dose of 50 mg/kg*

Time of collection[a] (min)	Midpoint (min)	Amount excreted[a] (μg)	Excretion rate (μg min^{-1})	Cumulative total (μg)	A_{ex}^{∞}-cumulative total (ΔA_{ex}) (μg)
0–5	2.5	7,518	1,503.6	7,518	18,247
5–15	10.0	6,275	627.5	13,793	11,972
15–30	22.5	4,989	332.6	18,782	6,983
30–45	37.5	2,580	172.0	21,362	4,403
45–60	52.5	1,485	99.0	22,847	2,918
60–75	67.5	861	57.4	23,708	2,057
75–90	82.5	561	37.4	24,269	1,496
90–105	97.5	363	24.2	24,632	1,133
105–120	112.5	300	20.0	24,932	833
120–∞[b]	—	833[b]	—	25,765[b]	—

[a] Raw data from Table 10.

[b] The additional amount excreted from the last data point to infinity can be calculated as the excretion rate (last) divided by the terminal slope. The graph of rate against time (Fig. 17; Table 13) gives a terminal slope of 0.024 min^{-1}; therefore the amount excreted 120–∞ equals 20.0 μg min^{-1}/0.024 min^{-1} = 833 μg.

a prolonged $\alpha + \beta$ phase. This choice was necessary, as information on the initial ($\alpha + \beta$) phase is decreased when urine data are analyzed. For other animals, the $\alpha + \beta$ phase was apparent only during the first 30 min, and linearity occurred between 30 to 45 and 120 min, so that they could not be studied adequately by the methods used in Tables 13 and 14 (see below). Thus in the animal selected, the data are actually deficient in that the β phase is dependent on only four points. Thus it is apparent that more reliable results would have been obtained had the sampling period been extended for another 30 min in this animal, such that both the α and β phases were represented by five or six points. This observation emphasizes an important principle, i.e., that the more data points measured, the more reliable are the results (provided that it does not involve removal of too much blood).

Intravenous Bolus Dose: Urine Analysis

The urinary excretion data have been recalculated in Table 12 in a form suitable for analysis of the excretion rate against time. A graph of excretion rate against time, using the midpoint of the sample collection period (Fig. 17; Table 13) shows a biphasic decrease similar to that seen in plasma. Because of the scatter in the points of the terminal β phase, it is not clear whether the 52.5-min point should be included in the β or the $\alpha + \beta$ phase. However, from the plasma curve (Fig. 16), it seems that the β phase started after 60 min, and thus the 52.5-min point was not included in the analysis of β. The residuals line (Fig. 17) was analyzed with the omission of the 2.5-min point, as this value did not fit the line clearly shown by other points, possibly due to high initial elimination prior to mixing of the compound within the central compartment. The constants α and β may be derived from the excretion rate or using the sigma-minus method, which is described by Eq. 28. The total amount finally excreted (Table 12) is obtained by extrapolation of the cumulative total (column 5, Table 12) to infinity, which may be done either graphically or from the excretion rate data, as shown in Table 12. The amount remaining to be excreted (ΔA_{ex}) is calculated

by subtracting the running total from the final total, for each time point (column 6, Table 12). A graph of ΔA_{ex} against time (Fig. 18) clearly showed a biphasic decrease, although

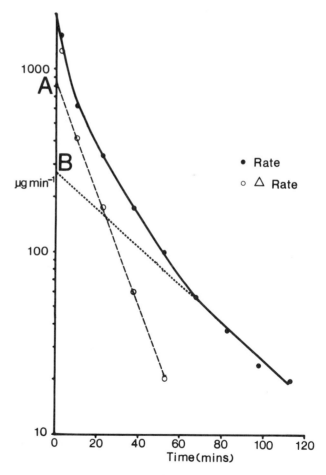

FIG. 17. Urinary excretion of saccharin after a single intravenous dose. The results are given as micrograms excreted per minute plotted against the time at the midpoint of the collection period. The data used are given in Table 12.

TABLE 13. *Data from Figure 17*

Analysis	Graphical	Linear regression
67.5–112.5 min		
β	$= \dfrac{(\log 270 - \log 20)}{110} \times 2.303 = 0.0237 \text{ min}^{-1}$	$\beta = 0.0240 \text{ min}^{-1}$
B'	$= 270 \ \mu g \ min^{-1}$	$B' = 277 \ \mu g \ min^{-1}$
Residuals		
	Time (min) *Rate (µg min⁻¹)*	*Rate (µg min⁻¹)*
	2.5 $1{,}503.6 - 256 = 1{,}247.6$	$1{,}503.6 - 260.5 = 1{,}243.1$
	10 $627.5 - 215 = \quad 412.5$	$627.5 - 217.6 = \quad 409.9$
	22.5 $332.6 - 160 = \quad 172.6$	$332.6 - 161.2 = \quad 171.4$
	37.5 $172.0 - 112 = \quad\quad 60.0$	$172.0 - 112.5 = \quad\quad 59.5$
	52.5 $99.0 - \ \ 79 = \quad\quad 20.0$	$99.0 - \ \ 78.5 = \quad\quad 20.5$
10–52.5 min		
α	$= \dfrac{(\log 830 - \log 20)}{52.5 - 0} \times 2.303 = 0.0710 \text{ min}^{-1}$	$= 0.0705 \text{ min}^{-1}$
A'	$= 830 \ \mu g \ min^{-1}$	$= 833 \ \mu g \ min^{-1}$
	(using the 2.5 min point, $\alpha = 0.0784$ and $A' = 1{,}138$)	

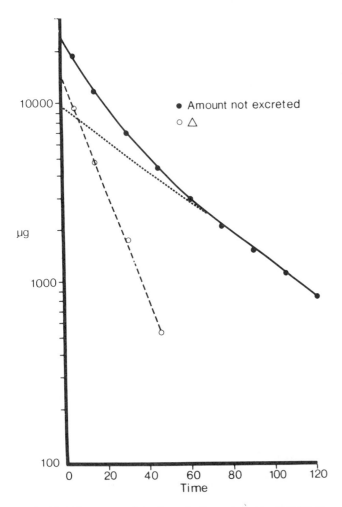

FIG. 18. Urinary excretion of saccharin analyzed by the sigma-minus method. The results are the amount remaining to be excreted (ΔA_{ex}) plotted against time. The data used are given in Table 12.

the β phase appeared to have started slightly earlier, at 60 min. Analysis of this curve by the method of residuals gave values of α, β, A'', and B'' (Table 14).

The renal clearance of the compound can be determined by Eq. 7 using the excretion rate during individual collection periods and the plasma concentrations at the middle of the collection period. These values are given in Table 15 and show a clearance of 5.0 ml min⁻¹ ± 10% for seven of the nine time points. The clearance adjusted for body weight was 8.82 ml min⁻¹ kg⁻¹. As an alternative to averaging the values derived during the experiment, Cl_R may be calculated also from the time averaged values A_{ex} and AUC (Table 15).

Intravenous Bolus Dose: Rate Constants

The values α, β, A, B, A', and so on, derived from plasma and urine, are given in Table 16. Using the six values for each constant given in Table 16, it is interesting that the value of β (0.0222 ± 0.0017 SD ± 7.5%) and α (0.0691 ± 0.0023 SD ± 3.3%) show much less variability than the values of k_{21}, k_{10}, and k_{12} derived by Eqs. 38, 39, and 40 (i.e., ±12%, 16%, and 19%, respectively).

Another important parameter that can be derived from the raw data is the plasma clearance, which is given by Eq. 22. The AUC may be measured by the trapezoid rule, as shown in Table 17, or by plotting the graph on linear paper and cutting out and weighing the area under the curve (as well as a rectangular area of suitable size and known area in $\mu g \ ml^{-1}$ min). Comparable results were obtained with the two methods, and the plasma clearance was calculated using the cut-and-weigh figure to be 10.18 ml min⁻¹ kg⁻¹.

With the trapezoid method the data points are joined by straight lines; thus after oral dosing the area during the increase is underestimated and that after the peak is overestimated—and the errors tend to cancel. After intravenous dosing, however, the AUC for each segment is overestimated,

TABLE 14. *Data from Figure 18*

Analysis		Graphical	Linear regression
60–120 min			
β		$= \dfrac{(\log 9{,}700 - \log 830)}{120} \times 2.303 = 0.0205$ min^{-1}	0.0199 min^{-1}
B″		$= 9{,}700$ μg	9,115 μg
Residuals			
	Time (min)	*Amount (μg)*	*Amount (μg)*
	5	$18{,}247 - 8{,}800 = 9{,}447$	$18{,}247 - 8{,}251 = 9{,}996$
	15	$11{,}972 - 7{,}200 = 4{,}772$	$11{,}972 - 6{,}760 = 5{,}212$
	30	$6{,}983 - 5{,}270 = 1{,}713$	$6{,}983 - 5{,}013 = 1{,}970$
	45	$4{,}403 - 3{,}870 = \;\;533$	$4{,}403 - 3{,}717 = \;\;686$
α		$= \dfrac{(\log 14{,}100 - \log 800)}{40} \times 2.303$ $= 0.0717$ min^{-1}	0.0668 min^{-1}
A″		$= 14{,}100$ μg	14,159 μg

Note: A″ + B″ is equivalent to the total amount excreted; it equals 23,800 μg by graphical and 23,274 μg by linear regression analysis.

the total extent of which depends on the number of time points available. These points are shown in Table 17; the clearance value calculated using the cut-and-weigh method gives good agreement with that obtained using the two-compartment equivalent of Eq. 21, i.e.,

$$Cl = k_{10}V_1$$

with the plasma values given in Table 16 (i.e., 10.17 ml min^{-1} kg^{-1}). Table 17 also illustrates the derivation of model-independent parameters MRT and V_{ss}.

Because the terminal half-life (β phase) from plasma was 30.8 min (0.693/0.0225), the duration of the study was the minimum necessary to adequately define the curve. Ideally, the data collection should have been extended for another

30 min to give five half-lives, which was borne out by the fact that the β phase was dependent on only four data points. Because the duration of the experiment was four half-lives, a total of about 94% of the dose should have been eliminated, which is in good agreement with that predicted from the urinary data, as the urinary clearance, 8.82 ml min^{-1} kg^{-1} (Table 15), represented 87% of the plasma clearance, and the total urinary recovery in 2 hr (24.9 mg) represented 87% of the dose administered (28.5 mg, or 50 mg/kg), or 93% of that eliminated in four half-lives (28.5 $\times$ 0.94). The urinary elimination rate constant k_R may be calculated by a number of methods using the data obtained, and these figures show good agreement (Table 17).

It is clear from these results that low doses of saccharin fit a two-compartment open model with a terminal half-life of

TABLE 15. *Renal clearance of saccharin after an intravenous bolus dose*

Time of collection (min)	Midpoint (min)	Excretion rate (μg min^{-1})	Midpoint plasma concentration[a] (μg ml^{-1})	Cl_R[b] (ml min^{-1})
0–5	2.5	1,503.6	225	6.68
5–15	10.0	627.5	138	4.55
15–30	22.5	332.6	71	4.68
30–45	37.5	172.0	35.5	4.84
45–60	52.5	99.0	18.8	5.27
60–75	67.5	57.4	10.6	5.42
75–90	82.5	37.4	6.9	5.42
90–105	97.5	24.2	4.8	5.04
105–120	112.5	20.0	3.4	5.88
			Mean value (5–105 min) =	5.03

[a] Data are from Fig. 16.
[b] Renal clearance, calculated using Eq. 7. Mean renal clearance = 5.03 ml min^{-1} (per 570 g) = 8.82 ml min^{-1} kg^{-1}. Cl_R may be calculated also from A_{ex} (Table 12) and AUC (Table 17) between 0 and 120 min:

$$Cl_R = \frac{A_{ex}}{AUC} = \frac{24{,}932 \; \mu g}{4{,}895 \; \mu g \; ml^{-1} \; min} = 5.09 \; ml \; min^{-1}$$

TABLE 16. *Summary of kinetic data after intravenous saccharin*

Parameter	Plasma		Urine (excretion rate)		Urine (sigma minus)	
	Graphical	Regression	Graphical	Regression	Graphical	Regression
β (min^{-1})	0.0224	0.0226	0.0237	0.0240	0.0205	0.0199
B or B' or B"	42	43.7	270	277	9,700	9,115
α (min^{-1})	0.0664	0.0683	0.0710	0.0705	0.0717	0.0668
A or A' or A"	198	204.5	830	833	14,100	14,159
V_1 (ml kg^{-1})	208	201				
k_{21} (min^{-1})	0.0301	0.0307	0.0353	0.0356	0.0414	0.0383
k_{10} (min^{-1})	0.0494	0.0503	0.0477	0.0475	0.0355	0.0347
k_{12} (min^{-1})	0.0093	0.0099	0.0117	0.0113	0.0153	0.0137

$$V_1 = \frac{\text{dose (50 mg/kg)}}{A + B}$$

$$k_{21} = \frac{A\beta + B\alpha}{A + B} \text{ or A', B', or A", B"}$$

$$k_{10} = \frac{\alpha\beta}{k_{21}}$$

$$k_{12} = \alpha + \beta - k_{21} - k_{10}$$

The constants were derived by graphical analysis or by least-squares linear regression analysis applied to β phase and residuals.

about 30 min, a plasma clearance of 10.1 ml min^{-1} kg^{-1}, and a renal clearance of about 8.8 ml min^{-1} kg^{-1}. The latter value is considerably higher than the glomerular filtration rate in the rat (3.4 ml min^{-1} kg^{-1}). Because glomerular filtration removes only the nonprotein-bound drug, and saccharin is about 80% protein-bound (74), the clearance due to filtration would be only about 0.7 ml min^{-1} kg^{-1}. It is therefore apparent that extensive secretion and negligible reabsorption must be occurring in the renal tubule, and we can conclude that the major route of elimination of saccharin is by renal tubular secretion. In cases where the renal clearance is close to the average glomerular filtration rate (i.e., about 3 ml min^{-1} kg^{-1}), it is necessary to measure inulin clearance simultaneously to quantify the extent of renal tubular secretion. However, for saccharin, renal tubular secretion is responsible for about 80% [$(8.8 - 0.7/10.1) \times 100$] of total elimination. This finding was confirmed by studies in which the plasma clearance of saccharin was reduced to about 30% by the drug probenecid, which inhibits renal tubular secretion (74).

Because renal tubular secretion is a saturable process, it was possible that the nonlinearity of plasma levels, seen on dietary administration, arose from saturation of this major route of elimination. This possibility was investigated by giving a range of intravenous bolus doses of saccharin (1–1,000 mg kg^{-1}) and calculating the plasma clearance. The plasma concentration–time curves for high doses (Fig. 19) reflected nonlinear kinetics (Fig. 12) being superimposed on the two-compartment pattern seen at low doses (Fig. 16). It resulted in high doses appearing to be a simple one-compartment system during the course of the experiment. Obviously, better data would have been obtained if the collection period was extended (74). These data illustrated well that the terminal half-life, which is derived at low plasma levels, does not show

a dose-dependent increase and that the best indication of saturation kinetics is given by plasma clearance, which was decreased at doses of 300 mg kg^{-1} or more (Fig. 20). The increased half-life at the highest dose is probably a reflection of the duration of the study rather than a true value.

Intravenous Infusion

Saturation kinetics apparent at doses of about 300 mg kg^{-1} (shown by the decreased plasma clearance and altered plasma concentration–time curve) could not be related closely to a particular plasma concentration, as the levels fell from about 500 to 30 μg ml^{-1} during the 2-hr study period. Infusion studies were used to relate altered clearance to a particular plasma level, as at steady state the rate of infusion equals the rate of elimination for a *fixed* plasma concentration. *Cl* can be calculated using Eq. 20, i.e.,

$$Cl = \frac{\text{rate of infusion}}{C_{pss}}$$

The rats were anesthetized and infused at a rate of 9.6 μl/min with [^{3}H]saccharin solution in isotonic saline via the jugular vein using a Harvard infusion pump. The infusion rate was selected because it approximates 14 ml/day and is therefore not an excessive fluid intake. Each animal was infused at a constant rate, within the range 50 to 2,000 μg min^{-1}, and the plasma was analyzed every 30 min from 90 min onward until three consecutive samples showed the same concentration (i.e., C_{pss}). The clearance for that animal was calculated using the equation given above. A graph of clearance against steady-state plasma concentration (Fig. 21) clearly shows that at plasma concentrations below 200 μg

TABLE 17. *Plasma clearance and renal elimination of saccharin*

Plasma clearance: $Cl = \dfrac{\text{dose}}{\text{AUC}}$

Trapezoid rule: $\text{AUC} = \text{sum of } \dfrac{(t_2 - t_1)}{2}(C_{p1} + C_{p2})$, etc.

where t_1 and t_2 are the first two time points and C_{p1} and C_{p2} are the corresponding plasma levels, i.e., for 0–5 min $= \dfrac{5-0}{2}(242 + 184.3) = 1,065.5$

time (min) (t)	C_p (μg ml^{-1})	AUC (μg ml^{-1} min)	$t \cdot C_p$ (μg ml^{-1} min)	AUMC (μg ml^{-1} min^2)
0	242.0[a]	1,066	0	2,305
5	184.3	1,432	922	12,260
15	102.0	1,144	1,530	22,838
30	50.5	566	1,515	19,770
45	24.9	293	1,121	14,753
60	14.1	166	846	10,845
75	8.0	103	600	8,348
90	5.7	73	513	6,998
105	4.0	52	420	5,760
120	2.9	129[b]	348	21,195[c]
Total		5,024 μg ml^{-1} min		125,072 μg ml^{-1} min^2

AUC measured by cut-and-weigh technique = 4,910 μg ml^{-1} min

Plasma clearance = 50,000 μg kg^{-1}/4,910 μg ml^{-1} min = 10.18 ml min^{-1} kg^{-1}

$Cl = k_{10}V_1 = 208 \times 0.0494 = 10.27$ ml min^{-1} kg^{-1} or $201 \times 0.0506 = 10.17$ ml min^{-1} kg^{-1} (Table 16)

Renal clearance (Cl_R) = 8.82 ml min^{-1} kg^{-1} (Table 15)

Renal excretion = $\dfrac{25,765}{50,000 \times 0.57} \times 100 = 90.4\%$ of dose (0.57 = body wt. in kilograms)

Renal elimination rate constant (k_R)

$$k_R = \frac{A' + B'}{\text{dose}} = \frac{277 + 833}{28,500} = 0.039 \text{ min}^{-1}$$

$$k_R = \frac{A_{ex}^{\infty} \times k_{10}}{\text{dose}} = \frac{25,765 \times 0.050}{28,500} = 0.045 \text{ min}^{-1}$$

$$k_R = \frac{Cl_R}{V_1} = \frac{8.82}{201} = 0.044 \text{ min}^{-1}$$

$$\text{MRT} = \frac{\text{AUMC}}{\text{AUC}} = \frac{125,072}{5,024} = 25 \text{ min}$$

$$V_{ss} = \frac{\text{dose} \cdot \text{AUMC}}{\text{AUC}^2} = \frac{50,000 \times 125,072}{5,024^2} = 248 \text{ ml kg}^{-1}$$

[a] By extrapolation of plasma concentration–time curve.
[b] Calculated by $C_p/\beta = 2.9/0.0225$.
[c] Calculated by $t \cdot C_p/\beta + C_p/\beta^2 = 348/0.0225 + 2.9/0.000506 = 15,467 + 5,728$.

ml^{-1} the clearance was about 8 to 12 ml min^{-1} kg^{-1}, whereas at concentrations above 300 μg ml^{-1} the clearance decreased to 4 to 8 ml min^{-1} kg^{-1} (a value similar to that seen after an intravenous bolus dose of 600 mg kg^{-1}).

Thus based on these studies, the renal tubular secretion of saccharin appears to be saturated by doses giving plasma concentrations of 200 to 300 μg ml^{-1} or more. This value correlates well with the concentration in the plasma of rats fed 7.5% saccharin diet, which animals showed elevated levels in the plasma and most organs (Fig. 15) (74).

Oral Studies

Because saccharin has a rapid terminal half-life (30 min), it is possible that there are rapid fluctuations in plasma concentrations during chronic dietary administration. This possibility was investigated by studies on the plasma concentration–time curve for animals maintained on a 5% saccharin diet for an extended period. The diurnal variation showed relatively small changes, with a peak at around 6 a.m. and a minimum at 6 p.m. (Fig. 22). The extent of variation was

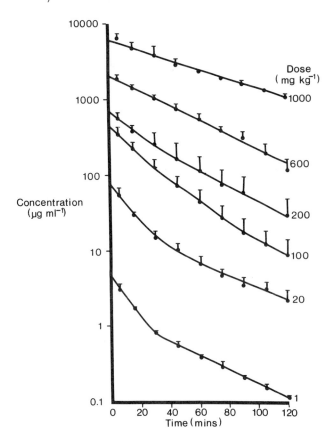

FIG. 19. Plasma concentration–time curves for rats given bolus intravenous doses of saccharin. Adult male rats were given [³H]saccharin (1–1,000 mg/kg i.v.) by bolus dose, and plasma levels were measured by liquid scintillation counting. (From ref. 74.)

less than might have been expected from the half-life and the fact that little saccharin-containing food was consumed between 6 a.m. and 6 p.m. It therefore seemed probable that the rate of absorption from the gut was low and blunted any large change in plasma level. The plasma concentration–time curve after oral administration was studied and showed much lower levels than after similar doses given intravenously (Fig. 23). The peak concentration was at the time of the first sample, followed by a slow and variable decrease. The decrease in concentration was obviously not related to the value of β, and thus saccharin is a good example of a compound for which the decrease after oral administration is related to k_a and not to k or β (see Mathematical Principles, above). The decrease was clearly slow and complex, emphasizing that if absorption from the gut is slow a single rate constant cannot be derived to apply to the many rates occurring simultaneously at different sites within the gastrointestinal tract. The duration of sample collection was inadequate for definition of the $AUC_{0-\infty}$, and thus the bioavailability could not be calculated from these plasma data. The methods for deriving simple absorption rate constants are described above under Mathematical Principles.

In summary, these studies have been used to illustrate the derivation of kinetic data and the insights they can give into the handling of the compound during chronic toxicity studies.

The possibility of saturation of one pathway revealing a second pathway of elimination could result in saccharin (which is not metabolized normally) undergoing metabolism in rats fed high saccharin diets. However, this phenomenon has not been detected for saccharin (73), although Gehring and co-workers (23) showed that metabolism of 2,4,5-T was revealed by doses resulting in saturation of renal tubular secretion.

Computation

The use of computer programs to derive rate constants and so on from plasma and urinary levels can greatly simplify data handling. Because data handling is also optimized, computer usage is the method of choice. There are a number of suitable programs available for nonlinear least-squares regression analysis, which is the most appropriate method (i.e., BLIN, SAAM, NONLIN), and readers are referred to Gibaldi and Perrier (26) and Wagner (79) for further details. The use of such a program would automatically put the best fit line through the data presented in Figs. 16 to 18 and would avoid a possibly erroneous decision as to the time at which the α component was exerting an insignificant influence and the line was described by β alone. In the analysis of data by computer program it is common to apply a suitable weight to each data point to ensure the most appropriate fit. The weights that can be applied to the concentration data include (a) all weights equal, which is applicable if the errors in measurement are a constant amount, e.g., ±2 µg/ml; (b) weighted by $1/y$, which is applicable if the errors of measurement are a constant proportion, e.g., ±2%; (c) weighted by $1/y^2$, which can be used to force the fit through the later time points at the expense of the early higher values. The second option, $1/y$, closely represents the accuracy of most assay procedures and is used most frequently. It is important with computer fitting of data that some indication of appropriateness of fit is obtained by either a graphical representation or analysis of the deviation between observed and calculated concentrations (error analysis). With the latter approach a consistent positive or negative deviation is more important than wider but randomly distributed deviations, as it indicates an inadequate fit. Reasons for this situation could be the choice of an inappropriate model to fit the data or incorrect weighting. Another factor to consider is that although adoption of a more complex model may give a closer fit to the data, the sampling times may be inadequate to provide accurate parameter estimates.

However, it should be realized that although kinetic constants derived from sophisticated computerized line fitting contain the minimum possible errors due to data handling, any errors in the raw data, due to methodological problems, will still be present. Indeed, the adage "rubbish in, rubbish out" is particularly pertinent to the use of sophisticated data handling to analyze inaccurate or badly designed animal pharmacokinetic experiments.

Interpretation of Pharmacokinetic Data

There are three principal aims of pharmacokinetic studies as applied to toxicology. First, pharmacokinetics can provide

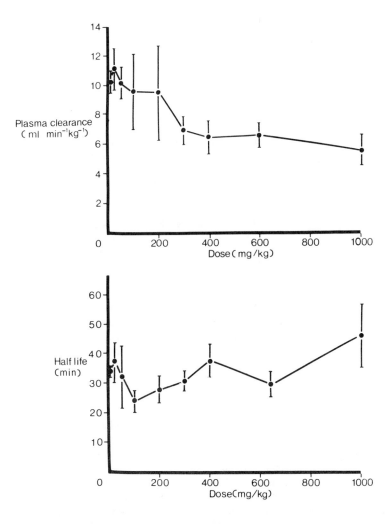

FIG. 20. Influence of dose on the plasma clearance and half-life of saccharin in male rats following an intravenous bolus dose. (From ref. 74, with permission.)

an understanding of the physiological processes that are involved in the fate of the chemical in the body. Second, the relation between dose and pharmacokinetics may be the key

to either the establishment of appropriate dose levels for chronic studies or the interpretation of such studies. Third, comparative pharmacokinetics may be used to assess poten-

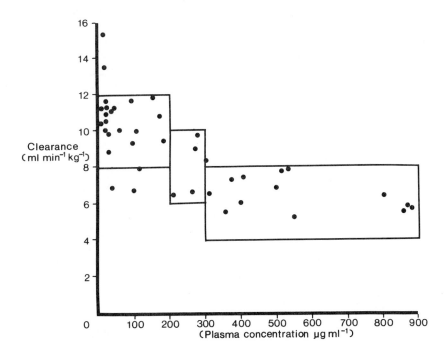

FIG. 21. Plasma clearance of saccharin at steady-state plasma concentrations. Adult male rats were given [³H]saccharin in isotonic saline by intravenous infusion (0.0096 ml/min) until a constant plasma [³H] was obtained. The plateau saccharin concentration was calculated from the specific activity of the dose solution, and the plasma clearance from the infusion rate and plasma concentration. (From ref. 74, with permission.)

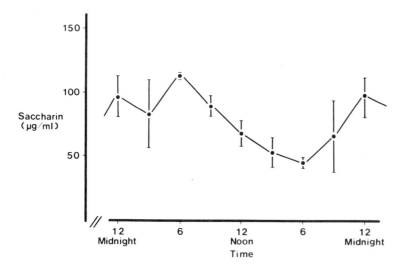

FIG. 22. Diurnal variation in the concentration of saccharin in the plasma of rats given a 5% saccharin diet. Adult male rats were given a 5% saccharin (sodium saccharin dihydrate) diet for 66 days *ad libitum,* and plasma samples were collected during a 24-hr period and analyzed for saccharin content by HPLC. The results given are the mean concentrations ± SD (as sodium saccharin dihydrate) for three animals. (From ref. 74, with permission.)

tial human risks with a more secure basis by reducing the number of unknown variables involved in the extrapolation from animal to man.

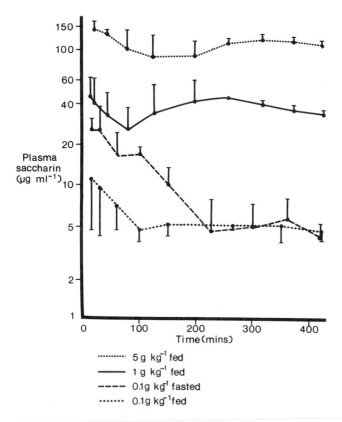

FIG. 23. Concentration of saccharin in the plasma of rats given [³H]saccharin orally. Adult male rats were given a single oral dose of [³H]saccharin, and the plasma ³H content was determined by liquid scintillation counting. The saccharin (5, 1, and 0.1 g/kg) was given in aqueous solution (20, 10, and 0.5 ml/kg). The plasma concentration–time curve for 0.1 g/kg was not altered by giving the dose in a large volume (10 ml/kg). The results given are the mean of three animals ± SD. (From ref. 74, with permission.)

A good example of the physiological insights that may be obtained is provided by the data on saccharin discussed above. In summary, these data showed that the sweetener is slowly absorbed from the gut. Thus during chronic feeding of saccharin diets there are only slight diurnal fluctuations due to the absorption rate producing "flip-flop" kinetics. The absorbed saccharin has a low volume of distribution so that the concentrations in most tissues are similar to or lower than those in plasma. The urinary bladder tissue is part of the central compartment (74). The sweetener is cleared rapidly from plasma, mostly as a result of renal clearance via active renal tubular secretion. This process is saturated at the high dietary intakes necessary to produce an increase in bladder tumors. Renal tubular secretion is a general mechanism for the elimination of organic acids, including the metabolites of tryptophan, which has been linked to bladder cancer in both animals and man. Saturation of renal clearance of saccharin has been confirmed at high dietary concentrations, accompanied by decreased renal clearance of indican, a major urinary metabolite of tryptophan (65). Subsequent studies demonstrated that not only does the absorbed saccharin interfere with the excretion of aromatic amino acid metabolites, but also the slow absorption of saccharin from the gut results in altered metabolism of these essential nutrients within the gastrointestinal tract (35,65,66). Thus the dietary levels necessary throughout life (≥3%) to increase the incidence of bladder tumors in male rats produced profound perturbations of the physiology and biochemistry of the test animal. The relevance of these findings to tumor formation is unclear at present, but other factors are almost certainly involved, as these changes were found also in female rats, which are less susceptible to bladder tumor development. Neither saturation of renal clearance (49) nor altered excretion of amino acid metabolites (55) has been found in man following doses equivalent to the highest likely human intake. Therefore doubts must exist about the relevance to man of phenomena observed at such grossly elevated dietary levels.

The relationship between kinetics, dose, and toxicity is probably the single most important contribution that pharmacokinetics can make to the field of toxicology. Although a few therapeutic chemicals show nonlinear kinetics at the doses normally given to man [notable examples being salicylates, phenytoin (diphenylhydantoin) and ethanol], the plasma levels of foreign chemicals in man are usually well below those necessary to saturate any protein-mediated reactions. However, in toxicology, when the maximum dose tested on chronic administration is designed to show some degree of toxicity, nonlinear kinetics are a distinct possibility and should be fully and carefully investigated. At doses above saturation, the body load of free drug increases steeply with an increase in dose. Under such circumstances, effective tissue concentrations of drug will also be considerably higher than predicted by extrapolation of doses showing first-order kinetics. The presence of dose-dependent kinetics may result in an extremely steep dose-response curve for the toxic effect observed. In such circumstances, the nonlinearity in pharmacokinetics shown in animal toxicity testing must be taken into account when extrapolating the effects to man.

A possible cause of toxicity associated with large saturating doses of chemicals is that normally minor pathways of metabolism may become of major significance. Thus if a chemical undergoes metabolism by two routes, one with a low K_m (high affinity) and one with a high K_m (low affinity), at low doses most chemical in the cell is eliminated by the former route. However, if the levels increase to saturate the high affinity enzyme, any further input will exceed removal and levels will rise such that the low-affinity enzyme will metabolize the excess. (A useful analogy is that of water pouring into a bucket that has two holes in the side at different heights.

Little escapes through the upper hole until the rate of input exceeds the rate of removal by the lower hole.)

There have been some notable examples of toxicity occurring largely at saturating doses of foreign chemicals. In a series of papers by Brodie and co-workers (33,42,43,47) it was shown that the hepatotoxicity of paracetamol (acetaminophen) was related to the metabolism of the compound and occurred only at high doses, which were associated with extensive covalent binding of the compound to tissue components. Little binding occurred at low doses or if the metabolism of toxic doses was inhibited by treatment with piperonyl butoxide. The binding at high doses arose from saturation of the capacity of the hepatocytes to protect themselves from the reactive metabolite produced. The protective mechanism was conjugation with glutathione, and saturation of this system at toxic doses was caused by depletion of the available glutathione.

Another example of saturation in toxicology is seen in the studies of Gehring and co-workers on the herbicide 2,4,5-trichlorophenoxyacetic acid (2,4,5-T) (23,61). This compound showed a higher toxicity in dogs than in rats because the former species exhibits a longer half-life, reduced renal and increased biliary elimination, and the presence of metabolites. In the rat, embryotoxicity is seen with doses of 100 mg kg^{-1}, and nonlinear pharmacokinetics were seen at similar doses due to saturation of elimination by renal tubular secretion. Metabolites for 2,4,5-T were detected in the urine

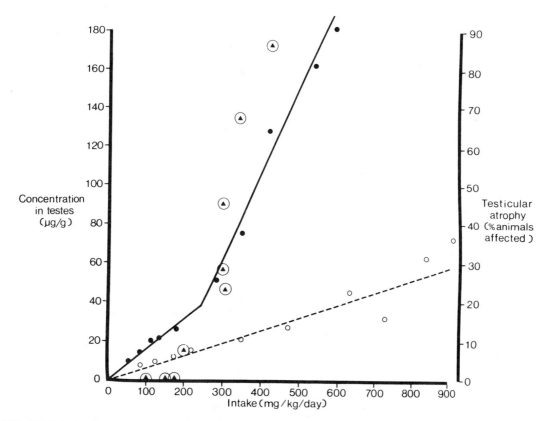

FIG. 24. Relation between dose, toxicity, and target organ concentrations of cyclohexylamine during chronic administration; (●) concentration in rat testes; (○) concentration in mouse testes; (▲) testicular toxicity in rats. (Data from ref. 57.)

of rats given saturating doses (i.e., 100 or 200 mg kg^{-1}). Saturation of the metabolism of 1,4-dioxane has also been shown at doses associated with toxicity (23). Saturation of biliary excretion of FPL 57787 in the dog has been demonstrated at toxic doses of this antiallergy compound (67).

A good example is provided by studies on the metabolism and pharmacokinetics of cyclohexylamine (56). This compound produces testicular toxicity when given chronically to rats, but not to mice (7). Pharmacokinetic studies indicated that the plasma clearance was higher in mice than in rats, whereas rats but not mice showed evidence of nonlinear kinetics at high doses (57). The steady-state concentrations in the plasma and testes during chronic administration confirmed dose-dependent kinetics in the rat (Fig. 24), which coincided with the dose-response for testicular atrophy in this species (57). These pharmacokinetic data thus provide a possible explanation for the steepness of the dose-response curve in the rat and the apparent species difference in sensitivity.

Finally, pharmacokinetic data can be invaluable for the interpretation of animal toxicity with respect to possible human risk. This analysis may be made in the absence or the presence of human pharmacokinetic data. In the absence of human data, extrapolation may be by either physiological or compartmental modeling methods. The physiological approach relies on the scale-up between animals and man of such parameters as tissue volume and blood flow (Fig. 3) and by their relation to body weight. Assuming that the uptake from blood to tissue (extraction ratio) is a function of the chemical and therefore independent of species, it is possible to derive complex models involving all the major tissues of the body (24). These models may then be scaled up from known animal data to man based on the known physiological differences. Alternatively and more pragmatically, the plasma pharmacokinetics in various species may be fitted by compartmental modeling and then scaled up empirically according to the body mass of the species studied and extrapolated to man (44).

The most secure comparison is when pharmacokinetic data are available in animals and man, allowing direct analysis of the potential risk. In any such analysis the species difference in basic physiological processes such as cardiac output and relative tissue weight usually result in lower clearances and longer half-lives in man than in animals. Thus comparisons of animals and man on the basis of plasma levels or AUC values, rather than intake or exposure data, results in a decreased apparent safety margin compared with intake data. However, by removing important variables from interspecies comparisons, such an approach provides a more secure basis for the safety assessment.

The increasing use of *in vitro* test systems facilitates a quantitative analysis of the dose–toxicity curve and studies on the mechanisms of action (18). The logical interpretation of such data with respect to human risk requires information on the steady-state concentrations of the active chemical species in the target organ and plasma of the test animal during chronic toxicity testing combined with knowledge of the pharmacokinetics of the chemical in the test animal at toxic doses and in man at the likely exposure level. It must be emphasized that large safety factors have been introduced to protect us from our own ignorance. The increased use of

pharmacokinetic data, especially when combined with knowledge of the mechanism of toxicity, will allow the future use of potentially toxic chemicals to be based on scientific principles and understanding.

REFERENCES

1. Andersen, M. E., Gargas, M. L., Jones, R. A., and Jenkins, L. J. (1979): The use of inhalation techniques to assess the kinetic constants of 1,1-dichloroethylene metabolism. *Toxicol. Appl. Pharmacol.*, 47:395–409.
2. Anderson, M. W., Hoel, D. G., and Kaplan, N. L. (1980): A general scheme for the incorporation of pharmacokinetics in low-dose risk estimation for chemical carcinogens: example—vinyl chloride. *Toxicol. Appl. Pharmacol.*, 55:154–161.
3. Bakar, S. K., and Niazi, S. (1983): Simple reliable method for chronic cannulation of the jugular vein for pharmacokinetic studies in rats. *J. Pharm. Sci.*, 72:1027–1029.
4. Bard, P. (1956): In: *Medical Physiology*, 10th ed., p. 221. Henry Kimpton, London.
5. Bauer, L. A., and Gibaldi, M. (1983): Computation of model-independent pharmacokinetic parameters during multiple dosing. *J. Pharm. Sci.*, 72:978–979.
6. Benet, L. Z., and Galeazzi, R. L. (1979): Noncompartmental determination of the steady state volume of distribution. *J. Pharm. Sci.*, 68:1071–1074.
7. Bopp, B. A., Sonders, R. C., and Kesterson, J. W. (1986): Toxicological aspects of cyclamate and cyclohexylamine. *CRC Crit. Rev. Toxicol.*, 16:213–306.
8. Bourgoignie, J. J., Hwang, K. H., Espinel, C., Klahr, S., and Bricker, N. S. (1972): A natriuretic factor in the serum of patients with chronic uremia. *J. Clin. Invest.*, 51:1514–1527.
9. Butler, T. C. (1971): The distribution of drugs. In: *Fundamentals of Drug Metabolism and Drug Disposition*, edited by B. N. LaDu, H. G. Mandel, and E. L. Way, pp. 44–62. Williams & Wilkins, Baltimore.
10. Caldwell, J., and Varwell Marsh, M. (1982): Metabolism of drugs by the gastrointestinal tract. In: *Presystemic Drug Elimination*, edited by C. F. George, D. G. Shand, and A. G. Renwick, pp. 29–42. Butterworth, Boston.
11. Chan, K. K. H., and Gibaldi, M. (1985): Assessment of drug absorption after oral administration. *J. Pharm. Sci.*, 74:388–393.
12. Clinical implications of drug protein binding (1984): *Clin. Pharmacokinet.*, 9(Suppl. 1):1–104.
13. Cocchetto, D. M., and Bjornsson, T. D. (1983): Methods for vascular access and collection of body fluids from the laboratory rat. *J. Pharm. Sci.*, 72:465–492.
14. Cohn, V. H. (1971): Transmembrane movement of drug molecules. In: *Fundamentals of Drug Metabolism and Drug Disposition*, edited by B. N. LaDu, H. G. Mandel, and E. L. Way, pp. 3–43. Williams & Wilkins, Baltimore.
15. Colburn, W. A., and Matthews, H. B. (1979): Pharmacokinetics in the interpretation of chronic toxicity tests: the last-in, first-out phenomenon. *Toxicol. Appl. Pharmacol.*, 48:387–395.
16. Davison, C. (1971): Protein binding. In: *Fundamentals of Drug Metabolism and Drug Disposition*, edited by B. N. LaDu, H. G. Mandel, and E. L. Way, pp. 63–75. Williams & Wilkins, Baltimore.
17. Despopoulos, A. (1965): A definition of substrate specificity in renal transport of organic anions. *J. Theor. Biol.*, 8:163–192.
18. Flamm, W. G., and Lorentzen, R. J. (1987): The use of in vitro methods in safety evaluation. *In Vitro Toxicol.*, 1:1–3.
19. Garattini, S. (1986): Toxic effects of chemicals: difficulties in extrapolating data from animals to man. *CRC Crit. Rev. Toxicol.*, 16:1–29.
20. Gardner, D. M., and Renwick, A. G. (1978): The reduction of nitrobenzoic acids in the rat. *Xenobiotica*, 8:679–690.
21. Garrett, E. R. (1978): Pharmacokinetics and clearance related to renal processes. *Int. J. Clin. Pharmacol.*, 16:155–172.
22. Gehring, P. J. (1979): Chemobiokinetics and metabolism. In: *Environmental Health Criteria, 6. Principles and Methods for Evaluating the Toxicity of Chemicals Part I*, pp. 116–177. WHO, Geneva.

23. Gehring, P. J., and Young, J. D. (1978): Application of pharmacokinetic principles in practice. In: *Proceedings of the First International Congress on Toxicology. Toxicology as a Predictive Science,* edited by G. L. Plaa and W. A. M. Duncan, pp. 119–141. Academic Press, New York.

24. Gerlowski, L. E., and Jain, R. K. (1983): Physiologically based pharmacokinetic modelling: principles and application. *Pharm. Sci.,* 72: 1103–1127.

25. Gibaldi, M., and Perrier, D. (1974): Route of administration and drug disposition. *Drug Metab. Rev.,* 3:185–199.

26. Gibaldi, M., and Perrier, D. (1982): *Pharmacokinetics,* 2nd ed. Marcel Dekker, New York.

27. Goldstein, A., Aranow, L., and Kalman, S. M. (1974): *Principles of Drug Action: The Basis of Pharmacology.* Wiley, New York.

28. Guy, R. H., Hadgraft, J., and Maibach, H. I. (1985): Percutaneous absorption in man: a kinetic approach. *Toxicol. Appl. Pharmacol.,* 78:123–129.

29. Hiles, R. A., and Birch, C. G. (1978): Nonlinear metabolism and disposition of 3,4,4'-trichlorocarbanilide in the rat. *Toxicol. Appl. Pharmacol.,* 46:323–337.

30. Hirom, P. C., Millburn, P., and Smith, R. L. (1976): Bile and urine as complementary pathways for the excretion of foreign organic compounds. *Xenobiotica,* 6:55–64.

31. Hirom, P. C., Millburn, P., Smith, R. L., and Williams, R. T. (1972): Species variations in the threshold molecular-weight factor for the biliary excretion of organic anions. *Biochem. J.,* 129:1071–1077.

32. Huang, C. H., Kimcera, R., Nassar, R. B., and Hussain, A. (1985): Mechanisms of nasal absorption of drugs. 1. Physicochemical parameters influencing the rate of in situ nasal absorption of drugs in rats. *J. Pharm. Sci.,* 74:608–611.

33. Jollow, D. J., Mitchell, J. R., Potter, W. Z., Davis, D. C., Gillette, J. R., and Brodie, B. B. (1973): Acetaminophen-induced necrosis II. Role of covalent binding *in vivo. J. Pharmacol. Exp. Ther.,* 187: 195–202.

34. Keen, P. M. (1971): Effect of binding to plasma proteins on the distribution, activity, and elimination of drugs. In: *Handbook of Experimental Pharmacology,* edited by B. B. Brodie and J. R. Gillette, Vol. 28, pp. 213–233. Springer-Verlag, New York.

35. Lawrie, C. A., Renwick, A. G., and Sims, J. (1985): The urinary excretion of bacterial amino-acid metabolites by rats fed saccharin in the diet. *Food Chem. Toxicol.,* 23:445–450.

36. Lien, E. J., and Tong, G. L. (1973): Physicochemical properties and percutaneous absorption of drugs. *J. Soc. Cosmet. Chem.,* 24:371–384.

37. Light, H. G., Witmer, C., and Vars, H. M. (1959): Interruption of the enterohepatic circulation and its effects on rat bile. *Am. J. Physiol.,* 197:1330–1332.

38. Lindup, W. E. (1975): Drug-albumin binding. *Biochem. Soc. Trans.,* 3:635–640.

39. McDougal, J. N., Jepson, G. W., Clewell, H. J., and Andersen, M. E. (1985): Dermal absorption of dihalomethane vapours. *Toxicol. Appl. Pharmacol.,* 79:150–158.

40. McKenna, M. J., Zempel, J. A., Madrid, E. O., and Gehring, P. J. (1978): The pharmacokinetics of [14C]vinylidene chloride in rats following inhalation exposure. *Toxicol. Appl. Pharmacol.,* 45:599–610.

41. Meyer, M. C., and Guttman, D. E. (1968): The binding of drugs by plasma proteins. *J. Pharm. Sci.,* 57:895–918.

42. Mitchell, J. R., Jollow, D. J., Potter, W. Z., Davis, D. C., Gillette, J. R., and Brodie, B. B. (1973): Acetaminophen-induced hepatic necrosis. I. Role of drug metabolism. *J. Pharmacol. Exp. Ther.,* 187: 185–194.

43. Mitchell, J. R., Jollow, D. J., Potter, W. Z., Gillette, J. R., and Brodie, B. B. (1973): Acetaminophen-induced hepatic necrosis. IV. Protective role of glutathione. *J. Pharmacol. Exp. Ther.,* 187:211–217.

44. Mordenti, J. (1985): Pharmacokinetic scale up: accurate prediction of human pharmacokinetic profiles from animal data. *J. Pharm. Sci.,* 74:1097–1099.

45. Ochsenfahrt, H., and Winne, D. (1972): Solvent drag influence on the intestinal absorption of basic drugs. *Life Sci.,* 11:1115–1122.

46. Piafsky, K. M., Borga, O., Odar-Cedelof, I., Johansson, C., and Sjoqvist, F. (1978): Increased plasma protein binding of propranolol and chlorpromazine mediated by disease-induced elevations of plasma α_1 acid glycoprotein. *N. Engl. J. Med.,* 299:1435–1439.

47. Potter, W. Z., Davis, D. C., Mitchell, J. R., Jollow, D. J., Gillette, J. R., and Brodie, B. B. (1973): Acetaminophen-induced hepatic necrosis. III. Cytochrome P-450-mediated covalent binding *in vitro. J. Pharmacol. Exp. Ther.,* 187:203–210.

48. Renwick, A. G. (1982): First pass metabolism within the lumen of the gastrointestinal tract. In: *Presystemic Drug Elimination,* edited by C. F. George, D. G. Shand, and A. G. Renwick, pp. 3–28. Butterworth, Boston.

49. Renwick, A. G. (1985): The disposition of saccharin in animals and man—a review. *Food Chem. Toxicol.,* 23:429–435.

50. Renwick, A. G. (1986): Gut bacteria and the enterohepatic circulation of foreign compounds. In: *Microbial Metabolism in the Digestive Tract,* edited by M. J. Hill, pp. 135–153. CRC Press, Boca Raton, Florida.

51. Renwick, A. G., and Sweatman, T. W. (1979): The absorption of saccharin from the rat urinary bladder. *J. Pharm. Pharmacol.,* 31: 650–652.

52. Rescigno, A., and Segre, B. (1966): *Drug and Tracer Kinetics.* Blaisdell, London.

53. Riegelman, S., and Collier, P. (1980): The application of statistical moment theory to the evaluation of in vivo dissolution time and absorption time. *J. Pharmacokinet. Biopharm.,* 8:509–534.

54. Riegelman, S., Loo, J. C. K., and Rowland, M. (1968): New method for calculating the intrinsic absorption rate of drugs. *J. Pharm. Sci.,* 57:918–928.

55. Roberts, A., and Renwick, A. G. (1985): The effect of saccharin on the microbial metabolism of tryptophan in man. *Food Chem. Toxicol.,* 23:451–455.

56. Roberts, A., and Renwick, A. G. (1985): The metabolism of 14C-cyclohexylamine in mice and two strains of rat. *Xenobiotica,* 15: 477–483.

57. Roberts, A., and Renwick, A. G. (1988): The fate of cyclohexylamine in rat and mouse in relation to testicular toxicity. *Hum. Toxicol.,* 7:229.

58. Rowland, M., and Tozer, T. N. (1980): *Clinical Pharmacokinetics: Concepts and Applications.* Lea & Febiger, Philadelphia.

59. Rowland, M., Benet, L. Z., and Graham, G. G. (1973): Clearance concepts in pharmacokinetics. *J. Pharmacokinet. Biopharm.,* 1:123–136.

60. *Saccharin; Technical Assessment of Risks and Benefits* (1978): Institute of Medicine, National Research Council–National Academy of Science, Washington, D. C.

61. Sauerhoff, M. W., Braun, W. H., Blau, G. E., and Gehring, P. J. (1976): The dose-dependent pharmacokinetic profile of 2,4,5-trichlorophenoxy acetic acid following intravenous administration to rats. *Toxicol. Appl. Pharmacol.,* 36:491–501.

62. Scheline, R. R. (1973): Metabolism of foreign compounds by gastrointestinal microorganisms. *Pharmacol. Rev.,* 25:451–523.

63. Schoenig, G. P., Goldenthal, E. I., Geil, R. G., Frith, C. H., Richter, W. R., and Carlborg, F. W. (1985): Evaluation of the dose response and in utero exposure to saccharin in the rat. *Food Chem. Toxicol.,* 23:475–490.

64. Shen, S. K., Williams, S., Onkelinx, C., and Sunderman, F. W. (1979): Use of implanted minipumps to study the effects of chelating drugs on renal 63Ni clearance in rats. *Toxicol. Appl. Pharmacol.,* 51:209–217.

65. Sims, J., and Renwick, A. G. (1983): The effects of saccharin on the metabolism of dietary tryptophan to indole, a known cocarcinogen for the urinary bladder of the rat. *Toxicol. Appl. Pharmacol.,* 67: 132–151.

66. Sims, J., and Renwick, A. G. (1985): The microbial metabolism of tryptophan in rats fed a diet containing 7.5% saccharin in a two-generation protocol. *Food Chem. Toxicol.,* 23:437–444.

67. Smith, D. A. (1979): Differences in toxicity due to species variation in the metabolism of an oral antiallergy agent. *Br. J. Pharmacol.,* 66:422P–423P.

68. Smith, J. W. (1965): Observations on the flora of the alimentary tract of animals and factors affecting its composition. *J. Pathol. Bacteriol.,* 89:95–122.

69. Smith, R. L. (1973): *The Excretory Function of Bile. The Elimination of Drugs and Toxic Substances in Bile.* Chapman & Hall, London.

70. Solomon, S. (1977): Developmental changes in nephron number, proximal tubular length and superficial glomerular filtration rate of rats. *J. Physiol. (Lond.),* 272:573–589.

71. Strong, H. A., Renwick, A. G., and George, C. F. (1984): The site of reduction of sulphinpyrazone in the rabbit. *Xenobiotica*, 14:815–826.

72. Su, K. S. E., Campanale, K. M., and Gries, C. L. (1984): Nasal drug delivery system of a quaternary ammonium compound: clofilium tosylate. *J. Pharm. Sci.*, 73:1251–1254.

73. Sweatman, T. W., and Renwick, A. G. (1979): Saccharin metabolism and tumorigenicity. *Science*, 205:1019–1020.

74. Sweatman, T. W., and Renwick, A. G. (1980): The tissue distribution and pharmacokinetics of saccharin in the rat. *Toxicol. Appl. Pharmacol.*, 55:18–31.

75. Taylor, A. E., and Gaar, K. A. (1970): Estimation of equivalent pore radii of pulmonary capillary and alveolar membranes. *Am. J. Physiol.*, 218:1133.

76. Upton, R. A. (1975): Simple and reliable method for serial sampling of blood from rats. *J. Pharm. Sci.*, 61:112–114.

77. Veng-Pedersen, P., and Gillespie, W. (1985): The mean residence time of drugs in the systemic circulation. *J. Pharm. Sci.*, 74:791–792.

78. Wagner, J. G. (1975): Do you need a pharmacokinetic model and, if so, which one? *J. Pharmacokinet. Biopharm.*, 3:457–478.

79. Wagner, J. G. (1975): *Fundamentals of Clinical Pharmacokinetics.* Drug Intelligence Publications, Hamilton, Illinois.

80. Waynforth, H. B. (1980): *Experimental and Surgical Technique in the Rat.* Academic Press, New York.

81. Weiner, I. M. (1967): Mechanisms of drug absorption and excretion: the renal excretion of drugs and related compounds. *Annu. Rev. Pharmacol.*, 7:39–56.

82. Weiner, I. M. (1971): Excretion of drugs by the kidney. In: *Handbook of Experimental Pharmacology,* edited by B. B. Brodie and J. R. Gillette, Vol. 28, pp. 329–353. Springer-Verlag, New York.

83. Wilkinson, G. R. (1976): Pharmacokinetics in disease states modifying body perfusion. In: *The Effect of Disease States on Drug Pharmacokinetics,* edited by L. Z. Benet, pp. 13–32. American Pharmaceutical Association, Academy of Pharmaceutical Sciences, Washington, D. C.

84. Wilkinson, G. R. (1987): Clearance approaches in pharmacology. *Pharmacol. Rev.,* 39:1–47.

85. Withey, J. R. (1978): Pharmacokinetic principles. In: *Proceedings of the First International Congress on Toxicology. Toxicology as a Predictive Science,* edited by G. L. Plaa and W. A. M. Duncan, pp. 97–117. Academic Press, New York.

86. World Health Organization (1986): Principles of toxicokinetic studies. In: *Environmental Health Criteria,* Vol. 57. WHO, Geneva.

Principles and Methods of Toxicology, Second Edition, edited by A. Wallace Hayes, Raven Press, Ltd., New York © 1989.

CHAPTER 31

Extrapolation to Man

Michael D. Hogan and David G. Hoel

National Institute of Environmental Health Sciences, National Institutes of Health, Research Triangle Park, North Carolina 27709

In recent years the number of new chemicals entering the environment has grown at an impressive rate. Paralleling this growth there has been increasing interest in the development of rational procedures for assessing human health risks associated with environmental exposures to potentially hazardous agents. Due to a lack of relevant human information, individuals concerned with this assessment process have often been forced to rely solely on experimental animal data when evaluating possible human health effects. Therefore, the question of how to extrapolate the results of laboratory studies to man in a meaningful way has become a matter of growing concern in modern toxicology.

Ideally, an investigator would like to be able to appeal to a universal species conversion factor that, when applied to results obtained from a given animal toxicity test, would yield a realistic estimate of the risk to man at environmental exposure levels. Unfortunately, no such simplistic conversion factor exists. Instead, the investigator in question usually resorts to one of two methodological approaches when addressing the issue of species extrapolation, i.e., the traditional safety factor procedure or actual effect estimation based on some presumed "mathematical model" of the toxic response under study.

This chapter presents a review of the status of carcinogenesis risk estimation covering both the issues of low-dose extrapolation and species-to-species extrapolation. A similar but more abbreviated summary is also given for mutagenesis and teratogenesis. These three areas of general toxicology currently represent the main focus of public health concern in assessing adverse human health effects resulting from chronic environmental exposure to potentially toxic chemicals. In addition, a discussion of the rationale behind the use of the safety factor approach is included along with some

recommendations regarding its employment. Finally, a synopsis is presented of ongoing and possible future research activities that could have a significant impact on the ability of toxicologists to extrapolate the results of laboratory animal studies to man in a quantitative and realistic fashion.

THE SAFETY FACTOR APPROACH

We begin the discussion with the original approach to determining acceptable exposure levels of chemicals, namely the safety factor approach. This method of interpreting animal toxicity data was introduced in the mid-50s in response to legislative guideline needs in the area of food additives (70). Under this approach an allowable human daily intake level (ADI) of the compound of interest is determined by dividing the no observable effect level (NOEL) established in chronic[1] animal toxicity studies by some safety factor that presumably reflects the uncertainties inherent in the extrapolation process. The NOEL is defined (69) as ". . . that level of a substance administered to a group of experimental animals at which those effects observed at higher levels are absent and no other significant differences between the exposed animals and the unexposed control group are observed. (The effects observed need not be severely toxic or even adverse.)" Traditionally, a safety factor of 100 has generally been as-

---

[1] Zielhuis and Van Der Kreek (77) cite research by McNamara, Weil, and others in support of the use of subchronic (3–6 months) exposure tests for the determination of the NOEL, noting, e.g., that toxic effects expressed in terms of body weight, liver weight, liver pathology, food intake and/or blood chemistry are usually in evidence within 3 months or less of exposure.

sumed in the calculation of ADIs. This figure of 100 is itself a combination of two separate safety factors—a factor of 10 to reflect a hypothesized increased sensitivity of man relative to laboratory test animals and an additional factor of 10 to take into account the presumed range in toxicological sensitivity to be found in the heterogenous human population.

While the safety factor approach certainly has the appeal of simplicity, it is subject to a number of potentially serious limitations that raise genuine concern about its utility. In the first place the observance of a "no effect" level will depend, at least in part, on the sample size employed in the experimental design. That is, at any given (true) nonzero level of toxicity an investigator is more likely to see one or more affected animals with a sample, e.g., of 100 or 1,000 than with a sample of 10. Thus, the indiscriminate use of the safety factor approach to safe dose level estimation may actually reward the investigator who uses too few animals to detect a toxic response. Furthermore, an experimentally observed no effect level is not necessarily equivalent to a true no effect level. For example, if the actual probability of an animal having a toxic response to some specified exposure was between 6 and 7%, and if 10 animals were exposed to the agent under study, then there would be a 50–50 chance that *all* of the exposed animals would fail to exhibit the response in question. Even if the underlying response rate were as high as 26%, the probability of observing no effect in the study sample would be 0.05. Also, there is the problem that the safety factor approach, as it is commonly applied, fails to take into account the shape of the dose-response curve. Intuitively, it seems that the size of the safety factor employed should be dependent to some extent on the responses observed at the higher dose levels. Finally, there is no real biological justification for the routine use of any given safety factor including the traditional factor of 100.

In partial response to some of these criticisms, a number of modifications of the safety factor approach have been proposed. For example, many investigators now advocate the use of the highest *no-adverse* effect level or possibly the minimal-adverse-effect level rather than the NOEL when calculating an ADI. If the lowest observed effect level is used as the basis for these calculations, it would seem reasonable to increase the magnitude of the associated safety factor; and values as high as 5,000 (28) have been suggested in this instance.

A case has also been made for increasing the flexibility of the safety factor approach so as to better depict the quality of the underlying data base in any given ADI determination. This sentiment was reflected to some degree in the 1977 report of the NAS Safe Drinking Water Committee (64) that proposed the following guidelines for selecting safety or, more appropriately, "uncertainty" factors to be used in combination with no-adverse effect level data.

1. An uncertainty factor of 10 should be used when valid human data based on chronic exposure are available.
2. An uncertainty factor of 100 should be employed when human data are inconclusive (e.g., limited to acute exposure histories) or absent, but when long-term, reliable animal data are available for one or more species.
3. An uncertainty factor of 1,000 should be utilized when no long-term or acute human data are available, and the experimental animal data are scanty.

Even with these modifications, many investigators would still argue against the use of the safety factor approach for certain types of toxicological responses. There seems to be, for instance, a broadly shared opinion among scientists concerned with the issue of species-to-species extrapolation that the safety factor approach should not be applied to cancer data (28,69,70,77). Others feel that this restriction should be extended to mutagenesis and teratogenesis as well, although in the latter case there are no widely accepted alternatives to the safety factor approach. Some investigators (69) have even proposed that tolerance levels for compounds producing reversible toxic effects be calculated using mathematical dose-response curves in much the same manner as they are currently employed to generate carcinogenic risk estimates.

CARCINOGENESIS

The introduction to this chapter indicated that individuals interested in risk assessment are increasingly being forced to seek information outside the normal channels of epidemiology when estimating human cancer risk. This search for supplemental information has been brought about by the lack of adequate human cancer data for many of the compounds that have been or are about to be introduced into the environment. Because of the relatively long latency periods typically associated with cancer, waiting for the appearance of epidemiological data would incur the risk of possibly exposing a significant segment of the population to the irreversible effects of some carcinogenic agent.

At the present time the main source of usable supplemental information is the lifetime animal cancer bioassay. However, the cancer bioassay is usually designed as a screening procedure with primary focus on detection of the carcinogenic potential of a compound and not human risk estimation. In addition to this emphasis on cancer detection, economic and logistic constraints on overall experimental size have led to a policy within the typical bioassay program of exposing animals at doses that approximate the animal's maximum tolerated level—a level that is often orders of magnitude higher than those encountered in man's ambient environment. As a result, investigators interested in assessing human cancer risk using animal bioassay-generated data are confronted not only with the problem of species scale-up, but also with the issue of low-dose extrapolation.

Low-Dose Extrapolation

When extrapolating the results observed in the experimental dose range down to the appropriate environmental level, investigators are forced to rely on some assumed mathematical model relating the probability of tumor onset to exposure because of their lack of knowledge about the actual form of the dose-response curve. Among the various types of mathematical models that have been proposed for low-dose extrapolation and risk estimation, the most commonly employed include the tolerance distribution models, simple linear extrapolation, the various "hit" models such as the one-hit, multistage and Gamma multi-hit formulations, and the time-to-tumor models.

Under the tolerance distribution model(s) it is assumed (70) that each individual has some threshold level below which he or she will be unaffected by exposure to the toxic agent of interest; that these threshold levels vary among the individual population members; and that this variation can be characterized in terms of some probability distribution function, F. While the distribution of tolerances will typically be skewed in the direction of individuals with unusually high tolerances, it is commonly presumed that a simple transformation such as the logarithmic transformation will make the distribution approximately symmetric. If a location parameter, α, and a scale parameter, β, are also introduced into the model, then the probability that a given individual will develop a tumor as a result of exposure to a dose d of some specified compound can be written as:

$$P(d) = F(\alpha + \beta \log d)$$

[It should be noted that with this particular format the probability of a response at zero dose which corresponds to the spontaneous or background rate is itself zero, i.e., $P(0) = 0$.] If it is assumed that F is the cumulative normal distribution, $P(d)$ becomes the familiar log-probit model of dose-response used in bioassays for median lethal dose estimation (70). (Other tolerance distribution models like the logistic model can be obtained by assuming different functional forms for F.)

The log-probit model also serves as the basis for the Mantel-Bryan extrapolation procedure (52,53), which was one of the first techniques to be employed in low-dose risk estimation. This procedure is perhaps most readily described in terms of the linearized version of the log-probit model that is obtained by plotting the experimental data on a probit vs. $\log_{10}$ dose scale. Given this framework, the dose associated with some predetermined "acceptable" level of risk, such as 10^{-6}, is estimated by extrapolating from an upper confidence limit on the observed proportion of animals with tumors at the experimental exposure level along a straight line with a slope of one. (Based on their empirical knowledge of experimental carcinogenesis data, Mantel and Bryan concluded that a fixed slope of one would generally lead to a conservative estimate of the acceptable dose level.) Alternatively, the procedure can be inverted to solve for an upper limit on the cancer risk at some specified low level of exposure.

Although the Mantel-Bryan procedure is regarded as one of the pioneering techniques in low-dose risk estimation, it has been subjected to a number of criticisms as research and methodological developments in this area of risk assessment have progressed. For example, it has been noted (20) that the Mantel-Bryan procedure often leads to a poor fit to the observed, experimental data, which would certainly raise questions about its suitability for low-dose risk estimation. Furthermore, the assumption of an underlying log-probit distribution has no particular biological justification, since there is no mechanistic model of carcinogenesis that logically leads to its use (20,35). In addition, the probit model approaches the origin more rapidly than any of its competitors, so it will typically generate an estimate of low-dose risk that falls well below any produced by these competitive techniques in spite of the fact that those who advocate its use often characterize it as a conservative procedure (20). Finally, since the log-probit model assumes that $P(0) = 0$, the Mantel-Bryan procedure needs to be modified to correct for spon-

taneous or background cancer whenever it is present. Traditionally, Abbott's correction factor (47,52) has been employed in these instances. Unfortunately, this approach makes certain mechanistic assumptions about the stochastic independence of background and the induced carcinogenesis that are usually unrealistic (e.g., see ref. 37).

Another type of heuristic model for low-dose extrapolation that has enjoyed a great deal of popular appeal is the simplistic computational procedure known as linear extrapolation. Linear extrapolation also attempts to place an upper-bound on the unknown cancer risk associated with exposure at some specified low-dose level. However, it is less restrictive than the Mantel-Bryan procedure, since it only requires that experimental dose range fall in the convex portion of the true dose-response curve in order to generate a bound on the unknown, underlying cancer risk.

With this approach a straight line is drawn from an upper confidence limit p^* on the observed proportion $\hat{p}_t$ of animals who developed tumors after being exposed at dose level d to the origin. (Drawing the extrapolation line through the origin reflects an assumption of no spontaneous or background rate.) Then, for any given dose level d' within the range $[0,d]$, an estimate of an upper limit on the associated probability of tumor onset is given by

$$p' = (d'/d)p^*$$

If background is present and known, then the extrapolation line would be drawn from the upper confidence limit to the point p_c on the y-axis that corresponds to this known spontaneous probability. On the other hand, if background has only been observed experimentally, then the upper $(1 - \alpha)\%$ confidence limit on the *excess* tumor rate at dose d would be approximately (40)

$$\hat{p}^* = (\hat{p}_t - \hat{p}_c) + z_{(1-\alpha)}[(\hat{p}_c)(1 - \hat{p}_c)/n_c + (\hat{p}_t)(1 - \hat{p}_t)/n_t]^{1/2}$$

where $z_{(1-\alpha)}$ is the normal deviate corresponding to the desired confidence level, and n_c and n_t are, respectively, the sample sizes for the control and treated groups. Having determined the value of $\hat{p}^*$, the investigator would, once again, extrapolate to the low-dose region along a straight line from $\hat{p}^*$ to the origin.

This rather simplistic approach to low-dose extrapolation obviously has a great deal of intuitive appeal because of both its relative lack of assumptions (other than the crucial assumption of convexity of the underlying dose-response curve), and the ease with which it can be applied to a given set of experimental data to produce an upper limit on low-dose risk. Nevertheless, there are many investigators who are critical of its unrestricted use, since they feel that it may be unduly conservative, i.e., may generate an upper limit that markedly exceeds the actual risk associated with a given level of exposure. Furthermore, while linear extrapolation (as described above) presumes the use of a single treated group of animals, the typical experiment will often include two or more exposure levels in addition to background.

The next major category of models employed in low-dose extrapolation is composed of what are commonly known as "hit" models, a title that refers to a mechanistic characterization of carcinogenesis which they attempt to depict. Basic to each of these models is the assumption that cancer originates within a single cell that undergoes a finite number of stages or transitions (that can be thought of as somatic mutations) or incurs a finite number of "hits" or interactions with the chemical under study before becoming a clinically expressible tumor.

The simplest of the various "hit" models is the so-called one-hit model which assumes that cancer can be induced after a single susceptible target or receptor has been hit by (or interacted with) a biologically effective unit of dose. Under the one-hit model the probability of developing a tumor as a result of exposure to a dose d of the chemical of interest is given by

$$P(d) = 1 - \exp(-\lambda d)$$

where λ is an unknown model parameter and λd is the expected number of hits at dose d. When λd is small (as, e.g., would be expected in the low-dose region), it can be shown mathematically that $P(d)$ is approximated by λd, i.e., in the low-dose region the one-hit model is equal to a simple linear model.

The one-hit model, like the linear model, is very appealing because of its basic simplicity. In addition, it has the advantage of using all of the experimental data simultaneously in the estimation of its model parameter λ. However, since the model does involve only a single parameter, it may not provide an acceptable fit to the observed responses in the experimental dose range.

A more complex "hit" model, commonly known as the multistage model of carcinogenesis, has been developed by Armitage and Doll (7). Under this model it can be shown that the probability of incurring a tumor after a (continuous) exposure to some specified chemical at dose rate d for time period T is given by (31):

$$P(d, T) = 1 - \exp[-F(T) \prod_{i=1}^{k} (a_i + b_i d)]$$

where a_i and b_i are non-negative constants, F is an increasing function of time, and k is an unknown integer corresponding to the number of stages in the carcinogenic process.

Although the multistage model is generally regarded as the most biologically defensible of the various models that have been proposed for low-dose extrapolation in carcinogenesis, it has also been criticized. One of the most commonly expressed doubts about the multistage model focuses on its dependency on the assumption of additivity. Critics have asserted (66) that the mechanistic hypothesis underlying the additivity assumption (i.e., ". . . that all carcinogens operate by a common mechanism and that any one increases some part of an ongoing process") is far from compelling and have cited arguments as to why it might not be expected to apply in general.[2] Still others have questioned the general appropriateness of the "hit" concept upon which the multistage model is based, noting that it certainly would not seem to be applicable in the case of nonalkylating carcinogens like

arsenic and saccharin. This latter criticism is obviously not limited to the multistage model alone but applies equally to all of the "hit" models.

The last of the "hit" models to be considered in this section is the Gamma multi-hit model, developed primarily by Cornfield and Van Ryzin (16,58,59). Basically, this model is an extension of the familiar one-hit model which assumes that at least k hits are required at the cellular level in order to initiate the process of carcinogenesis. Under this model, the probability of developing a tumor given exposure at some specified dose level d is

$$P(d) = \int_0^d \theta^k t^{k-1} \exp(-\theta t) \, dt / \Gamma(k)$$

where θ is a model parameter and $\Gamma(k)$ denotes the gamma function. Spontaneous cancer incidence is incorporated into the model through the use of Abbott's correction factor, giving the revised probability of developing a tumor of

$$P'(d) = p + (1 - p)P(d)$$

where $P(d)$ is defined as above, $P(0) = 0$, and $p = P'(0)$ is the background tumor probability.

Although the Scientific Committee of the Food Safety Council specifically recommended the use of the Gamma multi-hit model (66) for quantitative risk assessment, some investigators have taken exception both to this recommendation and to the statistical calculations upon which it was based. Haseman et al. (32) re-evaluated the data presented in the report and found enough problems associated with the Gamma multi-hit approach to conclude that it, at least in its present stage of development, should not be employed as a risk assessment procedure.

All of the preceding extrapolation procedures assume that the experimental data generated from the cancer bioassay will essentially be binary in nature (i.e., tumor incidence over the duration of the study). Occasionally, however, additional information concerning the length of time between the initial exposure and the detection of the tumor in question (which is often referred to as the latency period) will also be available. When such information exists, it may be possible to fit mathematical models to the experimentally generated plots of cumulative tumor incidence over time, and then to employ these models to obtain estimates of low-dose risk. Two mathematical functions are typically proposed for modeling time-to-occurrence cancer data, namely, the log-normal and the Weibull distributions (40).

Originally it was hoped that the inclusion of additional information such as data on time-to-tumor occurrence would lead to improved risk estimates in the low-dose exposure region. In fact it was hypothesized that at sufficiently low doses, the median time-to-tumor occurrence might well exceed the normal lifespan of the species under test, thereby implying a practical threshold level for the chemical of interest. Unfortunately, from a regulatory viewpoint, Schneiderman et al. (42) have been able to show that a sizable proportion of the exposed population can still potentially develop tumors during their lifetime, even when the median time-to-tumor substantially exceeds the normal life expectancy. Furthermore, in most instances the experimental data may not be of sufficient quality to allow the investigator to

---

[2] Recent work by Hoel (37), however, certainly suggests that as long as background is not completely independent from the effects of the agent under investigation, i.e., as long as some degree of additivity can be assumed, linearity in the low-dose region (which is typically associated with the multistage approach) is likely to be attained regardless of the extrapolation model employed.

distinguish between the "experimental fits" provided by the competing models (see, e.g., refs. 36 and 72), even though the corresponding estimates of low-dose risk may differ by orders of magnitude. Nevertheless, the limited time-to-tumor modeling that has actually been conducted on either animal or epidemiological data bases has clearly demonstrated the importance of taking duration of exposure into account when predicting low-dose risk (see, e.g., ref. 35).

This brief review of low-dose extrapolation procedures clearly indicates that there is no unanimity of opinion as to the method of choice for cancer risk assessment. Furthermore, as has already been noted, some investigators (see, e.g., ref. 11) have begun to question the general applicability of the somatic mutational theory that implicitly underlies the various "hit" models most commonly employed in low-dose extrapolation. Therefore, given the present state of knowledge, the best approach for the moment may be to rely on simple linear extrapolation or, at most, a linear-quadratic model in combination, if possible, with the pharmacokinetic characterization of the data base under analysis. In fact, an adequate description of the pharmacokinetics of the chemical under study, with a particular emphasis on metabolism, may be one of the most significant steps that can be taken in developing a realistic model for low-dose extrapolation.

Gehring et al. (29,30) and others (6) have explored the effects of including pharmacokinetics in the low-dose extrapolation process for a limited number of chemical carcinogens. In the case of vinyl chloride, a compound for which the relationship between the administered dose and the amount of covalent binding to cellular DNA is distinctly nonlinear, their findings (6) indicated that for either the probit or multistage model, an improved fit to the experimental data was obtained with the introduction of pharmacokinetic considerations.

Species Scale-Up

If one has been able to obtain relevant pharmacokinetic data for the experimental test species in question and to incorporate this information into a reasonable low-dose extrapolation model to generate environmental-level risk estimates, the resulting projections must still be scaled up to man. Given the current state of scientific knowledge concerning the process of carcinogenesis, many investigators feel that this problem of species scale-up is even more difficult to address adequately than the issue of low-dose extrapolation (see, e.g., ref. 35). The difficulty arises because there are a multitude of factors that can directly influence the extrapolation process that need to be taken into account by anyone attempting to obtain a quantitative estimate of human cancer risk from laboratory based data. These factors range from species-related pharmacokinetic effects (60) to temporal (60), size (60,61), population structure, and exposure regimen differences between the laboratory test species employed and man. While any one of these factors may play a significant role in accurately assessing the degree of human risk associated with a given exposure, species differences in metabolism will often constitute the greatest impediment to the meaningful extrapolation of laboratory animal test data to man.

In attempting to control for the various factors that contribute to interspecies variation in response to a potentially toxic insult such as a chemical carcinogen, scientists have long sought to establish a common biological baseline for extrapolating across species. One of the earliest efforts in this area was a paper published in 1949 by Adolph (5). In this article, Adolph correlated a number of anatomical, biochemical, and physiological properties of mammals with their body weights using the relationship:

$$\text{Property} = a(\text{body weight})^k$$

While the fitted exponents ranged from a low of 0.08 (diameter renal corp.) to a high of 1.31 (myoglobin weight), most estimates of k tended to be less than one. This result was particularly true for relationships depicting physiologic functions, indicating that as body weight increased, the physiologic function per unit of body weight decreased. However, the most significant finding of Adolph's research was the empirical demonstration that a large number of physiologic characteristics apparently could be extrapolated across a wide range of mammalian species if they were first standardized in terms of some power of body weight.

Many subsequent research articles have pursued this theme of establishing a body weight or mass dependent baseline for species scale-up. One of the most widely cited of these articles is by Freireich et al. (27). In this article, toxicity data for 18 anticancer agents tested subchronically in several different species of laboratory animals were used to estimate maximum tolerated doses (MTDs) in man. The results were then compared with clinically observed human toxicity data, after first adjusting the daily dosing schedules for both animals and man to a common basis. (In making dosage adjustments the authors assumed that effects were cumulative, i.e., that one unit of a drug given daily for a period of 10 days was equivalent to two units per day administered for 5 days.) When the daily dose was expressed in terms of mg of agent per m^2 of body surface area, the MTD in man and the various animal species were approximately equivalent for all anticancer agents under consideration. (None of the projected human MTDs differed from the clinically observed values by more than an order of magnitude; and in the majority of cases, they agreed within a factor of two.) Furthermore, Freireich et al. concluded that the results would not be altered substantially if body surface area was approximated by body weight raised to the two-thirds power.

In spite of the apparent accuracy of the projections generated by Freireich and his coworkers, standardization of risk estimates on the basis of body surface area is not universally accepted as the best approach to the estimation of subchronic toxicity. For example, Krasovskii (46) claims that expressing dosage in mg/m^2 in order to adjust for species differences in extrapolation only seemed to be appropriate in about half of the instances he considered.

When the response of interest is lifetime cancer risk rather than subchronic toxicity, this same lack of agreement as to the best choice of the scale for dose standardization has been observed. Among the various dosage units that have been proposed for species scale-up in carcinogenesis, the most commonly employed are mg/kg body weight/day, parts per million (ppm) in the diet, mg/m^2 body surface area/day, and mg/kg body weight/lifetime. The effects of using these different dose units to scale risks based on lifetime exposures from various animal species to man have been estimated by Crump and Guess (21) and are summarized in their Table III.2. The entries in Table III.2 are all based on "average" species' body weights, food consumption, and lifespans, and represent the dosages on various measurement scales that correspond to a dose of 1 mg/kg body weight/day in each of the designated species. These results indicate that if experimentally generated rat data were used to estimate human cancer risk and if risk were assumed to be proportional to dose (i.e., if a linear extrapolation model was employed), then the projected human risk given a dose rate measured on a mg/kg/day basis would be 25,500/730 = 35-fold less than that which would be obtained if a mg/kg/lifetime scale were adopted. (This factor of 35 is merely a reflection of the difference in relative average lifespans of man and the rat, i.e., 70 years vs. 2 years.) Similarly, if a mg/m^2/day scale had been employed, then the estimated human risk would have been

$$\frac{(25,500/37.0)}{(730/5.2)} = 4.9$$

fold less than the corresponding projection based on a mg/kg/lifetime standard.

In order to realistically choose among these competing dosage scales, it is necessary to compare actual human cancer risks derived from epidemiologic studies with the various animal-based estimates that would be produced with the different dosage scales under consideration. Unfortunately, very little data are available for making these types of comparisons.

One of the earliest published attempts to use epidemiologic information to evaluate the accuracy of animal-generated cancer estimates was contained in a 1975 National Academy of Science subcommittee report (15) on the health hazards of chemical pesticides. This report compared human cancer risk data with estimates derived from laboratory animal studies of six known human carcinogens using the mg/kg body weight/lifetime approach to dosage standardization. (As can readily be seen from Table III.2 (21), this particular conversion procedure yields higher human risk estimates than any of the other approaches commonly employed in species scale-up.) Based on the results of this comparison, the report concluded that if the data on the most sensitive published animal test were used to predict human cancer risk, the findings for benzidine, chlornaphazine, and cigarette smoking were approximately correct. On the other hand, the estimated human cancer risks for aflatoxin B$_1$, DES, and vinyl chloride exceeded the epidemiologically observed risks by factors of 10, 50, and 500, respectively.

In a Banbury Conference paper, Hoel (35) presented the results of a reanalysis of the NAS data using both a mg/kg/day and a mg/m^2/day approach to dose standardization. These results indicated that a more accurate prediction of human cancer risk was obtained when either of these dosage scales was used in place of the mg/kg/lifetime procedure employed in the original NAS analysis. More specifically, when identical sites of action were compared (where possible) and either a mg/kg/day or a mg/m^2/day dosage scale was used, the projected and the observed human cancer risks tended to agree within an order of magnitude for the compounds under consideration. Furthermore, the mg/kg/day-based animal projections always generated the lower estimate of human cancer risk and, in some instances, actually appeared to underestimate the observed human risk. However, all of these findings need to be interpreted cautiously because of the many inherent deficiencies in the NAS data set.

Crouch and Wilson (17) examined these same data as well as results for nine additional compounds. They essentially employed a linear model for low-dose extrapolation, expressed dose in terms of mg/kg/day, and made interspecies comparisons on the basis of a carcinogenic potency index that corresponded to the least squares estimate of the slope of the fitted linear model. Like Hoel they concluded that their results were ". . . consistent with the possibility of extrapolation between species, in particular between animals and humans, within a factor of 10."

Thus, the relatively few animal-human comparisons that have been made to date suggest that extrapolations of lifetime animal cancer risk estimates on a mg/kg body weight/day or a mg/m^2 body surface area/day dosage scale may lead to reasonable projections of the corresponding cancer risk for man. Alternatively, a range of potential human cancer risk could be estimated by employing both of these dosage scales (in turn) in the species extrapolation process. Regardless of the procedure that is adopted, however, it must be stressed that experience with species extrapolation is very limited and scale-up on any standardized dosage basis is at best a crude attempt to adjust for interspecies variability in pharmacokinetic parameters and the many other factors that can affect the extrapolation process.

MUTAGENESIS

Many of the submammalian test systems or assays employed in mutagenesis screening allow the researcher to experiment at much lower dose levels than are typically encountered in the standard cancer bioassay. Therefore, the problem of low-dose extrapolation in mutagenesis historically has not received the same degree of attention that has been given to this issue by investigators interested in cancer risk evaluations. Instead, much of the research effort in this area has centered on the question of species-to-species extrapolation of mutagenic responses—an emphasis that is reflected in the following discussion. However, this focus on species scale-up should certainly not be regarded as implying that the problem of low-dose extrapolation never arises when attempting to assess human mutagenic risk from laboratory generated data.

One of the first attempts to develop a general procedure for extrapolating the results of germinal cell mutation tests across species was presented in what is commonly referred to by geneticists as the ABCW (i.e., Abrahamson, Bender, Conger, and Wolff) paper (4). In this work, the authors reexamined published data on forward mutation rates induced by acute ionizing irradiation in test systems employing a variety of organisms (e.g., bacteria, yeast, fruit fly, mouse, tomato, barley). They concluded that when the reported specific locus mutation rates per rad were normalized to the corresponding amount of DNA per haploid genome, the experimentally observed three orders of magnitude variability in induced mutation rates among species could be essentially eliminated. Although they were not able to specify unequivocally the biological mechanism underlying such an association, they concluded that this apparent proportionality between mutations per locus per rad and DNA per haploid genome greatly increased one's confidence in the use of lower order test systems for estimating human genetic damage.

Shortly thereafter, Heddle and Athanasiou (33,34) attempted to extend the ABCW hypothesis to the field of chemical mutagenesis. For their model compound they selected a widely used chemical mutagen, ethyl methanesulfonate (EMS). After an extensive search of the EMS literature, they were able to abstract what they regarded as adequate mutation data for nine different test systems in organisms ranging from *E. coli* to the mouse. However, there were no data describing the effective amount of EMS actually reaching the specific target in each of the test systems considered. They therefore made the critical assumption that the chemical was uniformly distributed within the test organism at the level of the grossly administered dose. Next, they standardized the various specific locus mutation rates (per mole of EMS) under consideration to reflect relative DNA content per haploid genome. This adjustment to a common biological baseline appeared to reduce markedly the observed variation in the experimentally-based rates and to indicate a functional relationship between genome size and induced mutation rate that was very similar to the result given in the ABCW paper. Like Abrahamson et al., they advanced a number of hypotheses to explain this empirically observed relationship, including the possibilities that the additional DNA found in larger genomes is associated with larger rather than more genes (33) and/or that the effectiveness of gene repair is inversely related to genome size (34). Finally, they concluded that if ". . . similar correlations are found for other mutagens, rough extrapolations from the simple, rapid microbiological screens to human risk can be made to provide a quantitative evaluation."

A number of researchers have taken exception to the ABCW hypothesis in either its original, radiation-based formulation or in its extension to chemically induced mutations. Schalet and Sankaranarayanan (65) examined the ABCW paper and its supporting references in some detail, and raised a number of objections to its major conclusions. For example, they noted that since the various test systems considered differed markedly in their relative detection sensitivities, the genetic endpoints compared in the ABCW paper indiscriminately included intragenic changes, changes involving several genes or loci, and gross chromosomal abnormalities. As a result, they concluded that the radiation mutable target was not necessarily the same in all of the test organisms, which led them to question the basis for the interspecies comparison of mutation rates. They also noted that the cell stage irradiated was not always consistent from one test system to another (e.g., meiotic stages in barley as compared to spermatogonia in the fruit fly and mouse); but this was probably not a major source of error. Finally, they reevaluated the entire data base, and found that if they restricted their attention to *intralocus* forward mutations, there was no longer a tightly consistent relationship between genome size and mutation frequency. Russell (62,63) has also taken issue with the work of Abra-

hamson et al., claiming that their calculations for the mouse (which were based on a single cell stage in males) ignored the significant variability in mutagenic response seen in mice when both sexes and all cell stages are taken into consideration. He also noted that the important relationship between dose rate and mutation frequency observed in the mouse was essentially absent in drosophila, suggesting that factors other than nuclear DNA content have an important bearing on cell mutability.

Obviously, many of these same criticisms could also be levied against the ABCW-type association reported by Heddle and Athanasiou for the chemical mutagen EMS. In addition, their assumption that the effective dose at the site of action was equivalent to the applied dose in each species considered has already been shown not to hold for either the mouse or drosophila (51). Therefore, when all of these criticisms are viewed collectively, it seems that the universality and quantitative sensitivity of the hypothesized ABCW relationship have been seriously challenged. Although some correlation between mutational frequency and DNA/haploid genome does exist, the uncertainties in the correlation are probably strong enough that its practical usefulness in *quantitative* interspecies extrapolation is questionable without further, extensive verification and modification.

One of the next major efforts to address the topic of species extrapolation and genetic risk estimation was a *Science* article (14) entitled "Environmental Mutagenic Hazards." Because it was prepared by a committee appointed by the Council of the Environmental Mutagen Society, and the appointment was subsequently noted in item 17 of the minutes, the paper is known as the Committee 17 Report. This report raised a variety of issues that are pertinent to the question of species extrapolation and offered a number of specific suggestions as to how these issues might be addressed. For instance, the report's authors stated that extrapolations from curvilinear (convex) dose-response curves should be based on a straight line from the lowest test dose generating reliable data to the spontaneous mutation rate. They also suggested that all mutagens be regarded as producing simple additive effects in the absence of specific evidence of synergism. They recommended that whenever possible, extrapolations should be based on those test systems that are closest to man, such as mammalian cytogenetic and mouse specific locus tests. Furthermore, they asserted that when an investigator is attempting to extrapolate chemically induced mutation rates across species, every effort should be made to determine the amount of active compound actually penetrating to the genetic material, i.e., the genetically effective dose. Finally, in apparent recognition of the problem of dealing explicitly with species-specific genetic endpoints, the Committee 17 Report suggested that quantitative extrapolations might be expressed in terms of either the rate-doubling concentration or the rem-equivalent (REC) dose. The rate-doubling concentration was defined as that concentration of chemical that would be required to produce the same amount of mutational activity in a given unit of time as would have been expected to occur spontaneously in the particular test system under consideration. Similarly, the REC was described as that dose (or product of concentration times length of exposure) that would produce the same amount of genetic damage as would be generated by one rem of chronic ionizing irradiation.

Most criticisms of the Committee 17 Report that have appeared in the scientific literature have focused on the use of the REC. For example, Russell (62,63), has asserted that the range of potential genetic damage in an organism exposed to a chemical mutagen can be so qualitatively different from that induced by radiation that it is essentially meaningless to try to quantify chemically based mutation in terms of a radiation-standardized effect ratio. To illustrate his claim, Russell noted that the REC values for X-chromosome loss in the offspring of female mice exposed to hycanthone (which was one of the three chemicals considered in the appendix of the Committee 17 Report) varied from 0.026 to $+\infty$, depending on whether conception occurred within five days of maternal exposure or in the following week.

In spite of the lack of widespread support for the use of the REC, there are some investigators, such as Ehrenberg (23), who still advocate the expression of chemically induced genetic damage in terms of a basic unit of radiation risk. Using ethylene oxide as a model compound, Ehrenberg relates the mutational damage associated with the *biochemically* determined dose to the target cells to a corresponding level of damage that would be generated by some specified amount of radiation. More specifically, he develops a model in which chemical risk (in rad equivalents) is expressed as the product of (1) the time-integral of the concentration of the ultimate electrophilic form of the chemical under study, (2) a reaction rate constant from the kinetic equation that characterizes the association between the electrophilic agent, the nucleophilic compound, and the alkylated products, (3) a conversion constant relating chemically induced alkylation to ionizing radiation, and (4) a series of chemical-specific correction factors.

Unfortunately, while Ehrenberg provides what, at least on the surface, seems to be a reasonable biochemical framework for developing projections of genetic risk that can presumably be scaled up to man, there are undoubtedly many instances in which some of his essential model parameters (e.g., the dose of the ultimate electrophilic form of the chemical of interest) cannot be determined. Furthermore, even though Ehrenberg is careful to distinguish between his concept of rad-equivalence and the REC, it seems likely that his procedure will be subject to many of the same criticisms that have been levied against the REC with regard to the lack of correspondence between chemical and radiation induced mutation.

While these shortcomings undoubtedly limit the overall effectiveness of Ehrenberg's procedure, his model clearly underscores the importance of being able to determine the amount of a chemical mutagen that reacts with a selected target molecule and then to relate this amount or dose to genetic damage. One of the more promising approaches to this problem is a procedure commonly known as "molecular dosimetry" that has been investigated in detail by Lee (49,50,51), Aaron (1,2,3), and their co-workers. Under their approach, the determination of the genetically effective dose is based on radioactive labeling techniques [details of which are provided, e.g., in (2,50)]. Because of their particular focus, their research to date has been limited to alkylating agents that can be readily and appropriately labeled.

If an investigator were to attempt to estimate the potential human genetic damage associated with a specific chemical exposure utilizing molecular dosimetry, he might proceed in the following manner. First, given the current state of the art, he would probably expose the same germ-cell stage of two separate test systems, such as drosophila and a standard rodent, to the chemical of interest. [The choice of the specific germ-cell stage has important genetic and biochemical implications (1,50) that need to be considered carefully.] For each test system he would employ radiobiological procedures to determine the relationship between external exposure, expressed in mg/kg, and effective target dose, expressed in alkylations per nucleotide. [Lee (51) suggests that if the genetic endpoint of interest is chromatin loss or interchromosomal translocations rather than point mutations, then alkylations per haploid genome might be a more appropriate dosage scale.] For the drosophila, he would also determine the relationship between exposure and mutation frequency. Combining the data from the drosophila experiments, the investigator could obtain an estimate of the drosophila doubling dose for the germ-cell stage under consideration. Next, by applying the appropriate conversion factor derived from radiation research (which could be obtained from the BEIR or UNSCEAR reports), he could estimate the equivalent doubling dose in the mouse. Then, given the observed or presumed level of human exposure, the investigator could estimate the corresponding effective human dose from the mouse data, and ultimately express this estimate as a fraction of the projected doubling dose.

As with each of the other techniques already considered, the molecular dosimetry approach to species extrapolation has a number of potential limitations of varying significance. In addition to the requirement that the chemical under investigation be readily radioactively labeled, the procedure itself is very expensive and time consuming to apply. Furthermore, it crucially assumes that both the cellular labeling pattern and the cellular processing of the alkylation is the same in each of the test systems involved in the species scale-up.

Finally, there are some researchers who feel that there are too many deficiencies in our current knowledge of the mechanisms which govern species differences to allow us to have much confidence in quantitative extrapolations from lower organisms. For the present they advocate the estimation of human genetic damage based primarily if not entirely on mutation data generated from mammalian test systems. Of the various mammalian systems available, the one that is generally regarded as the most productive with respect to human risk estimation (26) is the specific locus test. Under this procedure a treated, wild-type mouse strain, which is homozygous for some dominant (or functional) alleles at a particular locus (loci), is mated with a stock strain known to be homozygous for the recessive (nonfunctional) alleles at the same locus. If the exposure has produced a mutation at the locus in question, then the effect will be detectable in the first generation offspring. However, germinal cell mutation rates scored at only a select number of loci will often be quite low. As a result, the specific locus test can be prohibitively expensive from a screening viewpoint because of the large number of animals it may require to ensure a reasonable level of sensitivity. On the other hand, Russell (63), the originator of the procedure, claims that if the test chemical can be administered to the mouse at much higher (i.e., orders of magnitude) levels than would typically be encountered by man, then the specific locus test can be an inexpensive and efficient means of estimating potential human genetic damage. In support of this contention, he cites his studies of 5-chlorouracil. Noting the absence of mutations among the 314 offspring of 11 male mice given drinking water containing a concentration of 5-chlorouracil that exceeded the anticipated human drinking water levels by a factor of 10^6, Russell estimated that the 95% upper confidence limit on the underlying mutation frequency to be 3.3/314. Subtracting the known (historical) spontaneous mutation rate of 28/531,500 and adjusting the mouse dose to reflect the 3-month to 30-year differential in mouse-to-man generation time exposure, he then concluded that at the human exposure level, the estimated induced mutation rate would be no more than

$$\left[\frac{(3.3/314) - (28/531,500)}{10^6[3/(30 \times 12)]} \middle/ \frac{28}{531,500} \right] \times 100 = 2\%$$

of the spontaneous rate.

While this particular example of the use of the specific locus test for human risk estimation may have intuitive appeal, one should not lose sight of the various assumptions that were made in the application of this procedure to the species extrapolation issue. For instance, it was assumed that the response of interest is linear in (the externally administered) dose over the broad range from the human exposure level to the highest dose tested in the mouse. In addition, it has been assumed that human and mouse exposures can be compared directly by considering the product of concentration times length of exposure or number of cell generations during the exposure interval. Neither of these assumptions will necessarily hold in general. Furthermore, any experimental dose level that is high enough to render the risk estimation procedure economically feasible from a sample size viewpoint may also produce undue toxicity in the test animals.

Given the diversity of opinion that exists among geneticists concerning the most appropriate approach to the species scale-up issue as well as the already noted limitations of the various techniques currently in vogue, it does not seem advisable to endorse any single procedure as the method of choice. A more prudent course would be to proceed, at least for the present, on a case-by-case basis, making full use of all available information. This approach would also seem to reflect the spirit of the recently published EPA Proposed Guidelines for Mutagenicity Risk Assessments (24). These guidelines indicate that when appropriate laboratory data are available, quantitative estimates of human risk are generally obtained through one of two alternative approaches. Either risk projections derived from intact mammalian systems are extrapolated directly to man, or the relationship between induced mutations and exposure is estimated by combining mutagenicity data obtained in lower organisms with biochemical data from whole rodent experiments. The guidelines also suggest that in the absence of appropriate mutagenicity data for quantitative risk estimation that some assessment of the extent of human risk can be derived by carefully weighing the evidence that the compound in question has mutagenic potential, affects or at least reaches the gonadal organs, and poses a meaningful exposure risk for some segment of the general population.

In conclusion, it should be noted that each of the procedures reviewed in this section, whether based solely on a mammalian test system, lower organisms, or some combination of the two, only generates an estimate of the potential increase in the human mutation rate associated with exposure to some environmental agent. However, genetic or inherited disease can be affected both by new mutation and by natural selection. Thus, knowledge of the estimated increase in the human mutation rate does not necessarily provide direct insight into either the nature of the specific health hazards or the overall dimension of the public health problem potentially associated with this increase.

TERATOLOGY

Of the three major areas of toxicology considered in this chapter, teratogenesis is perhaps the most difficult to address in terms of species extrapolation and quantitative risk assessment. Considerably less is understood about the biological mechanisms underlying a teratogenic response than is known, or at least hypothesized, about the corresponding processes that result in the onset of a tumor or in the expression of a mutagenic event. Furthermore, in the case of a potential teratogen there are a number of additional factors that can significantly affect species extrapolation besides the various anatomical, biochemical, and physiological characteristics already discussed in preceding sections. Many of these factors arise because the basic experimental unit in teratologic investigations is really the entire maternal-fetal complex rather than the individual fetus. As a result, questions about such issues as intralitter correlations in response, the potentially modulating effect of the placental transfer mechanism on the ultimate dose in the fetal target tissue, and the relationship(s) between developmental alterations and maternal toxicity need to be resolved when scaling laboratory results up to man. In addition, the possibility of a threshold effect and intra-/interspecies differences in the timing of developmental events (74) must also be taken into account.

As was noted earlier, the complexity of the species extrapolation problem has inhibited the development of standard, quantitative methods for species scale-up. Instead, individuals concerned with human teratogenic risk estimation have tended to rely on the safety factor approach for setting "acceptable" exposure limits. Unfortunately, few guidelines have been specifically established for the selection of safety factors in this area of toxicology, even though certain logical principles are generally accepted by most investigators [e.g., the concept that the margin of safety between the maternally administered and the embryotoxic dose levels needs to be considerably greater for non-essential exposures than for therapeutic drugs (13)].

This lack of widely accepted guidelines for safety factor selection, as well as the controversy that it can provoke, are both well illustrated, e.g., by the EPA "Notice to Cancel Registration" for the pesticide Endrin (57). The notice indicated that members of the independent Science Advisory Panel had informally concluded that a safety factor of 100–1,000 should provide ample protection against the potential teratogenic effects of Endrin but could offer no scientific basis for choosing the actual value to be employed. EPA investigators, on the other hand, estimated that humans might be 50 times more sensitive to the convulsive effects of Endrin than were dosed hamsters, and they hypothesized that this same level of increased sensitivity might also apply to teratogenic endpoints like the meningoencephaloceles observed in the treated animals. As a result, they concluded that a safety factor of 500 or less would be cause for concern. This conclusion, however, was in marked contrast to the findings of the manufacturer who argued that a safety factor of 100 would be appropriate for Endrin and even implied that the use of any safety factor might be unnecessary.

While safety factor methods are often employed in regulatory situations involving teratogenic risk assessment like the example described above, there is a growing concern [see, e.g., ref. (28)] that this branch of toxicology is far too complex to be adequately addressed by such a simplistic procedure. A number of investigators are currently attempting to develop more sophisticated approaches to the problem of quantitatively modeling teratogenic responses and/or extrapolating such effects across species.

Biddle (8,9,10), for example, has studied the effects of cortisone- and 6-aminonicotinamide-induced cleft palate in a variety of inbred and hybrid mouse strains using a probit model. For each compound he was able to fit[3] a separate family of linear, parallel dose-response curves to the experimental data generated by the various genotypes under study. Based on his analyses, Biddle concluded that when different genotypic dose-response curves have the *same slope,*[4] ratios of estimated ED_{50}'s provide the most reasonable measures of relative strain sensitivities to cleft palate induction.

While this result suggests a more quantitative approach to the characterization of strain or species differences in response to a teratogenic exposure, it suffers from a number of potential limitations. Even though Biddle's analysis was restricted to a single teratogenic endpoint for a small number of genotypes, significant lack of fit to the hypothesized model was noted in more than one instance. Furthermore, the observed interstrain parallelism was certainly dependent, to at least some extent, on the use of the probit model for which there is no particular biological justification. In addition, probit analysis, as it was applied by Biddle, ignored possible litter effects in the experimental data. [This is probably not a serious deficiency in terms of ED_{50} estimation (25) and can be corrected by using an approach similar to that proposed by Segreti and Munson (67).] Finally, while the observance of at least approximately parallel dose-response curves for different strains of mice exposed to the same teratogen is certainly interesting, the apparent relationships are clearly restricted to the experimental dose range. There is no assurance that they will persist in the low-dose region near the origin where the probit model is often poorly behaved.

Other investigators concerned with the regulatory aspects of the risk assessment issue have focused on the development of a quantitative index for comparing teratogenic activity across species that adjusts for concurrent maternal toxicity. Underlying this approach is the perceived need to distinguish between compounds that are uniquely teratogenic like tha-

lidomide (44) and those that only induce terata at dose levels that are also toxic or lethal to adults.

Johnson (43,44) was one of the first researchers to employ such an index. He defined his measure of "teratogenic hazard potential" as the ratio of adult to embryonic toxicity, i.e., as

$$\log\left[\frac{\text{lowest adult toxic (lethal) dose}}{\text{lowest developmental toxic dose}}\right]$$

However, his main concern was with the establishment of a practical screening system for teratogenic hazards, and he devoted relatively little attention to the quantitative details of his index.

Fabro et al. (25), on the other hand, have extensively explored the quantitative characteristics of this type of relative potency index. Like Biddle they employed a probit model to describe both maternal lethality and fetal toxicity (teratogenicity). Their analysis of the data for eight structurally related anhydrides and imides indicated that the slope of the probit dose-response line for maternal lethality was always steeper than the corresponding slope for teratogenicity. As a result, they concluded that a simple ratio of median effective doses would not be appropriate for describing teratogenic potency because of the lack of parallelism between the response curves of interest. Instead, they chose to define a "Relative Teratogenicity Index" as the ratio of maternal LD_{01} to the fetal tD_{05} (i.e., the dose required to induce an additional 5% malformation rate above background). They defended their selection of these particular dose levels on the grounds that both values typically can be estimated with a reasonable degree of confidence, that induced malformations often exhibit an incidence of 1 to 20% in laboratory studies, and that the use of a low LD value is necessary to guard against compounds that have a very shallow response curve for adult lethality. However, none of these arguments alters that fact that the observed probit dose response lines for lethality and teratogenicity were not parallel. Therefore, the Relative Teratogenic Index will not be invariant to the selection of other LD and tD values that some investigators might argue are equally or even more appropriate for evaluating teratogenic potency. Furthermore, the index will also be subject to all of the already enumerated deficiencies that accompany the use of the probit model in species scale-up and risk assessment. Finally, in some regulatory situations the maternal exposure level is likely to be predetermined; and interest will center solely on the estimation of (absolute) teratogenic potential at the predetermined exposure level.

In addition to the various mathematically-based modeling approaches advocated by investigators like Biddle and Fabro, there is a growing interest in the use of pharmacokinetics (74) to characterize the relationship between exposure and the effective dose in the fetal target tissue in order to facilitate the interspecies comparison of teratogenic outcomes. Jusko (45), who was one of the initial researchers to be concerned with the kinetics of teratogenic effects, constructed a general pharmacodynamic model for a class of teratogens that have no minimum effective embryopathic dose. Using this model he was able to show, e.g., that if the absorption and metabolism rates of the teratogen under study were not dose-dependent, then a linear relationship should exist between the logarithm of the fraction of normal or unaffected fetuses and

---

[3] On a probit, log-dose scale.
[4] A situation which he interpreted as implying a common mechanism of induction.

the externally administered dose. He also postulated that the same relationship would hold for "threshold" teratogens at large doses once a critical number of compound-receptor interactions had occurred. In support of his theory, he plotted data from different published studies and obtained dose-response curves that seemed to conform to his model predictions. While the usual doubts about the ability to experimentally determine threshold levels have been raised in response to Jusko's work (9), his findings at least illustrate the plausibility of developing pharmacokinetic models for teratogenic activity.

More recently, Young and his co-workers (41,75,76) have conducted a series of studies on the potential correlation of kinetically determined embryo exposure levels and teratogenicity/fetotoxicity using salicylic acid as a study compound. They developed a two-compartment pharmacokinetic model from which they were able to generate estimates of various kinetic parameters including the maternal overall elimination rate constant, the exposure area under the blood concentration-time curve, and the 45-min and 24-hr blood concentrations. (Maternal blood concentration was used to measure dosimetry in the fetus since the two levels seem to be equivalent after an initial equilibration lag period of approximately 45 min.) When these parameters were correlated with different measures of embryopathology, the strongest association was observed for 24-hr maternal blood concentration and the percent of affected fetuses (i.e., dead, resorbed, or abnormal) in the corresponding litter. Furthermore, repetitive studies indicated that there was much less between animal variability in the pharmacokinetically determined parameters than in the related estimates of fetotoxicity. However, since these results are limited to a single species and strain of laboratory animal as well as a single chemical agent, they obviously must be regarded as preliminary, even though they offer some indication of the potential importance of taking pharmacokinetics into consideration when extrapolating teratogenic outcomes across species. Therefore, it seems likely that until pharmacokinetic procedures are perfected and perhaps combined with some form of mathematical modeling, individuals interested in assessing human teratogenic risk will continue to rely on a safety factor approach or, possibly, on results obtained from the linear extrapolation of the experimental data expressed in terms of some appropriate standard dosage scale.

FUTURE RESEARCH DIRECTIONS

Future advances in quantitative species extrapolation and risk estimation will obviously be heavily dependent on the generation of laboratory research results that provide new insights into the biological mechanisms underlying toxicologic responses. Moreover, there are a number of statistical/mathematical issues associated with these processes that still need to be resolved.

It has already been noted that the main source of information for estimating human cancer risk is the life-time rodent bioassay. However, in many instances human exposure to potential carcinogens is for considerably less than a normal lifespan. (For example, in most occupational settings exposure will be limited to a maximum of 45 years.) Therefore,

there is the very real question of how most effectively to use lifetime animal exposure data to estimate the corresponding human risk associated with an exposure of possibly much shorter duration. Both Whittemore (71) and Day and Brown (22) have investigated various theoretical aspects of this issue within the framework of the multistage model. Whittemore was concerned with changes in the excess risk curve that would be expected to result from different temporal patterns of exposure when exactly one stage of the carcinogenic process is affected by the test chemical. Day and Brown attempted to extend her results, focusing particularly on the behavior of the excess risk curve following cessation of exposure. In addition to these two research efforts, the recently released data tapes from the National Center for Toxicologic Research ED_{01} study of 24,000 mice exposed to the known carcinogen 2-AAF (12) have provided investigators with a unique opportunity to empirically evaluate the relationship between lifetime and less-than-lifetime exposure. Specifically, parameter estimates derived from modeling of lifetime exposure data can be used to develop risk predictions for a subset of the study population for which dosing was discontinued several months prior to sacrifice. These predictions can then be compared to the results actually observed in the study.

The ED_{01} study has also renewed interest in the incorporation of time-to-tumor information into the low-dose extrapolation process [see, e.g., ref. (68)]. In response to this renewed interest, Hoel (38) has critically evaluated a number of measures of carcinogenic risk that encompass time-to-tumor concepts in their definition and found that there is no univariate measure of risk that adequately takes time into account. As a result, he has suggested that for the present the most reasonable approach to this problem may be to consider a bivariate index that combines the traditional lifetime probability measure of risk with some measure of time such as the adjusted mean time-to-tumor.

Another issue that is receiving increasing attention from researchers interested in species scale-up is the quantification of the biological model errors associated with human risk estimates. Crouch and Wilson (18), for example, have attempted to introduce a measure of the error resulting from species extrapolation into the modeling process. While their particular approach to this problem has been criticized (39,48,73) for a number of different reasons, their primary objective is generally regarded as being well worth pursuing. It has even been proposed (39) that this type of modeling research be expanded to incorporate the biological variability associated with the selection of a *specific* mathematical model to characterize the underlying dose-response relationship as well as that related to extrapolation across species.

The tremendous cost in terms of both resources and time that are involved in the conduct of the typical rodent bioassay and the resulting need to find a less expensive, shorter term alternative to this cancer screening procedure have stimulated interest in the reported association [see, e.g., refs. (54) and (55)] between Ames Test results and corresponding findings obtained from the lifetime cancer bioassay. However, even if this association holds for a broad range of chemical compounds, there are a number of important statistical issues that need to be addressed before a quantitative relationship useful for species scale-up and risk estimation can be established. For instance, there is the critical question of what response level in the cancer bioassay is biologically most appropriate for comparison with the selected index of mutagenic activity (such as the doubling dose), given the well-known potential for nonlinearity in the carcinogenic dose-response curve. Then, both the cancer test species and the tester strain in the microbial assay must be carefully selected in order to avoid introducing bias into the estimation of the quantitative relationship that presumably exists between these two screening systems.

As was mentioned earlier in this chapter, there is also the very basic issue of determining what effect (if any) on human health results from some specified increase in the mutation rate. This particular problem, which is clearly central to the entire process of mutagenic risk estimation, has been investigated via a number of different approaches. Newcombe (56), for example, discusses various methods for obtaining epidemiological data pertaining to the amount of mutation-maintained ill health in the general population. Crow and Denniston (19), on the other hand, use an empirical, population genetics-based argument to show that an estimate of the mutational component of genetic damage can often be determined by considering either the mode of inheritance or various measures of heritability.

Finally, in the area of teratogenesis there is an urgent need for the development of a biologically meaningful potency index or measure that can be used to make quantitative comparisons of teratogenic activity across species. Such an index should be stable over a broad range of the dose-response curve including the exposure levels of interest for risk estimation.

REFERENCES

1. Aaron, C. S. (1976): Molecular dosimetry of chemical mutagens: selection of appropriate target molecules for determining molecular dose to the germ line. *Mutation Res.*, 38:303–309.
2. Aaron, C. S., and Lee, W. R. (1978): Molecular dosimetry of the mutagen ethyl methanesulfonate in *Drosophila Melanogaster* spermatozoa: (dose) to sex-linked recessive lethals. *Mutation Res.*, 49: 27–44.
3. Aaron, C. S., Van Zeeland, A. A., Mohn, G. R., Natarajan, A. T., Knapp, A. G. A. C., Tates, A. D., and Glickman, B. W. (1980): Molecular dosimetry of the chemical mutagen ethyl methanesulfonate: Quantitative comparison of mutation induction in *Escherichia Coli*, V79 Chinese hamster cells and L5178Y mouse lymphoma cells, and some cytological results *in vitro* and *in vivo*. *Mutation Res.*, 69:201–216.
4. Abrahamson, S., Bender, M. A., Conger, A. D., and Wolff, S. (1973): *Nature*, 245:461–462.
5. Aldoph, E. F. (1949): Quantitative relations in the physiological constitutions of mammals. *Science*, 109:579–585.
6. Anderson, M. W., Hoel, D. G., and Kaplan, N. L. (1980): A general scheme for the incorporation of pharmacokinetics in low-dose risk estimation for chemical carcinogenesis: Example—vinyl chloride. *Toxicol. Appl. Pharmacol.*, 55:154–161.
7. Armitage, P., and Doll, R. (1961): Stochastic models for carcinogenesis. In: *Proceedings of the Fourth Berkeley Symposium on Mathematical Statistics and Probability, Vol. 4*, edited by L. Lecam and J. Neyman, pp. 19–38. University of California Press, Berkeley, California.
8. Biddle, F. G. (1977): 6-Aminonicotinamide-induced cleft palate in the mouse: The nature of the difference between the A/J and C57B1/6J strains in frequency of response and its genetic basis. *Teratology*, 16:301–312.
9. Biddle, F. G. (1978): Use of dose-response relationships to discrim-

10. inate between the mechanisms of cleft-palate induction by different teratogens: An argument for discussion. *Teratology*, 18:247–252.
10. Biddle, F. G., and Fraser, F. C. (1976): Genetics of cortisone-induced cleft palate in the mouse—embryonic and maternal effects. *Genetics*, 84:743–754.
11. Cairns, J. (1981): The origin of human cancers. *Nature*, 289:353–357.
12. Cairns, T. (1980): The ED$_{01}$ study: Introduction, objectives, and experimental design. *J. Environ. Pathol. Toxicol.* (special issue), 3(3): 1–7.
13. Collins, T. F. X., and Collins, E. V. (1976): Current methodology in teratology research. In: *Advances in Modern Toxicology (Volume 1, Part 1): New Concepts in Safety Evaluation*, edited by M. A. Mehlman, R. E. Shapiro, and H. Blumenthal, pp. 155–175. John Wiley & Sons, New York.
14. Committee 17 of the Environmental Mutagen Society (1975): Environmental mutagenic hazards. *Science*, 187:503–514.
15. Consultative Panel on Health Hazards of Chemical Pesticides (1975): *Pest Control (Volume 1): An Assessment of Present and Alternative Technologies*, National Academy of Sciences, Washington, D.C.
16. Cornfield, J., Carlborg, F. W., and Van Ryzin, J. (1978): Setting tolerances on the basis of mathematical treatment of dose-response data extrapolated to low doses. In: *Proceedings of the First International Congress on Toxicology*, edited by G. L. Plaa and W. A. M. Duncan, pp. 143–164. Academic Press, New York.
17. Crouch, E., and Wilson, R. (1978): Interspecies comparison of carcinogenic potency. *J. Toxicol. and Environ. Health*, 5:1095–1118.
18. Crouch, E., and Wilson, R. (1981): Regulation of carcinogens. *Risk Analysis*, 1:47–57.
19. Crow, J. F., and Denniston, C. (1981): The mutation component of genetic damage. *Science*, 212:888–893.
20. Crump, K. S. (1977): Response to open query: Theoretical problems in the modified Mantel-Bryan procedure. *Biometrics*, 33:752–757.
21. Crump, K. S., and Guess, H. A. (1980): *Drinking Water and Cancer: Review of Recent Findings and Assessment of Risks*. Science Research Systems, Inc., Ruston, Louisiana. CEQ Contract No. EQ10AC018.
22. Day, N. E., and Brown, C. C. (1980): Multistage models and primary prevention of cancer. *JNCI*, 64:977–989.
23. Ehrenberg, L. (1979): Risk assessment of ethylene oxide and other compounds. In: *Banbury Report No. 1: Assessing Chemical Mutagens: The Risk to Humans*, edited by V. K. McElheny and S. Abrahamson, pp. 157–190. Cold Springs Harbor Laboratory, New York.
24. Environmental Protection Agency (1980): Mutagenic risk assessments; proposed guidelines. *Fed. Register*, 45(221):74984–74988.
25. Fabro, S., Shull, G., and Brown, N. A. (1981): The relative teratogenic index: An approach to the estimation of teratogenic potency. *TCM* (in press). Laboratory of Reproductive and Developmental Toxicology, NIEHS, Box 12233, Research Triangle Park, N.C., 27709.
26. Fahrig, R. (1978): The mammalian spot test: A sensitive *in vivo* method for the detection of genetic alterations in somatic cells of mice. In: *Chemical Mutagens: Principles and Methods for Their Detection (Volume 5)*, edited by A. Hollander and F. J. de Serres, pp. 151–176. Plenum Press, New York and London.
27. Freireich, E. J., Gehan, E. A., Rall, D. P., Schmidt, L. H., and Skipper, H. E. (1966): Quantitative comparison of toxicity of anticancer agents in mouse, rat, hamster, dog, monkey, and man (1966): *Cancer Chemother. Rep.*, 50:219–243.
28. Gaylor, D. W., and Shapiro, R. E. (1979): Extrapolation and risk estimation for carcinogenesis. In: *Advances in Modern Toxicology (Vol. 1): New Concepts in Safety Evaluation (Part 2)*, edited by M. A. Mehlman, R. E. Shapiro, and H. Blumenthal, pp. 65–87. John Wiley & Sons, New York.
29. Gehring, P. J., and Blau, G. E. (1977): Mechanisms of carcinogenesis: Dose response. *J. Environ. Pathol. Toxicol.*, 1:163–179.
30. Gehring, P. J., Watanabe, P. G., and Park, C. N. (1978): Resolution of dose-response toxicity data for chemicals requiring metabolic activation: Example—vinyl chloride. *Toxicol. Appl. Pharmacol.*, 44: 581–591.
31. Guess, H., Crump, K., and Peto, R. (1977): Uncertainty estimates for low-dose-rate extrapolations of animal carcinogenicity data. *Cancer Res.*, 37:3475–3483.
32. Haseman, J. K., Hoel, D. G., and Jennrich, R. I. (1981): Some practical problems arising from the use of the gamma multihit model for risk estimation. *J. Toxicol. and Environ. Health*, 8:379–386.

33. Heddle, J. A., and Athanasiou, K. (1975): Mutation rate, genome size, and their relation to the rec concept. *Mutation Res.,* 31:333.

34. Heddle, J. A., and Athanasiou, K. (1975): Mutation rate, genome size, and their relation to the rec concept. *Nature,* 258:359–361.

35. Hoel, D. G. (1979): Low-dose and species-to-species extrapolation for chemically induced carcinogenesis. In: *Banbury Report No. 1: Assessing Chemical Mutagens: The Risk to Humans,* pp. 135–145. Cold Spring Harbor Laboratory, New York.

36. Hoel, D. G. (1979): Animal experimentation and its relevance to man. *Environ. Health Perspect.,* 32:25–30.

37. Hoel, D. G. (1980): Incorporation of background in dose-response models. *Federation Proc.,* 39:73–75.

38. Hoel, D. G. (1981): Statistical measures of risk. Presented at the Symposium on Metabolism and Pharmacokinetics of Environmental Chemicals in Man, Sarasota, Florida, June 7–12, 1981. Biometry and Risk Assessment Program, NIEHS, Box 12233, Research Triangle Park, N.C., 27709.

39. Hoel, D. G. (1981): Comment: Carcinogenic risk. *Risk Analysis,* 1: 63–64.

40. Hoel, D. G., Gaylor, D. W., Kirschstein, R. L., Saffiotti, U., and Schneiderman, M. A. (1975): Estimation of risks of irreversible delayed toxicity. *J. Toxicol. and Environ. Health* 1:133–151.

41. Holson, J. F., Kimmel, C. A., and Young, J. F. (1980): The precision of pharmacokinetic parameters for predicting embryotoxicity endpoints. Presented as a poster at the 19th Annual Meeting of the Society of Toxicology, Washington, D.C., March 10, 1980. Division of Teratogenesis Research, NCTR, Jefferson, Arkansas, 72079.

42. Interagency Regulatory Liaison Group, Work Group on Risk Assessment (1979): Scientific bases for identification of potential carcinogens and estimation of risks. *Fed. Register,* 44(131):39858–39879.

43. Johnson, E. M. (1980): A subvertebrate system for rapid determination of potential teratogenic hazards. *J. Environ. Pathol. Toxicol.,* 4:153–156.

44. Johnson, E. M. (1981): Screening for teratogenic hazards: Nature of the problems. *Ann. Rev. Pharmacol. Toxicol.,* 21:417–429.

45. Jusko, W. J. (1972): Pharmacodynamic principles in chemical teratology: dose-effect relationships. *J. Pharmacol. Exp. Ther.,* 183: 469–480.

46. Krasovskii, G. N. (1976): Extrapolation of experimental data from animals to man. *Environ. Health Perspect.,* 13:51–58.

47. Krewski, D., and Van Ryzin, J. (1981): Dose-response models for quantal response toxicity data. In: *Current Topics in Probability and Statistics,* edited by M. Csorogo, D. Dawson, J. N. K. Rao, and E. Saleh, (in press). North-Holland, Amsterdam.

48. Lave, L. B. (1981): Comment: Estimating the risk of carcinogens. *Risk Analysis,* 1:59–60.

49. Lee, W. R. (1976): Molecular dosimetry of chemical mutagens: Determination of molecular dose to the germ line. *Mutation Res.,* 38: 311–316.

50. Lee, W. R. (1978): Dosimetry of chemical mutagens in eukaryote germ cells. In: *Chemical Mutagens: Principles and Methods for Their Detection (Volume 5),* edited by A. Hollander and F. J. de Serres, pp. 177–202. Plenum Press, New York and London.

51. Lee, W. R. (1979): Dosimetry of alkylating agents. In: *Banbury Report No. 1: Assessing Chemical Mutagens: The Risk to Humans,* edited by V. K. McElheny and S. Abrahamson, pp. 191–200. Cold Spring Harbor Laboratory, New York.

52. Mantel, N., and Bryan, W. R. (1961): "Safety" testing of carcinogenic agents. *J. Nat. Cancer Inst.,* 27:455–470.

53. Mantel, N., Bohidar, N. R., Brown, C. C., Ciminera, J. L., and Tukey, J. W. (1975): An improved "Mantel-Bryan" procedure for "safety testing" of carcinogens. *Cancer Res.,* 35:865–872.

54. McCann, J., Choi, E., Yamasaki, E., and Ames, B. N. (1975): Detection of carcinogens as mutagens in the *Salmonella*/microsome test: assay of 300 chemicals. *Proc. Natl. Acad. Sci.,* 72:5135–5139.

55. Meselson, M., and Russell, K. (1977): Comparisons of carcinogenic and mutagenic potency. In: *Origins of Human Cancer: (Book C) Human Risk Assessment,* edited by H. H. Hiatt, J. D. Watson, and J. A. Winsten, pp. 1473–1481., Cold Spring Harbor Laboratory, New York.

56. Newcombe, H. B. (1977): Methods of obtaining epidemiological data for mutation risk estimation. In: *Handbook of Mutagenicity Test Procedures,* edited by B. J. Kilbey, M. Legator, W. Nichols, and C. Ramel, pp. 461–476. Elsevier Scientific Publishing Company, Amsterdam, New York, and Oxford.

57. Office of Pesticide Programs, Environmental Protection Agency (1979): Endrin; intent to cancel registrations and denial of applications for registration of pesticide products containing endrin, and statement of reasons. *Fed. Register,* 44(144):43632–43657.

58. Rai, K., and Van Ryzin, J. (1979): Risk assessment of toxic environmental substances based on a generalized multi-hit model. In: *Energy and Health,* edited by N. Breslow and A. Whittemore, pp. 99–117. Siam Press, Philadelphia.

59. Rai, K., and Van Ryzin, J. (1981): A generalized multi-hit dose-response model for low-dose extrapolation. *Biometrics,* 37:(in press).

60. Rall, D. P. (1974): Problems of low doses of carcinogens. *J. Wash. Acad. Sci.,* 64:63–68.

61. Rall, D. P. (1977): Species differences in carcinogenesis testing. In: *Origins of Human Cancer: (Book C) Human Risk Assessment,* edited by H. H. Hiatt, J. D. Watson, and J. A. Winsten, pp. 1383–1390. Cold Spring Harbor Laboratory, New York.

62. Russell, W. L. (1977): The role of mammals in the future of chemical mutagenesis research. *Arch. Toxicol.,* 38:141–147.

63. Russell, W. L. (1979): Comments on mutagenesis risk assessment. *Genetics,* 92(1):s187–s194.

64. Safe Drinking Water Committee (1977): *Drinking Water and Health.* National Academy of Sciences, Washington, D.C.

65. Schalet, A. P., and Sankaranarayanan, K. (1976): Evaluation and reevaluation of genetic radiation hazards in man, *Mutation Res.,* 35:341–370.

66. Scientific Committee of the Food Safety Council (1978): Quantitative risk assessment. *Fd. Cosmet. Toxicol.,* 16(Supplement 2):109–136.

67. Segreti, A. C., and Munson, A. E. (1981): Estimation of the median lethal dose when responses within a litter are correlated. *Biometrics,* 37:153–156.

68. Society of Toxicology ED_{01} Task Force (1981): Risk assessment using time. *Fundam. Appl. Toxicol.,* 1:88–123.

69. Study Group on Pesticide Tolerances (1979): *Review of EPA's Tolerance Setting System.* (Draft report) U.S. Environmental Protection Agency, Washington, D.C.

70. Subcommittee on Risk Assessment of the Safe Drinking Water Committee (1980): Problems of risk estimation. In: *Drinking Water and Health (Volume 3).* National Academy of Sciences Press, Washington, D.C.

71. Whittemore, A. S. (1977): The age distribution of human cancer for exposures of varying intensity. *Am. J. Epidemiol.,* 106:418–432.

72. Whittemore, A., and Altschuler, B. (1976): Lung cancer incidence in cigarette smokers: Further analysis of Doll and Hill's data for British physicians. *Biometrics,* 32:805–816.

73. Wodicka, V. O. (1981): Comment: Discussion of the regulation of carcinogens. *Risk Analysis,* 1:61–62.

74. Young, J. F., and Holson, J. F. (1978): Utility of pharmacokinetics in designing and improving interspecies extrapolation. *J. Environ. Pathol. Toxicol.,* 2:169–186.

75. Young, J. F., Holson, J. F., and Kimmel, C. A. (1979): Utilization of pharmacokinetic principles in extrapolation from animal data to man. Presented at the 39th International Congress of Pharmaceutical Sciences, Brighton, England, September 5, 1979. Division of Teratogenesis Research, NCTR, Jefferson, Arkansas, 72079.

76. Young, J. F., Kimmel, C. A., and Holson, J. F. (1979): Validation of a pharmacokinetic model for rat embryonal dosimetry of salicylates during a teratogenically susceptible period. Presented at the 18th Annual Meeting of the Society of Toxicology, New Orleans, Louisiana, March 14, 1979. Division of Teratogenesis Research, NCTR, Jefferson, Arkansas, 72079.

77. Zielhuis, R. L., and Van Der Kreek, F. W. (1979): The use of a safety factor in setting health-based permissible levels for occupational exposure. *Int. Arch. Occup. Environ. Health,* 42:191–201.

Subject Index

Hemoglobin, 494–495
 and heme synthesis, 496
  lead affecting, 95
 mean corpuscular, 497
 mean corpuscular concentration, 497–498
 stability of, 488
 statistical tests for, 475
Hemoglobinuria, in chronic toxicity studies, 249
Hemolytic anemia, drugs and chemicals inducing, 746
Hemoproteins
 microsomal, detection of by SDS gels, 827
 synthesis/degradation of, 827–828
Henle, loop of, 633
Heparin, effects and use of, 487
Hepatitis, aflatoxins causing, 87
Heptane
 classification of, 116
 properties of, 113
Herbicides, 149–153
 bipyridal, 152–153
 chlorophenoxy, 149–151
 dicamba, 151–152
 2,4-dichlorophenoxyacetic acid, 149–150
 diquat, 153
 oncogenic risk from, 156
 paraquat, 152–153
 2,4,5-trichlorophenoxyacetic acid, 150–151
Heroin, isolated perfused intestine preparations in study of, 730
Hexachlorobenzene, 156–158
 carcinogenic potential of, 157
 detoxification pathways for, 158
 immunotoxicity of, 157, 751, 752
 structure of, 156
 symptoms of exposure to, 157
 teratogenicity of, 157–158
Hexachlorocyclohexane, 139. See also Lindane
Hexane
 classification of, 116
 purification and characterization of, 802
n-Hexane
 isolated perfused heart preparations in study of, 708
 neurotoxicity of, 131
 properties of, 113
Hexobarbital, purification and characterization of, 802
Hexone, properties of, 113
Hexyldimethylamine, in gas chromatographic determination of acetylcholine, 583
Hexylene glycol, classification of, 117
5-HIAA. See 5-Hydroxy-3-indoleacetic acid
High density lipoprotein cholesterol, organs associated with, 504
High performance liquid chromatography-electrochemical assay
 for acetylcholine, 584

equipment for, 584
 procedures for, 584
 reagents for, 584
 of biogenic amines, 576–577
 equipment for, 576
 procedures for, 576
 reagents for, 576
 turnover rates and, 576–577
High risk groups, 19–22
 noncancer endpoints and, 20
 standards for cadmium in drinking water and, 21–22
 standards for carcinogens and, 22
 standards for nitrates in drinking water and, 20–21
Histamine, prolactin levels affected by, 684
Histocompatibility antigens, in cell membrane, 761
Histology. See also Histopathology
 for endomyocardial biopsy in drug-related heart disease, 651
 in evaluation of liver injury, 620–623
 gastrointestinal tract integrity studied with, 659
Histopathology. See also Histology
 in chronic toxicity studies, 250
 in male reproductive toxicity studies, 293–294
 statistical analysis of data from, 473–476
HLA. See Human leukocyte antigen
HPLC-EC assay. See High performance liquid chromatography- electrochemical assay
5-HT. See Serotonin
Human chorionic gonadotropin, measurement of by immune or nonimmune assays, 679
Human leukocyte antigen, in cell membrane, 761
Humoral immunity, 742, 744–745
Hydralazine, systemic lupus erythematosus induced by, 746
Hydration, in xenobiotic metabolism, 30
Hydrocarbons
 aliphatic, solvents classified as, 116
 aromatic
  immunotoxicity of, 751
  solvents classified as, 116
 chlorinated insecticides, 138–140
 cyclic, solvents classified as, 116
 halogenated aromatic
  immunotoxicity of, 752
  solvents classified as, 117
 nitro-, solvents classified as, 117
 polycyclic aromatic
  immunotoxicity of, 751–752
  oocyte toxicity and, 315
 polyhalogenated aromatic, immunotoxicity of, 751
Hydrocortisone, 688. See also Cortisol
Hydrogen cyanide, and toxic effects of cyanogenic glycosides, 69–70
Hydrolysis, 57–59
 amidases in, 58–59

epoxide hydrolase in, 57–58
 esterases in, 58–59
 in xenobiotic metabolism, 30
Hydrolytic enzymes, microsomal, toxic agents affecting, 830
5-Hydroxy-3-indoleacetic acid determination, 574
 procedures for, 574
 reagents for, 574
7-α-Hydroxy-4-cholesten-3-one, purification and characterization of, 802
β-Hydroxy-GABA, prolactin levels affected by, 684
Hydroxybutyric dehydrogenase analysis
 statistical tests for, 475
 target organ action and, 474
4-Hydroxymephenytoin, formation of, TLC analysis of, 790
Hydroxysteroid sulfotransferase, in xenobiotic metabolism, 48
Hydroxytoluene, butylated, isolated perfused heart preparations in study of, 706
5-Hydroxytryptamine. See Serotonin
Hydroxyzine, corticosteroids and ketosteroids affected by, 689
Hygienists, American Conference of Governmental, 3
Hyperglycemia, 694
Hypersensitivity diseases, 746–747
 immunological classification of, 746
Hypersensitivity myocarditis, 652–654
 drugs associated with, 653
 incidence of, 652
 morphological changes in, 652
Hypochlorite, thyroid function affected by, 686
Hypoglycemia, growth hormone affected by, 682
Hypoglycemics, oral, morphologic classification of liver injury caused by, 601
Hypoglycin, in food, toxicity of, 73
Hypothalamic-pituitary-uterine-ovarian axis, alterations in female reproductive toxicology, 315–317

I

IARC. See International Agency for Research on Cancer
Ibotenic acid, mushroom poisoning and, 71
ICG. See Indocyanine green
ICSH. See Interstitial cell stimulating hormone
Ig. See Immunoglobulins
IgM plaque-forming cell assay, 750–751
 materials for, 750
 procedure for, 750–751
 reagents for, 750
 sources of error and variability in, 751
Imipramine
 hepatic excretory function evaluated with, 610